D1219077

VOLUME
ONE

VOLUME
ONE

Neurosurgery

Editors

Robert H. Wilkins, M.D.
Professor and Chief
Division of Neurosurgery
Duke University Medical Center
Durham, North Carolina

Setti S. Rengachary, M.D.
Professor, Section of Neurological Surgery
University of Kansas Medical Center
Kansas City, Kansas;
Chief, Neurosurgery Section
Veterans Administration Medical Center
Kansas City, Missouri

McGraw-Hill Book Company

New York St. Louis San Francisco Auckland Bogotá Guatemala Hamburg
Johannesburg Lisbon London Madrid Mexico Montreal New Delhi Panama
Paris San Juan São Paulo Singapore Sydney Tokyo Toronto

Notice

Medicine is an ever-changing science. As new research and clinical experience broaden our knowledge, changes in treatment and drug therapy are required. The editors and the publisher of this work have checked with sources believed to be reliable in their efforts to provide drug dosage schedules that are complete and in accord with the standards accepted at the time of publication. However, readers are advised to check the product information sheet included in the package of each drug they plan to administer to be certain that the information contained in these schedules is accurate and that changes have not been made in the recommended dose or in the contraindications for administration. This recommendation is of particular importance in connection with new or infrequently used drugs.

Neurosurgery

Copyright © 1985 by McGraw-Hill, Inc. All rights reserved. Printed in the United States of America. Except as permitted under the United States Copyright Act of 1976, no part of this publication may be reproduced or distributed in any form or by any means, or stored in a data base or retrieval system, without the prior written permission of the publisher.

1234567890 HALHAL 8987654

ISBN 0-07-079790-0

This book was set in Plantin by York Graphic Services, Inc.; the editors were Robert E. McGrath and Stuart D. Boynton; the production supervisor was Avé McCracken; the designer was Caliber Design Planning.
Halliday Lithograph Corporation was printer and binder.

Library of Congress Cataloging in Publication Data
Main entry under title:

Neurosurgery.

Includes bibliographies and index.
1. Nervous system—Surgery. I. Wilkins, Robert H.
II. Rengachary, Setti S. [DNLM: 1. Neurosurgery.
WL 368 N4951]
RD593.N417   1985   617'.48   84-17188
ISBN   0-07-079790-0 (set)

This book is dedicated to
our wives and children:

Gloria Wilkins and
Michael, Jeffrey, and Elizabeth Wilkins;

and Dhanalakshmi Rengachary and
Dave Anand and Usha Rengachary

CONTENTS

List of Contributors *xiii*
Foreword *xxvii*
Preface *xxix*

VOLUME I

Part I   Historical Aspects of Neurosurgery

1   History of Neurosurgery   *Robert H. Wilkins*   3
2   Two Giants: Harvey Cushing and Walter Dandy
    Paul C. Bucy   16
3   History of Microneurosurgery
    R. M. Peardon Donaghy   20

Part II   Clinical Examination of the Nervous System and Correlative Neuroanatomy

4   The Art of History Taking   *Barrie J. Hurwitz*   29
5   Clinical Examination of Cognitive Functions
    Samuel H. Greenblatt   32
6   Psychological Assessment of Intelligence and
    Personality   *Patrick E. Logue,*
    Frederick A. Schmitt   42
7   Cranial Nerve Examination   *Setti S. Rengachary*   50
8   Neuro-ophthalmology   *Michael Rosenberg*   71
9   Nystagmus and Related Ocular Movements
    Nancy M. Newman   102
10 Neurotology   *Robert W. Baloh*   111
11 Gait and Station; Examination of Coordination
    Setti S. Rengachary   117
12 Examination of the Motor and Sensory Systems and
    Reflexes   *Setti S. Rengachary*   122

Part III   Ancillary Diagnostic Tests

Section A   Cerebrospinal Fluid Examination

13 Techniques of Ventricular Puncture
    Timothy B. Mapstone, Robert A. Ratcheson
    151
14 Intracranial Pressure Monitoring   *Gerald D. Silverberg*
    156
15 Cerebrospinal Fluid: Techniques of Access and
    Analytical Interpretation   *James H. Wood*   161

Section B   Electrodiagnostic Tests

16 Electromyography   *Didier Cros, B. Shahani*   174
17 Electroencephalography   *William P. Wilson*   184
18 Electronystagmography   *Robert A. Schindler,*
    Vivian D. Weigel   196
19 Evoked Potentials from the Visual, Auditory, and
    Somatosensory Systems   *C. William Erwin,*
    Andrea Brendle, Miles E. Drake   211

Section C   Some Evolving Neurodiagnostic Tests

20 Computed Tomography: Recent Trends
    Burton P. Drayer, G. Allan Johnson, C. Roger Bird
    224
21 Positron Emission Tomography   *Myron D. Ginsberg*
    255
22 Single Photon Tomography   *Allan H. Friedman,*
    Burton P. Drayer, Ronald J. Jaszczak   265

23 Brain Imaging with Nuclear Magnetic
    Resonance   *Michael Brant-Zawadzki*   268
24 Ultrasonic Brain Imaging in Pediatric Neurosurgery
    Philip R. Weinstein, Kai Haber   274
25 Digital Subtraction Angiography   *Meredith A. Weinstein,*
    Michael T. Modic, Anthony J. Furlan, William Pavlicek,
    John R. Little   280

Section D   Brain Biopsy

26 Diagnostic Brain Biopsy   *Howard H. Kaufman,*
    Peter T. Ostrow, Ian J. Butler   289

Part IV   General and Perioperative Care

27 Evaluation of the Patient in Coma   *Allen D. Roses*
    297
28 Seizure Disorders and Their Medical Management
    J. Scott Luther   304
29 Evaluation of the Patient with Dementia and Treatment
    of Normal Pressure Hydrocephalus   *Robert G. Ojemann,*
    Peter McL. Black   312
30 Blood-Brain Barrier; Cerebral Edema   *Michael Pollay*
    322
31 Increased Intracranial Pressure, Brain Herniation, and
    Their Control   *Donald O. Quest*   332
32 Induced Barbiturate Coma   *Warren Selman,*
    Robert Spetzler, Joseph Zabramski   343
33 Pseudotumor Cerebri   *Frederick H. Sklar*   350
34 Neurourology   *George D. Webster, Jorge L. Lockhart*
    354
35 Preoperative Evaluation of a Neurosurgical Patient
    Ted S. Keller   366
36 Blood Coagulation   *Salvatore V. Pizzo*   369
37 Blood Transfusion   *Fred V. Plapp, William L. Bayer*
    372
38 Neuroanesthesia   *Maurice S. Albin*   384
39 Intensive Care   *Allan B. Levin*   396
40 Prevention and Treatment of Thromboembolic
    Complications in a Neurosurgical Patient
    Stephen K. Powers, Michael S. B. Edwards   406
41 Spasticity and Spasm   *Wesley A. Cook, Jr.*   411
42 Principles of Rehabilitation of the Disabled Patient
    E. Wayne Massey   416

Part V   Neurosurgical and Related Techniques

43 Principles of Neurosurgical Operative Technique
    Robert H. Wilkins   427
44 Instrumentation for Microneurosurgery   *John M. Tew, Jr.,*
    Hans Jacob Steiger   439
45 Prophylactic Antibiotics   *Stephen J. Haines*   448
46 Patient Positioning   *Donald H. Stewart, Jr.,*
    John Krawchenko   452
47 Intraoperative Diagnostic Ultrasound
    George J. Dohrmann, Jonathan M. Rubin   457
48 Self-Retaining Retractors   *I. M. Greenberg*   463
49 Automated Cutting and Suction   *Martin L. Lazar*
    473
50 Ultrasonic Dissection   *Fred Epstein*   476
51 Application of the Laser to Neurological Surgery
    Leonard J. Cerullo   478

52 Interventional Neuroradiology *Fernando Viñuela,
    Allan J. Fox*   484

Part VI Neuro-oncology

Section A Neuro-oncology: An Overview
53 Genetic Factors in Brain Tumors *Robert L. Martuza*
    505
54 Neurofibromatosis and Other Phakomatoses
    Robert L. Martuza   511
55 Virus-Induced Brain Tumors *Jeffrey S. Walker,
    Darell D. Bigner*   522
56 Radiation-Induced Brain Tumors *Jeffrey S. Walker,
    Darell D. Bigner*   525
57 Chemically Induced Brain Tumors, Primary and
    Transplanted *Jeffrey S. Walker, Darell D. Bigner*
    528
58 Cell Kinetics of Brain Tumors *Takao Hoshino*   531
59 Biochemistry of Brain Tumors *C. J. Cummins,
    B. H. Smith, P. L. Kornblith*   535
60 Immunology of Brain Tumors *Michael L. J. Apuzzo*
    538
61 Tissue Culture Techniques in the Study of Human
    Gliomas *Joseph Bressler, Barry H. Smith,
    Paul L. Kornblith*   542
62 Tumor Markers *Dennis E. Bullard, S. Clifford Schold, Jr.*
    548

Section B Gliomas
63 Gliomas: Pathology *Peter C. Burger*   553
64 Supratentorial Gliomas: Radiology *Kenneth R. Maravilla*
    564
65 Supratentorial Gliomas: Clinical Features and Surgical
    Therapy *Michael Salcman*   579

Section C Metastatic Brain Tumors
66 Factors That Govern the Metastatic Process
    Leonard Weiss   591
67 Metastatic Brain Tumors *Joseph H. Galicich,
    Narayan Sundaresan*   597
68 Meningeal Carcinomatosis *John R. Little,
    Maurice R. Hanson*   610

Section D Meningiomas
69 Meningiomas: Pathology *Venkata R. Challa,
    William R. Markesbery*   613
70 Meningiomas: Radiology *Dixon M. Moody*   623
71 Meningiomas: Clinical Features and Surgical
    Management *Robert G. Ojemann*   635

Section E Epidermoid and Dermoid Tumors
72 Epidermoid and Dermoid Tumors: Pathology
    Jere W. Baxter, Martin G. Netsky   655
73 Epidermoid and Dermoid Tumors: Radiology
    Dennis R. Osborne   662
74 Epidermoid and Dermoid Tumors: Clinical Features and
    Surgical Management *Frances K. Conley*   668

Section F Tumors in the Region of the Pineal Gland
75 Pineal Tumors: Classification and Pathology
    Maie Kaarsoo Herrick   674
76 Pineal Region Masses: Radiology *Robert A. Zimmerman*
    680
77 Pineal Masses: Clinical Features and
    Management *Henry H. Schmidek, Alan Waters*
    688

Section G Cerebellopontine Angle Tumors
78 Tumors of the Cerebellopontine Angle: Pathology
    F. Stephen Vogel   694
79 Tumors of the Cerebellopontine Angle: Neurotologic
    Aspects of Diagnosis *Patrick D. Kenan*   698
80 Tumors of the Cerebellopontine Angle: Radiology
    Philip Dubois   704
81 Tumors of the Cerebellopontine Angle: Clinical Features
    and Surgical Management *William A. Buchheit,
    Tomas E. Delgado*   720

Section H Posterior Fossa Tumors
82 Radiology of Posterior Fossa Tumors
    Shelley B. Rosenbloom, Arthur E. Rosenbaum   730
83 Cerebellar Astrocytomas *David G. McLone*   754
84 Medulloblastomas *Luis Schut, Derek A. Bruce,
    Leslie N. Sutton*   758
85 Brain Stem Gliomas *Mark S. O'Brien, Mary M. Johnson*
    762
86 Ependymomas *George J. Dohrmann*   767
87 Hemangioblastomas *Setti S. Rengachary*   772
88 Choroid Plexus Papillomas *Hector E. James*   783
89 Chemodectomas *James T. Robertson*   785

Section I Sellar and Parasellar Tumors
90 Hypothalamic Control of Anterior Pituitary Function:
    Surgical Implications *Robert B. Page*   791
91 Anatomy and Physiology of the Neurohypophysis
    William A. Shucart, Ivor M. D. Jackson   805
92 Microsurgical Anatomy of the Sellar Region
    Albert L. Rhoton, Jr.   811
93 Radiology of Sellar and Parasellar Lesions
    James C. Hoffman, Jr.   822
94 Classification and Pathology of Pituitary Tumors
    Kalman Kovacs, Eva Horvath, Sylvia L. Asa
    834
95 Endocrine Diagnosis in Neurosurgery *Nicholas T. Zervas*
    843
96 Prolactinomas *George T. Tindall, Daniel L. Barrow*
    852
97 Cushing's Disease and Nelson's Syndrome
    James E. Boggan, Charles B. Wilson   859
98 Acromegaly and Gigantism *Edward R. Laws, Jr.*
    864
99 Perioperative Endocrine Management of Patients with
    Pituitary Tumors *Kalmon D. Post, William Cobb*
    868
100 Bromocriptine *William S. Evans, Michael O. Thorner*
    873
101 Pituitary Apoplexy *Richard L. Rovit*   879
102 Empty Sella Syndrome *Peter W. Carmel*   884
103 Trans-sphenoidal Approach to the Pituitary Gland
    J. Hardy   889
104 Stereotactic Treatment of Pituitary Tumors
    Robert W. Rand   899
105 Subfrontal Approach to the Pituitary Gland
    Russel H. Patterson, Jr.   902
106 Craniopharyngiomas *Peter W. Carmel*   905
107 Optic Gliomas *Edgar M. Housepian, Merlin D. Marquardt,
    Myles Behrens*   916
108 Suprasellar Germinomas *John W. Walsh*   921
109 Diencephalic Syndrome *John E. Kalsbeck*   925
110 Cranial Chordomas *Edward R. Laws, Jr.*   927
111 Parasellar Granular Cell Tumors *Dennis H. Becker*
    930
112 Benign Pituitary Cysts *Howard M. Eisenberg,
    Richard L. Weiner*   932

Section J Third Ventricular Tumors
113 Masses of the Third Ventricle *J. Lobo Antunes*
    935
114 Operative Approaches to the Third Ventricle
    Albert L. Rhoton, Jr., Isao Yamamoto   938

Section K Tumors of the Orbit
115 Radiology of the Orbit and Its Contents
    Richard E. Latchaw, William E. Rothfus   952
116 Tumors of the Orbit *Joseph C. Maroon,
    John S. Kennerdell*   964

Section L Tumors of the Scalp and Skull
117 Noninvasive Tumors of the Scalp *B. Thomas Harter, Jr.,
    Kathleen C. Harter, Donald Serafin*   977
118 Tumors of the Skull *Rand M. Voorhies,
    Narayan Sundaresan*   984
119 Craniofacial Resection for Advanced Head and Neck
    Cancers *James P. Neifeld, Harold F. Young*   1002

Contents ix

120 **Surgical Resection of Tumors of the Skull Base**
Leonard I. Malis 1011

Section M   Miscellaneous Intracranial Tumors
121 **Primary Lymphoma of the Central Nervous System**
*Milam E. Leavens, John T. Manning, Sidney Wallace,
Moshe H. Maor, William S. Velasquez* 1022
122 **Intracranial Sarcomas** *J. F. Ross Fleming,
John H. N. Deck, Mark Bernstein* 1030
123 **Lipoma of the Corpus Callosum** *Doyle G. Graham*
1036

Section N   Spinal Tumors
124 **Radiology of Spinal Canal Neoplasia** *Andrew L. Tievsky,
David O. Davis* 1039
125 **Spinal Intradural Tumors** *Bennett M. Stein* 1048
126 **Spinal Epidural Tumors** *Perry Black* 1062
127 **Spinal Chordomas** *Narayan Sundaresan,
Ralph C. Marcove* 1069
128 **Vertebral Hemangiomas** *David C. Hemmy* 1076
129 **Masses of the Sacrum** *Setti S. Rengachary* 1079

Section O   Adjunctive Therapy of CNS Tumors
130 **Principles of Radiotherapy of CNS Tumors**
K. Thomas Noell, Arnold M. Herskovic 1084
131 **Conventional Radiotherapy of Specific CNS
Tumors** *Steven R. Plunkett* 1096
132 **Heavy Particle Irradiation of Intracranial Lesions**
*John H. Lawrence, Cornelius A. Tobias, John A. Linfoot,
Joseph R. Castro, William M. Saunders, George T. Chen,
J. Michael Collier, Devron Char, Grant Gauger,
Kay Woodruff, Sandra Zink, Jacob I. Fabrikant,
John T. Lyman, Yoshio Hosobuchi* 1113
133 **Fast Neutron Irradiation of Malignant
Gliomas** *Alexander M. Spence* 1132
134 **Interstitial Brachytherapy of Primary Brain
Tumors** *Philip H. Gutin* 1136
135 **Immunotherapy of Human Gliomas**
Michael L. J. Apuzzo 1139
136 **Chemotherapy of Primary Brain Tumors**
*S. Clifford Schold, Jr., J. Gregory Cairncross,
Dennis E. Bullard* 1143
137 **Blood-Brain Barrier Modification in Delivery of
Antitumor Agents** *Edward A. Neuwelt* 1153
138 **Hyperthermia in the Treatment of Intracranial
Tumors** *Robert G. Selker* 1159

VOLUME II

Part VII   Vascular Diseases of the Nervous System

Section A   Occlusive Cerebrovascular Disease
139 **Cerebral Blood Flow** *Thomas W. Langfitt,
Walter D. Obrist* 1167
140 **Measurement of Cerebral Blood Flow** *Howard Yonas*
1173
141 **Normal Cerebral Energy Metabolism**
Michael J. O'Connor, Steven J. Barrer, Frank A. Welsh
1179
142 **Pathophysiological Consequences of Brain Ischemia**
Jewell L. Osterholm 1185
143 **Atherosclerosis** *Jack C. Geer, Julio H. Garcia* 1189
144 **Pathology of Ischemic Cerebrovascular Disease**
John Moossy 1193
145 **Clinical Syndromes of Brain Ischemia**
David G. Sherman, J. Donald Easton 1199
146 **Noninvasive Tests in the Diagnosis of Carotid Vascular
Disease** *Robert M. Crowell, J. Philip Kistler*
1212
147 **Radiology of Ischemic Cerebrovascular Disease**
Herbert I. Goldberg 1219
148 **Extracranial Carotid Artery Atherosclerosis**
Robert G. Ojemann 1236

149 **Vertebral Artery Atherosclerosis** *James I. Ausman,
Fernando G. Diaz, R. A. de los Reyes* 1248
150 **Moyamoya Disease** *David G. Piepgras* 1254
151 **Medical Treatment of Ischemic Cerebral Vascular
Disease** *H. J. M. Barnett* 1258
152 **Potential Role of Perfluorocarbons in Neurosurgery**
S. J. Peerless 1264
153 **Surgery for Acute Brain Infarction with Mass Effect**
Setti S. Rengachary 1267
154 **Extracranial to Intracranial Bypass Grafting: Anterior
Circulation** *Jack M. Fein* 1272
155 **Extracranial to Intracranial Bypass Grafting: Posterior
Circulation** *Thoralf M. Sundt, Jr., David G. Piepgras*
1281
156 **Fibromuscular Dysplasia** *L. N. Hopkins,
James L. Budny* 1293
157 **Arterial Dissections** *Allan H. Friedman* 1297
158 **Nonseptic Venous Occlusive Disease** *John P. Kapp*
1300

Section B   Intracranial Aneurysms
159 **Intracranial Aneurysms and Subarachnoid Hemorrhage:
An Overview** *Bryce Weir* 1308
160 **Microsurgical Anatomy of Saccular Aneurysms**
Albert L. Rhoton, Jr. 1330
161 **Radiology of Intracranial Aneurysms** *Eugene F. Binet,
Edgardo J. C. Angtuaco* 1341
162 **Intracranial Arterial Spasm** *Robert R. Smith,
Junji Yoshioka* 1355
163 **Timing of Aneurysm Surgery** *Neal F. Kassell,
David J. Boarini* 1363
164 **Patients with Ruptured Aneurysm: Pre- and
Postoperative Management** *Neal F. Kassell,
David J. Boarini* 1367
165 **Aneurysm Clips** *John M. Tew, Jr., Hans Jacob Steiger*
1372
166 **Middle Cerebral Artery Aneurysms** *Roberto C. Heros*
1376
167 **Distal Anterior Cerebral Artery Aneurysms**
Alan S. Fleischer, Daniel L. Barrow 1383
168 **Carotid-Ophthalmic Artery Aneurysms**
Gary G. Ferguson 1385
169 **Aneurysms of Internal Carotid and Anterior
Communicating Arteries** *Eugene S. Flamm* 1394
170 **Giant Intracranial Aneurysms** *Yoshio Hosobuchi*
1404
171 **Carotid Ligation** *Richard A. Roski,
Robert F. Spetzler* 1414
172 **Posterior Circulation Aneurysms** *S. J. Peerless,
Charles G. Drake* 1422
173 **Surgery for Unruptured Intracranial Aneurysms**
Duke Samson 1437
174 **Inflammatory Intracranial Aneurysms** *John G. Frazee*
1440
175 **Aneurysm Treatments Other Than Clipping**
John F. Alksne 1444

Section C   Vascular Malformations and Fistulas
176 **Intracranial Arteriovenous Malformations**
H. D. Garretson 1448
177 **Vein of Galen Aneurysms** *A. Loren Amacher* 1459
178 **Other Cranial Intradural Angiomas** *Setti S. Rengachary,
Uma P. Kalyan-Raman* 1465
179 **Dural Arteriovenous Malformations** *Alfred J. Luessenhop*
1473
180 **Surgical Anatomy of the Cavernous Sinus**
Dwight Parkinson 1478
181 **Carotid-Cavernous Fistulas and Intracavernous
Aneurysms** *Sean Mullan* 1483
182 **Spinal Arteriovenous Malformations** *Ayub Khan Ommaya*
1495
183 **Spontaneous Intraspinal Hemorrhage** *Hugh S. Wisoff*
1500

Section D Hypertension
184 Neurogenic Hypertension *Jack M. Fein*   *1505*
185 Spontaneous Intracerebral Hemorrhage
     Thomas B. Ducker   *1510*

Section E Coagulopathies and Vasculopathies
186 Coagulopathies Causing Intracranial Hemorrhage
     Justin W. Renaudin, Ralph P. George   *1518*
187 Vasculopathies *Setti S. Rengachary*   *1521*

Part VIII Trauma

Section A Cranial Trauma
188 Biomechanics of Head Injury *Thomas A. Gennarelli,*
     Lawrence E. Thibault   *1531*
189 Pathophysiology of Head Injury *A. John Popp,*
     Robert S. Bourke   *1536*
190 Pathology of Closed Head Injury *William F. McCormick*
     1544
191 Neurological Evaluation of a Patient with Head Trauma:
     Coma Scales *Victoria Neave, Martin H. Weiss*   *1570*
192 Computed Tomography in Head Trauma *Chi-Shing Zee,*
     Hervey D. Segall, Jamshid Ahmadi, Michael L. J. Apuzzo,
     Steven L. Giannotta   *1578*
193 Resuscitation of the Multiply Injured Patient
     Paul R. Cooper   *1587*
194 Intensive Management of Head Injury *Donald P. Becker,*
     Stephen Gardner   *1593*
195 Pediatric Head Injury *Derek A. Bruce, Luis Schut,*
     Leslie N. Sutton   *1600*
196 Outcome Prediction in Severe Head Injury
     Lawrence F. Marshall, Sharon A. Bowers   *1605*
197 Minor Head Injury: Management and Outcome
     Rebecca W. Rimel, John A. Jane   *1608*
198 Scalp Injuries *William J. Barwick*   *1612*
199 Cephalhematoma and Subgaleal Hematoma
     Derek A. Bruce, Luis Schut, Leslie N. Sutton   *1622*
200 Skull Fractures *L. M. Thomas*   *1623*
201 Growing Skull Fractures of Childhood
     Timothy B. Scarff, Michael Fine   *1627*
202 Facial Fractures *Ronald Riefkohl, Gregory S. Georgiade,*
     Nicholas G. Georgiade   *1629*
203 Cerebrospinal Fluid Fistula *Ayub Khan Ommaya*
     1637
204 Cranial Defects and Cranioplasty *Donald J. Prolo*
     1647
205 Traumatic Intracranial Hematomas *Paul R. Cooper*
     1657
206 Delayed and Recurrent Intracranial Hematomas and
     Post-Traumatic Coagulopathies *Michael E. Miner*
     1666
207 Penetrating Wounds of the Head *Griffith R. Harsh, III,*
     Griffith R. Harsh, IV   *1670*
208 Vascular Lesions with Head Injury *Steven L. Giannotta,*
     Jamshid Ahmadi   *1678*
209 Sequelae of Head Injury *Byron Young*   *1688*

Section B Spinal Trauma
210 Experimental Spinal Cord Injury *Arthur I. Kobrine,*
     Jerald J. Bernstein   *1694*
211 High Cervical Spine Injuries *Richard C. Schneider*
     1701
212 Mid- and Lower Cervical Spine Injuries
     Martin H. Weiss   *1708*
213 Psychological Aspects of Whiplash Injury *Henry Berry*
     1716
214 Cervical Traction *Albert B. Butler*   *1719*
215 Halo Immobilization of Cervical Spine Injuries
     William T. Hardaker, Jr.   *1723*
216 Anterior Approach in Cervical Spine Injuries
     Edward L. Seljeskog   *1727*
217 Diaphragm Pacing *Ronald F. Young*   *1733*
218 Injuries to the Thoracic and Lumbar Spine
     Wesley A. Cook, Jr., William T. Hardaker, Jr.   *1735*
219 Injuries to the Sacrum and Pelvis *Barth A. Green,*
     Ignacio Magana   *1744*

220 Penetrating Wounds of the Spine *Carole A. Miller*
     1746
221 Posterior Lumbar Spinal Fusion *J. Leonard Goldner*
     1749
222 Post-Traumatic Syringomyelia *Joseph H. Piatt, Jr.*
     1761

**Part IX Disorders of Peripheral and Cranial Nerves
     and the Autonomic Nervous System**

Section A Entrapment Neuropathies
223 Thoracic Outlet Syndromes *Russell W. Hardy, Jr.,*
     Asa J. Wilbourn   *1767*
224 Entrapment Neuropathies *Setti S. Rengachary*   *1771*

Section B Acute Nerve Injuries
225 Anatomy and Physiology of Peripheral Nerves
     Robert M. Worth   *1796*
226 Peripheral Nerve Injuries: Types, Causes, Grading
     F. Gentili, Alan R. Hudson   *1802*
227 Pathophysiology of Peripheral Nerve Trauma
     Thomas B. Ducker   *1812*
228 Brachial Plexus Injuries *Alan R. Hudson, B. Tranmer*
     1817
229 Diagnostic Approach to Individual Nerve Injuries
     David G. Kline   *1833*
230 Surgical Exposure of Peripheral Nerves
     Charles L. Branch, Jr., David L. Kelly, Jr.,
     George C. Lynch   *1846*
231 Management of the Neuroma in Continuity
     David G. Kline, Earl R. Hackett   *1864*
232 Techniques of Nerve Repair *John E. McGillicuddy*
     1871
233 Clinical Signs of Peripheral Nerve Regeneration
     Irvine G. McQuarrie   *1881*
234 Painful Neuromas *Suzie C. Tindall*   *1884*
235 Causalgia; Sympathetic Dystrophy (Sudeck's Atrophy)
     William H. Sweet   *1886*

Section C Nerve Tumors
236 Neoplasms of Peripheral Nerves *Humberto Cravioto*
     1894
237 Ganglion Cysts of Peripheral Nerves *Suzie C. Tindall*
     1900

Section D Neurovascular Compression Syndromes
238 Posterior Fossa Neurovascular Compression Syndromes
     Other than Neuralgias *Peter J. Jannetta*   *1901*

Section E Miscellaneous
239 Techniques of Diagnostic Nerve and Muscle
     Biopsies *Edward S. Connolly*   *1907*
240 Nontraumatic Brachial Plexopathy *E. Wayne Massey*
     1909
241 Surgical Sympathectomy *Janet W. Bay, Donald F. Dohn*
     1912

VOLUME III

Part X Infections

Section A Bacterial Infections
242 Acute Bacterial Meningitis *David T. Durack,*
     John R. Perfect   *1921*
243 Brain Abscess *Richard H. Britt*   *1928*
244 Inflammatory Thrombosis of Major Dural Venous
     Sinuses and Cortical Veins *Frederick S. Southwick,*
     Morton N. Swartz   *1956*
245 Cranial Epidural Abscess and Subdural Empyema
     Justin W. Renaudin   *1961*
246 Infections of the Scalp and Osteomyelitis of the Skull
     Stephen J. Haines, Shelley N. Chou   *1964*
247 Pituitary Abscess *James E. Boggan, Charles B. Wilson*
     1967
248 Spinal Cord Abscess *Arnold H. Menezes,*
     John C. VanGilder   *1969*

249 Spinal Epidural and Subdural Abscesses
     Marshall B. Allen, Jr., Wayne D. Beveridge   1972
250 Osteomyelitis of the Spine   *Donald E. McCollum*
     1975
251 Chronic Granulomatous Lesions: Tuberculosis, Leprosy,
     Sarcoidosis   *Mark L. Rosenblum*   1980

Section B   Viral Infections
252 *Herpes simplex* Virus Infections   *Richard J. Whitley,*
     Richard B. Morawetz   1987
253 Creutzfeldt-Jakob Disease   *Clarence J. Gibbs, Jr.*
     1994

Section C   Fungal and Parasitic Infections
254 Fungal Infections   *Allan H. Friedman, Elizabeth Bullitt*
     2002
255 Parasitic Infestations   *W. Eugene Stern*   2010

**Part XI   Developmental Anomalies and Neurosurgical
            Diseases of Childhood**

256 Neurological Evaluation of the Newborn and
     Child   *Andrew K. Hodson*   2019
257 Genetics of Developmental Defects   *David D. Weaver*
     2025
258 Spinal Dysraphism   *Robin P. Humphreys*   2041
259 Occult Spinal Dysraphism and Related Disorders
     Larry K. Page   2053
260 Diastematomyelia   *A. Norman Guthkelch*   2058
261 Intraspinal Cysts   *Robert H. Wilkins*   2061
262 Lateral and Anterior Spinal Meningoceles
     Robert H. Wilkins   2070
263 Sacral Agenesis   *Dachling Pang*   2075
264 Sacrococcygeal Teratomas   *Howard C. Filston*   2077
265 Congenital Dermal Sinus   *J. Gordon McComb*   2081
266 Congenital Defects of the Scalp and Skull   *Dan Fults,*
     David L. Kelly, Jr.   2084
267 Encephaloceles   *E. Bruce Hendrick*   2087
268 Craniopagus Twins   *Theodore S. Roberts*   2091
269 Craniovertebral Junction Anomalies   *John C. VanGilder,*
     Arnold H. Menezes   2097
270 Chiari Malformations, Hydromyelia, Syringomyelia
     W. Jerry Oakes   2102
271 Physiology of Cerebrospinal Fluid   *Humbert G. Sullivan,*
     Jerry D. Allison   2125
272 Hydrocephalus: Pathophysiology and Clinical
     Features   *Thomas H. Milhorat*   2135
273 Hydrocephalus: Treatment   *David C. McCullough*
     2140
274 Double Compartment Hydrocephalus   *Eldon L. Foltz*
     2151
275 Dandy-Walker Syndrome   *Robert L. McLaurin*   2153
276 Antenatal Diagnosis and Treatment of
     Hydrocephalus   *Robert A. Brodner*   2156
277 Intracranial Arachnoid and Ependymal Cysts
     Setti S. Rengachary   2160
278 Craniosynostosis   *Ken R. Winston*   2173
279 Craniofacial Anomalies   *Harold J. Hoffman*   2192
280 Neonatal Intracranial Hemorrhage   *Herbert Lourie*
     2203
281 Strokes in Children   *Mel H. Epstein*   2205
282 Subdural Hematomas and Effusions in Children
     Robert L. McLaurin   2211
283 Control of Increased Intracranial Pressure in Reye's
     Syndrome   *Joan L. Venes*   2215

**Part XII   Intervertebral Disc Disease and Selected
             Spinal Disorders**

284 Biomechanics of the Spine   *Manohar M. Panjabi,*
     Richard R. Pelker, Augustus A. White, III   2219
285 Osteoporosis   *John M. Harrelson*   2228
286 Cervical Disc Disease and Cervical Spondylosis
     Julian T. Hoff   2230
287 Rheumatoid Arthritis of the Cervical Spine
     Chitranjan S. Ranawat   2240

288 Ossification of the Posterior Longitudinal Ligament
     Louis Bakay   2243
289 Thoracic Disc Disease   *Phanor L. Perot, Jr.*   2245
290 Lumbar Disc Disease   *Frederick A. Simeone*   2250
291 Chemonucleolysis   *Clark Watts*   2260
292 Lumbar Intradural Disc Rupture   *Charles J. Hodge, Jr.*
     2264
293 Postoperative Intervertebral Disc Space Infections
     Charles E. Rawlings, III, Robert H. Wilkins   2266
294 Lumbar Spondylosis and Spinal Stenosis
     Joseph A. Epstein, Nancy E. Epstein   2272
295 The Lateral Recess Syndrome   *Ivan Ciric,*
     Michael A. Mikhael   2279
296 Redundant Nerve Root Syndrome of the Cauda Equina
     Setti S. Rengachary   2283
297 Lumbar Spondylolisthesis   *John M. Cuckler,*
     Richard H. Rothman   2285
298 The Failed Back   *Charles V. Burton*   2290
299 Postlaminectomy Kyphosis   *Eben Alexander, Jr.*
     2293
300 Neurological Complications of Scoliosis
     Shelley N. Chou   2298
301 Spinal Bracing   *James M. Morris*   2300
302 Neural Dysfunction in Paget's Disease of Bone
     Henry H. Schmidek, Alan Waters   2305

Part XIII   Pain

Section A   Basic Science
303 Anatomy and Physiology of Pain   *Donlin M. Long*
     2313
304 Gate Control Theory   *Ronald Melzack, Patrick D. Wall*
     2317

Section B   Clinical Evaluation
305 Psychological Factors in the Assessment and
     Management of Chronic Pain   *Randal D. France*
     2320
306 Multidisciplinary Pain Clinic   *Bruno J. Urban*   2323

Section C   Certain Specific Pain Syndromes
307 Craniofacial Pain Syndromes: An Overview
     Robert E. Maxwell   2327
308 Trigeminal Neuralgia: Introduction   *Robert H. Wilkins*
     2337
309 Trigeminal Neuralgia: Treatment by Percutaneous
     Electrocoagulation   *G. Robert Nugent*   2345
310 Trigeminal Neuralgia: Treatment by Glycerol
     Rhizotomy   *L. Dade Lunsford*   2351
311 Trigeminal Neuralgia: Treatment by Microvascular
     Decompression   *Peter J. Jannetta*   2357
312 Glossopharyngeal Neuralgia   *Burton M. Onofrio*   2363
313 Postherpetic Neuralgia   *Allan H. Friedman,*
     Blaine S. Nashold, Jr.   2367
314 Pain Following Spinal Cord Injury   *Charles H. Tator*
     2368
315 Phantom Limb Pain   *John D. Loeser*   2371

Section D   Management of Chronic Intractable Pain
316 Drug Therapy of Chronic Pain   *Nelson Hendler*
     2374
317 Diagnostic and Therapeutic Nerve Blocks
     Bruno J. Urban   2382
318 Intraspinal Infusion of Narcotic Drugs
     Dennis W. Coombs, Richard L. Saunders   2390
319 Physical Medicine and Physical Therapy   *John Mennell*
     2397
320 Conservative Management of Lumbar and Cervical
     Pain   *Marcia Sirotkin-Roses*   2404
321 Acupuncture   *Terence M. Murphy*   2408

Section E   Electrical Stimulation
322 Transcutaneous Electrical Stimulation for Pain Relief
     Donlin M. Long   2410
323 Peripheral Nerve Stimulation for Pain Relief
     James Gardner Wepsic   2415

324 **Percutaneous Spinal Epidural Stimulation for Pain Relief** *Bruno J. Urban* 2417
325 **Deep Brain Stimulation for Pain Relief** *Donald E. Richardson* 2421

Section F Ablative Procedures
326 **Percutaneous Radio-Frequency Denervation of Spinal Facets** *Douglas E. Kennemore* 2427
327 **Dorsal Rhizotomy** *A. Basil Harris* 2430
328 **Dorsal Root Entry Zone Lesions for Pain Relief** *Blaine S. Nashold, Jr., Alfred C. Higgins, Bennett Blumenkopf* 2433
329 **Commissural Myelotomy for Pain Relief** *Robert B. King* 2438
330 **Open Surgical Cordotomy** *Bruce L. Ehni, George Ehni* 2439
331 **Percutaneous Spinothalamic Cordotomy** *Hubert L. Rosomoff* 2446
332 **Medullary Tractotomy for Pain Relief** *Robert B. King* 2452
333 **Stereotactic Ablative Procedures for Pain Relief** *Ronald F. Young, Luciano M. Modesti* 2454
334 **Hypophysectomy** *George T. Tindall, Suzie C. Tindall* 2458

Part XIV Stereotactic and Functional Neurosurgery
335 **Stereotactic Surgery: Principles and Techniques** *Ronald R. Tasker* 2465
336 **CT Stereotactic Guidance Systems** *M. Peter Heilbrun, Theodore S. Roberts* 2481
337 **Methods of Making Nervous System Lesions** *Eric R. Cosman, Bernard J. Cosman* 2490
338 **Medical Therapy of Movement Disorders** *C. Warren Olanow* 2499
339 **Surgical Therapy of Movement Disorders** *Philip L. Gildenberg* 2507
340 **Surgical Treatment of Epilepsy** *George A. Ojemann* 2517
341 **Neurosurgery for Behavioral Disorders** *H. Thomas Ballantine, Jr.* 2527

342 **Chronic Cerebellar Stimulation in Humans** *Richard D. Penn* 2537
343 **Neural Prostheses** *John P. Girvin* 2543
344 **Central Nervous System Grafting** *Richard Jed Wyatt, William J. Freed* 2546

Part XV Miscellaneous Topics
345 **Practice Management** *Phillip Earle Williams, Jr.* 2555
346 **Disability Evaluation** *Byron C. Pevehouse* 2561
347 **The Informed Consent** *William E. Hunt* 2569
348 **The Professional Liability Insurance Crisis** *William H. Mosberg, Jr.* 2571
349 **Clinical Research** *Donlin M. Long* 2579
350 **The Medical Determination of Death** *Roy Selby* 2585
351 **Transplantation of Cadaver Tissues and Organs** *Donald J. Prolo* 2598
352 **Methods and Techniques of Intraoperative Microphotography** *Ronald I. Apfelbaum* 2601

Part XVI Appendix

Appendix A Drugs Commonly Used in Neurological Surgery
Table A1 **Drug Dosages** 2611
Table A2 **Drug Dosage Adjustments in Renal Insufficiency** 2634
Table A3 **Therapeutic and Toxic Dosage Ranges of Commonly Used Drugs** 2636

Appendix B Range of Values for Commonly Performed Laboratory Tests
Table B1 **Reference Ranges: Hematologic, Serologic, and Coagulation Studies** 2637
Table B2 **Reference Ranges: Clinical Chemistry** 2638

Index 2643

LIST OF
CONTRIBUTORS

Jamshid Ahmadi, M.D.
Assistant Professor, Department of Radiology, University of Southern California School of Medicine, Los Angeles, California

Maurice S. Albin, M.D., M.Sc. (Anes.)
Professor, Department of Anesthesiology and Director, Neuroanesthesia Service, University of Texas Health Science Center at San Antonio, San Antonio, Texas

Eben Alexander, Jr., M.D.
Professor, Section on Neurosurgery, Bowman Gray School of Medicine, Winston-Salem, North Carolina

John F. Alksne, M.D.
Professor and Chairman, Division of Neurological Surgery, University of California, San Diego, San Diego, California

Marshall B. Allen, Jr., M.D.
Professor and Chief, Section of Neurosurgery, Medical College of Georgia, Augusta, Georgia

Jerry D. Allison, Ph.D.
Assistant Professor, Department of Radiology, Medical College of Georgia, Augusta, Georgia

A. Loren Amacher, M.D., F.R.C.S.(C)
Associate Professor, Division of Neurosurgery, University of Connecticut, Hartford, Connecticut

Edgardo J. C. Angtuaco, M.D.
Department of Radiology, University of Arkansas for Medical Sciences, Little Rock, Arkansas

J. Lobo Antunes, M.D.
Professor and Chairman, Department of Neurological Surgery, University of Lisbon, Lisbon, Portugal

Ronald I. Apfelbaum, M.D.
Associate Professor, Leo M. Davidoff Department of Neurological Surgery, Albert Einstein College of Medicine, Bronx, New York

Michael L. J. Apuzzo, M.D.
Professor, Department of Neurosurgery, University of Southern California School of Medicine, Los Angeles, California

Sylvia L. Asa, M.D.
Department of Pathology, St. Michael's Hospital, University of Toronto, Toronto, Ontario, Canada

James I. Ausman, M.D., Ph.D.
Chairman, Department of Neurological Surgery, Henry Ford Hospital, Detroit, Michigan

Louis Bakay, M.D.
Professor and Chairman, Department of Neurosurgery, School of Medicine, State University of New York at Buffalo, Buffalo, New York

H. Thomas Ballantine, Jr., M.D.
Clinical Professor of Surgery Emeritus, Harvard Medical School, and Senior Neurosurgeon, Massachusetts General Hospital, Boston, Massachusetts

Robert W. Baloh, M.D.
Professor of Neurology and Surgery (Head and Neck), Department of Neurology, University of California Center for the Health Sciences, Los Angeles, California

H. J. M. Barnett, M.D., F.R.C.P.(C), F.R.C.P.
Richard and Beryl Ivey Professor, Department of Clinical Neurological Sciences, University of Western Ontario, London, Ontario, Canada

Steven J. Barrer, M.D.
Assistant Professor, Division of Neurosurgery, School of Medicine, University of Pennsylvania, Philadelphia, Pennsylvania

Daniel L. Barrow, M.D.
Resident, Division of Neurological Surgery, Emory University School of Medicine, Atlanta, Georgia

William J. Barwick, M.D.
Assistant Professor, Division of Plastic and Maxillofacial Surgery, Duke University Medical Center, Durham, North Carolina

Jere W. Baxter, M.D.
Assistant Professor, Department of Pathology, Vanderbilt University School of Medicine, Nashville, Tennessee

Janet W. Bay, M.D.
Department of Neurological Surgery, Cleveland Clinic Foundation, Cleveland, Ohio

William L. Bayer, M.D.
Community Blood Center of Greater Kansas City, Kansas City, Missouri

Dennis H. Becker, M.D.
Chief, Division of Neurosurgery, Santa Clara Valley Medical Center, San Jose, California

Donald P. Becker, M.D.
Professor and Chairman, Division of Neurological Surgery, Medical College of Virginia, Virginia Commonwealth University, Richmond, Virginia

Myles Behrens, M.D.
Associate Professor of Clinical Ophthalmology, College of Physicians & Surgeons, Columbia University, New York, New York

Jerald J. Bernstein, Ph.D.
Chief, Laboratory of Central Nervous System Injury and Regeneration, Veterans Administration Medical Center, Washington, District of Columbia

Mark Bernstein, M.D.
Division of Neurosurgery, University of Toronto, Toronto, Ontario, Canada

Henry Berry, M.D., D.Psych., F.R.C.P.(C)
Head, Department of Neurology, St. Michael's Hospital, Toronto, Ontario, Canada

Wayne D. Beveridge, M.D.
Associate Professor, Section of Neurosurgery, Medical College of Georgia, Augusta, Georgia

Darell D. Bigner, M.D., Ph.D.
Professor, Department of Pathology, Duke University Medical Center, Durham, North Carolina

Eugene F. Binet, M.D.
Professor and Vice Chairman, Department of Radiology, University of Arkansas for Medical Sciences, Little Rock, Arkansas

C. Roger Bird, M.D.
Assistant Professor, Department of Radiology, Stanford University Medical Center, Stanford, California

Perry Black, M.D., C.M.
Professor and Chairman, Department of Neurosurgery, Hahnemann University School of Medicine, Philadelphia, Pennsylvania

Peter McL. Black, M.D., Ph.D.
Assistant Professor of Surgery, Harvard Medical School; Assistant Visiting Neurosurgeon, Massachusetts General Hospital, Boston, Massachusetts

Bennett Blumenkopf, M.D.
Major, Medial Corps, U. S. Army; Assistant Chief, Neurosurgery Service, Brooke Army Medical Center, Fort Sam Houston, Texas

David J. Boarini, M.D.
Resident, Division of Neurosurgery, University of Iowa, Iowa City, Iowa

James E. Boggan, M.D.
Assistant Clinical Professor, Department of Neurological Surgery, School of Medicine, University of California, San Francisco, San Francisco, California

Robert S. Bourke, M.D.
Professor and Chairman, Division of Neurosurgery, Albany Medical College, Albany, New York

Sharon A. Bowers, B.S.N.
Division of Neurological Surgery, University of California, San Diego, San Diego, California

Charles L. Branch, Jr., M.D.
Resident, Section on Neurosurgery, Bowman Gray School of Medicine, Winston-Salem, North Carolina

Michael Brant-Zawadzki, M.D.
Associate Professor, Department of Radiology, School of Medicine, University of California, San Francisco, San Francisco, California

Andrea Brendle, B.A.
Evoked Potential Laboratory, Duke University Medical Center, Durham, North Carolina

Joseph Bressler, Ph.D.
Surgical Neurology Branch, National Institute of Neurological and Communicative Disorders and Stroke, Bethesda, Maryland

Richard H. Britt, M.D., Ph.D.
Assistant Professor, Division of Neurosurgery, Stanford University Medical Center, Stanford, California

Robert A. Brodner, M.D.
Assistant Professor, Department of Neurosurgery, Hahnemann University School of Medicine, Philadelphia, Pennsylvania

Derek A. Bruce, M.B., Ch.B.
Division of Neurosurgery, Children's Hospital of Philadelphia, Philadelphia, Pennsylvania

William A. Buchheit, M.D.
Professor and Chairman, Department of Neurosurgery, Temple University Health Sciences Center, Philadelphia, Pennsylvania

Paul C. Bucy, M.D.
Clinical Professor Emeritus of Neurology and Neurological Surgery, Bowman Gray School of Medicine, Winston-Salem, North Carolina

James L. Budny, M.D.
Dent Neurologic Institute, Buffalo, New York

Dennis E. Bullard, M.D.
Assistant Professor, Division of Neurosurgery, Duke University Medical Center, Durham, North Carolina

Elizabeth Bullitt, M.D.
Clinical Instructor, Department of Neurological Surgery, University of Cincinnati Medical Center, Cincinnati, Ohio

Peter C. Burger, M.D.
Associate Professor, Department of Pathology, Duke University Medical Center, Durham, North Carolina

Charles V. Burton, M.D.
Medical Director, Institute for Low Back Care, Minneapolis, Minnesota

Albert B. Butler, M.D.
Professor and Chairman, Department of Neurological Surgery, Health Sciences Center, State University of New York at Stony Brook, Stony Brook, New York

Ian J. Butler, M.B., F.R.A.C.P.
Professor, Department of Neurology, University of Texas Medical School at Houston, Houston, Texas

J. Gregory Cairncross, M.D.
Assistant Professor, Departments of Clinical Neurological Sciences and Radiation Oncology, University of Western Ontario, London, Ontario, Canada

Peter W. Carmel, M.D., D.Med.Sci.
Associate Professor, Department of Neurological Surgery, College of Physicians & Surgeons, Columbia University, New York, New York

Joseph R. Castro, M.D.
Lawrence Berkeley Laboratory and Donner Laboratory, University of California, Berkeley, Berkeley, California

Leonard J. Cerullo, M.D.
University Neurosurgeons, Chicago, Illinois

Venkata R. Challa, M.D.
Assistant Professor, Department of Pathology, Bowman Gray School of Medicine, Winston-Salem, North Carolina

Devron Char, M.D.
Lawrence Berkeley Laboratory and Donner Laboratory, University of California, Berkeley, Berkeley, California

George T. Chen, Ph.D.
Lawrence Berkeley Laboratory and Donner Laboratory, University of California, Berkeley, Berkeley, California

Shelley N. Chou, M.D. Ph.D.
Professor and Chairman, Department of Neurosurgery, University of Minnesota Medical School, Minneapolis, Minnesota

Ivan Ciric, M.D.
Department of Neurosurgery, Evanston Hospital, Evanston, Illinois

William Cobb, M.D.
Assistant Professor, Department of Medicine, Tufts University School of Medicine, Boston, Massachusetts

J. Michael Collier, Ph.D.
Lawrence Berkeley Laboratory and Donner Laboratory, University of California, Berkeley, Berkeley, California

Frances K. Conley, M.D.
Associate Professor, Division of Neurosurgery, Stanford University Medical Center, Stanford, California

Edward S. Connolly, M.D.
Head, Department of Neurosurgery, Ochsner Clinic and Alton Ochsner Medical Foundation, New Orleans, Louisiana

Wesley A. Cook, Jr., M.D.
Associate Professor, Division of Neurosurgery, Duke University Medical Center, Durham, North Carolina

Dennis W. Coombs, M.D.
Assistant Professor of Surgery (Anesthesiology), Dartmouth-Hitchcock Medical Center, Hanover, New Hampshire

Paul R. Cooper, M.D.
Associate Professor, Department of Neurosurgery, New York University Medical Center, New York, New York

Bernard J. Cosman, M.S.
Radionics, Inc., Burlington, Massachusetts

Eric R. Cosman, Ph.D.
Department of Physics, Massachusetts Institute of Technology, Cambridge, Massachusetts

Humberto Cravioto, M.D.
Professor, Department of Pathology, New York University Medical Center, New York, New York

Didier Cros, M.D.
Assistant Professor, Department of Neurology and Psychiatry, Tulane Medical Center, New Orleans, Louisiana

Robert M. Crowell, M.D.
Professor and Head, Department of Neurosurgery, University of Illinois at Chicago, Chicago, Illinois

John M. Cuckler, M.D.
Clinical Assistant Professor of Orthopaedic Surgery, School of Medicine, University of Pennsylvania, Philadelphia, Pennsylvania

C.J. Cummins, Ph.D.
National Institute of Neurological and Communicative Disorders and Stroke, National Institutes of Health, Bethesda, Maryland

David O. Davis, M.D.
Professor and Chairman, Department of Radiology, The George Washington University Medical Center, Washington, District of Columbia

John H. N. Deck, M.D., F.R.C.P.(C)
Associate Professor, Division of Neuropathology, University of Toronto, Toronto, Ontario, Canada

Tomas E. Delgado, M.D.
Assistant Professor, Department of Neurosurgery, Temple University Health Sciences Center, Philadelphia, Pennsylvania

R. A. de los Reyes, M.D.
Department of Neurological Surgery, Henry Ford Hospital, Detroit, Michigan

Fernando G. Diaz, M.D., Ph.D.
Department of Neurological Surgery, Henry Ford Hospital, Detroit, Michigan

Donald F. Dohn, M.D.
Singing River Neurological Surgery, Pascagoula, Mississippi

George J. Dohrmann, M.D., Ph.D.
Associate Professor, Section of Neurological Surgery, University of Chicago Medical Center, Chicago, Illinois

R. M. Peardon Donaghy, M.D.
Professor Emeritus, Division of Neurosurgery, College of Medicine, University of Vermont, Burlington, Vermont

Charles G. Drake, M.D., F.R.C.S.(C)
Professor and Chairman, Department of Surgery, University of Western Ontario, London, Ontario, Canada

Miles E. Drake, M.D.
Assistant Professor, Department of Neurology, Ohio State University College of Medicine, Columbus, Ohio

Burton P. Drayer, M.D.
Associate Professor, Section of Neuroradiology, Department of Radiology, Duke University Medical Center, Durham, North Carolina

Philip Dubois, M.B., B.S., F.R.C.R., F.R.A.C.R.
Department of Radiology, Mater Misericordiae Private Hospital, South Brisbane, Queensland, Australia

Thomas B. Ducker, M.D.
Clinical Professor, Division of Neurological Surgery, University of Maryland School of Medicine, Baltimore, Maryland

David T. Durack, M.B., B.S., D.Phil., F.R.C.P.
Professor and Chief, Division of Infectious Diseases, Duke University Medical Center, Durham, North Carolina

J. Donald Easton, M.D.
Professor and Chief, Division of Neurology, University of Texas Health Science Center at San Antonio, San Antonio, Texas

Michael S. B. Edwards, M.D.
Associate Professor, Departments of Neurological Surgery and Pediatrics, School of Medicine, University of California, San Francisco, San Francisco, California

Bruce L. Ehni, M.D.
Clinical Instructor, Department of Neurosurgery, Baylor College of Medicine and Affiliated Hospitals, Houston, Texas

George Ehni, M.D., M.S.
Professor, Department of Neurosurgery, Baylor College of Medicine and Affiliated Hospitals, Houston, Texas

Howard M. Eisenberg, M.D.
Professor and Chief, Division of Neurosurgery, University of Texas Medical Branch, Galveston, Texas

Fred Epstein, M.D.
Professor, Department of Neurosurgery, New York University Medical Center, New York, New York

Joseph A. Epstein, M.D.
Professor of Clinical Surgery (Neurosurgery), State University of New York at Stony Brook, Stony Brook, New York

Mel H. Epstein, M.D.
Associate Professor, Department of Neurological Surgery, Johns Hopkins University School of Medicine, Baltimore, Maryland

Nancy E. Epstein, M.D.
Lecturer in Neurosurgery, New York University Medical Center, New York, New York

C. William Erwin, M.D.
Professor, Division of Biological Psychiatry, Department of Psychiatry, Duke University Medical Center, Durham, North Carolina

William S. Evans, M.D.
Research Assistant Professor, Department of Internal Medicine, University of Virginia Medical Center, Charlottesville, Virginia

Jacob I. Fabrikant, M.D., Ph.D.
Lawrence Berkeley Laboratory and Donner Laboratory, University of California, Berkeley, Berkeley, California

Jack M. Fein, M.D.
Associate Professor, Leo M. Davidoff Department of Neurological Surgery, Albert Einstein College of Medicine, Bronx, New York

Gary G. Ferguson, M.D., Ph.D., F.R.C.S.(C)
Professor, Division of Neurosurgery, University of Western Ontario, London, Ontario, Canada

Howard C. Filston, M.D.
Professor, Departments of Surgery and Pediatrics, Duke University Medical Center, Durham, North Carolina

Michael Fine, M.D.
Associate Professor, Department of Radiology, Loyola University Medical Center, Maywood, Illinois

Eugene S. Flamm, M.D.
Professor and Vice Chairman, Department of Neurosurgery, New York University Medical Center, New York, New York

Alan S. Fleischer, M.D.
Professor and Chief, Section of Neurosurgery, University of Arizona Health Sciences Center, Tucson, Arizona

J. F. Ross Fleming, M.D., M.S., F.R.C.S.(C)
Associate Professor, Division of Neurosurgery, University of Toronto, Toronto, Ontario, Canada

Eldon L. Foltz, M.D.
Professor, Division of Neurological Surgery, University of California, Irvine Medical Center, Orange, California

Allan J. Fox, M.D., F.R.C.P.(C)
Associate Professor, Departments of Diagnostic Radiology and Clinical Neurological Sciences, University of Western Ontario, London, Ontario, Canada

Randal D. France, M.D.
Assistant Professor, Department of Psychiatry, Duke University Medical Center, Durham, North Carolina

John G. Frazee, M.D.
Assistant Professor, Division of Neurosurgery, University of California Center for the Health Sciences, and Wadsworth Veterans Administration Hospital, Los Angeles, California

William J. Freed, Ph.D.
Adult Psychiatry Branch, National Institute of Mental Health, Saint Elizabeth's Hospital, Washington, District of Columbia

Allan H. Friedman, M.D.
Assistant Professor, Division of Neurosurgery, Duke University Medical Center, Durham, North Carolina

Dan Fults, M.D.
Resident, Section on Neurosurgery, Bowman Gray School of Medicine, Winston-Salem, North Carolina

Anthony J. Furlan, M.D.
Director, Cerebrovascular Program, The Cleveland Clinic Foundation, Cleveland, Ohio

Joseph H. Galicich, M.D.
Chief, Neurosurgery Service, Memorial Sloan-Kettering Cancer Center, New York, New York

Julio H. Garcia, M.D.
Professor, Department of Pathology, University of Alabama in Birmingham, Birmingham, Alabama

Stephen Gardner, M.D.
Head Injury Fellow, Division of Neurological Surgery, Medical College of Virginia, Virginia Commonwealth University, Richmond, Virginia

H. D. Garretson, M.D., Ph.D.
Professor and Director, Division of Neurological Surgery, University of Louisville School of Medicine, Louisville, Kentucky

Grant Gauger, M.D.
Lawrence Berkeley Laboratory and Donner Laboratory, University of California, Berkeley, Berkeley, California

Jack C. Geer, M.D.
Professor and Chairman, Department of Pathology, University of Alabama in Birmingham, Birmingham, Alabama

Thomas A. Gennarelli, M.D.
Associate Professor, Division of Neurosurgery, School of Medicine, University of Pennsylvania, Philadelphia, Pennsylvania

F. Gentili, M.D., M.Sc., F.R.C.S.(C)
Assistant Professor, Division of Neurosurgery, University of Toronto, Toronto, Ontario, Canada

Ralph P. George, M.D.
Associate Clinical Professor, Department of Medicine, University of California, San Diego, San Diego, California

Gregory S. Georgiade, M.D.
Assistant Professor, Divisions of General and Cardio-thoracic Surgery, Duke University Medical Center, Durham, North Carolina

Nicholas G. Georgiade, D.D.S., M.D.
Professor and Chief, Division of Plastic and Maxillofacial Surgery, Duke University Medical Center, Durham, North Carolina

Steven L. Giannotta, M.D.
Assistant Professor, Department of Neurological Surgery, University of Southern California School of Medicine, Los Angeles, California

Clarence J. Gibbs, Jr., Ph.D.
Laboratory of Central Nervous System Studies, National Institute of Neurological and Communicative Disorders and Stroke, National Institutes of Health, Bethesda, Maryland

Philip L. Gildenberg, M.D., Ph.D.
Clinical Professor, Division of Neurosurgery, University of Texas Health Science Center at Houston, Houston, Texas

Myron D. Ginsberg, M.D.
Professor, Department of Neurology, School of Medicine, University of Miami, Miami, Florida

John P. Girvin, M.D., F.R.C.S.(C)
Professor and Chairman, Department of Clinical Neurological Sciences, University of Western Ontario, London, Ontario, Canada

Herbert I. Goldberg, M.D.
Professor, Department of Radiology and Division of Neurosurgery, School of Medicine, University of Pennsylvania, Philadelphia, Pennsylvania

J. Leonard Goldner, M.D.
James B. Duke Professor and Chief, Division of Orthopaedic Surgery, Duke University Medical Center, Durham, North Carolina

Doyle G. Graham, M.D., Ph.D.
Associate Professor, Department of Pathology, Duke University Medical Center, Durham, North Carolina

Barth A. Green, M.D.
Associate Professor, Department of Neurological Surgery, University of Miami School of Medicine, Miami, Florida

I. M. Greenberg, M.D.
Associate Professor of Clinical Neurosurgery, Department of Neurological Surgery, State University of New York at Stony Brook, Stony Brook, New York

Samuel H. Greenblatt, M.D.
Associate Professor, Division of Neurological Surgery, Department of Neurosciences, Medical College of Ohio, Toledo, Ohio

A. Norman Guthkelch, F.R.C.S.(Eng)
Professor, Department of Neurological Surgery, School of Medicine, University of Pittsburgh, Pittsburgh, Pennsylvania

Philip H. Gutin, M.D.
Assistant Professor, Department of Neurological Surgery, School of Medicine, University of California, San Francisco, San Francisco, California

Kai Haber, M.D.
Professor, Department of Radiology, University of Arizona Health Sciences Center, Tucson, Arizona

Earl R. Hackett, M.D.
Professor and Head, Department of Neurology, Louisiana State University Medical Center, New Orleans, Louisiana

Stephen J. Haines, M.D.
Assistant Professor, Department of Neurosurgery, University of Minnesota Medical School, Minneapolis, Minnesota

Maurice R. Hanson, M.D.
Department of Neurology, Cleveland Clinic Foundation, Cleveland, Ohio

William T. Hardaker, Jr., M.D.
Assistant Professor, Division of Orthopaedic Surgery, Duke University Medical Center, Durham, North Carolina

Jules Hardy, M.D., F.R.C.S.(C)
Professor and Chairman, Division of Neurosurgery, Faculty of Medicine, University of Montreal, Montreal, Quebec, Canada

Russell W. Hardy, Jr., M.D.
Department of Neurological Surgery, Cleveland Clinic Foundation, Cleveland, Ohio

John M. Harrelson, M.D.
Associate Professor, Division of Orthopaedic Surgery, Duke University Medical Center, Durham, North Carolina

A. Basil Harris, M.D.
Professor, Department of Neurological Surgery, University of Washington School of Medicine, Seattle, Washington

Griffith R. Harsh, III, M.D.
Professor and Director, Division of Neurosurgery, University of Alabama in Birmingham, Birmingham, Alabama

Griffith R. Harsh, IV, M.D.
Resident, Department of Neurological Surgery, School of Medicine, University of California, San Francisco, San Francisco, California

B. Thomas Harter, Jr., M.D.
Resident, Division of Plastic and Maxillofacial Surgery, Duke University Medical Center, Durham, North Carolina

Kathleen C. Harter, M.D.
Division of Plastic and Maxillofacial Surgery, Duke University Medical Center, Durham, North Carolina

M. Peter Heilbrun, M.D.
Professor and Chairman, Division of Neurosurgery, University of Utah School of Medicine, Salt Lake City, Utah

David C. Hemmy, M.D.
Associate Professor, Department of Neurosurgery, Medical College of Wisconsin, Milwaukee, Wisconsin

Nelson Hendler, M.D., M.S.
Clinical Director, Mensana Clinic, Stevenson, Maryland

E. Bruce Hendrick, M.D., F.R.C.S.(C)
Professor, Division of Neurosurgery, University of Toronto; The Hospital for Sick Children, Toronto, Ontario, Canada

Roberto C. Heros, M.D.
Director of Cerebrovascular Surgery, Massachusetts General Hospital, Boston, Massachusetts

Maie Kaarsoo Herrick, M.D.
Neuropathologist, Santa Clara Valley Medical Center, San Jose, California

Arnold M. Herskovic, M.D.
Associate Professor, Radiation Oncology Center, Wayne State University, Detroit, Michigan

Alfred C. Higgins, M.D.
Hickory, North Carolina

Charles J. Hodge, Jr., M.D.
Professor, Department of Neurological Surgery, State University of New York, Upstate Medical Center, Syracuse, New York

Andrew K. Hodson, M.B., Ch.B., M.R.C.P.(UK)
Chief, Division of Child Neurology, University Hospital of Jacksonville, Jacksonville, Florida

Julian T. Hoff, M.D.
Professor and Head, Section of Neurosurgery, University of Michigan Medical Center, Ann Arbor, Michigan

Harold J. Hoffman, M.D., F.R.C.S.(C)
Professor, Division of Neurosurgery, University of Toronto; The Hospital for Sick Children, Toronto, Ontario, Canada

James C. Hoffman, Jr., M.D.
Associate Professor, Department of Radiology, Emory University School of Medicine, Atlanta, Georgia

L. N. Hopkins, M.D.
Chairman, Department of Neurosurgery, Dent Neurologic Institute, Buffalo, New York

Eva Horvath, Ph.D.
Department of Pathology, St. Michael's Hospital, University of Toronto, Toronto, Ontario, Canada

Takao Hoshino, M.D., D.M.Sc.
Department of Neurological Surgery and Brain Tumor Research Center, School of Medicine, University of California, San Francisco, San Francisco, California

Yoshio Hosobuchi, M.D.
Professor, Department of Neurological Surgery, School of Medicine, University of California, San Francisco, San Francisco, California

Edgar M. Housepian, M.D.
Professor of Clinical Neurological Surgery, College of Physicians & Surgeons, Columbia University, New York, New York

Alan R. Hudson, M.B., Ch.B., F.R.C.S.(C)
Professor and Chairman, Division of Neurosurgery, University of Toronto, Toronto, Ontario, Canada

Robin P. Humphreys, M.D., F.R.C.S.(C)
Associate Professor, Division of Neurosurgery, University of Toronto; The Hospital for Sick Children, Toronto, Ontario, Canada

William E. Hunt, M.D.
Professor and Director, Division of Neurologic Surgery, Ohio State University College of Medicine, Columbus, Ohio

Barrie J. Hurwitz, M.B., M.R.C.P., F.C.P.(SA)
Assistant Professor, Division of Neurology, Duke University Medical Center, Durham, North Carolina

Ivor M. D. Jackson, M.D.
Professor, Department of Medicine, Tufts-New England Medical Center, Boston, Massachusetts

Hector E. James, M.D.
Associate Professor, Division of Neurological Surgery, and Department of Pediatrics, University of California, San Diego, San Diego, California

John A. Jane, M.D., Ph.D., F.R.C.S.(C)
Professor and Chairman, Department of Neurosurgery, University of Virginia Medical Center, Charlottesville, Virginia

Peter J. Jannetta, M.D.
Professor and Chairman, Department of Neurological Surgery, School of Medicine, University of Pittsburgh, Pittsburgh, Pennsylvania

Ronald J. Jaszczak, Ph.D.
Associate Professor, Department of Radiology, Duke University Medical Center, Durham, North Carolina

G. Allan Johnson, Ph.D.
Associate Professor, Department of Radiology, Duke University Medical Center, Durham, North Carolina

Mary M. Johnson, M.D.
Attending Neurosurgeon, Henrietta Egleston Hospital for Children and Scottish Rite Hospital for Children, Atlanta, Georgia

John E. Kalsbeck, M.D.
Professor, Section of Neurological Surgery, Indiana University School of Medicine, Indianapolis, Indiana

Uma P. Kalyan-Raman, M.D.
Associate Professor, Department of Pathology, University of Illinois College of Medicine at Peoria, Peoria, Illinois

John P. Kapp, M.D., Ph.D.
Professor, Department of Neurosurgery, University of Mississippi Medical Center, Jackson, Mississippi

Neal F. Kassell, M.D.
Professor, Division of Neurosurgery, University of Iowa, Iowa City, Iowa

Howard H. Kaufman, M.D.
Professor, Department of Neurosurgery, School of Medicine, West Virginia University, Morgantown, West Virginia

Ted S. Keller, M.D.
Assistant Professor, Division of Neurosurgery, University of Colorado Health Sciences Center, Denver, Colorado

David L. Kelly, Jr., M.D.
Professor and Head, Section on Neurosurgery, Bowman Gray School of Medicine, Winston-Salem, North Carolina

Patrick D. Kenan, M.D.
Associate Professor, Division of Otolaryngology, Duke University Medical Center, Durham, North Carolina

Douglas E. Kennemore, M.D.
Greenville, South Carolina

John S. Kennerdell, M.D.
Professor, Departments of Ophthalmology and Neurology, School of Medicine, University of Pittsburgh, Pittsburgh, Pennsylvania

Robert B. King, M.D.
Professor and Chairman, Department of Neurological Surgery, State University of New York, Upstate Medical Center, Syracuse, New York

J. Philip Kistler, M.D.
Associate Professor of Neurology, Harvard Medical School, Boston, Massachusetts

David G. Kline, M.D.
Professor and Chairman, Department of Neurosurgery, Louisiana State University Medical Center, New Orleans, Louisiana

Arthur I. Kobrine, M.D., Ph.D.
Professor, Department of Neurological Surgery, George Washington University Medical Center, Washington, District of Columbia

Paul L. Kornblith, M.D.
Chief, Surgical Neurology Branch, National Institute of Neurological and Communicative Disorders and Stroke, Bethesda, Maryland

Kalman Kovacs, M.D., Ph.D., F.R.C.P.(C)
Professor, Department of Pathology, St. Michael's Hospital, University of Toronto, Toronto, Ontario, Canada

John Krawchenko, M.D.
Clinical Assistant Professor, Department of Neurological Surgery, State University of New York, Upstate Medical Center, Syracuse, New York

Thomas W. Langfitt, M.D.
Charles Harrison Frazier Professor and Director, Division of Neurosurgery, School of Medicine, University of Pennsylvania, Philadelphia, Pennsylvania

Richard E. Latchaw, M.D.
Associate Professor, Departments of Radiology and Neurological Surgery, University of Pittsburgh Health Centers, Pittsburgh, Pennsylvania

John H. Lawrence, M.D.
Lawrence Berkeley Laboratory and Donner Laboratory, University of California, Berkeley, Berkeley, California

Edward R. Laws, Jr., M.D.
Professor, Department of Neurologic Surgery, Mayo Clinic and Mayo Medical School, Rochester, Minnesota

Martin L. Lazar, M.D.
Department of Neurological Surgery, Texas Neurological Institute at Dallas, Dallas, Texas

Milam E. Leavens, M.D.
Associate Professor and Chief, Neurosurgery Service, M.D. Anderson Hospital and Tumor Institute, Houston, Texas

Allan B. Levin, M.D.
Associate Professor, Division of Neurological Surgery, University of Wisconsin Center for Health Sciences, Madison, Wisconsin

John A. Linfoot, M.D.
Lawrence Berkeley Laboratory and Donner Laboratory, University of California, Berkeley, Berkeley, California

Vicki Lea Linman, B.S., M.T.
Senior Medical Technologist, Duke University Medical Center Laboratories, Durham, North Carolina

John R. Little, M.D.
Department of Neurological Surgery, Cleveland Clinic Foundation, Cleveland, Ohio

Jorge L. Lockhart, M.D.
Associate Professor, Division of Urology, University of Miami School of Medicine, Miami, Florida

John D. Loeser, M.D.
Professor, Department of Neurological Surgery, University of Washington School of Medicine, Seattle, Washington

Patrick E. Logue, Ph.D.
Associate Professor, Division of Medical Psychology, Department of Psychiatry, Duke University Medical Center, Durham, North Carolina

Donlin M. Long, M.D., Ph.D.
Professor and Chairman, Department of Neurological Surgery, Johns Hopkins University School of Medicine, Baltimore, Maryland

Herbert Lourie, M.D.
Clinical Professor, Department of Neurological Surgery, State University of New York, Upstate Medical Center, Syracuse, New York

Alfred J. Luessenhop, M.D.
Professor and Chief, Division of Neurosurgery, Georgetown University Hospital, Washington, District of Columbia

L. Dade Lunsford, M.D.
Assistant Professor, Department of Neurological Surgery, School of Medicine, University of Pittsburgh, Pittsburgh, Pennsylvania

J. Scott Luther, M.D.
Assistant Professor, Division of Neurology, Duke University Medical Center, Durham, North Carolina

John T. Lyman
Lawrence Berkeley Laboratory and Donner Laboratory, University of California, Berkeley, Berkeley, California

George C. Lynch
Professor of Medical Illustration, Department of Audiovisual Resources, Bowman Gray School of Medicine, Winston-Salem, North Carolina

Ignacio Magana, M.D.
Fellow, Department of Neurological Surgery, University of Miami School of Medicine, Miami, Florida

Leonard I. Malis, M.D.
Professor and Chairman, Department of Neurosurgery, The Mount Sinai Medical Center, New York, New York

John T. Manning, M.D.
Assistant Professor, Department of Pathology, M.D. Anderson Hospital and Tumor Institute, Houston, Texas

Moshe H. Maor, M.D.
Associate Professor, Department of Radiotherapy, M.D. Anderson Hospital and Tumor Institute, Houston, Texas

Timothy B. Mapstone, M.D.
Assistant Professor, Division of Neurological Surgery, Case Western Reserve University School of Medicine, Cleveland, Ohio

Kenneth R. Maravilla, M.D.
Associate Professor, Department of Radiology, University of Texas Health Science Center at Dallas, Dallas, Texas

Ralph C. Marcove, M.D.
Orthopedic Service, Memorial Sloan-Kettering Cancer Center, New York, New York

William R. Markesbery, M.D.
Professor of Neurology and Pathology, University of Kentucky Medical Center, Lexington, Kentucky

Joseph C. Maroon, M.D.
Professor, Department of Neurological Surgery, School of Medicine, University of Pittsburgh, Pittsburgh, Pennsylvania

Merlin D. Marquardt, M.D.
Assistant Professor, Department of Pathology, College of Physicians & Surgeons, Columbia University, New York, New York

Lawrence F. Marshall, M.D.
Associate Professor, Division of Neurological Surgery, University of California, San Diego, San Diego, California

Robert L. Martuza, M.D.
Assistant Professor of Surgery, Harvard Medical School, and Director of the Neurofibromatosis Clinic, Massachusetts General Hospital, Boston, Massachusetts

E. Wayne Massey, M.D.
Assistant Professor, Division of Neurology, Duke University Medical Center, Durham, North Carolina

Robert E. Maxwell, M.D., Ph.D.
Associate Professor, Department of Neurosurgery, University of Minnesota Medical School, Minneapolis, Minnesota

Donald E. McCollum, M.D.
Professor, Division of Orthopaedic Surgery, Duke University Medical Center, Durham, North Carolina

J. Gordon McComb, M.D.
Associate Professor, Department of Neurological Surgery, University of Southern California School of Medicine; the Childrens Hospital of Los Angeles, Los Angeles, California

William F. McCormick, M.D.
Professor and Chief, Division of Neuropathology, University of Texas Medical Branch, Galveston, Texas

David C. McCullough, M.D.
Chairman, Department of Neurosurgery, Children's Hospital National Medical Center, Washington, District of Columbia

John E. McGillicuddy, M.D.
Associate Professor, Section of Neurosurgery, University of Michigan Medical Center, Ann Arbor, Michigan

Robert L. McLaurin, M.D.
Professor, Department of Neurological Surgery, University of Cincinnati Medical Center and Children's Hospital Medical Center, Cincinnati, Ohio

David G. McLone, M.D., Ph.D.
Chairman, Division of Pediatric Neurosurgery, Children's Memorial Hospital, Chicago, Illinois

Irvine G. McQuarrie, M.D., Ph.D.
Departments of Anatomy and Surgery (Division of Neurological Surgery), Case Western Reserve University School of Medicine, Cleveland, Ohio

Ronald Melzack, Ph.D.
Professor, Department of Psychology, McGill University, Montreal, Quebec, Canada

Arnold H. Menezes, M.D.
Associate Professor, Division of Neurosurgery, University of Iowa Hospitals and Clinics, Iowa City, Iowa

John Mennell, M.D.
Vero Beach, Florida

Michael A. Mikhael, M.D.
Department of Radiology, Evanston Hospital, Evanston, Illinois

Thomas H. Milhorat, M.D.
Professor and Chairman, Department of Neurosurgery, State University of New York, Downstate Medical Center, Brooklyn, New York

Carole A. Miller, M.D.
Associate Professor, Division of Neurologic Surgery, Ohio State University College of Medicine, Columbus, Ohio

Michael E. Miner, M.D., Ph.D.
Associate Professor and Chief, Division of Neurosurgery, University of Texas Health Science Center at Houston, Houston, Texas

Luciano M. Modesti, M.D.
Professor, Department of Neurological Surgery, State University of New York, Upstate Medical Center, Syracuse, New York

Michael T. Modic, M.D.
Division of Radiology, The Cleveland Clinic Foundation, Cleveland, Ohio

Dixon M. Moody, M.D.
Professor, Department of Radiology, Bowman Gray School of Medicine, Winston-Salem, North Carolina

John Moossy, M.D.
Professor, Departments of Pathology and Neurology, School of Medicine, University of Pittsburgh, Pittsburgh, Pennsylvania

Richard B. Morawetz, M.D.
Professor, Division of Neurosurgery, School of Medicine, University of Alabama in Birmingham, Birmingham, Alabama

James M. Morris, M.D.
Associate Professor, Department of Orthopaedic Surgery, School of Medicine, University of California, San Francisco, San Francisco, California

William H. Mosberg, Jr., M.D.
Clinical Professor, Division of Neurological Surgery, University of Maryland School of Medicine, Baltimore, Maryland

Sean Mullan, M.D., D.Sc., F.R.C.S.(Eng)
Professor and Chairman, Section of Neurological Surgery, University of Chicago Hospitals, Chicago, Illinois

Terence M. Murphy, M.D., F.F.A.R.C.S.
Professor, Department of Anesthesiology, University of Washington School of Medicine, Seattle, Washington

Blaine S. Nashold, Jr., M.D.
Professor, Division of Neurosurgery, Duke University Medical Center, Durham, North Carolina

Victoria Neave, M.D.
Resident, Department of Neurological Surgery, University of Southern California School of Medicine, Los Angeles, California

James P. Neifeld, M.D.
Associate Professor, Division of Surgical Oncology, Medical College of Virginia, Virginia Commonwealth University, Richmond, Virginia

Martin G. Netsky, M.D.
Professor, Department of Pathology, Vanderbilt University School of Medicine, Nashville, Tennessee

Edward A. Neuwelt, M.D.
Associate Professor, Division of Neurosurgery, The Oregon Health Sciences University, Portland, Oregon

Nancy M. Newman, M.D.
Associate Professor and Chief, Neuro-ophthalmology Division, Department of Ophthalmology, Pacific Medical Center, San Francisco, California

K. Thomas Noell, M.D.
Ramagosa Radiation Oncology Center, Lafayette, Louisiana

G. Robert Nugent, M.D.
Professor and Chairman, Department of Neurosurgery, West Virginia University School of Medicine, Morgantown, West Virginia

W. Jerry Oakes, M.D.
Assistant Professor, Division of Neurosurgery, Duke University Medical Center, Durham, North Carolina

Mark S. O'Brien, M.D.
Professor, Division of Neurological Surgery, Emory University School of Medicine, Atlanta, Georgia

Walter D. Obrist, Ph.D.
Professor of Research in Neurosurgery and Neurology, University of Pennsylvania, Philadelphia, Pennsylvania

Michael J. O'Connor, M.D.
Associate Professor, Division of Neurosurgery, School of Medicine, University of Pennsylvania, Philadelphia, Pennsylvania

George A. Ojemann, M.D.
Professor, Department of Neurological Surgery, University of Washington School of Medicine, Seattle, Washington

Robert G. Ojemann, M.D.
Professor of Surgery, Harvard Medical School and Visiting Neurosurgeon, Massachusetts General Hospital, Boston, Massachusetts

C. Warren Olanow, M.D.
Assistant Professor, Division of Neurology, Duke University Medical Center, Durham, North Carolina

Ayub Khan Ommaya, M.D., F.R.C.S.
Clinical Professor, Department of Neurological Surgery, George Washington University Medical Center, Washington, District of Columbia

Burton M. Onofrio, M.D.
Professor, Department of Neurologic Surgery, Mayo Clinic and Mayo Medical School, Rochester, Minnesota

Dennis R. Osborne, M.D.
Associate Professor, Department of Radiology, Duke University Medical Center, Durham, North Carolina

Roger H. Ostdahl, M.D.
Camp Hill, Pennsylvania

Jewell L. Osterholm, M.D.
Professor and Chairman, Department of Neurosurgery, Jefferson Medical College of Thomas Jefferson University, Philadelphia, Pennsylvania

Peter T. Ostrow, M.D., Ph.D.
Associate Professor, Department of Pathology, The University of Texas Medical School at Houston, Houston, Texas

Larry K. Page, M.D.
Professor, Department of Neurological Surgery, University of Miami School of Medicine, Miami, Florida

Robert B. Page, M.D.
Associate Professor, Division of Neurosurgery, Milton S. Hershey Medical Center of the Pennsylvania State University, Hershey, Pennsylvania

Dachling Pang, M.D., F.R.C.S.(C)
Assistant Professor, Department of Neurological Surgery, School of Medicine, University of Pittsburgh, Pittsburgh, Pennsylvania

Manohar M. Panjabi, Ph.D., D.Tech.
Professor and Director, Biomechanics Research, Section of Orthopaedic Surgery, Yale University School of Medicine, New Haven, Connecticut

Dwight Parkinson, M.D.
Professor and Chairman, Section of Neurosurgery, University of Manitoba Health Sciences Centre, Winnipeg, Manitoba, Canada

Russel H. Patterson, Jr., M.D.
Professor and Chief, Division of Neurosurgery, The New York Hospital-Cornell Medical Center, New York, New York

William Pavlicek, M.S.
Diagnostic Physicist, The Cleveland Clinic Foundation, Cleveland, Ohio

S. J. Peerless, M.D., F.R.C.S.(C)
Professor and Chairman, Division of Neurosurgery, University of Western Ontario, London, Ontario, Canada

Richard R. Pelker, M.D., Ph.D.
Assistant Professor, Section of Orthopaedic Surgery, Yale University School of Medicine, New Haven, Connecticut

Richard D. Penn, M.D.
Associate Professor, Department of Neurosurgery, Rush Medical School, Chicago, Illinois

John R. Perfect, M.D.
Assistant Professor, Division of Infectious Diseases, Duke University Medical Center, Durham, North Carolina

Phanor L. Perot, Jr., M.D., Ph.D.
Professor and Chairman, Department of Neurosurgery, Medical University of South Carolina, Charleston, South Carolina

Byron C. Pevehouse, M.D.
Clinical Professor, Department of Neurological Surgery, School of Medicine, University of California, San Francisco, San Francisco, California

Joseph H. Piatt, Jr., M.D.
Resident, Division of Neurosurgery, Duke University Medical Center, Durham, North Carolina

David G. Piepgras, M.D.
Assistant Professor, Department of Neurologic Surgery, Mayo Clinic and Mayo Medical School, Rochester, Minnesota

Salvatore V. Pizzo, M.D., Ph.D.
Associate Professor, Department of Pathology, Duke University Medical Center, Durham, North Carolina

Fred V. Plapp, M.D., Ph.D.
Assistant Medical Director, Community Blood Center of Greater Kansas City, Kansas City, Missouri

Steven R. Plunkett, M.D.
Instructor, Section of Radiation Therapy, Bowman Gray School of Medicine, Winston-Salem, North Carolina

Michael Pollay, M.D.
Professor and Chief, Division of Neurosurgery, University of Oklahoma College of Medicine, Oklahoma City, Oklahoma

A. John Popp, M.D.
Associate Professor, Division of Neurosurgery, Albany Medical College, Albany, New York

Kalmon D. Post, M.D.
Associate Professor, Department of Neurological Surgery, College of Physicians & Surgeons, Columbia University, New York, New York

Stephen K. Powers, M.D.
Assistant Professor, Division of Neurological Surgery, School of Medicine, University of North Carolina at Chapel Hill, Chapel Hill, North Carolina

Donald J. Prolo, M.D.
Director, Neuroskeletal Transplantation Laboratory, Institute for Medical Research, San Jose, California

Donald O. Quest, M.D.
Associate Professor, Department of Neurological Surgery, Columbia University College of Physicians & Surgeons, New York, New York

Chitranjan S. Ranawat, M.D.
Professor of Orthopaedic Surgery, Cornell University Medical Center and the Hospital for Special Surgery, New York, New York

Robert W. Rand, Ph.D., M.D.
Professor, Division of Neurosurgery, School of Medicine, University of California, Los Angeles, Los Angeles, California

Robert A. Ratcheson, M.D.
The Harvey Huntington Brown, Jr. Professor and Chairman, Division of Neurological Surgery, Case Western Reserve University School of Medicine, Cleveland, Ohio

Charles E. Rawlings, III, M.D.
Resident, Division of Neurosurgery, Duke University Medical Center, Durham, North Carolina

Justin W. Renaudin, M.D.
Assistant Clinical Professor, Division of Neurological Surgery, University of California, San Diego, San Diego, California

Setti S. Rengachary, M.D.
Professor, Section of Neurological Surgery, University of Kansas Medical Center, Kansas City, Kansas; Chief, Neurosurgery Section, Veterans Administration Medical Center, Kansas City, Missouri

Albert L. Rhoton, Jr., M.D.
R. D. Keene Family Professor and Chairman, Department of Neurological Surgery, University of Florida College of Medicine, Gainesville, Florida

Donald E. Richardson, M.D.
Professor and Chairman, Department of Neurologic Surgery, Tulane University School of Medicine, New Orleans, Louisiana

Ronald Riefkohl, M.D.
Assistant Professor, Division of Plastic and Maxillofacial Surgery, Duke University Medical Center, Durham, North Carolina

Rebecca W. Rimel, B.S.N., M.B.A.
Assistant Professor, Department of Neurosurgery, University of Virginia Medical Center, Charlottesville, Virginia

Theodore S. Roberts, M.D.
Professor, Division of Neurosurgery, University of Utah School of Medicine, Salt Lake City, Utah

James T. Robertson, M.D.
Professor and Chairman, Department of Neurosurgery, University of Tennessee Center for the Health Sciences, Memphis, Tennessee

Arthur E. Rosenbaum, M.D.
Professor, Departments of Radiology and Radiological Science, and of Neurosurgery, The Johns Hopkins Medical Institutions, Baltimore, Maryland

Michael Rosenberg, M.D.
Associate Professor, Department of Ophthalmology, Northwestern University, Chicago, Illinois

Shelley B. Rosenbloom, M.D.
Assistant Professor, Department of Radiology and Radiological Science, The Johns Hopkins Medical Institutions, Baltimore, Maryland

Mark L. Rosenblum, M.D.
Associate Professor, Department of Neurological Surgery, School of Medicine, University of California, San Francisco, San Francisco, California

Allen D. Roses, M.D.
Professor and Chief, Division of Neurology, Duke University Medical Center, Durham, North Carolina

Richard A. Roski, M.D.
Assistant Professor, Division of Neurological Surgery, University of Louisville School of Medicine, Louisville, Kentucky

Hubert L. Rosomoff, M.D., D.med.Sc.
Professor and Chairman, Department of Neurological Surgery, University of Miami School of Medicine, Miami, Florida

William E. Rothfus, M.D.
Assistant Professor, Department of Radiology, University of Pittsburgh Health Centers, Pittsburgh, Pennsylvania

Richard H. Rothman, M.D., Ph.D.
Professor of Orthopaedic Surgery, School of Medicine, University of Pennsylvania, Philadelphia, Pennsylvania

Richard L. Rovit, M.D., M.Sc.
Director, Department of Neurological Surgery, St. Vincent's Hospital and Medical Center, New York, New York

Jonathan M. Rubin, M.D., Ph.D.
Assistant Professor, Department of Radiology, and Chief of Ultrasound Services, University of Chicago Medical Center, Chicago, Illinois

Michael Salcman, M.D.
Professor and Head, Division of Neurological Surgery, University of Maryland School of Medicine, Baltimore, Maryland

Duke Samson, M.D.
Associate Professor and Vice Chairman, Division of Neurological Surgery, University of Texas Health Science Center at Dallas, Dallas, Texas

Richard L. Saunders, M.D.
Associate Professor of Clinical Surgery and Chairman, Section of Neurosurgery, Dartmouth-Hitchcock Medical Center, Hanover, New Hampshire

William M. Saunders, M.D., Ph.D.
Lawrence Berkeley Laboratory and Donner Laboratory, University of California, Berkeley, Berkeley, California

Timothy B. Scarff, M.D.
Associate Professor, Division of Neurological Surgery, Loyola University Medical Center, Maywood, Illinois

Robert A. Schindler, M.D.
Associate Professor, Department of Otolaryngology-Head and Neck Surgery, School of Medicine, University of California, San Francisco, San Francisco, California

Henry H. Schmidek, M.D.
Professor and Chairman, Section of Neurosurgery, University of Vermont College of Medicine, Burlington, Vermont

Frederick A. Schmitt, Ph.D.
Center for the Study of Aging and Human Development, Duke University Medical Center, Durham, North Carolina

Richard C. Schneider, M.D.
Professor Emeritus, Section of Neurosurgery, University of Michigan Medical Center, Ann Arbor, Michigan

S. Clifford Schold, Jr., M.D.
Assistant Professor, Division of Neurology, Duke University Medical Center, Durham, North Carolina

Luis Schut, M.D.
Chief, Neurosurgical Services, Children's Hospital of Philadelphia, Philadelphia, Pennsylvania

Hervey D. Segall, M.D.
Professor, Department of Radiology, University of Southern California School of Medicine, Los Angeles, California

Roy Selby, M.D.
La Crosse, Wisconsin

Edward L. Seljeskog, M.D., Ph.D.
Professor, Department of Neurosurgery, University of Minnesota Medical School, Minneapolis, Minnesota

Robert G. Selker, M.D.
Professor, Department of Neurological Surgery, School of Medicine, University of Pittsburgh, Pittsburgh, Pennsylvania

Warren Selman, M.D.
Assistant Professor, Division of Neurological Surgery, Case Western Reserve University School of Medicine, Cleveland, Ohio

Donald Serafin, M.D.
Professor, Division of Plastic and Maxillofacial Surgery, Duke University Medical Center, Durham, North Carolina

Bhagwan T. Shahani, M.D., D.Phil.(Oxon)
Department of Neurology and Clinical Neurophysiology Laboratory, Massachusetts General Hospital, Boston, Massachusetts

David G. Sherman, M.D.
Associate Professor, Division of Neurology, University of Texas Health Science Center at San Antonio, San Antonio, Texas

William A. Shucart, M.D.
Professor and Chairman, Department of Neurosurgery, Tufts-New England Medical Center, Boston, Massachusetts

Gerald D. Silverberg, M.D.
Associate Professor, Division of Neurosurgery, Stanford University Medical Center, Stanford, California

Frederick A. Simeone, M.D.
Professor, Division of Neurosurgery, School of Medicine, University of Pennsylvania, Philadelphia, Pennsylvania

Marcia Sirotkin-Roses, M.A., L.P.T.
Division of Neurology and Department of Physical Therapy, Duke University Medical Center, Durham, North Carolina

Frederick H. Sklar, M.D.
Director of Pediatric Neurosurgery, Children's Medical Center, Dallas, Texas

Barry H. Smith, M.D., Ph.D.
Surgical Neurology Branch, National Institute of Neurological and Communicative Disorders and Stroke, Bethesda, Maryland

Robert R. Smith, M.D.
Professor and Chairman, Department of Neurosurgery, University of Mississippi Medical Center, Jackson, Mississippi

Frederick S. Southwick, M.D.
Assistant Professor of Medicine, Harvard Medical School, Boston, Massachusetts

Alexander M. Spence, M.D.
Associate Professor, Department of Medicine (Neurology), University of Washington School of Medicine, Seattle, Washington

Robert F. Spetzler, M.D.
J. N. Harber Foundation Chairman of Neurological Surgery, Barrow Neurological Institute, Phoenix, Arizona

Hans Jacob Steiger, M.D.
Clinical Fellow, Department of Neurological Surgery, University of Cincinnati Medical Center, Cincinnati, Ohio

Bennett M. Stein, M.D.
Byron Stookey Professor and Chairman, Department of Neurological Surgery, Columbia University College of Physicians & Surgeons, New York, New York

W. Eugene Stern, M.D.
Professor of Neurosurgery and Chairman, Department of Surgery, School of Medicine, University of California, Los Angeles, Los Angeles, California

Donald H. Stewart, Jr., M.D.
Clinical Assistant Professor, Department of Neurological Surgery, State University of New York, Upstate Medical Center, Syracuse, New York

Humbert G. Sullivan, M.D.
Associate Professor, Section of Neurosurgery, Medical College of Georgia, Augusta, Georgia

Narayan Sundaresan, M.D.
Assistant Attending Surgeon, Memorial Sloan-Kettering Cancer Center, New York, New York

Thoralf M. Sundt, Jr., M.D.
Professor and Chairman, Department of Neurologic Surgery, Mayo Clinic and Mayo Medical School, Rochester, Minnesota

Leslie N. Sutton, M.D.
Division of Neurosurgery, Children's Hospital of Philadelphia, Philadelphia, Pennsylvania

Morton N. Swartz, M.D.
Professor of Medicine, Harvard Medical School, and Chief, Infectious Disease Unit, Massachusetts General Hospital, Boston, Massachusetts

William H. Sweet, M.D., D.Sc., D.H.C.
Senior Neurosurgeon, Massachusetts General Hospital, Boston, Massachusetts

Ronald R. Tasker, M.D., F.R.C.S.(C)
Professor, Division of Neurosurgery, University of Toronto, Toronto, Ontario, Canada

Charles H. Tator, M.D., Ph.D., F.R.C.S.(C)
Professor, Division of Neurosurgery, University of Toronto, Toronto, Ontario, Canada

John M. Tew, Jr., M.D.
Professor and Chairman, Department of Neurological Surgery, University of Cincinnati Medical Center, Cincinnati, Ohio

Lawrence E. Thibault, Sc.D.
Assistant Professor of Bioengineering, University of Pennsylvania, Philadelphia, Pennsylvania

L. M. Thomas, M.D.
Professor and Chairman, Department of Neurosurgery, Wayne State University School of Medicine, Detroit, Michigan

Michael O. Thorner, M.B., M.R.C.P.
Professor, Department of Internal Medicine, University of Virginia Medical Center, Charlottesville, Virginia

Andrew L. Tievsky, M.D.
Assistant Professor, Department of Radiology, The George Washington University Medical Center, Washington, District of Columbia

George T. Tindall, M.D.
Professor and Chief, Division of Neurological Surgery, Emory University School of Medicine, Atlanta, Georgia

Suzie C. Tindall, M.D.
Assistant Professor, Division of Neurological Surgery, Emory University School of Medicine, Atlanta, Georgia

Cornelius A. Tobias, Ph.D.
Lawrence Berkeley Laboratory and Donner Laboratory, University of California, Berkeley, Berkeley, California

B. Tranmer, M.D.
Resident, Division of Neurosurgery, University of Toronto, Toronto, Ontario, Canada

Bruno J. Urban, M.D.
Professor, Department of Anesthesiology, Duke University Medical Center, Durham, North Carolina

John C. VanGilder, M.D.
Professor and Chairman, Division of Neurosurgery, University of Iowa Hospitals and Clinics, Iowa City, Iowa

William S. Velasquez, M.D.
Associate Professor, Department of Medicine, M.D. Anderson Hospital and Tumor Institute, Houston, Texs

Joan L. Venes, M.D.
Assistant Professor, Section of Neurosurgery, University of Michigan Medical Center, Ann Arbor, Michigan

Fernando Viñuela, M.D., F.R.C.P.(C)
Assistant Professor, Departments of Diagnostic Radiology and Clinical Neurological Sciences, University of Western Ontario, London, Ontario, Canada

F. Stephen Vogel, M.D.
Professor, Department of Pathology, Duke University Medical Center, Durham, North Carolina

Rand M. Voorhies, M.D.
Department of Neurosurgery, Ochsner Clinic, New Orleans, Louisiana

Jeffrey S. Walker, M.D.
Chief Resident, Division of Neurosurgery, Duke University Medical Center, Durham, North Carolina

Patrick D. Wall, M.D.
Professor, Department of Anatomy, University College London, London, England

Sidney Wallace, M.D.
Professor, Department of Diagnostic Radiology, M.D. Anderson Hospital and Tumor Institute, Houston, Texas

John W. Walsh, M.D., Ph.D.
Associate Professor, Division of Neurosurgery, University of Kentucky Medical Center, Lexington, Kentucky

Alan Waters, F.R.C.S.
Senior Registrar in Neurosurgery, New Addenbrooke's Hospital, Cambridge, England

Clark Watts, M.D.
Professor and Chief, Division of Neurosurgery, University of Missouri-Columbia Health Sciences Center, Columbia, Missouri

David D. Weaver, M.D.
Associate Professor, Department of Medical Genetics, Indiana University School of Medicine, Indianapolis, Indiana

George D. Webster, M. B., F.R.C.S.
Associate Professor, Division of Urologic Surgery, Duke University Medical Center, Durham, North Carolina

Vivian D. Weigel, B.S.
Department of Otolaryngology-Head and Neck Surgery, School of Medicine, University of California, San Francisco, San Francisco, California

Richard L. Weiner, M.D.
Assistant Professor, Division of Neurosurgery, University of Texas Medical Branch, Galveston, Texas

Meredith A. Weinstein, M.D.
Section of Neuroradiology, Division of Radiology, The Cleveland Clinic Foundation, Cleveland, Ohio

Philip R. Weinstein, M.D.
Professor and Vice Chairman, Department of Neurological Surgery, School of Medicine, University of California, San Francisco, San Francisco, California

Bryce Weir, M.D., M.Sc., F.R.C.S.(C)
Clinical Professor and Director, Division of Neurosurgery, University of Alberta, Edmonton, Alberta, Canada

Leonard Weiss, M.D.
Director, Department of Experimental Pathology, Roswell Park Memorial Institute, Buffalo, New York

Martin H. Weiss, M.D.
Professor and Chairman, Department of Neurological Surgery, University of Southern California School of Medicine, Los Angeles, California

Frank A. Welsh, Ph.D.
Associate Professor of Biochemistry, Division of Neurosurgery, School of Medicine, University of Pennsylvania, Philadelphia, Pennsylvania

James Gardner Wepsic, M.D.
New England Baptist Hospital, Boston, Massachusetts

Augustus A. White, III, M.D., D.Med.Sci.
Professor of Orthopaedic Surgery, Harvard Medical School; Surgeon-in-Chief, Department of Orthopaedic Surgery, Beth Israel Hospital, Boston, Massachusetts

Richard J. Whitley, M.D.
Professor, Department of Pediatrics, School of Medicine, University of Alabama in Birmingham, Birmingham, Alabama

Asa J. Wilbourn, M.D.
Department of Neurology, Cleveland Clinic Foundation, Cleveland, Ohio

Robert H. Wilkins, M.D.
Professor and Chief, Division of Neurosurgery, Duke University Medical Center, Durham, North Carolina

Phillip Earle Williams, Jr., M.D.
Clinical Associate Professor, Division of Neurological Surgery, University of Texas Health Science Center at Dallas, Dallas, Texas

Charles B. Wilson, M.D.
Professor and Chairman, Department of Neurological Surgery, School of Medicine, University of California, San Francisco, San Francisco, California

William P. Wilson, M.D.
Professor, Department of Psychiatry, Duke University Medical Center, Durham, North Carolina

Ken R. Winston, M.D.
Senior Associate in Neurosurgery, The Children's Hospital, Boston, Massachusetts

Hugh S. Wisoff, M.D.
Associate Professor and Acting Chairman, Leo M. Davidoff Department of Neurological Surgery, Albert Einstein College of Medicine, Bronx, New York

James H. Wood, M.D.
Assistant Professor, Division of Neurological Surgery, Emory University School of Medicine, Atlanta, Georgia

Kay Woodruff
Lawrence Berkeley Laboratory and Donner Laboratory, University of California, Berkeley, Berkeley, California

Robert M. Worth, M.D.
Section of Neurological Surgery, Indiana University School of Medicine, Indianapolis, Indiana

Richard Jed Wyatt, M.D.
Chief, Adult Psychiatry Branch, National Institute of Mental Health, Saint Elizabeth's Hospital, Washington, District of Columbia

Isao Yamamoto, M.D.
Department of Neurosurgery, University of Florida Health Center, Gainesville, Florida

Howard Yonas, M.D.
Associate Professor, Department of Neurological Surgery, School of Medicine, University of Pittsburgh, Pittsburgh, Pennsylvania

Junji Yoshioka, M.D.
Mississippi Heart Association Fellow, University of Mississippi Medical Center, Jackson, Mississippi

Byron Young, M.D.
Professor and Chairman, Division of Neurosurgery, University of Kentucky Medical Center, Lexington, Kentucky

Harold F. Young, M.D.
Professor, Division of Neurological Surgery, Medical College of Virginia, Virginia Commonwealth University, Richmond, Virginia

Ronald F. Young, M.D.
Professor, Division of Neurosurgery, School of Medicine, University of California, Los Angeles, Los Angeles, California

Joseph Zabramski, M.D.
Resident, Division of Neurological Surgery, Barrow Neurological Institute, Phoenix, Arizona

Chi-Shing Zee, M.D.
Assistant Professor, Department of Radiology, University of Southern California School of Medicine, Los Angeles, California

Nicholas T. Zervas, M.D.
Professor of Surgery, Harvard Medical School, and Chief, Neurosurgical Service, Massachusetts General Hospital, Boston, Massachusetts

Robert A. Zimmerman, M.D.
Professor, Department of Radiology, Hospital of the University of Pennsylvania, Philadelphia, Pennsylvania

Sandra Zink
Lawrence Berkeley Laboratory and Donner Laboratory, University of California, Berkeley, Berkeley, California

FOREWORD

Drs. Wilkins and Rengachary are neurosurgeons; they have written original papers; they have trained residents; and they keep up with current developments. I can think of no two better qualified to be the editors of this text.

Drs. Wilkins and Rengachary have obviously thought long and hard about this project, for they have covered all aspects of the field of neurosurgery in a comprehensive manner. Their talents for knowing the best authors to write the various sections, and for assembling and editing the material without incurring wrath, and for doing all that while remaining active in neurosurgery, are nothing short of impressive.

The introductory chapters dealing with neurosurgical history which begin this three-volume text, with the delightful authoritative section on Cushing and Dandy by Dr. Bucy (who was there), are themselves valuable contributions. But there is more, much more. Almost all details of neurosurgery and all of the neurosciences as they relate to neurosurgery are included. This text is not for the referring physician or the occasional surgeon. It is for the student, the graduate student, the neurosurgery resident, and the practicing neurosurgeon the world over. It will answer most questions on a given subject or refer the reader to the proper authority on that subject.

To have been asked to write this foreword is an honor, for this text is indeed an awesome compilation of neurosurgical knowledge.

Eben Alexander, Jr., M.D.

PREFACE

Advances in neurological surgery are occurring at such a rapid pace that attempts to capture a static image of the subject give a blurred picture at best. Ever-new diagnostic methodologies, advances in treatment, refinements in surgical technique, improvements in surgical instrumentation, and breakthroughs in the basic understanding of disease processes overwhelm even the most enthusiastic neurosurgeon. It has become impossible for any single individual to keep pace with all the advances and to be adept in all the techniques. We have thus resorted to a multiauthored text for a broad contemporary overview of the subject that is as up to date as we could make it.

The book is directed toward a wide readership, including residents in training in neurological surgery and neurosurgeons in an academic setting or in community practice. Since it is a reference text, medical students and specialists in related fields may find it useful as well.

Certain aspects of this text that reflect the philosophy of the editors deserve emphasis:

It deals with established as well as evolving aspects of neurological surgery. The reader will find such mundane topics as cranial nerve examination interspersed with esoteric ones like central nervous system grafting.

Subjects such as neuroradiology and neuropathology, which often are discussed in isolation in the beginning chapters of a text, are interwoven with related clinical material. This permits a meaningful correlation between clinical, radiographic, and pathological features instead of simply providing minitexts on neuroradiology or neuropathology.

An appropriate blend of "bench" and "bedside" is maintained. For example, in Part VI, which deals with neurooncology, each section begins with a discussion concerning the pathology of a tumor by a neuropathologist with particular interest in that area.

A judicious balance of basic and clinical sciences is kept throughout the book, and the historical aspects of neurological surgery are presented, especially in the beginning of the book. We hope that the historical material will be both informative and inspirational to our readers.

Clinical examination of the nervous system with correlated neuroanatomy is discussed in some depth, reflecting our conviction that newer diagnostic methodologies, however promising they may appear, will assist but can never replace the human mind.

To conserve space, the reference list at the end of most chapters is not comprehensive but contains the most pertinent and, to the extent possible, the most recent references. Any student exploring a particular topic in depth will be able to use the list as a good starting point for a search of the literature.

Important topics dealing with certain social, ethical, and legal issues, which are generally ignored in standard texts, are included in this work.

The contributors have been encouraged to follow their individual styles in writing and presentation to avoid monotony in exposition.

Finally, we have strived, wherever possible, to allow only healthy overlap, not undue repetition, throughout the text.

We thank all the contributors who volunteered to share their time, knowledge, and expertise, and especially Dr. Eben Alexander, Jr. who prepared the foreword and Dr. Eugene S. Flamm, who provided the historical woodcuts that introduce the various parts of the text. We also thank Mrs. Gloria K. Wilkins and Mrs. Yvonne Ellis for providing secretarial help, Mrs. Paula N. Ecklund for reading the proof, and Mrs. Elizabeth Adams and Mr. David K. Donlon for checking all of the references in the Duke Medical Center Library. Finally, we express our appreciation for the people at the McGraw-Hill Book Company, especially Mr. Stuart Boynton, Mr. Robert P. McGraw, and Mr. Robert E. McGrath, who enthusiastically supported this project from its very inception and worked very hard to complete it within the shortest possible time.

Robert H. Wilkins, M.D.
Setti S. Rengachary, M.D.

Part I

Historical Aspects of Neurosurgery

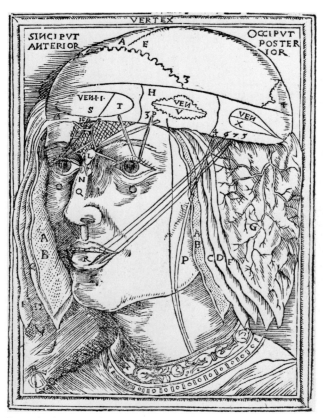

Dryander J. *Anatomiae, Hoc Est, Corporis Humani Dissectionis* . . . . Marpurgi, E Cervicornus, 1537. First illustrated work devoted to the anatomy of the brain. An early illustration of the cerebral ventricles.

1
History of Neurosurgery

Robert H. Wilkins

The student of neurosurgery does well to spend time reading the important early works in the field and the historical accounts that put them in perspective. In this way, he or she develops an understanding of the roots of current neurosurgical practice and an appreciation of the enormous amount of effort that has been expended to advance neurosurgery to its present level. In addition, by studying the great works of the past, the student is better able to sort the wheat from the chaff of current neurosurgical literature.

The development of neurosurgery has taken place primarily during the past century, and many of the key developments have occurred in English-speaking countries. For these reasons, the English-speaking student of neurosurgery has a unique access to the classical works in the field.[1,4,10,11,17,22,23,29,34,40,48,49,53,54,57–59] In addition, there are several excellent reviews of neurosurgical history[3,5,6,15,16,18,20,24,36,39,41–45,47,50–52,55,56] and related publications[7,8,12–14,19,30,32,33,35,38,46] that are written in English.

Neurosurgery in Antiquity

These and other sources reveal that, although most neurosurgical procedures have been developed within the past 100 years, trephination dates back to the Neolithic Period (about 7000 B.C. to 3000 B.C.).[25,27,28,50,51] Archeologists have discovered human skulls with craniectomy defects, apparently made with sharpened stones, in France, Peru, and other widely separated geographical locations around the world (Figs. 1-1 and 1-2). The rationale for these procedures is not known because there are no written records from the New Stone Age. However, it is conceivable that localized cranial deformities, headaches, or mental changes might have been the symptoms that led to this drastic form of treatment. In some of these skulls there are evidences of healing along the bony edges, indicating that the individual survived the operation and that the piece of skull was not removed post mortem as an amulet. That "patients" may survive such procedures has also been demonstrated in modern times in primitive civilizations in different parts of the world, e.g., in East Africa.[27]

The earliest trephined skulls in America were found in the burial caves of Paracas and probably belonged to the people of a civilization that existed along the southern Peruvian coast five hundred or more years before Christ . . . . From the instruments found in the burial caves of Paracas it may be deduced that the trephining was done with an obsidian, triangular, knife-like instrument fixed in a wooden handle . . . . With this blade a straight or curved groove could be made in the skull by repeated cuttings. Probably a longer pointed obsidian blade was used for making small perforations by rapidly rotating the handle. Such holes, closely spaced in a circle, were made for outlining a large bone fragment which was then removed by cutting the intervening bone. The bony defect was occasionally filled with a sheet of gold. The scalp margins were approximated and in some cases held together by tying the hair on either side across the wound. A large dressing of rolls of cotton was placed over it . . . . Healing occurred apparently without infection for the skulls rarely had evidence of osteomyelitic reaction.[50]

A dressing from one of the skulls is shown in Fig. 1-3.

The oldest known writing dealing with surgical topics, the Edwin Smith papyrus, is of special interest to the neurosurgeon.[4,53,54] This treatise dates back to the seventeenth century B.C. and represents a partial copy of an older work (in content, probably more than 1000 years old at the time it was transcribed). It contains the first descriptions of the cranial sutures, the meninges, the external surface of the brain, the cerebrospinal fluid, and the intracranial pulsations. Brain injuries are related to changes in the function of other parts of the body, and hemiplegic contractures are well described. In addition, quadriplegia, urinary incontinence, and priapism are noted to occur in association with cervical vertebral dislocation.

The Edwin Smith papyrus is unique in that it is a systematically organized treatise, consisting of 48 hypothetical cases of different types, with an indication of the prognosis and management of each. The treatment is rational and has a surgical orientation, although trephination is not mentioned. The cases presented begin with various types of head injury and proceed down to the spine and thorax, but the transcription ends abruptly in the middle of the forty-eighth case, in the middle of a sentence, as though the scribe stopped copying for some reason and then never returned to it.

The following two illustrative cases are taken from the translation of the papyrus by J. H. Breasted:

Case 10: . . . *Examination.* If thou examinest a man having a wound in the top of his eyebrow, penetrating to the bone, thou shouldst palpate his wound, (and) draw together for him his gash with stitching. *Diagnosis.* Thou shouldst say concerning him: "[One having] a wound in his eyebrow. An ailment which I will treat." *Treatment.* Now after thou hast stiched it, [thou shouldst bind] fresh meat upon [it] the first day. If thou findest that the stiching of his wound is loose, thou shouldst draw (it) together for him with two strips (of plaster), and thou shouldst treat it with

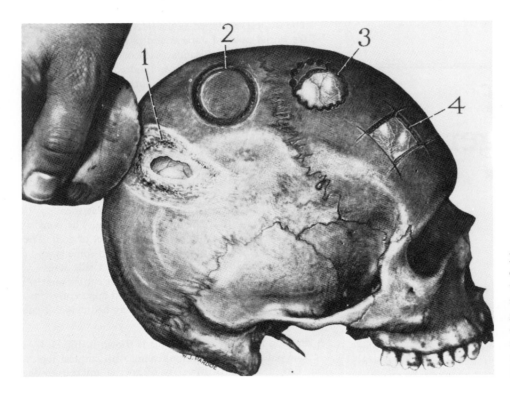

Figure 1-1 Different methods of trepanation (trephination) with a sharpened stone: (1) scraping, (2) grooving, (3) boring and cutting, and (4) using intersecting incisions to remove a rectangular piece of skull. (From Lisowski.[25])

grease and honey every day until he recovers. *Gloss A.* As for: "Two strips of linen," it means two bands of linen, which one applies upon the two lips of the gaping wound, in order to cause that one (lip) join to the other.[2]

Case 6: . . . *Examination.* If thou examinest a man having a gaping wound in his head, penetrating to the bone, smashing his skull, (and) rending open the brain of his skull, thou shouldst palpate his wound. Shouldst thou find that smash which is in his skull [like] those corrugations which form in molten copper,

(and) something therein throbbing (and) fluttering under thy fingers, like the weak place of an infant's crown before it becomes whole . . . . (and) he suffers with stiffness in his neck . . . . *Diagnosis.* [Thou shouldst say concerning him]: "An ailment not to be treated." *Treatment.* Thou shouldst anoint that wound with grease. Thou shalt not bind it; thou shalt not apply two strips upon it: until thou knowest that he has reached a decisive point. *Gloss A.* As for: "Smashing his skull, (and) rending open the brain of his skull," (it means) the smash is large, opening to the interior of his skull, (to) the membrane enveloping

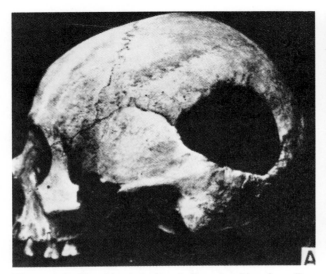

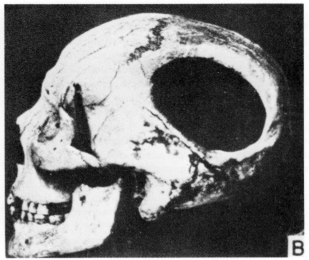

Figure 1-2 Trephined skulls. *A.* Precolumbian from Peru. *B.* Neolithic from France. (From O'Connor DC, Walker AE: Prologue, in Walker.[50])

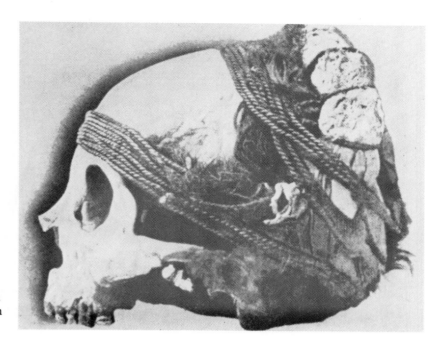

Figure 1-3 Dressing found on a trephined skull from Paracas, Peru. (From O'Connor DC, Walker AE: Prologue, in Walker.[50])

his brain, so that it breaks open his fluid in the interior of his head. *Gloss B*. As for: "Those corrugations which form on molten copper," it means copper which the coppersmith pours off (rejects) before it is forced into the mould, because of something foreign upon it like wrinkles. It is said: "It is like ripples of pus."[4]

The writings of Hippocrates (born 460 B.C.) contain the first recorded descriptions of trephination, and his instruments and methods were very similar to their modern counterparts.[1,35,53,54] Hippocrates also dealt with other subjects of neurosurgical interest. He discussed epilepsy, the coexistence of spinal deformity with pulmonary tubercles, and the functional effects of compression of the spinal cord. He devised a method for reducing vertebral dislocations, and he described permanent and transient facial paralyses, sciatica, and the complex of headache, visual disturbances, and vomiting. The astute observations of Hippocrates include the descriptions of various signs associated with disorders of the brain, such as aphasia, unconsciousness, respiratory and cardiac irregularities, carphologia, pupillary inequality, and ophthalmoplegia. He realized that a blow on one side of the head is occasionally followed by convulsions or paralysis of the contralateral limbs, and he recognized the poor prognosis of the patient with a head injury complicated by a dural laceration. These and other observations made the works of Hippocrates a beacon to surgeons for more than 2000 years (Fig. 1-4) until the development of anesthesia, asepsis, and cerebral localization in the nineteenth century established the foundation of modern neurosurgery.

Prerequisites

The introduction of anesthesia (1846), antisepsis (1867), and asepsis (1891) vastly increased the scope of surgery in general, and made surgery of the nervous system feasible. However, operations on the nervous system were not performed often because neurological knowledge had not advanced sufficiently to allow the preoperative localization of lesions affecting the brain and spinal cord that did not also deform the cranial or spinal surface. Therefore, the other main prerequisite to the development of surgery of the nervous system was the concept of the localization of function within the nervous system.

During the first half of the nineteenth century, debates occurred in medical meetings about the localization of function within different areas of the brain. At that time the brain was thought to act as a whole, with no focal areas of importance for specific functions. But a few clinicians such as Jean Bouillaud challenged this traditional view.

At the meetings of the Société d'Anthropologie de Paris in February and March 1861, a discussion of the localization of cerebral function grew out of a talk relating intelligence to the volume of the skull. Pierre Paul Broca, a 36-year-old general surgeon, was secretary of the society and listened to the debate with great interest. Then, by coincidence, in the next month a man was admitted to Broca's surgical service with a severe infection in his right leg. Twenty-one years previously he had suddenly lost the power of speech, except for one syllable, "tan." The patient died 6 days after admission to the hospital, and a lesion of the posterior half of the second and third left frontal convolutions was found. Six months later, a second patient was admitted to Broca's service with a fractured femur. He previously had been made aphasic as the result of a stroke. This man died, and a similar lesion was found in his brain. These two cases stimulated Broca to find additional cases and to advance the idea that the "center" for expressive speech is localized in the posterior inferior portion of the left frontal lobe. Thus an alert general surgeon made one of the basic discoveries in the field of neurology.

In 1870 two Germans, Gustav Fritsch and Eduard Hitzig, stimulated various points on the surface of the dog's

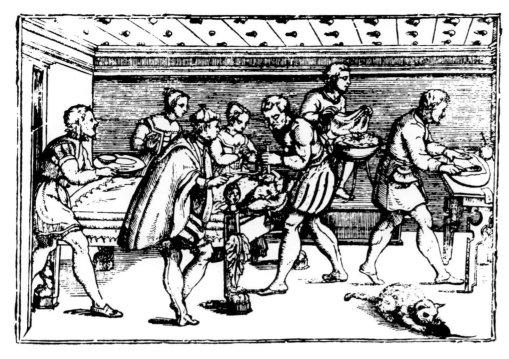

Figure 1-4 Trephination in the sixteenth century. (From della Croce GA: *Chirurgiae Universalis Opus Absolutum.* Venice, Robertus Meietus, 1596, obtained through the courtesy of Dr. Peter D. Olch.)

brain electrically, and at certain spots they were able to produce motor activity in the limbs. Then 4 years later, Roberts Barthalow, a professor of medicine at the Medical College of Ohio, took advantage of a peculiar set of circumstances to prove that similar areas exist in the human. He had under his care a girl dying of a malignant ulcer of the scalp that had exposed a portion of her cerebral surface. With her permission, Barthalow inserted fine insulated wires and stimulated the motor cortex electrically, producing contralateral movements.

These and other individuals who reported chance clinical observations or carefully planned animal experiments established the concept of cerebral localization as well as the broader concept of functional organization within the central and peripheral components of the human nervous system.[7,53,54] This information, coupled with the development of techniques that permitted the surgical exploration of larger areas of the nervous system (such as the osteoplastic craniotomy flap introduced by Wilhelm Wagner in 1889), opened the new field of neurological surgery to any surgeon who was foolhardy enough to try.

Many did try, but most were soon discouraged by the innumerable difficulties and poor results that they encountered. For example, between 1886 and 1896 more than 500 different surgeons reported brain operations that they had performed, but between 1896 and 1906 this number fell below 80. Fortunately, some neurologists and surgeons persevered, and a few began to devote their full attention to neurosurgery.

Neurosurgery at the Turn of the Century

British surgeons were among the first to become involved with the new field, and they guided neurosurgery through its infancy in the last two decades of the nineteenth century. William Macewen (1848–1924), regius professor of surgery at the University of Glasgow and a powerful figure in international surgical circles, was a pioneer in surgery of the brain and spinal cord. Macewen was a pupil of Joseph Lister, and he strongly believed in Lister's principles of antisepsis. His phenomenal success in treating intracranial abscesses, reported in 1893, established a record rarely equaled during the next 80 years despite the introduction of antibiotics.

Rickman Godlee also applied Lister's principles of antisepsis to neurosurgery in 1884, when he exposed and resected an intracranial tumor that had been localized solely by neurological means. William Bennett was another of these pioneering British surgeons. In 1888 he introduced the operation of posterior rhizotomy for the relief of pain.

However, the most outstanding surgeon in the field at that time was Victor Horsley of London (Fig. 1-5). Horsley devoted the majority of his efforts to clinical and experimental neurosurgery, with exceptional results. Although he made many contributions, Horsley is best remembered today for removing a neoplasm from the spinal canal in 1887 and attempting a retrogasserian neurotomy for tic douloureux in 1890. He also described, with Robert Clarke, a stereotactic apparatus for experimental intracranial procedures in 1908.

During the early development of modern neurosurgery it was common for neurologists to diagnose the disease, devise the operation, and direct the surgeon in its performance. For example, Hughes Bennett localized the brain tumor removed in 1884 by Rickman Godlee, and William Gowers diagnosed the spinal cord tumor removed in 1887 by Victor Horsley. In the United States, similar situations occurred. Charles Dana at the Cornell University Medical College proposed posterior rhizotomy as performed a short time later by William Bennett in London and Robert Abbe in New York.

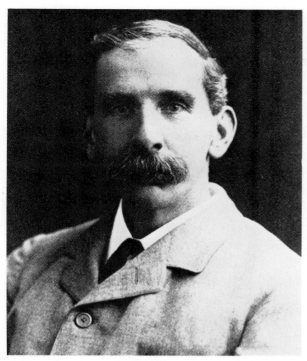

Figure 1-5 Dr. Victor Alexander Haden Horsley, 1857–1916. (From Haymaker and Schiller.[19])

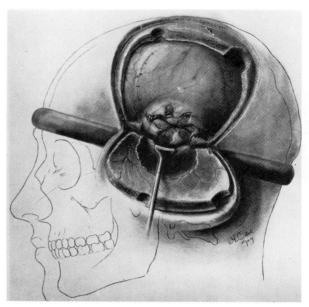

Figure 1-6 An illustration, drawn by Dr. Harvey Cushing, of his method of combining a subtemporal decompression with an exploration of the hemisphere. (From Cushing H: A method of combining exploration and decompression for cerebral tumors which prove to be inoperable. Surg Gynecol Obstet 9:1–5, 1909.)

William Spiller, at the University of Pennsylvania, directed Charles Frazier in the performance of a successful retrogasserian neurotomy in 1901, and 10 years later directed Edward Martin in the performance of the first cordotomy.

The latter event exemplifies Pasteur's remark that chance favors the prepared mind. In 1905, William Spiller, neurologist at the Philadelphia General Hospital, had under his care a 23-year-old man with a loss of the normal ability to perceive pain and temperature sensations in the lower extremities, but with preservation of the ability to appreciate touch. The patient died, and at autopsy was found to have bilateral tuberculomas involving the anterolateral portions of the spinal cord, as Spiller had predicted on the basis of emerging information about the existence of a spinothalamic tract important in pain transmission. In January 1911, a man with a 2-year history of progressive, painful paraplegia due to an irresectable spinal malignancy was admitted to Spiller's service. Spiller then proposed that the anterolateral columns be divided bilaterally, and the first cordotomy was performed under Spiller's direction by Edward Martin, John Rhea Barton Professor of Surgery at the University of Pennsylvania.

Harvey Williams Cushing (1869–1939) and Walter Edward Dandy (1886–1946)

As mentioned above, at the turn of the century neurosurgery was largely being done by surgeons with little understanding of neurology and neurophysiology, and the overall results were poor. Even Victor Horsley, who devoted his full attention to the nervous system, reported in 1890 ten deaths in a series of 44 brain operations that he had performed.

Fortunately, during this time a young surgeon at Johns Hopkins Hospital took an interest in neurosurgery and decided to make it his life's work. With the help of his associates and his many pupils, Harvey Cushing advanced neurosurgery from its infancy through its childhood. By the end of his career, Cushing's name was attached to 14 operations, techniques, diseases, syndromes, and laws.

Probably Cushing's major achievement was the development of a system of operating on the nervous system that in large part is still followed today (Fig 1-6). He standardized neurosurgical operating technique, and by firmly applying the principles of William Halsted to neurosurgical procedures, Cushing was able to achieve major reductions in operative morbidity and mortality. For example, his operative mortality figure by 1915 was 8.4 percent, compared with the 35 to 50 percent rates reported by other experienced surgeons performing brain operations.

Before Cushing's time, hemorrhage had presented an almost insurmountable problem during brain surgery.[24] In his typically thorough manner, Cushing mastered the techniques of others for compressing the scalp, waxing the bone edges, etc., and then he introduced the hemostatic clips and electrocautery that have become virtually indispensable for the control of intracranial and intraspinal bleeding.

Brain tumors attracted Cushing's attention, and during the course of his career, over 2000 patients with brain tumors were seen in his clinic (Fig. 1-7). With the aid of several brilliant assistants such as Percival Bailey and Louise Eisenhardt, Dr. Cushing classified these tumors morphologically, described their biological behavior, and formulated their surgical treatment.

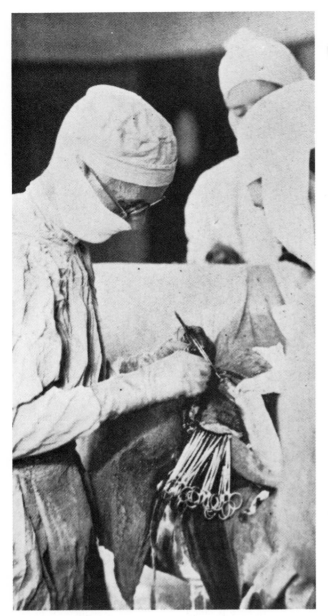

Figure 1-7 Dr. Harvey Cushing operating upon the two-thousandth brain tumor in his series, April 15, 1931. (From Fulton.[16])

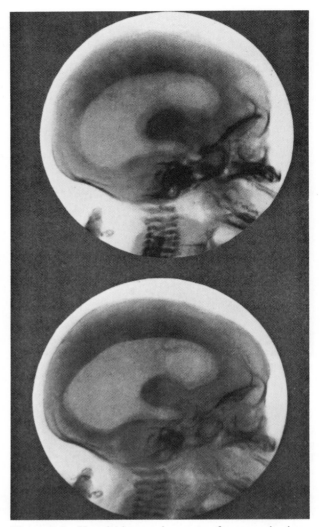

Figure 1-8 Ventriculogram in a case of communicating hydrocephalus. (From Dandy WE: Ventriculography following the injection of air into the cerebral ventricles. Ann Surg 68:5–11, 1918.)

The standardization of operative technique, the classification of brain tumors, and the training of a number of individuals who then developed neurosurgery in their own countries were only three of Harvey Cushing's many contributions. There are few areas of modern neurosurgical interest that are not based to some extent on the important clinical and experimental experience of this one man.

Another such giant was Walter Dandy, who worked with Cushing for a short time at the Johns Hopkins Hospital before Cushing moved to Boston and the Peter Bent Brigham Hospital. Dandy stayed at Johns Hopkins, and before he had finished his residency in surgery, he had made two important discoveries.

In association with Kenneth Blackfan, he established the

modern concept of hydrocephalus in studies reported in 1913. Based on these studies, he subsequently developed the operations of choroid plexectomy, third ventriculostomy, and catheterization of the aqueduct of Sylvius.

A few years after his work with Blackfan, in 1918 and 1919, Dandy introduced pneumoventriculography and pneumoencephalography, which were based in part on his chance observation of air under the diaphragm of a patient with intestinal perforation. On January 3, 1917, he had seen a patient with a suspected intestinal perforation. A roentgenogram of the chest had been made to exclude miliary tuberculosis, and Dandy had noticed air under the patient's diaphragm. This sign has been useful ever since in the diagnosis of intestinal perforation. Of more importance, however, was the fact that Dandy had been searching for a technique for visualizing the cerebral ventricles by radiographic means. This case stimulated him to inject air into the ventricular system, first directly (Fig. 1-8) and later by lumbar puncture. Thus, the chance observation by a prepared mind

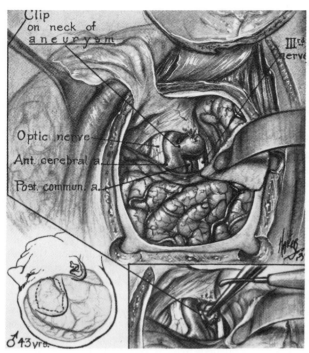

Figure 1-9 Clip ligation of an aneurysm of the internal carotid artery by Dr. Walter Dandy on March 23, 1937. The inset on the left shows the operative approach with the author's concealed incision. The inset on the right shows the clip on the neck of the aneurysm and the cautery shriveling the sac. (From Dandy WE: Intracranial aneurysm of the internal carotid artery, cured by operation. Ann Surg 107:654–659, 1938.)

led to two diagnostic techniques that were of daily importance in neurosurgical practice for over 50 years.

Dandy later developed ways to expose and resect a pineal tumor, to totally remove an acoustic neurinoma, to divide the sensory root of the fifth nerve at the pons for treatment of tic douloureux, to identify and remove a tumor from the third ventricle, to treat Ménière's disease by sectioning the eighth nerve, to clip the neck of an intracranial aneurysm (Fig. 1-9), etc. As was true of Cushing, Dandy's contributions to neurosurgery were legion, and his many pupils have strongly influenced the subsequent course of modern neurosurgery.

Serendipity

Neurosurgery has developed largely by the patient efforts of many people. On occasion, however, a discovery has been made by accident, usually by an individual who encounters an unexpected finding and who has the wit to recognize its potential value and to capitalize on it.[37] I have already mentioned Pierre Paul Broca, Roberts Barthalow, William Spiller, and Walter Dandy in this regard, but there have been others.

For example, in 1921 Jean Sicard, a French clinician, and his pupil, Jacques Forestier, reported their use of poppy

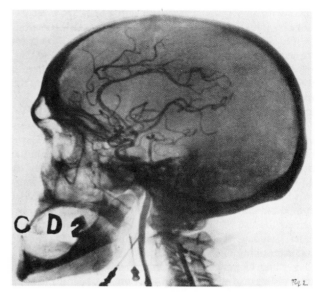

Figure 1-10 Intra-arterial injection of 30% sodium iodide in a human cadaver, showing the intracranial arborization of the internal carotid and vertebral arteries. (From Moniz E: L'encéphalographie artérielle, son importance dans la localisation des tumeurs cérébrales. Rev Neurol 2:72–89, 1927.)

seed oil as a pain-relieving medication. They injected it into the back to treat low back pain and sciatica. The oil, Lipiodal, was iodized and could be visualized on x-ray films. Sicard and Forestier found that if they injected the Lipiodol into the epidural space, they could outline intraspinal lesions radiographically. They also noted that if the Lipiodol was accidentally injected into the subarachnoid space, they could visualize structures in that compartment as well. Thus myelography was born in 1921 in a somewhat roundabout manner.

Also, in the 1920s the Portuguese neurologist, Antonio Caetano de Abreu Freire Egas Moniz (a man who was unusually talented in a number of fields other than medicine but who still found time to produce more than 300 medical publications) worked long and hard to perfect cerebral angiography (first presented in 1927). He overcame many technical obstacles and persevered despite the high initial morbidity and mortality of the procedure. After developing the procedure in cadavers (Fig. 1-10), he tried it in his patients. He attempted percutaneous carotid arteriography in four patients without success, but then was able to perform carotid arteriography after the carotid artery had first been exposed surgically. Egas Moniz used strontium bromide as the contrast medium at first, and then switched to sodium iodide. Of the first nine patients in whom carotid arteriography was attempted, one died and six had temporary neurological deficits. However, with further experience and appropriate modifications, the procedure became safer and more valuable diagnostically.

Therefore, Egas Moniz had already demonstrated his ingenuity and his ability to overcome obstacles in the pursuit of an idea when he attended the Second International Neurological Congress in London in 1935 to report his experiences with angiography. At that meeting he heard presentations by John Fulton and others about frontal lobe function.

This chance occurrence struck a spark. Egas Moniz returned home and, with his colleagues in psychiatry and neurosurgery (Pedro Manuel de Almeida Lima), began prefrontal leukotomy as an operative approach to the modification of abnormal behavior. For the initiation of psychosurgery, Egas Moniz was awarded a Nobel prize in 1949.

Another example of neurosurgical advancement by serendipity involved an American neurosurgeon, W. Gayle Crutchfield. In 1932, Crutchfield was a house officer on the neurosurgical service at the Medical College of Virginia. A 22-year-old woman was admitted following an auto accident. In addition to her C2-C3 fracture dislocation, she also had a compound comminuted fracture of the mandible that prevented the use of halter traction. At the suggestion of his chief, Claude C. Coleman, Dr. Crutchfield inserted Edmonton extension tongs into the patient's skull for cervical traction. Later he perfected the Crutchfield tongs, which came into widespread use. Skeletal traction has been called the greatest single advancement in the treatment of cervical spine injuries, and it originated because of a coincidental broken jaw.[26]

In 1952, an American neurosurgeon, Irving Cooper, accidentally discovered another technique that found widespread usefulness.[9] Before that time, the tremor and rigidity of parkinsonism had been treated by a number of different surgical procedures, none of them very effective. In October 1952, during a craniotomy for a proposed section of the left cerebral peduncle in a 39-year-old man incapacitated by right-sided tremor and rigidity, Cooper accidentally tore the left anterior choroidal artery and had to occlude it. The operation was stopped and the pedunculotomy was not performed. Surprisingly, the patient had an excellent result. Cooper then began clipping the anterior choroidal artery intentionally in these patients. Because the results were varia-

ble, presumably because of the individual variations in the distribution of the anterior choroidal artery, Cooper then began to destroy more directly certain portions of the deep gray matter supplied by that artery. His first target was the globus pallidus. Through a temporal burr hole, Cooper inserted a catheter as far in as the globus pallidus. He then injected a local anesthetic through the catheter. If a good response was achieved, he then created a permanent lesion by injecting alcohol. The resulting operation of chemopallidectomy was a major step in the development of effective surgical therapy for parkinsonism, which subsequently involved the stereotactic destruction of targets within the thalamus.

Painstaking Effort

Yet, despite these and other chance occurrences that resulted in significant progress, the majority of the advancements in neurosurgery have come slowly as the result of orderly observations, planned experiments, and hard work by numerous individuals from many countries. Such painstaking effort characterized the career of Otfrid Foerster of Breslau (1873–1941), a neurologist who later became a neurosurgeon to facilitate patient care and clinical investigations. Independently he devised the operations of posterior rhizotomy for spasticity and cordotomy for pain. However, Foerster's most notable achievement was his elucidation of the organization and function of the nervous system through meticulous clinical observations. Many of his craniotomies and spinal rhizotomies were performed under local anesthesia, and Foerster took the opportunity to study and record the results of electrical stimulation and of division or extirpation of neural tissue. Thus he added considerably to our understanding of cerebral cortical localization and the distribution of the human dermatomes (Fig. 1-11).

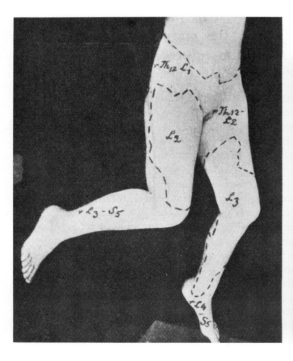 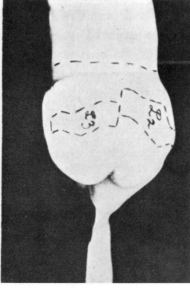

Figure 1-11 The second lumbar dermatome is shown on the right, as demonstrated following surgical division of the right T12, L1, and L3 to S5 nerve roots. The third lumbar dermatome is shown on the left following division of the left T12, L1, L2, and L4 to S5 nerve roots. On comparison of the legs, the great extent of dermatomal overlap is evident. (From Foerster O: The dermatomes in man. Brain 56:1–39, 1933.)

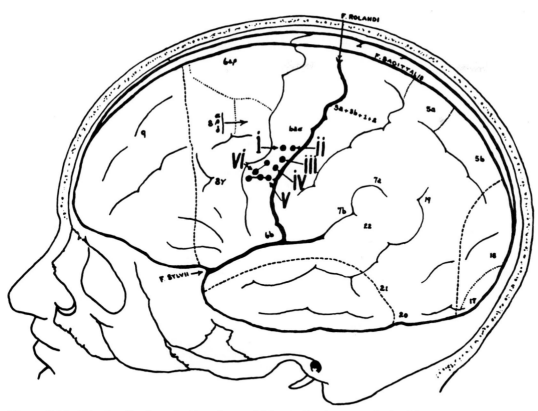

Figure 1-12 The localization of points from which vocalization was obtained by electrical stimulation of the cerebral cortex in six different cases. (From Penfield W: The cerebral cortex and consciousness. Harvey Lect. 32:35–69, 1937.)

Another person of this caliber with a similar interest in clinical neurophysiology was Wilder Penfield, who used his knowledge in many related fields, especially neural histology and histopathology, to develop a unique school of neurosurgery. The Montreal Neurological Institute was established according to Penfield's specifications, and there he and his colleagues carried out their important investigations, including studies relating to epilepsy and the function of the cerebral cortex (Fig. 1-12).[34] These investigations were a team effort that involved a succession of neurosurgical residents, many of whom have continued similar types of studies in other institutions. Thus, although Penfield was a prime mover in the field, advancements in the understanding of cerebral cortical function and of epilepsy have involved many small contributions by thousands of individuals, both before and since Penfield's time.

The history of the treatment of hydrocephalus is another example of slow and painstaking progress.[36,43,50] After the relative safety of intracranial operations was established in the late nineteenth century, a myriad of ingenious operations were devised to treat hydrocephalus. I have already mentioned Dandy's work with choroid plexectomy, third ventriculostomy, and catheterization of the aqueduct of Sylvius. Many other individuals developed operations to shunt cerebrospinal fluid from the ventricles or subarachnoid space into the subgaleal, subdural, subarachnoid, or spinal epidural space, or the pleural or peritoneal cavity, and into the intracranial or extracranial venous system, thoracic duct, ureter, fallopian tube, mastoid antrum, stomach, gallbladder, bone marrow, and other sites. However, shunt occlusion and infection proved to be two major obstacles.

In 1939, Arne Torkildsen of Oslo introduced his ventriculocisternostomy. This has remained an effective method because the shunt is a simple tube without valves and the cerebrospinal fluid is shunted from and to spaces that normally contain CSF. Yet the indications for this type of shunt remain limited, and it has not been of value in most types of hydrocephalus. It wasn't until the 1950s that reasonably reliable ventriculovenous shunting techniques were introduced (by Frank Nulsen and Eugene Spitz of the University of Pennsylvania in 1952 and by Robert Pudenz and his colleagues from the Huntington Institute of Medical Research in 1957). Key to the success of these operations were functional one-way valves constructed of inert materials, and several types were introduced. The Holter valve was developed in 1956 in response to an urgent personal need. The infant son of an industrial technician, John Holter, was being treated for hydrocephalus by Dr. Spitz at the Children's Hospital of Philadelphia. Ventriculoperitoneal shunting was not proving successful because of repeated shunt obstructions. As a result, Holter was stimulated to turn his inventive talents to designing a valve that permitted ventriculojugular shunting for his son's condition. This initial Holter valve and its subsequent modifications have been beneficial to neurosurgical patients for more than 25 years. Many other technical advancements have also been made, and these successive developments have progressively improved the outlook for patients with hydrocephalus.

It has also taken years to refine the surgical treatment of tic douloureux. Prior to the present century a number of operations had been devised for the extracranial interruption of the various branches of the trigeminal nerve. Since these operations seldom gave permanent relief, attempts were then made to attack the gasserian ganglion and its connections intracranially. Victor Horsley attempted a retrogasserian neurotomy unsuccessfully in 1890, but this was quickly followed by the successful development of an extradural temporal approach to the ganglion. Frank Hartley of New York employed this approach in 1891 to section the second and third trigeminal divisions, and Fedor Krause of Berlin a short time later independently introduced the same approach for excision of the ganglion. Then, in 1901, Charles Frazier of Philadelphia employed the Hartley-Krause approach for the first successful retrogasserian neurotomy. Later surgeons introduced the principle of differential section of the trigeminal root so that corneal sensation and trigeminal motor function are spared. Other operations, such as percutaneous trigeminal rhizolysis (with a radio-frequency current or with glycerol) and surgical division or microvascular decompression of the trigeminal sensory root at the pons, have been developed subsequently for the treatment of tic douloureux, and the quest for better procedures continues.

Carotid endarterectomy is now a frequently performed operation. Its initiation in 1953 was dependent upon the simultaneous extension of several lines of clinical and postmortem investigation by many individuals. By that year it had been established by angiographic and postmortem examinations that atherosclerosis frequently involves the proximal portion of the internal carotid artery and may give rise to arterial stenosis or occlusion. The clinical syndromes associated with such lesions were being defined, and reconstruction of arteries in other parts of the body were being carried out. The stage was set for the next logical step, carotid endarterectomy, and this was reported by Kenneth Strully, Elliott Hurwitt, and Harry Blankenberg in the *Journal of Neurosurgery* in 1953. That particular procedure did not yield vascular patency because it was done in a patient who had had a complete thrombosis of the internal carotid artery. However, in 1954, H. H. G. Eastcott, G. W. Pickering, and C. G. Rob reported the successful reconstruction of the internal carotid artery in a patient with carotid stenosis. Within a few years these and other groups established the clinical indications and surgical techniques of carotid endarterectomy.[39]

The definition and surgical treatment of intervertebral disc disease has evolved over many years. Sciatica as a symptom has been known to physicians for more than 2000 years. The anatomical presence of the intervertebral disc has also been known for centuries. However, although isolated cases of traumatic rupture of the intervertebral disc were reported in the nineteenth century, it has not been until relatively recent times that the syndrome of the herniated nucleus pulposus has been recognized. In 1911, Joel Goldthwait of Boston predicted that such a syndrome might occur, and from 1927 to 1934 a number of investigators added supportive evidence to this concept. But the problem escaped exact def-

inition until 1934 when two physicians from the Massachusetts General Hospital, William Jason Mixter, a neurosurgeon, and Joseph Barr, an orthopedic surgeon, presented their classical description (Fig. 1-13).[2] Since that time the surgical removal of herniated discs has become one of the most common operations that a neurosurgeon performs.

In addition, the surge of interest in disc disease that followed this report was a definite stimulus to the development of modern myelography. In 1891, Heinrich Quincke had laid the groundwork for myelography when he had introduced the technique of lumbar puncture. By 1922, Jean Sicard and Jacques Forestier had introduced positive contrast myelography. However, when the syndrome of the herniated nucleus pulposus finally was recognized, the need for a better contrast medium became apparent. This need was met by the development of Pantopaque (ethyl iodophenylundecylate) by Theodore Steinhausen and his colleagues at the University of Rochester during World War II. Pantopaque myelography subsequently became a frequently performed procedure.

The introduction of myelography, ventriculography,

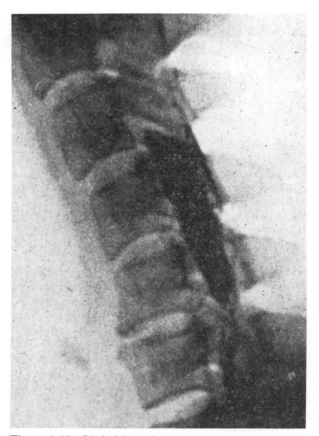

Figure 1-13 Lipiodol myelogram in a 28-year-old man with a progressive cervical myelopathy. After cisternal injection the iodized oil showed a partial block at the level of the C5-6 disc. Through a laminectomy an extradural encapsulated fibrocartilaginous mass 1.5 × 0.8 × 0.3 cm in size was removed. (From Mixter WJ, Barr JS: Rupture of the intervertebral disc with involvement of the spinal canal. N Engl J Med 211:210–214, 1934.)

pneumoencephalography, and cerebral angiography has been mentioned. Brain scanning with radioisotopes was heralded by the discovery by George Moore and his associates at the University of Minnesota (as reported in 1947) that intravenously administered fluorescein will concentrate in brain tumors and other lesions of the central nervous system.[31] This group then investigated the possibility that they could add a radioactive tag to the fluorescein that would permit localization of an abnormality through the intact skull by means of an external radiation detector. They first used radioactive diiodofluorescein and a Geiger-Müller tube, which yielded 41 correct positive (24) or negative (17) results among 66 patients. With improvements in technique and equipment they achieved a 76 percent correct diagnosis rate among 57 patients tested between September 15, 1950, and April 1, 1951. The entire field of radionuclide imaging enlarged rapidly after these and other pioneering efforts, and nuclear medicine as a specialty was begun.

Recent Developments

A parallel situation existed with the development of computed axial tomography scanning. One individual and one group did the key early work, which then led quickly to the explosive development of a new area of medical diagnosis. In 1967, Godfrey Hounsfield was investigating pattern recognition techniques at the Central Research Laboratories of EMI Limited in Hayes, Middlesex, England, and was working specifically on the interpretation of data derived from x-ray transmission through an object.[21] He perceived that the mathematical interpretation of such data could be simplified by dividing the object into a series of "slices," which would then collectively give a three-dimensional representation of the object.

Calculations showed that:

> . . . it would be possible to measure the absolute values of the absorption coefficient of areas within the slice with an accuracy approaching one hundred times greater than by conventional methods . . . . To test the practical feasibility of the technique . . . a simple laboratory machine was built on a lathe bed, the lead screw being driven in steps by an electric motor and the specimen rotated in one degree steps, at the end of each linear scan . . . . Because of the low intensity of gamma radiation, the machine had to be left operating for at least nine days to produce one picture. It took a large computer two and a half hours to process the readings. The computer had to solve 28,000 simultaneous equations and was programmed in Fortran . . . . The method of interpolation between picture points was modified and subsequent experiments were carried out using x-rays . . . . Results much closer to the theoretical maximum of $\frac{1}{2}$ percent accuracy were eventually achieved, although the process was still unacceptably slow, requiring at least one day to produce a picture.

In the course of this work, and in co-operation with Dr. James Ambrose, Consultant Radiologist at

Atkinson Morley's Hospital, Wimbledon, readings were taken of a specimen of human brain . . . . There was considerable elation when pictures processed from these readings revealed that not only were the tumors in the specimen clearly isolated, but it was possible also to discriminate between gray and white matter . . . . A specification for a brain machine, incorporating the new technique, was submitted to the Department of Health and Social Security; with their co-operation, design and development work began in August 1970 . . . . The first machine was installed at Atkinson Morley's Hospital in September 1971, under the guidance of Dr. Ambrose. The processing time for each picture was reduced to twenty minutes on an ICL 1905 computer, by using machine code instead of Fortran . . . .[21]

The subsequent rapid developments in this field have yielded a safe, accurate, and sensitive technique for detecting abnormalities throughout the human body, including the brain and spinal cord. Now the additional techniques of single photon tomography, positron emission tomography, and nuclear magnetic resonance scanning give us the means of assessing the function as well as the morphology of the human nervous system, in vivo and with little hazard and little discomfort.[32,33] Recent years have also seen the development of intravenous digital subtraction angiography and the introduction of safe water-soluble agents for myelography and cisternography. Interventional neuroradiological techniques are being applied to the treatment of carotid-cavernous fistulas and arteriovenous malformations. In fact, the entire field of neuroradiology has appeared and grown from its roots in radiology, neurosurgery, and neurology into a separate and rapidly advancing field.

For years, neurosurgeons throughout the world have been expanding and updating neurosurgery in their cities and countries according to their local circumstances.[3,44] The development of ideas and techniques, expansion and dissemination of knowledge, and creation of neurosurgical organizations continue at an ever increasing rate. Individual pioneers are being replaced by groups, teams, and institutions. Neurosurgeons now work frequently in conjunction with people from other disciplines. Furthermore, neurosurgeons are tending to subspecialize and are thus learning more and more about progressively narrower areas of interest. With this increase in manpower, knowledge, and techniques, and with the more sharply focused topics of investigation, advancements are being made at a remarkable rate.

Evoked potential measurements are proving their value in diagnosis and intraoperative monitoring, and ultrasound scanning is similarly being used both for diagnosis and for the intraoperative localization of intracranial lesions. The intracranial pressure is being monitored in a variety of clinical settings and by several techniques. Microneurosurgery has been developed and extracranial-intracranial bypass grafting procedures are performed frequently. Stereotactic techniques are being mated to computed tomography for the accurate biopsy and treatment of deep brain lesions. Complex methods of tissue retraction and tissue removal (e.g., laser, ultrasonic emulsification and suction) are being introduced into daily neurosurgical practice.

Ingenious pumps are being implanted to supply chemical agents such as morphine and heparin on a continuous, low-dose basis for the treatment of pain, occlusive cerebrovascular disease, and other conditions. Other clever techniques have also been devised for treating pain, and methods of electrical stimulation of numerous portions of the nervous system have been employed for a variety of reasons. The combination of sophisticated advancements in neuroendocrinology and neuroradiology with the rebirth of trans-sphenoidal operative techniques has permitted significant developments in the understanding and treatment of pituitary disorders. The same types of advancements in neuro-otology and neuroradiology have revolutionized the care of patients with acoustic neuroma. Reliable methods have evolved for measuring cerebral blood flow and other hemodynamic and metabolic parameters. Basic investigations have been made into the nature of intracranial arterial spasm. The treatment of hydrocephalus in utero and the transplantation of brain tissue are just beginning.

The Future

What of the future of neurosurgery? What challenges remain for the students of today? Undoubtedly more advanced surgical techniques remain to be developed. However, neurosurgeons have had, and will continue to have, a unique opportunity to add to the understanding of the central nervous system. Dr. Penfield summarized this idea in an address to the American Academy of Neurological Surgery in 1948:

> Young surgeons who have learned to use the scalpel so expertly that they can take anything out of anywhere without a fatality, to cut the pathways of the currents of the intellect and leave a man who is still capable of walking, may be tempted to look upon the performance of the pioneers in the earlier period with unjustified contempt.
>
> Elaboration of surgical technique is an important mechanical achievement. But beware of vainglory; for it may be that our intellectual maturity is yet far off, and to be acquired only after years of further pioneering.

What a study of the history of neurosurgery tells us is that advancements are made in steps, either by the planned extension of an existing line of inquiry or by the recognition of the importance of a chance occurrence. Furthermore, when the time and circumstances are right for a development, it may be thought of, discovered, created, or performed by more than one individual in different parts of the world simultaneously. Neurosurgeons are part of a dynamic and constantly changing field, and each of us has the opportunity to contribute to its present and eventual nature. Even those of us who are not involved in research activities must not forget the potential value of a chance observation. Our patients are providing us the clues to the understanding and control of their illnesses. It is up to us to recognize these clues and act in accordance with them.

References

1. Adams F: *The Genuine Works of Hippocrates.* New York, Wood, 1886, vols 1 and 2.
2. Ballantine HT: "Sciatica" and the neurosurgeon: Historical perspectives and personal reminiscences. Clin Neurosurg 27:541–552, 1980.
3. Black P: Perspectives in international neurosurgery. Neurosurgery 1:160–167, 1977 et seq.
4. Breasted JH: *The Edwin Smith Surgical Papyrus.* Chicago, University of Chicago Press, 1930, vols 1 and 2.
5. Bucy PC: The Journal of Neurosurgery: Its origin and development. J Neurosurg 21(7):1–14, 1964.
6. Bucy PC, Clark WK: The American Board of Neurological Surgery: A historical summary. Surg Neurol 7:304–311, 1977.
7. Clarke E, Dewhurst K: *An Illustrated History of Brain Function.* Berkeley, University of California Press, 1972.
8. Clarke E, O'Malley CD: *The Human Brain and Spinal Cord.* Berkeley, University of California Press, 1968.
9. Cooper IS: *The Neurosurgical Alleviation of Parkinsonism.* Springfield, Ill, Charles C Thomas, 1956.
10. Cushing H: Surgery of the head, in Keen WW (ed): *Surgery: Its Principles and Practice.* Philadelphia, Saunders, 1908, vol 3, pp 17–276.
11. Dandy WE: The brain, in Lewis D (ed): *Practice of Surgery.* Hagerstown, Md, WF Prior, 1932, vol 12, pp 1–682.
12. De Jong RN: *A History of American Neurology.* New York, Raven Press, 1982.
13. Denny-Brown D, Rose AS, Sahs AL: *Centennial Anniversary Volume of the American Neurological Association 1875–1975.* New York, Springer, 1975.
14. Elsberg CA: *The Story of a Hospital: The Neurological Institute of New York: 1909–1938.* New York, Paul B. Hoeber, Inc, 1944.
15. Feindel W: Highlights of neurosurgery in Canada. JAMA 200:853–859, 1967.
16. Fulton JF: *Harvey Cushing: A Biography.* Springfield, Ill, Charles C Thomas, 1946.
17. Gloor P: *Hans Berger on the Electroencephalogram of Man.* Electroencephalogr Clin Neurophysiol Suppl 28, 1969.
18. Gurdjian ES: *Head Injury from Antiquity to the Present with Special Reference to Penetrating Head Wounds.* Springfield, Ill, Charles C Thomas, 1973.
19. Haymaker W, Schiller F: *The Founders of Neurology,* 2d ed. Springfield, Ill, Charles C Thomas, 1970.
20. Horrax G: *Neurosurgery: An Historical Sketch.* Springfield, Ill, Charles C Thomas, 1952.
21. Hounsfield GN: Historical notes on computerized axial tomography. J Can Assoc Radiol 27:135–142, 1976.
22. Jefferson G: *Selected Papers.* Springfield, Ill, Charles C Thomas, 1960.
23. Kelly EC: *Classics of Neurology.* Huntington, NY, Robert E Krieger, 1971.
24. Light RU: Hemostasis in neurosurgery. J Neurosurg 2:414–434, 1945.
25. Lisowski FP: Prehistoric and early historic trepanation, in Brothwell D, Sandison AT (eds): *Diseases in Antiquity: A Survey of the Diseases, Injuries and Surgery of Early Populations.* Springfield, Ill, Charles C Thomas, 1967, pp 651–672.
26. Loeser JD: History of skeletal traction in the treatment of cervical spine injuries. J Neurosurg 33:54–59, 1970.
27. Margetts EL: Trepanation of the skull by the medicine-men of primitive cultures, with particular reference to present-day native East African practice, in Brothwell D, Sandison AT (eds): *Diseases in Antiquity: A Survey of the Diseases, Injuries and Surgery of Early Populations.* Springfield, Ill, Charles C Thomas, 1967, pp 673–701.

28. Massarotti M: Le origini della neurochirurgia nei documenti preistorici e protostorici. Minerva Neurochir 14:56–78, 343–359, 1970; 15:29–60, 1971.

29. Matson DD, German WJ, Committee of The American Association of Neurological Surgeons: *Harvey Cushing: Selected Papers on Neurosurgery.* New Haven, Yale University Press, 1969.

30. McHenry LC Jr: *Garrison's History of Neurology.* Springfield, Ill, Charles C Thomas, 1969.

31. Moore GE: *Diagnosis and Localization of Brain Tumors.* Springfield, Ill, Charles C Thomas, 1953.

32. Oldendorf WH: *The Quest for an Image of Brain.* New York, Raven Press, 1980.

33. Oldendorf WH: Nuclear medicine in clinical neurology: An update. Ann Neurol 10:207–213, 1981.

34. Penfield W: *No Man Alone.* Boston, Little, Brown, 1977.

35. Phillips ED: The brain and nervous phenomena in the Hippocratic writings. Irish J Med Sci, 381:377–390, 1957.

36. Pudenz RH: The surgical treatment of hydrocephalus: An historical review. Surg Neurol 15:15–26, 1981.

37. Remer TG: *Serendipity and the Three Princes: From the Peregrinaggio of 1557.* Norman, Okla, University of Oklahoma Press, 1965.

38. Riese W: *A History of Neurology.* New York, MD Publications, 1959.

39. Rob C: Occlusive disease of the extracranial cerebral arteries: A review of the past 25 years, J Cardiovasc Surg 19:487–498, 1978.

40. Rottenberg DA, Hochberg FH: *Neurological Classics in Modern Translation.* New York, Hafner, 1977.

41. Sachs E: *The History and Development of Neurological Surgery.* London, Cassell, 1952.

42. Scarff JE: Fifty years of neurosurgery, 1905–1955. Int Abstr Surg 101:417–513, 1955.

43. Scarff JE: Treatment of hydrocephalus: An historical and critical review of methods and results. J Neurol Neurosurg Psychiatry 26:1–26, 1963.

44. Scoville WB: The World Federation of Neurosurgical Societies: A brief history. Surg Neurol 7:185–188, 1977.

45. Society of Neurological Surgeons: *The Society of Neurological Surgeons 1920–1970.* Privately printed by the Society, 1970.

46. Spillane JD: *The Doctrine of the Nerves: Chapters in the History of Neurology.* Oxford, Oxford University Press, 1981.

47. Spurling RG, Woodhall B: *Medical Department, United States Army. Surgery in World War II: Neurosurgery.* Washington, DC, Office of the Surgeon General, Department of the Army, vol 1, 1958; vol 2, 1959.

48. Toyokura Y: A list of original and classical descriptions of neurological diseases, signs and syndromes with their historical notes. Shinkei Kenkyu No Shimpo 14:232–260, 1971; 15:1051–1070, 1971; 16:745–770, 1972.

49. Troland CE, Otenasek FJ: *Selected Writings of Walter E. Dandy.* Springfield, Ill, Charles C Thomas, 1957.

50. Walker AE: *A History of Neurological Surgery.* Baltimore, Williams & Wilkins, 1951.

51. Walker AE: The dawn of neurosurgery. Clin Neurosurg 6:1–38, 1959.

52. Wertheimer P, David M: Naissance et croissance de la neurochirurgie. Neurochirurgie 25:247–363, 1979.

53. Wilkins RH: Neurosurgical classics I–XXXVIII. J Neurosurg 19:700–710, 1962; 23:241–261, 1965.

54. Wilkins RH: *Neurosurgical Classics.* New York, Johnson Reprint Co, 1965.

55. Wilkins RH: *History of the American Association of Neurological Surgeons founded in 1931 as The Harvey Cushing Society, 1931–1981.* Chicago, American Association of Neurological Surgeons, 1981.

56. Wilkins RH: Birth of a journal: The origin and early years of *Neurosurgery.* 10:820–826, 1982.

57. Wilkins RH, Brody IA: Neurological classics I–XLI. Arch Neurol 17:331–333, 1967; 26:91–93, 1972.

58. Wilkins RH, Brody IA: *Neurological Classics.* New York, Johnson Reprint Co, 1973.

59. Wolf JK: *The Classical Brain Stem Syndromes.* Springfield, Ill, Charles C Thomas, 1971.

2

Two Giants: Harvey Cushing and Walter Dandy

Paul C. Bucy

No one in the neurosurgical world would deny that Cushing and Dandy were the outstanding giants in this field. Why is this true? They were by no means the first neurosurgeons, neither were they the only outstanding neurological surgeons. Their contribution was that they resurrected neurological surgery, which at the beginning of the twentieth century was a dying specialty. They put it on its feet. They demonstrated that neurosurgical procedures could be performed without a high mortality and with patients in improved condition, and that brain tumors previously regarded as inoperable could be operated upon safely and successfully.

Neurological surgery had begun almost a quarter of a century earlier when William Macewen in Glasgow removed the first brain tumor successfully and when Victor Horsley similarly removed the first tumor of the spinal cord in 1886. Following their examples, Fedor Krause in Germany, Von Eiselberg in Austria, and W. W. Keen in the United States began doing neurological surgery. Their surgical mortality was high, often estimated as high as 65 percent, and the condition of the patients following their operations left much to be desired. Neurological surgery was a dying specialty. Cushing and Dandy brought it back from the dead, breathed life into it, and ultimately made it into a vigorous surgical specialty.

Cushing and Dandy were not the only great men in neurological surgery. Charles Elsberg in New York established the means of diagnosis and treatment of tumors of the spinal cord. Frazier pointed the way to operate successfully on the preganglionic root of the trigeminal nerve for the relief of trigeminal neuralgia. Jefferson, Dott, and Cairns (the latter two were pupils of Cushing) revitalized neurological surgery in Great Britain. A neurologist, Otfrid Foerster, in Breslau, Germany, put cerebral cortical localization and the sensory distribution of the various spinal nerve roots on a firm basis. He also demonstrated that epilepsy with a focal origin could be relieved by removing the cortical scar that gave rise to the attacks. Olivecrona in Stockholm established neurosurgical technique in Europe and trained many of the neurosurgeons of Europe, and de Martel began neurological surgery in

France and added many innovations to neurosurgical technique. Clovis Vincent, also a neurologist, became the leading neurological surgeon of France, the true father of French neurological surgery, and trained many of the neurosurgeons of France and other countries. Sachs, Adson, and Peet established neurological surgery in the middle western part of the United States. Carl Rand and Howard Naffziger did the same for the far western part of the country. Jason Mixter with his orthopedic colleague, Barr, established that the herniated lumbar intervertebral disc was by all odds the most common cause of sciatica and that the condition could be relieved by removal of the herniated disc. Percival Bailey, working with the tumors that Cushing had removed, established a classification of gliomas and correlated their microscopic characteristics with their biological behavior. He also classified the vascular malformations and tumors of the brain. Wilder Penfield created the great Montreal Neurological Institute, the first true institute of the neurosciences in the world. He expanded Foerster's work on epilepsy and on cerebral localization, and he trained many of the leaders in neurological surgery in the United States and elsewhere. These men and others were all truly great, though not the initiators and innovators that Cushing and Dandy were. Their names are given here to point out that there were others and that our progress in neurological surgery over the years is dependent upon many people in many countries.

In many ways Cushing and Dandy were alike. They were both difficult, proud men. Of both it has been said that they could not bear to be surpassed. This is not surprising nor is it peculiar to these two men. Others were also difficult, proud men. All were determined and often temperamental. This was true because of the circumstances under which they toiled. Their patients were difficult. The diagnosis was difficult. They were confronted with a tightly enclosed box and had to try to determine what was going on inside that was making the patient ill. They had little to help them with their diagnoses. The x-ray that Cushing had brought to neurological surgery was of help in only a small percentage of the cases. They had no means of reducing the increased intracranial pressure from which most of their patients suffered. They had only inadequate means of controlling hemorrhage during neurosurgical procedures. Their neurological colleagues belittled them and their efforts and often discouraged the patients from having a neurosurgical operation. The administrators of their hospitals were unhappy with them because they demanded much and, in their opinions, damaged the reputation of the hospitals by raising the mortality rates. The young people under their training suffered most from their tyrannical outbursts. It is a wonder that any of them stayed to complete their training. Many of them did so only because the period of hell on earth was relatively short. For most of those who trained with Cushing, it was only 1 year. Bailey, who stayed longer, found that from time to time it was necessary for him to get away and work in more pleasant surroundings. Only Horrax, a master surgeon and a gentle soul, stayed with Cushing and bore his unpleasant outbursts. Dandy was not too different. However, from time to time he would recognize that he had gone too far and would seek to make amends by tickets to a ball game or by a dinner.

For most of their adult lives Cushing and Dandy conducted a feud.[2] Their antagonism was more reminiscent of the Appalachian Mountains than it was of Baltimore and Boston. A similar feud occurred in France between de Martel and Vincent, but that feud is not our concern here. The antagonism between Cushing and Dandy was not the result of a single episode. It began almost as soon as they first met, but not quite. There was a brief happier period, which is illustrated in the photograph, shown in Fig. 2-1, of the two men after a friendly tennis match.

Their antagonism arose out of many encounters. When they first worked together at the Johns Hopkins Hospital in Baltimore, the sparks flew. Cushing was operating, Dandy was his assistant. Dandy held a retractor with his left hand. Cushing told him not to operate with his left hand as he was awkward enough with his right. When Dandy began his work on hydrocephalus in the laboratory, work that was ultimately to lay the anatomical foundation for the understanding of hydrocephalus, Cushing belittled it. When Cushing was leaving Hopkins to go to Boston, he packed Dandy's research material with his own. When Dandy discovered this, he removed his things and told Cushing that they were his. Cushing remarked that they didn't amount to anything anyhow. A few years later when Dandy published his preliminary paper on the total removal of acoustic neuromas, "the fat was really in the fire." Dandy had not mentioned Cushing's earlier monograph on this subject. Cushing

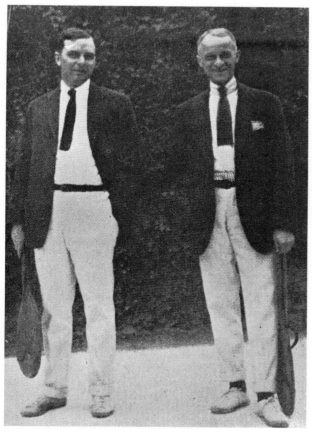

Figure 2-1 Dandy (left) and Cushing (right) in 1921 following a tennis match.

wrote a letter in which he called Dandy a liar, although not in those words. What he said was that it was not possible to remove one of these tumors completely without either killing the patient or rendering the patient hopelessly crippled if he or she should survive. Of course Dandy was paving the way to the modern treatment of these tumors. The differences between these two men was not limited to harsh words but at times to handicaps in their own surgical procedures. Dandy for some time refused to use the electric cautery that Bovie and Cushing had developed and the silver clips that McKenzie and Cushing had invented. Cushing, on the other hand, refused to utilize ventriculography for diagnosis. It must be admitted that Cushing was usually the aggressor in these disagreements, but Dandy expressed his feelings in ways that did him no credit either. Dandy refused to join the Society of Neurological Surgeons that Cushing had initiated and the Harvey Cushing Society (later the American Association of Neurological Surgeons) because it bore Cushing's name. But enough of this disgraceful episode, which hung like a pall over American neurological surgery for many, many years.

Harvey Cushing (1869–1939)

Cushing was born in Cleveland, Ohio and died in New Haven, Connecticut, 70 years later.[3,4] He came from a distinguished family of physicians. He attended Yale University. His highest grades at Yale were in mathematics and science, and his poorest in languages, particularly in Latin. He also played on the baseball team but does not seem to have distinguished himself in this area very much. Later in life he engaged in tennis and croquet. In these games he was known as a poor loser who was never satisfied unless he won. Following his graduation from Yale he entered Harvard Medical School (1891–1895) and then entered upon an internship at the Massachusetts General Hospital. In the autumn of 1896 Cushing moved to the Johns Hopkins Hospital to work with William S. Halsted, one of the greatest surgeons and teachers of surgery that the world has ever seen. This was the turning point in Cushing's career, from which he went on to become the father of neurological surgery. He gave evidence of his innovative bent, which was to characterize the rest of his professional career. He introduced the diagnostic use of x-rays into the Johns Hopkins Hospital. Following his training under Halsted, Cushing decided that he might be interested in the surgical treatment of lesions of the brain.

In July 1900 he arrived in England determined to learn about neurological surgery from Victor Horsley. The day after his arrival he accompanied Horsley to the home of a patient with tic douloureux. Horsley operated upon the patient in her own house. He "made a great hole in the woman's skull, pushed up the temporal lobe—blood everywhere, gauze packed into the middle fossa, the ganglion out, the wound closed." This so distressed Cushing that he rapidly changed his mind about working with Horsley and left England for the continent.

It is interesting that the operation that turned Cushing against the idea of working with Horsley, and almost turned him away from neurological surgery, was for trigeminal neuralgia. In the ensuing years neither Cushing nor Dandy became experts in operating upon the trigeminal nerve in the temporal fossa. This particular operation and its mastery remained for Frazier and more particularly for Max Minor Peet. Cushing's inadequacy in this surgical procedure became apparent to me early in my neurosurgical career. I had gone to Chicago with Percival Bailey in the summer of 1928. Shortly after our arrival, Bailey, with me as assistant, attempted to operate on the gasserian ganglion using the same technique as Cushing had used. Bailey's experience with this in Boston was less than satisfactory, as he attempted to operate although the head-light was on Cushing's head. In Chicago we operated with the patient lying down and his head on the side. Blood constantly ran down into the operative field, obscuring our vision. As a result the operation was soon terminated. It was obvious that we had to acquire a better technique. Accordingly we went to Ann Arbor, and Max Peet operated upon several cases for us and demonstrated how these operations should be performed with the patient in a sitting position. Thereafter our attempts proceeded more favorably. Neither was Dandy an expert in exposing the trigeminal nerve in the temporal fossa. Raphael Eustace Semmes of Memphis, Tennessee, was a close friend of Dandy. They had attended college in Missouri and the Johns Hopkins Medical School together and retained a close, friendly relationship thereafter. Semmes did not like the operation through the posterior fossa for exposure of the trigeminal nerve that Dandy had devised. On one occasion Semmes remarked to Dandy, "Walter, if you had only learned to operate upon the trigeminal nerve in the temporal fossa you would never have thought of that damn-fool operation of yours." Obviously even our greatest surgeons have their inadequacies and deficiencies. We should never place those we admire on a pedestal. If we do, we will all too often observe that they have clay feet.

After Cushing decided not to work with Horsley, he spent a short time in France and then went to Switzerland, first to Theodor Kocher, one of the most distinguished surgeons of his time. However, Kocher had little for Cushing to do and sent him to Kronecker, the physiologist. Here Cushing's interest in the nervous system reappeared. His experimental work in that laboratory led to his classical demonstration of the effects of increased intracranial pressure on respiratory rate, pulse rate, and blood pressure.

During a relatively brief visit to Italy in 1901 Cushing visited a number of cities, museums, and hospitals. In Pavia he saw the device for measuring blood pressure that had been designed by Riva-Rocci. When he returned to the Hopkins, he introduced the use of this instrument for following the blood pressure during surgical operations.

Another milestone in Cushing's career occurred immediately after he left the European continent. He went to Liverpool, where he worked with Sir Charles Sherrington. At that time Sherrington was studying the electrical excitability of the cerebral cortex of subhuman primates. Cushing was asked to assist in these experiments by exposing the cerebral cortex of apes. Although Cushing has not clearly said so, there appears to be little doubt that this brief experience in Sherrington's laboratory reversed Cushing's thinking back to neurological surgery.

When Cushing returned to Baltimore in the autumn of 1901, he soon indicated his desire to engage in neurological surgery in spite of the efforts of Halsted to dissuade him. Cushing was still doing general surgery, but in addition to operating upon exophthalmic goiter, he was operating upon children with meningoceles and upon brain tumors. Between 1901 and 1912 Cushing was primarily concerned with training himself to become a neurological surgeon. During the latter part of that period he had other pupils—Dandy and Howard Naffziger. At first he wrote more papers on general surgical subjects, but gradually those having to do with neurological surgery replaced the others. His book on the pituitary, his first monograph, appeared in 1912.

In 1910 Cushing operated upon General Leonard Wood and successfully removed a meningioma. This was another turning point in Cushing's career. Not only was this the first time that he had successfully removed such a tumor, but the patient was a most distinguished military officer. Dr. Arthur Tracy Cabot, a member of the Corporation of Harvard University, witnessed the operation and was so impressed with Cushing's surgical ability that he urged his appointment as professor of surgery at Harvard. In April of the same year Cushing received the invitation to become chief surgeon of the Peter Bent Brigham Hospital and professor of surgery at Harvard. When he was first appointed, the Brigham Hospital was not yet off the drawing board and far from being built. The hospital opened on April 30, 1912. Although some operations were performed in the first couple of years at the Brigham, Cushing's work as a surgeon, writer, and teacher had scarcely begun when the world was thrown into the shattering World War I. Nevertheless the training of some distinguished future neurological surgeons—Gilbert Horrax, E. B. Towne, and Carl Rand—had begun. In August 1914 a military hospital and ambulance service had been sponsored by the American ambassador to France. The following year a Harvard unit to that hospital was organized. In March 1915 Cushing arrived in Paris and took up his duties. Although during the next four years he made great contributions to the treatment of penetrating wounds of the brain and in 1917 his monograph on acoustic nerve tumors appeared, it is obvious that his career was interrupted. On May 11, 1917, Cushing again set sail for Europe, this time as a medical officer in the American Army. The following year he developed a debilitating polyneuritis. He returned to Boston in February 1919. Thirteen years later on September 1, 1932 Cushing retired from the Brigham and Harvard. Without a doubt these were the most productive years of his life.

During this short period of 13 years Harvey Cushing taught the general medical profession how to recognize the possibility that their patients might be suffering from brain tumors. He taught the neurosurgeons of the world how to operate upon brain tumors without the terrifying surgical mortality of those who had gone before him. He had reduced the operative mortality from the 65 percent of many of his predecessors to an unbelievable 10 percent. He and his pupil, Kenneth McKenzie, invented the silver clip for the control of bleeding vessels within the brain. He and Professor W. T. Bovie, a physicist, had invented the equipment and demonstrated the usefulness of electrocautery for controlling bleeding and removing brain tumors. He had proposed the development of a National Institute of Neurology in Washington, D.C. Although his suggestion did not bear fruit until almost 35 years later, it does indicate his wisdom and interest in promoting neurological and neurosurgical research. He wrote *The Life of Sir William Osler*, probably Cushing's greatest literary accomplishment. He initiated the organization of the Society of Neurological Surgeons, the first such organization in the world.

Having begun with such men as Walter Dandy, Howard Naffziger, Charles Bagley, Jr., Carl Rand, E. B. Towne, and Gilbert Horrax, he now proceeded to extend the list. Those who were trained by Cushing after World War I included Percival Bailey, Howard Fleming, Charles E. Locke, Paul Martin of Belgium, Kenneth G. McKenzie of Canada, Dimitri Bagdazar of Romania, Tracy Putnam, W. P. Van Wagenen, Norman M. Dott of Scotland, George Armitage of England, Loyal Davis, Carl F. List, Leo M. Davidoff, Hugh W. B. Cairns of England, Robert A. Groff, Louise Eisenhardt, John F. Fulton, Franc D. Ingraham, John E. Scarff, Frederic Schreiber, Richard C. Buckley, Eric Oldberg, Richard H. Meagher, Thomas I. Hoen, William deG. Mahoney, Bronson Ray, and Richard U. Light. There were also neurologists who sought to learn from Cushing. Their numbers included Charles P. Symonds of London, Frederic Brémer of Belgium, and Georges Schaltenbrand of Germany. There were others, too, who spent variable periods of time in his clinic and laboratory. What is truly striking about this list is not only that these people benefited so tremendously from their work with Cushing and returned to their homes to become the leaders in neurosurgery and neurology, but that Cushing exerted this influence in such a short time. With the exception of Horrax and Bailey, almost none of these people spent more than a year with Cushing, and many were in Boston for much shorter periods. Only a really great person could have had such a profound influence so quickly.

Cushing was a meticulous surgeon. Loyal to his training with Halsted, he handled tissues with great care. He was a slow operator, sometimes unbelievably so. He could be a most demanding, unreasonable, and irritating man. He was also extremely gracious when he wished to be. There are many stories illustrating the many facets of his character and behavior but there is no space in which to relate them here.

Walter Dandy (1886–1946)

Walter Dandy was in many ways similar to Cushing and in many others vastly different. There was one fundamental difference in the goals each of these men set for themselves. Cushing was determined to lower the surgical and postoperative mortality. As a result he was often less aggressive in attempting a total removal of the tumors upon which he operated than he might have been. Dandy, on the other hand, was determined to try to cure the patient of the tumor even though the aggressive surgical treatment that was necessary carried with it a higher risk. This difference is well indicated by the approach of these two surgeons toward acoustic neuromas. Cushing's operative mortality of 10 percent or less is well documented. Dandy's operative mortality is

more difficult to assess. However, a number of years ago a young neurological surgeon from Europe visited Max Peet's clinic in Ann Arbor, Michigan, Percival Bailey's at the University of Chicago, and Dandy's. He spent several months in each place and during his stay kept records of the patients operated upon and the results. The actual figures during these relative brief visits are of no significance except that Dandy's postoperative mortality during that time was considerably higher than either Peet's or Bailey's. It must be recognized that Dandy took the position that if brain tumors were not completely removed they were ultimately going to kill the patient and thus a higher risk was justified.

Walter E. Dandy was born in Sedalia, Missouri.[1,5,6] His parents had both immigrated from England only 2 years before. Dandy's father was a railroad engineer on the Missouri-Kansas-Texas Railroad. He was obviously very good at his job as he was the engineer on the railroad's crack passenger train. Dandy enrolled at the University of Missouri, where he was elected to both Phi Beta Kappa and Sigma Xi. At Missouri he attracted the attention of Professor W. C. Curtis of the department of zoology and Professor George Lefevre of the department of biology. He did additional work with these men, and they advised him to go to the Johns Hopkins Medical School for his professional education. He entered there in 1907. While at Missouri Dandy was selected for a Rhodes scholarship but did not accept it because of his desire to get on with his medical education. At the Hopkins he was admitted to the sophomore class because of the excellence of his work at Missouri. He attracted the attention of Professor Halsted during his years as a medical student, and upon graduation was offered a position on Halsted's house staff. The first year of that training was spent in the surgical research laboratory, and it was here that he had his first encounter with Harvey Cushing. Clashes between the two men continued on into the next year when Dandy became a member of the house staff. When Cushing left Hopkins for the Brigham in Boston, Dandy was sorely disappointed that Cushing did not invite him to go along. In retrospect this was probably very fortunate. Obviously the personalities of the two men would have ensured continuing clashes, and Cushing, being the chief, would probably have severely limited Dandy in his research and in his clinical work. As Campbell has said, their personalities were such that conflict was inevitable.

Dandy's contributions to neurological surgery are numerous and of great importance. They began with his study under the embryologist and anatomist, Mall, of a 2-mm human embryo. This work was the basis for his master's degree. Soon after beginning his surgical training, he began his work on hydrocephalus with Dr. Kenneth Blackfan. This work provided, for the first time, an anatomical understanding of hydrocephalus and its causes. Out of this work on hydrocephalus came one of Dandy's greatest contributions, the discovery of ventriculography and soon thereafter of pneumoencephalography. These two contributions were the first real breakthroughs in the accurate diagnosis and localization of brain tumors. Until then such diagnoses were dependent upon the often limited and at times inaccurate neurological manifestations of these tumors and the little help that x-ray studies of the skull could provide. Further contributions followed in rapid succession. The complete removal of acoustic neuromas, previously regarded as impossible, has now become the standard neurosurgical procedure. Then came the approach to the trigeminal nerve at its origin from the pons in the posterior fossa and shortly thereafter the section of the glossopharyngeal nerve, section of the eighth cranial nerve for Ménière's disease, removal of intraventricular tumors, surgical treatment of intracranial aneurysms, and the transcranial removal of orbital tumors. Dandy wrote many scientific papers. Probably his most valuable and best known surgical literary contribution was his section in Lewis's *Practice of Surgery* entitled "The Brain" in which he dealt with many aspects of brain surgery. For many years, and even today to some extent, this was the neurosurgeon's "bible."

Dandy's residents regarded him highly as a technical surgeon. Rizzoli, one of his trainees, classifies him as a "superb and dexterous technician." This was not my impression. Dandy was not the careful, meticulous technician that Cushing was. His removal of cerebral gliomas was often a massive extirpation with his finger and the prompt filling of the resulting cavity with a mass of cotton soaked in relatively hot saline to control the bleeding.

It also always seemed to me that Dandy suffered from an inferiority complex. I know that this is not the general impression, but how else does one explain his reluctance to have other neurosurgeons observe him operating. Both Glen Spurling and I had similar experiences at different times. We each went to Baltimore and called Dr. Dandy on the telephone and said that we would like to come to the Hopkins and watch him operate. Spurling was told that he was very sorry but that he was just taking off for a consultation in Virginia. I was also told that he was very sorry but that he did not have any cases on for operation that morning. Both

Spurling and I went to the hospital to visit other friends. On each occasion we found that he was actually in the operating room performing operations. My friend, Frank Walsh, said that Dandy was operating upon two of his patients and that we should go and watch him. So far as that experience is concerned I found him to be a less than expert diagnostician. Both patients were thought to be harboring cerebellar tumors. The signs of cerebellar involvement were minimal. The ventriculograms that were on the view-box showed minimal dilatation of the ventricular system. Not surprisingly the operations disclosed no evidence of tumors.

Obviously these examples are single experiences of two other neurosurgeons. They do not detract from the fact that Dandy was a great man, a great investigator and innovator who made outstanding contributions to neurological surgery.

References

1. Campbell E: Walter E. Dandy, surgeon:1886–1946. J Neurosurg 8:249–262, 1951.
2. Fox WL: The Cushing-Dandy controversy. Surg Neurol 3:61–66, 1975.
3. Fulton, JF: *Harvey Cushing: A Biography*. Springfield, Ill, Charles C Thomas, 1946.
4. Harvey Cushing Society: *A Bibliography of the Writings of Harvey Cushing: Prepared on the Occasion of his Seventieth Birthday, April 8, 1939*. Springfield, Ill, Charles C Thomas, 1939.
5. Rizzoli HV: Walter E. Dandy, 1886–1946. Surg Neurol 2:293–294, 1974.
6. Woodhall B: Neurosurgery in the past: The Dandy era. Clin Neurosurg 18:1–15, 1971.

3
History of Microneurosurgery
R. M. Peardon Donaghy

The history of surgery is brief if viewed against the human experience, but it is longer than a history of neurosurgery, which in turn far exceeds in length a history of microneurosurgery. Presented here is a partial listing of events more or less in order of their happening. No claim is made that these

events were more important than others not even mentioned.

It is not difficult to see why surgery itself was not commonly practiced for hundreds of years, for it had to await the passing of attitudes that prohibited the acquisition of knowledge of human anatomy and physiology, and it had to await the arrival of a period of investigation as well as an age of antisepsis. Once surgery arrived, it is also logical that microsurgery would remain a long way off, for there was far too much to learn about what one could readily see to worry about what was needed to work upon a structure so small as to require magnification. It is not so easy to understand why more than half a century elapsed between the introduction of magnification to surgery (in the field of ophthalmology) and its incorporation into neurosurgery, where the surgeon so often must deal with fine fragile structures at great depths—a situation for which the principle of magnification seems so admirably suited.

The term *microsurgery* was used as early as 1892, but then it referred to the study of neurological pathways in amphibia. In these studies the neural crest was removed just after closure of the neural tube, thus eliminating the development of spinal ganglia, dorsal roots, and sensory components of the spinal nerves and sheath cells.[24] It was surgical to be sure, but destructive.

It would seem that when microsurgery did appear in neurosurgery, it was not because of foresight and planning by someone who had come to the conclusion that the lack of sufficient visual acuity was one handicap of the neurosurgeon that could be at least partially overcome by finding a new instrument based on the use of magnification. Rather, chance played a major part: Lougheed and Tom[17] began work with a microscope in the mid 1950s in response to their feeling that they were "missing something," i.e., failing to satisfactorily note and follow changes in structure, in their attempts to study the effects of subarachnoid blood on vessels at the circle of Willis (Fig. 3-1). Someone suggested the use of a microscope, and one trial led to its use thereafter.

Also in the mid 1950s, Leonard Malis found the microscope helpful in his experiments on the cerebral cortex of cats at the Mount Sinai Hospital in New York City. His objective was to scarify the cerebral cortex and then correct matters by resecting the scar. Malis found that surgical trauma to the cortex could be lessened by using a microscope to identify small bands of tissue adherent to the cortical vessels. (Incidentally, along the way he experienced enough difficulty with bleeding to warrant a search for a method of improved hemostasis. He found such an instrument in the bipolar coagulator developed by James Greenwood.[7] This instrument he modified into the Malis bipolar coagulator, which has been responsible for so much of benefit to microneurosurgeons and their patients.)

Again in the 1950s, Theodore Kurze, of the University of Southern California, became interested in attempting to develop an improved route for operating upon difficult acoustic neuromas (Fig. 3-2). He and William House, his collaborator at that time, recognized the surgical microscope as an important instrument in such surgery, in which it was nec-

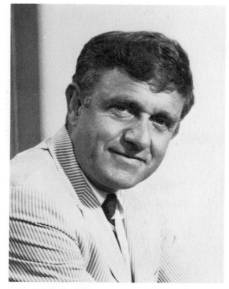

Figure 3-2 Theodore Kurze of Los Angeles, who performed a craniotomy in 1957 using the operating microscope, probably the first clinical microneurosurgical procedure.

essary to see small, fragile structures in difficult-to-illuminate corners or canals. They came to rely on the microscope regardless of the route traversed or the location or size of the tumor. Robert Rand has said that Kurze performed a craniotomy under the microscope on a human being in 1957, probably the first clinical microsurgical experience by a neurosurgeon (personal communication).

Use of the surgical microscope at the University of Vermont took hold as a result of frustration experienced in dealing with a case of embolus in 1959. A patient on the neurosurgical service suffered an embolus to the right middle cerebral artery following an open carotid angiogram. Embolectomy was considered but dismissed because of lack of neurovascular experience on the part of the neurosurgical staff and because the only reference to such a procedure in the literature was to two such operations by Keasley Welch[29] of the University of Colorado, who in 1955 had performed two embolectomies without the aid of a microscope. In neither case was patency maintained. It was later learned that David Scheibert performed an embolectomy of the middle cerebral artery in 1959 without the aid of a microscope and the vessel remained patent until the patient's death from coronary thrombosis several months later. The frustration experienced in this situation led to the beginning of microneurovascular research in the Neurosurgical Laboratory at the University of Vermont. Within a matter of days from the opening of this section of the laboratory, Julius Jacobson of the vascular service at that institution, who with Suarez was to publish in 1960 the tremendously influential paper "Microsurgery in Anastomosis of Small Vessels" in *Surgical Forum*,[11] suggested the use of the surgical microscope to the neurosurgeons. Once used, it became indispensable and was the centerpiece of instrument development at that institution thereafter (Fig. 3-3).

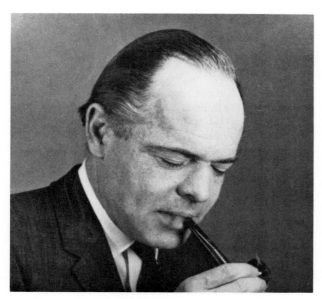

Figure 3-1 William Lougheed of Toronto, who used the operating microscope in his laboratory in the mid 1950s for the study of subarachnoid hemorrhage.

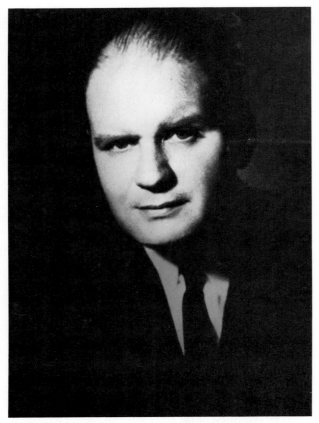

Figure 3-3 Julius Jacobson, pioneer vascular surgeon, who suggested the operating microscope for vascular anastomosis to neurosurgeons at the University of Vermont in 1959.

Treatment of Cerebrovascular Occlusive Disease

Indirect Approach

The history of attacks upon occlusive cerebrovascular disease by an indirect approach is interesting because of the early work on such procedures.

In 1939 in a laboratory at Yale University, William German and Max Taffel laid temporal muscle upon the cerebral hemisphere of dogs.[3] They noted the formation of new vessels passing over adhesions that developed between the temporal muscle and the cortex. In 1941, German and Taffel placed occipital muscle on the cerebellum of dogs for the same purpose and succeeded in demonstrating the development of new blood supply.[4] In 1942, Kredel[15] operated on three patients and performed temporal muscle–to–temporal cortex interface, and in 1950, Henschen[9] reported his work on temporal muscle–to–temporal cortex attachment. Although the microscope was not used in any of these procedures, they were precursors to later attempts at revascularization of the brain.

The direct application of temporal muscle to the cerebral cortex has been essentially abandoned because of the high incidence of postoperative seizures. The cerebellum–

occipital muscle interface was revived at the University of Vermont in 1980 for a case of vascular insufficiency of the posterior fossa with poor perfusion of the middle fossa and multiple evidences of small vessel disease throughout the posterior fossa without angiographic demonstration of any vessel that could receive the occipital artery.

In 1973, Goldsmith et al.[6] placed omentum with its vascular supply intact upon the cerebral cortex of dogs and reported the development of vascular channels to the cortex. Yasargil et al.[32] placed autogenous omentum that had its vascular pedicle anastomosed to the superficial temporal artery and vein on the cerebral cortex of dogs in 1974, and in 1978 Goldsmith[5] reported the first operation on a human being in which omentum with its original vascular base intact was laid upon the cerebral cortex in an effort to create a new cerebral blood supply. The omentum–cerebral cortex interface procedure is one of the later developments in the field of indirect cerebral revascularization and is still being investigated actively.

Direct Approach

The first microvascular neurosurgical procedure in a human was a middle cerebral artery embolectomy, which was done August 4, 1960, at the University of Vermont. The vessel exposure was performed by neurosurgeons, and the embolectomy under the microscope was performed by Jacobson.[12] Patency was not re-established except in a single branch of the middle cerebral artery. Eight other embolectomies or endarterectomies were performed in the next 6 years with two successes. Both of these patients had been the only ones operated upon within 4 h of onset. Neither of these cases was totally successful since one patient had a branch that did not refill and the other patient died subsequently as a complication of a follow-up angiogram. The first totally successful case of embolectomy of this type was recorded by Shelley Chou of the University of Minnesota in 1963.[1]

Revascularization via Vascular Grafts

Woringer and Kunlin[30] in 1963 sutured a saphenous vein graft between the internal carotid artery in the neck and the supraclinoid carotid artery and found the graft remained open at the time of the patient's death from coronary artery disease a few days after surgery. Lougheed et al.[16] successfully performed this procedure in 1970, and in this case the graft remained patent for 9 months. Charles Neblett of Houston, Texas, attained a patency rate of 50 percent over 12 months in a series of 22 patients (personal communication). Many others have had some experience with the procedure, but no one has acquired a series that is sufficiently large to be truly significant.

Revascularization via Extracranial-Intracranial Anastomosis

In 1965, M. Gazi Yasargil of the University of Zürich performed an anastomosis between the superficial temporal artery and a branch of the middle cerebral artery in a dog at the Microsurgical Laboratory at the University of Vermont (Fig. 3-4). The anastomosis remained patent, as did anastomoses in a series of such procedures. An end-to-side anastomosis was deemed proper because one could introduce a blood supply into both the proximal and distal segments of the recipient vessel if the circulation pressure was favorable in the donor supply.

The first clinical application of this procedure, the so-called extracranial-intracranial blood flow diversion, or EC-IC, was performed by Yasargil in Zürich on October 30, 1967. The second such procedure was performed at the University of Vermont on October 31, 1967. In both cases the anastomosis remained patent. The procedure has since been adapted to a variety of situations by a number of surgeons. At first it was performed only in cases of vascular insufficiency caused by atherosclerosis, but it has since been used to replace the blood supply in a vessel inadvertently damaged at the time of an operation and has been applied by Sidney Peerless of the University of Western Ontario to provide a blood supply to an essential vessel beyond a giant aneurysm, thus preserving blood flow in the essential vessel while allowing for occlusion of the aneurysm. Currently, patency rates for the procedure are reported at 80 to 90 percent.

Microvascular Neurosurgery to Prevent Potential Hemorrhage

Aneurysms

Although procedures directed toward the restoration of blood flow in an occluded or stenotic vessel were used relatively early in microvascular surgery, microsurgeons were not unmindful of the promise of better visibility in defining the base of a fragile aneurysm, and they foresaw an improvement in complication rates if important branches at the aneurysm site could be dissected free and preserved.

Pool and Colton in 1966 published their experience with the use of the microscope in aneurysm surgery.[22] Robert Rand[23] of the University of California at Los Angeles operated upon an aneurysm under the microscope in 1964 but did not publish a report of this case until 1967 (Fig 3-5). Adams and Witt gave a paper on intracranial aneurysm surgery in 1964 in which the use of the microscope was included. Charles Drake[2] of the University of Western Ontario published his experience on aneurysms of the posterior fossa in 1965 and has continued to carefully document his consistently enlarging successful series since that time.

Arteriovenous Malformations and Communications

In 1965, Yasargil was invited by Robert Rand to visit Los Angeles and join in an operation on a patient with an arteriovenous angioma in the spinal canal involving the spinal cord (personal communication). This procedure was performed with the aid of a surgical microscope and a Malis bipolar coagulator. These instruments so increased the ease of the

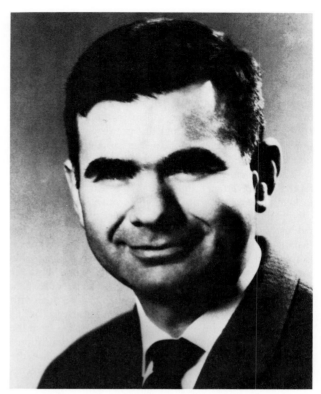

Figure 3-4 M. Gazi Yasargil of Zürich, microsurgeon of wide experience, who performed the first EC-IC procedure on a human being, on October 30, 1967.

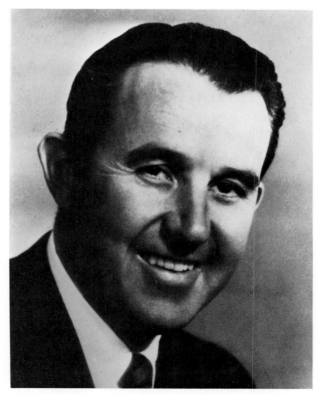

Figure 3-5 Robert Rand of Los Angeles, an early writer on microneurosurgical techniques.

operation that they still are regarded as essential to any surgical attack on an arteriovenous malformation of the spinal cord.

A large number of microsurgeons from Europe, Japan, and the Americas have made contributions to the techniques for treating intracranial malformations. These include surgeons such as Yasargil, Feindel, and Malis. The last named microsurgeon has presented a plan for following a venous structure back to its origin at the arteriovenous malformation, a technique that has helped in certain difficult situations.

The problem of an arteriovenous communication at the level of the cavernous sinus (usually post-traumatic) was attacked in the early part of the 1930s by ligation of the cervical carotid artery. More recently embolization via the internal carotid artery with skeletal muscle was considered, (Mixter W J: Personal communication), and later embolization with a number of other materials such as absorbable gelatin sponge and plastic have been tried.[18] The blindness of the procedure, however, has severely limited its use. Closure of the arteriovenous communication has been done with the use of balloon-carrying catheters from the arterial side as reported by Serbinenko[28] of the Soviet Union, and from the venous side by Mullan,[20] Wright (personal communication), and others. None of these procedures, however, requires the use of the microscope. Again, however, they were precursors to the approach described by Dwight Parkinson in which the sinus is directly opened and the arterial rent is closed directly.[21] This was done by Parkinson under conditions of cardiac arrest in order to control bleeding during the opening of the sinus. Dolenc in Yugoslavia has now per-

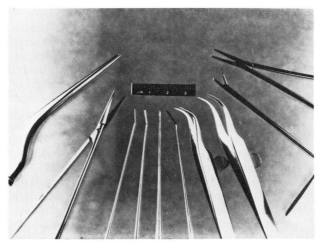

Figure 3-7   Early microsurgical instruments, 1959.

formed this procedure using the direct approach with microsurgical technique by interrupting the carotid supply intracranially during the procedure, thus making cardiac arrest unnecessary.

Peripheral Nerve Surgery

For some reason, not many neurosurgeons have played a great role in the development of microsurgical technique in peripheral nerve surgery, even though Chaffee and Numoto in 1964 (personal communication) were able to demonstrate a more complete return of motor units (as demonstrated by electromyography) in muscles innervated by the sciatic nerve in rats when the nerve was sutured under the microscope than when the nerve was sutured by naked eye. Madjid Samii[25,26] in Europe has been an outstanding exception and has beautifully demonstrated high recovery rates in small nerves meticulously sutured under the microscope.

The poor success rates noted in nerve grafting in World War I caused many neurosurgeons in World War II to pay scant attention to this technique. Samii's brilliant work in Europe and the work of David Kline[14] in America together with the research of many plastic and orthopedic surgeons have shown the importance of this technique, however. Much can be accomplished by grafting, especially in small nerves.

Facial nerve surgery has been an exception to the rule noted above, for here neurosurgeons have led the way in demonstrating innovative methods of repair, both intracranially and peripherally.

In 1967 Jannetta and Rand[13] pioneered work on compression of trigeminal nerve roots by vascular structures as a mechanism for the production of trigeminal neuralgia and have used microsurgical techniques to decompress the nerve. Jannetta has extended this work to include the treatment of hemifacial spasm and glossopharyngeal neuralgia. At present, nearly all neurosurgery performed in proximity to the neurological structures of the posterior fossa is performed by microsurgical techniques.

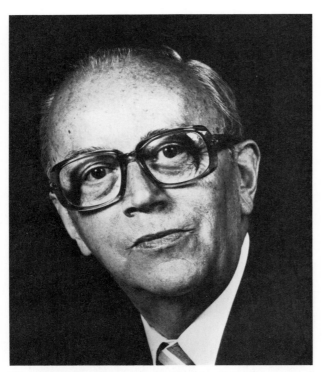

Figure 3-6   Dr. Hans Littmann of the Zeiss Company of Oberkochen, Germany, who is principally responsible for the development of the operating microscope.

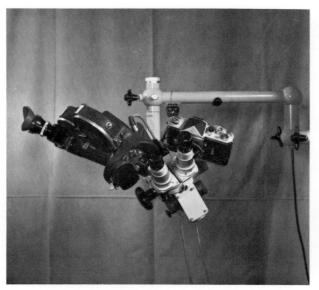

Figure 3-8 Operating microscope with Aireflex movie camera (left) and Nikon still camera (right), 1960.

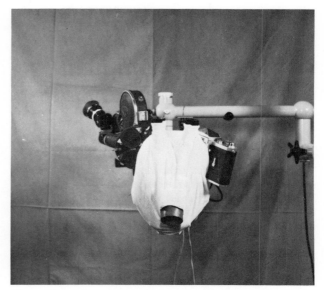

Figure 3-9 Operating microscope with first-generation drape, 1960.

Trans-sphenoidal Hypophysectomy

Oscar Hirsch,[10] an otorhinolaryngologist, developed his trans-septal approach to the pituitary fossa in 1910. Harvey Cushing considered this a superior approach in some situations, but was deterred from promoting it because of the high possibility of infection. Walter Dandy was uncomfortable with the limited operative field and the poor visibility. The trans-septal approach was revived by Gerard Guiot in Paris in 1958. It was Guiot's student, Jules Hardy[8] of Montreal, who conceived of the application of the surgical microscope in the approach. This he did in 1962. At first he used microsurgery for the introduction of yttrium 90, but the complications were unacceptable.

Much of the problem with the trans-sphenoidal approach had been the crudity of the available instruments. Hardy set about to revise the entire procedure, including the position of the patient, the position of the surgeon, instruments to match the operative situation, intraoperative x-ray monitoring of instrument position and the position of intraventricular air introduced by the usual techniques of pneumoencephalography, immediate inspection of the removed tissue, and reconstitution of the sphenoidal floor. He was eminently successful, and much of today's technique in this procedure stems from his innovative mind.

Instrumentation (Figs. 3-6 to 3-10)

The advent of microneurosurgery necessitated a review of instrumentation. First, of course, the microscope itself required adaptation to the requirements of neurosurgery: improved illumination, versatility in maneuverability so that the microscope could be set up for surgery in several

positions (posterior fossa, anterior fossa, spine, etc.). Hans Littman of the Carl Zeiss Company of Oberkochen, Germany, dedicated himself to the task and, more than anyone, has been responsible for the marked improvements of the microscope. More sophisticated microscopes have now been developed, such as that used by Yasargil, which has a freely movable head that is so neatly balanced as to follow the pressure of the lips, or that of the ophthalmologist John Beale, which consists of a microscope and attached chair so that the microscope and surgeon move as one unit into almost any position. These are but a beginning.

From the very beginning of microneurosurgery new instruments have been developed yearly. A large number of surgeons have played a role in this process. Yasargil, Rhoton, Maroon, Hardy, and a host of others have added

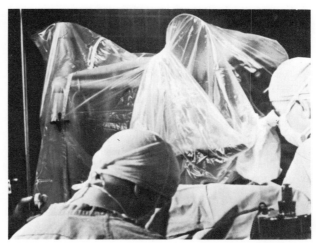

Figure 3-10 Operating microscope with third-generation drape, 1967.

one, two, or a dozen instruments to the armamentarium to perform a task better. It is certain, however, that the most important instruments in the development of microneurosurgery have been the minds of microscopists, surgeons, and surgical neurologists. Time has reserved for herself the final decision as to importance, and time has a way of being right.

Laser

The laser (acronym for *light amplification by stimulated emission of radiation*) was introduced by Maiman in 1960.[19] He developed the ruby laser, which first found application in ophthalmological problems such as retinal photocoagulation. In neurosurgery the laser most commonly used has been the CO_2 laser, which can be accurately aimed at abnormal tissue by visual guidance through the microscope and, if need be, effectively aimed by micromanipulative technique.[27] The CO_2 laser has found its early use in the surgical excision of a variety of benign and malignant brain and cord tumors. The neodymium-YAG laser has been used experimentally in performing vascular coagulative surgery in vessel anastomosis.[31]

References

1. Chou SN: Embolectomy of the middle cerebral artery: Report of a case. J Neurosurg 20:161–163, 1963.
2. Drake CG: Surgical treatment of ruptured aneurysms of the basilar artery: Experience with 14 cases. J Neurosurg 23:457–473, 1965.
3. German WJ, Taffel M: Surgical production of collateral intracranial circulation: An experimental study. Proc Soc Exp Biol Med 42:349–353, 1939.
4. German WJ, Taffel M: Surgical production of collateral intracranial circulation: An experimental study. Yale J Biol Med 13:451–459, 1941.
5. Goldsmith HS: Omental transposition to human brain (Letter to the editor). Stroke 9:272, 1978.
6. Goldsmith HS, Chen WF, Duckett SW: Brain vascularization by intact omentum. Arch Surg 106:695–698, 1973.
7. Greenwood J Jr: Two point coagulation: A new principle and instrument for applying coagulation current in neurosurgery. Am J Surg 50:267–270, 1940.
8. Hardy J, Provost J: Microneurochirurgie. Union Med Can 98:187–196, 1969.
9. Henschen C: Operative Revaskularization des zirkulatorisch geschädigten Gehirns durch Auflage gestielter Muskellappen (Encephalo-myo-synangiose). Langenbecks Arch Chir 264:392–401, 1950.
10. Hirsch O: Über Hypophysentumoren und deren Behandlung. Klin Monatsbl Augenheilkd 85:609–640, 1930.
11. Jacobson JH II, Suarez EL: Microsurgery in anastomosis of small vessels. Surg Forum 11:243–245, 1960.
12. Jacobson JH II, Wallman LJ, Schumacher GA, Flanagan M, Suarez EL, Donaghy RMP: Microsurgery as an aid to middle cerebral artery endarterectomy. J Neurosurg 19:108–115, 1962.
13. Jannetta PJ, Rand RW: Vascular compression of the trigeminal nerve at the pons in patients with trigeminal neuralgia, in Donaghy RMP, Yasargil MG (eds): *Micro-Vascular Surgery*. Stuttgart, Georg Thieme Verlag, 1967, p 150.
14. Kline DG, Hudson AR, Bratton BR: Experimental study of fascicular nerve repair with and without epineurial closure. J Neurosurg 54:513–520, 1981.
15. Kredel FE: Collateral cerebral circulation by muscle graft: Technic of operation with report of 3 cases. South Surg 11:235–244, 1942.
16. Lougheed WM, Marshall BM, Hunter M, Michel ER, Sandwith-Smyth H: Common carotid to intracranial internal carotid bypass venous graft: Technical note. J Neurosurg 34:114–118, 1971.
17. Lougheed WM, Tom M: A method of introducing blood into the subarachnoid space in the region of the circle of Willis in dogs. Can J Surg 4:329–337, 1961.
18. Luessenhop AJ, Spence WT: Artificial embolization of cerebral arteries: Report of use in a case of arteriovenous malformation. JAMA 172:1153, 1960.
19. Maiman TH: Stimulated optical radiation in ruby. Nature 187:493–494, 1960.
20. Mullan S: Treatment of carotid-cavernous fistulas by cavernous sinus occlusion. J Neurosurg 50:131–144, 1979.
21. Parkinson D: Carotid cavernous fistula: Direct repair with preservation of the carotid artery: Technical note. J Neurosurg 38:99–106, 1973.
22. Pool JL, Colton RP: The dissecting microscope for intracranial vascular surgery. J Neurosurg 25:315–318, 1966.
23. Rand RW, Jannetta PJ: Microneurosurgery for aneurysms of the vertebral-basilar artery system. J Neurosurg 27:330–335, 1967.
24. Rudnick D: Ross Harrison (1870–1959), in Haymaker W, Schiller F (eds): *The Founders of Neurology*, 2d ed, Springfield, Ill, Charles C Thomas, 1970, pp 123–128.
25. Samii M: Die operative Wiederherstellung verletzter Nerven. Langenbecks Arch Chir 332:355–362, 1972.
26. Samii M, Wallenborn R: Tierexperimentelle Untersuchungen über den Einfluss der Spannung auf den Regenerationserfolg nach Nervennaht. Acta Neurochir (Wien) 27:87–110, 1972.
27. Saunders ML, Young HF, Becker DP, Greenberg RP, Newlon PG, Corales RL, Ham WT, Povlishock JT: The use of the laser in neurological surgery. Surg Neurol 14:1–10, 1980.
28. Serbinenko FA: Balloon catheterization and occlusion of major cerebral vessels. J Neurosurg 41:125–145, 1974.
29. Welch K: Excision of occlusive lesions of the middle cerebral artery. J Neurosurg 13:73–80, 1956.
30. Woringer E, Kunlin J: Anastomose entre le carotide primitive et la carotide intra-cranienne ou la sylvienne par greffon selon la technique de la suture suspendue. Neurochirurgie 9:181–188, 1963.
31. Yahr WZ, Strully KJ, Hurwitt ES: Non-occlusive small arterial anastomosis with a neodymium laser. Surg Forum 15:224–226, 1964.
32. Yasargil MG, Yonekawa Y, Denton I, Piroth D, Benes I: Experimental intracranial transplantation of autogenic omentum majus. J Neurosurg 40:213–217, 1974.

Part II

Clinical Examination of the Nervous System and Correlative Neuroanatomy

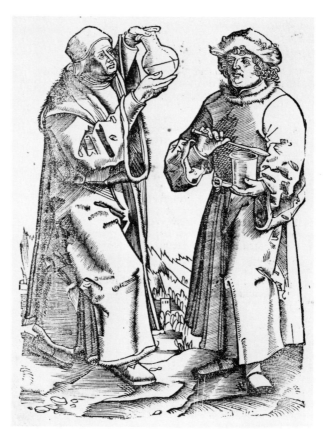

von Gersdorff H. *Feldtbuch der Wundartzney*. Strassbourg, J Schott, 1517. St. Cosmas and St. Damian, patron saints of the physician and apothecary. The illustration comes from the title page of the first book to illustrate operative procedures. St. Cosmas is shown carrying out the ancient diagnostic procedure of uroscopy.

4

The Art of History Taking

Barrie J. Hurwitz

The correct diagnosis of neurological disease is dependent upon an accurate interpretation of the patient's symptoms as well as the physical findings. At the conclusion of a detailed and relevant history taking, the neurosurgical consultant should have a good working diagnosis in mind. An accurate description of the patient's symptoms should point the examiner toward the appropriate site of the pathological process. The mode of occurrence and progression of symptoms should suggest the possible underlying etiology. Subsequent physical examination will often establish the anatomical area of disease and allow the physician to further evaluate the disease process by appropriate procedures such as computed tomography, electrodiagnostic studies, a myelogram, or an arteriogram. An inaccurate or inadequate history will result not only in misuse of the physician's and patient's time, but may result in the patient being subjected to an unnecessary array of expensive and, in some cases, potentially hazardous procedures. In addition, this could lead to a wrong diagnosis and incorrect treatment.

The first step in arriving at a diagnosis is thus the orderly gathering of a detailed history. The experienced physician soon realizes that an accurate history is of paramount importance. While the neurological history usually does not differ from the general medical history, it may in many cases be more difficult to obtain. An alert, intelligent patient will often relate the history in a clear and coherent manner, but many neurological conditions may result in alterations of mood and mental status, which may significantly impair the patient's ability to relate symptomatology accurately and coherently. In such situations, the physician often has to rely on a corroborating history from relatives, friends, referring physicians, or neighbors. A conscientious physician would not hesitate to contact any such person for supporting information.

Eliciting the history is a very personal matter for the patient. The conduct of the examiner, including demeanor, mood, behavior, and even dress, may have a profound influence on the patient's behavior during this interview. It may significantly alter the way in which a patient gives the history as well as its content. One patient may give a lucid, flowing history; another may seem quite unable to give any coherent account of what seems to be wrong. It is important to recognize that such a patient may not appreciate the need

for accurate information, but may feel that if only the doctor can be impressed with the urgency of the distress, he or she will be able to get relief for it—hence the patient's evasiveness. In such a situation the manner of questioning may make a significant difference to a nervous, suspicious, or very apprehensive patient. The physician must therefore encourage, reassure, and instill confidence in the patient. This implies a friendly, sympathetic, and reassuring approach from the beginning of the patient-physician encounter.

It is important to avoid leading questions, as these in themselves may suggest symptoms to the patient that the examiner in turn may expect to find. This is particularly true of suggestible patients who often present very circumstantial accounts of their symptoms. Such a patient can often be led back to the subject by intermittent, pertinent questions. It is important to avoid asking the same question twice, because this may convey an impression to the patient that the physician is not very attentive. It may be important, however, to have the patient repeat certain aspects of the history. In this situation, a word of explanation to the patient as to why it is important to go over this aspect of the history again is useful, if only to reassure the patient that the physician has been listening to the previous account.

All symptoms are not of equal importance. There is usually one symptom that troubles the patient more than any other, and it is around this chief complaint that the patient usually focuses the history. Special attention should always be given to this symptom. As the history proceeds, one may have to ask for corroborating symptoms in relation to the chief complaint that the patient may have failed to mention, and in this regard the physician should employ great skill in the choice of words in these leading questions. This art comes with experience, and an open-ended question is frequently of value at this point.

The mode of onset of the symptoms and their progression is of great importance. One should attempt to define the patient's symptoms in relation to the date and time of onset in a sequential manner. The locality and spread of the symptom together with its character, intensity, and severity helps further in defining the problem. There are frequently aggravating or relieving factors, and the effects of previous treatments should be noted.

Perhaps the most important aspect of the history taking, however, is clarification of the symptoms themselves. The physician must be absolutely certain that he or she understands the terminology used by the patient in describing the symptoms. Apart from colloquialisms that may be peculiar to certain geographic areas, the patient's understanding of common medical terms such as dizziness, seizures, or blackouts may be totally different from current medical usage of these terms. One frequently has to explain this to the patient with an example in order to obtain clarification of these frequently misleading terms. Thus, although the patient should be allowed to relate the history in his or her own words, at some point the patient must be made to be precise about the nature and duration of these symptoms. In addition, one should never be satisfied with generalizations or vague terminology. This is of particular importance when one is dealing with pain as a symptom. Sensory symptoms (and this includes pain) are subjective, and the patient's description of them may vary according to past experience or cultural background as well as the nature of accompanying symptoms. The words used may in fact amplify the patient's reaction to the pain or sensory dysfunction rather than truly categorize the pain with appropriate descriptors of radiation or aggravating and relieving factors. In this context, mistakes in history taking are as frequently the fault of the physician as of the patient. Besides an accurate account of the symptoms, immediate recording of the history at the bedside will tend to decrease any mistakes on the part of the physician.

Mechanics of the Interview

After the introduction, the physician should ask a few general questions to set the patient at ease and provide useful background information. Such questions include the patient's age, address, occupation, and marital status. The patient's handedness is vitally important to the neurosurgeon and should be established early in the interview. The patient should then be allowed to relate the symptomatology with particular emphasis being maintained on the chief complaint. Its mode of onset, duration, and progression should be elicited in detail. The location and associated symptomatology together with precipitating or relieving factors need to be inquired after. Once the patient has narrated his or her story, the experienced clinician learns to probe in order to clarify the symptoms according to the patient's description. It is important in this regard to obtain a detailed history of the progression and accompaniments of the chief complaint together with aggravating and relieving factors, the effect of any treatment, and any temporal relationship to occupation, activities, or time of day.

Once the main complaint has been evaluated in detail, a chronological notation of past illnesses and treatments and then a comprehensive neurological as well as general medical review of systems must be made. In this regard, general screening questions can be asked to cover all areas of nervous function. Inexperienced and overzealous examiners will sometimes ask detailed questions related to every area of function, which in turn will rapidly exhaust the patient, confuse the physician, and usually obscure any serious complaints that may be present in a mass of extraneous and irrelevant detail. On the other hand, the experienced clinician, in a brief period of time, can inquire about difficulties of thinking, memory, speech, and writing. Has the patient had a blackout, seizure, or head injury? Have headaches or pain occurred anywhere at any time? Alterations of smell, vision, hearing, facial sensation, and swallowing should be noted. Weakness, clumsiness, and sensory alterations in limbs together with any disturbance of gait should not be overlooked. Has the patient had any involuntary movements? Inquiry after bowel, bladder, and sexual function should not be left out because of embarrassment on the part of the examiner or patient. If the patient answers in the affirmative or has difficulties in any of these areas, the physician then proceeds with a detailed exploration of the characterization and accompaniments of these symptoms. It may be necessary to proceed here in as much detail as with the chief complaint, but this in turn will depend upon the nature of these symp-

toms and their possible relationship to the chief complaint. This neurological review of symptoms should be followed by a general medical review of illnesses and symptoms referrable to major organ systems in the body. Family history is most important because of the inherited nature of many neurological diseases. A history from a relative of the patient may be most useful at this part of the interview. Brief inquiry into the patient's social background, activities, and habits is frequently illuminating in terms of drug use or abuse as well as in the patient's psychological relationship to family, work, and friends.

Interpretation of Symptoms

The patient's symptoms are an expression of the pathophysiology, and the physician's interpretation of them is in turn dependent upon his or her knowledge of neuroanatomy, physiology, biochemistry, and pathological processes. A learned physician automatically keeps this in mind when inquiring after the characterization and mode of progression of the patient's symptoms. Although the characterizations of certain symptoms are definitive in and of themselves, this is not always immediately obvious. Such an example is the brief lancinating localized pain of trigeminal neuralgia. This may initially be erroneously described by the patient as being continuous, and it is only after careful inquiry as to the meaning of the patient's term "continuous" that the physician may in fact elicit that the pain is not actually continuous but is rapidly repetitive. Headache and pain are frequent and initially often difficult symptoms to the neurosurgical consultant, and characterization here is often not definitive. The associations will however frequently reveal the cause. Consider that while a severe tension headache may be as painful to the patient as that experienced with a subarachnoid hemorrhage, it is the abrupt onset of the latter or its association with a stiff neck or other focal neurological symptoms that will enable the astute clinician to arrive at a correct diagnosis prior to examination of the patient. The presence of premonitory presyncopal as opposed to focal neurological symptoms may frequently help the physician distinguish between a true syncope and a seizure disorder. With such a complaint of seizures or blackouts, the most pertinent information, however, is often obtained from firsthand observers of the episode rather than from the patient, who is often unaware of the exact evolution of the attack. To adequately elicit the history of a convulsive disorder as compared with vasovagal syncope, the physician must be familiar with the patterns and types of seizures and the findings of syncope. This knowledge is equally important in evaluating other neurological symptoms, as for example disorders of speech. In speech disorders the distinction between expressive aphasia and dysarthria is frequently not readily apparent to the patient or even to the observer of this symptom. A careful explanation of these differences to the patient at this point will frequently lead to immediate clarification. The object of a detailed history taking is therefore (1) to ascertain whether there is indeed a pathological process present, (2) to localize anatomically the pathological process, and (3) to consider the underlying etiologic possibilities.

Bizarre symptoms or unduly prolonged or multiple symptom complexes may suggest psychological dysfunction to the physician. This interpretation must be avoided. In this regard, first impressions are often invaluable, but if they are allowed to develop into instant diagnosis, this often leads to disaster. Many disease processes can present in an unusual fashion, and the patient's emotional demeanor should not unduly influence the physician in the interpretation of the symptoms at this point in the evaluation. Hysteria is not a diagnosis of exclusion, but should be based upon observed or recounted behavior that is in itself contradictory in terms of known pathophysiological principles. Malingering implies a conscious attempt to defraud, and such a diagnosis cannot be based on an unusual or disjointed history alone.

Last, it is necessary in certain instances, such as with the patient in coma and the patient in status epilepticus, to proceed with immediate examination and treatment. Even in these situations, though, one must not neglect to obtain a history. This may be obtained from relatives, friends, or authorities accompanying the patient or by a prompt telephone call to the patient's home or to neighbors, and may in turn obviate the need for numerous time-consuming and unrewarding investigations.

Recording the History

In all instances, a narrative record should be obtained. This is best obtained at the bedside and when complete should be critically studied by the physician. Jargon, which is frequently peculiar to one medical institution or another and which often changes with time, should be avoided at all costs. A coherent, well-organized narrative history is one that readily paints a clear picture of the problem to any other physician, health care professional, or intelligent layperson who reads the document. Although checklists can save time, they cannot document the subtleties of neurological symptoms that are so frequently essential to an accurate assessment of the patient's symptoms. The physician's interpretation of the symptom complex is important, but the recorded history should clearly identify the patient's symptoms from the physician's interpretation of them. Clarity of script should be pursued with the same detail as microvascular surgery.

The Examination and Beyond

It is important to realize that the neurological examination in fact starts at the beginning of history taking. The emotional state of the patient and any alteration in intellectual, hearing, and speech processes are readily apparent at this time, and the gait as well as mobility or lack of it can be studied during history taking. A movement disorder, such as parkinsonism, chorea, or athetosis, in fact is often best appreciated at this time. Severe skeletal deformities such as acromegaly or macrocrania should be looked for, and the unkempt dress and flattened affect of the depressed patient are frequently readily observable.

The history as well as the observations during the interview should enable the physician to direct and sequence subsequent examinations of the patient. Although every patient with neurological complaints should receive a detailed neurological examination, there are various degrees of detail to which the examination can be tailored. A patient with a history of low back pain radiating into one leg with accompanying foot weakness who gives a coherent concise history will require a detailed motor, sensory, and reflex examination of the lower limbs but will not require a detailed assessment of mental status. Likewise, a patient with a history of episodic speech disturbance with transient left monocular blindness will need a detailed assessment of mental status and speech together with careful assessment of cranial nerves, motor, and sensory systems and a detailed evaluation of the vascular system, but he would not need a detailed assessment of mechanical findings related to the lower back. Such tailoring of the examination is totally dependent upon the physician's ability to elicit a coherent and meaningful history as well as his or her understanding of the pathophysiology of the patient's symptom complex.

The young clinician must remember that a neurological diagnosis always takes time. The most important clues are always to be found in the history, which must be approached with confidence and precision. This part of the clinical encounter should therefore never be rushed.

5

Clinical Examination of Cognitive Functions

Samuel H. Greenblatt

The word *cognition* refers to the state or process of knowing. In its contemporary context, the term *higher cognitive functions* refers to those functions of the brain that require the conscious manipulation of knowledge, where "knowledge" is understood as mental content in the broad sense. Since the purpose of this chapter is to outline the clinical examination of these functions and the interpretation of their abnormalities, this presentation will be decidedly anatomical in orientation. This approach is consistent with the usual order in which the cognitive functions are examined and recorded in clinical practice. In general, the functions listed first in Table 5-1 are least well localized in the present state of the art, and those listed later are more clearly associated with specific cortical structures.

There are some important methodological points about the conduct and analysis of the mental status and language examination. The first is to determine and consider the patient's level of education and socioeconomic experience. The results of the examination must be interpreted in light of these factors. Second, one must accept the patient's best response as the most valid, because that is the only response against which repeat testing can be compared. Therefore, the examiner must make every reasonable effort to assure a proper environment for testing. The testing should be stopped if the patient becomes noticeably fatigued.

The final point relates to the technical aspects of the examiner's behavior. To avoid confused thinking and muddled results, one must keep one's modalities straight. In fact, there are two different kinds of modalities to keep in mind, the psychological and the physiological. *Psychological modalities* are those basic mental processes that are scientifically and clinically separable from each other, such as affect, attention, memory, and perception. For example, a test of short-term memory may be quite meaningless if the patient's attention span is inadequate. The clinically important *physiological modalities* are auditory, motor, tactile, and visual. These modalities of input and output are especially important in language testing, which usually involves audi-

TABLE 5-1 Clinical Examination of Cognitive Functions

I. General intellectual functions—not well localized
   A. Orientation: to person, place, and time
   B. Reasoning: insight, judgment, and abstraction
   C. General fund of knowledge
   D. Global attention
   E. Disorders of perception
      1. Generalized confusion, delirium
      2. Specific disorders: delusions, illusions, and hallucinations
II. Memory and affect—bilaterally mediated functions
   A. Memory: immediate recall, recent and remote memory
   B. Affect
III. Language and related functions—with lateralized localizations
   A. Cerebral dominance
   B. Auditory language
      1. General characteristics of normal and disordered speech
         a. Spontaneous speech: fluency
         b. Naming
         c. Repetition
         d. Comprehension
      2. Classical perisylvian aphasias
         a. Broca
         b. Conduction
         c. Wernicke
         d. Global
         e. Anomic
      3. Transcortical aphasias
      4. Thalamic aphasias
      5. Aprosodias
   C. Alexia and agraphia: disorders of written language
IV. Other lateralized or localized cognitive functions
   A. Dominant parietal functions: Gerstmann's syndrome
   B. Agnosias: auditory, visual, tactile
   C. Apraxias: ideational and ideomotor
   D. Neglect and denial syndromes

tory input and auditory response. But a nod of the head is a motor response. In many situations it may be necessary to use nonauditory modalities of input or output in order to get a response or to be sure that the given response is the best that the patient can do.

General Intellectual Functions

In the process of taking a history, the examiner acquires a wealth of information about the patient's general mental status and specific cognitive abilities or disabilities. This is especially true for those general intellectual functions that are not presently known to be well localized. However, casual conversation can be deceptive. Asking the patient for specific information allows repeatable assessment of the patient's general intellectual functions.

Orientation

It is traditional and useful to ask the patient about orientation in person, place, and time. In the absence of language impairment, an otherwise normal person should know (1) his or her own name, (2) location (address or name of institution and city), and (3) the day of the week, the month (or season), and the year, but not necessarily the exact date. In effect, knowledge of orientation may be a function of memory if nurses and other hospital personnel are constantly reinforcing this information for the patient.

Reasoning

It is not customary to test patients' reasoning abilities in the sense of pure socratic logic. Such testing would require the use of semantic relationships that are actually functions of educational level and/or language abilities. The following categories of reasoning require mental abilities that should be available to anyone who is in the normal range and not otherwise impaired:

1. **Insight** This is best evaluated by finding out if the patient understands the circumstances of the illness. "Why are you in the hospital?" is a good leading question. At a more sophisticated level, one can probe the patient's understanding of how the illness has affected his or her family or workplace relationships.
2. **Judgment** For clinical purposes, judgment implies the ability to make reasonable decisions in light of circumstances. Again, this ability can be tested in relation to the patient's illness. It can also be tested with such questions as, "If you smelled smoke in a movie theater, what would you do?"
3. **Abstraction** The ability to generalize the meaning of a specific statement is usually tested by asking the patient to interpret common proverbs, such as, "People who live in glass houses shouldn't throw stones." Asking about word similarities is another approach: "Are apples and oranges both fruits?"

General Fund of Knowledge

In our media-blitzed society, it is reasonable to assume that the average person has some knowledge of current affairs. This can be tested by asking the patient for the name of the President of the United States, the governor of the state, and a brief description of whatever events the national news broadcasts are covering at the time. Educational level and memory functions are important factors to consider in deciding about the meaning of the results.

Global Attention

There is increasingly strong evidence that attentional functions, as measured by the laboratory psychologist, are mediated in the parietal and (to a lesser extent) frontal lobes. Some of the clinical correlates of this information will be described at the end of this chapter under Neglect and Denial Syndromes. But it is still legitimate and useful to think about global attention as a generalized brain function. Decreasing attention span may be the first subtle sign of metabolic encephalopathy[32] or diffusely increased intracranial pressure. One can usually get a good initial impression of the patient's global attention span merely by observing his or her attentiveness to the other tasks in the examination. A semiquantitative assessment can be made at the bedside by asking the patient to do the serial 7s test, wherein the patient is told to subtract 7 from 100 and then to keep subtracting 7 from each result. In the absence of left (dominant) parietal damage, which can cause the specific syndrome of acalculia, this is really a test of attention span, not arithmetic ability. The mathematical accuracy of the final result is highly dependent on educational level. One can quantitate attention span by simply counting how many separate arithmetic operations the patient performs before his or her attention wanders, but this is legitimate only if prompting is avoided. To avoid practice effects, the patient can be asked to start at 101 or 99 on some occasions.

Disorders of Perception

In the process of examining general intellectual functions, the examiner may become aware that the patient is "confused" or "delirious." There is sufficient confusion about the term *confused* so that it probably should be dropped from the medical lexicon. The deplorable tendency is to apply the term to any patient who seems to be mentally aberrant. For example, many patients who actually have very specific aphasic syndromes have been described in chart notes as simply "confused." *Delirium*, on the other hand, has a more clearly defined meaning. It refers to a previously alert and coherent patient who becomes restless, agitated, fearful, depressed, labile, or any combination of the above.[32] A variety of cognitive deficits may be found in such patients, if they can be adequately examined, including disorientation, impaired reasoning, and poor attention span. Broadly speaking, the usual cause is either metabolic encephalopathy or sensory deprivation (e.g., the intensive care unit syndrome).

Among the specific phenomena observed in acutely delirious patients are delusions, illusions, and hallucinations. A *delusion* is a clearly false statement or belief that cannot be corrected by reason or evidence. An *illusion* is a misinterpretation of perfectly valid sensory data. An *hallucination* is an apparent perception of unreal sensory stimuli. Visual illusions and hallucinations are usually associated with cortical disorders, not with psychiatric disturbances.[20] Theoretically, visual illusions might masquerade as visual agnosias (see below), or vice versa, but the distinction can usually be made on the basis of the clinical context in which they occur.

Memory and Affect

It is a little artificial to say that memory and affective functions are bilaterally represented in the brain, because some types of amnesic and affective disorders are associated with unilateral lesions.[9,20] However, these disorders are usually specific to certain modalities or materials. At a more elementary level, reasonable practicality justifies the following brief presentation.

Disorders of Memory—the Amnesic Syndromes

Since memories are time-locked, it is important to try to establish the time of the onset of the patient's ictus. This may be difficult in cases of slowly growing tumors, but the moment of impact in a head injury or the time of onset of a stroke can often be determined with considerable accuracy. Obviously, if the patient was known to be unconscious for a certain period of time (as in a concussion), it cannot legitimately be said that the patient was amnesic for that period. If the moment of onset is assumed to be time 0, *retrograde amnesia* refers to lost recollection of events before time 0 and *anterograde amnesia* to absence of memory for events thereafter. This is a very fundamental distinction, because it implies a different pathophysiology for each type. In retrograde amnesia, the patient has lost the brain's record of events that have already been registered, whereas in anterograde amnesia the brain is unable to record ongoing events.

Although the terminology is somewhat confusing, there probably are different brain mechanisms for different durations of memory registration.[20] The following categorization is clinically based and easily testable, although it is not entirely consistent with models derived from laboratory experiments:

1. **Immediate recall** Strictly speaking, this term refers to memory traces that decay in seconds if rehearsal is not allowed. The closest clinical approximation to physiological reality is obtained in the digit span test, in which the patient is asked to repeat progressively longer strings of single digits until his or her limit is reached. The patient can also be asked to repeat the digits in reverse order, but this latter task invokes many abilities beyond simple short-term memory. Auditory digit span testing is not valid in aphasic patients with repetition deficits (see below).
2. **Short-term (recent) memory** The time duration of this category of memory is quite vague, since it does not have a substantial experimental basis. In this chapter it will be arbitrarily defined as lasting from several minutes to a few days. In a commonly applied test, the patient may be asked to remember three words, such as "chair, red, and Broadway." The patient is then asked to repeat these words immediately and is told that he or she will be asked for them later. After a period of distraction (usually 3 to 5 min) the patient is then asked to say the words again. The results can be quantitated as a fraction in time, e.g., ⅔ after 5 min. For aphasic patients with auditory output problems, one can present two or three objects from among a larger group and ask the patient to pick them out manually after an appropriate delay. To test a slightly longer time span, one can ask the patient to enumerate the items eaten at breakfast or at the previous evening's meal.
3. **Remote memory** There is a clear physiological distinction between short-term memory and long-term (remote) memory, but the time boundary between them is not well defined. For our purposes, remote memory refers to events that are at least some weeks away from the ictus and generally much longer. It is hardly necessary to test a patient who has already given a detailed and accurate history of his or her prolonged illness. In more acute situations, the patient can be asked about earlier life events (e.g., present address and previous residences) or about past events in local or national history.

Localization of Memory

The cerebral substrate of memory is essentially a bilateral inner circuit of the limbic system, including the hippocampal gyri, Ammon's horns, the fornices, the mammillothalamic tracts, the mammillary bodies, the anterior thalamic complexes and dorsomedial thalamic nuclei, and the cingulate gyri.[20] Unilateral damage to this system may cause some limited amnesic syndromes in specific modalities (e.g., auditory amnesia with left medial temporal lesions), but global memory dysfunction generally occurs only with bilateral lesions. There is good clinical and experimental evidence that this anatomical system is responsible for laying down new memories and for consolidating them to some extent. Long-term memories are more diffusely represented; they are often preserved in the presence of severe bilateral medial temporal damage. However, such patients are devastatingly disabled because they are totally unable to learn anything new.

Affect

In approaching a patient who may have a neurological disorder, one must first distinguish between the affective components of the disease and the patient's emotional reaction to the illness. The presence of an appropriate emotional reaction to disease speaks well for the integrity of those cerebral structures that mediate affective behavior. On the other hand, a change in affect may be the initial or predominant manifestation of a neurological disorder. A full discussion of the psychiatric aspects of neurological disease is beyond the scope of this chapter.[3,27] The following discussion summarizes some of the common types of affective change in relation to the relevant cerebral anatomy.

The main cerebral structures involved in emotional tone and expression are the limbic system, the frontal lobes, and the basal ganglia. A *flattening of affect* (emotional blunting) is usually associated with bilateral dysfunction of the dorsolateral frontal lobes. This is the classic, chronic result of the original, unlimited bifrontal lobotomy procedure, but some limbic lesions may produce the same effect.[34] Acute unilateral frontal or anterior callosal lesions commonly produce the same clinical picture, but it usually clears if the lesion is truly unilateral. These patients are apathetic, but they are not necessarily mute, especially in the chronic phase. The affective component of speech can also be disturbed by unilateral, nondominant hemispheric lesions; these syndromes are discussed below (see Aprosodias).

A more difficult problem may be to distinguish flattening of affect from a state of *deficient arousal*. The clinical spectrum of arousal disorders is very large. At one end it includes the akinetic mute states,[32] which are not really cognitive abnormalities. At the other end, it encompasses subcortical and thalamoreticular dysfunctions that influence the level of responsiveness in patients who are awake but seemingly unresponsive to most environmental stimuli. Partial *akinesia* (lack of initiation) is phenomenologically common to both flattening of affect and deficient arousal. However, the emotionally blunted patient does not express emotion even with flatly expressed words, whereas patients with hypoarousal will say that they feel emotions even if they do not modulate the tone of their language to express it. The best example of the latter phenomenon is the parkinsonian patient, who expresses emotions with well-chosen but uninflected words.

If flattening of affect and hypoarousal can be called "negative" psychological changes, because something normal has been lost, then we can also speak of "positive" psychological changes, in which something is gained, albeit something abnormal. Broadly speaking, these abnormal psychological gains are characterized by superficial euphoria, irritability, and/or lability. A superficial *euphoria* is frequently associated with frontal lesions. This phenomenon might better be called *pseudoeuphoria*, because its external appearance is not indicative of genuine emotional feelings. *Irritability* is characteristic of orbitofrontal or medial temporal (limbic) disorders. The sudden and often unprovoked outbursts of rage or anxiety (agitation) in these states have been analogized to the behavior of the Klüver-Bucy syndrome in monkeys.[34] While the basic analogy is undoubtedly valid, it should not be pushed too far in the ordinary clinical setting. Displays of irritability in humans are usually more muted and self-limited. Overt sexual hyperactivity is also quite rare, although inappropriate sexual references in language are not uncommon.

Almost by definition, *emotional lability* is an invariable accompaniment of euphoria or irritability, since the latter states do not usually persist ad infinitum. In fact, they often come and go rather suddenly and without apparent reason. This characteristic may serve to distinguish them from more genuine displays of the same emotions, but this distinction can be difficult to make during the early stages of cerebral disease. Labile irritability and impulsiveness are also seen in patients who have partial complex (psychomotor) seizures, which usually have medial temporal or orbitofrontal foci. There is a huge controversy about the true extent of this problem and its relationship to seizure activity.[3,23,27]

Language and Related Functions

The word *language* refers to any symbol system that conveys meaning between people. *Speech* is language in the auditory modality. The terminology of language disorders is much more confusing, because the prefixes *a* and *dys* are not used consistently. Etymologically, the prefix *a* should refer to complete absence of some behavior and *dys* should refer to its partial absence. Nonetheless, for the sake of consistency,

the prefix *a* will be used throughout this chapter in reference to acquired neurobehavioral disorders, both partial and complete. *Dys* is then reserved for development disorders. However it should not be assumed that all neurobehavioral problems in children are congenital. A 5- or 10-year-old child whose language abilities are deteriorating has an acquired disorder whose cause should be vigorously pursued.

In addition to the importance of remembering physiological modalities in language testing, one must also remember that there is a *physiological hierarchy of neurobehavioral functions*. For want of better terms, we can refer to (1) precognitive, (2) primary neurobehavioral, and (3) secondary neurobehavioral functions. The term *precognitive* will be applied to the functions of those sensory and motor structures that are used to receive and express language in its various modalities. Thus, the anatomical substrates of the precognitive language functions include all those skeletal, muscular, special sensory, and neural structures that participate in the performance of cognitive behavior, up to and including the primary motor and sensory areas in the cortex. A primary neurobehavioral function is any cognitive skill whose presence is necessary for the performance of a secondary function. For example, the primary neurobehavioral function of language comprehension must be present to some degree before one can test for agnosia or apraxia (see below). Therefore, the cortical structures subserving comprehension must be at least partially intact.

Cerebral Hemispheric Dominance

The concept of cerebral dominance is simply empirical. It conveys the idea that one cerebral hemisphere has a strongly observed relationship with some particular behavior. Thus, the left hemisphere is usually dominant for language and for other tasks that involve temporal sequencing, but the right hemisphere has a predominant influence on visuospatial functions and on some affective components of speech.[17,20] *Hemispheric specialization* refers to the presence of anatomical or physiological asymmetries that can be correlated with dominance.[14,17] Current clinical techniques of arteriography [24] and computerized tomography (CT)[26] are able to demonstrate these asymmetries, although there is some dispute about the reliability of CT in children.[13] However, clinical studies show that at least 96 percent of the adult population is left-brain-dominant for speech, whereas only about two-thirds can be shown to have the appropriate anatomical asymmetries.[14]

Definitive clinical demonstration of cerebral dominance for language requires the intracarotid injection of amobarbital (Wada test).[6] For clinical situations that do not justify this undertaking, other measures are available. Some of the formalized neuropsychological measures of dominance are described in Chap. 6. At the bedside, one can simply ask the patient which hand is used for writing or for other highly skilled, cognitive tasks. In dextrals who have no family history of left-handedness, fewer than 1 percent will actually be right-brain-dominant or bilaterally represented. In sinistrals, however, the genetic situation must be investigated more closely. Familial sinistrality is present when the patient has (1) a left-handed parent, sibling, or child *or* (2) two other left-handed relatives (cousins, aunts, uncles, or grandparents). About half of all familial left-handers actually have right or bilateral cerebral dominance for language.[21] Nonfamilial sinistrals are generally left-brain-dominant, as is the majority of the population. People may also have clinical preferences for *eyedness* ("With which eye would you sight a gun or telescope?") and *footedness* ("With which foot would you kick a ball?"), but these behaviors do not necessarily correlate with true hemispheric dominance for language.

Aphasia

In addition to the precognitive structures for hearing and sound production, the reception, processing, and emission of speech depends upon the functions of several cortical and subcortical areas in the dominant hemisphere (Fig. 5-1). These areas include Wernicke's area in the superior posterior temporal lobe (planum temporale), Broca's area at the foot of the third frontal gyrus, the arcuate fasciculus connecting Wernicke's and Broca's areas, and the inferior parietal lobule (supramarginal and angular gyri), lateral and posterior to the arcuate fasciculus at the posterior end of the sylvian fissure. The specific syndromes associated with lesions in each of these areas (and others) are listed in Tables 5-2 and 5-5. Definitive diagnosis of the aphasic syndromes cannot usually be made until at least a few weeks after an acute ictus, ostensibly because recovery and reorganization of language processes is very slow compared with motor reorganization, for example. Also listed across the top of Table 5-2 are the specific speech functions whose examination allows one to distinguish among the various syndromes. The following discussion is necessarily foreshortened; more detailed explanations will be found in the writings of Benson and Geschwind.[2,4]

The most important aspect of *spontaneous speech* is *fluency*. The latter term is defined by a number of characteristics, the most salient of which is rate of speech output in terms of words per minute.[2,25] The vast majority of acute (and almost all childhood) aphasics are nonfluent. They produce an abnormally low number of words with great effort, many hesitations, and obvious agrammatisms. However, some initially nonfluent aphasics may turn out later to be fluent or even hyperfluent. These patients produce speech at

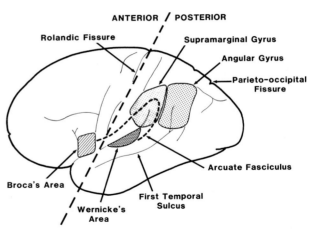

Figure 5-1 The principal perisylvian structures associated with language functions in the left hemisphere.

a normal or increased rate, but it may be quite meaningless or even incomprehensible. The presence or absence of fluency has localizing value (Fig. 5-1). Chronic nonfluent aphasics generally have "anterior" lesions, more or less restricted to the left frontal lobe. Chronically fluent aphasics usually have "posterior" lesions in the left parietal and/or temporal lobes. The terms *anterior aphasia* and *posterior aphasia* are derived from these localizations. *Paraphasias* are mistakes in words. They are commonly produced by nonfluent and fluent aphasics. The mistakes may involve an improperly substituted syllable, resulting in a phonetic paraphasia (e.g., "clorange" for "orange"); substitution of an entire word, which is a literal or semantic paraphasia (e.g., "apple" for "orange"); or a neologism (e.g., "flooflap" for "orange"). Speech that consists almost entirely of paraphasias, especially neologisms, is called *jargon*.

Naming is the ability to find and produce the auditory symbol for an object. Thus, a mistake in naming results in a paraphasia. Although abnormalities of naming can be observed in spontaneous speech, formal testing of this ability is usually done by showing the patient an object and asking for its name. This is a visual-auditory task, but other modalities of input may be needed in some circumstances. Most anomic patients who understand the task will indicate that they know what the object is by describing the object or its use or by producing a paraphasia that is close to the correct

TABLE 5-2   The Classical Perisylvian Aphasias

Type	Spontaneous Speech	Naming	Repetition	Comprehension	Usual Localization
Broca	Nonfluent	Poor	Usually poor	Good	Broca's area and beyond
Conduction	Fluent	Poor	Very poor	Good	Arcuate fasciculus
Wernicke	Fluent	Poor	Poor	Poor	Wernicke's area
Global	Nonfluent	Poor	Poor	Poor	Entire perisylvian cortex
Anomic	Fluent	Poor	Good	Good	Usually non-localizing; may be angular gyrus

name. Severely anomic or nonfluent patients may produce no response at all. If they have understood, they will often indicate this by obvious or even colorful expressions of frustration.

Repetition is the ability to exactly reproduce a word or phrase given by the examiner. Patients with mild repetition defects may simply omit small connecting words but repeat nouns correctly. Thus, one of the best ways to test repetition is to ask the patient to say, "No ifs, ands, or buts." Tongue twisters (e.g., "Round the rugged rock the ragged rascal ran") are not appropriate; they are meant to test for dysarthria. Nonfluent patients should be tested for repetition, but it may not be valid to draw localizing conclusions from the results if the nonfluency is severe.

Comprehension of auditory input can be assessed by starting with simple questions or commands and increasing their complexity until the patient's limits are discovered. One can begin with "Is there a nurse in this room?" and go on to "Is the nurse standing in front of the doctor?", and so on. In the second example just given, correct comprehension depends on the patient's ability to understand the semantic meaning of "in front of." One can also increase complexity by using less common words in a sentence, e.g., by asking for the source of the illumination in the room, rather than just asking where the light is.

The Classical Perisylvian Aphasias (Table 5-2)

The predominant clinical characteristic of *Broca aphasia* is poor naming in a nonfluent patient who also has poor repetition and good comprehension. It is now abundantly clear that the left lateral frontal lesion that produces Broca aphasia extends well beyond the boundaries of Broca's area.[25,30] Since Broca's area is immediately adjacent to the lateral aspect of the motor strip, most chronic Broca patients have contralateral paralysis of the arm and face but not leg. *Conduction aphasia* is characterized by strikingly poor repetition in a fluent patient with defective naming and relatively good comprehension. The essential lesion involves the arcuate fasciculus, generally under the supramarginal gyrus.[11,25] Conduction aphasia is quite rare as an isolated syndrome, but conduction defects (abnormalities of repetition) are commonly found in the other perisylvian aphasias. *Wernicke aphasia* is characterized by fluency or even hyperfluency (pressure of speech) in a patient who is otherwise devastated by poor naming, poor repetition, and very poor comprehension. The size of the associated lesion is quite variable. Smaller lesions, relatively restricted to Wernicke's area, may produce very few other clinical abnormalities. Larger le-

sions, extending into the adjacent parietal lobe, may produce many other cortical deficits, but most chronic Wernicke aphasics do not have severe contralateral hemiplegias.

Global aphasia is complete loss of all auditory language as a result of complete perisylvian tissue loss, usually associated with large infarctions in the territory of the left middle cerebral artery. These patients generally do not retain language abilities in any other modality. Syndromes of incomplete global aphasia in patients who retain some functions of Broca's and Wernicke's areas should be described as "mixed" perisylvian aphasias. *Anomic aphasia* describes patients who have naming difficulties but no other aphasic symptoms. This syndrome may be seen during recovery from more severe aphasias of any type. Although anomic aphasia is occasionally seen in patients who have small lesions of the dominant angular gyrus, it is usually nonlocalizing. This is consistent with cortical stimulation studies, which show that naming can be disrupted by electrical exploration of wide areas in the dominant hemisphere.[31]

The Transcortical Aphasias (Table 5-3)

These syndromes are associated with lesions in the cerebrovascular "watershed" zones between the middle cerebral artery laterally and the anterior and posterior cerebral arteries medially. The lesions are usually caused by hypoxic states, such as drowning or carbon monoxide poisoning. The important clinical characteristic of the patients is their striking ability to perform repetition in the face of otherwise major deficits. The presence of preserved repetition therefore implies that the perisylvian structures are intact, including the deep white matter containing the arcuate fasciculus. *Echolalia* is the phenomenon in which the patient repeats (echoes) much of what is said. Transcortical aphasics often repeat commands or questions rather than answering them.

Thalamic Aphasia

This term is currently used generically to refer to disorders of auditory language associated with lesions of the left basal ganglia. There is a major controversy about the nature of these disturbances. Are they truly aphasic in the sense of being primary neurobehavioral disorders, or are they simply precognitive?[2,7,8] Much of the clinical difficulty stems from the fact that basal ganglia lesions are often associated with hypoarousal states. The anatomical problem arises from the fact that cortical lesions often extend into the adjacent basal

TABLE 5-3 The Transcortical Aphasias

Type	Spontaneous Speech	Naming	Repetition	Comprehension	Usual Localization
Motor	Nonfluent	Fair	Good	Good	Frontal watershed zone
Sensory	Fluent, echolalic	Poor	Good	Poor	Parietotemporal watershed zone
Mixed	Nonfluent, echolalic	Poor	Good	Poor	Entire watershed zone

ganglia[8] and vice versa. At present it seems safe to say that (1) the basal ganglia do have an important role in the reception and production of auditory language, (2) distinctly aphasic phenomena are observed in patients with restricted basal ganglia lesions, and (3) categorization and localization of the thalamic aphasias is not yet clinically reliable.

The Aprosodias

Since the nineteenth century some astute clinical observers have felt that the nondominant hemisphere contributes an affective component to speech. One of the features of normal fluency is *prosody*. This term refers to the normal rhythm and inflection of speech, which conveys emotional intent. Ross[33] has shown recently that lesions of the nondominant hemisphere in areas homologous to the language areas on the dominant side will produce corresponding defects of prosody. For example, patients with lesions of the nondominant Broca's area do not inflect their speech normally, although they do understand the affective component of other people's speech (motor aprosodia). Similarly, patients with lesions of the nondominant Wernicke's area do not understand the emotional intent of others' speech, but they inflect their own speech quite well (sensory aprosodia). These observations have been extended to all of the aphasia types listed in Tables 5-2 and 5-3.

Alexia and Agraphia

Reading and writing are language functions in the visual modality. The central common pathway for reading and writing is the dominant angular gyrus.[18,19] Lesions of this area produce the syndrome of *alexia with agraphia*. Although the exact size of the lesions required to produce this syndrome is not really known, there is some evidence that the lesion usually extends into the posterior end of the first temporal gyrus.[19] More extensive posterior perisylvian lesions are generally associated with severe posterior aphasias, in which case the term *alexia with agraphia and aphasia* is more appropriate. *Alexia without agraphia* ("pure" alexia) describes patients who can write but not read. The presence of this syndrome implies that the dominant angular gyrus has been spared. The usual cause is an infarction in the territory of the left posterior cerebral artery, which produces dominant occipital and splenial infarction. These patients thus have right (dominant) hemianopsias; the lexic signals in the left visual field are seen by the right hemisphere, but they cannot get to the cerebral language apparatus in the left hemisphere because of the splenial lesion. Variants of this syndrome may be seen in surgical patients with left occipital tumors or vascular malformations.[18,19]

A "third alexia" has been well documented by Benson[1,2] in patients with anterior lesions and predominantly Broca aphasias. Broca patients can usually read text, but they have difficulty reading single letters. This fascinating but unexplained fact points up the importance of examining alexic patients properly. Patients should be tested with single letters, single words, and single sentences. The sentences can be commands written on plain paper or text taken from some handy bedside material, such as a newspaper or magazine. Patients should be asked to interpret what they have read to be sure that they can comprehend it. Reading aloud without comprehension is an interesting but futile exercise.

Writing can be tested briefly by first asking the patient to write his or her name. Name writing is a very automatic task, but it is useful to get the patient into the set of testing, especially if the nondominant hand must be used. If this can be done successfully, the patient is asked to write a few single words, followed by a dictated sentence or a sentence to command ("Write a sentence about the weather"). Isolated ("pure") *agraphia* does occur, but its localization is quite imprecise.[2,28]

Other Lateralized or Localized Cognitive Functions

In addition to reading and writing, the region of the dominant angular gyrus is associated with several other cognitive functions that may be disturbed by lesions in this area. *Gerstmann's syndrome* is the clinical combination of isolated agraphia, acalculia, right-left disorientation, and finger agnosia. Since it often occurs in conjunction with alexia and/or aphasia, there is some dispute about its reality as an isolated syndrome.[2,5,20] In any case, the clinical presence of its components points to the existence of a dominant parietal lesion. Bedside testing of writing has been discussed in the preceding paragraph, but tests for the other components of Gerstmann's syndrome require further explanation.

Acalculia should be sought in the auditory and visual modalities. A good auditory approach is to ask about an everyday task, such as shopping: "If you went to the store and bought a loaf of bread for 59 cents, how much change would you get from a dollar?" The patient can also be given simple arithmetic problems on paper. *Right-left orientation* is tested first on the patient and then on the examiner: "Show me your left eye. Now show me my right hand." This sequence can be made more complex by intermingling one's fingers and asking the patient to point to specific right or left fingers on the examiner. *Finger agnosia* is sought by asking the patient to move the same finger that the examiner moves or by asking the patient to point to a named finger on him- or herself, on the examiner, or on an outline drawing of a hand. Asking the patient to supply the name of a finger that is pointed out may not be useful if there is also anomia. In addition, systems of finger naming may be different for different individuals.

Agnosia

A patient is agnosic for some stimulus if he or she does not recognize the meaning or use of the stimulus, despite the presence of an intact precognitive sensory apparatus for the specific modality *and* appropriately intact language abilities. This definition is rather strict, because there has been much controversy about the role of aphasia in the agnosias, especially in the auditory modality. However, one may hope that the virtue of a strict definition is its contribution to clarity.

Agnosias can then be classified according to sensory modality such as auditory, tactile, and visual. Some localizing information is available for each of these types.[7,20] Within each modality, it is usually some particular kind of stimulus that is poorly understood by the patient. An interesting example of this is *prosopagnosia*, which is the inability to recognize faces. This syndrome is associated with bilateral, medial occipitotemporal lesions.[10]

The visual agnosias have also been classified according to their apparent mechanisms as *apperceptive* or *associative*.[4,7,20] In the apperceptive type, the image is apparently distorted; the patient cannot identify, describe, draw, or copy simple objects or line drawings. In the associative type, the patient can draw the object and identify it in other modalities, but cannot give its name, its use, or a description when it is presented visually.[7] Suffice it to say that an agnosia can be diagnosed only after an extensive workup of precognitive and primary neurobehavioral functions.

Apraxia

An apraxia is an inability to perform a requested motor act when the patient has (1) intact precognitive motor and sensory systems, (2) adequate comprehension, and (3) adequate cooperation and attention. Although it is not necessary to see the patient perform the act spontaneously at other times, such an observation does help to confirm the diagnosis. In testing for apraxia, one must be careful not to give the patient multiple stimuli. It is generally best to start with an oral command. A written command can be given if it is more appropriate. If this is not successful, the examiner can try to get the patient to mimic the movement. Although there are no known localizing differences, it is usually thought that mimicry is a lower order (or at least an easier form) of response. For example, in asking the patient to protrude the tongue, the examiner should not demonstrate the movement while giving the command, because the examiner's performance of the act would obviate the conclusion that the patient understood the oral command.

The example of tongue protrusion is an instance of *ideomotor* praxis, i.e., the performance of a commanded single motor act. A patient who can perform single actions but cannot do a series of them in sequence has *ideational* apraxia.[4] The latter implies a dominant parietal localization. However, some authors use the term *ideational apraxia* to refer to patients who can perform ideomotor praxis but cannot use actual objects to command.[7,12] This difference in terminological usage remains unresolved in the current literature on the subject.

Aside from the ideomotor versus ideational classification of the apraxias, there are more practical nomenclatures that are less confusing. These terms are based simply on the type of motor action being tested. *Limb-kinetic (body movement) apraxias* may be specific to face, tongue, limbs, or body axis. They can be elicited by asking the patients to do simple movements (e.g., protrude the tongue, make a fist) and by asking the patient to demonstrate more skilled movements with imaginary objects ("Show me how you would use a hammer"). *Dressing apraxia* describes a patient who cannot organize the activity of putting on clothing. This deficit can often be seen in the patient who cannot put on a hospital bathrobe. The definition and testing of *constructional apraxia* is more complex, because this syndrome includes a number of variants, depending on the details of the task and the localization of the associated lesions.[4,7,20] A common form of constructional apraxia is an inability to copy drawings (Fig. 5-2), which may be seen with lesions of either hemisphere.

Our understanding of the neural mechanisms of the apraxias has been significantly improved by contemporary advances in cerebral disconnection theory. The details of these clinically applicable theories are available in the writings of Geschwind.[15,16] To give just one example, consider a patient who can perform a commanded movement with the dominant hand but not with the nondominant limb. This finding is not uncommon. It indicates the presence of a lesion of the body of the corpus callosum or in other parts of the pathway from the left motor association cortex to the right. Such a lesion disconnects the nondominant limb from the language apparatus in the left hemisphere. The patient understands the command, but cannot transfer it internally from the left to the right hemisphere.

Neglect and Denial Syndromes

There is a broad spectrum of neglect and denial syndromes, ranging from simple sensory extinction to denial of illness altogether. Unilateral *extinction* of bilaterally applied tactile or visual stimuli (double simultaneous stimulation) is a form of imperception that might best be thought of as an attentional defect. The diagnosis presupposes the presence of intact primary sensory systems. It is associated with unilateral parietal or occipitoparietal lesions. *Neglect* refers to spontaneous inattention to one side of body or space. Although neglect can occur in otherwise intact patients, this need not be the case, because most hemiplegics and some hemianopics know that they have deficits. Hemispatial (visual) neglect is usually associated with nondominant parietal lesions (Fig. 5-2), but the dorsolateral frontal and cingulate areas have also been implicated.[22,29] The possible existence of dominant-side neglect is problematic, because the associated language difficulties are usually overwhelming.

Active *denial* of illness is called *anosognosia*. Unlike the hemiplegic with neglect, who will acknowledge the paretic limb when attention is drawn to it, the anosognosic patient actively denies that there is an abnormality. Such patients may make excuses to explain away the abnormality, or they may displace the ownership of the limb to the examining doctor. They may even claim that the limb really belongs to the nurse who is standing at the foot of the bed! Localization of the lesion for this extreme form of denial is not well established.[22,35]

Suggested Minimal Neurological Examination of Cognitive Functions

It is always a bit dangerous to suggest minimal standards. Nonetheless, screening examinations will be done, and it seems worthwhile to make some reasonable suggestions in

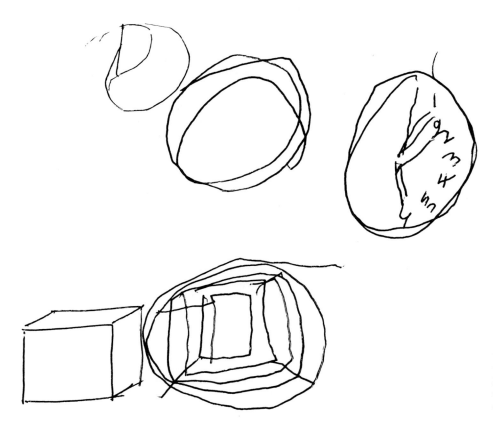

Figure 5-2 Drawings by a 52-year-old right-handed woman with a large, malignant right parietal astrocytoma. The upper group of three circular figures shows the patient's response to examiner's request that she draw a clock. Note her neglect of the left side in her final production on the right. At the bottom is the patient's response (on the right) to examiner's request that she copy his drawing of a cube. The patient's perseverative production of circles around the square in the center is unusual.

this regard. The emphasis in Table 5-4 is on the large amount of cognitive information that can be gained from other parts of the interview and examination. This information becomes directly relevant to the patient's cognitive status when it is analyzed carefully and coherently. Any hint of an abnormality should lead to a more thorough investigation of the suspected deficit.

Table 5-5 is presented as a summary of some of the locali-

zation information that has been discussed in this chapter. It can be used accurately only if three caveats are kept in mind:

1. Many different areas of both hemispheres participate in the normal performance of every cognitive function, but specific syndromes of cognitive dysfunction are usually associated with lesions in only one or two locations. Therefore, one may occasionally see rather well-defined

TABLE 5-4   Suggested Minimal Neurological Examination of Cognitive Functions in a Patient with No Apparent Cognitive Abnormalities

  I. General intellectual functions
    A. Record behavior observed during history taking and examination
      1. Reasoning: insight, judgment
      2. Disorders of perception: delirium, delusions, illusions, hallucinations.
    B. Determine by formal testing
      1. Orientation to person, place and time
      2. Global attention: serial 7s
 II. Memory and affect
    A. Record behavior observed during history taking and examination
      1. Memory: recent and remote
      2. Affect
    B. Determine by formal testing
      1. Immediate recall: digit span
III. Language and related functions

  A. Record behavior observed during history taking and examination
    1. Spontaneous speech, including fluency and prosody
    2. Auditory comprehension
    3. Attention to both sides of space and body
    4. Ability to perform commanded movements of face, limbs, and body axis
  B. Determine by questions or formal testing
    1. Hand preference for writing and family history of sinistrality
    2. Naming
    3. Repetition
    4. Reading: letters, words, simple sentences aloud and interpreted
    5. Writing: name and a dictated or spontaneous sentence

TABLE 5-5 Summary of Localization of Cognitive Dysfunctions

Lobe	Left	Right	Bilateral
Frontal			
Orbitomedial			Short-term amnesia; irritability
Dorsolateral	Transcortical motor aphasia		Flattening of affect
Posterolateral	Broca aphasia	Motor aprosodia	
Parietal			
Dorsolateral	Transcortical sensory aphasia		
Supramarginal	Conduction aphasia; fluent aphasia	Conduction aprosodia	
Angular	Anomic aphasia; alexia with agraphia; Gerstmann's syndrome	Hemineglect of body and space	
Temporal			
Medial	Auditory amnesia		Irritability; global short-term amnesia
Posterior-superior	Wernicke aphasia	Sensory aprosodia	
Occipital			
Dorsolateral		Spatial hemineglect	
Ventral	Alexia without agraphia		Prosopagnosia

cognitive deficits associated with lesions that are not in the "classic" locations.

2. A single brain area almost always participates in the performance of many different functions, but the specific functions of any particular area may be different from one person to another.[31] Therefore, lesions with exactly the same boundaries in two individuals may produce strikingly different clinical syndromes.

3. The rather precise localizations listed in Table 5-3 represent only the spatial centers of the lesions associated with the listed dysfunctions. The actual lesions may be considerably more extensive.

References

1. Benson DF: The third alexia. Arch Neurol 34:327–331, 1977.
2. Benson DF: *Aphasia, Alexia, and Agraphia.* New York, Churchill Livingstone, 1979.
3. Benson DF, Blumer D (eds): *Psychiatric Aspects of Neurological Disease.* New York, Grune & Stratton, 1975.
4. Benson DF, Geschwind N: Chapter 8. The aphasias and related disturbances, in Baker AB, Baker LH (eds): *Clinical Neurology.* Philadelphia, Harper and Row, 1976; rev ed, 1981, vol 1, pp 1–28.
5. Benton A: Body schema disturbances: Finger agnosia and right-left disorientation, in Heilman KM, Valenstein E (eds): *Clinical Neuropsychology.* New York, Oxford University Press, 1979, pp 141–158.
6. Blume, WT, Grabow, JD, Darley FL, Aronson AE: Intracarotid amobarbital test of language and memory before temporal lobectomy for seizure control. Neurology (NY) 23:812–819, 1973.
7. Brown, JW: *Aphasia, Apraxia and Agnosia. Clinical and Theoretical Aspects.* Springfield, Ill, Charles C Thomas, 1972.
8. Brunner RJ, Kornhuber, HH, Seemüller E, Suger G, Wallesch C-W: Basal ganglia participation in language pathology. Brain Lang 16:281–299, 1982.
9. Butters N: Amnesic disorders, in Heilman KM, Valenstein E (eds): *Clinical Neuropsychology.* New York, Oxford University Press, 1979, pp 439–474.
10. Damasio AR, Damasio H: Localization of lesions in achromatopsia and prosopagnosia, in Kertesz A (ed): *Localization in Neuropsychology.* New York, Academic, 1983, pp 417–428.
11. Damasio H, Damasio AR: Localization of lesions in conduction aphasia, in Kertesz A (ed): *Localization in Neuropsychology.* New York, Academic, 1983, pp 231–243.
12. De Renzi E, Faglioni P, Sorgato P: Modality-specific and supramodal mechanisms of apraxia. Brain 105:301–312, 1982.
13. Deuel RK, Moran CC: Cerebral dominance and cerebral asymmetries on computed tomogram in childhood. Neurology (NY) 30:934–938, 1980.
14. Galaburda AM, LeMay M, Kemper TL, Geschwind N: Right-left asymmetries in the brain. Science 199:852–856, 1978.
15. Geschwind N: Disconnexion syndromes in animals and man. Brain 88:237–294, 585–644, 1965.
16. Geschwind N: The apraxias: Neural mechanisms of disorders of learned movement. Am Sci 63:188–195, 1975.
17. Geschwind N: Specializations of the human brain. Sci Am 241:180–199, 1979.
18. Greenblatt SH: Neurosurgery and the anatomy of reading: A practical review. Neurosurgery 1:6–15, 1977.
19. Greenblatt SH: Localization of lesions in alexia, in Kertesz A (ed): *Localization in Neuropsychology.* New York, Academic, 1983, pp 323–356.
20. Hécaen H, Albert ML: *Human Neuropsychology.* New York, Wiley, 1978.
21. Hécaen H, Sauguet J: Cerebral dominance in left-handed subjects. Cortex 7:19–48, 1971.
22. Heilman, KM: Neglect and related disorders, in Heilman KM, Valenstein E (eds): *Clinical Neuropsychology.* New York, Oxford University Press, 1979, pp 268–307.

23. Hermann BP: Deficits in neuropsychological functioning and psychopathology in persons with epilepsy: A rejected hypothesis revisited. Epilepsia 22:161–167, 1981.

24. Hochberg FH, Le May M: Arteriographic correlates of handedness. Neurology (NY) 25:218–222, 1975.

25. Kertesz A: *Aphasia and Associated Disorders: Taxonomy, Localization, and Recovery.* New York, Grune & Stratton, 1979.

26. Le May M, Kido DK: Asymmetries of the cerebral hemispheres on computed tomograms. J Comput Assist Tomogr 2:471–476, 1978.

27. Lishman WA: *Organic Psychiatry: The Psychological Consequences of Cerebral Disorder.* Oxford, Blackwell, 1978.

28. Marcie P, Hécaen H: Agraphia: Writing disorders associated with unilateral cortical lesions, in Heilman KM, Valenstein E (eds): *Clinical Neuropsychology.* New York, Oxford University Press, 1979, pp 92–127.

29. Mesulam M-M: A cortical network for directed attention and unilateral neglect. Ann Neurol 10:309–325, 1981.

30. Mohr JP, Pessin MS, Finkelstein S, Funkenstein HH, Duncan GW, Davis KR: Broca aphasia: Pathologic and clinical. Neurology (NY) 28:311–324, 1978.

31. Ojemann GA, Whitaker HA: Language localization and variability. Brain Lang 6:239–260, 1978.

32. Plum F, Posner JB: *The Diagnosis of Stupor and Coma,* 3d ed. Philadelphia, Davis, 1980.

33. Ross ED: The aprosodias: Functional-anatomic organization of the affective components of language in the right hemisphere. Arch Neurol 38:561–569, 1981.

34. Valenstein E, Heilman KM: Emotional disorders resulting from lesions of the central nervous system, in Heilman KM, Valenstein E (eds): *Clinical Neuropsychology.* New York, Oxford University Press, 1979, pp 413–438.

35. Weinstein EA, Kahn RL: *Denial of Illness: Symbolic and Physiological Aspects.* Springfield, Ill., Charles C Thomas, 1955.

6
Psychological Assessment of Intelligence and Personality

Patrick E. Logue
Frederick A. Schmitt

Psychological testing can best be conceptualized as a systematic attempt to measure human behavior within an objective and standardized framework. The benefit of objective test data over such methods as the case history and clinical observation is that subjective elements in the patient assessment process are minimized. When these test methods are used in conjunction with the case history and clinical observation, the health professional can combine clinical impressions pertaining to each patient with test patterns that provide objective comparisons with other cases. Therefore, these tests yield reliable quantitative indices of present functioning that can be compared with population normative data. With repeated testing an assessment of even subtle intraindividual change can be obtained.

The measurement of human abilities originated with the work of Galton in the late nineteenth century and was based on his assumption that human abilities could be assessed through the use of scientific methods. The largest impetus for psychological test use came with the world wars and the need to assess the emotional and intellectual abilities of very large numbers of military personnel. Since that time the science of psychological assessment has shown a rapid expansion into other areas as well.

Test Construction

Test construction procedures are designed to minimize the effects of irrelevant personal and environmental variables on the final test score. One must also bear in mind that the statements made about a person's intellectual and/or personality structure will be based on a behavioral sample that represents but does not encompass all the possible behaviors of interest. Since no assessment device can measure all of the possible aspects of an intellectual or emotional domain, a specific methodology is vital for effective test construction and use.

The concepts of validity and reliability are fundamental in test construction. Validity relates to the connections that theoretically exist between a given test and the behavior of interest. (Does the test measure what it purports to measure?) The simplicity of the term *validity* may be misleading however. Many different types of validity are important for psychological testing. If a test "appears" to measure what we expect it to measure, at least on the surface, we are assessing the instrument's *face validity*. More empirically, when attempts are made to ensure that test items are truly representative of the behavior domain of interest, then we are attempting to ensure the test's *content validity*. Once test items have been selected, the test has been administered to representative populations (to establish normative performance), and scoring has been standardized, then three other types of validity become important.

When we ask such questions as "Does this neuropsychological test battery predict the possible location of lesions?" or "Does this test battery predict the patient's response to treatment?" we are concerned respectively with *concurrent* and *predictive validity*. Predictive validity, therefore, is an attempt to obtain indices of how well test scores predict performance on independent criterion measures (response to therapy). On the other hand, when our concerns deal with established criteria available at the time that the test is used, we are dealing with concurrent validity. Finally, when we attempt to assess how well the test mirrors a given trait (depression) theoretically assumed to underlie performance (e.g., memory loss), then we are concerned with the test's *construct* validity.

Validity relates test scores to behaviors and future outcomes of behavior; reliability involves the assessment of a test's consistency, replicability, and generalization of the test scores. In brief, test stability (test-retest reliability) can be measured by repeated administrations over time. Split-half reliability, or equivalence, is often assessed by administering parallel halves of a single test form and then correlating performance on each half. Reliability of a given test is especially important for diagnosis. Generally, if the same test or other forms of the test do not yield similar scores on separate occasions, then it is difficult to attribute changes in a patient's test results to actual changes in behavior as a result of disease processes or treatments. Space limitations do not allow for a more in-depth treatment of these important issues. The reader can, however, turn to texts by Anastasi[1] and Cronbach[5] for a more in-depth discussion of psychometrics.

While it is important to note that there are many uses for psychological test data such as evaluation, selection, and hypothesis testing, we will briefly discuss the diagnostic utility of the Wechsler Adult Intelligence Scale (WAIS) as a measure of general intelligence and the Minnesota Multiphasic Personality Inventory (MMPI) as a popular personality measure. Each test will be described in detail, relevant problems with each measure will be discussed, and research using these instruments will be summarized. Where appropriate, other related tests will also be mentioned.

Intelligence

Over the past few decades, intelligence has become a familiar concept. Yet, even though intelligence is a common term, there is no popular consensus as to a meaningful construct of "intelligent behavior" and no satisfactory definition of intelligence, per se. Part of the problem appears to be the multiplicity with which the term is used, and so the term becomes misleading. Historically, definitions of intelligence have concerned mental processes such as judgment, reasoning, comprehension, learning capacity, adaptive ability, problem solving, and so on. However, intelligence does not always appear to involve these processes alone, but also appears to encompass a more general capacity that reflects the functioning of the whole person. Therefore, the best defini-

tion appears to be one that recognizes the multidimensionality of intelligence and so reflects the interaction of numerous cognitive skills as well as personal variables. Interestingly, intelligence as a multidimensional construct is best reflected in over 100 published tests of intelligence (from general to specific abilities) found in Buros's *Mental Measurements Yearbook*.[4] Buros's texts are perhaps the most informative source about published tests. These yearbooks also include critical reviews and references for each test.

Rather than entering into a detailed review of intelligence testing, we will highlight two of the major approaches in this area. The first major test of intelligence was developed by Binet and Simon in an effort to determine which students in the Parisian school system required special instruction and which should attend regular classes. The important concept of intelligence quotient (IQ) that arose out of the test developed by Simon and Binet involved the ratio of mental age (MA) to chronological age (CA), where IQ = MA/CA × 100. In this case the IQ score has meaning in that an individual's performance is assessed relative to the performance of others of the same chronological age. Two criticisms of the Binet test arose, however. The first concerned the meaningfulness of the mental age concept for adults. The second criticism was that beyond age 12 or so, the test depended heavily on verbal ability. In response to these issues, David Wechsler developed the Wechsler-Bellevue scales (1939), which later became the Wechsler Adult Intelligence Scale (WAIS, 1955). It was recently revised and is called the WAIS-R (1981).[24,25,26]

The WAIS-R intelligence quotient is based on verbal and nonverbal performance subtests. WAIS IQ scores are obtained from a direct comparison of the individual's score with scores of persons of similar age. Therefore, a person's IQ represents the relative standing of that person's intellectual abilities with regard to persons who have had equal life and learning experiences. An additional benefit of the WAIS is that one can evaluate an individual's performance regardless of age by comparing the subtest scaled scores of different individuals. The WAIS scaled scores are based on a selected sample of adults in their "prime" between the ages of 20 and 34 years. Perhaps the most useful application of these scaled scores arises in evaluating elderly subjects' abilities in areas that might show age-related decrements by comparing their performance against a metric of test performance reflected by "adults at the height of their mental capacity."[25]

Administration of the WAIS-R is standardized. Items within each subtest are administered sequentially (as are the subtests themselves). Since the items are arranged in increasing order of difficulty, testing on each subscale is halted after a given number of failures to minimize failure experiences. Going beyond this point is also useful in testing the limits of a subject's cognitive skills. Depending on the subtest, items will be untimed, have time limits, or have bonus credits for rapid solutions. Item scoring is accomplished by comparing the examinee's responses to listings of appropriate answers found in the test manual. Administration of the WAIS to normal adults requires approximately 75 to 90 min.

Once points have been awarded for correct answers, raw scores for each subtest are converted into standard scores. These scaled scores are based on the reference group's performance. Scaled scores are then summed separately for the verbal and performance scales. This yields IQ scores that can be compared with the distributions of IQ scores for each age group. Given that the distribution of IQ scores at each age was set at a mean of 100 and a standard deviation of 15 IQ points, IQ scores always have the same meaning with regard to the individual's standing relative to his or her peers. Further, using the scaled scores, any subject's performance (regardless of age) on specific tasks can be compared with that of other age groups of interest.

A brief description of the verbal and performance scales of the WAIS-R as well as their respective subtests follows. (For a more detailed discussion of each subtest in terms of scores and response styles, the reader is referred to texts by Matarazzo and Wechsler,[18] Wechsler,[26] and Zimmerman and Woo-Sam.[27])

Verbal scale (six subtests):

1. **Information.** This is made up of 29 questions assessing general knowledge, retention of learned material, and culturally acquired information (e.g., "What is a thermometer?").
2. **Comprehension.** This is made up of 16 questions designed to measure judgment, "common sense," and conventional wisdom (e.g., "Why do we wash clothes?").
3. **Arithmetic.** In this test there are 14 mental arithmetic items assessing elementary arithmetic abilities, problem solving, and concentration.
4. **Similarities.** In this there are 14 item pairs requiring judgments of how the items are alike. Logical thinking as well as conceptual ability are assessed (e.g., "How are an apple and a pear alike?").
5. **Digit span.** Orally presented digit lists for forward and backward recall are designed to assess immediate memory along with attention.
6. **Vocabulary.** This is made up of 35 words of increasing difficulty. By supplying the meanings of these words, the subject's range of semantic knowledge and acculturation are measured. This scale is the best single correlate of general intelligence.

Performance scale (five subtests):

1. **Digit symbol.** This is a 90-second code-substitution task involving 93 items and measures a subject's flexibility and capacity for new learning. This subtest is the most reliable index on the WAIS of changes secondary to CNS involvement.
2. **Picture completion.** This is made up of 20 pictures of common objects from which some part is missing. The task is to identify the missing element; it assesses visual alertness and the ability of the subject to differentiate between relevant and irrelevant details.
3. **Block design.** This is considered to be the best single performance test. In this test, nine geometric designs of colored blocks are to be reproduced within time limits. This task assesses the ability to analyze, organize and develop problem-solving strategies. It tests perceptual and visual-motor coordination while providing a measure of constructional apraxia.
4. **Picture arrangement.** This utilizes 10 sets of line drawings that must be arranged to tell a coherent story, thereby testing the ability for logical sequencing and comprehension of a total situation.
5. **Object Assembly.** This is a timed test of perceptual ability involving four puzzles that must be assembled to form flat pictures of common objects.

The large impact of the Wechsler scales on the development of psychometric assessment cannot be readily summarized. Literally hundreds of studies have involved the W-B or the WAIS in the diagnosis of psychopathology. The importance of the Wechsler scales is best stated in surveys indicating that the WAIS ranked first in frequency among all tests used in clinical settings.[17] Given such widespread usage of the WAIS, a pertinent question concerns the significance of WAIS scores for the clinical practitioner.

IQ data obtained from the Wechsler scales can provide insights into intellectual level, while the pattern of test scores and test-taking behavior provides insights into intellectual strengths, weaknesses, problem solving skills, brain-behavior relationships, educational attainment, and qualitative indices of personality processes. For example, WAIS scores have been found to correlate rather well with measures of personal and social adjustment, educational attainment, occupational level, and even MCAT scores.[18] Wechsler IQ scores in combination with measures of social functioning are also efficient in diagnosing retardation. Additionally, given the numerous correlations between the WAIS and such criteria as those mentioned above, we can gain some insight into such issues as school failure, rehabilitation potential, foster home placement success, further diagnostic procedures, and treatment efficacy as a result of the WAIS IQ score.

Two main areas of research have been directed toward assessing the usefulness of the WAIS as a diagnostic instrument. The first area involved attempts to find WAIS correlates of the presence or absence of brain pathology.[19] The second area attempted to assess the usefulness of intelligence test data for exploring personality.[20]

Generally, the theoretical rationale behind the early work in brain-intelligence associations assumed that the brain-impaired person would show deficits in the ability to use well-learned information, often termed "crystallized intelligence."[14] Research, however, has shown that these deficits also occur in the learning of new information and problem solving, better known as "fluid" intellectual abilities.[14] As the WAIS is indicated in most neuropsychological assessments as an index of general intelligence and specific abilities, a brief mention of brain impairment–WAIS correlations is warranted.

Generally, full-scale IQ (FSIQ) decrements are consistently found between matched (age and education) groups of normal subjects and cerebrally impaired adults such as epileptics, chronic alcoholics, and patients with multiple sclerosis, Parkinson's disease, and Alzheimer's disease. The severity of intellectual impairment reflected by the WAIS is also related to the extent and type of impairment, lateralization, and age of onset. Numerous attempts to derive formulas for the WAIS subtest scores as a reliable measure to separate brain-impaired subjects from normal controls have appeared in the research literature. Probably as a result of the multidimensional nature of intelligence and/or sampling and research design problems, these formulas have not met with consistent success. For instance, a fairly reliable difference between verbal (VIQ) and performance (PIQ) scores has often been reported in the literature. In general, VIQ scores will exceed PIQ scores in cases of right hemisphere or diffuse brain damage. Left hemisphere lesions tend to be associated with PIQ exceeding VIQ scores. Individual cases can be considered to imply some form of brain damage and deserving of further diagnostic work when the VIQ-PIQ difference is roughly 15 points or greater. Problems with this index exist too. This verbal-performance split is often found in acute but not chronic cases. Also, interpretation of this index in persons with superior scores is not warranted.[16,20]

Other research in this area that has shown some promise involves indices such as deterioration quotients (ratios between constant performance and impaired subtest performance) and methods computing premorbid IQ for an individual based on educational, occupational, and socioeconomic data. At present, these measures are most useful as signs for further neuropsychological and medical assessment. Another interesting area derived from longitudinal studies of aging twins concerns the concept of "critical loss."[15] Here, WAIS data (similarities, digit symbol, vocabulary) have shown abrupt changes in intellectual ability for older adults, which have further been shown to signal imminent death. One hypothesis holds that the changes in WAIS scores could be associated with vascular changes that potentially precede death in these subjects.

The second area in which WAIS scores were hypothesized to provide clinically meaningful data was in the exploration of personality.[19] This concept was originally suggested by Binet and received a great deal of attention in the research literature given the early lack of adequate personality tests and theories. Assumptions in this research area have argued that personality differences could be reflected in the patterning of intellectual function and therefore could be observed in intelligence test data. Later, the hypothesis that one could identify pathological personality characteristics from test performance prompted increased interest in the WAIS. Research in this area does not support the utility of a differential diagnosis using the quantitative data from the WAIS.[20] However, many clinicians use both intertest and intratest scatter on the WAIS subscales as potential indices of personality disorders. For example, anxiety tends to selectively lower arithmetic and digit span scores, whereas alcoholism lowers block design performance and depression has been reported to lower performance IQs. However, no single pattern of test scores from the WAIS has been demonstrated for any disorder such as schizophrenia or depression.[20] These results are not surprising given the definition of intelligence as a multidimensional construct and that the purpose of the WAIS is to provide an index of intelligence, not personality.

An additional reason for the failure of tests such as the WAIS to provide information with regard to personality concerns the wide range of factors that affect performance on the WAIS. Both normal and abnormal personality factors might influence test performance, but when these factors are considered in conjunction with other variables, the picture becomes even more complex. Given the correlations that exist between WAIS performance and other variables, such as education, mentioned above, it is not surprising to find that interpretations of IQ data need to consider such variables as age, education, socioeconomic status, etc. in order to arrive at a clear picture of an individual's intellectual ability. If one considers what each of the WAIS subtests is designed to assess, it becomes clear that education, cultural background, and even occupation will serve to either raise or lower IQ scores to some extent. In fact, one of the major issues in developmental psychology and gerontology has been whether or not intelligence as measured by the WAIS and similar instruments declines with increasing age.[3] Longitudinal studies would indicate that performance does not decline until advanced age. Yet cross-sectional data show clear age differences in performance. One explanation of these data points to differences in performance. Another explanation points to differences in education, culture, life experiences, and so on that are due to generational differences. Succeeding generations are becoming increasingly more educated, sophisticated, and "test wise." These generational or birth cohort differences could account for the differences found in the literature that indicate that intelligence declines with age.

In summary, given that intelligence is a multidetermined concept, it is perhaps not surprising that different physical and mental states often lead to different results on the WAIS. The information obtained from the WAIS is useful given the proven correlation between IQ scores and many other predictors.[18,27] Further, the WAIS provides an excellent index of a person's problem solving skills and intellectual strengths and weaknesses. In the context of diagnosis, however, data from the WAIS are perhaps best viewed in the general context of other and perhaps more specific assessment data.

Neuropsychology

Often, it becomes necessary to assess more specific intellectual functions. Generally speaking, the examiner might wish to assess more directly receptive functions such as perceptual organization, the integration of sensory input, or various forms of agnosia. Further assessment might require focusing on attention, concentration, or expressive functions such as speaking, writing, and drawing. Finally, the examiner may wish to assess the patient's memory functioning, which may be central to the person's total intellectual functioning. The WAIS provides an initial measure of many of these cognitive activities. For example, items on the information and digit span subtests tap the memory store and working memory. However, more specific assessments may be required for adequate diagnosis of a person's capabilities and shortcomings. As a result of these needs and a concern with the intellectual and emotional expression of brain dysfunction, much of what is commonly recognized as clinical psychological assessment is slowly being complemented by neuropsychological testing.

Neuropsychological testing and research in this country could be divided into three major approaches: (1) Halstead-Reitan, (2) Luria, and (3) eclectic. The Halstead-Reitan (H-R) battery of tests was developed by Ward Halstead at the University of Chicago and later refined by Ralph Reitan. The Halstead-Reitan battery is the result of a collaborative effort by neuropsychologists, neurologists, and neurosurgeons and was originally intended to be a study of the frontal lobes. The H-R battery is a lengthy (up to 8 h), complex, and fixed battery with perhaps the most complete investigative history in the field of neuropsychology. The H-R often serves as the standard against which the reliability and validity of other instruments are judged. The cognitive domains tested by the H-R include problem solving, expressive and receptive language, attention, concentration, the ability to reproduce simple designs, complex motor performance, simple motor skills, and incidental learning.[2,22] As a test battery, the H-R is very demanding of patients and is difficult to interpret. However, the utility of the H-R battery has been demonstrated repeatedly. For example, Filskov and Goldstein[9] have shown the H-R to be more accurate for diagnosing type of damage and laterality than brain scans, EEGs, angiograms, pneumoencephalograms, or skull x-rays in patients with known etiology.

Luria's work in Russia is well known in the medical and psychological literature and provides the basis for the second neuropsychological approach. Until recently, the subjective and complex nature of Luria's technique has precluded its widespread acceptance among professionals in this country. Charles Golden has recently presented a shortened (3 h), quantified version of the Luria technique that is presently receiving widespread attention in the psychological literature.[10] The shorter nature of Golden's instrument when compared with the H-R and the simplicity of some of the test items appear to be a major advantage with certain patient groups.

Finally, the eclectic approach is best exemplified by the work of the Boston Aphasia Center group and is more traditionally clinical in its approach. Techniques such as the Bender Gestalt Test or the Benton Visual Retention Test are individually chosen for administration depending on patient characteristics, the clinical question, and experience of the clinician. Such an approach is a familiar one to the medical practitioner. In this approach, the reliability and validity of the evaluation are more clearly dependent on the expertise of the examiner in choosing and integrating test data.

Since diagnosis, patient care, and the study of the organization of brain function as it relates to behavior are the hallmarks of neuropsychology, it is perhaps not surprising that neuropsychological techniques can provide information regarding the often subtle changes in behavior that result from metabolic changes, head injury, and neurosurgical procedures. In this fashion, serial testing of the patient during recovery or where a progressive condition is suspected possibly constitutes the most useful aspect of psychological testing. Typically, because of the nature of the test and the subtlety of sequelae in certain conditions (e.g., closed head injury), serial testing can focus on cognitive aspects other than general intelligence such as memory (New York Memory Test; Buschke-Fuld Selective Reminding) or speed of processing (e.g., Gronwall procedure). Clinical and research experience suggests that a patient may show recovery to almost premorbid IQ levels and still be severely debilitated by cognitive dysfunction. With appropriate tests, the patient can be prevented from prematurely returning to school or work and suffering unnecessary and often traumatic failures. The key factor in this approach is to assess whether or not the patient can function under the speed and complexity

demands of the real world. In such cases, neuropsychological testing is useful in predicting future behavior as well as assessing the efficacy of any intervention efforts geared toward restoring lost functioning.

Personality

A second area in which psychological testing provides relevant data is in the assessment of personality. As is the case for intelligence, the hypothetical construct of personality can be assigned many different meanings, even though everyone has an intuitive notion about personality. Generally, we refer to the combination of a person's stable attitudes, habits, preferences, talents, values, etc. when we attempt a description of personality. Still, this multidimensionality has helped foster numerous definitions of personality where even intelligence is seen as a personality characteristic. Practically, however, it is perhaps best to conceptualize personality as reflecting a person's unique and enduring behavior patterns.

Given that personality, like intelligence, is a function of a great number of different factors, it is not surprising that there are numerous definitions of the concept and that different theories tend to focus on different factors or groups of factors in explaining personality. In general, five major approaches emphasizing the biological, psychodynamic, social, cognitive, and humanistic aspects of personality can be found in the literature. Attempts to elaborate on these theoretical approaches or to verify various elements of these theories have relied on one or more personality inventories or tests. The need for the evaluation of the emotional fitness for warfare that paralleled the need for intellectual assessment during the world wars also prompted the development of objective and projective analogues to the psychiatric interview. The objective and projective inventories that developed can generally be differentiated on the basis of the test's stimulus ambiguity and the nature of the response requested from the subject. Projective techniques such as the Rorschach test are classified as unstructured in that there are essentially an unlimited number and type of responses that can be elicited by the inkblot stimuli. Further, given that there is no single set of standard principles for test administration and scoring, a great deal of clinical expertise is required to interpret a projective test. Structured (objective) tests such as the MMPI are based on standardized principles where the subject is required to make some choice from a set of responses. Historically, objective tests have been constructed by statistically selecting items that differentiate between known groups (MMPI), starting with a set of hypotheses in advance and constructing items based on the hypotheses, or using factor analytic techniques.

Objective and projective personality tests differ in philosophy as well as in method. Projective techniques employ ambiguous stimuli not only to give the person a greater freedom in response, but also to allow the individual to impose a "projection" of his or her own personality. Many clinicians also assume that the symbolic quality of projective techniques circumvents an individual's automatic psychological defenses that might be invoked by more direct questions.

Further, projective tests appear to place less of an emphasis on a person's intellect. For an interesting model of what aspects of a person various personality and cognitive tests measure, the reader may refer to Wagner's[23] discussion of structural analysis, which provides a framework for selecting and interpreting psychological test data. Most of the common projective techniques such as the Rorschach test, thematic apperception test, hand test, etc. all contain stimuli that appear to elicit reliable and interpretable responses. These responses are in turn scored and then interpreted as an analogue to personality.

Objective personality tests are more standardized than are projective techniques and therefore can be handled more objectively and statistically. Further, objective tests are more easily administered and scored than their projective counterparts. Early objective measures did have some disadvantages, however. First, many relied on single personality traits and so were inadequate in describing personality. Also, many of the answers on a test could be faked in attempts to avoid issues or to present a very positive or negative picture of oneself. Also, some persons were unable to accurately respond to the test questions on an inventory because of an apparent lack of insight, while cultural factors appeared to have undetermined effects on the results of the inventories. One inventory, however, that attempted to deal with some of the problems evident in the early objective personality tests was the MMPI.[13]

As an objective personality measure, the MMPI provides a multidimensional approach to personality. In comparison to other objective inventories, the MMPI also ranks first in the amount of research activity and is the most widely used inventory of its type in clinical settings.[17] The MMPI was published in 1943 as a test to differentiate between normal subjects and a wide range of psychiatric groups.[13] Originally, a group of over 500 self-reference statements were chosen from psychiatric interviews and given to the criterion groups mentioned below. Once the items were administered to the criterion groups, item analyses were conducted to determine which items would show consistent group differences between normal subjects and the diagnostic categories of hypochondriasis, depression, hysteria, psychopathic deviate, paranoia, psychasthenia, schizophrenia, and hypomania. Later, items that appeared to discriminate between these groups were administered to new groups of individuals who also fit into the various criterion groups in order to validate the test. Additional scales were later added to identify homosexual males (later to differentiate normal males and females) and to identify outgoing versus socially withdrawn individuals. Four additional scales were added to detect deviant test taking and to minimize faking. The final result was an inventory of 566 true-false items represented as the 14 scales (4 validity and 10 clinical) described below.

The first of the four validity scales is the "cannot say" scale. This scale simply reflects the number of items that the subject has omitted or keyed both true and false. Usually when over 30 items are omitted, the test protocol is suspect and often is not interpreted. Problems with item omission can be reduced by encouraging the subject to try to respond to all of the items and by a quick visual check by the examiner for omissions. Items are usually omitted as a result of carelessness, a lack of information, or attempts to avoid

admission of undesirable personal characteristics. The L scale is the second validity scale, and high scores tend to reflect a person's attempt to look good by denying minor weaknesses that most people are willing to acknowledge. Low L scores tend to reflect higher socioeconomic status as well as frank responses to the items. High scores on the third validity, or F scale, may also indicate an invalid profile. Originally this scale was created to detect atypical or deviant responses to test items. Therefore, if the MMPI profile still appears to be valid, an elevated F score becomes a good index of psychopathology. Low F scores tend however to indicate social conformity or an attempt to look good. The last validity scale is the K scale. This scale was developed as a more subtle version of the L scale in order to detect defensive and inhibited response styles (high scores), exaggeration of problems (low score), and as a statistical correction factor.

Traditionally, the clinical scales of the MMPI were labeled for the criterion groups for which the test was originally developed. Recent trends in psychology, however, have tended to de-emphasize diagnostic labels. Attempts to lessen the impact of stereotypes associated with diagnostic labels has led to the adoption of scale numbers instead of the original scale names of the MMPI. For discussion purposes, however, both the old scale name and scale number will be presented.

Scale 1 (hypochondriasis) was developed to identify persons who showed excessive somatic complaints. High scale 1 scores tend to be associated with persons complaining of chronic pain, fatigue, and weakness affecting diverse bodily systems. Scale 1 scores also increase with age, physical illness, and somatic depression. Low scores will indicate persons who are fairly free of these concerns.

Scale 2 originally was intended to assess symptomatic depression. Characteristics of persons who show high scale 2 (depression) scores include dissatisfaction, irritability, lack of self-confidence, and a depressive state. Low scale scores reflect self-confidence, emotional stability, impulsiveness, and a freedom from psychological tension, guilt, and depression.

Scale 3 (hysteria) was constructed to identify individuals who showed involuntary losses of physical function in reaction to stressful situations. High scale 3 scores therefore suggest that the person may react to stress by developing somatic problems including headaches, chest pains, tachycardia, and attacks of anxiety. Additionally, high scores tend to indicate a person who lacks insight into his or her problems and is passive, immature, and often resistant to treatment. Low scores on scale 3 are usually seen as indicative of untrusting and unadventurous persons.

The fourth clinical scale was designed to identify asocial or amoral personalities more commonly referred to as sociopaths. High scorers on scale 4 are usually rebellious, tend to engage in a wide variety of antisocial behaviors, and often show excessive alcohol and drug usage problems. Additionally, these persons appear to be free of any psychosocial guilt or turmoil with regard to their actions while demonstrating aggressive tendencies and often sexual acting out behavior. Lower scale 4 scores reflect persons who accept authority but who may also be passive, conventional, and noncompetitive.

The masculinity-femininity scale, or scale 5, was initially

designed to detect homosexual males. However, high scale 5 scores for males are interpreted as indicating unstereotyped masculine interests, creativity, sensitivity, self-control, and high education. Low scores for males tend to reflect an over-emphasis on physical prowess and stereotyped male interests in work, sports, and hobbies. High scores for females tend to reflect masculine interests, assertiveness, and a rejection of the traditional female role. Low scores on the other hand indicate the acceptance of traditional female values. If the low scorer is a hospitalized female psychiatric patient, she is unlikely to be psychotic.

The sixth scale, or paranoia scale, tends to identify persons who have feelings of persecution, are suspicious, and may exhibit psychotic behavior. Very low scores on scale 6 also indicate a person who may have delusions and is shy, secretive, and withdrawn. Mild elevations or moderately low scores on this scale are usually seen as fairly balanced and emotionally healthy individuals.

Scale 7 (psychasthenia) was intended to identify persons whose thoughts reflected unreasonable fears and doubts and closely resembled the diagnostic category of obsessive-compulsive neurosis. This scale appears to be a good index of psychological turmoil, anxiety, agitation, and tension. Lowered scores reflect self-confidence and good adjustment.

Schizophrenia was the eighth scale to be included in the MMPI. Scores on scale 8 reflect a wide range of behaviors, including bizarre thoughts, hallucinations, sexual concerns, and other psychotic symptoms. Scores on this scale also appear to reflect adolescent turmoil. Extremely high scores are usually not generated by psychotics but by persons who are in acute turmoil or are crying out for help. Otherwise, a high score reflects psychotic behavior, confusion, feelings of isolation, and so on. Low scale 8 scores usually are obtained by individuals who are friendly, trustful, but who also may avoid deep emotional commitments.

Scale 9, or hypomania, attempted to identify irritability, elevated mood, grandiosity, and the likelihood of impulsive behavior in patients. High scores are indicative of excessive activity, low tolerance of frustration, and depressive episodes. Low scores reflect apathy, overcontrol, and a lack of self-confidence.

The last scale on the MMPI was designed to assess social introversion and extroversion. High scorers on scale 0 tend to be socially introverted, reserved, and unlikely to openly display their feelings. Low scores are indicative of persons who are socially extroverted, competitive, impulsive, and highly expressive.

Numerous other subscales of the MMPI have been developed over the years by combining test items in different fashions in an effort to identify social maladjustment, poor morale, organic symptoms, phobias, family problems, and heterosexual discomfort, just to mention a few.[8] Subscales of the ten standard clinical scales have also been developed. For example, scale 2, or depression, has five subscales for subjective depression, psychomotor retardation, physical malfunctioning, mental dullness, and brooding. Nearly 500 scales of these types have been developed.[7] Many of these scales have been constructed for very specific populations (i.e., alcoholics) and research purposes. Interested readers can refer to any of the many MMPI guides and handbooks for specific scales and research on particular populations.[6,7,11]

The MMPI is usually administered to patients who are at least 16 years of age and have at least a sixth grade reading level, although a tape-recorded form is also available. Once the subject's answers are scored, a K-scale correction is added to the raw scale scores, and then the results are converted into standard scores with a mean of 50 and a standard deviation of 10. Interpretation of these scores, however, has shifted from the predictive validity of the MMPI to a construct validity emphasis as a result of a large number of research studies.[12] Therefore, when a person obtains a score on a given scale, the practitioner can infer that the patient is indicating characteristics or behaviors that are similar to those shown by other persons with similar scores on that scale.

According to Graham[12] proficient interpretation of the MMPI requires a good knowledge of the research involving the MMPI. A general interpretive strategy of the MMPI looks at (1) the patient's test-taking attitude, (2) the general level of the patient's adjustment, (3) the behaviors that can be inferred from the test scores, (4) which psychological dynamics underlie the patient's behaviors, (5) which appropriate diagnostic labels apply, and (6) the implications for treatment. In general one must also consider demographic information in the interpretation of test scores. More educated subjects tend to score higher on scales K, 3, and 5 and score lower on L than do less educated subjects. Older adults show higher scores on scales 1, 2, and 0, and younger patients show elevated scores on scales F, 4, 8, and 9 when compared with each other. Racial differences are also evidenced. Compared with white patients black patients score higher on scales F, 4, 8, and 9.

Reliability (test-retest) for the MMPI is very high for short time intervals of 1 month or less. This reliability is substantially lower for periods greater than 1 month even though the general pattern of scores is reliable. These data, of course, are more likely to reflect the changes that occur in the many dimensions of personality over time rather than problems with the MMPI as a measurement instrument. The validity of the MMPI has been demonstrated in literally thousands of studies, and has led Graham[12] to suggest that the MMPI might be the most valid instrument available for personality assessment. Clearly, when used with other test data such as the WAIS, case history, and observational data, the MMPI proves to be a most valuable tool. What is most intriguing about the MMPI as an instrument is that it has not fared well in meeting the purpose for which it was constructed, namely the diagnosis of psychotic patients. The validity of the MMPI appears to rest in its construct validity, its success with neurotics, and the sheer number of nontest correlates of the various scales and items.

For example, numerous subscales of the MMPI have been developed over the years in efforts to detect various types of problems. One such area has been the detection of alcohol- and drug-related problems. Research in this area has shown that subscales of the MMPI reliably differentiate (55 to 82 percent hit rates) alcoholics from normal subjects and psychiatric patients. These same subscales do not, however, fare well in the differentiation of alcoholics and drug abusers, although the test is highly successful (69 to 94 percent hit rate) in differentiating alcoholics and/or drug abusers from groups of psychiatric patients.[7,11]

The MMPI has also received extensive use with medical

patients. Some of the areas in which the MMPI has served as a research instrument include the prediction of surgery outcome, speed of recovery from various illnesses, the delineation of psychosomatic disorders, and the differentiation of organic from psychosomatic problems. To date, much of this type of research has been inconclusive however. Some of the more promising data have shown elevations on scale 2, obtained before the diagnosis of cancer, to be correlated with findings of malignancy. On the other hand, Reitan in a review of the research on the neurological and physiological bases of psychopathology concluded that the localization of brain damage was not reflected by patterns or specific MMPI items.[20] More recent research, however, employed a key approach to successfully differentiate patients with organic disorders from psychiatric patients with a 78 percent accuracy rate.[21]

References

1. Anastasi A: *Psychological Testing*, 4th ed. New York, Macmillan, 1976.
2. Boll TJ: The Halstead-Reitan neuropsychology battery, in Filskov SB, Boll TJ (eds): *Handbook of Clinical Neuropsychology*. New York, Wiley-Interscience, 1981, pp 577–607.
3. Botwinick J: Intellectual abilities, in Birren JE, and Schaie KW (eds): *Handbook of the Psychology of Aging*. New York, Van Nostrand Reinhold, 1977, pp 580–605.
4. Buros OK: *The Seventh Mental Measurements Yearbook*. Highland Park, NJ, Gryphon Press, 1972.
5. Cronbach LJ: *Essentials of Psychological Testing*, 3d ed. New York, Harper & Row, 1970.
6. Dahlstrom WG, Welsh GS, Dahlstrom LE: *An MMPI Handbook, vol I: Clinical Interpretation*. Minneapolis, University of Minnesota Press, 1972.
7. Dahlstrom WG, Welsh GS, Dahlstrom LE: *An MMPI Handbook, vol II: Research Applications*. Minneapolis, University of Minnesota Press, 1975.
8. Davison AL, Reitan RM: *Clinical Neuropsychology: Current Status and Applications*. Washington, DC, Wiley, 1974.
9. Filskov SB, Goldstein SG: Diagnostic validity of the Halstead-Reitan Neuropsychological battery. J Consult Clin Psychol 42:382–388, 1974.
10. Golden CJ: A standardized version of Luria's Neuropsychological Tests: A quantitative and qualitative approach to neuropsychological evaluation, in Filskov SB and Boll TJ (eds): *Handbook of Clinical Neuropsychology*. New York, Wiley-Interscience, 1981, pp 608–642.
11. Graham JR: *The MMPI: A Practical Guide*. New York, Oxford University Press, 1977.
12. Graham JR: The Minnesota Multiphasic Personality Inventory (MMPI), in Wolman BB (ed): *Clinical Diagnosis of Mental Disorders*. New York, Plenum, 1978, pp 311–331.
13. Hathaway SR, McKinley JC: *The Minnesota Multiphasic Personality Inventory Manual*. New York, Psychological Corporation, 1967.
14. Horn JL, Cattell RB: Age differences in fluid and crystallized intelligence. Acta Psychol (Amst) 26:107–129, 1967.
15. Jarvik LF, Falek A: Intellectual stability and survival in the aged. J Gerontol 18:173–176, 1963.
16. Lezak MD: *Neuropsychological Assessment*. New York, Oxford Univ Press, 1976.
17. Lubin B, Wallis RR, Paine C: Patterns of psychological test usage in the United States: 1935–1969. Prof Psychol 2:70–74, 1971.
18. Matarazzo JD, Wechsler D: *Wechsler's Measurement and Appraisal of Adult Intelligence*, 5th ed. Baltimore, Williams & Wilkins, 1976.
19. Rapaport D, Gill MM, Schafer R: *Diagnostic Psychological Testing*. Holt RR (ed)., New York, International Universities Press, 1979.
20. Reitan RM: Neurological and physiological bases of psychopathology. Ann Rev Psychol 27:189–216, 1976.
21. Russell EW: Validation of a brain-damage versus schizophrenia MMPI key. J Clin Psychol 31:659–661, 1975.
22. Russell EW, Neuringer C, Goldstein G: *Assessment of Brain Damage: A Neuropsychological Key Approach*. New York, Wiley-Interscience, 1970.
23. Wagner EE: Personality dimensions measured by projective techniques: A formulation based on structural analysis. Percep Mot Skills 43:247–253, 1976.
24. Wechsler D: *Wechsler Adult Intelligence Scale Manual*. New York, Psychological Corporation, 1955.
25. Wechsler D: *The Measurement and Appraisal of Adult Intelligence*, 4th ed. Baltimore, Williams & Wilkins, 1958.
26. Wechsler D: *Wechsler Adult Intelligence Scale—Revised Manual*. New York, Psychological Corporation, 1981.
27. Zimmerman, IL, Woo-Sam JM: *Clinical Interpretation of the Wechsler Adult Intelligence Scale*. New York, Grune & Stratton, 1973.

7

Cranial Nerve Examination

Setti S. Rengachary

Introduction

Cranial nerves are generally examined sequentially. A thorough working knowledge of the peripheral distribution and central connections of the cranial nerves is essential for a meaningful interpretation of abnormalities found on clinical examination. The amount of time a clinician spends in clinical neurological assessment of a patient is to a degree inversely proportional to his or her grasp of anatomy and pathology of the nervous system.

The cranial nerves II, III, IV, VI and VIII are discussed elsewhere in this textbook. The remaining cranial nerves are discussed in this chapter.

Olfactory Nerve

Anatomy

Olfactory sensation is phylogenetically among the oldest of sensory functions. In primitive mammals this system is highly developed, constituting a major portion of their cerebral hemispheres. With evolution, higher primates, including humans, are less dependent on this function, yet the basic architecture of the olfactory system and its intricate central connections with the limbic system and certain brain stem nuclei are conserved. The olfactory system in the human is thus intimately associated with structures that subserve emotional expression and visceral function.

The olfactory epithelium or membrane (that part of the nasal mucous membrane containing the peripheral receptors for olfaction) is located in the roof of the nasal cavity and the adjacent lateral wall and septum. The olfactory receptors are bipolar nerve cells that are surrounded by non-neural supporting cells. The peripheral processes of the neurons extend to the surface, where they project as multiple ciliary processes (Fig. 7-1). The latter are covered with mucus. Odorant gaseous particles go into solution in this mucus and stimulate the bipolar neurons by a molecular mechanism whose details are as yet uncertain. The central unmyelinated processes collected approximately in 25 filaments constitute the true olfactory nerves. The olfactory nerves penetrate the

openings in the cribriform plate and synapse with the dendrites of the mitral cells contained in the olfactory bulb, forming the glomerulus. The axons of the mitral cells course posteriorly to form the olfactory tract. They give off occasional collaterals in the olfactory bulb that end on small granule cells, which in turn project back to the glomerulus forming a reinforcing circuit (Fig. 7-1).

The olfactory tract courses back to the anterior perforated substance. The anterior olfactory nucleus is a minor relay nucleus formed by a group of scattered cells located at the base of the olfactory tract. A small fraction of the olfactory tract axons end in the anterior olfactory nucleus. The nucleus in turn sends fibers into the olfactory tract. At the rostral limit of the anterior perforated substance, the olfactory tract divides into medial and lateral olfactory striae. A few fibers of the tract synapse on the cells of the anterior perforated substance, which in macrosmatic animals is highly developed and forms the olfactory tubercle (Fig. 7-2).

Each olfactory stria is associated with a thin band of gray matter, the lateral and medial olfactory gyri. The lateral olfactory stria courses along the rostrolateral border of the anterior perforated substance and enters into the temporal lobe. Its fibers terminate in the lateral olfactory gyrus, periamygdaloid area, parts of the amygdaloid nucleus, and the rostral segment of the parahippocampal gyrus. These structures represent the primary olfactory cortex and are known collectively as the pyriform lobe. The lateral olfactory gyrus is synonymous with the prepyriform area and with the remainder of the pyriform lobe is often referred to as the entorhinal cortex.

The majority of the fibers in the medial olfactory stria enter the medial surface of the cerebral hemisphere and terminate in the parolfactory area, septum pellucidum, and the subcallosal area. These latter structures collectively constitute the septal area. The remaining fibers in the medial olfactory stria cross in the anterior commissure to the opposite hemisphere to terminate in the anterior olfactory nucleus and olfactory bulb, forming another reinforcing circuit. There are three important discharge pathways from the various central olfactory areas mentioned above to lower centers that may be involved in mediating olfactory reflexes. They are the (1) medial forebrain bundle, (2) stria medullaris thalami, and (3) stria terminalis.

Method of Testing

The test substance chosen for evaluating the sense of smell should be a mild perfume or aromatic substance such as oil of cloves, cinnamon, peppermint, lemon, wintergreen, lavender, almonds, or chocolate or freshly ground coffee. A deodorant soap or a package of cigarettes readily available at bedside are acceptable substitutes. Pungent or irritating substances such as ammonia or strong acetic acid stimulate the endings of the trigeminal nerve and are thus not appropriate substances for testing the olfactory function.

A brief inspection of the nose is made to determine if there are any obvious local conditions that may interfere with testing of the olfactory sense such as the common cold, deviated nasal septum, occlusive nasal polyps, chronic atrophic rhinitis, etc. With the patient's eyes closed, the test

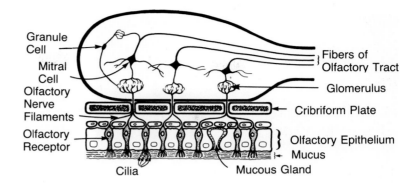

Figure 7-1 Anatomy of the olfactory nerves and the olfactory bulb.

odor is placed under one nostril, while the other is occluded. The patient is asked to sniff and indicate whether he or she can smell something and if so to identify it. The test is repeated with the opposite nostril. Quantitative methods for testing smell are available for research purposes but have no practical diagnostic value at the bedside.

Clinical Significance

Anosmia or inability to perceive olfaction denotes impairment of peripheral olfactory pathways—receptors, olfactory nerves, or olfactory bulb or tract. Lesions that are more central do not produce anosmia. Anosmia should be clearly distinguished from failure to identify the odor. The latter depends on other factors such as previous familiarity with the odor and ability to recall, and is thus a higher cortical function. Impairment or loss of sense of smell, especially when unilateral, is not apparent to the patient and may be missed unless tested objectively. Bilateral anosmia is more frequently seen than unilateral anosmia. It is not uncommon for a patient with bilateral anosmia to complain of loss of taste (ageusia) as well, although objective testing may not show any loss of elementary taste sensations. It underscores the fact that we tend to customarily combine the sense of taste and smell into one common sensation, that of flavor. The common cold is the most frequent cause of bilateral anosmia.

Head injury with fracture across the cribriform plate may result in tearing of olfactory nerve filaments, resulting in anosmia. The clinical triad, in the acute stage, indicative of a fracture across the anterior cranial fossa, are cerebrospinal fluid rhinorrhea, anosmia, and bilateral periorbital ecchymosis (raccoon eyes) (Fig. 7-3). Occasionally a surprisingly minor blow to the occipital area may result in anosmia, probably from shearing of the olfactory nerve filaments. The olfactory nerves and tracts are at risk during bilateral subfrontal intradural explorations using a bicoronal flap.

The gradual development of unilateral anosmia is most significant clinically, and is generally representative of a subfrontal tumor. An olfactory groove meningioma involves the olfactory tract and produces unilateral anosmia in the early stages. As the tumor extends posteriorly, the optic nerve may be compressed, resulting in ipsilateral optic atrophy. With further growth, there is increased intracranial pressure resulting in papilledema on the contralateral side. This rare clinical triad consisting of ipsilateral anosmia, ipsilateral optic atrophy, and contralateral papilledema constitutes the Foster Kennedy syndrome. In this condition, compression of the frontal lobes by the massive tumor may induce certain characteristic changes in behavior such as apathy, lack of initiative, lack of insight, and loss of social inhibitions.

Congenital anosmia occurs in albinos. This is thought to be due to the absence of olfactory pigment.

Olfactory hallucinations may represent the aura of a par-

Figure 7-2 Central connections of the olfactory pathways.

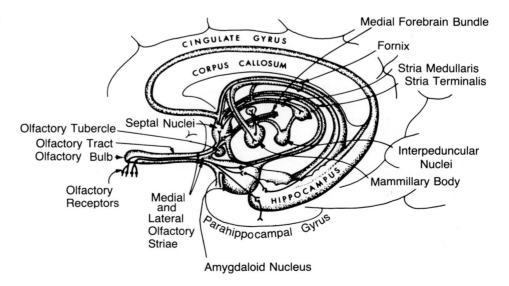

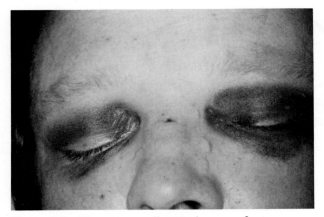

Figure 7-3 "Raccoon eyes" secondary to a fracture across the anterior cranial fossa.

tial complex seizure. The seizure focus is usually in the region of uncus and hence the term *uncinate fits*. The patient describes a powerful and unpleasant smell or taste such as that of rotten eggs, burnt rag, gasoline, or paint, etc. This may be followed by loss of consciousness, smacking of the lips, or chewing movements.

Parosmia or perverted sense of smell may be noted in suppurative infections of the upper airway such as empyema of the paranasal sinuses. Trauma to the olfactory nerves or bulbs may result in parosmia. Elderly individuals who are depressed may complain of parosmia without an apparent organic basis.

Trigeminal Nerve

Anatomy

The trigeminal nerve is a mixed sensorimotor nerve and is the largest of the cranial nerves. It is the principal somesthetic nerve of the head and innervates the muscles of mastication.

The majority of the cell bodies of its sensory neurons are located in the trigeminal (semilunar, gasserian) ganglion. A few subserving exclusively proprioceptive function are located in the mesencephalic nucleus of the trigeminal nerve. The sensory neurons are unipolar, giving rise to fibers that bifurcate. The peripheral processes are distributed via the three divisions of the nerve, namely ophthalmic, maxillary, and mandibular. The central processes constitute the sensory root or portio major. It enters the pons through the middle of the brachium pontis (middle cerebellar peduncle) and divides into short ascending and long descending fibers (Fig. 7-4). The descending root is concerned primarily with pain, temperature, and poorly localized touch, while the ascending root serves light touch, two-point discrimination, and proprioception. The descending root courses through the pons and the lateral aspect of the medulla and blends with the zone of Lissauer in the upper cervical segments of the cord. The fibers in the descending root terminate in the adjoining descending nucleus at multiple levels. The descending nucleus is functionally continuous with the substantia gelatinosa of the cervical cord. It has three subdivisions: subnucleus caudalis, interpolaris, and oralis.

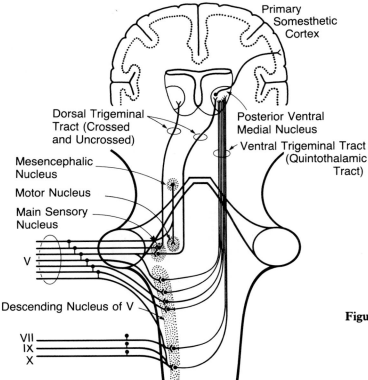

Figure 7-4 Central connections of the trigeminal nerve.

Sensory representation of the face in the descending nucleus is concentric, with the fibers carrying sensation from further out on the face entering the descending nucleus at progressively lower levels. This arrangement of pain and temperature fibers from the face in the brain stem is denoted as representing an "onion-skin" pattern and may be of value in localizing lesions in the brain stem and upper cervical cord (Fig. 7-5A). The second order of fibers arising from the descending nucleus cross the midline and ascend in a diffuse tract called the ventral trigeminal tract to terminate in the ventral posterior medial nucleus of the thalamus. Tertiary fibers from this nucleus project via the internal capsule to the inferior portion of the postcentral gyrus. Fibers subserving light touch and tactile discrimination in the ascending root terminate in the main sensory nucleus. Secondary fibers from this nucleus constitute the dorsal trigeminal tract and project to the ventral posterior medial nuclei of both sides. Central connections to the postcentral gyrus are similar to those of the ventral trigeminal tract.

The mesencephalic nucleus contains unipolar neurons. Their peripheral processes carry proprioceptive sensation from the muscles of mastication, and their central processes project to the motor nucleus of the trigeminal nerve. This is the anatomical substrate for the jaw jerk, which is a monosynaptic reflex similar to other muscle stretch reflexes.

The facial, glossopharyngeal, and vagus nerves each have a general somatic afferent component. The cell bodies of these sensory neurons are unipolar and are located in the geniculate ganglion of the facial, superior ganglion of the glossopharyngeal, and jugular ganglion of the vagus nerves. Their peripheral processes are distributed to the meninges of the posterior cranial fossa and the skin over the pinna and external auditory meatus. All of their central processes terminate in the descending nucleus of the trigeminal nerve (Fig. 7-4). Thus the trigeminal sensory nuclear system receives all of the general somatic afferents of the cranial nerves.

The peripheral distribution of the trigeminal nerve is as follows (Fig. 7-5B): the *ophthalmic division* passes forward in the cavernous sinus close to its outer wall and below the oculomotor and trochlear nerves. Immediately before entering the orbit through the superior orbital fissure it divides into three branches: lacrimal, frontal, and nasociliary. They carry sensations from the forehead, eyes, nose, temples, meninges, paranasal sinuses, and part of the nasal mucosa.

The *maxillary division* passes through the foramen rotundum into the pterygopalatine (sphenomaxillary) fossa. The nerve then passes through the inferior orbital fissure, crosses the floor of the orbit, and emerges through the infraorbital foramen. The sensory input from the upper jaw, teeth, and lip, cheeks, hard palate, maxillary sinuses, and nasal mucosa is carried through this division.

The *mandibular division* leaves the skull through the foramen ovale. It contains sensory and motor components. The motor component has its origin in the midpons; the fibers (portio minor) pass underneath the gasserian ganglion and become incorporated into the mandibular nerve. It innervates the following muscles: masseter, temporalis, medial and lateral pterygoids, mylohyoid, anterior belly of the digastric, tensor tympani, and tensor veli palatini. The sensory component receives input from the lower jaw, teeth, lip, and buccal mucosa, anterior two-thirds of the tongue, and parts of the external auditory meatus and meninges.

Clinical Testing

Sensory Testing

The patient is instructed to close his or her eyes and respond (1) when touched with a wisp of cotton, (2) when stuck with a pin, and (3) when touched with test tubes filled with warm and cold water. The representative areas chosen for preliminary evaluation are the forehead for the ophthalmic division, the malar region for the maxillary division, and the chin for the mandibular division. Any anesthetic zone is carefully mapped out. An assessment should be made if the anesthetic pattern corresponds to a peripheral division of the trigeminal nerve (Fig. 7-5B) or segmental distribution (onion-skin pattern) of the descending tract or nucleus (Fig. 7-5A) and if the sensory loss involves all modalities or only the sensations of pain and temperature with preservation of light touch (dissociated anesthesia). It is well to remember that the skin over the angle of the mandible is not supplied by the fifth nerve but by the greater auricular nerve from the second cervical segment. Contrary to the significant overlap one observes between adjacent dermatomes over the rest of the body (especially the trunk), overlap between cutaneous zones of major divisions of the trigeminal nerve tend to be minimal. Sensory defects in the face therefore tend to be better defined.

In patients with suspected trigeminal neuralgia, "trigger zones" that precipitate pain when touched lightly may be detected. The most common trigger area is on the lower lip near the angle of the mouth. The trigger zones tend to be located at the terminal distribution of one of the trigeminal divisions (usually the third), and not along the border of an adjacent dermatomal area. Neuropathic keratitis (Fig. 7-6) or erosion of the alae nasi, two of the trophic changes seen in the face, are hallmarks of trigeminal sensory loss.

Corneal Reflex

The afferent pathway for this reflex is through the ophthalmic division of the trigeminal nerve, and the efferent component that produces the blink response is through the facial nerve. The reflex is evoked by gently touching or strok-

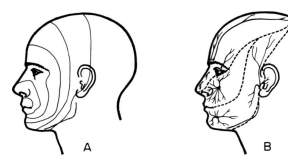

Figure 7-5 *A.* "Onion-skin" pattern of sensory representation of the face (pain and temperature) in the brain stem. *B.* Peripheral distribution of the three major divisions of the trigeminal nerve.

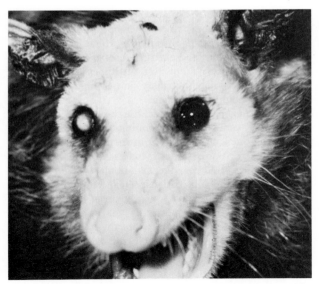

Figure 7-6 Experimentally induced neuropathic keratitis in an opossum.

ing the cornea with a wisp of moistened cotton. To avoid reflex blinking from visual threat, the stimulus is applied from the side while the patient is looking in the opposite direction (Fig. 7-7). It is important that the cornea be touched, not just the bulbar conjunctiva. Although conjunctival stimulation frequently produces a blink response, the conjunctival blink reflex may be absent in normal individuals, especially those with a high sensory threshold. A normal corneal reflex consists of an immediate blink response bilaterally. When the corneal reflex appears asymmetric, it is worthwhile asking the patient if the stimulus is felt equally on both sides before any interpretation is made. In the presence of trigeminal nerve impairment, the direct and consensual response will be absent when stimulated on the affected side, but the normal response is elicited on stimulation of the contralateral side. With facial paralysis, blinking will occur only on the nonparalyzed side when either cornea is stimulated.

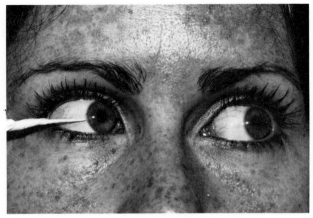

Figure 7-7 Method of eliciting corneal reflex.

The corneal reflex is an extremely sensitive reflex. Not infrequently, a decreased corneal reflex may be the sole evidence of trigeminal nerve impairment. Cerebellopontine angle masses may produce a decrease in the corneal reflex well before there is any subjective or objective evidence of sensory loss in the face. The depth of general anesthesia or depth of coma from any cause may be gauged from the corneal reflex response.

A blink reflex elicited by electrical stimulation of the supraorbital nerve with oscilloscopic recording of the motor response in the orbicularis oculi allows quantitative analysis of the reflex pathway. This technique is of diagnostic value in trigeminal and facial nerve lesions and lesions intrinsic to the brain stem. Modern sophisticated brain imaging techniques, however, offer sufficiently comprehensive and precise anatomical information as to limit the practical usefulness of this electrodiagnostic technique in neurosurgical practice.

Motor Examination

The temporalis and the masseter muscles are examined by inspection and palpation. Wasting of these muscles from lower motor neuron lesions causes noticeable hollowing above the zygoma and along the angle of the jaw. Palpable hardening of these muscles when the patient firmly clenches the teeth is compared on each side. The patient cannot bite when there is bilateral weakness, and the mouth tends to hang open.

The pterygoid muscles arise from the pterygoid process and the adjacent base of the skull and are attached to the inner surface of the mandible (Fig. 7-8A). When the pterygoid muscles of one side contract, the mandible is deviated toward the opposite side. When the pterygoids of both sides contract, they help to elevate or depress the jaw. In unilateral trigeminal motor lesions, the key movement to be tested is the lateral movement of the jaw. For instance, in a patient with a right-sided pterygoid weakness the following sequence of observations may be made (Fig. 7-8B to E). At rest the jaws are aligned and no obvious abnormality is noted. When the patient is asked to open the mouth widely, the jaw deviates to the right as a result of the unopposed action of the left pterygoid muscles. When asked to move the jaw to the right, the patient will be able to do so; when asked to move the jaw to the left, the patient will be unable to do so.

Jaw Jerk

The patient is asked to open the mouth partly and let the jaw muscles relax. The examiner places his or her forefinger on the patient's chin and percusses in a downward direction. The response is a reflex contraction of the masseter muscles with an upward jerk of the jaw. It is a monosynaptic muscle stretch reflex. An absent jaw jerk is not as helpful as a hyperactive one in clinical localization. The jaw jerk may be absent in healthy individuals. A hyperactive jaw jerk indicates an upper motor neuron lesion above the level of the midpons. In a patient with a pathological exaggeration of the deep tendon reflexes in the limbs and spasticity, a hyperactive jaw jerk denotes a suprapontine lesion rather than a

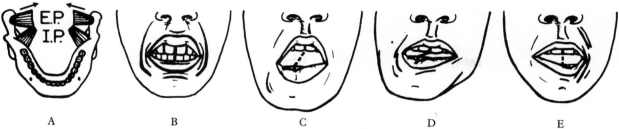

A   B   C   D   E

Figure 7-8 *A.* Anatomy of the pterygoid muscles; the direction of pull by the muscles is indicated by the arrows. E.P., external pterygoid; I.P., internal pterygoid. *B* to *E* show paralysis of the right pterygoid muscles: *B.* At rest the jaw does not deviate. *C.* When the patient attempts to open the mouth, the jaw deviates to the right as a result of the unbalanced action of the left pterygoid muscles. *D.* When asked to move the jaw toward the right, the patient is able to do so. *E.* When asked to move the jaw to the left, the patient is unable to do so.

cervical cord lesion. An increase in the jaw jerk is commonly observed in pseudobulbar palsy, motor neuron disease, and multiple sclerosis.

Localization of Lesions Based on Sensory Loss in the Face

Total loss of sensation over one or two sensory divisions but not involving the entire trigeminal nerve suggests a lesion peripheral to the trigeminal ganglion or a partial lesion of the ganglion or root. For instance, the ophthalmic division may be involved in cavernous sinus and superior orbital fissure syndromes, and the maxillary division may be involved by nasopharyngeal carcinoma invading the base of the skull. Fractures of the maxilla involving the infraorbital nerve leave a characteristic area of sensory loss over the malar region. Herpes zoster frequently involves the ophthalmic division; the delayed onset of contralateral hemiplegia in herpes zoster ophthalmicus suggests extension of inflammation into the carotid siphon. The Tolosa-Hunt syndrome is a benign, self-limiting, steroid-sensitive, indolent granuloma about the orbital apex, superior orbital fissure, and anterior cavernous sinus resulting in painful ophthalmoplegia and sensory loss in the ophthalmic (V_1) distribution.

Total loss of sensation over the entire distribution of the trigeminal nerve suggests a lesion in the ganglion or root or a more extensive lesion peripherally.

Loss of pain and temperature with preservation of touch (dissociated anesthesia) suggests a lesion in the descending root or nucleus of the trigeminal nerve. The sensory loss tends to follow an onion-skin pattern in the face. Syringobulbia and cervicocephalic junction anomalies and tumors produce this type of sensory loss. In vertebral or posterior inferior cerebellar artery thrombosis (Wallenberg syndrome), there is ipsilateral loss of pain and temperature in the face and the loss of the same sensations in the opposite half of the body.

Loss of touch with preservation of pain and temperature suggests a lesion involving the main sensory nucleus in the pons. Vascular diseases and pontine tumors produce this type of deficit.

Specific Syndromes

Trigeminal Neuralgia, Atypical Facial Pain, and Other Facial Pain Syndromes

These are discussed elsewhere in the textbook.

Raeder's Paratrigeminal Syndrome

Described by Raeder in 1924, the syndrome consists of unilateral oculosympathetic paresis and evidence of trigeminal involvement on the same side. The trigeminal involvement may be represented by neuralgic pain, sensory loss, or motor weakness. The associated Horner's syndrome is incomplete in that facial anhydrosis or ptosis of the lid may be absent. The syndrome is of localizing value, representing a lesion adjacent to the trigeminal nerve in the middle cranial fossa. Patients with Raeder's syndrome may have involvement of other adjacent cranial nerves such as the abducens nerve.

Unilateral vascular headaches (not true neuralgic pain from trigeminal nerve involvement) associated with an incomplete Horner's syndrome is of no localizing value, although it is often incorrectly reported as Raeder's syndrome in the literature.

Auriculotemporal Syndrome (Frey's Syndrome)

This syndrome usually results from injury to the auriculotemporal nerve. Regenerating secretomotor fibers in the auriculotemporal nerve become misdirected to the sweat glands and the vasodilator endings. This results in flushing, warmth, and excessive sweating over the cheek and pinna on ingestion of highly seasoned food.

Sturge-Weber Syndrome (Fig. 7-9)

In patients with this syndrome there are facial nevi or angiomas over the face in the trigeminal nerve distribution associated with calcified angiomatous lesions in the occipital cortex ("railroad track calcification"). The patient is generally subject to frequent seizures.

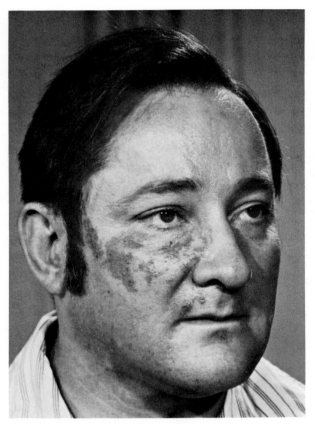

Figure 7-9   Sturge-Weber syndrome.

Facial Nerve

Anatomy

The facial nerve innervates principally the muscles of facial expression (special visceral efferent fibers). In addition it carries in its sensory and parasympathetic root (nervus intermedius of Wrisberg) the following fibers: (1) secretomotor (general visceral efferent) fibers to the submandibular and sublingual salivary glands, the lacrimal gland, and the mucous glands of the nose, nasopharynx, palate, and pharynx, (2) taste (special visceral afferent) fibers from the anterior two-thirds of the tongue, (3) visceral sensory (general visceral afferent) fibers from the salivary glands and the mucosa of nose and pharynx, (4) somatic sensory (general somatic afferent) fibers from the external ear.

The motor nucleus is located deep in the pons (Fig. 7-10) in the special visceral efferent column, in line with the motor nucleus of the trigeminal nerve and the nucleus ambiguus. The motor fibers course dorsomedially, looping around the nucleus of the abducens nerve, forming the internal genu. The internal genu is marked by an elevation on the floor of the fourth ventricle, the facial colliculus. The fibers then pass ventrally and laterally through the pons to emerge at the pontomedullary junction. The facial nerve traverses the subarachnoid space in the posterior cranial fossa and enters the internal acoustic meatus. In the depths of the meatus, the nerve enters the facial canal. In this canal the nerve is first directed laterally up to the epitympanic recess where it

turns sharply posteriorly (forming the external genu) and arches inferiorly behind the tympanic cavity to emerge from the stylomastoid foramen. A branch to the stapedius muscle arises from the facial nerve as the nerve courses along the posterior wall of the tympanic cavity. After leaving the skull, the nerve runs forward within the substance of the parotid gland to be distributed to the muscles of facial expression and the posterior belly of the digastric muscle (Fig. 7-11).

The sensory fibers arise from unipolar cells in the geniculate ganglion. Peripheral fibers that subserve the sensation of taste arise from the anterior two-thirds of the tongue and pass via the lingual and chorda tympani nerves to the geniculate ganglion; the central fibers terminate in the nucleus of the tractus solitarius; the visceral sensory fibers carrying sensation from the salivary glands terminate in a similar manner. Sensory fibers carrying general somatic sensation from the tympanic membrane and the external auditory canal terminate in the descending tract and nucleus of the trigeminal nerve.

The secretomotor fibers from the superior salivatory nucleus pass to the lacrimal gland and mucous glands of the palate, nose, and pharynx via the greater superficial petrosal nerve and the pterygopalatine ganglion, and to the submaxillary and sublingual glands via the chorda tympani and lingual nerves and the submaxillary ganglion.

Clinical Testing

Unilateral facial paresis may be suspected or detected on mere inspection of the patient's face at repose and while the patient is talking or smiling. Absence of wrinkles in the forehead, a widened palpebral fissure, slowness in blinking, upward rolling of the eye during blinking (Bell's phenomenon), and flattening of the nasolabial fold are easily observable signs of facial paresis. Finer degrees of facial paresis are ascertained by formal testing of individual groups of muscles in the face. The patient is asked to wrinkle the forehead by looking upward; to frown; to close the eyes tightly and resist the attempts by the examiner to open them; to show the teeth; to whistle; to blow out the cheeks against resistance by the examiner; to smile; and to bare the teeth with the mouth slightly open to allow contraction of the platysma.

In stuporous or comatose patients, facial musculature may be tested grossly by applying firm pressure on the supraorbital notch and observing for asymmetry in the wincing response. In addition, hypotonia of the buccal musculature may be evident from the puffing of the cheek with expiration and the blowing of air through the affected corner of the mouth.

In bilateral facial paralysis (of the nuclear or infranuclear type) the face may appear symmetric but the entire face remains immobile. Bell's phenomenon is readily observed.

There are two types of facial paralysis: the upper motor neuron and the lower motor neuron. In the upper motor neuron type (Fig. 7-12A), which results from a lesion in the corticobulbar pathway, the function of the muscles of the forehead is preserved but the musculature of the lower face is paralyzed. The palpebral fissure may be wider and there may be some degree of weakness in eye closure. This results from the fact that the facial nucleus in the pons subserving forehead muscle function receives bilateral innervation from the motor cortex, whereas the part of the facial nucleus subserving musculature of the lower face receives only contralateral innervation from the motor cortex (Fig. 7-13). In the lower motor neuron type, which results from a lesion in the facial nerve or its nucleus, there is paralysis of the entire ipsilateral half of the face (Fig. 7-12*B*).

Taste is tested with sugar, salt, or acetic acid. It is crucial that the test substance be placed with a moistened applicator stick only on the anterior two-thirds of one-half of the tongue. The patient should not be allowed to retract the tongue or speak during the test to prevent the flow of the test substance to other areas. The words *sweet*, *salty*, and *sour* are written on a piece of paper, and the patient is asked to point to the word that corresponds to the taste he or she perceives.

Hyperacusis or an abnormal increase in auditory acuity occurs with paralysis of the stapedius muscle.

The secretion of tears is assessed by Schirmer's test, which consists of placing a small piece of filter paper on each lower eyelid and comparing the degree and rate of moistening on each side. Salivary secretion is assessed by placing a very spicy substance on the tongue and noting the flow of saliva from the submaxillary duct. This test is seldom done in clinical practice.

Anatomical Localization of the Lesion in a Patient with Facial Paralysis (Fig. 7-11)

Lesion in the Corticobulbar Pathway (Supranuclear Type of Facial Palsy)

A lesion in this pathway produces a volitional type of central facial paralysis. The facial paresis is most marked on volitional movement, affecting the lower half of the face.

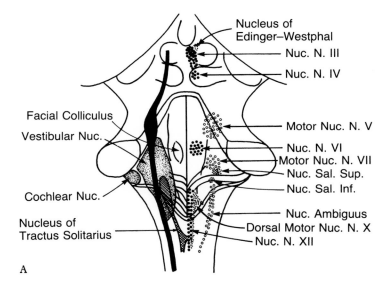

A

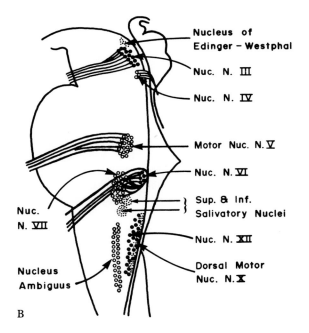

B

Figure 7-10 Anatomy of the cranial nerve nuclei in the brain stem. *A*. Coronal view. *B*. Sagittal view.

ANATOMY OF THE FACIAL NERVE AND CLINICAL LOCALIZATION OF FACIAL NERVE DYSFUNCTION

Anatomical Site	Course and Distribution of the Facial Nerve	Clinical Examination	Clinical Syndrome
Supranuclear (a) Supranuclear control from the motor cortex for volitional movements. (b) Supranuclear control from the basal ganglia and the thalamus for involuntary movements.		Facial muscle testing	Upper motor neuron type of facial palsy (a) Volitional type (b) Mimetic type
Nuclear (pons)		Examination of facial muscles, extraocular muscles, and motor examination of the extremities; brain stem auditory evoked potentials.	Millard-Gubler syndrome Raymond's syndrome Foville's syndrome
Cerebellopontine angle and internal auditory canal		Corneal sensation, facial muscle testing, tests for hearing loss including audiometry, cerebellar testing, brain stem auditory evoked potentials.	Cerebellopontine angle syndrome
Geniculate ganglion		Schirmer test for tearing.	Ramsay Hunt syndrome
Tympanomastoid region		Examination for taste in the anterior two-thirds of the tongue, test for hyperacusis.	Basal skull fracture Bell's palsy
Face		Facial muscle testing	Traumatic facial paralysis

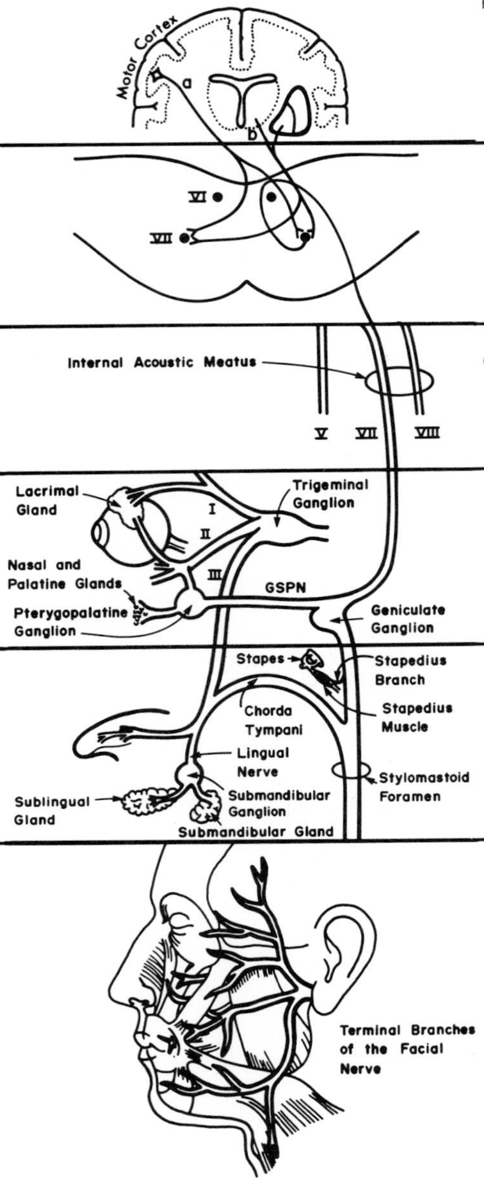

Figure 7-11 Central connections and peripheral distribution of the facial nerve. Anatomical localization of facial nerve lesions is also shown.

The frontalis function is retained (Fig. 7-12A). During involuntary emotional expression, such as smiling or weeping, the paresis may disappear.

The patient usually has a hemiparesis due to associated involvement of the corticospinal tract. Large frontal mass lesions compressing posteriorly on the facial area of the motor cortex may produce frontal lobe signs as well. A dominant hemisphere lesion may be associated with expressive speech impairment from involvement of Broca's area. Irritative lesions in the facial area of the motor cortex may produce focal motor seizure involving the face; in such instances one usually observes rapid blinking motion of both eyelids and twitching only in the contralateral angle of the mouth, further demonstrating the bilateral cortical control of the upper face and contralateral cortical control of the lower face (Fig. 7-13).

Deep Frontal Lobe Lesions

A lesion involving the basal ganglia or thalamus or their connections with the frontal lobe produces an emotional or mimetic type of facial palsy. In this type, the paresis of the

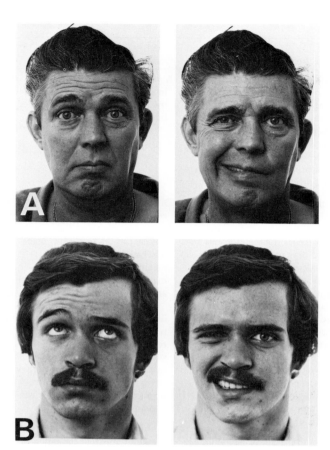

Figure 7-12 *A.* Upper motor neuron type of facial palsy showing paralysis mainly of the left lower face. *B.* Lower motor neuron type of facial palsy showing paralysis of the entire left half of the face.

angle of the mouth is most evident during involuntary emotional expression such as smiling or weeping but disappears during volitional movements. Thus the patient may readily retract the lips to show the teeth or blow out the cheeks on command, but when the patient is observed during smiling the facial paresis is evident. This phenomenon is thought to be due to loss of involuntary control of facial movements mediated through the connections from basal ganglionic structures to the facial nucleus.

Lesions in the Pons (Nuclear Type of Facial Palsy)

Lesions in the pons affecting the facial nerve nucleus produce ipsilateral peripheral facial paralysis. This is frequently associated with ipsilateral abducens paralysis and contralateral hemiplegia (Millard-Gubler syndrome). Other variants of this syndrome are described in Table 7-1.

Infranuclear Facial Palsy

Cerebellopontine Angle Lesion The most common lesion in this location is an acoustic neuroma. Although compression of the facial nerve within the internal auditory canal

occurs early, facial paralysis rarely occurs in the early stages of tumor growth. The patient presents with tinnitus and deafness (especially loss of word discrimination). Clinically observable facial paralysis occurs late. There may be evidence of involvement of the nervus intermedius with impairment of taste in the anterior two-thirds of the tongue and diminution of tear secretion. In the late stages evidence of ipsilateral fifth nerve and cerebellar hemispheric impairment is present.

Lesion in the Geniculate Ganglion Region There is a peripheral type of facial palsy, ipsilateral loss of taste in the anterior two-thirds of the tongue, decreased lacrimation in the ipsilateral eye, and hyperacusis. The Ramsay Hunt syndrome (geniculate neuralgia) is characterized by herpetic eruptions on the ear drum and external ear and pain in the ear. This syndrome is thought to result from herpes zoster infection of the geniculate ganglion.

Lesion Distal to the Geniculate Ganglion but Proximal to the Origin of the Nerve to the Stapedius There is a peripheral type of facial palsy, ipsilateral loss of taste in the anterior two-thirds of the tongue, and hyperacusis. Lacrimation is not affected.

Lesion Distal to the Nerve to the Stapedius but Proximal to the Chorda Tympani Branch There is a peripheral type of facial palsy and ipsilateral loss of taste in the anterior two-thirds of the tongue. Lacrimation is not affected, nor is there hyperacusis.

Lesion in the Facial Canal Distal to the Chorda Tympani Branch There is a peripheral type of facial palsy without impairment of taste, lacrimation, or hearing.

Lesion in the Parotid Gland or Face Lesions in these locations may selectively affect certain peripheral branches of the facial nerve with incomplete facial paralysis.

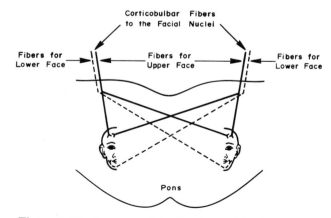

Figure 7-13 Anatomy of the facial nuclei in the pons and their supranuclear control. The facial nuclei in the pons are figuratively represented by one-half of the face. Upper parts of the facial nuclei receive bilateral cortical control, whereas the lower parts receive control only from the contralateral side.

TABLE 7-1 Cranial Nerve, Brain Stem, and Related Syndromes

Syndrome	Anatomy and Pathology of the Lesion	Clinical Features	Comments
Foster Kennedy syndrome	A large olfactory groove or medial third sphenoidal wing tumor, usually a meningioma.	Ipsilateral anosmia due to pressure on the olfactory tract; ipsilateral central scotoma and optic atrophy due to pressure on the optic nerve; contralateral papilledema due to increased intracranial pressure; occasionally ipsilateral proptosis due to invasion of the orbit by the tumor.	A very rare syndrome, especially in view of early detection of intracranial masses with computed tomography.
Tolosa-Hunt syndrome (painful ophthalmoplegia)	An indolent granuloma of unknown etiology about the anterior cavernous sinus, superior orbital fissure, and orbital apex.	Presents with steady "gnawing" or "boring" pain behind the eye and in the forehead. Pain usually precedes ophthalmoplegia by several days or may not appear until sometime later. Neurological involvement may begin in any of the nerves passing through the cavernous sinus: the third, fourth, sixth, or the first division of the fifth cranial nerves. Periarterial sympathetic fibers and the optic nerve may be involved. Spontaneous remission occurs, sometimes with residual neurological deficit. Attacks may occur at intervals of months or years.	Differential diagnosis includes collagen diseases (temporal arteritis, periarteritis nodosa), cavernous carotid aneurysm, diabetes, lymphoma, carcinoma, meningioma, specific granulomata such as syphilitic periostitis and ophthalmoplegic migraine. Diagnosis of Tolosa-Hunt syndrome is established through a process of exclusion and rapid response to administration of steroids. Carotid angiography may show irregular narrowing of the carotid siphon. Orbital venography may show venous occlusions.
Duane's syndrome	Etiology obscure. Aplasia of the abducens nerve with anomalous innervation of the lateral rectus by the oculomotor nerve or fibrosis of the lateral rectus and levator muscles are postulated as possibilities.	There is limitation of lateral gaze, widening of the palpebral fissure on abduction, and narrowing of the fissure during adduction.	In spite of apparent limitation of lateral gaze in the affected eye, the patient does not complain of diplopia.
Weber's syndrome (superior alternating hemiplegia)	Lesion in the cerebral peduncle of the midbrain affecting the pyramidal tract and the exiting fascicles of the third cranial nerve.	Ipsilateral oculomotor palsy and contralateral hemiplegia.	
Benedikt's syndrome	Lesion in the tegmentum of the midbrain involving the red nucleus, brachium conjunctivum, fascicles of the oculomotor nerve, and corticospinal tract.	Oculomotor palsy with contralateral hyperkinesia, ataxia, and intention tremor involving the arm only. There is contralateral hemiparesis.	
Claude's syndrome	Lesion in the tegmentum of the midbrain involving the red nucleus, brachium conjunctivum, and fascicles of the oculomotor nerve.	Ipsilateral oculomotor palsy and contralateral cerebellar ataxia and tremor.	A minor variant of Benedikt's syndrome.
Nothnagel's syndrome	Lesion in the tectum of the midbrain.	Unilateral oculomotor palsy combined with ipsilateral cerebellar ataxia due to involvement of oculomotor nerve and brachium conjunctivum.	
Parinaud's syndrome (Sylvian aqueduct syndrome)	Lesion around the tectum (superior colliculi) of the midbrain such as a pineal or posterior third ventricular tumor; may also result from vascular lesion or demyelinating disease.	Paralysis of conjugate movements of the eyes in the vertical plane. There is inability to elevate the eyes voluntarily or to elevate and depress the eyes. The pupils may be dilated and fail to react	The syndrome is often associated with convergence spasm and nystagmus retractorius. Skew deviation may represent a unilateral variant of Parinaud's syndrome. Passive head movements

TABLE 7-1 Cranial Nerve, Brain Stem, and Related Syndromes (*continued*)

Syndrome	Anatomy and Pathology of the Lesion	Clinical Features	Comments
		to light. Papilledema may be present from obstructive hydrocephalus.	may induce vertical eye movements in a patient who may be unable to look upward voluntarily. This confirms the clinical notion that Parinaud's syndrome results from supranuclear vertical gaze palsy.
Gradenigo's syndrome	The initial lesion is usually an acute mastoiditis. If uncontrolled, the infection spreads to involve the petrous temporal bone up to its apex (apical petrositis); epidural abscess may form at this location. Infection may then extend into the intradural space.	In patients with known acute mastoiditis, onset of pain about the eye and forehead suggests irritation of the gasserian ganglion. Corneal anesthesia may be present. Diplopia results from abducens palsy. The facial nerve may be involved infrequently.	Rarely tumors at the petrous apex (meningioma, trigeminal neurinoma) may give rise to this syndrome.
Millard-Gubler syndrome	A lesion in the ventral paramedian pons, usually an ischemic infarct, affecting the sixth and seventh nerve nuclei and the corticospinal tract.	Ipsilateral lateral rectus weakness and facial paralysis of lower motor neuron type with contralateral hemiplegia.	
Raymond's syndrome	A lesion in the ventral paramedian pons, usually an ischemic infarct, affecting the sixth nerve nucleus and the corticospinal tract.	Ipsilateral lateral rectus weakness and contralateral hemiplegia.	A minor variant of the Millard-Gubler syndrome.
Foville's syndrome (anterior inferior cerebellar artery syndrome)	A lesion in the dorsolateral pontine tegmentum.	Ipsilateral paralysis of lateral gaze due to involvement of the para-abducens area, ipsilateral lower motor neuron type facial palsy due to involvement of the facial nucleus, ipsilateral Horner's syndrome due to involvement of the descending sympathetic pathways in the reticular formation, ipsilateral analgesia of the face due to involvement of descending tract of the trigeminal nerve, and ipsilateral deafness due to involvement of auditory pathways.	Incomplete expression of this clinical syndrome frequently occurs.
Steele-Richardson-Olszewski syndrome (progressive supranuclear palsy)	Degenerative changes in the basal ganglia, brain stem, and cerebellum.	Supranuclear ophthalmoplegia especially for down gaze. With progression of the disease, there is supranuclear paresis of other eye movements and muscles of facial expression, speech, and deglutition. There may be dystonia of neck muscles, masklike facies, and rigidity in muscles. Progressive dementia may occur.	Thought to be related to Parkinson's syndrome.
Locked-in syndrome (pseudocoma)	Lesion in the basis pontis from basilar artery thrombosis, trauma, or neoplasm. Such a lesion spares the pathways for somatic sensation and the reticular activating system responsible for consciousness but disrupts the corticobulbar and corticospinal pathways.	All motor functions are absent except for ocular and eyelid movements. The patient is speechless and motionless, yet may respond to simple questions requiring "yes" and "no" answers by blinking once or twice when instructed to do so.	The terms *coma vigil* and *akinetic mutism* have been used synonymously with locked-in syndrome. Unfortunately, however, the former terms have also been used to describe patients with large bifrontal lesions (butterfly glioblastoma) or bilateral cingulate lesions who remain speechless and immobile although the motor and sensory pathways are intact.

TABLE 7-1 Cranial Nerve, Brain Stem, and Related Syndromes (*continued*)

Syndrome	Anatomy and Pathology of the Lesion	Clinical Features	Comments
Syndrome of central pontine myelinolysis	Selective noninflammatory demyelination with relative sparing of the axons and neurons in a variable area in the basis pontis.	Rapid onset of flaccid quadriplegia, with paralysis of bulbar muscles with inability to talk, chew, or swallow. Pupillary reflexes, movements of eyes, and lids, and corneal reflexes may be normal. Patients generally are critically ill. The clinical picture may simulate locked-in syndrome. Computed tomogram may show a hypodense lesion in the pons.	The etiologic factors are diverse. Nutritional deficiency in alcoholism is the most common cause. Severe hyponatremia has been shown to induce the syndrome clinically and experimentally.
Wallenberg's syndrome (lateral medullary syndrome)	Infarction of the dorsolateral medulla from atheromatous occlusion of the vertebral artery or the posterior inferior cerebellar artery—more commonly the former. Rarely results from aneurysms, intramedullary hematomas, or metastatic neoplasms.	Onset is acute with ipsilateral facial pain and paresthesias due to involvement of the descending tract and nucleus of the trigeminal nerve. Intense vertigo and vomiting may occur from involvement of the inferior vestibular nucleus and its central connections. Impairment of swallowing and hoarseness of voice results from involvement of nucleus ambiguus and motor paralysis of cranial nerves IX, X, and XI. Involvement of the spinocerebellar tract, inferior cerebellar peduncle, and inferior vestibular nuclei may result in nystagmus, ipsilateral dysmetria, intention tremor, and ataxia with a tendency to fall toward the side of the lesion. Ipsilateral Horner's syndrome results from destruction of descending sympathetic pathways in the medullary reticular formation. Loss of pain and temperature sensation in the ipsilateral half of face and contralateral half of body results from destruction of descending trigeminal pathways and spinothalamic tract.	The syndrome has also been reported from vertebral artery occlusion following chiropractic manipulation, yoga exercises, and trauma to the head and neck.
Avellis's syndrome	Vascular infarction of the tegmentum of the medulla from vertebral artery thrombosis.	Ipsilateral paralysis of the soft palate, pharynx, and vocal cord from involvement of the nucleus ambiguus; contralateral loss of pain and temperature sense from involvement of the lateral spinothalamic tract; occasionally contralateral hemianesthesia from involvement of the medial lemniscus. Horner's syndrome may be present from involvement of descending sympathetic pathways.	
Jackson's syndrome	Vascular infarction of the tegmentum of the medulla.	Involvement of cranial nerve nuclei X, XI (nucleus ambiguus), and XII, resulting in ipsilateral paralysis of the palate, pharynx, larynx, tongue, and sternocleidomastoid and trapezius muscles.	

TABLE 7-1 Cranial Nerve, Brain Stem, and Related Syndromes (*continued*)

Syndrome	Anatomy and Pathology of the Lesion	Clinical Features	Comments
Collet-Sicard syndrome	Lesions in the retropharyngeal and retroparotid space in the high neck such as tumors of the parotid gland or metastatic tumor in the lymph nodes; invasive tumors at the base of the skull near the jugular foramen and anterior condylar canal.	Paralysis of cranial nerves IX, X, XI, and XII.	
Villaret's syndrome	Same as Collet-Sicard syndrome.	In addition to the cranial nerve paralyses described in the Collet-Sicard syndrome, there is cervical sympathetic paralysis resulting in Horner's syndrome as well.	
Vernet's syndrome (jugular foramen syndrome)	Tumors (glomus jugulare tumor, metastatic tumor, meningioma); basilar skull fracture across the jugular foramen.	Paralysis of cranial nerves IX, X, and XI. There may be occlusion of the jugular bulb.	
Tapia's syndrome	Parotid or other tumors or penetrating injuries to the high cervical region.	Vagal and hypoglossal paralysis with or without involvement of the accessory nerve.	Tapia's syndrome or vagohypoglossal palsy may also result from an intrinsic lesion in the medulla.

Clinical Conditions

Bell's Palsy or Idiopathic Facial Paralysis

Bell's palsy is the most common type of facial paralysis and accounts for 80 percent of all peripheral facial paralysis. It affects 150 to 200 people out of 1 million in a year. Few topics in neurology are as controversial as the etiology and treatment of Bell's palsy. Although originally thought to result from ischemia of the facial nerve, the weight of current evidence points to a viral etiology. Some have presented evidence to suggest that Bell's palsy is part of a polyneuropathy syndrome induced by the herpes simplex virus; in this syndrome in addition to the facial nerve, the trigeminal nerve and certain branches of the vagus nerve may be involved as well. Heredity, pregnancy, diabetes, and exposure to cold have been implicated as contributing factors.

Typically a previously healthy individual awakens with unilateral stiffness and pain in the face associated with facial palsy. The paralysis is complete at onset in half the cases; in the remainder the paralysis is incomplete and may progress to completion over a period of a week. A viral prodrome consisting of upper respiratory tract infection, stuffy nose, sore throat, muscle aching, nausea, vomiting, or diarrhea may be observed in many cases. Since viral inflammation of the facial nerve is thought to occur in a distal-to-proximal direction, the chorda tympani branch becomes involved after the motor branches of the facial nerve, resulting in loss of taste and decreased salivary secretion. Next to be involved is the stapedial branch, resulting in hyperacusis, and lastly the geniculate ganglion, which results in decreased tearing. Such a caudorostral march of symptoms may not always be demonstrable, but as a general rule, the more proximal the

involvement, the worse the prognosis. Concurrent inflammation of the trigeminal nerve may be manifest as an impaired corneal reflex and decreased sensibility in the face. Causes other than Bell's palsy should be sought for under the following clinical settings: (1) recurrent unilateral paralysis, (2) bilateral facial paralysis, (3) slow progressive paralysis over several weeks, (4) slow progressive paralysis with facial hyperkinesias.

Of patients afflicted with Bell's palsy, 75 to 80 percent show a complete recovery, 10 percent have partial recovery, and the remainder have poor recovery. Some recovery of function is the rule even in patients showing poor recovery; if virtually no recovery occurs by six months, other etiologic factors must be explored.

The time of onset of recovery and the pattern of facial motor recovery are considered to be prognostic indicators. If recovery begins between the tenth day and the third week, recovery tends to be complete. If recovery does not begin until after 3 weeks but before 2 months, fair recovery may be expected. Improvement beginning 2 to 4 months after onset predicts poor recovery.

Patients with complete paralysis at onset have a 50 percent chance of having incomplete recovery. Those patients with incomplete paralysis at the onset and in whom the palsy does not progress will recover completely. Those patients with incomplete paralysis that progresses but not to complete paralysis will have complete recovery. Those patients that present with incomplete paralysis that progresses to complete paralysis will have an incomplete recovery in 75 percent of the cases. Electroneuromyography is helpful in detecting reinnervation potentials and may assist in prognostication.

Steroids are the mainstay in the initial management, although the efficacy of such drugs has not been proved conclusively in clinical trials. Faradic or galvanic stimulation of the facial muscles is neither necessary nor useful. Indications for surgical decompression of the facial nerve remain controversial, although there is some consensus to the following guidelines: (1) evidence of complete degeneration of the facial nerve without any response during nerve stimulation testing, (2) evidence of a progressively deteriorating response to nerve stimulation testing, (3) no improvement in clinical and objective nerve testing after 8 weeks.

Facial Myokymia

This is an uncommon and interesting involuntary facial movement disorder seen in patients with intrinsic organic lesions in the pons. It is characterized by unilateral, spontaneous, fine, continuous, undulating waves of muscle contraction spreading across the face. In well-established cases, there is persistent narrowing of the palpebral fissure and persistent drawing of the angle of the mouth, described as spastic paretic facial contracture. The muscle flickering is quite unique and different from fasciculations seen in lower motor neuron disease in that the flickering motion proceeds in a slow, wavelike, orderly, nonrandom manner. Local anesthetic block of the facial nerve at the stylomastoid foramen will eliminate the facial contracture and myokymic movements, indicating that the lesion responsible for this phenomenon lies central to this level. The two most common lesions in the pons that induce facial myokymia are glioma and multiple sclerosis. In patients with glioma, the myokymia persists unremittingly until death, whereas in multiple sclerosis, the abnormal movements have a self-limiting course and generally subside in a few weeks. Rarely a tuberculoma in the pons has been known to cause facial myokymia. Crucial pathological studies have indicated that the structural lesion is situated rostral to the facial nucleus and not in the nucleus itself. This lends support to the hypothesis that facial myokymia results from isolation of the facial motoneurons from their central inhibitory connections. Electromyography shows a pattern of continuous potentials resembling those of normal motor units; occasionally these potentials may assume a rythmic pattern. Fibrillation potentials and positive waves, however, are conspicuous by their absence.

Benign facial myokymia is a much more common condition seen in normal people after fatigue. The twitching motions are confined to the lower eyelids.

Blepharospasm

This condition consists of repeated, involuntarily forceful closure of the lids on both sides associated with lowering of the eyebrows. Blepharospasm may be either symptomatic (related to an irritative or painful eye disease) or idiopathic. Idiopathic blepharospasm occurs in elderly individuals, and is worse under stress.

Facial Tic (Habit Spasms)

This disorder is commonly seen in children and adolescents. There are recurrent, brief, stereotyped movements of the face consisting of sniffing, blinking, grimacing, or clearing of the throat. These movements may be briefly inhibited on will but soon recur when the person's attention is diverted. The affected individuals tend to be hyperactive and anxious.

Hemifacial Spasm (Fig. 7-14)

This condition is characterized by involuntary, paroxysmal clonic and tonic contractions of the facial muscles. At the onset, the paroxysmal contractions may be confined about the eye, but later other muscles innervated by the facial nerve may be affected. The condition is intensified by nervousness and stressful conditions but may be present during sleep. Although it is a benign condition, the persistent and involuntary nature of the syndrome is distressing to the patient. Occasionally, the patient may have ipsilateral tinnitus or hearing loss; association with trigeminal neuralgia has also been reported. Janetta has championed the idea that hemifacial spasm occurs from vascular compression of the facial nerve at its root exit zone from the pons.

Hemifacial spasm must be differentiated from focal motor seizures, habit spasms, blepharospasm, facial nerve dysfunction following Bell's palsy, and facial myokymia. In focal motor seizures, the patient has associated conjugate

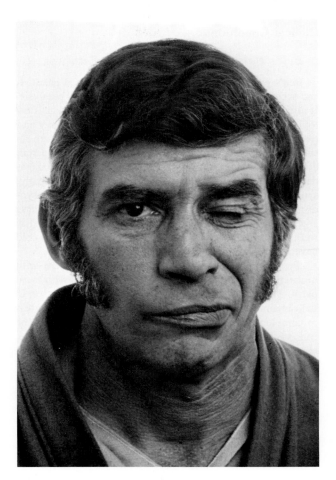

Figure 7-14 Left hemifacial spasm.

deviation of the head and eyes to the opposite side; both eyelids blink because of bilateral control of the facial nuclei by the contralateral motor cortex. Habit spasms are absent during sleep. They may be unilateral or bilateral, and may be associated with movements that are not served by the facial nerve, such as sniffing and clearing the throat. Blepharospasm primarily affects the orbicularis oculi muscles and is invariably bilateral; it disappears during sleep. Facial myokymia is characterized by an undulating movement of the facial muscles that is quite different from the tonic-clonic movements seen in hemifacial spasm.

Crocodile Tear Syndrome

This syndrome is seen in individuals with peripheral facial palsy from a lesion in the facial nerve proximal to the geniculate ganglion. Aberrant regeneration of the nerve may result in growth of nerve filaments subserving salivary secretion into the pathway to the lacrimal gland (greater superficial petrosal nerve). Clinically this is manifest as an abnormal gustatory-lacrimal reflex, characterized by ipsilateral excessive lacrimation during eating.

Glossopharyngeal Nerve

The glossopharyngeal and vagus nerves are closely related anatomically, functionally, and clinically. The same disease process frequently involves both nerves. Clinical evaluation of these two nerves is thus appropriately done together.

Anatomy

The glossopharyngeal nerve has the following components:

1. Motor (general visceral efferent) fibers arising from the rostral portion of the nucleus ambiguos. These fibers innervate a single muscle in the pharynx—the stylopharyngeus.
2. Visceral sensory (general visceral afferent) fibers. The cell bodies of the unipolar cells subserving this function are located in the inferior (jugular) ganglion. Centrally they terminate in the tractus solitarius and its nucleus. Peripherally they convey impulses concerned with tactile, thermal, and pain sensations from the mucous membrane of the posterior one-third of the tongue, pharynx, palate, fauces, auditory tube, and tympanic cavity. Through the carotid sinus nerve, they are connected to the special receptors in the carotid sinus and carotid body concerned with reflex control of blood pressure and heart rate.
3. Taste (special visceral efferent) fibers from the posterior one-third of the tongue. They terminate in the rostrolateral portions of the solitary nucleus called the *gustatory nucleus.*
4. General somatic sensory fibers from cutaneous areas in the external auditory meatus. The primary sensory neurons subserving this sensation lie in the superior or jugu-

lar ganglion. Central processes terminate in the descending tract and nucleus of the trigeminal nerve.
5. Parasympathetic or secretomotor (general visceral efferent) fibers arise from the inferior salivatory nucleus and pass via the tympanic nerve (nerve of Jacobson), tympanic plexus, and lesser superficial petrosal nerve to the otic ganglion situated below the foramen ovale and medial to the mandibular division of the trigeminal nerve. Postganglionic fibers arising from this ganglion are distributed to the parotid gland through the auriculotemporal nerve (Fig. 7-15).

Clinical Testing

The gag reflex is elicited by depressing the tongue with a wooden tongue depressor, and touching the palate, fauces, or the oropharyngeal wall with an applicator stick. The response consists of elevation of the palate, retraction of the tongue, and contraction of the pharynx. In some sensitive individuals retching or vomiting may be induced. The sensitivity of the gag reflex varies among individuals. The gag reflex may be absent in hysterics. The afferent component of the reflex arc is mediated through the glossopharyngeal nerve, and the efferent component through the vagus nerve.

Following unilateral surgical section of the glossopharyngeal nerve for glossopharyngeal neuralgia, there is usually no evidence of paralysis of the pharynx or impairment of the gag reflex. This indicates that the stylopharyngeus plays only a minor role in the motor function of the pharynx and that it is impossible to test this muscle in isolation. Normal pharyngeal sensation and an intact gag reflex after nerve section implies that there is a significant contribution from the vagus to the sensory innervation of the oropharynx and that the sensory function of the ninth cranial nerve is dispensable in the presence of an intact vagus nerve.

Testing the taste sensation in the posterior one-third of the tongue is awkward. It is seldom done in clinical practice.

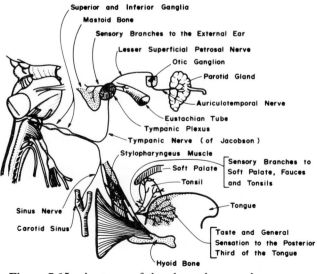

Figure 7-15 Anatomy of the glossopharyngeal nerve.

Vagus Nerve

Anatomy

The vagus is the longest of the cranial nerves, and it has a more extensive course and distribution than any of the other cranial nerves. The most significant functions of the nerve with respect to neurological diagnosis are those subserving sensation and movement of the palate, pharynx, and larynx (Fig. 7-16).

Components of the Vagus Nerve

1. The motor (special visceral efferent) fibers arise from the nucleus ambiguus and supply all muscles of the soft palate, except the tensor veli palatini (supplied by the trigeminal nerve); of the pharynx, except the stylopharyngeus (supplied by the glossopharyngeal nerve); and of the larynx.
2. Visceral motor (general visceral efferent) fibers arise from the dorsal motor nucleus of the vagus and are distributed to the thoracic and abdominal viscera.
3. Somatic sensory (general somatic afferent) fibers of unipolar cells in the jugular ganglion (superior ganglion) are distributed peripherally via the auricular branch to the external auditory meatus and via the recurrent meningeal branch to the dura of the posterior fossa. The central branches terminate in the descending tract and nucleus of the trigeminal nerve (Fig. 7-4).
4. Visceral sensory (general visceral afferent) fibers of the unipolar cells in the ganglion nodosum (inferior ganglion) are distributed peripherally to the pharynx, larynx, trachea, and esophagus, and to the thoracic and abdominal viscera. Central fibers terminate in the nucleus solitarius.
5. Taste (special visceral afferent) fibers from the epiglottic region likewise terminate in the nucleus solitarius.

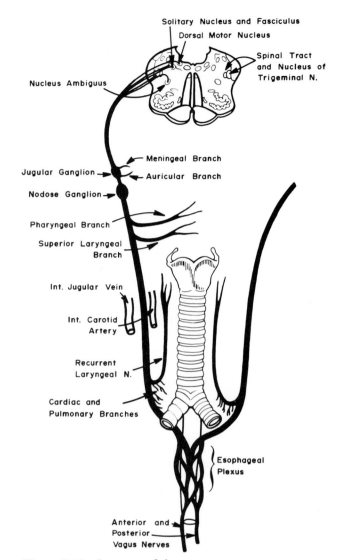

Figure 7-16 Anatomy of the vagus nerve.

Clinical Testing

Motor Functions of the Soft Palate and Pharynx

Elevation of the palate is tested by asking the patient to open the mouth widely and to say "ah." The uvula rises and stays in the midline. At the same time pharyngeal constrictor muscles may be seen at the back of the pharynx moving like a curtain toward the midline from the side of the pharynx. With unilateral vagal paralysis, the uvula deviates to the opposite side; with bilateral vagal paralysis, the palate remains immobile and does not elevate on phonation. The voice has a nasal quality, and on swallowing, fluids may regurgitate through the nose and induce coughing. The gag reflex is absent.

Motor Functions of the Larynx

Patients with laryngeal motor weakness present with a hoarse, husky voice. Laryngoscopic examination is essential

to determine the nature and extent of the vocal cord paralysis. In a slowly evolving recurrent laryngeal paralysis, initially there is a failure in abduction of the vocal cord with hoarseness of voice and mild inspiratory stridor. With the onset of complete paralysis, the cord takes a cadaveric position midway between abduction and adduction. The uninvolved cord may cross over the midline to meet the paralyzed cord during phonation. In bilateral recurrent laryngeal nerve paralysis loss of abduction of vocal cords may result in severe respiratory distress.

Lesions affecting the superior laryngeal nerve cause paralysis of the cricothyroid muscle, which results in loss of higher tones in speaking and singing. This impairment is brought out by asking the patient to say "eee." The disability from superior laryngeal paralysis is much less severe than that associated with recurrent laryngeal paralysis. Most patients will have a voice satisfactory for their daily needs.

A vast array of lesions produce laryngeal paralysis (Table 7-2). When confronted with a patient with laryngeal paralysis, a systematic approach should be used to arrive at a diag-

TABLE 7-2 Causes of Laryngeal Paralysis

Congenital	Trauma	Neoplasms	Neuropathies	Inflammation	Vascular	Cause Unknown
Cervicocephalic junction anomalies	Surgical	Intrinsic tumors of the medulla oblongata	Diabetic neuropathy	Chronic basal meningitis (TB, fungus, sarcoid)	Wallenberg's syndrome (lateral medullary syndrome)	Progressive bulbar palsy
Chiari's malformation	Anterior interbody fusion	Astrocytoma, ependymoma, hemangioblastoma	Alcoholic neuropathy	Guillain-Barré syndrome	Vertebral aneurysm	
Platybasia and basilar invagination	Thyroidectomy	Jugular foramen region	Toxic neuropathy (lead, mercury, arsenic)	Radiation neuropathy	Aortic aneurysm	
Syringobulbia	Removal of neck masses	Glomus jugulare tumor, metastatic carcinoma, meningioma, neurilemmoma, meningeal carcinomatosis	Serum sickness	Diphtheria		
	Scalene node biopsy	Neck				
	Accidental	Thyroid				
	Basilar skull fracture through the jugular foramen	Goiter, adenoma, carcinoma				
	Penetrating wounds of the neck	Cervical lymph nodes				
	Blunt trauma to the neck	Metastatic carcinoma, malignant lymphoma				
	Fracture of the clavicle	Neurogenic tumors				
		Neurilemmoma, neurofibroma, ganglioneuroma				
		Carotid body tumor				
		Mediastinum				
		Thymus tumors, malignant lymphoma, metastatic carcinoma				
		Lung				
		Bronchogenic carcinoma				

nosis, keeping in mind the origin, course, and distribution of the vagus nerve. Intrinsic lesions of the medulla are usually associated with Horner's syndrome, ipsilateral cerebellar signs, and loss of pain and temperature sensation over the ipsilateral face and contralateral arm and leg. Jugular foramen lesions result in paralysis of the glossopharyngeal and spinal accessory nerves. If the movements and sensation of the palate and pharynx are spared, the lesion is distal to the origin of pharyngeal branches.

Dysarthria

Dysarthria refers to the difficulty in articulating speech. Articulation is a complex motor process requiring the concerted action of muscles supplied by different lower cranial nerves controlled through higher motor centers. The type of dysarthria thus varies depending upon the neural element affected.

1. *Labial dysarthria* occurs in patients with facial paralysis. Weakness and lack of tone of the lip musculature results in difficulty in pronouncing the consonants *b* and *p*.
2. *Nasal voice* is characteristically observed with palatal weakness, and is especially noticeable with bilateral weakness of the palate from vagal paralysis. Difficulty is most noticeable in the pronunciation of *k*, *q*, and *ch*.
3. *Hoarseness* of voice is seen in patients with vocal cord paralysis.
4. *Lingual dysarthria* occurs in patients with paralysis of the tongue. They have particular difficulty in pronouncing *d* and *t*.
5. *Scanning speech* with an explosive dysrhythmic quality is observed in patients with cerebellar disease.
6. In *pseudobulbar palsy*, the speech is slow, spastic, and grunting in nature.

Accessory Nerve

Anatomy

The accessory nerve is a purely motor nerve. It consists of a cranial root and a spinal root; the cranial root is for practical purposes a part of the vagus nerve (Fig. 7-17).

The cranial root is the smaller of the two roots. It arises from the caudal segment of the nucleus ambiguus. The nerve emerges from the side of the medulla as four or five delicate rootlets just caudal to the roots of the vagus. The nerve runs laterally toward the jugular foramen and becomes united with the spinal root. It leaves the jugular foramen, separates from the spinal portion, and blends with the vagus nerve. It is distributed principally in the pharyngeal and recurrent laryngeal branches of the vagus, supplying the muscles of the soft palate and the intrinsic muscles of the larynx.

The spinal root arises from the spinal accessory nucleus, an elongated column of motoneutrons located in the lateral part of the ventral gray column of the spinal cord that extends as far as the fifth cervical segment. The fibers pass

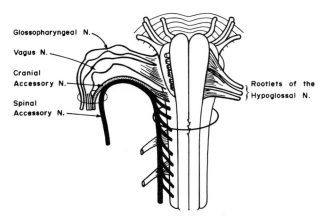

Figure 7-17   Anatomy of the accessory nerve.

through the lateral white column of the cord and unite to form a single trunk that ascends between the dorsal roots of the spinal nerves and the dentate ligament. On each side, the nerve enters the posterior cranial fossa through the foramen magnum where it joins the cranial portion of the nerve for a short distance and exits the skull through the jugular foramen. It descends in the neck, reaches the upper part of the sternocleidomastoid muscle, penetrates its inner surface, joins branches of the second cervical nerve, and supplies the muscle. The latter nerve subserves only proprioceptive function. Emerging a little above the middle of the posterior border of the sternocleidomastoid, the nerve crosses the posterior triangle of the neck to reach a point that is 5 cm above the clavicle, where it disappears into the trapezius muscle. It is joined by the third and fourth cervical nerves, which are thought to supply some motor fibers to the lower half of the trapezius.

Method of Testing

Since the cranial part of the accessory nerve is an integral part of the vagus nerve, it is tested along with the vagus nerve. Examination of the spinal accessory nerve is done by testing the sternocleidomastoid and trapezius muscles.

The sternocleidomastoid is tested by the inspection and palpation of the muscle as the patient turns the head forcibly against resistance. The test is repeated in the opposite direction, and the two sides are compared for muscle bulk and strength. Both sternocleidomastoids may be tested simultaneously by resting the hand of the examiner on the patient's forehead and asking the patient to bend the neck forward against resistance.

Wasting of one sternocleidomastoid is easily observed on inspection, especially when the patient turns the head to the opposite side; the patient will fail to turn against resistance to the opposite side. When both sternocleidomastoids are wasted, the neck appears thin and elongated with prominence of the thyroid cartilage and gland. When the patient sits up, the head tends to fall backward.

The trapezius muscles are tested by asking the patient to shrug the shoulders against resistance. Muscle power is compared on both sides. In unilateral paralysis of the trapezius, the contour of the neck becomes asymmetric. The shoulder on the involved side tends to droop, and the scapula tends to be displaced downward and outward. There may be slight winging of the scapula when the arm is forward-flexed at the shoulder; but this winging is not as prominent as seen after serratus anterior palsy. When both trapezius muscles are paralyzed, there is weakness of extension of the neck.

Common Lesions

Infranuclear or peripheral lesions are the most common. Congenital cervicocephalic junction anomalies, foramen magnum tumor, and glomus jugulare tumor may involve the spinal accessory nerve. Stab and gunshot wounds and surgical procedures in the posterior triangle of the neck may result in damage to the nerve in the neck. Infiltrating tumors or inflammatory adenopathy may affect the nerve in the neck. Trapezius paralysis in the absence of involvement of the sternocleidomastoid suggests a lesion of the peripheral segment of the nerve in the posterior triangle of the neck. Atrophy of both sternocleidomastoid muscles is a prominent sign in myotonic dystrophy.

Nuclear involvement may be seen in syringomyelia, syringobulbia, intrinsic neoplasms of the high cervical cord, and motoneuron disease.

Hypoglossal Nerve

Anatomy

The hypoglossal nerve is a pure motor nerve supplying the extrinsic and intrinsic muscles of the tongue. The hypoglossal nucleus in the medulla lies adjacent to the midline directly under the floor of the fourth ventricle and ventrolateral to the central canal. It lies in series with the general somatic efferent column of cells represented by the oculomotor and trochlear nuclei in the midbrain, the abducens nucleus in the pons, and the anterior horn cells in the spinal cord (Fig. 7-10). The rootlets of the hypoglossal nerve emerge from the anterolateral surface of the medulla between the olive and the pyramid, pierce the ventral dura, and pass through the anterior condylar canal (hypoglossal canal) to emerge from the skull as a single bundle. The nerve descends vertically through the neck to the level of the angle of the mandible and then passes forward to supply the extrinsic muscles (genioglossus, hyoglossus, chondroglossus, and styloglossus) and intrinsic muscles of the tongue (Fig. 7-18). In the neck the hypoglossal nerve is joined by motor fibers from cervical roots that leave as the ansa hypoglossi. The ansa hypoglossi supplies certain strap muscles of the neck (omohyoid, sterohyoid, sternothyroid), but it is not important in neurological localization.

The hypoglossal nerve controls all movements of the tongue. The extrinsic muscles of the tongue participate in forward protrusion, retraction, side-to-side movement, elevation, and depression of the tongue. The intrinsic muscles primarily alter the shape of the tongue, especially curling of the tongue in different directions.

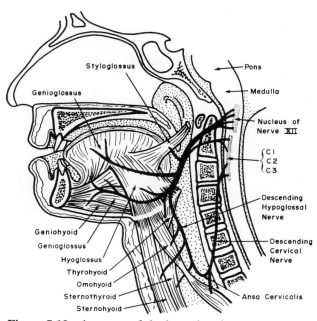

Figure 7-18 Anatomy of the hypoglossal nerve.

The hypoglossal nucleus receives its supranuclear control from the lowest part of the precentral gyrus of both sides, but predominantly from the contralateral side. The supranuclear fibers pass through the genu of the internal capsule.

Clinical Examination

The patient is asked to open the mouth widely, and the tongue is inspected for atrophy and fasciculations. Fasciculations are best observed when the tongue is at rest on the floor of the mouth because it is very common to see some degree of tremulousness of the tongue on sustained protrusion in many normal individuals. The patient is then asked to protrude the tongue and rapidly move it from side to side. An estimate of the motor strength of the tongue may be made by asking the patient to push the tongue against the cheek against resistance by the examiner. In unilateral nuclear or infranuclear lesions, the ipsilateral half of the tongue shows atrophy and fasciculations. The tongue is wrinkled, furrowed, and wasted on the affected side. The median raphe shows a sickle-shaped curvature. On protrusion, the tongue deviates to the paralyzed side due to the unbalanced action of the genioglossus muscle of the normal side (Fig. 7-19). Diffuse bilateral atrophy with generalized fasciculations in the tongue resembling a "bag of worms" is seen in bilateral nuclear involvement in motor neuron disease. The patient may be unable to protrude the tongue in bilateral paralysis. A unilateral upper motor neuron lesion may cause deviation of the tongue to the contralateral (hemiparetic) side, but this deviation is not as pronounced as is seen with nuclear or infranuclear lesions because of the bilateral supranuclear control of the hypoglossal nerve. The tongue is not atrophic. In bilateral upper motor neuron lesions, the tongue is tight and compact, the alternate motion rate of the tongue is slow, and in advanced stages the patient may be

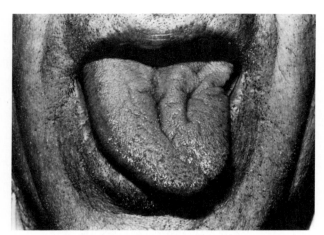

Figure 7-19 Hematrophy and deviation of the tongue as a result of left hypoglossal nerve paralysis.

unable to protrude the tongue. In motor neuron disease, features of nuclear and supranuclear lesions may coexist.

A coarse tremor of the tongue may be present in Parkinson's disease. Irregular jerky movements of the tongue with alternate protraction and retraction is seen in chorea. Abnormal dystonic tongue movements are frequently seen as part of orofacial tardive dyskinesia due to long-term phenothiazine therapy.

Clinical Conditions

Nuclear or Infranuclear Lesion

Primary tumors of the brain stem, such as hemangioblastoma, infiltrative glioma, or ependymoma may involve the hypoglossal nucleus of one or both sides. Syringobulbia is an infrequent cause of hypoglossal paralysis. Common traumatic lesions that involve the hypoglossal nerve are basilar skull fractures involving the anterior condylar canal and stab

and gunshot wounds of the neck. The hypoglossal nerve is at risk in carotid vascular surgery, during tumor dissection in the neck, or during clipping of an intracranial vertebral artery aneurysm. Large jugular foramen tumors and metastatic deposits in the base of the skull or upper cervical lymph nodes may involve the hypoglossal nerve. Paralysis of the tongue may be manifestation of certain congenital anomalies of the cervicocephalic junction such as platybasia or Chiari's malformation. The rare Collet-Sicard syndrome is characterized by unilateral involvement of the ninth, tenth, eleventh, and twelfth cranial nerves. This variant of the jugular foramen syndrome was described in victims of World War I who had sustained penetrating wounds. The syndrome may also be due to neoplastic, inflammatory, or vascular lesions.

In progressive bulbar palsy (a variant of amyotrophic lateral sclerosis), there is usually hypoglossal involvement bilaterally.

Upper Motor Neuron Lesion

In patients with hemiplegia due to massive ischemic infarction, the hemiplegic side may show weakness of the tongue as well. Bilateral upper motor neuron lesions are seen in amyotrophic lateral sclerosis and in bilateral ischemic vascular lesions causing pseudobulbar palsy.

Multiple Cranial Nerve and Brain Stem Syndromes

In clinical neurological practice one often encounters syndromes in which a cranial nerve or a group of cranial nerves and adjacent brain structures are involved from a single pathological process. Recognition of these syndromes is helpful in neurological diagnosis. They are summarized in Table 7-1.

8

Neuro-ophthalmology

Michael Rosenberg

Neuro-ophthalmic History

The neuro-ophthalmic history begins with a careful ophthalmologic history. Particular attention must be paid to the specific characteristics of the patient's chief complaint, which may provide clues to the pathophysiology of any disease process. When patients with complaints of visual loss are being interviewed, specific consideration must be given to the circumstances of the visual loss. Was the visual loss acute or chronic? Did the person note a specific event that brought his or her attention to the fact that there was a visual problem or was the observation incidental, i.e., when the "good" eye was inadvertently covered? If the patient cannot give a certain answer to this question, the clinician must attempt to document whether the visual loss is acute or progressive. In patients with transient visual symptoms, the chronology of the symptoms is important. How long do they last? Do they occur at any specific time of the day? Is there an initiating cause? Is there a prodrome? Are there associated neurological symptoms? Did the patient alternately cover each eye to confirm whether the visual loss was monocular or binocular? Is the vision loss worse during the day or night? Is color vision abnormal?

Patients complaining of diplopia must be questioned as to the mode of onset of the diplopia. Does diplopia disappear when either eye is covered? What does the patient mean by diplopia? Many patients with "ghost images" secondary to refractive errors or media abnormalities may complain of diplopia. This diplopia is often monocular and bilateral. Has the patient alternated closing one eye and the other to see if the diplopia disappears? Monocular diplopia in most cases implies ocular disease. Is the diplopia greater at distance or at near? Is the diplopia greater at one time of the day or the other? Is the diplopia present in primary positions of gaze or eccentric positions of gaze? How does the patient accommodate to the diplopia? A patient who complains of disabling diplopia but who has not spontaneously covered or closed one eye and functions with both eyes open must be suspected of having a chronic motility disorder. Does the patient have a childhood history of strabismus or treatment of an eye muscle problem?

Review of old photographs is an important adjunct to the history. Patients with presumably acquired anisocoria (unequal pupils) or ptosis may in fact have photographic evidence of having these findings at a time significantly previous to the current episode.

Review of old records and radiological studies is frequently important. It is preferred that the clinician review the actual roentgenogram with a neuroradiologist rather than relying on the official radiological interpretation. This is particularly important when x-rays are done at smaller hospitals without the advantage of subspecialty radiologists. If the clinician must review old visual fields, it is important to be able to evaluate whether the visual field was done in a proper and correct manner. The neurologist or neurosurgeon evaluating an ophthalmic evaluation should know enough about the neuro-ophthalmic aspects of the examination to judge whether the ophthalmologist is a credible source of information.

A careful family history is helpful. Are there unexplained instances of visual loss in other family members? If so, what is their relationship to the patient? Patterns of inheritance may provide important clues for specific diagnosis. If there family history of migraine? Is there family history of other neurological disease?

Neuro-ophthalmologic Examination

The normal ophthalmologic examination includes the following: (1) determination of visual acuity; (2) examination of visual fields; (3) external examination, including quantification of exophthalmos, quantification of lid position, presence or absence of ptosis or lid retraction, description of conjunctival vasculature, examination of facial and corneal sensation, and examination of seventh nerve function (orbicularis strength, tearing); (4) pupillary examination; (5) examination of extraocular motility; (6) measurement of intraocular pressure; (7) slit lamp examination; and (8) direct and indirect ophthalmoscopy.

Additional features of the examination required for neuro-ophthalmic evaluation may include: (1) color vision testing; (2) optokinetic nystagmus; (3) photostress test; (4) examination of the retinal nerve fiber layer; (5) ophthalmodynamometry; (6) fluorescein angiography; (7) electrophysiological testing: electroretinography, electro-oculography, and visual evoked response.

Determination of Visual Acuity

Visual acuity refers to the resolving power of the eye, i.e., the ability of the eye to distinguish one object from another. Standard methods of testing visual acuity require that the chart be 20 ft away from the patient and that the patient be wearing the best refractive correction. This is termed the *best corrected visual acuity*. The 20/20 line on an eye chart contains letters that subtend a visual angle of 5 minutes of arc. This letter size was determined in previous studies to be the smallest resolvable object by the vast majority of "normal" individuals. The letter E on the 20/20 line has each of the horizontal arms subtending a visual angle of 1 minute of arc. The space between each horizontal line is an additional minute of arc resulting in a letter subtending 5 minutes of arc. A patient who can read the 20/20 line therefore can resolve objects that differ from each other by a size of 1 minute of arc. The numerator of the fraction 20/20 indicates that the testing distance is 20 ft. If the patient reads the 20/20 line while the chart is held 10 ft away, his or her visual acuity is 10/20, which is equivalent to 20/40. Each line on the eye vision chart has an arithmetic relation to the standard 20/20 letter. The letters on the 20/40 line subtend a visual arc of 10 minutes. The 20/200 letter subtends a visual arc of 10 times 5 minutes or 50 minutes of arc. The visual acuity may be expressed as a single decimal value. In this case, a patient with normal visual acuity has a visual acuity of 1. A patient with a visual acuity of 20/40 has a visual acuity of 0.5.

If the patient cannot see any letters on the vision chart, vision may be recorded as an ability to count fingers (FC), to see hand movement (HM), to perceive light (LP), to barely perceive light (BLP), to perceive no light (NLP).

In the absence of corrective lenses, a pinhole may be used to determine the patient's visual acuity at 20 ft. The pinhole may obviate the necessity of lenses for testing except in patients with opacities of the media (lens, vitreous). In patients with media opacities, the use of a pinhole with the subsequent reduction of illumination may result in a false reduction of visual acuity.

The 20-ft testing distance is important because as an object is brought closer a person may accommodate (focus) in order to see it. Accommodation results in magnification of the object so that the visual arc subtended is greater than it would be if it were 20 ft away. Children who can only see the 20/200 letter 20 ft away may be able to read the 20/20 letters 4 in. away from their eyes as they use accommodation and therefore magnification to increase the image size. In addition, patients with unrecognized myopia may see normally when the near acuity is tested and abnormally at a distance. In patients with significant retinal or optic nerve disease, there is usually a good correlation between a drop in distance visual acuity and near visual acuity. If there is a disproportionate loss, i.e., distance visual acuity poor, near visual acuity good, one must strongly suspect ocular disease.

Near visual acuity is tested on a standard reading card held 14 in. away. Patients with loss of accommodation as a result of advancing age (presbyopia) must wear the proper reading correction for accurate quantification. Near visual acuity may be tested at the bedside and may be useful if the patient is wearing the correct spectacles, but it is not as accurate as distance visual acuity.

Examination of the Visual Fields

The techniques generally used to measure the visual field result in a two-dimensional representation of an area representing the peripheral limits of ocular perception. These methods include using the tangent screen, autoplot, projector light, and various manual and computerized perimeters. These apparatuses are all examples of kinetic techniques.

Kinetic visual field testing consists of moving a stimulus (the object) to different areas and plotting the points at which it is seen by the patient. The size and brightness of the objects may be varied. The line connecting the points as seen by the patient and generated by one specific object is called an *isopter* (Fig. 8-1). Outside the isopter the retina is not sensitive to objects equal to or smaller than the test object. Within the area of visual field, the retina is sensitive to the object or objects bigger than the test stimulus. Smaller areas of depressed sensitivity (inability to detect the object) surrounded by areas of normal sensitivity are called *scotomas*. Formal visual field testing requires the use of several objects and the graphing of several isopters.

The absolute borders of the kinetic visual field are 90 degrees temporally, 60 degrees nasally, 60 degrees superiorly, and 75 degrees inferiorly. The foreshortened nasal field is due to anatomical differences between temporal and nasal retina and not to obstruction by the nose. Visual fields may be tested with white or colored objects. The main advantage of colored objects is that patients are more readily able to detect subtle differences in their perception of the color, enabling the examiner to more easily detect a depression of the visual field. This is particularly useful in patients with optic nerve disease.

The simplest technique for visual field examination is confrontation fields. This is useful as a screening device. The patient is asked to cover one eye and fixate on the examiner's opposite eye. One, two, or five fingers are presented separately in each of the quadrants of the visual field. These numbers do not require a complicated cognitive response by the patient. If the patient correctly identifies the number of fingers, then the test is repeated with simultaneous presen-

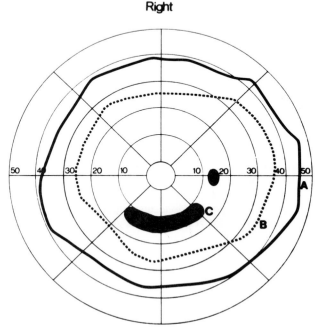

Figure 8-1   Kinetic visual field. *A*. Isopter of a large target. *B*. Isopter of a smaller target. *C*. An absolute scotoma. Visual acuity is 20/20.

tation in two quadrants. If the patient correctly identifies the number of fingers in each quadrant simultaneously, he or she is asked if there is any subjective difference between the two. The test may be brought to greater levels of sensitivity by presenting two identical colored objects in adjacent quadrants and asking the patient whether there is any subjective difference in the perception of color. If the visual acuity is normal and the confrontation field is normal, it is extremely unlikely that any field defect will be detected in more formal examinations. In patients with diminished visual acuity, confrontation field testing does not adequately measure the central visual field and more formal field examination is needed.

Slit Lamp Examination

Slit lamp examination will identify patients with corneal, lenticular, or vitreous disease. The slit lamp is also used to detect morphological changes in the iris and muscle of the iris and must be used to identify inflammatory cells in the anterior or posterior segments of the globe.

Intraocular Pressure

Intraocular pressure must be checked by any one of a number of techniques in all patients since visual loss secondary to increased ocular pressure (glaucoma) is not invariably associated with classic glaucomatous changes of the optic nerve.

Ophthalmoscopy

Examination of the ocular fundi, optic nerve, retinal vessels, and retina should be performed through a dilated pupil. The best agent for routine dilatation of the pupil is 1% tropicamide (1% Mydriacyl, Alcon Laboratories, Fort Worth, Tex.), which causes moderate pupillary dilatation lasting only 1 to 1½ h. The danger of causing an acute angle glaucoma attack is overemphasized, and ultimately the patient is well served should such an event occur under physician observation. An examination of the ocular fundus through an undilated pupil is fraught with the danger of misinterpretation even by the most skilled observer. Ideally, the patient should be examined with the conventional direct ophthalmoscope and the indirect ophthalmoscope. The indirect ophthalmoscope allows a three-dimensional view of the fundus, giving more accurate estimation of optic nerve swelling or cupping. The indirect ophthalmoscope is also necessary to examine the peripheral retina and retinal blood vessels. Retinal detachments, ocular tumors, retinal hemorrhages, and retinal degenerations may all simulate neuro-ophthalmic pathology and by their location be visible only with an indirect ophthalmoscope.

Color Vision

The most common abnormality of color vision is an inherited sex-linked disease occurring in males resulting in varying degrees of red-green color blindness. Color vision abnormalities may occur in hereditary retinal degenerations and acquired neuro-opthalmologic disorders. Color vision abnormalities usually indicate diffuse involvement of the optic nerve, such as that caused by compression or by demyelination. Color vision is not significantly affected in patients with segmental diseases of the optic nerve such as vascular infarction. Color vision abnormalities are a sensitive indicator of optic nerve disease and may be present in a person with normal visual acuity. Persons with reduced vision secondary to local pathology of the anterior segment of the eye usually maintain normal color perception. Preservation of color vision in a patient with optic nerve disease virtually excludes the possibility of a compressive lesion.

Standard color plates are available in book form as designed by a variety of clinicians. The Hardy-Rand-Rittler (American Optical Co.) series of color vision plates is best but is no longer being produced. A simple qualitative test of color vision may be done by having the patient compare perception of a red-colored object by one eye with that by the other eye.

Opticokinetic Nystagmus

Opticokinetic nystagmus is stimulated by asking the patient to look at a series of regularly presented targets. Usual stimuli include a rotating drum with alternate dark and light stripes or a similarly constructed long, narrow piece of cloth. Opticokinetic nystagmus may be elicited by moving the stimulus horizontally or vertically. It is present in all persons with normal vision and ocular motility. Normal opticokinetic nystagmus indicates some degree of visual acuity. However, varying the sizes of opticokinetic stimuli will not give precise visual acuity. Normal opticokinetic nystagmus is not compatible with vision of hand motion or worse.

Opticokinetic stimulation may be used to study ocular motility in infants, young children, and in adults who have difficulty with cooperation.

Photostress Test

The photostress test may differentiate unilateral visual loss secondary to optic nerve disease from visual loss caused by subtle retinal abnormalities. Each eye is tested separately. A bright light is shined directly into the eye being examined for a period of 60 s. The patient is then asked to read the smaller lines on the eye chart as soon as possible while the amount of time for visual recovery is measured. The procedure is repeated with the contralateral eye. The period of time for retinal readaptation should be symmetrical in patients with asymmetric vision due to unilateral optic nerve disease. If retinal disease is present, the readaptation time in the affected eye will be prolonged compared with that in the normal eye.

Ophthalmodynamometry

Ophthalmodynamometry indirectly measures ophthalmic artery blood pressure. It may be performed by one person using a direct ophthalmoscope or by two persons, one of whom uses an indirect ophthalmoscope. The ophthalmodynamometer is an instrument designed to apply a linearly increasing force onto the globe that is transmitted to the intraocular fluid. The instrument is placed on the eye, and the pressure is gradually increased while the central retinal vessels are observed. Diastolic blood pressure is noted as the point at which the central retinal artery begins to pulsate. Systolic blood pressure is the amount of pressure required to cause total collapse and blanching of the central retinal artery. The systolic pressure of the ophthalmic artery is approximately 80 percent of the brachial artery systolic pressure, while the diastolic pressure is 70 percent. A discrepancy between values of the two eyes of 20 percent for diastolic pressure above 50 units and 10 percent for diastolic readings below 40 units may be evidence of significant occlusion. Systolic pressures must differ by 20 percent to be significant.[11] Unfortunately, occlusion in the carotid artery less than 80 percent of the total lumen may be clinically significant yet not cause a change in ophthalmodynamometric measurements. Patients with bilateral disease may have a symmetric decrease of ophthalmic artery pressure that is not recognized. Ophthalmodynamometry may be most useful to verify asymmetric pressures and blood flow in persons with signs and symptoms signifying the same.

Examination of the Nerve Fiber Layer[24]

In 1972, William Hoyt and his associates re-emphasized the importance of ophthalmoscopic observations of the retinal nerve fiber[18] layer that had been made in the early part of this century in Europe. To evaluate the retinal nerve fiber layer, it is important to use a well-focused ophthalmoscope with a green light through a well-dilated pupil. A normal retinal nerve fiber layer is seen as a homogenous, slightly opaque striated layer.

Diffuse loss of the retinal nerve fiber layer parallels the development of optic atrophy in patients with severe optic nerve disease. Segmental loss of retinal nerve fiber layer may occur similarly in patients with segmental optic nerve disease, e.g., ischemic optic neuropathy. Slitlike defects in the nerve fiber layer are seen as an early sign of glaucomatous damage. Multiple slitlike defects in the retinal nerve fiber layer present bilaterally in patients with no subjective or objective evidence of visual loss but with neurological abnormalities is suggestive of multiple sclerosis. The preservation of normal retinal nerve striations in a patient with elevation of the optic nerve head indicates pseudopapilledema rather than true papilledema. Patients with congenital or long-standing or acquired defects in the retrochiasmal visual system show hemianopic patterns of retinal nerve fiber loss in each eye. Recognition of these patterns is important to diagnose a long-standing disease process.

Fluorescein Angioscopy and Angiography

If the retinal and choroidal vessels are observed through a blue filter after fluorescein dye is injected intravenously, the passage of the dye may be observed and/or recorded photographically. In normal patients, the retinal blood vessels do not leak dye since the normal blood-brain barrier is present. In patients with some types of retinal pathology and optic nerve pathology, the blood-brain barrier is not intact and fluorescein dye may be seen leaking from vessels. Fluorescein angiography may distinguish persons with true papilledema from patients with pseudopapilledema. In patients with pseudopapilledema, the blood-brain barrier is intact and no leakage of dye from the blood vessels on the optic nerve can be noted. Patients with true papilledema or nerve swelling from other causes show leakage of fluorescein dye in the area of the optic nerve[23] (Fig. 8-2).

Fluorescein angiography may show photographic evidence of retinal disease in patients with apparently normal ophthalmoscopic examinations. In patients with optic nerve disease or retinal vascular disease secondary to generalized vascular pathology such as vasculitis, fluorescein angiography may provide the clue to the presence of systemic disease. Fluorescein angiography may aid in the diagnosis of retinal angiomas in patients with suspected von Hippel–Lindau disease.

Electrophysiological Testing

Electroretinography uses an electrode mounted in a contact lens to measure the electrical potential of the globe following a flash of light. Electroretinography will be abnormal in patients with retinal receptor disease, i.e., retinitis pigmentosa. The electroretinogram differentially shows the integrity of inner and outer retinal layers and is an additional method for selectively studying choroidal and retinal circulations. The most common application for the electroretinogram in neuro-ophthalmology is the evaluation of visually handicapped infants. Many of these patients have Leber's congenital amaurosis, a type of hereditary retinal degeneration with minimal if any ophthalmoscopic signs. These patients may be diagnosed as having cortical blindness or optic nerve disease. The electroretinogram is normal in the latter cases and unequivocally abnormal in the former.

Electro-oculography measures retinal pigment epithelial function and may indicate abnormalities in patients with few ophthalmoscopic findings.

The visual evoked response (VER) is a wave appearing in the electroencephalogram following a change in visual stimulus. In the usual testing situation, a patient has electrodes placed over the occipital cortex and either a bright light is flashed repetitively into the patient's eyes or an alternating

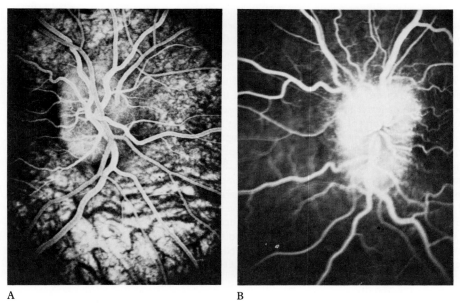

A   B

Figure 8-2 *A*. Fluorescein angiogram of normal optic disc, demonstrating normal capillaries on the disc surface without leakage. (Courtesy of Michael Rosenberg.) *B*. Fluorescein angiogram of papilledema demonstrating diffuse leakage of capillaries on the disc surface.

pattern of checkerboard squares is presented to the patient. A computer averages the resulting electrical activity recorded over both occipital cortexes. Random EEG activity slowly approximates zero, and the remaining wave, the VER, is the direct result of stimulation. The latency and amplitude of the various components of the visual evoked response as well as the form and timing are used to intimate the type and location of pathology within the visual system.

When the stimulus for a VER is a bright flash, approximately 50 percent of the resulting wave is generated by neurons arising from the central retina and 50 percent from neurons arising from the peripheral retina. If a patterned stimulus is used, the central neurons are responsible for approximately 70 percent of the resulting electrical wave.[26] Pupils must be dilated to assure a reproducible stimulus, and when a patterned target is used, the patient's refractive error must be controlled so that the stimulus is in focus.

The pattern of the normal visual evoked response is constant. The latency is the period of time between the stimulus and a selected peak of the visual evoked response. The amplitude is the height of the recorded response.

The usual clinical applications of visual evoked responses are identification of optic nerve disease, localization of pathology in the visual pathways, diagnosis of multiple sclerosis, and intraoperative monitoring of optic nerve functions.

Patients with acute optic neuritis show increased latency and decreased amplitude of the evoked response when compared with normal. This may be present when there is no clinical evidence of optic nerve disease. If recovery occurs normally, the amplitude may return to normal but the latency continues to be prolonged.[13] In a patient with total blindness, the evoked response generated from the involved eye should be flat.

Patients with diffuse demyelinating disease, i.e., multiple sclerosis, frequently show bilateral abnormal evoked responses whether or not the patient has subjective or objective visual difficulties or findings. The presence of bilateral optic nerve dysfunction as evidenced by abnormal evoked responses in a patient with neurological dysfunction in other pathways strongly suggests a diagnosis of multiple sclerosis.[14] For localization, asymmetry of evoked response amplitudes over both hemispheres indicates a hemianopic visual loss. Abnormal evoked responses recorded over the contralateral hemisphere when each eye is stimulated separately suggest bitemporal visual deficiency and indicate chiasmal pathology.

Evoked responses have been used to monitor optic nerve and chiasmal function during neurosurgical procedures.[39] A fiberoptic light source implanted in a scleral contact lens is placed on the patient's eye prior to surgery. Electrodes are placed in the usual locations. The visual evoked response is recorded sonically through the procedure to prevent excessive manipulation. In some patients with tumors, it may be difficult to distinguish optic nerve and chiasm from nonneural tissues and evoked response monitoring may aid in tissue identification.

Correlative Interpretation of Visual Field Defects

Accurate localization of pathology within the visual pathways may be determined by the pattern of field defect produced by that lesion. Topographic localization of field defects requires an understanding of the basic anatomy of the visual pathways.

Vision begins in the outermost retinal layer of receptors, the rods and cones. Fibers from the rods and cones synapse with a layer of bipolar cells in the middle retinal layer. Fibers from the bipolar cell synapse with the ganglion cells in the innermost retinal layer. The retinal ganglion cell is the nerve body for axons that originate in the retina and pass without synapse through the optic nerve, optic chiasm, and optic tract to the lateral geniculate bodies. The majority of axons in the visual pathways, more than 90 percent, subserve the central 25 degrees of vision. For this reason, the visual pathways may be considered as largely macular structures (corresponding to the macula of the retina). Retinal fibers from the macular area are small and thinly myelinated. The remaining fibers in the anterior visual pathways originate from peripheral retina and are thicker and more heavily myelinated. There are no ganglion cells directly in the fovea, and resolution is greatest in this area of densely packed cones without overlying retinal elements.

Axons originating from macular ganglion cells (the papillomacular bundle) pass in a straight line to the temporal portion of the optic nerve (Fig. 8-3). Peripheral retinal fibers arc around the papillomacular bundle and enter the optic disc superiorly and inferiorly. These are arcuate fibers. An imaginary vertical line drawn through the fovea of the retina separates nasal from temporal visual field. Fibers originating temporal to this imaginary line (noncrossing fibers) subserve vision in the nasal visual field. Fibers originating nasal or temporal to the optic nerve but nasal to the fovea (crossing fibers) subserve vision in the temporal visual field. Nasal retinal fibers (temporal field) will cross in the chiasm. Temporal retinal neurons (nasal field) will not cross in the chiasm. Within the arcuate bundles there is no separation of crossing from noncrossing fibers. Fibers from peripheral retina nasal to the optic nerve pass in a straight line to the nasal border of the optic disc.

An irregular horizontal line through the retina (the horizontal raphe) bisects the fovea and indicates the uneven separation of upper and lower peripheral fibers.

Within the optic nerve, posterior to the optic disc, macular fibers are central while peripheral fibers are located peripherally (Fig. 8-4A). Crossing and noncrossing fibers are mixed in the temporal periphery of the nerve while the nasal portion of the nerve contains primarily crossing fibers from peripheral retina nasal to the disc. There is no segregation of crossed from uncrossed fibers until they have passed several millimeters into the optic chiasm. An arcuate field defect may be produced by an anterior chiasmal lesion if the fibers are disturbed before the crossed and uncrossed fibers separate.

Within the optic chiasm nasal retinal fibers cross and pass to the contralateral optic tract (Fig. 8-4B). Inferonasal retinal fibers pass to the lateral portions of the contralateral tract while superonasal fibers are medial. After crossing in the chiasm, the inferonasal retinal fibers representing the superior temporal visual field loop for a short, variable distance into the contralateral optic nerve before passing to the optic tract. A lesion at the junction of the optic nerve and chiasm may cause an ipsilateral optic nerve field defect and

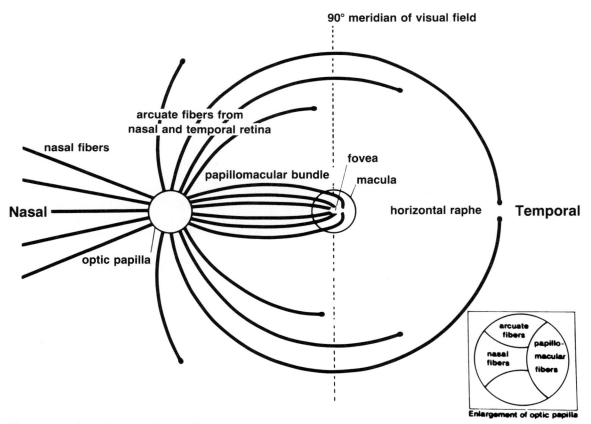

Figure 8-3 Organization of nerve fibers in the retina of the left eye.

contralateral superotemporal field defect by interfering with these looping fibers. These looping fibers are termed *von Willebrandt's knee*. There is no looping of superonasal retinal fibers in the ipsilateral optic tract. Central and peripheral fibers originating temporal to the fovea (uncrossed) pass to the optic tract on the ipsilateral side. As with crossing fibers, the noncrossing fibers originating in the inferior half of the retina are lateral in the tract while fibers originating in the superior retina are medial in the optic tract. Central or macular fibers are spread diffusely throughout the chiasm. The retinal nerve fibers passing in the nerves, chiasm, and optic tracts synapse within the lateral geniculate bodies.

The lateral geniculate body is a triangular structure with six laminae (Fig. 8-4C). Three of the laminae receive crossed fibers from the contralateral optic nerve and three laminae receive uncrossed fibers from the ipsilateral optic nerve. Superior retinal fibers project to the medial aspect of the geniculate body and inferior retinal fibers to the lateral aspect.

The optic radiation (Fig. 8-4D) starts in the lateral geniculate body, passes forward in the temporal lobe anterior to the lateral ventricle (Meyer's loop), sweeps posteriorly and laterally around the lateral ventricle, and terminates in area 17 of the occipital lobe (striate cortex). As has been described elsewhere, in the visual pathways the central and predominant portion of the optic radiations contain fibers subserving the central visual field. Within the optic tracts, axons from corresponding retinal elements of each eye are spatially separated. Within the optic radiations, fibers representing corresponding retinal areas move closer to one another until corresponding retinal fibers from each eye end on virtually adjacent cells in the visual cortex. The conglomeration of fibers from corresponding retinal areas occurs variably so that some lesions affecting the anterior visual radiations result in symmetric field defects in the two eyes while others result in asymmetric field defects.

Within the striate cortex the central visual field (macular fibers) are represented at the tip of the occipital lobe (Fig. 8-4E). More peripheral fibers terminate rostrally at the calcarine fissure. The most peripheral fibers, which serve the unilaterally represented temporal crescent, are located in the most anterior portion of the occipital lobe at the rostral end of the calcarine fissure. Superior retinal fibers (inferior visual field) are superior in the calcarine fissure and inferior retinal fibers (superior visual field) are inferior in the fissure.

Characteristics of Visual Field Defects

It is necessary to understand certain general characteristics of visual field defects in order to make inferences regarding the location and type of pathology. Retrochiasmal field defects may be congruous or incongruous. Visual field defects are congruous when the visual field defect measured in one eye is identical or nearly identical to the visual field defect in the other eye. If the visual field defects are very dissimilar, they are incongruous. The more posterior a lesion is in the visual pathways, the more congruous is the visual field de-

fect. Incongruous visual field defects are caused by lesions of the anterior retrochiasmal visual pathways.

Visual field defects may have great depth or be shallow. A deep visual field defect is one in which even large bright targets are not detected. A shallow defect is one which is present for small or dim targets but not for brighter or larger targets. A defect in which no object can be seen is absolute.

The margins of a visual field defect may be steep or sloping (Fig. 8-5). When the margins of a field defect are identical or nearly identical with different isopters, the border of the defect is considered steep. When the margins of the visual defect are widely disparate from one isopter to another, the borders are said to be sloping. Defects with steep borders are usually caused by discrete destructive processes such as a vascular infarction. Sloping defects indicate a gradation of structural damage, i.e., edema and reaction surrounding infective processes.

A scotoma is an area of decreased visual sensitivity surrounded by an area of normal or increased sensitivity. If the person is aware of the scotoma or area of decreased visual sensation, usually as a gray or black spot, the scotoma is positive. If the patient is unaware of the scotoma, the scotoma is negative. A patient with a retinal hole who sees a gray spot on a piece of paper is experiencing a positive scotoma. A patient with a homonymous hemianopsia who sees nothing to one side is experiencing a negative scotoma. If no object can be seen within the scotomatous area, the scotoma is absolute. If some objects may be seen in the scotomatous area but not other objects, the scotoma is relative. Most scotomas are defined by their position (Fig. 8-6). A central scotoma is a depressed area in the visual field that includes the point of fixation. A paracentral scotoma is a scotomatous area within the central 25 degrees of vision but not including fixation. A cecocentral scotoma is a scotoma that includes the blind spot and point of fixation. A ring or annular scotoma simply describes a scotoma surrounding and surrounded by areas of normal sensitivity.

Altitudinal field defects are areas of visual field depression occurring primarily in the upper or lower half of the visual field. Altitudinal field defects usually have one border corresponding to the 180 degree meridian. Hemianopic field defects are visual field depressions involving temporal or nasal halves of the visual field in one or both eyes. If the laterality of the hemianopic field defect in each eye is corresponding, the defect is considered a homonymous hemianopic field defect. Field defects confined to one quadrant of the visual field are quadrantanopic field defects.

Most neurological lesions of the chiasm or retrochiasmal visual pathways produce field defects with one border along the vertical (90 degree meridian). The main exceptions to this rule are field defects caused by lesions of the occipital lobe. Anterior to the occipital cortex the visual pathways are composed primarily of macular fibers. Virtually all visual field defects produced by lesions of the chiasm, optic tract, geniculate body, and optic radiations are apparent at least in the central 25 degrees of vision. Lesions of the occipital lobe, where the visual representation is spread over a large geographic area and the macular fibers are segregated, can cause visual field defects confined to peripheral areas of the visual field without central involvement.

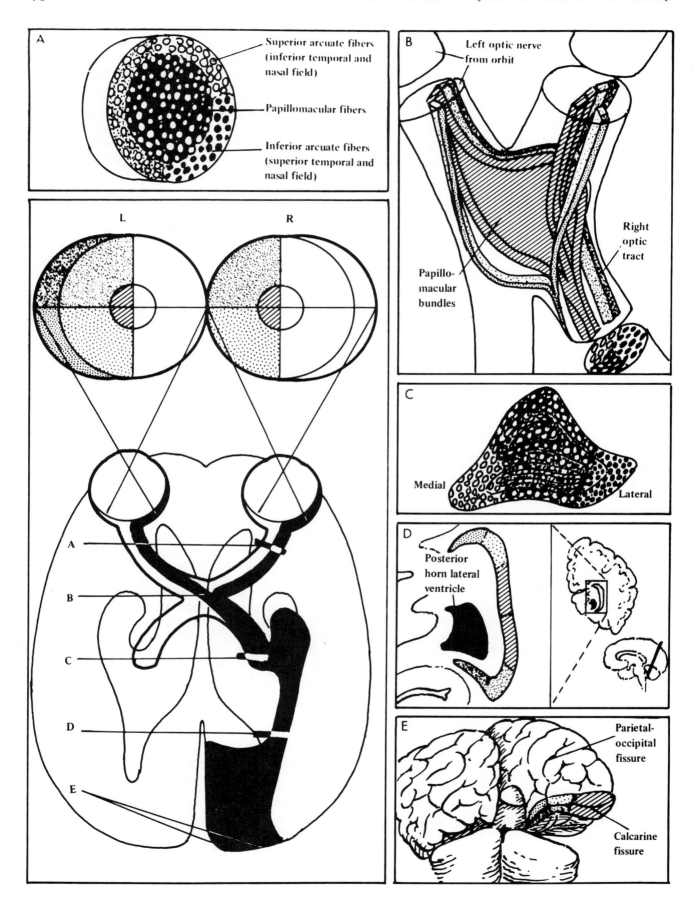

A

Superior arcuate fibers (inferior temporal and nasal field)

Papillomacular fibers

Inferior arcuate fibers (superior temporal and nasal field)

L   R

A
B
C
D
E

B

Left optic nerve from orbit

Right optic tract

Papillo-macular bundles

C

Medial   Lateral

D

Posterior horn lateral ventricle

E

Parietal-occipital fissure

Calcarine fissure

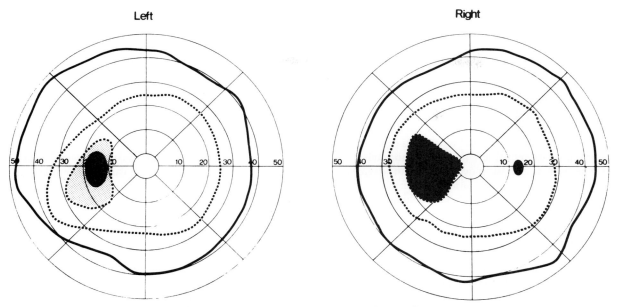

Figure 8-5 Left, sloping field defect, e.g., disc edema. Right, steep field defect, e.g., chorioretinitis. Visual acuity is 20/20 for both.

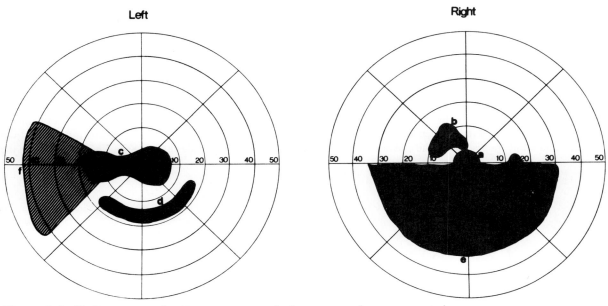

Figure 8-6 Various types of scotomas: *a*, central; *b*, paracentral; *c*, cecocentral; *d*, arcuate; *e*, inferior (altitudinal heminanopsia); and *f*, sector.

Figure 8-4 Arrangement of nerve fibers in the visual pathways. Fibers supplying the extreme temporal visual field (temporal crescent) are represented in one hemissphere only (contralateral). Pictured are an overall diagram in the lower left and sections through *A*, the optic nerve; *B*, optic chiasm and right optic tract; *C*, right lateral geniculate body; *D*, optic radiations; and *E*, striate cortex (area 17).

Diagnosis of Visual Field Defects

Visual field defects caused by retinal lesions that affect the rods and cones have the same morphology as the causative lesion. A round retinal lesion, i.e., choroidal tumor with overlying retinal detachment, causes a round visual field defect. The location of the visual field defect is opposite to the retinal localization. A round superior nasal melanoma will cause a round inferior temporal visual field defect. The scotoma produced by retinal lesions affecting the rods and cones may be absolute or relative depending on the degree of receptor damage. Patients with chorioretinal scars, i.e., following laser photocoagulation, will have absolute scotomas. Patients with incomplete destruction of the rods and cones, i.e., retinal detachments, have relative scotomas. Progression of the visual field defect may be used to follow retinal tumors.

If the retinal lesion results in destruction of the overlying retinal nerve fibers arising from the ganglion cells, the visual field defect produced consists of two parts. One part corresponds to the retinal lesion and destruction of rods and cones. A second component of the visual field defect results from interruption of the retinal fibers passing from more distal portions of the retina. If the overlying nerve fibers are arcuate, the resulting field defect will be an arcuate scotoma. If the interrupted neurons are running in a straight course, a sector field defect will result.

An enlarged blind spot is an example of a retinal lesion. A normal blind spot extends from 12 to 18 degrees temporal to fixation. It usually extends 5 to 6 degrees above and below the horizontal meridian. An enlarged blind spot is usually the result of pathology of the optic disc or adjacent to the optic disc. With rare exceptions, the cause of an enlarged blind spot is always apparent on ophthalmoscopic inspection. In the case of persons with swollen discs from any cause, the enlarged blind spot is due to the edematous disc displacing adjacent retinal receptors distally. In patients with inflammatory lesions of the optic nerve, there may be destructive changes of the receptors or pigment epithelium around the nerve. Many patients with old or congenital inflammatory disease have chorioretinal scarring adjacent to the nerve that results in permanent enlargement of the blind spot. Accurate determination of the blind spot requires a moderately bright object. Use of an excessively small or dim object may result in an inaccurately measured enlarged blind spot, since the normal decreased density of rods and cones adjacent to the optic nerve renders them incapable of responding to such stimulation. An enlarged blind spot with a normal appearing optic nerve and peripapillary retina suggests a flaw in the testing procedure.

Lesions of the prechiasmal optic nerve produce characteristic visual field defects. These field defects are (1) central scotoma; (2) cecocentral scotoma; (3) arcuate and paracentral scotoma; and (4) altitudinal and sector defects. A central scotoma is the most common visual field defect occurring from lesions that affect the optic nerve diffusely such as optic neuritis and extrinsic compressing masses. The thinner and less myelinated central fibers are more sensitive. Peripheral fibers are affected to some degree, causing peripheral depression as well. A cecocentral scotoma occurs primarily as a result of toxic amblyopia, certain hereditary forms of optic neuropathy (Leber's hereditary optic atrophy), and occasionally from inflammatory conditions. Arcuate and paracentral scotomas result from pathological processes interrupting arcuate fibers. These visual field defects suggest optic nerve pathology of vascular origin such as glaucoma, vasculitis, and migraine. An altitudinal field defect is an extreme example of an arcuate type of field defect. Lesions affecting the optic nerve near its junction with the chiasm produce a typical visual field defect. Traquair's junctional scotoma is an optic nerve defect in one eye, i.e., a central scotoma, associated with a superotemporal field defect in the contralateral eye (Fig. 8-7). The field defect in the

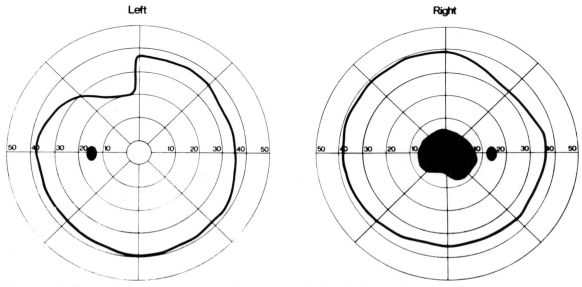

Figure 8-7 Traquair's junctional scotoma. Superotemporal field defect in left eye due to involvement of von Willebrandt's knee in right nerve. Visual acuity is 20/20. Central scotoma in right eye due to involvement of macular fibers in right optic nerve. Visual acuity is 20/80.

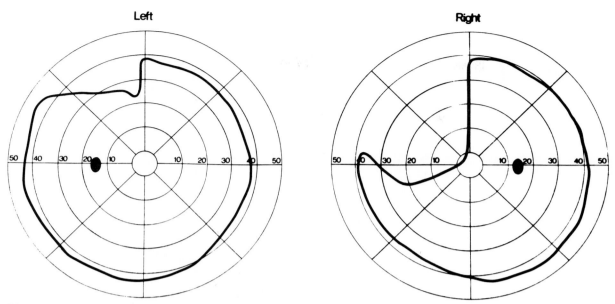

Figure 8-8 Incongruous homonymous hemianopsia from lesion of optic tract. Visual acuity is 20/20.

contralateral eye results from interruption of inferonasal retinal fibers in von Willebrandt's knee. Traquair's junctional scotoma is invariably caused by an extrinsic mass lesion.

Lesions of the optic chiasm cause bitemporal hemianopsia. Most chiasmal lesions are midline and involve the central crossing fibers initially. Bitemporal hemianopic field defects are noted initially in the central visual field when proper visual field examination is performed. Bitemporal field defects secondary to chiasmal pathology do not occur as isolated peripheral defects. As the lesion progresses, involvement of the more lateral noncrossing fibers ensues, resulting in additional depression of nasal portions of the visual field. It is likely that the primary mechanism of visual field dysfunction at the chiasmal area is interruption of the normal blood supply rather than direct compression and stretching of the neurons. Evidence for this is the rapid,

sometimes instantaneous, recovery of visual field following chiasmal decompression and the virtually instantaneous recovery of evoked responses during intraoperative recordings.

Incomplete lesions of the optic tract cause markedly incongruous homonymous visual field defects (Fig. 8-8). Complete destruction of the optic tract results in total homonymous hemianopsia. Total homonymous hemianopsia is not useful as a localizing sign, and the clinician must depend on accompanying signs and symptoms for more accurate localization.

Lesions of the geniculate body producing field defects are rare and usually associated with pathology near the thalamus. Visual field defects produced by geniculate lesions are incongruous and involve primarily the central visual field (Fig. 8-9).

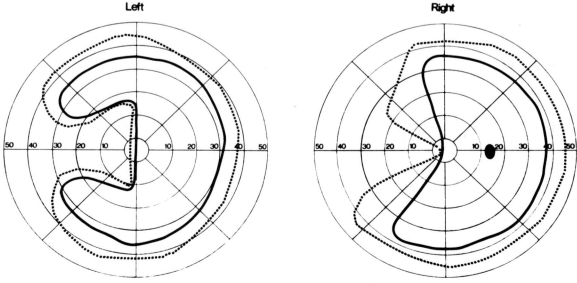

Figure 8-9 Incongruous geniculate field defect. Visual acuity is 20/20.

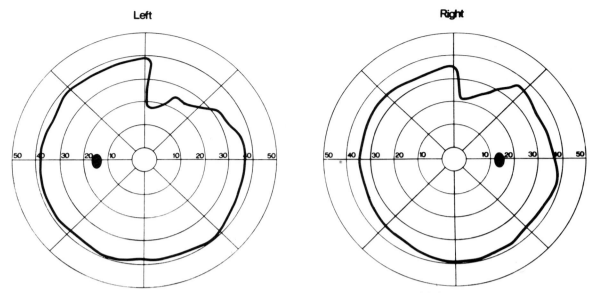

Figure 8-10 Superior quadrantanopia ("pie in the sky") caused by a temporal lobe lesion. Visual acuity is 20/20.

Lesions of the optic radiations cause typical patterns of visual field defects according to their location. Lesions of the temporal lobe usually involve inferior fibers in the optic radiation and cause a homonymous superior quadrantanopia ("pie in the sky") (Fig. 8-10). The hemianopsia is fairly congruous unless the underlying pathology is very anterior in the temporal lobe (Meyer's loop). Parietal lobe lesions produce congruous inferior quadrantanopia (Fig. 8-11). Lesions in either temporal or parietal lobe may cause a total homonymous hemianopsia.

The hallmarks of occipital cortical lesions are extreme congruity and complexity (Fig. 8-12).[35] There may be peripheral scotomatous lesions without central involvement. True macular sparing indicates an occipital lobe lesion. Mac-

ular sparing refers to a hemianopic field defect that lines up along the vertical meridian except in the central 5 degrees of vision. Most instances of apparent macular sparing are due to poor fixation. Macular sparing, when it occurs, may be due to sparing of neurons over a great area, dual blood supplies to the occipital pole, incomplete segregation of crossed and uncrossed fibers, or double innervation of macular areas. Bilateral hemianopic lesions without other neurological signs or symptoms usually indicate occipital lobe disease. Visual field defects caused by occipital lobe defects are associated with normal opticokinetic nystagmus. A lesion localized to the most anterior portion of the calcarine fissue may result in isolated unilateral loss of the temporal crescent (the temporal 30 degrees of the visual field). Sparing of this area

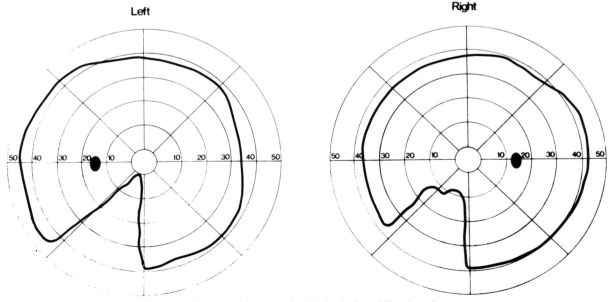

Figure 8-11 Inferior quadrantanopia caused by a parietal lobe lesion. Visual acuity is 20/20.

may result in preservation of the temporal crescent despite an otherwise hemianopic field defect. Either preservation or loss of the temporal crescent indicates an occipital cortical lesion.

The most common abnormality of recorded visual fields is generalized constriction. In the vast majority of cases, this is due to poor visual field examination techniques by the examiner or poor understanding and cooperation by the patient. The most usual causes of true constriction of the visual fields are quite distinct. These include glaucoma, retinal degeneration (retinitis pigmentosa), bilateral occipital lobe infarction, quinine toxicity, syphilitic perineuritis, chronic disc edema, and functional nonorganic visual loss. Patients with functional field loss show contraction or no change of the visual field when the testing distance is increased and the size of the test object is kept constant.

Ophthalmoscopic Correlates of Neurological Disease

Papilledema

Papilledema is a term that describes optic disc edema secondary to increased intracranial pressure. Unfortunately, many ophthalmologists use this term to describe optic disc edema secondary to local ocular and orbital disease. It is important for the neurologist or neurosurgeon to understand this when evaluating any ophthalmologic consultation and description. Optic disc swelling secondary to causes other than increased intracranial pressure should simply be described with the general term *optic disc edema* or with the specific pathogenetic mechanism, for example, disc edema secondary to central vein occlusion. The term *choked disc* is used by some clinicians in lieu of the phrase *optic disc edema*. The description of a choked disc should not be construed to indicate a specific cause of disc swelling.

The development of papilledema requires transmission of increased intracranial pressure to the vaginal sheaths surrounding the optic nerves.[38] A variable degree of communication between the vaginal sheaths of the optic nerve and the subarachnoid space and a variability of patency of the vaginal sheaths may partially explain instances of asymmetric papilledema. The increased pressure within the vaginal sheaths results in a series of complex hemodynamic and axoplasmic changes.[38] Axoplasmic flow is abnormal.[16] Axonal swelling that is initially secondary to the accumulation of intracellular material produces venous congestion and extracellular edema. Venous congestion also leads to increased blood flow with resulting capillary dilatation. The combination of axonal swelling, venous congestion, accumulation of metabolic by-products, and varying degrees of hypoxia cause varying degrees of visual dysfunction.

The ophthalmoscopic characteristics of papilledema may be inferred from the pathophysiological changes within the nerve. The ophthalmic characteristics of papilledema are (1) elevation of the optic disc; (2) venous distension; (3) dilation of optic nerve capillaries; (4) retinal hemorrhages; (5) preservation of the central cup; and (6) loss of spontaneous venous pulsation. Loss of venous pulsation in a person with no other signs of disc edema is not a significant finding.

Approximately 20 percent of normal persons have a spontaneous venous pulse. The presence of a spontaneous venous pulse indicates that at the moment of the observation the central venous pressure is greater than the intracranial venous pressure. Since the intracranial pressure may fluctuate even in patients with papilledema, it is not impossible to see a spontaneous venous pulse in a patient with well-developed papilledema. Elevation of the optic nerve as a result of axonal swelling requires the presence of functioning neurons. Patients with optic atrophy and loss of neurons will not develop papilledema. Patients with partial or segmental optic atrophy and increased intracranial pressure will develop edema only in the area of surviving neurons. Since the vast volume of large neurons enters the optic disc at the superior and inferior poles, patients with early papilledema have blurred margins in these areas initially. Patients with sharp margins at the inferior and superior poles and blurred nasal and/or temporal margins are not likely to have true papilledema. In patients with minimal ophthalmoscopic signs, serial observation is necessary to document the diagnosis.

The clinical characteristics of papilledema are (1) bilaterality; (2) normal visual acuity; (3) normal color vision; (4) normal pupillary reactions; and (5) visual field defects of enlarged blind spot. Unilateral disc swelling is rarely caused by increased intracranial pressure unless there is optic atrophy of the nonedematous nerve or a unilateral abnormality of the vaginal sheaths of the optic nerve. If visual acuity is reduced, one must reconsider the diagnosis of simple papilledema and consider the possibility of other types of optic nerve disease. Patients with a high degree of papilledema may develop spread of edema into the retina in the macular area of the eye, causing reduced central visual acuity. This is invariably a reversible phenomenon and does not indicate the need for urgent intervention. Chronic papilledema may progress to atrophy of the optic nerve with late loss of visual field, in the periphery initially, and ultimate loss of visual acuity.

As chronic papilledema progresses to optic atrophy, the reddish discoloration of the optic disc disappears and the optic disc appears grayish-white. Associated with this may be proliferation of connective tissue on the disc surface, with sheathing of the retinal vessels and permanent irregular blurring of the margins.

Optic Neuritis[22]

Optic neuritis implies involvement of the optic nerve by an inflammatory process. Involvement of the optic disc by such an inflammatory process is termed *papillitis*. Involvement of the retrobulbar portions of the optic nerve is termed *retrobulbar neuritis*. The clinical signs and symptoms of papillitis and retrobulbar neuritis and their implications are similar. The primary difference is that patients with papillitis have ophthalmoscopically visible changes at the optic nerve head.

Inflammatory optic neuritis may be caused by a diverse number of etiologic processes. Involvement of the optic nerve may occur as part of a local or diffuse demyelinating process. Patients with various viral infections may have demyelination secondary to direct invasion of the nerve by an infectious agent or indirectly by an autoimmune demyelination induced by an infectious agent.

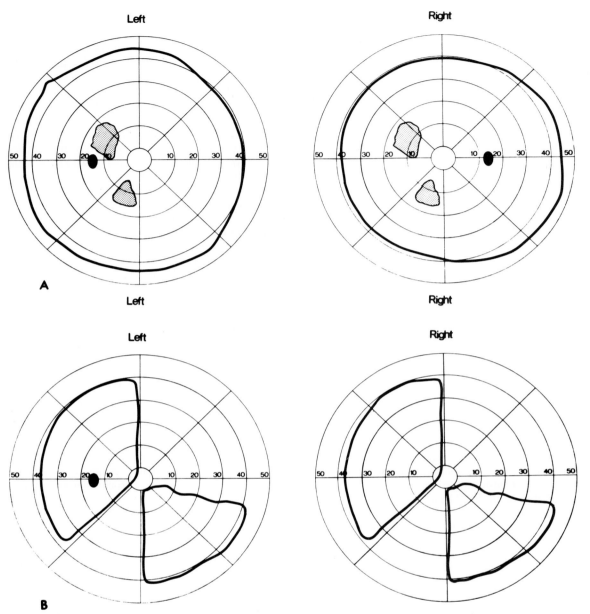

Figure 8-12 Field defects of the occipital lobe. *A.* Jigsaw field defect, very congruous. *B.* Bilateral congruous quadrantanopia caused by bilateral defects of occipital lobe. *C.* Left homonymous hemianopsia with sparing of macula. *D.* Right homonymous hemianopsia with preservation of right temporal crescent, secondary to sparing of most anterior calcarine cortex on the left side. Visual acuity in each example is 20/20.

The typical clinical characteristics of optic neuritis are (1) reduced vision in the involved eye; (2) decreased color perception in the involved eye; (3) presence of an afferent pupillary defect in the involved eye, presuming the contralateral eye is normal; (4) typical visual field defects, generally central scotoma with peripheral depression; and (5) evidence of intraocular inflammation, i.e., inflammatory cells in the vitreous.

Individuals with papillitis will show an edematous hyperemic disc possibly with vascular congestion and hemorrhages but less than that observed in persons with papilledema. Optic neuritis is usually unilateral. Optic neuritis may be present in the face of normal visual acuity, but color vision testing and pupillary testing are invariably abnormal. Loss of vision in patients with optic neuritis is usually acute. Recovery, at least from an initial attack, is usually complete with regard to visual function, though varying degrees of optic atrophy may ensue within a 10- to 21-day period. Recurrent optic neuritis strongly suggests a diagnosis of multiple sclerosis.

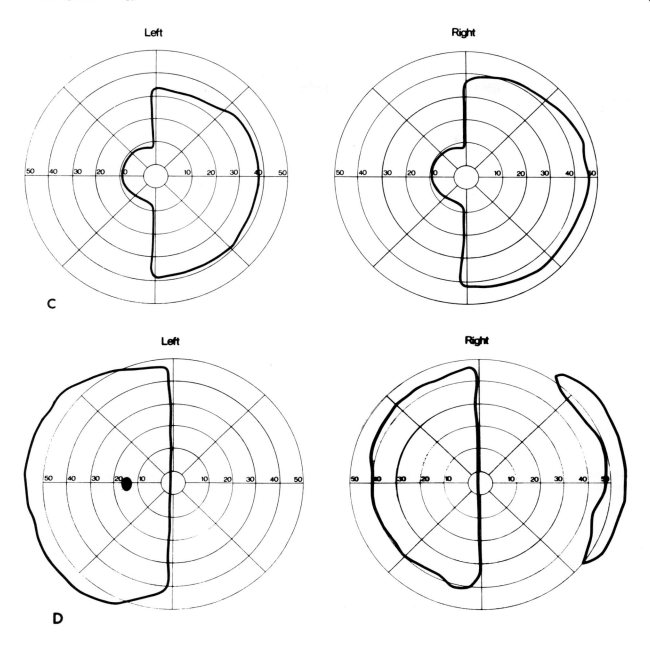

Ischemic Optic Neuropathy[3,15,17,20]

Ischemic optic neuropathy is a clinically recognizable entity caused by segmental or total interference of the blood supply to anterior portions of the optic nerve. The clinical characteristics of optic neuropathy are (1) acute loss of visual acuity; (2) pale edema of the optic nerve, which may be diffuse or segmental; (3) associated attenuation of arterioles on the optic nerve head; (4) visual field defects indicating segmental optic nerve damage, i.e., arcuate field defects, altitudinal field defects, and sector field defects; (5) afferent pupillary defect in the involved or more involved eye; and (6) preservation of color vision in persons with segmental involvement. The most common forms of ischemic optic neuropathy are the nonarteritic and arteritic types.

The arteritic type of ischemic optic neuropathy is infarction of the optic nerve associated with temporal arteritis. While most patients have involvement of the optic disc with appropriate ophthalmoscopic changes, a few patients may have retrobulbar involvement with little visible pathology. Patients with arteritic ischemic optic neuropathy are older, usually 65 years of age or greater. They complain of generalized fatigue, weakness, headache, proximal muscle pain (polymyalgia rheumatica), and jaw claudication. Visual complaints include transient or permanent visual loss and/or diplopia. The Westergren sedimentation rate is elevated to levels greater than 40 mm/h. Bilateral involvement within a short period of time is common, and the visual loss may be stabilized or improved by local and/or systemic steroid administration.

Persons with nonarteritic anterior ischemic optic neuropathy invariably have involvement of the optic disc. Patients with the nonarteritic form of ischemic optic neuropathy are middle-aged, 40 to 55 years of age, and approximately 50 percent of the patients have evidence or history of systemic vascular disease, i.e., diabetes and hypertension. The sedimentation rate is normal, and steroid treatment is not effective. Usually one eye is involved, but approximately 40 percent of patients develop involvement of the second eye at some time in their life. Unlike the arteritic forms of ischemic optic neuropathy, each optic nerve usually is involved on only one occasion. In both forms of ischemic optic neuropathy, arteritic and nonarteritic, the combination of optic atrophy from previous involvement in one eye with disc edema associated with present involvement in the other eye may suggest a Foster Kennedy syndrome. The history and typical clinical characteristics should distinguish this pseudo Foster Kennedy syndrome from the true Foster Kennedy syndrome. The true Foster Kennedy syndrome describes persons with unilateral optic atrophy and contralateral papilledema secondary to an increasing intracranial mass lesion causing initial compression of one optic nerve.

Other less common causes of ischemic optic neuropathy include syphilis, collagen vascular disease, hyperviscosity syndrome, and migraine.

Optic Atrophy

Optic atrophy denotes loss of neurons within the optic nerve usually secondary to a pathological process. The loss of neurons may occur as a result of destruction by compressing lesions, inflammatory lesions, chronic disc edema, and infarction, and from degeneration and destruction secondary to toxins. The ophthalmoscopic correlates of optic atrophy are pallor and loss of the retinal nerve fiber layer. The normal color of the optic nerve is probably related primarily to the color of the small capillaries and arterioles within the optic nerve. The architecture of the nerve fibers traversing the optic nerve is indirectly responsible for how the color of the blood vessels is transmitted. The diagnosis of optic atrophy should not be made on the basis of the appearance of disc color only. The presence or absence of a normal retinal nerve fiber layer, the configuration and size of the optic cup, and careful examination for defects in visual function are all necessary to diagnose optic atrophy with certainty. Connective tissue elements of the optic nerve (glial cell) show varying degrees of proliferation in persons with optic atrophy. When there is a relative absence of glial proliferation, the atrophic nerve looks white and flat and has sharp borders. This is termed *primary optic atrophy*. The surrounding retina is normal, and the retinal vessels are not sheathed. Secondary optic atrophy describes a gray-white appearance of the atrophic nerve, frequently with irregularity of the optic disc margins, heaped-up tissue on the surface of the disc, and vascular sheathing. Secondary optic atrophy is usually the result of processes causing edema of the optic disc antecedent of the axonal loss. Compressing lesions typically cause primary optic atrophy if there is no disc edema, and inflammatory lesions cause secondary optic atrophy.

This distinction is probably simplistic and is not a reliable distinguishing characteristic for accurate diagnosis.

Patients with glaucomatous optic atrophy show significant enlargement of the normal optic cup. Besides increased size, characteristics of the pathological optic cup are asymmetry between both eyes, vertical enlargement of the cup, and edge irregularities ("notching") of the rim. Patients with certain forms of acute optic disc damage such as ischemic optic neuropathy and methanol toxicity may show extreme degrees of nonglaucomatous cupping. An important distinguishing feature between glaucomatous optic atrophy and nonglaucomatous optic atrophy with cupping is that patients with glaucoma usually have good color of the remaining rim of neural tissue. Patients with optic atrophy and nonglaucomatous cupping usually show pallor of the neural rim.[37]

Retinal Pathology in Patients with Neurological Disease

Perivascular Sheathing

Sheathing of the retinal arterioles may be observed in patients with systemic vasculitis. Perivenous sheathing has been reported in some patients with multiple sclerosis.

Von Hippel–Lindau Disease

The characteristics of von Hippel–Lindau disease are (1) autosomal dominant heredity; (2) retinal angiomas; (3) central nervous system angiomas (cerebellar hemangioblastoma); (4) visceral angioma; (5) renal cell carcinomas; and (6) pheochromocytomas. The retinal lesions may be present as an isolated finding or may precede the development of neurological signs and symptoms by many years. Indirect ophthalmoscopy is necessary for the retinal evaluation of patients with suspected von Hippel–Lindau disease. An early retinal lesion appears as a small red dot similar to a microaneurysm but usually presents in the midperiphery of the retina. This gradually enlarges and develops a single feeding artery and tortuous draining vein. The lesion may remain stable or grow. Growth of the lesion may be associated with exudation along the abnormal vessels and beneath the retina. In severe cases, exudation may be severe and cause profound visual loss and retinal detachment. Fluorescein angiography is necessary to discover initially small lesions.

Subhyaloid Hemorrhage

Subhyaloid hemorrhage describes intraocular hemorrhage that is anterior to the retinal surface but posterior to the lamina of the vitreous body. The subhyaloid hemorrhage occurs as a result of rupture of a small capillary or venule on the inner retinal surface, which causes blood to pool in the potential space between the vitreous and the retina. Such hemorrhage may occur as the result of an acute elevation of venous pressure, i.e., any Valsalva maneuver, stress trauma, or subarachnoid hemorrhage. The degree and rapidity of venous elevation is proportional to the volume of hemorrhage. In severe cases, the hemorrhage may break through the posterior vitreous lamina (posterior hyaloid) and fill the vitreous cavity.

In typical cases, a defect in visual acuity or visual field occurs secondary to obstruction of light to the underlying rods and cones. In most patients, the hemorrhage will absorb over a period of weeks following the initial occurrence, leaving no visual sequelae.

Retinal Emboli

A number of types of retinal emboli may be observed. A cholesterol crystal (Hollenhorst plaque) is a crystalline refractile object usually noted at the bifurcation of retinal vessels. They do not interfere with blood flow and produce no visual symptoms. Their presence indicates an ulcerating atheroma on the side of the embolus. Fibrin platelet emboli have a creamy, pluglike consistency and usually extend over some segment of an arteriole. They are initiated by elements of the blood (RBCs, platelets) damaged during flow past atherosclerotic lesions of major arteries. They do cause obstruction of blood flow and cause transient or permanent retinal ischemia or damage.

Ocular Motor System

Supranuclear Control of Eye Movements[6,36]

There are four types of eye movements: saccades, smooth pursuit movements, vergence movements, and vestibulo-ocular movements. Each type of ocular movement is generated by a specific neural subsystem that can be differentiated anatomically and physiologically.

Saccades are rapid conjugate eye movements. Random eye movements and the fast component of nystagmus generated by any stimulus are examples of saccades. Saccades are present at birth. They are the fastest eye movements, with velocity as great as 400 degrees per second. The latency between the stimulus for saccadic eye movement and the onset of eye movement is 200 ms. Saccades are ballistic. A saccadic eye movement once generated cannot be modified until the original saccade is complete.

Saccadic eye movements are initiated in the frontal cortex. The greatest concentration of sites capable of initiating saccadic eye movement is in area 8 of the frontal cortex. Electrical stimulation of either cerebral hemisphere results in a saccadic eye movement to the opposite side. Stimulation of a single hemisphere may initiate a saccade with a vertical component, but pure vertical saccades probably require bilateral hemispheral involvement in normal persons. Neurons mediating saccadic eye movements pass from the frontal cortex in the internal capsule through the reticular formation adjacent to the cerebral peduncles. Pathways are probably polysynaptic. Neurons capable of generating horizontal saccades end in the paramedian pontine reticular for-

mation. Neurons capable of generating vertical eye movements end in the pretectal area. There is a decussation of the fibers for horizontal eye movements within the brain stem occurring between the third and fourth cranial nerve nuclei (Fig. 8-13). The brain stem gaze center for horizontal saccades is the paramedian pontine reticular formation (PPRF). From this area, signals are sent to the sixth nerve nucleus and the appropriate third nerve nucleus by way of the medial longitudinal fasciculus. The right PPRF generates horizontal eye movements to the right, and the left PPRF generates horizontal eye movements to the left. The brain stem gaze centers for vertical saccadic eye movements are located in the pretectum ventral to the periaqueductal gray matter. The gaze center for upward saccades is located dorsal and rostral to the gaze center for downward saccades. From the vertical gaze center, signals are sent to the appropriate ocular motor nuclei by way of the medial longitudinal fasciculus (MLF).

Smooth pursuit movements are slow conjugate movements that occur when the object of regard moves slowly. Pursuit eye movements are accurate and smooth to velocities of 30 degrees per second. If the object is moving faster than 30 degrees per second, smooth pursuit disappears and is replaced by multiple small-amplitude saccadic eye movements (saccadic pursuit). Smooth pursuit movements are not present until 6 weeks of age. They have a latency period of 120 ms but may be modified during active pursuit. While saccadic eye movements are not very sensitive to drugs or diffuse central nervous system dysfunction, smooth pursuit eye movements are. Smooth pursuit eye movements originate in anterior occipital and posterior callosal areas. The right hemisphere generates smooth pursuit movements to the right, and the left hemisphere generates smooth pursuit movements to the left. Both hemispheres are required to generate pure vertical smooth pursuit movements in normal

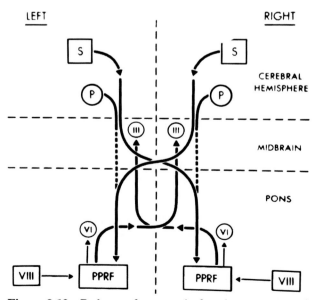

Figure 8-13 Pathways for control of ocular movement. S indicates saccade; P, pursuit; and PPRF, paramedian pontine reticular formation.

persons. Neurons mediating smooth pursuit eye movements pass from the occipital area in the internal sagittal striatum (the medial part of the lateral ventricular wall) to the internal capsule and through the reticular formation to the brain stem gaze centers in the PPRF and pretectum (Fig. 8-13).

Vergence eye movements are dysconjugate. The stimulus for convergence or divergence is disparity of retinal images. Vergence movements are slow, 20 degrees per second, and have a latency of 160 ms. Vergence movements are probably generated from the anterior occipital or posterior callosal areas. Brain stem gaze centers for convergence and divergence receive neurons from this area. The brain stem centers are ventral in the tegmentum of the midbrain.

Sensory organs for vestibular eye movements are the semicircular canals, utricle, and saccule. Vestibular eye movements maintain visual fixation during changes of body position. The right horizontal semicircular canal drives the eyes to the left, and the left horizontal semicircular canal drives the eyes to the right. Vestibular ocular movements have a short latency and may attain speeds of 300 degrees per second. They may be observed clinically after caloric stimulation. Cold water instilled in one external auditory meatus generates nystagmus with a slow movement (vestibulo-ocular movement) to the ipsilateral side and a fast component (saccade) to the contralateral side. The opposite response will occur after stimulation with warm water. Neurons pass from the vestibular end organs through the vestibular nuclei to the PPRF and subsequently to the appropriate ocular motor nuclei (Fig. 8-13).

Ocular Motility Abnormalities Associated with Defects of the Supranuclear Control System[2,7,8,21,29]

Conjugate gaze in any direction may be absent (gaze palsy) or weak (gaze paresis). In most clinical situations, there is symmetrical involvement of gaze for both smooth pursuit and saccadic eye movements. A gaze paresis may be manifest in several ways. Persons with gaze paresis may be able to move their eyes in a limited manner in one direction or may move their eyes fully but be unable to sustain gaze in that direction. If the patient is asked to look in one direction and there is a gaze paresis, the eyes may move appropriately, fatigue, and drift back to the primary position and move quickly again eccentrically as effort is expended. The resulting irregular jerky eye movements are called *gaze-paretic nystagmus*.

Gaze palsies may result from lesions anywhere along the supranuclear ocular motor pathways. A lesion involving a cerebral hemisphere usually results in gaze palsy or gaze paresis to the opposite side. An acute cerebral lesion initially causes gaze palsy with deviation of the eyes to the side of the lesion as a result of the unopposed action of the contralateral intact central ocular motor centers. As recovery occurs, the gaze palsy becomes a gaze paresis. Recovery in patients with hemispheral lesions is usually complete. Lesions of the paramedian pontine reticular formation cause gaze palsy or paresis to the same side. A lesion of the left paramedian pontine reticular formation results in a left gaze abnormality. Gaze palsies or paresis caused by brain stem lesions require ex-

tended periods of time for recovery and are more likely to be permanent.

It is rare to have a single hemispheral lesion cause an abnormality of pure vertical eye movements. Lesions in the pretectal or tectal areas cause abnormalities of vertical gaze. Upward gaze is most commonly disturbed, but isolated abnormalities of downward gaze may occur also. The syndrome of the Sylvian aqueduct (Parinaud's syndrome, Koerber-Salius-Elschnig syndrome) consists of (1) disturbances of vertical gaze, (2) pupillary abnormalities (light-near dissociation), (3) disturbances of accommodation, (4) convergence insufficiency, (5) lid retraction, and (6) retraction nystagmus. This syndrome is usually caused by mass lesions in the region of the posterior third ventricle, i.e., pinealoma, but has been observed in patients with vascular disease, multiple sclerosis, chronic alcohol intoxication, and trauma. In children and infants with hydrocephalus, bilateral lid retraction associated with paralysis of upward gaze ("sunset sign") may be the earliest sign of shunt decompensation. This occurs secondary to dilatation of the aqueduct with subsequent involvement of the pretectal gaze centers.

Abnormalities of vergence movements are difficult to diagnose. Normal convergence is dependent on patient effort and motivation and ought not to be considered abnormal unless associated with other signs of midbrain neurological abnormality. Divergence insufficiency is rare. Spasm of the near reflex that consists of apparent involuntary convergence, miosis, and accommodation should be considered secondary to psychiatric disease until proved otherwise.

Internuclear ophthalmoplegia is an ocular motor disturbance resulting from a lesion of the medial longitudinal fasciculus. It consists of total or partial weakness of adduction on the side of the lesion and nystagmus of the abducting (contralateral) eye. Internuclear ophthalmoplegia may be anterior or posterior.[32] Posterior internuclear ophthalmoplegia is associated with intact convergence. In patients with posterior internuclear ophthalmoplegia, the lesion in the medial longitudinal fasciculus lies between the paramedian pontine reticular formation and the third nerve nuclear complex. The lesion is usually caudal in the pons. Anterior internuclear ophthalmoplegia is associated with loss of convergence. The lesion causing anterior internuclear ophthalmoplegia must be present in the small group of fibers passing from the medial longitudinal fasciculus to the third oculomotor nerve subnucleus controlling the medial rectus muscle. Patients with unilateral internuclear ophthalmoplegia have straight eyes. Patients with bilateral internuclear ophthalmoplegia show divergent eyes.

The combination of an internuclear ophthalmoplegia and gaze palsy on the same side is called the "1½ syndrome"[9] or *paralytic pontine exotropia*.[30] This syndrome results from a lesion affecting the paramedian pontine reticular formation and median longitudinal fasiculus on the same side. The patient is not able to gaze with either eye toward the side of the lesion and is unable to adduct the eye ipsilateral to the lesion to the opposite side. Common causes of internuclear ophthalmoplegia and paralytic pontine exotropia are vascular disease, demyelinating disease, intraparenchymal neoplastic lesions, and trauma. Bilateral internuclear ophthalmoplegia is considered secondary to demyelinating disease until proved otherwise.

Anatomy of the Ocular Motor Nerves

The oculomotor nucleus (third nerve) is located in the peri-aqueductal gray matter at the level of the superior colliculus (Fig. 8-14). The oculomotor nuclei on each side are adjacent to one another. Each oculomotor nucleus is divided into subnuclei. A single caudal midline subnucleus innervates the levator muscle of both eyes and an anterior midline group of cells (Edinger-Westphal subnucleus) supplies the parasympathetic innervation to each eye. The medial rectus, inferior rectus, and inferior oblique muscles receive their innervation from the appropriate ipsilateral subnucleus while the superior rectus muscle receives innervation from the contralateral superior rectus subnucleus.

Fibers of the oculomotor nerve passing through the parenchyma of the midbrain make up the fascicular portion of the nerve. Fibers exit from the third nerve nucleus ventrally and pass laterally through the red nucleus and superior aspects of the cerebral peduncles into the interpeduncular fossa. The fibers of the oculomotor nerve exit from the midbrain as a series of discrete rootlets and coalesce into a single nerve trunk. Involvement in the area of the oculomotor nerve rootlets may result in asymmetric involvement of the ocular muscles supplied by the nerve. The oculomotor nerve passes through the subarachnoid space between the superior cerebellar artery and the posterior cerebral artery and is located inferior medial to the posterior communicating artery (Fig. 8-15). The nerve pierces the dura lateral to the posterior clinoid process, traverses the cavernous sinus, where it is located superiorly, and enters the orbit through the supe-

rior orbital fissure. Within the orbit, the nerve divides into superior and inferior divisions. The superior division innervates the levator and superior rectus muscles. The inferior division innervates the medial rectus, inferior rectus, and inferior oblique muscles and, in addition, contains parasympathetic fibers from the Edinger-Westphal subnucleus.

The trochlear nucleus (fourth nerve) is found in the peri-aqueductal gray matter at the level of the inferior colliculus (Fig. 8-16). The fascicular portion of the nerve exits the nucleus laterally and passes dorsal to the nucleus converging with the fascicular portion of the contralateral trochlear nerve above the aqueduct. This is the only cranial nerve exiting the brain stem dorsally. Each trochlear nerve nucleus innervates the contralateral superior oblique muscle. The trochlear nerve exits the brain stem at the edge of the tentorium. The nerve passes rostral in the subarachnoid space, pierces the dura, traverses the cavernous sinus lateral and inferior to the third nerve, and enters the orbit through the superior orbital fissure passing to the superior oblique muscle (Fig. 8-15).

The abducens nucleus (sixth nerve) is located in the pons ventral to the floor of the fourth ventricle (Fig. 8-17). Each abducens nucleus is slightly lateral to the midline. The paramedian pontine reticular formation is medial to the nucleus, and the medial longitudinal fasciculus is superior and medial to the sixth nerve nucleus. The fascicular portion of the abducens nerve exits from the nucleus ventrally and passes superior to the facial nucleus (seventh nerve). It exits the brain stem in a groove between the pons and medulla, passing upward along the base of the pons on either side of the

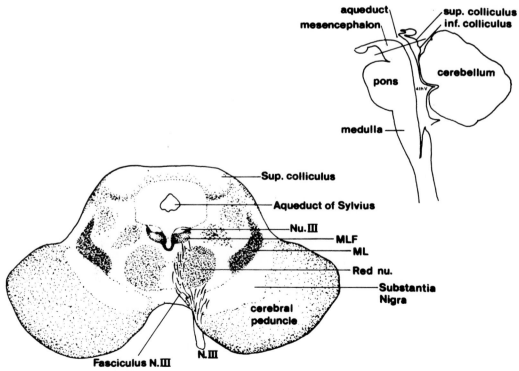

Figure 8-14   Midbrain section shows the origin of the third nerve at the level of the superior colliculus. MLF indicates medial longitudinal fasciculus; ML, medial lemniscus.

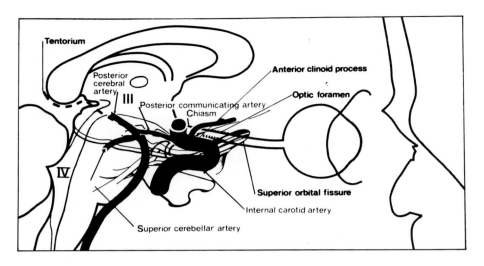

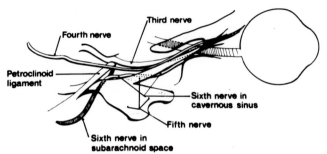

Figure 8-15 Subarachnoid, intracavernous, and orbital pathways of ocular motor nerves.

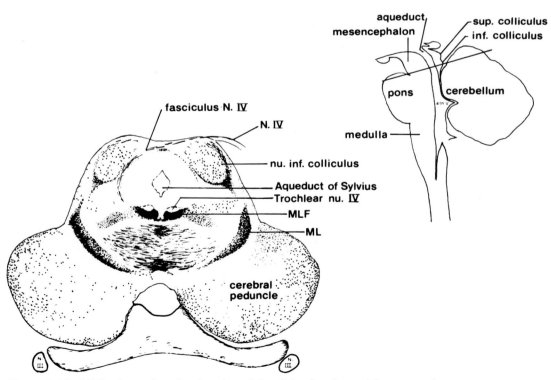

Figure 8-16 Midbrain section showing the origin of the fourth cranial nerve at the level of the inferior colliculus. MLF indicates medial longitudinal fasciculus; ML, medial lemniscus.

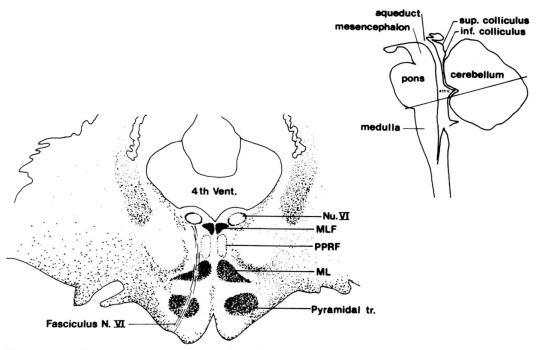

Figure 8-17 Pontine section shows the origin of the sixth nerve and demonstrates the medial longitudinal fasciculus (MLF) and paramedian pontine reticular formation (PPRF). ML indicates medial lemniscus.

basilar artery. It lies adjacent to or passes through the inferior petrosal sinus and through Dorello's canal, piercing the dura and transversing the cavernous sinus, where it is the most medial of the cranial nerves within the sinus (Fig. 8-15). The abducens nerve enters the orbit through the superior orbital fissure and innervates the lateral rectus muscle.

Examination of the Ocular Motor System

Versions describe the movement of both eyes together. Ductions describe the movement of each eye separately. Vergence describes the simultaneous movement or attempted movement of the eyes in opposite directions. A tropia is a manifest deviation of the eyes which is not overcome by fusion, i.e., the visual axis of each eye is not the same under binocular conditions. A cross-eyed child is an example of a person with a tropia. A phoria is a manifest deviation of the eyes that is overcome by fusion. A patient with a phoria may have an ocular motility imbalance or tendency for the eyes not to have the same visual axis but this tendency is overcome by fusional reflexes in the binocular state. A child whose eyes appear straight most of the time but tend to become cross-eyed when he is fatigued or ill is probably an individual with a phoria that will occasionally become a tropia (cross-eyed). Phorias and tropias refer to the state of ocular muscle balance. The direction of "drift" in patients with phorias and tropias is indicated by the prefixes *eso*, *exo*, and *hyper*. An *eso*tropia or *eso*phoria indicates a tendency for an eye to move *inward*. An *exo*tropia or *exo*phoria indicates a tendency for an eye to move *outward*. A

*hyper*tropia or *hyper*phoria indicates a tendency for an eye to move *upward*. All of these terms refer to the direction of the nonfixing eye when the person is asked to fixate a specific target. While the patient may prefer to use one eye for fixation, the fixating eye may alter simply by occluding the appropriate eye. A cross-eyed child is esotropic and a wall-eyed child is exotropic. If the amount of dysconjugacy of the eyes is the same in all positions of gaze, the deviation is said to be comitant. If the dysconjugacy of the eyes is different in various positions of gaze, the deviation is said to be noncomitant.

When a patient with a right lateral rectus palsy gazes in the primary position of gaze, the left eye fixes and the right eye is deviated inward; the patient has an esotropia. When the patient looks to the left, both eyes move normally because the left lateral rectus muscle and right medial rectus muscle are normal. In left gaze, the eyes are straight (orthophoric). When the patient is asked to look to the right, the left eye moves fully because the left medial rectus is intact. The right eye does not abduct because the right lateral rectus is defective. On right gaze, the patient has an esotropia that is more marked than the esotropia present in the primary position. Since the deviation varies in varying positions of gaze (none in left gaze, medium in primary gaze, and marked in right gaze), the deviation is said to be noncomitant. Ocular deviations caused by paralysis or paresis of individual ocular muscles are noncomitant.

Persons with paralytic strabismus have greater deviations of the eyes when the paretic eye is fixing than when the nonparetic eye is fixing. This is due to overaction of the normal yoke muscle of the uninvolved eye. The deviation observed when the nonparetic eye is fixing is termed the *primary deviation*, and the deviation observed when the paretic eye is fixing is the *secondary deviation*. Patients with paralytic strabismus show a secondary deviation during the acute phase.

When a patient with a right lateral rectus palsy fixes a distant object with the left eye, the right eye is deviated inward as a result of a weak lateral rectus muscle. If the patient is made to fix the distant object with the paretic eye, extra impulses will be sent to the right lateral rectus muscle in an attempt to make the eye move outward. The yoke muscle, the medial rectus muscle on the opposite side, receives equal innervation, which is greater than normal, and thus turns inward, causing a marked inward deviation. This is the secondary deviation.

Examination of the ocular motor system for the detection of muscle weakness requires an understanding of the preceding principles. If the clinician simply observes the versions and ductions, he or she will only be able to detect marked abnormalities of ocular muscle weakness, i.e., total paralysis of a single muscle. Many patients have mild paresis of a single ocular muscle. The paresis may be minimal so that the fusional reflexes can overcome the tendency of the paretic eye to move and the eyes will appear straight and move in concert with one another. To detect mild ocular muscle weakness, one must test for muscle balance. The tests for muscle balance may be objective or subjective. The former does not require patient response, while the latter does.

The objective test for ocular muscle balance is the alternate cover test and the cover-uncover test. The patient is asked to fixate a stationary object, preferably in the distance. Either eye is covered and the cover is moved from one eye to the other while the movement of the uncovered eye is noted. The direction of movement of the uncovered eye as it takes up fixation is opposite the direction of the underlying deviation. If the uncovered eye moves inward to take up fixation, it was deviated outward under the cover. That patient, therefore, has an exodeviation. If the uncovered eye moves outward to take up fixation, the eye was deviated inward under the cover and the patient has an esodeviation. The alternate cover test defines the direction of the underlying ocular motor imbalance. In order to determine whether a phoria or a tropia is present, the second step is to do a cover-uncover test. The patient is asked to fixate a stationary object. The eyes are alternately covered, and the direction of the deviation is ascertained. If a deviation is present, then while the patient is fixating the distant object, the cover is removed from the nonfixating eye without covering the fixating eye. If the uncovered eye moves to the point of fixation while the fixating eye remains fixating, a phoria is present, since the fusional reflex was enough to overcome the underlying deviation. If the uncovered eye does not move to take fixation but remains deviated, a tropia is present since the fusional reflex has not been able to overcome the underlying deviation. The alternate cover and cover-uncover test must be done in all of the directions of gaze to determine in which direction any deviation is greatest. From this analysis, the paretic muscle may be determined.

Consider the case of a patient with a right lateral rectus palsy. A cover-uncover test while the patient is gazing straight ahead may show a small esophoria. On gaze left at a distant object, the alternate cover test shows orthophoria (no deviation). In right gaze at a distant object, the alternate cover test shows a large eso deviation. A patient with a very mild lateral rectus weakness may be orthophoric on left gaze, be orthophoric on primary gaze, and show a small esophoria on right gaze.

The common subjective test for determination of ocular muscle imbalance is the red glass test. A red glass is placed in front of one eye, and the patient is asked to look at a stationary light source. The red glass test is only useful in patients with a tropia and overt diplopia. If a patient is phoric, the introduction of a red glass in front of one eye usually is not sufficient to depress the fusional reflex enough to make a phoria become a tropia. The patient is asked to describe the diplopia. What is the laterality of the red light and the white light? How does the amount of deviation vary in varying positions of gaze? The image seen is opposite the direction of the deviation. An eso deviation gives uncrossed diplopia. An exo deviation gives crossed diplopia.

Consider a patient with a right lateral rectus palsy. The red glass is placed in front of the patient's right eye. The patient is asked to fixate a distant light source. In the primary position of gaze, the patient reports diplopia with the red object to the right (the same side as the eye with the red glass). When the patient looks to the right, the diplopia increases. When the patient looks to the left, the diplopia disappears. The main problem with subjective tests of ocular motility balance is that they require a minimum level of intelligence and verbal ability by the patient.

Skew Deviation

Skew deviation[33] is a dysconjugate vertical deviation of the eyes that has been attributed to a disturbance of supranuclear pathways for vertical gaze. The characteristics of skew deviation are (1) sudden onset of vertical diplopia; (2) a significant vertical deviation, as revealed by a screen and cover test; (3) no history of pre-existing ocular motility disturbances; (4) associated signs and symptoms of neurological disorders; and (5) exclusion of third and fourth nerve disease, orbital pathology, and myopathy. Skew deviation may be comitant, i.e., the same in all directions of gaze, laterally comitant, i.e., present on gaze to one side only, both up and down, or noncomitant. Typically, the lower eye is ipsilateral to the lesion. Originally, skew deviation was attributed to lesions of the brachium pontis, but in recent years it has become apparent that skew deviation may result from lesions anywhere in the pathways for vertical gaze.

Ocular Motor Apraxia[5]

Congenital ocular motor apraxia is a specific disorder occurring in children. It is characterized by an absence of ocular pursuit and saccades. The child substitutes vestibulo-ocular movements in order to refixate. To change fixation, the child closes the eyes and thrusts the head rapidly in the desired direction. The head movement is greater than required, and the subsequent vestibulo-ocular reflexes slowly drive the eyes back to the original direction of gaze, until the new direction of fixation is established. Horizontal movements are most severely disturbed. The ocular motor apraxia is less apparent as the child matures. It is not clear whether this represents adaptation or a self-limiting disorder.

In adults, patients with acquired neurological lesions may show ocular motor apraxia. There may be selective loss of saccades or pursuit in some circumstances, with preservation of these eye movements in others. For example, a patient may be unable to saccade right when asked but may be noted to have normal saccades to the right during random eye movements. Acquired ocular motor apraxia is interesting primarily for its insights into the organization of the ocular motor pathways and is less useful for specific diagnosis.

Topographic and Etiologic Diagnosis of Ocular Motor Cranial Nerve Palsies

The determination of etiology of ocular motor nerve abnormalities requires localization of the lesion along the pathway of the cranial nerve. Since specific types of pathology tend to occur at specific anatomical locations, topographic diagnosis is important.

Third Cranial Nerve

Nuclear involvement of the third nerve is rare. Nuclear involvement of the third nerve occurs in several patterns. If the entire third nerve nuclear complex is affected, the result is absent adduction, elevation, and depression of the eye ipsilateral to the involved nuclear complex. There is bilateral ptosis due to involvement of the single levator nucleus. There is defective elevation of the eye contralateral to the lesion secondary to involvement of the ipsilateral superior rectus subnucleus (crossed innervation). A second pattern of the third nerve nuclear involvement is bilateral ptosis without ophthalmoplegia secondary to a small lesion at the caudal end of the nuclear complex affecting the unpaired levator subnucleus. The levator subnucleus may be spared in incomplete nuclear lesions, resulting in unilateral or bilateral ophthalmoplegia without ptosis. Vascular lesions of the perforating arteries in the midbrain, metastatic lesions, and demyelination are the most common causes of third nerve nuclear pathology.

Involvement of the fascicular portion of the ocular motor nerve results in several typical neurological syndromes. Benedikt's syndrome consists of ipsilateral third nerve palsy and contralateral ataxia. It is caused by involvement of the third nerve as it passes through the red nucleus. Weber's syndrome consists of ipsilateral third nerve palsy and contralateral hemiplegia. It is caused by an involvement of the third nerve adjacent to the cerebral peduncle. Benedikt's syndrome is most commonly caused by intraparenchymal pathology including vascular lesions, neoplasm, and demyelination. Weber's syndrome may be caused by intraparenchymal pathology and, additionally, by extrinsic mass lesions within the interpeduncular fossa compressing the peduncle and exiting third nerve rootlets.

Involvement of the third nerve within the subarachnoid space with one exception results in symmetric involvement of all divisions of the third nerve. The exception is ocular motor palsy with normal pupils (pupil sparing) resulting from intrinsic vascular lesions. Patients with systemic vascular disease such as diabetes, hypertension, temporal arteritis, and atherosclerosis develop occlusion of the vaso nervorum, resulting in a central ischemic infarction. The more peripherally placed parasympathetic fibers are spared. Within the subarachnoid space, the most common tumors affecting the third nerve are chordomas and clival meningiomas. The third nerve may be affected by infectious processes such as meningitis. The most important lesions affecting the third nerve within the subarachnoid space are aneurysms of the posterior communicating artery or basilar artery. Aneurysm causes third nerve paralysis with involvement of the pupillary fibers causing internal ophthalmoplegia. Pupillary sparing with aneurysmal lesions occurs in less than 1 percent of cases.

The third nerve may be affected by trauma, herniation, or compression as it passes through the dura at the posterior margin of the cavernous sinus. Patients with laterally expanding pituitary adenomas develop third nerve palsy rather than visual field defects commonly seen in patients with suprasellar extension. Within the cavernous sinus, lesions causing third nerve palsy usually cause accompanying abnormalities of the fourth, fifth, and sixth cranial nerves. Common vascular lesions include carotid-cavernous fistulas and intracavernous aneurysms. Neoplastic lesions in this area include meningiomas, nasopharyngeal tumors, and metastatic tumors. Inflammatory lesions include cavernous sinus thrombosis and granulomatous inflammation in the cavernous sinus.

Lesions of the third nerve within the orbit are more likely to affect various branches asymmetrically. If the superior division alone is affected, the patient will show ptosis and decreased elevation. Involvement of the inferior division results in defects of depression, adduction, and pupillary reaction. Orbital meningiomas, hemangiomas, and schwannomas are the most commonly occurring intraorbital tumors. Pseudotumor of the orbit is a diffuse granulomatous inflammation within the orbit that may cause abnormalities of any of the branches of the third nerve. It is usually associated with pain and ocular signs of inflammation.

Aberrant Regeneration of the Third Nerve

Aberrant regeneration of the third nerve consists of one or more of the following characteristics: (1) elevation of the affected lid on attempted adduction and depression of the lid on attempted abduction; (2) elevation of the affected lid on attempted down gaze; (3) elevation or depression of the globe on attempted adduction; (4) retraction of the globe on attempted adduction, elevation, or depression; (5) limitation of elevation and depression; (6) pupillary constriction on attempted adduction; (7) elevation or depression of the globe on attempted adduction; and (8) unilateral vertical optokinetic nystagmus. These patterns of ocular motor findings result from aberrant regeneration of fibers of the third nerve. Fibers that originally are intended for one muscle regenerate and terminate on another. Weakness of elevation and depression and retraction of the globe are due to cocontraction of the muscles innervated by the third nerve. Fibers originally intended for the medial rectus and ending instead at the pupillary sphincter cause pupillary constriction on attempted adduction. Lid abnormalities are caused by fibers originally intended for the rectus muscles ending instead in the levator.

Aberrant regeneration occurs most often following trauma and aneurysms. If the eye is examined carefully in patients recovering from posterior communicating aneurysm, virtually all patients will show some mild degree of aberrant regeneration. Aberrant regeneration occurs rarely with tumors and syphilis. With the former, the ocular motor findings occur following treatment. Aberrant regeneration never occurs as a result of diabetic neuropathy.

Fourth Nerve

Fascicular involvement of the fourth nerve cannot be distinguished from peripheral involvement. Patients with fourth nerve palsies complain of vertical and torsional diplopia. It is seldom possible to note decreased fourth nerve function by simply observing versions and adductions of the eye. Tests for ocular motility imbalance must be employed.

The most common cause of fourth nerve palsy is trauma. The fascicular portion of the fourth nerve and its exit from the brain stem are located at the level of the incisura. Contusions of the fourth nerve against the edge of the tentorium result from acceleration and deceleration of the head and the subsequent fluid movements of the brain. Fourth nerve palsy may occur after seemingly mild head trauma. Bilateral fourth nerve palsies are not rare. In patients with severe head trauma, fourth nerve weakness may be overlooked because the associated severe neurological abnormalities prevent careful examination. In patients with these problems, the weakness may not be apparent until late in recovery. The fourth nerve is rarely affected by cerebellopontine angle tumors and meningiomas. Demyelination and vascular infarctions affect the fourth nerve less often than they do the third and sixth cranial nerves. Within the cavernous sinus and orbital fissure, the fourth nerve is rarely involved as an isolated cranial nerve.

Sixth Nerve

Sixth nerve palsies are the most common isolated ocular motor palsy. Lesions affecting the sixth nerve nucleus usually affect the adjacent paramedian pontine reticular formation. Patients with lesions in this area show a gaze palsy or paresis ipsilateral to the lesion. While the gaze palsy is easy to diagnose, it obscures any weakness of the lateral rectus muscle. The fascicular portion of the seventh nerve passes over the sixth nerve nucleus. Facial weakness associated with a sixth nerve palsy indicates a lesion very close to the sixth nerve nucleus.

Involvement of the fascicular portion of the sixth nerve usually occurs as part of a more extensive brain stem syndrome. Foville's syndrome is characterized by ipsilateral paralysis of gaze, ipsilateral facial palsy, loss of taste from the anterior two-thirds of the tongue, ipsilateral Horner's syndrome, ipsilateral analgesia of the face, and ipsilateral deafness. Millard-Gubler syndrome is characterized by ipsilateral sixth nerve palsy, contralateral hemiplegia, and ipsilateral seventh nerve palsy. Raymond-Cestan syndrome includes ipsilateral seventh nerve palsy and contralateral hemiplegia.

The subarachnoid portion of the sixth nerve may be affected by a vast number of lesions. These lesions include ischemic infarcts associated with systemic vascular disease, tumors, inflammatory conditions including mastoiditis, intracavernous aneurysms, migraine, trauma, infection, and increased intracranial pressure. The mechanism of sixth nerve palsy associated with increased intracranial pressure may be related to the resulting downward displacement of the brain stem. The sixth nerve may be stretched and distorted, particularly as it passes through Dorello's canal. A resulting abnormality of axoplasmic flow is responsible for the dysfunction.

Syndromes of Multiple Ocular Motor Nerve Involvement

The third, fourth, fifth, and sixth cranial nerves are adjacent to each other within the cavernous sinus and superior orbital fissure. At the apex of the orbit they are joined by the optic nerve. A number of pathological processes tend to occur within this limited area from the cavernous sinus to the orbital apex. Most notable are inflammatory lesions and neoplastic lesions.

Lesions in the cavernous sinus cause involvement of the third, fourth, and sixth ocular motor nerves in association with the first and second divisions of the fifth cranial nerve. Lesions in the anterior cavernous sinus and superior orbital fissure (superior orbital fissure syndrome) cause lesions of the third, fourth, and sixth cranial nerves and the first division of the fifth cranial nerve. Lesions at the orbital apex (orbital apex syndrome) cause involvement of the second, third, fourth, and sixth cranial nerves and partial involvement of the first division of the fifth cranial nerve.

Painful ophthalmoplegia[34] describes a clinical condition characterized by pain and some combination of dysfunction of the third, fourth, fifth, and sixth cranial nerves. In early reports of this condition, Tolosa and Hunt described a granulomatous inflammation of the anterior cavernous sinus. As a result, the eponym Tolosa-Hunt[10] is frequently applied to this clinical syndrome. In fact, however, the granulomatous inflammation may occur in the superior orbital fissure or the orbital apex. This type of inflammation probably represents an entity that may occur at any one of a number of sites at the junction of the cavernous sinus and orbit. I prefer to consider these as variations of an orbital inflammatory disease. Persons with this problem should be evaluated for specific granulomatous inflammation such as sarcoid, tuberculosis, syphilis, fungal infections, and collagen vascular disease. Nevertheless, in most patients the only abnormal laboratory study is an elevated Westergren erythrocyte sedimentation rate. Treatment with systemic steroids results in a rapid and significant improvement, so much so that a prompt response is considered diagnostic.

Anatomy of the Pupillary Pathways

The pupil constricts in response to two different stimuli. The pupillary light reflex is the constriction that occurs when light enters a sighted eye. The pupillary near reflex is the constriction that occurs when gaze is directed to an object close to the eyes. The response of the pupils to such a close object is part of a central synkinesis that includes convergence and accommodation. When they occur together, there is a linkage of these phenomena that makes up the near reflex. Pupillary miosis (constriction), accommodation (focusing), and convergence of the eyes occur simultaneously. The pupillary constriction in response to light and near objects is mediated by the parasympathetic nervous system. Accommodation is likewise mediated by this portion of the autonomic nervous system.

Pupillary dilatation is mediated by the sympathetic portion of the autonomic nervous system. Active dilatation of the pupil caused by contraction of the dilator muscle of the iris, as opposed to the pupillary dilatation caused by relaxation of the constrictor muscle of the iris, occurs when the level of illumination on a sighted eye is reduced. In addition, acute pupillary dilatation may occur as a reflex phenomenon in conjunction with neural transmissions and humoral changes occasioned by acute excitement.

The Pupillary Light Reflex

The afferent arm of the pupillary light reflex originates in retinal receptors, rods, and cones. It is not clear whether there is a separate population of rods and cones mediating the light reflex or whether there are simply branching axons from rods and cones that, in addition, mediate visual imaging. The primary afferent neuron originates in the retinal ganglion cell and passes with the neurons subserving vision through the optic nerve, chiasm, and optic tract. While a pupillary light reflex may be generated from receptors anywhere in the retina, a stronger light reflex will occur from central retinal stimulation than will occur from peripheral retinal stimulation. This reflects the increased density and number of retinal receptors and, therefore, neurons in the central macular area. Neurons that mediate the light reflex and that originate from the temporal half of the retina, like neurons subserving vision, do not decussate in the chiasm and travel in the optic tract on the ipsilateral side (Fig. 8-18). Neurons from the nasal half of the retina decussate and travel to the midbrain in the contralateral optic tract. While the visual fibers terminate in the lateral geniculate body on each side, the pupillary fibers exit the optic tract anterior to the lateral geniculate body and pass to the pretectum, where they synapse in the paired pretectal nuclei. Each pretectal nucleus sends neurons to the Edinger-Westphal subnucleus in the third nerve nuclear complex on both sides of the brain stem. This neuron is the internuncial neuron and may be considered part of the afferent pathway. The normal decussation of pupillary fibers in the chiasm and representation of each pretectal nucleus in both Edinger-Westphal subnuclei is the anatomical basis for the symmetry of pupillary constriction in both eyes in response to the light entering either pupil. The efferent or motor pathway to the constrictor of the iris is the usual two-neuron pathway of the parasympathetic portion of the autonomic nervous system. The first

Figure 8-18 Pupillary pathways for the light reflex.

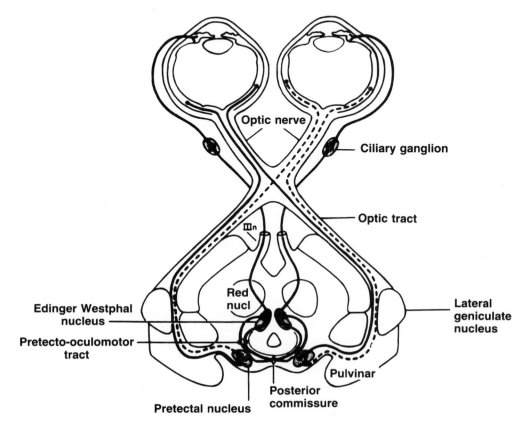

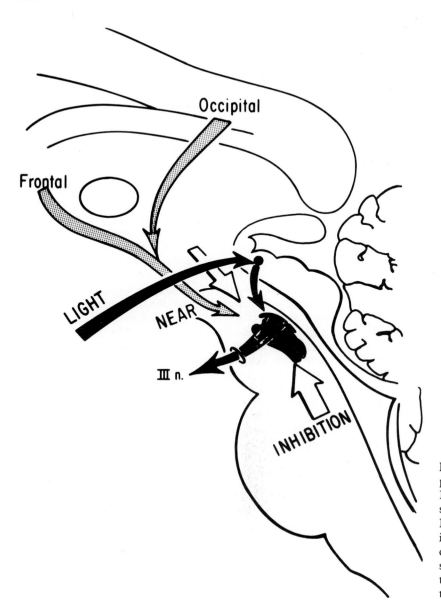

Figure 8-19 Separation of light and near pupillary reflexes in the pretectal area. Light and near inputs stimulate the sphincter nucleus and constrict the pupil. Excitement and mental activity result in inhibition of the sphincter nucleus with dilation of the pupil. In sleep and narcosis, this inhibitory activity is diminished, the sphincter nucleus becomes more active, and the pupils constrict.

efferent neuron (preganglionic) originates in the Edinger-Westphal subnucleus on each side and travels with motor fibers within the third nerve. The pupillary fibers are peripheral in the superior medial portion of the third nerve as it leaves the brain stem. During the course of the third nerve within the subarachnoid space, the pupillary fibers descend through the ocular motor nerve until, as the nerve enters the orbit, these fibers are located in an inferior peripheral position. Within the third nerve, the preganglionic neuron passes through the subarachnoid space, cavernous sinus, and superior orbital fissure into the orbit. Within the orbit the third nerve divides into a superior and inferior division. The pupillary fibers, along with other fibers from the Edinger-Westphal subnucleus, are in the inferior division and end in the ciliary ganglion, which is located just posterior to the eye. The second efferent neuron (postganglionic) passes from the ciliary ganglion to the sphincter of the iris within the long anterior ciliary nerves.

Ninety percent of the parasympathetic fibers originating in the Edinger-Westphal subnucleus and traveling in the third nerve will terminate on receptors in the ciliary body. The ciliary body contains the muscle controlling accommodation of the eyes, and the vast majority of parasympathetic fibers supply this function. Approximately 3 percent of the parasympathetic fibers will terminate in the constrictor muscle of the pupil. The remaining fibers innervate blood vessels and lacrimal glands.

Afferent fibers for the pupillary near response originate in the rostral portion of the occipital lobe (Fig. 8-19). Neurons from this area pass monosynaptically or polysynaptically to the area of the pretectum and terminate in the area of the Edinger-Westphal subnucleus. It is significant in considering certain pupillary abnormalities to note that the neurons for the light reflex are located ventral to the fibers for the light reflex in the mesencephalon. From the Edinger-Westphal subnucleus, the efferent arm of the near reflex is identical to that of the light reflex.

There are important supranuclear influences on pupillary

constriction. There is an active inhibition of the Edinger-Westphal subnucleus originating in the reticular activating system of the pons and medulla (Fig. 8-19). During periods of increased reticular activating system activity, i.e., excitement, the Edinger-Westphal subnucleus is actively inhibited and pupillary size is relatively large. In states of depressed consciousness, such as sleep or stupor, there is disinhibition by the reticular activating system and pupillary size is relatively small. This disinhibition, resulting from destruction of fibers in the reticular activating system in patients with pontine hemorrhage, intraparenchymal pontine tumors, and syphilis, is partially responsible for the relative miosis noted in persons with these disorders.

Sympathetic Pathways

The sympathetic pathway to the dilator muscle of the iris is a three-neuron pathway (Fig. 8-20). The first neuron (central neuron) originates in the area of the hypothalamus and travels in the tegmentum of the brain stem and in the intermediate column of gray of the spinal cord to the ciliospinal center of Budge at levels C7, C8, and T1. The second neuron (sympathetic preganglionic) passes through the ventral spinal roots and white rami to the lateral sympathetic chain. It ascends to the superior cervical ganglion and synapses. The third neuron (postganglionic) leaves the superior cervical ganglion and traveling on the walls of the carotid vessels, enters the skull. Sympathetic fibers to the sweat glands of the face travel with the external carotid vessels. Sympathetic fibers to the pupil travel with the internal carotid vessels. Within the cavernous sinus, the plexus of sympathetic neurons leaves the carotid artery and pass to enter the orbit with other cranial nerves. The majority of sympathetic fibers travel with the first division of the trigeminal nerve and enter the orbit with the nasociliary branch of the ophthalmic division of this nerve. Other sympathetic fibers travel with the sixth cranial nerve, and perhaps the third and fourth, to the orbit. Within the orbit, pupillary fibers pass through the ciliary ganglion into the dilator of the iris through the long anterior ciliary nerves.

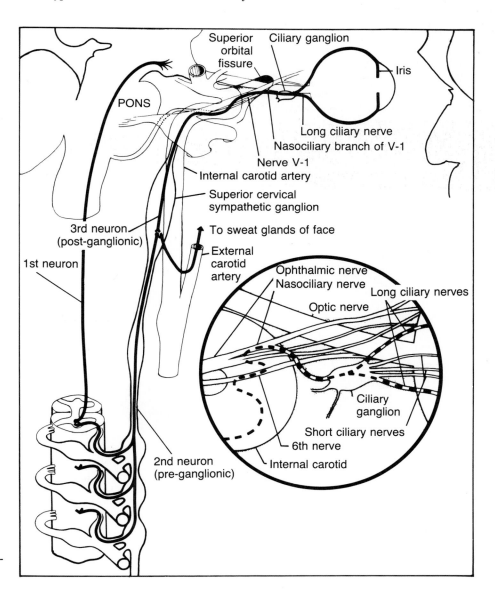

Figure 8-20 Sympathetic pathways to the eye.

Examination of the Pupil

Proper interpretation of pupillary responses requires accurate and careful observation. In addition, intelligent recording of the results of pupillary examination is necessary so that proper conclusions may be drawn from serial observations by more than one examiner. The pupils should be examined in a room of medium illumination. Pupillary size on each side is noted and recorded. Initially, a millimeter rule is necessary to gauge pupillary size, but with some experience the examiner will generally be able to estimate it accurately without specific quantitation in each case. Besides pupillary size, some note should be made of the regularity of the pupil, i.e., whether it is round, oval, or displaced. The light response is tested by shining a light upon each eye. A bright fresh light source is essential. The briskness of the light response is graded from 0 to 4 + , with 4 + considered normally brisk. If the light response is 4 + , then the examiner may assume that the motor pathways to the pupil are intact and the near reflex may be ignored. If the light response is sluggish, then the near response must be tested since a sluggish pupillary response to light may be caused by a defect in the afferent or efferent arm of the reflex. To test the near reflex, the patient's own index finger is placed approximately 6 in. in front of the eyes while the patient is asked to fix a distant object. The patient is then asked to fix his or her own finger and must be exorted to do this in a continual fashion by the observer. The near response is a direct function of patient effort, and the patient will not be motivated to make one without urging by the examiner. The near response is also graded from 0 to 4 + . If the near response is 4 + , the integrity of the efferent or motor arm of the reflex is verified. The situation in which the response to near stimulation is greater than the response to light stimulation is termed *light-near dissociation*. This is an abnormal situation and is associated with a number of pathological conditions, which will be discussed. Because the near response is so dependent on patient effort, the converse situation of near-

light dissociation in which the light response is greater than the near response is not considered to be a reliable indicator of pupillary abnormality. The consensual pupillary response is the constriction occurring in the pupil in the eye contralateral to that which is being directly stimulated. It is not necessary to specifically evaluate the consensual response. The consensual response is evaluated indirectly during the next portion of the pupillary exam, the swinging flashlight test.

The swinging flashlight test is used to determine the presence of a Marcus-Gunn pupil (afferent pupillary defect). When a light is shined into either eye, both pupils will constrict equally. When the flashlight is quickly moved to shine from one eye into the other, the pupillary size will remain the same since the intensity of the light stimulus entering the system has not changed. If some slight pupillary dilation occurs as the light is moved to the second eye, a small amount of constriction may be seen. If a pathological condition interferes with the transmission of the light reflex from one eye to the central pupillary centers, then the pupil in the affected eye will be seen to dilate when the flashlight is moved from the unaffected eye (Fig. 8-21). This apparent paradoxical dilation of the pupil when the light is moved to the affected eye is a Marcus Gunn pupil. A Marcus Gunn pupil is indicative of an optic nerve or retinal lesion. Occasionally, a dense vitreous hemorrhage will reduce the intensity of the ambient light to a degree sufficient to cause a Marcus Gunn pupil. Significant refractive errors, corneal diseases, and even dense cataracts do not interfere with the transmission of light sufficient to cause a Marcus Gunn pupil. Since an ophthalmoscope is available to identify retinal disease, the presence of a Marcus Gunn pupil is a good indicator of optic nerve disease in a patient with an otherwise normal ocular examination. Conversely, in most cases the absence of a Marcus Gunn pupil in a patient with severe unilateral visual dysfunction excludes the possibility of an optic nerve lesion as the cause for the decreased visual function. The exception to this rule would be in a patient with symmetric loss of neurons within both optic nerves but

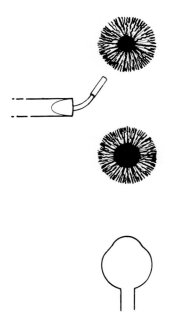

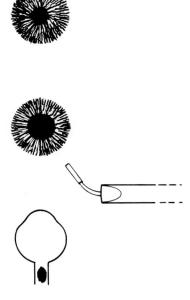

Figure 8-21 Marcus Gunn pupil. The optic nerve of the involved eye conducts light impulse less effectively than that of the normal eye. Pupillary dilatation occurs when changing from consensual to direct stimulation of the involved eye.

asymmetric loss of vision because of the differences in the patterns of neuronal loss. The swinging flashlight test is a comparison of one eye to the other. A bilateral Marcus Gunn pupil is not possible. A patient with bilateral optic nerve disease will not show a Marcus Gunn pupil if the optic nerve disease is symmetric. The presence of a Marcus Gunn pupil is one of the most sensitive indicators of optic nerve dysfunction. A Marcus Gunn pupil may be present in a patient with a compressive lesion of the optic nerve or inflammatory lesion of the optic nerve (old or new) despite normal visual acuity and normal visual fields. Retinal lesions severe enough to cause a Marcus Gunn pupil are generally large lesions. The absence or presence of a Marcus Gunn pupil correlates most closely with the presence or absence of a significant visual field difference between the two eyes of the patient.

Persons who have a nonreactive pupil on one side due to cycloplegic or miotic drops may still be tested for an afferent pupillary defect. If the normal eye is nonreactive, the test is done in the usual manner. No pupillary reaction will occur when the light is shined in the normal eye. When the light is moved to the abnormal eye (without iridoplegia) the expected pupillary dilation will occur. In patients with iridoplegia of the affected eye, a reverse Marcus Gunn may be noted. In these persons, when the light is shined in the abnormal eye, no pupillary action will occur. When the light is moved to the normal eye, a significant pupillary constriction will be noted since this pupil was previously larger due to the weaker light stimulus to the abnormal eye. This brisker constriction of the normal eye is the reverse Marcus Gunn, and this observation has the same implication with regard to the presence of retinal or optic nerve disease.

In some patients, a Marcus Gunn pupil may be difficult to interpret because of the presence of hippus. Hippus is the normal continuous alternating pupillary constriction and dilation occurring in most normal individuals. In some persons, this physiological pupillary movement may be of such an amplitude that it is difficult to judge whether dilation is significant. In patients with marked hippus, one may decide about the presence of a Marcus Gunn pupil either by using an extremely strong light source, which will tend to dampen the normal pupillary oscillations, or by simply noting the average pupillary size around which the physiological constriction and dilation are occurring.

Pharmacologic Cycloplegia

Persons with inadvertent or purposeful contact with atropine-like drugs may present with unilateral or bilateral fixed dilated pupils. Persons with pharmacologic cycloplegia have a moderately dilated pupil (6 to 7 mm) without any reaction to light or near stimulation and normal extraocular motility. Pharmacologic blockade should be suspected in any patient with these findings in otherwise good health. The unadmitted use of these agents to purposely paralyze pupillary reactions is a common example of a functional neuro-ophthalmologic problem. Persons who have family members who are being treated with atropine-like drugs, either topically or systemically, may accidentally come in contact with the agent and transfer it to their eye. This is not infrequent

among health personnel. There are a number of reports of patients who have developed a fixed dilated pupil as a result of wearing a scopolamine patch on the affected side for the symptomatic relief of motion sickness.[4] Persons who work in agricultural areas may be innoculated with plant material from the Jimson weed, the source of scopolamine. This plant grows wild in corn fields. The diagnosis of a pharmacologically paralyzed pupil requires a high index of suspicion. Once suspected, it may be verified using a simple pharmacologic test. A weak solution of 1% pilocarpine (acetylcholine) is instilled in the affected eye. In a normal person or in a person with a parasympathetic paresis of the pupil, there will be normal pupillary constriction since the drug acts directly at the neuromuscular junction. If no pupillary constriction occurs, it may be assumed that there is blockade at the neuro-effector junction by an atropine-like substance.

Traumatic Mydriasis

Traumatic mydriasis is pupil dilatation occurring after ocular trauma. Patients with traumatic mydriasis show a moderately dilated pupil (6 to 7 mm) that does not respond or responds only slightly to light and near stimulation. There are two possible mechanisms for traumatic mydriasis. Some patients are simply manifesting an analogue of spinal shock. In these persons, weak miotics will cause pupillary constriction. A larger group of patients probably have traumatic mydriasis secondary to multiple ruptures of the pupillary sphincter. Patients with this type of traumatic mydriasis will not respond to weak miotics but may be identified because of the marked irregularity or scalloping of the pupillary margin. The ophthalmologist may observe the areas of sphincter rupture using the slit lamp.

Tonic Pupil

Characteristics of a tonic pupil are (1) unilateral (80 percent) or bilateral involvement; (2) mild dilatation, usually 5 to 6 mm; (3) no reaction or minimal reaction to direct light stimulation; (4) tonic (slow) constriction to near stimulation; (5) tonic (slow) redilation; and (6) parasympathetic supersensitivity (pupillary constriction to normally ineffective concentrations of parasympathetic drugs such as $\frac{1}{8}$% pilocarpine).

Patients with tonic pupils are usually not observed acutely. When such an opportunity arises, the pupil is nonreactive to light and near stimulation. As recovery occurs, there is a recovery of pupillary movement predominantly to near stimulation.

A tonic pupil results from injury to the ciliary ganglion, usually inflammatory, resulting in an initial pupillomotor and accommodative paralysis. As recovery occurs, aberrant regeneration occurs within the ciliary ganglion. Since the parasympathetic fibers destined for the ciliary body predominate, there is a misconnection between these fibers and the pupillary constrictor. A lesser degree of aberrant regeneration occurs in the opposite direction. As the aberrant regeneration occurs, the tonic pupillary response to near stimulation may be noted. This tonic response is a slow irregular constriction that may occur over a period of several seconds as the patient fixates a near object. It is, in fact, the result of impulses meant to subserve accommodation. If the original injury is severe, the patient may retain a total internal ophthalmoplegia.

In most cases, the cause of the ciliary ganglionitis is obscure. Tonic pupils have been associated with a wide variety of viral disorders, collagen vascular disease, granulomatous inflammations, ischemic episodes, and physical injuries. A tonic pupil is more frequent in women. Adie described tonic pupils associated with absent deep tendon reflexes in the lower extremities.[1]

The diagnosis of a tonic pupil is most easily made by careful observation of the light and near response. In patients who have had parasympathetic denervation for some period of time $\frac{1}{8}$% pilocarpine will cause pupillary constriction, but it causes no pupillary constriction in normal persons. Pupillary constriction in response to these agents confirms the diagnosis of tonic pupil.

Hutchinson's Pupil[25]

Pupillary dilatation in patients with suspected or known supratentorial mass lesions may indicate the onset of a central cerebral herniation syndrome. As intracranial pressure rises, the third nerve may be compressed between the tentorial edge and the uncus. Because the pupillary motor fibers are peripheral, they are more sensitive to pressure and disturbances of circulation, and pupillary dilatation may occur before other signs of a third nerve palsy. Hutchinson's pupil implies severe central nervous system damage.

Syphilis

The classic, but least common, pupillary abnormality seen in patients with neurosyphilis is the Argyll Robertson pupil.[27,28] Characteristics of the Argyll Robertson pupil are (1) normal vision in the affected eye; (2) unilateral or bilateral involvement; (3) no reaction to light stimulation but brisk reaction to near stimulation; (4) miotic pupils; (5) irregular pupils; and (6) poor pupillary dilatation after instillation of atropine-like drugs.

The sites of pathology in pupillary pathways in patients with Argyll Robertson pupils are (1) the internuncial neuron, (2) the pontine reticular formation, and, questionably, (3) the iris. Interruption of the internuncial neurons causes a disturbance of light stimulation without interfering with near stimulation, causing the typical light-near dissociation. Diffuse disease of the pontine tegmentum and reticular formation causes loss of inhibition of the Edinger-Westphal subnucleus, resulting in relative pupillary miosis. The irregular pupillary margins and inability of the pupil to dilate well with atropine-like drops may implicate direct involvement of iris structures within the eye.

The majority of patients with syphilis and pupillary abnormalities simply have light-near dissociation. The pupils are of normal size, and the pupillary response to light stimulation may be sluggish but not absent. These patients presumably have disease only in one area and are therefore much less likely to have disseminated neurosyphilis.

Midbrain Pupillary Abnormalities

Light-near dissociation may occur as a result of lesions in the area of the posterior third ventricle. Classically, those lesions involve the area of the sylvian aqueduct. Gradual dilation of the sylvian aqueduct or increase in size of a posterior third ventricular mass will cause initial pathological effects on the dorsal aspect of the brain stem interfering with the light response but not affecting the pupillary near response. As the pathological process continues, ventral fibers in the pretectum may be affected and eventually the patient will develop loss of the pupillary near response. These pupillary abnormalities are usually seen as part of a Parinaud's syndrome. Trophic changes are rarely seen in the iris or sphincter.

Diabetes

Persons with diabetes have light-near dissociation due to parasympathetic denervation of the iris.[31]

Amaurotic Pupil

An amaurotic pupil may be observed in an eye that has no light perception. Characteristics of an amaurotic pupil are (1) no reaction to light stimulation in the affected eye; (2) no consensual pupillary constriction in the unaffected eye when the light is shined in the affected eye; (3) normal pupillary constriction when the light is shined in the normal eye; and (4) normal pupillary constriction in the affected eye when the light is shined in the nonaffected eye. If these criteria are not met, then there may be pathology in the pupillomotor system and no conclusions may be drawn about blindness.

Pupillary Miosis

The most common causes of pupillary miosis are (1) eye drops; (2) narcotics; (3) pontine disease, i.e., pontine hemorrhage; and (4) some cases of ocular inflammation or trauma. Pupillary constriction due to eye drops must be diagnosed on the basis of history. Pupils of patients with a history of taking topical glaucoma medication do not react to light or near stimulation. Persons using narcotics may have miotic pupils secondary to pharmacologic depression of the reticular activating system and secondary disinhibition of the Edinger-Westphal subnucleus. Patients with miosis secondary to narcotics do not have pupils quite as small as patients who have been receiving eye drops, and frequently a pupillary reflex may be noted despite miosis. Patients with pontine disease, classically pontine hemorrhage, have pinpoint pupils. The cause for the pupillary abnormalities is presumably secondary to destruction of inhibitory fibers to the Edinger-Westphal subnucleus. In addition, there is destruction of the sympathetic fibers in the tegmentum of the brain stem, resulting in loss of function of the iris dilator muscle. In some patients with ocular inflammation, such as iritis or following mild ocular trauma, there may be a spasm of the pupillary constrictor rather than paralysis and the pupil may be noted to be miotic in the affected eye.

Horner's Syndrome (Sympathetic Paresis)[12,19]

The classic features of a Horner's syndrome of the eye are ptosis and miosis on the involved side. There may be apparent enophthalmos due to narrowing of the fissure. If the lesion occurs below the bifurcation of the carotid, ipsilateral facial sweating is impaired. Other ocular findings include hyperemia of the involved eye and increased amplitude of accommodation. In a patient without classic findings, a Horner's syndrome may be diagnosed using cocaine. A drop of 10% cocaine is instilled in each eye. A second drop is instilled approximately 10 min after the first. The pupils are observed periodically over 30 min. Cocaine blocks the reuptake of norepinephrine by the postganglionic nerve endings at the neuroeffector junction. If the pupil dilates normally, Horner's syndrome is not present. In a patient with a Horner's syndrome, there is no normal release of norepinephrine at the neuroeffector junction, and therefore no accumulation can occur and no pupillary dilatation results. In patients with a partial Horner's syndrome, pupillary dilatation on the affected side may be delayed. The absence or delay of pupillary dilatation following the instillation of cocaine drops establishes the presence of a first, second, or third neuron lesion causing a Horner's syndrome. In most patients, a good clinical history and examination are sufficient to identify which of the three neurons are involved. Patients with first neuron lesions causing a Horner's syndrome usually have other signs and symptoms of brain stem disease. Vascular occlusive disease, syringobulbia, and intraparenchymal neoplasms are examples of lesions causing first neuron Horner's syndrome. Horner's syndrome caused by lesions of the second neuron occur in patients who have had lateral sympathectomies, significant chest trauma, or pulmonary neoplasms involving the sympathetic plexus. The largest group of persons with Horner's syndrome have lesions of the third neuron. Preservation of sweating on the ipsilateral side of the face indicates a lesion of the third neuron. Neck trauma, carotid vascular disease, carotid vascular studies, cervical bony abnormalities, migraine, and neoplasms at the base of the skull are common causes of third neuron abnormalities. Hydroxyamphetamine 1% (Paradrine, Smith, Klein and French, Philadelphia, Pa.) is a pharmacologic agent that acts directly on the neuroeffector junction and causes release of norepinephrine from vesicles at postganglionic nerve endings. Paradrine causes dilatation of normal pupils. Paradrine will not cause dilatation of pupils in patients with lesions of the third neuron.

Horner's syndrome, with no other neurological signs or symptoms, is observed frequently. Sophisticated neurological and neuroradiological evaluations are usually fruitless. A thorough history, neurological examination, review of old photographs, and skull and chest roentgenograms are reasonable diagnostic procedures.

NOTE: Figures 8-1 to 8-17, 8-20, and 8-21 are from Rosenberg MA: Neuro-ophthalmology, in Peyman GA, Sanders DR, Goldberg MF: *Principles and Practice of Ophthalmology*. Philadelphia, Saunders, 1980, pp 1917–1981. Figures 8-18 and 8-19 are from Ophthalmology Basic and Clinical Science Course, Sect. 5, *Neuro-ophthalmology*. Rochester, Minn., American Academy of Ophthalmology and Otolaryngology, 1981–82.

References

1. Adie WJ: Complete and incomplete forms of the benign disorder characterized by tonic pupils and absent tendon reflexes. Br J Ophthalmol 16:449–461, 1932.
2. Bird AC, Sanders MO: Defects in supranuclear control of horizontal eye movements. Trans Ophthalmol Soc UK 90:417–432, 1970.
3. Boghen DR, Glaser JS: Ischaemic optic neuropathy: The clinical profile and natural history. Brain 98:689–708, 1975.
4. Carlston J: Unilateral dilated pupil from scopolamine disk. JAMA 248:31, 1982.
5. Cogan DG: Congenital ocular motor apraxia. Can J Ophthalmol 1:253–260, 1966.
6. Daroff RB: Control of ocular movement. Br J Ophthalmol 58:217–223, 1974.
7. Daroff RB, Hoyt WF: Supranuclear disorders of ocular control systems in man, in Bach-y-Rita P, Collins CC (eds): *The Control of Eye Movements*, New York, Academic, 1971, pp 175–235.
8. Daroff RB, Troost BT: Supranuclear disorders of eye movements, in Duane TD (eds): *Clinical Ophthalmology*, New York, Harper and Row, 1976, vol 2, chap 10, pp 1–13.
9. Fisher CM: Some neuro-ophthalmology observations. J Neurol Neurosurg Psychiatry 30:383–392, 1967.
10. Fowler TJ, Earl CJ, McAllister VL, McDonald WI: Tolosa-Hunt syndrome: The dangers of an eponym. Br J Ophthalmol 59:149–154, 1975.
11. Gay AJ: Clinical ophthalmodynamometry. Int Ophthalmol Clin 7:729–744, 1967.
12. Giles CL, Henderson JW: Horner's syndrome: An analysis of 216 cases. Am J Ophthalmol 46:289–296, 1958.
13. Halliday AM, McDonald WI, Mushin J: Delayed visual evoked response in optic neuritis. Lancet 1:982–985, 1972.
14. Halliday AM, McDonald WI, Mushin J: Visual evoked reponse in diagnosis of multiple sclerosis. Br Med J 4:661–664, 1973.
15. Hamilton CR Jr, Shelley WM, Tumulty PA: Giant cell arteritis: Including temporal arteritis and polymyalgia rheumatica. Medicine 50:1–27, 1971.
16. Hayreh SS: Blood supply of the optic nerve head and its role in optic atrophy, glaucoma, and oedema of the optic disc. Br J Ophthalmol 53:721–748, 1969.
17. Hayreh SS: Anterior ischemic optic neuropathy. Arch Neurol 38:675–678, 1981.
18. Hoyt WF, Schlicke B, Eckelhoff RJ: Fundoscopic appearance of a nerve-fibre-bundle defect. Br J Ophthalmol 56:577–583, 1972.
19. Jaffe NS: Localization of lesions causing Horner's syndrome. Arch Ophthalmol 44:710–728, 1959.
20. Keltner JL: Giant cell arteritis. Contemp Ophthalmol 20:1–5, 1981.
21. Lemmen LJ, Davis JS: Horizontal conjugate gaze in brain stem lesions. Neurology 8:962–964, 1958.
22. Miller NR: Optic neuritis, in Miller N (ed): *Walsh and Hoyt's Clinical Neuro-ophthalmology*, 4th ed. Baltimore, Md, Williams & Wilkins, 1982, pp 227–247.
23. Miller SJH, Sanders MO, Ffytche TJ: Fluorescein fundus photography in the detection of early papilloedema and its differentiation from pseudo-papilloedema. Lancet 2:651–654, 1965.
24. Newman NM, Tornambe PE, Corbett JJ: Ophthalmoscopy of the retinal nerve fiber layer: Use in detection of neurologic disease. Arch Neurol 39:226–233, 1982.
25. Norris FH Jr, Fawcett J: A sign of intracranial mass with impending uncal herniation. Arch Neurol 12:381–386, 1965.
26. Regan D: *Evoked Potentials in Psychology, Sensory Physiology, and Clinical Medicine*, New York, Wiley-Interscience, 1972.
27. Robertson DA: Four cases of spinal myosis: With remarks on the action of light on the pupil. Edinburgh Med J 15:487–493, 1869.

28. Robertson DA: On an interesting series of eye-symptoms in a case of spinal disease with remarks on the action of belladonna on the iris, etc. Edinburgh Med J 14:1696–1702, 1869.

29. Sanders MO, Bird AC: Supranuclear abnormalities of the vertical ocular motor system. Trans Ophthalmol Soc UK 90:433–450, 1970.

30. Sharpe JA, Rosenberg MA, Hoyt WF, Daroff RB: Paralytic pontine exotropia. Neurology 24:1076–1081, 1974.

31. Sigsbee B, Torkelson R, Kadis G, Wright JW, Reeves AG: Parasympathetic denervation of the iris in diabetes mellitus. J Neurol Neurosurg Psychiatry 37:1031–1035, 1974.

32. Smith J, Cogan DG: Internuclear ophthalmoplegia. Arch Ophthalmol 61:687–694, 1959.

33. Smith JL, David NJ, Klintworth G: Skew deviation. Neurology 14:96–105, 1964.

34. Smith JL, Taxdal DSR: Painful ophthalmoplegia: The Tolosa-Hunt syndrome. Am J Ophthalmol 61:1466–1472, 1966.

35. Spector RH, Glaser JS, David NJ, Vining DQ: Occipital lobe infarctions: Perimetry and computed tomography. Neurology 31:1098–1106, 1981.

36. Spector RH, Troost BT: The ocular motor system. Ann Neurol 9:517–525, 1981.

37. Trobe JD, Glaser JS, Cassady J, Herschler J, Anderson DR: Nonglaucomatous excavation of the optic disc. Arch Ophthalmol 98:1046–1050, 1980.

38. Tso MOM, Hayreh SS: Optic disc edema in raised intracranial pressure: IV. Axoplasmic transport in experimental papilledema. Arch Ophthalmol 95:1458–1462, 1977.

39. Wright JE, Arden G, Jones BR: Continuous monitoring of the visually evoked response during intraorbital surgery. Trans Ophthalmol Soc UK 93:311–314, 1973.

9
Nystagmus and Related Ocular Movements

Nancy M. Newman

Nystagmus is a rhythmic biphasic oscillation of the eyes. Usually, both eyes move together (conjugately) and the two phases of the nystagmus are equal in amplitude. In true nystagmus the initial deviation is a slow eye movement; the corrective or return phase may be fast (jerk nystagmus) or slow (pendular nystagmus). Commonly, however, the term *nystagmus* has been used to describe a multitude of ocular movements. These other types of eye movements (such as opsoclonus and convergence retraction nystagmus) are best classed as *other ocular oscillations* when they do not result from slow eye movement abnormalities, even if they are nystagmoid in appearance.

Nystagmus has many forms and many causes. Some nystagmus is considered physiological (end-point nystagmus), and some is the result of visual pathology (visual deprivation nystagmus) or associated with strabismus (latent nystagmus); some nystagmus may be disconjugate (abducting nystagmus in internuclear ophthalmoplegia) or dissociated (see-saw nystagmus). Nystagmus may be named by its gross appearance on examination (upbeat nystagmus), its pre-

sumed anatomical substrate (vestibular nystagmus), its general configuration (jerk nystagmus), analysis of eye movement recordings (decreasing-velocity exponential nystagmus), the patient's age at onset (congenital nystagmus), or how it is elicited (positional nystagmus). (See Table 9-1.)

Anatomical Substrates

Since all nystagmus and all ocular oscillations have eye movement in common, their analysis must rest upon a thorough knowledge of the underlying anatomical substrates and appropriate methods for their examination.

Infranuclear Control Mechanism

The globes are moved in their orbits by six extraocular muscles; for each globe there are four rectus muscles (medial, lateral, superior, and inferior recti) and two oblique muscles (inferior and superior obliques). As discussed in the previous chapter, the extraocular muscles are innervated by cranial nerves III, IV, and VI, which arise from the oculomotor, trochlear, and abducens nuclei, respectively. The nuclei lie within the brain stem from the pretectal region to the pontomedullary junction.

Lesions of these brain stem areas, the cranial nerves, oculomotor muscles, or orbit cause nuclear and infranuclear disorders of eye movement that are associated with disconjugate (nonparallel) eye movements and are accompanied by deviation of the eyes in the primary position. These patients complain of diplopia.

Supranuclear Inputs to the Oculomotor Nuclei

Several major CNS systems significant to the generation of nystagmus and related ocular oscillations converge upon the oculomotor nuclei. These systems include the visual afferent

TABLE 9-1 Classification of Nystagmus

I. Jerk nystagmus
  A. Induced
    1. Optokinetic
    2. Vestibular
    3. Drug-induced
  B. Gaze evoked nystagmus
    1. Physiological end-point
    2. Common gaze evoked
    3. Gaze paretic
    4. Muscle paretic, myasthenia gravis
    5. Brun's nystagmus
    6. Internuclear ophthalmoplegia (INO)
    7. Rebound
  C. Primary position nystagmus
    1. Down-beat
    2. Up-beat
    3. Periodic alternating (PAN)
II. Pendular nystagmus
  A. Convergence and convergence evoked
  B. Seesaw
  C. Circular, elliptic, oblique
  D. Dissociated
III. Nystagmus of infancy
  A. Motor imbalance nystagmus
    1. Congenital
    2. Nystagmus associated with strabismus
      a. Latent
  B. Spasmus nutans
  C. Visual deprivation
IV. Other ocular oscillations
  A. Convergence, retraction
  B. Ocular bobbing
  C. Ocular dysmetria, ocular flutter, opsoclonus
  D. Square wave jerks and macro square wave jerks
  E. Macro saccadic oscillations
  F. Ocular myoclonus
  G. Voluntary "nystagmus"
  H. Superior oblique myokymia

systems, eye movement subsystems, cerebellar pathways, vestibular apparatus, and proprioceptive inputs. Nystagmus results from an imbalance either within these inputs to the oculomotor system, between one input and another, or in the oculomotor output itself. Only the supranuclear oculomotor control subsystems are considered in this chapter.

Supranuclear Oculomotor Control Subsystems

The eyes are controlled by five subsystems: the saccadic, pursuit, vergence, nonoptic reflex (vestibular, etc.), and position maintenance systems.

Rapid Eye Movements (Fast Eye Movements, Saccades)

All fast eye movements are generated by the saccadic or frontomesencephalic system. These movements are primar-

ily refixation movements utilized to place an object of interest on the fovea. The fast phases of all types of nystagmus are saccades. Saccadic eye movements are thought to be mediated by the frontal cortex and descending frontomesencephalic pathways. For horizontal saccades, the fibers descend in the paramedian pontine reticular formation (PPRF) after decussating at the level of the oculomotor nuclei. For vertical saccades they pass bilaterally to the pretectal area of the midbrain. Within the brain stem they are influenced by cerebellar control mechanisms.

Smooth Pursuit (Following)

The smooth pursuit system is used to follow a slowly moving target. Normally, a fixed relationship between the eye and target is maintained. The slow phase of optokinetic nystagmus (OKN) is a smooth pursuit movement.

Smooth pursuit eye movements are mediated by the cortex of the anterior occipital lobes. These occipitomesencephalic pathways descend near the internal sagittal stratum and pass to the pretectal area (for vertical pursuit) and the PPRF (for horizontal pursuit). There is some controversy as to whether the control is ipsilateral or contralateral, with the bulk of recent writing reflecting the belief that it is ipsilateral.

Vergence (Convergence and Divergence)

The vergence system controls the visual axes of the eyes, enabling foveal fixation on targets both near and far by turning the eyes toward each other or away from each other. Thus, vergence eye movements are disconjugate (nonparallel) movements of the eyes in contrast to most other eye movements, which are conjugate (parallel). These movements are represented in the occipitoparietal area with pathways that descend to presumed vergence centers in the pretectal area.

Nonoptic Reflex Systems

The nonoptic reflex systems (labrynthine, otolithic, and neck receptors) integrate body movements with eye movements. These systems feed directly into pontine and medullary nuclei via the eighth nerve, medial longitudinal fasciculus, and reticular formation. Their stimulation or imbalance results in vestibular nystagmus. A rotary component is frequent in vestibular nystagmus.

Position Maintenance

The position maintenance or fixation system keeps the object of interest on the fovea. It is thought to be subserved by both the occipitomesencephalic and frontomesencephalic pathways. It makes use of a system of microsaccades, and micro slow movements so fine they can be observed only by using special equipment.

Lesions of these supranuclear systems are not associated with diplopia, strabismus, or disconjugate eye movements. Exceptions are lesions of the pathways for vergence, lesions of the medial longitudinal fasciculus, and lesions producing skew deviations or dissociated or seesaw nystagmus.

Lesions frequently affect one or more of these subsystems, sparing the others. Thus, it is important to examine each of the supranuclear subsystems separately. In this way, those that are intact are detected and may be used to evaluate the nuclear and infranuclear mechanisms.

Clinical Examination of the Patient with Nystagmus

The examination of the patient with nystagmus begins with a thorough examination of ocular motility, evaluating each of the eye movement subsystems as well as the range of eye movement, the binocular coordination of the eyes, and the presence of any abnormal eye movements.

When the patient is asked to gaze at a target steadily, the *position maintenance system* is evaluated. Any interruptions of steady fixation should be noted and described. If fixation is poor, the patient should be asked to look steadily at his or her own thumb. The additional proprioceptive input will often aid an uncooperative, ill, or somewhat obtunded patient to maintain eye position.

If the patient is having difficulty cooperating or if there is a question of malingering, have the patient fix on a target and hold the eyes steady; slowly and smoothly rotate the head horizontally and/or vertically (doll's head maneuver). In obtunded patients, the proprioceptive input will help to maintain fixation by moving the eyes normally within the orbits; however, malingerers will frequently not realize that the eyes move when the head is turned with the eyes fixed, just as when the eyes are moved with the head fixed, and will execute more normal eye movements than when voluntary eye movements are tested.

Next, the *smooth pursuit system* is tested at the same time as the range of ocular movement by asking the patient to follow a slowly and smoothly moving target into the diagnostic positions of gaze; that is, the gaze positions that best isolate the action of a single extraocular muscle (Fig. 9-1). The eyes should move fully and conjugately into all extremes of gaze. If there is a lesion of the smooth pursuit system, the result is a jerky eye movement, "saccadic pursuit," or "cogwheeling" due to intrusion of fast eye movements (saccades). Saccadic pursuit may be associated with parietal lobe lesions, anxiety or fatigue, drug effects, or lesions of the cerebellar pathways.

If the eyes are not able to move fully into all positions of gaze, it should be noted whether the deficit affects both eyes equally (a gaze deficit) or only one eye. If one eye is limited, diplopia results and will be maximum in the field of action of a paretic muscle. The presence of diplopia almost always indicates a nuclear or infranuclear lesion, and, conversely, absence of diplopia suggests a supranuclear lesion. There is no diplopia in supranuclear lesions because the eyes remain conjugate. Exceptions are internuclear ophthalmoplegia (INO) and skew deviation, which result from supranuclear lesions but produce disconjugate eye movements.

With many brain stem lesions, the usually simple examination of ocular motility may become quite confusing, because gaze palsies, nystagmus, oculomotor paresis, and disconjugate or dissociated eye movements may coexist. Evaluation is simplified by examining the movements of each eye alone (ductions). Full horizontal movements of either eye signify intact horizontal gaze and thus an intact horizontal gaze center at the pontomedullary junction. Full vertical movements of either eye similarly signify an intact vertical gaze mechanism and, by implication, a relatively intact pretectal region. Thus, when either eye is able to make complete gaze movements, supranuclear mechanisms for that type of gaze are intact.

At this point, the *saccadic system* is tested by having the patient make rapid refixation movements between one target and another in the several positions of gaze. It is important to have a mental image of a normally rapid saccade, as defective saccades may be abnormally slow and, in the absence of apparatus for recording eye movements, must be judged against an internalized standard. Noting a lag or "floating" of the eye in adduction during horizontal saccades may be an important sign of internuclear ophthalmoplegia. Tests that cause repeated saccades such as optokinetic nystagmus and caloric stimulation may make obvious a lagging adducting eye and can be an important part of the clinician's armamentarium.

Normally, one or both eyes may undershoot the target and make a small catch-up movement. However, large errors and repetitive movements are definitely abnormal. A large overshoot or oscillation at the end of a saccade is termed *ocular dysmetria* and, like limb dysmetria, is a symptom of disturbed cerebellar pathways.

The *vergence system* is tested by bringing a target toward the eyes or away from the eyes and watching the eyes turn in or out, respectively. Vergence is quite sensitive to levels of

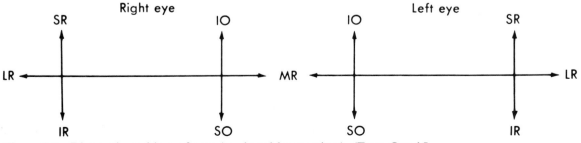

Figure 9-1 Diagnostic positions of gaze (as viewed by examiner). (From Gay AJ, Newman NM, Keltner JL, Stroud MH: *Eye Movement Disorders*. St. Louis, Mosby, 1974.)

cooperation and attention. Thus, if the patient does not converge well, the examiner must be sure that the patient is really trying. This may be done by observing the pupils for constriction that also occurs as part of the near synkinesis (miosis, convergence, and accommodation), even if there is a defect in the convergence system.

The normal response to caloric stimulation is a jerk nystagmus. Briefly, the mnemonic COWS may be used to help recall that with *c*old irrigation the fast phase is toward the side *o*pposite the side stimulated; with *w*arm irrigation, the fast phase is toward the *s*ame side. Simultaneous bilateral caloric stimulation produces vertical movements, fast phase up with cold stimulation and fast phase down with warm stimulation.

In a more complete evaluation of eye movements, or to clarify any abnormalities that have been found, eye movements may be elicited by an optokinetic stimulus, the oculocephalic (doll's head) maneuver, or vestibular stimulation. These tests may also be of value in evaluating malingering and obtunded or comatose patients who will not or cannot make voluntary eye movements.

If nystagmus has been noted during the examination of ocular motility, it should be described accurately. Is it conjugate? If not, is it disconjugate (involving one eye exclusively or significantly more than the other) or dissociated (with each eye moving in somewhat different direction)? Nystagmus is most frequently of the jerk variety, with both fast and slow components, but may also be pendular or rotary. The examiner should note the direction of slow and fast phases, any changes with different gaze positions, the amplitude of the nystagmus, and whether or not it is conjugate or dissociated.

The easiest way to describe all this information is graphically (Fig. 9-2). If the nystagmus is of the jerk variety, the fast phase is indicated by a single arrow pointing in the direction of the fast phase. Pendular nystagmus can be indicated by arrows of equal magnitude pointing in different directions. If the amplitude is indicated by the length of the arrows, the frequency can be indicated by the number of "feathers."

As pointed out above, it is important to go through all these steps in the patient suspected of having a neurological or neurosurgical disorder. For example, attempts at upward saccades may be the only manner in which the characteristic convergence retraction "nystagmus" of Parinaud's syndrome can be elicited. On the other hand, a very fine congenital nystagmus may be masked if the patient is only examined with near targets as convergence may block or dampen nystagmus, especially nystagmus of congenital origin.

This chapter deals almost exclusively with the clinical observation of nystagmus that may be made in the office or at the bedside. Accurate evaluation of eye movements and, in particular, abnormal eye movements, can be made only by quantitative clinical oculography such as electronystagmography and electro-oculography with dc recording. In order to accurately ascertain whether or not the movements are disconjugate, each eye must be recorded separately, allowing accurate measurement of velocity and precise characterization of waveforms. Thus, jerk nystagmus has been characterized by the form of the slow phase, either linear, decreasing velocity exponential, or increasing velocity expo-

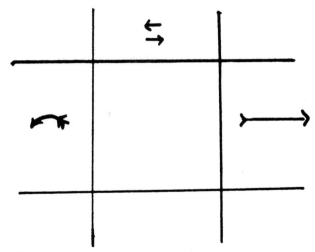

Figure 9-2 Graphic representation of nystagmus: arrows indicate direction of fast phase; length of arrows indicates amplitude; "feathers" indicate frequency (all from observer's view). This graph illustrates rotary nystagmus on right gaze of intermediate frequency and amplitude; rapid, small-amplitude pendular nystagmus on up gaze and large-amplitude, slow-frequency jerk nystagmus to the left on left gaze. (From Gay AJ, Newman NM, Keltner JL, Stroud MH: *Eye Movement Disorders*. St Louis, Mosby, 1974.)

nential. When eye movement recording is combined with careful examination of the eye movement subsystems, a much more complete description of eye movement abnormalities, including nystagmus, is obtained. Thus, upbeat nystagmus, for example, may be seen to result from defective pursuit, while the slow phase of vestibular nystagmus remains intact.

Classification of Nystagmus

While the recent advances in eye movement physiology have produced a great deal of information about nystagmus, there is still no complete classification of nystagmus that satisfies the needs of both the clinician and the control system engineer. The classification that follows (Table 9-1) is a pragmatic one. It is necessarily incomplete and touches only briefly on the mechanistic and control system attributes of nystagmus. (For those interested in pursuing those aspects further, the bibliography may be used as a guide.[1-4])

Jerk Nystagmus

Most acquired forms of nystagmus have definite slow and fast phases, hence, the appellation *jerk nystagmus*. The slow phase is the abnormal deviation, and the fast phase a corrective return. The nystagmus is named for the direction of the fast phase, which beats in the direction of defective gaze, and it is increased in amplitude by attempts to gaze further in this direction.

Induced Nystagmus

Optokinetic Nystagmus Optokinetic nystagmus is elicited by moving repetitive visual stimuli through the visual field. The slow phase is a pursuit movement with the eyes following the moving target. The fast phase is a saccadic movement in the opposite direction. Presumably, the slow phase is initiated by the occipital lobe and the fast phase by the frontal area. The connections from the occipital lobes to the frontal areas are via pathways lying deep in the parietal lobe. Thus, deep parietal lesions cause a deficit in the fast phase of optokinetic nystagmus. This deficit occurs when the tape is moved toward the side of the lesion. Thus, with a left parietal lesion, movement of the tape from right to left will demonstrate a decreased optokinetic response with the deficit of the fast phase to the right. The associated nystagmus results from a type of dysconnection syndrome. It is important to realize that the optokinetic deficit is due to damage to interconnections between the oculomotor pathways. Any hemianopsia present is incidental, occurring only because the optic radiations are adjacent to the oculomotor connections in the parietal lobe. Thus, while homonymous hemianopsias are frequently present when the optokinetic response is defective, patients with complete hemianopsia may have normal optokinetic nystagmus and patients without hemianopsia can have abnormal optokinetic nystagmus. Conversely, when the optokinetic response is normal in the presence of a homonymous hemianopic defect, the lesion is rarely in the parietal lobe.

The optokinetic response will override many voluntary eye movements and vestibular nystagmus. Thus, it can be used to gain an estimate of visual acuity in infants, as it is present within a few months of birth, and may be useful in establishing the presence of vision in patients who are hysteric or malingering. By varying the size of the targets presented, a rough estimate of visual acuity may be obtained. Since optokinetic nystagmus tests both saccadic and pursuit systems as well as their interconnections through the parietal lobes, it is an extremely useful part of the examination of ocular motility.

Vestibular Jerk Nystagmus Normally, both vestibular nuclei send balanced impulses to the pontine horizontal gaze centers. The gaze centers send the impulses to the ipsilateral lateral rectus via the sixth nerve nucleus and to the contralateral medial rectus through the medial longitudinal fasciculus and reticular formation. Any alteration in the inputs from the vestibular system whether within the ear, the cerebellopontine angle, or intramedullary portions of the pathway will result in a jerk nystagmus with a slow phase to the side opposite the lesion. Much vestibular nystagmus has a rotary component, and when this rotary component is present, it almost always indicates a vestibular origin of the nystagmus. Vestibular nystagmus may be induced by caloric stimulation or rotation. The details of caloric testing and its interpretation will be discussed in another chapter, as will positional testing and the differentiation of central and peripheral vestibular nystagmus.

Oscillopsia is a symptom and not a type of eye movement. It is the subjective sensation that the environment is moving. It is seen most frequently with disorders of the vestibular system or other brain stem systems where there are repetitive slow phases. This sensation occurs in nystagmus only when the nystagmus is of quite large amplitude. Since vision is suppressed during fast phases, the sensation of oscillopsia is due to the experience of environmental motion during the slow phase of nystagmus with the environment appearing to move in the direction opposite to that of the slow phase.

Drug-Induced Nystagmus The most common cause of nystagmus seen in clinical practice is drug intake. The most common drugs producing nystagmus are alcohol, phenytoin (Dilantin), barbiturates, or other central nervous system depressants. This nystagmus is usually a horizontal jerk gaze evoked nystagmus that may be associated with vertical up-gaze nystagmus and, rarely, down-gaze nystagmus. With increasing intoxication, especially with barbiturates, there is a degeneration of slow smooth pursuit movements resulting in saccadic pursuit or cogwheeling.

Even higher levels of intoxication with barbiturates will eliminate saccadic eye movements so that patients in a light barbiturate coma will show only tonic conjugate responses to caloric irrigation. More profound intoxication will cause an absence of caloric responses. Thus, a patient with absent caloric responses and an intact pupillary light reflex is probably in metabolic coma related to barbiturate overdose.

Additionally, in any given patient, one can roughly quantitate the degree of phenytoin toxicity with the degree of nystagmus.

Gaze Evoked Nystagmus

This is the most common form of nystagmus seen clinically; it is a jerk nystagmus that occurs when the patient attempts to maintain an eccentric position of gaze.

Physiological End-Point Nystagmus Three types of end-point nystagmus are described. The first, *fatigue nystagmus*, begins when sustaining gaze in the extreme of the gaze position. As fatigue usually doesn't occur until gaze is maintained for more than 60 s, this nystagmus is rarely seen on the routine evaluation of eye movements.

The most frequently encountered end-point nystagmus is termed *unsustained end-point nystagmus*. It is of fine amplitude and intermediate frequency, although the rhythm and amplitude may be variable. The fast phase of end-point nystagmus is in the direction of gaze. Not infrequently, horizontal end-point nystagmus may be dissociated, usually with the larger amplitude nystagmus in the abducting eye.

The third type of end-point nystagmus is *sustained end-point nystagmus*. This occurs in approximately 60 percent of patients tested, may occur at only 30 to 40 degrees of deviation, is of relatively fine amplitude, and has a linear slow phase.

Where there is uncertainty whether nystagmus is physiological or gaze paretic (see below), eye movement recording can be used to differentiate between the linear slow phases of physiological nystagmus and the descending velocity slow phase of gaze paretic nystagmus.

Common Gaze Evoked Nystagmus Gaze evoked nystagmus that is not induced by drugs usually occurs in the presence of brain stem or cerebellar pathway dysfunction. This nystagmus is fairly rapid and increases in amplitude with increasing eccentricity of gaze. Frequently, when there is bilateral horizontal gaze evoked nystagmus, there is also an associated gaze evoked nystagmus on up gaze, but rarely a down-beating nystagmus on down gaze.

Gaze Paretic Nystagmus   Patients who have lesions in the oculomotor areas of the hemispheres (frontal mesencephalic and occipitomesencephalic areas) or brain stem show a gaze paretic nystagmus when the deficit is subtotal. These patients seem unable to hold gaze, resulting in the eyes drifting slowly back toward primary position, the nystagmus occurring when a corrective saccade returns the eye to the eccentric position of gaze. This nystagmus is a relatively low frequency nystagmus with a decreasing velocity slow phase.

Muscle Paretic Nystagmus   A special type of paretic nystagmus occurs when a muscle is paretic whether on a neurogenic basis, because of muscular contraction associated with long-standing strabismus or thyroid orbitopathy, or as a result of eye muscle surgery or orbital trauma. In this case the nystagmus occurs almost exclusively in the eye with the paretic muscle when it moves into that muscle's field of action. When the lateral or medial rectus muscles are paretic, the muscle paretic nystagmus may mimic an intranuclear ophthalmoplegia (see below). This same type of nystagmus also occurs with myasthenia gravis. Thus, it is important to elicit a complete history from your patient, including a history of orbital injury or previous strabismus surgery. Patients having a muscle paretic type of nystagmus, no other evidence of central nervous system disease, and no history of strabismus or orbital trauma or other orbital disease should have a Tensilon test.

Brun's Nystagmus   Brun's nystagmus is a combination of gaze paretic nystagmus and vestibular nystagmus that is characteristic of cerebellopontine angle tumors. It is a horizontal jerk nystagmus with large-amplitude gaze paretic nystagmus when gaze is directed toward the side of the lesion. When gaze is directed to the side opposite the lesion, there is a small-amplitude vestibular nystagmus. With eyes closed, the nystagmus beats in the direction opposite the side of the lesion. Brun's nystagmus occurs when the cerebellopontine angle lesion is large enough to cause both a vestibular lesion and brain stem compression.

Internuclear Ophthalmoplegia   Lesions of the medial longitudinal fasciculus between the third and sixth nerve nuclei produce internuclear ophthalmoplegia. This is an apparent medial rectus paresis ipsilateral to the lesion associated with nystagmus of the abducting eye on lateral gaze to the side opposite the lesion. In the most common type of intranuclear ophthalmoplegia there is normal medial rectus activity on convergence. In an anterior internuclear ophthalmoplegia, convergence may be absent.

As mentioned above, the medial longitudinal fasciculus syndrome is a typical supranuclear disorder since the "paretic" medial rectus is able to produce normal convergence and there is no diplopia in primary position.

When the internuclear ophthalmoplegia is subtle or even subclinical, the abducting nystagmus may be elicited or magnified by asking the patient to converge (asymmetric convergence) on a target brought toward the abducting eye or stimulating or producing repetitive fast phases in the direction of the abducting nystagmus with either optokinetic or caloric stimulation.

The medial longitudinal fasciculus syndrome is characteristic of a pontine lesion and is frequently seen with multiple sclerosis in younger patients or ischemic lesions in elderly patients.

Rebound   Rebound nystagmus is a horizontal jerk nystagmus that appears to fatigue and then change direction when lateral gaze is sustained or with refixation to primary position. It is a manifestation of cerebellar pathway disease and is similar to periodic alternating nystagmus as it changes direction (see below).

Primary Position Nystagmus

Down-beat Nystagmus   This is a vertical jerk nystagmus present in primary position; thus it differs from gaze evoked down-beat nystagmus, which occurs only with gaze away from primary position. It has a slow phase that beats upward and fast corrective phases in the downward direction. It is usually associated with lesions in the region of foramen magnum such as the Arnold-Chiari malformation and with cerebellar lesions. Contrary to gaze evoked nystagmus, the nystagmus is not maximum in the extreme position of gaze. In fact, down-beat nystagmus is frequently of greater amplitude when the eyes are positioned laterally and slightly downward.

Up-beat Nystagmus   Up-beat nystagmus, again as differentiated from gaze evoked up-beat nystagmus, is a vertical nystagmus present in primary position with the fast phases upward. One form of up-beat nystagmus is of large amplitude increasing in intensity with increased upward gaze. Another type has smaller amplitude and decreases in intensity with increased upward gaze. Both types of up-beat nystagmus are usually seen with medullary lesions or Wernicke's encephalopathy.

Periodic Alternating Nystagmus   This dramatic nystagmus is a horizontal jerk nystagmus that periodically changes direction. Typically the nystagmus will beat in one direction for 60 to 90 s, begin to slow down, reach a neutral phase in which no nystagmus may be detected or in which there are apparently pendular oscillations, and then begin to beat in the opposite direction for a similar period of time. Periodic alternating nystagmus has many causes, but is also frequently associated with lesions in the region of the foramen magnum and cerebellum. Because at any given moment it may appear to be a rather ordinary jerk or pendular nystagmus, the alternating pendular nature will become evident only if the eyes are observed over a period of several minutes. Its presence is suggested when each notation in the patient's chart seems to describe a different nystagmus!

Pendular Nystagmus

Convergence and Convergence Evoked Nystagmus

Convergence nystagmus is a disconjugate, acquired convergent nystagmus. Sometimes it is present spontaneously, and other times it is evoked by convergence efforts.

Convergence evoked nystagmus is evoked when an effort is made to converge. Both congenital and acquired cases have been reported.

Seesaw Nystagmus

Seesaw nystagmus is a dramatic disconjugate nystagmus. One eye rises and intorts, while the opposite eye falls and extorts. It is usually associated with disorders of the diencephalon or thalamus, and many cases occur when chiasmal lesions produce a bitemporal hemianopsia. Congenital cases have also been reported.

Circular, Elliptic, and Oblique Nystagmus

These forms of pendular nystagmus are also very dramatic in appearance because the globes themselves are moving in a path around the orbit caused by simultaneous horizontal and vertical pendular nystagmus. When the oscillations are out of phase, the eyeball appears to roam around the orbit. Oblique nystagmus may also have a jerk component. All of these types of nystagmus may be disconjugate and either congenital or acquired.

Dissociated Nystagmus

In this nystagmus, each eye moves differently. It is characteristic of medullary lesions.

Nystagmus of Infancy

These types of nystagmus usually begin at birth (congenital nystagmus) or begin in the first year of life.

Obviously, all types of nystagmus discussed above may occur in infants as well as adults with lesions of the same underlying pathways. However, when they occur in very young infants who have not established strong patterns of oculomotor behavior, lesions may not always produce the typical patterns of disordered eye movements. Thus, the result of central nervous system disease in the young infant can produce very bizarre abnormal eye movements. The types of nystagmus described below are those that do not appear to be related to known disease processes affecting the oculomotor system or its supranuclear inputs.

Motor Imbalance Nystagmus

Congenital Nystagmus Congenital nystagmus is a binocular and conjugate nystagmus that is present at birth or very soon thereafter. It is noted in the first few weeks of life and may be hereditary. Several different patterns of congenital nystagmus waveform have been described. Perhaps, the most common kind is a nystagmus that tends to be relatively pendular near primary gaze or the null point, becoming a jerk nystagmus of increasing amplitude with gaze away from these points. The null point (a point of minimum eye movement) is characteristic of congenital nystagmus. Another important characteristic of congenital nystagmus is that it is

usually horizontal, and remains horizontal in up gaze. In contrast, acquired horizontal nystagmus is associated with vertical nystagmus on up gaze.

As has been mentioned above, convergence may damp several forms of nystagmus, especially congenital nystagmus, partially explaining why the patient with congenital nystagmus has poor distance visual acuity when the eyes are moving substantially, but perfectly normal near visual acuity when convergence is brought into play. In fact, patients with congenital nystagmus are often found to read at a very close distance in order to make best use of this effect.

On the other hand, efforts to fixate accurately frequently increase the severity of the nystagmus.

With congenital nystagmus, there may be an associated head nodding or "head nystagmus" that is the result of the same disordered motor outflow and not a compensatory head movement as has been thought previously.

The hereditary congenital nystagmus may be X-linked, recessive or dominant, as well as occurring spontaneously. In about 50 percent of patients spontaneous improvement occurs as the patient grows older.

It is not unusual for the families of patients and even the patients themselves to be entirely unaware of the presence of the nystagmus. Thus, these patients at times are admitted to neurosurgical services for evaluation of presumed brain stem disease. Awareness of the characteristics of congenital nystagmus will prevent this in most cases. In cases that remain doubtful, eye movement recordings may be helpful in identifying the slow components as increasing velocity exponentials and identifying clearly several of the distinct waveforms that are typical of congenital nystagmus and rarely found in any other kind of nystagmus.

These patients may adopt a head turn in order to keep their eyes near the null point and thus maximize visual acuity. When the head turn is excessive, or the nystagmus seems to be significantly interfering with the child's development, treatment may be considered. Phenobarbital and other medications that appear to work by their effect on the reticular formation can occasionally have a dramatic effect. Prisms may displace the null point, or surgery may be performed to place the eyes in a position that is cosmetically acceptable and improves vision.

Nystagmus Associated with Strabismus *Latent nystagmus* is a congenital nystagmus that appears or is made more apparent when one eye is covered. The eyes move conjugately with the fast phase directed toward the uncovered or fixing eye. Strabismus is present in 95 percent of patients with latent nystagmus, and conversely, about 20 percent of patients with strabismus will have latent nystagmus. This nystagmus may be hereditary, but the mode of inheritance is unclear. Latent nystagmus may also be a component of a congenital nystagmus, or, conversely, patients with latent nystagmus and strabismus may be thought to have congenital nystagmus because the latent nystagmus is made manifest by the monocular viewing associated with strabismus.

It is important when testing visual acuity in these patients that the nonfixing eye is not covered, thus inducing the nystagmus in the fixing eye and decreasing its visual acuity. The nonfixing eye may be blurred with plus lenses or a pencil held in front of fixation.

Spasmus Nutans

This is a syndrome seen in infants that usually develops between the second and twelfth months of life, disappearing spontaneously by the time the patient is 3 to 4 years old. It is a clinical triad: head nodding (87 percent), nystagmus (80 percent), and head turning (38 percent). The nystagmus is frequently monocular or predominantly monocular and may be pendular, jerk, rotary, horizontal, or vertical. It is a very fine and rapid nystagmus. The etiology is unclear, usually unassociated with any recognizable central nervous system deficit. However, a few cases associated with optic nerve glioma and other central nervous system diseases have been reported.

Visual Deprivation Nystagmus

This type of nystagmus is the result of a visual afferent deficit usually resulting in loss of central vision. Frequently this nystagmus associated with a visual loss is indistinguishable from congenital nystagmus in appearance. It is unknown whether the visual deprivation and the congenital nystagmus are associated or whether the visual loss is causative. Thus, visual deprivation nystagmus frequently appears much the same as congenital nystagmus, being pendular in the primary position and becoming a jerk nystagmus on gaze to either side. The nystagmus seems to vary proportionately with the degree of visual loss such that with profound visual loss the oscillations can be so irregular that the eyes appear to drift aimlessly. This nystagmus appears at 3 to 4 months of age, even if the visual deficit is congenital, distinguishing it from congenital nystagmus, which is present at birth (but not always noted then). The abnormal eye movements may be the first indication that a baby cannot see. Visual loss later in life rarely results in similar eye movements. As with congenital nystagmus, head oscillations are frequently present.

When the nystagmus is the result of congenital blindness or severe visual loss, the eye movements are usually wandering in character, slow, and large in amplitude. Other causes of visual deprivation nystagmus are ocular albinism and achromotopsia (total color blindness). Miner's nystagmus has been thought to be related to the lack of light in the coal mines and has been described almost exclusively in Great Britain. In the few cases that have been reported in relatively recent literature, there is some suspicion that some miner's nystagmus may really be voluntary "nystagmus" (see below) or a congenital nystagmus reported for reasons of secondary gain.

Other Ocular Oscillations

Convergence Retraction "Nystagmus"

Convergence retraction nystagmus is a frequent component of the dorsal midbrain syndrome (Parinaud's syndrome, sylvian aqueduct syndrome, Koerber-Salus-Elschnig syndrome). Attempted up gaze, especially attempts at fast movements upward, results in jerky bilateral eye movements of retraction, or convergence, or both. The movement that predominates depends on which ocular muscles are maximally stimulated. The movement is generated by cocontraction of normally antagonistic extraocular muscles producing the retraction of the globe. These are saccadic movements and thus this is not a true nystagmus in the limited definition adopted here.

Clinically, this dramatic eye movement is seen with compression of the upper midbrain by pinealomas, vascular accidents in this area, and compression by upward herniation of the cerebellum. This latter phenomenon occurs not infrequently in youngsters with obstructed shunts and may be present before other signs of decompensation or papilledema develop. Thus, any child who has had hydrocephalus and has been treated with a shunt of any sort should be observed carefully for this phenomenon.

Ocular Bobbing

Massive lesions of the pons may be associated with a distinctive oculomotor phenomenon that has been termed *ocular bobbing*. It consists of rapid downward movements of the eyes with a very slow return to primary position. These movements are generally conjugate, but may be disconjugate or even uniocular. Some other oculomotor function may be present, but commonly when bobbing is seen, it represents the only possible oculomotor response and is thus present when the patient attempts to make voluntary gaze movements in other directions or, since these patients are frequently obtunded or comatose, when the doll's head maneuver or caloric stimulation is utilized.

Ocular Dysmetria, Ocular Flutter, Opsoclonus

These three ocular movements are a saccadic decompensation of eye movements, and may occur in isolation, simultaneously, or sequentially in the same patient.

Ocular dysmetria occurs when refixation saccades are made and followed by a series of undershooting and overshooting saccades before the eyes come to rest. It is analogous to limb dysmetria and, like the other saccadic decompensations, is frequently seen in disease of the cerebellar pathways.

Ocular flutter is a series of small saccades occurring with efforts at fixation.

Opsoclonus (saccadomania) is chaotic, repetitive saccadic movements in all directions, preventing fixation. Opsoclonus has also been termed *dancing eyes* and *lightning eye movements*.

All three movements are back-to-back saccades with no intersaccadic interval as occurs in normal eye movements. They are all seen with disruption of the cerebellar pathways.

In an adult or an older child, opsoclonus is commonly associated with a postinfectious encephalopathy. In younger children, opsoclonus has been described in association with neuroblastoma. Thus, any young child with opsoclonus should be evaluated for neuroblastoma. Opsoclonus has also been described as a remote effect of tumor in adults, most frequently with carcinomas of the breast or lung, and is sometimes associated with histopathological changes in the dentate nucleus.

Square Wave Jerks and Macro Square Wave Jerks

These are pairs of saccades that cause deviation from fixation, and, after a short latency, a return to fixation. They are involuntary, and their name derives from the characteristic appearance on eye movement tracings. Square wave jerks are of small amplitude (a few degrees) and occur in normal subjects as well as patients with cerebellar disease. Macro square wave jerks are almost always related to pathological states, where they more frequently occur in bursts.

Macro Saccadic Oscillations

Macro saccadic oscillations are bursts of to-and-fro saccades similar to those seen in square wave jerks in that they have normal intersaccadic latencies. However, macro saccadic oscillations differ from macro square wave jerks in that their amplitudes gradually increase and then decrease, and in straddling fixation, rather than consisting of movements away from and back toward fixation. Like macro square wave jerks, they are frequently associated with cerebellar pathway disease.

Ocular Myoclonus

Ocular myoclonus is possibly a true nystagmus with a continuous, rhythmic oscillation, frequently vertical and frequently dissociated. It can only be termed myoclonus when it is associated with similar movements of the branchial musculature, most frequently the palate, but also (in order of descending frequency) the pharynx, larynx, face, mouth, eyes, tongue, diaphragm, extremities, and intercostal muscles. The frequency is quite rapid, varying from 400 to 200 beats per minute. Thus, in any patient who is suspected of having an acquired pendular nystagmus, particularly if it is rapid and dissociated, myoclonic movements of the palate and other branchial musculature should be sought for. Myoclonic movements are seen with lesions involving the myoclonic triangle (the Guillain-Mollaret triangle: the red nucleus, the ipsilateral inferior olive, and the contralateral dentate nucleus) and is associated with pseudohypertrophy of the inferior olive. These structures are connected by the central tegmental track, inferior cerebellar peduncle, and the superior cerebellar peduncle. It is interesting that the myoclonus may not have its onset until several months after the insult that caused the damage.

Voluntary "Nystagmus"

Voluntary nystagmus is a series of rapid, possibly saccadic, movements that are pendular and brought on at will. They are very rapid and pendular with the frequency of approximately 90 to 400 beats a minute. Because of the effort necessary, they can be sustained for only a few seconds. The oscillations are almost always horizontal.

TABLE 9-2 Nystagmus and Eye Movements with Localizing Value

Type of Eye Movement	Location
Seesaw nystagmus	Diencephalon
Convergence retraction "nystagmus"	Dorsal midbrain
Abducting nystagmus in internuclear ophthalmoplegia	Pons
Brun's nystagmus	Ponto medullary junction
Vestibular nystagmus	Ponto medullary junction
Ocular myoclonus	Myoclonic triangle
Up-beat nystagmus	Medulla
Down-beat nystagmus	Foramen magnum and cerebellum
Periodic alternating nystagmus (PAN)	Foramen magnum and cerebellum
Rebound nystagmus	Cerebellar pathways
Ocular flutter, dysmetria, opsoclonus	Cerebellar pathways
Square wave jerks, macro square wave jerks, macro saccadic oscillations	Cerebellar pathways

Superior Oblique Myokymia

Superior oblique myokymia is a uniocular, high-frequency, microtremor that is torsional and of small amplitude. It evokes oscillopsia and occurs apparently spontaneously in otherwise healthy individuals. The movement may be subclinical and not easily observed (it is sometimes best seen by noting torsional movements of small perilimbal vessels) and thus sometimes is documented only with the use of the slit lamp or ophthalmoscope, whose magnification makes the movement detectable.

The tremor may be self-limiting and, when persistent and troublesome, frequently responds to carbamazepine (Tegretol). Superior oblique tenotomy is also curative.

Many of the eye movements described above are typically associated with lesions in specific areas or in specific pathways within the central nervous system. These correlations are listed in Table 9-2.

References

1. Daroff, RB, Troost, BT, Dell'Osso LF: Nystagmus and related ocular oscillations, in Duane TD: *Clinical Ophthalmology*, Philadelphia, Harper & Row, 1982, vol 2, Chap 11, pp 1–25.
2. Dell'Osso, LF: Nystagmus and other ocular motor oscillations, in Lessel S, van Dalen JTW (eds), *Neuro-ophthalmology*, Amsterdam, Excerpta Medica, 1980, vol 1, pp 146–177.
3. Dell'Osso, LF: Nystagmus and other ocular motor oscillations, in Lessel S, van Dalen, JTW (eds), *Neuro-ophthalmology*, Amsterdam, Excerpta Medica, 1982, vol 2, pp 148–171.
4. Miller NR: *Walsh and Hoyt's Clinical Neuro-ophthalmology*, 4th ed. Baltimore, Williams & Wilkins, section 4: *Disorders of Ocular Motor System*, 1983 vol 2.

10
Neurotology
Robert W. Baloh

Background

The Labyrinth

The bony labyrinth is a series of hollow channels within the petrous portion of the temporal bone.[1] It consists of an anterior cochlear part, a posterior vestibular part, and a central chamber, the vestibule. Medial to the bony labyrinth is the internal auditory canal, a cul-de-sac housing the seventh and eighth cranial nerves and internal auditory artery. The membranous labyrinth is enclosed within the channels of the bony labyrinth. A space containing perilymphatic fluid, a supportive network of connective tissue, and blood vessels lies between the periosteum of the bony labyrinth and the membranous labyrinth; the spaces within the membranous labyrinth contain endolymphatic fluid.

Cerebrospinal fluid (CSF) directly communicates with the perilymphatic space through the cochlear aqueduct, a narrow channel 3 to 4 mm long with its inner ear opening at the base of the scala tympani. In most instances this channel is filled by a loose net of fibrous tissue continuous with the arachnoid. The size of the bony canal varies from individual to individual. Infection and blood within the CSF can make their way to the inner ear via the cochlear aqueduct.

Resorption of endolymph takes place in the endolymphatic duct and sac; the latter is located in a slitlike aperture of the dura on the posterior face of the pyramid of the temporal bone halfway between the opening of the internal auditory canal and the sigmoid sinus. Destruction of the epithelium lining the sac or occlusion of the duct results in an increase of endolymphatic volume in experimental animals.[4] The first change is an expansion of cochlear and saccular membranes, which may completely fill the perilymphatic spaces. The anatomical changes resulting from this experiment are comparable to those found in the temporal bones of patients with Ménière's syndrome (either idiopathic or secondary to known inflammatory disease).

The Inner Ear Sensory Receptors

The basic element of the inner ear that transduces the mechanical forces associated with sound and head acceleration to nerve action potentials is the hair cell.[2] In the vestibular labyrinth the hair cells are mounted in the macules and cristae, and in the cochlea they are mounted in the organ of Corti (Fig. 10-1). The hair cells function in the same way in each of these organs (as force transducers) yet the biological signals generated are quite different. This difference is due to the mechanical properties of the supporting structures (as described in Fig. 10-1).

Organization of Vestibular and Auditory Reflexes

The basic elements of a vestibular or auditory reflex are the hair cell, an afferent bipolar neuron, an interneuron or interneurons, and an effector neuron.[2] The terminal fibers of the primary afferent neuron make synaptic contact with the hair cell and transmit nerve signals to the nervous system where, by means of secondary neurons in the vestibular and auditory nuclei, a connection is made with the effector neuron. The effector neuron in turn controls the activity in appropriate muscles (e.g., the extraocular muscles, the stapedius muscles) or makes connections with neurons from other sensory reflex arcs (vision, proprioception) to coordinate orienting behavior.

Clinical Evaluation of Hearing

Types of Hearing Loss

Hearing loss can be classified as conductive, sensorineural, and central based on the anatomical site of lesion.[3]

Conductive hearing loss results from lesions involving the external or middle ear. The tympanic membrane and ossicles act as a transformer, amplifying airborne sound and efficiently transferring it to the inner ear fluid. If this normal pathway is obstructed, transmission can occur across the skin and through the bones of the skull (bone conduction), but at the cost of significant energy loss.

Sensorineural hearing loss results from lesions of the cochlea and/or the auditory division of the eighth cranial nerve. The spiral cochlea mechanically analyzes the frequency content of sound. For high-frequency tones only hair cells in the basilar turn are activated, while for low-frequency tones all or nearly all hair cells are activated. Therefore, with lesions of the cochlea and its afferent nerve the hearing levels for different frequencies are usually unequal and the phase relationship (timing) between different frequencies may be altered. Distortion of sounds is common with sensorineural hearing loss. A pure tone may be heard as noisy, rough, or buzzing, or it may be distorted so that it sounds like a complex mixture of tones. Binaural diplacusis occurs when the two ears are affected unequally so that the same frequency has a different pitch in each ear, i.e., the patient hears double. Monaural diplacusis occurs when two tones or a tone and noise are heard simultaneously in one ear. With recruitment there is an abnormally rapid growth in the sensation of loudness as the intensity of a sound is increased so that faint or moderate sounds cannot be heard while there is little or no change in the loudness of loud sounds.

Central hearing disorders result from lesions of the central auditory pathways. These consist of the cochlear and dorsal olivary nuclear complexes, inferior colliculi, medial genicu-

MACULE

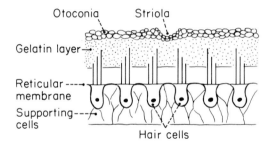

CRISTA

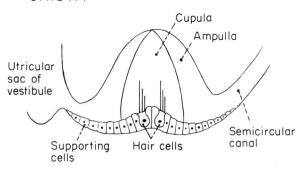

ORGAN OF CORTI

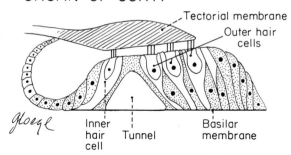

Figure 10-1 Inner ear receptor organs. In the macule the weight of the otolithic membrane produces a shearing force on the underlying hair cells that is proportional to the sine of the angle between the line of gravitational force and a line perpendicular to the plane of the macule. The hair cell cilia in the cristae of the semicircular canals are embedded in the cupula, a jelly-like substance of the same specific gravity as that of the surrounding fluids. Angular head acceleration results in a displacement of the cupula and bending of the hair cells of the crista. In the cochlea the hair cells are mounted on the flexible basilar membrane in the organ of Corti. A small acoustically induced pressure difference across the basilar membrane causes the organ of Corti and hair cells to vibrate at the frequency of sound.

late bodies, auditory cortex in the temporal lobes, and interconnecting afferent and efferent fiber tracts. As a rule patients with central lesions do not have impaired hearing

levels for pure tones and they understand speech as long as it is clearly spoken in a quiet environment. If the listener's task is made more difficult with the introduction of background or competing messages, performance deteriorates more markedly in patients with central lesions than in normal subjects. Lesions involving the eighth nerve root entry zone or cochlear nucleus, however, can result in unilateral hearing loss for pure tones. Since approximately 50 percent of afferent nerve fibers cross central to the cochlear nucleus, this is the most central structure in which a lesion can result in a unilateral hearing loss.

Rapid Qualitative Tests of Hearing

A quick test for hearing loss in the speech range is to observe the response to spoken commands at different intensities (whisper, conversation, shouting). The examiner must be careful to prevent the patient from reading his or her lip movement. A high-frequency stimulus such as a watch tick or coin click (approximately 4000 cycles per second) should also be used since sensorineural disorders often involve only the higher frequencies. Tuning fork tests permit a rough assessment of the hearing level for pure tones of known frequency. The clinician's own hearing level can be used as a reference standard. The Rinne test compares the patient's hearing by air conduction with that by bone conduction. The fork (preferably 512 cycles per second) is first held against the mastoid process until the sound fades. It is then placed 1 in. from the ear. Normal subjects can hear the fork about twice as long by air as by bone conduction. If bone conduction is greater than air conduction, a conductive hearing loss is suggested. The Weber test compares the patient's hearing by bone conduction in the two ears. The fork is placed at the center of the forehead or on a central incisor, and the patient is asked where the tone is heard. Normal subjects hear it in the center of the head, patients with unilateral conductive loss hear it on the affected side, and patients with unilateral sensorineural loss hear it on the side opposite the loss.

Clinical Evaluation of the Vestibular System

Symptoms and Signs of Vestibular Loss

At rest the afferent nerves from the macules and cristae maintain a balanced tonic rate of firing into the vestibular nuclei.[2] This tonic activity and its modulation with head movements is passed on to cortical centers and to the vestibulo-ocular and vestibulospinal reflexes. Vestibular symptoms and signs result from either an imbalance in the tonic activity or a loss of reflex activity.

Imbalance in the baseline activity originating from the labyrinths typically leads to vertigo (an illusion of rotation), nystagmus, and unsteadiness. If a patient slowly loses vestibular function on one side only over a period of months to years (e.g., with an acoustic neuroma), symptoms and signs are minimal or may even be absent. On the other hand, a sudden unilateral loss of labyrinthine function is a dramatic event. The patient complains of severe vertigo and nausea, is pale and perspiring, and usually vomits repeatedly. The patient prefers to lie quietly in a dark room but can walk if forced to (falling toward the side of the lesion). A brisk spontaneous nystagmus interferes with vision. These symptoms and signs are usually transient, and the process of compensation begins immediately. Within 1 week of the lesion a young patient can walk without difficulty and with fixation can inhibit the spontaneous nystagmus. Within 1 month most young patients return to work with few, if any, residual symptoms. By contrast, elderly patients compensate for a unilateral loss of vestibular function much more slowly (weeks to months) and may never return to their prior level of function.

Patients who lose vestibular function bilaterally in a symmetrical fashion (e.g., secondary to ototoxic drugs) usually do not develop vertigo or nystagmus since their tonic vestibular activity remains balanced. However, they do complain of unsteadiness and visual distortion due to loss of vestibulospinal and vestibulo-ocular reflex activity, respectively. Characteristically, when walking, such patients are unable to fixate on objects because the surrounds are bouncing up and down (oscillopsia). In order to see the faces of passersby, they learn to stop and hold their head still. Their imbalance is typically worse at night, when they are less able to use vision to compensate for the loss of vestibular function.

Caloric Testing

The caloric test uses a nonphysiological stimulus to induce endolymphatic flow in the horizontal semicircular canal and thus horizontal nystagmus by creating a temperature gradient from one side of the canal to the other.[2] With a warm caloric stimulus the column of endolymph nearest the middle ear rises because of its decreased density (Fig. 10-2). This causes the cupula to deviate toward the utricle (ampullopetal flow) and produces horizontal nystagmus with the fast phase directed toward the stimulated ear. A cold stimulus produces the opposite effect, causing ampullofugal endolymph flow and nystagmus directed away from the stimulated ear (COWS—*c*old *o*pposite, *w*arm *s*ame). Because of its ready availability, iced water (approximately 0°C) is usually used for bedside caloric testing. To bring the horizontal canal into the vertical plane the patient lies in the supine position with the head tilted 30 degrees forward. Infusion of 10 ml of iced water induces a burst of nystagmus usually lasting from 1 to 3 min. In a comatose patient only a slow tonic deviation toward the side of stimulation is observed. In normal subjects the duration and speed of induced nystagmus varies greatly depending on the size of the external canal, the thickness of the temporal bone, the circulation to the temporal bone, and the subject's ability to use fixation to suppress the nystagmus. Greater than a 20 percent asymmetry in nystagmus duration suggests a lesion on the side of the decreased response.

With bithermal caloric testing each ear is irrigated for a fixed duration (30 to 40 s) at a constant flow rate of water that is 7° below body temperature (30° C) and 7° above body

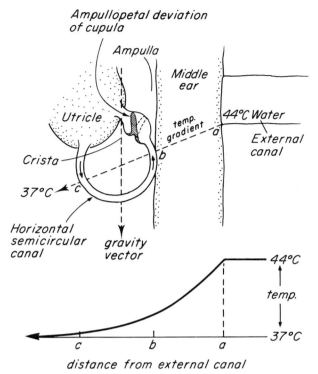

Figure 10-2 Caloric stimulation of the horizontal semicircular canal with 44°C water. (From Baloh and Honrubia.[2]).

temperature (44° C). Electronystagmography (ENG) is used to measure the maximum slow-phase velocity after each of the four nystagmus responses (Fig. 10-3). The four responses of a bithermal caloric test are routinely compared with two standard formulas. The vestibular paresis formula

$$\frac{(R\ 30° + R\ 44°) - (L\ 30° + L\ 44°)}{R\ 30° + R\ 44° + L\ 30° + L\ 44°} \times 100$$

compares the right-sided responses with the left-sided responses, and the directional preponderance formula

$$\frac{(R\ 30° + L\ 44°) - (R\ 44° + L\ 30°)}{R\ 30° + L\ 44° + R\ 44° + L\ 30°} \times 100$$

compares nystagmus to the right with nystagmus to the left in the same subject. In both of these formulas the difference in response is reported as a percentage of the total response. This is important because the absolute magnitude of caloric response is dependent on several factors. Dividing by the total response normalizes the measurements to remove the large variability in absolute magnitude of normal caloric responses. In our laboratory the upper normal value for vestibular paresis is 22 percent, while that for directional preponderance is 28 percent (using maximum slow-phase velocity in the above equations). As a general rule a significant vestibular paresis on bithermal caloric testing indicates a peripheral vestibular lesion while a significant directional preponderance is nonlocalizing (i.e., it can occur with peripheral and central lesions). The latter is often associated with spontaneous nystagmus, in which case the velocity of the slow components of the spontaneous nystagmus adds to

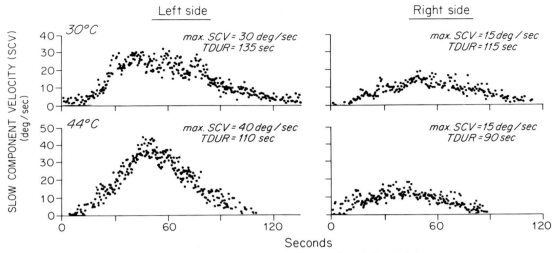

Figure 10-3 Results of a bithermal caloric test in a patient with a right viral laby-rinthitis. Each dot represents the average velocity of one nystagmus slow phase (SCV). TDUR indicates duration of response. (From Baloh and Honrubia.[2])

that cf caloric-induced nystagmus in the same direction and subtracts from that of caloric-induced nystagmus in the opposite direction.

Rotatory Testing

With rotatory testing, the patient is seated in a chair that rotates about its vertical axis. The head is fixed so that angular rotation occurs in the plane of one of the semicircular canal pairs (usually with the head tilted 30 degrees forward so that rotation occurs in the plane of the horizontal canals). The patient's eyes are opened in complete darkness, and the induced nystagmus is recorded with ENG. The gain of the response defined as the peak slow-phase eye velocity divided by the peak chair velocity is calculated for nystagmus in each direction. An asymmetry in rotatory-induced nystagmus has the same significance as a directional preponderance on bithermal caloric testing; it indicates an imbalance of the vestibulo-ocular reflex but is nonlocalizing. Patients with a highly significant unilateral vestibular paresis to caloric stimulation may have symmetrical rotatory-induced nystagmus since the remaining intact labyrinth is able to compensate for the damaged side.[2] For this reason rotatory testing is not particularly useful for identifying unilateral peripheral vestibular lesions.

Rotatory testing is very useful for evaluating patients with bilateral peripheral vestibular lesions (e.g., ototoxic exposure) since both labyrinths are stimulated simultaneously and the degree of remaining function is accurately quantified. Patients with absent caloric responses may have decreased but measurable rotatory-induced nystagmus, particularly at higher stimulus velocities. The ability to identify remaining vestibular function, even if minimal, is an important advantage of rotatory testing, particularly when the physician is contemplating ablative surgery or monitoring the effects of ototoxic drugs.

Evaluation of the Dizzy Patient

Detailed History Taking

Although the presence of vertigo indicates a lesion within the vestibular system (including visual-vestibular and nuchal-vestibular pathways), its absence does not rule out a vestibular lesion. Other less specific descriptions of the dizzy sensation associated with vestibular dysfunction include giddiness, swimming in the head, floating, and drunkenness. Rarely a patient will complain of an illusion of linear movement, suggesting an isolated involvement of a macule or its central connections. Dizziness caused by vestibular lesions is usually worsened by rapid head movements since the new stimulus is sensed by the intact labyrinth and existing asymmetries are accentuated. Episodes may be precipitated by turning over in bed, sitting up from the lying position, extending the neck to look up or bending over and straightening up. Symptoms of autonomic dysfunction (e.g., sweating, nausea, and vomiting) nearly always accompany vestibular lesions, and occasionally vegetative symptoms are the only manifestation of such a lesion.

The description of vestibular symptoms alone does not differentiate peripheral from central lesions. For this one must rely on the associated symptoms (Table 10-1). Lesions of the labyrinth usually produce hearing loss, tinnitus, and a sensation of pressure, fullness, or pain in the ear. Involvement of the eighth nerve also produces hearing loss and tinnitus but not the latter symptoms. If the lesion is in the internal auditory canal, there may be associated ipsilateral facial weakness; if it is in the cerebellopontine angle, ipsilateral facial numbness and weakness and ipsilateral extremity ataxia commonly occur.

Because of the close approximation of other neuronal centers and fiber tracts, it is unusual to find lesions in the brain stem and cerebellum that cause isolated vestibular

TABLE 10-1 Symptoms Commonly Associated with Vertigo Caused by Lesions at Different Neuroanatomical Sites

Labyrinth	Brain stem
Hearing loss	Diplopia
Tinnitus	Visual hallucinations
Pressure	(unformed)
Pain	Dysarthria
	Drop attacks
	Extremity weakness and
Internal auditory canal	numbness
Hearing loss	Cerebellum
Tinnitus	Imbalance
Facial weakness	Incoordination
	Temporal lobe
Cerebellopontine angle	Absence spells
Hearing loss	Visual hallucinations
Tinnitus	(formed)
Facial weakness and	Visual illusions
numbness	Olfactory or gustatory
Extremity incoordination	hallucinations

symptoms. Lesions of the brain stem are invariably associated with other cranial nerve and long tract symptoms. For example, with transient vertebrobasilar insufficiency vertigo is associated with other brain stem and occipital lobe symptoms such as diplopia, hemianopic field defects, drop attacks, weakness, numbness, dysarthria, and ataxia. Lesions of the cerebellum (e.g., infarction or hemorrhage) may be relatively silent but are always associated with extremity and truncal ataxia in addition to vertigo. As previously noted, hearing loss for pure tones is unusual with brain stem lesions, even in the late stages.

Vertigo can occur as part of the aura of temporal lobe seizures. The cortical projections of the vestibular system are activated by a focal discharge within the temporal lobe. Such vertigo is nearly always associated with other typical aura symptoms such as an abnormal taste or smell and distortion of the visual world (hallucinations and illusions). Occasionally, however, vertigo can be the only manifestation of the aura. In such cases the association with typical "absence" spells should lead one to the correct diagnosis.

Differential Diagnosis of Common Vestibular Disorders

Viral labyrinthitis is often part of a systemic viral illness such as an upper respiratory tract infection, measles, mumps, and infectious mononucleosis, or it may be an isolated infection of the labyrinth without systemic involvement. In the latter case, the infecting agent is rarely identified, but substantial pathological evidence exists to indicate that the sudden onset of hearing loss and vertigo can be caused by an acute isolated viral infection of the labyrinth. The pathological findings of atrophy of the organ of Corti and atrophy of the vestibular end organs are similar to those seen with labyrinthitis associated with well-documented viral illnesses (such as mumps or measles).[4] In such cases the vasculature remains intact and the cochlear and vestibular neuronal population is unaf-

fected. As a general rule a sudden onset of hearing loss and vertigo in an otherwise healthy patient is likely due to a viral labyrinthitis.

Viral mononeuritis of the vestibular nerve typically presents with the acute onset of severe vertigo, nausea, and vomiting unassociated with auditory or neurological symptoms. Most of these patients gradually improve over 1 to 2 weeks, but some develop recurrent episodes. Laboratory studies usually reveal spontaneous vestibular nystagmus, unilateral caloric hypoexcitability, and normal hearing. A large percentage of such patients report an upper respiratory tract illness within 1 to 2 weeks prior to the onset of vertigo. This syndrome frequently occurs in epidemics (epidemic vertigo), may affect several members of the same family, and erupts more commonly in the spring and early summer. All of these factors suggest a viral origin, but attempts to isolate an agent have been unsuccessful except for occasional findings of a herpes zoster infection. Pathological studies showing atrophy of one or more vestibular nerve trunks with or without atrophy of their associated sense organs support a vestibular nerve site and probable viral etiology for this syndrome.[4]

Patients with *benign paroxysmal positional vertigo* develop brief episodes of vertigo (<30 s) with position change typically when turning over in bed, bending over and straightening up, or extending the neck to look up. Studies of the temporal bones of patients who manifested typical paroxysmal positional nystagmus revealed basophilic deposits on the cupulae of the posterior canals.[4] These deposits were present only on one side, the side that was undermost when paroxysmal positional nystagmus and vertigo were induced. These cupular basophilic deposits are apparently otoconia released from a degenerating utricular macule. The otoconia settles on the cupula of the posterior canal (situated directly under the utricular macule), causing it to become heavier than the surrounding endolymph and thus sensitive to changes in the gravity vector. When the patient moves from the sitting to head-hanging position (provocative test for paroxysmal positional nystagmus), the posterior canal moves from an inferior to superior position, a utriculofugal displacement of the cupula occurs, and a burst of nystagmus is produced. This nystagmus usually has a latency of a few seconds and fatigues on repeated testing. The latency could be due to the period of time required for the otoconial mass to be displaced, and fatigability may be caused by the dispersing of particles in the endolymph. Consistent with this theory, the burst of rotatory paroxysmal positional nystagmus is in the plane of the posterior canal of the "down" ear with the fast component directed upward, as would be predicted from ampullofugal stimulation of the posterior canal.[2] Additional support for this concept has come from reports showing disappearance of fatigable paroxysmal positional nystagmus after the ampullary nerve has been sectioned from the posterior canal on the diseased side.

Ménière's syndrome is characterized by fluctuating hearing loss and tinnitus, episodic vertigo, and a sensation of fullness or pressure in the ear. Typically the patient develops a sensation of fullness and pressure along with decreased hearing and tinnitus in one ear. Vertigo rapidly follows, reaching a maximum intensity within minutes and then slowly subsiding over the next several hours. The patient is usually left with a sense of unsteadiness and dizziness for days after the acute vertiginous episode. In the early stages the hearing loss is completely reversible, but in later stages a residual hearing loss remains. Although the pathological findings of a distended endolymphatic system have been well described, the mechanism for the fluctuating symptoms and signs of Ménière's syndrome are not well understood.[4] A leading theory is that the episodes of hearing loss and vertigo are caused by ruptures in the membranes separating endolymph from perilymph, producing a sudden increase in potassium concentration in the latter. As the potassium is slowly cleared over several hours, the symptoms and signs subside. Another possible explanation is mechanical deformation of the end organ that is reversible as the endolymphatic pressure decreases. The infrequent but dramatic sudden falling attacks seen in patients with Ménière's syndrome are most likely due to sudden deformation or displacement of one of the vestibular sense organs.

The *ototoxicity* of the aminoglycosides is due to hair cell damage in the inner ear. Unlike other antibiotics, the aminoglycosides are concentrated in the perilymph and endolymph, increasing their ototoxic potential. Of the common aminoglycosides, streptomycin primarily damages the hair cells of the cristae with relative sparing of the hair cells of the macules and cochlea. Because of this highly selective effect on the vestibular end organ, streptomycin has been used to produce a chemical vestibulectomy in patients with Ménière's syndrome.

Vestibular schwannomas (acoustic neuroma, neurinoma, neurilemmoma) usually begin in the internal auditory canal, producing symptoms by compressing the nerves in the narrow confines of the canal. As the tumor enlarges, it protrudes through the internal auditory meatus, producing a funnel-shaped erosion of the bone surrounding the canal, stretching adjacent nerve roots over the surface of the mass, and deforming the brain stem and cerebellum. Vestibular schwannomas account for approximately 10 percent of intracranial tumors and over 75 percent of cerebellopontine angle tumors. By far the most common symptoms associated with vestibular schwannomas are slowly progressive hearing loss and tinnitus from compression of the cochlear nerve. Rarely an acute hearing loss occurs, apparently from compression of the labyrinthine vasculature. Vertigo occurs in less than 20 percent of patients, but approximately 50 percent complain of imbalance or dysequilibrium. Next to the auditory nerve, the most commonly involved cranial nerves (by compression) are the fifth and seventh, producing facial numbness and weakness, respectively.

Vertebrobasilar insufficiency (VBI) is a common cause of vertigo in patients over the age of 50. Whether the vertigo originates from ischemia of the labyrinth, brain stem, or both structures is not always clear since the circulation to both the labyrinth and the vestibular nuclei originates from the vertebrobasilar system. Vertigo with VBI is abrupt in onset, usually lasts several minutes, and is frequently associated with nausea and vomiting. The key to the diagnosis is to find associated symptoms resulting from ischemia in the remaining territory supplied by the posterior circulation. Common associated symptoms include formed and unformed visual hallucinations, diplopia, drop attacks, dysarthria, and weakness. These symptoms occur in episodes either in combination with the vertigo or in isolation. Vertigo may be an isolated initial symptom of VBI, but repeated episodes of vertigo without other symptoms suggest a disorder other than VBI. The cause of VBI is usually atherosclerosis of the subclavian, vertebral, and/or basilar arteries.

Although the *lateral medullary syndrome* (Wallenberg's syndrome) is commonly known as that of the posterior inferior cerebellar artery, it usually occurs from occlusion of the ipsilateral vertebral artery, and only rarely with occlusion of the posterior inferior cerebellar artery. The zone of infarction producing the lateral medullary syndrome consists of a wedge of the dorsolateral medulla just posterior to the olive. The medial and descending vestibular nuclei are usually included in this zone. Major symptoms include vertigo, nausea, vomiting, and intractable hiccuping. Patients with Wallenberg's syndrome suffer a prominent motor disturbance that causes their body and extremities to deviate toward the lesion side as if being pulled by a strong external force. This so-called lateropulsion also affects the oculomotor system, causing excessively large voluntary and involuntary saccades directed toward the side of the lesion while saccades away from the lesion side are abnormally small. Spontaneous nystagmus away from the side of the lesion is present with fixation, and occasionally the spontaneous nystagmus changes direction with eye closure.

References

1. Anson BJ, Donaldson JA: *Surgical Anatomy of the Temporal Bone and Ear*, 2nd ed. Philadelphia, Saunders, 1973.
2. Baloh RW, Honrubia V: *Clinical Neurophysiology of the Vestibular System*. Philadelphia, Davis, 1979.
3. Davis H, Silverman SR (eds): *Hearing and Deafness*, 4th ed. New York, Holt, 1978.
4. Schuknecht HF: *Pathology of the Ear*. Cambridge, Mass. Harvard University Press, 1974.

11

Gait and Station; Examination of Coordination

Setti S. Rengachary

Gait refers to the way a person walks, and stance or station refers to the way a person stands. Although they appear to be effortless and automatic, the bipedal stance and normal human gait are indeed expressions of complex integrated neural activity at all levels of organization in the nervous system. It is common knowledge that the gait and stance of a given person are as individualistic as facial appearance or fingerprints. Lesions in the nervous system affecting certain specific pathways produce a predictable alteration in the gait pattern. Experienced clinicians gather a great deal of information from a seemingly casual but educated look at the patient's station and gait long before they begin their formal neurological examination.

Minimal energy is utilized in the maintenance of upright posture. The proprioceptive input originating from the muscles, tendons, and joints are carried through the peripheral nerves and the posterior columns. Integrative mechanisms within the spinal cord initiate tonic contraction of antigravity muscles. This simple reflex mechanism is modulated by input from the vestibular system, reticular nuclei, basal ganglia, cerebellum, and motor cortex. When the system is suddenly perturbed by, say, a sudden jostling, compensatory muscular activity restores poise.

When a person starts to walk, certain dynamic reflexes become superimposed against a background of static reflex activity. The weight is alternately shifted from one extremity to the other. Propulsion is achieved by the non-weight-bearing extremity being carried forward in a rhythmic, alternate fashion. At the same time the contralateral arm swings forward in unison with forward propulsion of the leg. The trunk tends to remain upright.

Examination of Station

Station is examined by inspection and by performing Romberg's test.

On inspection, certain gross abnormalities of the neuromuscular or skeletal system may be obvious. A patient with Parkinson's disease typically has a rigid forward stoop with flexion of the trunk, limbs, and head with inability to make the necessary postural adjustments to being pushed or shoved. Patients with chorea or athetosis are unable to stand still and may appear to be restless and fidgety. Individuals with midline cerebellar lesions tend to sway in all directions and may not be able to stand unsupported. Those with cerebellar hemispheric disease or vestibular impairment tend to fall toward the side of the lesion when standing. Hemiplegic patients stand with the affected arm flexed at the elbow, wrist, and fingers and the leg extended at the knee, plantar flexed and inverted at the foot. Patients with cerebellar or posterior column disease tend to stand with feet far apart to give them a broader base of support to compensate for their static ataxia.

Romberg's test is done by asking the patient to stand erect with the feet together and arms extended, first with the eyes open, then closed. Unsteadiness and the tendency to sway or fall, if present, are noted. Romberg's sign is said to be present if there is an appreciable increase in unsteadiness with a tendency to fall with eye closure; it is characteristically seen in posterior column disease with proprioceptive loss. Patients with cerebellar disease remain unsteady with the eyes open or closed. One should be aware that normal individuals may show slight swaying and the unsteadiness in cerebellar disease may get somewhat worse with eye closure but not to the extent seen in individuals with posterior column disease. Thus, the cerebellar and posterior column functions should be evaluated in more detail should Romberg's test be positive to make meaningful interpretation of the latter test. Hysterical patients may show a false-positive Romberg's sign in that they may dramatically sway with eye closure although they may not fall. They may be distracted by asking them to perform a simultaneous mental or motor task such as counting backwards from 10 or sequentially touching the fingertips with the thumb.

Examination of Gait

Formal examination of gait should be tailored to the clinical circumstance. The age of the patient, degree of alertness and cooperation, presence or absence of severe pain, nature of the suspected clinical illness (e.g., gait testing may be contraindicated in a patient with suspected subarachnoid hemorrhage from a ruptured cerebral aneurysm), etc. are factors to be taken into account in deciding the rigor of testing.

One gleans as much or perhaps more valuable information from observation of gait as the patient enters the examining room as from formal testing. One should observe the patient as a whole, paying particular attention to associated movements of the arms, trunk, and face.

A systematic sequence should be developed in formal gait testing. The patient is first asked to walk at his or her usual pace for about 15 to 20 ft, stop, turn, and return to the starting point. Cerebellar ataxia may become more apparent with sudden stopping or turning than during walking. In certain instances asking the patient to walk backward or sideways may bring out the gait disturbance that was not apparent during walking forward. The patient is then asked to walk on tiptoes and heels. This maneuver may reveal ataxia, spasticity in the legs, or weakness in the gastrocnemius-soleus or anterior tibial groups. Heel-to-toe tandem walking may be difficult or impossible in patients with ataxia. If cerebellar hemispheric disease is suspected, the patient may be asked to walk around a chair. The patient will veer into it if the affected side is toward the chair and will go around farther and farther away from it if the lesion is on the opposite side. Minimal degrees of spasticity that are barely apparent during walking at a normal pace may become more evident when the patient is asked to walk swiftly or trot. Having the patient hop on one foot and then the other is an especially good way of comparing each side for ataxia, motor weakness, or spasticity.

Certain non-neurological conditions may affect walking and simulate gait disturbances from neurological disorders. Common conditions include painful calluses on the sole of the foot, flat feet, a shortened lower limb, bony or joint deformities secondary to previous trauma, operation, or arthritis, and intermittent claudication from ischemic vascular disease. The problem becomes compounded if these disorders are superimposed on a neurological disorder.

Disorders of Gait

The following are some of the most common gait disturbances seen in clinical practice.

Spastic Gait

A spastic gait may result from either unilateral or bilateral upper motor neuron lesions.

Spastic Hemiplegic Gait

This type of gait results from a unilateral upper motor neuron lesion; it is frequently seen following a completed stroke. There is spasticity of all muscles on the involved side, but it is more marked in certain muscle groups. This results in spastic extension of the lower limb with plantar flexion and inversion of the foot associated with flexion at the elbow, wrist, and fingers. During walking, the leg tends to circumduct, rotating outward and describing a semicircle. The foot drags and scrapes the floor. Associated swinging movement of the arm on the affected side is conspicuously absent even with a mild hemiparesis.

Spastic Paraplegic or Quadriplegic Gait

This condition results from bilateral upper motor neuron lesions. The most common lesion that gives rise to bilateral spastic gait is cervical spondylotic myelopathy in adults and cerebral palsy in children. The gait can be equated with a bilateral hemiplegic gait but only affecting the lower limbs. The patient ambulates in a slow, stiff, and jerky manner, often accompanied by compensatory movements of the trunk and upper extremities. There is spastic extension at the knees with adduction of the hips with a resultant

scissor-like gait. Minimal spasticity may become evident if the patient is asked to trot or to tap with the foot rapidly on the floor.

Ataxic Gait

Ataxic gait is seen in two principal disorders: cerebellar disease and posterior column disease.

Cerebellar Ataxic Gait

The cerebellar ataxic gait is seen in patients with disorders of the cerebellum or its connections. The nature of the abnormality in gait is dependent on whether the midline vermis or cerebellar hemisphere is predominantly involved.

In *vermal lesions*, the gait is broad-based, unsteady, staggering, and lurching with an irregular sway. There may be titubation of head or trunk. The patient is unable to walk in tandem, or on a straight line. The ataxia may be associated with other signs of cerebellar incoordination such as intention tremor, past pointing, etc., but this is not always the case. The latter signs are dependent on involvement of the cerebellar hemisphere. The ataxia of gait gets worse on attempting to stop suddenly or turn, with a tendency to fall to the floor. On occasion the ataxia may be too severe to allow standing without support. Cerebellar ataxia is present with the eyes open or closed, although the swaying may be slightly worse on eye closure.

In *hemispheral lesions* the ataxia tends to be less severe. There is persistent lurching or deviation toward the involved side. When asked to walk around a chair in a clockwise or counterclockwise direction, the patient tends to fall toward the involved side. The patient, in addition, shows signs of unilateral hemispheric disease such as intention tremor, finger-to-nose ataxia, dysdiadochokinesis, muscular hypotonia, and pendular reflexes on the involved side.

Sensory Ataxia

This results from deprivation of proprioceptive input in disorders involving the posterior columns, dorsal roots, or peripheral nerves. The patient is unaware of the position of the limbs. The gait is broad-based, and the patient tends to lift the feet too high and slap on the floor in an incoordinate and abrupt manner. The patient tends to watch the floor and the feet to maximize attempts at visual correction of the proprioceptive deficit, and may have difficulty walking in the dark. When asked to stand with the feet together and eyes closed, the patient shows greatly increased swaying or actual falls (Romberg's sign).

Spastic-Ataxic Gait

Combined involvement of the corticospinal tracts and the posterior columns or cerebellum results in a spastic-ataxic gait. The gait is described as jiggling or bobbing. The weight-bearing limb shows clonic dancing or bouncing movements that are transmitted to the trunk.

Steppage Gait

This occurs in patients with a foot drop. The patient lifts the leg high enough to clear the flail foot off the floor by flexing at the hip and knee, and then slaps the foot on the floor. Foot drop may occur unilaterally or bilaterally.

Apraxia of Gait

Apraxia of gait is seen in patients with bilateral frontal lobe disease such as degenerative disorders (Alzheimer's disease) or tumors ("butterfly" glioblastoma of the corpus callosum). It is also typically seen in normal-pressure hydrocephalus.

Despite lack of impairment of motor strength or sensation in the legs, the patient has difficulty walking. The most difficulty is with initiation of walking. The patient appears reluctant or unable to step forward as though the foot is attracted to the floor as steel is to a magnet (magnetic apraxia). When the patient does walk, it is in small, shuffling hesitant steps. Each time the patient stops walking, he or she can resume only with great effort. On turning, the patient pivots with one foot on the floor and the other foot taking small shuffling steps. In late stages the patient may be unable to stand.

Parkinsonian Gait

A typical parkinsonian patient stands somewhat stooped forward with flexion at the elbows, metacarpophalangeal joints, hips, and knees. The patient has difficulty initiating movements and walks in short steps. The feet barely clear the ground as the patient shuffles along. As the patient gets going, he or she leans forward, tends to pick up speed, and even starts to run as though chasing his or her center of gravity (propulsive gait or festinating gait). Less commonly, deviation of the center of gravity to one side or backward may produce lateropulsion or retropulsion, respectively. There is lack of associated arm movements as the patient walks, and the typical picture is completed by the masklike facies, infrequent blinking, drooling of saliva, and "pill rolling" tremor involving the index finger and thumb.

Hysterical Gait

The hysterical gait tends to be nonspecific and bizarre and does not conform to a specific organic pattern. The abnormality may vary from moment to moment and from one examination to another. There may be ataxia, spasticity, inability to move, or other types of abnormality. There are bizarre superfluous movements, with swaying from side to side, but the patient does not usually fall. The abnormality is minimal or absent when the patient is unaware of being watched or is distracted. The gait may suggest monoplegia, paraplegia, or hemiplegia, yet the patient may be able to move the limb, especially when distracted. One should be cautious, however, not to interpret a gait of unusual pattern as hysterical, unless there are other signs of functional illness. All hysterical gaits are bizarre, but all bizarre gaits are not hysterical.

Coordination

Motor coordination refers to the smooth, precise, and harmonious muscular activity that is an expression of complex integrated neural activity. *Equilibratory coordination* is the maintenance of stance in the upright position; it is dependent upon proprioceptive, cerebellar, and vestibular antigravity mechanisms. *Nonequilibratory coordination* is concerned with fine movements of the extremities, especially the fingers, and is a reflection of intact cerebellar and proprioceptive activity.

All movements, however simple they may appear, require the coordinated contraction of many groups of muscles. This can be illustrated by analyzing a simple movement such as a hand grasp. Here the primary movement is contraction of flexor muscles of the fingers (agonists or prime movers). To allow flexion of the fingers, the extensors of the fingers (antagonists) must relax concurrent with contraction of finger flexors. The finger flexors have a tendency to flex the wrist as well; to counteract this, the extensors of the wrist contract synergistically (synergists). And finally, during the hand grasp, the elbow, wrist, and shoulder joints need to be stabilized by the appropriate muscles acting on these joints (fixators). Although the coordination of agonists, antagonists, synergists, and fixators is brought about by reciprocal innervation and segmental spinal reflex activity, smooth, gracefully performed complex muscular activity requires complicated neural interaction at multiple levels of the neuraxis. These include the motor and premotor cortex, basal ganglia, cerebellum and its connections, vestibular system, posterior columns, and peripheral nerves. From a practical clinical viewpoint, however, incoordination refers to the nonharmonious movement that is *not* secondary to paresis, alterations in muscular tone, or the presence of involuntary movements.

It is customary and useful to classify disorders that result in motor incoordination into three groups: (1) cerebellar syndrome, (2) syndrome of the vestibular system, and (3) posterior column syndrome. The distinguishing features of these three major disorders of equilibrium are summarized in Table 11-1.

Syndrome of the Cerebellar System

The cerebellum is the central integrative organ that controls muscular coordination. The afferent input enters the cerebellum principally through the middle (brachium pontis) and the inferior (restiform body) cerebellar peduncles. Sensory input from the muscles, tendons, and joints that does not reach consciousness enters through the dorsal (from the lower limbs) and ventral (from the upper limbs) spinocerebellar tracts to the anterior vermis and parts of the posterior vermis ("spinocerebellum"). Information regarding volun-

TABLE 11-1 Differentiation of the Disorders of Equilibrium

Symptom or Sign	Cerebellar Syndrome	Posterior Column Syndrome	Vestibular Syndrome
Sensory disturbances	Absent	Striking loss of vibration and position sense	In peripheral lesions, may have associated deafness; in central (brain stem-vestibular nuclear) lesions, hearing usually unaffected
Vertigo	Absent	Absent	Hallmark of vestibular disease
Nausea and vomiting	Present only when there is increased intracranial pressure due to fourth ventricular obstruction, or from direct irritation of the vagal nucleus by a vermian mass (medulloblastoma)	Absent	Nausea and vomiting accompany vertigo especially in an acute peripheral vestibular lesion
Nystagmus	Pure cerebellar lesions may not produce nystagmus; presence of nystagmus in cerebellar syndrome implies involvement of the vestibulocerebellar pathways or direct pressure on the vestibular nuclei	Absent	Nystagmus may be horizontal, vertical, or rotary. Positional changes may have a substantial effect on the nature and degree of nystagmus
Influence of vision	Symptoms and signs unchanged or only made slightly worse with removal of visual cues	Dramatic increase in ataxia with removal of visual cues	Illusion of the floor of the room rising or sinking, walls tilting; illusion of to-and-fro or up-and-down movement of the body
Romberg's sign	Absent	Present	Absent
Tremor	Intention tremor	Pseudoathetoid movements	Absent
Dysmetria	Present	Present especially with the eyes closed	Absent
Gait	In vermis lesions: wide-based gait, considerable difficulty in standing or walking, tendency to fall in any direction. In hemispheral lesion: tendency to veer toward the side of the lesion	Wide-based steppage gait with eyes watching the feet and ground; difficulty in ambulating in the dark or with eyes closed	Ataxic with a feeling of impulsion, an uncontrollable sensation of being pulled to the ground or to one side or the other

tary activity originating from the cerebral motor cortex enters the cerebellar hemispheres, the neocerebellum (pontocerebellum), through the brachium pontis. The major efferent pathway is the superior cerebellar peduncle (brachium conjunctivum) carrying the dentatorubrothalamic fibers, which ultimately return to the cerebral cortex.

The vermis of the cerebellum is primarily concerned with the maintenance of posture and equilibrium and influences the truncal musculature principally. The cerebellar hemisphere is concerned with the coordinated skilled activity in the ipsilateral extremities.

Cardinal features of cerebellar disease are muscular incoordination, disturbances in posture and gait, muscular hypotonia, and disordered equilibrium. *Dys-synergy*, typical of cerebellar disease, is defined as a lack of coordinated action of various groups of muscles (agonists, antagonists, synergists, and fixators). Thus, patients are unable to carry out movements in a smooth or harmonious manner; instead the movements are jerky, irregular, and uncoordinated, resembling those of a puppet or robot; a complex act is thus de-

composed and carried out as a series of simpler movements. Impairment of judgment of distance, range, speed, and force of movement is described as *dysmetria*. Hypotonia of muscles and a resultant hypermotility of joints is seen only in acute cerebellar disease. Methods of testing cerebellar function follow.

Finger-to-Nose Test

While sitting, standing, or reclining, the patient is instructed to abduct and extend the arm completely and touch the tip of the index finger to the tip of the nose. It is important that the upper arm is fully abducted and not braced against the chest. Normal individuals should be able to do this maneuver with precision with the eyes open or closed. In cerebellar disease, an intention tremor becomes evident during this test, the tremor becoming coarser as the finger approaches the nose. The patient may overshoot the target but may try to correct it with undue force and speed, indeed overcorrecting the error (dysmetria). The movements are irregular, wavering, and jerky, becoming more so as the target is approached. The degree of ataxia may vary from mild ataxia with mild tremor noticeable only as the target is approached to extreme incoordination with wild flinging motions of the arm.

Nose-Finger-Nose Test

The patient is instructed to touch the tip of the nose with the tip of the index finger and then the tip of the examiner's finger, repetitively, while the examiner moves his or her finger to different positions at random.

Finger-to-Finger Test

The patient is asked to bring the abducted, extended arms through a forward hemicircle to the midline and touch the tips of the index fingers together. This maneuver is done repetitively, with increasing speed each time.

Holmes Rebound Phenomenon

The patient is asked to flex the arm at the elbow against firm resistance, and the resistance is suddenly released. In the normal individual, abrupt flexion of the forearm is checked by contraction of the antagonist, the triceps muscle (check reflex). In a patient with cerebellar disease, however, this check reflex is impaired, such that the arm may strike the patient's face.

Heel-to-Knee Test

This test is performed with the patient recumbent. The patient is asked to place the heel of one foot on the opposite knee and slide it downward over the shin toward the great toe. In cerebellar disease, the heel is carried towards the knee in a wavy or jerky manner, overshoots the knee sideways, and develops a circular oscillatory motion as it approaches it, a movement that resembles an intention tremor in the upper extremity. As the heel moves down the shin, it wobbles from side to side and may uncontrollably drop off the opposite foot without ever touching the big toe.

Figure-of-Eight or Circle Test

While recumbent, the patient is asked to draw either a figure of eight or circle in the air with the great toe. In cerebellar disease, the movements are jerky, coarse, and unsteady and figures are irregular.

Toe-Finger Test

The patient, while recumbent, is asked to touch the examiner's finger with the great toe. The examiner then moves the target finger randomly to varying positions within the range of the patient's leg, and the patient is asked to pursue it with the big toe. This test is analogous to the finger-nose-finger test in the upper extremity.

Dysdiadochokinesis

Dysdiadochokinesis is characterized by the difficulty in performing rapid alternating movements. The ability to abruptly stop one movement and follow it immediately by an exactly opposite movement is impaired. Although this phenomenon may be demonstrated in several ways, the following three methods are most frequently used. While sitting, the patient is asked to (1) pat the knee alternately with the palm and the dorsum of one hand or pat the palm with the palm or dorsum of the other hand; (2) open and close the fists alternately; or (3) rapidly tap the foot against the floor. One should note the rate, rhythm, amplitude, and the smoothness of movement, all of which are affected in cerebellar disease. Patients with spasticity or rigidity will show a decrease in the rate of rapid alternating movements, but they do not exhibit the ataxia seen characteristically in cerebellar disease.

Ocular Dysmetria

Analogous to the dysmetria in the extremities, dysmetria in eye movements may occur. Jerkiness and oscillations, superficially resembling nystagmus, occur during attempts at conjugate gaze fixation. This results from the eyes overshooting or undershooting the target with subsequent oscillations through several cycles until accurate fixation is obtained.

Ataxic Dysarthria

Changes in the clarity, rhythm, and rate of speech characterize cerebellar ataxic dysarthria. In the parlance of speech pathologists, the normal rhythm, variability in loudness and pitch, rate of speech, phrasing, and pauses contribute collectively to the prosody of speech. In patients with cerebellar disease, the grammar and the meaning of the sentences are intact but the melodic elements of the speech are deranged; there is prosodic excess or dysprosody. Common clinical descriptions of dysprosodic speech include speech that is scanning, tremulous, slurred, staccato, explosive, hesitant, slow, or garbled, or has an altered accent. Thus, unnatural separation of words with excessive stress on parts of speech that are normally unstressed (scanning), imprecise enunciation, monotony, and slowness characterize cerebellar dysarthria. The patient speaks as though there is not enough breath to utter certain words or syllables while others are uttered with greater force than necessary (explosive speech).

Syndrome of the Vestibular System

Vestibular disorders may simulate the cerebellar syndrome, but the presence of true vertigo is the hallmark of vestibular disease, and this helps to distinguish it from the cerebellar syndrome. Vertigo is a purely subjective sensation characterized by a disturbance of equilibrium with illusory movement of either the patient or the patient's environs. Frequently the feeling may be described as an up-and-down or to-and-fro movement of the body. The floor or walls may seem to rise up, sink, or tilt. A feeling of impulsion, an uncontrollable sensation of being pulled to the ground or to one side or other, is characteristic of vestibular disease. Nausea and vomiting may accompany vertigo in acute cases. Nystagmus is frequently present; it may be horizontal, vertical, or rotary. The nature and the degree of nystagmus may be affected by posture. It is doubtful whether pure cerebellar lesions can cause nystagmus. Presence of nystagmus in cerebellar disease implies involvement of the vestibulocerebellar pathways rather than the cerebellum itself. Ataxia, especially of the trunk, is often striking in vestibular disease, but true dysmetria or dys-synergy in the extremities is lacking.

Syndrome of the Posterior Column System

Symptoms and signs of the posterior column syndrome result primarily from deprivation of proprioceptive input.

Regardless of the pathological lesion causing the deficit or the location of the lesion along the proprioceptive pathway from the cord to the cortex, the symptoms and signs tend to be similar. A distinguishing characteristic of this syndrome is the worsening of symptoms with eye closure.

Ataxia is the dominant symptom. The patient walks with a broad base and slaps the foot to the ground. He constantly has to watch the feet while walking and the arms while reaching. On finger-to-nose testing, the patient may do reasonably well with the eyes open; but with the eyes closed the finger is unable to find the nose and after groping around the face, the patient ultimately touches the nose with tactile guidance. Similarly on heel-to-knee testing the patient clumsily places the heel on the opposite leg at the approximate position of the knee and thereafter slides it down guided only by tactile input but not by proprioception. Errors in the range of movement of the extremities (dysmetria) are evident during these maneuvers. In cortical lesions, astereognosis and disturbance in two-point discrimination may be present as well.

12
Examination of the Motor and Sensory Systems and Reflexes
Setti S. Rengachary

Motor System

Examination of the motor system, like other aspects of a physical examination, follows a systematic order. Muscle contour and abnormal movements, if any, are carefully inspected; the motor tone and strength are evaluated; and the coordination is tested. Assessment of reflex activity completes the examination.

Motor Atrophy

Muscular development varies with a person's build, occupation, training and conditioning, handedness, age, sex, and state of health. Atrophy or loss of muscle bulk may result from systemic causes, such as malignant disease, endocrinopathy, or malnutrition, and from focal neurological disease. The latter is significant in neurological localization. Focal neurogenic atrophy is typically associated with weakness in the corresponding muscle, whereas in a systemic wasting illness the muscle strength may be disproportionately good.

Focal atrophy is generally seen in disorders of the lower motor neuron (which includes the anterior horn cell, motor root, plexus, and peripheral nerve) or muscle. The distribution of wasting varies with the anatomical location of the lesion. With lesions that affect the spinal cord (anterior horn cells), such as syringomyelia (Fig. 12-1), cord tumor, spondylosis, disc disease, or motor neuron disease, the wasting tends to be segmental in distribution, especially if the pathological lesion is very localized. Fasciculations (see below) are generally associated with anterior horn cell disease. The distribution of wasting with plexus lesions varies greatly with the extent and the level of involvement. In nontraumatic brachial plexopathy, for instance, the wasting primarily involves the shoulder girdle muscles. In peripheral nerve disorders, the wasting is distal in the limb if it is a diffuse disorder (peripheral neuropathy), but in localized lesions of nerves, the atrophy closely follows the distribution of the nerve; in addition, the associated sensory loss when mixed nerves are involved gives additional clues in localization.

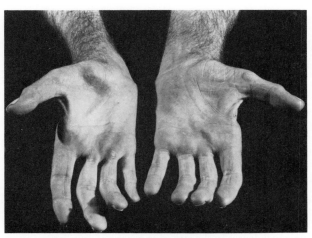

Figure 12-1 Bilateral wasting of the thenar and the hypothenar muscles in a patient with syringomyelia involving the lower cervical spinal cord.

The wasting in myopathies, at least in the initial stages, most generally involves the proximal muscles in the limbs.

Upper motor neuron lesions are not usually associated with atrophy, except from disuse, such as in long-standing hemiplegia from a cerebral lesion. Indeed, hemiatrophy, with poor development of muscles and bones, may occur in infantile hemiplegia. Certain parietal lobe lesions involving the primary sensory cortex may lead to a curious atrophy on the contralateral side; it may or may not be associated with hemiplegia.

Intrinsic Movements in Muscles

Fasciculations

Fasciculations are spontaneous, irregular, randomly distributed twitchings or flickers of contraction of muscle fascicles occurring within a resting muscle. Each fascicle represents a group of a hundred or more muscle fibers supplied by a single motor neuron (the motor unit) (Fig. 12-2). Although fasciculations are observed in diseases affecting any component of the lower motor neuron except the muscle (anterior horn cell, motor root, plexus or peripheral nerve), they appear particularly with involvement of the anterior horn cell, as in amyotrophic lateral sclerosis, spinal cord tumor, herniated cervical disc, spondylosis, or syringomyelia.

Fasciculations are frequently observed in larger muscles such as the pectoralis, deltoid, quadriceps femoris, and gastrocnemius-soleus. They are best seen with oblique lighting. Tapping the muscle or placing the muscle under slight tension intensifies the muscle twitches. Excessive adipose tissue may obscure the fasciculations. Fasciculations tend to disappear with advanced muscle atrophy.

Contraction fasciculations are fasciculations that appear on weak contraction of a muscle but disappear on relaxation. They are observed in otherwise healthy anxious individuals and in some patients with amyotrophic lateral sclerosis.

Fasciculations sometimes observed in individuals without any other evidence of neurological disease are called *benign fasciculations*. This condition may occur as a familial disorder.

Fibrillations

Fibrillations are spontaneous independent contractions of individual muscle fibers occurring after denervation. They are thought to occur from denervation hypersensitivity. The contractions are too minute to be seen through the skin. They can be detected however with electromyography. Fibrillations last for several months, occasionally even years, after denervation.

Myokymia

Myokymia is a benign form of muscle twitching most commonly seen in the orbicularis oculi muscle in highstrung individuals or after fatigue. It consists of rapid rippling movement of contiguous muscle fibers. *Facial myokymia* is discussed elsewhere in the text.

Muscle Tone

Muscle tone is the degree of tension in a muscle at rest. Resistance to passive movement of a fully relaxed extremity is a function of the tone in its muscle. There are several ways

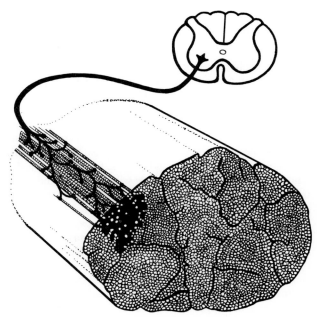

Figure 12-2 Diagrammatic representation of a motor unit. A motor unit consists of a motor neuron supplying a group of a hundred or more muscle fibers (a muscle fascicle). Fasciculation consists of spontaneous random contractions of muscle fascicles from anterior horn cell irritation or degeneration, whereas fibrillation represents independent contraction of individual muscle fibers from denervation hypersensitivity.

to assess the tone of muscles in clinical practice; all require that the patient be as fully relaxed as possible.

The tone in the neck muscles is tested by passively moving the cervical spine through its full range or by the head-dropping test. To elicit the later, the patient lies supine without a pillow, the head is flexed and supported with one hand and allowed to drop unexpectedly on the other hand. In patients with extrapyramidal rigidity the head may drop slowly.

The tone in the distal upper extremity muscles is tested by grasping the forearm and briskly shaking it, allowing passive flexion and extension of the hand at the wrist. The range and speed of the flexion-extension movement are noted. With the patient supine, the patient's arms are briskly raised and then dropped; the rate of fall is determined by the tone in the proximal shoulder muscles. Alternately, with the patient standing, the examiner briskly shakes the patient's shoulders in a forward and backward direction. The speed and range of the to-and-fro swinging motion of the arms are observed.

The tone of the muscles in the lower extremities is appraised by having the patient sit at the edge of the examining table with the legs dangling freely. The leg is lifted and suddenly released. Or, the leg may be pushed back to initiate the swing. With hypotonus, there is a prolonged pendular motion of the limb, whereas with hypertonus the swing amplitude is decreased. As an alternative method, with the patient in the recumbent position, the examiner lifts the patient's leg and then, supporting the back of the knee, releases the leg. The rate of fall of the leg is a function of tone in its muscles.

Spasticity

Spasticity is a state of increased tonus in the muscles resulting from hyperactivity of stretch reflexes. The increase in tonus is not generally uniformly distributed, but involves opposing groups of muscles to differing degrees. As a rule, the increase in tonus is most marked in the flexor muscles of the arms and the extensor (antigravity) muscles of the legs, resulting in a characteristic posture seen in a hemiplegic individual: the arm is held adducted against the chest with flexion at the elbow, wrist, and fingers, while the leg is extended at the hip, knee, and ankle with inversion and plantar flexion of the foot. There is an increase in resistance to a rapidly performed passive movement, followed by a sudden release, referred to as *clasp-knife phenomenon*, best demonstrated at the elbow and knee. The dual phases in this phenomenon are thought to be mediated by two types of stretch receptors, the muscle spindles in the resistive phase and the Golgi tendon organs in the abrupt-release phase.

Spasticity is seen in lesions that abolish the inhibitory influence of the upper motor neuron on the anterior horn cell. It should be emphasized that the term *upper motor neuron* includes the pyramidal (corticospinal) and the extrapyramidal (corticostriate, corticothalamic, corticopontine, and corticoreticular) systems. Thus, in certain rare discrete lesions that affect the corticospinal system selectively (such as a focal lesion in the motor cortex or a lesion in the pyramid of the medulla), flaccidity rather than spasticity may result. Also, in the acute phases of upper motor neuron impairment, such as after a cerebrovascular accident or traumatic

transverse lesion of the spinal cord, there is a temporary reduction in the tonus of the affected muscles (shock reaction) lasting for a few days to a few weeks. This phase is followed by spasticity in the muscles. In certain clinical conditions, such as in some cases of spondylotic myelopathy, one finds an imperfect correlation between the degree of spasticity and the degree of motor weakness; there may be an extreme degree of spasticity, yet testing for muscle power may show surprisingly good strength. This may imply that voluntary motion and spasticity are mediated through separate neural networks.

Rigidity

Rigidity results from diseases of the extrapyramidal system, especially the basal ganglia. The tonus is increased to an equal degree in the opposing groups of muscles, resulting in a uniform resistance to passive movement, from the beginning to the end of the movement. After being moved, the limb may retain its new position, offering equal resistance to fall back to the starting position. Uniform resistance to passive motion has been likened to the sensation of bending a lead pipe, and hence the term *lead-pipe rigidity*. The resistance during passive motion, unlike in spasticity, does not seem to vary the speed of motion or its direction. There is no associated paresis, or alteration of muscle stretch reflexes, unless the corticospinal tract is also affected in the disease process. In some instances, a rhythmic give in the resistance is felt, presumably due to the underlying tremor, and hence the term *cog wheel rigidity*.

Gegenhalten

In frontal lobe disease, the patient may be unable to relax a group of muscles on command; indeed, the muscles stiffen increasingly with attempts at passive motion. This phenomenon is called *gegenhalten*.

Hypotonia (Flaccidity)

Hypotonia or flaccidity typically results from lesions that affect the spinal reflex arc. The lesion may interrupt the afferent component such as the posterior root or the efferent component such as the anterior horn cell, anterior root, plexus, peripheral nerve, myoneural junction, or muscle. The muscle stretch reflex is decreased. There is muscular weakness and wasting. Muscle tone may also be decreased in cerebellar diseases and in chorea.

Muscle Strength

The systematic testing (and grading) of muscle strength is perhaps the most rewarding element in neurological localization. One should first ascertain whether the patient is able to move a body part voluntarily. With advanced weakness, movement against gravity may not be possible, but with gravity eliminated, movement may still be possible through the full range of the joint. With lesser degrees of weakness, movement against resistance should be tested. This may be done in one of two ways: in testing the flexion at the elbow, the patient first completely flexes the elbow, and tries to keep the muscle maximally contracted while the examiner tries to overcome it; or the examiner applies resistance throughout the flexion movement. The latter method tends to detect earlier degrees of weakness.

The standardized grading of muscle strength (Table 12-1) is desirable for comparing the results of neurological evaluation by various examiners, for assessing the course of a neurological illness involving motor weakness, and for assessing the effects of therapy. The methods of testing individual muscles are illustrated in Figs. 12-3 to 12-6, and the clinical localization of motor lesions is summarized in Table 12-2.

From time to time the clinician encounters a patient with hysterical or feigned weakness. Among many methods of clinical evaluation, motor examination often offers the most clues in diagnosing a hysteric. When the hysteric is asked to perform a specific motion, the movement is seen to be slow,

TABLE 12-1 Grading of Muscle Strength

Grade 0:	No voluntary muscle contraction
Grade 1:	Flicker or trace of muscle contraction; no joint motion
Grade 2:	Active movement, but only with gravity eliminated
Grade 3:	Active movement against gravity but not against resistance
Grade 4−:	Active movement against minimal resistance
Grade 4:	Active movement against moderate resistance
Grade 4+:	Active movement against strong resistance
Grade 5:	Normal strength

jerky, and tremulous because of the simultaneous contraction of agonists and antagonists. The muscle contractions are brief and poorly sustained. At times the patient may

TABLE 12-2 Clinical Localization of Motor Lesions

Clinical Syndrome	Clinical Characteristics
	Upper Motor Neuron
Pyramidal (corticospinal) syndrome	Paralysis involves the opposite arm, leg, and side of the face, but the distribution of paralysis varies with the site of interruption of the corticospinal tract. Unilateral lesions in the cerebral hemisphere produce hemiplegia; if only a part of the corticospinal pathway is affected, monoplegia (e.g., faciobrachial monoplegia) may result. Bilateral lesions in the brain produce diplegia (e.g., infantile diplegia). Quadriplegia or paraplegia results from bilateral pyramidal lesions in the brain stem or spinal cord. Occasionally bilateral supratentorial lesions (e.g., parasagittal meningioma) may give rise to paraplegia.
	In pyramidal tract lesions, muscles are affected in groups, never as individual muscles. A clasp-knife type of spasticity is present, more marked in the flexor muscle groups of the upper limb and extensor muscle groups of the lower limb. Distal muscles and finer movements are involved to a greater extent than proximal muscles and coarser movements. Muscle stretch reflexes are increased on the paralyzed side, and clonus may be elicited. Cutaneous reflexes, notably the abdominal and cremasteric reflexes, are lost on the side of paralysis in hemiplegics and bilaterally in paraplegics. Pathological reflexes such as the Babinski response may be elicited. Muscular fasciculation and fibrillations are absent. Nerve conduction velocities are normal, and no denervation potentials are recorded in the electromyogram.
Extrapyramidal syndromes: Akinetic or bradykinetic syndromes	Parkinson's disease epitomizes this syndrome. The muscle strength is unaffected, but there is slowness of volitional movements. Muscle tonus is equally increased in agonists and antagonists, resulting in "lead-pipe" rigidity. Resistance to passive movement is present throughout the range of motion. Masklike facies and infrequent blinking are indicative of the poverty of movements seen throughout. Resting tremor is present. Gait is slow and shuffling.
Hyperkinetic syndromes Choreiform syndrome	Chorea appears in typical form in Huntington's disease (a chronic, progressive hereditary disease due to degeneration of the striatum), Sydenham's chorea (rheumatic chorea), and chorea gravidarum. It may be unilateral (hemichorea or hemiballismus). This movement disorder is characterized by arrhythmic, forcible, jerky, irregular, rapid, random, purposeless motions. Facial grimacing is common.
Athetoid syndrome	Athetoid movements are irregular, slow, purposeless, and sinuous, and are most pronounced in the digits, hands, face, tongue, and pharynx.
Dystonic syndrome	Dystonia musculorum deformans or torsion spasm best exemplifies the dystonic syndrome. The dystonic movements affect the trunk and girdle. They are slow, agonizing, writhing, and virtually reptilian. Facial grimacing is a common accompaniment.
	Lower Motor Neuron
Anterior horn cell syndrome	This is typically seen in amyotrophic lateral sclerosis (ALS), syringomyelia, and poliomyelitis. Paralysis is flaccid in type and segmental in distribution. Atrophy is invariably present. Fasciculation is a hallmark of the anterior horn cell syndrome. Muscle stretch reflexes are diminished or absent as a result of interruption of the reflex arc. Sensory disturbances are conspicuously absent unless the sensory tracts in the spinal cord are involved as well. Denervation potentials are demonstrated by electromyographic testing. Muscle biopsy shows neurogenic atrophy.

TABLE 12-2   Clinical Localization of Motor Lesions (*continued*)

Clinical Syndrome	Clinical Characteristics
Anterior root syndrome	Disc disease, spondylosis, intradural extramedullary tumors (neurilemmomas and meningiomas) are common causative lesions. All the clinical features are similar to those of the anterior horn cell syndrome except for certain subtle differences: (1) The posterior root is involved concurrently, resulting in "root" pain (radiating pain around the trunk or down a limb along a dermatome). (2) There may be sensory loss in a dermatomal distribution for the same reason. (3) Root lesions of neurosurgical significance tend to be localized, affecting only one or two roots.
Plexus syndromes: Brachial plexus syndrome	Common etiologic factors that lead to brachial plexus paralysis are birth injury in the neonate, traction injury in the adult, penetrating wounds, primary neoplasms (neurofibrosarcoma), metastatic tumors of the lung with contiguous spread (Pancoast tumor), and idiopathic brachial plexopathy. The upper brachial plexus (Erb-Duchenne), the lower brachial plexus (Kumpke), or the entire brachial plexus may be involved. When the T1 root leading to the brachial plexus is avulsed, Horner's syndrome may result. Avulsion of the root in close proximity to the spinal cord is confirmed by the presence of arachnoid diverticula on myelography. Upper plexus lesions of the Erb-Duchenne type involve the C5-6 roots of the upper trunk. The resulting deformity is characterized by adduction and medial rotation of the shoulder, extension at the elbow, pronation, flexion at the wrist, and extension of the fingers ("policeman tip" position; see figure). A lower plexus lesion of the Klumpke type is caused by injury to the C8-T1 roots of the lower trunk. The patient has an ipsilateral Horner's syndrome and weakness and atrophy of the intrinsic muscles of the hand, with a claw hand deformity. There may be a sensory deficit in the medial two fingers, hand, and forearm. A complete plexus lesion, caused by interruption of all roots to the plexus, leaves a flail arm with absent motor power, sensation, and reflexes.

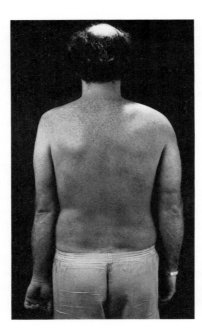

Brachial plexus injury of the Erb-Duchenne type. Note atrophy of the left deltoid and spinati muscles.

Lumbosacral plexus syndrome	Involvement of the lumbosacral plexus most commonly occurs with pelvic fractures and infiltrating retroperitoneal tumors. Variable paralysis and sensory loss involving the pelvic girdle and the leg result.
Peripheral nerve syndrome	Peripheral nerve disorders of neurosurgical interest include acute nerve injuries, chronic entrapment syndromes, and primary neoplasms of the nerve. These are discussed in detail in respective chapters elsewhere in the text. Since most peripheral nerves are mixed nerves, in addition to motor paralysis and atrophy, sensory loss occurs in a characteristic peripheral nerve distribution.
Myoneural junction and primary muscle diseases	These disorders are outside the domain of clinical neurosurgery.

produce a motion opposite to what is asked for because of contraction of antagonists. The strength of voluntary movement is proportional to the resistance offered by the examiner; thus the extent of weakness may vary from total paralysis to near normal strength depending upon the resistance offered. The motor performance tends to improve with coaxing. With much coaxing, a strong contraction is produced momentarily followed by sudden relaxation ("give-away weakness"), or, when the resistance is suddenly withdrawn by the examiner, there is no "follow-through" or rebound. When unaware of being watched, the patient will perform motor acts that are inconsistent with the claimed weakness. Motor tone and muscle stretch reflexes remain unaltered. Hysterics with "paraplegia" may not have sphincter disturbance.

Hoover's sign is helpful in differentiating hysterical weakness of a leg from organic paralysis. To elicit this sign, the examiner places his or her hands under the heels of the recumbent patient. With true weakness of a leg, when the patient attempts to lift the paralyzed leg, increased downward pressure from the sound leg is felt by the examiner (Hoover's sign). In the hysterical patient the downward pressure of the normal leg will be absent.

Abnormal Movements

Tremor

Tremor may be defined as an involuntary, rhythmic, nonpurposeful to-and-fro oscillatory motion about a joint or joints. The distal parts of the limbs are usually affected, although the head, tongue, or jaw may participate.

Parkinsonian (resting or static) tremor is a coarse alternating tremor that averages 3 to 7 cps (cycles per second) and is of moderate to large amplitude. It particularly affects the distal segments of the extremities. The tremor is characteristically present in the resting position and momentarily decreases or stops with volitional movement, only to resume after the limb assumes a new position or rests again. Alternate flexion-extension at the metacarpophalangeal joint of the index finger with synchronous adduction-abduction of the thumb results in a typical pill-rolling movement. The tremor may also involve the feet, jaw, lips, or tongue. In Wilson's disease (hepatolenticular degeneration) a similar resting tremor may be encountered. However, when the arms are held extended, the tremor becomes greatly exaggerated, resembling wing-beating motions of birds, and hence the term *wing-beating tremor*.

Intention (kinetic, ataxic, or cerebellar) tremor is absent at rest but becomes evident on initiation of voluntary movement. It increases in amplitude in a crescendo manner as the target is reached (Fig. 12-7). This tremor is best elicited with the finger-to-nose test; in mild cases it appears as a few oscillations as the nose is approached, but in advanced instances, the amplitude of the tremor may exceed 12 in. Cerebellar tremor is typically seen in lesions involving the dentate nucleus or the superior cerebellar peduncle. Common clinical examples are cerebellar hemispheric tumors and multiple sclerosis.

Rubral tremor is a slow coarse tremor present at rest and accentuated during volitional movements. The tremor is present only on one side, contralateral to the involved red nucleus. The tremor is not sufficiently unique in itself to lend a diagnosis, but often an impression of rubral tremor is surmised if there are other associated signs of involvement of the midbrain tegmentum. Some have questioned the justification of classifying rubral tremor as a separate entity.

Postural (tension) tremor is absent at rest and appears only when the arms are held outstretched in a sustained posture against gravity. In contrast to the parkinsonian tremor, which is caused by alternate contractions of agonist and antagonist muscles, postural tremor results from simultaneous but unequal contractions of the opposing group of muscles. Postural tremor is best exemplified by certain toxic-metabolic conditions. Thus, fine tremors (best brought out by balancing a piece of paper on the patient's fingers) of the extended fingers and hands are seen (1) in thyrotoxicosis, (2) in certain physiological conditions such as fatigue, anxiety, and nervousness among normal individuals (physiological tremor), (3) after the administration of epinephrine, ephedrine, amphetamine, cocaine, or morphine, (4) during periods of alcohol withdrawal in a chronic alcoholic, and (5) in lithium toxicity.

Familial tremor is generally absent at rest but becomes manifest as a coarse tremor of the outstretched fingers and is exaggerated during volitional movements. It is inherited as an autosomal dominant trait, and the tremor may make its appearance as early as adolescence. In sporadic cases, where there is no family history, the term *benign essential tremor* is used. When the onset is delayed until late in life, the term *senile tremor* is appropriate. Men are affected more often than women. The upper extremities are predominantly affected, although in later stages titubation of the head appears and the voice becomes quavering. Even in the advanced cases, the muscle tone remains normal and there is no other neurological abnormality. The tremors of the hands may cause considerable disability and embarrassment as a result of spillage of food or drink. Skilled manual vocation becomes impossible. The tremors are temporarily suppressed by the ingestion of alcohol. Therapy by a beta-adrenergic blocking agent such as propanolol may be beneficial.

Asterexis

In certain toxic-metabolic states such as impending hepatic failure, uremia, or phenytoin intoxication, a coarse wrist flapping appears that may be mistakenly called a tremor. On close scrutiny, instead of an alternate contraction of the flexors and the extensors of the wrist, the wrist flap actually results from intermittent sudden relaxation of the wrist extensors. The flap occurs at irregular intervals and lacks the rhythmicity of a true tremor. The term *asterexis* (inability to maintain a fixed posture) is more appropriate for this movement disorder.

Chorea

Choreic movements are quick, forcible, jerky, arrhythmic, asymmetric, nonpurposeful, and unsustained. Grotesque grimacing with jerking up and down of one or both

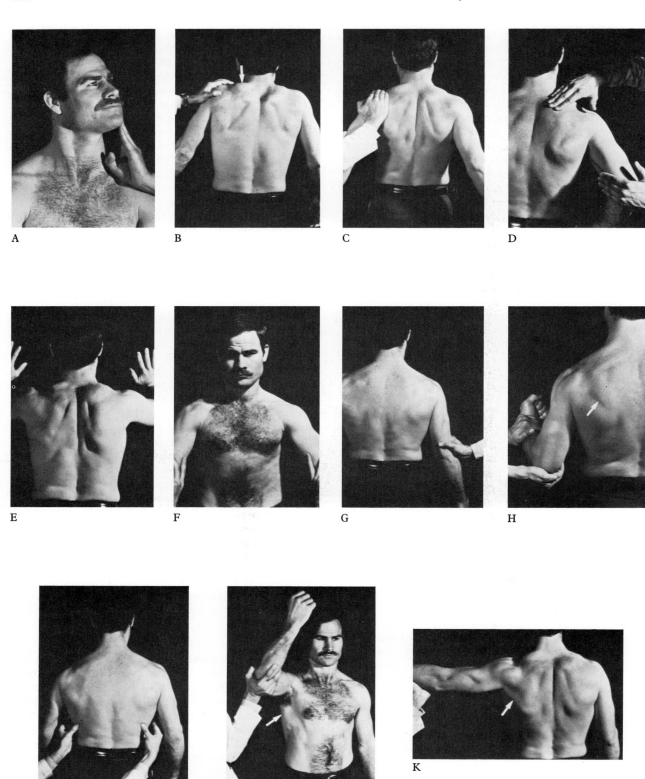

A   B   C   D

E   F   G   H

I   J   K

eyebrows, twitching of the corners of the mouth, rapid protrusion and retraction of the tongue, puckering of the mouth, and movement of the chin forward or sideways is seen typically in advanced cases of Sydenham's or Hunting-ton's chorea. Respirations are irregular and peculiar respiratory sounds may be made. Speech may be slurred. Chewing and swallowing may be difficult. The trunk and extremities appear to undergo constantly changing movements at irregular intervals. Sustained maintenance of a given position becomes impossible. This phenomenon may be clinically demonstrated in various ways: inability to keep the tongue protruded; inability to maintain the outstretched arms above the head; and inability to sustain a firm grip on the examiner's fingers ("milk-maid's grip"). The muscles are hypotonic and the knee jerks tend to be pendular. In the milder or early forms of this movement disorder, the patient may simply appear restless and fidgety, and the diagnosis may be missed.

Hemiballismus (hemichorea)

Violent choreic movements limited to one side of the body are seen in elderly individuals with a vascular lesion (ischemic infarct or hemorrhage) in the opposite subthalamic nucleus of Luys. Wild, rapid flinging movements of large amplitude and wide radius, generally involving the proximal joints of the limb, are seen. The movements are forcible and flail-like. The constant involuntary motion may lead to exhaustion and even precipitate congestive heart failure in some individuals. The movements are absent during deep sleep. The movement disorder runs a self-limited course. Tranquilizing drugs may be of benefit, but stereotactic lesions may need to be made in resistant cases.

Figure 12-3 Individual muscle testing: *A.* Sternocleidomastoid (spinal accessory nerve and C3,4). The patient turns his head forcibly against the examiner's hand away from the muscle being tested. The contraction of the muscle is observed. *B.* Trapezius, upper fibers (spinal accessory nerve and C3,4). The patient shrugs his shoulders upward against resistance. The arrow points to the upper part of the muscle. *C.* Trapezius, middle fibers (spinal accessory nerve and C3,4). The patient braces his shoulder backward against resistance. *D.* Rhomboids (dorsal scapular nerve; C5). With hand on hip, the patient tries to force the elbow backward against resistance while the examiner palpates the muscle belly. *E.* Serratus anterior (long thoracic nerve; C5,6,7). The patient pushes outstretched arms forward against a wall. *F.* Pectoralis major (lateral and medial pectoral nerves; C5,6,7,8). The patient adducts his arms against resistance. *G.* Supraspinatus (suprascapular nerve; C5). The patient initiates abduction against resistance. *H.* Infraspinatus (suprascapular nerve; C5). The patient rotates the upper arm at the shoulder against resistance, with the elbow flexed. The arrow points to the infraspinatus muscle. *I.* Latissimus dorsi (thoracodorsal nerve; C7). The muscle bellies are palpated as the patient coughs. *J.* Latissimus dorsi (thoracodorsal nerve; C7). Alternative method: The patient's arm is placed in abduction to the horizontal position; then adduction and backward movement are made against resistance applied to the elbow. The arrow points to the muscle belly. *K.* Teres major (subscapular nerve; C6). The patient adducts his horizontally elevated arm against resistance. The arrow points to the muscle.

Athetosis

In contrast to chorea, athetoid movements are slower, more continuous, and sustained. They may involve the head, neck, limb, girdles, and especially the distal portions of the extremities. Facial grimacing, if present, is slower and more sustained. In the distal extremities, there may be hyperextension of the fingers associated with writhing, twisting, and turning movements of the limbs. There is usually increased tone in the muscles with spasticity and some weakness due to associated involvement of the corticospinal tract. Voluntary movements are impaired, and graceful coordinated movements may be impossible. Although acquired athetosis may follow disease or trauma in adult life, most commonly athetosis results from an insult to the basal ganglia, such as anoxic encephalopathy, kernicterus, or encephalitis, in the neonatal period or infancy.

Pseudoathetosis denotes the athetoid movements seen in patients with profound proprioceptive sensory loss. Athetoid movements are increased with closure of the eyes, and there may be marked hypotonia.

Dystonia

Dystonic movements resemble athetoid movements to a large extent, but the former involves larger portions of the body, especially the truncal muscles and the proximal muscles in the extremities. The movements are slow, writhing, and twisting, resembling reptilian movement. Arching of the back and neck and extreme torsion of neck and arms into grotesque positions occur. Such distorted postures may be held tonically for a few seconds before a random change to a new position occurs. The muscle tone is markedly increased. In the end stages, muscle contractures occur.

Dystonia musculorum deformans, an uncommon heredofamilial disease starting in childhood, exemplifies dystonic movements the best. Dystonic movements may also be seen on long-term administration of phenothiazines. Spasmodic torticollis is thought to represent a focal form of dystonia.

Myoclonus

Myoclonus is a brief, abrupt, jerky, asynergic shocklike contraction involving part of a muscle or more generally a whole muscle or groups of muscles regardless of their functional association. The extent of muscle contraction in a myoclonic jerk may vary from a contraction ineffective in moving a joint to one so widespread as to throw the patient to the floor. Myoclonic jerks may occur paroxysmally at a slow or rapid rate at irregular intervals and may involve the face, trunk, or extremities. In certain clinical syndromes, myoclonic jerks may be provoked by extraneous stimuli (stimulus-sensitive myoclonus) such as a flickering light, loud sounds (as in Tay-Sachs disease), or an abrupt tactile stimulus. A myoclonic jerk represents a symptom and has no localizing value in itself. It may be seen in diseases that affect widely differing parts of the neuraxis such as the cerebral cortex, thalamus, substantia nigra, basal ganglia, dentate nucleus, brain stem, or spinal cord. Myoclonus may be associated with certain types of epilepsy (idiopathic epi-

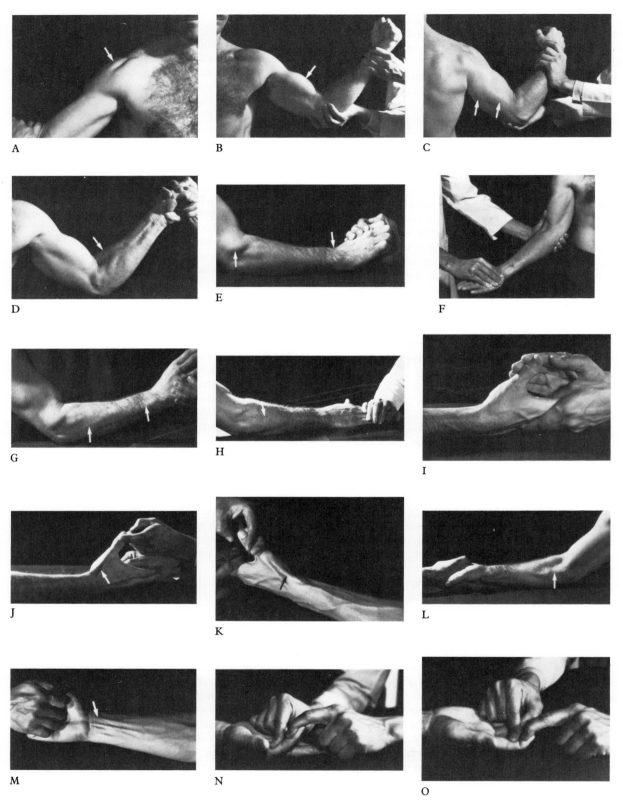

lepsy, salaam or jackknife seizures of infancy, familial myo-clonus epilepsy of Unverricht and Lundborg) or dementing illnesses (Creutzfeldt-Jakob disease, subacute sclerosing panencephalitis, progressive poliodystrophy, and advanced Alzheimer's disease). Intention or action myoclonus (Lance-Adams syndrome) is characterized by a myoclonic jerk pre-cipitated by discrete volitional movement. It may be seen as a late sequel of anoxic encephalopathy. Myoclonic move-ments that occur as one is about to fall asleep are considered physiological.

Palatal myoclonus (which is a rhythmic tremor affecting the palate, rather than a myoclonus) is a well-defined syndrome that results from hypertrophic degeneration of the inferior olive. The primary pathological process is in the central tegmental fasciculus or contralateral dentate nucleus. Muscles of a branchial origin (namely those of the soft palate and, less commonly, the pharynx, face, tongue, and vocal cords) and the diaphragm may be involved. Rhythmic movement of the uvula and other affected muscles at a rate of 50 to 240 per minute may be seen. The movements persist during sleep. The intrinsic rhythmicity of the movement is comparable to respiratory activity, which is of brain stem origin.

Figure 12-4 Individual muscle testing: *A.* Deltoid (circumflex or axillary nerve; C5). The patient abducts his elevated arm against resistance. The arrow points to the muscle belly. *B.* Biceps (musculocutaneous nerve; C5,6). The patient flexes his supinated forearm against resistance. The arrow points to the muscle belly. *C.* Triceps (radial nerve; C7). The patient extends the forearm at the elbow against resistance. Arrows point to the long and lateral heads of the triceps muscle. *D.* Brachioradialis (radial nerve; C6). The patient flexes his forearm against resistance with the forearm midway between pronation and supination. The arrow points to the muscle belly. *E.* Extensor carpi radialis longus (radial nerve; C6,7). The forearm is in nearly complete pronation. The patient extends and abducts the wrist against resistance. Arrows point to the muscle belly and its tendon. *F.* Supinator (posterior interosseous nerve; C6,7). The patient supinates the forearm against resistance with the forearm extended at the elbow. *G.* Extensor carpi ulnaris (posterior interosseous nerve; C7). With the forearm in complete pronation, the patient dorsiflexes and adducts the wrist against resistance. Arrows point to the muscle belly and its tendon. *H.* Extensor digitorum (posterior interosseous nerve; C7). With the forearm in pronation and the wrist stabilized in the straight position, the patient extends the fingers at the metacarpophalangeal joints against resistance applied to the proximal phalanges. The arrow points to the muscle belly. *I.* Abductor pollicis longus (posterior interosseus nerve; C7,8). The patient abducts the thumb at the carpometacarpal joint in a plane at right angles to the palm. *J.* Extensor pollicis longus (posterior interosseous nerve; C7). The patient extends the thumb at the interphalangeal joint against resistance. The arrow points to the tendon. *K.* Extensor pollicis brevis (posterior interosseous nerve; C7,8). The patient extends the thumb at the metacarpophalangeal joint against resistance; the distal phalanx is in flexion to minimize the action of the extensor pollicis longus. An arrow points to the tendon. *L.* Pronator teres: (median nerve; C6,7). The patient pronates the forearm against resistance. The arrow points to the muscle. *M.* Flexor carpi radialis (median nerve; C6,7). The patient is flexing and abducting the hand against resistance; the arrow points to the tendon. *N.* Flexor digitorum sublimis (median nerve; C8). The patient flexes at the proximal interphalangeal joint against resistance with the proximal phalanx stabilized by the examiner. *O.* Flexor digitorum profundus I and II (median nerve and its anterior interosseus branch; C8,T1). The patient flexes the distal phalanx stabilized by the examiner.

The Sensory Examination

Testing of sensory function is perhaps the most difficult and the least objective component of the neurological evaluation. To be reliable, it requires an alert, cooperative, intelligent patient who should remain objective and not be amenable to suggestions. Such an ideal is rarely met in clinical practice, yet it is possible to make some meaningful conclusions in most patients, indeed even in some who are comatose. The degree of reliability of test results varies depending upon the said conditions, and this should be so recorded in the chart. Detailed and systematic testing of all modalities of sensations in all patients from head to foot may convince a novice of his or her thoroughness, but seasoned neurologists tailor the testing to the clinical circumstance, keeping the patient's history and complaints constantly in mind. Explaining to the patient briefly the objective and nature of the test just before each test improves the reliability of test results and expedites the procedure.

It is customary to classify sensations into three major categories:

1. *Exteroceptive (superficial) sensations* are those that originate in the sensory receptors in the skin and mucous membrane in response to an environmental stimulus. Examples are pain, light touch, heat, and cold.
2. *Proprioceptive (deep) sensations* are those that arise from the deeper tissues of the body, namely, joints, ligaments, tendons, and muscles. Examples are sense of position, passive movement, vibration, and deep pain.
3. *Cortical sensations* are those that require integrative cerebral function for their recognition. Examples are stereognosis, graphesthesia, and two-point discrimination.

Testing of Exteroceptive (Superficial) Sensations

Light Touch

Tactile sensation is tested with a wisp of cotton, paper tissue, or a camel's hair brush. The patient is asked to close the eyes and is requested to say "yes" whenever the stimulus is felt and to indicate the area stimulated. A systematic "no" response after each stimulus exposes a malingerer. The areas stimulated are varied at random and are compared with the opposite half of the body. The stimulus applied should be quite light. Heavily cornified areas of the skin such as the palms and soles may require a heavier stimulus. Hairy skin requires a lighter stimulus than glabrous skin since the hair roots are rich in cutaneous nerve endings.

Superficial Pain Sensation

The superficial pain sensation is tested with a safety pin. To ensure a uniform stimulus, the pin is held lightly between the fingers. This allows the pin to slide if too much of

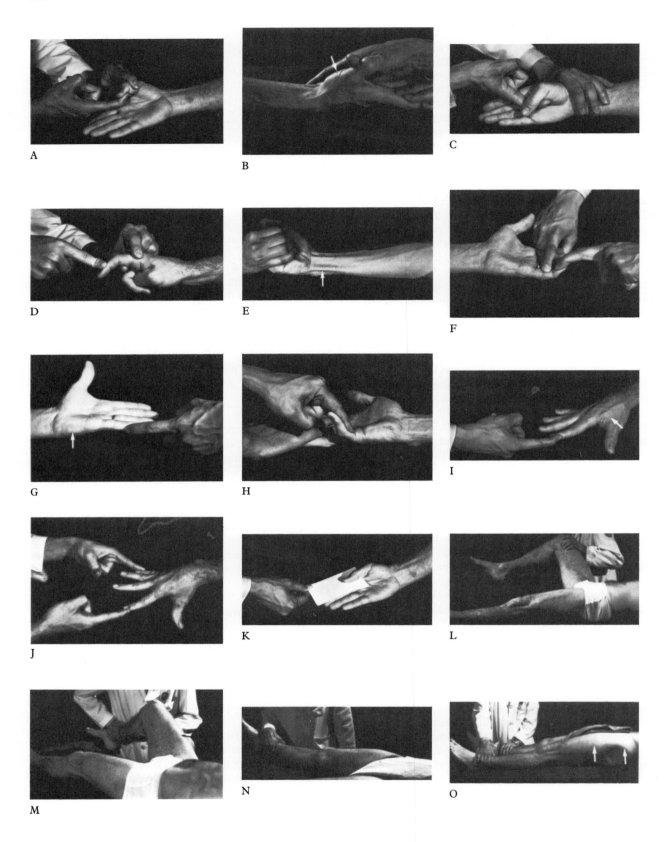

A

B

C

D

E

F

G

H

I

J

K

L

M

N

O

a pressure is applied on the pin. The patient is instructed to close his eyes and indicate what he feels. The accuracy of the patient's response may be grossly tested by alternately using the sharp and dull ends of the pin. The patient should be

urged to give the answers "sharp" or "dull" as quickly as the sensations are perceived. The patient should also be asked to indicate relative differences in pain perception in different areas of the skin. Painful stimuli should not be applied in too rapid a sequence lest they summate and produce an erroneous response; also, if there is a conduction delay, the patient's response may refer to the previous stimulation. It is well to remember that sensory threshold to pinprick (as is true for other primary sensations) varies in different areas of the body.

Various areas of the skin should be examined systematically, preferably following a sequential dermatomal pattern. The two halves of the body are compared for any differences. If an area of impaired sensation is found, an attempt is made to define this area by first proceeding from the analgesic zone to the normal area. The test is repeated by proceeding in the reverse direction. In complete destructive lesions of the nervous system, the zones of sensory loss will tend to be sharply defined, whereas in incomplete lesions, the transition zones tend to be broad.

Figure 12-5 Individual muscle testing: *A.* Flexor pollicis longus (anterior interosseous nerve: C8,T1). The patient flexes the distal phalanx of the thumb against resistance with the proximal phalanx stabilized by the examiner. *B.* Abductor pollicis brevis (median nerve; C8,T1). The patient abducts the thumb against resistance. The arrow points to the muscle belly. *C.* Opponens pollicis (median nerve; C8,T1). The patient touches the base of the little finger with his thumb against resistance. *D.* First lumbrical, interosseous muscles (median and ulnar nerves; C8,T1). The patient extends the finger at the proximal interphalangeal joint against resistance, with the metacarpophalangeal joint hyperextended and stabilized by the examiner. *E.* Flexor carpi ulnaris (ulnar nerve; C8,T1). The patient flexes and adducts the hand at the wrist against resistance. The arrow points to the tendon. *F.* Flexor digitorum profundus III and IV (ulnar nerve; C8, T1). The patient flexes the distal phalanx of the little finger against resistance with the middle phalanx stabilized by the examiner. *G.* Abductor digiti minimi (ulnar nerve; T1). The patient abducts the little finger against resistance. *H.* Flexor digiti minimi (ulnar nerve; T1). The patient flexes the little finger at the metacarpophalangeal joint against resistance with the interphalangeal joints held extended. *I.* First dorsal interosseous muscle (ulnar nerve; T1). The patient abducts the index finger against resistance. *J.* Interossei (ulnar nerve; T1). The patient abducts the fingers against resistance with the fingers extended. *K.* Adductor pollicis (ulnar nerve; T1). The patient attempts to hold a card between the thumb and index finger while the examiner pulls on the card. *L.* Iliopsoas (lumbar plexus and femoral nerve; L1,2,3). The patient flexes the thigh at the hip against resistance. *M.* Quadriceps femoris (femoral nerve; L3,4). The patient extends the leg at the knee against resistance. *N.* Adductors (adductor magnus, adductor longus, and adductor brevis) of the thigh (obturator nerve; L2,3). The patient adducts the thigh against resistance. *O.* Abductors (gluteus medius, gluteus minimus, tensor fascia lata) of the thigh (superior gluteal nerve; L4,5). The patient abducts the thigh against resistance. The arrows point to the muscle bellies of gluteus medius and tensor fascia lata.

Temperature

Temperature sensation is tested by using two large test tubes, one containing ice-cold water and the other hot water (45°C). The patient closes the eyes and identifies the warm or cold sensation as the test tubes are applied in random sequence to the skin surface on different parts of the body. Extreme degrees of hot and cold stimuli should not be used since they induce a pain response. Inability to differentiate warm and cold sensation, with no loss of touch sensation, is seen in patients with syringomyelia (dissociated anesthesia).

Testing of Proprioceptive (Deep) Sensations

The sense of position is a conscious awareness of the position of the body or its parts in space. The sense of motion is awareness of active or passive motion about a joint. These two sensations are closely inter-related; both modalities are usually tested together.

Sense of Passive Movement

The patient's finger or the big toe is grasped firmly on each side and is carried through a wide range of movement; the patient is instructed which movement is to be called "up" and which "down." With the patient's eyes now closed, the test is repeated carrying the digit through progressively smaller excursions. The movements should be slow, deliberate, and precise. Care should be taken to avoid touching the adjacent digits. If the sense of passive movement is impaired in the digits, the same may be carried out at the proximal joints (the wrist, elbow, and knee).

Position Sense

The position sense may be tested in one of different ways (all tests are done with the eyes closed):

1. The patient may be asked to extend the arms forward. With a loss of position sense, the arm tends to drift (Fig. 12-8) and the fingers move constantly ("piano-playing" movements).
2. The patient may be asked to touch the tip of the index finger of one hand with that of the other.
3. The patient may be asked to touch the tip of the nose with the tip of the index finger.

Sense of Vibration

Vibration sense is tested with a tuning fork of 128 Hz. The tuning fork is struck and applied firmly to the skin over bony prominences of digits, ankles, knees, anterior superior iliac spine, ribs, sternum, clavicles, wrists, and elbows and the spinous processes of vertebrae, starting peripherally in the extremities and moving toward the trunk. The patient is asked if the vibration is felt and to report immediately when it ceases. (The patient should be clearly instructed at the outset that what should be observed is the vibration and not just pressure from the tuning fork or the humming sound.) If the vibratory sense is impaired, the examiner may still feel the vibration, after the patient has failed to appreciate it.

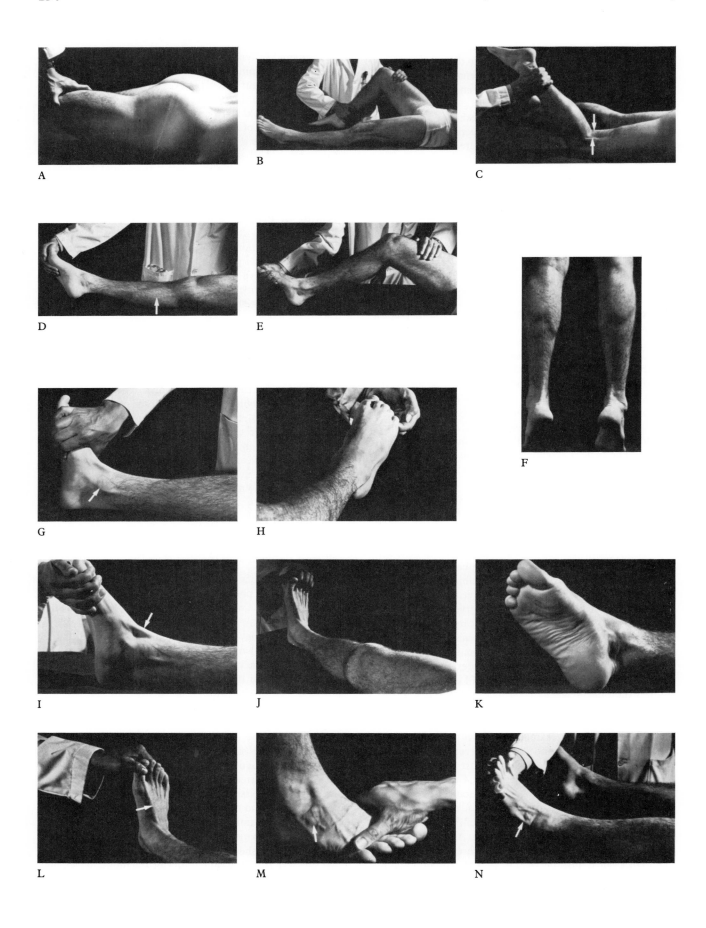

During the examination it is wise to randomly stop the vibrations from time to time by grasping the prongs of the tuning fork and observe the patient's response to the stimulus. This constitutes a good control.

Vibratory sensation is thought to be a composite sensation consisting of light touch and rapidly alternating deep pressure sense. Although it is traditionally taught that this sensation is conducted through the dorsal columns of the spinal cord, some have suggested that it may be conducted in part through the lateral column as well. This explains the occasional dissociation one finds between the loss of position and vibration sense in some patients with spinal lesions. Vibratory sensation is perceived at the thalamic level, but the position sense requires the functioning of the parietal sensory cortex; thus lesions involving thalamocortical connections or the sensory cortex itself may affect the position sense more than the vibratory sense.

Loss of vibration sense in the ankles with graded preservation at the knees and the anterior superior iliac spines suggests polyneuropathy. In spinal lesions, impairment of vibratory sensation extends to more proximal levels. Indeed in

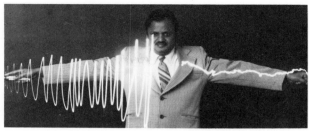

Figure 12-7 Contrast between cerebellar tremor (right arm) and parkinsonian tremor (left arm) in executing the finger-to-nose test. The cerebellar tremor is absent at rest but increases in amplitude in a crescendo manner as the target is reached. The parkinsonian tremor is present at rest but virtually disappears during volitional movement.

spinal lesions one may be able to detect a level of sensory impairment by testing vibration sense over successive spinous processes.

Figure 12-6 Individual muscle testing: *A.* Gluteus maximus (inferior gluteal nerve; L5,S1). The patient extends the thigh against resistance. *B.* Hamstring muscles (semitendinosus, semimembranosus, and biceps femoris) (sciatic nerve; L4,5, S1,2). The patient, in the supine position, flexes the knee against resistance. *C.* Hamstring muscles (semitendinous, semimembranosus, and biceps femoris) (sciatic nerve; L4,5, S1,2). The patient in the prone position flexes the knee against resistance. Arrows point to the tendons of the biceps and semitendinosus. *D.* Gastrocnemius (posterior tibial nerve; S1). With the leg extended at the knee, the patient plantar flexes the foot against resistance. The arrow points to the muscle belly. *E.* Soleus (posterior tibial nerve; S1). With the leg flexed at the knee and hip, the patient plantar flexes the foot against resistance. *F.* Gastrocnemius-soleus (posterior tibial nerve; S1). Alternate method: The patient stands on tiptoes. *G.* Tibialis posterior (posterior tibial nerve; L4,5). With the foot in plantar flexion, the patient inverts the foot against resistance. The arrow points to the tendon. *H.* Long flexors of the toes (posterior tibial nerve; S1,2). The patient flexes the toes against resistance. *I.* Tibialis anterior (deep peroneal nerve; L4,5). The patient dorsiflexes and inverts the foot against resistance. The arrow points to the tendon. *J.* Extensor digitorum longus (deep peroneal nerve; L5). The patient extends the lateral four toes against resistance. *K.* Intrinsic muscles of the foot (medial and lateral plantar nerves; S1,2). The patient cups the sole of the foot. *L.* Extensor hallucis longus (deep peroneal nerve; L5,S1). The patient extends the big toe against resistance. The arrow points to the tendon. *M.* Extensor digitorum brevis (deep peroneal nerve; L5,S1). The patient dorsiflexes the proximal phalanges of the toes against resistance. The muscle is visible (*arrow*). *N.* Peroneus longus and brevis (superificial peroneal nerve; L5,S1). The patient everts the foot against resistance. The arrow points to the tendon of the peroneus brevis.

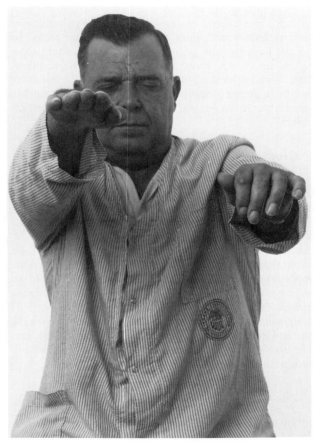

Figure 12-8 Drift of the extended left arm. This may denote either proximal muscle weakness in the arm or a lack of position sense.

Deep Pain

Elicitation of deep pain sensation is a rather crude test; one does not look for minor abnormalities but for gross changes such as the absence of deep pain sensation (e.g., in peripheral neuropathy or tabes dorsalis) or exaggerated muscle pain response (e.g., in polymyositis). Deep pain is tested in the lower extremities by squeezing the tendo Achillis or calf muscles, and in the upper extremities by hyperextending the finger joints.

Testing of Cortical Sensations

Stereognosis

Stereognosis is the ability to recognize common objects placed in the hand, purely from the feel of their size, shape, and texture. Coins of various denominations, keys, safety pin, pencil, comb, or pocket knife are generally utilized as test objects. The patient is asked to close the eyes, and the test object is placed first into the hand suspected to have a cortical sensory loss; the same object is then transferred to the opposite hand. Patients with paresis of the hand may be unable to manipulate the test object; in such instances, the examiner may manipulate the object as it lies in the patient's fingers. The patient's response in recognizing the object in the affected hand is compared with that in the normal hand. Astereognosis is defined as the inability to recognize objects by feel in the absence of impairment of primary sensations such as light touch, joint sense, and pressure sense. In reality, however, the primary sensations are rarely completely intact. An operational definition of astereognosis then is the impairment of the ability to identify objects by feel by a degree disproportionate to the loss of primary sensations. Astereognosis is observed in parietal cortical lesions.

Graphesthesia

Graphesthesia is the ability to identify traced figures on the skin. The inability to do so in the presence of intact tactile sensibility indicates parietal lobe dysfunction.

The test is carried out by writing, with a blunt point, letters or Arabic numerals on the palm of the hand. The examiner stands beside the patient in order to present the traced figures in a familiar orientation. After being given the opportunity to watch one or two traced figure samples, the patient is asked to close the eyes and to identify the traced figures. The figures drawn should be at least 4 cm in height. A simpler variation of this test is to draw a simple straight line and have the patient indicate the direction of the line. The basis of this test is precise tactile localization, which is a parietal lobe function.

Two-point Discrimination

Two-point discrimination is the ability to identify two separate but identical cutaneous stimuli applied simultaneously and close together. Different regions of the body vary widely in their ability to perceive two points applied simultaneously. For instance, at the tip of the tongue and on the lip a separation of as little as 2 to 3 mm between the points of stimuli may be sufficient; at the fingertips, approximately 5 mm; and on the dorsum of the hands or feet, 20 to 30 mm. On the trunk, a separation of 4 to 7 cm may be necessary.

A compass with dull points (so as not to inflict a pain stimulus) or a paper clip bent to varying distances between its points may be used. With the patient's eyes closed, the stimuli are applied starting far apart and then approximated until the patient starts to make errors, thus determining the threshold of perception of two-point stimulation.

Integrity of the posterior columns and the parietal cortex is essential for two-point discrimination. Intact or nearly intact tactile sensibility with impairment of two-point discrimination suggests parietal lobe dysfunction.

Anatomical Localization of Sensory Disorder

The normal segmental sensory distribution and cutaneous innervation are shown in Fig. 12-9. Anatomical localization of sensory disorders is illustrated in Fig. 12-10 and is summarized in Table 12-3.

Examination of the Reflexes

Reflexes, in a neurological sense, are quick involuntary motor responses to sensory stimuli. Being involuntary, they represent the most objective of the neurological tests. It is customary to classify reflexes into three categories:

1. *Muscle stretch reflexes* (deep tendon, periosteal, and myotatic reflexes) are segmental reflexes induced by sudden stretch of the muscle.
2. *Superficial reflexes* are motor responses induced by stimulation of superficial structures (cornea, skin, or mucous membrane).
3. *Pathological reflexes* are complex responses to certain stimuli seen only with organic diseases of the nervous system but not in normal adults.

Muscle Stretch Reflexes

Muscle stretch reflexes are simple monosynaptic reflexes consisting of an afferent sensory pathway synapsing on motor neurons innervating a muscle or muscles in a segmental distribution. This reflex arc is influenced by cortical and subcortical input. Absence of a reflex signifies an interruption of the reflex arc, either its afferent or efferent component. Hyperactive reflexes denote a release from cortical inhibitory influences. It is customary to grade the reflex response as follows:

0:	*no reflex*
1 + :	*hypoactive reflex*
2 + :	*normally active reflex*
3 + :	*hyperactive reflex*
4 + :	*markedly hyperactive reflex*

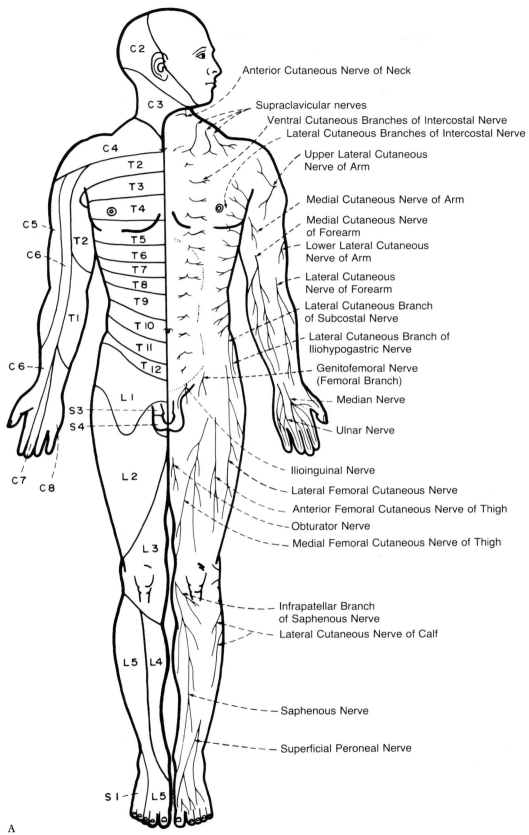

Figure 12-9 Segmental sensory distribution and cutaneous innervation in the human, shown in anterior (*A*) and posterior (*B*) views. For *B*, turn the page.

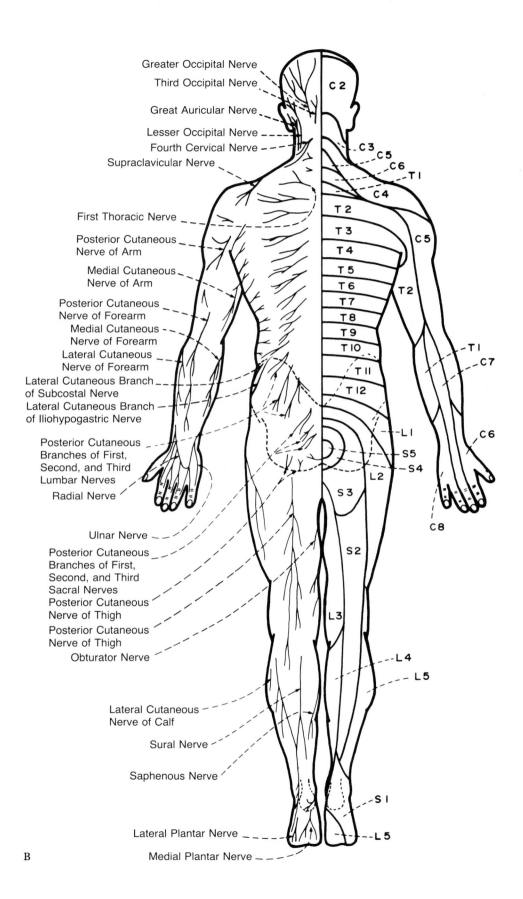

Greater Occipital Nerve
Third Occipital Nerve
Great Auricular Nerve
Lesser Occipital Nerve
Fourth Cervical Nerve
Supraclavicular Nerve
First Thoracic Nerve
Posterior Cutaneous Nerve of Arm
Medial Cutaneous Nerve of Arm
Posterior Cutaneous Nerve of Forearm
Medial Cutaneous Nerve of Forearm
Lateral Cutaneous Nerve of Forearm
Lateral Cutaneous Branch of Subcostal Nerve
Lateral Cutaneous Branch of Iliohypogastric Nerve
Posterior Cutaneous Branches of First, Second, and Third Lumbar Nerves
Radial Nerve
Ulnar Nerve
Posterior Cutaneous Branches of First, Second, and Third Sacral Nerves
Posterior Cutaneous Nerve of Thigh
Posterior Cutaneous Nerve of Thigh
Obturator Nerve
Lateral Cutaneous Nerve of Calf
Sural Nerve
Saphenous Nerve
Lateral Plantar Nerve
Medial Plantar Nerve

B

C 2
C 3
C 5
C 6
T 1
C 4
T 2
T 3
C 5
T 4
T 5
T 6
T 2
T 7
T 8
T 9
T 10
T 1
C 7
T 11
T 12
L 1
C 6
S 5
S 4
L 2
C 8
S 3
S 2
L 3
L 4
L 5
S 1
L 5

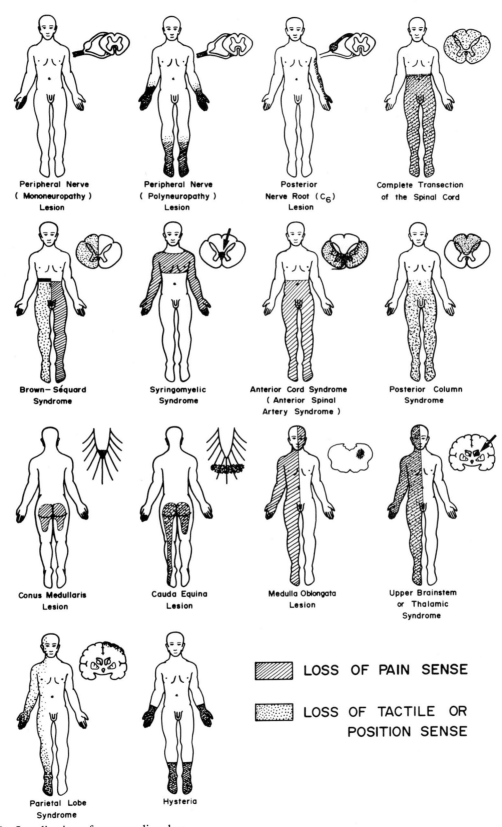

Figure 12-10 Localization of sensory disorders.

Grades 3 + and 4 + may be associated with transient or sustained clonus. It should be emphasized, however, that mere absence of muscle stretch reflexes or the presence of hyperactive reflexes even with sustained clonus in themselves are not pathological. Interpretation should be governed by the presence or absence of asymmetry of responses and other associated neurological signs.

Muscle stretch reflexes are ideally elicited in an adequately relaxed patient by placing the muscle in question under optimal tension (usually in a position midway between the greatest and shortest lengths of the muscle) and applying an adequate but abrupt stretch stimulus. In individuals in whom the reflexes are not easily elicited, reinforcement techniques may be used. The reflexes in the upper extremities may be reinforced by the patient clenching the teeth, and in the lower extremities by asking the patient to pull apart the firmly hooked fingers held in front of the chest.

The technique of elicitation of specific muscle stretch reflexes, their segmental and peripheral nerve innervation, and certain remarks in their interpretation are included in Table 12-4.

TABLE 12-3   Localization of Sensory Disorders (Fig. 12-10)

Clinical Syndrome	Clinical Characteristics
	Peripheral Nerve
Single peripheral nerve (mononeuropathy or mononeuropathy multiplex)	The signs will vary depending upon whether the involved nerve is a motor, sensory, or mixed nerve. Sensory loss is in a peripheral nerve distribution and generally involves all modalities of sensation, although joint sense is rarely abolished by interruption of a single peripheral nerve. The intensity and the nature of sensory loss varies with the extent and nature of involvement of the nerve. Extrinsic compression of the nerve (entrapment neuropathy) affects the large touch and pressure fibers in preference to small, thinly myelinated pain fibers. Flaccid paralysis with atrophy may be associated in mixed nerve involvement. Painful burning dysesthesia (causalgia) may be seen in patients with partial injury to a peripheral nerve.
Multiple peripheral nerves (polyneuropathy)	The sensory impairment is generally symmetrical. The feet, legs, and hands are especially affected (glove-and-stocking anesthesia), with sparing of the trunk because the longest nerve fibers tend to be affected. The boundaries of sensory loss are poorly defined. All modalities of sensation are impaired, although not to an equal degree. Intense burning dysesthetic pain may be present in diabetic and alcoholic neuropathies. The muscle stretch reflexes are hypoactive or absent. There may be associated flaccid motor weakness.
	Posterior Nerve Root
Root syndrome	This syndrome is most commonly seen with cervical or lumbar disc disease or spondylosis. It may also be seen with a metastatic epidural tumor or an intradural extramedullary tumor. Patients present with radiating pain along a root, which is aggravated with the Valsalva maneuver. The sensory loss is in a root distribution. There may be associated motor weakness if the anterior root is involved as well.
	Spinal Cord and Cauda Equina
Complete transection or transverse myelopathy	All modalities of sensation are lost below the level of the lesion; in some instances a narrow band of hyperesthesia may be found at the upper margin of the anesthetic zone. Total paralysis of all muscles occurs below the level of the lesion. In the acute phase, the muscles are flaccid and areflexic (stage of spinal shock); later spasticity and hyper-reflexia develop. There is retention of urine with overflow incontinence in the acute phase, but in later stages automatic reflex emptying occurs. Trophic lesions occur in long-standing cases.
Brown-Séquard syndrome (hemisection of the spinal cord)	This syndrome may occur with trauma, an intra- or extramedullary tumor, or a hematoma. Ipsilateral paralysis and loss of proprioceptive sensation occur as a result of involvement of the corticospinal tract and posterior column, and contralateral loss of pain and thermal sense occurs due to involvement of the spinothalamic tract. A pure form of this syndrome is rarely encountered, minor variations being quite frequent.
Syringomyelic syndrome (commissural, central gray, and central cord syndromes)	Although typically associated with syringomyelia, this syndrome may result from trauma, hematomyelia, or an intramedullary tumor. Since the fibers carrying pain and thermal sense cross in the anterior white commissure, a longitudinal spinal lesion in this location results in multisegmental loss of these sensations bilaterally and often symmetrically. The sense of touch is preserved (dissociated sensory loss). Because of insensitivity to pain, the patient may not be aware of cuts or burns in the fingers. Charcot's neuropathic arthropathy may result (see figure). Involvement of the ventral gray matter results in segmental weakness and atrophy (Fig. 12-1). With progression of the lesion, the white matter is involved, resulting in impairment of corticospinal, spinothalamic, and posterior column function. Lamellar organization of these tracts (see figure) accounts for early paralysis of the arm and sacral sparing of pain sensation.

TABLE 12-3 Localization of Sensory Disorders (Fig. 12-10)(*continued*)

Clinical Syndrome	Clinical Characteristics

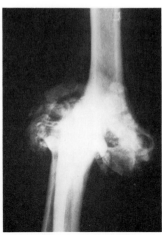

Roentgenogram of the elbow of a patient with syringomyelia demonstrating Charcot's neuropathic arthropathy.

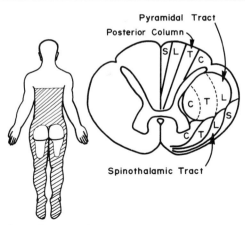

Lamellar organization of the long tracts.

The central cord contusion syndrome occurs in acute hyperextension injury to the cervical spine from simultaneous squeezing of the cord anteriorly (by spondylotic ridges) and posteriorly (by redundant ligamentum flavum). This lesion may occur without apparent fracture or dislocation of the vertebrae. The syndrome is characterized by a disproportionate weakness of the upper limbs compared with the lower limbs. This is because pyramidal tract fibers to cervical segments are more medial than those to lumbar segments (see figure). Varying degrees of sensory disturbances below the level of the lesion as well as sphincter disturbances may occur.

Posterior column syndrome

Position and vibration senses are impaired below the level of the lesion, but pain, thermal, and tactile senses are unaffected. Sensory ataxia and rombergism are hallmarks of this syndrome. In many clinical situations (e.g., subacute combined degeneration of the cord, pernicious anemia, Friedreich's ataxia, and multiple sclerosis) the corticospinal tracts are involved as well.

Anterior cord syndrome (anterior spinal artery syndrome)

Infarction in the distribution of the anterior spinal artery results in paraplegia, loss of pain and thermal sensation, and preservation of posterior column function. This syndrome may also result from ventrally situated compressive lesions.

Conus medullaris and cauda equina syndromes

Conus and cauda lesions generally produce sensory loss in the saddle distribution: with *conus* lesions, the sensory loss is usually bilaterally symmetrical and there may be dissociation in sensory loss. Spontaneous pain is significantly absent. Motor weakness also tends to be symmetrical. There is early loss of sphincteric and sexual functions. The knee jerks tend to be preserved, and a Babinski response may be present. With *cauda equina* lesions, radiating pain is a cardinal feature. The sensory and motor deficits are asymmetric; sphincter disturbances occur late and tend to be incomplete.

Brain Stem

Medullary syndrome

Infarction in the distribution of the posterior inferior cerebellar artery involving the tegmentum of the medulla (Wallenberg syndrome) is a typical example. In this syndrome, a crossed sensory disturbance occurs characterized by loss of pain and temperature sense on the ipsilateral side of the face and the contralateral side of the body. This results from involvement of the descending tract or nucleus of the trigeminal nerve, which carries pain and temperature fibers from the ipsilateral face, and of the spinothalamic tract, which carries the same information from the opposite half of the body.

Pons and midbrain syndromes

Above the level of the medulla the pain and temperature fibers from the opposite half of the body and the face run together since the fibers originating from the descending trigeminal nucleus decussate and assume a position in the quintothalamic tract closely applied to the spinothalamic tract itself. Thus lesions in the brain stem above the level of the medulla result in impairment of pain and temperature sense in the opposite side of the face and the body.

TABLE 12-3 Localization of Sensory Disorders (Fig. 12-10)(*continued*)

Clinical Syndrome	Clinical Characteristics
	Thalamus
Thalamic syndrome	Because the thalamus is the main sensory nucleus that receives all crude forms of sensibility, a lesion in the nucleus ventralis posterolateralis and posteromedialis causes diminution or loss of all forms of sensation in the opposite half of the body and face. The cause is usually vascular occlusion, but an infiltrating glioma may also be responsible. In some patients with ischemic infarcts affecting the thalamus, severe spontaneous dysesthetic burning pain may be experienced in the anesthetic area. The pain is usually intractable (thalamic pain; syndrome of Déjerine-Roussy). The pathophysiology of this syndrome is poorly understood.
	Parietal Cortex
Parietal lobe syndrome	In parietal cortical lesions, all modalities of sensation on the opposite side of the body are affected, but discriminative sensations are especially impaired. Pain, touch, and vibration senses are impaired to a lesser degree. Loss of position sense, impairment of two-point discrimination, astereognosis, and agraphesthesia are hallmarks of involvement of the primary sensory cortex. In addition, if the adjacent parietal associative cortex is involved, constructional apraxia and directional disorientation may be manifest. Postrolandic cortical lesions may induce sensory jacksonian seizures.
	Psyche
Nonorganic sensory syndrome (hysteria and malingering)	Hysterical sensory loss rarely conforms to any defined anatomical pattern. A glove-and-stocking type of distribution is sometimes seen, but in contrast to peripheral neuropathy, the proximal limits of the sensory loss tend to be abrupt. There are no associated neurological changes such as an alteration in muscle strength or tone or change in reflexes. Sometimes the sensory loss may be confined to one-half of the body, without any alteration in the dexterity of motor acts. It is difficult to conceptualize normal skilled motor function in the absence of proprioceptive input. Repeated examination done in a random, confusing manner will show the inconsistencies in the distribution of sensory impairment. In the conversion reaction of hysteria, patients may remarkably be able to psychically inhibit pain.

Superficial Reflexes

Abdominal Reflexes

The abdominal skin reflex is elicited by lightly scratching the skin over the abdomen and lower chest with a semisharp pointed object such as a split tongue blade, applicator stick, or dull pin. There is a reflex contraction of the abdominal musculature beneath the stimulated skin with resultant drawing of the umbilicus toward the stroked side. Heavy stroking should be avoided for two reasons; first, it induces a muscle stretch reflex of the abdominal muscles rather than a reflex contraction to a true cutaneous stimulus; second, heavy stroking often leaves lasting scratch marks from superficial abrasion, a reflection of an unpolished neurological examination.

An optimal response is obtained if the patient is fully relaxed in a recumbent position with the arms by the sides, head down, and knees slightly flexed. The reflex is best elicited after the patient has taken a few deep breaths and when the stimulus is applied at the end of expiration. The epigastric (T6-T9), midabdominal (T9-T11), and lower abdominal or hypogastric (T11-L1) reflexes are elicited by scratching the lower costal, midabdominal and lower abdominal areas, respectively, and observing for muscle contraction in the corresponding areas (Fig. 12-11). The strokes should be directed toward the umbilicus; stroking in the reverse direction may result in mechanical deviation of the umbilicus that may be mistaken for a muscular response.

The abdominal reflexes are difficult to elicit in obese patients with a pendulous abdominal wall, multiparous women with lax abdominal musculature, and patients who have undergone multiple laparotomies with consequent scarring and denervation of the abdominal muscles. A hyperactive abdominal reflex has no localizing value; it is seen in anxious and nervous individuals. Diminished or absent superficial abdominal reflexes when associated with hyperactive deep tendon reflexes and positive pathological reflexes are suggestive of a corticospinal tract lesion above the upper level of the segmental innervation of the reflex. This is seen in spinal lesions (ipsilaterally or bilaterally) or cerebral lesions (contralaterally). Unlike muscle stretch reflexes, the cutaneous reflexes are not simple monosynaptic reflexes mediated segmentally through the spinal cord; their reflex arc is more complex and includes the corticospinal tract and motor cortex. Superficial abdominal reflexes are frequently lost in early stages of multiple sclerosis, although their presence in no way negates this diagnosis.

Cremasteric Reflex (L1, 2)

In men, elevation of the ipsilateral testicle from contraction of the cremasteric muscle occurs upon stroking the inner surface of the thigh near the groin (Fig. 12-14). This reflex must not be mistaken for the dartos response, which is slow and vermicular. The cremasteric reflex is absent in corticospinal tract lesions above the first lumbar segment.

TABLE 12-4 Muscle Stretch Reflexes

Reflex	How Elicited	Segmental Innervation	Peripheral Nerve	Comments
Pectoralis reflex	With the patient's arm partly abducted, the examiner places his or her thumb on the patient's pectoralis tendon near its insertion onto the humerus and strikes the blow toward the axilla.	C5,6	Medial and lateral pectoral nerves	Normally this reflex is not easily elicited, but in upper motor neuron lesions above the fifth cervical segment the pectoral contraction may be very brisk.
Biceps reflex	The arm is flexed to about 90 degrees and the forearm is pronated. The biceps tendon is palpated just above the crease of the elbow and gently pressed with the thumb. The thumb is briskly tapped. There is contraction of the biceps with flexion at the elbow.	C5,6	Musculocutaneous nerve	In advanced upper motor neuron lesions with severe spasticity, there may be associated flexion of the wrist and fingers and adduction of the thumb.
Brachioradialis reflex (radial periosteal reflex, supinator reflex)	The tendon of the brachioradialis is struck just above the wrist joint with the forearm in semipronation. There is flexion at the elbow.	C5,6	Radial nerve	In upper motor neuron lesions, if the reflex is hyperactive, there may be associated flexion of the wrist and fingers and adduction of the thumb. In lesions of the cervical spinal cord involving the C5 segment, a phenomenon called the *inverted brachioradialis (supinator) reflex* is demonstrated. When one attempts to elicit the brachioradialis reflex, only the finger flexor or response is obtained, without flexion at the elbow. The biceps reflex may be absent as well. The finger flexor reflex and the triceps reflex are exaggerated. This phenomenon results from a lower motor neuron deficit in the C5 segmental level and an upper motor neuron pattern caudal to this level. The inverted brachioradialis reflex may be seen with cervical disc disease, cervical spondylosis, cervical cord neoplasms, and syringomyelia.
Triceps reflex	The triceps reflex is elicited with the arms flexed or akimbo on the hips. The triceps tendon is tapped just above the olecranon process.	C7,8	Radial nerve	

TABLE 12-4 Muscle Stretch Reflexes (*continued*)

Reflex	How Elicited	Segmental Innervation	Peripheral Nerve	Comments
Finger flexor reflex	With the patient's hand resting on the table in a supine position, and with the fingers in slight flexion, the examiner places his or her middle and index fingers on the palmar surfaces of the patient's four fingers and strikes his or her own fingers briskly. The response consists of brisk flexion of all fingers.	C7,T1	Median and ulnar nerves	This reflex is difficult to elicit in normal individuals. Usually there is little or no response. The reflex may be reinforced by having the patient flex his fingers as the blow is being applied. In upper motor neuron lesions, the finger flexor reflex is very brisk; there may even be finger flexor clonus.
Knee reflex (quadriceps femoris reflex, patellar reflex, knee jerk)	Extension at the knee occurs when the patellar tendon is struck. This reflex may be elicited with the patient in either the sitting position with the legs dangling over the edge of the examining table, or in the dorsal decubitus position with the examiner's hand lifting the knee from the bed.	L3,4	Femoral nerve	In upper motor neuron lesions, the knee reflexes are not only hyperactive but may be associated with adduction of the thighs.
Ankle jerk (tendo Achillis reflex, gastrocnemius-soleus reflex)	Plantar flexion of the foot occurs when the Achilles tendon is struck. This reflex may be elicited in one of several ways: (1) *Sitting position:* The patient sits with the feet dangling. The foot is passively dorsiflexed and the tendo Achillis is struck. (2) *Dorsal decubitus position:* The leg is flexed at the knee and externally rotated slightly. The foot is dorsiflexed, and the tendo Achillis is struck. (3) *Prone position:* The knee is flexed, the foot is gently dorsiflexed, and the tendo Achillis is struck. (4) *Kneeling position:* With the patient kneeling on a chair, with the feet and ankles extending unsupported over the front edge of a chair, the foot is gently dorsiflexed and the tendo Achillis is struck.	L5,S1	Tibial nerve	

NOTE: The jaw jerk is described under the fifth cranial nerve.

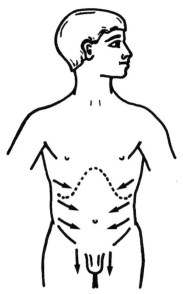

Figure 12-11 Technique of eliciting abdominal and cremasteric reflexes.

Superficial Anal Reflex (S3-5)

When the skin around the anus is scratched or pricked with a pin, there is reflex contraction of the external anal sphincter that can be seen ("anal wink") or felt by a gloved finger in the rectum. This reflex is absent in lesions of the lower sacral segments and is associated with a patulous insensitive anus. The reflex is especially helpful in evaluating anal sphincter function in an infant with a meningomyelocele.

Bulbocavernosus Reflex (S3, 4)

This reflex is elicited by pinching or pricking the foreskin of the penis or glans penis. The bulbocavernous muscle contracts, and this can be seen or felt in the perineum at the root of the penis. In patients who have an indwelling Foley catheter, a gentle tug on the catheter will induce reflex contraction of the bulbocavernosus muscle. The presence of this reflex in a paraplegic patient after acute spinal trauma indicates that he has passed the stage of spinal shock.

Plantar Reflex (L5-S2)

The plantar reflex is elicited by stroking the outer aspect of the sole of the foot from the heel toward the toes. Normally, there is flexion of the foot and toes in response to this stimulus. The extensor plantar response, the sign of Babinski, is described under pathological reflexes.

Pathological Reflexes

Certain reflexes are demonstrable only with organic diseases of the central nervous system and are designated as pathological reflexes. These generally are primitive reflexes that

are physiological in infancy but are later suppressed with the maturation of cortical control of the spinal segmental system. Demonstration of such reflexes in an adult is thus considered to be a release phenomenon due to impairment of the cortical inhibitory control resulting from disease processes affecting the upper motor neuron. For descriptive purposes it is customary to classify pathological reflexes into two major categories: (1) frontal lobe release signs and (2) pyramidal tract responses.

Frontal Lobe Release Phenomena

These phenomena are generally demonstrable in patients with diffuse dementing illnesses due to widespread nonlocalized bilateral hemispheric lesions, especially in the frontal lobes. Etiologic processes include degenerative disease, extensive infiltrating neoplasm, low-pressure hydrocephalus, closed head injury, and toxic-metabolic encephalopathy.

The glabellar reflex is elicited by gently tapping the forehead between the eyebrows with the finger. Normally there is a blinking response, but this response attenuates on repeated tapping. In lesions involving corticobulbar pathways from the frontal cortex to the facial nucleus in the pons, the reflex is hyperactive and the blinking response persists after repeated tapping (Myerson's sign). This reflex is present most frequently in patients with Parkinson's disease, "butterfly" glioblastoma of the corpus callosum, and degenerative diseases.

The snout reflex is elicited by briskly tapping the upper or lower lip with a percussion hammer; a pursing response is obtained (Fig. 12-12). Like the glabellar reflex, it is seen with bilateral corticobulbar lesions. It is most frequently seen in pseudobulbar palsy and amyotrophic lateral sclerosis.

The sucking reflex is a physiological reflex present in infancy, but it disappears after weaning. It reappears in adults with diffuse bifrontal disease. It is elicited by stroking the lip with a finger or a tongue blade. The lips pout and the patient makes sucking, tasting, chewing, or swallowing movements.

The grasp reflex is elicited by stroking the palm of the hand (between the thumb and index finger) with the examiner's fingers. The patient grasps the examiner's hand and is unable to release the grasp. Alternatively, if the patient's flexed fingers are slowly extended, they will flex against the resistance offered by the examiner; the stronger the resistance, the stronger is the flexor response. If the dorsum of the patient's fingers is stroked, the reflex may be inhibited, and the patient may release the examiner's fingers. A *groping response* with rhythmic, oscillating reaching movements may be seen after withdrawal of the examiner's fingers from the patient's grasp. The patient may attempt to grope and reach for any object presented in his or her visual field.

The grasp reflex is thought to represent a body righting or postural reflex and is normally seen in infants up to 4 months of age, after which this reflex is inhibited by the frontal lobes. Demonstration of this reflex in adults represents a release phenomenon. If it is unilateral, it is indicative of involvement of the contralateral frontal lobe, especially the premotor cortex. Bilateral grasp reflexes indicates a more diffuse bifrontal disorder.

Pyramidal Tract Responses: Hoffmann Reflex, Clonus, and Babinski's Sign

The *Hoffmann reflex* is not a pathological reflex in a strict sense but is only an alternative way of eliciting a finger flexor reflex. It is not pathognomonic of pyramidal tract disease but is simply reflective of hyper-reflexia, be it on an organic or emotional basis. If it is unilateral and associated with hyper-reflexia and spasticity on that side, it suggests pyramidal tract involvement. The Hoffmann reflex is elicited as illustrated in Fig. 12-13. The wrist of the patient is held dorsiflexed, and the middle phalanx of the long finger is grasped firmly. The distal phalanx is flicked downward abruptly. After the release, the terminal phalanx recoils into extension, stretching the tendon of the flexor digitorum profundus, initiating a stretch reflex. The degree of the stretch of the tendon, however, is inadequate to induce a finger flexor reflex, but if the latter is elicited, it is indicative of a hyper-reflexic state. When the distal phalanx of the long finger is flicked, flexion of the thumb also indicates hyper-reflexia.

Clonus is defined as a series of rhythmic involuntary muscle contractions induced by sudden stretching of a spastic muscle. Clonus may be elicited under different situations, but the common denominator is the sudden stretch of a spastic muscle. The patient may observe the clonus during everyday activities (e.g., ankle clonus when pressing on the brake pedal of an automobile). At times clonus may be demonstrable on examination of deep tendon reflexes; conventionally, clonus is elicited by suddenly stretching the muscle in question during the neurological evaluation. Although any muscle may show clonus, three areas are most frequently tested: ankle, knee, and wrist. Depending upon the degree of spasticity, the clonus may be sustained or unsustained. Although sustained clonus along with hyper-reflexia and spasticity are indicative of pyramidal tract involvement, occasionally a few beats of unsustained clonus may be seen in some normal individuals without any evidence of organic disease of the central nervous system.

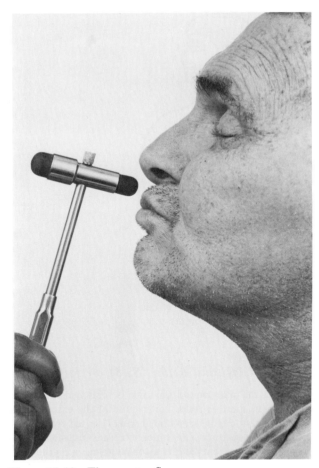

Figure 12-12   The snout reflex.

Babinski's sign is another illustration of a release phenomenon, the loss of inhibitory control of the pyramidal system over the lower motor neurons. To be specific, the Babinski sign represents the primitive flexion reflex, a defensive re-

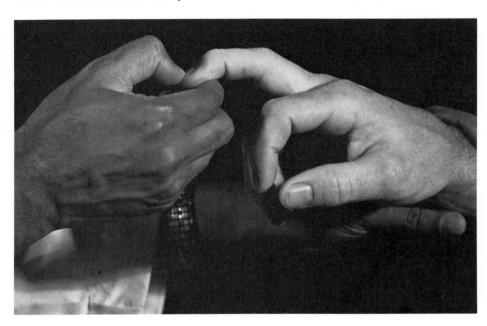

Figure 12-13   Technique of eliciting the Hoffmann reflex.

flex withdrawal of the lower extremity from a painful stimulus. It is characterized by flexion of the hip, knee, ankle, and toes (dorsiflexion). (At this point, it is worthwhile pointing out that the terminology for the movements at the ankle and toes used by physiologists are exactly the opposite of what the anatomists use. Flexion of the ankle and toes in a physiologist's parlance refers to dorsiflexion about these structures, but the anatomist would call these movements an extension.) This defensive movement is normally suppressed by the motor cortex through its projections on the lower motor neuron. In healthy individuals, this flexion reflex cannot be induced by stimuli that are ordinarily used to elicit the plantar reflex. In patients with lesions in the pyramidal system, be it structural (stroke, trauma, tumor, demyelination) or functional (impaired consciousness, metabolic disturbances), the flexion reflex is released from inhibitory control, and is manifest clinically as the Babinski sign. The Babinski response is elicited by stimulation of the plantar surface of the foot with a blunt point (key, end of the handle of a percussion hammer, wood applicator). A painful stimulus with a pin should be avoided since it will induce a rapid withdrawal response. The stimulus is directed from the heel forward toward the metatarsophalangeal joints in a slow, deliberate manner. The patient should be relaxed, and the examiner may prefer to hold the patient's ankle firmly against the bed. The typical response is one of abduction ("fanning") of the toes and slow dorsiflexion of the great toe. In some instances the smaller toes may fail to fan out, and may actually flex. In extreme cases, the great toe may be in persistent dorsiflexion even without a stimulus applied to the sole of the foot. Because of these variations, it is better to describe the response rather than merely stating that the Babinski response is present, absent, or equivocal. The extensor plantar response is normally present during infancy but gradually converts to a flexor response concurrent with myelination of the pyramidal axons.

Part III

Ancillary Diagnostic Tests

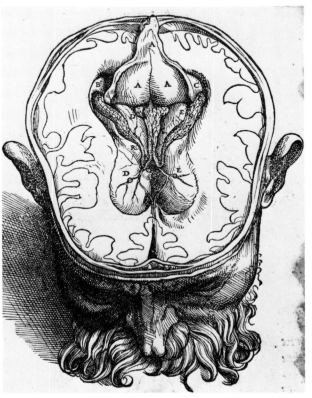

Vesalius A. *De Humani Corporis Fabrica Libri Septem.* Basel, J Oporini, 1543. A 16th century view of the brain, reintroduced today by means of CT scanning.

SECTION A

Cerebrospinal Fluid Examination

13

Techniques of Ventricular Puncture

Timothy B. Mapstone
Robert A. Ratcheson

History

Puncture of the lateral ventricles, a technique developed early in the course of modern neurological surgery, remains a basic tool of the neurological surgeon. Brain puncture via trephine opening dates to the time of Hippocrates.[21] However, it is unlikely that the ancients knowingly punctured the cerebral ventricles, as their premorbid existence was not accepted until the eighteenth century. "Paracentesis hydrocephali" was described by Hill in 1850 but was "not generally recommended—even as a last resort."[9] The first edition of Keen's *An American Textbook of Surgery*[13] cited the use of ventricular puncture for hydrocephalus using landmarks that Keen had outlined in 1890.[12] Although ventricular puncture was used sporadically for ventricular decompression, a major clinical use was not realized until 1918 when Walter Dandy described injection of air into the lateral ventricles for the purpose of radiographic localization of cerebral masses, thus beginning the era of interpretive neuroradiology.[5] Despite its clinical value, not all early neurological surgeons adopted this technique. Most notably, Harvey Cushing was reported to be unenthusiastic because he feared ventriculography would circumvent a thorough neurological examination.[8]

Pressure measurement and drainage of CSF were occasionally performed by ventricular puncture in the early twentieth century, but since the rigid needles used could not be adequately stabilized to prevent migration through the brain and the risk of infection was high, continuous cannulation of the ventricles was not possible. Ventriculostomy drainage via a burr hole was first reported by Adson in 1927.[1] Utilizing a prethreaded piece of animal bone to stabilize his equipment, he continuously monitored intracranial pressure (ICP) in a patient until death 4 days later. However, little was added concerning the use of external ventricular drainage until the seminal report of Ingraham and Campbell in 1941.[10] They described their experience utilizing a sterile closed system with a silver cannula left in the lateral ventricle for the emergent management of obstructive hydrocephalus. By building upon the initial concepts of Ingraham and Campbell and adding pliable catheters as suggested by Robinson and others,[2,20] neurosurgeons now undertake long-term external ventricular drainage, with a low incidence of complications.[7,22]

Indications

The major indications for performing ventricular puncture or drainage—diagnostic and therapeutic—have not changed significantly through the history of neurological surgery.

Diagnostic indications include the collection of ventricular CSF for chemical or cytological evaluation, the introduction of contrast agents to allow radiographic imaging of the anatomy of the CNS and CSF pathways, measurement of intracranial pressure, and ventriculoscopy. Therapeutic modalities generally concern the relief of increased intracranial pressure through CSF drainage and the introduction of chemotherapeutic agents.

Landmarks and Trajectories

The most frequently chosen sites for ventricular puncture are coronal (Kocher's point), posterior parietal (Keen's point), and occipital. However, a number of other sites have been safely used and include the supraorbital region, orbital roof, and fontanelles.[19]

Coronal placement is in many respects ideal for ventricular catheter placement in that the tip of the catheter remains anterior to, and above, the foramen of Monro and choroid plexus, thus decreasing the likelihood of blockage of the tip by migration into the plexus or third ventricle. Through a burr hole placed 1 cm anterior to the coronal suture and 2 to

3 cm from the midline over the nondominant hemisphere (Fig. 13-1*a*), a premeasured catheter is introduced approximately in the coronal plane and angled toward the medial canthus of the ipsilateral eye.[19] At a depth of 4 to 5 cm CSF should flow freely from the tip. Advancement, *after removal of the stylet*, another 1 cm should ensure placement in the frontal horn.

Keen's point, 2.5 to 3 cm superior to and 2.5 to 3 cm posterior to the superior aspect of the pinna, allows placement into the trigone of the lateral ventricle (Fig. 13-1*b*).[12] During posterior fossa surgery, through a separate incision 4 cm lateral to the midline and 6 cm above the inion, a burr hole may be placed for cannulation of the posterior aspect of the lateral ventricle (Fig. 13-1*c*). Some surgeons feel that placement here is less likely to damage the visual pathways than a puncture at Dandy's point, which is located 2 cm from the midline and 3 cm above the inion (Fig. 13-1*d*).[5,14]

Other placements have been suggested but offer little advantage. Even in emergent situations cannulation of a normal or enlarged ventricle can be readily performed via the coronal, posterior parietal, or occipital route.

Two alternative techniques for emergency cannulation take advantage of the thin bone present in the infant and in the orbital roof of older patients. Navarro has described the use of a large-bore (18- or 16-gauge) spinal needle placed in the anterior third of the orbital roof after elevating the upper lid and depressing the globe.[16] Penetration of the bone is accomplished by firm, gentle pressure 1 to 2 cm behind the orbital rim, aiming the needle toward the coronal suture at the midline. The frontal horn is usually reached within 4 cm (Fig. 13-1*e*).

In infants, because of their open sutures and thin calvarium, either coronal or occipital entrance can be carried out with an 18- or 20-gauge spinal needle inserted just lateral to the anterior fontanelle or lateral to the posterior fontanelle and immediately above the lambdoid suture. With firm but controlled pressure and a 16-gauge needle, this technique can be utilized in young children and on occasion has been employed in patients up to 10 to 12 years of age.

Finally, cannulation of the frontal horn can be attempted via a twist drill hole placed approximately 4 cm above the orbital rim in the plane of the pupil. The needle is aimed at a point on the midline posteriorly and 3 cm above the inion (Fig. 13-1*f*).[11]

When any of the landmarks described above are used, free-flowing CSF should be encountered at a depth of 4 to 5 cm after puncture of the cortex. Failure to cannulate the ventricle using these criteria should direct the surgeon to re-evaluate the chosen external landmarks and perhaps to consider another puncture site.

Technique and Preparation

Although it is usually performed in the operating room, ventricular puncture can be performed in the emergency room and intensive care unit when necessary. Except for very uncooperative patients and frightened children, a local anesthetic is adequate. If necessary, this can be supplemented with intravenous administration of an analgesic or anxioly-

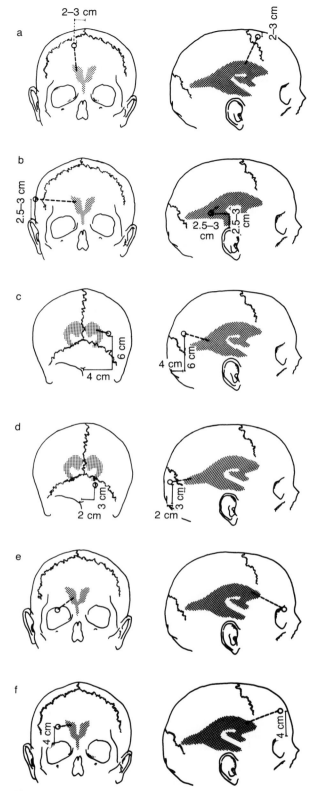

Figure 13-1 *a.* Kocher's point, 2 to 3 cm from the midline and just anterior to the coronal suture. *b.* Keen's point, 2.5 to 3 cm posterior and superior to the pinna. *c.* Occipital-parietal, 4 cm from the midline and 6 cm above the inion. *d.* Dandy's point, 2 cm from the midline and 3 cm above the inion. *e.* Orbital, 1 to 2 cm behind the orbital rim. *f.* Supraorbital, 4 cm above the orbital rim in the plane of the pupil.

tic. In most instances, a patient requiring external ventriculostomy is taken to the operating room and a Rickham-type reservoir is connected to the ventricular catheter. A generous field that includes not only the burr-hole site but also the path and site of exit of a subcutaneous tunnel is prepared. A C-shaped incision is made to avoid the incision crossing over the reservoir or connecting tubing. The skin flap should be large enough to enable a tension-free closure if a large reservoir is used. A burr hole is placed and the dura is opened with a fine-tipped blade after cauterizing the dural surface. A hole only slightly larger than the diameter of the catheter is made to ensure a snug fit and provide a seal against CSF leakage. A premeasured catheter with stylet is then passed into the ventricle. Often a distinctive "give" can be appreciated when the ventricle is entered. At this time pressure should be measured since if even small amounts of fluid are lost, an artificially low value will be obtained. After the pressure has been measured and fluid collected, the premeasured catheter is slowly advanced to the appropriate depth without the stylet, care being taken that CSF continues to flow. Before the connecting tubing or a reservoir to the trimmed catheter is attached, 3 cc of air is injected into the ventricle, allowing x-ray confirmation of catheter placement. The drainage tube is tunneled subcutaneously approximately 3 to 5 cm and brought out through a stab incision, secured with a single stitch and attached to the collecting system. The incisions are irrigated with an antibacterial solution and closed in layers. This system uses commercially available catheters and reservoirs and is especially versatile, providing separate sterile sites for sampling CSF, measuring ICP, and injecting medications or radiographic contrast agents and thus maintaining a closed system. It can be converted into a ventriculoperitoneal or ventriculoatrial shunt without repositioning the ventricular catheter. If there is no need to place a subcutaneous reservoir, the procedure is modified by cannulating the ventricle via a small incision and twist drill hole. As before, to provide stabilization of the catheter and prevent infection, the connecting tube is tunneled subcutaneously. Use of a rigid ventricular needle for anything other than brief, intermittent ventricle puncture to obtain ICP and CSF is dangerous, and should not be attempted. If a need for long-term access is anticipated, a pliable ventricular catheter is always used.

Drainage Systems

The connecting tube is attached to an external collection and measuring system via a series of three-way stopcocks. Disconnection of any external connection is done using sterile technique. Utilizing three or more stopcocks provides flexibility while maintaining a sterile, closed system. One stopcock can be used for monitoring ICP. The second stopcock is connected to a container of sterile IV solution used as an irrigating solution to clear the ventriculostomy line of debris or medications. The third stopcock is connected to a sterile syringe that is used to inject medications, to sample CSF, or to draw irrigation fluid via the second stopcock to flush the ventriculostomy without removing the syringe, thus minimizing the number of times connections are broken for maintenance. ICP and the amount of drainage can be varied by raising or lowering the drainage bottle. Alternatively, a Y connector can be placed in the drainage tube; one limb is connected directly to an ICP monitor while the second limb goes to the drainage bottle and contains a pressure-regulated valve. This system allows close regulation of CSF pressure, helps prevent siphoning, and retards retrograde travel of bacteria from the closed collection bottle (Fig. 13-2). With either system CSF can be collected for volume measurement and chemical, bacteriologic, or cytological studies. Appro-

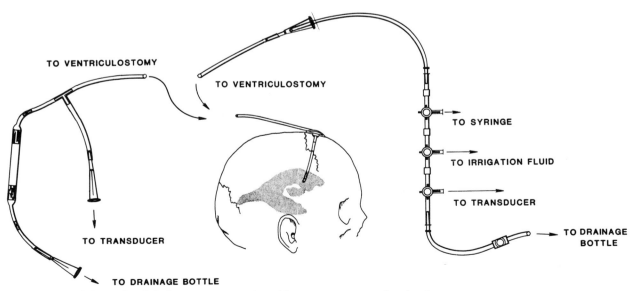

TO VENTRICULOSTOMY

TO VENTRICULOSTOMY

TO SYRINGE

TO IRRIGATION FLUID

TO TRANSDUCER

TO TRANSDUCER

TO DRAINAGE BOTTLE

TO DRAINAGE BOTTLE

Figure 13-2 Schematic of drainage systems using either a pressure-regulated valve and Y connector or a series of stopcocks to regulate input and output from the closed system.

priate oral or systemic antibiotics are administered.[23] If the system is completely internal (i.e., an Ommaya or Rickham reservoir), antibiotics are given for 24 h after insertion. This technique provides an acceptably low infection rate, permitting external drainage systems to function without evidence of CSF or wound infection for greater than 7 days and on rare occasions for longer than 3 weeks.

Reservoir Placement

Placement of an Ommaya reservoir is useful for long-term intermittent ventricular puncture. A generous C-shaped incision, concave posteriorly, is made and a subgaleal pocket constructed. A burr hole is placed at Kocher's point and the dura incised. A right-angled ventricular catheter is used for the puncture, and the catheter is connected to a large, straight sidearm reservoir placed in the subgaleal pouch. The wound is closed in layers. Since no part of the incision is over the reservoir, puncture can be performed immediately after insertion.[18]

Conversion to Shunt

If placement of the ventricular drain has been carefully planned, appropriate equipment used, and strict aseptic technique adhered to, it is feasible to convert an external ventriculostomy of short duration into an internal shunt.

In the operating room the patient is prepared for a peritoneal or atrial shunt. The exit site is prepared but excluded from the sterile field by draping. The C incision is reopened and the drainage tube connected to the reservoir removed. An unscrubbed assistant can grasp the drainage tube near the exit site and remove it from the field with a sharp tug. The reservoir is also removed and a new reservoir is attached to the original ventricular catheter. Free flow of CSF or irrigating fluid indicates continued placement of the catheter tip in the proper location. If there is doubt, air should be injected and placement checked with an intraoperative AP roentgenogram. The wound and subcutaneous tunnel of the removed drainage tube are copiously irrigated with an antibacterial solution. The remainder of the shunt system is installed in the usual manner, taking care not to allow the track of the shunt to cross the subcutaneous tunnel. This technique is particularly useful in patients whose ventricles have become quite small during drainage, thus making placement of a new ventricular catheter difficult.

It is noteworthy that some neurological surgeons prefer not to utilize parts of an external drainage system for an internal shunt because of the potential for increased infection. An alternative method of management would be to raise the collecting system, allowing the ICP to rise in order to expand the ventricles before placing an entirely new shunt on the opposite side of the head. The external system is totally removed. If it is clear that a permanent shunt will be needed and there is no need to have control of CSF drainage with an external ventriculostomy, an internal shunt should be placed initially.

Technical Variations

At times aberrant intracranial anatomy secondary to congenital defects or mass lesions make direct puncture of the lateral ventricles difficult and even dangerous. Modifications of two current radiological techniques, CT scanning and real-time ultrasonography, have provided improved safety in these circumstances. There are a number of commercially available head holders for stereotactic procedures that have been designed for use with CT scanners. These devices, in addition to minimizing imaging artifacts, can be adapted to take advantage of the CT scanner's data base to precisely locate the appropriate ventricle and to assign to the target internally consistent instructions utilizing x, y, and z axes to determine a trajectory with no more than a 1-mm error.[17] This procedure offers no advantage in routine catheter placement.

Recent advances in real-time ultrasonography have made this imaging modality available in the operating room. Although it requires a small craniectomy (3×3 cm) for imaging, this technique allows rapid visualization of both the catheter and ventricles. Recent models produce the image instantaneously, thus allowing the surgeon to place the catheter virtually under direct vision.[3]

Complications

With appropriate attention to detail, complications as a result of ventricular puncture will be quite rare. The most common is CSF infection. As would be expected, the strongest predictor of infection is the length of time an external system is in place. The common pathogens are *Staphylococcus epidermidis* and *Staphylococcus aureus*, which are generally sensitive to second generation cephalosporins or penicillinase-resistant synthetic penicillins. Placements of less than 3 days are usually free of infection. The incidence rises with time, although as previously mentioned meticulous care and antibiotic coverage can maintain a sterile system for weeks. Recent reports of techniques utilizing a subcutaneous tunnel and local wound care cite infection rates of less than 1 percent.[7]

Less commonly subdural, intraparenchymal, or intraventricular hemorrhage has occurred in association with ventricular puncture, either as a result of direct vascular trauma or secondarily as a result of rapid drainage of an enlarged ventricular system. These complications can be minimized by utilizing the sites of entry previously described and avoiding the procedure in patients with abnormal clotting mechanisms. A treacherous problem can arise through the use of a rigid cannula such as a ventricular needle. Because of the difficulty in stabilizing such a needle, especially in a thrashing infant, the needle may be torqued about its pivotal point at the skull, sweeping a wide arc through the brain. Because of its communication with the ventricular system, the needle track can become permanent and even enlarge as a result of CSF pulsation, giving rise to so-called needle porencephaly. Seizures due to ventricular puncture are rare, and prophylactic anticonvulsants are not recommended in general, although many patients undergoing ventricular puncture may be taking anticonvulsants for other reasons. If the ventricular catheter is utilized for instillation of chemotherapeutic agents, it is mandatory that the exit ports of the catheter are placed in CSF pathways and not intraparenchymal, as many antineoplastic agents are cytotoxic. We have had personal experience with an intense inflammatory response around the intraparenchymal catheter ports that mimicked a mass lesion in a patient receiving intraventricular methotrexate. A final complication, rarely seen, may occur in patients who undergo ventricular decompression for hydrocephalus due to a large posterior fossa mass. Pathological and clinical experience suggests that the pressure differential between supra- and infratentorial compartments is enough to cause upward herniation of the cerebellum through the incisura.[4]

Uses of Ventricular Puncture

Although access to the ventricles is required for both diagnostic and therapeutic purposes, the measurement and/or treatment of increased intracranial pressure is the most common goal. The standard range of ICP is 50 to 200 mm H_2O with the patient in the lateral recumbent position. In addition to the waveforms described by Lundberg[15] there are rhythmic variations of CSF pressure with pulse and respiration. Ventricular puncture provides direct measurement of ICP variations. In most cases drainage of small amounts of CSF will temporarily restore elevated ICP to near normal levels.[6]

Another diagnostic use of ventricular puncture is the placement of radiographic contrast agents into the third and lateral ventricles. Air was the first contrast agent used, but it often requires significant manipulation of the patient and does not always provide high-quality films. Water-soluble iodinated contrast agents (e.g., 60% methylglucamine iothalamate, metrizamide) provide better contrast for both plain radiography and CT scanning but have been associated with occasional transient neurological defects (e.g., cortical blindness) and seizures when allowed to collect over the cerebral cortex.

CNS chemotherapy often requires ventricular instillation because medications placed in the lumbar subarachnoid space may be present in very low concentrations in the ventricles as a result of poor retrograde circulation of CSF or mechanical obstruction. This is an important consideration in the treatment and laboratory follow-up of infections or malignancies involving the ventricular system and mandates direct access to ventricular CSF.

References

1. Adson AW, Lillie WL: The relationship of intracranial pressure, choked disc, and intraocular tension. Trans Am Acad Ophthalmol 30:138–154, 1927.
2. Bering EA Jr: A simplified apparatus for constant ventricular drainage. J Neurosurg 8:450–452, 1951.
3. Chandler WF, Knake JE, McGillicuddy JE, Lillehei KO, Silver TM: Intraoperative use of real time ultrasonography in neurosurgery. J Neurosurg 57:157–163, 1982.
4. Cuneo RA, Caronna JJ, Pitts L, Townsend J, Winestock DP: Upward transtentorial herniation: Seven cases and a literature review. Arch Neurol 36:618–623, 1979.
5. Dandy WE: Ventriculography following the injection of air into the cerebral ventricles. Ann Surg 68:5–11, 1918.
6. Fleischer AS, Patton JM, Tindall GT: Monitoring intraventricular pressure using an implanted reservoir in head injured patients. Surg Neurol 3:309–311, 1975.
7. Friedman WA, Vries JK: Percutaneous tunnel ventriculostomy: Summary of 100 procedures. J Neurosurg 53:662–665, 1980.
8. Fulton JF: *Harvey Cushing: A Biography*. Springfield, Ill, Charles C Thomas, 1946, p 490.
9. Hill BL: *American Eclectic System of Surgery*. Cincinnati: W Phillips and Co, 1850, p 608.
10. Ingraham FD, Campbell JB: An apparatus for closed drainage of the ventricular system. Ann Surg 114:1096–1098, 1941.
11. Kaufmann GE, Clark K: Emergency frontal twist drill ventriculostomy: Technical note, J Neurosurg 33:226–227, 1970.
12. Keen WW: Surgery of the lateral ventricles of the brain. Med News 57:275–278, 1890.
13. Keen WW, White JW (eds): *An American Textbook of Surgery for Practitioners and Students*, Philadelphia: Saunders, 1892, p 490.
14. Kempe LG: *Operative Neurosurgery*. New York, Springer-Verlag, 1970, vol 2, p 1.
15. Lundberg N: Continuous recording and control of ventricular fluid pressure in neurosurgical practice. Acta Psychiatr Scand [suppl] 149:1–193, 1960.
16. Navarro IM, Renteria JAG, Peralta VHR, Castilli MAD: Transorbital ventricular puncture for emergency ventricular decompression. J Neurosurg 54:273–274, 1981.
17. Ratcheson RA, Heilbrun MP: Computerized tomographic stereotaxic guidance systems, in Haaga JR, Alfidi RJ (eds): *Computed Tomography of the Whole Body*. St. Louis, Mosby, 1983, pp 1005–1008.
18. Ratcheson RA, Ommaya AK: Experience with the subcutaneous cerebrospinal-fluid reservoir: Preliminary report of 60 cases. N Engl J Med 279:1025–1031, 1968.
19. Robertson JT, Denton IC Jr: Surgical considerations of ventriculography, in Youmans JR (ed), *Neurological Surgery*, 2d ed. Philadelphia, Saunders, 1982, pp 375–381.
20. Robinson F: An apparatus for continuous ventricular drainage and intraventricular therapy. J Neurosurg 5:320–323, 1948.
21. Tillmanns H: Something about puncture of the brain. Br Med J 2:983–984, 1908.
22. White RJ, Dakters JG, Yashon D, Albin MS: Temporary control of cerebrospinal fluid volume and pressure by means of an externalized valve-drainage system. J Neurosurg 30:264–269, 1969.
23. Wyler AR, Kelly WA: Use of antibiotics with external ventriculostomies. J Neurosurg 37:185–187, 1972.

14
Intracranial Pressure Monitoring

Gerald D. Silverberg

Intracranial pressure (ICP) normally varies between 100 and 180 mmH$_2$O (10 to 15 mmHg) when measured from a lumbar puncture with a patient in the lateral decubitus position. Intracranial pressure, however, is posture-dependent, and when one is standing up, the intracranial pressure may be negative when compared with atmospheric pressure.

In many neurological conditions, intracranial pressure may be elevated. This elevation may be generalized or have a focal origin, depending upon the cause. In toxic or metabolic disorders, such as Reye's syndrome, brain swelling is diffuse and ICP may be elevated equally throughout the cranium. In focal brain lesions, such as tumors or hematomas, pressure may be higher in the region of the tumor compared with other areas within the skull, creating a pressure gradient. Raised intracranial pressure may cause neurological dysfunction by interfering with cerebrovascular perfusion (increasing the resistance to blood flow) and by herniation of brain tissue along a pressure gradient. Raised intracranial pressure is a common cause of death in neurosurgical cases.

Although Cushing reported the changes in vital signs seen with cerebral compression in experimental animals,[3] interest in the clinical measurement of ICP began much later. In 1951, Guillaume and Janny studied continuous ICP monitoring,[5] and in 1953, Ryder et al. showed that changes in cerebrospinal fluid (CSF) volume changed the ICP.[9] Lundberg in 1960 reported his observations on continuous ICP monitoring in 130 neurosurgical patients, the measurements being made via an indwelling catheter within the lateral ventricle.[6] He meticulously noted the variety of pressure phenomena associated with intracranial mass lesions and sought to correlate pressure wave patterns with clinical conditions. He described three waveforms: A waves occurred upon a background of raised pressure. The amplitude of the A wave would vary from 50 to 100 mmHg and persist for 5 to 20 min. The longer A waves have also been called *plateau waves*. Symptoms thought to be due to raised intracranial pressure, such as headache, decreasing level of consciousness, nausea, vomiting, visual blurring, pupillary changes, decerebrate posturing, blood pressure elevation, bradycardia, and hyperventilation, seemed to be temporally related

to the appearance of plateau waves. Resolution of the plateau waves by hyperventilation, osmotic diuresis, or CSF drainage was accompanied by improvement in the patient's condition. Lundberg also described oscillations of 0.2 to 2 cycles per minute (cpm) that appeared to be related to respirations. He termed these B waves, and 4 to 8-cpm waves, related to systemic pulse fluctuations, were termed C waves. B and C waves have not proved to be of value in clinical situations. The close correlation between a worsening clinical picture and the appearance of plateau waves, however, made it evident that monitoring ICP could predict somewhat the clinical course of a patient suffering from intracranial hypertension (Fig. 14-1).

It was a short step then from being able to predict which patients were getting into trouble to an attempt at altering the outcome of conditions associated with raised ICP by controlling intracranial tension within defined limits. A number of neurosurgical centers studied a wide variety of conditions, such as head trauma, brain tumors, subarachnoid hemorrhage, occult hydrocephalus, Reye's syndrome, and other toxic-metabolic encephalopathies, and did routine monitoring of all craniotomy cases in an effort to define which patients would be benefited by ICP monitoring and careful control of intracranial pressure. Some differences of opinion have arisen concerning the value of constant ICP monitoring in several of the above conditions. With the attendant risks of the more invasive monitoring systems, a reappraisal of the various methods of monitoring as well as a more careful patient selection became necessary.

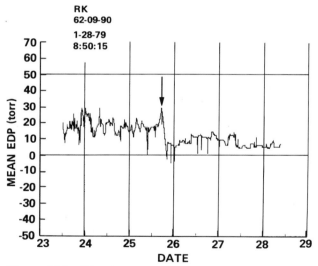

Figure 14-1 Five-day trace of the mean ICP in a patient suffering the effects of a severe closed head injury. Over the first 48 h, a number of pressure waves occurred. These could be resolved with hyperventilation and osmotic diuresis. During the evening of January 25, however, the patient's ICP continued to rise despite these maneuvers. The patient was taken to the operating room and a large decompression was done. ICP from then on remained below 20 torr, although the patient did not regain consciousness. The arrow marks the point of surgical decompression.

Methods of Measuring Intracranial Pressure

An ideal system for measuring intracranial pressure should be accurate, free of risk to the patient, and simple to use. Unfortunately, no monitoring system presently available meets these criteria. All are invasive to some degree. Usually the less invasive the technique, the less accurate and more complicated it is to use. The majority of systems require some connection between the intracranial space and an external pressure-sensitive transducer or recording system, but newer systems utilizing an implantable, telemetered transducer are being developed.

Presently available monitoring systems can be divided into fluid- and nonfluid-coupled systems. The fluid-coupled systems have either a fluid-filled catheter or hollow bolt in communication with the lateral ventricle, the cerebrospinal fluid over the cerebral convexity, or the subdural space. The sensing element is connected to a manometer or a pressure-sensitive transducer. The transducer converts the hydraulic pressure to an electrical signal that may then be displayed on an oscilloscope or digital readout and recorded on a strip chart or onto magnetic tape. Non-fluid-coupled units depend upon a pressure-sensitive transducer mounted in the skull with the pressure-sensing surface either open to the subdural space or external to the dura.[8] These units then transmit the pressure as an electrical signal via wires to a display and recording device. The majority of these units are some variant of a Wheatstone bridge, but inductive and capacitative-coupled oscillating circuits as well as an optical transducer have been described.

The intraventricular catheter is placed through a twist drill hole or burr hole usually positioned on the nondominant side anterior to the coronal suture. Under rigidly aseptic conditions, the catheter is passed into the frontal horn of the ipsilateral lateral ventricle and connected to a pressure transducer zeroed to the atmosphere at the level of the frontal horn. A three-way stopcock is positioned at the pressure transducer to allow for irrigation of the catheter by a tuberculin syringe. Usually no more than 0.1 ml of fluid is required to unblock the catheter should it become occluded. The distal end of the catheter is best tunneled under the scalp and exited at some distance from the twist drill incision to avoid a CSF leak around the catheter and to retard infection. The catheter must be securely sutured to the scalp to prevent its migration. Ventricular catheters are presently available with a sliding flange that facilitates securing the catheter without kinking or occluding it with the suture. A closed drainage system is also available from the same company to minimize the risk of infection in patients that require CSF drainage to control elevated ICP (Cordis Corporation, Miami, Fla.).

The subarachnoid bolt is also inserted through a twist drill hole, again placed on the nondominant side anterior to the coronal suture. The bolt has self-tapping screw threads that seat into the skull. The dura and arachnoid are opened to allow continuous fluid coupling between the subarachnoid space over the cerebral convexity and an external pressure transducer through the hollow bolt. The device is modified on top to provide a standard intravenous tubing connection. With all hydraulic systems, rigid arterial pressure tubing is preferred over standard intravenous tubing to minimize damping of the pressure signal by tube capacitance. Infant-size and pediatric-size bolts are now available for infants and small children who require ICP monitoring (Philadelphia Medical Specialties, Inc., Laurel Springs, N.J.).

Monitoring ICP from the subdural space is accomplished by a silastic catheter with a recessed cup at its distal end. The catheter is fluid-filled and connected to any pressure-sensitive transducer and recording-display system. It is a fairly bulky catheter and would not be easily inserted through a burr hole, particularly if the brain were swollen. It is more suited to placement beneath the dura following a craniotomy in order to monitor ICP postoperatively. With all fluid-coupled systems, the presence of an undamped pulse wave assures the physician that the intracranial end is patent. The external transducer may be checked easily for zero-point drift, sensitivity, and hysteresis, and may be recalibrated at any time while a patient is being monitored.

All the above monitoring techniques have significant drawbacks, which will be discussed later. All suffer from the risk of infection, brain damage, and occlusion of the sensing device with increasing brain swelling. The patient is also confined to bed. Therefore, over the past 10 to 15 years, an effort has been made to perfect an implantable electronic transducer that could be telemetered through the intact scalp, eliminating a good deal of the risk of infection, reducing the risk of brain injury, and eliminating the risk of catheter or bolt occlusion. Ideally, such a device would be positioned in a burr hole epidurally and be completely implantable, being energized and recorded from through an intact scalp. Because of its inaccessibility once implanted, it would have to be very stable both electrically and mechanically. It would need to have no significant zero drift, minimal hysteresis, and negligible change in sensitivity. It would need to be impervious to the variety of electronic and radiofrequency signals prevalent in intensive care units and operating rooms as well as inert to tissue fluids. Myriad attempts have been made by many biomedical engineering teams to perfect such a device, but the majority have not reached fruition. Several hard-wired units are available, but none have met with uniform acceptance. Here at Stanford, we have had a long experience with such a unit. Using NASA technology, we succeeded in fabricating an acceptable prototype telemetered unit and have had a commercial firm succeed in working out an assembly line production technique. The first group of units has been produced, and they are presently undergoing rigorous testing for stability and biocompatibility.

Indications for Intracranial Pressure Monitoring

Since the general acceptance of intracranial pressure monitoring as a clinically useful tool by the neurosurgical community, a spectrum of neurosurgical problems have been monitored and a great variety of pathological conditions have perhaps been better understood and treated more appropriately. If raised intracranial pressure exerts its ill effects by increasing resistance to blood flow and, therefore, reducing cerebral perfusion as well as by causing brain injury from herniation, it would seem reasonable that the earlier the pressure was brought down to normal, the less likely it would be that the patient would suffer permanent harm.

As many clinicians have learned to their sorrow, patients may harbor an expanding intracranial lesion without manifesting clinical signs of raised pressure until late in the course of their illness. The more attention-getting symptoms, such as decreasing level of consciousness, paralysis, and changing vital signs may not occur until just prior to fatal herniation. The frequent lack of close correlation between the size of a lesion and its symptoms can be best understood if one appreciates the pressure-volume-time relationships within the skull. The skull is a rigid container in the adult, though the intracranial space is not a completely fixed volume since it communicates through the foramen magnum with the spinal subarachnoid space. The intracranial contents may be looked at as three compartments: brain tissue, blood volume, and CSF volume. These three compartments exist in dynamic equilibrium normally at a pressure of 10 to 15 torr (mmHg). Enlargement of any compartment must be at the expense of another compartment if ICP is to remain at normal levels. Initially, an expanding mass is compensated for by displacement of CSF out of the intracranial cavity primarily into the spinal subarachnoid space and perhaps by decreased production and increased absorption of CSF. Compression of the blood volume may also contribute added space, mainly on the capillary and venous side of the circulation. Compression and, over time, atrophy of normal brain tissue also occurs to accommodate a mass lesion.

The ability of the intracranial cavity to absorb an increase in volume without a significant increase in pressure is termed *compliance*. This is a time-dependent function. The slower growing the lesion, the more readily the brain, CSF, and blood compartments can be compressed to make room for the mass without a rapid increase in intracranial pressure. Decreasing compliance occurs when the intracranial space is "tight." This usually occurs in neurosurgical practice because of an increase in brain volume, frequently from tumor mass or edema or increased blood volume secondary to loss of vascular tone. It may also occur from obstruction to the pathways of CSF flow and absorption. When compliance decreases, a small increment of volume added to the intracranial space causes a significant rise in pressure (Fig. 14-2). Compliance curves can be constructed for any patient with an ICP monitor by adding mock CSF or saline at known volume increments over a specified time. The heart also adds a volume of blood to the brain with each cardiac output. The resultant expansion of the brain produces the pulse wave seen in ICP tracings. Computer programs are being devised to assess the change in amplitude and the slope of the rising phase of the pulse wave as a function of compliance.

Head-injured patients have provided a fertile ground for research in raised intracranial pressure.[1,4] Various monitoring techniques, therapeutic regimens, and statistical analyses of outcome have led to some conflict of opinion concerning the value of ICP monitoring and aggressive therapy in controlling elevated ICP in the patient with severe head injuries. Initial studies seemed to suggest that (1) most patients who die following severe head injuries suffered from raised ICP, (2) ICP monitoring could predict which patients

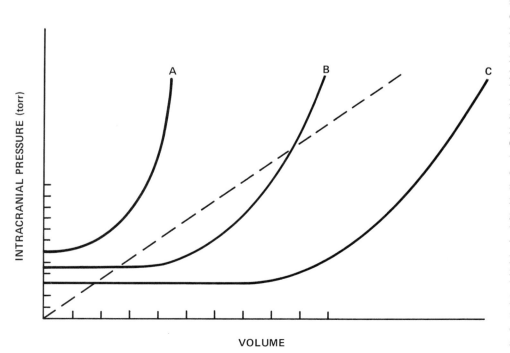

Figure 14-2 Hypothetical pressure-volume relationships in various states of compliance. If curve B represents the normal state, then curve A would represent decreased compliance, where a given volume added to the intracranial compartment results in a greater pressure rise than in the normal state. Curve C would represent a situation of greater than normal compliance and might be seen in a patient with significant brain atrophy. A greater than normal volume of intracranial CSF would then have to be displaced from the intracranial space before pressure began to rise. The dashed line represents a theoretical system of a closed, rigid container being filled with a compressible substance.

were in the severe-risk group, and (3) aggressive therapy aimed at reducing ICP to less than 20 torr significantly reduced mortality and morbidity in these patients. Other investigators, however, could not confirm the last finding, and, indeed, some investigators seemed to suggest that patients treated with an aggressive multimodal therapeutic regimen aimed at reducing ICP actually had increased morbidity and mortality. What seems to be closest to the truth is that the single most influential factor in the head-injured patient is the extent of the biostructural injury. If the injury is severe enough, the patient will die or remain in a vegetative state regardless of what is done to the ICP, while if it is less severe, the patient will survive with or without some neurological deficit with standard supportive care. Between these two subgroups there probably exists a relatively small number of patients, not sufficient to influence the statistical evaluation of the whole group, that are potentially salvageable if ICP is brought down to normal and kept there, whereas such a patient might die or end up severely crippled neurologically if ICP were not carefully controlled. At the present time, it is not possible to define the "vulnerable" group that would benefit from ICP monitoring, so one is obliged to monitor all head-injured patients that are comatose and treat elevated ICP aggressively.

In certain neurosurgical problems, the indications for ICP monitoring are more clear-cut. For instance, in children with CNS manifestations of Reye's syndrome, ICP monitoring and very aggressive ICP control clearly seems beneficial. In our experience, the majority of these patients now recover without significant neurological deficit. In patients suffering from the syndrome of occult hydrocephalus (gait apraxia, dementia, nocturnal incontinence, and large ventricles as seen on CT scan), shunting appears to improve the neurological deficit. When the syndrome is complete and there is some underlying cause for hydrocephalus, such as a prior head injury, meningitis, or subarachnoid hemorrhage, the patient should probably simply be shunted. However, not unusually, the clinical presentation can be less straightforward, particularly when the patient presents with just dementia and large ventricles. The differential diagnosis also includes a number of degenerative brain diseases that are not benefited by shunting. In these cases, ICP monitoring as a diagnostic test is helpful.[10] Patients that display pressure waves (usually nocturnal) will most likely be helped by a functioning shunt. If, over 1 or 2 days of monitoring, there is no elevation of CSF pressure, one can be fairly certain that a shunt will do no good.

Several neurosurgical centers have reported that ICP monitoring is of value in patients suffering from subarachnoid hemorrhage.[7] ICP elevation may predict rebleeding, and ICP monitoring will allow an estimate of cerebral perfusion pressure (CPP). Since one can probably decrease the rate of rebleeding by lowering systemic arterial pressure (SAP), it is desirable to keep such patients at as low a blood pressure as they can tolerate until surgical correction of the bleeding source (aneurysm or arteriovenous malformation) can be accomplished. It may not be necessary to monitor those patients that are awake and without significant neurological deficit since the patient's clinical condition can be used to titrate the blood pressure. Systemic pressure can then be lowered to levels consistent with maintaining the patient's neurological state intact. However, in those patients who are obtunded, where rigid control of systemic arterial pressure may be more hazardous, ICP monitoring can be helpful to ensure a reasonable cerebral perfusion pressure (CPP = SAP − ICP).

The use of high-dose barbiturate therapy in a number of neurosurgical cases has provided a measure of cerebral protection from ischemia and anoxia. Barbiturates are also used for decreasing intracranial pressure.[2] In those cases where barbiturates may be necessary to lower ICP, such as severe head injury or in Reyés syndrome, monitoring the ICP provides an end point for therapy. In cases where barbiturates in high doses are used as an adjunct to neuroanesthesia, particularly where blood flow to some or all of the brain may have to be stopped for a time, postoperative monitoring of ICP is important until the patient recovers consciousness and can be followed in the usual way. During the 24 h or so after high-dose barbiturates have been administered, the patient may remain in barbiturate coma and not be accessible to the usual postoperative testing. ICP elevation has alerted us to such surgical complications as a postoperative hematoma or brain swelling before irreversible damage has occurred.

ICP monitoring of all craniotomy cases will probably become routine only when the risks of monitoring are significantly less than the complication rate for which one is monitoring and when monitoring can be made simple and easy for both the patient and the surgeon. With the continued improvements in pre- and postoperative care, neuroanesthesia, and operative technique, complications requiring re-exploration have become gratifyingly uncommon. Presently the extra time required, the added risk attendant upon invasive monitoring, and the added inconvenience to the patient, tying him or her to a hard-wired or hydraulic pressure system, makes the value of routine monitoring questionable in many surgeons' minds. When a completely implantable, telemetered system capable of being easily placed in one of the craniotomy burr holes at the end of the procedure becomes available, then routine monitoring of ICP will probably become as prevalent as arterial pressure and central venous pressure monitoring in the postoperative care of craniotomy cases.

Risks of ICP Monitoring

The risks of ICP monitoring are directly related to the degree of invasiveness of the monitoring system used. The risks are primarily those of infection and brain injury. There is also, particularly in the case of implantable transducers, the risk of poor therapeutic choices based on inaccurate data.

Hydraulic-coupled systems are most prone to infectious complications. Indeed, most neurosurgeons fear infection so much that they will only maintain the patient on these monitoring systems for 72 h. Infection of a subarachnoid bolt usually means meningitis for the patient, while infection of a ventricular cannula results in ventriculitis and occasionally brain abscess as well. The actual incidence of infectious complications varies from center to center and probably is directly related to how carefully one looks for it and inversely related to how organized and specialized the critical care units are that care for these patients. Anywhere from 5 to 15 percent infection rates have been reported for fluid-coupled systems. The varying figures in the main reflect the criteria set by the authors for documenting infection: clinical signs, temperature, blood counts, CSF cell counts, protein and glucose determinations, and cultures. Since many neurosurgeons treat patients on monitoring systems with prophylactic antibiotics either systemically or into the monitoring system or both, patients may be infected yet not grow out any organisms on culture. If infection occurs, the outcome may be lethal, considering the already compromised brain. Frequently the monitoring device must be discontinued, and if ventricular drainage were critical, one has to maintain ICP control by frequent ventricular taps.

Brain injury probably occurs more frequently than one can assess, particularly if the patient is already severely injured. Multiple passes through an already damaged, friable brain in an attempt to locate a small, perhaps shifted, lateral ventricle cannot be terribly beneficial. With the advent of more frequent high-resolution CT scanning, small hemorrhages along the tract of the ventricular cannula are becoming a more commonplace finding. In order to avoid penetration of the brain, many neurosurgeons use the subarachnoid bolt. However, there are hazards associated with this device as well. Subdural hematomas have been reported following bolt placement, and I have seen edematous brain extruded from the bolt in cases of severe brain swelling from head injury and from Reyés syndrome.

Poor therapy based on inaccurate data can occur with any monitoring system. Intraventricular catheters can occlude, subarachnoid bolts may become obstructed by meninges or brain, and external transducers may malfunction. These problems are usually obvious and are reasonably easy to correct. Damping of the CSF pulse waveform denotes obstruction of the catheter or bolt. Irrigation will usually clear the obstruction. External transducers may be easily recalibrated or exchanged. Completely implanted transducers, however, may provide an acceptable waveform while the zero point drifts into unacceptable error ranges or the sensitivity changes. Such units will require many months of testing in the laboratory and many hours of monitoring patients before one can place any confidence in them. Eventually, I believe they will replace all the presently available systems.

Practical Considerations in ICP Monitoring

There are probably now sufficient data to warrant the use of ICP monitoring in any neurosurgical case where intracranial pressure elevation is a potential or actual threat. Head-injury patients in coma, subarachnoid hemorrhage patients who are hypertensive and obtunded, children with Reye's syndrome, surgical cases that may be prone to ventricular obstruction or cerebral swelling, and patients being evaluated for occult hydrocephalus may all be considered reasonable candidates for ICP monitoring.

The choice of monitoring systems will depend upon the experience of the surgeon and the available equipment. At present, there is no clear-cut advantage to any one system. The choice of device may well be dictated by the particular circumstances of each case. Patients harboring a tumor obstructing the ventricles are probably best served by an intraventricular catheter, allowing pressure monitoring as well as ventricular drainage should it be required. Patients with massive edema of the brain and slitlike ventricles might be best managed by a subarachnoid bolt or epidural transducer. Postoperative monitoring of more routine craniotomy cases could be managed by a subdural catheter.

ICP monitoring should aid in the early detection of potentially dangerous elevations of intracranial pressure. It should be safe and simple to use. Effective and reliable ICP measurement should provide a measure of reassurance that all is going well or alert the neurosurgeon that something may be amiss before irretrievable damage occurs to the patient.

References

1. Becker DP, Miller JD, Ward JD, Greenberg RP, Young HF, Sakalas R: The outcome from severe head injury with early diagnosis and intensive management. J Neurosurg 47:491–502, 1977.
2. Bruce DA, Raphaely RA, Swedlow D, Schut L: The effectiveness of iatrogenic barbiturate coma in controlling increased ICP in 61 children, in Shulman K, Marmarou A, Miller JD, Becker DP, Hochwald GM, Brock M (eds), *Intracranial Pressure IV*. New York, Springer-Verlag, 1980, pp 630–632.
3. Cushing H: Concerning a definite regulatory mechanism of the vaso-motor center which controls blood pressure during cerebral compression. Johns Hopkins Med J 12:290–292, 1901.
4. Fleischer AS, Payne NS, Tindall GT: Continuous monitoring of intracranial pressure in severe closed head injury without mass lesions. Surg Neurol 6:31–34, 1976.
5. Guillaume J, Janny P: Manométrie intracranienne continue: Intérêt de la méthode et premiers résultats. Rev Neurol (Paris) 84:131–142, 1951.
6. Lundberg N: Continuous recording and control of ventricular fluid pressure in neurosurgical practice. Acta Psychiatr Scand [Suppl] 149:1–193, 1960.
7. Nornes H, Magnaes B: Intracranial pressure in patients with ruptured saccular aneurysm. J Neurosurg 36:537–547, 1972.
8. Ream AK, Silverberg GD, Corbin SD, Schmidt EV, Fryer TB: Epidural measurement of intracranial pressure. Neurosurgery 5:36–43, 1979.
9. Ryder HW, Espey FF, Kimbell FD, Penka EJ, Rosenauer A, Podolsky B, Evans JP: The mechanism of the change in cerebrospinal fluid pressure following an induced change in the volume of fluid space. J Lab Clin Med 41:428–435, 1953.
10. Symon L, Dorsch NWC: Use of long-term intracranial pressure measurement to assess hydrocephalic patients prior to shunt surgery. J Neurosurg 42:258–273, 1975.

15

Cerebrospinal Fluid: Techniques of Access and Analytical Interpretation

James H. Wood

The physiological compartmentalization of the central nervous system not only provides protection of its delicate function from aberrant peripheral influences but also impedes its diagnostic evaluation.[29] The cerebrospinal fluid (CSF) bathes the brain and spinal cord, is in physiological continuity with their extracellular fluid,[19] and reflects the state of health or disease of the central nervous system.[32] Chemical and cellular analysis of CSF has become increasingly important in neurosurgical patient evaluations. The purpose of this chapter is to review the techniques of CSF access[30] and the interpretation of CSF findings associated with neurological disorders. For further information concerning more experimental and research-oriented topics dealing with the neurochemistry of CSF, readers are referred to other reviews by the author.[9,29,30,31,32,33]

Historical Background

Although Corning first performed spinal subarachnoid injections of cocaine in patients in 1885, Quincke is given credit for the development of the percutaneous technique of lumbar puncture with needles containing stylets in 1891. Quincke also measured the intrathecal pressure employing a manometer and determined the cellular, glucose, and protein content of CSF. In that same year, Wynter drained spinal CSF through a trocar using a cutdown incision in patients with meningitis. Froin, in 1903, described the CSF coagulation, and Queckenstedt, in 1916, described the manometric findings associated with spinal subarachnoid blockage. In 1918, Dandy described the ventricular puncture,

and 2 years later Ayer introduced the technique of cisternal puncture. (See reviews by Fishman[5] and Tourtellotte and Shorr.[26])

Indications for CSF Analysis

Following funduscopic and computed tomographic (CT) examination, CSF analysis is indicated in patients suspected of having central nervous system bacterial, fungal, or viral infections as well as subarachnoid hemorrhage (SAH). As in cases of suspected brain abscess, the use of CSF examination in the detection of hemorrhagic infarctions in stroke patients has been supplanted by CT. CSF analysis is useful in the diagnosis of demyelinating and degenerative disorders. Cytological examination of CSF often enables identification of desquamated cells from central primary or metastatic tumors and meningeal cancer.

CSF pressure recordings are useful in the diagnosis of pseudotumor cerebri and normal-pressure hydrocephalus as well as in the monitoring of head-injured patients. CSF drainage is often used therapeutically in cases of communicating hydrocephalus and CSF fistulas. Access to the CSF compartment is required for neuroradiological procedures such as ventriculography, pneumoencephalography, cisternography, and myelography. In addition, intrathecal administration of antimicrobial and antineoplastic agents normally excluded by the blood-brain barrier enables the achievement of therapeutic central concentrations.

Technique of Lumbar Puncture and Chronic Spinal CSF Drainage

The patient is usually placed in the horizontal knee-chest position with the site of spinal needle insertion at the same level as the external occipital protuberance. An 18- or 20-gauge spinal needle is preferred when manometric recordings are to be obtained so as not to dampen respiratory variations in CSF pressure. A 22-gauge needle should be employed to avoid large dural holes in patients suspected of having increased intracranial pressure. Small-gauge needles also decrease the incidence of post-lumbar puncture headache. Spinal needles should always be inserted with stylet or obturator in place so as to ensure patency, to avoid the transfer of skin or subcutaneous tissue into the subarachnoid space, and to prevent iatrogenic intraspinal epidermoid tumors.

The optimum puncture site in adults lies in the midline beneath the spinous process at the third and fourth lumbar interspace. This level is located on an imaginary line extending between the superior iliac crests and avoids the conus medullaris, which may extend as low as the second lumbar level. Lumbar punctures should be performed at the fourth and fifth lumbar interspace in children and between the fifth lumbar and first sacral spinous processes in infants so as to avoid the conus medullaris, which may lie as caudal as the third and fourth lumbar interspace.

The skin is cleansed with antiseptic solution and then infiltrated with a local anesthetic agent. The bevel of the lumbar puncture needle point should enter the dura parallel to the longitudinal fibers of the dura mater. This needle orientation will minimize the size of the dural hole by spreading rather than cutting the dural fibers. A tactile sensation may be experienced during dural penetration, and the initiation of CSF flow may be prompted by performing a half-turn of the needle hub so that the bevel faces rostrally. The manometer should be attached to the needle hub immediately after CSF flow is established, and an opening pressure in millimeters of water recorded with the patient's legs partially extended. Needle patency is documented by abdominal-compression–induced or respiration-evoked fluctuations in CSF pressure. The presence of CSF pressure above 240 mm H_2O in a relaxed patient using this technique[30] is considered abnormally elevated[7] and precludes further CSF drainage. The CSF within the manometer should then be used for diagnostic analysis.

In obese patients, lumbar punctures may be difficult and the sitting position may be an aid in needle orientation. Immediately after the initiation of CSF flow, sterile plastic tubing should be attached to the spinal needle hub. The CSF pressure should normally cause the CSF within the tubing to rise only to the level of the foramen magnum.[16]

Chronic spinal CSF drainage has classically been accomplished by passing a fine catheter through a 14-gauge Touhy spinal needle (Becton-Dickinson Company, Rutherford, N.J.) and removing this needle over the catheter. Despite care being taken to secure this catheter to the skin without kinking, this standard technique has been plagued by diffi-

culty in maintaining patency. An alternative method[21] involves placing a no. 5 French Stamey ureteral catheter (American Latex Corporation, Sullivan, Ind.) with mutiple side holes at the tip in the lumbar subarachnoid space. A 14-gauge Touhy needle is inserted into a low lumbar interspace, and thereafter the bevel is turned cephalad. The Stamey ureteral catheter is advanced through the bore of the Touhy needle to the first lumbar level. The catheter stylus and needle are then removed, and a blunt-ended 20-gauge needle with Intramedic Luer Stub Adapter (Clay Adams Division of Becton-Dickinson Company, Parsippany, N.J.) is connected to the catheter. This Luer adapter facilitates the connection of the ureteral catheter to a closed drainage system[28]. Patients undergoing prolonged spinal drainage usually receive prophylactic antibiotics.

Spinal Subarachnoid Blockage

Manual compression of both jugular veins (Queckenstedt's test) induces cerebral venous engorgement and a rapid rise of intracranial pressure that normally is transmitted to the lumbar subarachnoid space.[25] A prompt elevation of CSF pressure on light or deep jugular vein compression with rapid return to baseline after the release of compression indicates the absence of spinal canal blockage (Fig. 15-1). A prompt rise but a slow fall in CSF pressure after deep jugular vein compression and a failure of CSF pressure to return to the baseline level after release suggests an incomplete subarachnoid obstruction (Fig. 15-2). With complete spinal canal blockage, the elevation in CSF pressure is greater following straining or abdominal compression than after deep

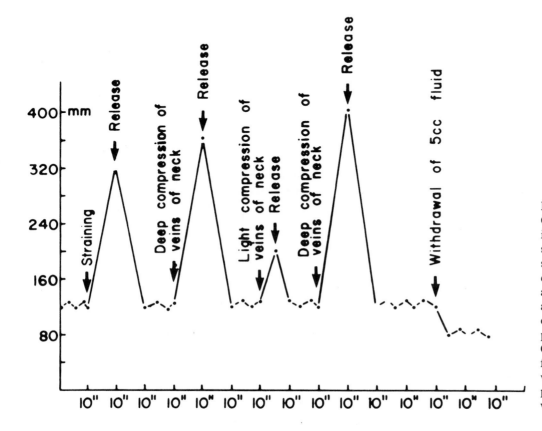

Figure 15-1 Lumbar CSF manometric chart in patient with normal spinal subarachnoid space. Note normal oscillations of respiration and pulse, rapid rise and fall of CSF pressure on straining, and prompt rise and fall of CSF pressure on superficial and deep jugular vein compression. (Reprinted from Wood,[30] with permission.)

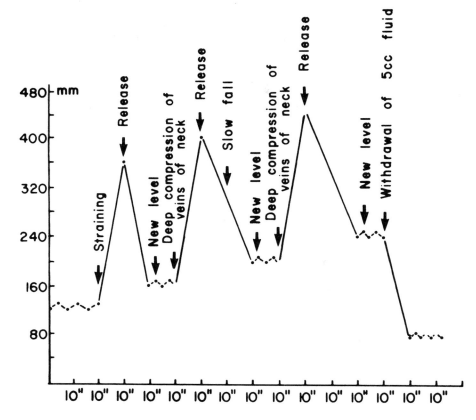

Figure 15-2 Lumbar CSF manometric chart in patient with incomplete spinal subarachnoid block. Note higher CSF pressure level after each trial of straining or jugular compression. Also note prompt rise and slow fall of CSF pressure after deep compression of jugular veins. (Reprinted from Wood,[30] with permission.)

jugular vein compression (Fig. 15-3). More accurately quantified manometric evaluations may employ a cervical pressure cuff for graded jugular vein compression. The presence of a complete spinal block precludes further removal of CSF and indicates the need for the intrathecal injection of positive contrast medium and immediate myelography.

Contraindications to Lumbar Puncture

Lumbar punctures are to be avoided if evidence of infection is present in the region of the puncture site. This procedure is generally avoided in the presence of known or suspected increased intracranial pressure or posterior fossa mass lesions if CSF data will not alter therapy, even though reports[12] have documented complications following lumbar puncture in only 1.2 percent of patients with papilledema. Elective lumbar punctures are contraindicated in the presence of known spinal canal blockage in patients with neurological function below the obstruction. This procedure should also be avoided in patients with blood dyscrasias or known spinal cord arteriovenous malformations and those receiving anticoagulants.[30] Contrarily, previous lumbar laminectomy is not a contraindication for lumbar puncture.

Complications of Lumbar Puncture

Lumbar punctures may be complicated by backache, damage to intervertebral discs, nerve root or spinal cord injury, and subarachnoid bleeding from epidural veins. Pain-

ful contact with sensory roots of the cauda equina occurs in about 13 percent of procedures. Post-lumbar puncture headaches occur in approximately 20 percent of patients; they usually remit after 2 to 5 days, but may persist for 8 weeks. The incidence of this headache syndrome may be decreased by employing small-bore needles and draining only the minimum amount of CSF required for study. Maintenance of the prone position for several hours, bed rest, adequate hydration, and mild analgesics reduce the patient's discomfort.

Approximately 9 percent of patients with spontaneous SAH may dramatically deteriorate after lumbar puncture.[3] As many as 60 percent of SAH patients with cerebral dislocation as visualized on CT scanning worsen, whereas patients without mass effect have no neurological deterioration after lumbar puncture.[3] Thus, lumbar puncture, if necessary, should be avoided until a CT scan has been undertaken in patients with SAH. Similarly, patients at risk of harboring brain tumors, abscesses, or empyemas should undergo CT scanning initially instead of lumbar puncture.

Cisternal Puncture

Cisternal punctures are performed with the patient in the lateral decubitus position with shoulders vertical and head flexed. The spinal needle is marked 7.5 cm from its point prior to insertion into the anesthetized scalp in the midline just above the spinous process of the axis. The needle is

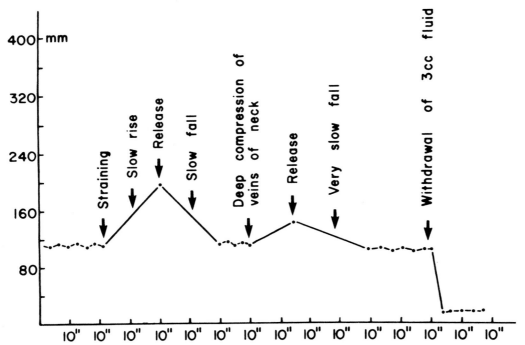

Figure 15-3 Lumbar CSF manometric chart in patient with complete spinal subarachnoid block. Note that rise in CSF pressure is greater on straining than after deep jugular vein compression. (Reprinted from Wood,[30] with permission.)

passed in an upward direction toward the midpoint of an imaginary line through both external auditory meatuses. After it strikes the occipital bone, the needle is redirected slightly downward and passed under the occiput into the cisterna magna. The needle should not be advanced more than 7.5 cm so as to prevent injury to the medulla. If no CSF flow is observed at this depth, an alternative method such as lateral cervical puncture should be employed.

Complications of Cisternal Puncture

This technique for puncture of the cisterna magna is generally safe for cooperative patients, but reported major complications include large-vessel perforation, medullary injury with vomiting or cessation of breathing, and compromise of the vertebral arterial blood supply in elderly patients.[30]

Lateral Cervical Puncture

The lateral cervical approach to the spinal subarachnoid space, initially developed for percutaneous cordotomy, does not require fluoroscopic control.[34] The patient is placed in the supine position, without a pillow and with neck straightened. The puncture site, localized 1 cm caudal and 1 cm dorsal to the tip of the mastoid process (Fig. 15-4), is infiltrated with local anesthetic. The interspace between the atlas and axis lacks bony overlap laterally at the atlantoaxial joint and creates a reasonably wide intervertebral space. A 20-gauge spinal needle is inserted perpendicular to the neck and parallel to the plane of the bed. The stylus must be

removed frequently to check for CSF flow because tactile sensations are experienced as a number of tissue planes are traversed.

Complications of Lateral Cervical Puncture

Slow, careful needle advancement avoids overpenetration of the subarachnoid space and injury to the spinal cord. If the vertebral artery is advertently entered, then the needle should be removed and local pressure applied. Infrequently, a nerve root may be irritated, producing local pain, or the procedure may be followed by headache. Generally, the rate of traumatic taps employing this procedure has been less than 20 percent.[34]

Ventricular Puncture, External Ventricular Drainage, and Subcutaneous CSF Reservoir Installation

These procedures[15,22] are discussed in a previous chapter.

Physiological Neurochemical Composition of CSF

The solute composition of CSF is determined by several factors: (1) metabolism, production, or uptake of solutes by cells of the central nervous system; (2) restriction of intracel-

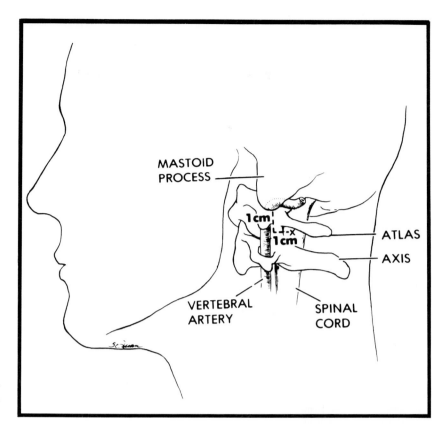

Figure 15-4 Diagram of relationships of major structures and landmarks in the lateral cervical region. Lateral cervical puncture target lies 1 cm caudal and 1 cm dorsal to tip of mastoid process. (Reprinted from Wood,[30] with permission.)

lular diffusion coupled with special transport mechanisms at both the blood-brain and blood-CSF barriers; (3) rates of CSF production and excretion by bulk flow. Interpretation of CSF solute data may be complicated by pharmacological or disease-related alterations in central metabolism, blood-brain-CSF barriers, CSF circulation, or CSF concentration gradients.[32] The steady-state concentrations of various solutes in plasma and lumbar CSF of humans are listed in Tables 15-1 to 15-5.[32]

Glucose

The glucose content in CSF originates from that in plasma and is dependent on the blood glucose level.[32] Glucose transfer from plasma to CSF occurs by carrier-facilitated diffusion. The CSF/plasma ratio for glucose is normally 0.60 to 0.80 but may decrease by saturation kinetics after elevations in blood glucose. The glucose content of CSF is relatively increased in both premature and newborn infants, whose CSF/plasma ratio for glucose is 0.8 or greater. These ratios imply that the rate of glucose removal from CSF is greater than that of its entry into CSF. The concentration of glucose in brain is approximately 20 mg/dl; thus, the brain serves as a sink for both blood and CSF glucose.

Perturbations in plasma glucose content are reflected in parallel changes in CSF glucose concentrations. However, the peak glucose level in CSF may lag 2 h behind that in blood following rapid intravenous glucose infusions, and the CSF level may not return to baseline concentrations for 4 to 6 h after the hyperglycemic episode. Thus, for diagnostic purposes, simultaneous CSF and plasma glucose levels should be compared, preferably with patients in the fasting state.

Hypoglycorrhachia may be masked by hyperglycemia and caused by hypoglycemia, neoplastic or inflammatory infiltrations of the meninges, subarachnoid bleeding, or chemical meningitis. The low CSF glucose levels in meningeal disorders reflect increased glucose utilization by nervous tissue or leukocytes and inhibition of glucose transport. Increased CSF lactate levels always occur with hypoglycorrhachia from any cause except hypoglycemia, reflecting increased anaerobic glycolysis. Contrarily, elevations in CSF glucose do not have diagnostic significance but may reflect hyperglycemia.

Lactic and Pyruvic Acids

The lactic acid content of brain varies with the rate of brain lactate formation but is not related to the blood lactate concentration. Since a blood-CSF barrier exists for lactic acid, the lactate levels in CSF primarily reflect brain lactate content.[32]

The lactate/pyruvate ratio reflects the redox state in the brain and depends in part on lactate dehydrogenase activity. Whenever central glycolysis is augmented during hypoxia, SAH, ischemia, seizures, or nonviral meningitis, both the lactate and pyruvate levels in brain and CSF as well as the lactate/pyruvate ratio are increased.

TABLE 15-1 Solute Composition of Plasma and Lumbar CSF in Humans

Constituent	Units	Plasma	CSF	CSF/Plasma Ratio
Osmolarity	mosm/liter	295	295	1.0
Water content		93%	99%	
Sodium	meq/liter	138	138	1.0
Potassium	meq/liter	4.5	2.8	0.6
Calcium	meq/liter	4.8	2.1	0.4
Magnesium	meq/liter	1.7	2.3	1.4
Phosphorus	mg/dl	4.0	1.6	0.4
Chloride	meq/liter	102	119	1.2
Bicarbonate	meq/liter	24★	22	0.9
P_{CO_2}	mmHg	41★	47	1.1
Ph		7.41★	7.33	
P_{O_2}	mmHg	104★	43	0.4
Glucose	mg/dl	90	60	0.67
Lactate	meq/liter	1.0★	1.6	1.6
Pyruvate	meq/liter	0.11★	0.08	0.73
Lactate/pyruvate ratio		17.6★	26	
Total protein	mg/dl	7000	35	0.005
Total free amino acids	μmol/dl	228	81	0.4
Ammonia	μg/dl	37★	24	0.6
Urea	mmol/liter	5.4	4.7	0.9
Creatinine	mg/dl	1.8	1.2	0.67
Uric acid	mg/dl	5.50	0.25	0.05
Iron	μg/dl	15.0	1.5	0.01
Putrescine	pmol/ml		184	
Spermidine	pmol/ml		150	
Total lipids	mg/dl	750	1.5	0.002

★Arterial plasma.
Source: Derived from review of Fishman.[5]

TABLE 15-2 Amino Acid Composition of Plasma and Lumbar CSF in Humans

Constituent	Units	Plasma	CSF	CSF/Plasma Ratio
Alanine-citrulline	μmol/liter	488.5	34.3	0.08
2-Aminobutyric acid	μmol/liter	29.8	3.5	0.14
Arginine	μmol/liter	80.9	22.4	0.31
Asparagine	μmol/liter	111.7	13.5	0.12
Glutamic acid	μmol/liter	61.3	26.1	0.40
Glutamine	μmol/liter	641.0	552.0	0.86
Glycine	μmol/liter	282.7	5.9	0.02
Histidine	μmol/liter	79.8	12.3	0.16
Isoleucine	μmol/liter	76.7	6.2	0.09
Leucine	μmol/liter	155.3	14.8	0.10
Lysine	μmol/liter	170.7	20.8	0.12
Methionine	μmol/liter	27.7	2.5	0.10
Ornithine	μmol/liter	73.5	3.8	0.06
Phenylalanine	μmol/liter	64.0	9.9	0.17
Phosphoethanolamine	μmol/liter	5.1	5.4	1.05
Phosphoserine	μmol/liter	8.3	4.2	0.58
Serine	μmol/liter	139.7	29.5	0.23
Taurine	μmol/liter	77.2	7.6	0.11
Threonine	μmol/liter	165.5	35.5	0.25
Tyrosine	μmol/liter	73.0	9.5	0.14
Valine	μmol/liter	308.6	19.9	0.07

Source: Data from McGale et al.[18]

TABLE 15-3 Protein Composition of Plasma and Lumbar CSF in Humans

Constituent	Units	Plasma	CSF	CSF/Plasma Ratio
Prealbumin	mg/liter	238	17.3	0.07
Albumin	mg/liter	36,600	155.0	0.004
Transferrin	mg/liter	2,040	14.4	0.007
Ceruloplasmin	mg/liter	366	1.0	0.003
IgG	mg/liter	9,870	12.3	0.001
IgA	mg/liter	1,750	1.3	0.0007
α_2-Macroglobulin	mg/liter	2,220	2.0	0.0009
Fibrinogen	mg/liter	2,964	0.6	0.0002
IgM	mg/liter	700	0.6	0.0009
β-Lipoprotein	mg/liter	3,728	0.6	0.0002

Source: Data from Felgenhauer.[4]

TABLE 15-4 Neurotransmitter, Metabolite, and Cyclic Nucleotide Composition of Lumbar CSF in Humans

Constituent	Units	CSF
Acetylcholine	μM	0.07
	pmol/ml	187
γ-Aminobutyric acid	pmol/ml	233
Norepinephrine	pg/ml	373
3-Methoxy-4-hydroxyphenylethylene glycol	ng/ml	8.1
Homovanillic acid	ng/ml	35.1
5-Hydroxyindoleacetic acid	ng/ml	17.1
Cyclic adenosine 3′,5′-monophosphate	pmol/ml	19.6
Cyclic guanosine 3′,5′-monophosphate	pmol/ml	2.4

Source: Reprinted from Wood.[32]

Protein

The low protein content of normal CSF with respect to plasma protein levels suggests its relative exclusion by the blood-brain or blood-CSF barrier. Since the total protein concentration in CSF is less than 0.5 percent of that of plasma, the exit rate of protein is about 200 times the entry rate.

The characteristic pattern of separation of proteins by electrophoresis depends on their molecular weight and electric charge. Albumin constitutes about 56 to 76 percent of total CSF protein but only 52 to 67 percent of total serum protein. The albumin in CSF originates from plasma. Albumin elevations are relatively greater when the total CSF protein is increased and leads to a rise in the CSF albumin/total protein ratio.

The normal source of the γ-globulin present in CSF is plasma γ-globulin. Immunoglobulin G (IgG) is the major γ-globulin in both plasma and CSF, accounting for 15 to 18 percent of total plasma protein but only 5 to 12 percent of total CSF protein. Most antibodies against bacteria and viruses are IgG. The IgG response to central inflammation or demyelination must be related to that of other CSF proteins in order to assess whether elevations in CSF IgG represent increased blood-brain barrier permeability of plasma IgG or local central nervous system IgG synthesis.

TABLE 15-5 Hormone Composition of Plasma and Lumbar CSF in Humans

Constituent	Units	Plasma	CSF	CSF/Plasma Ratio
Thyrotropin-releasing hormone	pg/ml		4.9–40.2	
Thyrotropin	μU/ml	4.0–5.95	0.1–2.65	0.025–0.44
Thyroxine				
Total	ng/dl	7400	185	0.025
Free	ng/dl	2.4	5.8	2.4
Tri-iodothyronine				
Total	ng/dl	168	17.4	0.1
Free	ng/dl	0.32	1.77	5.53
Luteinizing hormone–releasing hormone	pg/ml		11.2	
Luteinizing hormone	mIU/ml		2.39–5.7	
Follicle-stimulating hormone	mIU/ml		1.67–5.3	
Testosterone				
Female	ng/dl	58	1.4	0.024
Male	ng/dl	504	11.1	0.022
Estradiol				
Female	pg/ml	68	2.4	0.035
Male	pg/ml	56	3.9	0.070
Progesterone				
Female	ng/dl	66	4.5	0.07
Male	ng/dl	33	3.9	0.12
Prolactin	ng/ml	7–25	0.4–1.2	0.02–0.17
Somatostatin	pg/ml		35.4–130	
Growth hormone	ng/ml	1.95–6.7	0.35–0.5	0.07–0.17
β-Lipotropin	pg/ml	78.2	89.3	1.14
β-Endorphin	ng/ml		6.1	
	pg/ml	5.5	17.9	3.25
	fmol/ml		22.3	
Methionine-enkephalin	ng/ml		26.8	
	pg/ml	69.3	13.3	0.19
	pmol/ml		3.12	
β-Melanocyte-stimulating hormone	ng/liter	16.1	60.1	3.73
Adrenocorticotropin	pg/ml	65–74	27–98	1.12–1.32
	fmol/ml		14.4	
Cortisol	μg/dl		0.68 (A.M.)	
			0.38 (P.M.)	
Substance P	pg/ml		1–45	
	fmol/ml		7.0	
Arginine vasopressin	pg/ml	2.8	1.8–2.4	0.86
Calcitonin	pg/ml	89	28	0.31
Cholecystokinin	pM		14.0	
Gastrin	pM	23	3.4	0.15
Vasoactive intestinal polypeptide	pmol/ml	6.8	49.9	7.3
Insulin	μU/ml	19.8–38.0	4.0–11.0	0.20–0.29
Melatonin	pg/ml	63	59	0.94
Bombesin	fmol/ml		34.43	

Source: Modified from Wood.[31,33]

Discrimination between blood-brain barrier dysfunction and inflammation may be accomplished by evaluation of the CSF protein profile. The *IgG-albumin index* may be used to correct the CSF IgG level for the contribution of plasma IgG that penetrates a damaged blood-brain barrier:

$$\text{IgG-albumin index} = \frac{\text{IgG}_{\text{CSF}} \times \text{albumin}_{\text{plasma}}}{\text{IgG}_{\text{plasma}} \times \text{albumin}_{\text{CSF}}}$$

Alternatively, the contribution of *locally synthesized IgG* to the total CSF IgG content may be calculated as follows:[26]

$$\textit{de novo} \text{ IgG synthesis in mg/day} = 5\left[\left(\text{IgG}_{\text{CSF}} - \frac{\text{IgG}_{\text{plasma}}}{369}\right) \right.$$
$$\left. - \left(\text{albumin}_{\text{CSF}} - \frac{\text{albumin}_{\text{plasma}}}{230}\right)\left(\frac{\text{IgG}_{\text{plasma}}}{\text{albumin}_{\text{plasma}}}\right)(0.43)\right]$$

The IgG molecule may be dissociated into two heavy and two light polypeptide chains. The two types of light chains, κ and λ, are about equal in concentration in both normal CSF and plasma. The CSF κ/λ ratio elevates during central inflammation or demyelination.

The CSF/serum protein and albumin ratios increase with age, whereas the IgG-albumin index remains constant. Total protein content in lumbar CSF normally varies with the patient's age according to the equation:

Total lumbar CSF protein
$= 23.8 + 0.39 \times$ age ± 15.0 mg/dl

Generally, total protein concentrations in the ventricle are 6 to 12 mg/dl, whereas those in the cisterna magna and lumbar sac are 15 to 25 and 20 to 50 mg/dl, respectively.[5]

The true total protein content of CSF obtained by a traumatic puncture can be calculated assuming a normal cellular profile and protein level in the blood; 1 mg/dl of protein is subtracted from the total protein concentration of the bloody CSF for every 1000 erythrocytes per cubic millimeter counted. This correction is valid only if the cell count and the total protein content are determined from the same aliquot of CSF.[5]

An increase in the total protein content is the single most useful alteration in the chemical composition of CSF that serves as an indicator of central disease.[5] Despite its lack of specificity, an elevated CSF protein content is usually a reliable index of a pathological process that increases endothelial cell permeability. Generally, a slight increase in CSF total protein is common in many diseases, but elevations to more than 500 mg/dl are usually associated with meningitis, intraspinal tumor with spinal block, or bloody CSF. Occasionally, such high protein levels are observed in polyneuritis and brain tumor.

Profoundly high CSF protein concentrations (>1000 mg/dl) are found in patients with intraspinal tumors having complete obstruction of the spinal subarachnoid space. The loculated CSF below the block coagulates when drained from the spinal needle (Froin's syndrome) because of the large amounts of serum fibrinogen crossing the capillary endothelial cells. The lower the level of the blocking intraspinal tumor, the higher the CSF protein concentration and the more likely the clotting of the CSF below the block. Any lesion causing complete spinal block may cause Froin's syndrome.

Contrarily, low protein levels (3 to 20 mg/dl) may occur in young children between ages 6 months and 2 years, following removal of large volumes of lumbar CSF or CSF leaks, in 30 percent of patients with pseudotumor cerebri, during acute water intoxication, and in hyperthyroid or leukemic patients.[5]

Physiological Cellular Composition of CSF

Precise identification and quantification of the cells in CSF are critical to neurological diagnosis. Aside from automated methods, cell counting is usually performed employing a Fuchs-Rosenthal hemocytometer having a volume of 3.2 mm³. Normally, no erythrocytes should be present in CSF. Leukocyte counts in thoroughly mixed CSF are made by adding vital dye solution containing acetic acid (to lyse erythrocytes) to make a 0.9 dilution of CSF. After it is mixed, this prepared solution is examined in the hemocy-

tometer under a light microscope. The differential leukocyte count is made by centrifuging at least 3 ml of CSF at 4°C at 900 revolutions per minute (rpm) for 15 min and smearing the resuspended sediment to which 5 μl of 2% albumin solution has been added on a glass slide. After drying, about 250 consecutive cells should be counted for a valid differential leukocyte determination.[26]

Methylene blue or Wright's staining of dried CSF smears permits identification of the various types of leukocytes, erythrocytes, bacteria, cryptococci, and neoplastic cells.[26]

In normal adults, no more than 5 leukocytes per cubic millimeter should be present in CSF and no more than 2 of them should be polymorphonuclear leukocytes. The CSF in young children should contain less than 10 lymphocytes per cubic millimeter. A pleocytosis of 5 to 50, 50 to 200, or more than 200 leukocytes per cubic millimeter is clinically graded as mild, moderate, or marked, respectively.[5]

An approximation of the leukocyte count can be made in case of a traumatic puncture. If a normal blood cellular profile is assumed, the number of leukocytes in the CSF before the addition of blood is obtained by subtracting 1 leukocyte per cubic millimeter for every 700 erythrocytes from the actual CSF leukocyte count. In the presence of significant anemia or leukocytosis, Fishman[5] has developed the following formula for the appropriate correction:

$$W = WBC_F - \frac{WBC_B \times RBC_F}{RBC_B}$$

where W is the leukocyte count of the CSF before the blood was added; WBC_F is the total leukocyte count in the bloody CSF; WBC_B is the leukocyte count in the blood; RBC_F and RBC_B are the erythrocytes per cubic millimeter in the CSF and the blood, respectively.

Cytolysis of cells in CSF occurs rapidly after puncture, therefore the CSF specimen should be fixed as quickly as possible. Although refrigeration at 4°C preserves cellular structure for 48 h, cytological studies should be performed soon after CSF sampling for accuracy.

CSF Alterations in Selected Disease States

Central nervous system pathology is indicated by high CSF pressures, abnormal manometric (Queckenstedt) testing, xanthochromia, spontaneous clotting, pleocytosis, abnormal differential leukocyte counts, microorganisms, positive serological tests, or elevated total protein, albumin, or immunoglobulin levels[26] provided valid CSF sampling and analysis techniques have been employed.[30]

Subarachnoid Hemorrhage and other Cerebrovascular Disorders

By definition, the presence of a single erythrocyte in the CSF is technically a SAH. However, 100 erythrocytes per cubic millimeter has been suggested by Laurent[14] to be diagnostic of clinical SAH. The number of erythrocytes in lumbar CSF does not always correlate with that contained in the cephalic subarachnoid CSF. The CSF will be uniformly bloodstained or pink to red in the majority of symptomatic patients at the time of initial puncture. Occasionally, blood from an intracranial bleeding source will not extend to the lumbar subarachnoid space for 6 to 12 h, and, sometimes, intraparenchymal bleeding will not extravasate into the subarachnoid space.

Normal CSF should be crystal clear; however, it may contain as many as 500 erythrocytes per cubic millimeter and appear clear. Gross evidence of bleeding (erythrocytes >4000 per cubic millimeter) may disappear within 24 h, but usually persists for 7 to 14 days. If the CSF is bloody, the specimen should be centrifuged and the supernatant examined for the presence of color.

Differentiation of Traumatic from Atraumatic Subarachnoid Hemorrhage

Traumatic punctures will be associated with a decline in the number of erythrocytes as more CSF is serially drained from the spinal needle, and the proportion of leukocytes to erythrocytes will be similar to that in blood (Table 15-6). Crenated erythrocytes, if present, do not indicate an earlier bleeding episode. After CSF centrifugation, if the supernatant exhibits yellow discoloration (xanthochromia), true SAH likely antedated the puncture. However, caution should be exercised in this interpretation since three other conditions may cause xanthochromia. Protein contents exceeding 150 mg/dl may tinge CSF. High erythrocyte contamination (>1,500,000 per cubic millimeter) may be associated with true coloration of CSF secondary to the plasma component of the contaminating blood. Lastly, necrotic tissue causing high lipid levels in CSF may yield xanthochromia. Traumatic puncture is usually indicated if a clot forms in the specimen vial when the erythrocyte count exceeds 200,000 per cubic millimeter. Bleeding from any source will elevate the CSF protein content about 1 mg per 1000 erythrocytes. If the actual total CSF protein level exceeds the sum of this calculated protein elevation and the upper limit of normal CSF protein, then true SAH has likely occurred. The presence of CSF leukocytosis, e.g., leukocyte/erythrocyte ratios greater than that in blood (>2 leukocytes per 1000 erythrocytes), dates the SAH to at least 24 h before the CSF sampling.

Differential Diagnosis

Xanthochromia is produced by the pigmented degradation products of hemoglobin that are released during erythrocyte lysis: red, oxyhemoglobin; yellow, bilirubin; brown, methemoglobin. Detection of these pigments can be accomplished by biochemical methods: benzidine test for oxyhemoglobin, Van den Bergh test for bilirubin, and potassium cyanide test for methemoglobin.[14] Pigmental quantitation in CSF can be made utilizing spectrophotometry.[11]

Xanthochromia appears in the CSF supernatant within 2 h after SAH in a few cases, within 6 h in 70 percent of cases, and within 12 h in 90 percent of cases after the onset of clinical symptoms. The initial pigment is oxyhemoglobin; its red coloration of CSF peaks within 2 to 3 days and diminishes over the next 7 to 10 days.[14] Oxyhemoglobin is enzy-

matically degraded to bilirubin, the iron-free derivative of hemoglobin. Although the initial SAH releases both bound bilirubin and unbound bilirubin into the subarachnoid space, *de novo* bilirubin accounting for the yellow color of the CSF appears within 2 to 4 days of the ictus and may persist for 2 to 4 weeks. The detection of these pigments in CSF leukocytes or macrophages can be used to diagnose SAH as late as 17 weeks after the ictus in the presence of clear CSF.[10] Methemoglobin, the oxidized form of hemoglobin in which the iron atom is in the ferric form, is produced when blood has been encapsulated, as in a subdural hematoma, and is usually not found in SAH (see Table 15-6).

If lumbar puncture is performed within 1 week of the onset of neurological deficits from either cerebral hemorrhage or cerebral infarction, the assessment of CSF color and erythrocyte count are more useful than pressure, protein, and leukocyte values. With intracerebral hemorrhage, 75 percent of patients will present with bloody or xanthochromic CSF (Table 15-6). The CSF in patients with cerebral infarction is never grossly bloody, but it can be xanthochromic if hemorrhagic infarction has occurred.[14] Spectrophotometric analysis of the CSF approximately 1 week after symptom onset increases the accuracy of detecting intracerebral hematomas or hemorrhagic infarctions to greater than 95 percent.[11]

Migraine attacks characterized by focal transient ischemic neurological deficits followed by headache and nausea are rarely associated with CSF abnormalities. Mildly elevated opening pressures, mononuclear pleocytosis ranging from 40 to 233 leukocytes, elevated peak protein levels ranging from 70 to 184 mg/dl, and normal glucose levels have been reported in CSF following migraine episodes in seven patients, five of whom had abnormal electroencephalograms.[1]

Seizure Disorders

Postictal pleocytosis is uncommon, occurring in about 3 percent of seizure patients, but it may follow a single prolonged seizure as well as repetitive seizures. Abnormal postictal CSF findings include maximal leukocyte counts of a varied cell type ranging from 9 to 80 per cubic millimeter and reaching a maximum on the day after cessation of convulsions, erythrocyte counts up to 650 per cubic millimeter, and mildly elevated protein (<100 mg/dl).[23]

Bacterial Infections

Purulent meningitis is usually associated with increased pressure due to a concomitant increase in CSF outflow resistance, marked pleocytosis ranging from 500 to 10,000 leukocytes per cubic millimeter (predominantly polymorphonuclear cells in the acute stages), increased protein from 50 to 1000 mg/dl and hypoglycorrhachia (glucose < 50 mg/dl). Staining of CSF smears or clots may identify the infecting microorganism. Previous treatment with antibiotics may result in negative CSF cultures and milder derangements of the CSF profile, thereby necessitating polysaccharide antigen and bacterial endotoxin testing for diagnosis. Chronic

TABLE 15-6 CSF Alterations in Cerebrovascular Disorders

Disorder	Appearance	WBCs/mm³	Protein	Comments
Traumatic puncture	Streaked; clearing; no xanthochromia	2 WBCs per 1000 RBCs	1 mg per 1000 RBCs	Crenated RBCs not significant
Subarachnoid hemorrhage	Bloody; 90% have xanthochromia in less than 12 h	Initially proportional to RBCs; Leukocytosis in 24–48 h	Initially proportional to RBCs; Increased by 24–48 h	Oxyhemoglobin and bilirubin content determined spectrophoto-metrically
Intracerebral hemorrhage	Bloody; xanthochromia	Initially proportional to RBCs; Leukocytosis in 48–72 h; Confirmation with CT scan	Increased	None
Cerebral thrombosis	Normal	Normal, increased in 30%; Leukocytosis in 48–72 h	Normal, increased in 40%	Hemorrhagic infarction may produce bloody CSF
Subdural hematoma	Normal; bloody if brain is lacerated	Normal	May increase	Methemoglobin may be present in CSF

Source: Reprinted from Laurent[14], with permission. RBCs, erythrocytes; WBCs, leukocytes; CSF, cerebrospinal fluid; CT, computed tomography.

meningitis usually has the same CSF profile except that the pleocytosis involves lymphocytes predominantly.

Acute syphilitic infections of the meninges are rare, but they produce turbid CSF, increased pressure, elevated protein, hypoglycorrhachia, and either a neutrophilic or lymphocytic pleocytosis ranging from 100 to 500 cells per cubic millimeter. Gamma globulin levels are elevated and VDRL titers in CSF are greater than 1:32.

The CSF profile is abnormal in about 35 percent of cases of secondary syphilis, usually exhibiting a pleocytosis of 500 leukocytes and elevated protein. Approximately 60 percent of symptomatic patients have an increased percentage of CSF IgG and oligoclonal IgG bands on agarose gel electrophoresis.[5] CSF is always abnormal in the various central forms of tertiary syphilis and tests positive during serological examination.

CSF pressures are abnormally high in 60 percent of patients with brain abscess; lumbar puncture in this patient population is associated with an 8 percent mortality. Although 70 percent of patients have pleocytosis and elevated protein, positive CSF cultures and hypoglycorrhachia are only present in patients with concomitant meningitis. Frequently, the organism growing in the CSF is different than that in the abscess. Thus, CSF analysis offers little diagnostic information in cases of brain abscess.

Aseptic CSF changes occurring in response to extradural septic foci (mastoiditis, petrosis, venous sinus thrombophlebitis, extradural abscess, or osteomyelitis) or subdural empyema are characterized by a polymorphonuclear pleocytosis (usually between 10 to 1000 per cubic millimeter) and elevated protein (ranging from 45 to 100 mg/dl) with normal glucose levels. Opening pressures are elevated with venous sinus thrombosis and intracranial empyemas, but CSF smears and culture usually reveal no organisms.

Although early in the course of tuberculous meningitis a polymorphonuclear reaction may occur, the classic CSF findings include a predominantly lymphocytic pleocytosis ranging from 100 to 500 cells per cubic millimeter, increased protein levels, hypoglycorrhachia, and, in severe cases, low chloride concentrations. Typically, the CSF is clear and colorless, but it may show a pellicle or cobweb clot on standing at room temperature or after refrigeration, reflecting the presence of fibrinogen.[5] Smears are positive in only 10 to 22 percent but cultures are positive in 38 to 88 percent of confirmed cases.[26]

Fungal Meningitis; Unusual Infections

The CSF findings of cryptococcal meningitis resemble those of tuberculous meningitis. The yeastlike organism can be visualized in India ink preparations in about 50 percent of cases or on Wright's staining of centrifuged sediment.[26] Cryptococcal capsular antigen can be detected in the CSF of 85 percent of active cases, but it disappears with successful treatment.

CSF cultures are more often positive than are smears in cases of coccidioidal meningitis. Fortunately, about 75 percent of patients with coccidioidal meningitis have serum complement-fixation titers greater than 1:32, which is considered diagnostic.[26]

Candida meningitis is associated with a CSF pleocytosis of less than 500 leukocytes per cubic millimeter, increased protein, and reduced glucose in half the cases. CSF cultures are required for diagnosis, since smears will be positive in only 50 percent of cases.

Central cysticercosis evokes a lymphocytic, granulocytic, or eosinophilic pleocytosis with hypoglycorrhachia. Recurrent aseptic meningitic syndrome has been associated with repeated leakage of an echinococcal cyst. Blastomyces meningitis causes a lymphocytic pleocytosis and elevated protein level but may not always depress the CSF glucose level. CSF cultures are frequently negative. Meningoencephalitic toxoplasmosis often presents in a fulminant form, but chronic courses are not infrequent. Although serological testing is supportive, brain biopsy is required for diagnosis.

Viral Meningoencephalitis

Since central viral infections often involve both the brain and meninges, the CSF findings are similar in viral encephalitis and meningitis. Following the elimination of bacterial, tuberculous, fungal, and carcinomatous meningitis from the differential diagnosis, the specific offending virus in many cases of meningoencephalitis is never identified. Other than the usually self-limited "aseptic meningitis" caused by enteroviruses, herpes simplex accounts for the majority of sporadic central viral infections.

Commonly, the CSF pressure is elevated to 200 to 400 mmHg in acute phases, the protein is mildly increased to 50 to 80 mg/dl (sometimes with increased immunoglobulins), but the glucose level is usually normal. Although in a few cases CSF glucose may be depressed, the finding of hypoglycorrhachia should not be presumed to be viral-induced until more common causes have been excluded. The cellular response to central viral infections varies with the degree of meningismus. Usually the prdominantly lymphocytic and mononuclear pleocytosis is in the range of 5 to 10 leukocytes per cubic millimeter for parenchymal disease but may be intensely polymorphonuclear when associated with acute viral meningitis.

The CSF is abnormal in most cases of herpes simplex encephalitis but may initially be normal in 10 percent of confirmed cases.[5] At first examination, the CSF usually contains 50 to 100 leukocytes per cubic millimeter, predominantly lymphocytes. The leukocyte count and, to a lesser extent, the protein tend to increase during the course of the illness. A few erythrocytes and xanthochromia is observed in 40 percent and 10 percent of cases of herpes simplex encephalitis, respectively, and this finding helps to distinguish herpes simplex from other types of viral encephalitis. Signs of meningismus occur in about half of cases, usually appearing 4 to 11 days after the onset of the encephalitis. Unfortunately, the CSF alterations do not correlate with the course of the illness, and the overall mortality is 70 percent regardless of age of the patient. Open brain biopsy is usually required for early diagnosis.

During the preparalytic stage of acute poliomyelitis, a polymorphonuclear pleocytosis predominates, but by the fifth day of the illness, this cellular reaction becomes lymphocytic, averaging about 200 leukocytes per cubic millimeter. The CSF glucose levels are usually normal, with the protein level ranging from 50 to 100 mg/dl during a mild rise in gamma globulins. CSF pressure elevations are observed in cases with paralytic respiratory insufficiency and are related to hypercapnia.[5]

Herpes zoster infections may cause alterations in CSF during the eruptive phases. Similar CSF changes are seen with Reye's syndrome, except that the pressure elevations are more pronounced. The CSF profile is usually normal in central rabies infections; however, the virus can be isolated from CSF.[5]

Guillain-Barré Syndrome

The syndrome of acute idiopathic polyneuritis evokes progressive protein elevations for the first 2 to 3 weeks of the illness, peaking as high as 1000 mg/dl. All protein fractions including gamma globulins are increased, but only about 15 percent of patients have a leukocytosis (albuminocytological dissociation). Both central synthesis of immunoglobulins and oligoclonal bands have been observed in 60 percent of cases. The severity of the CSF immunoglobulin alterations does not correlate with that of the illness.[26] Unlike multiple sclerosis, the κ/λ ratio in this form of polyneuritis is normal (about 1.0). Opening pressures may be elevated secondary to protein-induced elevations in CSF outflow resistance or the hypercapnia associated with respiratory dysfunction.

Multiple Sclerosis

The central demyelinating disorder, multiple sclerosis, is associated with a mild lymphocytic pleocytosis in only 30 percent of cases,[26] with leukocyte counts rarely exceeding 50 per cubic millimeter. Although total CSF protein or albumin concentrations are mildly elevated in only 20 percent of patients with "definite" cases,[26,27] approximately 70 percent and 90 percent have elevations in *de novo* IgG and electrophoretic oligoclonal bands, respectively, in CSF.[17] Among monosymptomatic patients with "possible" multiple sclerosis having only a chronic myelopathy, optic neuritis, or brain stem disease undergoing CSF electrophoresis, only 8 percent without oligoclonal bands and 16 percent with oligoclonal bands develop "definite" multiple sclerosis after 28 to 29 months of follow-up.[20]

These CSF findings are not pathognomonic and can be seen in cases of neurosyphilis, subacute sclerosing panencephalitis, and viral infections.[26] Similarly, the CSF κ/λ ratio elevations (>1.0) observed in multiple sclerosis have also been reported in central inflammations.[32]

Immunoreactive myelin basic protein has been found to be transiently increased after acute episodes of central demyelination, but may be normal in cases with only optic neuritis.[2] Elevations of this myelin component have been reported in 90 percent of patients with confirmed multiple sclerosis if CSF is obtained within 1 week of the exacerbation.[17,27] Myelin basic protein levels return to normal (<4.5 ng/ml) over the subsequent 2 weeks in most patients. Patients with chronic forms of multiple sclerosis tend not to have CSF myelin basic protein elevations. Since raised CSF concentrations of myelin basic protein appear to reflect active demyelination, the elevations in this component associated with ischemic infarction, encephalitis, leukodystrophies, metabolic encephalopathies, and methotrexate toxicity probably reflect generalized nervous tissue destruction.

Diabetes Mellitus

Total protein elevations associated with diabetic neuropathy may range from 50 to 400 mg/dl. However, the magnitude of these elevations is not related to the severity of the symptoms. Unless neuropathy is prominent, the CSF protein in patients with diabetes mellitus is unlikely to be greater than 60 mg/dl.[5] The cell count is normal and, as discussed previously, the CSF glucose level depends upon its concentration in plasma.[5]

Pseudotumor Cerebri

Patients with benign intracranial hypertension have elevated CSF pressures, a normal neurological exam except for possible abducens nerve palsies and papilledema, and normal to small ventricles on CT. Generally the cell count and glucose levels are normal, but the total protein concentration is commonly *reduced* in the CSF.

Meningeal Carcinomatosis

Neoplastic infiltration of the subarachnoid space and ventricles may result in elevated CSF pressure secondary to increased CSF outflow resistance. However, greater than 50 percent of patients have normal pressure during the initial lumbar puncture.[5] Low pressures may be observed if measured below a spinal block.

Approximately one-quarter of patients with central nervous system malignant tumors have positive premortem cytological examinations of the CSF.[8] Malignant cells are found in only about 2 percent of patients whose tumors do not reach the leptomeninges. Among patients with leptomeningeal tumor at autopsy, CSF cytology is positive in about 60 percent. Thus, a positive cytological finding of malignant cells in CSF is a reliable indicator of central nervous system cancer and almost always reflects leptomeningeal tumor. In addition, repeated CSF sampling can raise the percentage of diagnosis to about 80 percent.[5]

In addition to the presence of malignant cells in the CSF, meningeal carcinomatosis evokes a polymorphonuclear leukocytosis up to 500 per cubic millimeter. Although the total protein concentration may be as high as 1200 mg/dl, approximately 25 percent of patients will have a normal CSF protein level during the first lumbar puncture. Hypoglycorrhachia has been suggested to indicate *diffuse* meningeal involvement rather than focal cerebral or meningeal metastasis.[5]

Brain Tumors

Patients with brain tumors are being examined earlier in the course of their disease as diagnosis becomes more accurate with the advent of CT scanning. Fewer patients found to have brain tumors undergo CSF examination so as to avoid possible uncal or tonsillar herniation. Tumors may elevate intracranial pressure by their mass effect or may increase the CSF outflow resistance at the arachnoid villi by the elevation of CSF protein levels or blockage with desquamated cells.

The CSF is usually clear, but may be xanthochromic secondary to bleeding, high protein concentrations, or serum bilirubin transudation. Heavy pleocytosis may cloud the CSF and increase its viscosity. Although the leukocyte count is usually normal, predominantly polymorphonuclear pleocytosis has been associated with large necrotic tumors. Abundant macrophages found within some primary brain tumors may serve as a source for the leukocytes observed in the CSF. Neoplastic cells are found preoperatively in lumbar CSF of about 15 percent and 20 percent of primary and metastatic brain tumors, respectively. Higher percentages of positive cytologies are obtained postoperatively and in ventricular CSF.

The most common CSF abnormality associated with brain tumors is elevated total protein concentrations, probably secondary to increased endothelial cell permeability. Highly vascular gliomatous or metastatic tumors are more likely to cause higher protein extravasation. Patients with cerebellopontine angle syndrome and CSF protein levels greater than 200 mg/dl are more apt to harbor an acoustic neuroma than a meningioma.[5] The electrophoretic pattern of the CSF proteins in the CSF of brain tumor patients usually resembles that of plasma. The CSF glucose levels are usually normal, and the presence of hypoglycorrhachia tends to indicate diffuse meningeal involvement with tumor.

Recent research has been aimed at the verification of biochemical "markers" that may aid in diagnosing and in monitoring treatment in patients with brain and meningeal neoplasms.[24] CSF human chorionic gonadotropin levels are elevated in patients with central choriocarcinoma, often prior to clinical evidence of neurological disease. Elevated CSF levels of carcinoembryonic antigen (CEA) have been reported in cases of metastatic breast, lung, and bladder cancer as well as melanoma. Although CSF α-fetoprotein has been found to be present in patients with metastatic testicular carcinoma and hepatoma, the detection of this glycoprotein is more valuable in diagnosing central primary germ cell tumors.

The levels of the polyamines spermidine and spermine and their precursor, putrescine, in CSF are elevated in patients with central neoplasms.[6] Spermidine, but not putrescine, may be increased in CSF in the presence of meningiomas. CSF polyamine elevations are frequently found in patients with central metastasis and leukemia prior to the detection of malignant cells in the CSF and may be useful in monitoring disease progression or response to therapy. Polyamine levels have diagnostic significance in patients with malignant gliomas adjacent to the ventricular system or subarachnoid space but not with deep hemispheric gliomas. CSF polyamine levels have been correlated with the clinical status of patients with medulloblastomas and elevations may be the earliest indication of tumor recurrence or progression. Increased CSF polyamine levels have also been associated with brain abscesses, arteriovenous malformations, functional pituitary adenomas, and SAH.[6]

The increased desmosterol in the CSF after the administration of triparanol, an inhibitor of enzymatic conversion of desmosterol to cholesterol, prior to CSF sampling has inconsistently been reported in patients with gliomas.[24] Lactate dehydrogenase (LDH_4 and LDH_5) alterations are associated with those tumors that directly invade the subarachnoid pathways. β-Glucuronidase, a lysosomal enzyme, has been found to be elevated in the CSF of patients with leptomeningeal spread of cancer and tends to return to normal following therapy, paralleling the clinical course.[24]

Spinal Disorders

Among spinal cord tumors, intradural extramedullary (meningiomas and neurofibromas) and extradural (sarcomas and metastasis) varieties more often have elevated CSF protein

TABLE 15-7 CSF Total Protein Content and Leukocyte Count Associated with Spinal Tumors and Disorders

Diagnosis	Total Number of Cases	Protein, mg/dl			Leukocytes/mm³	
		<50	50–100	>100	<10	>10
Meningioma, neurofibroma	31	16	23	61	81	19
Extradural tumor (metastasis or sarcoma)	25	24	16	60	80	20
Intramedullary tumor	17	35	18	47	82	18
Syringomyelia and other anomalies	59	83	15	2	90	10
Multiple sclerosis	598	86	13.5	0.5	80	20
Amyotrophic lateral sclerosis	83	87	13	0	99	1
Cervical spondylosis with myelopathy	193	82	16.5	1.5	97	3
Lumbar disc disorder	350	84	15	1	98	2

Source: Data derived from Laterre.[13]

greater than 100 mg/dl with less than 100 leukocytes per cubic millimeter (Table 15-7). These tumors may be associated with Froin's syndrome if a complete block is present, especially if the tumor is more caudally placed. Intraspinal neurofibromas have been associated with elevated CSF pressure and papilledema secondary to the increased CSF outflow resistance caused by the associated high CSF protein levels. In the absence of meningeal cancer, CSF glucose concentrations are usually normal.

Interestingly, syringomyelia with craniocervical junction malformations, amyotrophic lateral sclerosis, multiple sclerotic myelopathy, lumbar disc herniations, and even cervical spondylosis with myelopathy do not usually cause major total protein or cellular CSF abnormalities. In fact, if the total CSF protein is greater than 100 mg/dl in a myelopathic patient with cervical spondylosis, another diagnosis such as a foramen magnum meningioma should be investigated.

References

1. Bartleson JD, Swanson JW, Whisnant JP: A migrainous syndrome with cerebrospinal fluid pleocytosis. Neurology 31:1257–1262, 1981.
2. Cohen SR, Brooks BR, Jubelt B, Herndon RM, McKhann GM: Myelin basic protein in cerebrospinal fluid: Index of active demyelination, in Wood JH (ed): *Neurobiology of Cerebrospinal Fluid 1*. New York, Plenum, 1980, pp 487–494.
3. Duffy GP: Lumbar puncture in spontaneous subarachnoid haemorrhage. Br Med J 285:1163–1164, 1982.
4. Felgenhauer K: Protein size and cerebrospinal fluid composition. Klin Wochenschr 52:1158–1164, 1974.
5. Fishman RA: *Cerebrospinal Fluid in Diseases of the Nervous System*. Philadelphia, Saunders, 1980.
6. Fulton DS, Levin VA, Lubich WP, Wilson CB, Morton LJ: Clinical correlations of cerebrospinal fluid polyamine levels, in Wood JH (ed): *Neurobiology of Cerebrospinal Fluid 2*. New York, Plenum, 1983, pp 441–452.
7. Gilland O, Tourtellotte WW, O'Tauma L, Henderson WG: Normal cerebrospinal fluid pressure. J Neurosurg 40:587–593, 1974.
8. Glass JP, Wertlake PT: Malignant cells in cerebrospinal fluid and their clinical significance, in Wood JH (ed): *Neurobiology of Cerebrospinal Fluid 2*. New York, Plenum, 1983, pp 411–425.
9. Hare TA, Wood JH: Pathological neurochemistry of cerebrospinal fluid: Neurotransmitters and neuropeptides, in Lajtha A (ed): *Handbook of Neurochemistry*, vol 10, 2d ed. New York, Plenum, 1983.
10. Ito U, Fukumoto T, Inaba Y: Cerebrospinal fluid cytology after subarachnoid hemorrhage, in Wood JH (ed): *Neurobiology of Cerebrospinal Fluid 2*. New York, Plenum, 1983, pp 541–557.
11. Kjellin KG: Xanthochromic compounds in cerebrospinal fluid: Quantitative spectrophotometry and electromigration, in Wood JH: *Neurobiology of Cerebrospinal Fluid 2*. New York, Plenum, 1983, pp 559–570.
12. Korein J, Cravioto H, Leicach M: Re-evaluation of lumbar puncture, a study of 129 patients with papilledema or intracranial hypertension. Neurology (NY) 9:290–297, 1959.
13. Laterre EC: Cerebrospinal fluid, in Vinken PJ, Bruyn GW (eds): *Handbook of Clinical Neurology*, vol. 19. *Tumours of the Spine and Spinal Cord*. Amsterdam, North Holland, 1975, pp 125–138.
14. Laurent JP: Subarachnoid hemorrhage, in Wood JH (ed): *Neurobiology of Cerebrospinal Fluid 1*, New York, Plenum, 1980, pp 279–286.
15. Leavens ME, Aldama-Luebert A: Ommaya reservoir placement: Technical note. Neurosurgery 5:264–266, 1979.
16. Magnaes B: Body position and cerebrospinal fluid pressure, in Wood JH (ed): *Neurobiology of Cerebrospinal Fluid 2*. New York, Plenum, 1983, pp 629–642.
17. McFarlin DE, McFarland HF: Multiple sclerosis. N Engl J Med 307:1183–1188, 1982.
18. McGale, EHF, Pye IF, Stonier C, Hutchinson EC, Aber GM: Studies of the inter-relationship between cerebrospinal fluid and plasma amino acid concentrations in normal individuals. J Neurochem 29:291–297, 1977.
19. Milhorat TH, Hammock MK: Cerebrospinal fluid as reflection of internal milieu of brain, in Wood JH (ed): *Neurobiology of Cerebrospinal Fluid 2*. New York, Plenum, 1983, pp 1–23.
20. Moulin DW, Paty DW, Ebers GC: The predictive value of cerebrospinal fluid electrophoresis in "possible" multiple sclerosis. Ann Neurol 12:104, 1982.
21. Post KD, Stein BM: Technique for spinal drainage. Neurosurgery 4:255, 1979.
22. Robertson JT, Denton IC Jr: Surgical considerations of ventriculography in Youmans JR (ed): *Neurological Surgery*. Philadelphia, Saunders, 1973, pp 229–234.
23. Schmidley JW, Simon RP: Postictal pleocytosis. Ann Neurol 9:81–84, 1981.
24. Schold SC, Bullard DE: Cerebrospinal fluid analysis in central

nervous system cancer, in Wood JH (ed): *Neurobiology of Cerebrospinal Fluid 1*. New York, Plenum, 1980, pp 549–559.

25. Spurling RG: *Practical Neurological Diagnosis*, 6th ed. Springfield, Ill, Charles C Thomas, 1960, pp 204–206.

26. Tourtellotte WW, Shorr RJ: Cerebrospinal fluid, in Youmans JR (ed): *Neurological Surgery*, 2d ed. Philadelphia, Saunders, 1982, pp 423–486.

27. Walsh MJ, Tourtellotte WW, Potvin AR: Central nervous system immunoglobulin synthesis in neurological disease: Quantitation, specificity and regulation, in Wood JH (ed): *Neurobiology of Cerebrospinal Fluid 2*. New York, Plenum, 1983, pp 331–368.

28. White RJ, Dakters JG, Yashon D, Albin MS: Temporary control of cerebrospinal fluid volume and pressure by means of an externalized valve-drainage system. J Neurosurg 30:264–269, 1969.

29. Wood JH: Physiology, pharmacology and dynamics of cerebro-

spinal fluid, in Wood JH (ed): *Neurobiology of Cerebrospinal Fluid 1*. New York, Plenum, 1980, pp 1–16.

30. Wood JH: Technical aspects of clinical and experimental cerebrospinal fluid investigations, in Wood JH (ed): *Neurobiology of Cerebrospinal Fluid 1*. New York, Plenum, 1980, pp 71–96.

31. Wood JH: Neuroendocrinology of cerebrospinal fluid: Peptides, steroids and other hormones. Neurosurgery 11:293–305, 1982.

32. Wood JH: Physiological neurochemistry of cerebrospinal fluid, in Lajtha A (ed): *Handbook of Neurochemistry*, 2d ed. New York, Plenum, 1982, vol 1, pp 415–487.

33. Wood JH: Physiology and pharmacology of peptide, steroid and other hormones in cerebrospinal fluid, in Wood JH (ed): *Neurobiology of Cerebrospinal Fluid 2*. New York, Plenum, 1983, pp 43–65.

34. Zivin JA: Lateral cervical puncture, an alternative to lumbar puncture. Neurology (NY) 28:616–618, 1978.

SECTION B

Electrodiagnostic Tests

16

Electromyography

Didier Cros
B. Shahani

Clinical Electromyography

A variety of electrophysiological techniques are used to evaluate patients with disorders of the peripheral and central nervous systems. These techniques include electromyography (EMG) and electroneurography in which electrical activity produced by skeletal muscles and peripheral nerves is studied. In most modern clinical EMG laboratories, in addition to conventional EMG and motor and sensory nerve conduction studies, single fiber EMG (SFEMG), somato-

sensory evoked potentials, reflex studies (H reflex, blink reflexes), and other late response studies such as F response studies are also performed. In this chapter a brief overview of some physiological and pathophysiological concepts relevant to clinical EMG will be presented first. A description of the techniques commonly used in the EMG laboratory will follow. Finally, the approach to common clinical problems, especially those encountered in surgical practice, will be reviewed.

The Motor Unit: Anatomy and Physiology

The motor unit (MU) represents the quantum element of the motor system. The concept of motor unit was introduced by Liddell and Sherrington in 1925.[8] To date, most physiologists define the MU as the entity including a motoneuron, its axon, and the population of muscle fibers innervated by it. All motor activity, including voluntary movement, postural adaptation, and reflexes, results from the combination of the activity of several MUs organized through spinal and/or supraspinal mechanisms.

The axon of an alpha motoneuron supplies a number of muscle fibers within a single muscle. These muscle fibers belonging to a given motor unit have the same histochemical properties. The number of muscle fibers in a MU varies from muscle to muscle. MUs in the strong postural muscles such as the gastrocnemius or quadriceps muscles may include more than 1000 fibers. The fibers belonging to individual MUs are distributed in a large volume of the muscle which represents the MU territory. Only occasionally are several fibers of the same MU contiguous in normal muscle. At any given point within a muscle, such as the area sampled by an EMG needle electrode, there is an overlap of different MUs.

Most muscles are composed of a heterogenous population of muscle fibers, and hence of MUs. Histochemical reactions reveal three types of muscle fibers in human muscle: Types I, IIa, and IIb. The three fiber types appear in a cross section as a random, mosaic pattern. Morphologically, type II (pale) fibers have high concentrations of glycogen, a low density of mitochondria, and relatively few surrounding capillaries. These fibers are adapted to function anaerobically and therefore require less blood supply and fewer mitochondria, but they are dependent on their glycogen as a source of energy. Type II fibers are suited for brief periods of high-frequency activity, and fatigue rapidly as soon as the glycogen is depleted. On the other hand, type I (red) fibers contain a large number of mitochondria and are supplied by an abundant network of capillaries bringing the oxygen needed for aerobic metabolism. These fibers are extremely resistant to fatigue and are adapted to prolonged tonic activity.

Physiologically, three types of MUs have been individualized in mammals. They are the FF (fast-fatiguing), FR (fatigue-resistant), and S (slow) MUs. The FF and FR MUs are characterized by a short contraction time and a high tetanic force. The S MUs, on the other hand, have a longer contraction time and a lower tetanic force. The FF and FR MUs are composed of type II fibers, and the S MUs of type I muscle fibers.

The slow and fast MUs tend to be innervated by motoneurons with distinct properties. The slow MUs are supplied by motoneurons with a smaller perikaryon and a thinner axon than the motoneurons supplying fast-twitch MUs. The number of fibers innervated by a motor axon also correlates with its diameter, and thus the fast-twitch MUs are on the average larger than the slow-twitch MUs. The difference in size of the cell body between the individual alpha motoneurons provides a physiological basis for the recruitment of MUs in a graded contraction. The smaller motoneurons corresponding to the slow-twitch MUs are recruited first, larger motoneurons being recruited only later (Henneman's size principle). In the physiological range the mechanical output, which is the sum of the tensions developed by the active MUs, is a function of the temporal and spatial recruitment of MUs. Temporal recruitment involves modulation in the firing frequency of an individual MU. Spatial recruitment refers to an increased number of motor units being activated. The asynchrony in the firing of the various MUs and the relatively long contraction time compared with the duration of the action potential provide a fairly smooth mechanical output.

Reaction of Peripheral Nerve to Compression and Trauma

Focal damage to peripheral nerves is commonly seen in surgical practice. It may present acutely following acute compression, stretch, or open injury, or as a chronic compression or entrapment syndrome. In both instances, electromyography is an important step in the patient evaluation. EMG may help the clinician to localize the exact site(s) of lesions and may document the extent and severity of motor and/or sensory fiber dysfunction. When repeated during the follow-up, EMG provides clues about the final outcome. Many peripheral nerves are vulnerable to chronic mechanical injury at sites where they are anatomically exposed to external pressure or repeated microtrauma. The entrapment neuropathies are due to the narrowing of anatomical passageways.[6] The cervical and lumbosacral spinal roots are also commonly affected by compression due to herniated disc material or osteophytes.

Most of our knowledge of the pathology and pathophysiology of acute and chronic compression of peripheral nerves derives from animal studies.[1] Mechanical damage to peripheral nerves usually results in patchy lesions on a cross section. Knowledge of the intraneural anatomy may provide an explanation for its differential involvement. The nerve fibers are organized in fascicles that are surrounded and separated from each other by a relatively elastic connective tissue, which may provide some degree of protection from compression forces. In addition, the fascicles that are superficial with regard to the mechanical compression may protect those more deeply situated. Compression also affects different diameter nerve fibers to a different degree. It has been shown both experimentally and clinically that thick myelinated fibers (MF) are less resistant to pressure than thin MF, the unmyelinated fibers being relatively spared in cases of chronic compression.

Experimentally, the effect of pressure is to provoke a block of conduction in the segment of nerve actually compressed. The conduction remains normal distal to the compression site. The respective roles of increased mechanical pressure and ischemia induced by compression in this phenomenon are unknown. The Schwann cells and myelin sheath of MF are very susceptible to pressure. The histological changes following application of a pneumatic tourniquet have been studied by Ochoa et al. in the baboon.[9] In early stages of tourniquet conduction block, the nodes of Ranvier at the two edges of the compression site are obliterated by paranodal invaginations of myelin. These changes are limited to a short region centered by the node, the rest of the fiber showing no alteration. As compression progresses in time, however, the internodal segment of the myelin sheath may be thinned or disappear completely. When the compression is released, repair of the demyelinated segments occurs, resulting in internodes of shorter length than originally present. Even though the axons are less sensitive to pressure than Schwann cells and myelin sheaths, their resistance to stretch and compression may be surpassed. This leads to wallerian degeneration of the distal segment of the fibers. Such an axonal loss has been demonstrated in laboratory animals and with chronic entrapment in humans.

Thus, acute compression and chronic compression are characterized by a combination of conduction block and axonal loss. The conduction block is usually more marked in acute compression syndromes than in chronic compression neuropathies. In acute injury the electrophysiological evaluation may be difficult in the first days after the injury since conduction does not fail immediately in transected fibers below the site of injury. In chronic entrapment syndromes, the neurological deficit may be due more to axonal loss than to the conduction block, although the latter component is not completely lacking.[20]

The EMG Examination

Clinical electromyography (EMG) is performed by recording the electrical activity of muscle with a needle electrode inserted into it. Most commonly, a concentric needle electrode is used for bipolar recording, but monopolar electrodes are preferred by some electromyographers. The electrical signal detected is filtered, amplified, and displayed on the screen of an oscilloscope and played on a loudspeaker for simultaneous visual and auditory analysis.

Muscles and nerves are excitable tissues and as such maintain a potential difference across their membranes. In the resting state, this potential difference amounts to 70 to 90 mV, with the interior of the cell negative. The muscle resting potential is accounted for by restrictions of the movement of sodium and potassium ions across the sarcolemma, resulting in a high potassium and low sodium concentration inside the muscle fiber compared with the extracellular medium. Propagation of electrical impulses is an essential characteristic of muscle and nerve fibers. In both tissues, the action potential is initiated by depolarization of a specialized region above a critical level. This region is the node of Ranvier in myelinated nerve fibers and the motor end plate in muscle fibers. In muscle, depolarization of the motor end plate then propagates along the whole length of the fiber. All fibers in the same motor unit discharge almost synchronously in response to a single impulse in the motor axon. The resulting muscle potential (summated action potential of muscle fibers belonging to the same unit) recorded by the EMG needle is the motor unit potential (MUP).

The needle examination includes three essential steps: (1) examination of the muscle at rest; (2) examination of single MUPs on weak voluntary contraction; and (3) study of the MUP recruitment pattern on graded contractions, and of the EMG pattern on maximal effort.

EMG at Rest

Activity at rest or spontaneous activity is absent in normal muscle, with the exception of insertional activity that may follow electrode movements for brief periods of time. Insertional activity may become prominent in denervation states or in rapidly progressive muscle disease. In these cases, however, other features of denervation are always conspicuous. Other types of spontaneous activity include fibrillation potentials, positive sharp waves, fasciculations, myotonic discharges, bizarre repetitive potentials, and cramps.

Fibrillation potentials are the action potentials of single muscle fibers. They are seen when the motor supply to the muscle fibers has been interrupted. They are biphasic or triphasic potentials with an initial positive deflection. Their duration range is 1 to 5 ms, and their amplitude varies from 50 to 300 μV. The firing rate of fibrillation potentials is 2 to 30 Hz and may be regular or irregular. Fibrillation potentials are almost invariably accompanied by positive sharp waves, which have an initial sharp positive deflection followed by a long-duration negative phase. Fibrillation potentials and positive sharp waves are prominent in denervated muscle but are not pathognomonic of a lower motor neuron lesion. They are not uncommon in primary diseases of muscle such as polymyositis and dermatomyositis or Duchenne muscular dystrophy. In these diseases, it is suggested that segmental necrosis disconnects part of a muscle fiber from the neuromuscular junction, resulting in denervation of the isolated part of the fiber. In denervating diseases, the appearance of fibrillations is delayed by 2 to 4 weeks with respect to interruption of the motor supply. The shorter the length of the nerve from the site of injury to the muscle, the quicker is the appearance of fibrillations. For instance, in lumbar disc herniation, fibrillations may appear in the paraspinal muscles within a week, whereas it may take 3 weeks for these to appear in muscles of the lower limb. Therefore, absence of fibrillations a few days after a nerve injury does not exclude severe axonal loss.

Fasciculation potentials are produced by spontaneous activity of MUs or groups of muscle fibers in the MU. Unlike fibrillation potentials, fasciculations correlate with visible twitching of muscle. Fasciculation potentials have the characteristics of MUPs. Although fasciculations are commonly present in diseases affecting anterior horn cells and are a regular feature of amyotrophic lateral sclerosis, they can be seen in a number of relatively benign conditions such as cervical or lumbar radiculopathies, entrapment syndromes, and polyneuropathies. Isolated fasciculations in an otherwise normal study do not necessarily imply a disorder of the peripheral nervous system. There is a syndrome of benign fasciculations in which the fasciculation potentials have the shape, duration, and amplitude of normal MUPs and can usually be recruited on weak voluntary contraction. There are, however, no totally reliable criteria to distinguish benign fasciculations from "malignant" fasciculations.

Myotonic discharges consist of trains of single muscle fiber action potentials. The duration of the discharge is usually long, and typically the amplitude and firing frequency of the potential change from time to time. This characteristic waxing and waning produces the so-called dive-bomber sound on the loudspeaker. Myotonic discharges are seen in myotonic dystrophy and myotonia congenita, both primary disorders of muscle.

Bizarre repetitive potentials, also called bizarre high-frequency discharges or pseudomyotonic discharges, must be differentiated from true myotonic discharges. They consist of trains of action potentials that do not wax or wane and have an abrupt onset and termination. The single potentials usually have a complex polyphasic shape. These bizarre repetitive potentials are seen in a variety of disorders of the neuromuscular system, including denervating diseases.

Cramp discharges consist of a high-frequency discharge of MUPs with abrupt onset and termination. Cramps per se are not a pathological phenomenon, but they may be associated with several neurological disorders.

Single Motor Unit Potentials

Single MUPs can be easily studied during a weak voluntary effort. The MUP is defined by its duration, amplitude, and shape (number of phases). Most of the time, these parameters are assessed qualitatively by the electromyographer. In difficult cases, careful, quantitative studies are necessary. Prior to study of a single MUP, the needle electrode must be carefully positioned so that the rise time of the motor potential is less than 0.2 ms. Under this condition only are duration measurements meaningful. The mean duration should be estimated from at least 20 different MUPs in a given muscle. Normal values vary from muscle to muscle. Increased duration of the MUPs is a feature of chronic neurogenic disease and probably reflects enlargement of the MU following collateral reinnervation. Amplitude of MUPs is a somewhat less reliable parameter than duration, since it may vary greatly with only slight change in electrode position. Normal values again are different from muscle to muscle. An increase in the mean amplitude of MUPs is an indicator of chronic neurogenic disease. A normal MUP is bi- or triphasic. In normal muscle, usually less than 15 percent of MUPs have four or more phases. Increase in the number of polyphasic motor units may be seen in both neurogenic and myopathic diseases. It should be recognized that single MUP analysis provides information on low-threshold tonic motor units only. However, this bias is unavoidable since these MUs are the only ones recruited with the weak effort needed to isolate single potentials.

Motor Unit Recruitment Pattern

Study of behavior of single MUs and the pattern of recruitment during graded voluntary activity and maximal effort is one of the most important parts of the EMG examination. With weak effort, a low-threshold MU is recruited and fires at a frequency of 4 to 5 Hz. With increasing effort, increase in the frequency of the first unit is seen and a second, higher-threshold unit is recruited. It initially fires irregularly at a frequency of 1 to 3 Hz. Further increase in effort results in the increase in the firing frequency of both units. With strong contractions, many MUs are recruited, making it impossible for individual MUPs to be recognized. The normal recruitment pattern on maximal contraction is called a full recruitment pattern, i.e., the oscilloscope screen shows continuous EMG activity without electrical silence in the baseline. If only one MU is recruited on maximal voluntary effort, then the pattern is called a single unit recruitment pattern. There is further classification of the recruitment pattern: low-mixed (a few units), mixed (individual MUPs cannot be isolated but there are silent areas on the baseline), and high-mixed (intermediate between mixed and full). Reduction in the recruitment pattern indicates a loss of MUs and is a feature of denervation.

Abnormal EMG

Electromyographic changes are useful indicators of the degree and type of nerve pathology. Loss of motor axons leads to denervation of muscle fibers, which then exhibit spontaneous activity. The amount of spontaneous activity provides an estimate of the degree of current axonal loss and hence of the actual severity of denervation. Changes in the recruitment pattern on maximal effort also reveal the degree of axonal loss in neurogenic lesions. A reduced (mixed, low-mixed, or single unit) recruitment pattern is seen in these disorders and correlates with the clinical weakness. This is different from the full recruitment pattern despite weakness noted in myopathic disorders. In neurogenic disease, an important parameter during recruitment of MUPs is their firing frequency. The rate at which the MUP is recruited usually increases with increasing strength. Isolated single MUPs in normal muscle are rarely seen at frequencies of 15 to 20 Hz because at this level of contraction many MUs are recruited and interfere with the identification of single potentials. When the total number of MUs is reduced in denervation, it becomes possible to visualize the behavior of single MUs with strong effort. In these instances, a high firing frequency is often noted, suggesting that the patient is making a maximal effort in spite of clinical weakness. A reduced recruitment pattern with a rapid rate of firing of single MUPs suggests a lesion of the lower motor neuron. In hysterical subjects and patients with painful syndromes, a low-mixed recruitment pattern is associated with firing frequencies similar to those seen with weak effort in normal subjects.

Nerve Conduction Studies

These techniques are widely used to assess the function of motor and sensory nerve fibers. The numerical data provided are expressed as latency in milliseconds (ms) and conduction velocity in meters per second (m/s). Nerve conduction studies are more objective and reproducible than the results of needle electromyography. They also provide information that cannot be derived from needle examination. They have proved very useful in documenting and localizing entrapment neuropathies. In some instances, they make possible a distinction between neuropathies in which the primary feature is segmental demyelination and those with primary axonal degeneration. There are, however, several limitations in nerve conduction studies. The first one is that conventional methods determine conduction velocity in the largest motor fibers only and provide no information with regard to conduction velocity in the remaining fibers. These conduction studies may be normal in neuropathies in which the smaller myelinated fibers are predominantly affected. Similarly, in severe nerve injury, maximum motor conduction velocity may be normal across the lesion if a few large motor fibers remain intact. A second limitation arises from the wide range of normal values for conduction velocities. For example, in a given patient with a baseline motor conduction velocity in the median nerve of 70 m/s, a lesion in this nerve may impair conduction to 50 m/s, which is still in the normal range.

Any anatomically accessible nerve can be stimulated through the skin by surface electrodes. The resulting nerve action potential may be recorded (1) over the nerve more proximally (orthodromic sensory study, mixed nerve conduction study), (2) over the nerve or its branches distally (antidromic sensory studies), or (3) over a muscle distally (motor conduction studies). Motor conduction studies are most commonly performed in the median, ulnar, and radial nerves in the upper extremity, and in the peroneal and tibial nerves in the lower extremity. However, reliable studies can also be obtained with the facial, musculocutaneous, axillary, suprascapular, and femoral nerves. Sensory conduction studies are commonly recorded from the median, ulnar, and radial nerves in the upper extremity, and from the sural nerve in the lower extremity. They may also be obtained from other accessible nerves using averaging techniques. Stimulation is usually administered through a surface bipolar electrode, with the cathode proximal with respect to the recording electrode. Stimulus intensity is adjusted to produce a maximal-amplitude compound action potential, after which the stimulus intensity is increased by 25 percent to deliver a supramaximal stimulation. The conduction time measurement from the beginning of the stimulation artifact to the initial deflection of a compound muscle action potential or the beginning of the negative deflection of a nerve action potential is termed *distal latency*. Normal values for distal latency are directly related to the distance between the stimulating and recording electrodes if the temperature remains constant. Maximal motor conduction velocity is obtained through supramaximal stimulation of two points along the nerve (e.g., wrist and elbow for the median nerve, or ankle and fibular head for the peroneal nerve). The distance between these two points is divided by the conduction time, which is the difference between the latency on proximal stimulation and the distal latency, and is expressed in meters per second. For measurement of maximal sensory conduction velocity, sensory nerve action potentials are recorded at two sites. The velocity is similarly obtained by dividing the distance between the two recording sites by the conduction time.

In addition to conduction velocities, study of configuration, amplitude, and duration of compound muscle and nerve action potentials may be helpful. For motor studies, adequate placement of the recording electrode over the endplate zone provides a compound action potential with an initial negative deflection. The area of the negative wave and, to a lesser extent, its amplitude are roughly proportional to the number of alpha motor axons. Provided the duration is normal, these parameters may provide useful information regarding the number of alpha motor axons. Side-to-side comparison in unilateral disease is often needed to assess the significance of an amplitude difference. The duration of the compound muscle action potential (CMAP) is measured from the beginning of the M wave to the first baseline crossing. It reflects the synchrony of the volley elicited by the electrical stimulus, and may be extremely prolonged and asynchronous in demyelinating lesions.

Measurements of amplitude from the beginning to the peak of the negative deflection and duration of the whole potential must also be obtained from sensory studies. They also provide information regarding synchrony of conduction and number of large-diameter sensory fibers. Side-to-side comparison is often needed in localized nerve dysfunction.

Acute or chronic nerve damage will cause a combination of the following lesions: conduction block, conduction slowing, and loss of motor and sensory fibers distal to the injury. Conduction studies provide a direct evaluation of the extent of nerve damage. Slowing of motor or sensory conduction across the affected segment of nerve is due to demyelination-remyelination and is commonly detected. If this finding is lacking because some large myelinated fibers are intact across the lesion, study of the compound nerve action potential can be revealing. One of the earliest signs of entrapment neuropathies may be the abnormally prolonged duration of nerve action potentials when impulses have to travel through the affected segment of the nerve. Similarly, dispersion of the CMAP on proximal stimulation may reveal focal demyelination in some fibers at the site under investigation. A partial conduction block with a low-amplitude CMAP following stimulation above the level of injury documents block of conduction in motor fibers. This lesion is likely to recover following treatment. Axonal loss is responsible for a low-amplitude CMAP due to loss of motor axons and for low-amplitude or absent sensory potentials due to sensory fiber loss.

Late Responses

The limitations of routine motor and sensory conduction studies outlined above have prompted the development and clinical application of more sensitive techniques. Among these, the F-response and H-reflex studies significantly increase the diagnostic yield of the EMG examination. The term *late responses* refers to responses of longer latency than the direct (M) motor responses.[15,16] These responses explore conduction along the motor or motor and sensory axons from roots to peripheral segment. The F responses can be readily obtained from any distal muscle following a supramaximal stimulus of its motor nerve. F responses most likely represent centrifugal discharge of individual motoneurons initiated by antidromic volleys in their axons. They explore only the motor component of the peripheral nervous system. The H reflex evoked by stimulation of the tibial nerve in the popliteal fossa is recorded from the soleus muscle. It is a monosynaptic reflex elicited by electrical stimulation of the large-diameter muscle afferent fibers (IA). It is obtained with a relatively low intensity stimulus, and disappears when the stimulus intensity is supramaximal. The H reflex is dependent on the integrity of the monosynaptic arc of the S1 segment.

Late response minimal latency is the most commonly used parameter for clinical purposes. The minimal latency correlates well with body height and arm and leg length. The H-reflex latency is constant, whereas the F-response latency varies within a narrow range. This range, as well as the persistence of F responses in a series of stimulations are useful clinical indicators of conduction abnormalities in different diameter nerve fibers and/or excitability of the motoneuron pool.

Late responses have proved useful in the diagnosis of polyneuropathies (both axonal and demyelinating) and particularly in the diagnosis of the Guillain-Barré syndrome in its early stage.[10,11,14] The usefulness of late response studies has also been demonstrated in the assessment of entrapment neuropathies and root compression syndromes.[4,5] In entrapment syndromes, a search for prolongation of minimal F latencies is an important adjunct to routine motor and sensory conduction studies. Abnormalities have been noted with a high frequency in the carpal tunnel syndrome, ulnar entrapment neuropathies, and the thoracic outlet syndrome. Similarly, late responses are also useful in the evaluation of lumbosacral root compression syndromes.

Compression Syndromes in the Upper Extremity

Median Nerve

Carpal Tunnel Syndrome

A lesion of the median nerve at the wrist is the most common form of entrapment in the upper extremity. It occurs when the median nerve passes, along with the flexor tendons of the fingers, between the carpal bones and the transverse carpal ligament.

Sensory symptoms usually precede the motor manifestations. Complaints of bouts of pain at the wrist and paresthesias in the fingers, often occurring during the night, are common. Characteristically shaking or rubbing the hands provides some relief. Marked weakness or atrophy of the thenar muscles is uncommon at presentation, perhaps because of greater awareness of the syndrome. However, a slight motor deficit is often noted on examination. The carpal tunnel syndrome is often bilateral, usually more severe in the dominant hand. It may be associated with Colles' fracture, hypothyroidism, and rheumatoid arthritis, among other pathological conditions, and may also occur during pregnancy.

Abnormalities of motor conduction studies typically consist of prolonged distal latency to the abductor pollicis brevis muscle on stimulation of the median nerve at the wrist. If compression is severe, this finding may be associated with decreased amplitude and prolonged duration of the CMAP. Abnormal motor studies were present in 67 percent of cases in a large series.[19] This study revealed prolonged distal latency of more than 4.7 ms in 60 percent of cases, absence of an evocable motor response in 4.4 percent, and asymmetry of distal latencies by 1 ms or more between the symptomatic and asymptomatic sides, both latencies being in the normal range, in the remaining cases. Sensory abnormalities were present more often than motor abnormalities, reaching 85 percent of cases in the series of Thomas et al.[19] Fifty percent of these cases had absent median sensory potentials on stimulation of the index finger, while 35 percent had prolonged sensory latencies of 3.5 ms or more. Even though sensory studies are abnormal more often than motor studies, there are a few cases in which only motor abnormalities are detected. Therefore, both studies should be performed in all cases.[7]

Stimulation of the median nerve in the palm of the hand while recording at the wrist includes the distal segment unlikely to be affected and enhances the degree of demonstrable abnormality.[2] Double simultaneous recordings from wrist and index finger following stimulation of the palm is a convenient way to demonstrate a mild slowing through the carpal tunnel. A prolonged minimal latency and an in-

creased range of F responses may be useful findings in cases with mild abnormalities on routine studies. The maximal motor conduction velocity may be slightly slowed in the median nerve proximal to the wrist. This may be present in up to two-thirds of the patients. In such cases, as in patients with polyneuropathies and generalized slowing of nerve conduction, it is important to recognize the increase in the distal latency relative to the motor conduction velocity above the wrist. This is the purpose of the terminal latency index (TLI), which is the conduction time in the proximal segment over the same distance as the terminal distance divided by the terminal latency.[17] In control subjects, the TLI is always greater than 0.34. It becomes abnormal in patients with the carpal tunnel syndrome with or without neuropathy.

Needle EMG may show abnormalities in some patients, revealing chronic denervation or spontaneous activity, or both. Fasciculations may be noted in one-fifth of cases. Needle EMG examination must localize the lesion at the wrist by documenting normal findings in median innervated muscles in the forearm.

Pronator Syndrome

The median nerve may be damaged in the upper forearm where it passes between the two heads of the pronator teres muscle. There is usually a complaint of persistent nonlocalized forearm pain of several months' duration. On physical examination, the most consistent finding is tenderness over the pronator teres muscle. The spontaneous pain may be reproduced by pronation of the forearm against resistance. Sensory loss in the distribution of the median nerve in the hand and weakness of the flexor pollicis longus and abductor pollicis brevis are often found on examination.

The motor and sensory conduction studies may localize the lesion, but they are normal in more than 50 percent of cases. The needle examination seems much more reliable in this instance. Both flexor digitorum profundus and flexor pollicis longus muscles were denervated in all patients in the series of Buchthal et al.[3] although the abductor pollicis brevis was abnormal in three patients only.

Anterior Interosseous Nerve Syndrome

This nerve arises from the main trunk of the median nerve just distal to its passage through the two heads of the pronator teres. It is a purely motor nerve that supplies the flexor pollicis longus, the radial portion of the flexor digitorum profundus, and the pronator quadratus. A lesion of the anterior interosseous nerve causes a deficit of flexion of the distal phalanges of the thumb and index finger, resulting in the classic posture assumed during an attempted pinch (positive pinch test). Motor and sensory studies in the median nerve are normal. EMG abnormalities limited to the appropriate muscles are consistent with a lesion of the anterior interosseus nerve. However, since this nerve often participates in anomalous distribution (e.g., the Martin-Gruber anastomosis), abnormalities in intrinsic hand muscles may be found occasionally.

Ulnar Nerve

Aside from penetrating injuries, the ulnar nerve is most often damaged at or around the elbow, at the wrist and hand, and in the thoracic outlet.[12,13]

Lesions at the Elbow

Pressure neuropathies are extremely common at the elbow, where the ulnar nerve lies superficial in an osseous groove. In this region the nerve is vulnerable to direct trauma, and even more to indirect injury through being drawn tightly against the ulnar groove. Tightening may be secondary to conditions that disturb the angular relationship at the elbow, such as sequelae of fracture or dislocation.

The symptoms include tingling in the fourth and fifth digits with occasional pain in the hand, forearm, or elbow. Mild hollowing of the first dorsal interosseous space is often noted. In advanced cases, marked weakness of the ulnar-innervated muscles in the hand and the forearm may be present. Sensory abnormalities are found on the palmar and dorsal aspects of the ulnar side of the hand and on the fourth and fifth digits. The clinical manifestations may be delayed by several years following a local trauma, hence the term *tardy ulnar palsy.*

Maximal motor conduction velocities are usually performed in three segments: from the wrist to below the elbow, from below the elbow to above the elbow, and from above the elbow to the axilla. Slowing in the segment across the elbow relative to the segment in the forearm is often found. It is significant if such slowing is of 10 m/s or more. Slight slowing in the upper arm segment is also seen in some patients. Sensory action potentials in the ulnar nerve at the wrist following stimulation of the small finger are usually absent or of reduced amplitude, revealing loss of sensory axons. The mixed nerve conduction studies from below to above the elbow are usually impaired also, contrasting with normal studies from above the elbow to the axilla.

Conduction studies are helpful in localizing the lesion in a large proportion of cases. In mild cases in which conduction studies are not revealing, the F responses obtained from the abductor digiti minimi or first dorsal interosseus muscle usually show prolonged minimal latencies. The ulnar innervated muscles may show prolonged minimal latencies. The ulnar innervated muscles may show features of denervation, but several muscles must be sampled because of the frequent patchy involvement of the ulnar trunk. The flexor carpi ulnaris is frequently denervated when the lesion is at the elbow. Sparing of this muscle, however, has no localizing value since the branches supplying it may arise several centimeters above the medial epicondyle.

Lesions at the Wrist and Hand

Before entering the palm, the ulnar nerve passes in a narrow canal medial to the median nerve, limited by the carpal bones dorsally and by the volar portion of the carpal ligament anteriorly. In this canal the nerve divides into a superficial cutaneous branch and a deep muscular branch. Ulnar lesions in the wrist and hand are of three types according to the level of the lesion.[18] Type I is due to simultaneous involvement of both superficial and deep branches, usually within or proximal to the canal of Guyon. It results in both motor and sensory symptoms and signs. Type II involves motor symptoms or signs in the ulnar innervated intrinsic muscles of the hand, and may be due to a lesion limited to the deep branch. Type III is secondary to involvement of the superfical branch and includes only sensory manifestations. Occupational neuritis, ganglionic compression, and open injury are responsible for more than 60 percent of the lesions of the ulnar nerve at the wrist or hand. Motor conduction studies may demonstrate increased distal latency on stimulation of the ulnar nerve at the wrist, with normal velocity or mild slowing in the forearm. The sensory studies between the small finger and the wrist are abnormal if the superficial cutaneous branch is damaged. The EMG may show denervation in the ulnar innervated muscles; it may be misleading if there is a crossover from the median to the ulnar nerve at the forearm, with denervation appearing in median innervated muscles in the hand as well.

Thoracic Outlet Syndrome

This syndrome results from compression of the brachial plexus and the subclavian vessels between the first rib and the clavicle. It is a neurovascular syndrome, the symptoms of which are due to mechanical pressure on the vascular elements, the neural elements, or both. The lower part of the brachial plexus that lies in direct contact with the first rib is most frequently involved in the thoracic outlet syndrome. Thus the fibers originating in the C8 and T1 nerve roots, including motor and sensory components of the ulnar nerve and partly of the median nerve, are frequently damaged.

Sensory symptoms usually precede motor involvement. They include pain in the hand, forearm, and arm and/or paresthesias localized to the medial side of forearm and hand. Numbness in the same distribution may also be noted by the patient. Weakness and wasting may be prominent in the lateral part of the thenar eminence, and this can be easily mistaken for the carpal tunnel syndrome. However, involvement of other intrinsic muscles of the hand is usually demonstrated on testing. In severe cases, obvious weakness and atrophy of the hypothenar and interosseous muscles along with the thenar muscles is noted. Sparing of the muscles of the thenar eminence is the exception. Involvement of the forearm muscles (flexors or extensors), if present, is usually slight.

Needle electromyography discloses denervation in hand muscles and is of localizing value in establishing that motor fibers traveling in both median and ulnar nerves are affected. Sensory conduction studies in the hand are abnormal from the small finger to the ulnar nerve at the wrist, showing an absent or low-amplitude nerve action potential. Sensory conduction from the index finger to the median nerve at the wrist is, however, unimpaired, since these cutaneous fibers originate from the C6 and C7 nerve roots and travel in the upper and middle trunks and lateral cord of the brachial plexus. Motor conduction velocities in the median and ulnar nerves are normal in the upper and middle trunks and lateral cord of the brachial plexus. Motor conduction velocities in the median and ulnar nerves are normal in the upper extremity, yet the compound muscle action potentials may be of low amplitude when loss of motor units is pronounced. Many studies have reported the localizing value of studying the motor conduction across the thoracic outlet by stimulation of the brachial plexus at the supraclavicular region; there is a significant decrease in velocity in subjects with the thoracic outlet syndrome. This stimulation is, however, painful since a large current is needed for supramaximal stimulation, and measurement of the conduction distance is often inaccurate. F responses recorded from the abductor pollicis brevis and abductor digiti minimi muscles are often delayed and provide a clue to documentation of proximal motor involvement in the presence of normal motor conduction velocities distal to the axilla.[22]

Radial Nerve

The radial nerve is the continuation of the posterior cord of the brachial plexus after it has given off the axillary nerve. It includes fibers in the C5–8 distribution. The radial nerve winds around the shaft of the humerus and then passes anterior to the lateral epicondyle and the radiohumeral joint prior to entering the forearm. It enters the supinator muscle and then bifurcates into a superficial branch, which is a purely cutaneous twig, and a purely motor branch, the posterior interosseus nerve.

Common sites of compression are (1) the middle and lower third of the arm where the nerve lies first in the spiral groove in contact with the posterior aspect of the humerus, and then lateral and superficial to it; (2) the region immediately distal to the elbow in the forearm; and (3) the lower third of the forearm where the superficial cutaneous branch may be damaged in its subcutaneous location.

For motor conduction studies, the radial nerve is accessible for surface stimulation in the lower part of the arm and in the upper third of the forearm. It is convenient to record the CMAP from the extensor indicis, which is the most distal muscle innervated by the posterior interosseus nerve. Reliable F responses may also be recorded from this muscle. Sensory conduction studies are readily performed between the thumb and the superficial cutaneous branch in the lower forearm.

Aside from the localizing value of motor conduction studies, information concerning the site of the lesion may be easily derived from needle EMG examination. Branches to the triceps muscle originate in the upper arm proximal to the spiral groove. This muscle is thus spared in compression at the midarm level and involved only in lesions in the axilla such as those resulting from improper use of crutches (crutch paralysis). Branches originating proximal to the division of the radial nerve in the upper forearm innervate the brachioradialis and extensor carpi radialis longus and brevis muscles. These muscles are usually involved in lesions following fractures of the humerus, yet the brachioradialis may be spared in Saturday night palsies or sleep paralysis in which the site of injury may be more distal on the lateral aspect of the humerus. Injury due to external compression is characterized by localized slowing in the affected segment, and its prognosis is usually good.

1. Injury of the radial nerve at the forearm involves several mechanisms: The nerve is usually loosely tethered to the capsule of the radiohumeral joint. In some subjects this fibrous band is thick and constricting and may compress the nerve. The anatomical relationship of the nerve to the head of the radius explains why radial nerve lesions may be caused by a radiohumeral dislocation such as in the Monteggia fracture. Injury to the radial nerve at this site spares the brachioradialis and extensor carpi radialis but may damage the sensory fibers to the hand.
2. The deep radial nerve may be compressed at its entry into the supinator muscle by a fibrous arch called the arcade of Frohse. In this case the supinator muscle is spared, as are the sensory fibers.
3. The posterior interosseus nerve may be damaged within the supinator mass itself. Sensory studies between the thumb and wrist reveal axonal loss in the main trunk of the radial nerve or damage to the superficial cutaneous branch in the forearm.

Compression Syndromes in the Lower Extremity

Femoral Nerve

The femoral nerve is the longest branch of the lumbar plexus. It receives fibers from the second, third, and fourth lumbar roots. Within the pelvis it runs along the lateral border of the psoas muscle under its aponeurosis and enters the thigh deep to the inguinal ligament and lateral to the femoral artery. In its intrapelvic course it supplies branches to the iliopsoas muscle. Its main terminal branches in the thigh are (1) branches supplying sensation to the anterior aspect of the thigh and anteromedial aspect of the leg, (2) a branch providing motor innervation to three heads of the quadriceps muscle, and (3) the saphenous nerve, which innervates the skin of the anterior and medial side of the leg.

Femoral neuropathy manifests itself by wasting and weakness of the quadriceps muscle, a decreased or absent knee jerk, and sensory loss over the anterior aspect of the thigh. Spontaneous pain may also be found in this distribution. If weakness of hip flexion is also present, the lesion is intraabdominal, in the proximal part of the nerve or (more likely) in the lumbar plexus. Diabetes is the most frequent cause of femoral neuropathy. Diabetic femoral neuropathy is characterized by the sudden onset of pain and motor weakness in this distribution, although minor involvement of other nerves is frequently noted. The mechanism of this neuropathy is most probably vascular. Entrapment of the femoral nerve is uncommon but may occur in the inguinal region, associated with an inguinal hernia or resulting from scarring after surgery. Femoral nerve involvement is also seen following long surgical procedures in the pelvic region and may be due to prolonged compression by retractors; this syndrome is often bilateral. Compression of the femoral nerve in the pelvis may also be caused by a retroperitoneal hematoma, which has been described in patients on anticoagulant therapy and in hemophiliacs. The saphenous nerve may be damaged at Hunter's canal or against the medial condyle of the femoral bone. It may also be injured during or following stripping of a varicose saphenous vein.

There is a technique to measure the motor conduction velocity in the femoral nerve by stimulation above and below the inguinal ligament. This technique might be helpful in identifying compression of this nerve by the inguinal ligament, which occurs infrequently. Sensory conduction studies in the saphenous nerve may also reveal local dysfunction of this nerve, or loss of sensory axons in lesions of the trunk. In femoral neuropathy, needle EMG shows denervation in the quadriceps muscle. It is important to sample other muscles in the thigh and leg to exclude involvement of the plexus.

Sciatic Nerve

The sciatic nerve includes fibers of the L4, L5, S1, S2, and S3 spinal roots. The trunk is formed in the posterior region of the pelvis and passes in the gluteal region through the greater sciatic notch and then deep to the pyriformis muscle. The sciatic nerve then enters into the thigh where it is deeply situated along most of its course. Above the popliteal space, it divides into the peroneal and posterior tibial nerves.

Aside from penetrating injuries, direct trauma causing damage to the sciatic nerve is uncommon. In the gluteal region the nerve is exposed to misplaced intramuscular injections and may be damaged in disorders of the hip joint such as fractures of the posterior rim of the acetabulum or posterior dislocations of the hip. The sciatic nerve may also be injured during surgery on the hip joint, particularly hip arthroplasty. Compression neuropathies have also been described at the level of the sciatic notch by the pyriformis muscle, and in the thigh by a fibrous band between the biceps femoris and adductor magnus muscles. In lesions of the sciatic nerve, the common peroneal portion of the nerve is invariably more affected than the posterior tibial portion.

Electrophysiological evaluation of the sciatic nerve may include direct stimulation at the sciatic notch through needle electrodes. Loss of motor fibers may be demonstrated by conduction studies in the peroneal and posterior tibial nerves. It is useful to study F responses from foot muscles in the distribution of peroneal and posterior tibial nerves, both studies being frequently abnormal in a lesion of the trunk of the sciatic nerve. The H reflex recorded from the soleus muscle is also abnormal in this case, correlating with a decreased or absent ankle jerk. Sensory fiber loss is easily documented by studying the sural nerve conduction bilaterally. Needle electromyography discloses denervation in the foot and leg muscles, in the peroneal and posterior tibial distribution. Denervation in muscles supplied by branches originating in the thigh, such as the short head of the biceps femoris, is a good clue to a sciatic nerve lesion. Involvement of the roots of the plexus must be excluded by documenting normal findings in the glutei and adductor muscles.

Peroneal Nerve

The peroneal nerve travels down the popliteal fossa, reaches the lateral aspect of the neck of the fibula, and winds around it, passing through an opening in the origin of the peroneus longus muscle. At the neck of the fibula the nerve divides into its terminal branches, the superficial peroneal nerve supplying the peroneus longus and brevis muscles, and the deep peroneal nerve supplying other muscles of the anterolateral compartment of the leg and the extensor digitorum brevis in the foot.

Disorders of the common peroneal nerve are common. The nerve is vulnerable to compression in its superficial course around the neck of the fibula, where it lies in contact with the bone. Peroneal palsy may be caused by sitting with legs crossed or working in a squatting position for prolonged periods of time. Direct trauma, plaster casts, or the weight of the lower limb in a bedridden or comatose patient may also be responsible for its compression.

Motor conduction studies may help to localize the lesion if the examiner stimulates above and below the fibular head and at the ankle while recording from the extensor digitorum brevis muscle. A localized slowing in the segment, including the fibular head, is of obvious diagnostic value but is not always found. A decrease in amplitude of the evoked CMAP on stimulation at the popliteal fossa compared with stimulation below the fibular head may reveal a conduction block and be helpful particularly in the earliest stages of peroneal palsy. Abnormal F responses from the extensor digitorum brevis with normal F responses from the flexor hallucis brevis helps exclude sciatic nerve involvement, and abnormal F responses from the tibialis anterior muscle may be useful in localizing the lesion. If the conduction studies are nondiagnostic, the pattern of EMG abnormalities may help to establish the diagnosis, if they show changes limited to the distribution of branches arising below the fibular head.

Posterior Tibial Nerve

The course of the posterior tibial nerve is deep until it reaches the ankle. In this region the nerve passes through a fibro-osseous passageway, the tarsal tunnel, posterior and inferior to the medial malleolus. Within the tarsal tunnel or immediately distal to it the nerve divides into three branches, the medial, lateral, and calcaneal plantar nerves. The tibial nerve or any of its branches is liable to a compression neuropathy.

The tarsal tunnel syndrome is characterized by the gradual onset of symptoms often following local trauma such as ankle sprain or fracture about the ankle joint. The symptoms include pain, numbness, and paresthesias in the foot. Sensory symptoms always precede motor involvement (e.g., paresis or paralysis of the intrinsic muscles of the foot). Frequently, local tenderness or Tinel's sign is elicited by pressure on the tarsal tunnel.

The diagnosis is supported by motor conduction studies showing prolonged distal latencies to the abductor pollicis or the abductor digiti quinti. The findings of denervation in the intrinsic foot muscles with normal EMG findings in the calf muscles also point to a distal lesion in the posterior tibial nerve.

Electromyography in Radiculopathies

The EMG evaluation of root compression syndromes must be based on an accurate knowledge of the segmental innervation of the myotomes commonly involved in cervical and lumbosacral rediculopathies. Irritation of the motor fibers is probably the earliest change and expresses itself by increased insertional activity, repetitive discharges (doublets, triplets, or multiplets), fasciculations, or bizarre repetitive potentials. These changes have a high diagnostic value when seen in the distribution of a single spinal root with sparing of the adjacent myotomes. With increased severity of root compression, axonal degeneration occurs and fibrillation potentials and positive sharp waves are detected. Careful search for spontaneous activity in the paraspinal muscles is indicated, since these changes may be lacking in distal muscles while already present in axial muscles. When abnormalities are present, a diagnosis of root compression must be based on their distribution in the territory of a single root and in muscles supplied by different peripheral nerves. Denervation in the paraspinal muscles may be of critical value in differentiating a root lesion from a plexus lesion.

Motor conduction studies are usually normal. Only in cases severe enough to cause significant axonal degeneration is the amplitude of the CMAP significantly reduced. Sensory conduction studies are always normal, even in the presence of objective sensory loss. This is due to the fact that sensory axons do not degenerate after injury to the dorsal root if the lesion is proximal to the posterior root ganglion.

Late response studies are often useful in the diagnosis of root lesions, particularly in lumbosacral root disease.[21] H-reflex and F-response studies, when abnormal, help localize the lesion in the appropriate root distribution. Abnormalities of late responses, however, are rarely found in isolation.

Finally, it should be pointed out that a normal electromyographic examination does not rule out root compression but only shows the absence of motor dysfunction secondary to it. Root lesions, however, often cause only pain, the evaluation of which is not within reach of routine clinical electromyography.

References

1. Aguayo A, Nair CPV, Midgley R: Experimental progressive compression neuropathy in the rabbit. Arch Neurol 24:358–364, 1971.
2. Buchthal F, Rosenfalck A: Sensory conduction from digit to palm and from palm to wrist in the carpal tunnel syndrome. J Neurol Neurosurg Psychiatry 34:243–252, 1971.
3. Buchthal F, Rosenfalck A, Trojaborg W: Electrophysiological findings in entrapment of the median nerve at wrist and elbow. J Neurol Neurosurg Psychiatry 37:340–360, 1974.
4. Egloff-Baer S, Shahani BT, Young RR: Usefulness of late response studies in diagnosis of entrapment neuropathies. Electroencephalogr Clin Neurophysiol 45:16P, 1978 (abstr).
5. Eisen A, Schomer D, Melmed C: The application of F-wave measurements in the differentiation of proximal and distal upper limb entrapments. Neurology 27:662–668, 1977.
6. Gilliatt RW: Chronic nerve compression and entrapment, in Sumner AJ (ed): *The Physiology of Peripheral Nerve Disease*. Philadelphia, Saunders, 1980, pp 316–339.
7. Kopell HP, Goodgold J: Clinical and electrodiagnostic features of carpal tunnel syndrome. Arch Phys Med Rehabil 49:371–375, 1968.
8. Liddell EGT, Sherrington CS: Recruitment and some other features of reflex inhibition. Proc R Soc Lond [Biol] 97:488–518, 1925.
9. Ochoa J, Fowler TJ, Gilliatt RW: Changes produced by a pneumatic tourniquet, in Desmedt JE (ed): *New Developments in Electromyography and Clinical Neurophysiology*. Basel, S. Karger, 1973, vol 2, pp 174–180.
10. Shahani BT, Dominque J, Potts F, Ropper A: Serial electrophysiological studies in patients with acute Guillain-Barré syndrome undergoing plasmapheresis. Muscle Nerve 3:440, 1980 (abstr).
11. Shahani BT, Potts F, Dominque J: F response studies in peripheral neuropathies. Neurology 30:409–410, 1980 (abstr).
12. Shahani BT, Potts F, Juguilon A, Young RR: Maximal-minimal motor nerve conduction and F response studies in normal subjects and patients with ulnar compression neuropathies. Muscle Nerve 3:182, 1980 (abstr).
13. Shahani BT, Potts F, Juguilon A, Young RR: Electrophysiological studies in "thoracic outlet syndrome." Muscle Nerve 3:182–183, 1980 (abstr).
14. Shahani BT, Sumner AJ: Electrophysiological studies in peripheral neuropathy: Early detection and monitoring, in Stalberg E, Young RR (eds): *Butterworth's International Medical Reviews*, vol 1: *Neurology*. London, Butterworth, 1981, pp 117–144.
15. Shahani BT, Young RR: Studies of reflex activity from a clinical viewpoint, in Aminoff MJ (ed): *Electrodiagnosis in Clinical Neurology*. New York, Churchill Livingstone, 1980, pp 290–304.
16. Shahani BT, Young RR: Clinical significance of late response studies in infants and children. Neurology 31:66, 1981 (abstr).
17. Shahani BT, Young RR, Potts F, Maccabee P: Terminal latency index (TLI) and late response studies in motor neuron disease (MND), peripheral neuropathies and entrapment syndromes. Acta Neurol Scand [Suppl] 73:118, 1979 (abstr).
18. Shea JD, McLain EJ: Ulnar-nerve compression syndromes at and below the wrist. J Bone Joint Surg [Am] 51:1095–1103, 1969.
19. Thomas JE, Lambert EH, Cseuz KA: Electrodiagnostic aspects of the carpal tunnel syndrome. Arch Neurol 16:635–641, 1967.
20. Thomas PK, Fullerton PM: Nerve fibre size in the carpal tunnel syndrome. J Neurol Neurosurg Psychiatry 26:520–527, 1963.
21. Tonzola RF, Ackil AA, Shahani BT, Young RR: Usefulness of electrophysiological studies in the diagnosis of lumbosacral root disease. Ann Neurol 9:305–308, 1981.
22. Wulff CH, Gilliatt RW: F waves in patients with hand wasting caused by a cervical rib and band. Muscle Nerve 2:452–457, 1979.

17

Electro-encephalography

William P. Wilson

The first noninvasive technique developed to examine the central nervous system was the electroencephalogram (EEG). Even so, it is less accepted in the fields of neurology and neurosurgery than is noninvasive and invasive radiography. This probably derives from two factors, the first being that the physician who is well trained in gross anatomy easily transfers his or her anatomical knowledge to the statically visualized roentgenogram. In contrast, central nervous system physiology, a measurement of the process, activities, and phenomena incidental to and characteristic of living processes, does not receive as much attention in the medical curriculum. Even when it does attend to the nervous system, it focuses on subject matter that is not readily related to anatomical lesions of the brain. It is no small wonder that clinical neuroscientists prefer radiographic investigative techniques and do not exploit the full potential of electrophysiological techniques. Since electroencephalography is easily applied, causes the patient little inconvenience, is inexpensive, is without danger, is quite accurate, is very portable, and can be used to monitor intracranial physiological activity over long periods, it deserves wider application.

Technical

The electrophysiological activity of the brain can be recorded from the scalp, the exposed cortex, and the depths of the brain. The equipment used to record the electrical potentials from all these sites is inexpensive and utilizes "state of the art" electronic components, including integrated circuits and operational amplifiers. The miniaturization of the EEG machine is limited only by the necessity to make a cheap permanent record of the outputs of the amplifiers. This necessitates the use of ink-writing equipment that is heavy and bulky. It is required because the time base of the record must be sufficiently long and the amplitude sufficiently great to make visual analysis possible. Visual analysis is still necessary because we have not as yet developed computer techniques that make data extraction, summation, *and* interpretation possible.

Computer Analysis

Barlow[1] has summarized the current state of the art of computer analysis of the EEG. He observes that computer analysis can readily determine the spectrum of rhythmic activity of the EEG. The detection and classification of transients, especially fast spikes, has not progressed as satisfactorily, although techniques are available. Techniques for detecting and classifying complex transients has hardly begun. Much work remains to be done before computer analysis of the EEG will be a reliable clinical tool.

Electroencephalography

The major variant in recording the electrophysiological potentials from the brain is in the design of the electrodes and their application. Electrodes are usually fabricated of noble metals. Subdermal electrodes are made of platinum while surface electrodes are chlorided silver or silver plated with gold. Surface electrodes are held in place using an electrolytic paste and collodion or with an adhesive electrolytic paste. Their placement is determined using measurements that are derived from standard landmarks on the head. These are the nasion, the inion, and the points at which the tragus intersects the helix of the ears. This system makes it possible to accurately place electrodes on the head each time a recording is desired, and also makes certain the anatomical location of these electrodes over the various surface landmarks of the brain. The system that has been adopted by most electroencephalographers, the 10-20 system, provides for accurate reproduction and a high degree of certainty of anatomical placement.

Scalp recordings do not allow one to record from areas of the cortex that are on the inferior and mesial surfaces of the lobes of the brain, especially the areas in the sylvian and sagittal fissures. Special techniques are available to record from some of these areas. Nasopharyngeal electrodes made of insulated silver rods with the tip exposed can be introduced through the nares into the nasopharynx. These, when appropriately placed, will record from the region of the uncus and anterior hippocampus on the medial surface of the temporal lobe. Sphenoidal electrodes are long, insulated stainless steel needles that are inserted to touch the ala magna of the sphenoid bone near the foramen ovale. They record from the inferior surface of the temporal lobe. It is impossible to record from the insula, the cortex in the fissure of Sylvius, the sagittal fissure, or the orbital surface of the frontal lobe except by surgically implanting electrodes.

The details of deriving various montages or runs is not within the scope of this writing; however, it is well to note that there are two basic methods, both of which are used by competent electroencephalographers. Scalp-to-scalp or bipolar linkages are most effective in the localizing of abnormalities. They are also more useful for determining the frequency and symmetry of rhythmic activity in the various areas of the brain. With this technique, a grid of the head is derived using several montages (Fig. 17-1). If appropriate parameters of the electrical potentials are used, it is possible

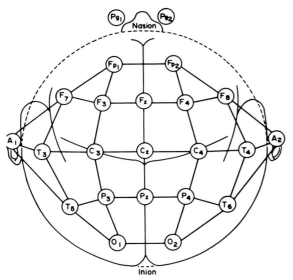

Figure 17-1 Distribution of scalp electrodes illustrating most of the standard derivations used in routine electro-encephalography.

to extract the information necessary for interpretation. The second technique is called the common reference or monopolar technique. It is used primarily to record the basic rhythms of the brain and to describe their distribution. It also best records generalized abnormalities, especially those that are rhythmic. It is not as effective in localizing lesions as the scalp-to-scalp or bipolar technique, but it is very useful when screening for abnormalities because the wide interelectrode distances cause abnormalities to be of greater amplitude.

Electrocorticography

Intracerebral recording in humans was first carried out by Hans Berger in 1931. A few years later, Foerster and Altenburger also successfully used the technique in their research. It was not, however, until A. E. Walker and W. Penfield with H. Jasper performed their classic researches that the technique became highly developed for the surgical treatment of epilepsy.[5] As with scalp recordings, a sufficiently large number of electrodes must be available to provide a recording grid over the exposed brain surface. Electrodes must be adjustable to allow flexibility of placement. This is achieved by using ball-and-socket joints on the frame of the holder, which is firmly attached to the skull at the margin of the craniotomy. Electrodes are fabricated of stainless steel rods to which are soldered silver wires. The end of this wire may be fused into a smooth ball of chlorided silver and then surrounded by a cotton ball, or the wire may have a woven cotton wick attached. Both the cotton and the cotton wick must be soaked in saline when placed on the cortex. Smooth balls or small buttons of carbon have been used as contacts by some workers. Flexible multicontact electrodes can be slipped extra- or subdurally into areas not exposed by the craniotomy. Acute depth recordings can be obtained

using rigid multicontact electrodes that are blunt needles with narrow silver chloride rings 10 mm apart separated by an area of insulation between each ring.

More recently, surgeons have implanted braided Teflon-insulated stainless steel electrodes with multiple recording points to record from the cortex to obtain corticograms over a prolonged period.[14] This technique has a distinct advantage in that the length and discomfort of a long operation can be avoided. In many instances, it is necessary to keep a heavily sedated patient awake and in one position for many hours while the electrographic mapping and surgery are carried out. This makes the procedure extremely stressful to the patient and operating room personnel. With chronic implanted electrode corticography, the brain is exposed, and then three to five electrodes, whose recording points are 10 to 15 mm apart, are placed over the cortical surface so that a recording grid can be derived (Fig. 17-2). They are held in place with Surgicel (oxidized regenerated cellulose; Surgikos, New Brunswick, N. J.). At the same time, electrodes may be placed stereotactically in subcortical structures if needed. All implanted electrodes are sutured to the dural edge and then to the scalp wound margin. The dura is closed, the bone flap replaced, and the wound closed. The ends of the electrodes with their plugs are pulled through the gauze dressing to be placed between the two layers of a head dressing. It is only necessary to remove the outer layer when the recordings are made. These may be left in place for periods of up to 3 weeks. After all studies are complete, the patient is taken to the operating room, the wound reopened, the electrodes removed, and surgery performed when indicated.

Depth Electrodes

Depth electrodes are used to investigate patients whose epilepsy is not sufficiently localized by conventional clinical and electroencephalographic techniques. In most instances

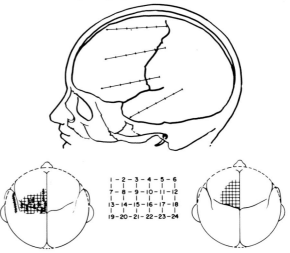

Figure 17-2 Distribution of transcortical implanted electrodes. Lower figure at left indicates sites of independent spiking; at center, electrode derivations; at right, lesion as delineated with scalp recording.

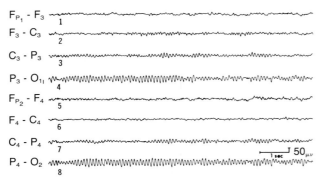

Figure 17-3   Normal waking EEG.

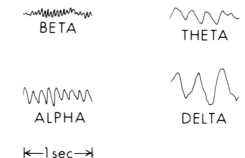

Figure 17-4   Basic rhythms seen in waking EEG.

these patients have intractable seizures that have not responded to medical regimes. If there is a chance that the patient can be helped by surgical treatment, it is wise to consider the implantation of multicontact electrodes in selected areas of the brain. As we have noted before, the most likely candidates are those patients whose possible lesions are in those areas of the brain inaccessible to scalp recording, i.e., the structures of the sagittal and sylvian fissures. Patients with bilateral abnormalities in which there is a possibility that a unilateral lesion is primary are also candidates.

The placement of implanted electrodes is a procedure that has a statistically small risk, but it should not be taken lightly. The complications most likely to occur are infection along the electrode track, meningitis, and hemorrhage caused by the rupture of a vessel by the penetrating electrode. These risks can be minimized by scrupulous attention to correct surgical and aseptic techniques as well as preoperative visualization of the individual's vascular tree by arteriography. There is no evidence that significant damage is done to the parenchyma of the brain by the introduction and removal of the electrodes. A detailed discussion of the subject can be found in Gloor's excellent review.[5]

Interpretation

The interpretation of the electroencephalogram is not simple. In the first place, there is a great mass of data now conventionally composed of 16 to 32 channels of information obtained over a minimum of 30 min up to a maximum of 2 to 3 days. Even at slow paper speeds, an 8-h recording will be composed of 1440 pages of information, so that intermit-

tent sampling is the preferred method for periods longer than 8 h. These recordings are read (1) by determining the frequency amplitude and the symmetry of rhythmic activity, (2) by determining the waveform, amplitude, and distribution of any transient activity that may occur, and (3) by determining the effects of activating procedures on both of these components (Fig. 17-3).[3] These activities are affected by the state of consciousness of the individual. Arousal elicited by stimuli from the environment increases the frequencies of the rhythmic activity, while natural sleep will cause a reduction in frequency. The age of the patient also determines the frequency of rhythmic activities. At the beginning of life the EEG is predominantly slow, but it shifts to faster frequencies until the early twenties. It then stabilizes, only to slow once again in the senium. Except in sleep, transient activity in the EEG is almost always evidence of abnormal function.

The spectrum of rhythmic (Fig. 17-4) activity of the brain is divided and classified as follows:[7]

1. Delta rhythms, 0.5 to 3 Hz (cycles per second)
2. Theta rhythms, 4 to 7 Hz
3. Alpha rhythms, 8 to 13 Hz
4. Beta rhythms, 14 to 40 Hz

One rarely sees cerebral rhythms slower than 0.5 Hz or faster than 40 Hz.

At birth the occipital rhythms of children in the waking state with eyes closed ranges from 3.5 to 4.5 Hz. By 9 years of age they will range from 7 to 10 Hz, and by 15 years they will reach their adult range of 8 to 11 Hz. There is a frequency spectrum of rhythms with large amounts of delta and theta rhythms at birth. These disappear most rapidly after 11 years of age.

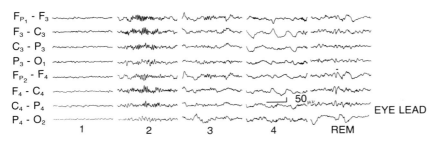

Figure 17-5   Sleeping EEG, all stages.

A. Spikes

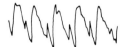

B. Sharp Waves

C. Paroxysmal Rhythmic Waves

D. PLEDS

E. Spike and Wave

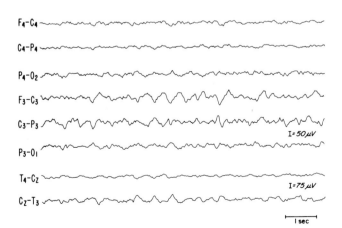

Figure 17-6 Types of epileptic discharge.

Sleep profoundly alters the normal rhythms of the EEG (Fig. 17-5). As a child goes to sleep, one often sees paroxysmal slow activity in the theta frequency. In other children and in adults, the resting waking rhythms (W stage) disappear and are replaced by beta rhythms, usually of low voltage (stage 1). As sleep deepens, spindles of 14-Hz rhythms occur in the central region. These may be associated with high-voltage waves known as *vertex sharp waves* (stage 2). Further deepening of sleep results in an increasing number of delta waves. If these are present 20 to 50 percent of the time, the stage of sleep is classified as stage 3; if present 50 to 100 percent of the time, it is classified as stage 4. A fifth stage of

sleep (REM sleep) is characterized by rapid eye movements and bursts of wicket-shaped delta waves punctuated by bursts of beta rhythms.

Epileptiform abnormalities (Fig. 17-6) are classified as follows:

1. Spikes, duration 20 to 70 ms
2. Sharp waves, 70 to 200 ms
3. Spike and slow wave complexes
4. Paroxysmal rhythmic waves (focal)
5. PLEDs (*p*eriodic *l*ateralized *e*pileptiform *d*ischarges)

These abnormalities are usually transient and may occur singly or in trains of discharge at variable frequencies lasting for brief periods. Spikes and spike and slow wave complexes can be generalized as well as bilaterally synchronous. PLEDs, which tend to be focal, are rhythmically continuous at 0.5 to 1 Hz but do not have a rigidly fixed rate.

Epileptic activity that arises in the cortical mantle most often is focal, except in children, where diffuse involvement of the cortex gives rise to a multifocal and/or generalized electrographic discharge known as *hypsarrhythmia*. Another type of discharge that seems to arise in the cortex is not associated with any pathological process. This disturbance, sometimes called rolandic spikes or polyphasic spikes, seems to have its origin in corticoreticular systems. Bilaterally synchronous and symmetrical forms of epileptic discharge are considered to be evidence of corticoreticular system disease.

Pathological processes in the brain tend to produce abnormalities of electrical activity that are related to the specific effects of the process on the cell. Processes that depress the metabolism of the cells will produce slowing of rhythmic activity in the affected area (Fig. 17-7). At the cortical level, this may be quite focal. If certain subcortical areas, especially the structures of the lower diencephalon, are affected, slowing will be generalized. Generalized disturbances of cerebral metabolism produce generalized slowing (Fig. 17-8). In contrast, processes that deafferentate cells but leave their metabolism intact render them hyperexcitable. If the aggregates of hyperexcitable cells are sufficiently large, epileptic

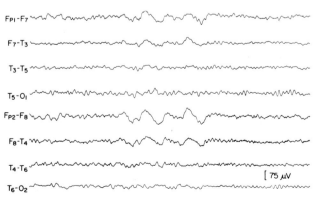

Figure 17-7 Focal delta wave abnormality in left frontal region (channel 4, F_3-C_3; channel 5, C_3-P_3 electrode pairs).

Figure 17-8 Bilaterally synchronous delta frequency slow wave abnormality. This is called frontal intermittant rhythmic delta activity (FIRDA).

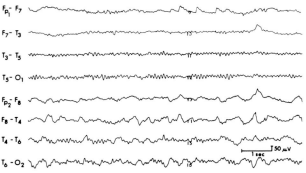

Figure 17-9 Lateralized slowing in patient with a glioblastoma multiforme of the right hemisphere.

discharge will occur anywhere in the central nervous system. Thus, we observe that a rapidly growing tumor like a glioblastoma, which severely injures cells, will most often produce slowing in the EEG (Fig. 17-9). An astrocytoma, which will deafferentate cells in certain areas but severely compromise the metabolism of cells in others, may give rise to both slow waves and epileptic discharge (Fig. 17-10). Oligodendrogliomas tend to deafferentate cells, which gives rise to epileptic discharge. In toxic withdrawal states, at certain stages there will be hyperexcitability of cells (Fig. 17-11) and epileptic discharge, whereas in metabolic disorders, such as hypothyroidism, liver failure, or uremia, there will be generalized slowing (Fig. 17-12). Interestingly, lesions, such as a meningioma, that do not depress the metabolism or cause deafferentation of cells but simply displace tissues produce few changes in the EEG.

Activation Procedures

In all patients it is desirable that latent abnormalities be activated.[5] This is especially true of epileptics, where it is imperative that an ictal record be obtained since the recording

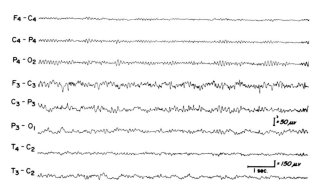

Figure 17-10 Mixture of epileptic discharge, potentiated beta activity, and epileptic discharge in left frontal region in a patient with an astrocytoma.

of a seizure may provide the best evidence for the localization of the lesion. Since spontaneous seizures are most often random events, special effort may be required to elicit a seizure. Sometimes, if one is fortuitously recorded, it may be obscured by muscle or movement artifact. There are methods that can help reduce the number of failures to record an ictus.

The method most commonly used to record an ictus is to obtain a prolonged recording. Here a patient may be recorded for 24 h using 16 or more channels of recording. The recording montage should provide maximum coverage of the brain areas accessible to recording and use derivations that minimize contamination by muscle artifact. Sphenoidal electrodes are highly desirable in most epileptics.

Telemetric recording is a second way to record an ictal event. The information can be stored by multiplexing the information onto magnetic tape, and once an ictus has occurred, that portion of the record can be demultiplexed into a standard EEG recording.

Activation procedures may be used to elicit seizures, as follows:

1. Hyperventilation is most commonly used as it is a very effective method of increasing the number or severity of abnormalities and frequently precipitates seizures.
2. Intermittent photic stimulation is not highly productive of useful information except in generalized epilepsies, but it is simple and harmless so it is usually presented.
3. One of the more effective methods of activating epilepsy is by inducing sleep. One can deprive the patient of sleep the night before the recording, record during their natural nocturnal sleep cycle, or induce sleep with drugs. The most useful drug is chloral hydrate as it produces fewer distortions of the natural rhythms and does not produce the beta rhythms that occur so commonly with other drugs. These beta rhythms can obscure spike discharge. Most abnormalities occur in stages 1 and 2 or in REM sleep. Epileptic discharges decrease in numbers or are masked by the high-voltage slow waves of stage 3 and 4 sleep. Intravenous methohexital has been used as an activation procedure, but there is some question as to whether it has any advantages over conventional methods of inducing sleep.
4. Intravenous pentylenetetrazol or bemigride are drugs that are used to elicit seizures in epileptic patients in a controlled situation. In most instances, the drug is given in a graded dose at a predetermined rate. The dose of pentylenetetrazol is usually 1 mg/kg given every 30 s to a total of 10 mg/kg. Some workers have put the patient to sleep with a barbiturate and given the entire dose in a single injection. One of the major objections to this technique is that patients with a normal brain can have a seizure if given these drugs. Another is that, as the threshold for generalized seizures vary, it is possible that the epileptic patient may have a generalized seizure before a habitual attack is precipitated. A second major objection is that the conscious patient almost always develops profound anxiety characterized by a terrifying sense of impending doom as a result of the injection of these

drugs. Although this can to some extent be ameliorated with the administration of a benzodiazepine, the patient may nevertheless find the anxiety intolerable. Many workers no longer use this technique since its yield is low in comparison with its risks.

5. The most efficacious activation procedure is withdrawal of anticonvulsant medication. This should be done gradually and wih careful observation of the patient. It is contraindicated in patients with a history of status epilepticus. It should be remembered that anticonvulsant blood levels do not drop quickly. In the brain, it is likely that there may be an even greater delay before there is a significant drop in phenytoin levels. Phenobarbital will decrease in the brain at about the same rate as in the blood.

EEG Technicians and Electroencephalographers

It is imperative that those persons who obtain the recording and those who interpret their efforts be adequately trained. Technicians should have 1 year of training in an approved program leading to certification. Physicians should be trained in clinical neuroscience and certified in their specialties and have the equivalent of 1 year of full-time training that qualifies them for the certification examination in electroencephalography. Although the American Board of Qualification in Electroencephalography is not approved as a subspecialty by the American Medical Association, the examination for certification is nevertheless a rigorous evaluation of related basic science and clinical knowledge as well as interpretative knowledge and skill. Certification does provide some assurance of competency in a field where inadequate training is all too common.

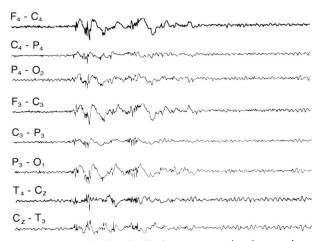

Figure 17-11 Epileptic discharges occurring in a patient who is withdrawing from chlordiazepoxide hydrochloride. The patient had seizures shortly after this EEG was obtained.

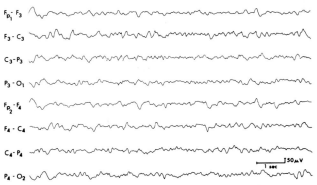

Figure 17-12 Severe metabolic encephalopathy in patient with chronic renal failure. Note the generalized random slowing.

General Usefulness of the EEG

Infancy and Childhood, Ages 0 to 5

1. Birth trauma
2. Infantile spasms or hypsarrhythmia
3. Cerebral palsy
4. Febrile seizures
5. Encephalitis
6. Cerebral abscess
7. Meningitis
8. Head injury other than birth trauma
9. Retarded development
10. Failure to thrive

Although obtaining an electroencephalogram from the newborn is difficult, there is no doubt that the procedure can be useful in investigating central nervous system symptoms and signs that may occur. When birth trauma is obvious, the electroencephalogram has its main value in delimiting, or at least attempting to delimit, the degree of involvement due to the injury. If the injury is localized, the EEG may help to delineate the extent and severity of the cerebral damage.

If patterns are characteristic of those that occur with the diffuse abnormality called hypsarrhythmia, it may be further predicted that the chances of the child being mentally deficient are quite high. Localized abnormalities may also aid in diagnosing cerebral palsy; however, generalized abnormalities are more common than focal abnormalities in more severely physically and mentally handicapped persons. There is some positive correlation between EEG abnormalities and epilepsy in cerebral palsy.

During and after the first year of life, the development of seizures, either focal or generalized, makes the utilization of electroencephalography imperative. Frequently, seizures may have their onset with febrile illness. A normal electroencephalogram occurring in patients with febrile convulsions is often a good prognostic sign and may indicate that the occurrence of seizures is secondary to the febrile episode rather than a result of the activation of a previously existing lesion by the fever.

In a manner similar to this, the occurrence of other central nervous system disease may be ruled out. As subclinical encephalitic processes are associated with the exanthemata, the occurrence of an abnormal EEG in a patient who has had seizures with the exanthemata is not expected; however, a persistently abnormal record would indicate that there is a likelihood that the patient has developed a secondary encephalitis as a complication of the disease.

Although brain abscesses are not as commonly seen as they were in the past, they still occur frequently and should be considered when central nervous system symptoms develop in association with fever. Such parenchymatous infections in the central nervous system are readily localized by electroencephalography. Meningitis is a diagnosis readily made by a lumbar puncture, and the utilization of the EEG is not imperative. However, when recovery is not as rapid as one would anticipate with antibiotic therapy, the EEG may be quite useful in indicating the occurrence of secondary complications of the meningitic process such as subdural hygroma or abscess.

Following head injuries, the EEG is useful in determining the extent of damage incurred and in evaluating residual damage even when symptoms resulting from the trauma have decreased or disappeared.

Although the EEG may only aid in determining the possible etiology of mental deficiency, it is often used. An abnormal record usually suggests pathophysiological disturbances or pathological lesions as bases for the retarded development or failure to thrive.

Late Childhood, Ages 5 to 10

1. Brain tumor
2. Epilepsy
3. Behavior problems
4. Recurrent abdominal pain or headaches
5. Neurotic disorders

As the child grows older, the incidence of brain tumors increases precipitously. Tumors of the posterior fossa constitute 65 to 75 percent of neoplasms occurring in childhood. Although the EEG may be useful, diseases of the brain in the posterior fossa are not readily localizable until neurological signs and symptoms have developed. A negative EEG will not rule out a subtentorial tumor, and other measures are necessary to further investigate the suspected occurrence of such a lesion. Tumors occuring above the tentorium can generally be demonstrated electroencephalographically.

Generalized seizures are not as common during this period as is focal cortical epilepsy. Most frequent among the focal lesions are those of the frontal lobe, which may be associated with seizures and disturbances in behavior. The seizures may be Jacksonian, minor, or major in their patterns. Focal temporal epilepsies do not occur with high incidence in this age group. Centrencephalic or corticoreticular epilepsy of the petit mal, myoclonic, and grand mal types begins to make its appearance and is readily diagnosed by

electroencephalographic techniques. The abnormality described by Gibbs and Gibbs, called 14 and 6 per second positive spikes and associated with pain, dysautonomia, and behavior disorder is now recognized with increasing frequency. This abnormality particularly is accompanied by headaches and abdominal pain and can be diagnosed only electroencephalographically. In most EEGs abnormalities occur only during sleep. The most common cause is cerebral trauma.

Rolandic epilepsy, also called the *polyphasic spike phenomenon*, is a benign seizure disorder in children and has a good prognosis—the seizures usually disappear at or before puberty. The rather characteristic EEG features help in differential diagnosis between this disorder and focal cortical epilepsy or cerebral damage.

Adolescence, Ages 10 to 15

1. Epilepsy
2. Behavior disorders
3. Supratentorial tumors
4. Encephalitis
5. Psychoses

In this age group an increasing incidence of epilepsy is observed and all types are seen. Although focal epilepsy has a rather high incidence in the 5- to 10-year-old age group, more seizures are observed in children 10 to 15 years old. Corticoreticular epilepsy appears with increasing frequency, as does temporal lobe epilepsy. The latter remains, however, a minor part of the problem of epilepsy in children. Quite frequently, behavior disorders may occur as the initial symptom of epilepsy, and it is only after this behavioral disturbance has manifested itself for a considerable length of time that seizures are observed. On the other hand, in some forms of epilepsy, notably corticoreticular, behavior disorders may be a minor part of the presenting symptomatology. In patients with this type of epilepsy, brief absences and generalized tonic-clonic seizures represent the major presenting symptoms. In all instances, a sleep EEG in addition to a waking tracing is extremely useful in determining the origin of the epileptic seizure or behavior disorder that the patient may have concomitant to the epilepsy.

The incidence of supratentorial tumors begins to increase, and the tumors may be readily detected by electroencephalography.

Encephalitis is accompanied by EEG abnormalities that are of great help in diagnosis. These may be the only positive accessory clinical findings. During convalescence the EEG is useful in determining how rapidly the process is clearing.

An abnormal EEG in a child with juvenile psychosis often indicates the occurrence of this entity as a result of either infectious or posttraumatic encephalopathy.

Finally, it is in the 10- to 15-year-old age group that the 14 and 6 per second positive spikes become more common in their occurrence. Indeed, it has been said that this abnormality is the most common form of abnormal cerebral electrical activity observed in an EEG laboratory that examines both adults and children.

Late Adolescence and Early Adulthood, Ages 15 to 20

1. Epilepsy
2. Brain tumors
3. Encephalitis
4. Endocrinopathies
5. Metabolic disease
6. Cerebral trauma

In late adolescence one begins to see an increasing incidence of temporal lobe epilepsy, which may occur in association with a number of symptoms referable either to the autonomic nervous system or to disturbances of consciousness and behavior. In contrast, the 14 and 6 abnormality begins to disappear, so that by the age of 21 very few individuals with this abnormality are observed.

Supratentorial brain tumors increase in incidence with maturation, with a corresponding reduction in the percentage of posterior fossa neoplasms seen. Glioblastoma multiforme begins to occur, although these tumors do not reach their peak incidence until later in life.

Infectious diseases of the central nervous system become less frequent but still occur.

Endocrinopathies with concomitant metabolic disease begin to appear more frequently, and the EEG may be quite useful in diagnosis. Generalized slowing of the cerebral rhythms frequently occurs in both hypo- and hyperthyroidism, as well as in diseases of the adrenal gland. Often an increase in frequency of alpha rhythm is seen in hyperthyroidism, whereas the alpha rhythm tends to be slow and poorly sustained in hypothyroidism. Abnormalities are particularly noted in disorders of the pituitary gland with associated Sheehan's syndrome or panhypopituitarism from any cause. Frequently, psychiatric symptoms may obscure the occurrence of these illnesses, and it is in differential diagnosis that the EEG may be quite useful. Abnormal records are seen in patients with hypoglycemic attacks due to islet cell adenomas; a prolonged fast may activate the record if it is otherwise normal.

EEG abnormalities are common in a wide variety of metabolic comas; however, they are nonspecific for the most part. Triphasic waves were first described as diagnostic of hepatic encephalopathy; however, it has been demonstrated since that "typical" triphasic waves are specific to hepatic encephalopathy only when prevalent and symmetrical anteriorly. "Atypical" triphasic waves also occur in other metabolic disorders. In general, the incidence of triphasic waves is higher in hepatic and renal encephalopathy than in any other metabolic encephalopathy.

As vascular disease does not occur with great frequency in this age group, it will be discussed later.

Adulthood and the Senium, Age 30 +

After the age of 30, there is an increasing incidence of vascular disease and cerebral tumors of metastatic origin. The EEG is of limited value in cerebral vascular disease. After thrombosis has occurred, the EEG adds little more than confirmation of the obvious. In those instances where it could be of greatest value, i.e., while the patient is having ischemic attacks, it seldom is abnormal and is of little help. After intracranial bleeding, the EEG may demonstrate intracerebral and other intracranial hematomas and may help to determine the site of bleeding in aneurysms.

Just as it aids in the diagnosis of intrinsic brain tumors, the EEG can be useful in diagnosing metastatic brain tumors, often indicating the occurrence of multiple lesions.

As toxic and metabolic disorders tend to increase in frequency in this age group, the occurrence of an abnormally slow EEG in patients with symptoms suggesting such syndromes may assist in further investigating the patient's illness.

In later life the EEG is useful in investigating and evaluating the mental aberrations that occur in the senium and presenium.[13] Its major usefulness is in differential diagnosis, for it behooves every physician to rule out brain tumor and the treatable metabolic or psychiatric illness before coming to a final diagnosis of arteriosclerosis or cerebral degeneration. The EEG may be helpful in establishing the diagnosis or may indicate a need for further investigation.

General

Of the subacute viral encephalopathies, subacute sclerosing panencephalitis reveals a highly characteristic EEG pattern. This consists mainly of periodic high-voltage bilaterally synchronous sharp wave complexes on a low-voltage background. The rate of repetition of these complexes is commonly between 6 and 16 times per minute; however, it may vary during the course of the illness. Subacute sclerosing panencephalitis is a disease of children and adolescents now recognized as caused by the measles virus.

Subacute spongiform encephalopathy, which affects mainly patients over 40 years of age, also reveals highly characteristic EEG abnormalities. With progression of the disease, high-voltage bilaterally synchronous polyphasic sharp wave complexes alternate with periods of lower-voltage slow activity. These complexes are not symmetrical and may show predominance in any locality; they may also show a marked periodicity. Some cases originally described as Creutzfeldt-Jakob syndrome are really those of subacute spongiform encephalopathy. The EEG in Creutzfeldt-Jakob syndrome shows a progressive loss of normal rhythms, which are replaced by generalized slow activity. In time, periodic sharp wave components will develop.

Another striking EEG pattern consists of periodic lateralized epileptiform discharges (PLEDs), which can be found in any age group. PLEDs are periodic or quasiperiodic epileptiform patterns that may be either localized or lateralized. A large majority of these patients have epileptic seizures, and the cause in most cases is either cerebral infarct, infection, or chronic cerebral seizure disorder.

The EEG in drug abuse is usually abnormal but nonspecific. Increase in REM sleep has been observed with withdrawal of amphetamines.

The EEG plays an important role in determining cerebral death, which in the case of organ transplantation becomes an important issue. A more detailed discussion of the various uses of the EEG described here can be found in the book edited by Klass and Daly.[7]

Specific Uses in Neurosurgery

In the foregoing, we have presented the general usefulness of the EEG. At this point it seems desirable to focus on those uses that are of greater value to the neurosurgeon.

Developmental Diseases

Developmental malformations and *perinatal injuries* that cause porencephaly and holoprosencephaly usually give rise to the absence of or reduction in voltage of electrical activity over the lesion with focal epileptic discharge along the margin of the lesion.

In *hydrocephalus*, the electroencephalogram is not of great use. No matter what the cause, the tracing is usually normal. Only in a rare case does one encounter either generalized slowing, focal slow waves, or spike foci. These abnormalities most often follow surgical intervention.

In *Chiari malformations, hydromyelia,* and *syringomyelia,* one seldom observes electroencephalographic abnormalities.

Infection

Meningitis will produce a generalized reduction in the amplitude of the rhythmic activity of the brain. Only rarely does it produce focal slowing or generalized slowing in the adult, but it may occasionally produce them in a child. PLEDs and focal spikes can occasionally occur if the infectious process extends into the brain, although early abscess formation is most often associated with focal slowing.

Abscesses of the brain in the acute stage are usually associated with focal slowing rather than other abnormalities such as unilateral slow waves, epileptic discharge, or reductions in amplitude. As the abscess becomes more chronic and scarring develops, epileptic discharge will occur with increasing frequency. Deeply located abscesses may produce generalized slowing. This is particularly true for those that develop in the cerebellum.

Subdural abscesses and *subdural empyemas* are usually associated with suppression of the electrical activity or lateralized slowing. If they are large, they may distort brain stem structure and give rise to bilateral slowing.

Encephalitis produces a kaleidoscopic array of changes in the EEG patterns. It may cause a reduction in amplitude but most often will produce generalized asynchronous slowing or focal slowing. Herpes simplex encephalitis, because of its proclivity to involve orbital frontal and temporal structures, may produce slowing that is more anterior, occasionally associated with sharp waves. Other epileptic discharges rarely occur in encephalitis except for PLEDs, which do occur on occasion.

Creutzfeldt-Jakob disease is associated with generalized periodic sharp wave complexes that may be localized to one part of the brain early in the course of the disease. In time, though, they do become generalized. These sharp waves are associated with a generalized slowing of the rhythmic activity. The sharp wave complexes are often associated with myoclonic twitches. They may be triggered by startle.

Subacute sclerosing panencephalitis (SSPE) is also associated with periodic discharges that are bilateral. These discharges differ from those of Creutzfeldt-Jakob disease in that they are more complex, usually consisting of a sharp wave with one or more slow waves following. Other epileptic discharges such as spikes and spike wave complexes occasionally occur. The rhythmic activity is also generally slowed and is either asynchronous or bisynchronous.

If there is marked mesencephalic involvement by the encephalitic process, then suppression burst activity may occur. Such a change carries a grave prognosis.

Chronic granulomatous infections of the nervous system usually produce generalized slowing. This is especially true in tuberculous meningitis.

Neuro-oncology

Prior to the advent of the CT scan, the EEG was the only noninvasive method useful in the localization of intracranial tumors. It was surprisingly accurate for it provided a good localization of the lesion in 60 to 70 percent of cases.[4] It was even more accurate if one divided the cases into those with supratentorial lesions and those with subtentorial lesions.

Almost all *supratentorial invasive tumors* can be localized accurately! This is especially true of the gliomas. These lesions have growth characteristics that frequently provide clues as to their histological characteristics. As noted above, glioblastomas usually produce focal or lateralized slowing; astrocytomas, a mixture of focal slowing and epileptic discharge; and oligodendrogliomas, mostly epileptic discharge.

Tumors of the pineal are not readily localizable in the EEG and only give rise to lateralized or generalized slowing in the EEG.

Supratentorial tumors of the ependyma, because they are usually deep and first invade the white matter of the brain, do not produce abnormalities in the EEG that are of diagnostic or localizing value.

Meningiomas, because they do not alter the cellular relationships of the cortex, do not produce alterations of EEG rhythms unless they interfere with the vascular supply to the brain. Lesions in the olfactory groove, on the sphenoid ridge, and on the floor of the middle fossa rarely produce changes that would suggest their presence.

In *subtentorial lesions*, the EEG is not a highly useful procedure. Cerebellopontine angle tumors, cerebellar astrocytomas, hemangioblastomas, and medulloblastomas rarely produce EEG changes unless they have distorted the brain stem structure and have produced hydrocephalus. When these things have happened, then generalized slowing is common.

Subtentorial axial tumors only produce changes in the EEG if they involve the structures above the level of the pons; thus, tumors of the aqueduct and third ventricle will always produce EEG changes. This will usually consist of bilaterally synchronous paroxysmal slowing. It is important to note that although these changes do occur, they are not highly diagnostic since many other conditions can produce similiar changes.

In *metastatic disease of the brain*, the EEG has proven to be quite useful. Both single and multiple metastases produce slow waves in the EEG. Multiple metastases usually produce more diffuse slowing.

Vascular Disease

In general, the EEG is not of great value diagnostically. The EEG is of value in patients with *transient ischemic attacks* in that it may provide evidence of other etiologic possibilities.[2] Indeed, if the EEG is abnormal in a patient with symptoms suggesting transient ischemic attack, then the lesion may not be a vascular one.

In those patients who have *occlusive vascular disease*, the EEG can only confirm the obvious. However, it can be of some help in the follow-up period because persistent slowing is usually associated with little neurological improvement.

In patients with *subarachnoid hemorrhage secondary to ruptured aneurysms or arteriovenous anomalies*, the EEG is often generally slowed because of the toxic effect of the degradation products of the blood on the cortex.[12] A focal lesion is evidence of an intracerebral hematoma. Unruptured aneurysms or anomalies do not produce EEG abnormalities. An occasional patient may have focal slowing or focal epileptic discharge if the lesion has scarring associated with it, perhaps due to previous subclinical hemorrhage.

Venous thrombotic disease will produce generalized, lateralized, or focal slowing. These abnormalities will depend on the extent of the venous occlusion. The EEG is not diagnostically useful in these problems.

Trauma

Significant trauma to the brain almost always gives rise to both anatomical and physiological changes. The anatomical change may be only slight edema, and the physiological change may be only a slight suppression of the cerebral electrical activity, but there is a need to be able to examine the change over time to determine its course. The EEG is an ideal way of meeting this need. That it has value is documented by the reports of numerous investigators.

One of the first and most significant of these was the report of Walker and Erculei concerning patients who had sustained missile-induced head injuries.[11] Their patients were examined electroencephalographically after head injuries that only lacerated the scalp, those with uncomplicated fractures, those with compound comminuted fractures of the skull, and those with perforating lesions. In these patients, the more severe the injury, the greater the incidence of generalized abnormality in the EEG. In a like manner, there was a higher incidence of generally abnormal EEGs in the patients with neurological deficits. Focal EEG abnormalities were much more frequent, however, in those patients with compound comminuted fractures and perforating wounds.

Epilepsy was relatively common in the series of Walker and Erculei as a complication of injury. They observed that there was a good correlation between the occurrence of abnormal EEGs and a history of seizures. Even so, one-third of the patients had normal or near normal EEGs. They concluded that the EEG is of great value from a diagnostic and prognostic standpoint especially when serial tracings are done.

Jennett and Van de Sande, on the other hand, are not as enthusiastic about the usefulness of the EEG in patients with closed head injuries who developed epilepsy.[6] They concluded that the EEG does not contribute materially to the problem of predicting late epilepsy in individual patients. Many patients with persisting abnormalities, either generalized or focal, do not develop epilepsy while some with normal EEGs do have seizures.

Stockard et al., in their excellent review, have observed that the EEG is a useful tool in the evaluation and follow-up of patients with head injury.[9] In the immediate phase of the uncomplicated head injury, a variety of changes can be observed. In one group of patients, there may be (1) a focal suppression of the normal rhythms that will progress to focal slowing to recovery, or (2) severe generalized slowing in the delta frequency that will progress to theta slowing then to recovery, or (3) alpha-like coma that may only progress to delta slowing in the subacute stage, or (4) spindle coma that can be followed by recovery, or (5) fluctuating rhythms with arousal that may also be followed by recovery.

There are, of course, many complications of closed head injuries that must be considered if focal or lateralized abnormalities are seen. These include subdural hematomas, epidural hematomas, and intracerebral hematomas. These lesions almost always give rise to focal abnormalities such as voltage suppression, slowing, or epileptic discharge.

The late phase of the head injury may be characterized by the persistence of an earlier EEG abnormality, or by abnormalities that are seen only as a late change. It is a fact that in time (6 months) the incidence of generalized abnormalities may drop from 93 percent to 3 percent. Focal abnormalities do not decrease as much because, after injury, 20 percent of patients who have such abnormalities early still have them 4 years later.

In general, it can be said that focal delta activity, if present 6 months after an injury, may improve but theta slowing will persist as random occasional waves. In the same way, bilaterally synchronous slowing may persist as mild dys-synchronous generalized slowing. An area of delta slowing present at 6 months can evolve into an area of focal epileptic discharge, while generalized slowing can develop into a typical generalized spike and wave discharge. The usual late complication of trauma is epilepsy.

Finally, the EEG has been shown to be of diagnostic and prognostic significance in patients with acute midbrain injuries who are in coma. In those patients with acute injuries to the midbrain, fast rhythms in the alpha frequency or in spindles in the frontal regions indicate a poor prognosis, whereas generalized slowing is associated with a better one.

Epilepsy

The neurosurgical treatment of epilepsy is only possible when it can be demonstrated that the patient's seizures originate in a circumscribed area of the brain. This area is almost always in the neocortex or in the limbic structures of the temporal lobe, i.e., the amygdala and hippocampus. In most instances, the clinical observation of seizures and radiographic examination is of little value. Only the electroen-cephalogram provides the necessary evidence that an ictus has a constant origin in a sufficiently circumscribed area of the brain to make surgery possible.

Evaluation of Patients for Surgery

Those patients who are selected for surgery are patients whose seizures have not responded to aggressive medical management and whose lesion is in an area of the brain where surgical ablation will not leave the patient with some other impairment.[8]

Although I have noted earlier that the clinical examina-tion and radiographic examination are of little value in local-izing the patient's lesion, it is important that the patient be carefully evaluated in both of these areas. Workers in the field do, of course, emphasize the need to evaluate the pa-tient's history to determine the possible cause of the seiz-ures. It is important to determine the age at the onset, the natural history of the development of seizures, the seizure pattern, the changes in seizure patterns, response to medica-tion, triggering mechanisms, and the psychological concom-itants of the seizures. Radiographic evaluation is necessary to determine the presence of parenchymal lesions or vascular anomalies of the brain.

Electrographic evaluation of the patient should include both ictal and interictal recordings. The techniques by which these recordings are obtained have been described, but the necessity of obtaining both ictal and interictal re-cordings must be emphasized. Adequate recording time is a must since seizures are, for the most part, random events; therefore, to obtain recordings of the seizure, and especially to obtain the onset of the seizures, a recording must be in process. The purpose of the preoperative recording is, of course, to demonstrate the discretely focal nature of the le-sion. In patients with temporal lobe lesions it is imperative that the lesion be unilateral; therefore, both temporal lobes must be carefully scrutinized for the occurrence of abnor-mality. These observations require the routine use of naso-pharyngeal and sphenoidal electrodes.

Withdrawal of medication is the first activation proce-dure to be used after hyperventilation and sleep. Sleep is desirable in all patients, especially if the patient has a history of nocturnal seizures. Once again, I emphasize the desirabil-ity of obtaining natural sleep recordings as opposed to re-cordings during drug-induced sleep. Obviously, all night sleep recordings will be most helpful as they are prolonged, and natural sleep can be most easily obtained in the patient's natural sleep cycle.

Stereotactic Investigation

This is sometimes undertaken prior to an operative crani-otomy. Here electrodes are placed stereotactically in either the limbic structures of the temporal lobe or in other deeper structures of the brain using conventional stereotactic tech-niques. In this instance, recordings can be made from the implanted electrodes as well as from the scalp simultane-ously to provide what has been called stereo-EEG studies. It is possible to obtain a three-dimensional view of the electri-cal activity of the brain using this method.

Electrocorticography

The technique for this investigative procedure has been previously described. However, it is important at this point to describe the clinical aspects of its use. Once the cortex is exposed, anatomical landmarks must be identified. Then functional areas of the brain can be clearly determined by stimulating the cortex. This is performed using a neuro-physiological stimulator that generates mono- or biphasic square wave pulses. These pulses should be controllable in their frequency, voltage, amperage, and duration. It is gen-erally accepted that the cortex responds best to a 30- to 60-Hz stimulus usually below 15 V with no greater current intensity than 1 mA and a pulse duration of less than 7 ms. Such stimuli are quite effective in producing motor and sen-sory responses in the awake patient.

The use of stimulation to activate seizure discharge in a lesion is not highly productive. Most authors have found that these discharges, called afterdischarge, are nei-ther highly reliable in delineating the extent of a lesion nor consistently useful in localizing the most excitable area of a lesion. There are, however, a few instances where prop-erly interpreted afterdischarge does provide useful infor-mation.

After a lesion has been excised, a postremoval cor-ticogram has been used, but it usually does not provide in-formation that is of prognostic significance. Postoperative electroencephalograms are usually abnormal for variable lengths of time because of the trauma of the surgery. Within 1 year, they usually have stabilized. Rather interestingly, many patients with abnormal EEGs have no seizures while others with the same amount of abnormality do have seiz-ures.

A normal or near normal postoperative EEG at 1 year is almost always associated with a good clinical result.

Brain Death

The cessation of life, or death, was never a problem for phy-sicians until the twentieth century, since the cessation of breathing and the cessation of the heartbeat provided an eas-ily determined end point. The development of modern re-suscitative techniques changed all of this, for many times persons were resuscitated whose brains had been deprived of oxygen for so long a period as to result in destruction of all or part of the brain. This gave rise to a situation in which there was a living body housing a dead brain. As a result, physicians began to try to define death using new criteria. These have evolved to those presently accepted by both medicine and the law.

In his most recent monograph on the subject, Walker[10] has developed an algorithm for cerebral death that reads as follows:

The patient, normothermic and normotensive, must be comatose, apneic and without cephalic reflexes
and
A case must meet the conditions specified in A, B, or C.
    A. This state must be present for 3 days
                    or

B. (1) The primary condition must be known to be an irreparable lesion of the brain.

   (2) The patient, by appropriate examination, must be shown to have for at least 30 minutes:

     a. Electrocerebral silence (ECS)

     b. Absence of cerebral blood flow

        or

     c. No cerebral metabolism

C. (1) The primary condition, not known to be an irreparable lesion of the brain, has not responded to appropriate treatment.

   (2) The patient's EEG must be isoelectric for 2 days.

        or

At least six hours after the ictus, the EEG must be isoelectric for 30 minutes and either there must be no evidence of cerebral blood flow or no cerebral metabolism for 30 minutes.

These criteria were developed from the results of a massive interdisciplinary study of brain death in which no person survived who met these criteria.

As the EEG is a pivotal accessory clinical finding, it is well to discuss this in detail. For a record to be acceptable for use in the determination of brain death, the following technical criteria must be met:

1. There must be a minimum of eight scalp and ear reference electrodes.
2. The interelectrode resistances must be under 10,000 Ω but over 100 Ω.
3. A test of integrity of the recording system by deliberate creation of electrode artifact should be made by manipulation.
4. Interelectrode distances should be at least 10 cm.
5. Gains must be increased during the recording from 7.0 uV to 2.0 uV/min.
6. Time constants of 0.3 or 0.4 s should be used during part of the recording.
7. Extracerebral potentials should be monitored with appropriate leads.
8. There should be tests for reactivity to pain, loud noises, or light.
9. The record should include 30 min of recording time.
10. Recordings should be made by a qualified technician.
11. The record should be repeated if there is any doubt about electrocerebral silence (ECS).
12. Telephonically transmitted EEGs are not appropriate for determination of ECS.

The isoelectric or flat electroencephalogram is presumptive evidence of brain death if there is no history or evidence of the ingestion of sedative drugs or alcohol and it remains flat for 2 or 3 h. No patients meeting these criteria are known to have recovered.

About 40 percent of apneic and comatose patients will have an initial record that is isoelectric. Another 22 percent will develop flat records over a period of several days. There are, however, no good predictive criteria for the development of a flat record if the initial record is not isoelectric.

It is important that the brain death record be interpreted by someone who has more than average experience in reading EEGs.

Comparative Usefulness

It is clear that the electroencephalogram is a method of choice in the evaluation of patients with epilepsy or with toxic and metabolic disorders, and in the determination of brain death. Radiographic techniques are of little value in these situations. In patients with infectious disease, the EEG may be helpful, especially when the patient has encephalitis or is suspected of having a brain abscess. If, however, the patient has a space-occupying lesion, radiographic techniques may be of greater value. It is true, however, that when computed tomography and EEG are used together, definite diagnostic findings are obtained in 98 percent of patients examined. In many studies, the EEG may be diagnostic when the CT scan is not.

In ischemic vascular lesions, the EEG may also be more useful than the CT scan since in some studies the latter has been shown to fail to demonstrate a lesion in 20 percent of the patients studied. When compared with the CT scan, the EEG is more useful in vascular disease than in space-occupying lesions.

In trauma, the EEG is more useful than the CT scan for serial evaluation of brain damage. They are, of course, both necessary for the initial evaluation, but once the acute effects of the trauma have subsided, only the EEG will provide evidence of continuing dysfunction and the development of epileptic activity in the brain.

References

1. Barlow JS: Computerized clinical electroencephalography in perspective. IEEE Trans Biomed Eng 26:377–391, 1979.
2. Birchfield RI, Wilson WP, Heyman A: An evaluation of electroencephalography in cerebral infarction and ischemia due to arteriosclerosis. Neurology (NY) 9:859–870, 1959.
3. Cobb, WA: The normal adult EEG, in Hill D, Parr G (eds): *Electroencephalography.* New York, Macmillan, 1963, pp 232–249.
4. Culebras A, Henry CE, Williams GH Jr: Evaluation of intracranial space-occupying lesions by computed tomography and electroencephalography. Cleve Clin Q 45:275–280, 1978.
5. Gloor P: Contributions of electroencephalography and electrocorticography to the neurosurgical treatment of the epilepsies. Adv Neurol 8:59–105, 1975.
6. Jennett B, Van de Sande J: EEG prediction of post traumatic epilepsy. Epilepsia 16:251–256, 1975.
7. Kellaway P: An orderly approach to visual analysis: Parameters of the normal EEG in adults and children, in Klass DW, Daly DD (eds): *Current Practice of Clinical Electroencephalography.* New York, Raven Press, 1979, Chap 5, pp 69–147.
8. Rasmussen T: Surgical aspects of temporal lobe epilepsy. Results and problems. Acta Neurochir (Wien) [Suppl] 30:13–24, 1980.
9. Stockard JJ, Bickford RG, Aung MH: The electroencephalogram in traumatic brain injury, in Vicken PJ, Bruyn, GW (eds): *Handbook of Clinical Neurology,* vol 23: *Injuries of the*

Brain and Skull. Amsterdam, North Holland. 1975, pp 317–367.
10. Walker AE: *Cerebral Death*, 2d ed. Baltimore, Urban & Schwarzenberg, 1981.
11. Walker AE, Erculei F: *Head Injured Men Fifteen Years Later.* Springfield, Ill, Charles C Thomas, 1969.
12. Wilkins RH: Update: Subarachnoid hemorrhage and saccular intracranial aneurysms. Surg Neurol 15:92–101, 1981.

13. Wilson WP, Musella L, Short MJ: The electroencephalogram in dementia, in Wells C (ed): *Dementia*, 2d ed, Philadelphia, Davis, 1977, pp 205–221.
14. Wilson WP, Nashold BS: The uses of an improved technique of chronic electrode implantation in the human brain. Presented at a meeting of the Southern EEG Society, Tulsa, Okla, October 1972.

18

Electro-nystagmography

Robert A. Schindler
Vivian D. Weigel

A very common medical complaint is the patient's vague reference to "dizzy spells," the causes of which are often difficult to diagnose and treat. The immediate problem is to determine if the patient has vertigo, which is the hallucination of motion, often described as turning, falling or spinning, or if the patient is merely light-headed or experiences syncopal attacks. Accurate definition of the patient's actual symptoms is important because true vertigo, which is associated with a jerk nystagmus, indicates a disturbance of either the central or peripheral vestibular system.

Often it is difficult to determine from the vertiginous patient's imprecisely recalled history if true vertigo exists or not. The physician can then attempt to determine this by observing the patient's eye movements during an attack or during visual and vestibular stimulation, trying thus to draw some conclusions concerning the anatomical location of the patient's disorder. Some of the eye movements noted will indicate a peripheral (inner ear) vestibular pathology, while others will characterize a central nervous system pathology. Jerk nystagmus, the repetitive slow deviation of the eye toward one side followed by the rapid or saccadic movement of the eye back to the center gaze, is characteristic of vestibular disorders. Simple visual observation of the eye movements in a clinical setting can be misleading, however, because jerk nystagmus can be reduced by as much as 90 percent in intensity when the patient visually fixates on an object.

Frenzel glasses, 20-diopter lenses mounted together with two small lights in a goggle-like frame that fits snugly against the patient's head, have been used to abolish patient fixation, but they do not completely eliminate it.

Complete elimination of visual fixation can only be assured by testing the patient with his or her eyes closed. The results of eyes closed testing can be seen by using electronystagmography, a method of electrically recording eye movements that is now widely used clinically to provide a record of eye movements with the patient's eyes both open and closed, in light and/or darkness. Further advantages of the electronystagmogram (ENG) are that it provides a permanent tracing of eye movements that can be examined at leisure, can be compared with previous or subsequent tests, and can allow quantitative measurements of nystagmus intensity.

Electronystagmography is possible because the eye is a dipole, with the cornea acting as a positive pole and the retina as a negative pole, with the potential difference being normally at least 1 mV. This corneoretinal potential creates an electric field in the front of the head that changes its orientation with eyeball rotation. Electrodes placed on the skin near the eyes can detect these electrical changes, which, when amplified 20,000 times without distortion, can be used to drive a dynograph recorder, thereby making a tracing of the eye movements. When the eyes are at midposition, there is a "resting" voltage between the electrodes that serves as a baseline. By convention, the recording system is such that horizontal eye movements to the right produce an upward pen deflection, and horizontal eye movements to the left produce a downward pen deflection. Vertical eye movements are recorded on a separate channel; upward movement causes the pen to deflect upward, and downward eye movement produces a downward pen deflection.

Physiology

The maintenance of equilibrium depends on the complex interaction between the visual-oculomotor, vestibular, and somatosensory systems (Fig. 18-1). The vestibular end organ consists of three semicircular canals oriented at 90° to each other. Each has an ampulla containing a crista and vestibular sensory epithelium (type I and type II hair cells). The sensory hair cells lie on the crista and project into the lumen of the endolymphatic space (Fig. 18-2). The hairs, the kinocilium and the stereocilia of each cell, are imbedded in a gelatinous mass, the cupula, which fills the ampulla and thereby prevents free flow of endolymph through it.

Major portions of this chapter have appeared in Aminoff MJ (ed): *Electrodiagnosis in Clinical Neurology.* New York, Churchill Livingstone, 1980, pp 468–495

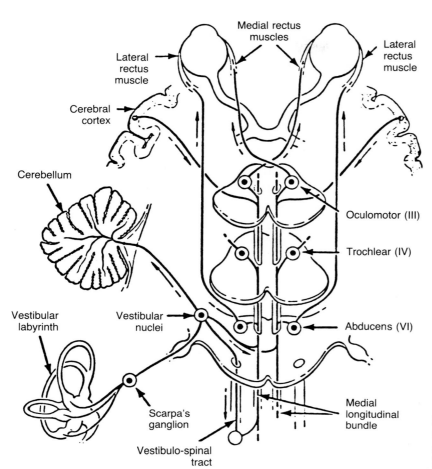

Figure 18-1 Central vestibular pathways. (From English GM: *Otolaryngology: A Textbook*. Hagerstown, Md, Harper & Row, 1976.)

In the healthy ear, the semicircular canals function in angular acceleration, each canal working in consort with its counterpart in the opposite ear. Gravitational and linear acceleration are perceived by the otolith organ, the macula of the utricle. Here, hair cells, similar in structure to those in the semicircular canals, are covered by an otolithic membrane into which the kinocilium and stereocilia are imbedded. The otolithic membrane is a gelatinous mass packed with calcium carbonate crystals called otoconia. Endolymph flows freely through the healthy utricle, and hair cell activation is achieved by shearing forces produced by the otolithic membrane relative to the surface of the hair cells. The function of the other otolith organ, the saccule, is still uncertain, but it may also function in linear acceleration.

The orientation of the kinocilium and stereocilia on the surface of the hair cell determines how that particular cell will respond to displacement of the cilia by either the cupula or otolithic membrane. A bending of the cilia toward the kinocilium results in an increase in the resting discharge rate of the efferent neuron innervating that cell; displacement of the hairs away from the kinocilium decreases the neural discharge rate (Fig. 18-3). The distribution of these cells on the cristae and utricular macula determines how that sense organ responds to shearing movements by the cupula and otolithic membrane.

The orientation of hair cells in the crista is uniform, with all cells polarized in the same direction. In the horizontal or lateral semicircular canal the kinocilia face the utricle. In the posterior and superior canals the kinocilia face away from the utricle. Thus, movement of endolymph and bending of the cupula toward the utricle (utriculopetal displacement) increases the resting discharge rate of afferent neurons in the horizontal crista while decreasing the discharge rate in vestibular nerve fibers from the posterior and superior cristae. Cupular displacement away from the utricle (utriculofugal displacement) decreases the activity in fibers from the horizontal crista while increasing the response of those from the posterior and superior canal cristae. On the utricular macula, hair cell kinocilia are oriented toward the organ's periphery and away from its central axis.

These physiological details permit the neural response produced by cupular movement to be predicted and help to explain the effect of caloric stimulation. With the patient positioned so that the horizontal canal is perpendicular (vertical) to the ground, cooling of the endolymph in the region of the ampulla increases its relative specific gravity and produces a downward (utriculofugal) deflection of the cupula, thereby decreasing the resting discharge rate. Conversely, hot water irrigation of the ear canal warms the fluid near the ampulla, reverses the direction of the endolymph flow, and produces a utriculolopetal deflection of the cupula, which increases neuronal activity. The ampulla, in effect, acts as a switch, increasing or decreasing vestibular neuronal responses.

The central integration of these peripheral vestibular responses in the brain stem gives rise to the characteristic jerk

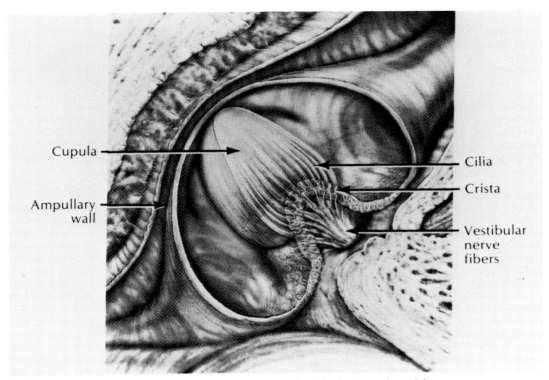

Figure 18-2 Structural anatomy of the ampullated end of the horizontal semicircular canal. (From English GM: *Otolaryngology: A Textbook*. Hagerstown, Md, Harper & Row, 1976.)

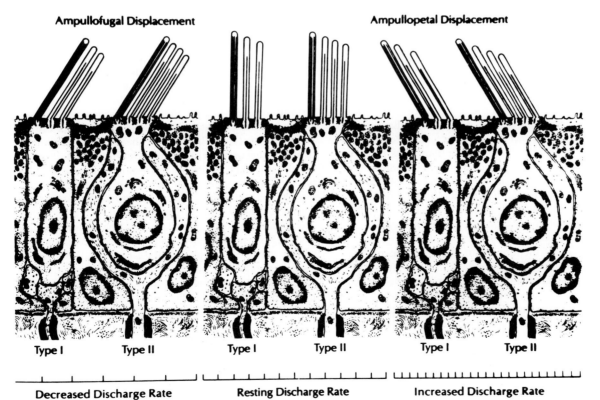

Figure 18-3 Diagram illustrating the effect of utriculofugal and utriculopetal displacement of cilia on the resting discharge rate of afferent vestibular neurons. (From English GM: *Otolaryngology: A Textbook*. Hagerstown, Md, Harper & Row, 1976.)

nystagmus seen with caloric irrigations and peripheral vestibulopathies. The direction of the nystagmus can often be helpful in determining the site of involvement. Destruction of the vestibular nerve on one side will evoke the same pattern of nystagmus as is seen with cold water caloric stimulation. Both produce a reduction in afferent neural activity on the involved side and a jerk nystagmus that beats toward the opposite ear. Since all peripheral vestibular responses are suppressed by visual fixation, ENG can be a useful means of detecting nystagmus that may only be present when the eyes are closed or in a darkened room.

The use of ENG is much broader than its application to vestibular stimulation. It may be applied to the study of eye movement systems, each of which may be tested during an ENG examination (Table 18-1). Lesions in the cerebellum, brain stem, and vestibular apparatus may produce abnormal eye movements that can be recorded by electronystagmography.

TABLE 18-1   Eye Movement Systems Tested by ENG

Eye Movement Systems	ENG tests
Saccadic	Calibration (refixation)
	Optokinetic (fast phase)
	Caloric (fast phase)
Smooth pursuit	Tracking
	Optokinetic (slow phase)
Vergence	Patient looks from near to far; not routinely tested
Nonoptic reflex	Caloric
	Positional
	Rotational
Position maintenance	Fixation
	Gaze—right and left

Preparations for Testing

A certain amount of screening is involved before proceeding with ENG testing; for example, no patient with an intracardiac catheter or pacemaker with exposed leads can be given an ENG since such a person is exquisitely sensitive to minute electric currents. Each patient's ears should be examined for tympanic perforations or other abnormalities such as mastoid cavities, cholesteatomas, or external canal infections. Such findings should be confirmed by an otologist, and air caloric testing should be performed instead of water caloric testing. Any excessive accumulation of cerumen or other debris should be removed before caloric irrigation.

The patient should be questioned carefully about any recent consumption of alcohol or drugs, since some patients fail to follow instructions to abstain from 48 to 72 h before testing, depending on the drugs concerned. Additional history should be taken regarding neck or back injury and/or surgery as these conditions might limit the examination by excluding positional tests.

No ENG recording can be obtained from patients with nonfunctioning retinas, because the corneoretinal potential is absent. Even when such a potential is present, ENG recordings on blind patients cannot provide quantitative data

because of the impossibility of accurately calibrating the nystagmograph, although a crude calibration can be performed by having the patient hold out the arms with thumbs extended and asking the patient to "look" back and forth from one thumb to the other.

Electrode placement will vary depending on which eye movements are to be recorded, i.e., vertical, bitemporal horizontal, or disconjugate. Horizontal eye movements may be recorded from two electrodes, the bitemporal pair, placed near the outer canthus of each eye; monocular horizontal eye movements may be recorded with a pair of electrodes for each eye, one near the outer canthus and one on the side of the nose bridge. Vertical movements are recorded from two electrodes placed above and below one eye. A ground electrode is usually placed on the forehead (Fig. 18-4).

A number of electrical artifacts may obscure the tracing, and some of these are shown in Fig. 18-5. These artifacts must be eliminated, if possible, before beginning testing. In addition, a number of non-nystagmic eye movements, called *square waves*, occur in many patients, but are most pronounced with nervous, apprehensive patients, who should be encouraged to relax. Such waves may, however, indicate brain stem–cerebellar pathology. Large, random eye movements generally are seen with children or with uncooperative patients, and again greater relaxation must be obtained. Slow, sinusoidal eye swings are a sign of patient drowsiness, and may be due to heavy sedation or organic brain damage.

The ENG Test

Calibration

The electronystagmograph is first calibrated so that 1 degree of eye movement is equal to 1 mm of pen deflection on the ENG graph paper. The patient is asked to look at fixation points placed 10 degrees, 20 degrees, and 30 degrees from the center in both the horizontal and vertical planes as the technician adjusts the gain controls. Figure 18-6A shows a standard dc calibration tracing. Horizontal and vertical tracings will look identical; ac system tracings will reflect pen drifts back toward the baseline. Calibration should be repeated frequently during the testing procedure, since patient alertness will change the magnitude of the corneoretinal potential, and should certainly be checked before each major test and before and after each caloric irrigation.

Gaze Testing

Gaze testing is accomplished by having the patient gaze at the center point, then 30 degrees right, 30 degrees left (and 30 degrees upward and 30 degrees downward if vertical nystagmus is recorded) both with eyes open and with eyes closed in each gaze position while a record of eye movement is obtained. It is necessary to alert the patient during gaze testing with the eyes closed since nystagmus usually becomes weaker and may disappear when the patient is not actively performing concentration tasks. Many normal peo-

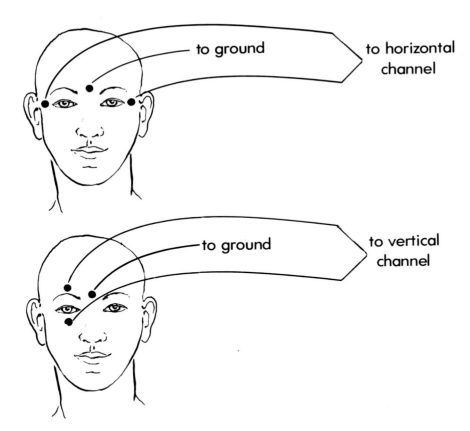

Figure 18-4 Electrode placement.

ple have a physiological gaze nystagmus if the eyes are deviated more than 30 degrees to the left or right, and the angle of gaze must, therefore, be carefully controlled.

Tests for Spontaneous Nystagmus

After calibration and gaze testing, and before the patient is moved, tests for spontaneous nystagmus are performed. The patient is first asked to hold a blank sheet of white paper approximately 4 in. from the eyes in order to reduce visual stimulation from the rest of the room, and to keep the eyes open without visual fixation while a further record of eye movement is obtained. Alertness must be maintained by a concentration task at this time and throughout the ENG test because nystagmus disappears in the absence of concentration. After recalibration, the patient is tested in a darkened room with the eyes open, then with the eyes closed.

Positioning Tests

The Hallpike-Dix maneuvers are used for positioning tests. The seated patient is made to lie down suddenly, with the head hanging to the right, unsupported below the horizontal, and the eyes closed, and to maintain the position for approximately 30 s, during which time the eye movements are recorded. The patient is asked to sit up and allowed to rest for 30 s. The test is then repeated with the head back and turned to the left. If positioning nystagmus is produced

by any such maneuvers, those that elicited the nystagmus are repeated since a vital characteristic of the Hallpike-Dix response is its fatigability with repeated testing.

Positional Tests

Calibration is again performed, and the patient is then asked to keep the eyes closed while moving into various head and body positions in order to see how postural changes affect the recorded eye movements. The patient's eyes may be taped closed in order to reduce movements from the eyelids and to ensure that they are not opened during this portion of the examination. The exact order in which tests are performed may vary, but the basic positions are recumbent (with the patient's head flat), body turned to the right (the head should be kept level with the body by using a small pillow beneath the patient's head), head turned to the right (the pillow is removed so that the head is flat), body to the left, head to left, and sitting up. Each position should be maintained for at least 60 s while a record of eye movement is obtained.

Tracking and Optokinetic Tests

The patient is asked to smoothly track a horizontally moving object with the eyes while the recording is continued. This tracking is performed first with both eyes, then with the right eye alone, and finally with the left eye only. During the

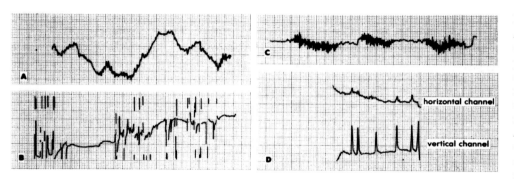

Figure 18-5 Artifacts. *A.* Baseline shift and 60-Hz "hum" caused by poor electrode contact, by a ground loop or uncommon ground, or by unusually intense radiation from nearby equipment. *B.* Broken electrode wire. *C.* Muscle potential from contraction of facial or neck muscles. *D.* Eye blink artifacts.

monocular tracking tests, the patient must keep both eyes open while the technician covers one, since closing the eye not used for tracking may cause muscle artifacts to appear on the recording.

The optokinetic (OPK) test is performed by having the patient sit under or in front of an optokinetic drum, or by moving an OPK stimulus horizontally on a wall or screen before the patient's eyes. The optokinetic stimulus is moved both to the left and to the right, using velocities of 20 degrees, 50 degrees, 80 degrees, 100 degrees, and 120 degrees visual angle per second. Vertical optokinetic responses can also be obtained at this time, if desired. Optokinetic nystagmus is an involuntary response and appears when the subject focuses on the stimulus pattern. If the patient is asked to count the strips, a tracking response is usually obtained instead of a true OPK response.

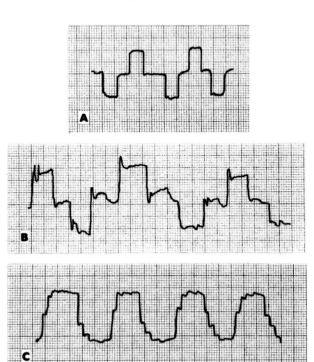

Figure 18-6 *A.* Normal calibration. By convention upward deflection represents eye movement to the right; downward, to the left. *B.* Ocular dysmetria. *C.* Calibration undershoots or hypometric saccades.

Caloric Testing

The caloric test is performed either with the patient sitting, head tilted back at 60 degrees, or, more commonly during ENG testing, with the patient supine, head ventroflexed 30 degrees so that the lateral semicircular canals are in the vertical plane perpendicular with the plane of the floor. The positioning of the lateral semicircular canal is crucial since it is the canal maximally stimulated by caloric irrigation. It is important for the patient to understand that light-headedness or vertigo may occur during the test in normal subjects, but will not continue for longer than 1 or 2 min. A careful record should be made of any symptoms that persist.

Standard caloric irrigations are 250 ml of water at 30°C and at 44°C introduced into the ear over a 30 s time period. If no nystagmus is elicited using the above standard irrigations, ice water may be used to determine whether vestibular function is present or not in the nonresponsive ear or ears. With ice water stimulation, the patient's head is turned so that the irrigated ear is upward; after 10 s, the patient's head is returned to the usual caloric test position. The amount of water used varies: as little as 2 ml of ice water can be used for this purpose, and, although up to 30 ml of ice water has been used by some workers, more than 5 ml is not recommended. For all practical purposes, the irrigated labyrinth (or its CNS connections) can be considered as nonfunctional if no nystagmus results from stimulating the ear with 5 ml of ice water. Irrigation with 30 ml of ice water may be used in the comatose patient to test the vestibulo-oculomotor connection similar to the doll's eyes nystagmus. Air caloric irrigations are performed in the same manner as water caloric irrigations, with air at temperatures of 24 and 50°C. If no response results from such irrigations, a Dundus-Grant coiled copper tube attached to the air hose and sprayed with ethyl chloride can be used to cool the air to about 14°C.

Interpretation and Clinical Application of ENG Test Results

Gaze Nystagmus

Nystagmus caused by peripheral vestibular lesions is nearly always horizontal or horizontal-rotatory, is direction-fixed (most often toward the normal side), is suppressed by ocular fixation, and is strongest when the gaze is toward the fast phase of the nystagmus. Since peripheral nystagmus results from an acute unilateral lesion that causes an imbalance in the normal input arising from the two labyrinths, this nystagmus will lose intensity with time due to central compensation. The terms first-, second- and third-degree gaze nystagmus relate to Alexander's law: nystagmus resulting from an acute peripheral lesion beats strongest when the eyes gaze in the direction of the quick component, less strongly with center gaze, and with least activity when the gaze is in the opposite direction of the fast component. Nystagmus present in all three directions is called *third-degree*, that seen with straight gaze and with gaze in the direction of the fast component is called *second-degree*, and that seen only with the gaze in the direction of the fast component is called *first-degree* nystagmus. Third-degree nystagmus is converted to second- and then to first-degree nystagmus as the CNS compensatory mechanisms become effective with time.

Nystagmus caused by CNS lesions may be horizontal, vertical, oblique, or rotatory, may vary considerably in amplitude, and usually declines slowly, if at all, with time. It may be enhanced by visual fixation and is usually not suppressed by it. Horizontal CNS nystagmus usually beats in the direction of the gaze, i.e., right-beating with gaze to the right and left-beating with gaze to the left.

Bilateral horizontal gaze nystagmus is the most common form of CNS nystagmus, with the nystagmus usually beating in the direction of the gaze. (Figure 18-7A and B). It is usually seen only when the patient's eyes are open, although occasionally it may be enhanced or occur only with the eyes closed. Gaze evoked nystagmus, increased by fixation and gaze-dependent for direction, implies interruption of volitional eye movements, which may be due to neuromuscular insufficiency or extravestibular brain stem or cerebellar lesions, but provides no information about its pathological basis. Only CNS lesions produce gaze nystagmus that is abolished by eye closure. Gaze nystagmus of low amplitude and high velocity may be obvious to the clinical observer yet difficult to discern on the ENG tracing. Separate eye recordings help to show this nystagmus since the abducting eye has stronger nystagmus than the adducting eye.

Rebound nystagmus, described by Hood, Kayan, and Leech,[15] is a horizontal gaze nystagmus associated with chronic cerebellar system disease. It can be seen on both clinical examination and with ENG testing. It is character-

ized by the appearance of nystagmus that is not present on center gaze but develops into a right-beating nystagmus on right gaze and reverses to a left-beating nystagmus as the eyes move from right gaze back to center gaze. Similarly, a left-beating nystagmus appears on left gaze and becomes right-beating when the eyes return to center gaze. Accordingly, when examining patients with gaze nystagmus due to suspected CNS pathology, lateral gaze should be observed for 20 s and center gaze should then be examined before gaze in the opposite direction, so that rebound nystagmus is not overlooked.

Periodic alternating nystagmus (PAN) is a persistent, horizontal-rotatory nystagmus that alternates in direction at regular intervals that may be as short as 1 min or as long as 6 min but will be constant for individual patients. The nystagmus begins beating weakly in one direction, builds up to a peak level, declines, and stops. This cycle is then repeated, with nystagmus beating in the opposite direction and so on. This periodic alternating nystagmus may be seen with eyes open and closed, but is usually enhanced with fixation and with alertness. Although not of specific diagnostic significance, periodic alternating nystagmus indicates a central disturbance, probably in the cerebellomedullary region.[6,22] PAN has also been associated with posterior fossa pathology, chronic otitis media with fistula, cerebral trauma, vertebrobasilar artery insufficiency, encephalitis, syphilis, demyelinating disease, cerebellar lesions, Friedreich's ataxia, tumors of the corpus callosum, Arnold-Chiari malformation, congenital nystagmus with or without albinism, and total amaurosis.[4]

Up-beating vertical nystagmus, seen with upward or downward gaze or in the primary position, is clinically important since it indicates an acquired lesion, either from drug intoxication or posterior fossa disease. Large-amplitude up-beating vertical nystagmus has been associated with vermis lesions, and small-amplitude up-beating vertical nystagmus with medullary lesions. Down-beating vertical nystagmus, especially when seen with lateral gaze, strongly suggests that the medullocervical region is the site of the responsible lesion. Causes of such pathology include basilar artery compression, Arnold-Chiari malformation, medullary infarction, and brain stem encephalitis.

Congenital nystagmus, which appears at birth or shortly thereafter in an otherwise normal individual, is important to recognize since it should not be confused with other varieties

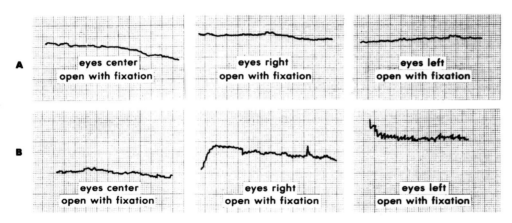

Figure 18-7 *A.* Gaze test result in normal subject. *B.* Gaze nystagmus.

of nystagmus that are of pathological significance. The nystagmus may be pendular or jerk or both, varying with gaze direction or position. Congenital nystagmus is usually distinctive for each patient. Nystagmus that is pendular is usually congenital or secondary to blindness, but it may be seen with a patient who has multiple sclerosis. Care must be taken to differentiate congenital nystagmus from lesional or drug-induced gaze nystagmus. The distorted character of the eyes open nystagmus strongly suggests a congenital origin. Congenital nystagmus will also have a null point at which nystagmus sharply declines or stops as the patient's eyes move slowly from about 30 degrees right lateral gaze to 30 degrees left gaze. At the null point, the right-beating nystagmus seen with 30 degrees right gaze will stop, after declining as the eyes move to the center, and then to the left. As the eyes continue to move to the left, the nystagmus will become left-beating. Another feature of congenital nystagmus is that it is rarely vertical, usually being horizontal or horizontal-rotatory. Thus, congenital nystagmus on upward gaze is virtually always horizontal, not vertical (persistent vertical nystagmus on upward gaze indicates a pathological or drug-induced condition). Congenital nystagmus can also be identified by its reduction or abolition on convergence (eye fixation at 6 ft will allow nystagmus to be clearly seen, but with fixation at 2 ft the nystagmus declines and may disappear for a few seconds). Since variability is the main trademark of congenital nystagmus, checks for null point, upward gaze, and convergence effect will help to determine whether the nystagmus is, indeed, congenital or not.

Internuclear ophthalmoplegia results from a medial longitudinal fasciculus lesion between the third and sixth nerve nuclei in the brain stem. Internuclear ophthalmoplegia is often caused by multiple sclerosis, but it may also be due to other more discrete lesions, e.g., vascular lesions. Bilateral internuclear opthalmoplegia in young adults strongly suggests multiple sclerosis. Internuclear ophthalmoplegia presents with two distinguishing patterns: delay in movement of the adducting eye with lateral gaze, and nystagmus only in the abducting eye. Medial rectus muscle weakness from defective innervation is responsible for the adduction lag, which is ipsilateral to the site of the lesion. ENG recording from each eye separately is the easiest way to identify internuclear ophthalmoplegia.

Saccades

Saccadic testing is performed as the patient moves the eyes left and right, looking at the lights or dots used for calibrating the ENG machine. Normal individuals can move their eyes rapidly and stop precisely on target, although some consistently undershoot or overshoot the target slightly, reaching it by making one or two small corrective saccades or by moving the eyes to the target in one slow movement called a *glissade*.

Ocular dysmetria is an abnormal saccadic eye movement characterized by the patient's eyes overshooting (hypermetric saccades) or undershooting (hypometric saccades) the target consistently by 150 to 200 ms before fixating on the target itself. Unilateral overshoots are more common than overshoots in both directions. Ocular dysmetria accompanies diseases of the cerebellum or its neural connections and

is the ocular counterpart of past pointing. Both result from the inability of the impaired cerebellar hemispheres to control smooth integration of body muscles that function in an agonist-antagonist relationship. Figures 18-6*B* and *C* illustrate ocular dysmetria seen as calibration overshoot and undershoot. The finding must be clearly and consistently seen throughout the ENG recording whenever saccadic movements are elicited for calibration before they are regarded as abnormal.

Saccadic slowing, eye movement slower than 188 degrees per second, indicates basal ganglia disease, especially associated with an inability to perform vertical saccadic movements, especially downward.

Internuclear ophthalmoplegia presents on saccadic testing as a rounding of one side of the upper plateau of the saccade, caused by the lag of the adducting eye. Separate recordings for each eye should be taken to confirm the diagnosis if such rounding is seen repeatedly.

In evaluating saccadic movements it is important to consider whether apparent abnormalities are due to superimposition of spontaneous or congenital nystagmus on the saccades; to a drug effect, especially when ocular dysmetria is a finding; or to eye blink artifacts. Eye blinks superimposed on saccades may resemble calibration overshoot on the ENG recording using bitemporal leads; the vertical eye movement tracing should be carefully examined since blinks will show up as spikes on the vertical channel, whereas calibration overshoots will not. Blinks also are usually spikelike on the horizontal tracing, unlike overshoots, which have flattened tops.

Spontaneous Nystagmus

Spontaneous nystagmus can be defined as a nystagmus that is present with the eyes open or closed, is direction-fixed, and has an intensity that does not change (or varies only slightly) with changes in head and body positions. Nystagmus that varies in intensity with position changes or that disappears in one or more positions may be called either *direction-fixed positional nystagmus* or may be referred to as a *latent spontaneous nystagmus*. Spontaneous jerk nystagmus, when strictly defined, is always pathological. Horizontal nystagmus is the most common and may result from vestibular lesions, posterior fossa lesions, or extraocular neuromuscular insufficiency. Both spontaneous and direction-fixed positional nystagmus result from either peripheral or central lesions; the direction of the nystagmus is not necessarily of localizing value. Dissociated nystagmus implies a lesion of the medial longitudinal fasciculus.

Another type of spontaneous nystagmus is block nystagmus, also called *square waves*. This type of nystagmus is sometimes seen in normal individuals as a result of nervousness, but it may also indicate a central pathology and has been associated with hydrocephalus, vertebrobasilar insufficiency, and postconcussion syndrome.[24]

All nystagmus is enhanced by attention-requiring tasks. Kileny, McCabe, and Ryu found that conversation was superior to mental arithmetic in engaging the cortex and preventing response decline and can even reverse caloric-induced habituation.[18] Hofferberth et al. used a tape with simple arithmetic problems, the answers to which are given after a 15-s interval.[14] The person being tested presses the button of an electric bell once or twice, depending on whether the solution is correct or not. These signals are seen as rectangular impulses on the ENG tracing, allowing control over patient cooperation. This method has proved valuable for increasing vigilance during ENG testing.

Positional Nystagmus

Positional nystagmus that is present when the eyes are open is always abnormal, but many normal people have horizontal positional nystagmus in one or more head positions if examined with the eyes closed. This nystagmus may be direction-fixed or direction-changing (but will not change direction within a given head position); it may be persistent or intermittent. Barber and Wright,[7] who tested 112 normal people and found nystagmus in at least one head position in 92 of them, established the following criteria of abnormality for positional nystagmus that is present when the eyes are closed:

1. It changes directions within a given head position.
2. It is persistent in three or more positions.
3. It is intermittent in four or more positions.
4. The slow-phase eye speed of the three strongest consecutive beats exceeds 6 degrees per second in any head position.

Ninety-five percent of their 112 normal subjects failed to meet any of these criteria.

Direction-fixed or direction-changing positional nystagmus that is present with the eyes open and continues as long as the head position is maintained is good evidence of pathology within the posterior fossa if positional, alcohol-induced nystagmus has been excluded.

The site of lesion cannot be determined with certainty from the direction of direction-fixed positional nystagmus, although the nystagmus usually beats toward the normal side, especially in patients with vestibular neuronitis. Such nystagmus is usually found in patients with peripheral pathology but may occur with CNS disease. Usually direction-changing positional nystagmus will beat toward the down ear in lateral head and body positions (geotropic) if the nystagmus has a peripheral origin (Fig. 18-8A and B). Ageotropic (beats away from the down ear) direction-changing positional nystagmus suggests a central lesion unless alcohol has been taken within 6 to 24 h of testing (Fig. 18-8C and D). Also indicative of a CNS lesion is nystagmus that changes direction within a given head or body position, or during one of the Hallpike-Dix maneuvers. This nystagmus often beats geotropically, declines to nothing, then, after a few seconds, beats in the opposite direction.

Positioning Nystagmus

Neither vertigo nor nystagmus results from the Hallpike-Dix maneuvers in normal subjects with open eyes, but a few nystagmoid beats are sometimes seen on the ENG tracing if the eyes are closed while recording.

Benign paroxysmal positioning nystagmus is most often seen with the Hallpike-Dix maneuvers and is important to identify since it localizes the lesion laterally and nearly always indicates harmless inner ear disease. The nystagmus appears most often in either head-hanging right (HHR) or left (HHL) positions, rarely in both. It beats in a horizontal-rotatory pattern toward the down ear, when this is the ear with the responsible peripheral vestibular lesion. Frequently, nystagmus beating in the opposite direction will be seen briefly when the patient sits up after performing those Hallpike-Dix maneuvers that provoked nystagmus. Benign paroxysmal positioning nystagmus always (1) is delayed in onset for 2 to 15 s after the patient's head is positioned; (2) is transient, lasting only 30 s or less; (3) is accompanied by vertigo, which lasts as long as the nystagmus; and (4) is fatigable, becoming weaker with each successive repetition of the maneuver. When benign paroxysmal positioning nystagmus is recorded by ENG, the nystagmus appears to beat in an "unexpected" direction, i.e., left-beating in HHR and right-beating in HHL. Baloh et al., using monocular and vertical eye tracings, found that the vertical component was up-beat in both eyes (fast phase toward the ground in the head-hanging position), whereas the horizontal component was dissociated with the ipsilateral eye beating away from the down ear and the contralateral eye beating toward the down ear.[5] The amplitude of the vertical component was larger in the contralateral eye, but that of the horizontal component was larger in the ipsilateral eye. This dissociated nystagmus profile is consistent with a burst of excitatory activity originating in the posterior canal of the ear that is undermost at the end of the positioning maneuver.

The Hallpike-Dix maneuvers may also provoke positional nystagmus that is not rotatory, has no measurable latency, gives the patient little or no vertiginous sensations, and does not fatigue with repetition of the test. This nystagmus may be horizontal, oblique, or vertical and is important because it strongly indicates significant CNS disease, although unidirectional positional nystagmus caused by an acute unilateral peripheral vestibular lesion may also be intensified by the Hallpike-Dix maneuver.

Tracking

Most normal individuals or patients with peripheral (end-organ) vestibular disease are able to visually track a moving object with little or no eye deviation from it, although this ability declines somewhat with age. A patient with brain stem disease involving the pursuit system will track a moving object imperfectly, producing saccadic movements instead of a smooth tracking record. As the eye repeatedly falls behind the movement of the target and catches up again with a saccade, a "cogwheeling" effect is recorded (Fig. 18-9).

Disorganized and disconjugate pursuit also indicates brain stem pathology. Monocular leads will allow the ENG tracing to show disconjugate eye movements, recording movement in one eye while the other remains momentarily stationary or drifts aimlessly. Bitemporal leads will record this type of eye movement as slow, wandering, inaccurate tracings. Disorganized pursuit may also be seen as rapid

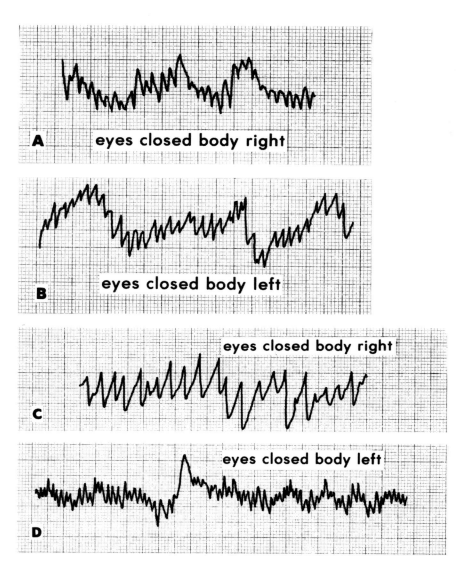

Figure 18-8 *A*. Geotropic right beating positional nystagmus seen in body right position. *B*. Geotropic left beating positional nystagmus seen in body left position. *C*. Ageotropic left beating positional nystagmus seen in body right position. *D*. Ageotropic right beating positional nystagmus seen in body left position.

overshoots to both right and left (blinks should be ruled out by observing the vertical channel tracing), or as a completely ataxic tracking record that is impossible to identify as tracking at all.

Benitez's classification of tracking is useful, and his findings regarding the localizing information derived from the test are worth reviewing here. Pattern I is a smooth sinusoidal tracing. Pattern II is a slightly irregular, sinusoidal curve with a few periodic non-nystagmic movements appearing intermittently on it. Pattern III is a sinusoidal curve with fast saccadic movements superimposed on it. Pattern IV is completely ataxic; the sinusoidal curve has been lost, and the pursuit eye movements are disorganized. These patterns are shown in Fig. 18-9. Patterns I and II are considered normal recordings. Ninety-seven percent of the patients with eye-tracking patterns I and II fell into the category of patients with peripheral pathologies; three percent were in the central category (all had multiple sclerosis). Pattern III had 35 percent of patients with peripheral abnormalities and 65 percent with central ones. Pattern IV had 97 percent of patients in the central category. The remaining 3 percent

(one case) was ocular with congenital strabismus. In a later study, Benitez and Bouchard found that 10 patients with tumors of the cerebellopontine recess showed impaired ocular pursuit movements when the eyes were moving toward the side of the lesion.[9] Standardization of the eye-tracking test, especially of the target velocity, is advocated by Umeda for the purpose of comparing abnormalities of eye-tracking patterns recorded in different clinics.[34] Umeda found that:

1. The minimum velocity of a target that normal subjects can follow without delay of the eye movement is about 20 degrees per second.
2. When pursuit eye movements of normal subjects are registered with the aid of electronystagmography, the eye-tracking patterns will remain normal at target velocities of up to 45 degrees per second.
3. In order to detect abnormalities of pursuit eye movement with the aid of electronystagmography, the target velocity should be as fast as possible, but not exceeding 45 degrees per second.

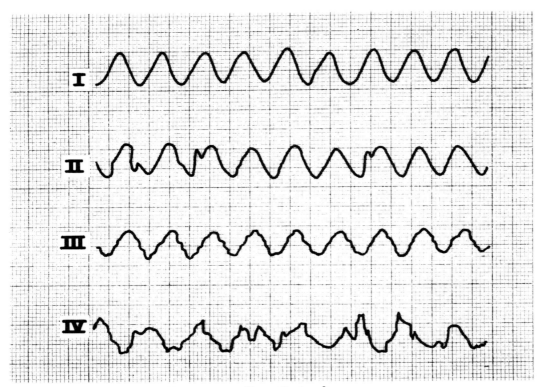

Figure 18-9 Benitez eye-tracking patterns. (From Benitez.[8])

Umeda recommends a circular eye-tracking test apparatus (amplitude 40 degrees, frequency 0.33 Hz, and target velocity 42 degrees per second) as ideal for the examination of pursuit eye movements.

Optokinetic Results

A normal OPK response is symmetrical, that is, the OPK nystagmus intensity will be the same for both left-beating and right-beating nystagmus provoked by a stimulus moving at a given speed to the right and left (Fig. 18-10A). OPK nystagmus is usually symmetrical, even when a unilateral peripheral lesion is present. A decidedly asymmetric OPK response denotes a CNS abnormality without necessarily indicating laterality, although Benitez and Bouchard found a unilateral diminution of OPK response toward the side of the tumor when testing 10 patients with tumors of the cerebellopontine recess[9] (Fig. 18-10B).

Brain stem pathology is indicated by nystagmus that does not increase in intensity with increasing stimulus velocities, but instead remains stable or declines in intensity. In this case, the nystagmus is symmetrical but is not appropriate to the stimulus speeds used.

A bidirectional reduced OPK response, symmetrical or asymmetric, indicates central disease, usually in the brain stem or the cerebellum. Two other central signs that may be elicited are dysrhythmia and "fatigue." Dysrhythmia is present when the saccades are of varying amplitude, the intersaccade interval is irregular, and the slow phase is of varying speed. Fatigue refers to pathological adaptation of the response; that is, the velocity of the slow phase decreases even though the drive speed remains unchanged.

Comparison of the OPK saccade with the caloric nystagmus saccade may suggest brain stem disease. Normally, the caloric saccade is slightly slower and of longer duration than the OPK saccade. Comparison should be made between OPK and caloric nystagmus signals of the same slow-phase velocity. With CNS disorders, the caloric saccade may be of abnormally slow velocity and long duration.[13]

In the presence of a strong spontaneous nystagmus or direction-fixed positional nystagmus, the OPK responses sometimes reflect a directional preponderance in the direction of the spontaneous nystagmus. This should not be considered as an abnormal OPK response. Drugs can affect the OPK response, making it appear abnormal, but a more common problem is patient suppression of the OPK response by staring through a drum or looking under it, allowing it to become a blur, or by tracking the stimulus. The OPK response has also been noted to be disturbed by poor adaptation to sudden acceleration in the stimulation.[12]

Calorics

As with the OPK test, symmetry of responses is the expected finding in normal subjects (Fig. 18-11 A, B, C, and D). Three parameters of the caloric response are measured: duration, frequency, and velocity of the slow component of the induced nystagmus, the latter being the most important of the three. Duration of the nystagmus is the time that elapses from the beginning of the irrigation until the nystag-

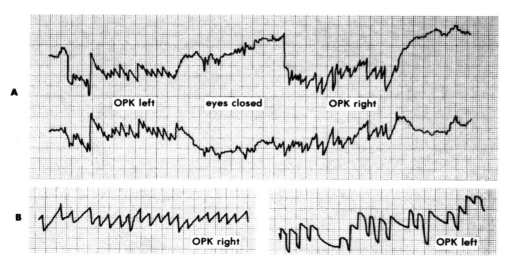

Figure 18-10 *A.* Normal optokinetic nystagmus. *B.* Asymmetric optokinetic responses.

mus ceases. Peak nystagmus frequency is the average frequency of beats per second within the 10-s interval of the most intense caloric nystagmus. The maximum slow-phase eye speed is the average slow-phase eye speed during the 10-s interval in which the caloric nystagmus is most intense (usually about 60 s after the beginning of the irrigation). Calculating slow-component velocity is simple if the machine has been calibrated so that 1 degree of eye movement equals 1 mm of pen deflection.

Unilateral weakness (UW) can be said to be present when the intensity of the nystagmus provoked by irrigation of the right ear differs from that elicited by irrigations of the left ear. Unilateral weakness is expressed as a percentage and is calculated by using the formula:

$$UW = \frac{(RW + RC) - (LW + LC)}{(RW + RC + LW + LC)} \times 100$$

where RW = peak slow-phase eye speed after 44 degree irrigation, right ear
RC = peak slow-phase eye speed after 30 degree irrigation, right ear
LW = peak slow-phase eye speed after 44 degree irrigation, left ear
LC = peak slow-phase eye speed after 30 degree irrigation, left ear

Directional preponderance (DP) is the difference between the intensity of the right-beating caloric nystagmus when compared with the left-beating caloric nystagmus. Using the same parameters as those used to determine unilateral weakness, we have the following formula for directional preponderance.

$$DP = \frac{(RW + LC) - (LW + RC)}{(RW + LC + LW + RC)} \times 100$$

The fixation index (FI) indicates the ability of the patient to effectively suppress the caloric nystagmus with visual fixation. The following formula is used to determine the fixation index.

$$FI = \frac{SPES\ (EO)}{SPES\ (EC)}$$

where SPES = slow-phase eye speed
EO = eyes open
EC = eyes closed

Normal caloric responses range from 6 degrees per second to 80 degrees per second, but all four irrigation responses will be approximately of the same intensity for any one individual. Normal variations for unilateral weakness is 25 percent; for directional preponderance, 30 percent. Alpert has reported the 95 percent limit of normal variation of the fixation index as 0.6.[1]

In the determination of directional preponderance, it is important to consider whether any spontaneous nystagmus or strong direction-fixed positional nystagmus may be affecting the caloric responses. If the caloric responses are being facilitated by a pre-existing nystagmus, the calorics should not be considered truly asymmetric. Even a significant directional preponderance is of little clinical importance since it indicates only that something is probably wrong but does not correlate well with either peripheral or central pathology.

A decided unilateral weakness is an important finding and usually suggests a peripheral vestibular lesion on the weak side (Figs. 18-12*B* and *C*). Bilateral weakness may be seen in patients treated with ototoxic drugs such as streptomycin or gentamicin. Other causes of bilateral weakness include various peripheral vestibular lesions as well as CNS lesions. Among peripheral vestibular lesions that cause bilateral weakness of caloric responses are bilateral eighth nerve tumors, bilateral temporal bone fracture, bilateral Ménière's disease, and Cogan's syndrome.

Simmons found 43 of 2500 consecutively tested patients to have no vestibular responses bilaterally to stimulation with 5 ml of ice water.[30] Of these 43, nine had CNS neoplasms (six in the midline posterior fossa), five had autoimmune or collagen disease, five had infections (otitis, meningitis, syphilis), five had congenital abnormalities involving only the ear, five had abnormalities that were drug-induced, and four had combined visual and eighth nerve hereditary disorders.

Karlsen et al. studied the effects of age, sex, hearing loss, and water temperature on caloric nystagmus.[17] They found

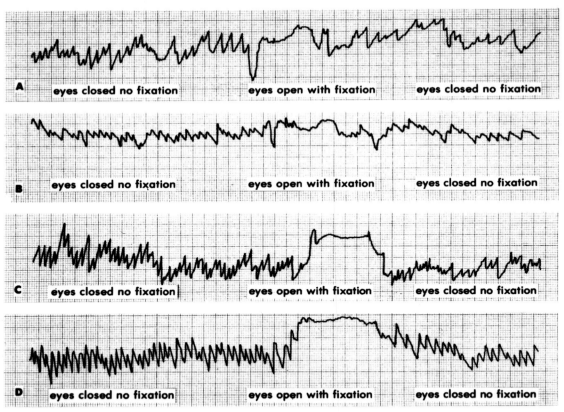

Figure 18-11 Normal caloric responses. *A*. Right cold. *B*. Left cold. *C*. Left hot. *D*. Right hot.

that hearing loss and sex are not related to the degree of caloric responsiveness to bithermal caloric stimulation. Age has no significant effect on cool water calorics with the exception of duration, which decreases with age. Warm water testing indicates that the speed of the slow component and the duration, frequency, and amplitude of nystagmus decrease with increasing age. Cool water calorics produced responses with shorter latencies than did warm water calorics. Response duration in cool water calorics is not significantly correlated to the speed of the slow component, while latency and frequency showed excellent correlation to the speed of the slow component.

Hyperactive caloric responses (above 50 degrees per second from cool stimulation and 80 degrees per second from warm stimulation) are uncommon unless the patient has a tympanic membrane perforation or a mastoidectomy cavity. Very alert or nervous patients sometimes have hyperactive caloric responses that have not been correlated with any pathogenic state.

Failure of fixation suppression will only be seen in patients with CNS disease (Fig. 18-12*A*). The caloric nystagmus intensity with eyes open will be nearly equal to, be equal to, or exceed that of nystagmus with eyes closed in one nystagmus direction or both. Normal individuals and patients with peripheral vestibular disorders will suppress caloric nystagmus with visual fixation. Some CNS pathology, such as Wernicke's metabolic encephalopathy or barbiturate intoxication, inhibits eyes closed caloric responses so that

the nystagmus is seen only with eyes open. With this sort of extreme failure of fixation suppression, it is important to be certain that the patient is alerted during testing since cases have been reported of nonalerted (often deaf) patients whose caloric nystagmus is suppressed except with visual fixation. Alerting such a patient when the patient's eyes are closed will elicit the suppressed nystagmus.

Congenital nystagmus superimposed on caloric responses sometimes makes interpreting these responses impossible. Congenital nystagmus that is abolished with eye closure will not, of course, affect caloric nystagmus interpretation except with regard to evaluating failure of fixation suppression, which may be difficult to discern.

Other Testing

The need for accurate and reliable diagnostic tests for the evaluation of vestibular function has stimulated investigation of rotational methods and, more recently, an evaluation of harmonic angular acceleration, variously called the *pendular rotation test* or the *sinusoidal harmonic acceleration test*. Initial studies using these techniques on humans demonstrated a linear input-output function from 0.24 cycle at 0.4 radian, but a reduction in the increase of response with an increase of acceleration or a decrease of frequency from this range. Nystagmic responses were symmetrical in these same normal individuals. In patients with vestibular disease input-

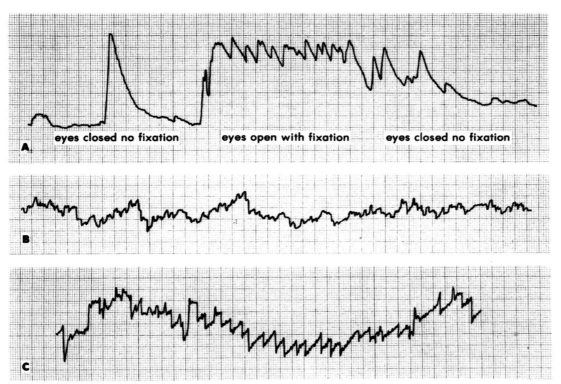

Figure 18-12 Abnormal caloric responses. *A.* Absence of fixation suppression. *B.* No labyrinthine responses to 5 ml ice water. *C.* No labyrinthine response; superimposed left beating spontaneous nystagmus seen with 5 ml ice water on the left.

output functions as well as symmetry were altered and appeared related to the degree of pathology. Evaluation of the test system in animals rendered ototoxic with streptomycin showed a depression in response similar to that from caloric tests. Many reports suggest that harmonic angular acceleration tests provide a reliable and sensitive method for evaluation of vestibular function and a useful and important confirmation to the other methods that are available for these evaluations.[10,16,20,25,28,31]

Drug Effects

All patients referred for ENGs are asked to discontinue all but life-supporting medications for 48 h before the test and to discontinue all vestibular medications for 72 h before the test. Drug-induced abnormal eye movements are most often seen with antihistamines, tranquilizers, barbiturates, alcohol, and phenytoin. Opium and demerol produce vertical nystagmus. Antihistamines and tranquilizers have a mild sedative effect, presumably from action on the CNS. Overall reduction of caloric responses is common with patients taking diazepam or other similar drugs. Alcohol will cause direction-changing positional nystagmus, abnormal tracking, and inadequate saccadic eye movements.

Barbiturates and phenytoin affect the CNS at times, causing bilateral gaze nystagmus and abnormal tracking. Aschan et al. reported that barbiturates produce positional nystagmus.[2] They may, in high doses, cause vertical (usu-

ally up-beating) nystagmus or oblique up-beating nystagmus. If it is impossible to discontinue all medications before ENG testing, as happens with hospital inpatients, medications being taken should be noted on the patient's ENG record.

Recent Clinical ENG Findings

Nystagmography was reported to have great sensitivity when applied in patients with multiple sclerosis.[23,32] This was confirmed in the Tackmann study.[33] Because of the long pathways of the oculomotor system, there is a high degree of probability that parts of these structures are involved in multiple sclerosis. Though multiple sclerosis may produce nearly every type of pathological nystagmus[5], acquired pendular nystagmus and dissociated nystagmus on lateral gaze are typical for multiple sclerosis[3,11] and rarely exist in other diseases.

Scarpaleozos et al. demonstrated the use of ENG in multiple sclerosis patients, revealing nystagmus in cases in which it was not detected by clinical examination.[29] In addition, nystagmus that was clinically apparent could be analyzed and the different components revealed. Spontaneous nystagmus was proved to be particularly multiform in this disease. Often a combination of two or three types of nystagmus was recorded in the same ENG. The most frequent type was the dissociated nystagmus of abduction and, secondly, the vertical type. The pendular rotation test appeared to be very use-

TABLE 18-2 Responses in Peripheral and
Central Vestibulopathies

ENG Tests	Peripheral (End-Organ) Vestibulopathy	Central Vestibulopathy
Calibration	Normal	Ocular dysmetria
Gaze	Symmetric	Asymmetric
Positional	Geotropic	Ageotropic
Tracking	Sinusoidal	Ataxic
Optokinetic	Symmetrical	Asymmetric
Caloric	Fixation suppression	Failure of fixation suppression

ful in revealing abnormalities mainly of the central type in cases in which spontaneous nystagmus was not recorded.

ENG has its widest surgical application in the evaluation of patients with peripheral vestibulopathies and acoustic neuroma. In Ménière's disease ENG examination during an attack can be extremely helpful in objectively localizing the involved ear. McClure et al. reported that all their Ménière's disease cases studied showed a contralateral beating nystagmus during the acute phase of the attack and ipsilateral beating nystagmus as the acute symptoms subsided.[21] Similarly, ENG can be helpful in the identification of a perilymphatic labyrinthine fistula or sudden changes in intracranial pressure. Maton, Gabersek, and Salel suggest the role of sudden variations in intracranial pressure and their influence on endolabyrinthine fluids when they studied the ENG recordings of sleeping patients who experience sudden vertigo when aroused.[19]

Rubenstein et al. reported that CT scans confirmed "benign" cerebellar infarctions in patients whose ENG findings mimicked peripheral vestibulopathies.[27] More recently, Proust et al. demonstrated that the ENG is useful in the identification of the central nature of the pathology in cases of "benign" cerebellar infarction when the test is performed early.[26] They noted that these patients frequently showed a rapidly disappearing spontaneous nystagmus that was both inconstant and multidirectional, suggesting the cerebellar nature of the lesion.

ENG testing has a particularly important role in providing valuable diagnostic information to the clinician who is attempting to determine whether a patient who complains of dysequilibrium has central or peripheral pathology. Table 18-2 summarizes the distinguishing features that may be seen in either instance with the various testing procedures in current use. In some cases, however, the findings may be inconclusive, and in all cases they need to be incorporated with the clinical and other laboratory data.

References

1. Alpert JN: Failure of fixation suppression: A pathologic effect of vision on caloric nystagmus. Neurology (NY) 24:891–896, 1974.
2. Aschan G, Bergstedt M, Stahl J: Nystagmography. Acta Otolaryngol [Suppl] (Stockh) 129:1–103, 1956.
3. Aschoff JC, Conrad B, Kornhuber HH: Acquired pendular nystagmus with oscillopsia in multiple sclerosis: A sign of cerebellar nuclei disease. J Neurol Neurosurg Psychiatry 37:570–577, 1974.
4. Babin RW: Periodic alternating nystagmus. Ann Otol Rhinol Laryngol 90:524–525, 1981.
5. Baloh RW, Sakala SM, Honrubia V: Benign paroxysmal positional nystagmus Am J Otolaryngol 1:1–6, 1979.
6. Barber HO: Positional vertigo and nystagmus. Otolaryngol Clin North Am 6:169–187, 1973.
7. Barber HO, Wright G: Positional nystagmus in normals. Adv Otorhinolaryngol 19:276–285, 1973.
8. Benitez JT: Eye-tracking and optokinetic tests: Diagnostic significance in peripheral and central vestibular disorders. Laryngoscope 80:834–848, 1970.
9. Benitez JT, Bouchard KR: Electronystagmography: Significant alterations in tumors of the cerebellopontine recess. Ann Otol Rhinol Laryngol 83:399–402, 1974.
10. Carre J: Apports et limites de l'electronystagmographie dans l'appréciation médicolegale des séquelles des traumatismes crâniens. Rev Otoneuroophtalmol 53:357–361, 1981.
11. Cogan DG: Internuclear ophthalmoplegia, typical and atypical. Arch Ophthalmol 84:583–589, 1970.
12. Gabersek V, Salel D: La réactivité optocinétique en électronystagmographie. Rev Otoneuroophtalmol 53:67–77, 1981.
13. Hart CA: The optokinetic test and ENG test battery. Ann Otol Rhinol Laryngol [Suppl] 86:2–6, 1981.
14. Hofferberth B, Moser M: Die Aufrechterhaltung eines gleichmässigen Vigilanzniveaus bei der Elektronystagmographie. Laryngol Rhinol Otol (Stuttg) 60:255–258, 1981.
15. Hood JD, Kayan A, Leech J: Rebound nystagmus. Brain 96:507–526, 1973.
16. Kanzaki J: Effects of ocular fixation on perrotatory nystagmus in clamped pendular rotation test. Arch Otorhinolaryngol 230:209–219, 1981.
17. Karlsen EA, Hassanein RM, Goetzinger CP: The effects of age, sex, hearing loss and water temperature on caloric nystagmus. Laryngoscope 91:620–627, 1981.
18. Kileny P, McCabe BF, Ryu JH: Effects of attention-requiring tasks on vestibular nystagmus. Ann Otol Rhinol Laryngol 89:9–12, 1980.
19. Maton P, Gabersek V, Salel D: Vertiges brusques au décours du sommeil: A propos de 76 enrégistrements électronystagmographiques. Rev Otoneuroophtalmol 52:351–358, 1980.
20. Mathog RH: Sinusoidal harmonic acceleration. Ann Otol Rhinol Laryngol [Suppl] 86:10–14, 1981.
21. McClure JA, Copp JC, Lycett P: Recovery nystagmus in Ménière's disease. Laryngoscope 91:1727–1737, 1981.
22. Money KE, Myles WS, Hoffert BM: The mechanism of positional alcohol nystagmus. Can J Otolaryngol 3:302–313, 1974.
23. Noffsinger D, Olsen WO, Carhart R, Hart CW, Sahgal V: Auditory and vestibular aberrations in multiple sclerosis. Acta Otolaryngol [Suppl] (Stockh) 303:1–63, 1972.
24. Olson JE, Wolfe JW: Block nystagmus. Ann Otol Rhinol Laryngol 89:286–287, 1980.
25. Olson JE, Wolfe JW: Comparison of subjective symptomatology and responses to harmonic acceleration in patients with Meniere's disease. Ann Otol Rhinol Laryngol [Suppl] 86:15–17, 1981.
26. Proust B, Abuet MJ, Courtin P, Andrieu-Guitrancourt J: Aspects vestibulaires cliniques et électronystagmographiques des accidents vasculaires cérébelleux bénins. Rev Otoneuroophtalmol 54:17–24, 1982.
27. Rubenstein RL, Norman DM, Schindler RA, Kaseff L: Cerebellar infarction: A presentation of vertigo. Laryngoscope 90:505–514, 1980.
28. Rubin W: Sinusoidal harmonic acceleration test in clinical practice. Ann Otol Rhinol Laryngol [Suppl] 86:18–25, 1981.
29. Scarpaleozos S, Tsakanikas C, Stamboulis E: Étude électronys-

tagmographique de la sclérose en plaques. Rev Neurol (Paris) 137:137–146, 1981.

30. Simmons FB: Patients with bilateral loss of caloric response. Ann Otol Rhinol Laryngol 82:175–178, 1973.
31. Simpson RA: Sinusoidal harmonic acceleration labyrinthine test: Clinical experience. Ann Otol Rhinol Laryngol [Suppl] 86:26–28, 1981.
32. Solingen LD, Baloh RW, Myers L, Ellison G: Subclinical eye

movement disorders in patients with multiple sclerosis. Neurology (NY) 27:614–619, 1977.
33. Tackmann W, Strenge H, Barth R, Sojka-Raytscheff A: Evaluation of various brain structures in multiple sclerosis with multimodality evoked potentials, blink reflex and nystagmography. J Neurol 224:33–46, 1980.
34. Umeda Y: The eye-tracking test. Ann Otol Rhinol Laryngol [Suppl] 71:1–12, 1980.

19

Evoked Potentials from the Visual, Auditory, and Somatosensory Systems

C. William Erwin
Andrea Brendle
Miles E. Drake

Evoked potentials are small electrical events arising from neural tissue occurring in response to abrupt sensory stimulation. In current clinical application this usually involves stimulation of the visual, auditory, or somatosensory systems.

Evoked potentials were first described by Richard Caton in 1875, who recorded spontaneous electrical potentials from the cortex of animals and noted that the spontaneous activity (EEG) changed in response to visual stimulation. He also applied electrical stimuli to peripheral nerves and recorded "evoked" electrical potentials from appropriate cortical regions. Among the early discoveries about the human EEG after Berger's 1929 report was that photic stimulation gives rise to small potentials in the occipital region (the driving response) and that potentials could be elicited by auditory stimulation during sleep (K complexes). Subsequent

work has shown that there are many types of responses to stimulation that are time-locked (have a fixed temporal relationship to the stimulus); however, most responses are too small to be distinguished from the ongoing EEG.

An early approach to resolving the inherent signal-to-noise problem was reported by George Dawson in 1947.[21] Responses to repetitive stimuli were displayed on an oscilloscope and superimposed on photographic film. Time-locked activity produced an overexposure in one area of the film as compared with random activity, which lightly exposed all of the film. The technique permitted the identification of low-amplitude potentials, time-locked to the stimuli. This superimposition is known as the *overtrace method*. Subsequently, the averaging of multiple responses by computer techniques facilitated the recording of evoked potentials; the random events of the ongoing activity are suppressed by the averaging process, and small evoked events that have a fixed temporal relationship to a stimulus are preserved for identification. Availability of commercial systems has facilitated the recording of sensory evoked potentials in a wide variety of clinical situations.

General Clinical Applications

Evoked potentials are principally useful in neurological practice for the evaluation of multiple sclerosis, which in the early stages often has signs and/or symptoms of one clinical lesion but one or more subclinical lesions that may be demonstrable by evoked potential techniques.[15] Many degenerative disorders of the nervous system are associated with evoked potential abnormalities.[20] Visual evoked potentials are often useful in ophthalmologic assessment,[4,5] and brain stem auditory evoked responses provide an objective test of hearing[67] in addition to their value in the detection of intrinsic or extrinsic lesions of the brain stem.[66] Brain stem auditory and somatosensory evoked potentials are also useful in the assessment of coma[35,48] and brain death.[32,63]

Somatosensory evoked potentials have the capacity, at least in theory, to evaluate both the peripheral and central nervous system from the most distal peripheral nerve to the arrival of the evoked response at the cortex.[22]

Responses derived from all modalities have been used in monitoring of operative procedures in which specific neural tissue is in jeopardy. In such monitoring a stimulus is applied distally and responsive neural tissue is evaluated at a location proximal to the surgical procedure.[54] The serial responses are evaluated continuously in reference to baseline values. In theory, physiological alteration resulting in EP changes may warn of impending irreversible damage that may be averted by appropriate action.

Currently, the principal value of evoked potentials is in the detection of organic neurological impairment in patients with functional complaints that cannot be verified by clinical examination.

Evoked Potential Instrumentation and Techniques

The analog neural electrical activity is amplified, filtered, and converted to digital values for computation and storage. A trigger pulse is supplied by the stimulator or the computer triggers the stimulator to establish the time-locked relationship. Each epoch is stored and added to previously obtained digital values, and the sum is normalized. The average is then displayed on an oscilloscope, stored magnetically, or committed to paper by an X-Y plotter. The averaging process results in a marked improvement of the signal-to-noise ratio, in which the noise reduction factor can be estimated by calculating the square root of $1/N$, where N is the number of epochs taken to produce the average. The number of individual responses required to form an adequate average may vary from less than 10 to over 4000 depending on the relative amplitudes of the signal and noise. When the signal is large and the noise is small, few responses are required. Unfortunately, the opposite is more common, and more than 1000 stimuli may be needed.[30]

Visual Evoked Potentials

In the current practice of evoked potentials, stimulation of the visual system may be by flash or pattern (see below). Flash stimulation of the visual system affords a diffuse retinal stimulus, activating both the central and peripheral visual fields. Shifting checkerboard or grating patterns provide mainly macular stimulation, and the response is dependent upon the integrity of the central visual field.[14,29,62]

Stimulation to elicit a visual evoked potential requires light with abrupt onset, such as a stroboscopic light or an array of light-emitting diodes (LEDs). Flash evoked responses (Fig. 19-1) consist of a number of positive and negative peaks that vary greatly between individuals. This variability has limited their clinical utility. However, they are helpful in assessing patients whose visual acuity is too poor to generate evoked potentials to pattern reversal and in testing comatose patients and others unable to fixate on the pattern stimulus. In addition, flash evoked responses can be used for prognostic assessment of visual function before cataract surgery,[1] and for monitoring of the integrity of the optic nerve and chiasm during surgery in the pituitary region[33] (loss or distortion of the responses being associated with poor visual outcome). Changes in the latencies and morphology of the responses have been used to follow the

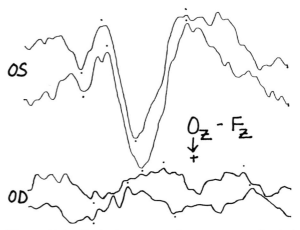

Figure 19-1 Evoked responses from separate stimulation of the left and right eyes (OS and OD) by an array of light-emitting diodes. Patient is a sedated 2-year-old with a later confirmed glioma of the right optic nerve. Behavior would not allow pattern reversal testing. Stimulus and recording parameters indicated.

course of hydrocephalus both before and after shunting, with improvement in the flash evoked potentials when shunting is successful and regression of the expected maturational change in the response if shunt failure occurs.[26] In general, absence of a flash response is indicative of poor or absent visual function, and failure to record such responses in children indicates a poor prognosis for visual development.

Pattern reversal techniques use several types of stimulators, all of which provide a checkerboard image. Stimulation occurs when the black (or colored) squares become white and vice versa. This is accomplished mechanically by pattern shift or electrically by pattern reversal. The patient is instructed to fixate on the shifting pattern. Recording electrodes are placed at scalp locations over the visual cortex (O_Z). Prechiasmal disturbances can be detected by abnormalities of the response from a midline occipital electrode, with each eye being stimulated separately (Fig. 19-2).[39,6,56,29] Retrochiasmal lesions require multiple simultaneous recording channels with electrodes placed over lateral occipital and posterior temporal regions. The practical utility of evoked potentials in the assessment of retrochiasmal lesions is open to debate and requires a high level of patient cooperation (Fig. 19-3).[9,41,46,57,49,36]

Response latency and amplitude are sensitive to alteration of technical parameters and are affected by size and intensity of the checkerboard pattern, rate of stimulation, and filter settings. The major events of clinical interest occur within one-fifth of a second (200 ms) following a pattern shift. The analysis time is generally 250 ms and an artifact-free response may rquire 200 to 400 stimuli.[29]

Criteria for abnormality related to prechiasmal lesions are statistically based, primarily on the latency of the P1 component, although N1 and N2 components are also compared with norms. Pattern reversal evoked responses have a consistent morphology. The latency of the principal positive component occurring at about 100 ms (P100 or P1) when

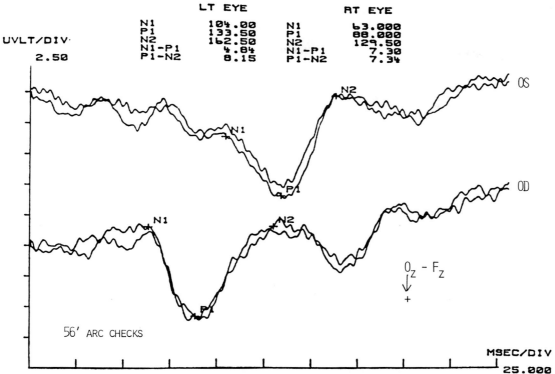

Figure 19-2 Pattern responses in a 39-year-old female with ataxia and an internuclear ophthalmoplegia. Replicated responses from the right eye are normal in morphology, amplitude, and latency of all components. Responses to left eye stimulation show good preservation of morphology and amplitude, but the P1 latency is grossly prolonged to 133.5 ms, indicating a conduction disturbance of the left anterior optic pathway. In the absence of macular disease this would indicate optic nerve involvement, providing physiological evidence of "a second lesion in space" compatible with multiple sclerosis.

subjected to statistical analysis yields a low standard deviation in the range of 3 to 4 ms. A normal pattern reversal response from right eye stimulation is shown in Fig. 19-2; the negative components occur around 75 and 135 ms, and are therefore called N75 and N135, or N1 and N2.

With prechiasmal lesions, abnormalities of pattern reversal responses consist primarily of a unilateral or bilateral prolongation in latency of the P1 component, or an asymmetry in latency between the eyes exceeding statistical norms. This is usually defined as the mean plus three standard deviations. A more appropriate statistical criterion is the tolerance limit (TL), in which the 99 percent TL is calculated from a sample of the normal population. Although often present, amplitude changes can be affected by nonneurological factors including simple errors of refraction. Evoked potential latency prolongation is often seen in multiple sclerosis (Fig. 19-4) and may be present bilaterally when symptoms are unilateral or even when the patient is visually asymptomatic.[38] The predilection of multiple sclerosis for the optic nerve is well known: autopsy series have suggested that as many as 90 percent of MS patients may have demyelination of the optic nerves even though there may have been no visual symptoms during life. EP testing reveals almost the same incidence of abnormality in end-stage MS. An acute attack of optic neuritis may not be associated with any

discernible abnormality of the eye on clinical examination, and visual acuity not uncommonly returns to normal, although an enlargement of the central blind spot, pallor of the optic disc, or impairment of color perception may be detectable. Early investigators reported that 100 percent of MS patients who had had optic neuritis showed prolongation of response latencies[37] even if they no longer had disturbances of visual acuity or fields. Although the actual figure may not be this high, it probably exceeds 90 percent. Moreover, it is estimated that less than 5 percent of abnormal responses subsequently return to the normal range. Approximately 60 percent of patients with MS have response abnormalities with no history or findings of optic nerve involvement.[38] Thus, visual evoked potentials are a useful diagnostic tool for detecting additional lesions of MS that are not evident clinically and for confirming that subjective complaints of visual disturbance are in fact due to organic visual dysfunction.

Compressive or destructive lesions in or around the optic nerve may prolong response latencies, but they are more likely to attenuate amplitude or distort morphology.[37] Prominent changes are caused by a glioma of the optic nerve. Such lesions are not uncommon in children, and occur less frequently in adults. They are often subtle in their clinical presentation and may present as visual complaints of

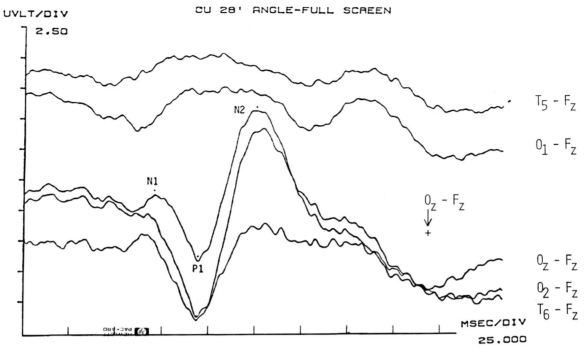

Figure 19-3 Pattern elicited responses recorded from five electrode placements on a line from the left posterior temporal through the occiput to the right occipital area. The five channels are recorded simultaneously. In normal controls with both eyes stimulated by a full screen, a symmetrical response would be expected from homologous regions. The asymmetry present is consistent with a left homonymous disturbance. The patient, asymptomatic at the time of testing, had recently had a left homonymous field defect on a migrainous basis.

possibly functional character. Diseases of the eye or optic nerve that primarily affect visual acuity will also cause diminution of response amplitudes.[55,60,61]

Brain Stem Auditory Evoked Potentials

Potentials evoked by stimulation of the auditory system develop within 2 ms after the stimulus with a cochlear microphonic and subsequent compound action potential from the auditory nerve. The later components are generally larger in amplitude and more variable in morphology. All the components occurring within the first 7 to 9 ms are of brain stem origin and are recorded as far-field events with the exception of wave I.[42] After the first 10 ms the exact neural generators are not known. Currently these responses have limited clinical applications, although much work is being done in this area of research.[7]

Click stimulation is supplied to the auditory system through headphones, generally unilaterally and with white noise masking of the contralateral ear. The electrical impulse is a square wave of very brief (100 μs) duration. The oscillations it creates in the headphone contain a broad-frequency spectrum with the major energy in the 3- to 4-kHz range. The latency of the responses are directly influenced by the intensity of the click. The clicks are generated by inward or out-

ward movement of the headphone diaphragm with respect to the tympanic membrane, and may have one of two polarities: rarefaction (R), in which the headphone diaphragm initial movement is away from the tympanic membrane, and condensation (C), in which movement is toward the tympanic membrane. An alternating polarity that is an interleaved mixture of the above R and C clicks is also employed.[13]

Short latency auditory evoked potentials are now widely used in neurology and audiology. Seven components may be recorded within the first 10 ms, and specific sites of origin have been suggested as follows (Fig. 19-5): wave I, the action potential of the acoustic nerve; wave II, the cochlear nucleus; wave III, the superior olivary complex; wave IV, the nucleus of the lateral lemniscus; wave V, the inferior colliculus; and waves VI and VII, the medial geniculate nucleus and the geniculocortical pathway. Subsequent work has indicated that these putative generators, with the exception of wave I, may not be entirely accurate and it is more likely correct simply to ascribe wave III to a pontine origin and wave V to a mesencephalic generation. Some workers interpret the data to indicate a nuclear origin, while others feel a tract origin is more likely. Waves II, IV, VI, and VII are more variable in terms of their presence and morphology; waves IV and V may be fused; and waves I and III may have more than one peak. With the exception of wave I, these are far-field responses, generated in the brain stem but

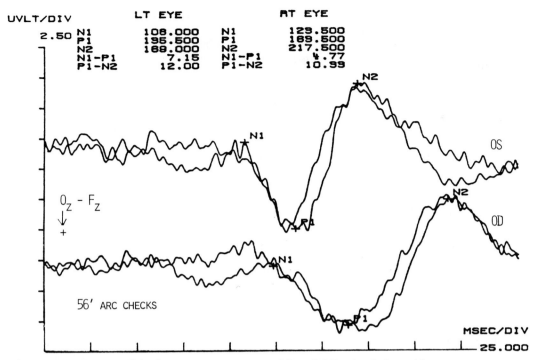

Figure 19-4 Pattern elicited responses to separate OS and OD stimulation with replications showing severe bilateral latency prolongations in a patient with suspected multiple sclerosis. The history indicated optic neuritis OD, but a Marcus Gunn pupil was absent. Evoked potentials suggested a subclinical disturbance OS in addition to corroborating the OD lesion.

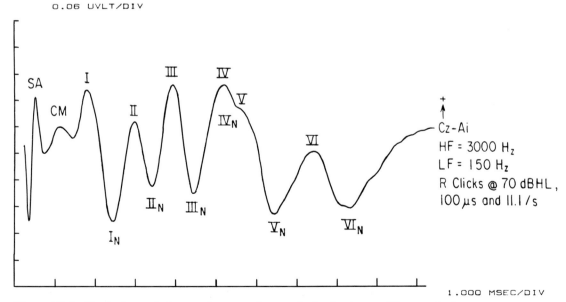

Figure 19-5 Typical morphology and nomenclature of a brain stem auditory evoked potential (BAEP). SA = stimulus artifact, CM = cochlear microphonic. Peaks labeled with roman numerals are described in the text as to their putative generators. Roman numerals subscripted by N are "negative" valleys. Stimulation and recording parameters are given with: R Clicks = rarefaction clicks, dBHL = decibels above hearing level (mean of control group), C_Z = vertex electrode of 10/20 electrode placement system, and A_i = ear lobe of the ear being stimulated (ipsilateral).

recorded at the scalp; wave I is near field, recorded by the ear or mastoid electrode and generated by the peripheral nervous system. Better-developed and earlier responses are more common with rarefaction clicks. Clicks are generally delivered at rates of 10 to 80 per second, with changes in responses engendered by faster rates of click presentation. Recordings are usually made from the Cz electrode with reference to ears. Analysis time is 10 ms, and as many as 4000 stimuli may be required to obtain an artifact-free response. These responses are influenced by a number of nonpathological factors. Lower stimulus intensities and more rapid rates of click presentation produce longer absolute latencies. Females have shorter latencies than males. Latencies lengthen with increasing age and decreasing brain temperature, and are prolonged in neonates, decreasing to adult values by 2 to 3 years of age. Latencies are also influenced by the acoustic phase of the click stimulus. Normality or abnormality is determined by the presence or absence of waves I, III, or V, and by the interpeak latencies between them as compared with statistical norms.[66,65]

Brain stem response audiometry is a technique of evaluating end-organ function in patients who cannot participate in behavioral testing. This is generally done by determining the wave V latency as a function of stimulus intensity. Relatively distinct patterns of response are produced by patients suffering conductive as opposed to sensorineural dysfunction. Deafness of functional origin is associated with normal responses, as is deafness produced by bilateral lesions of the auditory cortex and epileptic aphasia. Generally one cannot prove organic deafness on the basis of abnormal or absent responses, although it is often implied.[50] However, in multiple sclerosis and some posterior fossa structural lesions, unilaterally absent responses may be encountered in patients who have no audiologically detectable hearing deficit (Fig. 19-6).[65,64]

A major neurological application is in the diagnosis of multiple sclerosis. Roughly half of MS patients have brain stem auditory evoked response (BAER) abnormalities, including patients without signs or symptoms of brain stem dysfunction. Thus, as in visual EPs, the test may provide physiological evidence of areas of involvement that are silent clinically. This may take the form of complete or partial absence of waveforms, relative attenuation of wave V, or prolonged interpeak latencies (Fig. 19-7).[15,17,34] In a Mayo Clinic study,[65] a significant number of patients with brain stem evoked response abnormalities at the initial presentation, when only a single neurological lesion was suggested clinically, developed clinically definite MS within the next 3 years. Response abnormalities of similar character are also seen in other demyelinating diseases. Chief among these are the leukodystrophies of childhood, which are generally hereditary and involve developmental disturbance and motor dysfunction, and central pontine myelinolysis.[8,11,52]

Intrinsic or extrinsic tumors of the brain stem may pre-

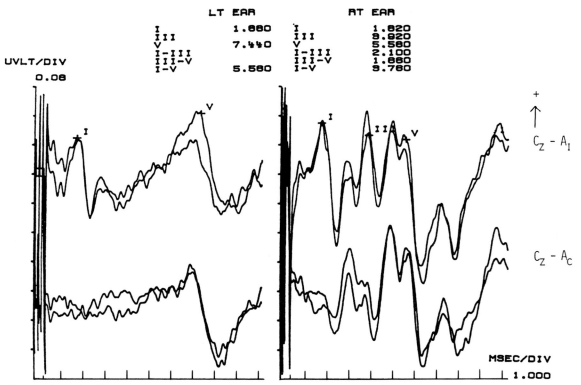

Figure 19-6 Replicated responses from left ear and right ear recorded from a vertex electrode (C$_Z$) and ipsilateral (A$_i$) and contralateral (A$_c$) ear electrode. Right-ear responses are entirely normal. Left-ear responses show loss of at least wave III and a marked I–V interpeak prolongation (5.58 ms). Audiogram and CT were normal. One month later, wave V was absent. A mass lesion was demonstrated on a subsequent rhombencephalogram. At operation there was a pathological diagnosis of a meningioma at the porus acusticus.

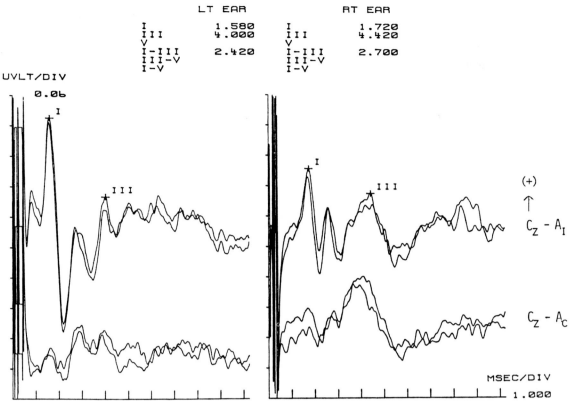

Figure 19-7 A 23-year-old female with findings suggestive of MS. BAEPs severely and bilaterally abnormal due to absence of major "waves" (V absent bilaterally), and severe I–III interpeak prolongation AD. Findings are etiologically nonspecific and have an inconsistent correlation with clinical severity of dysfunction.

sent clinically with various combinations of cranial nerve, motor tract, and sensory pathway dysfunction, although a functional diagnosis is often entertained until the neurological findings become blatant (Fig. 19-6). Currently, CT scan evaluation of the brain stem is less sensitive than that of cortical areas. EP abnormalities develop early in both intrinsic and extrinsic brain stem tumors. A wide variety of abnormalities may be produced by more slowly progressive extrinsic tumors, of which acoustic neuroma is the best example. Such abnormalities may not only involve prolongation of interpeak latencies or attenuation of responses on the side of the tumor, but may also include abnormalities on the opposite side because of brain stem compression from the neoplasm.[49,64] Evoked potential monitoring has been found helpful during surgical resection of such tumors, in which the facial and acoustic nerves may be damaged. Changes in evoked responses have been associated with intraoperative compromise of the acoustic nerve function, while identification of the facial nerve by electrophysiological techniques may help to avoid its sacrifice.[40]

Another major area of utility is the evaluation of coma. In patients unconscious as a result of bilateral cerebral cortical dysfunction, and in other diseases diffusely involving the cerebral cortex such as Alzheimer's disease, responses are generally normal. The same is true of psychogenic coma. In coma due to bilateral damage of brain stem structures, abnormality or absence of responses indicate a poor prognosis.[10,58] Brain stem auditory evoked potentials are resistant

to anesthesia, and normal responses can be recorded when the EEG is isoelectric, particularly from high barbiturate levels, even when the patient otherwise meets clinical criteria of brain death. Thus, preservation of BAER in a patient with coma, apnea, areflexia, and flat EEG may suggest an overdose if the history is not known when the patient presents in coma.[32,63] Alternately, profoundly abnormal or absent responses support an impression of irreversible brain insult. In both head-injured patients and those subjected to ischemia or anoxia, inability to record brain stem auditory evoked potentials is correlated with a poor outcome; however, one must be cautious in interpreting such data, as the patient may have pre-existing audiological disease. Prolonged deep barbiturate anesthesia is utilized in some centers in the treatment of severe cerebral trauma. BAERs have been used to monitor such patients, as they may be the only evidence of preserved neural function because vital signs may be suppressed by the anesthetic agents.[34]

Somatosensory Evoked Potentials

Stimulation to produce a somatosensory evoked response is usually electrical and is applied transcutaneously to a peripheral nerve, the amount of current being the level required to produce a clearly visible muscle twitch. Although intensity-dependent changes in the response are present at

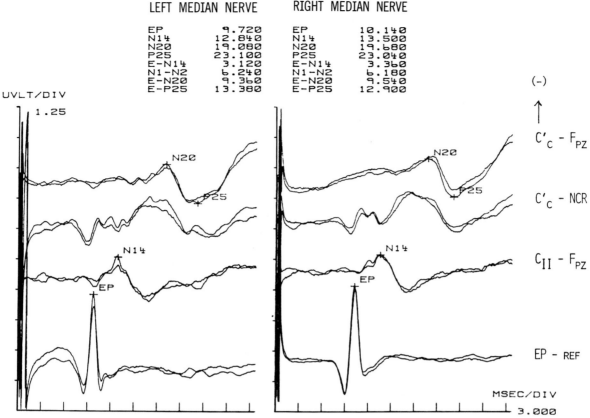

Figure 19-8 Somatosensory responses to electrical stimulation of the left and right median nerves at the wrist, sufficient to produce a thumb twitch (5.0 mA). Pulse rate of 5.4 per second and pulse duration of 100 μs. Bottom traces, left and right, show typical, triphasic action potentials from brachial plexus from electrodes at Erb's point (EP). Second from bottom shows medullary N14 and preceding cervical N11 derived from electrodes at the second cervical vertebra and a prefrontal placement. Third tracing from bottom is derived from electrodes overlying the contralateral rolandic area (C'$_c$) connected to a noncephalic reference (NCR, in this case hand). A series of far-field (subcortical) and near-field (cortical) components are present. The top channel reveals the cortically generated N20 and P25 components in a bipolar derivation. Analysis time is 30 ms with low and high filter settings at 30 and 3000, respectively. Upper field displays absolute and interpeak latencies (E = EP, N1 = N14, N2 = N20).

stimulus levels below motor threshold, there is little change in amplitude or latency of the response once the stimulus is above motor twitch threshold.[19] Electrical stimulation of peripheral dermatomes is also being used, and this has the advantage of specific root evaluation. In addition, mechanical stimulation of the nail bed has been reported, which may evaluate the spinothalamic pathways instead of the posterior column pathway utilized by electrical stimulation. These forms of stimulation may yield information not obtained from direct electrical stimulation of a peripheral nerve, but their application is not as yet widespread.[24]

Electrical stimulation, which is the most common clinical procedure, produces ascending volleys up both motor and sensory pathways in peripheral nerves. This action potential can be easily recorded by surface electrodes overlying the nerve at various locations. These peripheral action potentials are subject to a variety of unwanted variables such as age, temperature, limb length, and interindividual variation.

Stimulation of nerves at the wrist or ankle elicits peripheral and central nervous system (CNS) responses. CNS responses may be generated from the spinal cord, brain stem, thalamus, and cortex. The variability induced by peripheral factors mentioned above is minimized if not eliminated by determining the latency of the response just prior to entry into the CNS and calculating the interpeak latencies from this peripheral response to later, more rostrally generated responses. Such interpeak latencies indicate the central transmission time and provide the major criteria for normalcy of a somatosensory study. The peripheral response from Erb's point (brachial plexus)[24] or lower spinal (cauda equina) electrodes is analogous to wave I (auditory nerve) of the BAER (Figs. 19-8 and 19-9).[25]

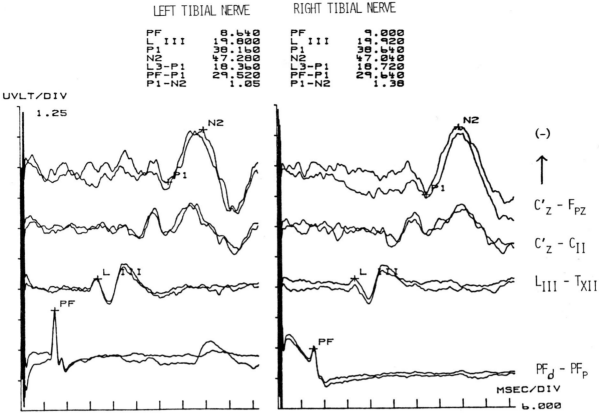

Figure 19-9   Somatosensory responses from electrical stimulation of left and right tibial nerves at the ankle. Intensity is sufficient to produce a toe twitch. Stimulation and recording parameters are similar to those in Fig. 19-8, with the exception of analysis time, which is extended to 60 ms. Bottom traces reveal action potential from common peroneal nerve at the popliteal fossa (PF). Second from the bottom is the "spinal" response from a bipolar derivation of electrodes at the third lumbar (L_{III}) and twelfth thoracic (T_{XII}) location. Third channel reveals probable subcortical components and fourth channel demonstrates the cortical response arising from the vertex. (P1 − N2 = amplitude in μV.)

The conduction velocity from the stimulated wrist (median nerve) to the brachial plexus (or lower extremity analogue) can and should be calculated, although because of its long length it is relatively insensitive to change caused by the acquired peripheral neuropathies, which primarily involve distal regions. Conduction changes caused by the various congenital neuropathies such as Charcot-Marie-Tooth disease are readily detected and often present as an unexpected finding in clinically asymptomatic individuals.[16]

Upon entry into the CNS the electrically elicited somatosensory evoked response is communicated primarily, if not exclusively, over the dorsal column and lemniscal pathways. Median nerve stimulation elicits subcortically generated components with mean absolute latencies of 11 and 14 ms. They may be recorded by several electrode derivations, which affects their polarity, and therefore they are sometimes referred to as N11 and N14 or P11 and P14. Regardless of the technical questions, data relating to the putative generators are fairly well accepted. According to most authors, the 11-ms component arises from cervical dorsal column pathways.[23] Unfortunately, in clinical practice over 30 percent of normal controls lack a definable response at this latency unless heavily sedated, which therefore limits its utility. The later 14-ms response is generally attributed to a lower medullary origin, with some workers feeling their data suggests a dorsal column nuclear generation. Other workers interpret similar data as implying a lemniscal origin.[16,23,3] Anatomically and clinically it is of small significance. Unfortunately, subcortical responses from lower extremity stimulation have been more elusive. However, there have been several recent reports describing techniques (electrode montage and filter setting) to record such subcortical responses following tibial and peroneal stimulation.[18,44]

The next series of components are generally considered to represent a mixture of subcortical (far-field) and cortical (near-field) events recorded from electrodes overlying the primary sensory cortex. The N20 is felt by many to be generated by cortical neuronal elements, with the preceding negative limb to be generated by thalamic nuclei or thalamocortical projections. Like the 14-ms component, the N20 is recorded in essentially all normal subjects. They both have definitive peaks, and statistical analysis reveals a low inter-individual variation in interpeak latency from the Erb's point action potential. There is a variable sequence of waveforms that follow the N20. The P25 is a stable component, but subsequent components follow the rule common to all evoked responses: The later the peak or valley, the greater the variability. This is true not only of morphology and latency but also of symmetry, as easily demonstrated by poor reproducibility. These later components are affected by alcohol, sedatives, tranquilizers, and analgesics as well as level of arousal and psychological factors. It is this latter fact that makes the later components of interest to the physiological psychiatrists and psychologists but limits their value in neurological diagnosis. Abnormality in these later components is usually produced by cortical disease, and other diagnostic procedures such as EEG and CT scan are usually of greater diagnostic value.[31]

Following median nerve stimulation, the Erb's point (EP) to N20 latency is calculated as the overall central conduction time from brachial plexus to primary sensory cortex. If this value is prolonged as compared with normative data, further analysis is required to determine if the prolongation is due to the more caudal EP to N14 segment or the more rostral N14 to N20. In severe lesions components may be entirely missing or grossly attenuated and altered in morphology.[16]

Numerous reports indicate that the somatosensory evoked potentials are similar to visual and auditory responses in the sense that they are sensitive to subclinical lesions. Evidence to support this contention may be found in the many cases of acute trauma with clear neurological signs of deficit that resolve with time but leave subclinical physiological residuals detectable by the above-described techniques. Somatosensory testing is reported to be only slightly less sensitive than visual EPs in the detection of occult lesions in MS and to have a higher incidence of abnormality than auditory brain stem responses in patients suspect for demyelinating disorders.[27]

The clinical utility of this class of responses includes those of auditory and visual EPs with some important additions. In MS, somatosensory responses are only slightly less likely to be abnormal than pattern reversal visual EPs and more sensitive than auditory brain stem responses.[15,35] Neoplasia of the spinal cord and brain stem usually produces major disturbances. An example of the effects of an occult brain stem lesion is illustrated in Fig. 19-10. Although rarely necessary in the evaluation of brain death, somatosensory evoked responses have a certain advantage over BAERs because the stimulus has direct access to the nervous system

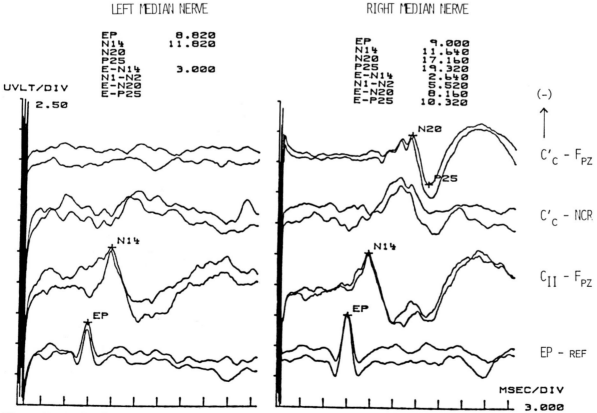

Figure 19-10 Median nerve somatosensory responses in a patient with an early mesencephalic glioma showing absence of thalamic and cortical responses following left median nerve stimulation. Stimulation and recording parameters are identical to those in Fig. 19-8.

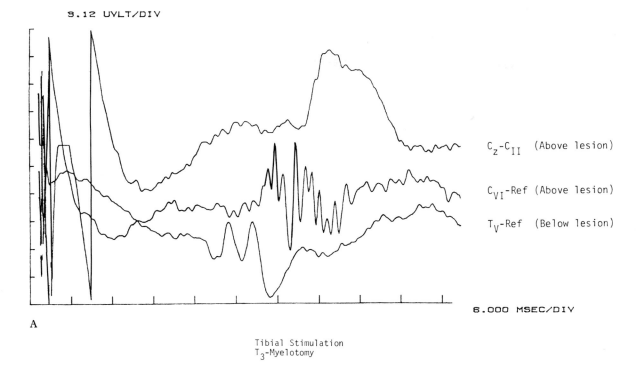

A

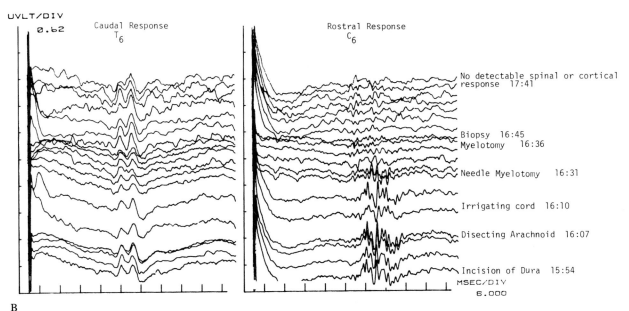

B

Figure 19-11   Monitoring of operative procedure during biopsy of a midthoracic spinal glioma. *A*. This illustrates a three-channel recording with one channel (T_V-Ref) recording from an interspinous needle electrode below the biopsy site. The second channel (C_{VI}-Ref) is obtained from an epidural electrode just above the biopsy site (skin reference). The top channel is recorded from bipolar scalp electrodes at the vertex (C_Z) and overlying the second cervical vertebra (C_{II}). Recording before biopsy. Bilateral tibial nerve stimulation with recording and stimulating parameters are similar to those in Fig. 19-9. Analysis time is 60 ms. *B*. Sequential responses during the course of surgery are indicated at the right. As the myelotomy and biopsy were performed on the dorsal column, the response was lost. Only a minimal and transient sensory loss was present on the day following surgery, and scalp evoked responses returned during the following week.

rather than being transduced by the cochlea, which may be defective for many reasons.[2]

Obviously, this form of stimulation is at least theoretically capable of evaluating both the peripheral and central nervous system from toe to cortex (at least some aspect of the sensory system). Peripheral neuropathies may be detected. Useful information may be obtained in patients suffering traumatic brachial plexopathies in which the degree of root involvement is unknown.[43,59,68]

Lastly, the use of evoked potentials in monitoring of operative procedures should be mentioned. The basic concept is that in any operative procedure in which neural tissue is in jeopardy, the physiological integrity of the tissue and the system it subserves can be monitored, even in deeply anesthetized patients. The system is evaluated by insertion of a signal that must traverse the area under threat; response changes are interpreted as altered physiology that is hopefully reversible. The most common use of this EP technique is in the treatment of scoliosis by fusion and instrumentation procedures. Frequently some distraction of the vertebral column and cord takes place (although it may be minimal), and permanent neurological sequelae are known. Prior to EP monitoring the "wake up" test was employed.[54]

Stimulation of common peroneal or tibial nerves and recording of responses from the spinal cord rostral to the area at risk, or from scalp electrodes reflecting cortical activity, is the most common technique. Figure 19-11 demonstrates such a procedure.[12,28]

Similar techniques have been reported in spinal operative procedures for neoplasms, AV malformations, thoracoabdominal aneurysms, and various acute and chronic defects leading to cord compression.[51]

Although less extensive, there have also been some reports on monitoring by EPs of visual responses in procedures involving the optic nerve(s) and/or chiasm. Brain stem auditory evoked potential responses have been utilized in procedures involving the posterior fossa.[47]

Several basic assumptions underlying these approaches have yet to be adequately documented. There appear to be few false-negative changes. That is, there are few if any reports of serious neurological complications related to an intraoperative event in which the evoked potentials remained stable and unchanged. Although neurological complications are uncommon, they are usually, but not universally, accompanied by major alteration in, if not complete loss of, the response.

References

1. Andreassi JL, Zalkind SS, Gallichio JA, Young NE: Monocular and binocular visual evoked potentials before and after cataract surgery. Percept Mot Skills 49:699–704, 1979.
2. Anziska B, Cracco RQ: Short latency somatosensory evoked potentials: Studies in patients with focal neurological disease. Electroencephalogr Clin Neurophysiol 49:227–239, 1980.
3. Anziska B, Cracco RQ, Cook AW, Feld EW: Somatosensory far field potentials: Studies in normal subjects and patients with multiple sclerosis. Electroencephalogr Clin Neurophysiol 45:602–610, 1978.
4. Arden GB, Barnard WM: Effect of occlusion on the visual evoked response in amblyopia. Trans Ophthalmol Soc UK 99:419–426, 1979.

5. Arden GB, Lewis DR: The pattern visual evoked response in the assessment of visual acuity. Trans Ophthalmol Soc UK 93:19–21, 1973.
6. Asselman P, Chadwick DW, Marsden CD: Visual evoked responses in the diagnosis and management of patients suspected of multiple sclerosis. Brain 98:261–282, 1975.
7. Battmer RD Lehnhardt E: The brain stem response SN_{10}, its frequency selectivity, and its value in classifying neural hearing lesions. Arch Otorhinolaryngol 230:37–47, 1981.
8. Black JA, Fariello RG, Chun RW: Brainstem auditory evoked response in adrenoleukodystrophy. Ann Neurol 6:269–270, 1979.
9. Blumhardt LD, Barrett G, Halliday AM, Kriss A: The effect of experimental 'scotomata' on the ipsilateral and contralateral responses to pattern-reversal in one half-field. Electroencephalogr Clin Neurophysiol 45:376–392, 1978.
10. Britt RH, Herrick MK, Mason RT, Dorfman LJ: Traumatic lesions of the pontomedullary junction. Neurosurgery 6:623–631, 1980.
11. Brown FR III, Shimizu H, McDonald JM, Moser AB, Marquis P, Chen WW, Moser HW: Auditory evoked brainstem response and high-performance liquid chromatography sulfatide assay as early indices of metachromatic leukodystrophy. Neurology (NY) 31:980–985, 1981.
12. Brown RH, Nash CL Jr, Lorig RA, Schatzinger LA: Spinal cord monitoring during operative treatment of the spine. Clin Orthop 126:100–105, 1977.
13. Cann J, Knott J: Polarity of acoustic click stimuli for eliciting brainstem auditory evoked responses: A proposed standard. Am J EEG Technol 19:125–132, 1979.
14. Celesia GG: Visual evoked potentials in neurological disorders. Am J EEG Technol 18:47–59, 1978.
15. Chiappa KH: Pattern shift visual, brainstem auditory, and short-latency somatosensory evoked potentials in multiple sclerosis. Neurology (NY) 30:110–123, 1980.
16. Chiappa KH, Choi SK, Young RR: Short-latency somatosensory evoked potentials following median nerve stimulation in patients with neurological lesions, in Desmedt JE (ed): *Clinical Uses of Cerebral, Brainstem and Spinal Somatosensory Evoked Potentials*. Basel, Karger, 1980, pp 264–281.
17. Chiappa KH, Norwood AE: A comparison of the clinical utility of pattern-shift visual evoked responses and brain stem auditory evoked responses in multiple sclerosis. Neurology (NY) 27:397, 1977 (abstr).
18. Cracco JB, Cracco RQ, Graziani L: The spinal evoked response in infants with myelodysplasia. Neurology (NY) 24:359–360, 1974 (abstr).
19. Cracco RQ: Scalp-recorded potentials evoked by median nerve stimulation: Subcortical potentials, traveling waves and somatomotor potentials, in Desmedt JE (ed): *Clinical Uses of Cerebral, Brainstem and Spinal Somatosensory Evoked Potentials*. Basel, Karger, 1980, pp 1–14.
20. d'Allest AM, Laget P, Raimbault J: Visual and somesthetic potentials in neurolipidosis, in Courjon J, Mauguiere F, Revol M (eds): *Advances in Neurology*, vol 32: *Clinical Application of Evoked Potentials in Neurology*. New York, Raven Press, 1982, pp 397–407.
21. Dawson GD: Cerebral responses to electrical stimulation of peripheral nerve in man. J Neurol Neurosurg Psychiatry 10:137–140, 1947.
22. Desmedt JE, Brunko E: Functional organization of far-field and cortical components of somatosensory evoked potentials in normal adults, in Desmedt JE (ed): *Clinical Uses of Cerebral, Brainstem and Spinal Somatosensory Evoked Potentials*. Basel, Karger, 1980, pp 27–50.
23. Desmedt JE, Cheron G: Prevertebral (oesophageal) recording of subcortical somatosensory evoked potentials in man: The spinal P_{13} component and the dual nature of the spinal generators. Electroencephalogr Clin Neurophysiol 52:257–275, 1981.

24. Desmedt JE, Cheron G: Recent progress in the understanding of subcortical somatosensory evoked potentials, in Courjon J, Mauguiere F, Revol M (eds): *Advances in Neurology*, vol 32:*Clinical Applications of Evoked Potentials in Neurology*. New York, Raven Press, 1982, pp 295–302.

25. Dorfman LJ, Perkash I, Bosley TM, Cummins KL: Use of cerebral evoked potentials to evaluate spinal somatosensory function in patients with traumatic and surgical myelopathies. J Neurosurg 52:654–660, 1980.

26. Ehle A, Sklar F: Visual evoked potentials in infants with hydrocephalus. Neurology (NY) 29:1541–1544, 1979.

27. Eisen A, Odusote K: Central and peripheral conduction times in multiple sclerosis. Electroencephalogr Clin Neurophysiol 48:253–265, 1980.

28. Engler GL, Spielholz NI, Bernhard WW, Danziger F, Merkin H, Wolfe T: Somatosensory evoked potentials during Harrington instrumentation for scoliosis. J Bone Joint Surg [Am] 60A:528–532, 1978.

29. Erwin CW: Pattern reversal evoked potentials. Am J EEG Technol 20:161–184, 1980.

30. Erwin CW: Signal averaging. Duke University Evoked Symposium, 1981, pp1–14.

31. Goff WR, Williamson PD, Vangilder JC, Allison T, Fisher TC: Cortical and far-field SEP components in normals: Neural origins of long latency evoked potentials recorded from the depth and from the cortical surface of the brain in man, in Desmedt JE (ed): *Clinical Uses of Cerebral, Brainstem and Spinal Somatosensory Evoked Potentials*. Basel, Karger, 1980, pp 126–145.

32. Goldie WD, Chiappa KH, Young RR, Brooks EB: Brainstem auditory and short-latency somatosensory evoked responses in brain death. Neurology (NY) 31:248–256, 1981.

33. Gott PS, Weiss MH, Apuzzo M, Van Der Meulen JP: Checkerboard visual evoked response in evaluation and management of pituitary tumors. Neurosurgery 5:553–558, 1979.

34. Green JB, Price R, Woodbury SG: Short-latency somatosensory evoked potentials in multiple sclerosis: Comparison with auditory and visual evoked potentials. Arch Neurol 37:630–633, 1980.

35. Greenberg RP, Newlon PG, Hyatt MS, Narayan RK, Becker DP: Prognostic implications of early multimodality evoked potentials in severely head-injured patients: A prospective study. J Neurosurg 55:227–236, 1981.

36. Haimovic IC, Pedley TA: Hemi-field pattern reversal visual evoked potentials: II. Lesions of the chiasm and posterior visual pathways. Electroencephalogr Clin Neurophysiol 54:121–131, 1982.

37. Halliday AM, Halliday E, Kriss A, McDonald WI, Mushin J: The pattern-evoked potential in compression of the anterior visual pathways. Brain 99:357–374, 1976.

38. Halliday AM, McDonald WI, Mushin J: Delayed visual evoked response in optic neuritis. Lancet 1:982–985, 1972.

39. Halliday AM, McDonald WI, Mushin J: Visual evoked potentials in patients with demyelinating disease, in Desmedt JE (ed): *Visual Evoked Potentials in Man: New Developments*. Oxford, Clarendon Press, 1977, pp 438–449.

40. Hashimoto I, Ishiyama Y, Totsuka G, Mizutani H: Monitoring brainstem function during posterior fossa surgery with brainstem auditory evoked potentials, in Barber C (ed): *Evoked Potentials*. Baltimore, University Park Press, 1980, pp 377–390.

41. Holder GE: Abnormalities of the pattern reversal visual evoked potential in patients with homonymous visual field defects, in Barber C (ed): *Evoked Potentials*. Baltimore, University Park Press, 1980, pp 285–291.

42. Jewett DL, Romano MN, Williston JS: Human auditory evoked potentials: Possible brainstem components detected on the scalp. Science 167:1517–1518, 1970.

43. Jones SJ: Somatosensory evoked potentials in traction lesions of the brachial plexus, in Barber C (ed): *Evoked Potentials*. Baltimore, University Park Press, 1980, pp 443–448.

44. Jones SJ, Halliday AM: Subcortical and cortical somatosensory evoked potentials: Characteristic waveform changes associated with disorders of the peripheral and central nervous system, in Courjon J, Mauguiere F, Revol M (eds): *Advances in Neurology*, vol 32:*Clinical Applications of Evoked Potentials in Neurology*. New York, Raven Press, 1982, pp 313–320.

45. Kjaer M: The value of a multimodal evoked potential approach in the diagnosis of multiple sclerosis, in Courjon J, Mauguiere F, Revol M (eds): *Advances in Neurology*, vol 32: *Clinical Applications of Evoked Potentials in Neurology*. New York, Raven Press, 1982, pp 507–512.

46. Kuroiwa Y, Celesia GG: Visual evoked potentials with hemifield pattern stimulation: Their use in the diagnosis of retrochiasmatic lesions. Arch Neurol 38:86–90, 1981.

47. Levine RA: Monitoring auditory evoked potentials during acoustic neuroma surgery, in Silverstein H, Norrell H (eds): *Neurological Surgery of the Ear*. Birmingham, Aesculapius 1979, pp 287–293.

48. Mackay AR, Hosobuchi Y, Williston JS, Jewett D: Brain stem auditory evoked response and brain stem compression. Neurosurgery 6:632–638, 1980.

49. Maitland CG, Aminoff MJ, Kennard C, Hoyt WF: Evoked potentials in the evaluation of visual field defects due to chiasmal or retrochiasmal lesions. Neurology (NY) 32:986–991, 1982.

50. Michel F, Peronnet F, Schott B: A case of cortical deafness: Clinical and electrophysiological data. Brain Lang, 10:367–377, 1980.

51. Nash CL Jr, Schatzinger LH, Brown RH, Brodkey J: The unstable stable thoracic compression fracture: Its problems and the use of spinal cord monitoring in the evaluation of treatment. Spine 2:261–265, 1977.

52. Ochs R, Markand ON, DeMyer WE: Brainstem auditory evoked responses in leukodystrophies. Neurology (NY) 29:1089–1093, 1979.

53. Pratt H, Starr A: Mechanically and electrically evoked somatosensory potentials in humans: Scalp and neck distributions of short latency components. Electroencephalogr Clin Neurophysiol 51:138–147, 1981.

54. Raudzens PA: Intraoperative monitoring of evoked potentials, in Bodis-Wollner I (ed): *Evoked Potentials*. New York, New York Academy of Sciences, 1982, pp 308–325.

55. Regan D: Rapid methods for refracting the eye and for assessing visual acuity in amblyopia, using steady-state visual evoked potentials, in Desmedt JE (ed): *Visual Evoked Potentials in Man: New Development*. Oxford, Clarendon Press, 1977, pp 418–426.

56. Rosén I, Bynke H, Sandberg M: Pattern-reversal visual evoked potentials after unilateral optic neuritis, in Barber C (ed): *Evoked Potentials*. Baltimore, University Park Press, 1980, pp 567–574.

57. Rowe MJ III: A sequential technique for half-field pattern visual evoked potential testing. Electroencephalogr Clin Neurophysiol 51:463–469, 1981.

58. Seales DM, Torkelson RD, Shuman RM, Rossiter VS, Spencer JD: Abnormal brainstem auditory evoked potentials and neuropathology in "locked-in" syndrome. Neurology (NY) 31:893–896, 1981.

59. Siivola J, Myllylä VV, Sulg I, Hokkanen E: Brachial plexus and radicular neurography in relation to cortical evoked responses. J Neurol Neurosurg Psychiatry 42:1151–1158, 1979.

60. Sokol S: Measurement of infant visual acuity from pattern reversal evoked potentials. Vision Res 18:33–39, 1978.

61. Sokol S: Pattern visual evoked potentials: Their use in pediatric ophthalmology. Int Ophthalmol Clin 20:251–268, 1980.

62. Sokol S: Visual evoked potentials, in Aminoff MJ (ed): *Electrodiagnosis in Clinical Neurology*. New York, Churchill Livingstone, 1980, pp 348–369.

63. Starr A: Auditory brainstem responses in brain death. Brain 99:543–554, 1976.

64. Starr A, Hamilton AE: Correlation between confirmed sites of neurological lesions and abnormalities of far-field auditory brainstem responses. Electroencephalogr Clin Neurophysiol 41:595–608, 1976.

65. Stockard JJ, Sharbrough FW: Unique contributions of short-latency auditory and somatosensory evoked potentials to neurologic diagnosis, in Desmedt JE (ed): *Clinical Uses of Cerebral, Brainstem and Spinal Somatosensory Evoked Potentials*. Basel, Karger, 1980, pp 231–263.

66. Stockard JJ, Stockard JE, Sharbrough FW: Brainstem auditory evoked potentials in neurology: Methodology, interpretation, clinical application, in Aminoff MJ (ed): *Electrodiagnosis in Clinical Neurology*. New York, Churchill Livingstone, 1980, pp 370–413.

67. Weber BA, Spaulding JP, Fletcher GL: Auditory brainstem response audiometry: Cautions and practical considerations. Hear Aid J 3:40–42, 1980.

68. Zverina E, Kredba J: Somatosensory cerebral evoked potentials in diagnosing brachial plexus injuries. Scand J Rehabil Med 9:47–54, 1977.

SECTION C

Some Evolving Neurodiagnostic Tests

20

Computed Tomography: Recent Trends

Burton P. Drayer
G. Allan Johnson
C. Roger Bird

Basic Principles

In the short time since its demonstration by Hounsfield,[16] computed tomography (CT) has become an indispensable tool in the diagnosis of disorders of the central nervous system. During this brief period, CT has undergone a rapid evolution, with new versions, upgrades, or options introduced by commercial interests every year. The modern CT scanner can do substantially more than produce individual slices. In addition, modern scanners accomplish the principal goal of CT, i.e., the computation of images representing axial anatomy, with much greater fidelity and reliability than early machines. Spatial resolution has improved tenfold, that is, from 1.5 lp/cm to more than 15 lp/cm (lp = resolved line pairs, a general parameter used to compare the spatial resolution of radiographic systems). Modern scanners can discern differences in tissue density of <0.3 percent.[4]

Historical Development

The dramatic improvements in CT are shown in Fig. 20-1, in which a scan from a first-generation machine is compared with one from a third-generation scanner. The term *generation* has been used to distinguish the various geometries of data acquisition in CT.

In first-generation machines (Fig. 20-2) a tube emitting a single collimated beam of x-rays was translated (moved in a straight line) in parallel with a single x-ray detector placed on the other side of the patient. At 160 discrete points during the translation transmitted x-ray intensity was measured at the detector and electrical signals proportional to the intensity were produced. This set of 160 measurements was the x-ray profile for that view. The x-ray tube and detector

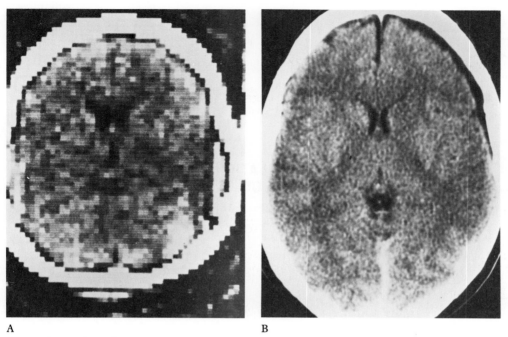

A   B

Figure 20-1 *A.* A CT scan with a first-generation machine employing an 80×80 matrix (6400 elements) of 3×3 mm pixels. Data acquisition (28,800 measurements) required 5 min. *B.* CT scan with a third-generation machine using a 320×320 matrix (102,400 elements) of 0.8×0.8 mm pixels. Data acquisition (1,400,000 measurements) required 2 s.

were then rotated 1 degree and another translation executed, producing a second view. The process was repeated until 180 views were obtained. The entire set of 180 views with 160 x-ray measurements per view (total of 28,800 x-ray transmission measurements) was then processed by the computer to generate the final image of one slice.

The final image displayed on a cathode ray tube is really a discrete set of picture elements (pixels) with the brightness of each element directly proportional to the x-ray attenuation of the elements. The Hounsfield unit (HU) has been adopted as the uniform scale:

$$HU = K\frac{\mu_{tissue} - \mu_{tissue}}{\mu_{water}}$$

where μ is the x-ray absorption coefficient. K is a constant chosen so that the HU of air equals -1000, that of dense bone equals $+1000$, and that of water equals 0. Figure 20-1A demonstrates the discrete nature of the picture matrix. Each row of the image has 80 elements, and there are 80 rows for a total of 6400 picture elements. Each picture element in the figure corresponds to a 3×3 mm area of the slice. The slice thickness is 13 mm. The image becomes less like a box as the size of the pixels is reduced. The pixels in Fig. 20-1B are 0.8×0.8 mm in size, requiring 320 pixels per row for 320 rows (total of 102,400 elements) to cover a similar field of view. The slice thickness is 5 mm. Newer systems use a 512×512 matrix (262,144 elements) with pixels less than 0.5 mm $\times$ 0.5 mm. A slice thickness of 1 mm is possible.

A complete description of the computations necessary to

generate the picture from the x-ray profiles is beyond the scope of this chapter.[15,28] However, Fig. 20-2 demonstrates conceptually the method of image reconstruction through back projection. Consider an idealized object, i.e., a solid rod in the center of the field of view. The detector response or view 1 is shown graphically in Fig. 20-2A. The data from this view tell the computer that at the center of the translation an object caused attenuation of the x-ray beam. The location of the object along the path between tube and detector is not defined by this single view, however, so the computer projects a uniform density back along that line. The uniform density (shaded area in Fig. 20-2B) when added to similar back projections from translations at other angles locates the point and produces the summed back-projected image (Fig. 20-2C). While the image is reasonable in the central darkest section of Fig. 20-2C, the star pattern (crosshatched area) resulting from overlap of back projections is not an accurate rendition of the initial object. A variant of the back-projection technique filters the initial input response, producing both negative and positive components. The filtering is done in such a fashion that the negative and positive components add to cancel the star pattern (Fig. 20-3).

Data acquisition in first-generation machines was extremely inefficient, requiring 5 min for a single slice. The majority of this time was necessary for the translation across the patient at each angle. Second-generation scanners addressed this problem by adding more detectors and collimating the x-ray field to produce multiple pencil beams. This array of 30 essentially parallel beams impinging on 30 x-ray

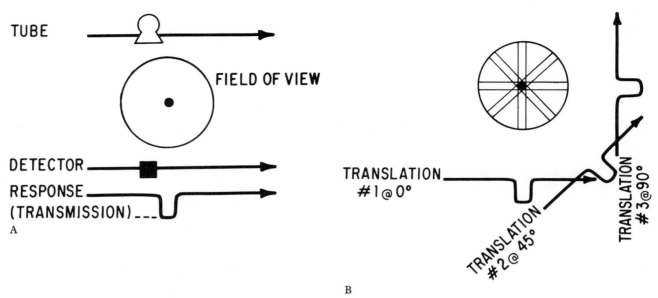

TUBE

FIELD OF VIEW

DETECTOR

RESPONSE
(TRANSMISSION)

A

TRANSLATION
#1 @ 0°

TRANSLATION
#2 @ 45°

TRANSLATION
#3 @ 90°

B

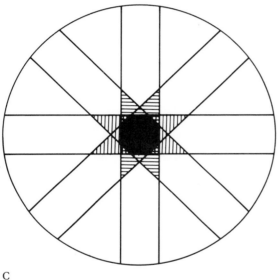

C

Figure 20-2 Image reconstruction of a single point using simple back projection. *A*. Tube and detector are translated in direction of arrow, the x-ray beam crossing the field of view. The detector locates the object someplace along the line defined by the translation. *B*. The computer projects back along the translation line a uniform density proportional to the x-ray transmission. *C*. Summing projections made at multiple angles produces a pattern approximating the original point. Note the star artifact produced by overlap of the back projections.

detectors could be translated across the patient much faster, reducing the data acquisition time for a single slice to less than 20 s. In recent years, one manufacturer has reconfigured a scanner to operate in the second-generation (translate-rotate) geometry with speeds of 5 s per slice.

The third-generation design, introduced in 1976, was a major improvement in technology since it permits data acquisition for a single slice in under 5 s. The impact on body imaging has been significant since the patient can hold his or her breath during the scan, thus reducing motion-induced artifacts that limited second-generation systems. Figure 20-4 demonstrates the third-generation geometry, which utilizes the detector array of more than 300 elements sufficient to cover the entire patient in one view. This eliminates the need for translation and requires only that the tube and detector rotate about the patient, an approach sometimes referred to as *rotate-rotate* geometry. Substantially more sophisticated software is required. The fan beam of x-rays required to cover the patient without translation cannot be

approximated as a series of separate parallel beams as it could in second-generation machines. For example, the distance between rays of the fan beam is much closer near their point of origin (the x-ray tube) than at their point of detection. This has some subtle but significant implications regarding variations in resolution across the field of view.[19,21]

Early versions of third-generation scanners were limited by ring artifacts stemming from the precision of the CT technique itself. A single detector element as it is rotated about the patient will always be sampling along a ring centered at the center of rotation. If for some reason that detector is slightly more or less sensitive than the rest of the array, a series of measurements will be presented to the computer that look like a ring of increased or decreased x-ray attenuation.[20] An example of the resulting ring artifact can be seen in Fig. 20-5*A*, a scan of a uniform 25-cm water bottle. What appears in the water bottle scan as a curiosity for the physicist could pose a serious problem in a scan of a patient (Fig. 20-5*B*). An error of 0.1 percent in a single detector is easily

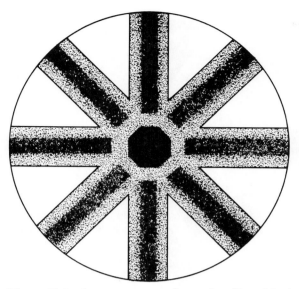

Figure 20-3 Image reconstructions using filtered back projection. The original detector response is convolved with a filter function to produce a back projection with both positive and negative components. Summation of the back projection produces a more accurate representation of the original point since the positive and negative components add in a manner that eliminates the star artifact.

seen. This leads to extraordinary requirements for the precision of detector fabrication. Improved detector design and fabrication have eliminated this problem in modern machines.

The fourth-generation scanner was developed as a solution to the problems noted above in the third-generation

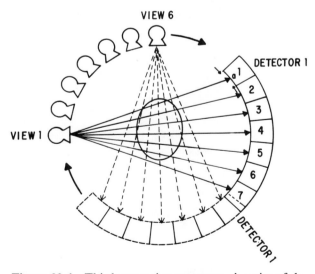

Figure 20-4 Third-generation geometry. A series of detectors rotating in synchrony with the x-ray tube defines the sampling rays. The detectors are sampled at discrete points (e.g., every 1 degree), producing one view (with seven rays per view in this example).

systems, and as a method for improving scan speed. The geometry depicted in Fig. 20-6 utilizes a fan beam from a rotating x-ray tube, as does third-generation geometry. However, the moving detector array is now replaced by a large number (>600) of fixed detectors. Since only the x-ray tube moves, this is sometimes called *rotate only* geometry. The ring artifact encountered with third-generation machines is no longer a problem since every point in the picture is sampled by every detector during a 360 degree scan. An imbalance between detectors is averaged out. However, early fourth-generation systems had a different set of artifacts. The severe demands placed on detector performance in third-generation machines is replaced by demands on the x-ray tube. The systematic variation of <1 percent in x-ray tube output produces a structured noise that can be detrimental. In fact, the fourth-generation geometry solved some of the problems of third-generation designs and generated an entirely new set of problems.[20] The third- and fourth-generation geometries have evolved with hardware and software improvements so that they are both competitive in the clinical arena.

CT Improvements

A complete catalog of improvements in CT since its inception is beyond the scope of this chapter. Instead, the focus will be directed at a qualitative description of major improvements. Improvements in spatial resolution lead this list.

Spatial Resolution

Spatial resolution of any imaging system is most accurately described by the modulation transform function (MTF), which describes the spatial resolution for any given difference in contrast. As a useful simplification the limiting spatial resolution for a system can be learned by determining the smallest resolvable structure with 100 percent contrast, for example, the smallest detail in the inner ear, where the contrast between the bone and the surrounding air is very high.

The limiting spatial resolution of a CT scanner is dependent on, among other things, (1) the detector geometry, (2) the reconstruction software, and (3) the display pixel. Consider Fig. 20-4. The spacing between rays (arrows from tube to detector) at a point in the scan area determines the resolution in that particular view.[19,21] The ray spacing is in turn fixed by the number of *detectors*, their dimension, and their distance from the tube. One could decrease the spacing between rays at the center of the field by packing more detectors closer together or by moving the detector array further from the patient. Moving the array produces problems since the radiation intensity falls off as $1/r^2$, where r is the detector tube distance. Thus, the better alternative is to increase the number of detectors. The earliest third-generation scanners used 300 detectors, each one measuring 2 mm across. Later versions used more than 500 detectors and a recent example uses 742 detector elements.

Fourth-generation scanners are limited in a similar fashion. Figure 20-6 shows the detector with collimating pins in

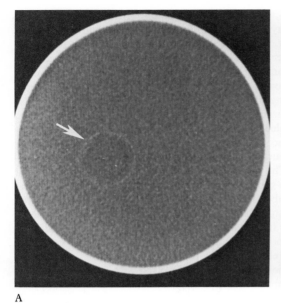

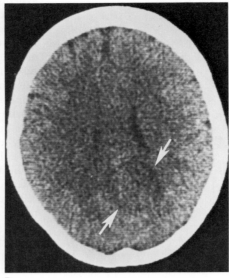

A

B

Figure 20-5 *A*. A scan of a 25-cm water bottle showing a ring artifact due to detector imbalance. *B*. A ring artifact as in *A* but appearing in a clinical scan. The resulting artifact could be mistaken for a lesion.

front defining the sampling aperture *a*. The distance between rays (individual samples) is defined by the movement of the x-ray tube, not the size of the detector. The size of the detector or aperture determines the width of each ray (its beam profile). The limiting resolution depends on a combination of the two.[20] These distances in turn define the resolution in the center of view. Two approaches have been utilized to reduce *a* and therefore improve resolution. The first approach, directed specifically at neurological studies, uses larger pins, thus reducing *a*. While the desired increase in resolution can be obtained, a dose penalty is imposed. The reduced aperture lets fewer x-rays through, wasting photons and increasing the noise (see below). A more efficient

method, albeit substantially more expensive, is to increase the number of detectors. The early fourth-generation machines used 600 individual detectors. One company has recently introduced a system using 1200 detectors. The resulting improvement in resolution (from 9 lp/cm to 12 lp/cm) is shown in Fig. 20-7.

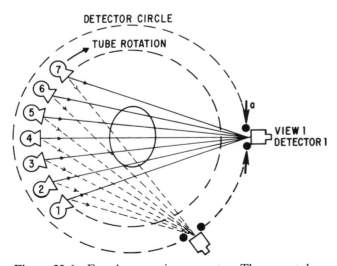

Figure 20-6 Fourth-generation geometry. The x-ray tube rotates about the patient, but the detectors are fixed. Now each detector defines a view. Rays contributing to the view are acquired as the x-ray tube moves. The detector aperture (*a*) is defined by collimating pins.

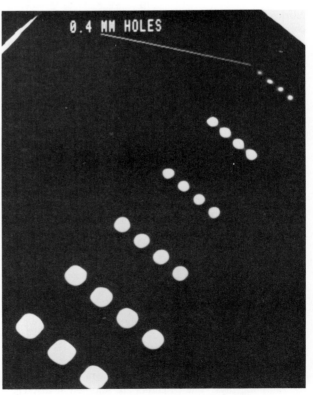

Figure 20-7 A high-resolution scan (1200 fixed detector fourth generation system) showing 0.4-mm holes.

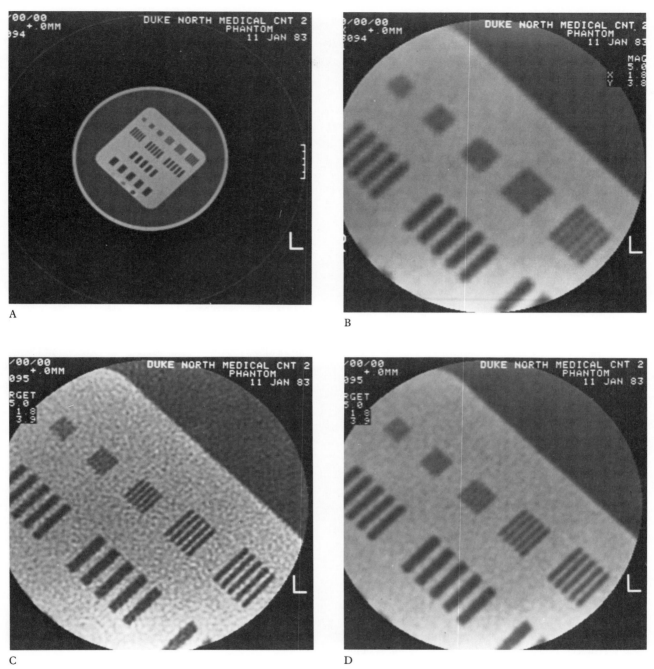

Figure 20-8 *A*. A full body scan (42 cm field of view) showing the resolution pattern with 1.3-mm pixels. *B*. A magnified view of (*A*) using 5X magnification of existing pixels. *C*. The reconstruction of raw data used for (*A*) with bone (high-resolution) enhancement and 0.26-mm pixels. *D*. The reconstruction of raw data for *A* with soft tissue enhancement and 0.26-mm pixels.

A second major improvement in resolution has been accomplished through effective use of the *pixels*. The early scanners used an 80 × 80 matrix of 3-mm pixels. Modern machines use up to 512 × 512 pixels with the option for choosing the size of the pixel to fit the field of view. Figure 20-8*A* demonstrates a resolution pattern reconstructed on a 320 × 320 matrix with a 42-cm field of view. The pixel size is 1.3 × 1.3 mm. One can magnify the reconstructed image, as is done in Fig. 20-8*B*. The image appears larger, and the pixels, which are now 0.26 × 0.26 mm, are smaller. There is now a 3 × 3 array of smaller pixels with the same value where there had been a single large pixel. In this situation the original pixel size determines the limiting resolution, and thus magnification of picture data does not improve the resolution. On the other hand, Fig. 20-8*C* demonstrates the improvements obtained with the same raw data used for Figs. 20-8*A* and 20-8*B* but now reconstructed onto a 10-cm field of view with a 320 × 320 matrix of 0.26-mm pixels. In this case the limit of resolution is fixed by the system geometry, and therefore the larger image also has improved spatial resolution.

Finally the *software* used in reconstructing the image can have a profound effect on the resolution. The filtering during back projection can be planned to enhance large low-contrast (e.g., soft tissue) structures or small high-contrast (e.g., bony) structures. Figure 20-8*D* has been reconstructed to optimize soft tissue structures and Fig. 20-8*C* to optimize bony structures.

Contrast Resolution and Noise

As noted above, the limiting spatial resolution is not sufficient to characterize a scanner's performance. A major strength of CT is its ability to discern small density differences, particularly in relatively large diameter objects. For example, tumors of moderate size (3 to 5 mm) can generally be shown with CT. Their clear demonstration is primarily dependent on the scanner's ability to distinguish the small (0.5 percent) difference in Hounsfield units of tumor and normal tissue.

CT is fundamentally a noise-limited imaging technique. Since a relatively small number of x-ray photons are used in each attenuation measurement, there is a certain statistical uncertainty in the measurement. If one uses more photons (e.g., higher doses or longer scan times), the uncertainty is reduced and the random variation of supposedly identical pixels is minimized. Scans of a uniform 25-cm bottle of water (Fig. 20-9) demonstrate the effect. Figure 20-9*A* was produced with a total exposure of 0.5 rad, Fig. 20-9*B* with a dose of 3.7 rad. The greater noise of the lower-dose exposure is easily seen. The impact of this noise on low-contrast resolution has been studied extensively.[4]

Artifacts

Early generations of scanners frequently suffered from various artifacts. Both third- and fourth-generation systems can be affected by artifacts generated by subtle minor machine malfunction or loss of calibration as shown in Fig. 20-5. Beyond that, the technique of computed tomography itself has some limitations when pressed to do certain imaging tasks. In the calculations for filtered back projection some assumptions are made to reduce the computation time for a single slice. Generally these simplifications assume that structures with spatial frequency components above some cutoff frequency are not really important. A pointed dense object such as a sharp bone makes this assumption invalid. The resulting streaks can severely degrade the image (Fig. 20-10).

A second limitation arises from the finite amount of data acquired. If, for example, one were to obtain a lateral and anteroposterior projection only, the fidelity with which the

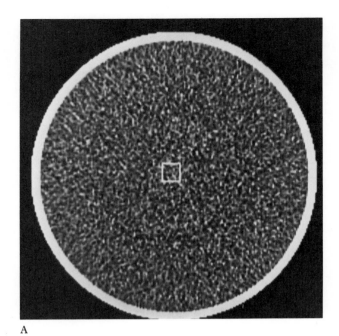

A

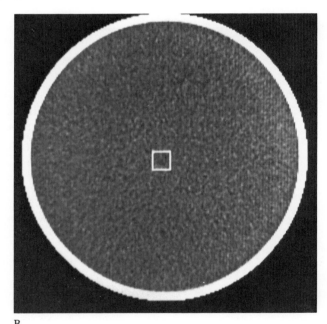

B

Figure 20-9 *A*. A scan of a 25-cm water bottle at low dose (0.5 rad). Note that the standard deviation of pixels in the central area is high (9.74). This large variation is evident in the "salt and pepper" texture of the scan. *B*. A scan of a 25-cm water bottle at high dose (3.7 rad). Note the reduction in noise demonstrated by the smoother image and the smaller standard deviation of the pixels in the sampled region (2.93).

cross section could be constructed would be limited. As the number of views taken around the object (Figs. 20-4 and 20-6) is increased, the fidelity is improved. In a similar fashion, problems with higher frequencies (sharp boundaries) in the image are reduced with more rays at each view. The

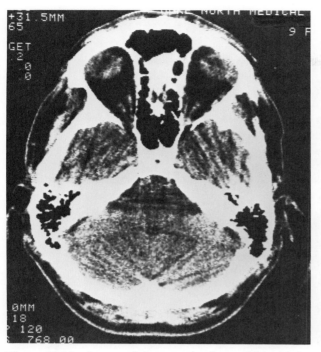

Figure 20-10 A scan of the posterior fossa with a third-generation CT scanner using 576 views. Note streak artifacts emanating from pointed bony structures.

details of these considerations have been discussed extensively.[29] Newer systems have taken this into account; as many as 742 rays with up to 7800 views are used, resulting in 5.7 million measurements. This compares to 300 rays for 576 views (0.2 million measurements) in early third-generation systems. This increase in data vastly increased demands for computation, and special-purpose computers (array processors) are incorporated in most new systems. These processors, capable of up to 100 million calculations per second complete the image reconstruction generally in less than 30 s.

Multiplanar Imaging

Shortly after the introduction of CT, it became evident that multiple axial slices obtained in a routine fashion could in some cases be displayed to advantage using reformatting software.[12,17,18] A series of two-dimensional matrices is "stacked" by the computer so as to create a three-dimensional array. Initial work concentrated on displaying sagittal and coronal slices. For example, axial slices (Fig. 20-11A) can be converted to a sagittal image (Fig. 20-11B) by displaying one column of data from each slice.

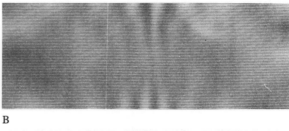
B

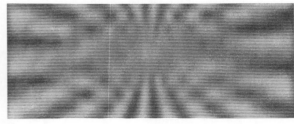
C

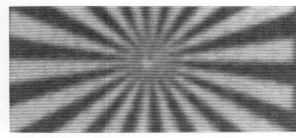
D

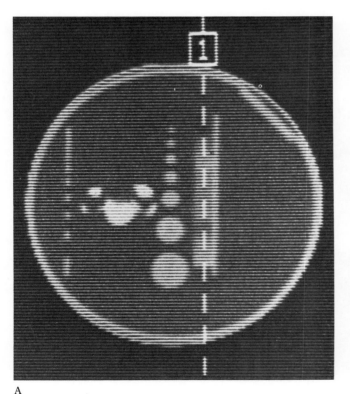
A

Figure 20-11 *A.* An axial scan of a multiplanar phantom showing cross sections of a vertebral body, a series of lucite spheres, and a lucite star pattern. The line indicates the location of the sagittal plane used to reformat images. *B.* The sagittal plane of the star reformatted from 10-mm slices. *C.* The sagittal plane of the star reformatted from 5-mm slices. *D.* The sagittal plane of the star reformatted from 1.5-mm slices.

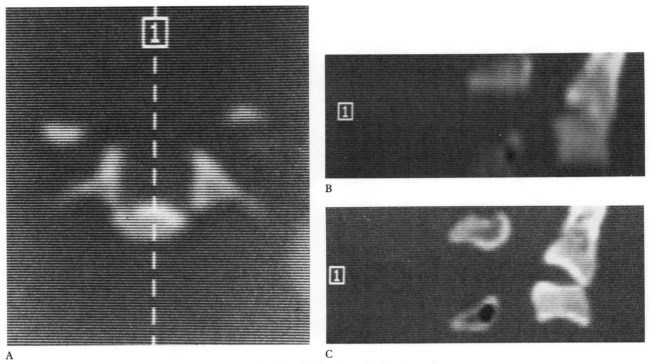

A   C

Figure 20-12 *A*. An axial plane through a vertebral body showing the location of the sagittal plane. *B*. The sagittal plane of the vertebral body reformatted from 5-mm slices. *C*. The sagittal plane of the vertebral body reformatted from 1.5-mm slices.

Multiplanar reformatting is not without difficulties. The slices used to generate the three-dimensional array are frequently 5 to 10 mm thick. The thickness determines the limiting resolution in the sagittal or coronal plane. For example, a phantom containing a lucite star pattern in the

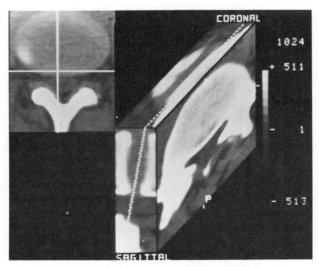

Figure 20-13 A simultaneous perspective display of axial, coronal, and reformatted slices. (Courtesy of Dr. David Hill, Siemens Corporation, Iselin, N.J.)

sagittal plane was imaged with 10-mm, 5-mm, and 1.5-mm-thick axial slices. Figure 20-11*A* shows the axial slice through the center of the phantom. The line indicates the position of the sagittal slice shown in Figs. 20-11*B* to 20-11*D*. Because the slices are thick, a boxlike image is produced. The computer can perform a smoothing operation to "round" the edges, but this is really just blurring the image. A more desirable method starts with the acquisition of thinner axial slices. When reformatted in the sagittal plane, the improvement is marked (Fig. 20-11*C* and *D*). Note that not only are the edges defined better in Fig. 20-11*D* but there is less geometric distortion. These effects are similarly demonstrated in Fig. 20-12, where vertebral bodies in the phantom are reformatted from 5-mm and 1.5-mm slices.

If narrow slices are used, the time necessary to cover the area of interest will increase (i.e., complete coverage of L5 and S1, which requires five 10-mm slices, needs 32 1.5-mm slices). However, most scanners will permit suppression of reconstruction and display during data acquisition, which then requires as little as 6 min. Afterward, reconstruction in any plane can proceed.

Display of these data sets is complex since the clinician frequently likes to synthesize a number of views at one time. Figure 20-13 demonstrates one example showing simultaneous axial, sagittal, and coronal sections displayed in perspective.

A true three-dimensional view is also possible. Several alternatives have been proposed. Figure 20-14 shows a

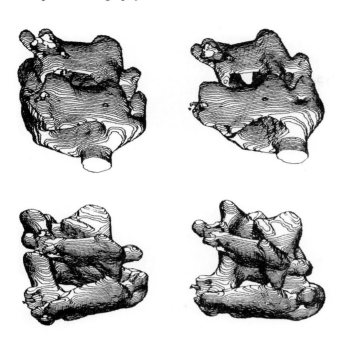

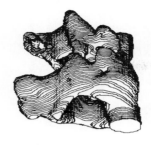

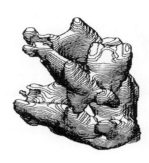

Figure 20-14 A three-dimensional display of vertebral bodies reformatted from 1.5-mm contiguous slices. (Courtesy of Dr. E.K. Fram, Duke University Medical Center, Durham, N.C.)

three-dimensional display from the data used to reformat Fig. 20-12C. The data have been transferred to a research computer and displayed on a special graphics terminal. Separate programs locate boundaries, stack the individual planes, and rotate the resulting array in space. Similar software has recently been developed for experimental use on clinical machines.

Advanced CT Applications

Anatomical Specificity

Spine CT

One of the major advances that has occurred with the development of high-resolution body CT scanners is the ability to study disorders of the spinal column with minimal invasiveness (Fig. 20-15). The accuracy of nonenhanced CT is equal or superior to conventional myelography in the diagnosis of lumbosacral herniated nucleus pulposus as well as canal stenosis, lateral recess stenosis, vertebral trauma, and extradural neoplasia.[1,35] The characterization of hydrosyringomyelia, cystic myelomalacia, and intramedullary neoplasm generally requires low-dose intrathecal enhancement prior to CT scanning.

By photographing the spine CT at "wide windows," one can obtain a detailed view of the vertebral bodies, pedicles, transverse processes, neural foramina, superior and inferior facets, laminae, and spinous processes. A narrower window width permits excellent visualization of disc material, epidural fat, ligamentum flavum, thecal sac, nerve root sleeves, and the dorsal root ganglia. Although it is usually not necessary, the CT data generated from axial scans may be reformatted in coronal, oblique, or sagittal projections.

A herniated disc in the lumbosacral region (Fig. 20-16) has a relatively straightforward CT appearance consisting of an eccentric, increased-density, soft tissue (disc) bulge that obliterates the adjacent epidural fat and may displace the adjacent nerve root sleeve and thecal sac. CT is superior to even conventional myelography in delineating a laterally placed disc herniation or determining the extent of a free disc fragment. Additional invaluable information is obtained concerning the vertebral canal diameter and whether overgrowth of the superior articular facet causes narrowing of the lateral recess. CT is often unable to resolve the diagnostic dilemma in the postoperative back as scarring distorts the normal tissue planes that are critical to definitive diagnosis.[31] Although it has been suggested that fibrous scarring will preferentially enhance as compared with herniated disc after the intravenous infusion of an iodinated contrast medium, definite discontinuity between the disc material and the scarred soft tissue is probably the only useful CT feature in distinguishing disc herniation from postoperative scar.

The intrathecal introduction of a nonionic, hydrosoluble, iodinated contrast medium is usually required to diagnose a herniated cervical disc, although a nonenhanced or intravenously enhanced CT scan will sometimes provide sufficient information, particularly above the level of the fifth cervical vertebra. Anatomical specificity is often not sufficient at the important C5-6, C6-7, and C7-T1 disc space levels where the shoulders are also in the scanning field. With the introduction of safer nonionic, hydrosoluble, intrathecal iodinated contrast agents such as Iopamidol (E.R. Squibb & Sons, Princeton, N.J.), Iotrol (Berlex Imaging, Wayne, N.J.), and Iohexol (Winthrop Laboratories, New York, N.Y.), the infusion of <1.5 g of contrast material for CT studies is extremely safe, without significant neurobehavioral adverse reactions, and therefore is useful for outpatient studies.[10] The currently used contrast medium, metrizamide, causes far greater neurotoxicity because it is a deoxyglucose ana-

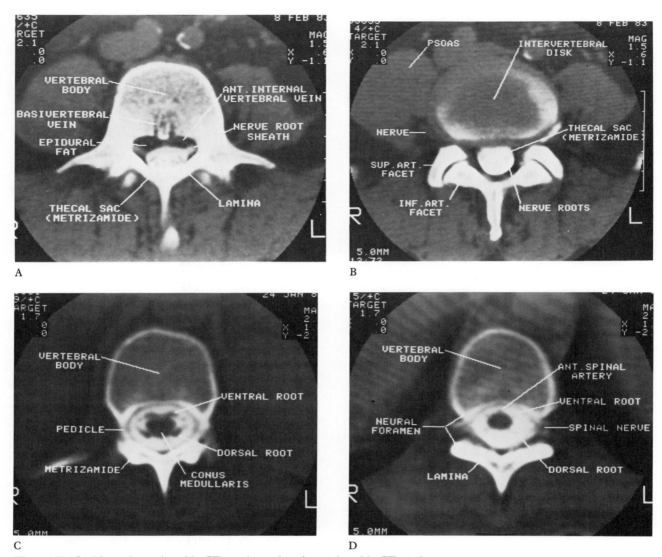

Figure 20-15 Normal metrizamide CT myelography. A metrizamide CT study performed 6 h after a conventional lumbosacral myelogram showing the normal appearance at the level of a lumbar vertebra (*A*), lumbar disc (*B*), conus medullaris (*C*), and thoracic spinal cord (*D*). Metrizamide permits excellent visualization of not only the subarachnoid spaces but also the spinal cord and cauda equina structures that appear as filling defects in the metrizamide.

logue that competitively inhibits glucose utilization and often results in an encephalopathic clinical picture that may last for up to a few days, although it usually resolves within 24 h. In suspected cervical disc disease, CT can therefore be used to determine whether an abnormality is present, to distinguish "soft" from "hard" disc disease, and to evaluate bony degenerative changes and bony canal dimensions (Fig. 20-17).

Although conventional radiography and complex motion tomography utilizing Pantopaque, metrizamide, or air have proved accurate in the diagnosis of intramedullary masses (e.g., neoplasm, hydrosyringomyelia), intrathecally enhanced CT scanning may better define the nature of a cord neoplasm and more accurately distinguish a syrinx, whether

of congenital, post-traumatic (i.e., cystic myelomalacia), or neoplastic origin. An unenhanced CT scan is generally not sufficient to definitively distinguish cord enlargement (Fig. 20-18). With hydrosyringomyelia, a CT study performed immediately after the intrathecal infusion of contrast medium shows cord widening, while a delayed CT examination (after 6 to 12 h) defines entry of iodinated contrast material into the syrinx cavity, giving a "bull's-eye" appearance (Fig. 20-19). The contrast medium will enter a cystic myelomalacia cavity on the immediate scan and will generally not enter a cord neoplasm.

CT scanning is becoming a primary diagnostic study in the evaluation of spinal cord trauma.[3] Thin-section CT studies directed at the level of trauma as well as at the spine

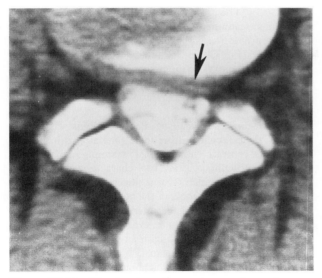

Figure 20-16 Herniated nucleus pulposus shown by Iopamidol CT myelography. The scan shows the eccentric bulging of a herniated disc (*arrow*) causing obliteration of the epidural fat and displacement of the thecal sac. In general, intrathecal contrast material is not necessary to make a diagnosis of a herniated disc. The performance of a CT scan following conventional myelography, however, often assists in better delineating the site and extent of a herniated disc and of a free disc fragment.

immediately above and below detect abnormal bone within the vertebral canal, hematoma, and fractures. Sagittal reformatting often assists in visualizing the vertical extent of the bony impingement on the vertebral canal. Although the nonenhanced CT examination generally provides the information necessary to determine the surgical or medical course of action, particularly when the spinal canal is severely narrowed by displaced bone, properly positioned air or nonionic, iodinated contrast medium may be introduced by lumbar or C1-2 puncture to definitively affirm the presence of a complete block.

Cervicomedullary Junction CT

Nonenhanced CT scanning generally provides excellent visualization of the upper cervical cord because of the widened subarachnoid space at this level (Figs. 20-20 and 20-21). The bony anatomy of the upper cervical vertebrae and skull base is also superbly delineated using bone target image processing. In contrast to the upper cervical spinal cord, the medulla, pons, and inferior cerebellum are poorly visualized using CT because of the transverse artifacts described above. A diagnosis of meningioma, neurilemmoma, and even a Chiari type I malformation is often obtainable without the use of contrast enhancement, although the intrathecal instillation of a hydrosoluble contrast medium generally improves the anatomical delineation of these pathological processes (Fig. 20-22).

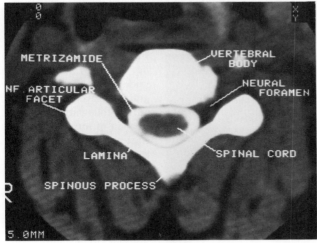

A

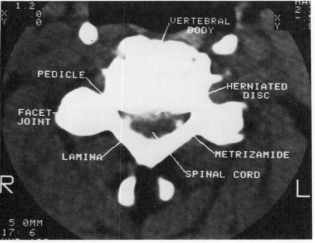

B

Figure 20-17 Cervical CT myelography. *A.* A normal metrizamide CT myelogram in the midcervical region. The use of intrathecal contrast material provides excellent contrast between the spinal cord and the surrounding subarachnoid space and adjacent structures. *B.* Cervical spondylosis with an associated herniated disc seen by metrizamide CT myelography. The CT findings include a decrease in density and homogeneity in the metrizamide ventral to the spinal cord and a compression and distortion of the spinal cord without an associated bony defect. On conventional myelography it is often difficult to distinguish herniated (soft) disc from degenerative (hard) spondylotic changes, and CT therefore provides important additional information.

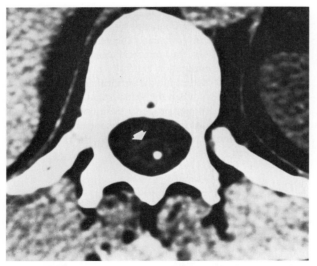

Figure 20-18 A thoracic CT scan showing syringomyelia. On this high-resolution, nonenhanced CT scan, the thin rim of spinal cord (*arrow*) can be seen surrounding a central cystic abnormality. A high-density droplet of Pantopaque that was previous placed in the central canal (endomyelogram) is also seen. Nonenhanced CT scanning is often not sufficient to see syringomyelia, and the introduction of intrathecal contrast material is required.

Petrous Bone CT

Complex motion tomography has been replaced by CT scanning as the method of choice for evaluating the petrous temporal bone, even when subtle inner ear pathology is sus-

pected.[33,34,37] The use of bone highlighting algorithms, axial and coronal scanning, and thin (1.5 to 2.0 mm) collimation greatly improves the pathoanatomical sensitivity and specificity of CT (Fig. 20-23). Scanning with intravenous contrast enhancement is also the preferred means for diagnosing glomus jugulare and tympanicum chemodectomas, although selective angiography is generally used to confirm the diagnosis.

The diagnosis of acoustic neurilemmoma and other masses in the cerebellopontine angle generally requires only intravenous contrast enhanced CT scanning. Small intracanicular neurilemmomas are best characterized by air CT cisternography, in which 6 ml is injected by lumbar puncture with proper positioning of the head to fill the cerebellopontine angle cistern and the internal auditory canal (Fig. 20-24). The soft tissue in the internal auditory canal should have a medial convexity highlighted by the air that does not fill or incompletely fills the canal. If this strict criterion is met, vascular structures and arachnoid adhesions will not be mistaken for a tumor.

Sella Turcica CT

High-resolution CT scanning has become the primary diagnostic technique in the evaluation of sellar and suprasellar masses.[30] Coronal CT with intravenous contrast enhancement is the currently popular method to delineate the presence of a pituitary microadenoma. The common findings include upward convexity of the dura overlying the sella, displacement of the infundibulum, a low density within the pituitary gland, and focal depression of the floor of the sella. Unfortunately, as with previous radiographic methods (e.g., complex motion tomography), false-positive results, false-negative results, and false localizations have all

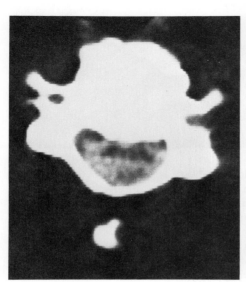
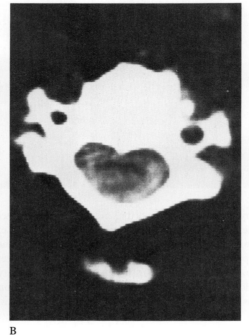

Figure 20-19 Syringomyelia, shown by a metrizamide CT cervical myelogram. Delayed CT scans (*A, B*) following the introduction of intrathecal contrast material reveal metrizamide within the spinal cord. This type of finding on a delayed scan is most consistent with syringomyelia; however, delayed filling may also be seen in unusual circumstances with neoplasms. It is important to realize that an abnormality must consist of a central "bull's-eye" appearance, because intrathecal contrast material will normally enter the spinal cord, causing a false-positive study.

A   B

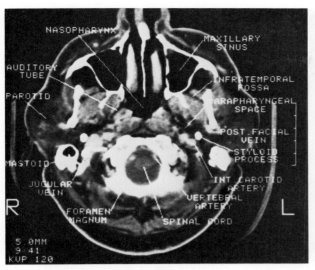

Figure 20-20 A normal CT scan at the level of the naso-pharynx shows the superb anatomical detail afforded by high-resolution CT scanning.

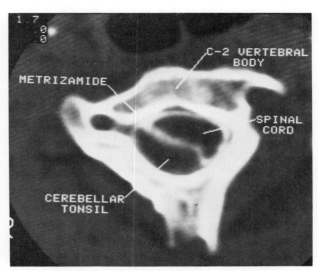

Figure 20-22 A metrizamide CT scan of a patient with a Chiari type I malformation. The introduction of intrathecal iodinated contrast material greatly assists in delineating the upper cervical spinal cord from abnormally low lying cerebellar tonsils.

too commonly occurred; thus caution is required when using this new "gold standard." High-resolution CT also provides excellent visualization of suprasellar structures and the cavernous sinus. Although intravenously enhanced CT is generally sufficient to exclude lesions in the suprasellar region, even greater pathoanatomical specificity can be obtained in selected cases with CT cisternography using metrizamide, Iopamidol, or some other hydrosoluble nonionic contrast medium (Fig. 20-25).

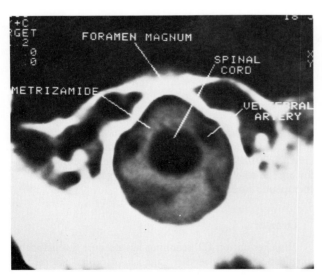

Figure 20-21 A normal metrizamide CT scan at the cervicomedullary junction. Although the spinal cord at the level of cervicomedullary junction is often well defined without intrathecal contrast material, the introduction of contrast medium further assists in delineating anatomical structures.

Intracranial Anatomy

Since the introduction of CT scanning, there have been significant advances in anatomical specificity. This has been of great benefit not only in terms of specialized region imaging (e.g., spine, sella, temporal bone), but also in our ability to image the brain substance, cerebrospinal fluid spaces, and even blood vessels. This improved spatial resolution is a double-edged sword in that an exquisitely defined normal anatomical structure may be mistaken for a pathological process.

This difficulty is most acutely noted when one is trying to distinguish normal from abnormal white matter in the cerebral hemispheres, the posterior limb of the internal capsule, the cerebellar hemispheres, or the superior cerebellar peduncles where they enter the midbrain in a patient with suspect ischemic or demyelinating disease who is otherwise normal (Figs. 20-26 and 20-27). The normal gray-white distinction becomes even more prominent following the intravenous infusion of iodinated contrast media as the gray matter has approximately four times the capillary density of the white matter (Fig. 20-28).

High-resolution CT also offers an improved view of the cortical sulci and basal subarachnoid spaces that should not be mistaken for "atrophy." Improved border detection has improved the accuracy of computer programs used to estimate ventricular volume. Normal anatomical variants such as an enlarged "incompetent" cisterna magna and a cavum septi pellucidi or Vergae are well seen and should not be misdiagnosed as arachnoid cysts.

Normal venous and arterial structures are also highlighted with high-resolution CT. An abnormal, linear high density in the cerebral or cerebellar white matter may represent a venous angioma. This is an important finding as the patients often have symptoms that are not referable to the

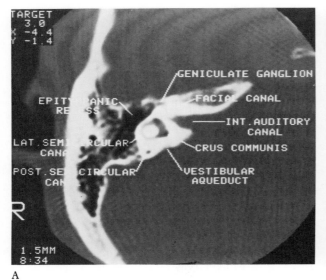

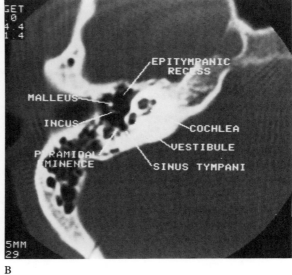

A

B

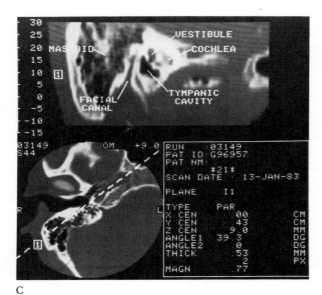

C

Figure 20-23 High-resolution CT scans of normal petrous temporal bone (*A–C*) showing the excellent anatomical detail provided by this technique. If consecutive thin sections (e.g., 1.5 mm) are obtained, the information derived from the axial CT scans can be reformatted in a coronal, oblique, or sagittal projection. CT is now the definitive imaging modality utilized in ENT radiology.

angioma and surgery may lead to worsening of or an initiation of a neurological deficit. Even with high-resolution CT, smaller saccular ("berry") aneurysms generally require angiography for definitive diagnosis as well as to search for additional lesions. The full extent of giant fusiform (atherosclerotic) aneurysms is underestimated at angiography as compared to the delineation afforded by CT. Finally, lesions that are both subtle and grossly apparent (e.g., in ischemic hypoxic brain damage), are either better delineated or only seen using high-resolution CT (Fig. 20-29).

Brain Edema

CT scanning provides an excellent tool for the in vivo determination of abnormalities in brain water content. The anatomical specificity of CT permits delineation of not only the presence but also the type of brain edema.[8,25] This dis-

tinction of edema type often assists in differentiating whether a CT abnormality represents infarction or neoplasm (Fig. 20-30). CT also provides an excellent method for following the resolution or extension of brain edema following therapeutic intervention.

Orbital CT

High-resolution CT scanning has become the definitive diagnostic modality in the diagnosis of orbital masses and thyroid ophthalmopathy.[26,32,36] The superb anatomical specificity of CT permits the routine distinction of the optic nerves, rectus muscles, lens, vitreous, and other venous and soft tissue structures (Fig. 20-31). Direct coronal imaging or oblique and coronal reformatting provides important information concerning the vertical dimension and boundaries of a lesion (Fig. 20-32).

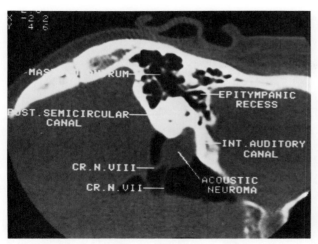

Figure 20-24 Air CT cisternography showing an acoustic neurilemmoma. Air in the cerebellopontine angle cistern highlights the visualization of an acoustic neurilemmoma. In addition, air often permits visualization of the seventh and eighth cranial nerves as well as vascular structures.

CNS Function

Intravascular Contrast Enhancement

The majority of head CT scans are now performed following the intravenous infusion of an ionic iodinated contrast medium. The dose is generally 42 g of iodine in a volume of 150 to 300 ml, infused just prior to scanning. The basic rationale for giving the intravenous contrast medium is to determine the integrity of the blood-brain barrier (Fig. 20-33), although additional information concerning arterial and venous structures is also obtained.[6,11] Some authors suggest using a double dose of contrast medium (for example, 80 to 84 g of iodine) when searching for more subtle barrier abnormalities.[5] Although the intracarotid infusion of an ionic contrast agent will produce a transient, reversible disruption of the blood-brain barrier, the degree of which correlates with osmolality, no study has definitively established that an intravenous infusion of even large doses of contrast material will adversely affect the barrier.

Another technique used to highlight abnormal contrast enhancement (i.e., blood-brain barrier disruption) involves obtaining a delayed (30 to 60 min after infusion) CT scan. Since contrast material in the intracranial vascular pool clears much faster than contrast material in abnormal tissue, the delayed scan increases the signal-to-background ratio and thereby increases the identification of barrier lesions.[13]

Current concepts suggest that the blood-brain barrier resides in the capillary endothelial cells of the central nervous system. These capillary endothelial cells differ from their peripheral counterparts in that they do not contain fenestrations or normally exhibit pinocytosis and they have zonulae occludens ("tight junctions") between one another. Barrier breakdown with increased permeability to an intravenously infused iodinated contrast medium is a nonspecific finding that may be seen with a neoplasm (primary or meta-

static, intra-axial or extra-axial), an abscess, demyelinating disease, and infarction.[6]

When intravenously enhanced CT scans are being analyzed, it is also important to recognize that certain areas of the brain have a peripheral type of capillary endothelial cell, permitting normal entry of iodinated contrast material. These regions are predominantly circumventricular and include the area postrema, the median eminence of the hypothalamus, the organ vasculosum of the lamina terminalis, the subfornical organ, the pineal gland and the lines of attachment of the choroid plexus. In addition, contrast medium leaks into the falx cerebri and falx cerebelli.

Blood-brain barrier disruption may also occur as a result of severe hypertension, seizures, acidosis, hypercapnia, concussion, and markedly increased intracranial pressure, and iatrogenically following the intracarotid infusion of hypertonic mannitol or iodinated contrast media. The mechanism of increasing barrier permeability likely differs depending on the insult. There may be a stimulation of pinocytosis through the capillary endothelial cells, an opening of the tight junctions, or an abnormal endothelial proliferation or development. A quantitative estimate of barrier integrity or abnormality may be derived from CT scanning using a contrast enhancement ratio (CER):

$$CER = \frac{C_i\,(T_E) - C_i\,(T_0)}{\displaystyle\int_{T_0}^{T_E} C_v\,dt}$$

where $C_i\,(T_E)$ equals the CT number in a specific brain locale (i, for gray or white matter) at a given time, T_E, after the intravenous infusion of contrast medium; $C_i(T_0)$ equals the CT number of this same region just prior to the infusion of contrast, and $\displaystyle\int_{T_0}^{T_E} C_v$ equals the venous concentrations of iodinated contrast medium from time T_0 to time T_E in CT units.

A large bolus of iodinated contrast medium may be rapidly infused intravenously with the subsequent performance of multiple, rapid CT scans every 1 to 4 s using a dynamic scan mode (Fig. 20-34). By plotting the change in CT number over a given time interval, a time-concentration curve is obtained that can be fitted and analyzed using a variety of methods to estimate a *mean transit time* $(\bar{t})$.[2]

Since intravenously infused iodinated contrast agents are confined to the plasma compartment, *regional cerebral blood volume* (rCBV) can be estimated by dividing the CT number in a selected brain region by the CT number in a simultaneously drawn venous blood sample scanned in a phantom.[22] The vein of Galen may be used as a substitute for venous blood, although partial volume averaging poses a potential problem. After correcting for cerebral to large vessel hematocrit (0.85) (as iodinated contrast media does not penetrate red blood cells) and also accounting for the decrease in hematocrit from contrast medium infusion (dilution factor, DF), we get the final operational equation for calculating rCBV:

$$rCBV = \frac{CT\ no.\ (brain) \times 0.85 \times 100}{CT\ no.\ (blood) \times DF \times g}\ ml/100\ g$$

Although resonable results have been achieved in the estimation of rCBV and $\bar{t}$, it is important to understand that

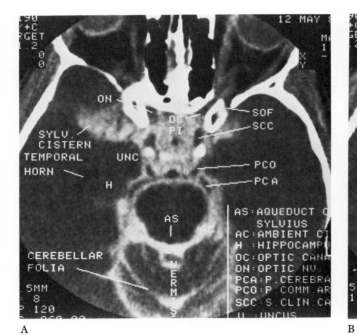

A

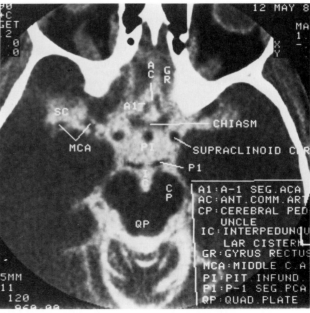

B

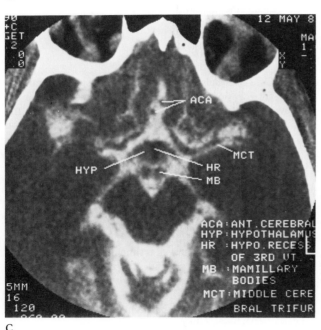

C

Figure 20-25 Normal metrizamide CT cisternogram. CT scans (*A–C*) performed after the introduction of 6 ml of metrizamide containing 190 mg of iodine per milliliter via lumbar puncture. *SOF,* superior orbital fissure; *OC,* optic canal; *ON,* optic nerve; *PI,* pituitary infundibulum; *SCC,* supraclinoid internal carotid artery; *POC,* posterior communicating artery; *PCA,* posterior cerebral artery; *AS,* aqueduct of Sylvius; *UNC,* uncus; *H,* hippocampus; *AC,* anterior communicating artery; *A1,* A1 segment of anterior cerebral artery; *GR,* gyrus rectus; *P1,* P1 segment of posterior cerebral artery; *MCA,* middle cerebral artery; *SC,* sylvian cistern; *IC,* interpeduncular cistern; *QP,* quadrigeminal plate; *CP,* cerebral peduncle; *ACA,* anterior cerebral artery; *MCT,* middle cerebral artery trifurcation; *HR,* hypothalamic recess of third ventricle; *MB,* mammillary bodies; *HYP,* hypothalamus.

limitations may exist. These include patient motion between the baseline and enhanced CT scans; limited enhancement in the brain capillary bed; variability of the cerebral to large vessel hematocrit correction; changes in blood volume, autoregulation, and blood pressure with contrast infusion; and inaccuracies that occur with blood-brain barrier disruption.

Inhalation Contrast Enhancement

CT scanning can also be used to accurately and reproducibly measure *regional cerebral blood flow* (rCBF) using diffusible indicator (e.g., xenon) methodology. Nonradioactive (stable) xenon is an inert gas with a *k*-edge and atomic number near that of iodine, permitting visualization using CT scanning if it is administered in sufficient concentrations (Fig. 20-35). The major advantages of the xenon CT technique are the high degree of anatomical specificity and the capability to directly measure the brain-blood partition coefficient (λ) in normal and pathological tissue.[6,22]

By obtaining CT scans every 30 to 60 s during the inhalation of stable xenon and continuously monitoring the arterial or end tidal xenon concentration (input function), one can use the operational equation set forth by Kety to calculate rCBF:

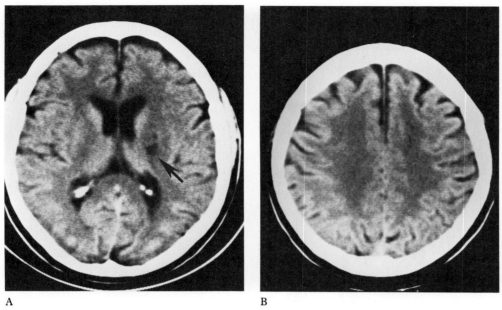

A   B

Figure 20-26 Two levels (*A, B*) from a high-resolution brain CT scan. The superb gray-white distinction seen on this nonenhanced CT scan suggests the possibility that diffuse ischemic white matter disease may be present, as is seen in subcortical arteriosclerotic encephalopathy. This high-resolution CT scan provides superb delineation of a small lacunar infarct (*arrow*) in the posterior limb of the internal capsule in the distribution of the lenticulostriate arteries.

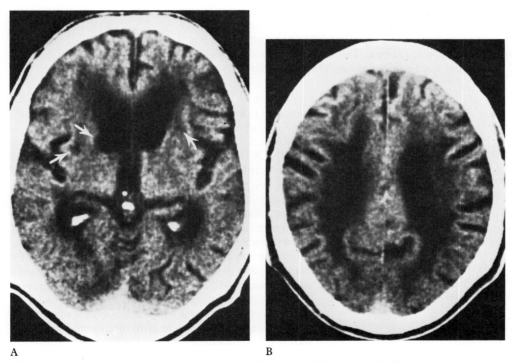

A   B

Figure 20-27 Subcortical arteriosclerotic encephalopathy (Binswanger's disease). Extensive low density involving the cerebral white matter adjacent to not only the frontal horns of the lateral ventricles but also the bodies of the lateral ventricles is shown on these two CT scan views (*A, B*). The involvement of the white matter adjacent to the bodies of the lateral ventricles distinguishes subcortical arteriosclerotic encephalopathy from communicating hydrocephalus. In association with the ischemic white matter disease, lacunar infarcts are seen in the basal ganglia region (*arrows*).

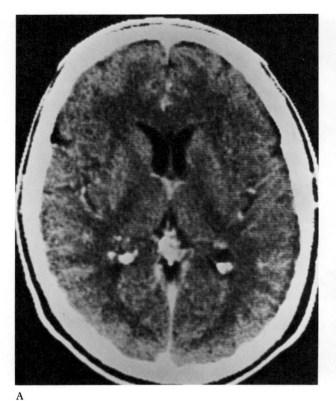 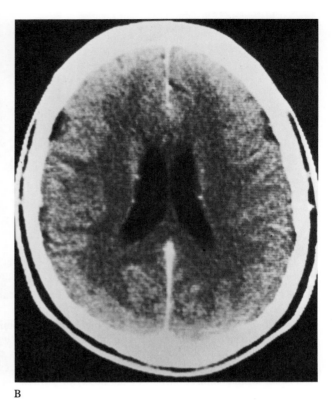

A   B

Figure 20-28 Two levels (*A, B*) of a normal intravenously enhanced CT scan. Excellent gray-white distinction is noted as a result of contrast enhancement in the cerebral capillary bed. The capillary density in the gray matter is approximately four times that in the white matter. For this reason, contrast enhancement greatly improves the distinction between gray and white matter. This normal gray-white delineation on an enhanced CT scan should not be mistaken for subcortical arteriosclerotic encephalopathy.

$$C_i(T) = \lambda_i k_i \int_0^T C_a(t) e^{-k(T-t)} \, dt$$

where λ_i is the xenon brain-blood partition coefficient and k_i is the flow rate constant. The λ for xenon may be calculated directly by dividing the increase in CT number in brain by the increase in CT number in blood when equilibrium is reached:

$$\lambda_i = \frac{\text{CT no. (brain)(at equil)} - \text{CT no. (brain)(baseline)}}{\text{CT no. (blood)(at equil)} - \text{CT no. (blood)(baseline)}}$$

If the end tidal xenon concentration is available using a mass spectrometer or thermoconductivity analyzer, the Ostwald solubility coefficient may be used to calculate using the following formula:

$$\Delta\text{CT no. (blood)} = \frac{5.15 \times \theta_{\text{Xe}} \times C(\%)}{\mu_p^w / \mu_p^{\text{Xe}} \times 100}$$

where $\theta_{\text{Xe}} = 0.0011 \times$ hematocrit (%) $+ 0.10$, $C(\%)$ equals the equilibrium xenon concentration, and $\mu_p^w / \mu_p^{\text{Xe}}$ is established by scanning varying concentrations of iodine (similar atomic number to xenon) at specific kilovoltage settings in a phantom.

Most groups use a single compartment model with a nonlinear least squares curve fit of the brain data (C_i) and a noise correction to calculate rCBF. The flow data may then be presented in a map format where the signal intensity on the derived image is seen in terms of λ, k (flow rate constant), or F (rCBF) as opposed to CT attenuation coefficient (Fig. 20-36). The rCBF can also be presented in terms of anatomically selected regions of interest. Although the xenon CT method has proved quite useful, the application of the technique requires a thorough understanding of its limitations. The shortcomings may be practical (patient motion, respiratory apparatus, end tidal xenon analyzer), quantitative (CT number instability, region of interest compromises, partial volume averaging, dose trade-offs), theoretical (limited brain CT data points, tissue inhomogeneity in this single compartment model, methods used for nonlinear, multivariate least squares fitting and noise analysis), and biological (anesthetic effects increase with changes in flow when higher doses of xenon are used to improve quantitative accuracy). Xenon CT studies have been used to show decreased rCBF with cerebral infarction, transient ischemic attack, cerebrocirculatory arrest, glioma, Alzheimer's disease, and hypometabolic interictal seizure foci.

Intrathecal Contrast Enhancement

If direct information concerning the cerebrospinal fluid (CSF) circulation or spaces is required, a nonionic, water-soluble iodinated contrast agent can be introduced by lum-

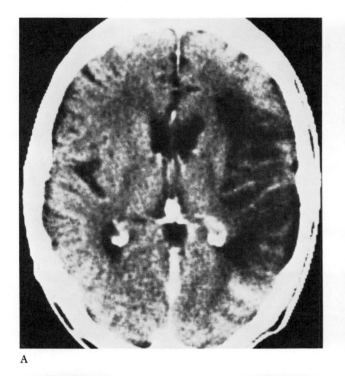

A

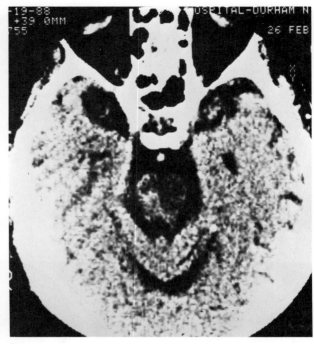

B

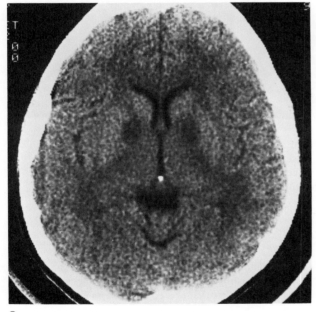

C

Figure 20-29 Cerebral infarction. *A.* Cerebral infarction in the distribution of the middle cerebral artery. *B.* Pontine infarction in the distribution of penetrating branches of the basilar artery. *C.* Bilateral infarctions in the globus pallidus secondary to carbon monoxide poisoning.

bar puncture, C1-2 puncture, or a ventricular shunt tube. It is only necessary to infuse 5 to 6 ml of a contrast medium of 170 to 200 mg of iodine per milliliter. When the contrast medium (e.g., metrizamide, Iopamidol, Iotrol) is introduced by lumbar puncture, the patient is tilted into the Trendelenburg (head down) position for 3 min and then carefully transferred to the CT scanner (CT cisternography).

Before the advent of high-resolution CT, CT cisternography was widely utilized in the diagnosis and characterization of subtle masses that impinged upon the basal subarachnoid

spaces (e.g., brain stem, cerebellopontine angle, and suprasellar masses) in place of pneumoencephalography.[9] With improved scanners, sellar and suprasellar masses are now generally best characterized using intravenous contrast enhancement and high-resolution coronal CT scanning.[30] CT cisternography continues to be of value in the depiction of subtle suprasellar germinomas and hypothalamic astrocytomas. Although optimal visualization of the upper pons and midbrain may often be obtained without intrathecal enhancement, transverse linear artifacts continue to degrade images of the pons, medulla, and cervicomedullary junction,

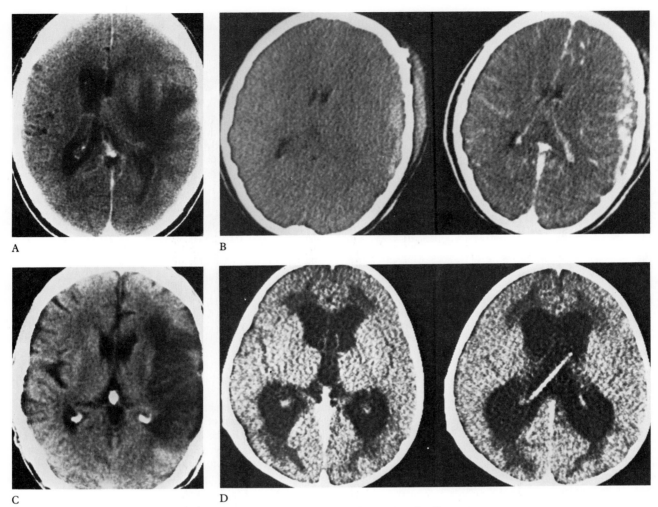

Figure 20-30 Brain edema. *A*. Vasogenic edema secondary to brain metastasis. *B*. Cytotoxic edema involving both cerebral hemispheres secondary to severe head trauma with subdural hematoma. *C*. Ischemic edema secondary to cerebral infarction in the middle cerebral artery distribution. *D*. Periventricular interstitial edema secondary to obstructive hydrocephalus.

and thus intrathecal enhancement is still required (Fig. 20-25).[23] The use of nonionic iodinated contrast media for intrathecal enhancement has been replaced by intrathecal air enhancement as the method of choice for diagnosing small, intracanalicular acoustic neurilemmomas (Fig. 20-24).

In order to obtain a dynamic assessment of an abnormality involving the CSF circulation, the intrathecal instillation of a nonionic, hydrosoluble contrast agent is still generally necessary. CT cisternography and ventriculography are especially helpful in the following conditions:[7]

1. **Extra-axial cyst** With a combination of nonenhanced, intravenously enhanced, and intrathecally (cisternography and/or ventriculography) enhanced CT scanning, the location, extent, dynamics, and type of brain cyst can generally be determined.[7] This distinction becomes most important in the posterior fossa (Table 20-1), where nor-

mal anatomical variants (e.g., a large cisterna magna) must be distinguished from developmental cysts, such as a Dandy-Walker cyst or a posterior fossa extra-axial cyst, and cystic neoplasms, for example, astrocytoma and hemangioblastoma (Fig. 20-37).

2. **CSF leak** The characterization of a CSF leak, especially when it is spontaneous, is an extremely perplexing diagnostic dilemma. Conventional radiography and radionuclide cisternography often prove unrevealing. The technique of choice has generally become intrathecally enhanced CT scanning because of the combination of morphological and functional information afforded by this method.[7] With high-resolution CT scanning, both the presence and bony site of leakage are often delineated (Fig. 20-38). The development of safer nonionic contrast media make CT cisternography an extremely safe and well-tolerated procedure.

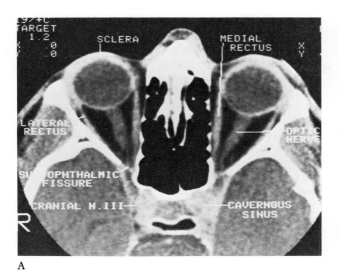
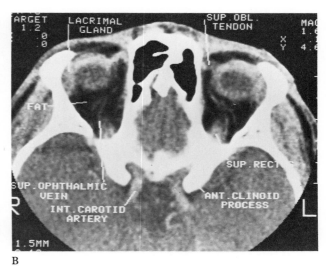

A   B

Figure 20-31 A high-resolution CT scan showing normal orbital contents. CT scanning provides superb delineation of the orbital contents and has become the definitive imaging modality utilized for defining orbital pathology.

3. **Communicating hydrocephalus** After a baseline CT scan is performed, the circulation of an intrathecally injected iodinated contrast medium can be followed by performing serial CT scans at 8, 24, and if necessary, 48 h.[7] As with radionuclide cisternography, the basic abnormalities consist of reflux of the contrast medium into the lateral ventricles, its persistence (stasis) within the ventricles for 24 h, and delayed transit of the contrast agent over the cerebral convexities as defined by a decreased or persistent "blush" of the adjacent brain substance (Fig. 20-39). Unfortunately, intermediate patterns of reflux with minimal stasis and normal convexity transit are also common. It has yet to be determined whether this intermediate circulation pattern reflects increased ventricular volume, Alzheimer's disease, or communicating hydrocephalus.

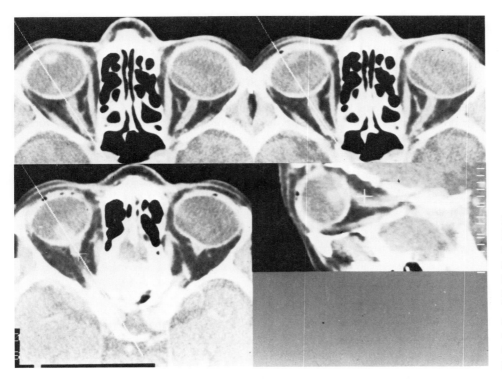

Figure 20-32 A high-resolution CT scan showing retinoblastoma. The high-density abnormality in the posterior right globe is consistent with retinoblastoma. Thin-section CT scans were obliquely reformatted in order to delineate the entire optic nerve in the sagittal plane.

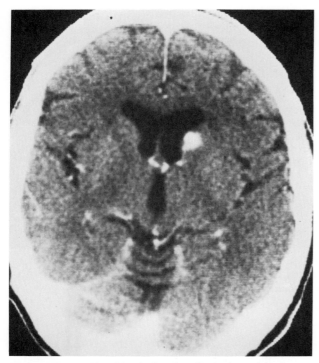

Figure 20-33 Blood-brain barrier disruption with abnormal contrast enhancement. There is a focal area of barrier breakdown in the caudate nucleus region. This abnormal enhancement was present in a patient with multiple infarcts secondary to arteritis.

Future Challenges

Expanded Applications

High-resolution CT scanning has achieved such a high degree of sophistication that future advances will likely involve new applications and convenience as opposed to improvements in image quality. With the development of x-ray tubes with better cooling characteristics and more rapid techniques and equipment for image processing, CT scan-

ning will become an even faster process than it is today. The increased speed of this method and its superb anatomical accuracy should permit the acquisition of more and thinner CT sections that can be quickly reformatted in coronal and sagittal planes covering extensive vertical dimensions, for example, the entire spine or the entire brain from the foramen magnum to the vertex. CT units with extremely rapid scanning times (e.g., 0.1 s) are now being developed for cardiac imaging. These may also prove extremely useful in the brain for measuring the transit time of contrast materials through the brain vasculature and for situations requiring extremely fast scanning times, for instance, for trauma victims or uncooperative patients.

Areas of potential new applications of CT scanning in the future include the following.

Extracranial Vascular Imaging

High-resolution CT scanners can provide extremely accurate information concerning the lumen of the carotid artery and thereby directly differentiate the patent lumen from the associated atheroma or ulcer.[14] Although intravenous contrast enhancement has generally been required, newer scanners give superb definition of the extracranial vasculature even without iodinated contrast. This superb anatomical specificity in combination with faster scanning times should permit the noninvasive acquisition of 30 axial scans 1.5 to 2.0 mm thick that can be reformatted as sagittal or oblique views to define the anatomical level (e.g., common carotid artery bifurcation, internal and external carotid arteries) and axial images to specifically and directly delineate the presence of atherosclerosis and the resultant ulceration and luminal stenosis.

Dual Kilovoltage Imaging

If CT scans are performed at two different kilovoltages (for example, 80 and 120 kV), it is possible to create a cross-sectional image of the effective atomic number of a tissue[24,27] rather than the attenuation coefficient relative to water, as is generally done in CT. Dual kilovoltage imaging has been used with limited success to analyze the degree of enhancement in different tumor types. Although initial attempts have not proved to be of clinical utility, further

TABLE 20-1 Differentiation of Posterior Fossa Cystic Abnormalities

Abnormality	Low Density	IV Enhanced CT			CT Cisternography		CT Ventriculography	
		Hydro-ceph-alus	Ventricle/SAS* Displacement	Abnormal Enhancement	Cystic Space Filling	Basal Cistern Filling	Cystic Space Filling	Basal Cistern Filling
Large cisterna magna	+	0	0	0	+	+	+	+
Extra-axial cyst	+	+	+	0	−	+	−	+
Dandy-Walker cyst	+	+	±	0	−	+	+	−
Cystic neoplasm (hemangioblastoma/astrocytoma)	+	+	+	+	−	+	−	+
Epidermoid cyst	+	±	+	0	−	+	−	+

*SAS, subarachnoid space.

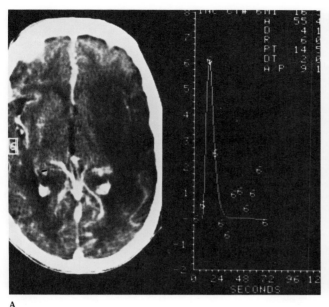

A

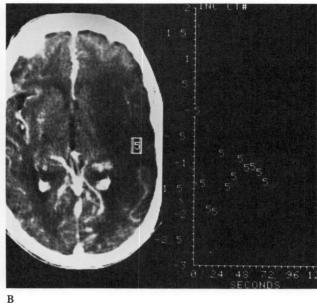

B

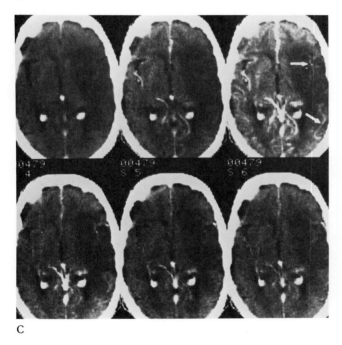

C

Figure 20-34 Dynamic intravenously enhanced CT scans. A series of rapid consecutive CT scans (*A–C*) were performed at 4.8-s intervals following the rapid intravenous infusion of iodinated contrast material. Even on visual inspection, the decrease in entry of contrast material into an area of cerebral infarction is readily apparent. Delayed entry of contrast material into sylvian and posterior parietal middle cerebral artery branches is noted in the region of infarction (*arrows*). In addition to visual inspection, a time-density curve can be obtained by defining regions of interest in consecutive CT scans. With this technique a transit time through normal or abnormal brain tissue can be calculated.

efforts to determine the value of dual kilovoltage imaging for in vivo tissue characterization and for quantitative assessments of brain or lesion enhancement are now in progress.

Cerebral Blood Flow

As CT technology continues to improve, the mapping of stable xenon enhancement in various lesions as well as normal activated and unactivated gray and white matter has become a relatively straightforward procedure.[6,22] Software is now available with commercial CT scanners to estimate from the increase in derived CT number and end tidal xenon

level both the brain-blood partition coefficient and the local cerebral blood flow. The information may be presented in the form of multiple selected regions of interest or as a flow map where each pixel represents calculated flow rather than the CT number. This will permit the measurement of nutritional cerebral blood flow on a routine basis at the local and community hospital level.

Tissue-Specific Enhancement

In addition to stable xenon, there is a definite need for the development of an intravenously administered, radiodense (e.g., iodinated) indicator that will normally cross the

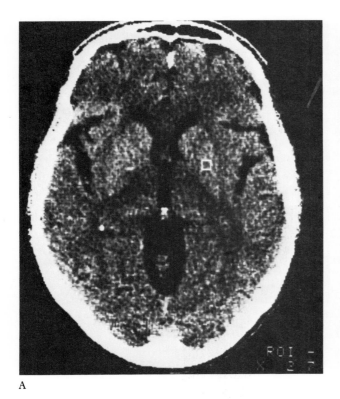

A

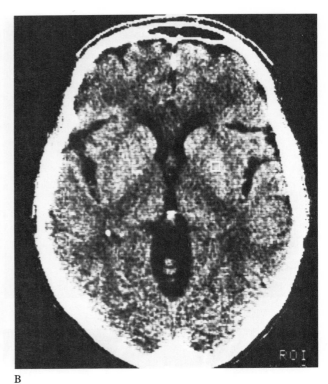

B

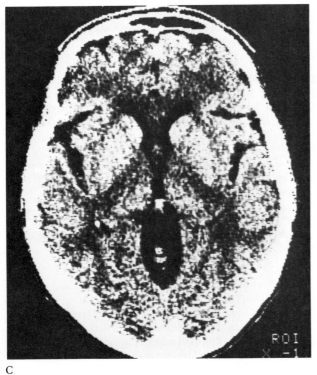

C

Figure 20-35 Normal xenon enhanced CT scanning. CT scans performed before (*A*), and 2 min (*B*), and 4 min (*C*) after the inhalation of 35 percent xenon. The far greater enhancement (whiteness) of the gray matter as compared with white matter structures coincides with the four times greater blood flow to the gray matter. As xenon has an atomic number similar to that of iodine, inhalation of this diffusible indicator in sufficient quantities will cause a sufficient increase in the brain attenuation coefficient to be readily monitored using CT scanning.

blood-brain barrier, remain in the brain for a sufficient time to permit equilibrium imaging, and define a specific brain function (e.g., glucose utilization, specific receptor binding). Unfortunately, relatively large concentrations of an iodinated metabolic indicator or ligand will be required to achieve sufficient CT enhancement, and thus the requirements for synthesis will be extremely stringent. Another approach is to enhance the brain via the CSF route, as there is ready transport of even large, hydrosoluble molecules from the CSF to the adjacent brain.

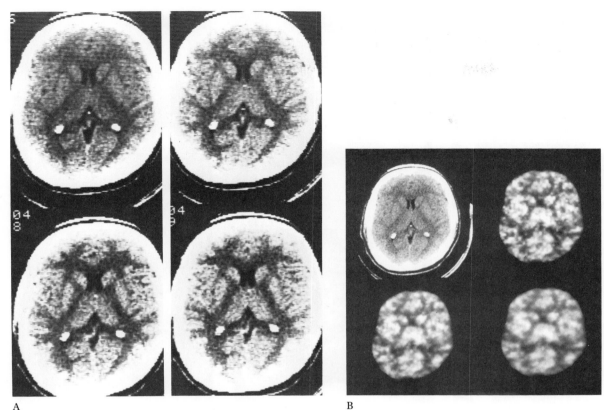

A
B

Figure 20-36 Normal xenon enhanced CT scanning. *A*. A series of xenon enhanced CT scans performed prior to and 2, 4, and 5 min following the inhalation of nonradioactive xenon. Once again, the prominent early enhancement of gray matter structures to a greater degree than white matter structures is apparent by visual inspection. *B*. The information derived from the consecutive CT scans obtained in (*A*) are displayed as flow maps with different degrees of smoothing. (The upper left scan is a baseline scan.) The greater the degree of whiteness, the greater is the cerebral blood flow. Rather than in CT numbers, the density seen on these flow maps is in terms of absolute flow in milliliters per 100 g per minute. (Courtesy of David Gur, University of Pittsburgh Medical Center, Pittsburgh, Pa.)

CT versus Magnetic Resonance Imaging

The rapid development of magnetic resonance imaging (MRI) as an anatomical and potentially metabolic modality has raised inevitable comparisons with the present "gold standard," CT scanning. There are various contraindications to MRI, including pacemakers, ferrous surgical clips, respirators, and poor patient cooperation. In addition, site specifications for the MRI equipment are extremely rigid and often require the construction of a separate, isolated building.

The major advantages of MRI involve (1) the excellent contrast differential between gray matter, white matter, CSF, and pathological tissue obtained with proton imaging (Fig. 20-40) and no contrast enhancement; (2) the absence of artifact when imaging neural structures adjacent to bone (e.g., spinal cord and spinal nerves, cervicomedullary junction, posterior fossa contents, pituitary gland, and temporal lobes); and (3) the ease of obtaining coronal and sagittal as well as axial images (Fig. 20-40). It has not yet been established that high field MR units can provide metabolic information concerning other nuclei (e.g., ^{31}P spectroscopy) with a sufficient degree of anatomical specificity to be of clinical value.

CT has definite advantages due to the high morphological specificity that is achieved using extremely short (subseconds to a few seconds) scan times. Our long experience analyzing CT images has permitted a deep understanding of the limitations and false-positive results, and at least initially both techniques may be required. Certain radiological landmarks, such as the presence of calcium, are far better observed using CT than MRI. In addition, intravenously enhanced CT provides a highly sensitive marker to the integrity of the blood-brain barrier. Although intravenous enhancement with nondiffusible paramagnetic compounds (e.g., transition metals, nitroxide stable free radicals) has been suggested to test the integrity of the blood-brain barrier using MRI, the safety and utility of these compounds

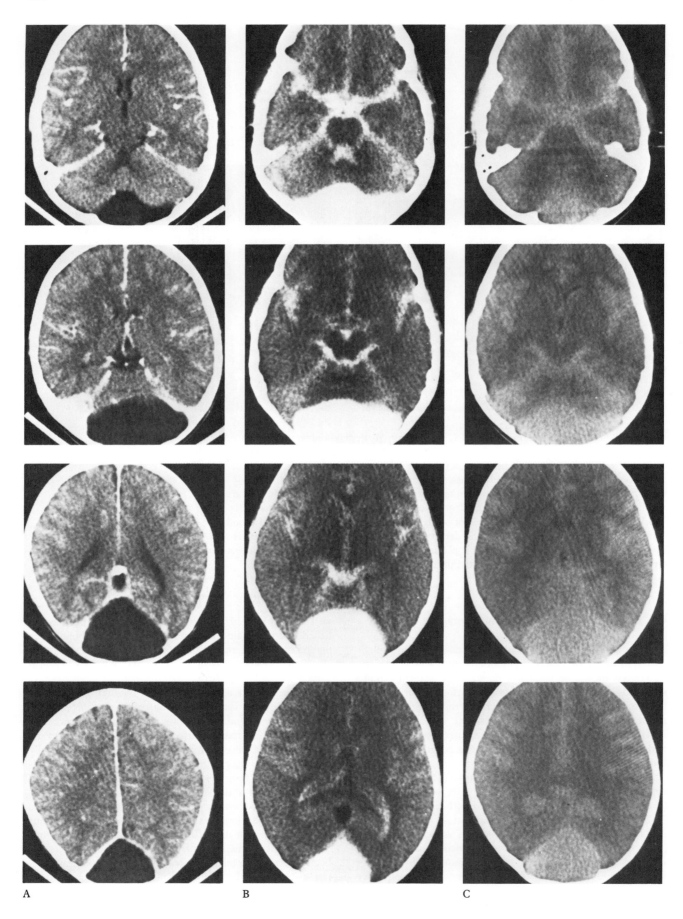

A   B   C

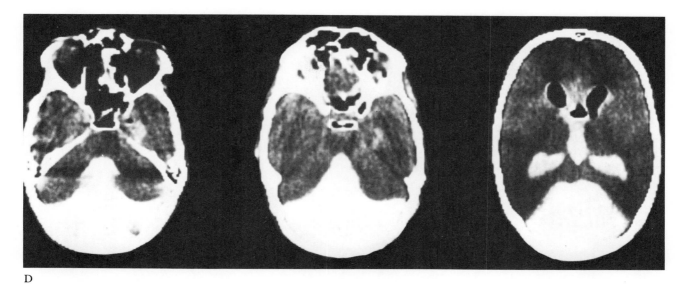

D

Figure 20-37   Metrizamide CT cisternograms demonstrating a large cisterna magna (normal anatomical variant) and a Dandy-Walker cyst. *A*. Intravenously enhanced CT scan defines a well-circumscribed, nonenhancing low-density area in the posterior fossa. The absence of displacement of the fourth ventricle and brain stem and the normal size of the ventricular system confirm that this is a benign anatomical variant. With chronicity, a large cisterna magna may cause scalloping in the occipital bone, as seen in this case. *B*. A metrizamide CT cisternogram shows that metrizamide fills the large cisterna magna and the basal subarachnoid spaces equally, confirming that this represents a large cisterna magna rather than a posterior fossa cyst. *C*. A delayed study performed 8 h after the introduction of metrizamide further confirms that this represents a large cisterna magna as the metrizamide in the cisterna magna clears at the same rate as the metrizamide in the basal subarachnoid spaces. *D*. A metrizamide CT ventriculogram of a patient with a Dandy-Walker cyst. As opposed to *A* to *C*, the posterior fossa abnormality involves the fourth ventricle and causes hydrocephalus. The metrizamide placed in the ventricles immediately fills the ventricular system as well as the cystic structure in the posterior fossa but does not fill the basal subarachnoid cisterns, confirming that this represents a Dandy-Walker cyst rather than a large cisterna magna.

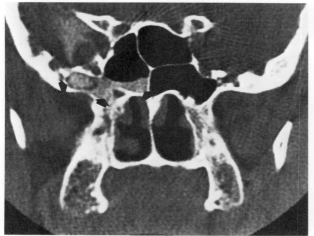

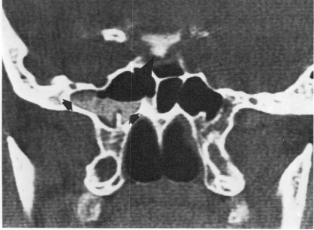

A   B

Figure 20-38   Metrizamide CT cisternograms demonstrating a cerebrospinal fluid leak into the sphenoid sinus. *A*. A patient with spontaneous CSF drainage through the right nostril. The lateral walls of the sphenoid sinus have a pitted appearance, as has been described with spontaneous CSF leaks into the sphenoid sinus. Metrizamide is noted to enter the sphenoid sinus (*arrows*) through the pitting in the lateral sphenoid sinus wall. A loculated collection in the sphenoid sinus represented a diverticulum from the intracranial sylvian subarachnoid space. *B*. The CSF leak into the right sphenoid sinus is again seen. In addition, an empty sella filled with metrizamide is noted (*arrowhead*). The CSF leak did not occur at the site of the empty sella, but rather the empty sella may represent a manifestation of a transient increase in intracranial pressure, which might also lead to spontaneous leakage of cerebrospinal fluid through the pitted lateral extension of the sphenoid sinus.

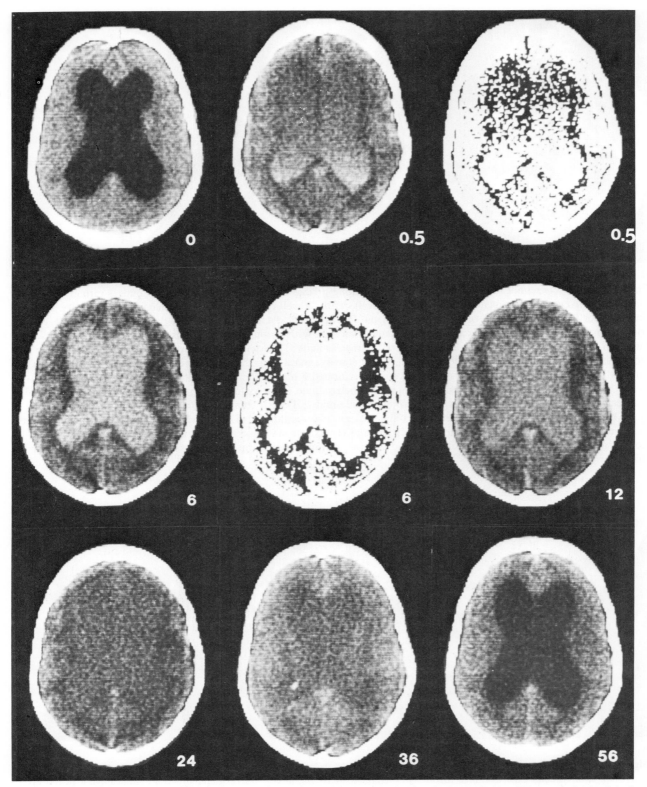

Figure 20-39 Metrizamide CT cisternography of a patient with communicating hydrocephalus. CT scans obtained before (0), immediately after (0.5), and 6, 12, 24, 36, and 56 h after the intrathecal introduction of metrizamide. On the unenhanced CT scan, there is prominent ventricular enlargement with normal-appearing sulci. There is reflux of metrizamide into the ventricular system and stasis of metrizamide within the ventricles for greater than 56 h. This combination of reflux and stasis beyond 24 h is consistent with the diagnosis of communicating hydrocephalus.

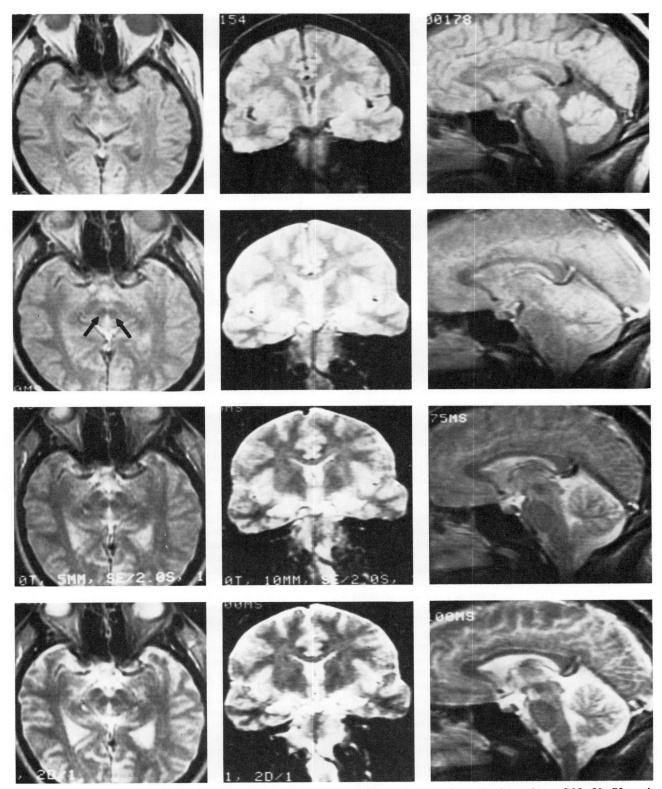

Figure 20-40 Multiple spin echo NMR scans of a normal patient. Scans were performed using values of 25, 50, 75, and 100 ms for tau (T_E). These axial (*left*), coronal (*middle*), and sagittal (*right*) NMR scans reflect the superb anatomical specificity associated with NMR imaging. Use of a multiple echo sequence also permits estimation of T2 relaxation times in absolute terms. Note the excellent gray-white distinction obtained without contrast enhancement. In the posterior fossa excellent delineation is obtained without artifacts. The red nuclei (*arrows*) are well delineated on the axial scans. Note the change in relative signal intensity that occurs depending on the T_E (for example, CSF is black at T_E of 25 ms and white at T_E of 100 ms).

are not yet understood. CT seems clearly superior at present for the moderately to severely ill patients in the hospital setting. The independent as well as integrated roles of CT and MRI imaging will certainly be delineated in the years to come.

References

1. Anand AK, Lee BCP: Plain and metrizamide CT of lumbar disk disease: Comparison with myelography. AJNR 3:567–571, 1982.
2. Axel L: Cerebral blood flow determination by rapid-sequence computed tomography. Radiology 137:679–686, 1980.
3. Brown BM, Brant-Zawadzki M, Cann CE: Dynamic CT scanning of spinal column trauma. AJNR 3:561–565, 1982.
4. Cohen G: Contrast-detail-dose analysis of six different computed tomographic scanners. J Comput Assist Tomogr 3:197–203, 1979.
5. Davis JM, Davis KR, Newhouse J, Pfister RC: Expanded high iodine dose in computed cranial tomography: A preliminary report. Radiology 131:373–380, 1979.
6. Drayer BP: Functional applications of CT of the central nervous system. AJNR 2:495–510, 1981.
7. Drayer BP, Rosenbaum AE: Studies of the third circulation; Amipaque CT cisternography and ventriculography. J Neurosurg 48:946–956, 1978.
8. Drayer BP, Rosenbaum AE: Brain edema defined by cranial computed tomography. J Comput Assist Tomogr 3:317–323, 1979.
9. Drayer BP, Rosenbaum AE, Riegel DB, Bank WO, Deeb ZL: Metrizamide computed tomography cisternography: Pediatric applications. Radiology 124:349–357, 1977.
10. Drayer BP, Vassallo C, Sudilovsky A, Luther JS, Wilkins RH, Allen S, Bates M: A double-blind clinical trial of Iopamidol versus metrizamide for lumbosacral myelography. J Neurosurg 58:531–537, 1983.
11. Gado MH, Phelps ME, Coleman RE: An extravascular component of contrast enhancement in cranial computed tomography: Part II. Contrast enhancement and the blood-tissue barrier. Radiology 117:595–597, 1975.
12. Glenn WV Jr, Johnston RJ, Morton PE, Dwyer SJ: Image generation and display techniques for CT scan data: Thin transverse and reconstructed coronal and sagittal planes. Invest Radiol 10:403–416, 1975.
13. Hayman LA, Evans RA, Bastion FO, Hinck VC: Delayed high dose contrast CT: Identifying patients at high risk of massive hemorrhagic infarction. AJNR 2:139–147, 1981.
14. Heinz R, Dubois P, Drayer B, Osborne D, Berninger W, Pizer S, Fuchs H, Barrett W: Intravenous carotid imaging utilizing the third dimension. AJNR 1:363, 1980 (abstr).
15. Herman GT, Lakshminarayanan AV, Naparstek A: Reconstruction using divergent ray shadowgraphs, in Ter-Pogossian MM, Phelps ME, Brownell EL, Cox JR Jr, Davis DO, Evens RG (eds): Reconstruction Tomography in Diagnostic Radiology and Nuclear Medicine. Baltimore, University Park Press, 1977, pp 105–117.
16. Hounsfield GN: Computerized transverse axial scanning (tomography): Part 1. Description of system. Br J Radiol 46:1016–1022, 1973.
17. Johnson GA, Korobkin M: Image techniques for multiplanar computed tomography. Radiology 144:829–834, 1982.
18. Johnson GA, Korobkin M, Heinz ER: An evaluation of multiplanar imaging capabilities of four current computed tomography (CT) scanners. Proc Soc Photo-opt Instrum Eng 273:318–325, 1981.
19. Joseph PM: Image noise and smoothing in computed tomography (CT) scanners. Opt Eng 17:396–399, 1978.
20. Joseph PM: The influence of gantry geometry on aliasing and other geometry dependent errors. IEEE Trans Nucl Sci 27:1104–1111, 1980.
21. Joseph PM, Spital RD, Stockham CD: The effects of sampling on CT images. Comput Assist Tomogr 4:189–206, 1980.
22. Ladurner G, Zilkha E, Iliff D, DuBoulay GH, Marshall J: Measurement of regional cerebral blood volume by computerized axial tomography. J Neurol Neurosurg Psychiatry 39:152–158, 1976.
23. Mawad ME, Silver AJ, Hilal SK, Ganti SR: Computed tomography of the brain stem with intrathecal metrizamide: Part 1. The normal brain stem. AJNR 4:1–11, 1983.
24. McDavid WD, Waggener RG, Dennis MJ, Sank VJ, Payne WH: Estimation of chemical composition and density from computed tomography carried out at a number of energies. Invest Radiol 12:189–194, 1977.
25. Monajati A, Heggeness L: Patterns of edema in tumors vs. infarcts: Visualization of white matter pathways. AJNR 3:251–255, 1982.
26. Peyster RG, Hoover ED, Hershey BL, Haskin ME: High resolution CT of lesions of the optic nerve. AJNR 4:169–174, 1983.
27. Rutherford RA, Pullan BR, Isherwood I: Measurement of effective atomic number and electron density using an EMI scanner. Neuroradiology 11:15–21, 1976.
28. Shepp LA, Logan BF: Fourier reconstruction of a head section. IEEE Trans Nucl Sci 21:21–43, 1974.
29. Shepp LA, Stein JA: Simulated reconstruction artifacts in computerized tomography, in Ter-Pogossian MM, Phelps ME, Brownell GL, Cox JR Jr, Davis DO, Evens RG (eds): Reconstruction Tomography in Diagnostic Radiology and Nuclear Medicine. Baltimore, University Park Press, 1977, pp 33–48.
30. Syvertsen A, Haughton VM, Williams AL, Cusick JF: Computed tomographic appearance of the normal pituitary gland and pituitary microadenomas. Radiology 133:385–391, 1979.
31. Teplick JG, Haskin ME: Computed tomography of the postoperative lumbar spine. AJNR 4:1053–1072, 1983.
32. Trokel SL, Hilal SK: Submillimeter resolution CT scanning of orbital diseases. Ophthalmology (Rochester) 87:412–417, 1980.
33. Virapongse C, Rothman SLG, Kier EL, Sarwar M: Computed tomographic anatomy of the temporal bone. AJNR 3:379–389, 1982.
34. Virapongse C, Sawar M, Kier EL, Sasaki C, Pillsburg H: Temporal bone disease: A comparison between high resolution computed tomography and pluridirectional tomography. Radiology 147:743–748, 1983.
35. Williams AL, Haughton VM, Daniels DL, Grogan JP: Differential CT diagnosis of extruded nucleus pulposus. Radiology 148:141–148, 1983.
36. Wilms G, Smits J, Baert AL: CT of the orbit: Current status with high resolution computed tomography. Neuroradiology 24:183–192, 1982.
37. Zonneveld FW: The value of non-reconstructive multiplanar CT for the evaluation of the petrous bone. Neuroradiology 25:1–10, 1983.

21

Positron Emission Tomography

Myron D. Ginsberg

Positron emission tomography (PET) is an exciting and innovative technology through which the spatial distribution of radiolabeled pharmaceuticals may be imaged noninvasively within the human brain and other organs.[4,24,26] The method resembles x-ray computed tomography in its use of reconstruction algorithms to produce an image, but it differs in that the source of radiation is in the form of an administered radiolabeled compound, rather than an external x-ray beam. The goal of PET is to provide insights into the biological functioning of the imaged organ. Thus, PET strategies hinge upon choosing radiolabeled compounds capable of "tracing" specific biological processes, as well as appropriate mathematical models with which to interpret the quantitative behavior of tracers in physiological terms. Thus, while PET yields tomographic images, it is not primarily an anatomical but rather a physiological method. Quantitation is essential to its success, and conclusions drawn from qualitative images alone are of limited significance and, at worst, may be erroneous. The particular power of PET derives from (1) the nature of the labeled compounds that may be employed, and (2) the advantages afforded to tomographic reconstruction by the nature of positron annihilation itself.

Isotopes (radionuclides) that decay by positron emission do so by the emission of a positron, or positively charged electron, from their nucleus. A positron is able to travel only a few millimeters in tissue, whereupon it loses its kinetic energy and interacts with a nearby electron, resulting in annihilation of both particles and the release of two gamma photons, each having an energy of 511 keV. The property of key importance is that the two annihilation photons travel in a direction 180 degrees from each other. Thus, if the organ to be imaged is surrounded by an array of external detectors, the location of each positron annihilation may be registered as a *coincident event* by the pair of opposing detectors in line with the annihilation photons (Fig. 21-1). This forms the basis of PET detection systems.

Among positron-emitting nuclides are several of crucial biological relevance: oxygen 15 (half-life 2.05 min), carbon 11 (half-life 20.4 min), and nitrogen 13 (half-life 9.96 min). These are isotopes of the constituent atoms of all organic molecules. Thus, with appropriate radiochemical strategies, these nuclides may be incorporated within compounds of biological interest. The isotope fluorine 18 (half-life 110 min) is also useful in that it may substitute for hydrogen atoms in organic molecules. In contrast, non-positron gamma-emitting nuclides of the type employed in conventional nuclear imaging (for example, ^{99m}Tc) represent "nonbiological" atoms. Table 21-1 lists important positron-emitting nuclides together with representative radiolabeled compounds and their uses. An advantage of the short half-life of these nuclides is the relatively low patient radiation dose per PET study and the ability to perform repeated studies in the same patient. An occasional disadvantage, however, is that the physical half-life of the tracer may be too short for the biological process being studied (for example, neurotransmitter receptor binding).

Instrumentation, Radionuclide Production, and Radiochemistry

Because of their short half-lives, positron-emitting radionuclides must generally be produced on site and rapidly synthesized into pharmaceuticals of interest. Thus, typical PET facilities include a cyclotron for nuclide production; a radiochemistry suite for synthesis and purification of radiopharmaceuticals; and an imaging area, housing the tomograph together with the high-speed computer facility needed for data acquisition, image reconstruction, and mathematical modeling. PET is thus a demanding collaborative effort requiring a team of skilled radiophysicists, radiochemists, computer specialists, applied mathematicians, engineers, physiologists, and physiologically oriented physicians.

Cyclotron

Instruments for this purpose are typically capable of accelerating protons (hydrogen nuclei) to greater than 14 meV and/or deuterons (heavy hydrogen nuclei) to 8 meV and above. Conventional cyclotron installations are generally characterized by thick concrete walls to provide the necessary radiation shielding. Recently, smaller self-shielded instruments for the production of positron-emitting nuclides have been manufactured. A variety of cyclotron targets is in use, each specially composed and designed for the production of a specific nuclide. For the synthesis of ^{15}O, for example, a $^{16}O_2$ target is bombarded by a proton beam; a proton and neutron are ejected. This reaction is abbreviated $^{16}O(p,pn)^{15}O$. Alternatively, ^{15}O may be produced by deuteron bombardment of a ^{14}N target: $^{14}N(d,n)^{15}O$. The most common scheme for synthesizing ^{11}C consists of irradiating a $^{14}N_2$ gas target with protons; an alpha particle is lost from the nucleus: $^{14}N(p,\alpha)^{11}C$.

Radiochemistry

Strategies for the incorporation of positron-emitting radionuclides into organic compounds vary widely in complexity; all must take place within the time constraints imposed by

255

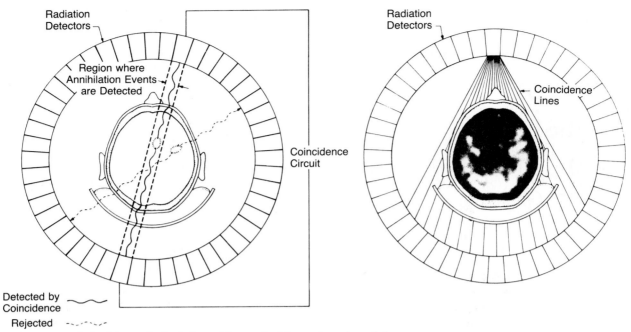

Figure 21-1 *Left*: Schematic depiction of how coincidence detection of the two annihilation photons resulting from radioactive decay of a positron-emitting nuclide is used to localize radioactivity within tissue. *Right*: Each radiation detector is in coincidence with many opposing detectors in order to increase the number of coincidence lines passing through the imaged object. (Reproduced from Raichle[26] by permission.)

the short physical half-life of the nuclides themselves. Molecular $^{15}O_2$ may be used directly from the cyclotron. ^{15}O-labeled CO_2 is readily formed from $^{15}O_2$ by combustion over charcoal and copper oxide at elevated temperature. ^{15}O-labeled water, used as a cerebral blood flow tracer, is synthesized from $^{15}O_2$ by reaction with hydrogen over a platinum catalyst. ^{11}C-labeled glucose may be isolated from Swiss chard leaves following a photosynthetic reaction using ^{11}C-labeled carbon dioxide as a reactant. [^{18}F] Fluoro-2-deoxyglucose (FDG), which has been widely applied to study cer-

ebral glucose utilization in humans, requires a complex synthesis. The reader is referred to a paper by Wolf[30] for an overview of radiopharmaceuticals.

Tomographs

The design of instruments for PET imaging has undergone extensive evolution in the past decade. Present-day instruments incorporate multiple (commonly 48 to 128) detec-

TABLE 21-1 Useful Positron-Emitting Nuclides and Their Compounds

Radionuclide	Half-Life, min	Nuclear Reaction	Representative Compounds	Use
Oxygen 15	2.05	$^{14}N(d,n)^{15}O$	$^{15}O_2$	Oxygen metabolism
		$^{16}O(p,pn)^{15}O$	$H_2^{15}O$	Blood flow
			$C^{15}O_2$	Blood flow
			$C^{15}O$	Blood volume
Carbon 11	20.4	$^{14}N(p,\alpha)^{11}C$	^{11}CO	Blood volume
		$^{10}B(d,n)^{11}C$	[^{11}C]2-deoxyglucose	Glucose metabolism
		$^{11}B(p,n)^{11}C$	[^{11}C] glucose	Glucose metabolism
			[^{11}C] iodoantipyrine	Blood flow
			[^{11}C] palmitate	Cardiac metabolism
			[^{11}C] methionine or leucine	Protein synthesis
			^{11}C alcohols	Blood flow
Nitrogen 13	9.96	$^{12}C(d,n)^{13}N$	$^{13}NH_3$	Ammonia metabolism
		$^{16}O(p,\alpha)^{13}N$		
Fluorine 18	110	$^{20}Ne(d,\alpha)^{18}F$	[^{18}F] fluorodeoxyglucose	Glucose metabolism
			[^{18}F] DOPA	Dopamine receptor
			[^{18}F] spiroperidol	Dopamine receptor
Gallium 68	68	Generator synthesis	[^{68}Ga] EDTA	Blood-brain barrier

tors ringed in a circular or hexagonal array around a central opening. In earlier instruments, sodium iodide crystals served as detectors, but bismuth germanate oxide offers the advantage of greater efficiency and higher spatial resolution and is being currently used in commercially produced instruments.[4,24] Tomographs using cesium fluoride detectors are capable of resolving differences in the respective detector arrival times of the two photons arising from a given positron annihilation (so-called time-of-flight), thus offering additional resolution particularly advantageous for body imaging.[4,24] Multiple-layer detector systems enable a tomographic image of several adjacent axial levels to be generated simultaneously. While detector rings may be stationary, the superimposition of phasic wobble and/or small-angle rotatory motions further enhances spatial resolution by increasing nonredundant sampling. A typical 48-detector sodium iodide circular tomograph is shown in Fig. 21-2.

Image Reconstruction

The circumferential array of detectors is electronically interconnected such that each detector forms a pair with several opposite detectors. The imaginary lines connecting a detector with the paired ones opposite thus form a *fan array* (Fig. 21-1). A pair of photons arising from positron annihilation within the imaged organ travel along one such line. Their arrival is registered as a coincident event in the appropriate detector pair. In contrast, annihilation events arising outside the imaged volume are not registered. The PET image is reconstructed from the raw data of the coincidence detectors (bank pairs) by a mathematical technique termed *filtered back projection*, in which data are represented as a series of parallel lines, filtered by the mathematical process of deconvolution, and "back-projected" to form the image. The final resolution of the reconstructed image, expressed as full width at half maximum for a line source, ranges typically from 10 to 20 mm in the image plane.[4]

Physiological Measurement Strategies

Local Cerebral Blood Volume (lCBV)

Measurement of lCBV is easily accomplished by the single-breath inhalation of trace amounts of labeled carbon monoxide, which, by binding tightly to hemoglobin, serves to label the intravascular space. CO may be labeled with either ^{11}C or ^{15}O, though the former is preferable because of its longer half-life. The large cerebral arteries and veins and the venous sinuses are clearly depicted on lCBV scans.[13] Quantitative lCBV scans may be used in conjunction with measurement of regional cerebral blood flow or metabolism to correct for the concentration of *intravascular* tracer contributing to the PET image. By so correcting, the accuracy of the latter studies may be enhanced.

Local Cerebral Blood Flow (lCBF)

Ideal tracers for the measurement of lCBF are small, metabolically inert molecules capable of diffusing from blood to brain at rapid rates relative to the rates of blood flow being measured, so that their extraction by the brain is virtually complete during a single transcapillary passage. The short-chain alcohols, notably *n*-butanol, have been shown to be the least diffusion-limited,[26] and a number of ^{11}C-labeled alcohols have been synthesized, although they are not being routinely employed for measuring blood flow. Iodoantipyrine has been fully validated as a CBF tracer in experimental animals, and its synthesis accomplished with the ^{11}C label, though not with sufficient ease to recommend its routine use. In contrast, ^{15}O-labeled water, though having a somewhat greater degree of diffusion limitation, is emerging as the most serviceable tracer for routine application since it can be synthesized easily in high yield and purity.

Conventional CBF measurement strategies, which rely

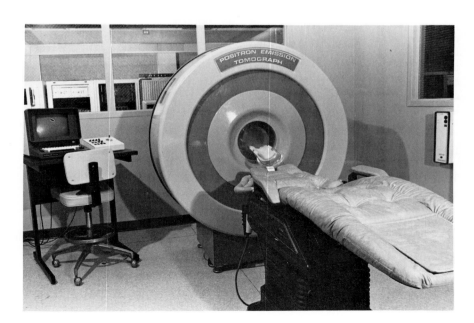

Figure 21-2 Typical PET facility, housing a 48-detector sodium iodide circular "PETT V" tomograph (foreground) and associated computer and image-processing hardware (background). (Positron Emission Tomography Center, University of Miami School of Medicine and Mt. Sinai Medical Center.)

on second-by-second measurement of the cerebral clearance of an inert tracer, are not well suited to PET since "instantaneous" cerebral count rates are inevitably too low for satisfactory statistical precision in the reconstructed image. A more suitable strategy is based upon the accumulation of a cerebral image over minutes and analysis by an in vivo autoradiographic strategy analogous to that used for experimental studies of lCBF.[11] The mathematical model derives from that of Seymour Kety, modified for the requirements of PET image accumulation and physical decay of short-lived tracers:

$$C = f \int_{T1}^{T2} \int_0^t A(t - \tau)e^{-k\tau} \, d\tau \, dt$$

where C represents activity in any pixel of the accumulated cerebral image; T1 and T2 are the start and stop times of the PET scan; A is the arterial activity function of the tracer; f is flow (ml/g per minute); and k is a rate constant equal to $f/\lambda + \alpha$, where λ is the brain/blood partition coefficient of the tracer and α is the physical decay constant of the nuclide. An optimal strategy is to administer 25 to 30 μCi of ^{15}O-labeled water as an intravenous bolus and to carry out the PET scan over the ensuing 1.5 to 2 min. Although the relationship between C and f is not fully linear, this method yields an excellent separation of flow values in the physiological range. Variants of this strategy are currently under evaluation in several PET centers.[11,24,26]

In another method of measuring lCBF by PET, ^{15}O-labeled carbon dioxide is administered by continuous inhalation.[9,29] This is converted to water by the action of carbonic anhydrase in the lungs and red cells. This water is then distributed in accordance with blood flow. At equilibrium,

$$B = \frac{Af}{f/\lambda + \alpha}$$

where A and B are the arterial and cerebral concentrations of ^{15}O-labeled water, respectively, and f, λ, and α are as defined above. This method, although widely used, suffers from a significant nonlinearity in the relationship between cerebral activity at equilibrium (B) and flow, which may result in progressively larger errors in the estimation of CBF in the high-normal and supranormal flow range. Quantitation of lCBF by all methods above requires that the arterial blood be sampled. However, a qualitative impression of regional CBF differences may be gained from the cerebral image alone.

Local Cerebral Glucose Metabolism (lCMRgl)

The most widely employed method to measure local cerebral glucose metabolism with PET derives from the highly successful method developed by Sokoloff and co-workers in animals, using as a tracer the glucose analogue 2-deoxyglucose (2-DG).[28] 2-DG differs from glucose in the absence of a hydroxyl group on the second carbon atom. 2-DG and glucose are transported from blood to brain by the same carrier system, and both compete at the phosphorylation step for the enzyme hexokinase. However, whereas glucose-6-phosphate continues to be metabolized via glycolysis and the Krebs cycle, 2-DG-6-phosphate cannot be further metabo-

lized and hence persists in tissue in that form. Sokoloff and co-workers have devised a mathematical model based upon these considerations, from which the rate of glucose metabolism may be computed from the knowledge of the arterial plasma concentration of glucose and the activity of the 2-DG label in plasma and brain.[28] Values for various constants must be assumed or else independently determined.

In the emission tomographic version of this method, the positron-emitting radiopharmaceutical [^{18}F] fluoro-2-deoxyglucose (FDG) has been used in place of 2-DG itself[15,27] and the mathematical model modified to take into account the small amount of dephosphorylation of FDG-6-phosphate to free FDG that may occur at the longer study times required for human PET studies.[15] More recently, 2-DG itself has been synthesized with the ^{11}C label.

The tracer is administered as an intravenous bolus at time zero. Over the next 30 to 45 min, samples of arterial blood (or "arterialized" venous blood taken from a limb warmed to 44°C) are drawn to define the arterial plasma concentration curve for 2-DG as well as glucose. During this period, the free tracer is taken up by brain and other organs and is phosphorylated; by 30 to 45 min, most of the tracer present in the brain is in the form of the 6-phosphate. The definitive PET image is carried out at that time. (A series of earlier PET scans may be performed if one wishes to evaluate the kinetic constants as well.) The mathematical model assumes that the brain's rate of glucose utilization is in a steady state throughout the study period.

An alternative strategy proposed for the measurement of lCMRgl involves the use of ^{11}C-labeled glucose itself, rather than a glucose analogue.[26] This method is complicated by the fact that ^{11}C-labeled glucose is metabolized rapidly within the brain and gives rise to a variety of labeled metabolites with subsequent egress from brain tissue. Although this strategy has been well studied in animals, it has not yet been used for the tomographic measurement of lCMRgl in humans.[26]

Local Cerebral Oxygen Metabolism (lCMRO$_2$)

The rate of local cerebral oxygen utilization in the brain may be measured with PET. The most widely used strategy consists of the continous inhalation of a stable inspired concentration of ^{15}O$_2$, which is continuously generated by a cyclotron.[9,29] Inhaled ^{15}O$_2$ is metabolized to ^{15}O-labeled water in the brain and other organs. After 8 to 10 min of inhalation, a steady-state concentration of ^{15}O-labeled water is achieved in the brain, wherein the amount of ^{15}O-labeled water being produced in the brain by the metabolism of ^{15}O$_2$ is counterbalanced by the amount leaving the brain via blood flow and physical decay. Thus:

$$C \cong \left(\frac{f}{f/\lambda + \alpha}\right) \times (A_w + A_O E)$$

where C represents the imaged cerebral activity per volume; A_w and A_O are the activities of radiolabeled water and oxygen, respectively, in the arterial blood; E is the cerebral exaction fraction for oxygen; f is CBF; α is the physical decay constant for the radionuclide; and λ is the brain/blood partition coefficient for water.[29] Thus, CMRO$_2$ = $E \times f \times$ arterial oxygen content. For quantitation of oxygen metabolic rate, it is thus necessary that local cerebral blood flow (f) also be measured and that the arterial tracer activities be known. An important advantage of this method is that the pixel-by-pixel division of the $^{15}O_2$ equilibrium image by the equilibrium $C^{15}O_2$ image yields an image in which the distribution of activity represents the *oxygen extraction fraction* (OEF). This method of lCMRO$_2$ does not take into account the small amount of ^{15}O present as oxyhemoglobin in the cerebral vascular compartment. Nonetheless, the method has proven highly serviceable.

Raichle and co-workers have proposed an alternative model for oxygen metabolism that requires only a single-breath inhalation of $^{15}O_2$. However, the mathematical model is complex and the validation not yet fully published.

PET Studies of Normal Cerebral Function

PET studies in normal volunteers have served to define patterns of regional cerebral metabolism in the resting brain as well as patterns of response to modality-specific sensory stimulation or deprivation. Mazziotta et al.,[22] using [18]FDG, demonstrated that normal subjects studied in the awake, resting state with eyes closed and patched and with a low ambient noise level showed no right-to-left metabolic differences. The mean value of glucose metabolic rate averaged over the whole brain was 5.9 ± 0.9 mg per 100 g per minute; the metabolic rate of the cerebral hemispheres themselves averaged 6.7 mg per 100 g per minute. Within the primary and associative visual cortex, the level of metabolic activity was found to depend upon the nature and complexity of the visual stimuli presented (Fig. 21-3).[23,25] Compared with the white light stimulated state, closing the eyes was found to reduce CMRgl by 10 percent in the primary and 12 percent in the associative visual cortex, whereas a monocular checkerboard stimulation produced a 17 percent increase in the primary and a 22 percent increase in the associative visual cortex.[25] A comparable binocular stimulation resulted in 28 percent and 27 percent mean increases, respectively. Complex visual stimuli (observing an outdoor scene) produced the greatest increases in CMRgl (mean 45 percent in the primary and 59 percent in the associative visual cortex). Thus, complex visual interpretations appear to require extensive recruitment of the associative visual cortex (Fig. 21-3).[23] Hemianopsia-producing lesions of the visual pathways were found to lower CMRgl of the affected visual cortex by one-third or more, compared with the contralateral side; in contrast, the degree of visual cortical metabolic rate reduction produced by congenital blindness associated with retrolental fibroplasia was no greater than that produced by eye closure in normal subjects.[25]

FDG studies of the normal auditory system have given rise to conflicting findings. Whereas Greenberg et al.[12] found that monaural auditory stimuli (a factual story) elevated the CMRgl of the temporal cortex contralateral to the stimulated ear (by about 7 percent), the findings of Mazziotta et al.[21] suggest that auditory metabolic responses are determined by the nature and content of the auditory stimulus rather than by the side of stimulation. Thus, monaural verbal stimuli increased CMRgl diffusely in the left hemisphere and caused bilateral increases in the transverse and posterior temporal lobes, whereas monaural nonverbal stimuli (musical chords) resulted in frontotemporal asymmetry, right greater than left. These workers found that the metabolic response to a tone sequence task reflected the analytic strategy employed: musically naive subjects showed right greater than left frontotemporal asymmetries, whereas musically sophisticated subjects employing "analytic" strategies had left greater than right *temporal* asymmetries. Regardless of the stimulus, the transverse temporal cortex showed the greatest metabolic response (34 to 40 percent above mean hemispheric values).[21]

In contrast to the above, auditory and visual deprivation, either singly or in combination, resulted in an overall decrease of CMRgl but with a redistribution of metabolic rate, favoring frontal over parietal and occipital cortex.[20] Interestingly, the normal left-right symmetry of metabolic activity was maintained with selective eye closure and ear blockage, whereas *combined* audiovisual deprivation caused a greater decrease in metabolic activity in the right than in the left hemisphere.[20]

PET Studies of Disease States

Cerebral Vascular Disease

Several groups have used PET to study patients with cerebral infarction and cerebral vascular insufficiency.[1,2,18] From these reports, it is evident that a variety of patterns of altered blood flow and metabolism may be observed, and that these physiological derangements typically precede, and in some instances may be used to predict, eventual structural tissue injury demonstrable by x-ray CT scans. When $^{15}O_2$ and $C^{15}O_2$ are used to image regional CMRO$_2$ and blood flow, respectively, an image of regional oxygen extraction fraction (OEF) may be derived (Fig. 21-4). The latter is a useful descriptor of disordered physiology in stroke. Normally, the OEF is rather uniform throughout the brain, exemplifying the normal flow-metabolism couple. In contrast, the great majority of patients with ischemic stroke studied during the first month show a focal abnormality of the OEF.[2] Most commonly, the OEF is decreased, implying that local blood flow is in excess of the local metabolic needs of the tissue (Fig. 21-4). This may occur even though the *absolute* level of CBF is decreased (as is most often the case in ischemic stroke), normal, or increased above the normal level. Thus, PET has allowed Lassen's concept of "luxury perfusion" to be generalized to the situation of flow-greater-than-metabolism uncoupling occurring in the absence of an absolute elevation of blood flow.[2]

In a smaller percentage of early infarcts, OEF is focally increased: this denotes a state in which local flow is insufficient to meet the demands of the tissue for oxygen consumption. Baron[2] has termed this condition "misery perfusion" and has found it to occur characteristically in the first several days following cerebral infarction and never in infarcts older than 2 weeks. It has been suggested that severe focal luxury perfusion may at times be an unfavorable sign as regards tissue survival; furthermore, when luxury perfusion is observed at 10 to 20 days, it is said to correlate best with local

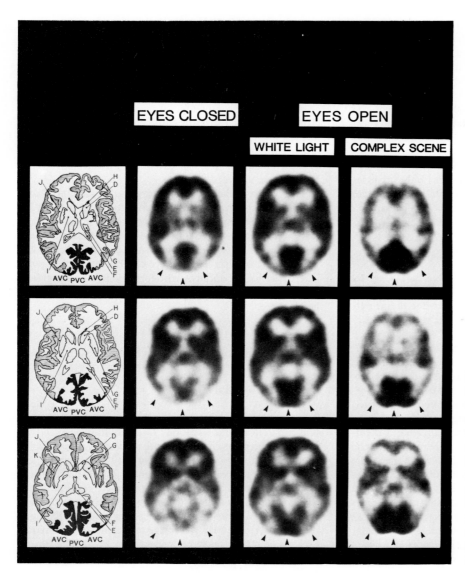

Figure 21-3 FDG scans at three horizontal levels, demonstrating reduced metabolic activity in the primary (PVC) and associative (AVC) visual cortex bilaterally during eye closure (second column); increased local metabolic rate during stimulation by white light (third column); and still greater increases in metabolic activity while viewing a complex scene (fourth column). Sketches of corresponding anatomical levels are shown on the left. (Reproduced from Phelps et al.[23] by permission.)

capillary hyperplasia and, thus, to connote tissue infarction.[24] In contrast, tissue zones exhibiting misery perfusion, although in a precarious hemodynamic state, are nonetheless capable of full recovery since the tissue so affected remains viable.[1,2] Combined FDG and blood flow studies in patients with acute stroke have shown that local CBF may be depressed disproportionately to the local metabolic rate for glucose; this is consistent with the occurrence of anaerobic glycolysis in marginally perfused tissue areas.[18] In early ischemic stroke, zones of physiological hypofunction demonstrable by PET are often larger than the structurally abnormal regions defined by CT scans.[18]

In patients with hemispheric infarcts of 6 to 8 weeks' duration or more, PET studies show marked *coupled* decreases in CBF and metabolism, which correlate well with zones of necrosis demonstrable by CT scans. Kuhl et al.[18] found that all zones having more than approximately 60 percent depression of local CMRgl had permanent infarcts on CT scan.

An interesting feature of cerebral infarction studied by PET is the occurrence of depressed tissue metabolism re-

mote from the ischemic lesion, constituting a form of *diaschisis*. Thus, transhemispheric diaschisis has been observed in hemispheric infarcts. Depressed tissue metabolism and perfusion may occur in the ipsilateral thalamus subjacent to a cortical infarct.[24] Finally, Baron et al.[2] have demonstrated "crossed cerebellar diaschisis" in the form of a transiently depressed metabolic rate in the cerebellar hemisphere contralateral to a supratentorial infarct.

Superficial Temporal–Middle Cerebral Artery (STA-MCA) Anastomosis

In a preliminary study, Grubb et al.[14] used the intracarotid injection of the positron emitters ^{15}O-labeled oxyhemoglobin and ^{15}O-labeled water together with a nontomographic multiple-detector system to study 1CBF and 1CMRO$_2$ in patients before and after STA-MCA anastomosis. Preoperative studies performed at the time of angiography showed either a coupled depression of both 1CBF and 1CMRO$_2$ or a depressed 1CBF with relative preservation of oxygen meta-

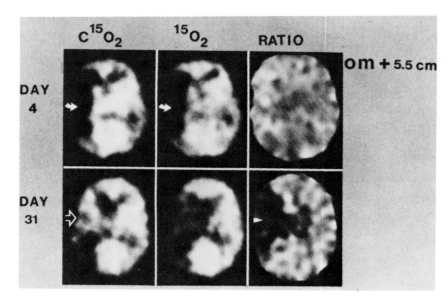

Figure 21-4 PET studies of 1CBF ($C^{15}O_2$), $1CMRO_2$ ($^{15}O_2$), and OEF (ratio image), at day 4 and day 31 following an infarction in the left middle cerebral artery territory. Both CBF and $CMRO_2$ are severely reduced within the infarct on day 4, and local OEF may be slightly increased; at day 31, perfusion has partially returned, but OEF is severely reduced within the infarct, signifying luxury perfusion. (Reproduced from Baron et al.[2] by permission.)

bolic rate (that is, increased OEF). These situations (in the absence of cerebral infarction) were viewed as favorable indications for surgery. In patients having a functional anastomosis, late postoperative studies showed significant improvement of both flow and oxygen utilization in several cases. Baron et al.[3] subsequently reported sequential PET studies performed by the ^{15}O continuous inhalation method in a single case of cerebral ischemia with internal carotid artery occlusion, before and after STA-MCA anastomosis. These workers documented misery perfusion (decreased CBF with increased OEF) involving the parieto-occipital watershed area, which resolved postoperatively. These preliminary observations provide further substantiation of the brain's ability to increase its degree of oxygen extraction when blood flow is primarily limited. PET studies appear to have an important contributory role in the preoperative evaluation of patients being considered for STA-MCA anastomosis and in the metabolic characterization of brain regions at potential risk for ischemic infarction.

Epilepsy

PET has contributed importantly to the understanding of altered cerebral function in epilepsy. Engel et al.[6-8] have recently reported an ambitious series of studies correlating emission tomographic observations with electrophysiological recordings and with pathological findings in patients undergoing temporal lobe resections. In a majority of patients with complex partial seizures studied in the *interictal* state, PET scans using FDG revealed one or more zones of cerebral *hypo*metabolism, estimated to range in degree from approximately 10 percent to 55 percent (Fig. 21-5). These zones were typically normal on conventional x-ray computed tomographic brain scans. In those patients undergoing anterior temporal lobe resection, 86 percent of those having hypometabolic zones on PET scans had corresponding focal pathological abnormalities, most commonly mesial temporal sclerosis. In general, the size of the focal abnormality as revealed by PET was larger than the corresponding area of

pathological involvement. Patients without focal PET abnormalities failed to show pathological changes in their resected specimens.[6] There was commonly a discrepancy between the site of focal hypometabolism and the locus suggested by individual ictal or interictal EEG recordings, and the degree of focal hypometabolism failed to correlate with the frequency of interictal EEG spikes.[8] However, the "best" combined impression gained from all electrophysiological studies tended to agree well with the PET localization of the hypometabolic focus. These authors view PET and EEG as complementary techniques in this setting, in that the former localizes lesions accurately whereas the latter determines whether they are epileptogenic.[24]

In cases in which FDG scans have been performed *during*

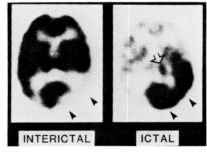

Figure 21-5 FDG scans performed in the interictal and ictal states in a patient with complex partial epilepsy. The patient had visual auras, consisting of formed numerals in the left hemifield. The primary and associative visual cortex and posterior temporal regions on the right demonstrate hypometabolism interictally and marked hypermetabolism (involving as well the right thalamus—open arrow) during the seizure. (Reproduced from Phelps et al.[25] by permission.)

partial seizures, focal *hyper*metabolism has been observed in zones that exhibited *hypo*metabolism interictally (Fig. 21-5). In other cases, the pattern of ictal hypermetabolism may be multifocal or generalized.[7] Patients undergoing induced electroconvulsive shock treatments exhibit generalized cerebral hypermetabolism during the ictus, and a generalized decrease in cortical metabolism when studied immediately postictally.[7] During petit mal seizures induced by hyperventilation, a two- to threefold global increase in cerebral metabolic rate has been described.[7]

Aging and Dementia

In normal volunteers aged 18 to 78 years old studied with FDG, the whole brain mean cerebral metabolic rate for glucose at age 78 was 26 percent less than at age 18.[17] While this mild decline in metabolic rate generally affected various brain regions in similar fashion, the CMRgl of the superior frontal cortex appeared to decline to a greater extent than that of the superior parietal cortex. PET scans in patients with various vascular and degenerative dementias were obtained by Frackowiak et al.[10] using the ^{15}O equilibrium inhalation method for CBF and $CMRO_2$. These workers observed a parallel decline in both blood flow and metabolic rate, the degree of which correlated with the severity of the clinical dementia. Among cortical areas, the parietal region appeared to be the most affected, the occipital cortex the least. In the degenerative dementias, the changes in the frontal and parietal regions were particularly severe. While the results of this study doubtless reflect the consequences of the dementing process, these data do not elucidate causal mechanisms. Interestingly, these authors found no evidence for a state of "chronic ischemia," i.e., marginal blood flow associated with an increased oxygen extraction fraction (OEF). Rather, OEF was unchanged. This finding would tend to discourage attempts to improve cerebral blood flow in an effort to treat the metabolic dysfunction of dementia.

Brain Tumors

In a series of patients with cerebral gliomas studied with PET using FDG, all high-grade (III and IV) astrocytomas contained zones of high metabolic activity, varying from large and occasionally multiple areas to barely discernible foci.[5] In contrast, regions of distinctly elevated metabolism were not observed within gliomas of lower grade (I and II). In that study, quantitation of glucose metabolic rate was based on an assumption of *normal* values for the lumped constant and rate constants of the mathematical model—an assumption that may not be valid for tumor tissue. Values so obtained were 8.6 ± 2.8 mg per 100 g per minute in the high-grade tumors compared with 3.6 ± 1.4 mg per 100 g per minute in gliomas of lower grade. In over one-half of the patients in that series, a zone of metabolic suppression was noted in cortical regions either adjacent to tumor tissue or having neural connections with the involved zone.[5] In several patients having large supratentorial tumors, hypometabolism was observed in the contralateral cerebellar hemisphere.

In other, preliminary studies of local oxygen utilization in tumors, decreased oxidative metabolism has been noted. PET studies combining measurements of both $CMRO_2$ and CMRgl are expected to offer insights into relationships between aerobic and anaerobic metabolism within brain tumors. PET is also able to provide excellent spatial localization of brain tumors when tracers sensitive to altered blood-brain barrier (for example, ^{68}Ga–labeled EDTA) are utilized. ^{11}C- or ^{13}N-labeled amino acids have also been used to image brain tumors.

Huntington's Disease

In a recent report, patients with documented Huntington's disease studied with FDG were found to have decreased glucose utilization involving the caudate nucleus and putamen; importantly, this focally depressed metabolism was noted to occur early in the disease and to precede CT scan evidence of tissue loss.[19] Even in clinically severely affected patients, glucose utilization in other brain areas tended to be normal. In subjects without clinical symptoms but genetically at risk for this inherited, autosomal dominant disease, a derived index reflecting metabolism of the caudate nucleus was found to have a much greater *range* of values than was observed in normal subjects, despite the fact that the mean values of the two groups did not differ significantly. In six of fifteen subjects at risk for the disease, values for the caudate metabolic rate index were increased beyond two standard deviations of the normal mean.[19] Whether emission tomography will prove to be a reliable means of diagnosing Huntington's disease in its presymptomatic state is not yet established but is the object of continuing study.

Comparison with Other Tomographic Imaging Methods

Transmission x-ray computed tomography (CT) has revolutionized neurological diagnosis by providing highly detailed images of cross-sectional brain anatomy. For the depiction of brain structure per se, PET appears to offer no advantage over CT scanning since the optimal resolution possible with PET (and not yet achieved in practice) appears to be limited to about 4 mm.[4] However, transmission CT scans provide little direct information regarding cerebral *function* (with the exception of blood-brain barrier alterations visible on contrast-enhanced scans). While a noninvasive method has been developed to measure lCBF by (stable) xenon-enhanced x-ray transmission computed tomography, inhalation of xenon in concentrations exceeding 40 to 50 percent is often associated with sedative or anesthetic effects, and use of lower concentrations greatly degrades the signal-to-noise ratio. The necessity for multiple scans in this technique may lead to significant radiation exposure to the patient.

Nuclear magnetic resonance (NMR) imaging entails physical principles entirely different from those of transmission or emission tomography, and utilizes neither x-rays nor radioactive substances. Rather, the subject is exposed to a strong static magnetic field together with a weaker, rapidly alternating (radiofrequency) magnetic field. The sensitivity of NMR is such that high-resolution imaging is presently possible only in the case of the proton (hydrogen nucleus), although it is possible to measure (but not to image) the relative concentrations of phosphorus-containing metabolites, including high-energy phosphate compounds (ATP, phosphocreatine) in selected brain regions.[4] A variety of NMR parameters may serve as the basis of an image; these include the concentration of hydrogen nuclei, the spin-lattice relaxation time (T1), and the spin-spin relaxation time (T2). A resolution of 2 mm is currently being achieved in human NMR images.[4] This is comparable to the resolution of CT scans and far better than that of PET. In addition, NMR T1 imaging is capable of much greater contrast sensitivity in differentiating cerebral gray and white matter than is possible with transmission CT. Subtle alterations of brain water content are easily visible. Among the striking successes already demonstrated with NMR imaging are the clear depiction of the lesions of human demyelinating disease and the detection of cerebral infarction within a few hours of its onset. In the future, it may prove feasible to measure cerebral blood flow with NMR.[4]

Single photon emission tomography (SPET) is a technique for the tomographic measurement of the tissue concentration of conventional gamma-emitting radionuclides. The goals of SPET are akin to those of PET. Its chief advantage is the ability to image the common gamma-emitting isotopes (^{133}Xe, ^{99m}Tc, ^{123}I, and so on), which are typically of longer half-life than positron-emitting nuclides and do not require an on-site cyclotron or an elaborate support staff for their production. Offsetting these advantages for daily clinical use are several important disadvantages: (1) Isotopes of "biological" atoms (oxygen, carbon, nitrogen) are unavailable for single photon imaging, and (2) electronic collimation afforded by coincidence detection of annihilation photons in PET is not possible with SPET, and mechanical collimation imposes significant limitations on the efficiency and sensitivity of radioactivity detection. Spatial resolution is nonuniform across the image plane. Scattered photons degrade image quality and interfere seriously with efforts to achieve quantitation. Nonetheless, SPET promises to be useful in the routine clinical setting, especially when used with paradigms not requiring dynamic imaging. Local cerebral blood volume is studied satisfactorily with SPET. The recent availability of the ^{123}I-labeled compound, *N*-isopropyl-*p*-iodoamphetamine (IMP), a substance having a high first-pass brain extraction and a prolonged persistence within brain tissue, has permitted SPET to achieve excellent imaging of local cerebral blood flow. Efforts to quantitate lCBF measurements with SPET have been recently reported.[16] Blood-brain barrier studies are also possible with SPET.

Future Directions

The application of an autoradiographic method of local brain protein synthesis first developed in Sokoloff's laboratory to human PET studies has already commenced, utilizing ^{11}C-labeled amino acids. A much wished for application of PET is the delineation of patterns of neurotransmitter receptor binding within the central nervous system. Success in this regard will depend upon (1) the synthesis of appropriate radiolabeled ligands in sufficiently high yield and specific activity, and (2) the development of mathematical and analytical strategies capable of interpreting the kinetics of these tracers and of distinguishing patterns of specific from nonspecific binding. Preliminary efforts have been directed toward the synthesis of ^{11}C- or ^{18}F-labeled ligands for the dopamine, opiate, benzodiazepine, and acetylcholine receptors. All of these efforts are still in the developmental stages.

Lipophilic substances have been used in preliminary studies to image brain myelin with PET. While this effort may bear clinical fruit, NMR proton imaging will probably prove to be far superior in this regard, e.g., in characterizing the lesions of human demyelinating diseases. The application of PET to the understanding of psychiatric disorders is still in its infancy. Tantalizing observations have been made using FDG, both in schizophrenia and, quite recently, in the major affective disorders. This is an area of great promise but one that demands scrupulously controlled experimental design in order to avoid misinterpretation arising from uncontrolled environmental stimuli, effects of concurrent medications, and instrumentation artifacts.

References

1. Ackerman RH, Correia JA, Alpert NM, Baron J, Gouliamos A, Grotta JC, Brownell GL, Taveras JM: Positron imaging in ischemic stroke disease using compounds labeled with oxygen 15. Arch Neurol 38:537–543, 1981.
2. Baron JC, Bousser MG, Comar D, Soussaline F, Castaigne P: Noninvasive tomographic study of cerebral blood flow and oxygen metabolism in vivo: Potentials, limitations, and clinical applications in cerebral ischemic disorders. Eur Neurol 20:273–284, 1981.
3. Baron JC, Bousser MG, Rey A, Guillard A, Comar D, Castaigne P: Reversal of focal "misery-perfusion syndrome" by extra-intracranial arterial bypass in hemodynamic cerebral ischemia: A case study with ^{15}O positron emission tomography. Stroke 12:454–459, 1981.
4. Brownell GL, Budinger TF, Lauterbur PC, McGeer PL: Positron tomography and nuclear magnetic resonance imaging. Science 215:619–626, 1982.
5. Di Chiro G, DeLaPaz RL, Brooks RA, Sokoloff L, Kornblith PL, Smith BH, Patronas NJ, Kufta CV, Kessler RM, Johnston GS, Manning RG, Wolf AP: Glucose utilization of cerebral gliomas measured by (^{18}F) fluorodeoxyglucose and positron emission tomography. Neurology (NY) 32:1323–1329, 1982.
6. Engel J Jr, Brown WJ, Kuhl DE, Phelps ME, Mazziotta JC, Crandall PH: Pathological findings underlying focal temporal lobe hypometabolism in partial epilepsy. Ann Neurol 12:518–528, 1982.
7. Engel J Jr, Kuhl DE, Phelps ME: Patterns of human local cerebral glucose metabolism during epileptic seizures. Science 218:64–66, 1982.
8. Engel J Jr, Kuhl DE, Phelps ME, Mazziotta JC: Interictal cerebral glucose metabolism in partial epilepsy and its relation to EEG changes. Ann Neurol 12:510–517, 1982.
9. Frackowiak RSJ, Lenzi G, Jones T, Heather JD: Quantitative measurement of regional cerebral blood flow and oxygen metabolism in man using ^{15}O and positron emission tomography: Theory, procedure, and normal values. J Comput Assist Tomogr 4:727–736, 1980.

10. Frackowiak RSJ, Pozzilli C, Legg NJ, du Boulay GH, Marshall J, Lenzi GL, Jones T: Regional cerebral oxygen supply and utilization in dementia: A clinical and physiological study with oxygen-15 and positron tomography. Brain 104:753–778, 1981.

11. Ginsberg MD, Lockwood AH, Busto R, Finn RD, Butler CM, Cendan IE, Goddard J: A simplified *in vivo* autoradiographic strategy for the determination of regional cerebral blood flow by positron emission tomography: Theoretical considerations and validation studies in the rat. J Cerebr Blood Flow Metab 2:89–98, 1982.

12. Greenberg JH, Reivich M, Alavi A, Hand P, Rosenquist A, Rintelmann W, Stein A, Tusa R, Dann R, Christman D, Fowler J, MacGregor B, Wolf A: Metabolic mapping of functional activity in human subjects with the (^{18}F) fluorodeoxyglucose technique. Science 212:678–680, 1981.

13. Grubb RL Jr, Raichle ME, Higgins CS, Eichling JO: Measurement of regional cerebral blood volume by emission tomography. Ann Neurol 4:322–328, 1978.

14. Grubb RL Jr, Ratcheson RA, Raichle ME, Kliefoth AB, Gado MH: Regional cerebral blood flow and oxygen utilization in superficial temporal-middle cerebral artery anastomosis patients: An exploratory definition of clinical problems. J Neurosurg 50:733–741, 1979.

15. Huang S, Phelps ME, Hoffman EJ, Sideris K, Selin CJ, Kuhl DE: Noninvasive determination of local cerebral metabolic rate of glucose in man. Am J Physiol 238:E69–E82, 1980.

16. Kuhl DE, Barrio JR, Huang S, Selin C, Ackermann RF, Lear JL, Wu JL, Lin TH, Phelps ME: Quantifying local cerebral blood flow by *N*-isopropyl-*p*-(^{123}I)iodoamphetamine (IMP) tomography. J Nucl Med 23:196–203, 1982.

17. Kuhl DE, Metter EJ, Riege WH, Phelps ME: Effects of human aging on patterns of local cerebral glucose utilization determined by the (^{18}F)fluorodeoxyglucose method. J Cerebr Blood Flow Metab 2:163–171, 1982.

18. Kuhl DE, Phelps ME, Kowell AP, Metter EJ, Selin C, Winter J: Effects of stroke on local cerebral metabolism and perfusion: Mapping by emission computed tomography of ^{18}FDG and ^{13}NH$_3$. Ann Neurol 8:47–60, 1980.

19. Kuhl DE, Phelps ME, Markham CH, Metter EJ, Riege WH, Winter J: Cerebral metabolism and atrophy in Huntington's disease determined by ^{18}FDG and computed tomographic scan. Ann Neurol 12:425–434, 1982.

20. Mazziotta JC, Phelps ME, Carson RE, Kuhl DE: Tomographic mapping of human cerebral metabolism: Sensory deprivation. Ann Neurol 12:435–444. 1982.

21. Mazziotta JC, Phelps ME, Carson RE, Kuhl DE: Tomographic mapping of human cerebral metabolism: Auditory stimulation. Neurology (NY) 32:921–937, 1982.

22. Mazziotta JC, Phelps ME, Miller J, Kuhl DE: Tomographic mapping of human cerebral metabolism: Normal unstimulated state. Neurology (NY) 31:503–516, 1981.

23. Phelps ME, Kuhl DE, Mazziotta JC: Metabolic mapping of the brain's response to visual stimulation: Studies in humans. Science 211:1445–1448, 1981.

24. Phelps ME, Mazziotta JC, Huang S: Review: Study of cerebral function with positron computed tomography. J Cereb Blood Flow Metab 2:113–162, 1982.

25. Phelps ME, Mazziotta JC, Kuhl DE, Nuwer M, Packwood J, Metter J, Engel J Jr: Tomographic mapping of human cerebral metabolism: Visual stimulation and deprivation. Neurology (NY) 31:517–529, 1981.

26. Raichle ME: Quantitative *in vivo* autoradiography with positron emission tomography. Brain Res Rev 1:47–68, 1979.

27. Reivich M, Kuhl D, Wolf A, Greenberg J, Phelps M, Ido T, Casella V, Fowler J, Hoffman E, Alavi A, Som P, Sokoloff L: The (^{18}F)fluorodeoxyglucose method for the measurement of local cerebral glucose utilization in man. Circ Res 44:127–137, 1979.

28. Sokoloff L, Reivich M, Kennedy C, Des Rosiers MH, Patlak CS, Pettigrew KD, Sakurada O, Shinohara M: The (^{14}C) deoxyglucose method for the measurement of local cerebral glucose utilization: Theory, procedure, and normal values in the conscious and anesthetized albino rat. J Neurochem 28:897–916, 1977.

29. Subramanyam R, Alpert NM, Hoop B Jr, Brownell GL, Taveras JM: A model for regional cerebral oxygen distribution during continuous inhalation of ^{15}O$_2$, C^{15}O, and C^{15}O$_2$. J Nucl Med 19:48–53, 1978.

30. Wolf AP: Special characteristics and potential for radiopharmaceuticals for positron emission tomography. Semin Nucl Med 11:2–12, 1981.

22

Single Photon Tomography

Allan H. Friedman
Burton P. Drayer
Ronald J. Jaszczak

Single photon emission computed tomography is a technique of quantitatively and qualitatively mapping a three-dimensional distribution of a radionuclide. Standard radionuclide scans, as obtained with a rectilinear scanner or gamma camera, are two-dimensional reductions of a three-dimensional radionuclide distribution. The third dimension of the distribution must be extrapolated by the observer from multiple two-dimensional images obtained at different angles. An area of interest deep within the organ may be obscured by superimposed radionuclide densities. Further hampering the imaging of the radionuclide distribution within the organ is the attenuation of photons emitted from the radionuclide as they pass through tissue prior to reaching the detector. This attenuation is obviously greatest for photons that originate deep within the organ. In order to produce clear images of radionuclide distributions within an organ, two obstacles must be overcome. First, images resulting from radionuclide densities superimposed on the plane of interest must be eliminated, and second, a correction for photon attenuation by tissue lying between the radionuclide and the detector must be made.

These problems have led to the development of longitudinal and transverse emission tomography.[5] Longitudinal tomographic scanning devices yield images of longitudinal tomographic planes parallel to the long axis of the patient. This is analogous to conventional x-ray planar tomography and is accomplished by fitting the scanner with a focused collimator so that only points at a predetermined distance from the scanner remain in focus. Photons from planes overlying and underlying the plane of focus are blurred, becoming a homogenous background of activity. Multiplaner longitudinal tomographic devices, rotating slant hole collimation, and multiple pinhole imaging techniques have been employed in the development of longitudinal tomography devices. This technique has been successful in imaging small organs such as the thyroid. When the technique has been applied to larger organs, the images of the focused plane are obscured by the excessive homogenous background derived from the out-of-focus planes.

Emission computed axial tomography images transverse sections or cross-sectional slices of the radionuclide distribution. Emission computed tomography (ECT) uses many of the same strategies utilized in x-ray computed tomography or transmission computed tomography, the essential difference being that with ECT the source of the radiation is within the transverse section being scanned. Transmission computed tomography measures a physical parameter, the radiodensity of the material between the x-ray source and the detector. Emission computed tomography measures a physiological parameter, the ability of the organ to concentrate a radiopharmaceutical. While the x-ray absorption of a brain lesion and the surrounding brain may be similar, their ability to concentrate a radiopharmaceutical may differ severalfold, making these two methods of imaging complementary.

Two separate lines of investigation have been pursued in emission computed tomography, positron emission tomography (PET), and single photon emission computed tomography (SPECT). These two techniques differ in the types of radiopharmaceuticals employed by each. PET incorporates positron-emitting isotopes such as ^{11}C, ^{13}N, ^{15}O, and ^{18}F. The positron released in the nuclear decay of these isotopes interacts with a nearby electron to release two photons that travel in opposite directions. The strategies employed in PET scanning are outlined in another chapter of this text. Since all organic compounds of biological importance contain one or more of these elements, there is great hope that biologically useful tracer substances can be synthesized for this mode of emission computed tomography. The short half-life of the positron-emitting isotopes necessitate isotope production at the site of the scanner. The primary limitation to the widespread application of PET are the high capital and maintenance costs of the particle accelerator necessary for this production.

Single photon emission tomography employs the same type of gamma-emitting isotopes routinely employed in most hospital nuclear medicine departments, such as ^{99m}Tc, ^{201}Tl, and ^{123}I. The half-life of these isotopes is long enough that they can be produced in commercial nuclear reactors or accelerators and shipped to the hospital for incorporation into radiopharmaceuticals.

The SPECT camera generates images from projection data gathered at over 100 different angles. Because the images are constructed only from data gathered within the plane of interest, there is no degradation of the image from radionuclide densities above or below the imaged plane. SPECT data-collecting devices can be divided into those that employ individually collimated detectors and those that employ a scintillation camera. The individually collimated detector system originated with the work of Kuhl and Edwards in 1963. This type of system employs an array of detectors that encircle the single transverse section to be imaged. The array is designed to optimize the resolution and sensitivity within a single transverse section. Several refinements of Dr. Kuhl's apparatus have led to the Mark IV scanner, which uses 32 individual NaI scintillation crystals mounted in a square array with eight detectors on a side. A similar technique has been employed in the development of the Aberdeen scanner and the Headtome by Hattorie et al. of Japan.

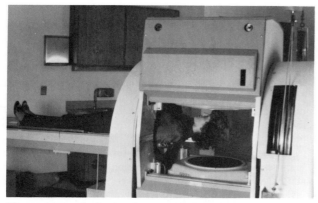

Figure 22-1 A single photon emission computed tomography (SPECT) system based on a rotating gamma camera. The Searle-Duke University SPECT system consists of two dual scintillation cameras mounted on a rotatable gantry.

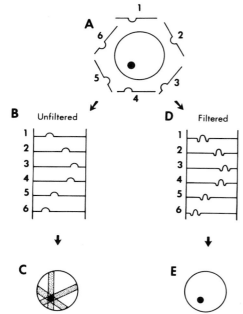

Figure 22-2 Reconstruction of a radionuclide density by SPECT techniques. *A, B.* The profile of the radionuclide density collected by the scanner in six positions around a transverse plane. *C.* The reconstruction of the image by projecting the six profiles back in the direction in which they were collected (note the star artifact). *D.* The collected profiles are manipulated by a mathematical function. *E.* The reconstruction of the image by projection of the filtered profiles back in the direction in which they were collected.

The rotating gamma camera devices (Jaszczak et al.; Keyer et al.) scan multiple transverse planes simultaneously (Fig. 22-1). One or two cameras are mounted on a gantry that rotates around the patient. The information gathered during a single revolution of the camera is used to construct multiple transverse, coronal, and sagittal section images (Fig. 22-2).

The image reconstruction process is similar in many respects to that employed in transmission computed tomography. Collimated radiation detectors (scintillation camera or individually collimated detectors) obtain count rate profiles at multiple angles around a transverse section of a defined thickness (Fig. 22-2A). The original image is then reconstructed using a simple back-projection algorithm. This method simply projects the count profile recorded at each angle back along its line of origin. The total number of events detected are then summed in a pixel-by-pixel fashion (Fig. 22-2B and C). Because the collected data only have positive values, pixels along the lines of the back projection receive a net positive value, giving rise to the star artifact. This artifact can be remedied by manipulating or following the original data with a mathematically derived correction factor (Fig. 22-2D and E). Radiation originating deep within the transverse section is attenuated by the tissue lying between the radionuclide and the detector. If no correction is made for this attenuation, the radionuclide densities deep within the transverse section will be interpreted as being of a lesser magnitude. Attenuation compensations are added at the time of reconstruction to correct for this observed decrease in count density from the central portion of the transverse section.[2]

SPECT scanning has been employed to measure local cerebral blood volume using ^{99m}Tc-labeled red cells.[3] En-

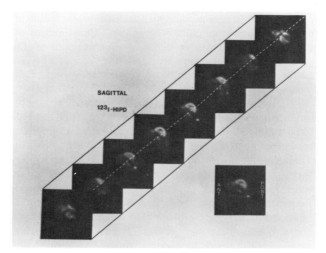

Figure 22-3 Cerebral blood flow in a baboon as measured by ^{123}I-labeled HIPD and imaged by SPECT. The multiple sagittal sections were reconstructed from a single scan. Serial coronal and axial images were obtained from the same scan. The baboon was given a single intravenous injection of ^{123}I-labeled HIPD. Quantitation of regional cerebral blood flow was obtained using microsphere methodology.

couraging reports have described the mapping of muscarinic cholinergic receptors and the scanning of myelin with single photon agents.

SPECT has been shown to be particularly useful in detecting areas of cerebral ischemia in the deep portions of the cerebral hemispheres that are difficult to evaluate in detail using traditional radionuclide methodology. Conventional ^{133}Xe-clearance techniques have incorporated SPECT scanning to produce three-dimensional flow maps of the brain. The accumulation of intra-arterially injected krypton 81m, a high-energy single photon–emitting radionuclide, can be monitored by SPECT scanning devices. Krypton 81m, which has a short half-life, can be generated in the hospital's nuclear medicine department from more stable ^{81}Rb. Although ^{81m}Kr infusion methods fail to provide accurate quantitation of cerebral blood flow, this method has demonstrated areas of relative ischemia in brain tissue that appeared normal on transmission computed tomography scans.

N,N,N'-Trimethyl-*N'*-(2-hydroxy-3-methyl-5-iodobenzyl)-1,3-propanediamine (HIPDm),[1] and *N*-propyl-*p*-iodoamphetamine (IMP)[4] have been used in conjunction with SPECT scanning to generate accurate flow maps of tomographic brain sections (Fig. 22-3). These lipophilic molecules are completely cleared during a single pass through the brain so that regional cerebral blood flow is proportional to the amount of ^{123}I locally deposited. These agents have a low toxicity and can be injected intravenously.

SPECT is a relatively low cost technique of imaging three-dimensional distribution of radionuclides. Its future applications in the imaging of brain metabolism rests on the development of appropriate radiopharmaceuticals.

References

1. Drayer BP, Jaszczak R, Friedman A, Kung H, Coleman E, Blau M, Trantosh K, Lischko M, Greer K: Tomographic measurement of regional brain perfusion using hydroxyiodopropyl-diamine and single photon-emission computed-tomography. Stroke 13:121, 1982 (abstr).
2. Jaszczak RJ, Coleman RE, Whitehead FR: Physical factors affecting quantitative measurements using camera-based single photon emission computed tomography (SPECT). IEEE Trans Nucl Sci 28:69–80, 1981.
3. Kuhl DE, Alavi A, Hoffman EJ, Phelps ME, Zimmerman RA, Obrist WD, Bruce DA, Greenberg JH, Uzzell B: Local cerebral blood volume in head-injured patients: Determination by emission computed tomography of ^{99m}Tc-labeled red cells. J Neurosurg 52:309–320, 1980.
4. Kuhl DE, Barrio JR, Huang S, Selin C, Ackermann RF, Lear JL, Wu JL, Lin TH, Phelps ME: Quantifying local cerebral blood flow by *N*-isopropyl-*p*-[^{123}I] iodoamphetamine (IMP) tomography. J Nucl Med 23:196–203, 1982.
5. Murphy PH, DePuey EG, Sonnemaker RE, Burdine JA: Emission computed tomography: A current status report, in Freeman LM, Weissmann HS (eds): *Nuclear Medicine Annual*. New York, Raven Press, 1980, pp 83–125.

23

Brain Imaging with Nuclear Magnetic Resonance

Michael Brant-Zawadzki

Just as the general medical community has attained a level of familiarity with the role of computed tomography (CT) in the diagnostic imaging armamentarium, a new modality capable of producing cross-sectional images has been introduced. Nuclear magnetic resonance (NMR) does not use ionizing radiation (x-rays), but is based on a known interaction of atomic nuclei placed in a static magnetic field and perturbed by radiowaves. The safety benefits derived from the method's use of low-level energy radiation represented by the radio-frequency waves and magnetic fields as well as the unprecedented level of information regarding tissue characteristics available from nuclear signals have combined to propel early research on the imaging potential of NMR to the point where clinical applicability is imminent.

Based on the Nobel prize–winning work of Bloch and Purcell done in the 1940s[1,10] NMR spectroscopy had become an accepted method of analysis for physical and biochemical samples. In the early 1970s, several investigators suggested the possibility that the principles of NMR could be used for medical purposes, and the first NMR images of the human body were produced.[6,9] Initial progress was slow, but over the past 2 years imaging with NMR has come of age.

Machines are now being installed and evaluated in the clinical setting so as to allow comparison with other techniques, and the results are proving quite favorable for the future implementation of NMR on a much greater scale.[2,3,7,8,11] Although its exact role remains to be defined, NMR has already demonstrated its superiority to CT in the detection of certain central nervous system (CNS) lesions and its complementary utility in the evaluation of others. The purpose of this chapter is to outline briefly the basic principles of NMR imaging and to illustrate its diagnostic capabilities in the evaluation of the CNS.

Basic Principles of NMR Imaging

Conventional radiographic techniques (including CT) rely on differences in electron density between tissues to variably affect x-ray attenuation. This differential transmission of x-rays is what effects differences in tissue density or contrast on the resulting images. Various radiographic contrast agents such as iodine or barium can be administered to enhance intrinsic contrast differences between tissues or their compartments. The NMR image is dependent on totally different tissue contrast parameters. Hydrogen density, the state of motion of the hydrogen, and the relaxation times T1 and T2, which represent the behavior of hydrogen protons within tissue that is placed in a strong magnetic field, all play a major role in the formation of an image.

Atomic nuclei with an odd number of protons or neutrons act like small magnets when placed in a strong magnetic field. The hydrogen nucleus with its single proton is the most ubiquitous of the body's elements to behave in this manner, and is thus the focus of current NMR imaging technology. An alignment of the hydrogen nuclei (protons) tends to occur in the magnetic field. A net magnetic vector or moment can be described for the population of nuclei so affected, one aligned with the magnetic field. Application of a radiofrequency (RF) pulse of a specific frequency (dependent on the strength of the magnetic field) introduces energy into the sample of protons and displaces the net magnetic vector by an amount determined by the amplitude and duration of the RF pulse. After the pulse is removed, the protons return to their original orientation and emit the absorbed energy in the form of an RF signal. This signal is detected and used to generate the NMR image. If the original magnetic field varies in a predetermined way, i.e., has a gradient introduced, the frequency of signals emitted by the irradiated protons will vary with their position in the gradient. In this manner, spatial information can be obtained.

The chemical state of the hydrogen atoms, and thus the nature of the surrounding tissue, dictates the time it takes for these protons to regain their original orientation, or to "relax," within the magnetic field after RF pulsation. Two basic forms of relaxation occur, T1 and T2 relaxation. Each can be measured. Each reflects a distinct physical characteristic of the tissue imaged. When protons are placed in a magnetic field, their magnetization and alignment (or realignment after an RF disturbance) occurs exponentially with the time constant T1, which reflects the interactions of the hydrogen nucleus with its molecular environment.

In forming an image, the RF pulses must be applied repetitively. After each pulse, the net proton alignment or magnetization of the sample is zero. Rapid repetition of the RF pulsation would not allow much magnetization to be re-established, and little signal would be seen. Thus, a certain time interval is necessary between successive RF pulses.

During exposure to the RF pulse, not only is the proton vector of magnetization altered, but coherent resonance of the protons is induced (a rapid, repetitive alteration of their energy state occurring in unison for all the protons). The magnitude of RF signal detected initially from a sample of protons during relaxation is dependent on the magnitude of their collective magnetization vector at the time of RF ir-radition (a T1 function), while the decay of this signal is dictated by the loss of coherent resonance induced by local inhomogeneities of the magnetic field. This decay of the signal as a result of loss of coherent resonance is characterized by the exponential function T2. Such local variations in magnetic field homogeneity are also related to tissue characteristics. It should be parenthetically noted that protons rapidly traversing the plane being imaged return relatively little signal during the acquisition sequence.

The characteristic tissue parameters (i.e., hydrogen density, the motion of hydrogen, and the T1 and T2 relaxation times of the particular tissue imaged) interact with certain parameters of the instrument to form the image, and the instrument parameters can be varied. For example, although the frequency of the pulse used to perturb the protons is characteristic for the magnet used, one can vary the strength and sequence of pulses, as well as the time between the application of the pulse and the point in time at which the signal from the excited nuclei is sampled. Because multiple tissue variables are encoded within the signal sampled, any one combination of instrument parameters, i.e., a single image, may produce a fortuitous similarity of the signal intensities from disparate tissues, causing lesions to be indistinguishable from their surrounding tissues. Therefore, the ability to vary the imaging sequence to highlight different combinations of T1 and T2 characteristics is an important flexibility to retain in an instrument. In our experience, the spin-echo technique as performed in our laboratory offers such flexibility.[5] We also use the inversion recovery technique, which emphasizes T1 tissue characteristics and highlights gray-white matter differences in the brain.

It should be noted that, although numerical values for T1 and T2 relaxation times for normal and abnormal tissues have been published, T1 and T2 relaxation values will vary from instrument to instrument since they depend on the particular imaging technique, method of calculation, and magnetic field strength used. Until some sort of standardization is accepted, it seems prudent to discuss T1 and T2 relaxation times in relative terms. In the same vein, even the clinical imaging results will vary somewhat from instrument to instrument, depending on the hardware and the sequences employed.

Our imager incorporates a 3.5 kG superconducting magnet and is currently capable of several imaging techniques. Up to 15 contiguous sections can be imaged in one of three planes in as little as 6.5 min, using the spin-echo technique. Each section includes several distinct images based on variable instrument parameters that encode differential contributions of T1 and T2, and allow calculation of these relaxation times. The particulars of our NMR imager and the techniques we employ have been the subject of a recent report,[4] and we refer the interested reader to that communication. We will next give a brief overview of our recent clinical experience in the evaluation of selected central nervous system (CNS) abnormalities with NMR. Because of the rapid evolution of NMR imaging techniques, the results herein, and others currently in publication, will likely be obsolete by the time they reach the reader. However, the clinical potential of NMR imaging is already apparent.

Clinical Applications

In illustrating the clinical use of NMR imaging of the CNS, it is worth remembering that the brain and spinal cord react nonspecifically to a broad spectrum of insults. Any cellular damage or breakdown of the blood-brain barrier is generally accompanied by an increase in the water content (edema) of the damaged tissue. Such edema represents probably the most common pathological alteration encountered in the CNS. The sensitivity of NMR in detecting disease in the CNS is strongly affected by its detection of brain edema.

Unlike CT, where the influx of water serves to decrease x-ray attenuation and produce low density on the image whether one is looking at brain edema or CSF, NMR detects the magnetic properties of protons, and these differ markedly in CSF as opposed to edematous brain. Hydrogen nuclei (protons) in a relatively pure fluid, such as cerebrospinal fluid (CSF), will behave differently during the NMR imaging sequence than those protons in impure fluids such as tissue edema, where water molecules attach to proteins. Also, the greater concentration of proteins in vasogenic as opposed to cytotoxic edema will differentially affect the signal characteristics of the tissue involved. Cerebral edema characteristically induces prolongation of T2 relaxation time and a less marked lengthening of T1 relaxation when compared with normal brain. This generally translates to high intensity on images obtained with spin-echo technique, when the signal from the "relaxing" protons is sampled 56 ms after their radiofrequency (RF) perturbation (Fig. 23-1).

Another frequent and nonspecific tissue alteration of the CNS is hemorrhage. This, too, is well detected with NMR as a result of the marked shortening of T1 relaxation seen in the involved brain.

Blood vessels are distinguished by virtue of the fact that rapidly moving protons return relatively little signal;[2] therefore, arteries are seen as tubular structures with very low intensity in their lumen. Slow or altered flow can be detected because of its characteristic intensity variation on images produced with variable instrument parameters.

Calcified tissue and dense bone have relatively little hydrogen, therefore little signal is seen from such normal structures as the pineal or the dense bone of the calvarium. Calcified brain lesions can be suspected when a focus of low intensity appears on an image, but a small fleck of calcium detectable with CT might be missed with NMR.

As stated above, the intensity of normal and abnormal tissue on a spin-echo image can be separated into contributions from either T1 or T2 relaxation, thus helping characterization. While the ability of NMR to distinguish one disease process from another is still being evaluated, it is worth remembering that CT's depiction of pathology is relatively nonspecific because of the nonspecific response of the CNS to a wide variety of insults. It is the accumulated experience in the appearance of certain lesions on CT before and after contrast injection, coupled with the clinical setting, that allows a concise differential diagnosis to be formulated. As experience with NMR is garnered, it is likely that a similar, or probably improved, ability to differentiate disease will be gained. This, together with the inherently greater sensitivity

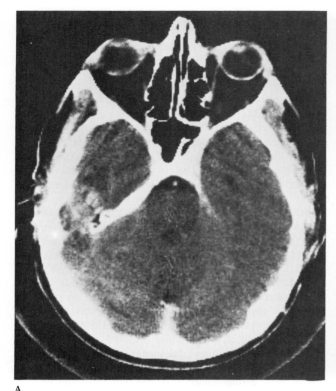

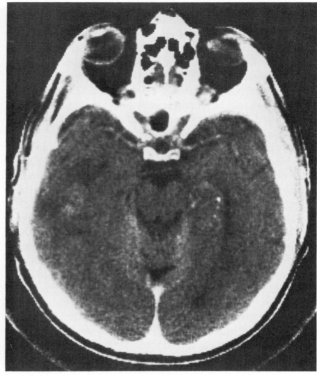

A

B

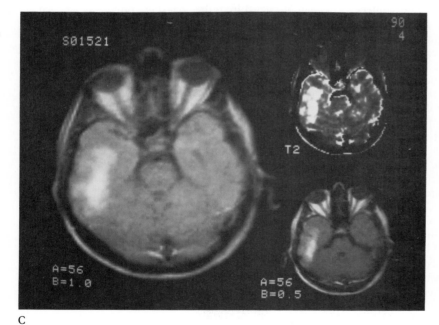

C

Figure 23-1 Brain edema, cerebral infarct. *A, B.* Contiguous CT sections (following IV contrast) at the petrous level and immediately above in a patient 17 days after right temporal infarction. Subtle edema with minimal contrast enhancement is seen on the higher section; bone streak artifact degrades the lower section. *C.* Axial spin-echo NMR image at level corresponding to *B* shows high-intensity signal from the infarcted brain. Inset (lower right) shows lower section, corresponding to *A.* Note absence of streak artifact. Upper inset is a synthesized image of the same section seen on the left in which each pixel is assigned a shade of gray based on the T2 relaxation time of that volume of tissue the pixel represents. By convention, long relaxation time is light, short is dark. The edematous brain exhibits very long T2 relaxation in this case.

of NMR to tissue contrast differences, should optimize the modality's diagnostic potential.

Over 75 patients with various brain and spinal cord images have been studied at our institution in the first 8 months of our experience. The spectrum of diseases included degenerative disorders, tumors, infarction, hemorrhage, arteriovenous malformations, and congenital abnormalities.

Degenerative Disease

Generalized degenerative disease usually manifests itself as regional or global brain atrophy, which is depicted with both NMR and CT as an ex vacuo enlargement of CSF spaces. More localized or focal disease processes, such as the demyelination plaque of multiple sclerosis, can be shown especially well with NMR.[12] The alteration of fat and consequent in-

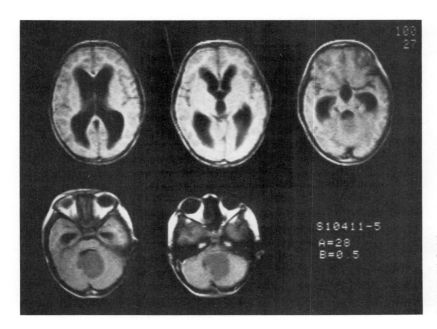

Figure 23-2 Medulloblastoma with hydrocephalus. Sequential axial spin-echo NMR images show the midline tumor in the posterior fossa (low intensity), compressing the fourth ventricle, causing hydrocephalus.

creased water content at the site of such a plaque correlates well with the high intensity seen in the lesions on spin-echo images. The inversion recovery images as currently performed on our instrument depict white matter as having a much higher intensity than gray matter, because of the former's shortened T1 relaxation characteristics. Hence a lesion in the white matter is seen as a low-intensity focus with the inversion recovery technique, and may be difficult

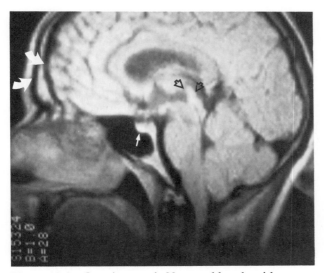

Figure 23-3 Germinoma. A 22-year-old male with Parinaud's syndrome shows a small focal tumor (*arrowheads*) just above the superior colliculus on a midline spin-echo NMR image. The cerebral aqueduct beneath the tumor is compressed. Biopsy verified the diagnosis. Incidentally, note the pituitary gland (*arrow*) and the high-intensity signal from the bone marrow in the clivus. Note too the diploe. The skull's cortical bone gives no signal, and is seen as black (*curved arrows*).

to distinguish from adjacent gray matter or CSF, which also have a low-intensity appearance on inversion recovery images.

Tumors

Whether primary or metastatic, most neoplasms in the brain sufficiently distort anatomy that their visualization with NMR is not difficult (Figs. 23-2 and 23-3). Even when the lesion is small and tissue distortion is subtle, intrinsic tumor characteristics or associated peripheral edema may help in the lesion's detection, although separation of tumor from edema with NMR may not be possible in certain instances.

The intrinsic tissue properties of some tumors allow a relatively specific characterization; for instance, NMR's sensitivity to fat (because of its short T1 relaxation) makes neoplasms with a lipomatous component easily discernible. The ability to obtain direct coronal and sagittal images with NMR is useful, especially in lesions involving the brain stem or spinal cord since the entire vertical extent of the abnormality and its anatomical relationships can be discerned (Figs. 23-4 and 23-5).

Further work in tumor diagnosis with NMR is needed. Questions have been raised regarding the capacity of NMR to separate benign from malignant tumors, but any such speculation is at best premature. The response of tumors to chemotherapy or radiation might be more sensitively evaluated with NMR than with current techniques.

Infarction

The earliest pathological change in an area of infarcted brain detectable with NMR is the increase in water content. Such an increase prolongs the T1 and especially the T2 relaxation time of protons in the tissue involved (Fig. 23-1).

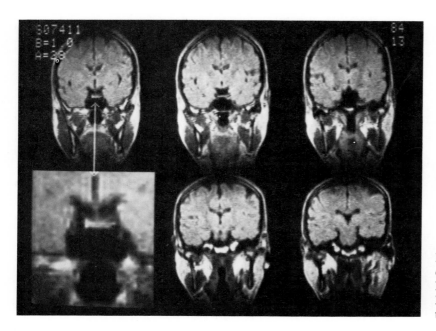

Figure 23-4 Normal volunteer, direct coronal imaging. Sequential spin-echo NMR images through the frontal horns. Inset shows magnification of the pituitary stalk and gland.

If a hemorrhagic component is present in the infarct, the resulting high-intensity component on the spin-echo images is due to the shortened T1 relaxation induced by blood. By proper use of instrument parameters and calculation of T1 and T2 relaxation times, the hemorrhagic and edematous components of an infarct (or other lesion; see below) can be separated. It is worth re-emphasizing that numerical T1 and T2 quantification is a function of both the tissue characteristics and the NMR instrument and methodology used for their calculation. Therefore, numerical tissue T1 and T2 values may vary in imagers from different institutions. It is useful to express T1 and T2 tissue differences in relative or analogue form. After calculating T1 and T2 times on an imaged section, our imager can then synthesize a T1 or T2 image or "map" of that section, on which each pixel has a gray scale representation corresponding to its numerical T1 or T2 value. In this manner, calculated T1 or T2 differences of a given tissue or lesion can be depicted with the surrounding brain as "control" (Fig. 23-1C inset).

Arteriovenous Malformation (AVM)

The rapidly flowing protons within the feeding and draining vessels associated with an AVM do not participate in the NMR imaging process of any given section for a long enough time to return a strong signal. Therefore, these or any rapidly flowing vessels appear prominently as tubular structures with a very low internal intensity. Hemorrhage from such a malformation is easily detected.

Cryptic arteriovenous malformations are a greater diagnostic challenge. They are not detectable with angiography and may present a very atypical appearance on CT. Subclinical hemorrhage may occur, and the resulting clot may develop granulation tissue at its borders, leading to peripheral enhancement on CT. An old clot will not attenuate x-rays as much as normal brain; therefore a low-density lesion with

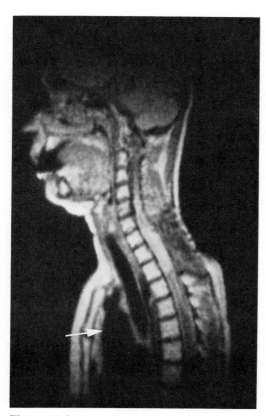

Figure 23-5 Recurrent ependymoma. Direct sagittal image shows the tumor at the cervicothoracic junction. Note the aortic arch and cervical pedicle (*arrow*) seen as black as a result of the rapidly flowing protons (see text).

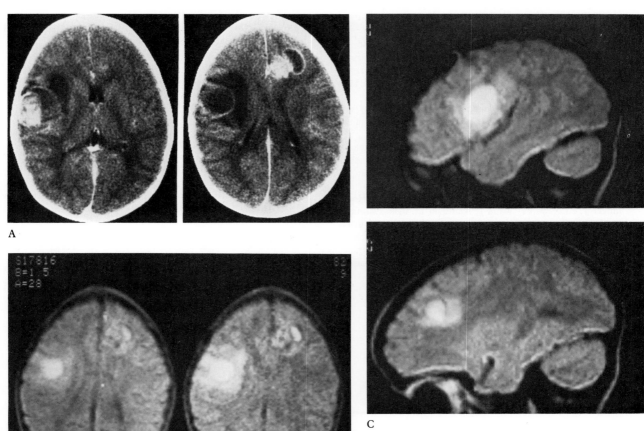

C

Figure 23-6 Cryptic AVM. *A.* Adjacent CT sections show bilateral intra-axial lesions with areas of ring enhancement, homogeneous enhancement, and edema. *B.* Axial spin-echo images of the same section, the first sampling the nuclear signal 28 ms after RF perturbation, the second sampling 56 ms after RF perturbation. The persistent central high intensity indicates a short T1 relaxation, suggesting a clot within the core of the lesion. The increase in peripheral intensity suggests edema in the surrounding tissue. *C.* Sagittal spin-echo NMR images of both the right-sided (top) and left-sided (bottom) lesions. Surgical excision verified the diagnosis.

ring enhancement may be seen on CT, simulating tumor (Fig. 23-6A). Peripheral edema may be present and indistinguishable from old thrombus by CT.

NMR, however, is better able to characterize such a lesion. It is able to identify hemorrhage (old or new) as a very high intensity signal, possibly because of the influence of the iron ion and/or its carrier molecule on the magnetic properties of the surrounding protons. The very short T1 relaxation time of hemorrhage distinguishes it from the slight prolongation of T1 relaxation and the more definite prolongation of T2 relaxation of edema, despite the similar high intensity that both produce on selected spin-echo images (Fig. 23-6B and C).

The clinical case material briefly illustrated in this communication suggests that NMR has already achieved a stage of development that allows clinical utility. Spatial detail rivals that of CT. Bone streak artifacts so prevalent on CT images of the posterior fossa and spine are not a problem for NMR. Tissue contrast resolution allows early detection of such processes as edema, hemorrhage, and alterations in lipid content. NMR studies can be performed efficiently,

and multiple planes can be imaged. The absence of ionizing radiation offers safety benefits. Currently, difficulties with metallic life-support equipment (e.g., respirators, pacemakers) limit the spectrum of patients who can be imaged, but such limitations can be overcome in future designs of the life-support equipment. Those institutions already using a CT scanner and considering a second one are beginning to consider an NMR imager instead.

The current role of NMR imaging with respect to CT is only now being evaluated. Its future potential in diagnosis has only begun to be explored. In the course of the next 5 years, the medical imaging field will change drastically because of the impact of NMR. For this reason, the astute clinician will start becoming familiar with this new modality.

References

1. Bloch F: Nuclear induction. Phys Rev 70:460–474, 1946.
2. Brant-Zawadzki M, Davis PL, Crooks LE, Mills CM, Norman D, Newton TH, Sheldon P, Kaufman L: NMR demonstration of cerebral abnormalities: Comparison with CT. AJNR 4:117–124, 1983.
3. Bydder GM, Steiner RE, Young IR, Hall AS, Thomas DJ, Marshall J, Pallis CA, Legg NJ: Clinical NMR imaging of the brain: 140 cases. AJR 139:215–236, 1982.
4. Crooks L, Arakawa M, Hoenninger J, Watts J, McRee R, Kaufman L, Davis PL, Margulis AR, DeGroot J: Nuclear magnetic resonance whole-body imager operating at 3.5 KGauss. Radiology 143:169–174, 1982.
5. Crooks LE, Mills CM, Davis PL, Brant-Zawadzki M, Hoenninger J, Arakawa M, Watts J, Kaufman L: Visualization of cerebral and vascular abnormalities by NMR imaging: The effects of imaging parameters on contrast. Radiology 144:843–852, 1982.
6. Damadian R: Tumor detection by nuclear magnetic resonance. Science 171:1151–1153, 1971.
7. Holland GN, Hawkes RC, Moore WS: Nuclear magnetic resonance (NMR) tomography of the brain: Coronal and sagittal sections. J Comput Assist Tomogr 4:429–433, 1980.
8. James AE Jr, Partain CL, Holland GN, Gore JC, Rollo FD, Harms SE, Price RF: Nuclear magnetic resonance imaging: The current state. AJR 138:201–210, 1982.
9. Lauterbur PC: Image formation by induced local interactions: Examples employing nuclear magnetic resonance. Nature 242:190–191, 1973.
10. Purcell EM, Torrey HC, Pound RV: Resonance absorption by nuclear magnetic moments in a solid. Phys Res 69:37–38, 1946.
11. Young IR, Burl M, Clarke GJ, Hall AS, Pasmore T, Collins AG, Smith DT, Orr JS, Bydder GM, Doyle FH, Greenspan RH, Steiner RE: Magnetic resonance properties of hydrogen: Imaging the posterior fossa. AJR 137:895–901, 1981.
12. Young IR, Hall AS, Pallis CA, Legg NJ, Bydder GM, Steiner RE: Nuclear magnetic resonance imaging of the brain in multiple sclerosis. Lancet 2:1063–1066, 1981.

24

Ultrasonic Brain Imaging in Pediatric Neurosurgery

Philip R. Weinstein
Kai Haber

Recent advances in diagnostic ultrasound technology have resulted in new applications in pediatric neurosurgery. These include imaging of brain ventricles, cystic lesions, and acute or chronic hematoma in the perinatal age group, where fontanelle and sutures remain patent or cranial bone thickness does not impede transmission of sound waves. Fetal examination with abdominal ultrasonography is becoming a routine method for early detection of developmental central nervous system anomalies in utero. Use of ultrasound for localization of brain lesions during craniotomy will be described in a later chapter.

Ultrasound Technology

Ultrasound imaging uses sound waves of a very high frequency (2 to 10 MHz), which is far above the level of the 15,000- to 20,000-cps (cycles per second) range of human hearing.[5] The physical principles are similar to those exploited by bats in the air and by porpoises and dolphins under water for navigation and food finding. Pulses of high-frequency sound waves are emitted by ultrasonic transducers. The sound wave is transmitted at a velocity that depends upon the density of the medium through which it is traveling. When the ultrasonic energy reaches an interface between two media of different densities, a portion of the pulse will be reflected back as an echo. The returning sound wave is received by the crystal in the transducer, which converts sonic energy to an electric impulse.

The earliest ultrasound devices applied to neurodiagnosis utilized A-mode (for amplitude-based) echo encephalography. This equipment registers large alterations in echo amplitude that correlates with the position of midline CSF–brain tissue interfaces occurring in relation to the third ventricle and thalamus. The amplitude and relative positions of the returning echoes vary with respect to the degree of density difference between the two media forming the interface and the distance that the reflecting interface is located from the transducer. When tissue densities and sound velocities are known, distance can be derived from the time required for reception of returning echoes, and a determination can be made as to whether or not there is a shift of midline brain structures as a result of the presence of an intracranial mass lesion. A-mode brain examinations are technically quite difficult, and the resultant display, even when accurate, is not in the form of a two-dimensional image. Today A mode has been supplanted in most modern centers by more sophisticated ultrasonic imaging techniques.

On the other hand, scanning by B (or brightness) mode, which translates information as to the amplitude and distance of returning echoes into levels of brightness or shades of gray on a two-dimensional image, has developed rapidly as an accurate diagnostic method that avoids ionizing radiation and causes no harmful biological effect.[5] The B-mode scanner displays images composed of 16 to 32 shades of gray with brightness and location in relation to the transducer determined by the integral of the amplitude function and the distance of the reflecting surface from the transducer.

There are two types of B-mode scanners currently in use. Static scanners obtain a series of discrete images that are of limited diagnostic value in the brain as resolution is often poor because of inadequate transducer-skull contact. Real-time scanners provide a rapid sequence of images useful for visualizing moving structures in the brain and other organs. Sector real-time transducers are mechanically or electronically moved through a given angle (usually 90 degrees) and provide a high-resolution image that is updated approximately 25 times per second (thus, the term *real-time*). Such scanners have relatively small transducer surfaces, which are most appropriate for positioning and aiming through the anterior fontanelle in infants (Fig. 24-1). Linear array real-time scanners utilize a much larger transducer, which has been most appropriate for transabdominal intrauterine visualization of fetal cranial and spinal structures.

The most sophisticated ultrasound scanning device currently in use for pediatric neurosurgical applications is the Octoson system (The Ausonics Corporation, New Berlin, Wis.), which is a fully automated tomographic scanner that interposes a water-filled mattress between the patient and an array of eight transducers to provide panoramic high-resolution images as coronal or axial tomographic sections similar to those obtained with CT scanners (Fig. 24-2).[6] The Octoson is not limited by perinatal skull bone thickness or contour, and it does not depend upon acoustic windows such as the fontanelle or sutures as does the realtime sector scanner.[6] However, increasing skull thickness after the age of 24 months often results in image degradation, and successful scans cannot be routinely obtained after the age of 2. Image orientation is simplified with this device since the entire circumference of the head is visualized on each section (Fig. 24-3). Unlike with CT scanning, sedation is rarely required, since most infants are calm or sleeping after positioning on the water bed mattress. Instantaneous screen monitoring of the processed images enables the radiologist to correct the position of the transducer arc in order to optimize visualization of normal or pathological anatomy. However, real-time sector scanners are less expensive and portable, providing a practical method for brain imaging in the neonatal intensive care unit or the community hospital.

In our initial series of patients studied with the Octoson unit, CT scans were also obtained in 19 cases.[6] Ventricular size and fluid cyst measurements demonstrated a high degree of correlation on linear regression analysis. Since scanning time is 0.5 to 2 s for each image, there was less problem due to patient motion with Octoson studies than with CT. In addition to hydrocephalus, other fluid-filled lesions such as arachnoid and porencephalic cysts and Dandy-Walker cysts as well as corpus callosum agenesis were clearly demonstrated. In a few cases neoplastic lesions such as midbrain

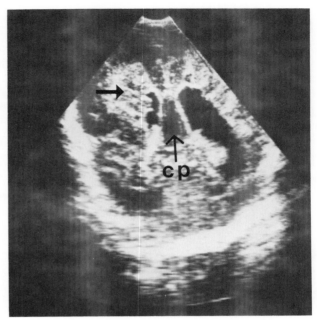

A

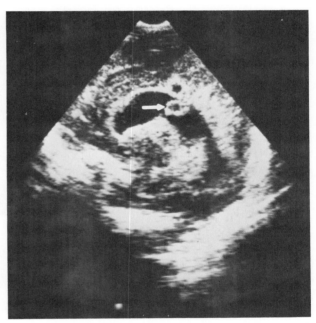

B

Figure 24-1 Coronal (*A*) and right parasagittal (*B*) real-time sector images of premature infant with right anterior parietal parenchymal hemorrhage showing some early liquefaction (*black arrow*). Cavum septi pellucidi (cp) is clearly seen between dilated lateral ventricles. The parasagittal section shows intraventricular blood clot (*white arrow*) and adjacent small posterior parietal intracerebral hematoma. Both have central lucencies also representing central liquefaction.

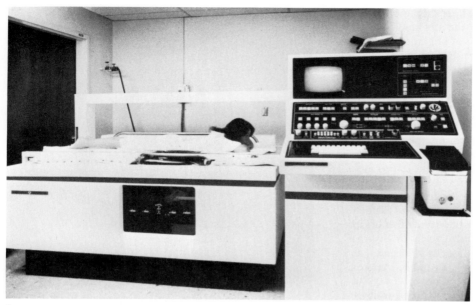

A

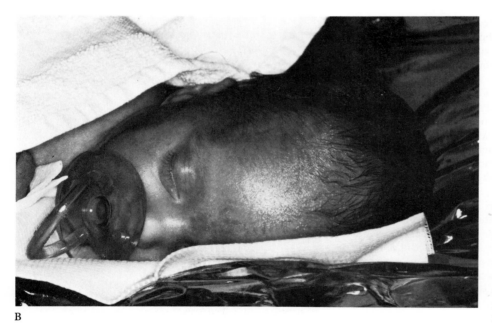

B

Figure 24-2 *A*. Octoson ultrasonic instrument showing patient lying upon water tank in which the eight transducers are submerged. They are steered by remote control by operator from console on the right. *B*. Positioning of infant's head for scanning.

glioma and cerebral lymphoma were identified with resolution equal to that on CT scans. False-negative results were obtained in only 6 of 54 patients in whom small germinal matrix hemorrhages were demonstrated on CT but not by Octoson. However, intraventricular or intracerebral hematoma, as well as associated mass effect shifting the ventricles, were clearly demonstrated in other patients.

Fluid-filled low-density structures transmit echoes with minimal reflection to the transducer. Accordingly, CSF-filled ventricles or cystic lesions of the brain appear anechoic. Brain tissue and blood clot, being relatively dense or echogenic, produce bright echoes.

Applications and Results

Intrauterine Diagnosis of CNS Anomalies

Since ultrasound examination presents no danger whatsoever to mother or fetus during pregnancy, scanning has become a routine screening procedure during pregnancy.[5] Real-time scanners provide an instantaneous image of fetal anatomy and activity.[4] Head size can be measured and antenatal diagnosis of hydrocephalus can be made based upon the ratio of ventricular size to that of the cerebral hemi-

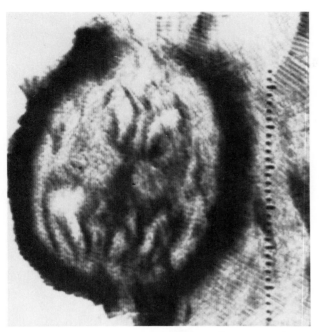

Figure 24-3 Octoson semiaxial image of premature infant with mild hydrocephalus and small area of germinal matrix hemorrhage in head of left caudate nucleus. Orientation is the same as for CT scan, with patient's right on reader's left.

spheres. Normal values for lateral ventricle and hemisphere size have been established for various stages of gestation. Lateral ventricular/hemispheric ratios as high as 50 to 60 percent are normal up to 20 weeks of gestation. However, extension of the lateral ventricles beyond a point midway between the falx and outer table of the skull after 17 weeks of gestation is indicative of developing hydrocephalus.[3] In cases of aqueductal obstruction, disproportionate or selective dilatation of the occipital horns may be observed, and it is therefore especially important to attempt to visualize the entire ventricular system sonographically. Although ventricular dilatation may precede increase in head circumference, both before and after delivery, eventually an increase in biparietal skull diameter as a measure of head circumference may be evident in utero. When the biparietal diameter exceeds the fetal abdominal diameter by more than 2 cm, it is considered to be indicative of cranial growth out of proportion to gestational age and body size as a result of hydrocephalus. Accordingly, high-risk pregnancies in women with a previous history of hydrocephalic infants should receive routine sonographic evaluation.

Other anomalies such as occipital encephalocele, hydranencephaly, and rachischisis have also been identified with antenatal ultrasound scanning.[9] Lesions characterized by poor developmental prognosis such as hydrocephalus with head circumference of more than 50 cm and cerebral mantle thickness of less than 0.5 cm can be identified with ultrasonography, providing a basis for appropriate antenatal counseling and planning for the parents. For example, vaginal delivery preceded by transvaginal ventricular aspiration would be more appropriate than cesarean section in a case of hydranencephaly. On the other hand, we have identified a large occipital meningoencephalocele antenatally that was not associated with hydrocephalus or significant brain deformity. After consultation with the parents, this child was delivered by cesarean section followed by immediate surgical repair without rupture of the giant, but delicate, meningocele sac. In this case advance diagnosis prevented possible contamination or rupture of the sac during delivery and delay of definitive surgical repair. Microcephalus is difficult to diagnose sonographically because gestational age may be unsure and comparison of cranial with abdominal diameters inaccurate.[4]

Spinal anomalies such as meningomyelocoele, which occur at a rate of 1 per 800 births, can also be diagnosed sonographically after 12 to 20 weeks of gestation by visualization of the cystic mass adjacent to the spinal column or the typical V-shaped diversion of the normally parallel sonographic spinal images.[7] However, lesions less than 2 cm in diameter may be missed. Again, advance warning based upon prenatal sonography may facilitate atraumatic vaginal delivery as well as reduce emotional difficulties experienced by parents.

When spina bifida with an open neural tube defect or anencephaly are present, elevated amniotic fluid α-fetoprotein levels may be obtained. However, ultrasound scanning will then be necessary to identify the nature and severity of the developmental anomaly as well as to rule out other diagnoses associated with this nonspecific finding, such as Turner's syndrome, duodenal atresia, congenital nephrosis, and impending fetal death.[4]

Intrauterine Treatment of Hydrocephalus

Use of ultrasound scanning to locate the optimum site for transcutaneous amniocentesis by visualizing the location of the placenta and fetus has suggested the possibility of intrauterine treatment of cystic lesions such as urinary outflow tract obstruction and hydrocephalus. Under real-time ultrasound control, serial bladder or ventricular aspiration can be accomplished with a reasonable degree of safety. Since ventricular size can be estimated with ultrasound scanning beginning in the second trimester and defective CNS embryogenesis should be detectable by 20 weeks of gestation, early diagnosis and treatment of hydrocephalus with serial CSF aspiration is possible.[1] Increased intracranial pressure, which develops as cranial ossification progresses, can be prevented in cases where a 1 cm cerebral mantle is present. Ventriculoamniotic shunting to drain CSF accumulation after percutaneous catheter placement under sonographic control has also been reported.[2] Although these procedures remain experimental at this time, there is reason to expect that antenatal treatment of hydrocephalus utilizing these techniques may promote more normal brain development or at least prevent severe cerebral atrophy due to in utero obstructive hydrocephalus.

Postnatal Ultrasound Scanning

Because of the decreased risk, expense, and disturbance to the infant as compared with CT scanning, serial ultrasound scans can be carried out on a routine basis after delivery in

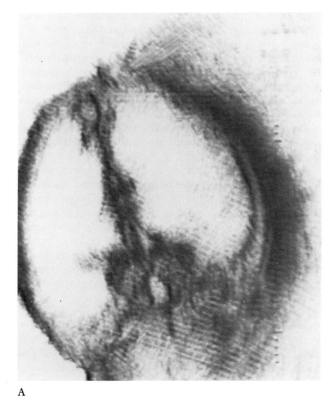

A

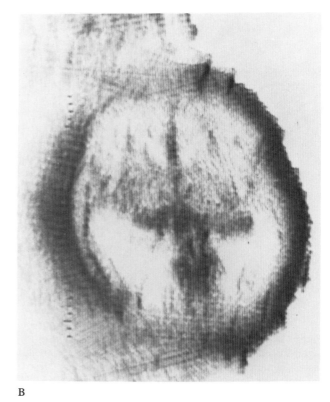

B

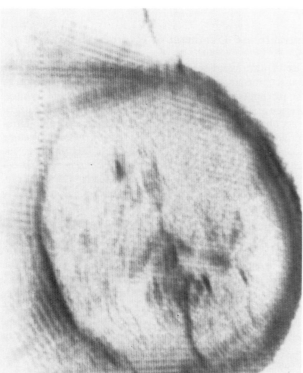

C

Figure 24-4 *A.* A ventriculoperitoneal shunt was placed in this neonate with marked hydrocephalus. Octoson examinations obtained 2 days (*B*) and 5½ months (*C*) postoperatively demonstrate dramatic response to surgical treatment. (From Smith et al.[8])

patients in whom the possibility of development of hydrocephalus is significant. Sequential scanning in premature infants can not only detect germinal matrix or intraventricu-lar hemorrhage but also provides an accurate method of documenting increase or stabilization of ventricular size. Results of serial lumbar or ventricular punctures can be monitored. Indication for ventricular shunting can be clearly and accurately defined. Following repair of meningomyelocele or encephalocele in children who initially demonstrate normal ventricular size, progressive enlargement requiring shunting has been demonstrated before the onset of increased intracranial pressure diagnosed by palpation at the anterior fontanelle or measurement of increase in head circumference. Postoperative evaluation of patients with Dandy-Walker cysts and either supratentorial or infratentorial arachnoid or ependymal cysts has been similarly helpful with respect to determining whether or not decompression of both the cysts and the ventricular system has been accomplished by surgery and shunting (Fig. 24-4).

We have routinely obtained daily ultrasound scans following shunt surgery and monthly scans after hospital discharge in an effort to evaluate the time course of response to shunting and its clinical significance.[8] In this study an average of 74 percent of the decrease in ventricular size seen within the first 6 postoperative days had occurred within the first 24 h after shunting. An average of 49 percent of the ultimate decrease in ventricular size had occurred by the end of the first postoperative week. Absence of early and rapid decrease in ventricular size after shunting appears to be associated with poor prognosis, although results of long-term follow-up in these cases are not yet available.

Complications or failure of ventricular shunting were often identified before symptoms developed or in association with minimal clinical signs and symptoms. Early recurrence of shunt obstruction, ventricular cysts, nondecompressed ependymal cysts, and subdural hygroma due to mantle collapse could also be clearly visualized (Fig. 24-5). Occasionally, subgaleal hygroma was demonstrated as a sign of obstruction of the distal shunt catheter. Ultrasound scans were also obtained to document adequacy of shunt function in children who later developed irritability, anorexia, or emesis, often in association with viral infections or other unrelated medical problems.

Information obtained from ultrasound examination in this setting duplicated or in some cases surpassed that provided by CT scanning. Since ultrasound examination is exquisitely sensitive to tissue-fluid interfaces, imaging of thin-walled ventricular cysts missed by CT scan without intraventricular contrast injection has been accomplished sonographically with the Octoson unit.

In patients with ventricular drainage established because of shunt infection or intraventricular hemorrhage, adequacy of ventriculostomy function can be monitored with serial ultrasound scans. In some cases, delayed onset of outflow obstruction in a lateral or fourth ventricle has been demonstrated and corrected with additional drainage procedures.

In a few cases, borderline ventriculomegaly associated with communicating hydrocephalus after neonatal hemorrhage or meningitis has been followed expectantly with serial outpatient ultrasound scans. When ventricular size stabilized or decreased, shunting was deferred with a diagnosis of satisfactorily compensated or resolving hydrocephalus.

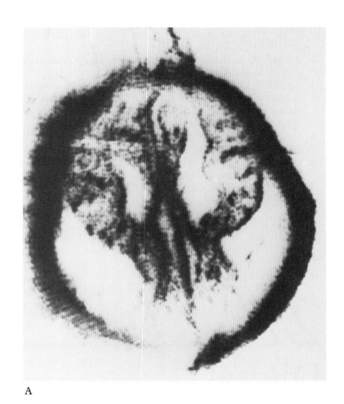

A

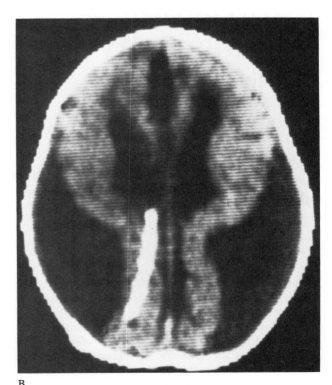

B

Figure 24-5 Octoson image (A) and CT scan (B) of a 7-month-old child with mild hydrocephalus after shunt placement, showing bilateral occipital subdural hygromas. Note visualization of the shunt tube in both images. (From Haber et al.[6])

References

1. Birnholz JC, Frigoletto FD: Antenatal treatment of hydrocephalus. N Engl J Med 304:1021–1023, 1981.
2. Brodner RA: Intracranial surgery in the fetus: Rat, dog and monkey models. Presented at the 51st Annual Meeting of the American Association of Neurological Surgeons, Honolulu, Hawaii, April 26, 1982.
3. Campbell S: Early prenatal diagnosis of neural tube defects by ultrasound. Clin Obstet Gynecol 20:351–359, 1977.
4. Dunne MG, Johnson ML: The ultrasonic demonstration of fetal abnormalities in utero. J Reprod Med 23:195–206, 1979.
5. Haber K: An introduction to B-scan ultrasonography: For the primary care physician. Ariz Med 35:322–326, 1978.
6. Haber K, Wachter RD, Christenson PC, Vaucher Y, Sahn DJ, Smith JR: Ultrasonic evaluation of intracranial pathology in infants: A new technique. Radiology 134:173–178, 1980.
7. Herzog KA: The detection of fetal meningocele and meningoencephalocele by B-scan ultrasound: A case report. J Clin Ultrasound 3:307–308 1975.
8. Smith JRL, Haber K, Reynolds AF, Weinstein PR: Ultrasonic evaluation of postventricular shunt dynamics in infants and young children. Radiology 145:133–138, 1982.
9. Weinstein P, Weinstein L, Dotters D, Bedrick A, Anderson C: Prenatal diagnosis of occipital encephalocoele by ultrasound scanning. Neurosurgery 12:680–683, 1983.

25

Digital Subtraction Angiography

Meredith A. Weinstein
Michael T. Modic
Anthony J. Furlan
William Pavlicek
John R. Little

Intravenous angiography is a safe, rapid procedure that can be performed on an outpatient basis and provide diagnostic information comparable to conventional angiography. Intravenous angiography is performed by obtaining a radiographic exposure of a portion of the body before and after the intravenous administration of contrast material. The image obtained prior to the administration of contrast material is subtracted from an image obtained after the administration of contrast material. Christenson et al. reported that a 2 to 3 percent concentration of contrast material can be visualized with digital intravenous subtration.[5] A 40 to 50 percent intra-arterial concentration is needed to produce images of equal contrast with unsubtracted film screen radiography.

Brief History of Intravenous Angiography, Analog and Digital

Robb and Steinberg performed "analog" intravenous angiography in 1939.[13] In spite of improvements by Bernstein et al.[2] and Steinberg et al.[17] in the late 1950s, intravenous angiography did not gain widespread acceptance because of the large amounts of contrast material that were needed and because of the poor quality of the vascular images. In 1982, Manelfe et al. reported 1000 examinations of the extracranial cerebral arteries by intravenous angiography using conventional film screens.[9] These studies were superior to earlier studies primarily because of improvements in radiographic film, film screens, film subtraction technique, and contrast media.

Major contributions to the development of digital subtraction angiography (DSA) were made by groups at the University of Wisconsin[6] and the University of Arizona[14] in the late 1970s. Recent improvements in computers, television systems, radiographic image intensifiers, and digital electronic storage devices have made DSA technology possible. Real-time subtraction with DSA is a result of the recent availability of low-cost computers with high-speed data acquisition systems.

Digital Versus Analog Radiography

When a beam of x-rays is transmitted through a patient in conventional angiography, the x-rays are absorbed in a film screen cassette. The film screen cassette is designed so that a scintillating screen absorbs the majority of the x-rays striking it. The light given off by this screen then exposes the film, which is developed. There are certain attributes of this system that are not optimum. The crystal in the scintillation screen does not absorb all the x-rays to which the screen is exposed. The amount of light given off by the screen is relatively small with little amplification. The film that is used to record the light has three major limitations. It has a fixed response to variations in radiation exposure. It has a fixed contrast, and small differences cannot be enhanced in their shades of gray. It has a major loss of contrast at either low or high regions of radiation exposure.

Digital radiography represents a new way to record radiographic data. A digital image is made by obtaining a fluoroscopic exposure of a portion of the body with the use of an image intensifier. The crystal in an image intensifier absorbs approximately 60 percent of the incident x-rays. Because of electronic amplification, the light emitted by an image intensifier is much brighter than that given off by conventional film screens. The light levels are sufficiently bright to be viewed by a television camera. The signal produced by the television camera is converted from analog to digital form.

In digital radiography, shades of darkness and degrees of contrast are assigned numbers. An infinite number of copies can be made of digitized data, each a perfect copy of the other. Previously, most radiographic data were recorded in an analog mode on either radiographic film or cine film. In analog recording, the numbers are represented by directly measurable quantities such as light or voltage. The density of radiographic films is analogous to the amount of light or x-rays to which they have been exposed. Once the film is exposed, there can be no further manipulation of the data.

With digital radiography, the x-rays are converted to a video signal. The image on the television monitor is completely variable and not fixed to one speed of film. The contrast is also variable within the limits of the information presented.

With analog or film recordings of a chest roentgenogram, one must decide before the exposure if one is going to examine the lungs or the bones. With a digital recording of a single chest x-ray, the data can be modified so that the lungs, the heart, and the bones can be optimally examined after a single exposure. Because this system is versatile and not fixed with respect to speed or contrast, there is virtually never a need to repeat the exposure because of improper technique. The ability to get a "perfect" exposure every time reduces x-ray exposure and increases the productivity of the x-ray technician and x-ray equipment.

Digital Angiography Versus Conventional Film Screen Angiography

Modern image intensifier tubes provide an essentially noiseless electronic amplification of the light signal from the cesium iodide crystals used as detectors. When these images are scanned with low-noise television cameras, small differences in radiation exposure can be more faithfully detected. This results in a better contrast sensitivity with DSA compared with conventional angiography. With DSA, the digital memory and electronic subtraction produce real-time images and the capability to remask instantly. This obviates the time-consuming and expensive process of manual film screen subtraction. The elimination of background information by subtraction results in a marked increase in the degree to which an area of interest stands out from its surroundings (conspicuity).

All film has an H and D curve, which is a graph of the optical density versus the log of exposure. Conventional film screens are limited by a fixed H and D curve. In the "toe" and "shoulder" regions of the H and D curve, the change in the optical density or contrast produced by an equal difference of radiation exposure is much less than that produced in the straight-line portion of the curve, since the slope of the curve is less in the toe and shoulder regions.

With digital radiography, the change in optical density has a linear relation to the logarithm of the exposure dose. The contrast changes of vessels overlying bone and air-containing structures are linear with DSA and nonlinear with conventional film screen because of their location in either the toe or shoulder regions of the H and D curve. Subtractions obtained with DSA are more accurate than conventional film screen subtractions, because the attenuation of iodine will be constant with DSA and will vary with conventional film screens depending on whether the iodine is located in the toe, on the slope, or in the shoulder region of the H and D curve.

The spatial resolution of conventional film screens is 5 to 6 line pairs per millimeter, and the spatial resolution of DSA is approximately 2 lines per millimeter. The spatial resolution of DSA is limited by the size of the matrix, by the number of lines of the television system, and the image intensifier blurr.

An intravenous (IV) DSA study can be stored on tape with hard copies at a cost of approximately $10 per examination. Conventional angiography requires $60 to $100 in film cost alone.

Contrast material is injected intravenously for digital subtraction angiography. This can be performed as an outpatient procedure. DSA requires significantly less material and staff than does conventional intra-arterial angiography. If the intravenous catheter is inserted while the patient is outside the DSA room, one examination can be performed every 20 to 30 min.

Because the contrast material is injected intravenously, there is no risk of stroke by embolic material. In our experience with more than 8000 IV DSA examinations, we have had no serious morbidity. Transient renal dysfunction occurred in one patient, underscoring the need for proper hydration and for routine assessment of kidney function prior to IV DSA. Arm vein cannulation has been associated with a very low incidence of venous extravasation (less than 1 in 1000 cases). We have not experienced problems with cardiac dysrhythmias and do not routinely monitor our patients undergoing IV DSA. Contrast reactions are the most serious potential complication of IV DSA. The risk of death parallels that of any intravenous contrast procedure and approximates 1 in 70,000 cases.

Technique

At our institution, DSA is performed with a 1300 mA x-ray generator. The x-ray generator supplies a water-cooled x-ray tube having a nominal focal spot selection of 0.6/1.2 mm with a heat capacity of 1.8 million heat units. X-rays are detected using a 9-, 6-, 4.5 in. cesium iodide image intensifying tube. An 8:1 grid with 40 line pairs per centimeter is used. The output phosphor of the image tube is scanned with a video camera with a lead oxide tube. The video signal from the camera is logarithmically amplified and digitized for storage in the imager, which currently has two 512 × 512 × 10 bit memories. A PDP 11/34 computer (Digital Equipment Co., Maynard, Mass.) is used for image processing.

Before the arrival of contrast media at the region of interest, an image is converted to digital form and stored in one of the memories. This image, termed the *mask image*, is subtracted from subsequent images containing contrast material, also digitized, and the resultant images are viewed in real time.

To expedite throughput an 8-in., 16-gauge intravenous catheter is inserted into an arm vein by a nurse in a holding area. The catheter is attached to a 50-ml solution of dextrose and water for constant infusion to maintain patency. A peripheral arm vein catheter is used to examine large vessels such as the carotid bifurcations and aortic arch. The advantages of injecting into a peripheral arm vein rather than into the superior vena cava are:

1. A nurse can insert the catheter, saving physician time.
2. The catheter can be inserted outside the room, saving room time and increasing patient throughput.
3. With this catheter, there is no need to use a sterile pack and angiographic wires.

To examine smaller vessels such as the intracranial vessels, a catheter is placed into the superior vena cava so that the contrast material can be injected more rapidly in a more compact bolus.

For peripheral injections, the catheter position is examined fluoroscopically with a small test injection. If the cannulated vein is tortuous or very small, the catheter is repositioned. In approximately 3.5 percent of cases where an arm vein cannot be cannulated, the catheter is inserted into the femoral vein. For extracranial studies, 40 ml of Renografin-76 (diatrizoate meglumine and diatrizoate sodium injection; E.R. Squibb & Sons, Inc., Princeton, N.J.) is layered over a 5 percent dextrose solution and injected at a rate between 12 and 20 ml/s, depending on the size of the arm vein. Contrast material may remain in the arm vein for up to 5 min after the completion of an injection if the layered dextrose solution is not used to flush the contrast material out of the vein. With careful loading of the dextrose and contrast in the inverted position, there is no mixing of the two solutions. For intracranial studies with the catheter in the superior vena cava, 50 ml of Renografin-76 is used. Up to five injections are performed depending on the patient's weight, age, and renal function. Because injecting both arms simultaneously doubles the amount of residual contrast material in the arm vein, better studies are obtained with the same amount of contrast material if only one arm is injected.

Carotid Arteries

Techniques

We examined the carotid bifurcations with different degrees of obliquity and determined that the 70 degree right posterior oblique (RPO) and left posterior oblique (LPO) projec-

tions most frequently show the separate origins of the internal and external carotid arteries without superimposition with the vertebral arteries. To study the carotid bifurcations, we first obtain 70 degree RPO and LPO views. We then obtain additional views of the carotid artery with lesser or greater degrees of obliquity until the separate origins of both internal and external carotid arteries are well visualized without overlap. With accurate positioning, both carotid bifurcations can be included within the 4.5 in. image intensifier diameter of examination (Figs. 25-1 and 25-2). Smaller image intensifier areas have less light scatter than large image intensifier areas. Light scatter decreases the perceived density of contrast material within vessels.

If not prohibited by contrast limitations, we obtain a 30 degree off-lateral view of the carotid siphons to evaluate for arteriosclerotic disease of the intracranial arteries (Fig. 25-3), and a view of the aortic arch (Fig. 25-4). The most frequent cause of a poor study of the carotid arteries is a misregistration artifact caused by the patient swallowing between the time the mask image is made and the time that the contrast-containing image is made. We have tried to prevent this by having the patient inhale through a straw, exhale through a straw, bite down on the tongue, or bite down on a cork, and by cooling the contrast material. None of these methods decreased swallowing artifacts. Consequently, we do not mention swallowing prior to the first injection. If the patient swallows during the first injection, then we ask the patient to try not to swallow on subsequent injections.

Others have reported decrease swallowing artifacts with the use of viscous lidocaine[9] and with the use of nonionic contrast material.[14] At the present time, the use of nonionic contrast material is prohibited by its cost.

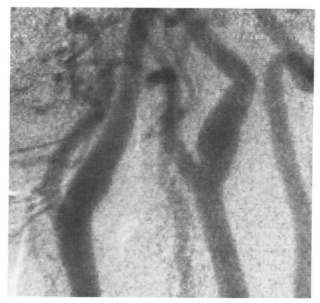

Figure 25-1 Both normal carotid bifurcations and both vertebral arteries are well visualized on this 70-degree RPO projection after injecting 40 ml of contrast material into a peripheral arm vein.

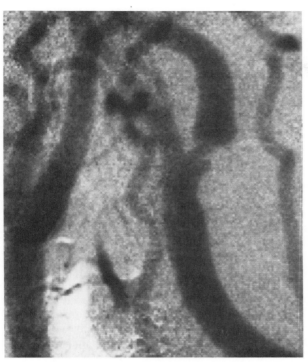

Figure 25-2 The origin of the left internal carotid artery is moderately narrowed and irregular on this RPO projection. The common carotid bifurcation is normal.

Comparison with Conventional Angiography

In order to establish the accuracy and clinical usefulness of DSA in the diagnosis of atherosclerotic disease of the carotid arteries, DSA examinations were compared with conventional carotid angiograms in 100 patients.[4] The degree of stenosis visualized with the DSA examination and with the conventional angiogram was classified into one of seven categories: 0, normal; 1, minimal stenosis (20 percent); 2, mild stenosis (20 to 40 percent); 3, moderate stenosis (40 to 60 percent); 4, moderate to marked stenosis (60 to 80 percent); 5, marked stenosis (80 to 99 percent); 6, occluded (100 percent). DSA examinations were rated as good or excellent quality if the separate origins of the internal and external carotid arteries were well visualized without superimposition and without overlap by the vertebral arteries, and when the arterial contrast density was good or excellent. In only 1 patient out of the 100 patients was a poor-quality DSA examination the result of poor contrast density within the carotid arteries. In this comparative study, the quality of the DSA examination was good or excellent 70 percent of the time. Currently, the carotid bifurcations are well visualized 85 percent of the time. There are several reasons for this improvement. In the comparative study, fewer injections of contrast material were made because the patients had already had a conventional angiogram. The patients currently being examined have as many injections as can be safely performed to clearly visualize the carotid bifurcation en face. In the comparative study, if an arm vein could not be

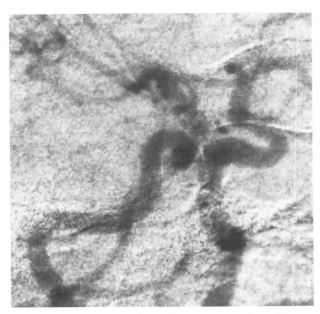

Figure 25-3 Both carotid siphons are normal on this 30-degree off-lateral view to exclude a "tandem lesion."

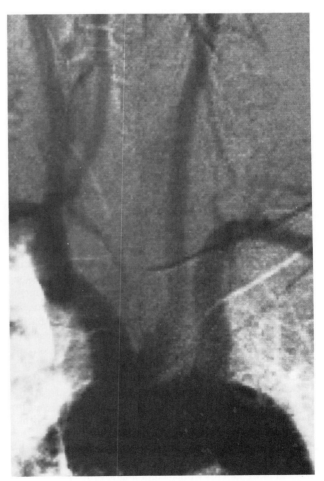

Figure 25-4 Normal aortic arch with visualization of the proximal portions of both vertebral arteries.

catheterized the study was considered unsuccessful. Currently, if an arm vein cannot be catheterized, as occurs in approximately 0.5 percent of patients, we will perform the study via the femoral vein. In the comparative study, venous reflux occurred in 1 to 2 percent of patients because of patients performing Valsalva maneuvers or because of compression of the superior vena cava. Currently, if the study is inadequate because of venous reflux, we will repeat the study on the following day via the femoral vein. As the technicians, nurses, and physicians have increased experience with DSA, their confidence in this procedure is sensed by the patients. This makes the patients less anxious, which is reflected in a decreased number of misregistration artifacts caused by patient swallowing during the examination.

The DSA interpretation was considered to be correct if it agreed with or was within one category of the interpretation of the degree of stenosis on conventional carotid angiography. When the carotid bifurcations were well visualized, there was excellent correlation of conventional and digital angiograms, with the sensitivity 95 percent, specificity 99 percent, and accuracy 97 percent. When the carotid bifurcations were not well visualized with DSA, there was a substantial chance for misinterpretation of the study, with the sensitivity 54 percent, specificity 70 percent, and accuracy 64 percent (Fig. 25-5). An important advantage of DSA over other indirect and direct methods of evaluating the carotid bifurcations is that it is immediately obvious when the DSA examination is of good or excellent quality and when the carotid bifurcations are not well visualized.

In the cooperative study, all four ulcerations that were visualized with conventional angiography and that occurred on DSA studies of good or excellent quality were identified with DSA. Four ulcerations occurred in patients whose carotid bifurcations were not well visualized with DSA examination.

Carotid Bifurcations, Vertebral Arteries

Asymptomatic Carotid Bruit

The management of patients with asymptomatic carotid bruits is controversial.[12] Although IV DSA provides a powerful tool for demonstrating asymptomatic internal carotid artery stenosis, the natural history of such patients is ill-defined. One recent study suggests that about 4 percent of people over age 65 will have a localized, asymptomatic carotid bifurcation bruit.[16] Many persons undoubtedly harbor asymptomatic internal carotid artery stenosis yet have no bruit. Considering the increasing age of our population, the potential for the indiscriminate use of IV DSA in asymptomatic patients is obvious. More optimistically, IV DSA provides a means of clarifying the natural history of patients with asymptomatic internal carotid artery stenosis, and for determining the best treatment approach for lowering stroke risks and improving longevity.

IV DSA appears to be the procedure of choice for demonstrating the present severity of internal carotid artery stenosis in most patients with asymptomatic bruit. IV DSA can clearly distinguish external carotid (Fig. 25-6) and subcla-

vian artery stenosis from internal carotid artery disease. All degrees of stenosis and ulceration can be demonstrated with IV DSA. If an adequate view of the major intracranial vessels is obtained with IV DSA, significant tandem stenosis can be ruled out, and such patients can safely undergo endarterectomy without conventional angiography (Fig. 25-3).

No studies are available comparing IV DSA with either direct or indirect noninvasive tests for detecting carotid artery disease. While IV DSA can provide accurate pictures of all degrees of carotid stenosis or ulceration, indirect noninvasive tests such as oculoplethysmography and supraorbital directional Doppler studies provide reliable inferential data only with stenoses greater than 60 percent. Direct noninvasive tests, such as the B-scan and Doppler imaging systems, also have several limitations.[1,15] Noninvasive tests may provide data regarding the physiological significance of a carotid artery lesion that is not obtainable with IV DSA or angiography. Some investigators think that ulcerations and arterial wall calcifications are better seen with the B scan.[8] The relation of such data to stroke risk and patient management requires further study. Since some carotid lesions can progress rapidly, it may be impractical to perform an IV DSA at very frequent intervals. A noninvasive test, supplemented by periodic IV DSA, may prove useful in such situations. However, in most asymptomatic patients, IV DSA obviates the need for a large battery of noninvasive tests designed merely to detect the presence of internal carotid artery stenosis.

Transient Ischemic Attacks (TIA) and Infarction

We currently recommend that patients with carotid territory TIA who are low-risk surgical candidates undergo conventional film screen angiography or intra-arterial digital subtraction angiography (IA DSA). In symptomatic patients, IV DSA may not clearly visualize the carotid bifurcations and cannot predictably provide sufficient visualization of the intracranial vessels to exclude tandem stenosis, small-vessel disease, or the need for an extracranial-intracranial arterial anastomosis. We have had the experience of having to do both an IV DSA and a conventional angiogram because of these problems. The small risk (at most institutions) of conventional angiography or IA DSA is certainly justified in symptomatic patients and provides optimal visualization of the cerebral circulation. In patients with carotid territory ischemia who are suboptimal surgical risks because of age or associated medical conditions, or in patients refusing conventional angiography, IV DSA is a useful means of evaluating for high-grade internal carotid artery stenosis. IV DSA may demonstrate nonsurgical internal carotid artery disease, thereby obviating the need for hospitalization.

The role of angiography in patients with vertebrobasilar insufficiency is uncertain.[3] The aortic arch, vertebral arteries, and basilar artery can often be well visualized with IV DSA, thereby avoiding the risks of selective vertebral catheterization (Fig. 25-7). Although surgically correctable lesions are less common in patients with vertebrobasilar TIA, IV DSA affords a safe means of assessing the cerebral circulation and collateral flow patterns in such patients.

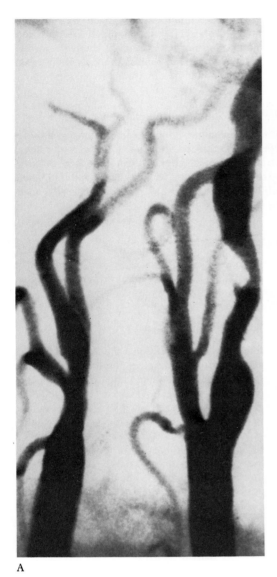

A

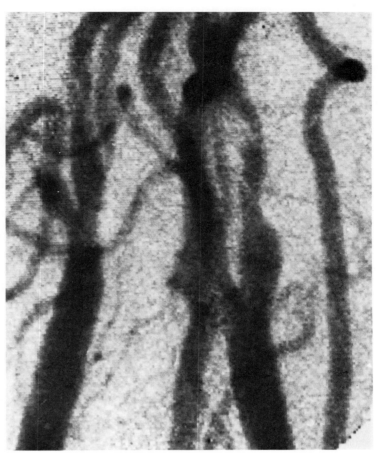

B

Figure 25-5 *A*. Composite subtraction of conventional carotid angiogram showing occlusion of the right internal carotid artery at its origin, and moderate stenosis and irregularity of the proximal 5 cm of the left internal carotid artery. *B*. IV DSA on same patient as in (*A*) shows identical findings.

Because of its safety and convenience, it is tempting to do outpatient IV DSA examinations on patients with nonspecific or nonfocal neurological symptoms. Occlusive disease in such patients may have little or nothing to do with symptoms, and IV DSA is not a substitute for a careful history and neurological examination.

In many patients with completed cerebral infarction, the circulation can be safely assessed with IV DSA, thus clarifying the stroke etiology while avoiding the hazards of conventional angiography. IV DSA is particularly useful in ruling out major-vessel stenosis in patients with apparent lacunar infarcts or presumed cardiac embolic infarcts. We have used IV DSA in patients with carotid reversible ischemic neurological deficits to help gauge the urgency of endarterectomy. IV DSA is extremely useful for screening patients with central retinal arterial occlusion or venous stasis retinopathy for carotid disease.

Intracranial Vessels

Technique

The major disadvantage of intracranial DSA is the simultaneous opacification of the carotid and vertebral arteries and their branches. Tailoring oblique views to the examination makes it possible to visualize areas of interest in most cases. Both carotid siphons can be visualized with a 30 degree off-lateral view (Fig. 25-3). To visualize the parasellar internal carotid arteries in patients with sellar and suprasellar mass lesions, a Water's view is most useful. Submentovertex views usually are not useful with DSA because misregistration subtraction artifacts are caused by patient swallowing and motion because of the discomfort of this position. To evaluate the basilar artery, the straight, lateral, and Water's

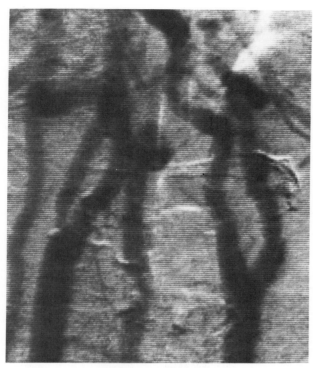

Figure 25-6 IV DSA demonstrates that this patient's right-sided asymptomatic bruit originated from the origin of the right external carotid artery and is not of clinical significance. The white area at the origin of the right internal carotid artery is caused by misregistration motion artifact of a calcified plaque.

views are used. To maximize spatial resolution, all intracranial examinations are performed with a 512 × 512 matrix with the smallest image intensifier diameter that includes the area of interest.

Comparison with Conventional Angiography

Intracranial vessels were examined in 55 patients with both conventional selective angiography and DSA.[10] The fourth-order intracranial vessels were visualized in all cases with conventional angiography and infrequently with DSA. In 65 percent of the patients, the DSA examinations provided as much information as the conventional angiogram. In 22 percent the DSA examination provided diagnostic information, but there was a significant chance of misinterpreting the results of this study. In 13 percent of cases, the DSA examination was not diagnostic.

Clinical Applications

Tumors

Although the small intracranial vessels are not as well visualized with IV DSA as with conventional angiography, combined with CT, IV DSA is usually sufficient for the pre-

operative evaluation of tumor patients. In the vast majority of tumor patients with a CT examination, IV DSA provides sufficient information on the location of the large vessels, the patency of the large sinuses, and the vascularity of the tumor.

Pituitary Tumors

DSA has replaced conventional cerebral angiography for the preoperative evaluation of the juxtasellar carotid arteries prior to trans-sphenoidal surgery because the large intracerebral vessels are consistently well visualized with DSA, and the possibility of a moderate- or large-sized juxtasellar aneurysm can be excluded with DSA.

Hemifacial Spasm

DSA can determine if hemifacial spasm in a patient is secondary to a dolichoectatic vertebral or basilar artery located adjacent to the facial nerve.

Aneurysms

DSA cannot replace conventional angiography for detecting small aneurysms because the resolution of DSA is not as good as that of conventional angiography, and because of vessel overlap with DSA. DSA can be used to detect large aneurysms, to evaluate arterial spasm, and to evaluate the results of aneurysm surgery. Intracranial aneurysms that are 1 cm or larger can be reliably demonstrated with IV DSA. Visualization is usually better for anterior circulation than posterior circulation aneurysms. Special views are sometimes necessary to adequately show aneurysms arising from the carotid siphon. However, the resolution of IV DSA is not adequate to demonstrate fine arterial detail, and conventional angiography remains a necessity prior to surgery.

Arteriovenous Malformations

In most cases, DSA does not replace conventional angiography for the evaluation of arteriovenous (AV) malformations because the simultaneous opacification of vessels makes it difficult to determine which vessels are feeding the AV malformation (Fig. 25-8). Therefore, conventional angiography is also necessary in most cases of arteriovenous malformation when surgery is planned. However, IV DSA is a useful screening procedure for patients suspected of having an AV malformation. After surgery and/or therapeutic embolization, DSA can be used to determine if the entire arteriovenous malformation has been occluded.

Extracranial-Intracranial (EC-IC) Arterial Bypass Surgery

With superior vena cava injections, IV DSA can usually demonstrate severe stenosis of the intracranial internal carotid artery, but the spatial resolution is often inadequate to detect middle cerebral artery stenosis. Conventional angiography or IA DSA remains the procedure of choice for evaluating the intracranial circulation for atherosclerotic disease.

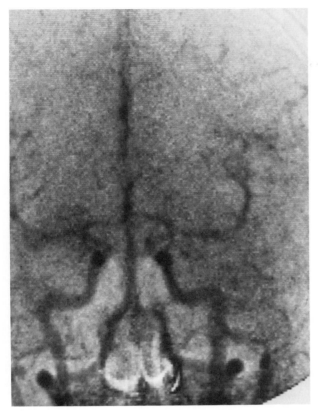

Figure 25-7 The normal basilar artery is well visualized between the internal carotid arteries. Both vertebral, anterior, and middle cerebral arteries are seen.

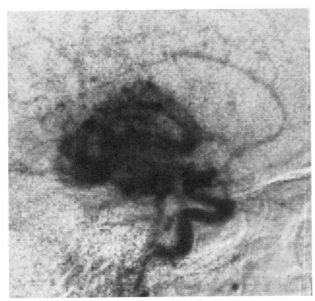

Figure 25-8 Large arteriovenous malformation with multiple feeding vessels arising from the middle and posterior cerebral arteries is visualized with IV DSA.

Intracranial IV DSA does provide a convenient means for demonstrating bypass patency. Initially our patients undergoing anastomosis of the superficial temporal artery to a branch of the middle cerebral artery were studied using anterior, posterior, and lateral views of the head. This technique proved unreliable in assessing bypass patency. Subsequent patients were studied using magnified, oblique views, which allowed demonstration of bypass patency in more than 90 percent of patients. All patients with a superficial temporal artery luminal diameter greater than 2 mm had bypass patency confirmed with IV DSA. Conventional angiography is not necessary in such patients.

Intracranial Veins

IV DSA appears to be the procedure of choice for studying the intracranial veins and dural sinuses because of the simultaneous opacification of all intracranial vascular structures.[11] Confusing filling defects due to unopacified blood entering the veins and sinuses is not a problem with IV DSA. The simultaneous opacification of vessels is advantageous for evaluation of compression of the dural sinuses by parasagittal meningiomas because the flow defects that occur in selective angiography from the mixture of opacified and unopacified blood are not present with DSA. IV DSA can be used preoperatively to evaluate anatomical variations of the venous outflow and help determine which sinuses may be safely occluded if necessary during surgery in the region of the temporal bone, jugular fossa, and base of the skull. IV DSA is an effective means of evaluating the superior sagittal sinus and of distinguishing a large jugular bulb from a neoplasm.

Postendarterectomy Evaluations

IV DSA clearly shows the carotid arteries after endarterectomy.[7] Many patients demonstrate mild irregularity at the bifurcation or slight narrowing at the distal end of the arteriotomy if studied within 1 week of surgery. Rarely, a silent internal carotid artery occlusion will be discovered. IV DSA is particularly useful in the evaluation of patients with neurological symptoms complicating carotid endarterectomy. Thrombosis at the operative site can be easily demonstrated, and if the operative site is patent, there is no need for re-exploration. IV DSA also provides an accurate means for following long-term patency after carotid endarterectomy.

In summary, DSA is useful for the evaluation of large intracranial arteries, for establishing the vascularity of lesions, and for the initial evaluation of AV malformations and aneurysms. It is not useful for the evaluation of small intracranial vessels.

Intra-arterial DSA (IA DSA)

IV DSA is diagnostic for the majority of neuroangiographic examinations. However, motion artifact, vessel overlap, or the need for improved spatial resolution may render the IV DSA examination inadequate. In these cases, IA DSA offers a faster, less costly alternative to conventional angiograpy.

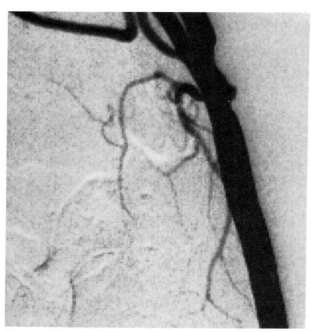

Figure 25-9 IA DSA after injection of 6 ml of contrast material shows ulcer in the posterior wall of the distal right common carotid artery.

Because of better contrast sensitivity, IA DSA requires less contrast than conventional angiography, although spatial resolution is slightly less. A representative IA DSA examination is shown in Fig. 25-9.

References

1. Ackerman RH: A perspective on noninvasive diagnosis of carotid disease. Neurology (NY) 29:615–622, 1979.
2. Bernstein EF, Greenspan RH, Loken MK: Intravenous abdominal aortography: A preliminary report. Surgery 44:529–535, 1958.
3. Caplan LR: Vertebrobasilar disease: Time for a new strategy. Stroke 12:111–114, 1981.
4. Chilcote WA, Modic MT, Pavlicek WA, Little JR, Furlan AJ, Duchesneau PM, Weinstein, MA: Digital subtraction angiography of the carotid arteries: A comparative study in 100 patients. Radiology 139:287–295, 1981.
5. Christenson PC, Ovitt TW, Fisher HD III, Frost MM, Nudelman S, Roehrig H: Intravenous angiography using digital video subtraction: Intravenous cervicocerebrovascular angiography. AJNR 1:379–386, 1980.
6. Crummy AB, Strother CM, Sackett JF, Ergun DL, Shaw CG, Kruger RA, Mistretta CA, Turnipseed WD, Lieberman RP, Myerowitz PD, Ruzicka FF: Computerized fluoroscopy: Digital subtraction for intravenous angiocardiography and arteriography. AJR 135:1131–1140, 1980.
7. Hertzer NR, Beven EG, Modic MT, Ohara PJ, Vogt DP, Weinstein MA: Early patency of the carotid artery following endarterectomy: Digital subtraction angiography after 262 operations. Surgery 92:1049–1057, 1982.
8. Johnson JM: Angiography and ultrasound in diagnosis of carotid artery disease: A comparison. Contemp Surg 20:79–93, 1982.
9. Manelfe C, Ducos de Lahitte M, March-Vergnes JP, Rascol A, Bonafé A, Guiraud B, Chambers E: Investigation of extracranial cerebral arteries by intravenous angiography: Report of 1,000 cases. AJNR 3:287–293, 1982.
10. Modic MT, Weinstein MA, Chilcote WA, Pavlicek W, Duchesneau PM, Furlan AJ, Little JR: Digital subtraction angiography of the intracranial vascular system: Comparative study in 55 patients. AJR 138:299–306, 1982.
11. Modic MT, Weinstein MA, Starnes DL, Kinney SE, Duchesneau PM: Intravenous digital subtraction angiography of the intracranial veins and dural sinuses. Radiology 146:383–389, 1983.
12. Mohr JP: Asymptomatic carotid artery disease. Stroke 13:431–433, 1982.
13. Robb GP, Steinberg I: Visualization of the chamber of the heart, the pulmonary circulation, and the great blood vessels in man. AJR 41:1–17, 1939.
14. Sackett JF, Strother CM: Contrast media for computerized fluoroscopy. Presented at the 66th Scientific Assembly and Annual Meeting of the Radiological Society of North America, Dallas, Texas, November 16–21, 1980.
15. Sandok BA: Noninvasive techniques for diagnosis of carotid artery disease. Stroke 9:427–429, 1978.
16. Sandok BA, Whisnant JP, Furlan AJ, Mickell JL: Carotid artery bruits: Prevalence survey and differential diagnosis. Mayo Clin Proc 57:227–230, 1982.
17. Steinberg I, Finby N, Evans JA: A safe and practical intravenous method for abdominal aortography, peripheral arteriography, and cerebral angiography. AJR 82:758–772, 1959.

SECTION D

Brain Biopsy

26

Diagnostic Brain Biopsy

Howard H. Kaufman
Peter T. Ostrow
Ian J. Butler

Indications for Brain Biopsy

Although open brain biopsies are usually accompanied by low morbidity and mortality, there is no question that they carry some risk and, of course, considerable expense. There is, accordingly, general agreement that two criteria must be fulfilled before such procedures are performed: first, that no alternative procedure can provide the information desired, and second, that this information serve a useful purpose. Of course, the operation must be done with informed consent.

As the pathogenesis of various diseases has been better understood, examination of blood, urine, and spinal fluid, biopsies of other tissues, and a variety of other tests such as computed tomography have provided diagnoses for many conditions that previously required brain biopsy. However, there are still a number of diseases that can only be identified by brain biopsy and that require diagnosis for purposes of treatment; prognostication; proper protection of families, friends, and medical personnel; and genetic counseling of family members. The need for fresh tissue to detect enzyme abnormalities or the presence of viral infections or to perform tissue cultures also requires fresh biopsy material. Even if such investigations are experimental, biopsy may be the only way of obtaining the appropriate specimens to study to increase understanding of a particular disease.[1, 6, 9]

Disease Entities

Diseases of the central nervous system in which a brain biopsy is often necessary for diagnosis and management can be categorized relative to the duration of the illness and clinical manifestations. Neurological disorders are usually judged to have an acute (days), subacute (weeks), or chronic (months or years) course. Based on clinical features, family history and ancillary investigations, differential diagnoses can be generated prior to brain biopsy in order that the specific investigation of the tissue will be optimal. Physicians involved in the decision of whether to perform a biopsy and how to examine the specimen may include internists, pediatricians, neuropathologists, infectious disease specialists, neurochemists, and neuroradiologists in addition to neurologists and neurosurgeons with a particular interest in evaluating different brain disorders and their management. Brain disorders in which ancillary investigations may be confusing or nondiagnostic but that require specific treatments include bacterial infections (antibiotics), herpes simplex encephalitis (adenine arabinoside), cerebral microgliomatosis (i.e., malignant lymphoma) and carcinomatous meningitis (radiation), fungal and tuberculous leptomeningitis (chemotherapy), and sarcoidosis and granulomatous angiitis (corticosteroids). An algorithm for decision making, based on clinical presentation and laboratory findings, has been developed (Table 26-1).

It is obvious from the relatively abbreviated list at the bottom of Table 26-1 that the number of disorders requiring brain biopsy for diagnosis is fairly small. This is because of a variety of new diagnostic techniques for many rare genetic, neurological disorders. For example, the general availability of amino acid quantitation of blood and urine and enzymatic analysis of body fluids, white blood cells, and cultured skin fibroblasts has reduced the need for brain biopsy for diagnosis of disorders of amino acid metabolism and the numerous lysosomal storage disorders. Such storage disorders include those affecting metabolism of sphingolipids (ganglioside G_{M2}, Tay-Sachs disease: hexosaminidase A deficiency), mucopolysaccharides (Hurler's disease: α-L-iduronidase deficiency), mucolipids (generalized G_{M1}, gangliosidosis: β-galactosidase deficiency) and glycogen (Pompe's disease: α-1, 4-glucosidase deficiency).

Some disorders affecting predominantly gray matter, such as cerebral ceroid lipofuscinosis, may only be definitively diagnosed by brain biopsy, although this disease can be strongly suspected from histological examination of various tissues, including skin, muscle, fibroblasts, bone marrow, conjunctiva, rectum, appendix, and testes.

TABLE 26-1   Indications for Brain Biopsy By Disease Course

Acute	Subacute	Chronic
Clinical Disturbances		
Conscious level	Conscious level	Conscious level
Confusion	Confusion	Confusion
Coma	Disorientation	Disorientation
Functional (local)	Functional (local)	Functional (local)
Aphasia	Aphasia	Aphasia
Paresis	Paresis	Ataxia
Visual field deficit	Blindness	Blindness
		Dystonia
	Functional (general)	Functional (general)
	Cognition deficit	Retardation
	Memory deficit	Memory deficit
	Psychiatric symptoms	Dementia
		Apraxia
Convulsions	Convulsions	Convulsions
Focal	Intermittent	Isolated
General	Myoclonic	Myoclonic
*Important Investigations**		
Radiological	Radiological	Radiological
CT scan (+)	CT scan (+)	CT scan (+)
Radionuclide scan (±)	Angiography (±)	Radionuclide scan (±)
Sinus films (+)	Chest films (+)	
EEG (+)	EEG (±)	EEG (+)
CSF (±)	CSF (+)	CSF (+)
		Other tissues
		Fibroblasts
		WBCs
		Conjunctiva
		Bone marrow
Anticipated Diagnoses†		
Infection	Sarcoidosis	Childhood dementia
Bacterial cerebritis	Granulomatous angiitis	Ceroid lipofuscinosis
Viral encephalitis	Microgliomatosis	Neuroaxonal dystrophy
	Leptomeningitis	Canavan disease
	Tuberculous	Alexander disease
	Carcinomatous	Lafora inclusion disease
	Fungal	Adult dementia
		Alzheimer disease
		Creutzfeldt-Jakob disease
		Pick disease

*(+) necessary, (±) often necessary.
†Primary or secondary brain tumors are possible in all three clinical categories.

Some of the genetic disorders affecting white matter (leukodystrophies) can be diagnosed by enzyme analysis (metachromatic leukodystrophy and Krabbe's globoid cell leukodystrophy), but several rare entities (Canavan's spongiform encephalopathy and Alexander's disease) can only reliably be diagnosed by brain biopsy. Computed tomography (CT) is frequently abnormal in the leukodystrophies and will strongly indicate both the diagnostic category and the best site for brain biopsy. New techniques in quantitating the ratio of $C_{26:0}$ to $C_{22:0}$ saturated unbranched fatty acids in cultured skin fibroblasts and other tissues have made unnecessary the need for brain biopsy to diagnose the various forms of X-linked adrenoleukodystrophy.[12]

In the diagnosis and management of several of the chronic epilepsies, brain biopsy may have a role both in diagnosis and treatment. In the ataxic myoclonic syndrome with Lafora body inclusions, a biopsy of the cerebellum may be necessary. The focal and progressive epilepsy of children in which there is pathological evidence of an encephalitis (Rasmussen) can be suspected clinically but diagnosed only by brain biopsy. In this condition, seizures may be controlled only by extensive brain resection (hemispherectomy).

Surgical Considerations

Preoperative evaluation should be comprehensive, especially since many of these patients have been ill for some time and may have the medical problems seen with debilitation and inanition. Pulmonary problems and malnutrition[13] as well as deep vein thrombosis[10] may occur in such patients and increase surgical risk, and they should be sought and treated appropriately.

An operative site is chosen based on the disease suspected and the results of such tests as computed tomography and electroencephalography to give the highest probability of yielding positive findings while removing tissue from "silent" areas of the brain.[6]

Configuration of incision and type of bone opening, whether small craniectomy, trephine craniotomy, or formal craniotomy, are optional but should provide adequate exposure of the brain surface. If meningeal biopsy is to be done, this membrane should not be cauterized and should be removed by sharp dissection. The volume of brain to be resected is determined by the range of studies for which tissue is required. This should be decided in advance in consultation with neuropathologists, virologists, and other specialists, and even with colleagues at other centers to whom tissue is to be sent. With careful planning, 1 to 1½ cm^3, including both gray and white matter and a sulcus, may be sufficient for all studies if the specimen is removed without damaging it and is divided carefully. Obviously removal must be done by sharp dissection, and coagulation is to be avoided until the specimen has been excised. Although bleeding is generally minor, it may be annoying, and blood may enter the subarachnoid space of the specimen. The use of the laser, which causes very little tissue trauma while providing improved hemostasis, rather than a knife, may aid in the dissection and prevent troublesome bleeding. If the bony defect is small, heavy wire mesh may be used to cover it for appearance with little increased risk of infection.

The use of prophylactic anticonvulsants and a short course of perioperative antibiotics is suggested, as are pulsating boots intra- and postoperatively, good pulmonary toilet, early mobilization, and adequate nutritional support when appropriate.

The secret of a successful biopsy is thus thorough planning, gentle handling of the specimen, and good postoperative care.

Tissue Preservation and Preparation

It is worthwhile to re-emphasize the importance of prior consultation with those who will be examining the tissue. In most cases, the specimen will have to be divided into several samples, each of which will require specific processing. Any delay in the initiation of these procedures or transportation in an inappropriate medium may reduce the likelihood of success.

The neuropathologist should be called to the operating room to view the specimen with the surgeon. After noting the site and orientation of the biopsy and any landmarks that may be present within it (sulcus, gray-white junction), the pathologist should then divide the specimen into appropriate samples. For example, a 1-cm^3 specimen taken from a patient with a tentative diagnosis of herpes simplex encephalitis might be divided as follows:

1. A 2-mm-thick slice, perpendicular to the surface, would be frozen for rapid examination and immunofluorescent study.

2. The adjacent slice, 3 mm thick, would be fixed in formalin for routine histology.

3. The next section, 1 to 2 mm thick, would be fixed in glutaraldehyde for electron microscopy. Since glutaraldehyde penetrates tissues slowly, adequate fixation requires that the sample be further subdivided into 1- to 2-mm cubes. It is usually worthwhile to separate the gray and white matter portions of the sample and fix them individually.

4. The remainder of the specimen would be placed in an appropriate transport medium to be used in an attempt to culture the virus.

Table 26-2 indicates the type of tissue preservation and time required for a variety of investigations.

Literature Review

General Series

The yield of cerebral biopsy in terms of immediate diagnosis and correlation with later autopsy findings will vary with the nature of the clinical material seen at any given institution and the criteria used to select the patients as well as the nature of the laboratory tests and the criteria used to categorize the pathological material. Biopsy findings have been divided into the categories of "diagnostic," "abnormal but not diagnostic," and "normal." But neuropathological judgment, particularly of what is diagnostic, makes these definitions somewhat imprecise.

Two recent articles have addressed these questions and are in general agreement, although the numbers of patients are probably not large enough for statistical analysis (Table 26-3). Of the 46 biopsies performed between 1960 and 1972 reviewed by Kaufman and Catalano, 37 percent were diagnostic, 48 percent were abnormal but not diagnostic, and 15 percent were normal. Several of the abnormal biopsies would now be considered diagnostic (e.g., Creutzfeldt-Jakob disease). Both autopsies performed on patients who had diagnostic biopsies confirmed the diagnoses. All six autopsies in the abnormal but not diagnostic group were compatible with biopsy findings (Creutzfeldt-Jakob disease, 2; reticulocytic encephalitis, i.e., microgliomatosis; Schilder's diffuse sclerosis, i.e., adrenoleukodystrophy; moderate acute encephalitis; and ischemia). Postmortem examinations in two patients with normal biopsies showed meningoencephalitis in one and a developmental anomaly in the other.[9] In 1971, Blackwood described follow-up data on 173 patients whose initial findings were reported in 1966, at which time 42 percent were considered diagnostic, 38 percent abnormal but not diagnostic, and 20 percent normal. All 24 autopsies in those with diagnostic biopsies confirmed the diagnoses. Seven of the ten autopsies in the abnormal but nondiagnostic group were revealing: postepileptic encephalopathy, pinealoma, basal glioma, cerebral glioma, acoustic neurofibroma, amaurotic familial idiocy, globoid body diffuse sclerosis. Postmortem examinations in two patients with normal biopsies showed cerebellar degeneration in one.[1]

Another important aspect of the findings on brain biopsy

TABLE 26-2 Tissue Preservation, Preparations, and Information Yielded

Study	Method of Preservation	Technique Used and/or Information Obtained	Time
Frozen section	Freeze on chuck as rapidly as possible	Hematoxylin/eosin for general morphology	Minutes
		Histochemical stains for lipids or metachromatic material	Same day
		Immunofluorescence, e.g. for viral antigens	Same day
Paraffin section	Fix in 10% neutral buffered formalin	Hematoxylin/eosin for general morphology	1 day
		Special histochemical stains for myelin, lipids, axons, neurofibrillary tangles, amyloid, bacteria, metachromasia, iron, calcium, etc.	1–2 days
		Immunoperoxidase technique for enzymes, viral antigens, myelin basic protein, glial fibrillary acidic protein, immunoglobulins, etc.	1–2 days
Electron microscopy	3% buffered glutaraldehyde	Ultrastructural features (viral particles, inclusions, lysosomal alterations, membranes, etc.)	3 days
Viral cultures	Viral transport medium	Presence of viable virus	5 days
Biochemistry	Frozen	Presence and quantitation of enzymes	Days

is that they may rule out a suspected disease and diagnose another disease that is indeed treatable. This has been noted in reports of series of biopsies for herpes encephalitis.[5,14]

The safety of the procedure must also be considered. Since many of the patients who undergo brain biopsy do have chronic, debilitating, and progressive diseases, it is sometimes difficult to separate postoperative complications from problems related to the natural history of their illness.

However a variety of complications have been related to surgery, including postanesthetic pulmonary difficulties, wound infection, spinal fluid leakage, systemic febrile reactions, seizures and transient hemiparesis, subdural hematomas or hygromas, intracerebral hematomas and porencephalic cysts, and even death.[6,9] In our experience with 50 biopsies performed between 1960 and 1972, there was one death (2 percent) due to aspiration and five major complica-

TABLE 26-3 Results of Biopsies

Study	Total	Diagnostic	Abnormal, Not Diagnostic	Normal
Kaufman and Catalano,[9] 1979	46	17 (37%)	22 (48%)	7 (15%)
	Died	8 (47%)	11(50%)	3 (43%)
	Autopsy results known	2	6	2
	Results	2/2 confirm	6/6 compatible	2/2 pathological findings
Blackwood,[1] 1971	173	72 (42%)	66 (38%)	35 (20%)
	Died	36 (50%)	17 (26%)	5 (14%)
	Autopsy results known	24	10	2
	Results	24/24 confirm	7/7 diagnostic	1/2 pathological findings

tions (10 percent), i.e., three cases of pneumonia, one of pulmonary embolus, and one episode of seizures believed to be related to the biopsy site.[9]

Another complication of brain biopsy relates to risk to operative personnel. It is now clear that kuru and Creutzfeldt-Jakob disease are transmissible and can be contracted by handling infected brain tissue. However, based on the work of Gajdusek and his co-workers, a recent review suggests that contaminated equipment can be sterilized by autoclaving for 1 h at 121°C under 15 lb/in² pressure or by immersion in 0.5% sodium hypochlorite for 1 h.[2] Of note is that appropriate precautions by Gajdusek's personnel have prevented transmission of the virus in a large group handling known infected tissue for many years.[7] Other diseases may be similarly transmitted.[4]

Research Potential and Future Prospects

The techniques currently used to diagnose degenerative disorders of the brain in children and adults may involve tissues and mechanisms far removed from the fundamental abnormalities in brain structure and function. Therefore, brain biopsy may be critical to eventually understanding these diseases.

For example, in the diseases having an excessive storage of ceroid lipofuscin material in neurons, there are a variety of different clinical disorders with different ages of onset, course, and systems involved. The adult form of ceroid lipofuscinosis (Kufs' disease) has decreasing amounts of storage material in peripheral tissue with advancing age and can only be reliably diagnosed by brain biopsy. In addition, the enzyme defect in this group of diseases has not been defined. Indeed, many of the known genetic and enzymatic disorders affecting children occur also in adulthood, but then show little in the way of peripheral tissue abnormalities. Clinical criteria in adults may be quite different from those exhibited in children with the same enzymatic deficit. Furthermore, the defect may be partial or an unusual variant not readily diagnosed by routine screening studies of enzyme function (variant forms of adult-onset metachromatic leukodystrophy). Analysis of brain tissue for stored material and demonstration of an enzyme defect may thus be the only method at this time to investigate adult patients having such unrecognized, progressive neurological disorders.

Since there is increased recognition of isoenzymes specific to particular tissues (cardiac and brain isoenzymes of creatine phosphokinase or liver and muscle forms of glycogen phophorylase), defects in isoenzymes in brain alone are possible causes of neurological disease and only diagnosable by analysis of brain biopsy material.

Disorders of neurotransmitters have been recognized and studied since the demonstration of low levels of dopamine in the basal ganglia in Parkinson's disease. Some other disorders may involve specific brain pathways not accessible to cortical biopsy. However, in disorders with a diffuse metabolic abnormality, a cortical biopsy may define a specific neurotransmitter defect (decreased biogenic amine levels in dihydropteridine reductase deficiency[3] and γ-aminobutyric

acid levels in Huntington's disease or low levels of choline acetyltransferase, the synthetic enzyme for acetylcholine in the cortex of patients with dementia). Biopsies will thus be necessary to define the different forms of dementia, some of which are currently diagnosed as Alzheimer's disease. Positron emission tomography (PET) scanning and nuclear magnetic resonance (NMR) scanning may help elucidate such disorders of neural transmission or intermediary metabolism, but confirmatory studies using fresh brain tissue at biopsy will be required.

PET scanning with [^{18}F] fluorodeoxyglucose administration is currently utilized in a few centers to localize abnormal brain metabolism in various physiological states and in the focal epilepsies[11] and may define the area to biopsy to determine a metabolic defect.

From these few examples it is obvious that the need for brain biopsy will continue but that the questions asked of and answers obtained from a biopsy will be very different from those sought previously. In the past the need was to define the histopathological nature of neurological disorders in which ataxia, dystonia, dementia, seizures, and abnormal behavior were prominent. Currently the questions asked are related to the subcellular or biochemical disturbances leading to brain dysfunction, including disorders of neural transmission, membrane structure and function, and immunology and virology.[8] Future studies involving brain biopsy may address other issues, such as interactions between genetic material and environment, as suggested by the recent demonstration that some dominantly inherited forms of Alzheimer's disease are transmissible.[4]

References

1. Blackwood W: Cerebral biopsy, in Vinken PJ, Bruyn GW (eds): *Handbook of Clinical Neurology*. Amsterdam, North-Holland, 1971, vol 10, pp 680–687.
2. Brown P, Gibbs CJ Jr, Amyx HL, Kingsbury DT, Rohwer RG, Sulima MP, Gajdusek DC: Chemical disinfection of Creutzfeldt-Jakob disease virus. N Engl J Med 306:1279–1282, 1982.
3. Butler IJ, Koslow SH, Krumholz A, Holtzman NA, Kaufman S: A disorder of biogenic amines in dihydropteridine reductase deficiency. Ann Neurol 3:244–230, 1978.
4. Cook RH, Austin JH: Precautions in familial transmissible dementia: Including familial Alzheimer's disease. Arch Neurol 35:697–698, 1978.
5. DiScalfani A, Kohl S, Ostrow PT: The importance of brain biopsy in suspected herpes simplex encephalitis. Surg Neurol 17:101–106, 1982.
6. Ellis WG, Youmans JR, Dreyfus PM: Diagnostic biopsy for neurological disease, in Youmans JR (ed): *Neurological Surgery*, 2d ed. Philadelphia, Saunders, 1982, Chap 12, pp 382–422.
7. Gajdusek DC, Gibbs CJ Jr, Asher DM, Brown P, Diwan A, Hoffman P, Nemo G, Rohwer R, White L: Precautions in medical care of, and in handling materials from, patients with transmissible virus dementia (Creutzfeldt-Jakob disease). N Engl J Med 297:1253–1258, 1977.
8. Johnson RT: The contribution of virologic research to clinical neurology. N Engl J Med 307:660–662, 1982.
9. Kaufman HH, Catalano LW Jr: Diagnostic brain biopsy: A series of 50 cases and a review. Neurosurgery 4: 129–136, 1979.
10. Kaufman HH, McConnell BJ, Costin BS, Gould KL, Borit A,

Satterwhite T, Pruesner JL, Bernstein D, Gildenberg PL: Deep vein thrombosis and pulmonary embolism in head injury. Angiology. (In press)

11. Mazziotta JC, Phelps ME, Carson RE, Kuhl DE: Tomographic mapping of human cerebral metabolism: Auditory stimulation. Neurology (NY) 32:921–937, 1982.

12. Moser HW, Moser AB, Kawamura N, Migeon B, O'Neill BP, Fenselau C, Kishimoto Y: Adrenoleukodystrophy: Studies of the phenotype, genetics and biochemistry. Johns Hopkins Med J 147:217–224, 1980.

13. Seltzer MH: Specialized nutrition support: The standard of care. JPEN 6:185–190, 1982.

14. Whitley RJ, Soong SJ, Hirsch MS, Karchmer AW, Dolin R, Galasso GJ, Dunnick JK, Alford CA: Herpes simplex encephalitis: Vidarabine therapy and diagnostic problems. N Engl J Med 304: 313–318, 1981.

Part IV

General and Perioperative Care

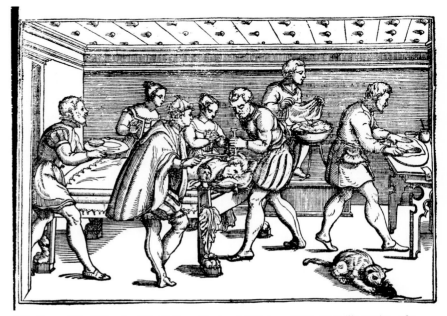

della Croce GA. *Chirurgiae Libri Septem*. Venice, J Zillettus, 1573. First illustration of a neurosurgical operation in progress.

27
Evaluation of the Patient in Coma

Allen D. Roses

Initial Evaluation and Treatment of the Comatose Patient

Coma can be defined as unarousable unresponsiveness. An extensive differential diagnosis may be responsible for coma in neurosurgical practice. Although the neurosurgeon may see a biased population of the various etiologies leading to coma, it is necessary to approach each patient with a clinical routine that expeditiously establishes the etiology yet protects the patient from any harm caused by either delay of proper treatment or unnecessary and inappropriate treatment.

The goal of any coma evaluation is to promptly stabilize the patient in order to be able to proceed with appropriate diagnostic procedures and specific therapy. A possible pitfall in dealing with comatose patients is to assume the obvious: for instance, that patients involved in accidents are comatose because of head trauma or that hospitalized patients receiving intravenous fluids cannot be hypoglycemic. By providing an algorithm (Table 27-1) for use in every coma encounter, one can avoid damaging patients because of an inaccurate initial etiologic assessment.

The rationale for using the systematic approach outlined in Table 27-1 develops from the pathological basis of coma. Coma results from either a lesion or dysfunction of the high brain stem, both cerebral hemispheres, or a combination of both. The initial neurological examination evaluates the structural integrity of the brain stem rostral to the vestibular nucleus (VIII) and provides necessary information to allow differentiation of eye signs due to herniation versus intrinsic brain lesions. As will be discussed, if a distinct brain stem lesion is not present, the subsequent approach to the patient's evaluation can be divided into several rational steps.

The initial strategy of dealing with any comatose individual is to protect the brain by providing it with oxygen and glucose as well as providing circulation to transport them. Thus, the initial approach to the patient involves protecting respiratory integrity, maintaining adequate blood flow, and assuring an adequate glucose supply.

Respiration

The initial concern in encountering any comatose patient is to protect the respiration. In practice this means to assure that the patient's airway is open. If an obstruction is present, prompt correction is mandatory. In all cases the rate and rhythm of respiration should be noted (and later recorded), since these data may be useful in determining the anatomy of the patient's coma.

Cerebral Blood Flow

Adequate perfusion of the brain depends on the functional integrity of the heart to maintain an adequate output. In practice, the pulse pressure is evaluated by checking the carotid pulses and noting rate and rhythm. Blood pressure can be measured in the upper extremities, but noting the presence of an adequate carotid pulse can be as valuable as measurement of the blood pressure in the arms. Both should be evaluated, however; circumstances are possible in which carotid pulses may be adequate but no blood pressure can be obtained. Examples would be a patient with subclavian thrombosis, a patient with upper extremity fractures, or an immobilized patient with multiple arterial and venous lifelines. The rate, rhythm, and strength of the carotid pulse provides good information quickly.

Glucose

All comatose patients should have an intravenous line instituted and an adequate supply of glucose provided. In practice, one usually obtains a small amount of blood for glucose measurement and injects at least 25 ml of 50% dextrose in water. There are no exceptions to this rule unless it is known with absolute certainty that the glucose levels are adequate. This knowledge is never available for patients entering the emergency room nor is it absolutely certain in hospitalized patients. There is no danger in administering intravenous dextrose to any comatose patient. The assumption that an adequate glucose level is present in a trauma patient or that an inpatient receiving intravenous 5% dextrose in water has a sufficient glucose level can lead to disastrous consequences if incorrect. It is an error of omission not to provide adequate glucose immediately.

Core Neurological Examination

The initial steps (airway, blood flow, glucose) result in a situation in which time is made available to establish the anatomy and cause of the coma. The brain now has adequate oxygen and glucose and a circulation to transport them there. The next 90 s can be used to perform the core neurological examination, evaluating primarily the midbrain and upper pons. It should be emphasized that this is a rapid, minimal examination that allows the next decisions to be made. A more complete neurological examination will cer-

297

TABLE 27-1 Step-by-Step Approach to the Evaluation of the Comatose Patient

    I. Establish airway and ensure respiration.
   II. Check circulation (carotid pulse, heartbeat, blood pressure)
  III. Intravenous glucose (usually after blood pressure measured and blood obtained for diagnostic studies)
  IV. Core neurological examination
      1. Rate and rhythm of respiration
      2. Pupillary size in millimeters, including light reactions
      3. Position of eyes
      4. Oculovestibular responses (ice water calorics after checking tympanic membranes and ear canals)
      5. Motor tone, including motor responses to painful stimuli, asymmetries of tone, and Babinski responses
      6. Ciliospinal responses
Then:
    V. If a herniation syndrome or signs of an expanding posterior fossa lesion with pressure on the brain stem exist, lower the intracranial pressure; CT for diagnosis, no LP
  VI. If meningitis is suspected, LP indicated for diagnosis and treatment should be instituted
 VII. Treat generalized convulsions (if present)
VIII. Treat metabolic abnormalities
      1. Restore acid-base balance
      2. Restore electrolyte balance
      3. Maintain body temperature
   IX. Administer thiamine
    X. Administer specific therapies. Once the vital functions have been protected, a complete history (from relatives, police, etc.) should be obtained and a complete physical examination completed.

tainly be performed following the notation and recording of the core examination. Table 27-1 lists the examination data necessary. The cranial nerve nuclei and pathways concerned with eye movement and pupil size are located in the midbrain. In general, the core examination, including everything except ice water calorics, takes less than 30 s to perform. In practice, the longest part of the evaluation may be the wait for ice water; therefore, every emergency room or inpatient unit dealing with possible coma patients should have available a handy supply of ice water. Table 27-2 lists some of the signs that may be helpful.

Pupillary Size

Pupillary pathways are relatively resistant to most causes of metabolic coma and the presence or absence of the light reflex is the most useful single sign in distinguishing metabolic coma from coma due to structural causes. The size of the pupils should be carefully measured in ambient light. In addition, the direct and consensual responses to light should be measured. These measurements should be recorded in millimeters on every coma chart, with six numbers appearing as in the following example:

	A	**D**	**C**	
R	5	5	5	**A** = ambient light
L	3	1	1	**D** = direct
				C = consensual

In this example, the right pupil is dilated compared with the left, with no direct or consensual response to light. The left pupil responds to direct light or to shone light into the right eye, which suggests a lesion involving the right oculomotor nerve. Should the rest of the examination be compatible

with an uncal herniation syndrome (lateral deviation of the right eye and/or motor system signs), the recognition of a 1-mm change may be crucial. Only if pupillary sizes are accurately and quantitatively recorded will such data be available and dependable.

Eye Position

When measuring pupillary size it is impossible not to note the position of the pupils. It is important to accurately record their position with respect to the midline and to each other. Any spontaneous movement or change in their position should also be noted and recorded in clear language that does not denote etiology. Examples are conjugate deviation of both pupils to the right, and midline position of the left pupil with deviation of the right pupil to the left. Other changes to be noted are spontaneous movements, whether roving, conjugate, dysconjugate, or orienting towards stimuli; patterned movements such as spontaneous nystagmus; ocular bobbing or other unclassified movements; and skew deviations (eyes not on the same horizontal plane).

Oculovestibular Responses

Eye movement can be tested by irrigating each external auditory canal with ice water, usually with the head elevated 30 degrees above the horizontal plane. Care should be taken in moving the head of any patient suspected of having sustained neck injury. The external canal and tympanic membrane should be examined prior to using a small catheter to irrigate the external auditory canal with up to 200 ml of ice water. Since the catheter may cause trauma to the canal or membrane, it should be recorded that this was not present before oculovestibular testing.

In coma, the normal fast component of nystagmus is not present so that the comatose patient in whom the oculovestibular response is preserved will have conjugate tonic devia-

TABLE 27-2 Clues on Physical Examination to the Cause of Coma

I. Respirations
    1. Cheyne-Stokes: usually bilateral cerebral dysfunction: early increased intracranial pressure or metabolic abnormality
    2. Bizarre patterns: usually subtentorial destruction; appear early rather than developing as herniation proceeds (ataxic, apneustic, hyperventilation)
    3. Absent: early respiratory arrest or hypoventilation may be present in metabolic coma
    4. Hyperventilation: with no other brain stem signs, suggests psychiatric unresponsiveness

II. Circulation
    1. Shock: blood loss, cardiac etiology, overwhelming meningitis, septicemia (especially meningococcemia)
    2. Blood pressure: usually maintained in early coma owing to supratentorial mass lesions

III. Pupils
    1. Toxic/metabolic coma: usually equal and reactive, may exhibit hippus
    2. Unequal pupils: suspect possible herniation, especially if larger pupil is associated with ipsilateral oculomotor signs

IV. Eye position
    1. Bilateral deviation: supratentorial lesions with brain stem compression, posterior fossa lesions with pressure on brain stem
    2. Bilateral deviation with spontaneous jerking or changes in direction: seizures
    3. Lateral deviation on side of larger pupil: uncal herniation
    4. Skew deviation: subtentorial lesion

V. Oculovestibular response
    1. No response: symmetrical, could be due to specific toxin (e.g., neuromuscular block) or metabolic cause, could be massive subtentorial lesion
    2. Asymmetric: subtentorial lesion, especially if responses are inconsistent with solely a peripheral third nerve palsy (herniation)
    3. Usually maintained in toxic/metabolic coma

VI. Motor tone
    1. Asymmetric: supratentorial lesions, usually increased
    2. Inconsistent, variable: psychiatric disorder, seizures
    3. Symmetrical: metabolic cause, usually decreased; asterixis, tremor, myoclonus may be present in metabolic coma

VII. Ciliospinal
    1. Bilaterally present: metabolic cause
    2. Unilaterally present: possible peripheral third nerve lesion (herniation) if on side of larger pupil; possible pre-existing Horner's syndrome if on side of smaller pupil
    3. Bilaterally absent: not usually helpful

tion of the eyes towards the side of the cold stimulus. It is possible to detect not only whether the oculovestibular response is present or absent but whether the eyes move conjugately, unilaterally, or partially.

Oculocephalic responses, or doll's eye responses, can be useful in obtaining similar information. Movement of eyes can be elicited by rapid turning of the head. There is a significant risk in patients who have sustained head trauma and possible spinal injury. Since the same information is usually available from testing ice water calorics, we have avoided oculocephalic testing of all trauma patients and those comatose patients with unknown history. Oculocephalic tests may be useful when there is hesitation in introducing ice water into the external auditory canal because of blood behind the tympanic membrane, but it is precisely these patients in whom the greatest danger of neck injury is also present. We have observed patients who have suffered unsuspected neck injury during difficult airway intubations without previous history of trauma and who have experienced spinal injury during oculocephalic testing.

Motor Responses and Tone

The initial evaluation of skeletal muscle tone is important, particularly if there are differences in spontaneous tone on either side. The presence of unilateral or bilateral abnormal motor responses to painful stimuli should be noted. Asymmetric decorticate or decerebrate responses are less likely to occur in coma with metabolic etiologies and more likely to occur in situations in which rostral-caudal herniations or structural etiologies are present.

Spontaneous movements of the extremities, particularly with respect to differences in the movements of either side, may be quite helpful. Alternating increased tone or rapid changes in tone from hypertonic to hypotonic, or vice versa, may indicate seizures.

Eliciting motor responses by applying a noxious stimulus, gently but firmly, to the supraorbital notch or to each extremity may bring out differences. Appropriate avoidance responses, nonstereotypical withdrawal responses, and abnormal flexion or extension responses should be noted.

Ciliospinal Reflexes Pupillary dilation may be evoked by noxious cutaneous stimuli in the lightly comatose (or sleeping) individual. Bilateral ciliospinal reflexes can test the integrity of the sympathetic pathways but are not very useful in evaluating brain stem function. They may be helpful in evaluating pupillary inequalities in comatose patients with a previous history of sympathetic nervous system dysfunction such as Horner's syndrome.

Funduscopic Examination Patients presenting in coma should not have pharmacologic dilation of their pupils. The detection of abnormalities such as subhyoid hemorrhages with subarachnoid hemorrhages or papilledema is not worth the loss of the pupillary responses for following the patient's course. Information concerning papilledema may be inferred from other neurologic signs, and if the fundus cannot be visualized, papilledema may be assumed to be present.

Computed tomography (CT) examination can be performed for suspected increased intracranial pressure to determine if there is a treatable etiology.

The purpose of the initial neurological examination is to determine whether or not there is a structural lesion located in the brain stem, e.g., pontine infarction. The question of whether or not the brain stem is destroyed can have one of three answers: yes, no, or uncertain. In most instances, the second or third answer will be most appropriate.

If indeed the brain stem is intact, then the emergency resolution of the differential diagnosis of other causes of coma can be determined by either a CT examination or a spinal tap. A patient with metabolic coma will not be hurt by these procedures. Table 27-3 lists the categories of coma causes. Once the patient's oxygenation, circulation, and glucose needs have been met, the general differential diagnostic considerations are whether there is increased intracranial pressure and an impending herniation and/or whether there is life-threatening meningoencephalitis.

It may be useful to briefly review the rationale of differentiating a potential herniation syndrome from meningoencephalitis. If the patient is in a coma with a metabolic etiology, neither a CT scan nor a lumbar puncture (LP) will contribute to the specific diagnosis, but neither will hurt the patient, since the brain's immediate needs are stabilized. Postseizure stupor or coma will usually resolve or, if status epilepticus is present, become obvious. While a CT scan may demonstrate a focal lesion responsible for a seizure focus, the treatment of the coma will be to control the seizures. An LP is less likely to yield useful information and could be risky if a focal lesion is present even if the coma is not secondary to increased intracranial pressure or herniation. Midline aneurysms and hemorrhage may be visualized on a CT scan or bloody cerebrospinal fluid (CSF) may be obtained from an LP; either can be useful and neither will damage the patient. Patients with metabolic encephalopathy, concussion, or hysterical coma will not be hurt by either test—hence the necessity for recognizing herniation syndromes and lesions of the posterior fossa leading to coma with brain stem compression.

TABLE 27-3 The Use of Computed Tomography and Lumbar Puncture in the Evaluation of the Comatose Patient with No Structural Brain Stem Lesion

Condition	Computed Tomogram	Lumbar Puncture
Lateralized lesion with increased intracranial pressure	4+	No
Posterior fossa lesion with brain stem compression	4+	No
Metabolic/toxic abnormality	±	±
Subarachnoid hemorrhage	2+	2+
Meningoencephalitis	±	4+
Hysteria	±	±
Seizures	±	±

± May not be helpful or may hurt the patient
2+ May provide useful data for diagnosis and not hurt the patient
4+ Indicate for diagnosis
No: Can potentially hurt the patient

Specific Processes Causing Coma

Herniation Syndromes

The two most common syndromes accompanying increased intracranial pressures are: (1) the syndrome of rostral-caudal deterioration, sometimes referred to as central herniation; and (2) the syndrome of uncal herniation and lateral brain stem compression.[2] Recognition of either should alert the examiner to the possible need for emergency neurosurgical intervention. An LP should not be performed. Increased intracranial pressure is covered in detail in Chap. 31. The abbreviated sections below refer to recognizing coma associated with herniation syndromes.

Rostral-Caudal Deterioration

The central syndrome can be understood as early bilateral central involvement exerting pressure on the diencephalon. Among the early characteristics of central herniation is the impairment of the level and content of consciousness. The patient may be less alert, and frequently confusion or behavioral abnormalities are present. There may be a normal respiratory pattern interrupted with deep sighs or yawns or Cheyne-Stokes respirations. If the patient is cooperative, posthyperventilation apnea can be demonstrated. In the early stages, the pupillary size may be small (<2 mm), but on close examination the light responses are present. Ice water calorics produce full conjugate responses, with nystagmus disappearing as the patient becomes comatose. Motor tone may be increased bilaterally with decorticate posturing to noxious supraorbital pressure. Bilateral Babinski signs may be present. The ciliospinal responses are present.

As central herniation progresses from the early stage affecting primarily the diencephalon to a stage involving the midbrain and upper pons, the examination begins to show sustained, regular hyperventilation. The pupils enlarge to 3 to 5 mm and lose their response to light. Previously present ciliospinal reflexes may disappear. Ice water caloric responses can become more difficult to obtain and if the high midbrain is involved, there may be dysconjugate eye deviation with only the abducting eye responding. Motor tone is increased and decerebrate posturing to noxious stimuli may be present.

As the herniation progresses to involve the midbrain and pons and to affect the medulla, rapid, shallow respirations or slow, irregular breathing may be present. The pupils are fixed at midposition, usually equal, but sometimes slightly unequal (1 to 2 mm). Caloric responses disappear and motor tone diminishes so that even reflexes disappear. Death is inevitable by the medullary stage.

Uncal Herniation

Expanding lesions in the lateral middle fossa or temporal lobe may push the medial edge of the uncus and hippocampal gyrus towards the midline. Since the diencephalon does not bear the brunt of the pressure early on, the patient may be alert with only mild confusion or headache. Post-traumatic lateralized injuries may therefore be quite insidious, with the patient appearing to have an unimpaired state of consciousness.

A unilaterally dilating pupil, due to pressure on the third nerve as it crosses over the tentorial edge, is the earliest sign of uncal herniation. Anisocoria with a sluggish light reaction of the dilated pupil may be present for several hours. However, it is critical that this be recognized since rapid progression to coma can be a common and alarming feature. During the early stages of uncal herniation there may be no other abnormalities of the core neurological examination (Table 27-1). However, asymmetric motor responses may be present with increased tone, reflexes, and an upgoing toe on the contralateral side. As the clinical syndrome of uncal herniation develops, the pupil continues to dilate, the light reaction can be lost, and the eye may deviate laterally—all effects due to pressure on the third nerve. Respiration can become Cheyne-Stokes in pattern or there can be sustained hyperventilation. Ice water caloric responses can be brisk in the opposite eye with only lateral deviation produced on the side of the dilating pupil. The ciliospinal response can disappear on the side of the dilating pupil. Bilateral increased tone and decorticate or decerebrate responses can be present, although usually asymmetrically. As the pressure pushes the brain stem laterally, the opposite cerebral peduncle becomes compressed against the opposite tentorial edge, which leads to motor changes ipsilateral to the dilated pupil. This is called *Kernohan's notch*. There may be bilateral increased tone and Babinski signs. By this time the patient is usually highly stuporous or comatose.

Unless the pressure is relieved, uncal herniation can progress to damage the pons and midbrain so that both pupils become fixed (usually asymmetrically) and caloric responses disappear. As in central herniation, progression to this stage carries a poor prognosis and continued pressure leads to death.

Although uncal herniation syndromes are more common than central syndromes, the two types may occur together, that is, features of each can occur simultaneously. As a general rule in evaluating a patient with coma of unknown etiology, unilateral pupillary dilation, lateral deviation of that eye, or bilaterally deviated eyes should elicit the choice of a CT scan (and/or emergency therapy for increased intracranial pressure). These signs are unusual for meningitis or metabolic coma, although hypoglycemia can produce almost any combination of signs. Since glucose has been administered, a lateralized lesion with increased intracranial pressure should be ruled out when these signs are present.

Posterior Fossa Lesions with Brain Stem Pressure

Lesions of the posterior fossa presenting with coma are extremely difficult to diagnose or even suspect, particularly if there is no history available for a patient presenting in coma. Since the rapid relief of pressure may prevent permanent brain stem damage, this particular syndrome should always be in the back of one's mind. The only objective physical sign may be bilateral eye deviation. Since this sign will usually lead to a CT scan, it is imperative to make sure that the posterior fossa is visualized.

The usual clinical picture associated with posterior fossa lesions such as cerebellar infarction, cerebellar hemorrhage, or posterior fossa subdural hematoma involves headache, nausea, vomiting, staggering gait, and dysarthria, followed by coma. Without a history there may be no localizing signs other than bilateral eye deviation. With increasing pressure on the brain stem, intrinsic brain stem signs may be produced. The syndrome can take minutes to days to develop. If the pressure can be relieved before the onset of coma, prognosis for a complete functional recovery is excellent. The longer the coma, the poorer the prognosis. If pressure can be relieved before intrinsic brain stem damage has occurred, the patient may still have a remarkable recovery. This cause of coma is frequently forgotten and should be kept in mind as a critical, treatable etiology.

Encephalomeningitis, Especially Due to Meningococcal Infection

A lumbar puncture is absolutely indicated in the evaluation of meningitis as an etiology of coma. In general, the patient will have no focal neurological signs, especially pupillary dilation or eye deviation. There may be fever or a stiff neck, but the latter may also be seen with the herniation syndromes or a posterior fossa lesion. Absence of a stiff neck does not rule out meningitis. Meningococcal meningitis is a particularly fulminant disease, which should be recognized. It is usually associated with the rapid onset of illness, with chills and fever, pain in the back, stiff neck, conjunctivitis, a petechial or hemorrhagic skin rash, stupor, and coma. Acute fulminating cases can result in severe circulatory collapse. Focal neurological signs are uncommon. Rapid specific treatment with antibiotics and steroids may be critical. Thus when evaluating a comatose patient with no known history, this etiology should be considered in a patient with a nonfocal examination but with fever, stiff neck, or a petechial skin rash. Meningitis is covered in more detail in another chapter.

Metabolic Encephalopathy

Metabolic encephalopathy is the most common etiology for coma in a general hospital. This includes patients with diseases prone to complications, such as diabetes mellitus with acidosis, as well as those suffering from drug overdoses or toxic exposures. There is usually a progression, with confusion and disorientation gradually proceeding to stupor or coma. Respirations may be affected early (hypoventilation or hyperventilation) with preserved pupillary reactions and oculovestibular responses. If motor signs develop, they are preceded by stupor or coma and are symmetrical unless superimposed on an existing motor asymmetry. Patients may exhibit tremors, myoclonus, or asterixis when stuporous, and coma may be associated with repetitive seizures. Occasionally, patients with metabolic coma (particularly due to uremia, hepatic coma, or hypoglycemia) may have asymmetric motor signs usually associated with intact pupillary and oculomotor responses. Rare patients, particularly those who are hypoglycemic, can develop focal pupillary signs that mimic structural lesions of the brain stem or even herniation syndromes. Since all patients will have received glucose during the initial encounter, evaluation of suspected herniation using CT scanning will not damage the patient. Treatment of other causes of metabolic coma can proceed once the patient is stabilized.

Blood for glucose, electrolytes, calcium, phosphate, creatinine, arterial gases, and CSF (cells, Gram stain, glucose) should be obtained immediately for evaluating metabolic encephalopathy. Samples for specific blood and urine tests for drugs or toxins, liver function tests, coagulation studies, and thyroid and adrenal function tests, can be obtained early and processed later, if appropriate, as well as blood, urine, and CSF cultures. In the presence of metabolic coma it has become routine to administer naloxone hydrochloride (0.4 mg) to comatose patients on the assumption that morphine (or a similar substance) may be the cause of the coma. Naloxone HCl (Narcan, Endo Laboratories, Inc., Garden City, N.Y.) is a morphine antagonist which does not further depress the state of consciousness of the patient and may rapidly reverse coma induced by morphinelike narcotics. Thiamine (50 to 100 mg) is also administered for coma due to Wernicke's encephalopathy (rare) in alcoholics or to safeguard an alcoholic patient from the precipitation of Wernicke's encephalopathy by the glucose load already administered. Certain sedative drugs, particularly the tricyclic antidepressants, have anticholinergic properties. Reversal of the depressant effects of these drugs is achieved by the intravenous injection of 1 mg physostigmine (Antilirium, O'Neal, Jones, and Feldman, St. Louis, Mo.) Because of its cholinergic effects on the nervous system, physostigmine can arouse patients who may not have overdosed on anticholinergic drugs, although complete reversal usually indicates that such a drug was taken.

Trauma; Head Injury

Coma in a setting of head trauma will be a frequent presentation to the neurosurgeon.[1] The approach to a patient with head injury involves the same steps as that used with any other comatose patient (Table 27-1). The importance of supplying oxygen, blood, and glucose to the brain remains. Management may be modified to deal with practical considerations of the traumatized head and the risk of herniation will be higher than in patients presenting without known head injury. This affects the management but does not change the specific order of considerations.

Respiration

Head trauma may present additional problems in evaluating the rate and rhythm of breathing. Severe facial injuries may make intubation impossible, especially if there are fractures of the maxillary or mandibular areas. An adequate airway must be provided for respiration; an emergency tracheostomy may be necessary. If chest trauma accompanies the injuries, it may be necessary to place a chest tube or treat a flail chest or hemopneumothorax by mechanical ventilation. In general, it is always advisable to aggressively assure ventilation in the early stages of treatment of trauma patients.

Patients who are stuporous owing to hypoxia or hypercarbia may be combative. Since a CT scan will usually be performed, any patient with unknown intracranial trauma who receives a neuromuscular blocking agent or sedation should be intubated.

Cerebral Blood Flow

Hypotension in a patient with head trauma can be assumed to be due to causes other than brain injury. The most frequently encountered cause of hypotension in trauma patients is blood loss or pooling due to hypoxia. If a proper airway and ventilation have been established, sources of bleeding from extremity, intra-abdominal, intrathoracic, or retroperitoneal injuries should be sought. Maintenance of adequate blood pressure should be assured by blood replacement or volume expanders. Comatose patients with no obvious site of bleeding should have peritoneal lavage. The abdominal examination in a comatose patient can be particularly unrewarding. Peritoneal lavage is an effective method to determine if intra-abdominal bleeding is a problem complicating obvious trauma.

Glucose

Provided that the ventilation and circulation of the patient are stabilized, glucose should always be administered to traumatized patients. Since the head injury may be obvious, this simple procedure is often neglected, to the patient's detriment. It is not uncommon, particularly in automobile accidents, for hypoglycemia to play a role in causing the accident. A simple precaution is to administer glucose by intravenous infusion to all patients with head injury.

Core Neurological Examination

CT examination will be part of virtually all evaluations of patients with head injury. This radiographic test does not preclude a careful core neurological examination. Evidence of a unilaterally dilating pupil should make the examiner think twice before placing the patient in a CT scanner and may require expeditious neurosurgical intervention. Frequent neurological examinations can provide information on the rate of herniation as well.

Thus, pupillary size and reaction to light and position of the eyes and their response to vestibular stimuli should be recorded. It is clearly dangerous to perform the doll's eye maneuver in a head-injured patient. The oculovestibular information obtained by quickly turning the head is not worth the possible risk of damaging the cord if a spinal injury is present. Ice water caloric examination can provide the same information at considerably less risk. Indeed, examination of the ear canals before caloric testing can frequently provide the initial sign of skull fracture with blood behind the tympanic membrane. Recognition of rapidly changing neurological signs such as a dilating pupil or lateral deviation of an eye should alert the examiner to the possibility of an epidural hematoma or acute subdural hematoma or intracerebral hemorrhage.

Management of patients with head injury requires an assessment system that can be used by medical and nursing

TABLE 27-4 Glasgow Coma Scale

Modality	Response	Score	Actual Patient Response over Time				
Eye opening	Spontaneous	4					
	To speech	3					
	To pain	2					
	None	1					
Best verbal response	Oriented	5					
	Confused	4					
	Inappropriate words	3					
	Incomprehensible sounds	2					
	None	1					
Best motor response	Obeys commands	6					
	Localizes pain	5					
	Flexion withdrawal	4					
	Abnormal flexion	3					
	Abnormal extension	2					
	None	1					
Total		15					

personnel. The assessments must be highly reproducible and easy. A number of systems have been devised, but the Glasgow Coma Scale provides information concerning three aspects of the patient's responsiveness: (1) eye opening; (2) best verbal response; (3) best motor response (Table 27-4). Each modality is described according to a defined series of neurological responses, each associated with a progressive degree of neurological impairment. The Glasgow Coma Scale does not take the place of careful neurological examination but may provide an effective means of following patients with head injury who are not frankly comatose. By following eye opening, verbal response, and motor response, deterioration can be noted by relatively unsophisticated personnel and the physician can be alerted. Such a procedure does not replace, but only supplements, careful periodic follow-up examination of vital signs, pupillary size (in millimeters), and reaction to light, eye position and movement, and limb tone and movement. It also becomes less useful if the patient's eyes are closed by swelling or if speech cannot be evaluated owing to an endotracheal tube or tracheostomy. As a reproducible system to follow the level of consciousness, the Glasgow Coma Scale can be valuable. It is not meant to be used in the absence of careful monitoring of vital and neurological signs.

Uncal herniation can develop in a patient with spontaneously open eyes who is oriented and can obey motor commands. Dilation of a pupil with spontaneous Cheyne-Stokes respirations or posthyperventilation apnea may precede stupor or coma and can obviously be missed unless vital and neurological signs are monitored.

The management of intracerebral lesions due to trauma and of herniation syndromes is covered elsewhere in this textbook. It is important to realize that appropriate treatment depends on accurate diagnosis. In comatose patients, an accurate diagnostic evaluation begins within seconds of a patient's presentation. A safe and efficient assessment with a CT scan or an LP can be decided upon in less than 2 min. In situations in which a herniation syndrome is suspected and no CT evaluation is available, arteriography or immediate surgical decompressive procedures can be instituted (for example, evacuation of an epidural or acute subdural hematoma). There is no substitute for a systematic approach to a comatose patient that protects the patient during evaluation.

References

1. Jennett WB, Teasdale G: *Management of Head Injuries* (Contemporary Neurology Series, vol 20). Philadelphia, Davis, 1981.
2. Plum F, Posner JB: *The Diagnosis of Stupor and Coma* (Contemporary Neurology Series, vol 19), 3d ed. Philadelphia, Davis, 1982.

28

Seizure Disorders and Their Medical Management

J. Scott Luther

Definition, Incidence and Prevalence

Seizure disorders (or epilepsy) rank second only to stroke as the most common chronic neurological disorder seen in developed countries. The term epilepsy, which is derived from the Greek *epilepsia* meaning a "taking hold of," refers to a disorder whereby abnormal neuronal excitability leads to the periodic and unpredictable occurrence of seizures. The term *seizure* refers to the clinical or behavioral changes which result from brain dysfunction due to excessive neuronal discharge.

The precise incidence and prevalence of seizure disorders in the general population is difficult to ascertain although epidemiologic studies indicate that when populations are considered as a whole, the incidence of seizure disorders is between 0.5 and 1 percent. Age specificity is important in that during the first 5 years of life the incidence of seizures, excluding febrile seizures, is approximately five times the rate for the general population. The incidence gradually decreases between the ages of 5 and 20 and then gradually increases again in the elderly. Prevalence data are even more difficult to obtain but are estimated at 3 to 5 per 1000.[2]

Pathophysiology of the Epileptic Discharge

Experimentally, many neuronal populations can be made to produce abnormal electrical discharges or seizures by either electrical or chemical induction. Certain neuronal populations seem to be more susceptible to induction of such discharges and seizures. In addition to the prefrontal and motor cortex, the limbic system, especially the limbic structures of the temporal lobe, is particularly susceptible to experimental induction of seizures. This correlates clinically with the most common seizure type seen in adults, namely, complex partial seizures. Ninety percent of these seizures appear to arise from either the amygdala or hippocampus.

Most electrical activity that can be recorded from the surface of the cortex or at the scalp presumably represents the summation and interaction of synaptic potentials generated by cortical neurons. Subcortical structures, most notably the thalamus, have a profound effect on electrical activity generated by the cortex but are not thought to be primarily responsible for the spike and spike-and-wave discharges that are the characteristic abnormalities generated from cortical neurons in patients with epilepsy.

Electroencephalographic recordings between seizures in both human and experimental epilepsy disclose the presence of sharp transients termed *interictal spikes*. Intracellular recordings from neurons presumably generating the interictal spikes disclose a large, prolonged membrane depolarization termed a *paroxysmal depolarizing shift* (PDS). These neurons fire numerous action potentials during this depolarization resulting in a train of action potentials which are subsequently conducted along the axon of the neuron. This depolarization is followed by a prolonged hyperpolarization, an *inhibitory postsynaptic potential* (IPSP). The transition from interictal to ictal activity is heralded by the disappearance of the hyperpolarization and repetitive neuronal firing.

Extensive investigations have sought to elucidate the mechanisms responsible for the PDS. Recent evidence supports the idea that the depolarization is triggered by an excitatory postsynaptic potential.[9] Whether the massive depolarization itself represents a giant excitatory postsynaptic potential or an intrinsic neuronal regenerative event is not clear. Equally unclear is whether the following hyperpolarization is a synaptic or nonsynaptic event. Identification of the factors governing transitions from interictal to ictal activity would likely provide clues for the development of new anticonvulsant medications.

The term *inhibitory surround* has been used to describe the region near the periphery of an epileptogenic focus in which only large hyperpolarizing IPSP's can be seen associated with the epileptic phenomena without any preceding depolarization. During the ictal phase, this inhibitory surround disappears and rhythmic depolarization is seen in the region. This phenomenon has been used as an explanation for mechanisms responsible for both the continued localization of interictal activity and the transition from interictal to ictal activity with spread of activity to other neurons. Clearly, the influences on an epileptic focus are complex and represent the combined effects of local membrane activity and remote neuronal populations, as well as the metabolic state of the patient.[8]

Etiological Factors

The term *idiopathic* is applied to seizure disorders or forms of epilepsy in which no identifiable cause can be found on either a biochemical or structural basis by using currently available investigational techniques. The majority of seizure disorders fall into this category whether they are generalized or partial in type. The highest percentage of idiopathic seizure disorders do occur in the generalized group, with less than 15 percent of patients having an identifiable cause for their seizures. Even in the group of patients with partial seizures, which implies a focal onset, 75 percent fall into the idiopathic category.[6,13] Patients with complex partial seizures constitute the largest subgroup in which no identifiable etiology is demonstrated. Idiopathic seizures may occur at any time during life; however, they appear most frequently between the ages of 2 and 7 years and also have a tendency to be manifested around puberty.

Genetic factors have their greatest role in the idiopathic epilepsies, predominantly in the generalized types. Electroencephalographic abnormalities, as well as clinical seizures, occur in a significant portion of siblings and first-degree relatives of patients with absence seizures, as well as of those with seizures associated with centrotemporal spikes.

When a specific cause, whether structural or biochemical, can be identified, the seizure disorder is referred to as *symptomatic* or *acquired*. Metabolic abnormalities are responsible for a significant number of symptomatic seizures, both generalized and focal, and are important to identify because treatment of the underlying metabolic disorder will frequently eliminate the seizures. In adults, uremia, hypoglycemia, anoxia, hypertensive encephalopathy, and hyponatremia are common causes of generalized and focal seizures. Myoclonic jerks are also frequently seen in the setting of metabolic imbalance, primarily with uremia and anoxia. Withdrawal or abstinence from sedative drugs and intoxicants (primarily barbiturates and alcohol) that have been used on a chronic basis can be associated with the appearance of generalized tonic-clonic seizures. In the setting of alcohol withdrawal, the seizures usually occur within the first 48 h following cessation of drinking and usually precede delirium tremens. Other metabolic conditions also associated with generalized seizures but less frequent in occurrence are porphyria, thyroid storm, and hypocalcemia. In neonates and infants manifesting seizures, pyridoxine deficiency, phenylketonuria, anoxia, and hypocalcemia need to be considered. Uncomplicated febrile convulsions in children, which usually occur before 3 years of age, are probably most appropriately considered in the toxic and metabolic category. These seizures usually occur with a rapid rise in temperature and are ordinarily not associated with any direct central nervous system infection. Approximately one-third of patients with febrile convulsions will develop seizure disorders later in life but most of these patients are those who have had complicated febrile convulsions.[7]

Infections of the central nervous system, whether acute or chronic, may be responsible for seizures during the period of maximum activity or as long-term sequelae. Meningitis, bacterial or viral, may cause generalized seizures. It is estimated that approximately 40 percent of cerebral abscesses are associated with recurrent seizures. Herpes simplex encephalitis, which has the propensity to affect the temporal lobes to a greater degree than other head regions, is often associated with focal seizures. The slow viral diseases, subacute sclerosing panencephalitis and Creutzfeldt-Jakob disease, characteristically have seizures as a prominent clinical feature. Schistosomiasis and cysticercosis are endemic in certain geographic areas and frequently cause seizures.

Head trauma has always been an important cause of acquired seizures. Despite improved first aid, methods of evacuation to a hospital, and neurosurgical techniques, the incidence of recurrent seizures following penetrating missile wounds to the head remains between 40 and 45 percent. The incidence of epilepsy following nonpenetrating missile head injuries is not as well defined but is thought to be approximately 5 percent. A severe head injury, as gauged by the presence of a contusion or hematoma, violation of the integrity of the dura, or amnesia for more than 24 h, carries approximately a 12 percent risk of recurrent seizures at 5 years.[1] Minimal head trauma (as defined by no associated structural abnormality or fracture as well as a period of amnesia of less than 30 min) is thought to carry no increased risk of seizures as compared with that of the general population.

Cerebral vascular disease (stroke) is an important cause of seizures, particularly in the elderly population. Seizures are unusual during the acute phase of thrombotic stroke although occasionally an embolic stroke may be associated with a focal seizure. Conversely, it is estimated that 20 percent of old cortical infarcts become epileptogenic. On the other hand, cortical vein thrombosis, which occurs primarily in the puerperium, frequently presents as repetitive focal seizures. Vasculitides that involve cerebral vessels, i.e., primarily systemic lupus erythematosus, produce seizures in approximately 20 percent of patients.

Both primary and metastatic tumors are an important cause of seizures in the adult population. Tumors in the supratentorial brain regions are particularly prone to cause focal seizures. Fifteen to twenty percent of patients with brain tumors will present with seizures as their initial symptom. It is estimated that 30 to 40 percent of all patients with brain tumors will experience seizures during the course of their illness. Gliomas, metastatic tumors (especially from the lung), and meningiomas are the tumor types most likely to produce seizures.

Several congenital, inherited, and degenerative diseases are associated with a significant incidence of seizures. The presence of seizures in the setting of a significant congenital anomaly usually reflects the degree of abnormality present on a gross structural as well as cellular basis. Inborn errors of metabolism in which seizures are a prominent component usually manifest themselves within the first several weeks of life. Tuberous sclerosis, which is inherited in an autosomal dominant pattern, has a high incidence of seizures (90 percent). Approximately 10 percent of patients with neurofibromatosis will have seizures. Lipid storage diseases are associated with a high incidence of seizures. Generalized or myoclonic seizures occur in presenile dementia of the Alzheimer type.

Classification and Clinical Manifestations

The classification of epileptic seizures is important for etiologic, therapeutic, and prognostic reasons. The current proposed international classification is summarized in Table 28-1.[5] The generalized seizures tend to begin at an earlier age, are more responsive to medications and overall carry a more favorable prognosis than do partial seizures.

TABLE 28-1   Classification of Epileptic Seizures

  I. Generalized seizures (bilaterally symmetrical and without local onset)
     A. Absences (petit mal)
     B. Tonic-clonic seizures (grand mal)
     C. Clonic seizures
     D. Tonic seizures
     E. Bilateral massive epileptic myoclonus
     F. Atonic seizures
 II. Partial seizures (seizures beginning locally)
     A. Partial seizures with elementary symptomatology (generally without impairment of consciousness)
        1. With motor symptoms (includes Jacksonian seizures)
        2. With special sensory or somatosensory symptoms
        3. With autonomic symptoms
        4. Compound forms
     B. Partial seizures with complex symptomatology (generally with impairment of consciousness)
        1. With impairment of consciousness only
        2. With cognitive symptomatology
        3. With affective symptomatology
        4. With psychosensory symptomatology
        5. With psychomotor symptomatology (automatisms)
        6. Compound forms
     C. Partial seizures evolving to secondarily generalized seizures
        1. Simple partial evolving to generalized seizures
        2. Complex partial evolving to generalized seizures
        3. Simple partial evolving to complex partial evolving to generalized seizures
III. Unclassified Epileptic Seizures

Generalized Seizures

Generalized seizures by definition have no evidence of focal onset either electrically or clinically. The two most common types of generalized seizures encountered in clinical practice are absence (petit mal) and tonic-clinic (grand mal) seizures. The age of onset for absence seizures is typically between the ages of 4 and 12 years. These seizures are never preceded by an aura (although the patients are often aware that they have had a seizure following the episode) and usually last less than 30 s. Immediately following the episode, the patient's mental status returns completely to normal. Behavioral ictal manifestations present a wide clinical spectrum. Simple absence consists of only a motionless stare unassociated with other motor activity. This occurs in less than 10 percent of patients with absence. The most commonly associated motor activity is bilateral symmetrical eye blinking or fluttering during the episode. Other complex motor manifestations as well as automatic behavior may also occur during absence and may be indistinguishable from the motor and automatic behavior seen in complex partial seizures. These complex motor manifestations may be present during brief seizure episodes but are much more common in prolonged absence seizures (10 to 15 s). It is not unusual for patients to have between 20 and 80 absence seizures per day. One clue that the patient may be having absence seizures is an unexplained decline in school performance in a previously normal child.[11]

Primary generalized tonic-clonic seizures (grand mal) present as dramatic events clinically. At the beginning of these seizures the patient often gives an audible cry which is followed by a variable period of generalized tonic posturing

lasting from 10 to 30 s. Subsequent to this, clonic activity supervenes, as evidenced by rhythmic motor activity, again without evidence of focal onset. During the period of tonic as well as tonic-clonic activity, patients often become cyanotic, exhibit tongue biting, and have urinary incontinence. Following the tonic-clonic phase of the seizure, muscle tone is markedly reduced and patients are unresponsive to any stimuli administered. The period of postictal confusion lasts anywhere from several minutes to as long as 12 h.

The other generalized seizure types occur primarily in childhood and adolescence and are rare in their occurrence in comparison with absence seizures and generalized tonic-clonic seizures. Purely clonic, tonic, or atonic seizures may imply severe underlying cerebral abnormalities, as seen in the clinical syndrome of infantile spasms, which often correlates with the EEG characteristics of hypsarrythmia. Myoclonic seizures, which usually also begin in childhood or adolescence, may be idiopathic but are also associated with Lafora's disease, Unverricht's disease, and other ganglioside storage diseases.

Partial Seizures

The term *partial* means that the seizure begins focally. Such focal seizures may or may not be associated with impairment of consciousness, which is the criterion for separating elementary from complex partial seizures. During an elementary partial seizure, the patient does not lose contact with his environment or exhibit impairment of consciousness, and if tested during and following the event will be able to process and remember all information given to him during the seizure. The behavioral manifestations of elementary partial seizures may be quite complex and very similar to the type of behavior seen during absence or complex partial seizures. Testing consciousness during a seizure may be necessary to differentiate these elementary partial seizures from complex partial seizures.

The sine qua non of complex partial seizures is impairment of consciousness, manifested as impairment in the degree of awareness or responsiveness to externally applied stimuli. Responsiveness refers to the ability of the patient to carry out a simple command or willed movement, whereas awareness refers to the patient's contact with events during the period of time in question and the patient's ability to recall this information. Persons aware and unresponsive will be able to recount the events that occurred during an attack and yet their ability to respond may be impaired by limitations of movement or speech. Complex partial seizures, in contrast to absence, are followed by a period of mental clouding or confusion, which may last a period of seconds to hours after cessation of electrical correlates of seizure activity by scalp EEG.

Automatisms are also characteristic of this seizure type. These may represent a continuation of activity that was going on when the seizure occurred or, conversely, a new activity developed in association with the ictal impairment of consciousness. Usually the activity is stereotyped in nature and often provoked by the patient's environment or by his sensations during a seizure. It is exceptional for fragmentary, primitive, infantile, or antisocial behavior to be seen. From a behavioral standpoint, the following automatisms can be distinguished: (1) eating (chewing, swallowing); (2) mimicry, expressing the patient's emotional state (usually fear) during the seizure; (3) gestural automatisms (either crude or elaborate), often directed toward either the subject or the environment; (4) ambulatory behavior; (5) verbal automatisms.[3] It should be noted that automatisms are not unique to complex partial seizures. They are observed following generalized tonic-clonic seizures and are also seen in association with absence seizures.

The clinical onset of a complex partial seizure is variable. The seizures may begin with impairment of consciousness only and not be associated with an aura. On the other hand, one of the more commonly encountered auras is that of a rising epigastric sensation. This feeling is often poorly described although it may be referred to as nausea or a nondescript discomfort in the epigastrium. Other frequently encountered auras include psychic symptoms such as flashbacks, déjà vu, fear, olfactory or gustatory hallucinations, and/or visual or auditory hallucinations. The mean duration of complex partial seizures is approximately 3 min, varying from less than 1 to 28 min.

A typical complex partial seizure often begins with a motionless stare for a few seconds, followed by stereotyped or unreactive automatisms for 15 to 60 s. This is followed by reactive automatisms and confusion for several minutes. Other complex partial seizures begin with the initial manifestation of stereotypic behavior without a motionless stare. Unusually, complex partial seizures may manifest themselves as a "drop attack" with complete loss of muscle tone by the patient. Recent data suggest that complex partial seizures that begin with a motionless stare followed by stereotyped automatisms have the greatest chance of arising from limbic structures in the temporal lobes.[3] In complex partial seizures which exhibit stereotyped behavior at onset, involvement of the limbic system is certain; however, it is thought that these seizures have a greater chance of involving limbic structures outside of the temporal regions. The site(s) of origin for complex partial seizures manifested as a loss of muscle tone are unclear. Approximately 75 percent of patients with complex partial seizures will also exhibit secondary spread to generalized tonic-clonic seizures at some time during their course. Elementary partial seizures may evolve to complex partial seizures, which may in turn evolve to generalized tonic-clonic seizures.

Differentiation of complex partial seizures from complex absence seizures may be difficult because both are associated with impairment of consciousness and yet may not have dramatic clinical behavioral correlates.[3] Differentiation is essential because of etiologic and pharmacologic considerations. Table 28-2 lists clinical and electroencephalographic criteria for differentiating these two seizure types.

Status Epilepticus

Major motor status epilepticus is defined as the occurrence of two or more primary or secondarily generalized tonic-clonic seizures without a return to normal consciousness between the ictal events. This is a neurologic emergency. Studies have indicated that the longer tonic-clonic status is allowed to continue, the more severe will be the residual neurologic

TABLE 28-2 Differentiating Features between Absence and Complex Partial Seizures

	Absence	CPS
Age of onset	4–12 years	Any age
Aura	Never	Often (50%)
Duration	Almost always <30 s	Rarely <30 s
Activated by hyperventilation	80–90%	10–20%
Mental clearing after seizure	Immediate	Slow
Interictal EEG	Normal	Focal spike wave, slowing
Ictal EEG	3/s spike wave	Varied

sequelae. Permanent brain damage has occurred after 60 min of continued status. Mortality approaches 10 percent in patients who remain in status for 12 h or more. Neurologic sequelae are much less likely to occur when status is broken within 90 min of its onset. Table 28-3 outlines an approach to treatment of generalized tonic-clonic status epilepticus.[4,6]

In addition to generalized tonic-clonic status epilepticus, several other forms of status epilepticus occur in which the clinical presentation is often more subtle. These forms may present behaviorally as fugue states, in which the patient may exhibit prolonged periods of confusion and impaired interaction with the environment, and as well as behavior that is out of character for that patient. Automatic behavior often allows the patient to interact with the environment in both appropriate and inappropriate manners. Absence status and complex partial status constitute this category of "nonconvulsive" status epilepticus. Differentiation between these two types of nonconvulsive status is important because of etiologic and pharmacologic considerations. Absence status (spike wave stupor) often occurs in adults who have not had a prior history of epilepsy. Patients are often able to carry on daily activities although they are usually not performing to the same degree or with the same accuracy when compared with their normal baseline. The electroencephalogram taken during this time should show bilateral and synchronous spike wave discharges although these frequently do not occur at the classic three per second rate typical of isolated absence seizures. Absence status may be terminated abruptly in a controlled situation with circulatory and respiratory support by the intravenous administration of diazepam. Simultaneous electroencephalographic monitoring is beneficial in determining the efficacy of the response. Cessation of absence status is often heralded by an abrupt return to normal behavior. During complex partial status epilepticus, behavior tends to be more variable than seen during absence status, and simultaneous electroencephalographic monitoring should help clarify the diagnosis. In addition to more variations in the patient's functional ability, complex partial status epilepticus is often followed by a period of prolonged postictal confusion.

Epilepsia partialis continua (EPC) refers to partial somatomotor status epilepticus in which consciousness is frequently preserved. EPC can be differentiated from a typical partial motor seizure both by the absence of progression from tonic to clonic phases and by the absence of a topo-

TABLE 28-3 Treatment of Generalized Tonic-Clonic Status Epilepticus

A. Immediate intervention (first 10 min)
   1. Support circulation
   2. Support respiration: most patients should be intubated
   3. Draw blood for anticonvulsant levels, glucose, electrolytes, complete blood count, calcium
   4. Draw arterial blood gas
   5. Administer 50 ml of 50% glucose intravenously
   6. Administer 100 mg thiamine intramuscularly
B. Intermediate intervention (second 10 min)
   1. Diazepam 10 mg intravenously at 2 to 4 mg/min until seizures stop or to a total of 30 mg
   2. Slow intravenous infusion of phenytoin (<50 mg/min) to a total of 20 mg/kg
   3. Perform general and neurologic exam with attention to evidence of primary or secondary trauma, pupils, fundi, extremity movements, pathological reflexes
C. Further intervention (next 40–60 min, if status epilepticus continues)
   1. Phenobarbital intravenously at 50 mg/min to total of 20 mg/kg
   2. General anesthesia to obtain burst suppression pattern on electroencephalogram, or
   3. 4% paraldehyde solution in normal saline

graphic march of the tonic phase from one group of muscles to another.

Treatment for generalized tonic-clonic, complex partial, or absence status epilepticus should be vigorous and instituted as soon after the diagnosis is made as possible. An outline for a systematic approach for the treatment of these conditions is presented in Table 28-3. Absence status is usually responsive to intravenous diazepam, followed by oral ethosuximide, valproic acid, or clonazepam. Intravenous diazepam will stop tonic-clonic status epilepticus within 5 min in 80 percent of patients. The combination of phenytoin and diazepam will stop the seizures of approximately two-thirds of patients who have secondarily generalized tonic-clonic status from partial seizures. Once observation of the patient's clinical behavior is impaired by anticonvulsant medications, neuromuscular blockade, or general anesthesia, continuous monitoring of brain activity by electroencephalography is necessary.

Diagnosis and Differential Diagnosis

The diagnosis of a seizure or seizure disorder depends primarily on historical information supplied by a reliable observer. Any patients who lose contact with the environment for whatever reason disqualify themselves as reliable historians and observers from the time of loss of contact until the time of full recovery. Behavioral observations made during the time when the patient has impairment of consciousness are crucial to establishing whether or not that impairment was due to a seizure or to some other cause.

Generalized seizures, with the exception of absence seizures, present the most dramatic behavioral changes in which motor features (e.g., tonic, clonic, myoclonic, atonic) predominate. Patients with syncope may demonstrate one or two tonic-clonic or myoclonic jerks at the beginning of the episode, but rarely are these sustained for the length of time seen during generalized seizures. Breath-holding spells in children may resemble generalized seizures.

Differentiation between complex partial seizures and absence seizures may be difficult because both are associated with impairment of consciousness, have stereotyped and reactive automatisms, and behaviorally may appear similar. Table 28-2 lists both the clinical and electroencephalographic criteria useful in this differentiation. In addition, absence seizures can be frequently induced in the clinical setting by hyperventilation for 4 to 6 min. Frequently, patients will demonstrate their typical clinical absence seizure during this activation but the changes can be as subtle as a mere break in the cadence of the patient's breathing pattern.

Certain other features of seizure disorders help distinguish them from other causes of impairment of consciousness. The age of onset of the clinical condition should serve as one clue. Generalized seizures begin primarily in childhood and are the seizures most easily controlled by anticonvulsant medication. Partial seizures may begin at any age, but are typically stereotyped in behavior from one event to the next. The patients often have clusters of seizures, occurring either several times in 1 day or several times in 1 week and separated by irregular but often prolonged seizure-free intervals. Episodes of presumed seizure activity that occur frequently, i.e., daily or several times per week, and are unresponsive to anticonvulsant therapy may be pseudo-epileptic in nature and should be investigated further in an attempt to precisely define their character and physiology.[10]

Medical Management

Of the large variety of anticonvulsant medications available, the most commonly used drugs are listed in Table 28-4. Identification of the patient's seizure type is an important consideration in the choice of medication. Carbamazepine (Tegretol, Geigy Pharmaceuticals, Ardsley, N.Y.) phenobarbital, phenytoin (Dilantin, Parke-Davis, Morris Plains, N.J.), and primidone (Mysoline, Ayerst Laboratories, New York, N.Y.) are all effective in the treatment of primary generalized tonic-clonic seizures as well as partial seizures; however, these drugs are ineffective in controlling absence seizures. Conversely, ethosuximide (Zarontin, Parke-Davis), valproic acid (Depakene, Abbott Laboratories, North Chicago, Ill.), and clonazepam (Clonopin, Roche Laboratories, Nutley, N.J.) are medications that are effective in the treatment of absence seizures but have variable if little effect on generalized tonic-clonic and partial seizures.[12]

In addition to the influence of a patient's seizure type on the choice of initial anticonvulsant therapy, consideration must also be given to the pharmacologic properties of the anticonvulsants listed in Table 28-4, the potential for both dose-related and idiosyncratic side effects, and the route of administration. Currently, phenytoin, phenobarbital, and diazepam are the only anticonvulsants available for intravenous administration.

In an attempt to achieve acceptable seizure control while

TABLE 28-4 Commonly Used Anticonvulsant Drugs

Drug	Indications	Average Daily Dosage, mg	Days to Achieve Steady State	Serum Half-Life, h	Therapeutic Blood Level, (μg/ml)	Dose-Related Side Effects	Idiosyncratic Side Effects
Phenytoin	Partial seizures; generalized tonic-clonic seizures	300–500	5–10	24 ± 12	10–20	Nystagmus, ataxis, lethargy	Rash, hepatitis, lymph node enlargement, systemic lupus erythematosus
Phenobarbital	Partial seizures; generalized tonic-clonic seizures	180–200	14–21	96 ± 12	15–40	Lethargy, nystagmus, ataxia	Exfoliative dermatitis
Carbamazepine	Partial seizures; generalized tonic-clonic seizures	1000–1200	2–4	12 ± 3	4–8	Diplopia, ataxia, blurred vision	Aplastic anemia (3 cases)
Primidone	Partial seizures; generalized tonic-clonic seizures	750–1000	4–7	12 ± 6	5–12	Lethargy, nystagmus, ataxia	Exfoliative dermatitis
Ethosuximide	Absences (petit mal)	750–1000	5–8	30 ± 6	40–100	Nausea, vomiting, drowsiness, hiccups	Stevens-Johnson syndrome, aplastic anemia (3 cases)
Valproic acid	Absences; generalized tonic-clonic seizures; myoclonic seizures	Start 15 mg/kg, maximum 60 mg/kg	2–4	12 ± 6	50–100	Nausea, vomiting, drowsiness	Hepatitis, alopecia, weight gain
Clonazepam	Absences; myoclonic seizures; atonic seizures	1.5–4.0, maximum 20	3–4 (unclear)	22–32	5–50	Sedation, tolerance, behavioral disturbance	Rash

avoiding adverse toxic side effects, several general principles of anticonvulsant drug administration need emphasis. Drug therapy should be initiated with the dosage gradually increased until the desired clinical effect is achieved, until the patient remains refractory with documented blood levels in the high therapeutic range, or until the patient develops significant side effects. The serum half-life is an important consideration in determining dosage schedules, appropriate timing for serum anticonvulsant level determination, and expected time to achieve a steady state following a change in dosage. When an initial loading dose has not been used, five half-lives are usually required for the patient to achieve a steady state following a change in dosage, either an increase or decrease. This means that following a change in the patient's dose of carbamazepine, one might expect to see an accurate reflection in the blood level in 3 days, whereas in the case of phenobarbital, the steady state may not be achieved for 2 weeks. Dosage schedules are also affected by the half-life of a particular anticonvulsant medication. In an attempt to achieve stable blood levels without wide fluctuations between peaks and troughs, most of the anticonvulsants are administered at intervals that approximate one-half of their serum half-life. On the basis of half-life, phenobarbital, clonazepam, and ethosuximide are the only anticonvulsants that can be administered in a single daily dose; however, the dose-related side effects of ethosuximide and clonazepam require that they be administered in divided doses throughout the day.

Two different anticonvulsant medications may be appropriate as initial therapy, especially when the patient manifests several distinct seizure types. This situation is commonly encountered in children with absence seizures, one-quarter to one-third of whom may also have concomitant generalized tonic-clonic seizures. When seizures are resistant to adequate single drug therapy, a second anticonvulsant should be added gradually while again trying to achieve clinical control or a high therapeutic level based on serum determinations. When patients require multiple anticonvulsant medications, changes should be made in a single drug with a sufficient interval to allow a steady state to be achieved again. Abrupt withdrawal or changes in medications may precipitate undesirable side effects as well as an increase in seizure activity.

The mechanisms by which anticonvulsants mediate their anticonvulsant effects are unknown. Much information is available regarding the biochemical, pharmacological, and electrophysiological actions of many of these drugs. Which, if any, of these actions is responsible for their anticonvulsant action is unclear. Several postulates regarding the action of the anticonvulsant medications have been proposed. Phenytoin reduces the spread of electrical activity from an active focus, reduces post-tetanic potentiation of synaptic transmission, and also abolishes post-tetanic hyperpolarization. Phenobarbital reduces excitatory postsynaptic potentials without changing resting membrane potential. It is postulated that carbamazepine has a depressant action on transmission through the nucleus ventralis anterior of the thalamus. Valproic acid is thought to increase gamma-aminobutyric acid (GABA) activity by reducing GABA-degradative enzyme activity. Perhaps the drugs whose action is best understood are the benzodiazepines.

These drugs interact with specific receptors in neuronal membranes and thereby increase neuronal responsiveness to synaptically released GABA.

At present there are no data that indicate that any one of the drugs used in the treatment of generalized tonic-clonic and partial seizures is far superior to the others for obtaining and maintaining seizure control. All the anticonvulsant medications have certain advantages that make the administration of that particular drug more desirable in a particular clinical setting. Likewise, they all have side effects and potential adverse reactions, which limit their usefulness clinically.

Phenobarbital is an effective anticonvulsant and is the only anticonvulsant medication that can be confidently administered in a single daily dose. This is a direct result of the extended half-life of phenobarbital, which allows maintenance of a steady-state concentration without utilizing divided doses. Phenobarbital is also inexpensive. The major disadvantages of this medication are its sedative properties, to which the patient may develop tolerance after 8 to 12 weeks of therapy, the need to begin the medication at low doses with a gradual buildup to a total effective dose because of its sedative side effects, and its potential for causing paradoxical hyperactivity, especially in children.

Phenytoin requires no buildup of the dosage administered and is effective when given twice daily to a total adult dose of 300 to 500 mg per day. Gingival hyperplasia and mild hirsutism are side effects; these are not dose-related and may be bothersome to patients, especially young females. This medication should never be used intramuscularly because it crystallizes in intramuscular sites before being absorbed and is extremely irritating because of the high pH of the vehicle.

The total adult daily dose of carbamazepine (usually 1000 to 1600 mg) should be administered in three or four divided doses in order to avoid large swings in serum anticonvulsant concentration and to maintain a steady state. The medication is usually well tolerated from the standpoint of not inducing significant sedative side effects, but complete blood counts need to be followed after institution of therapy at regularly spaced intervals because of potential leukopenia. Aplastic anemia has developed rarely.

Primidone has anticonvulsant properties similar to those of phenobarbital, and a portion of this medication is converted to phenobarbital by the liver. Active metabolites other than phenobarbital are also detectable. The side effects of primidone are very similar to those of phenobarbital. All the medications discussed above are capable of producing drowsiness, lethargy, nystagmus, and ataxia at toxic levels.

The medication of choice for absence seizures is ethosuximide. The average daily dose of 1000 to 1500 mg is usually divided into three or four daily doses because gastrointestinal irritation occurs when the medication is administered in a single dose. The medication should be given with meals to reduce the potential for gastrointestinal side effects. The adequacy of a particular dose of ethosuximide is determined more by the patient's clinical response than by absolute blood levels. Continued absence seizures dictate that the dose of medication is inadequate even in light of blood levels that may be in the therapeutic range. In many patients, absence seizures will be controlled completely at a particular dose of the medication but will return abruptly if the dosage is lowered even slightly. Complete blood counts should be monitored during the early phases of therapy. Hiccups, headaches, nausea, and vomiting are the most frequent dose-related side effects.

Valproic acid is an effective medication for primary generalized tonic-clonic seizures, absence seizures, and myoclonic seizures. In a patient with absence as well as primary generalized tonic-clonic seizures, valproic acid is considered the drug of choice because both seizure types may be controlled by a single medication. The short half-life of valproic acid necessitates that it be given in three or four divided doses a day. Therapeutic blood levels are not fully established, and as with ethosuximide, the total daily dose is determined in part by the patient's clinical response. Hepatotoxicity, which has been fatal in some cases, is the major potential side effect following institution of therapy. This has occurred primarily in children and may reflect an increased susceptibility to liver damage in young patients although it may also reflect the more widespread use of the medication in the pediatric population. Most of the adverse hepatic reactions have occurred within the first 12 weeks of therapy although several cases have occurred within the first 6 months. Monitoring of complete blood counts and liver function studies is recommended at regularly spaced intervals during the initial 4 to 6 months following the institution of therapy.

Clonazepam, a benzodiazepine, has shown efficacy in the treatment of absence, myoclonic, and photically induced seizure disorders. Its major limiting side effect early in therapy is sedation. An additional limitation is that some patients may develop tolerance to the anticonvulsant effects of the medication after 6 to 9 months of therapy.

Most of the anticonvulsant medications are metabolized by the hepatic microsomal enzyme systems. As a consequence, the serum level of an anticonvulsant that is in steady state may be increased or decreased by addition of another anticonvulsant or a change in the dose of that anticonvulsant. Valproic acid usually elevates the serum level of phenobarbital when it is added to a therapeutic regimen. The interactions of the other anticonvulsants are less predictable and close monitoring of serum blood levels is indicated during the institution of or a change in anticonvulsant medication.

Guidelines and Prognosis for Patients with Epilepsy

The primary goal of patients with seizure disorders and the physicians who treat them is to obtain complete control. Patients with epilepsy have an unemployment rate twice that of the normal population and are often viewed as unsatisfactory workers by employers. Two questions are ever present: (1) Will the patient ever be able to discontinue anticonvulsant medication? (2) What restrictions and guidelines should be given to the patients regarding limitations on their activity?

The issue of discontinuation of medications is not clear.

Most of the information available addresses the issue of discontinuation of medication in children with epilepsy but no specific information regarding the discontinuation of medication in adults is available. The chances of achieving a seizure-free state are directly related to the patient's age at the onset of the seizure disorder. Among patients with idiopathic seizures that begin before 10 years of age, 75 percent will have been seizure-free for 5 years or more 10 years after the onset of their seizures. In the 10- to 19-year-old age group, 68 percent will be seizure-free 10 years later. Above the age of 20 an even smaller percentage of patients will remain seizure-free at a 10-year follow-up interval. Factors responsible for reducing the success of complete control are the presence of partial seizures, both elementary and complex, the presence of underlying cerebral dysfunction in addition to seizures, and a lengthy period of time before seizure control is obtained. In a multicenter controlled study using single drug therapy, only 28 percent of patients with complex partial seizures were seizure-free after an interval of 1 year. Twenty percent of patients with elementary partial seizures were seizure-free, but by contrast 73 percent of patients with generalized tonic-clonic seizures experienced no recurrence. Additional epidemiologic data indicate that 65 percent of patients with complex partial seizures are seizure-free on medication after 20 years whereas only 35 percent of patients with complex partial seizures are seizure-free off medication at the 20-year follow-up interval.

A standard for the pediatric population has been to consider discontinuation of anticonvulsant medications after a seizure-free interval of 4 years. The time frame over which the patient's anticonvulsants are reduced has been variable and is currently being investigated as to whether withdrawal over an extended period of time (9 months) affords the patient any better protection against recurrent seizures than rapid withdrawal (6 weeks). Therefore, patients with partial seizures, seizures that begin later in life, poorly controlled seizures, and seizures associated with other evidence of underlying brain dysfunction are the least likely to remain seizure-free after anticonvulsant withdrawal.

Limitations placed on patients because of their seizure disorder are a major concern. Common sense should be utilized in recommending whether a patient with epilepsy may undertake certain activities. The question should be asked: If the patient had a seizure in this particular setting, would it endanger the health of the patient or other individuals? Most states have guidelines pertaining to the seizure-free interval necessary before a patient may begin operating a motor vehicle. This varies among states. Certain activities are considered prohibitive for patients with clearly documented seizures regardless of their interval of control, e.g., obtaining a pilot's license, scuba diving, or swimming alone. Other limitations that are usually imposed for the same interval of time as recommended for the avoidance of operating a motor vehicle include operating dangerous machinery both at work and at home and avoiding precarious situations such as climbing ladders or working on scaffolding. Regular sleep habits should be encouraged. Patients should be encouraged to continue in school or in their work environment provided no threat to their well-being exists. Organizations and support agencies are available to assist patients in attaining and maintaining as normal a lifestyle as possible.

References

1. Anneggers JF, Grabow JD, Groover RV, Laws ER, Jr, Elveback LR, Kurland LT: Seizures after head trauma: A population study. Neurology NY 30:683–689, 1980.
2. Anneggers JF, Hauser WA, Elveback LR: Remission of seizures and relapse in patients with epilepsy. Epilepsia 20:729–737, 1979.
3. Delgado-Escueta AV: Epileptogenic paroxysms: Modern approaches and clinical correlations. Neurology NY 29:1014–1022, 1979.
4. Delgado-Escueta AV, Wasterlain C, Treiman DM, Porter RJ: Current concepts in neurology: Management of status epilepticus. N Engl J Med 306:1337–1340, 1982.
5. Driefuss FE, Bancaud J, Henriksen O, Rubio-Donnadieu F, Seino M, Penry JK: Proposal for revised clinical and electroencephalographic classification of epileptic seizures. Epilepsia 22:489–501, 1981.
6. Engel J, Troupin AS, Crandall PH, Sterman MB, Wasterlain CG: Recent developments in the diagnosis and therapy of epilepsy. Ann Intern Med 97:584–598, 1982.
7. Freeman JM: Febrile seizures: A consensus of their significance, evaluation and treatment. Pediatrics 66:1009–1112, 1980.
8. Gabor AJ: *Physiological Basis of Electrical Activity of Cerebral Origin.* Quincy, Massachusetts, Grass Instrument Co., 1979.
9. Johnston D, Brown TH: Giant synaptic potential hypothesis for epileptiform activity. Science 211:294–297, 1981.
10. Luther JS, McNamara JO, Carwile S, Miller P, Hope V: Pseudoepileptic seizures: Methods and videoanalysis to aid diagnosis. Ann Neurol 12:458–462, 1982.
11. Penry JK, Porter RJ, Dreifuss FE: Simultaneous recording of absence seizures with video tape and electroencephalography. Brain 98:427–440, 1975.
12. Porter RJ, Penry JK: Efficacy and choice of antiepileptic drugs, in Meinardi H, Rowan AJ (eds): *Advances in Epileptology, 1977.* Amsterdam, Swets and Zeitlinger, 1978, pp 220–231.
13. So EL, Penry JK: Epilepsy in adults. Ann Neurol 9:3–16, 1981.

29

Evaluation of the Patient with Dementia and Treatment of Normal Pressure Hydrocephalus

Robert G. Ojemann
Peter McL. Black

Introduction to the Problem of Dementia

The term *dementia* does not have precise meaning but has been used to describe a clinical syndrome of failing memory and loss of other intellectual functions. Many specific illnesses may be associated with this syndrome; these are termed the *dementing diseases.*[2]

The criteria used for dementia by the American Psychiatric Association may serve as a useful guide to diagnosis.[3]

A. A loss of intellectual abilities of sufficient severity to interfere with social or occupational functioning
B. Memory impairment
C. At least one of the following:
   1. Impairment of abstract thinking, as manifested by inability to provide a reasonable interpretation of proverbs, inability to find similarities between related words, difficulty in defining words and concepts, and other similar tasks
   2. Impaired judgment
   3. Other disturbances of higher cortical function, such as aphasia, agnosia, constructional difficulty
   4. Personality change (i.e., alteration or accentuation of premorbid traits)
D. State of concentration not clouded (i.e., does not meet criteria for delirium, though these may be superimposed)
E. Either (1) or (2):
   1. Evidence of specific organic factor
   2. Presumption of an organic factor in the absence of such evidence if conditions other than organic mental disorders have been reasonably excluded and if the behavioral changes represent cognitive impairment in a variety of areas

Causes of dementia are traditionally classified as presenile (those occurring before age 65) and senile (those after age 65) but this division does not serve any specific purpose. Diseases producing dementia may occur at any age. It is useful to classify them according to whether dementia occurs alone, whether there are other neurological findings from a central nervous system disease causing the problem, or whether there are findings of a systemic illness associated with it (Table 29-1). To give some idea of the frequency of these diseases, Wells has summarized three

TABLE 29-1 Diseases Associated with Dementia

I. Diseases of the central nervous system in which dementia is the predominant manifestation
  A. Alzheimer's disease–senile dementia complex
  B. Pick's disease
II. Diseases of the central nervous system often causing neurological symptoms and signs in addition to dementia
  A. Vascular disease
    1. Subarachnoid hemorrhage
    2. Arteriovenous malformation
    3. Atherosclerosis
  B. Normal pressure hydrocephalus
  C. Intracranial masses
    1. Brain tumors
    2. Chronic infections
    3. Chronic subdural hematoma
  D. Huntington's chorea
  E. Creutzfeldt-Jakob disease
  F. Post-traumatic syndromes
  G. Infections
    1. Bacterial meningitis
    2. Fungal infection
    3. Syphilis
    4. Viral encephalitis
  H. Demyelinating diseases
    1. Schilder's disease
    2. Multiple sclerosis
  I. Parkinson's disease
  J. Lipid storage diseases
  K. Hypoxia
  L. Uncommon diseases
    1. Cerebral-basal ganglia degeneration
    2. Marchiafava-Bignami disease
    3. Myoclonic epilepsy
    4. Progressive multifocal leukoencephalopathy (PML)
    5. Spinocerebellar degeneration
    6. Subacute sclerosing panencephalitis (SSPE)
III. Diseases in which a systemic medical illness is associated with dementia
  A. Endocrine disorders
    1. Hypothyroidism
    2. Cushing's syndrome
    3. Hypoglycemia
    4. Hypopituitarism
  B. Hepatic disorders
    1. Cirrhosis
    2. Wilson's disease
  C. Nutritional disorders
    1. Alcoholism (Wernicke-Korsakoff syndrome)
    2. Pellagra
    3. Vitamin B_{12} and folate deficiency
  D. Renal disorders
    1. Uremia
    2. Dialysis
  E. Toxins
    1. Bromide
    2. Barbiturates
    3. Heavy metals
  F. Heat stroke
  G. Depression

reported series of dementia involving 222 patients (Table 29-2).[23]

The incidence of moderate to severe mental impairment in persons above age 65 is about 4 percent and over half of

TABLE 29-2 Common Causes of Dementia

Cause	Percent of Cases
Alzheimer's disease	50.0
Vascular disease	7.7
Normal pressure hydrocephalus	6.3
Alcoholism	5.9
Intracranial masses	5.4
Huntington's chorea	4.5
Depression	4.1
Drug intoxication	3.2
Creutzfeldt-Jakob disease	1.4
Other causes	1.0 (each)

From C.E. Wells.[23]

these individuals have dementia severe enough to require institutionalization.[18] It is estimated that by the year 2000 there will be 1.43 million demented elderly patients in the United States,[23] with the risk of Alzheimer's disease for a given individual being about 5 percent by age 80.[2] The management of dementia is, therefore, a major public health problem.

Major Dementing Diseases

Alzheimer's Disease—Senile Dementia Complex

The characteristic clinical and pathological changes of this condition have been called *Alzheimer's disease* or *presenile dementia* if they occur before age 65, and *senile dementia* if the patient is older than 65. The Alzheimer's disease–senile dementia complex is characterized clinically by a state of deteriorating intellect without evidence of either neurological or systemic disease known to be associated with dementia. The majority of patients have the onset of the illness in their late fifties or sixties but cases involving similar pathological changes have been reported in persons as young as 15 years.[2] In nearly all patients the cause is unknown and only a few familial cases have been documented. Males and females are equally affected.

The onset of the dementia is insidious. The first evidence of the disease may be the observation by a relative, friend, or employer of forgetfulness, lack of initiative, or loss of interest in work. Sometimes an unusual degree of confusion in relation to taking medication or a febrile illness is the first warning of the problem.

Gradual impairment in memory is the major symptom. Recent events are forgotten, names cannot be recalled, appointments are missed, possessions are lost, and questions are repeated. Other changes in mentation become apparent as time goes along. Speech may be halting as words cannot be recalled; comprehension of requests is lost. Dyscalculia develops and visual-spatial orientation fails. The patient takes the wrong direction, is unable to put clothes on correctly, or cannot set a table. Eventually, the patient forgets how to use common objects and tools while retaining normal motor power and coordination.

During the early phases of the illness, the patient seems unchanged in gait, motor function, behavior, temperament, and conduct, but later these areas may also deteriorate. Dressing, shaving, and bathing are neglected; hallucinations, paranoia, and inappropriate behavior may develop. The patient seems indifferent and unaware of what is happening. Late in the illness, frontal lobe signs are found, sphincter control is lost, and the patient becomes akinetic and mute.

The course of the disease usually extends over 5 or more years but during this time, motor, sensory, and visual function remain relatively intact. The sequence of the symptoms may vary somewhat but almost all intellectual functions deteriorate. However, memory impairment is the consistent and most prominent feature of the illness.

The pathological changes in this disorder consist of diffuse atrophy with narrowed cerebral convolutions and widened sulci.[2] The changes are usually most pronounced in the frontal and temporal lobes. Microscopically, there is widespread loss of nerve cells, most marked in the cerebral cortex; astrocytic proliferation; development of tightly knit extracellular aggregates of amorphous argentophilic material (senile plaques); a condensation of intraneural neurofibrils called *Alzheimer neurofibrillary change;* and granulovesicular degeneration of neurons in the hippocampus. The senile plaques have been shown to be areas of degenerated nerve processes with amyloid change. Although they occur in normally aging brains, the presence of more than 20 per high power field is associated with dementia. Alzheimer's neurofibrillary change involves loops or tangled masses of abnormal neurofibrils within neurons.

The neurochemistry of Alzheimer's disease has been an area of major recent advance. The enzyme choline acetyltransferase is deficient in the cortex of patients with pathologically proven Alzheimer's disease, and its absence correlates with the severity of dementia.[23] Much of the choline acetyltransferase in the cortex comes from the nucleus basalis of Meynert, whose cells have also been demonstrated to be deficient in Alzheimer's disease. The recently proposed *cholinergic hypothesis* suggests that "damage to the ascending cholinergic system is an important determinant of the functional deficits observed in Alzheimer's disease."[19]

The diagnosis of Alzheimer's disease may be made clinically when there is a chronic dementia with diffuse cerebral dysfunction, a CT scan that shows mild ventricular enlargement with marked cortical atrophy, and no evidence of another disease process. However, it can be made definitively only with cerebral biopsy. The major differential diagnosis is between Alzheimer's disease, depression, and normal-pressure hydrocephalus. Late life depression may be difficult to separate clinically from Alzheimer's disease; if poor appetite, sleep disturbance, psychomotor retardation, diminished interest, fatigue, feelings of worthlessness, subjective complaint of diminished ability to think or concentrate, or recurrent thoughts of death are a part of the clinical picture, the diagnosis of depression should be considered. A useful guide is that the person who complains of memory and concentration difficulty is more likely to be depressed than to have senile dementia. As depression is a treatable disease, it should be looked for carefully.

In the section on indications for shunting in normal-pressure hydrocephalus we discuss the differential diagnosis of that syndrome and Alzheimer's disease. It should be noted that most patients with senile dementia walk normally until relatively late in the illness when there is already a severe deterioration in mental function.

The term *atherosclerotic dementia* is often applied incorrectly to the Alzheimer's–senile dementia complex. When dementia is due to a major stroke, there are usually other signs of occlusive cerebrovascular disease. However, multi-infarct dementia may resemble Alzheimer's disease.

No treatment has been established as effective for Alzheimer's disease. Treatment with choline and lecithin may have promise, although early clinical trials have shown no effect.[19]

Pick's Disease

This is a special form of cerebral degeneration in which atrophy involves both gray and white matter and usually is most prominent in the frontal and temporal lobes.[2] The clinical syndrome is identical to that of Alzheimer's disease.

Wernicke-Korsakoff Syndrome

Wernicke's disease is characterized by nystagmus, abducens and conjugate gaze weakness or paralysis, ataxia of gait, and disturbance of mentation (usually a global confusional state).[2] The symptoms usually have an abrupt onset and may occur in various combinations and sequences. The disease is due to a deficiency in thiamine and is usually seen in alcoholics. Often it is associated with Korsakoff's psychosis.

Korsakoff's psychosis is a unique mental disorder in which memory is impaired out of all proportion to other cognitive functions. The patient is alert and otherwise attentive, responsive, capable of understanding written and spoken words, makes appropriate deductions and solves problems within the memory span. This disorder is also usually associated with alcoholism and malnutrition but may be caused by lesions of the diencephalon or hippocampal formation, such as third ventricle tumors or herpes simplex encephalitis. On occasion, the symptoms may be confused with Alzheimer's disease. Usually the onset is more abrupt and the widespread deterioration in mental functions of Alzheimer's disease is not seen.

Patients with Wernicke's disease who respond to treatment with thiamine recover. The most dramatic improvement is in the ocular manifestations, and recovery almost always begins within hours or days and is complete within a few weeks. Improvement in ataxia is less rapid and may not be complete. The global confusional state is also reversible, as are the symptoms of apathy and drowsiness, but the deficit in memory and learning recovers in only a small percentage of patients.

Huntington's Disease

This disease is characterized by the triad of dominant inheritance, choreoathetosis, and dementia.[2] The usual age of onset is the fourth or fifth decade but in 5 to 10 percent of patients symptoms begin before age 20. A gradual deterioration in mental function occurs over many years, with memory loss being among the first deficits to be recognized. This, together with development of movement disorder and the family history, usually makes the diagnosis apparent. However, the dementia may precede the movement disorder by a significant period. The diagnosis should be considered when there is progressive deterioration in cognitive powers without aphasia or visual symptoms and when there is prominent apathy. The CT scan may show alteration in the frontal horns because of atrophy of the caudate nucleus. A neurotransmitter defect is suspected.

Parkinson's Disease

Parkinson's disease is characterized by rigidity, slowness of voluntary movement, tremor at rest, festinating gait, and expressionless face. Dementia is a common accompaniment, occurring in 32 percent of patients in one series.[2]

Creutzfeldt-Jakob Disease

This term is now used to describe an illness characterized by rapidly progressive profound dementia, in association with ataxia and diffuse myoclonic jerks.[2] This disorder is quite different from the slow dementia and pyramidal-extrapyramidal symptoms described by Creutzfeldt and Jakob.

The illness affects men and women equally and occurs between the ages of 10 and 60 although it tends to be a disease of middle age. In the early stages of the disease the most frequent changes are in behavior, emotional response, memory, and reasoning, and there may be complaints of distorted vision. Myoclonic jerks develop. The disease progresses rapidly, with a median survival of 9 months.

On pathological examination the disease affects principally the cerebral and cerebellar cortex, with disappearance of nerve cells and extensive astroglial proliferation. The microscopic vacuoles that give the tissue its typically spongy appearance are located within the cytoplasmic processes of the glial cells. There is no evidence of an inflammatory reaction.

Occasionally, the neurosurgeon is called upon to do a brain biopsy in a patient with dementia.[7] It is important to recognize the possibility of Creutzfeldt-Jakob disease in such patients so that appropriate precautions can be taken with the tissue and instruments. It has been shown that brain tissue from patients with this disorder, when injected into subhuman primates, can transmit the disease, with an incubation period of about 1 year. This is due to the presence of a slow virus. The disease has been transferred from one patient to another by infected brain depth electrodes and human tissue has been found to be infective even after formalin fixation and routine sterilization.

Ellis et al. nicely summarize the problem of biopsy in patients with this disease and consider the risk to the neurosurgeon and operating room personnel.[7] They refer to reports that there has been no accidental human transmission among laboratory workers, surgeons, or pathologists and that a review of the operative procedures performed by a prominent neurological surgeon "who died with Creutzfeldt-Jakob disease revealed that none of his patients, either child or adult, were identified as having the disease." They conclude that with proper care, biopsy can be safely done.

Gajdusek et al. have outlined the methods for sterilization.[10] They found that the Creutzfeldt-Jakob agent is inactivated by autoclaving for 1 h at 250°F under 15 lb/in² pressure or by immersion for 2 h in 5 percent sodium hypochlorite, iodophore, or phenolic disinfectants. These procedures protect operating room personnel from accidental inoculation by soiled instruments prior to washing and resterilization. Disposable materials should also be decontaminated. The anesthesia equipment does not have to be sterilized and no special isolation procedures are needed since the disease is not spread by the respiratory tract.

Diagnostic Workup in a Patient with Dementia

At least 25 percent of patients with dementia from the causes listed in Table 29-1 may benefit from treatment. It is therefore imperative that an attempt be made to establish a diagnosis.

The first step is to obtain an adequate history. It may be necessary to verify the presence and details of intellectual deterioration by repeated evaluations or by obtaining information from relatives or employers. Questions are asked about all the areas of mental functions which have been outlined in the section on Alzheimer's disease: speech, behavior, motor performance, vision, and gait. An attempt is made to bring out any evidence of depression.

In the examination, neatness of dress, general demeanor, appearance, animation, and cooperation are noted. Language fluency and correctness, mood, and general intellect can be evaluated during conversation, with special attention paid to superficial response. Orientation and calculations should be tested by asking direct questions. Memory testing should include immediate recall (repeat digits forward and backward), recent memory (events of the day), remote memory, and general store of information. The general neurological examination looks for any evidence of focal abnormality.

Every patient with dementia should have a CT scan. In addition, hematologic tests, blood chemistry, serology, T4, vitamin B_{12}, and folate are checked. Other tests will be guided by the history and results of these initial studies. For example, if the CT scan and other studies do not establish a diagnosis or a chronic meningitis or fungal infection is considered, a lumbar puncture is done to examine the cerebrospinal fluid (CSF). Wilson's disease should be considered if dementia occurs before age 40, and then one looks for Kayser-Fleischer rings in the eyes, elevated serum copper levels, and increased urine copper values. Drug intoxication should be investigated if the patient begins to improve during hospitalization. A negative serologic test for syphilis in blood or CSF does not exclude a diagnosis of syphilis and if there is any suspicion of this disease, an FTA-ABS test (fluorescent treponemal antibody-absorption) should be performed.

In most patients the diagnosis of dementia is established on the basis of the history, examination, CT scan, and laboratory findings. Rarely, a brain biopsy may be indicated for an accurate diagnosis and prognosis if it can be safely obtained.[7]

Syndrome of Normal Pressure Hydrocephalus

Historical Review

The possibility that clinical symptoms could be associated with ventricular enlargement, despite normal intracranial pressure, was recognized in patients following subarachnoid hemorrhage; this history has been summarized by Barnett.[4] In 1964 Salomon Hakim presented a dissertation describing three patients (the first treated in 1958) with hydrocephalus and normal CSF pressure who had obtundation, gait disorder, and urinary incontinence.[12,13] Three patients having a syndrome of mild impairment of memory with slowness of thought and action, difficulty with gait, urinary incontinence, normal CSF pressure, and hydrocephalus were described by Adams, Fisher, Hakim, Ojemann, and Sweet in 1965, and with this paper the syndrome of normal pressure hydrocephalus (NPH) was established.[1] Fisher has summarized the details of how the problem came to be recognized at the Massachusetts General Hospital.[8] After recounting the history of the first patient seen by R.D. Adams in 1959 he states: "The author having a penchant for identifying any unusual clinical phenomenon or state by applying a name tag to it, one day, as Dr. Salomon Hakim and I left the patient's room the term symptomatic normal pressure hydrocephalus was proposed as a working label for the condition".[8] Other terms such as *occult hydrocephalus, low pressure hydrocephalus, normotensive hydrocephalus,* and *hydrocephalic dementia* have been used, but *normal pressure hydrocephalus* (NPH) has emerged as the best descriptive term.

There followed a period of enthusiasm about the syndrome of idiopathic NPH as a treatable cause of dementia. It was well-documented that several different pathological processes, particularly subarachnoid hemorrhage, could be followed by NPH.[16] However, a large number of reports dealt with the problem of idiopathic NPH. The expectation that tests such as CSF infusion, pneumoencephalography, and radioisotope cisternography would be diagnostic of the syndrome was slowly dispelled. The problem was well summarized by Stein and Langfitt in 1974 when they pointed out that many patients with idiopathic NPH did not improve with shunting and no combination of tests accurately predicted the results of treatment.[21] With the advent of the CT scan it was again hoped that specific criteria might be found to establish the diagnosis but this has not been the case. Even the finding of dilated cerebral sulci does not preclude the possibility of improvement with shunting.[6,17]

In 1977 Fisher emphasized that the history was possibly the best predictor of outcome.[8] He found that when the gait disturbance preceded impaired mentation or came at about the same time, there was a good chance of improvement after shunting whereas in those cases in which dementia came first or was not associated with a gait disturbance, the chances of improvement were low. Reports by Laws and

Mokri and by Black showed that the chances of a good response from shunting were 61 to 66 percent if the classical triad of idiopathic NPH was present.[5,15] Now, 20 years after the description of the syndrome, there is still hope that as we gain more understanding of the problem, a sophisticated physiological test may select shunt responders.

Pathogenesis

Certain disorders are characteristically associated with the subsequent development of NPH.[16] The most common is subarachnoid hemorrhage (SAH). In evaluation of 914 cases reported in the literature, Katzman found that in 33 percent there was no history of any preceding event (idiopathic NPH), 33 percent had a history of SAH, 11 percent had trauma, 4.7 percent had previous surgery, 3.7 percent had meningitis, 3.7 percent had aqueductal stenosis, 2.8 percent had a third ventricle tumor, and 2 percent had a fourth ventricle lesion.[14]

The various lesions associated with NPH have in common a blockade of CSF flow, not so much a blockade in absorption but rather in the pathways within the ventricles or around the base of the brain. This was often demonstrated on pneumoencephalography, and in two patients with idiopathic NPH who came to autopsy, there was evidence of fibrosis in the subarachnoid pathways.[16] It is an obstruction to CSF flow rather than a change in absorptive rate of CSF that is the first step in the development of NPH. Sklar et al. have demonstrated a significant absorptive reserve in patients with communicating hydrocephalus. For example, patients are able to absorb CSF well despite their ventriculomegaly.[20]

The development of hydrocephalus despite adequate CSF absorption can be best explained by increased resistance to outflow from the ventricular system or by other causes of increased pulse pressure of CSF. White et al. have presented clinical and theoretical evidence that limitation of flow through the aqueduct of Sylvius is an important component.[24] Foltz and Aine have demonstrated that an increase in pulse amplitude in humans may be associated with ventriculomegaly without an increase in mean CSF pressure.[9] It is perhaps these mechanisms rather than a compensation of high pressure by ventricular enlargement[13] that allows normal pressure despite ventriculomegaly.

Clinical Features

The syndrome is usually progressive but the rate of evolution is variable and symptoms may fluctuate. Mean age for the idiopathic patient is 68 years and men and women are equally afflicted.[5] When a specific etiologic factor is present, the problem can occur at any age. The onset may be within days of the event in some patients but in others the time interval may be months or years.[16] In the original reports of the syndrome the clinical picture was described as mild impairment of memory, slowness and paucity of thought and action, unsteadiness of gait, and unwitting urinary incontinence.[1] Numerous reports have confirmed that these are the clinical hallmarks of NPH.

Gait disturbance is an important clinical feature in idiopathic cases, helping to distinguish NPH from senile dementia, and is the best predictor of shunt success. This complaint may be the first and remain the most prominent symptom but can come on with or follow the onset of dementia. The gait varies from a mild imbalance to an inability to walk or even stand.[8,15] There is usually a history of frequent falls. The problem appears to be a matter of balance, with a slowness in correcting a potential instability. Progression leads to immobility. Occasionally, the gait disorder may be due to spasticity or resemble parkinsonism. On examination the steps are shortened, with a wide base, and the patient is unable to turn without losing balance and cannot do tandem walking.

The dementia may range from severe impairment in recent memory to a deficit revealed only by detailed psychological testing. Spontaneity and initiative are decreased and the patient may appear unconcerned, apathetic, lethargic, or depressed. Interest in conversation, reading, writing, hobbies, and recreational activities declines. On examination, tests are performed slowly and attention and concentration are impaired. This complex of abnormalities has been termed the *abulic trait* by Fisher.[8]

Urinary incontinence is usually a late symptom. In most patients it is of a frontal lobe type with a lack of awareness or concern.

In a few patients, aberrant behavior, delusions, hallucinations, paranoia, and irrational speech have been part of the clinical picture. Headache is not present. Occasionally, the presenting picture may resemble parkinsonism.

There are usually no focal signs unless there has been brain damage from an underlying disease process. The deep tendon reflexes may be increased and the plantar responses are variable. Frontal lobe signs usually appear late in the illness. Occasionally the patient may become quite obtunded.

Diagnostic Tests

A CT scan with contrast enhancement should be done in all patients suspected of having NPH to look for lesions that may be causing the hydrocephalus. Note is made of the ventricular size and sulcal atrophy. With the newest scanners, the presence of periventricular low density is often seen (Figs. 29-1 and 29-2). This finding has been associated with increased possibility of shunt success (Borgesen and Gjerris found that 16 out of 16 patients with it improved after shunting[6]). We do not know if nuclear magnetic resonance imaging will improve our ability to assess the periventricular region in these patients.

The presence of sulcal atrophy does not exclude the diagnosis of NPH and there may be a good response to shunting if there is also significant ventricular enlargement (Fig. 29-2). However, the chances of improvement with treatment are greater when there is little or no sulcal enlargement. Laws and Mokri found that when hydrocephalus without atrophy was seen on the CT scan in patients with idiopathic NPH, 75 percent (9 of 12) improved.[15] When atrophy was also present, 46 percent (6 of 13) were better after shunting. Black reported improvement in 85 percent (11 of 13) when

ventricular enlargement was associated with little or no sulcal enlargement and in 33 percent (3 of 9) when there was sulcal enlargement.[5] Severe sulcal atrophy with only slight to moderate ventricular enlargement on CT scan and a history of dementia with no gait disturbance is most likely due to Alzheimer's disease.

Isotope cisternography has been used in attempts to confirm the diagnosis of NPH. The normal pattern of flow is rapid ascent of the isotope to the basal cisterns and flow over the cerebral convexities within 24 h. In some patients there may be transient entry into the ventricular system. The most characteristic finding in NPH is ventricular entry of the isotope followed by ventricular stasis, with accumulation of the isotope within the ventricles for at least 48 h and delayed ascent of the isotope over the convexity. There is often a mixed pattern, with some ventricular stasis associated with varying degrees of flow in the subarachnoid spaces. The finding of a typical pattern for hydrocephalus does seem to increase the chances of having a good result from shunting, but even patients with a normal pattern may benefit from treatment. In one study, an excellent or good response to a shunt was found in 55 percent (6 of 11) with a "typical" NPH pattern, 23 percent (3 of 13) with a mixed pattern, and 11 percent (1 of 9) with a normal study.[5] However, these results were not statistically significant. Laws and Mokri found that 55 percent (14 of 25) of their patients with a positive cisternogram improved with treatment.[15]

Continuous monitoring of CSF pressure to attempt to ascertain a pattern of abnormal waves and the use of infusion tests to detect deficits in absorption of CSF have produced variable success in attempts to confirm the diagnosis of idiopathic NPH and predict the results of shunting.[6,16,22] Symon and Hinzpeter, while emphasizing that the clinical picture is most important, found that the presence of A waves or recurrent B wave activity, with radiographic evidence of hydrocephalus, seemed to confirm the diagnosis in a significant percentage of patients.[22] Borgensen and Gjerris found that all patients with B wave activity more than 50 percent of the time improved with shunting and no patients with fewer than 5 percent B waves did so.[6] They described a lumboventricular perfusion test to measure resistance to CSF outflow, and its reciprocal conductance was reported to have a high correlation with success of shunting in idiopathic NPH. In 49 of 51 patients with conductances below 0.08 ml/min per mmHg there was improvement after shunting, and no patients with conductance above 0.08 improved. However, since both lumbar and ventricular catheters are required, this test may not be practical on a routine basis. A single lumbar puncture pressure will not help in prognostication except to establish that such pressure is sometimes in the normal range. In Black's series good results from shunting were comparable for patients with an opening pressure above 100 mmH$_2$O and those with pressure below 100 mmH$_2$O.[5] C. Miller Fisher has found that one of the more reliable criteria is whether the gait disorder improves after draining CSF from the lumbar subarachnoid space.

Pneumoencephalography and angiography are no longer indicated for evaluating a patient suspected of having NPH. Measurements of regional cerebral blood flow (rCBF) have shown an increase following CSF drainage in patients with hydrocephalus but the same finding has been seen in pa-

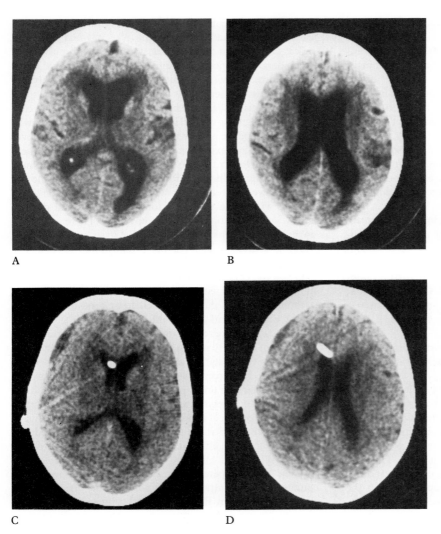

A   B

C   D

Figure 29-1 This 71-year-old woman had progressively increasing difficulty in walking for over a year. There was minimal impairment of memory. A CSF isotope flow study was equivocal. The lumbar puncture CSF pressure was 150 mmH$_2$O. Her gait improved temporarily after lowering of the CSF pressure. After placement of a vetriculovenous shunt there was marked improvement in her gait and her memory was normal. *A, B.* Preoperative CT scan. There is marked ventricular enlargement with prominent periventricular low density. There is some but not marked enlargement of the sulci. *C, D.* Postoperative CT scan. There is significant reduction in ventricular size. The shunt is well placed in the frontal horn of the lateral ventricle. Some of the periventricular low density persists. Note the small low-density collection in the right posterior frontal subdural region. This did not cause any focal neurological symptoms and resolved completely over several months.

tients with dementia.[17,22] Not enough patients have been studied to know if a certain percentage increase in rCBF can predict a good response to treatment. There is no EEG tracing that is of value in evaluating these patients, but the use of evoked responses has not been fully evaluated.

Indications for a Shunting Procedure

In considering this problem it is useful to separate those patients with idiopathic NPH from those in whom a specific etiologic factor is present. In this latter group it is well established that the patient who develops progressive dementia after subarachnoid hemorrhage and has large ventricles on the CT scan will almost always improve with a shunt if there is no underlying cerebral infarction. This is also true when a progressive gait disorder and dementia are associated with large ventricles on the CT scan and there has been a history of previous surgery or meningitis or when aqueduct stenosis or a mass lesion is found.[16] The problem following trauma is more difficult because of the underlying brain injury and because it is a rare complication. The onset of symptoms

may be delayed up to several months after the injury. If the post-traumatic patient develops a worsening gait disorder and/or dementia and the CT scan shows progressive or persistent ventricular enlargement, a shunt is indicated.[16]

The patient with possible idiopathic NPH presents a difficult problem. The neurosurgeon is commonly faced with a demented patient having cerebral atrophy and a family or referring physician who wishes a shunt placed. One must resist a tendency to insert a shunt "because there is nothing else to do." At worst, this may lead to anesthetic or postsurgical disaster in a fragile patient. Having said this, however, it is important to reiterate that there is no one test or combination of tests that will absolutely indicate what the response to a shunt will be.

What factors indicate that a shunt should be done? The most reliable predictor of a good response to shunting is the clinical history. The patient with a gait disorder alone or with mild to moderate dementia with or without urinary incontinence and showing large ventricles on the CT scan is a candidate for operation. The presence of sulcal atrophy should not deter surgery. Findings of periventricular low density and improvement in symptoms with CSF drainage

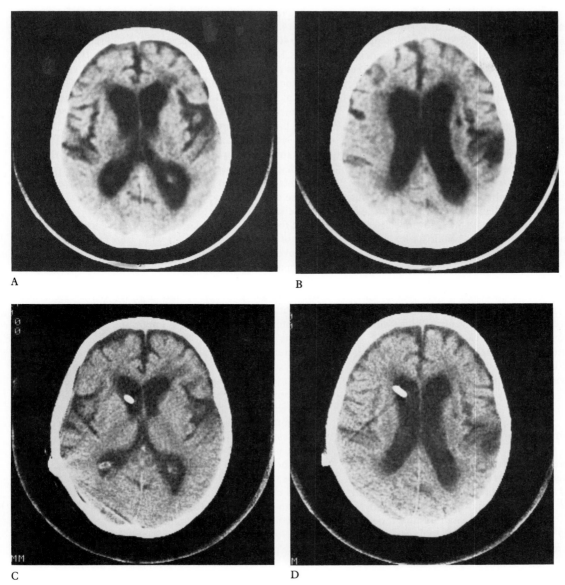

Figure 29-2 This 79-year-old woman noted over a 2-year period increasing difficulty with gait and a slowing down of her ability to function mentally and physically. Gradually she had increasing trouble with incontinence. Memory had become much worse over the 4 months prior to admission. An isotope CSF flow study showed entry of isotope into the lateral ventricle at 4 h but significant convexity flow at 24 and 48 h. Lumbar puncture showed a pressure of 130 mmH$_2$O. Some but not striking improvement occurred after draining CSF. After the ventriculovenous shunt she gradually improved. One year later her physician husband said "it is a miracle." Gait was nearly normal, incontinence was much less, she was more active, and her memory was improved. *A, B.* Preoperative CT scan. This showed marked ventricle enlargement, marked widening of the sulci, and a small area of periventricular low density at the anterolateral margins of the lateral ventricles. *C, D.* Postoperative CT scan. The ventricles are reduced in size and the sulci are not quite as prominent as before operation. The shunt is in good position.

improve the chances of success. In the patient in whom dementia is present with little or no gait disorder and in whom the CT scan shows only mild to moderate ventricular enlargement, other tests may be helpful. The finding of an abnormal cisternogram or plateau or B waves on overnight recording of CSF pressure indicates that a shunt may be beneficial.

Fisher has reviewed the problem of dementia as it relates

to separating NPH from Alzheimer's disease.[8] In a review of 25 consecutive personal cases of dementia presumed to be Alzheimer's disease, he found that none had a hydrocephalic disturbance of gait. Senile dementia may start with a memory disorder that mimics hydrocephalic dementia but the severe memory loss so common in Alzheimer's disease is seen with hydrocephalus only when walking is virtually impossible. Urinary incontinence is usually a late development in Alzheimer's disease. Dementia, beginning in the late fifties and early sixties and accompanied by dominant and nondominant hemispheric deficits results in patterns of dementia that have not been associated with hydrocephalus. There is a small group of Alzheimer's cases in which a disturbance of gait parallels the progression of the dementia but these cases have not been well documented. A shuffling, small-stepped gait can be associated with several different disease processes and is by no means specific for hydrocephalus. If the diagnosis of Alzheimer's disease seems likely, a shunt should not be done.

It should be emphasized that there is a difference between making a diagnosis of normal pressure hydrocephalus and predicting a good shunt response. It is possible that prolonged extensive dilatation of the ventricular system will ultimately result in damage that cannot be reversed even with shunting. Occasionally, Alzheimer's disease will become complicated by the unrelated development of hydrocephalus and shunting will only temporarily improve the symptoms.[8,16,17]

Results and Complications

An overall review of the literature indicates that improvement from shunting has occurred in about 65 percent of the patients with NPH from a known cause and 41 percent with idiopathic NPH.[14] Review of individual reports of significant series reveals remarkably consistent results for idiopathic NPH: 20 to 30 percent of patients will be markedly improved and 40 to 70 percent will be improved to some extent.[5,11,15,22] The length of follow-up must also be considered. Greenberg et al. found that 64.3 percent were improved at an average follow-up period of 9 months but this dropped to 42.8 percent at 3 years.[11] In all but one of the patients who deteriorated, the primary problem was dementia. It is important to remember that these patients may have medical problems, and careful preoperative evaluation, anesthesia, and postoperative evaluation are vitally important to the outcome.

The results of treatment in patients with idiopathic NPH done by several surgeons at the Massachusetts General Hospital between 1959 and 1977 have been considered in detail by Black.[5] In that group of 62 patients there were 32 women and 30 men; the median age was 68 years; 56 had some degree of memory impairment, 53 had gait disturbance, and 34 had urinary incontinence. The postoperative classification was as follows: excellent (resumed preillness activity without deficit); good (resumed preillness activity with moderate deficit); fair (improved but did not return to previous work); transient (temporary major improvement); poor (no change or worse); and death (died within 6 weeks of surgery). In the entire series, 46.7 percent of 62 patients

improved (excellent, 12.9 percent; good, 14.5 percent; fair, 14.5 percent; and transient improvement, 4.8 percent) while 40.3 percent were unchanged, 4.8 percent were worse, and 8.1 percent died. He did a statistical analysis of 15 factors as possible predictors of shunt outcome. A good indication for improvement from shunting was the presence of the clinical triad of mild memory difficulty, significant gait disturbance, and incontinence, with a total of 61.2 percent of these patients improving. When there was no incontinence, only 31.5 percent improved. Patients with dementia as the predominant symptom fared about the same as those in whom gait disturbance predominated, but more of the latter patients returned to normal activity. The age of the patient, degree of deficit, and duration of disability were irrelevant to the shunt outcome.

In the Mayo Clinic experience the presence of the classic triad of NPH was associated with a 66 percent chance of improvement.[15] In Fisher's personal series the presence of a predominant gait disturbance was associated with a good chance of improvement.[8] Greenberg et al. found that a predominant gait disturbance and large ventricles were associated with a favorable result in 84 percent of their patients.[11]

Postoperative evaluation is important. A CT scan should be done on every patient before discharge to have a baseline measurement of ventricular size and to detect the presence of any subdural fluid collection. In many patients who improve the ventricles will become smaller but some maintain large ventricles even with reduced CSF pressure.[6] Some patients will have a low-density subdural collection with no clinical symptoms and no evidence of ventricular or sulcal compression (Fig. 29-1C and D). Often this collection will persist unchanged or gradually resolve.

If the patient is not improved, a CT scan is done and if there is no hematoma or subdural collection, the CSF pressure is checked with a lumbar puncture. We usually use a medium-pressure Hakim valve with a ventriculoatrial or ventriculoperitoneal shunt and we like to have the pressure below 90 mmH$_2$O. If the ventricles are still large on CT scan and the pressure is above 100 mmH$_2$O, the shunt should be revised. On occasion we have replaced a medium-pressure with a low-pressure valve when symptoms did not improve and ventricles were still large with CSF pressures of 60 to 100 mmH$_2$O.

If the patient becomes worse, a CT scan should be done. The cause may be subdural collection. A solid hematoma will require a craniotomy and probably temporary ligation of the shunt. More often there is a subdural hygroma that may respond to drainage but if the patient has become dependent on the ventricular shunt, a subdural peritoneal shunt is required. If the CT scan does not show a reason for worsening, a lumbar puncture should be done to measure the pressure and look for meningitis. In the elderly patient, it may be difficult to recognize this diagnosis on clinical grounds. If the pressure is above 100 mmH$_2$O, the CSF is clear, and the ventricles are still large, it is likely that the shunt is not working and a revision is indicated.

Occasionally the patient complains of a low pressure problem with headache and neck discomfort on getting up and with relief when lying down. This problem usually resolves itself but occasionally a higher-pressure valve is placed.[11]

The incidence of shunt infection in the adult has been low, in the range of 1 to 2 percent. We give an intravenous, antistaphylococcal antibiotic just before making the incision and continue it for 24 h after operation. We also use one dose of gentamicin (4 mg) injected into the ventricular catheter during the operation.

In the Massachusetts General Hospital series, 4 of 62 patients developed seizures within 6 months of the shunt. All were easily controlled with anticonvulsant drugs.

References

1. Adams RD, Fisher CM, Hakim S, Ojemann RG, Sweet WH: Symptomatic occult hydrocephalus with "normal" cerebrospinal fluid pressure: A treatable syndrome. N Engl J Med 273:117–126, 1965.
2. Adams RD, Victor M: *Principles of Neurology*, New York, McGraw-Hill, 1977.
3. American Psychiatric Association: Task Force on Nomenclature and Statistics. *Diagnostic and Statistical Manual of Mental Disorders*, 3d ed. Washington, D.C., American Psychiatric Association, 1980.
4. Barnett HJM: Some clinical features of intracranial aneurysms. Clin Neurosurg 16:43–72, 1969.
5. Black P McL: Idiopathic normal-pressure hydrocephalus: Results of shunting in 62 patients. J Neurosurg 52:371–377, 1980.
6. Borgesen SE, Gjerris F: The predictive value of conductance to outflow of CSF in normal pressure hydrocephalus. Brain 105:65–86, 1982.
7. Ellis WG, Youmans JR, Dreyfus PM: Diagnostic biopsy for neurological disease, in Youmans J (ed): *Neurological Surgery*, 2d ed. Philadelphia, Saunders, 1982, pp 382–422.
8. Fisher CM: The clinical picture in occult hydrocephalus. Clin Neurosurg 24:270–284, 1977.
9. Foltz EL, Aine C: Diagnosis of hydrocephalus by CSF pulse-wave analysis: A clinical study. Surg Neurol 15:283–293, 1981.
10. Gajdusek DC, Gibbs CJ Jr, Asher DM, Brown P, Diwan A, Hoffman P, Nemo G, Rohwer R, White L: Precautions in medical care of, and in handling materials from patients with transmissible virus dementia (Creutzfeldt-Jakob disease). N Engl J Med 297:1253–1258, 1977.
11. Greenberg JO, Shenkin HA, Adam R: Idiopathic normal pressure hydrocephalus: A report of 73 patients. J Neurol Neurosurg Psychiatry 40:336–341, 1977.
12. Hakim S: Algunas observaciones sobre la presión del LCR sindrome hidrocefálico en el adulto con presión normal del LCR (presentación de un nuevo sindrome) (Tesis de grado). Facultad de Medicina, Universidad Javeriana, Bogota, Colombia, 1964.
13. Hakim S, Adams RD: The special clinical problem of symptomatic hydrocephalus with normal cerebrospinal fluid pressure: Observations on cerebrospinal fluid hydrodynamics. J Neurol Sci 2:307–327, 1965.
14. Katzman R: Normal pressure hydrocephalus, in Wells CE (ed): *Dementia*, 2d ed. Philadelphia, Davis, 1977, pp 29–92.
15. Laws ER Jr, Mokri B: Occult hydrocephalus: Results of shunting correlated with diagnostic tests. Clin Neurosurg 24:316–333, 1977.
16. Ojemann RG: Normal pressure hydrocephalus. Clin Neurosurg 18:337–370, 1971.
17. Ojemann RG, Black PM: Normal pressure hydrocephalus, in Youmans J (ed): *Neurological Surgery*, 2d ed. Philadelphia, Saunders, 1982, pp 1423–1435.
18. Pfeiffer E: A short portable mental status questionnaire for the assessment of organic brain deficit in elderly patients. J Am Geriatr Soc 23:433–439, 1975.
19. Rossor MN: Dementia. Lancet 2:1200–1203, 1982.
20. Sklar FH, Beyer CW Jr, Diehl JT, Clark WK: Significance of the so-called absorptive reserve in communicating hydrocephalus: A preliminary report. Neurosurgery 8:525–530, 1981.
21. Stein SC, Langfitt TW: Normal-pressure hydrocephalus: Predicting the results of cerebrospinal fluid shunting. J Neurosurg 41:463–470, 1974.
22. Symon L, Hinzpeter T: The enigma of normal pressure hydrocephalus: Tests to select patients for surgery and to predict shunt function. Clin Neurosurg 24:285–315, 1977.
23. Wells CE: Diagnostic evaluation and treatment of dementia, in Wells CE (ed): *Dementia*, 2d ed. Philadelphia, Davis, 1977.
24. White DN, Wilson KC, Curry GR, Stevenson RJ: The limitation of pulsatile flow through the aqueduct of Sylvius as a cause of hydrocephalus. J Neurol Sci 42:11–51, 1979.

30

Blood-Brain Barrier; Cerebral Edema

Michael Pollay

Blood-Brain Barrier

Introduction

The observation that vital dyes introduced into the bloodstream do not stain the nervous system provided the original basis for the concept of the blood-brain barrier (BBB). Even before these classic animal experiments were performed in the first quarter of this century, pathological anatomists had observed in jaundiced patients colorful staining within and around the periphery of metastatic brain tumors that left untouched the remaining white matter. The early view that this barrier was virtually impregnable and served only to protect the brain from harmful substances has been replaced by the concept that a single cell layer regulates selectively both the entry and exit of biologically important substances in order to rigorously control the neural environment and sustain normal function.[15,17]

Location of the Blood-Brain Barrier

It was once believed that the BBB was composed of both the endothelium of the cerebral capillary and the juxtaposed glial end feet. The demonstration by electron microscopy that the glial envelopment was incomplete and that tissue markers entered the endothelial clefts after circumventing the glial end feet firmly established the cerebral capillary as the site of the BBB.[4]

Electron-dense markers given either intravascularly or in the cerebrospinal fluid (CSF) are impeded from passage through the endothelial cleft by interendothelial tight junctions (Fig. 30-1). These tight junctions (zonulae occludentes) appear during development and are functionally complete before or shortly after birth in most species.[21] There are special small areas of the central nervous system located around the periphery of the ventricular system that have no BBB. These areas include the choroid plexus, area postrema, median eminence, neurohypophysis, pineal body, subfornical and commissural organs, and supraoptic crest.

The capillaries in these special structures have no tight junctions, but the epithelial cells that cover the choroid plexus, area postrema, and median eminence are connected by "less tight junctions." The easy access that these special structures have to the blood and cerebrospinal fluid and the presence of clear and dense-cored vesicles are indications of intracellular transport, secretion of neurohumoral or neurotransmitter substances, or CSF secretion.[21]

Permeability of the BBB

General Properties of the Cerebral Capillary

The structural differences between the capillaries generally found in the body and those of the brain are presented diagrammatically in Fig. 30-2. It is apparent that the tight junctions, lack of fenestrations, and pinocytosis (under normal circumstances) markedly restrict the passage of highly polar hydrophilic molecules while allowing virtually unrestricted transcellular movement (as do all capillaries) of lipid-soluble substances.[15] In addition, the cerebral capillary has by volume 2 to 4 times as many mitochondria as do most capillaries in the body. It is believed that active metabolic activity of cells is usually associated with an increase in mitochondrial volume. As will be seen, the large volume of these

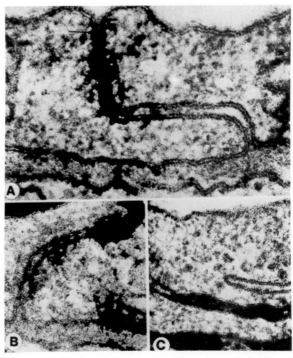

Figure 30-1 *A.* Electron micrograph of a cerebral capillary. Arrow indicates site of tight junction. The capillary lumen is at the top of the photomicrograph ($\times$ 340,000). *B.* Passage of lanthanum blocked by tight junctions (blood side) after intravenous infusion ($\times$ 250,000). *C.* Passage of peroxidase blocked at the endothelial junction (CSF side) after intraventricular injection ($\times$ 190,000). (From Brightman and Reese.[4])

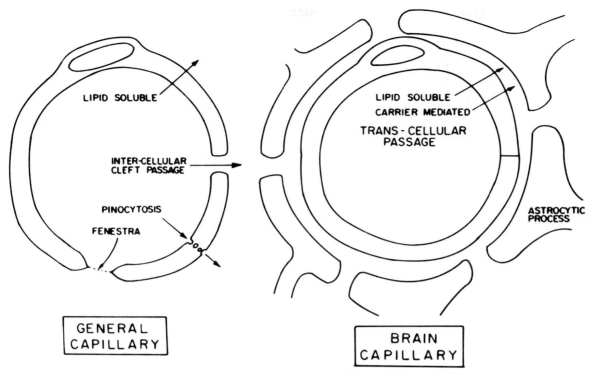

Figure 30-2 The structural differences between the general capillary and the central nervous system capillary. See text for details. (From Oldendorf.[15])

structures in the cerebral endothelial cell is associated with the energy-utilizing specialization of the cells that comprise the BBB.[15]

Remarkably, the cerebral capillary cell contains a wide assortment of biologically important enzymes, which include adenosine triphosphatase (ATPase), dehydrogenases (succinate, lactate, glutamate, and glucose), monamine oxidase, dopa decarboxylase, acid phosphatase, alkaline phosphatase, nicotinamide adenine dinucleotide (NAD), gamma-glutamyl transpeptidase, and others associated with glucose, amino acid, and neurotransmitter metabolism.[3,7,17] Some of these serve as the basis of transport across the BBB whereas others trap substrates and thereby inhibit transcapillary movement (Figs. 30-3 and 30-5). Recently the cerebral capillary (BBB) has been shown to possess insulin and alpha receptors.[6]

The BBB appears to have central innervation (cholinergic and aminergic) as well as peripheral innervation (sympathetic and parasympathetic). Beta receptors are found elsewhere in the cerebral circulation while alpha receptors are found at the BBB. The role of these innervations is poorly understood at the present time.

Carrier-Mediated BBB Movement

As mentioned earlier, substances that have high lipid solubility (high olive oil–water partition coefficent) rapidly penetrate the BBB.[15] Examples of this would be most anesthetic and analgesic agents. It is on this basis that heroin is taken up more easily by the brain and therefore has greater po-

tency than morphine, since the former drug is more lipid-soluble owing to substitution in the basic molecule of relatively nonpolar groups for the highly polar hydroxyl groups of morphine. Once in the brain, the heroin is hydrolyzed to morphine (the form which exhibits the analgesic property), and becomes less lipid-soluble so that its egress from the brain is more restricted.

There are some exceptions (circled in Fig. 30-4) to this relationship between lipid solubility and ease of penetration into brain.[15] These exceptions (such as glucose and certain amino acids) are usually metabolically active and penetrate easily not because of lipid solubility but because of their particular molecular configuration. The movement of these substances (some of which are shown in Fig. 30-5) satisfy the requirements for an active transport (uphill transport requiring the utilization of cellular energy) or a facilitated diffusion process. These processes demonstrate stereospecificity (e.g., D-glucose and not L-glucose), competitive inhibition (e.g., D-glucose and D-mannose), and saturation (limited transport capacity at high concentrations). The location of these transport systems (L-system for neutral amino acids, glucose, sodium, and potassium) in the endothelial cell are shown in Fig. 30-5. In some cases the transport process is bidirectional (glucose, large neutral amino acids, sodium?), but in others it is probably unidirectional (brain to blood: small neutral amino acids, potassium, iodide, protein, and prostaglandin $F_{2\alpha}$).[2] The kinetics of only six of the proposed carrier-mediated transport systems have been described in great detail: hexose; neutral, acidic, and basic amino acids; adenine; and short-chain monocarboxylic acids.[15]

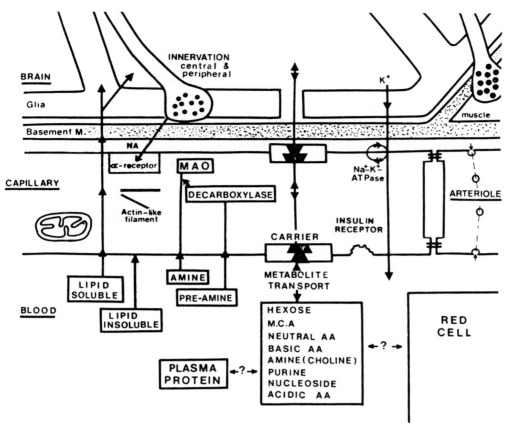

Figure 30-3 Diagrammatic representation of biological processes occurring within the BBB. (From Berry et al.[2])

Were it not for the hexose transport system, the brain would run out of its primary metabolic substrate. The maximal rate of glucose transport in mammals is in the range of 1.9 μmole per g brain per min. At the usual blood concentration (5 to 7 mM), the transport of glucose across the BBB is at half the maximal rate. Normally there is a 250 percent excess of extracellular glucose in relation to the usual cellular demands and this substrate is transported back across the BBB into the blood. In humans hypoglycemic symptoms occur when blood glucose falls to a level of 1.0 mM and coma is observed at half this level.[20,21] It might be anticipated that competitive inhibition between sugars would adversely influence cerebral metabolism. Clinically this is seen in galactosemia. Owing to an inborn error of metabolism, a high blood concentration of galactose occurs that blocks glucose transport by flooding (competitively inhibiting), the hexose carrier. This results in a functional hypoglycemia, which, together with the metabolic products of the preferentially transported glucose, leads to altered cerebral function.

The amino acid transport systems also play an important role in cerebral metabolism and function. In general, real and putative neurotransmitters are significantly restricted in passage across the BBB owing to relative lipid insolubility and/or enzyme trapping and degradation within the endothelial cell.[7] A number of amines are degraded by monoamine oxidase after penetrating the capillary cell membrane (Fig. 30-3). The metabolic precursors of these transmitters,

e.g., L-dihydroxyphenylalanine (L-dopa) L-tryptophan, L-tyrosine, penetrate the BBB without great restriction. The presence of dopa decarboxylase in the endothelial cell of the cerebral capillary results in the enzymatic trapping of the transported L-dopa and therefore limits its concentration in brain. The action of these enzymes in restricting amine movement across the BBB can be offset either by exceeding the capacity of the available intracellular enzyme or by the use of an enzyme inhibitor. Normally the concentration and metabolism of the transported amino acids in the brain depend on their concentration in plasma. The biologically important neutral amino acids tryptophan, phenylalanine, leucine, isoleucine, valine, and tyrosine compete for the same carrier system operating across the BBB. The ratio of the amount of any of these substances to the total amount of the others establishes the quantity entering the brain. The dietary intake of any of these essential amino acids (tyrosine is nonessential) will affect the plasma concentration and this plasma ratio and therefore will also affect substrate availability in the brain for maintenance of neurotransmitter and general cell metabolism.[21] It is this competition for entry into the brain coupled with an inborn error of metabolism that underlies the development of aminoacidurias.[11] In the case of phenylketonuria the deficiency of the appropriate hydroxylase does not allow the conversion of phenylalanine (PA) to tyrosine and its resulting accumulation in blood. The increase in the plasma concentration of PA and its ratio

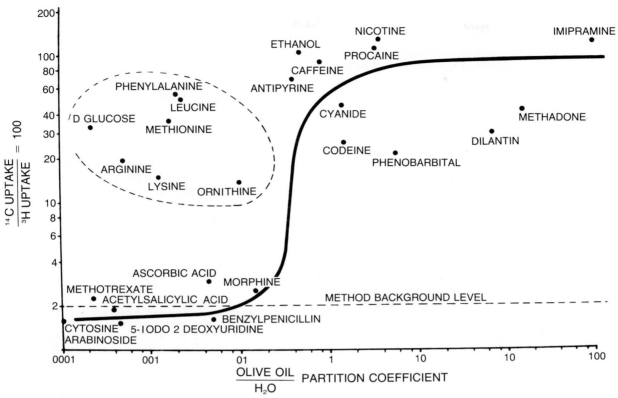

Figure 30-4 The relationship between the lipid solubility (oil/water partition coefficient) of a biological substance and the ease of passage across the cerebral capillary (extraction in a single pass through the brain—see text). (From Oldendorf.[15])

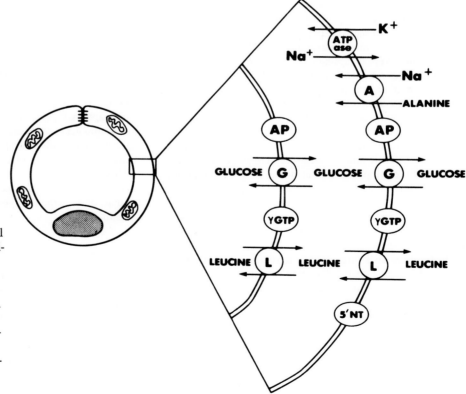

Figure 30-5 Model of a cerebral capillary demonstrating the distribution of enzyme and transport systems on the luminal and antiluminal membrane. ATPase-sodium, potassium ATPase. A = A system for neutral amino acid transport; γGTP = gamma-glutamyl transpeptidase; L = L system for neutral amino acid transport; 5'NT = 5'-nucleotidase. (From Betz and Goldstein.[3])

to the other amino acids results in a flooding of the transport system and a preferential entry of PA into the brain over the other competing amino acids. The excess of PA and its derivatives and the relative cerebral depletion of the other amino acids important in cerebral metabolism lead to the observed neurological abnormalities. This condition may be ameliorated by using a diet low in PA and high in the other neutral amino acids. A similar situation is seen in maple syrup disease, in which the defect is in the decarboxylation of ketoacids derived from leucine, isoleucine, and valine. These derivatives accumulate in brain and interfere with metabolic processes involved in myelination in addition to inhibiting (by competition) the entry of the other required amino acids. This disease as well as one in which there is a deficiency in tyrosine aminotransferase can also be treated by controlled dietary intake.[11]

Evaluation of BBB Function

The basis for most experimental and clinical tests for BBB integrity is the ability of the cerebral capillary to exclude most large, water-soluble molecules. Staining of the brain following introduction of a dye-protein complex into the vascular system is one of the earliest methods for indicating physical disruption of the BBB.[21] This method has been made more sensitive by substituting a radiolabeled marker for the vital dye. The evaluation of the architectural integrity of the cerebral capillary has been accomplished by ultrastructural localization of a tissue marker in relation to the endothelial cell and its intercellular junctions.[4] The carrier-mediated and diffusionary functions of the BBB can be evaluated quantitatively by a constant infusion or bolus injection into the carotid artery.[15] The latter method is that most commonly used in recent experimental work and is based on the extraction of the substance under study in a single pass through the cerebral capillary bed. The indicator diffusion technique uses a bolus injection containing a nondiffusible reference marker and the test molecule; frequent cerebral venous outflow samples make it unnecessary to sample brain tissue. The brain uptake method uses a highly diffusible marker and requires a sample of brain tissue. In both methods, the extraction of the test molecule as compared with the reference molecule and the measurement of cerebral blood flow allow the computation of an actual flux of the molecule per unit time and weight of tissue. This measurement at various blood concentration levels allows characterization of the transport system in terms of maximal rate of transcapillary movement (V_{max}) and concentration of substrate (K_m) at half the maximal rate.

In humans BBB integrity has most commonly been determined by the external detection of radionuclide activity with a sodium iodide crystal. This technique has been largely replaced by computed tomography (CT), in which the contrast enhancement is indicative of BBB breakdown.[12,16] Recently the use of intravascular rubidium-82 in conjunction with positron emission tomography (PET) has been shown to have great sensitivity in evaluating loss of BBB integrity.[23] Furthermore, the ability to perform dynamic scanning at 5-min intervals allows temporal changes in BBB permeability to be measured. A more comprehen-

sive evaluation of BBB transport function can be measured in humans by using the indicator diffusion technique mentioned above, but at the present time this method is only used in a clinical research setting.

Perturbation of the BBB

Anesthesia

It has been shown in rodents that although pentobarbital and halothane anesthesia do not affect total glucose influx into brain, the carrier-mediated portion falls with 1.5 to 2.0 percent halothane while the diffusionary component increases.[14] It has been suggested that this agent might compete with the glucose carrier. It appears more likely that the increase in the BBB permeability to glucose under these conditions is probably secondary and related to the effects of halothane on brain cyclic adenosine monophosphate (cAMP) concentrations.

Starvation and Hepatic Failure

In animals starved for up to 1 week, the transport of glucose across the cerebral capillary is enhanced by some 16 to 25 percent as compared with normal controls. In addition to this, ketone body uptake by the brain is greatly increased. It is unclear at the present time whether this represents accelerated transport or an increase in simple diffusion.[19] There is no anatomical evidence that the endothelial tight junctions are in any way modified in this condition that would explain an increase in the diffusionary component of ketone body movement across the BBB. Regardless of the mechanism, the net result is greater availability of these substances as a metabolic fuel during fasting. The human brain appears to depend more on this alternate source than the brain of most lower animals.[19]

The bulk of available evidence supports the notion that the encephalopathy associated with liver failure is primarily due to altered amino acid concentration in plasma and brain rather than to the toxic effects of ammonia, fatty acids, and mercaptans.[21] As noted earlier, an abnormal plasma pattern of amino acids interferes with the normal BBB transport of those compounds sharing the same BBB carrier. In addition, the neutral amino-acid-carrier protein seems to be modified. This leads to an abnormal accumulation of certain amino acids (e.g., phenylalanine, tryptophan) in brain with subsequent derangement of general and neurotransmitter metabolism.

Sepsis and Central Nervous System Infection

As noted with liver failure, patients with sepsis often demonstrate altered states of consciousness. There is recent evidence that sepsis induced by cecal rupture results in enhanced BBB transport of several neutral amino acids and their excessive accumulation in the brain in a manner previously described for liver failure.[8] When infection involves the central nervous system and its coverings, there seems to be a breakdown in the physical integrity of the BBB although the anatomical substrate in not known. It is believed that leukocytes can pass through the barrier during the acute untreated phase of bacterial meningitis and it is suspected that BBB glucose transport is also deranged under these same conditions.

Brain Tumors and Barrier Permeability

The growth of both primary and secondary brain tumors that are more than a few millimeters in diameter requires new capillary development. This stimulation of capillary growth is probably due to the presence of a tumor angiogenesis factor (TAF). A TAF has been found in human gliomas and is responsible for the abnormal capillaries found in the more malignant grades of these tumors.[17] These capillaries may demonstrate cellular fenestrations, wide intercellular junctions, pinocytotic vesicles, and infolding of luminal surfaces. Capillary abnormalities are also seen in the majority of the more malignant primary and metastatic brain tumors. It is not known whether these changes represent malignant degeneration of the endothelial cell or simply a response of the cerebral capillary to the metabolic requirements of the tumor. The overall decrease in the passage of glucose across the abnormal capillary and the usual increase in glucose utilization seem to support the latter view.

It is not suprising from the significant anatomical changes described above that normally excluded large molecules penetrate the BBB. This is the basis for the abnormal uptake of radionuclides and the contrast enhancement of lesions in radioisotope brain scans and CT brain scans, respectively.[12,16] It is difficult to equate exactly the abnormalities in the images with the alterations in the cerebral vessels since some enhancement has been seen in lesions with normal-appearing cerebral capillaries. The anatomical or biochemical basis for the inhibitory effect of steroids on the contrast enhancement of lesions observed on CT is also poorly understood at this time.

Microwave and X-Irradiation

The effects of microwave radiation on the BBB of humans appears to be primarily due to the hyperthermia associated with excessive exposure to this form of radiation.[17] The alterations in the BBB require an exposure of greater than 10 mW per cm^2. Below this level there is enough thermal regulation in brain to prevent cerebral "hot spots."

In all animal species studied, acute radiation injury to the nervous system results in disruption not only of the BBB but also of the usually more resistant cellular elements. The damage to the cerebral endothelial cell is dose-related and therefore is usually found in brains irradiated at the upper ranges for malignant tumors. The damage to the capillary is greatest in the adventitia and may be evident after a few months. The latent period, however, can be measured in years. The changes in the barrier can be great enough to result in the extravasation of plasma and a focal mass effect. The capillaries may also occlude, resulting in tissue necrosis. The neovascularization that usually follows this necrosis consists initially of leaky immature capillaries. The resulting mass effect often cannot be distinguished from a recurrent tumor. In recent years, with a more aggressive approach to radiotherapy, this complication is being seen more frequently. The spinal cord is also vulnerable to the effects of radiation, with an occasional tragic result.

Loss of Cerebral Autoregulation

The phenomenon of cerebral autoregulation can be described briefly as a compensatory change in cerebrovascular resistance in response to variations in vascular pressures. Usually regulation of resistance to flow occurs between 60 and 160 mmHg, although in the hypertensive patient this may be extended to 200 mmHg. These changes in vascular resistance are due in part or totally to myogenic, autonomic, and metabolic mechanisms. The conditions that produce loss of autoregulation and subsequent vasodilatation often lead to stretching of the capillary endothelium (and opening of the tight junctions?) and pinocytosis.[21] This occurs in prolonged hypercapnia, where the BBB opens to large molecules but reverts to normal after the blood P_{CO_2} is corrected.

In acute hypertension, normally excluded macromolecules easily enter the brain, primarily by pinocytotic activity in cerebral arterioles and capillaries.[9] It has been suggested that the alterations in neurological function in these cases are due to excessive entry of monoamines into the brain. BBB changes are not seen in chronic hypertension because of the increased vessel wall-lumen ratio in the cerebral resistance vessels.

The loss of autoregulation and changes in BBB permeability are also seen after cerebral seizure activity.[17] The rapid elevation of intravascular pressure is accompanied by an increase in cerebral blood flow by as much as 400 percent. Under these conditions the barrier opens transiently, although such a change may be more permanent in status epilepticus.

The ultrastructural effects of global ischemia are surprisingly modest because the cerebral capillary cell is so resistant to ischemic and hypoxic insults.[10,21] Even after 17 min of complete circulatory arrest, dye-protein markers are usually unable to traverse the BBB. The situation is quite variable when ischemia is prolonged since the opening of the BBB can be delayed up to 24 h after the ischemic episode. When the ischemia is nonglobal, the collateral circulation allows normal-appearing capillaries to be found in the same area as those showing gross disruption, even after many hours. The anatomical changes include the dehiscence of tight junctions as well as increased lucency of the basal lamina. In cerebral infarction there is also great variability in the damage to the neural tissue, especially along the periphery of a small lesion, because the altered blood flow may be sufficient to maintain the relatively hardy vascular endothelium. Intravascular pressure and hypercapnia also play a role in BBB disruption after restoration of blood flow. The more rapid and greater the elevation of blood pressure, alone or in combination with a high P_{CO_2}, the more likely the BBB disruption.

Cerebral Edema

It is appropriate to discuss the BBB in conjunction with cerebral edema (CE) because the most common type of CE is due to the breakdown of this barrier. *Cerebral edema* can be defined briefly as the excess accumulation of water in the intra- and/or extracellular spaces of the brain. As we shall see, this simple definition covers a wide range of causes.

Classification of Cerebral Edema

The presently recognized types of cerebral edema are presented briefly in Fig. 30-6 and will now be described in some detail.[6,10] Disruption of the cerebral capillary provides the underlying mechanism for the development of vasogenic edema. The changes in the BBB are gross enough to allow plasma or a filtrate of plasma to enter the extracellular space of the brain. In the white matter both the water and sodium contents are increased while the potassium content is diminished. Similar changes are seen in the cerebral cortex except that the increase in water content and fall in potassium content are of lesser magnitude. Histologically, the astrocytes are swollen in both white and gray matter, but only in the former is the extracellular space enlarged. This form of edema is the one most frequently seen in a clinical setting in response to trauma, primary and metastatic tumors, focal inflammation, and the later stages of cerebral ischemia.

Cytotoxic edema is due primarily to derangement of cellular metabolism, which results in inadequate functioning of the sodium and potassium pump in the glial cell membrane. This disturbance in the pump results in cellular retention of sodium and water. The content of water and these ions in white matter is similar to those noted for vasogenic edema, although in the cerebral cortex only the sodium content is elevated. The histological consequence is swollen astrocytes in both the cortex and white matter, and in the latter there

is often accumulation of fluid within myelinic vacuoles. This type of CE is seen in various intoxications (e.g., dinitrophenol, triethyltin, hexachlorophene, isoniazid), Reye's syndrome, severe hypothermia, and the early stages of ischemia.

The accumulation of excess water in the brain in response to an unfavorable osmotic gradient operating across the intact BBB has been labeled *osmotic cerebral edema*. Normally the osmolality of the CSF and the extracellular fluid of the brain is only slightly greater than that of plasma. When the plasma is diluted by pathological ingestion of water, inappropriate secretion of antidiuretic hormone, or severe hemodialysis of the uremic patient, the chemical potential of the plasma increases and water enters the brain down this abnormal gradient. Generally, only the water content in white and gray matter is elevated although it has been suggested that the reduction of potassium content may indicate a cellular adaptation to this process. In both the cortex and the white matter, the astrocytes are swollen, as is the extracellular space of the brain. The intraventricular fluid formation rate is also increased by the same causes given for the observed water movement across the cerebral capillary, although some of this excess fluid may be derived from the adjacent periventricular white matter.[21]

The last type of CE to be discussed has been reported to occur in acute hypertension, in which the elevated pressure is directly transmitted to the cerebral capillary. Pre-

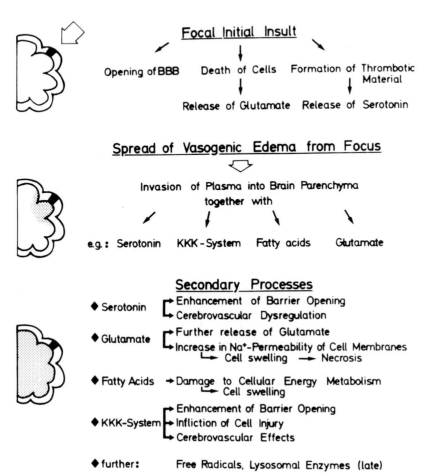

Figure 30-6 A concept of formation, release, and function of edema factors based on cold-induced vasogenic edema. (From Baethmann et al.[1])

sumably the vasodilatation of the capillary allows the movement of a protein-free transudate into the extracellular space. In acute hypertension marked increases in pinocytosis in the cerebral vasculature have been shown and it is likely that this mechanism is responsible in part for the fluid accumulation.[9] The periventricular edema associated with hypertensive hydrocephalus is another example of hydrostatic CE. In this case the hydrostatic gradient forces the CSF across the leaky ventricular ependyma into the extracellular space. The composition of the white matter fluid is similar to that seen in vasogenic edema except that the edema fluid has a low protein content.

Pathophysiology of Cerebral Edema

It is important to review some of the factors that influence the development and resolution of the most common type of edema seen in a clinical setting.[1,22] As mentioned earlier, vasogenic edema is initiated by loss of the integrity of the BBB. The prevailing vascular hydrostatic gradient is then responsible for the movement of the plasma (or its filtrate) into the extracellular space and by bulk flow to areas remote from the site of the BBB breakdown. In the region of the edema there is an increase in tissue pressure, loss of autoregulation, decrease in cerebral blood flow (CBF), and tissue acidosis. Edema formation will continue as long as capillary leakage and tissue pressure gradients persist. The rate and extent of the edema depend not only on hydrostatic forces but also on chemical changes in the involved tissues.[1] These chemical factors are shown in Fig. 30-7 and represent a partially documented model, which may not be fully operative in every case of vasogenic CE. In this model glutamate, serotonin, components of the kallikrein-kininogen-kinin (KKK) system, and fatty acids enter the tissue with the plasma, although some may be released with tissue damage. It has been proposed that these substances lead to the spread and the maintenance of the edema process by enhancing local and distal barrier permeability by stimulating pinocytosis (serotonin and the KKK system), or by deranging microcirculatory control, thereby increasing hydrostatic filtration through the damaged capillaries.[1] Presumably, glutamate and free fatty acids lead to cell swelling by increasing the cellular permeability to sodium. The large volume of edema seen with relatively small lesions may be due to the release of these secondary factors after the initial insult to the BBB.

The resolution of CE appears to be secondary to the uptake and degradation of edema fluid protein by glial cells.[21] This process, coupled with the repair of the damaged barrier, creates a favorable osmotic gradient (brain > blood) for water to move from the extracellular space of the brain into blood. The movement of the accumulated water out of the brain is also aided by the molecular transfer of osmotically active particles into blood by a pinocytotic process. There is evidence that edema fluid drains into the ventricular cavity down a hydrostatic gradient and ultimately is cleared from the CSF system by bulk flow through the arachnoid villi. At the present time the relative importance of each of these mechanisms in human CE is unknown.

In general the metabolic effects of CE are primarily due to the associated increased intracranial pressure (ICP), altered CBF, and release of substances that are toxic to the brain or adversely affect cerebral metabolism. It is apparent from this that by decreasing the mass effect of the edematous tissue these metabolic abnormalities will be reversed and normal neural function restored.

Diagnosis of Cerebral Edema

Clinical Features

Until the intracranial pressure (ICP) reaches a level that produces local ischemia, CE alone will not produce clinical neurological abnormalities. When this point is reached in the later stages of edema, the symptoms and signs are related to the location of the inciting lesion although remote effects are not uncommon. The important role of vascular insufficiency in the development of the clinical features is supported by the often remarkable and rapid reversal of both symptoms and signs when antiedema therapy is instituted.[13]

Radiological Imaging

The development of CT has for the first time allowed the visualization of CE.[12] The areas of edema appear as a low density on the unenhanced CT scan. This is due to the dilution of all the constituents of the white matter. The resulting changes in the CT numbers can be used to estimate the amount of water added to the brain tissue. The effects, however, of decreased lipids, increased protein, and electrolytes in the exudate lead to an underestimation of the amount of edema fluid based on the CT number printout. In general the more malignant primary tumors of the brain and metastatic tumors entail the greatest incidence of CE although CE can be seen with any intracranial tumor and therefore the presence of edema does not rule out benign lesions.[16] CE is also seen in about 90 percent of patients with brain abscesses. Only 15 percent of patients with spontaneous intracerebral hemorrhage have CE in the white matter whereas CE in acute vascular occlusive lesions can be demonstrated in both the cortex and underlying white matter. The CE seen on CT scan with acute epidural and intracerebral hematomas is typically limited to the white matter, but with acute subdural hematomas the CE extends into both the gray and white matter of the involved hemisphere.

PET scanning has been used to good advantage in evaluating the integrity of the BBB, as mentioned earlier in this chapter.[23] Its greatest potential, however, will be in providing a frequent assessment of disease processes as they develop and respond to therapy.[20] In the case of CE, PET is capable of measuring not only regional water content but regional cerebral blood volume (rCBV) as well. This allows estimation of the contribution of vascular engorgement to an area of regional brain swelling as well as estimation of the concentration of (radiolabeled) therapeutic agents in the intra- and extravascular compartments. The most exciting and useful capacity of PET scanning will be for measurement of regional cerebral blood flow (rCBF) and metabolism. Since CE alone does not influence cerebral function until the rCBF is markedly reduced, serial determinations of flow will allow the clinician to judge the stage of edema and its response to therapy.

Treatment of Cerebral Edema

The treatments of cerebral edema and of increased intracranial pressure are virtually the same but will be discussed here on the assumption that the CE, and not vasoparalysis or the focal inciting lesion, is primarily responsible for the mass effect.

Restoration or Improvement of BBB Breakdown

The surgical removal of the focal lesion responsible for CE usually results in the resolution of edema owing to the removal of the greater portion of the deranged BBB. The remaining edema fluid can then be reabsorbed by mechanisms described earlier without replenishment of the fluid. The decrease in lesion bulk may also improve rCBF and therefore enhance the process of edema resolution.[10] The effect of BBB disruption can also be diminished by decreasing the hydrostatic gradient by either lowering blood pressure or increasing cerebrovascular resistance. Blood pressure can be lowered with a nitroprusside infusion (0.1 μg/kg per min) while the resistance can be increased by hyperventilation or the use of barbiturates, which will be discussed later. Due care must be taken when manipulating cerebral hemodynamic factors that an adequate cerebral perfusion pressure is maintained. The only drugs that may exert their effect on ICP and CE by stabilizing cell membranes and restoring BBB integrity are the corticosteroids.[5,13] These substances may also inhibit those plasma and tissue substances that secondarily increase both local and distal cerebral vascular permeability (Fig. 30-7). The effect of steroids on ATPase activity will be discussed later. The clinical improvement following their use precedes CT evidence of loss of contrast enhancement (by restoring BBB function), increase in density numbers, or reduction of brain distortion. There is some evidence that high-dose dexamethasone therapy (150 to 400 mg per day) might be somewhat more effective than standard or low-dose therapy (10 to 20 mg loading dose and then 16 mg per day). In either case this form of therapy has been shown to be very effective in perifocal edema associated with focal infection or tumor and questionably effective for trauma, viral encephalitis, hypoxia-ischemia, and Reye's disease. The advocates of steroid use in head trauma believe that only high-dose therapy helps in this condition.

Removal of Tissue Water

The most rapid and effective means of decreasing tissue water and brain bulk is osmotherapy.[13] The most common agent used is mannitol (20% solution) in a dose varying between 0.25 and 1.0 g per kg body weight. There is some evidence that the lower doses are quite effective, with less chance of inducing hyperosmolar problems that have been noted with frequent high-dose therapy. It should be appreciated from the previous discussion in the BBB section of this chapter that water is being removed from those regions of the brain with an intact barrier. This osmotic effect can be prolonged by the use of loop diuretics (furosemide and ethacrynic acid) after the osmotic agent infusion.[18] Furosemide in a dose of 0.7 mg per kg has been shown to prolong the reversal of the blood-brain osmotic gradient established with the osmotic agents by preferentially excreting water over solute.[18] Oral glycerol has also been shown to effectively lower ICP by the removal of brain tissue water although its effectiveness appears to decrease after a few days.[12] It is used in a dose of 0.5 to 1.0 g per kg body weight. The solution can be made up in 5% dextrose in water or 0.4% NaCl. In the uncooperative or unconscious patient it can be given by a nasogastric tube, which is then clamped for 2 to 3 h. The effectiveness of decreasing brain bulk in the clearance of the edema fluid is thought to be due to the improvement in CSF outflow resistance, which initially is increased by the collapse of the subarachnoid space by the edematous brain tissue. It is assumed in this case that the cerebral ventricles serve as a "sink" for edema fluid.[22]

Compensation in Vascular and CSF Compartments

Another approach to dealing with increased ICP and CE is to decrease other components that fill the intracranial compartment. This can be accomplished by decreasing the

TABLE 30-1   Classification of Cerebral Edema Based on Pathogenesis*

Type	Pathogenesis	Compositions	Location	CSF Formation Rate	BBB
Vasogenic	BBB breakdown	Water, Na+ and plasma proteins	Primary extracellular, secondary intracellular	Not increased	Disturbed
Cytotoxic	Disturbance of cellular metabolism	Water, Na+	Intracellular	—	Undisturbed
Osmotic	Osmotic gradient	Water	Intracellular and extracellular	Increased	Undisturbed
Hydrostatic	Hydrostatic gradient	Water, Na+	Extracellular	—	Undisturbed

*From Go.[6]

rate of CSF formation or by decreasing the cerebral vascular volume. It appears that the secretion of CSF is adversely affected by those drugs that inhibit Na-K-ATPase activity namely, steroids (dexamethasone 16 mg per day), loop diuretics (furosemide 50 mg per kg), carbonic acid inhibitors (acetazolamide 20 to 50 mg per kg), glycerol (1.0 mg per kg), and dimethyl sulfoxide (DMSO). A 10% solution of DMSO has been used effectively in experimental animals in an intravenous dose of 1.0 g per kg.[5]

Clinical Approach to Cerebral Edema

By using the information given above it is possible with the continuous measurement of ICP to rationally and often effectively deal with CE. The use of hyperventilation to achieve a blood P_{CO_2} of about 25 mmHg is often effective in temporarily decreasing the ICP associated with CE. If needed, osmotic agents can be used alone or in combination with the loop diuretics. If these agents become less effective, barbiturate therapy (pentobarbital or thiopental) can be used. Pentobarbital is generally used as a loading dose of 3 to 5 mg per kg and then 100 to 200 mg every 30 to 60 min to produce the desired effect. The loading dose of thiopental is 20 mg per kg, with a constant intravenous infusion of 10 mg/kg per h for 6 h, after which the dose is decreased to 3 mg/kg per h. The effectiveness of barbiturate therapy is still in question, and this is often the treatment of last resort. It must be appreciated that the combination of therapies listed above can adversely affect cerebral perfusion pressure and this must be frequently computed from the mean arterial pressure and the ICP.

The progress in the understanding and treatment of CE over the past 25 years has been remarkable. There is every indication from the newer diagnostic techniques and experimental drug development that this progress will be continued.

References

1. Baethmann A, Oettinger W, Rothenfulsser W, Kempski O, Unterberg A, Geiger R: Brain edema factors: Current state with particular reference to plasma constituents and glutamate. Adv Neurol 28:171–195, 1980.
2. Berry DI, Paulson OB, Hertz MM: The blood-brain barrier: An overview with special reference to insulin effects on glucose transport. Acta Neurol Scand [Suppl] 78:147–156, 1980.
3. Betz AL, Goldstein GW: The basis for active transport at the blood-brain barrier, in Eisenberg HM, Suddith RL (eds): *The Cerebral Microvasculature: Investigation of the Blood-Brain Barrier*. New York, Plenum, 1980, pp 5–16.
4. Brightman MW, Reese TS: Junctions between intimately apposed cell membranes in the vertebrate brain. J Cell Biol 40:648–677, 1969.
5. Camp PE, James HE, Werner R: Acute dimethyl sulfoxide therapy in experimental brain edema: Part 1. Effects on intracranial pressure, blood pressure, central venous pressure, and brain water and electrolyte content. Neurosurgery 9:28–33, 1981.
6. Go GK: The classification of brain edema, in de Vlieger M, de Lange SA, Beks JWF (eds): *Brain Edema*. New York, Wiley, 1981, pp. 3–9.
7. Mardebo JE, Owman C: Barrier mechanisms for neurotransmitter monoamines and their precursors at the blood-brain interface. Ann Neurol 8:1–11, 1980.
8. Jeppsson B, Freund HR, Gimmon Z, James JH, von Meyenfeldt MF, Fischer JE: Blood-brain barrier derangement in sepsis: Cause of septic encephalopathy? Am J Surg 141:136–142, 1981.
9. Johansson BB, Linder LE: The blood-brain barrier in renal hypertensive rats. Clin Exp Hypertension 2:983–993, 1980.
10. Katzman R, Pappius HM: *Brain Electrolytes and Fluid Metabolism*. Baltimore, Williams & Wilkins, 1973.
11. Kindt E, Halvorsen S: The need of essential amino acids in children. An evaluation based on the intake of phenylalanine, tyrosine, leucine, isoleucine, and valine in children with phenketonuria, tyrosine amino transferase defect, and maple syrup urine disease. Am J Clin Nutr 33:279–286, 1980.
12. Lanksch W, Baethmann A, Kazner E: Computed tomography of brain edema, in de Vlieger M, de Lange SA, Beks JWF (eds): Brain Edema. New York, Wiley, 1981, pp. 67–98.
13. Marshall LF: Treatment of brain swelling and brain edema in man. Adv Neurol 28:459–469, 1980.
14. Nemoto EM: Blood-brain barrier transport during anesthesia, in Eisenberg HM, Suddith RL (eds): *The Cerebral Microvasculature: Investigation of the Blood-Brain Barrier*. New York, Plenum, 1980, pp. 167–178.
15. Oldendorf WH: Blood-brain barrier, in Himwich HE (ed): *Brain Metabolism and Cerebral Disorders*, 2d ed. New York, Spectrum Publications, 1976, pp. 163–180.
16. Penn RD: Cerebral edema and neurological function: CT, evoked responses, and clinical examination. Adv Neurol 28:383–394, 1980.
17. Pollay M, Roberts PA: Blood-brain barrier: A definition of normal and altered function. Neurosurgery 6:675–685, 1980.
18. Pollay M, Roberts PA, Fullenwider C, Stevens FA: The effect of mannitol and furosemide on the blood-brain barrier osmotic gradient and intracranial pressure. Presented at the 5th International Symposium on Intracranial Pressure, Tokyo, May 31, 1982.
19. Pollay M, Stevens FA: Starvation-induced changes in transport of ketone bodies across the blood-brain barrier. J Neurosci Res 5:163–172, 1980.
20. Raichle ME: Brain edema: Evaluation in vivo with positron emission tomography. Adv Neurol 28:423–427, 1980.
21. Rapoport SI: *Blood-Brain Barrier in Physiology and Medicine*. New York, Raven Press, 1976.
22. Reulen HJ, Tsuyumu M: Pathophysiology of formation and natural resolution of vasogenic brain edema, in de Vlieger M, de Lange SA, Beks JWF (eds): *Brain Edema*. New York, Wiley, 1981, pp. 31–48.
23. Yen CK, Budinger TF: Evaluation of blood-brain barrier permeability changes in rhesus monkeys and man using [82]Rb and positron emission tomography. J Comput Assist Tomogr 5:792–799, 1981.

31

Increased Intracranial Pressure, Brain Herniation, and Their Control

Donald O. Quest

Increased Intracranial Pressure

One of the commonest pathological phenomena encountered by the neurosurgeon is that of increased intracranial pressure. Attempts to understand the etiologic factors involved in producing intracranial hypertension have been an important aspect of laboratory and clinical research since the advent of neurosurgery as a specialty. In earlier days emphasis was placed on the clinical diagnosis of increased intracranial pressure, and methods of treatment evolved as experience with intracranial lesions and their surgical therapy increased. In the last 20 years intensive research into the pathophysiological effects of intracranial pressure on brain function, metabolism, blood flow, and other parameters has been undertaken.

Lundberg in 1960 first reported his landmark series of the direct continuous recording of intracranial pressure in a large number of patients.[43] Prior to this time intracranial pressure was measured only infrequently and usually indirectly via lumbar puncture. Lundberg's series was followed by laboratory investigation of the effects of a variety of experimental intracranial lesions on intracranial pressure in order to explain the clinical findings encountered in this series.

Anatomy and Physiology

The cranium can be thought of as a hollow, rigid sphere of constant volume. There is one large vent, the foramen magnum, and a number of smaller foramina for cranial nerves and blood vessels. There are three main components within the intracranial space: brain, cerebrospinal fluid, and blood (normal brain volume is approximately 1400 ml, intracranial cerebrospinal fluid volume about 75 ml, and cerebral vascular volume about 75 ml[38]). All these components are essentially noncompressible. The rigid cranial sphere provides the premise of the Monro-Kellie doctrine, introduced into neurosurgery in modified form by Cushing.[14] This doctrine states that a change in the volume of the brain causes a reciprocal change in the volume of one of the other intracranial components, i.e., either blood or cerebrospinal fluid.

Normal Intracranial Pressure

Normal intracranial pressure is pulsatile owing mainly to intracranial arterial pulsations[19] that reflect the cardiac and respiratory cycles.[2] The generally accepted normal lower limit of cerebrospinal fluid pressure via lumbar puncture is 50 mmH$_2$O and the upper limit is 200 mmH$_2$O.

Intracranial pressure is affected by a number of complicated physiological variables within the intracranial space.[61,89] Magnaes found that when a patient sat up, lumbar cerebrospinal fluid pressure transiently rose by several hundred millimeters, the blood pressure in the cerebral arteries transiently decreased, and the cerebral resistance vessels dilated as a manifestation of autoregulation. As cerebral arterial pressure increased toward normal, the resistance vessels constricted and cerebral blood volume decreased, thereby accounting for the transience of the cerebrospinal fluid (CSF) pressure rise.[45]

Methods of Measurement of Intracranial Pressure

The lumbar puncture method of measuring intracranial pressure was first published by Quincke in 1891.[63] Although this method is simple, there are problems associated with its use. There is the danger of precipitating acute brain stem compression from herniation either at the tentorial notch or at the foramen magnum. In addition it is by no means certain that the spinal fluid pressure via lumbar puncture is an accurate reflection of intracranial pressure. Any patient who has signs of brain herniation or papilledema should not undergo spinal puncture except in the most unusual circumstances. Lumbar puncture pressure *may* be equal to intracranial pressure, but if there is a failure of communication of pressure from the intracranial space to the spinal canal, the lumbar spinal fluid pressure will be incorrect and misleading. Incisural block or brain herniation into the tentorial notch or foramen magnum will prevent accurate measurement of intracranial pressure via the spinal puncture route.

Lundberg, the first to continously measure intracranial pressure, used a cannula in the frontal horn through a burr hole although the practice of ventricular cannulation for the relief of intracranial pressure is one of the oldest in neurological surgery.[43] The use of the intraventricular cannula continues to be one of the most reliable means of measuring pressure within the intracranial space. The problems with this method include the fact that the brain must be penetrated to insert the cannula, which can lead to hematoma, seizures, or neurological dysfunction—however, all these are rare. If the ventricles are shifted or are small, insertion of the cannula may be technically difficult. The most serious problem is that of the risk of infection; however, this can be minimized by tunneling the catheter beneath the skin prior to its exit from the scalp.

Another commonly used technique for measuring intracranial pressure is that of the subarachnoid screw or bolt.[87] The screw is placed in position via a twist-drill hole in the skull near the coronal suture 2 to 3 cm lateral to the midline on the nondominant side. The dura is opened through the twist-drill hole so that CSF is obtained and the screw is then inserted and attached to an external transducer. If pressure pulsations become damped because of brain swelling or obstruction of the orifice, this may be corrected by injection of a small amount of sterile saline into the screw. The subarachnoid screw may not be quite as reliable as the ventricular catheter—in particular, its use may lead to underestimation of high intracranial pressure.[49]

A number of other devices have been used to monitor intracranial pressure, including the subdural cup catheter[92] and the fiberoptic epidural sensor.[40] More sophisticated transducers, which require no outside connection, may be used as chronically implantable devices functioning via telemetry. Generally these devices are expensive and sufficiently complicated and unavailable so that the ventricular catheter or subarachnoid screw methods of measuring intracranial pressure are the most commonly used.

Intracranial Volume/Pressure Relationship

Reciprocal changes among the various components in the intracranial space occur when the volume of one of these components is changed. As an intracranial mass expands or the brain swells, the cerebrospinal fluid volume (the main buffer) is decreased. Reduction of cerebral blood volume may also occur, but later and with more serious sequelae. An important factor is the rapidity of mass expansion in relation to the compensating compartmental shifts. CSF may be driven out of the intracranial space relatively quickly in response to increasing intracranial pressure.

A common method of studying increased intracranial pressure in laboratory animals involves use of an extradural balloon, which is gradually expanded while pressure is measured. It has been demonstrated that the volume added to the balloon is compensated by a decrease in volume of the other intracranial components, thereby keeping pressure constant until a certain point is reached at which the pressure begins to rise rapidly. This point of rapid rise occurs when there is no further displaceable volume available. This relationship of intracranial volume and pressure, elucidated by Langfitt et al., is depicted in Fig. 31-1 and is an essential element in the understanding of intracranial pressure relationships.[37]

The concepts of compliance and elastance of the intracranial contents are also important.[42] *Compliance* (dV/dP) is that quality of distensibility available within the intracranial space and *elastance* (dP/dV) is the inverse of this, i.e., the resistance offered to expansion of an intracranial mass. A high degree of compliance is present when a large change in volume produces a small change in pressure. A high degree of elastance is present when a small change in volume produces a large change in pressure. On the vertical portion of the volume-pressure curve the compliance is low and the elastance is high. As pressure continues to rise, compliance progressively decreases no matter what the cause of the increased pressure. The entire curve may be shifted to the left if the mass is expanded rapidly or a pathological change has

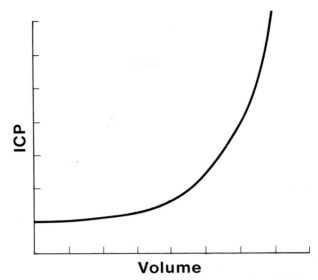

Figure 31-1 Volume-pressure relationship. This stylized volume vs. pressure curve demonstrates that as intracranial volume increases, a point is reached at which the intracranial pressure begins to rise exponentially. Added increments of volume (dV) cause larger and larger increases in pressure (dP). It can be seen that elastance (dP/dV) increases as intracranial pressure increases and, conversely, compliance (dV/dP) changes in a reciprocal fashion.

occurred within the intracranial space decreasing the amount of displaceable volume. The elastance and compliance of the intracranial space may be determined by measuring the change in intraventricular pressure after injection of 1 ml of sterile saline into the ventricle in 1 s.[52] This is called the *volume-pressure response*. How useful this measurement is in determining compensatory capacity has been questioned, and cerebrospinal fluid pulse amplitude and wave form analysis may be more helpful.[10,78] These relationships are complex and how much each of the three intracranial components contributes to the volume-pressure response is unknown.

In measurements of intracranial pressure the assumption is made that transmission of pressure is uniform throughout the intracranial space. There is evidence, however, that this is not so. The elastic properties of the cortex and the subdural network of blood vessels probably are different from those of the white matter and deep nuclei. Measurements of intraparenchymal pressure have been attempted experimentally with varying success; however, it is probable that pressure gradients do develop in the intracranial space, especially during rapid expansion of a mass, and these gradients probably dissipate rapidly as well.[90]

Pathology of Increased Intracranial Pressure

The cause of increased intracranial pressure is as important as the magnitude of that pressure in terms of brain function. With a diffuse increase in intracranial pressure, a patient may function normally even though the increase is marked. Patients with pseudotumor cerebri or hydrocephalus may have very thin intracranial pressures but no neurological sequelae. The reason is probably that autoregulation is intact and cerebral blood flow is adequate to maintain brain function. In patients with mass lesions, autoregulation is disturbed and cerebral blood flow may be decreased below the level necessary for normal brain function. Local tissue pressure may be higher than the measured intracranial pressure and regional cerebral blood flow may be more easily compromised, with a rise in intracranial pressure due to mass effect, edema, or hypercarbia. Increased intracranial pressure affects brain function adversely by decreasing cerebral blood flow below a critical level or by herniation of brain through the tentorial incisura or foramen magnum, which results in compression and ischemia of the brain stem.

Effects on Vital Signs

In earlier days changes in blood pressure, heart rate, and respiration were taken as indices of the onset and severity of increased intracranial pressure. Cushing emphasized the increase in blood pressure that occurs with increasing intracranial pressure, along with bradycardia and respiratory irregularities.[13] The relationship of these parameters to increased intracranial pressure is not so clear-cut. The vasopressor response present with increased intracranial pressure appears to arise in the medulla. Distortion and displacement of the brain stem appear to be important in determining the nature and degree of the cardiorespiratory changes produced by an expanding mass.[83] Experimentally, after the onset of brain stem compression blood pressure rises sharply, probably owing to a direct neurogenic effect on peripheral arterioles. A secondary rise is observed that may be due to release of pressor substances into the blood, and the final increase is attributed to increased circulating blood volume.[68]

Respiratory irregularities in response to increased intracranial pressure are well known and are thought to be due to damage to higher centers, which releases the respiratory mechanism within the brain stem from supranuclear control.[24,48] The changes that occur in experimental animals in response to an expanding supratentorial mass are, in sequence: decrease in respiratory rate, bradycardia, cardiac arrhythmia, pupillary constriction followed by unilateral dilatation, increase in pulse pressure, and finally an increase in arterial blood pressure.[16,23]

Intracranial Pressure and Cerebral Blood Flow

The cerebral vascular pressure falls from about 90 mmHg in the large extracranial cerebral arteries to 3 mmHg in the jugular veins in normotensive subjects. The greatest drop in pressure occurs across the arterioles. Cerebral blood flow is regulated to provide the brain with sufficient oxygen and glucose to carry out its normal metabolic processes. When the systemic arterial pressure falls, the cerebral resistance vessels dilate in an attempt to maintain normal cerebral blood flow. The opposite occurs when systemic arterial pressure increases. This is termed autoregulation and the re-

sponse occurs within a few seconds of the change in systemic arterial pressure.[38] When autoregulation is impaired, cerebral blood flow changes are slower and less complete, and when autoregulation is absent, cerebral blood flow passively follows the changes in systemic arterial pressure. The lower limit of autoregulation is at about 50 mmHg systemic pressure and the upper limit about 160 mmHg.[20] As systemic arterial pressure is decreased, the cerebral resistance vessels dilate until they are maximally dilated. When systemic arterial pressure is increased, the vessels constrict until the pressure exceeds 160 mmHg, at which point vasoconstriction is overcome, passive dilatation follows, and cerebral blood flow increases, with possible disruption of the blood-brain barrier.[15]

There are several theories as to how autoregulation takes place. One is the *myogenic theory*, which postulates a smooth muscle reflex within the resistance vessels. The increase in intraluminal pressure causes an increase in tone of the smooth muscle cells, producing shortening and a reduction in vascular diameter.[38] Decreasing intraluminal pressure has the opposite effect. Another is the *metabolic theory* according to which tissue tension of O_2 or CO_2 mediates the change in vessel diameter. There is some evidence of a sympathetic[21] and neural vasodilator[36] contribution to cerebral blood flow regulation as well.

Hypoxemia causes cerebral vasodilatation, which begins once Pa_{O_2} drops to a threshold of about 50 mmHg and becomes maximum at Pa_{O_2} around 20 mmHg.[32] It is unclear whether the hypoxic dilatation is mediated via the chemoreceptors in the carotid and aortic bodies,[62] via centers within the brain stem, or via local regulation by way of tissue pH or metabolic products.[32] An increase in Pa_{CO_2} is the most potent stimulus to cerebral vasodilatation and the response is linear in the Pa_{CO_2} range of 15 to 80 mmHg.[66] Thus, with hypoxia cerebral blood flow rises precipitously once the threshold value of 50 mmHg Pa_{O_2} is reached, whereas with hypercarbia cerebral blood flow rises in a gradual, linear fashion from 15 to 80 mmHg Pa_{CO_2}. As with hypoxia, the cerebral vascular response to hypercarbia may occur locally via the vascular smooth muscle[64] and/or via vasodilator pathways.

The demand of the brain for oxygen and glucose is closely coupled to the cerebral blood flow, and this is termed *metabolic autoregulation*.[80] It is achieved by changes in cerebral vascular resistance mediated most likely by changes in the local tissue hydrogen ion concentration.

As intracranial pressure rises, cerebral blood flow is maintained at a constant rate when autoregulation is intact. Cerebral blood flow equals carotid artery pressure minus jugular vein pressure divided by cerebrovascular resistance

$$CBF = \left(\frac{CAP - JVP}{CVR} \right)$$

Cerebral venous pressure is nearly equal to intracranial pressure and follows its elevation or decrease. Thus, as intracranial pressure increases, cerebrovascular resistance decreases to keep cerebral blood flow constant.[55] At very high levels of intracranial pressure the cerebral veins and sinuses collapse, which raises cerebrovascular resistance and decreases cerebral blood flow.[76]

As a mass lesion expands, cerebral blood flow remains

constant if the rate of expansion is slow; if it is fast, however, high tissue pressure and local ischemia around the mass probably occur, accounting for decreased flow. With slow expansion the plastic, deformable properties of the brain allow it to creep away from the mass, thereby decreasing local tissue pressure and preserving blood flow.[90] As intracranial pressure rises with autoregulation intact, vasodilatation occurs in order to maintain cerebral blood flow, thus increasing cerebral blood volume and producing further brain swelling. As this swelling becomes more severe, intracranial pressure rises to the point that maximal vasodilatation is present, vasomotor paralysis occurs, and the vessels no longer autoregulate or respond to arterial pressure or hypocapnia.[37]

Alteration or abolition of the normal responses of the cerebral vasculature contribute to the pathological effects of intracranial masses. Vascular congestion increases the mass effect and arterial vasodilatation may lead to more edema by increasing local capillary pressure. These changes increase local tissue pressure, which in turn causes intracranial structures to shift. The local tissue pressure may exceed capillary pressure, decreasing cerebral blood flow enough to cause ischemia.

Lundberg first described intracranial pressure waves in humans.[43] The B wave is a rhythmic variation related to various types of periodic breathing, with a frequency of $\frac{1}{2}$ to 2 per minute. The C waves are rhythmic variations related to the Traube-Hering-Mayer waves of the systemic blood pressure, which have a usual frequency of 6 per minute. These intracranial pressure waves are probably related to periodic fluctuations of pressure within the cerebral vascular bed. They are of low amplitude and are not harmful.

Type A waves, as originally described, have subsequently been termed *plateau waves* and are of considerable importance (Fig. 31-2). The plateau wave is an acute elevation in intracranial pressure lasting from 5 to 20 minutes followed by a rapid fall in pressure to the former resting level. The amplitude is variable but may reach very high levels (50 to 100 mmHg). Clinical signs of acute brain stem dysfunction, such as restlessness, impaired consciousness, rigidity of the limbs, and tonic-clonic movements, have been noted in conjunction with plateau waves. Lundberg noted that these waves were more prevalent in the advanced stages of in-

creased intracranial pressure. Invariably a rise in arterial blood pressure occurred concomitantly with the plateau waves. At times hypercarbia preceded the onset of plateau waves and hyperventilation usually preceded the decrease in intracranial pressure at the end of the wave. Plateau waves often occurred without visible cause but could happen coincident with bodily activity, emotional upset, or painful stimuli. Increased cerebral blood volume is thought to be related to the development of the plateau waves.

Paroxysmal increases in intracranial pressure or more sustained elevations can create pressure gradients between the intracranial compartments. Plateau waves create alarming, though temporary, neurological deterioration, which suggests transient vascular insufficiency. Plateau waves are found in intracranial hypertension, especially with parenchymal lesions, and most likely are due to episodic arterial dilatation, which promptly raises the pressure in an intracranial space that is already suffering from decreased compliance.

Symptoms and Signs of Increase Intracranial Pressure

Very high intracranial pressure can be present without symptoms or signs. Headache, which is commonly attributed to increased intracranial pressure, was not found in several studies with very high intracranial pressures as long as the pressure was diffuse, as in pseudotumor cerebri or after injection of saline experimentally into the lumbar subarachnoid space. Causes of head pain include venous dilatation, traction on the bridging veins, and stretching of the pain-sensitive meningeal and basal arteries of the brain.[94] With diffuse increased intracranial pressure there is insufficient traction on the vessels to cause headache. Patients with space-occupying lesions have headache because of invasion of pain-sensitive structures or compression or distortion of these by the mass or its attendant edema. The headache associated with increased intracranial pressure is often severest in the morning, perhaps because there is brain swelling from vascular dilatation secondary to hypercarbia during sleep. It is frequently relieved by vomiting, which probably decreases intracranial pressure by hyperventilation.[43] It may be that vomiting occurs without nausea in patients with increased intracranial pressure because of brain stem distortion.

Papilledema is the most reliable clinical sign of increased intracranial pressure. Other neurological signs generally associated with increased intracranial pressure are in fact due to brain herniation.

Incidence and Significance of Increased Intracranial Pressure

Intracranial pressure may not be elevated after head injury and a normal intracranial pressure is not necessarily a favorable prognostic sign. In compiling a large number of cases from several series, Langfitt found that about one-third of the patients had moderate to severe increase in intracranial

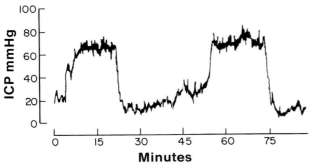

Figure 31-2 Type A or plateau waves. Typical acute elevations in intracranial pressure lasting 5 to 20 min, followed by rapid decline to resting level. Amplitudes of 50 to 100 mmHg are common.

pressure (over 30 mmHg) after head injury.[35] Patients with severe brain stem injury frequently have normal intracranial pressure but eventually die from their brain injury.

It has been found that elevated intracranial pressure is much more common in patients with space-occupying masses than those without and indeed those patients with head injury who have very high or uncontrollable intracranial pressure (over 40 mmHg) have a very poor survival rate.[51] It has been shown that early, aggressive treatment of even mild intracranial pressure elevations prevents intracranial pressure from getting out of control and reduces the number of patients suffering life-threatening events. Severely head-injured patients benefit from this early therapy, as mortality is reduced without increasing the number of those severely disabled.[72]

Cerebral blood flow is frequently decreased in those with head injury, as is cerebral metabolism.[5] Metabolic autoregulation is defective and cerebral blood flow is disconnected or unlinked from cerebral metabolism. It has been postulated that in children with head injury without a mass lesion the associated brain swelling is due to cerebrovascular dilatation rather than to cerebral edema, as on CT scan there is no decrease in density and cerebral blood flow may even be increased.[6] Although the relationships of intracranial pressure, cerebral blood flow, and outcome are not absolute after head injury, it is clear that with very high intracranial pressure cerebral blood flow decreases and mortality increases dramatically.

In brain tumor patients it has been shown that the headache, alterations in level of consciousness, and focal neurological findings are associated with increased intracranial pressure. Even with very high pressure, however, these clinical signs can be absent. Markedly increased intracranial pressure was found during sleep in these patients and plateau waves, which did not terminate spontaneously, could reach increasingly higher pressures and eventually cause coma, fixed dilated pupils, and respiratory arrest.[43]

In brain tumor patients it has been found that the prolonged plateau waves produce a rise in systemic arterial pressure. This rise in systemic blood pressure was found to produce a slight further increase in cerebral blood volume, raising the intracranial pressure further and thereby inducing a further increase in blood pressure. Eventually cerebral perfusion pressure decreased progressively as the plateau waves continued to develop and ultimately intracranial pressure reached the level of mean arterial pressure, in the form of either a succession of higher and higher plateau waves or a steady rise in intracranial pressure. This represents the state of cerebral vasomotor paralysis, and perfusion pressure could not be restored by increasing the arterial pressure or by decreasing the intracranial pressure by reducing the volume of any of the intracranial components.[37] In general, intracranial pressure monitoring has not proved necessary in brain tumor patients as the lesion is either removed or decompressed adequately to prevent harmful elevations of intracranial pressure.

When an aneurysm ruptures, there is an immediate severe rise in intracranial pressure, which then declines rapidly.[56] Cerebral blood flow decreases, as does cerebral metabolism in those patients who have suffered a subarachnoid hemorrhage.[18] It has been shown that the level of intracra-

nial pressure correlates well with the clinical grade of the patient after hemorrhage, and those with vasospasm have consistently elevated intracranial pressures.[86]

Brain Herniation

In the nineteenth century supratentorial lesions were thought to produce coma because of widespread or rapid involvement of the cortical mantle in the disease process. Cushing believed the major cause of coma in these patients to be ischemia of the medulla.[13] Transtentorial herniation of the temporal lobe was first observed in autopsy specimens,[50] and grooving of the cerebral peduncle at the edge of the tentorium[31] and displacement of the diencephalon and midbrain were noted. Spatz and Stroescu in 1934 published illustrations of the intracranial cisterns and how they were altered by various herniations.[81] The emphasis on transtentorial herniation as the cause of false localizing signs and brain stem dysfunction, previously thought to be due to herniation at the foramen magnum, was strongly advocated by Jefferson, who cited "vegetative storm," nuchal rigidity, bilateral motor signs including decerebrate rigidity, and anisocoria as important evidence of the tentorial pressure cone.[29]

The brain's ability to adjust to space-occupying masses is limited by the inelasticity of the skull, which allows only minimal expansion through the foramen magnum and smaller foramina that transmit blood vessels and nerves. The supporting dural septa (falx and tentorium), which divide the intracranial cavity into various compartments, protect the brain against excessive movement but limit the amount of compensatory shift and displacement that can develop in response to abnormal conditions.

The semioval opening of the incisura or tentorial notch measures from 50 to 70 mm in the fronto-occipital axis and 25 to 40 mm in the interparietal axis. The medial surfaces of the temporal lobe slightly overhang the tentorial incisura with the uncus protruding into the notch approximately 3 to 4 mm. The hippocampal gyrus as well as the uncus may be grooved by the medial edge of the tentorium.[74] The anterior portion of the notch is occupied by the midbrain, the posterior part by the cerebellum. The posterior cerebral artery circles around the midbrain in the cisterna ambiens within the tentorial notch. It crosses over the oculomotor nerve, coming to lie above the tentorium on the ventral surface of the hippocampal gyrus. The anterior choroidal artery runs between the dentate gyrus of the temporal lobe and the edge of the tentorium. The oculomotor nerve emerges from the midbrain to cross the interpeduncular cistern between the posterior cerebral and superior cerebellar artery, lying adjacent to the uncus, where it overhangs the tentorial edge.

The medulla, cerebellum, and vertebral arteries lie within the foramen magnum. The cerebellar tonsils protrude through the foramen and the inferior portion of the surface of the cerebellum is grooved against the foramen's posterior lip.

The hallmarks of transtentorial herniation include the dilated pupil and other oculomotor dysfunction. This may be due to direct pressure from herniating brain tissue, ischemia of the nerve or midbrain, or trapping of the nerve between the posterior cerebral and superior cerebellar arteries. Visual obscurations of an hemianopic nature or even total blindness are also well known and are ascribed to involvement of the posterior cerebral arteries or less likely involvement of the anterior choroidal artery or compression of the optic tracts. The hemiparesis seen with transtentorial herniation may be due to compression of the cerebral peduncle and when the Kernohan notch phenomenon of grooving the opposite peduncle against the tentorial edge is present, the false localizing ipsilateral hemiparesis appears. Compression of the posterior cerebral artery or anterior choroidal artery may also be a contributing factor with ischemia of the cerebral peduncle or internal capsule.

Decerebration, commonly seen in patients with supratentorial masses with herniation, is found more frequently at the peak of intracranial pressure waves[26] and has been ascribed to midbrain ischemia or distortion. The change in behavior and personality and the decrease in level of consciousness, progressing to coma, are the last of the cardinal signs of brain stem dysfunction produced by transtentorial herniation, as has been so well described by Sunderland.[82]

It may be that caudal displacement and distortion of the brain stem and possibly elongation and rupture of the paramedian arteries are directly responsible for the clinical signs.[21,25,83,90] In addition, spreading ischemia could be responsible for the orderly rostral to caudal brain stem dysfunction described by McNealy and Plum.[48]

Plum and Posner have clearly and authoritatively categorized the major supratentorial brain shifts as cingulate herniation, central transtentorial herniation, and uncal herniation (Fig. 31-3).[60] *Cingulate herniation* occurs when an expanding hemispheric mass forces the cingulate gyrus under the falx, which may displace or compress the internal cerebral vein and the anterior cerebral artery.[79]

Central transtentorial herniation results from the downward movement of the hemispheres and basal nuclei, which eventually shift the entire diencephalon and adjoining midbrain rostrocaudally through the tentorial notch.[73] The diencephalon may actually be buckled against the midbrain, and hemorrhages and edema are found within the diencephalon and paramedian region of the midbrain.[21,25,73]

Uncal herniation occurs when expanding lesions in the hemisphere push the edge of the uncus and hippocampus toward the midline over the incisural edge. The medial temporal lobe may encroach upon the midbrain and push it against the opposite tentorial edge. The third nerve and posterior cerebral artery on the side of the expanding temporal lobe may be caught by the uncus at the edge of the tentorium or the petroclinoid ligament.

One danger of herniation is that it may produce vascular obstruction, which aggravates the effects of the original expanding mass. Herniation under the falx compresses the anterior cerebral artery, accentuating the already existing ischemia and edema of the herniating hemisphere. Posterior displacement across the midline compresses the great cerebral vein, raising the pressure in the entire deep venous system. Central transtentorial and uncal herniation into the tentorial notch compresses the posterior cerebral artery, producing occipital ischemia and swelling, and the anterior choroidal artery, producing further diencephalic ischemia and swelling.

The subarachnoid cisterns and the aqueduct may be compressed as well, interfering with cerebrospinal fluid circulation.[74] This compression prevents the displacement of cerebrospinal fluid within the intracranial space by an enlarging mass. The resultant pressure increase in the supratentorial compartment will further aggravate herniation through the tentorial notch and will not be reflected in lumbar puncture pressure owing to the blockage at the incisura or aqueduct.

Tentorial herniation may produce brain stem ischemia and hemorrhage. Hemorrhage into the center of the brain stem and diencephalon occur and perforating branches of the basilar artery are stretched downward, producing paramedian ischemia, which advances down the brain stem in a rostral to caudal manner. Pathological changes in brains with supratentorial mass lesions are indicated by ischemia, vascular congestion, and edema, which spreads from the lesion at first radially and then rostrocaudally in a progressive manner.

Treatment of Increased Intracranial Pressure and Brain Herniation

Since increased intracranial pressure disturbs brain function by reducing cerebral blood flow or by brain herniation through the tentorial incisura or the foramen magnum, the goals of treatment are to reduce intracranial pressure in order to increase cerebral blood flow and relieve herniation. If the cause of increased intracranial pressure is a tumor or

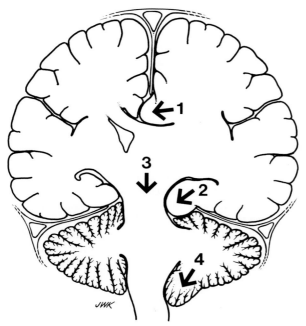

Figure 31-3 Patterns of brain herniation. (1) Cingulate herniation under the falx. (2) Uncal herniation through the tentorial incisura. (3) Central transtentorial herniation through the incisural notch. (4) Cerebellar tonsillar herniation through the foramen magnum.

mass lesion, removal or decompression is the best way of reducing intracranial pressure if the lesion is accessible. If the cause of the increased pressure is hydrocephalus, drainage of cerebrospinal fluid by intermittent or permanent drainage is the treatment of choice. If the increased pressure is due to edema or increased brain tissue fluid content, steroids and hypertonic solutions may be of value. Cerebral vascular volume can increase, producing raised intracranial pressure, and this too can be addressed via hyperventilation, positioning, and diuretics.

Increased intracranial pressure can be lowered by reducing the volume of any of the intracranial components even if that component is normal. Hypertonic solutions reduce the fluid content of normal brain, removal of CSF may be done via ventriculostomy, and hyperventilation may reduce cerebral blood volume. Unfortunately, with a defective blood-brain barrier, edema and brain swelling may not be effectively treated with hypertonic solutions. When vasomotor paralysis is present, a dilated cerebral vascular bed may not respond to hyperventilation.

The simplest and most rapid way of decreasing intracranial pressure is removal of CSF via a ventricular cannula. Hyperventilation is nearly as fast-acting when the cerebral vessels are responsive to changes in Pa_{CO_2}. Hypertonic mannitol takes somewhat longer but is relatively quick-acting.

The first step in the management of intracranial pressure is to quiet the patient, since voluntary movements or any type of straining frequently causes elevation of intracranial pressure. Tranquilization may be required and if necessary the patient may be paralyzed and artificially ventilated.

Patient positioning is also important and the head should be elevated at 20 degrees to ensure adequate venous drainage.

Hyperventilation, hypertonic solutions, and steroids are used as necessary, as described in detail in the following sections. If these measures fail, it must be kept in mind that an intracranial mass or hydrocephalus, not found on initial evaluation, could have developed. If intracranial pressure is not measured, the only criterion for judging the intracranial pressure is the clinical status of the patient, which can be quite misleading.

Hyperventilation

Hyperventilation is one of the most effective means of controlling increased intracranial pressure.[44] It achieves its effect by reducing cerebral blood flow and cerebral blood volume. Cerebral blood flow changes approximately 2 percent per mmHg change in Pa_{CO_2}.[66] In a normal patient hypercapnia produces cerebral dilatation without a rise in intracranial pressure, but when the CSF has been displaced and the vertical portion of the volume vs. pressure curve is reached, even the mildest respiratory insufficiency with hypercarbia can produce severely increased intracranial pressure. Many patients with increased intracranial pressure spontaneously hyperventilate, but when intubation is necessary, it should be done most expertly, as straining during intubation can cause a marked elevation in intracranial pressure.

Pa_{CO_2} should be reduced to 25 to 30 mmHg; if Pa_{CO_2} is reduced below 20 mmHg, the blood flow so decreases that the oxygen available to the brain is inadequate to maintain normal metabolism. Thus, the cerebral ischemia produced by increased intracranial pressure may be relieved only to be replaced by cerebral ischemia caused by cerebral vasoconstriction.[64]

When Pa_{CO_2} is reduced by hyperventilation, blood may be shunted from normal brain, where vessels are normally responsive to changes in Pa_{CO_2}, to areas of damaged brain, where vessels are already maximally dilated.[59] This phenomenon is of potential benefit since areas of ischemia would be better perfused.

Hyperventilation is not always effective in decreasing intracranial pressure.[27] Even in those patients who benefit from hyperventilation with resulting decrease in their intracranial pressure, there is no clear evidence that hyperventilation changes long-term outcome.[64]

Hyperbaric Oxygen

Hyperbaric oxygen therapy is not generally used nor is it commonly available.

The reduction of cerebral blood flow induced by increased intracranial pressure damages the brain because the supply of oxygen is insufficient to maintain normal metabolism. This ischemia may be alleviated by increasing cerebral blood flow or by increasing the oxygen content per unit volume of blood flowing through the brain. The hemoglobin in the blood is nearly fully saturated at normal atmospheric pressure. The rationale for treating with hyperbaric oxygen is to increase oxygen delivery by increasing the partial pressure of oxygen beyond 1 atm so that the volume of oxygen dissolved in plasma rises. In addition, hyperoxia lowers intracranial pressure by the same mechanism as hypocapnia, that is, vasoconstriction and reduction in cerebral blood flow.[53]

This is a rarely used and specialized area of medicine with its own set of complications. A beneficial effect of hyperbaric treatment on outcome in patients with increased intracranial pressure has not been convincingly demonstrated, perhaps because so many variables are involved in the therapy of these patients.

Hypothermia

Hypothermia has been shown to be somewhat successful in reducing increased intracranial pressure in a number of patients.[27] Cerebral blood flow and oxygen metabolism have been shown to decline with hypothermia.[69] At temperatures around 27°C cardiac arrhythmias occur, posing a problem with this type of therapy. In addition, seizures, drowsiness, coma, and hemiparesis frequently occur during rewarming, probably owing to increased intracranial pressure, increased cerebral blood volume, and cerebral edema.[1] These concerns have limited the use of this therapeutic modality.

Hypertonic Solutions

The osmolality of brain, cerebrospinal fluid, and intracranial blood is equal in normal subjects, i.e. about 300 mosmol per liter. For an agent to be effective as an osmotic diuretic it must have restricted access across the blood-brain barrier. Thus a defective blood-brain barrier limits the usefulness of hypertonic solutions since an osmotic gradient cannot be formed. An osmotic gradient must be set up to drive water from the brain to the plasma. Gradients as low as 10 mosmol per liter appear to be effective in reducing intracranial pressure. Osmotic agents have complex effects on brain metabolism as well as osmotic dehydrating effects. It has been shown that CSF formation is inhibited by hyperosmolar agents. The reduction of intracranial compliance appears to be one of the major attributes of osmotic therapy.

Gradients between brain and plasma disappear after a short period of time because the administered osmotic solute crosses the blood-brain barrier, dissipating the gradient, and adaptive responses of the brain occur with an increase of intracellular osmotically active solutes. It is essential that serum osmolality be monitored as a guide to therapy while these agents are being used. There are several theoretical reasons for the possibility of a "rebound phenomenon" with use of hypertonic agents. One is progressive entry of the osmotically active solute into the brain cells, which then draws water into those cells. Second, the solute reaches equilibrium in the CSF and disappearance from the cerebrospinal fluid is slower than from plasma. The presence of the rebound phenomenon has been questioned, and should a secondary rise in intracranial pressure occur after treatment, a search for the development of a new mass lesion should be considered.[41]

Urea

Use of hypertonic urea to treat elevated intracranial pressure was introduced by Javid in the 1950s.[28] The urea is slowly eliminated from the blood but it is not inert and does penetrate the blood-brain barrier. It rather rapidly equilibrates in the CSF and brain and thus the rebound phenomenon may occur.[34] Where the blood-brain barrier has been damaged, urea acts as do other hypertonic solutions, i.e., it is ineffective in removing water from edematous brain but instead dehydrates the normal brain tissue.[57] It has some epileptogenic properties and may be neurotoxic. Also it may produce hemoglobinuria and cause sloughing of the skin if the intravenous solution infiltrates. It has largely been replaced in clinical practice by mannitol.

Mannitol

In 1962 Wise and Chater reported the use of mannitol to treat increased intracranial pressure.[93] Mannitol is not metabolized and is excluded from the CSF and brain to a much greater degree than urea, which thus minimizes the potential for rebound. Mannitol decreases cerebrospinal fluid pressure as effectively as does urea and for longer periods of time. When 1 g mannitol per kg body weight is given over a period of 10 min, a rise in serum osmolality of approximately 20 to 30 mosmol per liter occurs, with return to control levels in about 3 h.[77] Studies with mannitol show a mean intracranial pressure reduction of 52 percent after 1 gram per kg was administered intravenously over 10 min. Maximal pressure reduction was obtained at an average of 90 min postinjection. The intracranial pressure returned to control levels about 4 h after the bolus injection.[27] Because of the possibility of rebound, the smallest effective dose should be used. Serum osmolality, electrolytes, urinary excretion, and intracranial pressure should be monitored during its use.

Mannitol almost always reduces increased intracranial pressure regardless of the cause. Marshall et al. showed that reduction of intracranial pressure with a dose of 0.25 g per kg was equal to the response obtained with doses of 0.5 to 1.0 g per kg. Considerable reductions in intracranial pressure occurred, with increases in osmolarity of as little as 10 mosmols.[46] Severe hyperosmolarity produces renal damage. Miller and Leech showed that mannitol improved compliance to a greater degree than its beneficial effect on intracranial pressure, thereby favorably influencing the slope of the volume vs. pressure relationship.[39,54] Other properties of mannitol include its ability to decrease CSF production, which might contribute significantly to its effectiveness in lowering intracranial pressure.[71] In addition the drug has been shown to possess antioxidant properties, which could theoretically provide added benefits by imparting a stabilizing effect on cell membranes.[9]

Mannitol increases cerebral blood flow and cerebral oxygen consumption in patients independently of its effects on intracranial pressure.[5,30] Therefore measuring intracranial pressure may not be an adequate guide to therapy. It is known that mannitol opens the blood-brain barrier, perhaps by dehydrating endothelial cells and thus causing separation of tight junctions.[65] If endothelial cells are swollen in areas of brain edema with increased intracranial pressure, mannitol may be effective by decreasing the cellular edema, thereby increasing capillary diameter and blood flow.[5] In addition mannitol has been shown to decrease blood viscosity, thereby enhancing tissue perfusion,[7] and it may have a benefical effect on cardiac function as well.[4]

With rapid infusion of a large dose of mannitol, plasma volume increases more rapidly than renal clearance of the additional fluid and a transient increase in cerebral blood volume and intracranial pressure is observed.[12] Mannitol has been shown experimentally to increase cerebral blood flow,[30] and hyperosmolar agents in general possess significant vasodilator properties, possibly causing increased cerebral blood volume and *increased* intracranial pressure on this basis.[33] Outside of the central nervous system the increased blood volume and loss of electrolytes associated with the obligatory osmotic diuresis can cause cardiac decompensation and arrhythmias.

Glycerol

Glycerol has been shown to reduce increased intracranial pressure; unlike mannitol, it is partially metabolized and has high caloric effects. An advantage of glycerol is that, in addition to intravenous administration, it may be given orally in doses of 0.5 to 2 g per kg body weight every 4 h[8] and it may produce less dehydration and electrolyte abnormalities than the other hypertonic agents.[88] It may be impossible to achieve a sustained decrease in intracranial pressure because osmotic equilibrium occurs, owing to leakage of glycerol into the brain and production of idiogenic osmoles.[70] There are major complications of glycerol therapy, including hemolysis, hemoglobinuria, renal failure, and hyperosmolar coma.[75, 85] Because of its sweet taste it may induce nausea and vomiting when given orally.

Furosemide

Cottrell et al. have demonstrated that furosemide decreases intracranial pressure without an initial rise as seen with mannitol, and it is effective without increasing serum osmolarity or causing hypokalemia or hyponatremia.[12] Experimentally marked reduction in cerebral edema has been found with furosemide, which has been shown to reduce CSF production as well.[84] In contrast to the osmotic agents, which are effective only where the blood-brain barrier is intact, furosemide decreases edema in the pathological areas as well, giving it a theoretical advantage.

Steroids

Glucocorticoids were introduced into neurosurgery as a treatment for brain edema in the early 1960s.[17] The mechanisms of the beneficial effects of steroids are still poorly understood. It is known that CSF production is reduced,[91] and a direct effect on endothelial cell function to restore normal permeability has also been suggested.[47] Experimental support has been increasing for neuronal membrane stabilization with steroids via an attenuation of free radical production,[3] inhibition of release of edema-producing polyunsaturated fatty acids from cellular membranes, and suppression of lysosomal activity. Free radicals may be involved in the peroxidation of membrane lipids.

The therapeutic effects of steroids on intracranial pressure appear to be secondary to their antiedema activity rather than direct effects. In addition glucocorticoids may facilitate bulk flow reabsorption through the ventricular system or improve CSF circulation where it is impaired by inflammatory changes in the subarachnoid space or at the arachnoid villi.

In 1964 French and Galicich reviewed 300 cases treated with dexamethasone and concluded that the drug was effective in the management of cerebral edema. It was found to be very safe with little in the way of fluid retention, hypertension, electrolyte abnormalities, wound healing problems, or gastrointestinal hemorrhage.[17] Dexamethasone is usually given in doses of 10 mg loading and 4 mg four times a day, which is 20 times the normal rate of endogenous cortisol production. It is most effective in the treatment of gliomas and metastatic tumors. Unfortunately it has not been shown to be consistently effective in reducing increased intracranial pressure or outcome in patients with head injury.[11] Dramatic effects of steroids have been seen in experiments in which white matter edema was produced by freezing lesions. Little change was noted in the first 24 h but thereafter reduction in edema was progressive.[58] Pretreatment was the most effective modality. In brain tumor patients reduction in intracranial pressure has been observed during steriod therapy and larger doses have proved useful where 4 mg four times daily has been ineffective.[67] Significant reduction in fluid content of both gray and white matter near tumors has been observed.

Barbiturate Coma

This therapeutic modality is discussed in the next chapter.

References

1. Bloch M: Cerebral effects of rewarming following prolonged hypothermia: Significance for the management of severe cranio-cerebral injury and acute pyrexia. Brain 90:769–784, 1967.
2. Bradley KC: Cerebrospinal fluid pressure. J Neurol Neurosurg Psychiatry 33:387–397, 1970.
3. Braughler JM, Hall ED: Correlation of methylprednisolone levels in cat spinal cord with its effects on (Na$^+$ + K$^+$)-ATPase, lipid peroxidation, and alpha motor neuron function. J Neurosurg 56:838–844, 1982.
4. Brown FD, Johns L, Jafar JJ, Crockard HA, Mullan S: Detailed monitoring of the effects of mannitol following experimental head injury. J Neurosurg 50:423–432, 1979.
5. Bruce DA, Langfitt TW, Miller JD, Schutz H, Vapalahti MP, Stanek A, Goldberg HI: Regional cerebral blood flow, intracranial pressure, and brain metabolism in comatose patients. J Neurosurg 38:131–144, 1973.
6. Bruce DA, Schut L, Bruno LA, Wood JH, Sutton LN: Outcome following severe head injuries in children. J Neurosurg 48:679–688, 1978.
7. Burke AM, Quest DO, Chien S, Cerri C: The effects of mannitol on blood viscosity. J Neurosurg 55:550–553, 1981.
8. Cantore G, Guidetti B, Virno M: Oral glycerol for the reduction of intracranial pressure. J Neurosurg 21:278–283, 1964.
9. Cederbaum AI, Dicker E, Rubin E, Cohen G: The effect of dimethylsulfoxide and other hydroxyl radical scavengers on the oxidation of ethanol by rat liver microsomes. Biochem Biophys Res Commun 78:1254–1262, 1977.
10. Chopp M, Portnoy HD: Systems analysis of intracranial pressure: Comparison with volume-pressure test and CSF-pulse amplitude analysis. J Neurosurg 53:516–527, 1980.
11. Cooper PR, Moody S, Clark WK Kirkpatrick J, Maravilla K, Gould AL, Drane W: Dexamethasone and severe head injury: A prospective double-blind study. J Neurosurg 51:307–316, 1979.
12. Cottrell JE, Robustelli A, Post K, Turndof H: Furosemide-and mannitol-induced changes in intracranial pressure and severe osmolality and electrolytes. Anesthesiology 47:28–30, 1977.
13. Cushing H: Some experimental and clinical observations concerning states of increased intracranial tension. Am J Med Sci 124:375–400, 1902.
14. Cushing H: Studies in Intracranial Physiology and Surgery. London, Oxford University Press, 1926, pp 19–23.
15. Ekström-Jodal B, Häggendal E, Johansson B, Linder LE, Nilsson NJ: Acute arterial hypertension and the blood-brain barrier: An experimental study in dogs, in Langfitt TW, McHenry LC Jr, Reivich M, Wollman H (eds): Cerebral Circulation and Metabolism. New York, Springer, 1975, pp 7–9.
16. Fitch W, McDowall DG, Keaney NP, Pickerodt VWA: Systemic vascular responses to increased intracranial pressure. J Neurol Neurosurg Psychiatry 40:843–852, 1977.
17. French LA, Galicich JH: The use of steroids for control of cerebral edema. Clin Neurosurg 10:212–223, 1964.
18. Grubb RL Jr, Raichle ME, Eichling JO, Gado MH: Effects of subarachnoid hemorrhage on cerebral blood volume, blood flow, and oxygen utilization in humans. J Neurosurg 46:446–453, 1977.
19. Hamer J, Alberti E, Hoyer S, Wiedemann K: Influence of systemic and cerebrovascular factors on the cerebrospinal fluid pulse waves. J. Neurosurg 46:36–45, 1977.
20. Harper AM: Autoregulation of cerebral blood flow: Influence

of the arterial blood pressure on the blood flow through the cerebral cortex. J Neurol Neurosurg Psychiatry 29:398–403, 1966.

21. Harper AM, Deshmukh VD, Rowan JO, Jennett WB: The influence of sympathetic nervous activity on cerebral blood flow. Arch Neurol 27:1–6, 1972.

22. Hassler O: Arterial pattern of human brainstem: Normal appearance and deformation in expanding supratentorial conditions. Neurology 17:368–375, 1967.

23. Hekmatpanah J: The sequence of alternations in the vital signs during acute experimental increased intracranial pressure. J Neurosurg 32:16–20, 1970.

24. Hoff HE, Breckenridge CG: Intrinsic mechanisms in periodic breathing. Arch Neurol Psychiatry 72:11–42, 1954.

25. Howell DA: Longitudinal brain stem compression with buckling. Arch Neurol 4:572–579, 1961.

26. Ingvar DH, Lundberg N: Paroxysmal symptoms in intracranial hypertension, studied with ventricular fluid pressure recording and electroencephalography. Brain 84:446–459, 1961.

27. James HE, Langfitt TW, Kumar VS Ghostine SY: Treatment of intracranial hypertension: Analysis of 105 consecutive, continuous recordings of intracranial pressure. Acta Neurochir (Wien) 36:189–200, 1977.

28. Javid M: Urea in intracranial surgery: A new method. J Neurosurg 18:51–57, 1961.

29. Jefferson G: The tentorial pressure cone. Arch Neurol Psychiatry 40:857–876, 1938.

30. Johnston IH, Harper AM: The effect of mannitol on cerebral blood flow: An experimental study. J Neurosurg 38:461–471, 1973.

31. Kernohan JW, Woltman HW: Incisura of the crus due to contralateral brain tumor. Arch Neurol Psychiatry 21:274–287, 1929.

32. Kogure K, Scheinberg P, Reinmuth OM, Fujishima M, Busto R: Mechanisms of cerebral vasodilatation in hypoxia. J Appl Physiol 29:223–229, 1970.

33. Krishnamurty VSR, Adams HR, Smitherman TC, Templeton GH, Willerson JT: Influence of mannitol on contractile responses of isolated perfused arteries. Am J Physiol 232:H59–H66, 1977.

34. Langfitt TW: Possible mechanisms of action of hypertonic urea in reducing intracranial pressure. Neurology 11:196–209, 1961.

35. Langfitt TW: The incidence and importance of intracranial hypertension in head injured patients, in Beks JWF, Bosch DA, Brock M (eds): *Intracranial Pressure III*. New York, Springer, 1976, pp 67–72.

36. Langfitt TW, Kassell NF: Cerebral vasodilatation produced by brain-stem stimulation: Neurogenic control vs autoregulation. Am J Physiol 215:90–97, 1968.

37. Langfitt TW, Weinstein JD, Kassell NF: Cerebral vasomotor paralysis produced by intracranial hypertension. Neurology 15:622–641, 1965.

38. Lassen NA: Cerebral blood flow and oxygen consumption in man. Physiol Rev 39:183–238, 1959.

39. Leech P, Miller JD: Intracranial volume-pressure relationships during experimental brain compression in primates: 3. Effect of mannitol and hyperventilation. J Neurol Neurosurg Psychiatry 37:1105–1111, 1974.

40. Levin AB: The use of a fiberoptic intracranial pressure monitor in clinical practice. Neurosurgery 1:266–270, 1977.

41. Levin AB, Duff TA, Javid MJ: Treatment of increased intracranial pressure: A comparison of different hyperosmotic agents and the use of thiopental. Neurosurgery 5:570–575, 1979.

42. Löfgren J, Von Essen C, Zwetnow NN: The pressure-volume curve of the cerebrospinal fluid space in dogs. Acta Neurol Scand 49:557–574, 1973.

43. Lundberg N: Continuous recording and control of ventricular fluid pressure in neurosurgical practice. Acta Psychiatr Neurol Scand [Suppl] 149:1–193, 1960.

44. Lundberg N, Kjallquist A, Bien C: Reduction of increased intracranial pressure by hyperventilation. Acta Psychiatr Neurol Scand [Suppl] 139:1–64, 1959.

45. Magnaes B: Body position and cerebrospinal fluid pressure. Part 1: Clinical studies on the effect of rapid postural changes. J Neurosurg 44:687–697, 1976.

46. Marshall LF, Smith RW, Rauscher LA, Shapiro HM: Mannitol dose requirements in brain-injured patients. J Neurosurg 48:169–172, 1978.

47. Maxwell RE, Long DM, French LA: The effects of glucosteroids on experimental cold-induced brain edema: Gross morphological alterations and vascular permeability changes. J Neurosurg 34:477–487, 1971.

48. McNealy DE, Plum F: Brainstem dysfunction with supratentorial mass lesions. Arch Neurol 7:10–32, 1962.

49. Mendelow AD, Rowan JO, Murray L, Kerr AE: A clinical comparison of subdural screw pressure measurements with ventricular pressure. J Neurosurg 58:45–50, 1983.

50. Meyer A: Herniation of the brain. Arch Neurol Psychiatry 4:387–400, 1920.

51. Miller JD, Butterworth JF, Gudeman SK, Faulkner JE, Choi SC, Selhorst JB, Harbison JW, Lutz HA, Young HF, Becker DP. Further experience in the management of severe head injury. J Neurosurg 54:289–299, 1981.

52. Miller JD, Garibi J: Intracranial volume/pressure relationships during continuous monitoring of ventricular fluid pressure, in Brock M, Dietz H (eds): *Intracranial Pressure*. Berlin, Springer, 1972, pp 270–274.

53. Miller JD, Ledingham IM: Reduction of increased intracranial pressure: Comparison between hyperbaric oxygen and hyperventilation. Arch Neurol 24:210–216, 1971.

54. Miller JD, Leech P: Effects of mannitol and steroid therapy on intracranial volume-pressure relationships in patients. J Neurosurg 42: 274–281, 1975.

55. Miller JD, Stanek A, Langfitt TW: Concepts of cerebral perfusion pressure and vascular compression during intracranial hypertension. Prog Brain Res 35:411–432, 1972.

56. Nornes H, Magnaes B: Intracranial pressure in patients with ruptured saccular aneurysm. J Neurosurg 36:537–547, 1972.

57. Pappius HA, Dayes LA: Hypertonic urea: Its effect on the distribution of water and electrolytes in normal and edematous brain tissues. Arch Neurol 13:395–402, 1965.

58. Pappius HM, McCann WP: Effects of steroids on cerebral edema in cats. Arch Neurol 20:207–216, 1969.

59. Paulson OB: Regional cerebral blood flow in apoplexy due to occlusion of the middle cerebral artery. Neurology 20:63–77, 1970.

60. Plum F, Posner JB: *The Diagnosis of Stupor and Coma*, 3d ed. Philadelphia, Davis, 1980, pp 88–101.

61. Pollock LJ, Boshes B: Cerebrospinal fluid pressure. Arch Neurol Psychiatry 36:931–974, 1936.

62. Ponte J, Purves MJ: The role of the carotid body chemoreceptors and carotid sinus baroreceptors in the control of cerebral blood vessels. J Physiol (Lond) 237:315–340, 1974.

63. Quincke H: Die Lumbalpunction des Hydrocephalus. Berl Klin Wochenschr 28:929–933, 1891.

64. Raichle ME, Plum F: Hyperventilation and cerebral blood flow. Stroke 3:566–575, 1972.

65. Rapoport SI, Hori M, Klatzo I: Testing of a hypothesis for osmotic opening of the blood-brain barrier. Am J Physiol 223:323–331, 1972.

66. Reivich M: Arterial P_{CO_2} and cerebral hemodynamics. Am J Physiol 206:25–35, 1964.

67. Renaudin J, Fewer D, Wilson CB, Boldrey EB, Calogero J, Enot, KJ: Dose dependency of Decadron in patients with partially excised brain tumors. J Neurosurg 39:302–305, 1973.

68. Rodbard S, Stone W: Pressure mechanisms induced by intracranial compression. Circulation 12:883–890, 1955.

69. Rosomoff HL, Holaday DA: Cerebral blood flow and cerebral oxygen consumption during hypothermia. Am J Physiol 179:85–88, 1954.

70. Rottenberg DA, Hurwitz BJ, Posner JB: The effect of oral glycerol on intraventricular pressure in man. Neurology 27:600–608, 1977.

71. Sahar A, Tsipstein E: Effects of mannitol and furosemide on the rate of formation of cerebrospinal fluid. Exp Neurol 60:584–591, 1978.

72. Saul TG, Ducker TB: Effect of intracranial pressure monitoring and aggressive treatment on mortality in severe head injury. J Neurosurg 56:498–503, 1982.

73. Scheinker IM: Transtentorial herniation of the brain stem: A characteristic clinicopathologic syndrome; pathogenesis of hemorrhages in the brain stem. Arch Neurol Psychiatry 53:289–298, 1945.

74. Schwarz GA, Rosner AA: Displacement and herniation of the hippocampal gyrus through the incisura tentorii. Arch Neurol Psychiatry 46:297–321, 1941.

75. Sears ES: Nonketotic hyperosmolar hyperglycemia during glycerol therapy for cerebral edema. Neurology 26:89–94, 1976.

76. Shapiro HM, Langfitt TW, Weinstein JD: Compression of cerebral vessels by intracranial hypertension: II. Morphological evidence for collapse of vessels. Acta Neurochir (Wien) 15:223–233, 1966.

77. Shenkin HA, Goluboff B, Haft H: The use of mannitol for the reduction of intracranial pressure in intracranial surgery. J Neurosurg 19:897–901, 1962.

78. Sklar FH, Elashvili I: The pressure-volume function of brain elasticity. Physiological considerations and clinical applications. J Neurosurg 47:670–679, 1977.

79. Sohn D, Levine S: Frontal lobe infarcts caused by brain herniation: Compression of anterior cerebral artery branches. Arch Pathol Lab Med 84:509–512, 1967.

80. Sokoloff L: Influence of functional activity on local cerebral glucose utilization, in Ingvar DH, Lassen NA (eds): *Brain Work: The Coupling of Function, Metabolism and Blood Flow in the Brain*. New York, Academic Press, 1975, pp 385–388.

81. Spatz H, Stroescu GJ: Zur Anatomie und Pathologie der äusseren Liquorräume des Gehirns. Nervenarzt 7:425–437, 1934.

82. Sunderland S: The tentorial notch and complications produced by herniations of the brain through that aperture. Br J Surg 45:422–438, 1958.

83. Thompson RK, Malina S: Dynamic axial brain-stem distortion as a mechanism explaining the cardiorespiratory changes in increased intracranial pressure. J Neurosurg 16:664–675, 1959.

84. Tornheim PA, McLaurin RL, Sawaya R: Effect of furosemide on experimental traumatic cerebral edema. Neurosurgery 4:48–52, 1979.

85. Tourtellotte WW, Reinglass JL, Newkirk TA: Cerebral dehydration action of glycerol: I. Historical aspects with emphasis on the toxicity and intravenous administration. Clin Pharmacol Ther 13:159–171, 1972.

86. Voldby B, Enevoldsen EM: Intracranial pressure changes following aneurysm rupture. Part I: Clinical and angiographic correlations. J Neurosurg 56:186–196, 1982.

87. Vries JK, Becker DP, Young HF: A subarachnoid screw for monitoring intracranial pressure: Technical note. J Neurosurg 39:416–419, 1973.

88. Wald SL, McLaurin RL: Oral glycerol for the treatment of traumatic intracranial hypertension. J Neurosurg 56:323–331, 1982.

89. Weed LH: Some limitations of the Monro-Kellie hypothesis. Arch Surg 18:1049–1068, 1929.

90. Weinstein JD, Langfitt TW, Bruno L, Zaren HA, Jackson JLF: Experimental study of patterns of brain distortion and ischemia produced by an intracranial mass. J Neurosurg 28:513–521, 1968.

91. Weiss MH, Nulsen FE: The effect of glucocorticoids on CSF flow in dogs. J Neurosurg 32:452–458, 1970.

92. Wilkinson HA: The intracranial pressure-monitoring cup catheter: Technical note. Neurosurgery 1:139–141, 1977.

93. Wise BL, Chater N: The value of hypertonic mannitol solution in decreasing brain mass and lowering cerebrospinal-fluid pressure. J Neurosurg 19:1038–1043, 1962.

94. Wolff HG: *Headache and Other Head Pain*. New York, Oxford, 1948.

32

Induced Barbiturate Coma

Warren Selman
Robert Spetzler
Joseph Zabramski

The first barbiturate was introduced into medicine by Fisher and von Mering in 1903. This drug and up to 50 of its analogs have seen extensive clinical use. Initially these drugs were used for their sedative and hypnotic effects and for the treatment of seizure disorders. More recently they have received attention for their role as protective agents during cerebral ischemia.

Interest in the protective effects of barbiturates during central nervous system (CNS) insults was generated by the work of Arnfred and Secher.[1] In 1962 they reported that barbiturates markedly increased the tolerance of the brain to anoxia. Since that time barbiturates have been examined for their therapeutic potential in a wide variety of cerebral insults. Although early enthusiasm for several of these applications has waned, their effectiveness as a treatment for focal cerebral ischemia has been repeatedly documented.[23,26]

Indications for Induced Barbiturate Coma

In general terms, barbiturate therapy has been utilized for brain protection from hypoxia or ischemia. The conditions responsible for the hypoxia or ischemia have included head trauma, cardiac arrest, raised intracranial pressure (ICP), and stroke. The established effect of barbiturates in increasing CNS tolerance to ischemia makes them a logical component of anesthesia in patients who are exposed to a risk of ischemia during surgery. Thus, barbiturates may be used as a component of general anesthesia in any patient in whom temporary vessel occlusion might be anticipated during surgery. Patients undergoing endarterectomy, extracranial-intracranial bypass, and intracranial aneurysm clipping and arteriovenous malformation removal are those in whom cerebral protection may be useful.

Rationale for Barbiturate Coma Therapy

Since ischemia or anoxia is a component of various CNS insults, it may be that barbiturates exert their protective effect at this level. The target of any therapeutic must be to preserve those cells which are nonfunctioning but still viable, the so-called idling neurons. Energy-requiring functions of the cell may be broadly categorized as those directed toward synaptic transmission and those directed toward membrane function. Functional disturbance is evidenced when blood flow falls below a critical level for electrical activity, while structural damage occurs only after a period of time with flow below a critical level for membrane failure.[3] Recent investigation has suggested that these flow thresholds are not absolute entities but vary with the type of ischemia, i. e., global versus focal, and are also time-dependent.[14] Astrup noted that membrane failure inevitably develops in all conditions of very severe ischemia.[2] Thus preservation of membrane function is a primary therapeutic goal. With global ischemia, membrane failure may be complete within minutes. In focal ischemia, membrane function depends on residual perfusion in the so-called ischemic penumbra. Astrup suggests that membrane failure develops only when blood flow falls below the critical level necessary to provide for the minimum energy required to sustain the sodium-potassium transport system and other activities such as calcium homeostasis.[2] Other theories invoked to explain the structural damage associated with ischemia include the generation of highly reactive compounds, formed during ischemia and recirculation, that can interact with membrane lipids.

The precise mechanism of barbiturate protection in CNS insults is not clearly defined. Several mechanisms of action have been suggested. One is a reduction of the cerebral metabolic rate of oxygen consumption. This alone is not sufficient to explain protection, however, since other anesthetics that lower the metabolic rate do not confer protection.[30] Moreover, barbiturates do not lower the metabolic rate after the attainment of an isoelectric EEG. The energy-requiring functions for cell membrane integrity must still be met. Branston et al. noted that barbiturates could not reduce the minimum blood supply required to support the sodium-potassium transport system.[4] Thus, other mechanisms of barbiturate action must be operative.

One possible mechanism is hemodynamic alterations. This is only true in cases of focal ischemia. In carefully controlled, nonhypotensive barbiturate therapy it is possible to document an increase in flow in the ischemic territory and a simultaneous decrease in flow in areas remote from the ischemic territory; thus a "reversed steal phenomenon" is produced.[4,27] While barbiturates may not alter the minimum flow requirements for structural integrity of the cell, they may provide enough increase in flow to allow viability of the marginally perfused neurons.

Barbiturates have also been characterized as having an antioxidant, or membrane sealing, effect.[9] With a decrease in blood flow or oxygen there is an accumulation of highly reactive radicals from the mitochondrial respiratory chain. These reactive molecules may initiate widespread alterations in membrane lipids with the liberation of fatty acid peroxidation products, which can further damage cell membranes and result in edema.[6] It is important to stress that local increases in tissue pressure, which may not be reflected in gross measures of ICP, may compromise local blood flow, leading to a vicious cycle of increased tissue damage.

Steen and Michenfelder have suggested that a specific anesthetic effect is necessary to explain the protective action of barbiturates.[35] Mice were made tolerant to the anesthetic effect of barbiturates, and this group and a nontolerant group were subjected to the same degree of hypoxia. Although both groups had a similar tissue level of drug, only the nontolerant anesthetized group showed evidence of brain protection. Therefore these investigators concluded that it is the specific anesthetic effect of barbiturates, not the presence of the barbiturate molecule alone as an antioxidant, that is necessary for protection.

Methodology, Monitoring, and Endpoint

Although barbiturates have been used in various experimental and clinical settings, the most controlled clinical environment is in the operating room and therefore the discussion of administration will center on this use.

Despite the established beneficial effects of barbiturates in ameliorating the deleterious consequences of focal cerebral ischemia, the apparent drawbacks of barbiturate anesthesia have previously prevented its more routine use during anesthesia for procedures with a high risk of cerebral ischemic injury. One of the major concerns of barbiturate anesthesia is cardiovascular depression. Our method of barbiturate administration is based on extensive laboratory investigation in our baboon model of middle cerebral artery occlusion, with modifications to permit practical use in the operating room. Initial experimentation in both ischemic and nonischemic primates demonstrated that the most consistent anesthetic effect with the least change in systemic arterial pressure could be achieved with continuous, as opposed to bolus, barbiturate infusion.[24]

The endpoint of barbiturate therapy is a 20- to 30-s burst suppression pattern of the EEG. This depth of anesthesia was based on several considerations. First, no further reduction of the cerebral metabolic rate of oxygen consumption would be expected below this point. Second, this would represent the maximum anesthetic effect, which has been suggested to be related to maximum protection.[24,35] Finally, this dose can be safely administered, while higher doses might lead to unnecessary cardiovascular compromise. In order to rapidly achieve and maintain the maximum anesthetic effect, it is necessary to saturate the various compartments of distribution of the lipid-soluble barbiturate. This can be most easily accomplished by a loading dose before initiation of continuous infusion.

Initial work with barbiturate protection from focal ischemia utilized preocclusion administration of barbiturate. Subsequent experimentation demonstrated that protection could still be obtained with the initiation of therapy after the onset of ischemia. There were, however, specific limitations on the timing of barbiturate therapy. In our baboon model of focal cerebral ischemia two conditions were necessary for protection.[25,28] The first was that recirculation had to be

established by 6 h. Those animals with permanent middle cerebral artery occlusion that were treated with barbiturates had more aggravated intracranial hypertension, more extensive infarction, and worse neurological scores and greater mortality than those animals not treated. In animals with recirculation, a second condition for protection was evident: barbiturate therapy initiated by ½ h after occlusion provided nearly complete protection. When barbiturate therapy was administered after 2 h, the animals did better than controls but still had significant neurological deficits. If barbiturate administration was delayed for 4 h, then the animals had earlier and more aggravated intracranial hypertension, more extensive infarction, worse neurological scores, and increased mortality when compared with controls (Figs. 32-1 and 32-2).

In the clinical setting, a thiopental infusion is started approximately 15 min before the anticipated time of vessel occlusion. A dose of 10 mg per kg is infused over an initial 10-min period.[36] The EEG is monitored and the infusion rate is titrated to maintain a burst suppression pattern of EEG activity. The infusion rate is limited by the need to prevent more than a 10 percent decrease in mean arterial pressure (MAP). The loading dose approximates a bolus infusion and loading is the most critical period for maintaining systemic arterial pressure. The highest priority is given to maintaining an adequate blood pressure. Thus in a patient with a particularly brittle vascular system, the necessity for blood pressure maintenance may prevent full suppression of the EEG. Sokoll et al. studied large-dose thiopental anesthesia in 20 patients undergoing aneurysm surgery.[31] All patients were monitored with the aid of a Swan-Ganz thermodilution cardiac output catheter. The results confirmed that thiopental causes a venous dilatation, which may be augmented by narcotic supplementation. They note, however, that even with a burst suppression EEG pattern, cardiovascular reflexes are preserved. Thus blood pressure remains stable because of the reflex interaction between cardiac output and peripheral vascular resistance, which acts to maintain a normal arterial blood pressure. These authors stated that with constant monitoring of the arterial blood pressure, the rate of thiopental administration can approach 200 mg per min. Our loading dose is, therefore, well within a safe range. In our experiments with 96 h of continuous barbiturate infusion in primates, there was no progressive decrement in either cardiac output or systemic pressure.[24] Although some authors have suggested that cardiovascular complications can be minimized by maintaining a specific blood barbiturate level, we found no level that could predict cardiovascular complications.[24] Sokoll et al. also found no correlation between blood barbiturate levels and cardiovascular parameters.[31] Moreover, in neither investigation was there a consistent correlation between the EEG pattern and blood barbiturate levels. These findings again suggest that MAP and the EEG pattern are the only parameters necessary for safely monitoring barbiturate administration.

Specific cases may, however, require more sophisticated monitoring. For example, Sokoll et al. studied the use of high-dose barbiturate anesthesia in two groups of aneurysm patients, those with early surgery and those with late surgery.[32] They noted no difference in blood pressure between the two groups, but there was a significant decrease in the

ICP RESPONSE

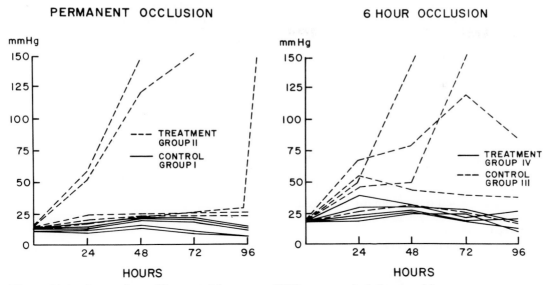

Figure 32-1 Comparison of intracranial pressure (ICP) response in baboons with permanent or temporary arterial occlusion to barbiturate therapy 0.5 h after occlusion.

cardiac index and increase in the total peripheral resistance in the late operation group. The authors thought that these differences were related to the relatively greater time of fluid restriction imposed on the late operation group. With barbiturate administration, the cardiac index decreased to the same extent in both groups, and MAP remained stable. This change is in agreement with experimental studies that indicate that barbiturates are associated with a decrease in central vasomotor activity but a preservation of baroceptor reflexes.[29] In light of these results, the authors suggest that partial volume expansion may contribute to greater safety of this anesthetic technique.

The total amount of barbiturate received and its distribution into the patient's particular body compartments will determine the rate at which clearance occurs and hence consciousness returns. Since in our regimen barbiturates are discontinued after constitution of vessel patency has occurred or the risk of occlusion has passed, brain stem responses are always present by the time the procedure is terminated. Patients often require ventilatory support for several hours postoperatively and occasionally overnight, but rarely longer. We feel that the relatively longer postoperative period during which the patient remains unconscious with barbiturates, as opposed to other anesthetic tech-

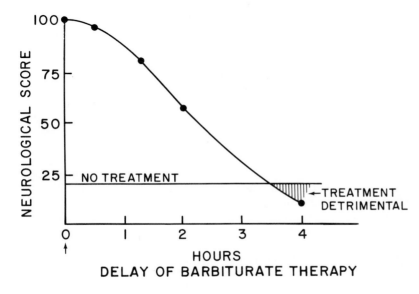

Figure 32-2 Comparison of neurological scores of baboons having temporary arterial occlusion and receiving barbiturate therapy begun at 30, 75, 120, and 240 min with those of baboons receiving no therapy.

niques, is acceptable since basic brain stem reflexes can be monitored. In critical situations ICP monitoring can provide further reassurance that there is neither a postoperative clot nor swelling.

Barbiturate Coma in Specific Situations

Intraoperative Use

Since the therapeutic window for effective barbiturate therapy is so small, its greatest use could be expected to be in situations of controlled focal ischemia, such as those encountered in the operating room. These laboratory results are well supported by clinical experience.

Hoff first reported encouraging clinical results with barbiturate administration during aneurysm surgery in which a major vessel required occlusion.[11] He reported results for seven patients, of whom three required only temporary vessel occlusion. Those three patients requiring only temporary occlusion recovered without postoperative neurological deficits. Of the four patients requiring permanent occlusion of a major intracranial vessel, three had a severe postoperative stroke. This report supports laboratory results demonstrating that revascularization is critical to prevent infarction following middle cerebral artery occlusion, and that barbiturates alone, without recirculation, are ineffective. In fact, the poor outcome of the patients with permanent vessel occlusion may have been in part a result of the treatment. As discussed previously, primates with permanent middle cerebral artery occlusion have a better prognosis without treatment than when treated with barbiturates. Barbiturates in that setting actually aggravate, rather than control, intracranial pressure changes and edema.[25]

The experience of Rockoff and his coworkers amplifies Hoff's report of the deleterious results of barbiturate therapy without revascularization.[20] This group reported four cases of intraoperative vessel occlusion treated for 5 days with barbiturate therapy. Although ICP could be maintained below 20 torr during the time of therapy, all patients died after a fatal ICP rise during withdrawal of barbiturate therapy.

The good results in Hoff's patient with temporary vessel occlusion and barbiturate therapy are supported by others. Lawner and Simeone reported a case requiring middle cerebral artery occlusion in the management of a meningioma.[17] Barbiturate administration and revascularization prevented infarction of the middle cerebral artery territory. Ditmore et al. reported good results in a case of revascularization of the middle cerebral artery under barbiturate protection in the treatment of a middle cerebral artery aneurysm.[8] We have also reported the successful treatment of three patients by barbiturate therapy and revascularization following the unanticipated occlusion of a major intracerebral vessel.[34]

The intraoperative risk from cerebral ischemia is perhaps best defined in patients who undergo temporary clipping of a cortical branch of the middle cerebral artery in a cerebral bypass procedure. There is up to a 20 percent incidence of temporary aphasia following this procedure on the dominant hemisphere. In our series, we have used barbiturate therapy in 100 bypass patients in 54 of whom the procedure was performed on the dominant hemisphere. In this group there were no postoperative neurological deficits attributable to intraoperative cerebral ischemia.

In our experience with over 300 patients operated on for extracranial-intracranial bypasses, aneurysms, arteriovenous malformations, endarterectomies, and difficult tumors by one surgeon, no ischemic deficits attributable to intraoperative temporary vessel occlusion were seen postoperatively despite several unanticipated and lengthy (up to 6 h) internal carotid, middle cerebral, and anterior cerebral artery occlusions. Furthermore, no cardiovascular complications attributable to barbiturate administration were encountered.

Thus the rationale for intraoperative barbiturate therapy is based on sound laboratory and clinical experience. For patients in whom temporary vessel occlusion is required, barbiturate therapy as an adjunct to general anesthesia can be recommended.

Strokes

Barbiturate therapy for strokes differs from the therapy for focal intraoperative ischemia in several important respects. As previously stressed, the timing of barbiturate therapy is critical. We have demonstrated in our primate model of middle cerebral artery occlusion that with the same 6-h occlusion time barbiturate therapy was protective only up to 2 h, and was actually deleterious after 4 h.[28] Another major consideration is the need to establish recirculation within 6 h. Patients with transient ischemic attacks would need to be distinguished from patients with completed strokes, a distinction which can be made only by time, in order to avoid treating those patients whose deficit is only temporary. Patients with completed strokes would also need to be differentiated with respect to etiology. Thus, patients with occlusion of a major vessel who would require a bypass procedure need to be distinguished from those suffering from temporary embolization or hypoperfusion. Whether all this evaluation could be completed in time to institute therapy during the safe therapeutic window remains to be determined. Modifications of barbiturate regimens that permit extension of the time constraints on barbiturate protection to allow time for evaluation of the extent and etiology of an ischemic event would be helpful in the clinical setting.

At present there are only anecdotal reports of the treatment of patients with focal ischemia. Rockoff, Marshall, and Shapiro reported the results of barbiturate therapy in four patients with acute strokes.[20] The cause of the strokes was intraoperative vessel occlusion without revascularization procedures. These four patients were all treated for 5 days by barbiturate therapy. Treatment was initiated immediately in two patients, after 1 h in another, and after 4 h in the final patient. During the time of barbiturate administration ICP was well controlled; however, all four died from massive cerebral edema with markedly elevated ICP following withdrawal of barbiturate therapy.

Woodcock and his colleagues reported the results of barbiturate therapy in the treatment of five patients with focal ischemia.[37] Three patients had a middle cerebral artery embolus, one had an internal carotid artery dissection, and one had middle cerebral artery spasm from an aneurysm. Barbiturates were administered as soon as possible after failure of standard measures to control ICP. Intravenous bolus doses of pentobarbital were administered (1.5 to 4.0 mg/kg per h) and modified according to ICP response and undesirable hypotension. All five patients died and ICP could be controlled in only one patient.

Global Ischemia

Interest in the protective effects of barbiturates in global ischemia is particularly relevant to the post–cardiac arrest situation. Initial pessimism, which regarded the upper limit of survival of the CNS without oxygen or blood supply to be only 5 min, is no longer supported by experimental evidence.[7] Thus, there may be time to administer therapeutics from 15 min to 1 h after a global ischemic insult.[13] This knowledge, coupled with the fact that up to 20 percent of patients surviving a cardiac arrest may have severe permanent brain damage, is a major impetus for evaluating therapeutics for global ischemia.

Safar and his colleagues have developed a primate model of global ischemia based on a neck tourniquet. They evaluated barbiturate therapy initiated 5 to 60 min after 16 min of global ischemia.[21] They were able to demonstrate a reduction of neurological deficit with 90 mg/kg of thiopental after a delay of 15 min. This protection was not evidenced with a delay of either 30 or 60 min. Larger doses of thiopental, 120 mg/kg, resulted in a lower neurological deficit score for these animals than for control monkeys when administered after a 60-min delay, but these results were not reproducible after only a 30-min delay. Although these results appear encouraging, they should be interpreted with caution for several reasons. First, these investigators also controlled for immobilization and ventilation and demonstrated that in all groups in which thiopental administration was delayed more than 15 min there was no difference in the neurological deficit scores between those receiving barbiturates and those just immobilized and ventilated. Second, animals that died were excluded from both the control and experimental groups. Third, the inconsistent protection with the barbiturate doses could not be explained. Finally, in a separate study by these authors, there was a great difference from the first study in the degree of neurological deficit in the control group, which suggests a degree of variation in the control model.

The results of barbiturate therapy for global ischemia are not in as much agreement regarding the beneficial effects as are those for focal ischemia. Steen and his coworkers examined the effect of pentobarbital loading before a global ischemic episode produced in dogs by ligation of the aorta. They reported that 30 to 45 mg/kg of pentobarbital provided no improvement in survival or neurological outcome.[36] These authors stress that many of the studies that have claimed protection after barbiturate administration in global ischemia have examined only specific variables such as cerebral vascular, metabolic, or electrical events without considering neurological function. Since many of these functions can be normal in animals with severe neurological deficit, they stressed that protection cannot truly be evaluated in models that do not assess neurological function.

The clinical application of barbiturate therapy in global ischemia is also anecdotal. Breivik, Safar, and coworkers reported on the clinical feasibility of trials of barbiturate therapy after cardiac arrest.[5] Forty cases were reported from a total of four institutions. They noted that most patients could tolerate 30 mg/kg of thiopental given rapidly intravenously. They stated that continuous ECG, MAP, and central venous pressure monitoring permitted titration of the barbiturate infusion and its discontinuance in time before the occurrence of rearrest. Although the authors note that brain damage–ameliorating effect of barbiturates could not be proved by the results of their study because comparable groups with and without therapy were not used in a randomized form, they state that several cases defy the concept of the 4- to 5-min limit of cardiac arrest with neurological recovery.

Rockoff and coworkers reported three children who suffered cardiac arrest secondary to near drowning.[20] Two patients had a documented period of anoxia not greater than 6 min, although the third child had an undocumented period of anoxia. Although ICP was initially controlled during barbiturate administration, all three patients died after removal of barbiturate therapy.

Head Injury

Since its introduction over 20 years ago, ICP monitoring has become more widely applied in the evaluation of head trauma. It has become well recognized that severe intracranial hypertension may be a component of head injury. Miller has warned, however, that the treatment of ICP must not become an end in itself.[19] He notes that the relationship between ICP and brain function is far from direct. In evaluating the effects of elevated ICP on cerebral blood flow and brain function and the expected benefit of controlling ICP, four factors need to be considered: (1) arterial pressure; (2) ICP; (3) the active component of cerebrovascular resistance that can respond to reduced perfusion pressure; (4) the passive component imposed by vasospasm, edema, and mechanical distortion. Thus reduction of ICP must be looked at in the broad range of therapeutic priorities. Despite this caveat, it should also be remembered that gross measurements of ICP may not reflect small changes at the microcirculatory level and that small reductions of ICP may improve circulation to marginally perfused neurons.

Standard regimens have been developed to counteract the increased ICP associated with head injury, including hyperventilation, CSF drainage, and osmotic diuresis. Some cases of elevated ICP have proved refractory to these standard measures. It is in this situation that barbiturates have been applied to the treatment of severe head injury. Horsley in 1936 reported the first systematic study of the effects of barbiturate anesthesia on ICP.[12] He noted that common to all barbiturates, including pentobarbital and pentothal, was the effect of lowering ICP. This effect was dependent on full narcosis and was absent with subhypnotic doses of barbital.

Marshall and colleagues initially reported the use of barbiturates for the treatment of severe head injury in 1979.[18] In a consecutive series of 100 patients, uncontrolled intracranial hypertension occurred in 25 patients. They reported that initial pentobarbital treatment reduced the ICP in 76 percent of these patients. Prolonged barbiturate administration was associated with a normalization of ICP in 52 percent. Thus, six patients were categorized as nonresponders, and five of these died while one remained vegetative. Of the 19 responders, 10 returned to productive life, 2 were moderately disabled, 2 severely disabled, 1 was vegetative, and 4 died. The authors stated that the high rate of good quality survival in a group of patients with otherwise uniform mortality indicated the usefulness of barbiturates for severe head injury.

An extension of this work was reported by Rockoff et al. These authors reported 45 patients with a Glasgow coma score scale of less than 7,[20] of whom 22 had a score of less than 4. Barbiturates were employed after the standard measures failed to reduce ICP. Pentobarbital sodium was initially administered intravenously in divided doses over a period of 10 to 20 min to a total of 3 to 5 mg/kg, followed by 1 to 2 mg/kg supplements every 1 to 2 h to maintain a mean blood pressure (BP) of 60 to 90 torr, an ICP less than 15 torr, a cerebral perfusion pressure greater than 50 torr, and a serum pentobarbital level of 2.5 to 4 mg/dl. Barbiturate therapy was withdrawn when there was a normalization of the intracranial volume-pressure response, an ICP less than 15 torr for 72 h, and a systolic BP less than 160 torr. Barbiturates were also withdrawn if there was no reduction of ICP or signs of neurological deterioration developed, or were arbitrarily withdrawn after 14 days. This group noted a mortality of 36 percent in patients with an ICP greater than 40 torr, whereas previously patients with an ICP of this magnitude all died. It must be noted, however, that this comparison is not between concurrent controls. Furthermore, more patients were declared resistant to standard therapeutic modalities and fewer patients had intracranial mass lesions than in other large series of head injuries. Thus it may well be that these patients would have done well without the addition of barbiturates.

It is also important to consider other variables that can reduce the mortality from severe head injury. Seelig et al. demonstrated a reduction in the mortality to 30 percent of comatose patients who underwent an evacuation of an acute subdural within the first 4 h, compared with 90 percent mortality in those who had surgery after 4 h.[22] Although postoperative management included standard regimens to reduce ICP and even the addition of barbiturate in some patients, the authors stress that early evacuation of clot was the only variable that influenced the reduction in mortality. This report emphasizes the fact that improvement in the management of head injury is dependent on many variables and that significant gains can be made without prematurely employing unproved therapies such as barbiturates.

Subarachnoid Hemorrhage (SAH)

It is well established that cerebral blood flow may be reduced in patients following subarachnoid hemorrhage (SAH). Ischemic lesions have been implicated as a major factor in the morbidity and mortality after SAH. ICP has been correlated with clinical grade after SAH and it is generally felt that ICP may be one important parameter determining outcome from SAH.[10] Grade III patients especially may benefit from lowering the ICP to 15 torr before surgery.[16]

Despite the theoretical advantages of barbiturates, this therapy should still be regarded as experimental in the treatment of SAH.[33] One series reported the use of barbiturates for life-threatening neurological deficits from vasospasm secondary to SAH that were refractory to other therapeutics.[15] Seven of eight patients died in this trial despite the fact that in only two patients was it not possible to control the ICP. While this trial used barbiturates only as a last resort and in addition used other therapeutics such as hypothermia, which may in itself have deleterious effects from prolonged use, the poor results should warrent caution before this therapy is applied to the treatment of SAH.

Woodcock and colleagues in another report employed barbiturate-induced coma in four patients with SAH.[37] Intravenous bolus pentobarbital was used in doses of 1.5 to 4 mg/kg per hr. The dose was modified in amount and timing according to ICP response and undesirable hypotension. Barbiturate therapy was continued for at least 12 h in all patients. Barbiturates were discontinued under three conditions: absence of ICP reduction after two consecutive doses, reappearance of increased ICP at maximum tolerated pentobarbital doses after an initial response (defined as *escape*), or 48 h or ICP less than 15 torr. With this regimen, one patient had a good ICP response and had a good recovery, being stated as ambulatory. Two other patients had no ICP response and died. The final SAH patient had escape of the ICP response and died.

Whether these statistics can be improved by earlier barbiturate administration, different barbiturate regimen, or different patient selection remains to be determined.

References

1. Arnfred I, Secher O: Anoxia and barbiturates: Tolerance to anoxia in mice influenced by barbiturates. Arch Int Pharmacodyn Ther 139:67–74, 1962.
2. Astrup J: Energy-requiring cell functions in the ischemic brain. J Neurosurg 56:482–497, 1982.
3. Astrup J, Siesjo BK, Symon L: Thresholds in cerebral ischemia—the ischemic penumbra. Stroke 12:723–725, 1981.
4. Branston NM, Hope DT, Symon L: Barbiturates in focal ischemia of primate cortex: Effects on blood flow distribution, evoked potential and extracellular potassium. Stroke 10:647–653, 1979.
5. Breivik H, Safar P, Sands P, Fabritius R, Lind B, Lust P, Mullie A, Orr M, Renck H, Snyder JV: Clinical feasibility trials of barbiturate therapy after cardiac arrest. Crit Care Med 6:228–244, 1978.
6. Butterfield JD Jr, McGraw CP: Free radical pathology. Stroke 9:443–445, 1978.
7. Cole SL, Corday E: Four-minute limit for cardiac resuscitation. JAMA 161:1454–1458, 1956.
8. Ditmore QM, Samson DS, Beyer CW: Traumatic middle cerebral artery aneurysm: Case report. Neurosurgery 6:293–296, 1980.
9. Flamm ES, Demopoulus HB, Seligman ML, Ransohoff J: Possible molecular mechanisms of barbiturate-mediated protection in regional cerebral ischemia. Acta Neurol Scand [Suppl] 64:150–151, 1977.
10. Hase U, Reulen HJ, Fenske A, Schürmann K: Intracranial pressure and pressure volume relation in patients with subarachnoid haemorrhage (SAH). Acta Neurochir (Wien) 44:69–80, 1978.
11. Hoff JT, Pitts LH, Spetzler R, Wilson CB: Barbiturates for

protection from cerebral ischemia in aneurysm surgery. Acta Neurol Scand [Suppl] 64:158–159, 1977.

12. Horsley JS: The intracranial pressure during barbital narcosis. Lancet 1:141–143, 1937.

13. Hossmann KA, Kleihues P: Reversibility of ischemic brain damage. Arch Neurol 29:375–384, 1973.

14. Jones TH, Morawetz RB, Crowell RM, Marcoux FW, FitzGibbon SJ, DeGirolami U, Ojemann RG: Thresholds of focal cerebral ischemia in awake monkeys. J Neurosurg 54:773–782, 1981.

15. Kassell NF, Drake CG, Peerless SJ, Adams HP, Gross CE: Cerebral vasospasm: Treatment with barbiturate coma. (Abstr.) Stroke 10:104, 1979.

16. Klafta LA Jr, Hamby WB: Significance of cerebrospinal fluid pressure in determining time for repair of intracranial aneurysms. J Neurosurg 31:217–219, 1969.

17. Lawner PM, Simeone FA: Treatment of intraoperative middle cerebral artery occlusion with pentobarbital and extracranial-intracranial bypass: Case report. J Neurosurg 51:710–712, 1979.

18. Marshall LF, Smith RW, Shapiro HM: The outcome with aggressive treatment in severe head injuries. Part II: Acute and chronic barbiturate administration in the management of head injury. J Neurosurg 50:26–30, 1979.

19. Miller JD: Barbiturates and raised intracranial pressure. Ann Neurol 6:189–193, 1979.

20. Rockoff MA, Marshall LF, Shapiro HM: High-dose barbiturate therapy in humans: A clinical review of 60 patients. Ann Neurol 6:194–199, 1979.

21. Safar P, Bleyaert A, Nemoto EM, Moossy J, Snyder JV: Resuscitation after global brain ischemia-anoxia. Crit Care Med 6:215–227, 1978.

22. Seelig JM, Becker DP, Miller JD, Greenberg RP, Ward JD, Choi SC: Traumatic acute subdural hematoma: Major mortality reduction in comatose patients treated within four hours. N Engl J Med 304:1511–1518, 1981.

23. Selman WR, Spetzler RF: Therapeutics for focal cerebral ischemia. Neurosurgery 6:446–452, 1980.

24. Selman WR, Spetzler RF, Anton AH, Crumrine RC: Management of prolonged therapeutic barbiturate coma. Surg Neurol 15:9–10, 1981.

25. Selman WR, Spetzler RF, Roessmann UR, Rosenblatt JI, Crumrine RC: Barbiturate-induced coma therapy for focal cerebral ischemia: Effect after temporary and permanent MCA occlusion. J Neurosurg 55:220–226, 1981.

26. Selman WR, Spetzler RF, Roski RA: Barbiturate resuscitation from focal cerebral ischemia: A review. Resuscitation 9:189–196, 1981.

27. Selman WR, Spetzler RF, Roski RA, Crumrine RC: Regional cerebral blood flow following middle cerebral artery occlusion and barbiturate therapy in baboons. J Cereb Blood Flow Metab 1 (Suppl 1):214–215, 1981.

28. Selman WR, Spetzler RF, Roski RA, Roessmann U, Crumrine R, Macko R: Barbiturate coma in focal cerebral ischemia: Relationship of protection to timing of therapy. J Neurosurg 56:685–690, 1982.

29. Skovsted P, Price ML, Price HL: The effects of short acting barbiturates on arterial pressure, preganglionic sympathetic activity and barostatic reflexes. Anesthesiology 33:10–18, 1970.

30. Smith AL, Marque JJ: Anesthetics and cerebral edema. Anesthesiology 45:64–72, 1976.

31. Sokoll MD, Kassell NF, Davies LR: Large dose thiopental anesthesia for intracranial aneurysm surgery. Neurosurgery 10:555–562, 1982.

32. Sokoll MD, Kassell NF, Gergis SD: Hemodynamic effects of N_2O, O_2, barbiturate anesthesia and induced hypotension in early versus late aneurysm clipping. Neurosurgery 11:352–355, 1982.

33. Spetzler RF, Selman WR: Barbiturate-induced coma for the treatment of subarachnoid hemorrhage, in Hopkins LN, Long DM (eds): Clinical Management of Intracranial Aneurysms. New York, Raven Press, 1982, pp 155–160.

34. Spetzler RF, Selman WR, Roski RA, Bonstelle C: Cerebral revascularization during barbiturate coma in primates and humans. Surg Neurol 17:111–115, 1982.

35. Steen PA, Michenfelder JD: Barbiturate protection in tolerant and nontolerant hypoxic mice. Anesthesiology 50:404–408, 1979.

36. Steen PA, Milde JH, Michenfelder JD: No barbiturate protection in a dog model of complete cerebral ischemia. Ann Neurol 5:343–349, 1979.

37. Woodcock J, Ropper AH, Kennedy SK: High dose barbiturates in nontraumatic brain swelling: ICP reduction and effect on outcome. Stroke 13:785–787, 1982.

33

Pseudotumor Cerebri

Frederick H. Sklar

Patients with pseudotumor cerebri have intracranial hypertension unrelated to tumor, hydrocephalus, or frank brain edema. Unfortunately, the term has been used to describe patients with a potpourri of clinical conditions. Unrelated disease mechanisms may share similar clinical presentations. Accordingly, pseudotumor cerebri likely represents multiple and different disease entities. This nonspecificity of pathophysiology has most certainly been a major contributing factor to confusion and controversy associated with this topic.

Moreover, pseudotumor cerebri is a diagnosis of exclusion; routine neuroradiological and laboratory tests serve to eliminate other diagnostic possibilities. For example, brain tumors can be identified with computed tomographic (CT) scans, arteriograms, nuclear brain scans, cytological evaluation of the cerebrospinal fluid (CSF), etc. In contrast, there is no single positive test result that would lead the clinician to a diagnosis of pseudotumor cerebri. Instead, a series of diagnostic negatives is required to make this diagnosis.

In most instances, the condition is self-limited, and there are no neurologic sequelae. However, there are occasional patients who suffer severe visual impairment. For these patients the often used term *benign intracranial hypertension* is a misnomer.

Pseudotumor cerebri occurs in both children and adults. There is likely an infantile presentation as well. From a management standpoint the therapeutic approaches of the clinician are different for each group, as are the prognostic considerations.

Clinical Manifestations

In children and adults pseudotumor cerebri presents with symptoms and signs of intracranial hypertension. Headaches, nausea and vomiting, dizziness, and visual dysfunction are common presenting symptoms. In children, diplopia is a frequent presenting symptom whereas visual obscurations rarely occur. The reverse is the rule for adult patients with pseudotumor cerebri, in whom transient visual disturbances such as brief obscurations, blurred vision, or sensations of looking through a gray film occur with frequency. On the other hand, infants rarely have symptoms at

all but present with a rapidly growing head, split sutures, and a tense fontanelle.

Aside from papilledema, the general and neurological examinations may be unremarkable. Lateralizing and focal neurological signs are not characteristic of the syndrome, although transient peripheral facial paralysis coincident with the onset of symptoms of intracranial hypertension has been reported in children. Children frequently show cranial nerve dysfunction as a secondary sign of the intracranial hypertension, and this is occasionally also seen in the adult population.

Unlike other conditions characterized by raised intracranial pressure, the absence of severe brain dysfunction is the rule in pseudotumor cerebri. These patients show no alteration in level of consciousness despite the presence of significant intracranial pressure (ICP) elevations.

Patient Population

The adult group is comprised mostly of women although the syndrome occasionally occurs in men. Most patients are obese, and disease activity may vary with the individual's weight status. The onset of symptoms can relate temporally to other disease processes, surgical procedures, administration and withdrawal of various drugs and medications, and dietary considerations. These associated conditions are listed in Table 33-1 and will be considered subsequently. But patients with identifiable factors of etiologic importance are in the distinct minority. In most patients no predisposing mechanism can be found and the syndrome must be considered idiopathic.

On the other hand, there is no apparent female predomi-

TABLE 33-1 Clinical Conditions and Factors Associated with Pseudotumor Cerebri

Hematological disorders
  Iron deficiency anemia
  Pernicious anemia
  Polycythemia vera
  Thrombocytopenia
Endocrine conditions and disorders
  Addison's disease
  Menstrual irregularities; menstrual cycle
  Pregnancy
Medical/surgical conditions with impaired cerebral venous drainage
  Otitis media, mastoiditis
  Idiopathic dural sinus thrombosis
  Radical neck surgery
  Chronic pulmonary disease with venous hypertension
  Heart failure with venous hypertension
  Congenital heart disease
Dietary considerations
  Hypervitaminosis A
  Hypovitaminosis A
  Obesity
Common drugs
  Systemic steroid withdrawal
  Topical steroid withdrawal (infants)
  Oral contraceptives
  Tetracycline
  Nitrofurantoin
  Sulfamethoxazole

nance in children. Many are obese. The association of a predisposing medical condition may occur with greater frequency than in the adult group, but patients with identifiable etiologies remain in the minority.

In infants there may actually be a male predominance. It is this group of patients to which the term benign intracranial hypertension best applies. These patients come to medical attention for evaluation of rapid head growth, split sutures, and a full fontanelle. These infants have normal developmental milestones and are generally asymptomatic of the raised intracranial pressure. Predisposing conditions are unusual, although topical steroid withdrawal has been reported.

Clinical Course

In many patients, children and adults, pseudotumor cerebri is a self-limited process, resolving without neurological residua. These patients seem to respond to the simplest of therapeutic measures. Rarely do visual obscurations play a prominent role in symptomatology.

In other patients symptoms may persist on a more chronic basis, and visual disturbances are more common. Approximately 10 percent of adult pseudotumor patients are left with permanent visual impairment. Accordingly, it is generally held that frequently recurring visual obscurations, prolonged attacks of blurred vision, and persistent problems with focusing necessitate aggressive therapeutic measures to forestall permanent visual damage. Nearly all patients with active disease show blind spot enlargement on visual field testing,[15,20] and these blind spot abnormalities seem to respond rapidly to therapeutic maneuvers.[9] On the other hand, in a retrospective analysis of 63 adult patients, Rush could find no clinical features that might serve to distinguish those patients who developed permanent visual damage from the rest of the group.[15] Obviously, visual prognosis is of primary consideration in the treatment of pseudotumor cerebri[3], and therapy is geared to this single factor.

In various series the recurrence rate ranges from 9 to 43 percent. Moreover, in another substantial group of patients the persistence or recurrence of asymptomatic intracranial hypertension also occurs. These data and observations speak against the self-limited nature of pseudotumor cerebri and lend support to the concept that the syndrome may encompass multiple clinical entities.

Associated Medical Disorders

In the minority of patients there appears to be an association between the occurrence of pseudotumor cerebri and systemic disorders, drug regimens, and dietary considerations. An abbreviated summary is listed in Table 33-1.

It is tempting to examine the list for clues to the pathophysiology of this symptom complex. The typical patient is an obese female. Frequently her symptomatology varies with her menstrual cycle. Pseudotumor occurs during pregnancy and has been related to taking oral contraceptives. Steroid withdrawal can cause pseudotumor cerebri. The syndrome occurs in addisonian patients, and in this group symptoms respond to steroid replacement. It would there-

fore be attractive to suggest an underlying hormonal mechanism but extensive endocrinological profiles in nonaddisonian patients have failed to demonstrate any abnormalities.

Pathophysiology

Evidence for primary involvement of the cerebrovascular bed, the brain parenchyma, and the CSF compartment can be found in the literature. Dandy hypothesized that the intracranial hypertension is secondary to vascular engorgement and impaired vasomotor control.[4] He observed that patients with subtemporal decompressions for pseudotumor show rapid variations in brain bulk, as indicated by the fullness of the decompression. Dandy noted that emotional stimulation could cause the decompression to become very tense over a brief time period. Indeed, isotope clearance techniques to measure regional cerebral blood flow and transit times document increased cerebral blood volume in patients with pseudotumor cerebri.[12,13]

On the other hand, Sahs and Joynt reported light microscopic evidence of brain edema in needle biopsy specimens from patients with pseudotumor cerebri.[16] A brain edema mechanism may fit with the more recent observations on the role vasopressin may play in conditions characterized by intracranial hypertension, and these studies will be considered in brief.

Hammer et al. reported elevated CSF vasopressin levels in patients with benign intracranial hypertension when compared with a group of normal controls.[8] Moreover, CSF vasopressin levels are generally lower than serum levels but this relationship appears to be reversed in pseudotumor cerebri. It seems possible, however, that these vasopressin abnormalities may be secondary to the intracranial hypertension and not the cause of the ICP elevations. Increases in serum vasopressin concentration have been documented in animals with acute ICP elevations.[7,14] Dóczi et al. have documented increased brain water content with intraventricular administration of vasopressin in rats.[6] These observations may indeed suggest a possible hormonal basis for the symptom complex.

CSF absorptive defects have been reported in patients with pseudotumor cerebri. Constant rate infusions are abnormal in these patients.[2,11] Absorptive defects have also been suggested by the data of variable rate lumbar infusions.[17] Isotope cisternography is abnormal in some patients and the clearance of tracer from over the brain convexities is significantly delayed, which is consistent with a problem in CSF absorption.[1,10]

It seems attractive to speculate why pseudotumor patients with impressive levels of intracranial hypertension remain clinically well. Aside from visual disturbances, neurological sequelae are uncommon. On the other hand, patients with the same degree of intracranial hypertension from hydrocephalus are typically very ill, frequently presenting with alterations in the level of consciousness. Differences in the pressure-volume relationship of brain elasticity may account for this apparent paradox.

It is a feature of physiology that the intracranial pulse pressure increases proportionally with the level of intracranial pressure. Adverse symptomatology may relate more to pulse pressure augmentation than to the actual level of pressure. Pseudotumor patients tend to have lower pulse pressures at a given level of intracranial pressure than do their counterparts with hydrocephalus.[18] Graded neck compression in dogs appears to be an acute laboratory model of pseudotumor cerebri. These animals develop intracranial hypertension and show the typical CSF absorptive defects characteristic of pseudotumor patients (Nichols J, Linder M, Sklar FH: unpublished observations). In this model pathological augmentation of pulse pressure under conditions of intracranial hypertension is not observed. Instead, pulse pressure reductions are the rule. It may be that patients with pseudotumor cerebri have lowered intracranial pulse pressures and therefore enjoy some neurological protection. Moreover, craniectomy reduces intracranial pulsations,[19] and this may explain why subtemporal decompression is occasionally effective in the treatment of pseudotumor. Obviously, further work is necessary to define how pulse pressure changes and the pressure-volume relationship relate to the symptom complex of pseudotumor cerebri.

Diagnosis and Treatment

The diagnosis of pseudotumor cerebri is one of exclusion. Brain tumors, hydrocephalus, and non-neoplastic space-occupying lesions are apparent on CT scans. Plain skull x-rays may suggest mastoid disease, which may have caused transverse sinus thrombosis. Although such an observation would warrant aggressive otolaryngologic management of the mastoid problem, arteriography is rarely indicated. Demonstration of the thrombosed sinus by arteriography is not required nor is direct surgical attack on the venous sinus. Eventually the sinus will recanalize without surgical interference. Spinal puncture provides a single pressure measurement and allows for laboratory evaluation of the CSF.

A complete ophthalmologic evaluation with careful perimetry testing and documentation of the size of the blind spot is indicated. Because the visual system is primarily at risk with this disease, ophthalmologic assessments must be repeated with frequency throughout therapy.

The infant with macrocephaly, a bulging fontanelle, and few if any symptoms of intracranial hypertension requires a CT scan to exclude space-occupying lesions and hydrocephalus. These children with the infantile form of pseudotumor cerebri typically have generously sized ventricles with enlarged fluid spaces over the surface of the brain. Their development is usually on the mark. The condition is typically self-limited and warrants no therapeutic intervention other than clinical follow-ups.

Therapeutic Considerations

Patients with intracranial hypertension induced by various drugs generally improve with discontinuance of the medication. Symptomatology associated with tetracycline, nitrofurantoin, or sulfamethoxazole usage or with hypervitaminosis-

A warrant discontinuation of the respective drug. Pseudotumor symptoms associated with steroid withdrawal may not necessarily respond to subsequent steroid administration, but this therapeutic tack should be tried. Obviously, when there is an associated underlying medical, hematologic, or endocrinologic disorder, treatment must also be directed to the concurrent systemic disease. For instance, patients with Addison's disease improve with steroid replacement. Pseudotumor cerebri associated with mastoiditis, otitis media, and secondary venous sinus thrombosis requires antibiotic therapy and aggressive otolaryngologic management of the mastoid infection. Classically, mastoidectomy is considered.

The patient with idiopathic pseudotumor cerebri requires aggressive medical management. In general, the symptomatology responds to medication alone. In this clinic, furosemide is the drug of first choice. Doses of 160 mg per day in adults are used, and the dosage is adjusted according to symptomatology and the visual examination, not according to the pressure as measured by lumbar puncture. The object is to halt visual symptomatology, relieve the headache, and avoid progressive visual deterioration as indicated by acuity, perimetry, and blind spot measurements. If symptomatology persists or visual deterioration occurs, the furosemide dosage is doubled. Clinical improvement would warrant halving the daily dose after several weeks of satisfactory progress. Dexamethasone at doses of 12 mg per day is additionally added in the few cases resistant to the 320 mg furosemide regimen.

The pharmacologic management of pseudotumor cerebri is directed at reducing intracranial pressure. The various diuretics such as furosemide and acetazolamide are thought to work by inhibiting CSF production. Dexamethasone may work by a similar mechanism, but the site of drug action may relate also to the drug's favorable effect on vasogenic edema and the blood-brain barrier. Although efforts are directed at reducing intracranial hypertension, it is clinically impractical to use pressure measurements obtained from either a lumbar puncture or an implanted monitoring device to help make management decisions. Frequently, the pressure does not come down despite a remarkable clinical or visual improvement. To modify therapy or abandon medical management entirely for a surgical procedure would be inappropriate. Similarly, asymptomatic pseudotumor patients off all medications occasionally have high pressures. These patients require careful follow-up of their visual examinations but should not otherwise be treated.

Serial lumbar punctures with CSF drainage have been advocated for the treatment of pseudotumor cerebri. In some patients this simple procedure is indeed effective. This therapeutic maneuver is worthy of clinical trial in the patient who cannot be controlled on medication alone.

Surgical management is reserved for the rare patient in whom medical management has failed. Persistent symptomatology or progressive visual deterioration warrants surgical intervention. Lumboperitoneal CSF shunting and subtemporal decompression are effective procedures done for patients with pseudotumor cerebri resistant to medical management. Each will be considered.

Lumboperitoneal shunts treat the intracranial hypertension. The patients are frequently obese, which makes the surgery difficult. Some shunt systems can be placed with percutaneous techniques but an effective valve mechanism must be used or the patient will complain of headache related to intracranial hypotension. Commercial valve systems are available specifically for lumboperitoneal shunts; some drain at two different pressures according to whether the patient is erect or supine. Occasionally patients will complain of sciatica, presumably related to nerve root irritation by the subarachnoid catheter. Usually this problem eventually requires removal of the shunt since conservative measures are frequently ineffective.

Subtemporal decompressions were advocated by Dandy to treat the symptom complex of pseudotumor cerebri.[4] This procedure is indeed effective in controlling the symptoms in some patients. It is attractive to postulate a pulse pressure damping effect as the underlying mechanism of action. The procedure is usually done bilaterally, although unilateral craniectomy can occasionally suffice. A silver dollar–sized bony defect is created beneath the temporalis muscle, extending down to the floor of the middle fossa. The dura is opened widely, and the brain is covered with absorbable gelatin sponge. The temporalis muscle and fascia are reapproximated in a watertight fashion. The patients are at risk for postoperative seizures and require anticonvulsant coverage.

Decompression of the optic nerve sheath has also been used in the treatment of pseudotumor cerebri.[5] The nerve sheath is incised in the orbit, and CSF is generally visualized as escaping. The procedure is reported to correct the visual disturbances, even those of the unoperated eye. Experience has shown a favorable effect on headache symptomatology as well. Escape of CSF into the orbit has been hypothesized as the mechanism of action for the effectiveness of this procedure. Certainly the orbit cannot accommodate large volumes of fluid, and this mechanism seems unlikely. Pulse pressure damping may play a role. Optic nerve decompression should be considered seriously in the rare patient with visual complaints but no headache symptomatology in whom medical therapy has failed.

References

1. Bercaw BL, Greer M: Transport of intrathecal ^{131}I RISA in benign intracranial hypertension. Neurology (Minneap) 20:787–790, 1970.
2. Calabrese VP, Selhorst JB, Harbison JW: Cerebrospinal fluid infusion test in pseudotumor cerebri. (Abstr.) Ann Neurol 4:173, 1978.
3. Corbett JJ, Savino PJ, Thompson HS, Kansu T, Schatz NJ, Orr LS, Hopson D: Visual loss in pseudotumor cerebri. Arch Neurol 39:461–474, 1982.
4. Dandy WE: Intracranial pressure without brain tumor: Diagnosis and treatment. Ann Surg 106:492–513, 1937.
5. Davies G, Zilkha KJ: Decompression of the optic nerve in benign intracranial hypertension. Trans Ophthalmol Soc UK 96:427–429, 1976.
6. Dóczi T, Szerdahelyi P, Gulya K, Kiss J: Brain water accumulation after the central administration of vasopressin. Neurosurgery 11:402–407, 1982.
7. Gaufin L, Skowsky WR, Goodmann SJ: Release of antidiuretic hormone during mass-induced elevation of intracranial pressure. J Neurosurg 46:627–637, 1977.
8. Hammer M, Sorensen PS, Gjerris F, Larsen K: Vasopressin in the cerebrospinal fluid of patients with normal pressure hydrocephalus and benign intracranial hypertension. Acta Endocrinol (Copenh) 100:211–215, 1982.
9. Jefferson A, Clark J: Treatment of benign intracranial hypertension by dehydrating agents with particular reference to the measurement of the blind spot areas as a means of recording improvement. J Neurol Neurosurg Psychiatry 39:627–639, 1976.
10. Johnston I, Paterson A: Benign intracranial hypertension: II. CSF pressure and circulation. Brain 97:301–312, 1974.
11. Martins AN: Resistance to drainage of cerebrospinal fluid: Clinical measurements and significance. J Neurol Neurosurg Psychiatry 36:313–318, 1973.
12. Mathew NT, Meyer JS, Ott EO: Increased cerebral blood volume in benign intracranial hypertension. Neurology (Minneap) 25:646–649, 1975.
13. Raichle ME, Grubb RL, Jr, Phelps ME, Gado MH, Caronna JJ: Cerebral hemodynamics and metabolism in pseudotumor cerebri. Ann Neurol 4:104–111, 1978.
14. Rap ZM, Chwalbińska-Moneta J: Vasopressin concentration in the blood during acute short-term intracranial hypertension in cats. Adv Neurol 20:381–388, 1978.
15. Rush JA: Pseudotumor cerebri: Clinical profile and visual outcome in 63 patients. Mayo Clin Proc 55:541–546, 1980.
16. Sahs AL, Joynt RJ: Brain swelling of unknown cause. Neurology (Minneap) 6:791–803, 1956.
17. Sklar FH, Beyer CW Jr, Ramanathan M, Cooper PR, Clark WK: Cerebrospinal fluid dynamics in patients with pseudotumor cerebri. Neurosurgery 5:208–216, 1979.
18. Sklar FH, Diehl JT, Beyer CW Jr, Clark WK: Brain elasticity changes with ventriculomegaly. J Neurosurg 53:173–179, 1980.
19. Sklar FH, Linder M, Johnston RA: The effect of craniectomy on the intracranial pressure-volume relationship and its relevance to the syndrome of shunt dependent ventricles. In press.
20. Weisberg LA: Benign intracranial hypertension. Medicine (Baltimore) 54:197–207, 1975.

34

Neurourology

George D. Webster
Jorge L. Lockhart

Neurourology is a relatively new science concerned mainly with the urinary and sexual difficulties resulting from neurological disease. It is a multidisciplinary endeavor drawing on the expertise of basic scientists (physiologists, pharmacologists, biochemists, engineers) as well as clinicians (urologists, neurologists, neurosurgeons, gynecologists, psychiatrists, pathologists). Because of this interdisciplinary origin the practicalities of neurourology have often escaped the clinician, and in this chapter we will attempt to gel current theoretical and practical concepts in an interpretable fashion.

The Neurophysiology of Micturition and Male Sexual Function

The neurophysiology of the vesicourethral unit is an evolving subject, many of the details of which remain unclear. Necessarily our abbreviated discussion must be simplistic, and the interested reader is referred to the well-referenced overview by Wein and Raezer.[21]

Central Nervous System Control of Micturition

Bradley et al. contend that micturition is controlled by a center in the pontomesencephalic portion of the brain stem and not in the sacral cord.[4] They have grouped neuronal input to this center from other parts of the central nervous system into four distinct neuroanatomical loops or circuits, and have suggested that the functional integration of these loops provides for coordinated detrusor-sphincter function during urine storage and evacuation.

Loop I

This consists of pathways between the frontal cortex, basal ganglia, thalamic nuclei, and cerebellum and the pontomesencephalic reticular formation. These are predominantly inhibitory pathways, and their interruption produces partial or complete loss of volitional control of the micturition reflex, resulting in uninhibited detrusor function. This loop is interrupted in cerebrovascular accident, brain tumor, head injury, multiple sclerosis, Parkinson's disease, etc.

Loop II

This pathway comprises sensory afferent neurons from the detrusor muscle traveling up the spinal cord in the posterior and lateral columns, "long routing" to the brain stem micturition center. Efferent neurons from this center travel down the spinal cord in the reticulospinal tracts, similarly "long routing" without synapse in the spinal cord area. Integrity of this loop is necessary in order to establish a detrusor reflex of adequate magnitude and duration to accomplish complete bladder emptying. Its partial interruption produces a low-threshold detrusor reflex (a hyper-reflexic detrusor) that will also be inadequate and poorly sustained, with resultant inefficient voiding. Its complete interruption causes detrusor hyper-reflexia after an initial period of spinal shock, and the patient is unable to generate a voluntary voiding contraction. Clinical situations in which such interruptions occur include spinal cord trauma, multiple sclerosis, spinal cord tumor, and arachnoiditis.

Loop III

This comprises the detrusor and pudendal motor nuclei and their interneurons in the sacral cord. They provide for coordination between detrusor contraction and striated urethral sphincter relaxation during voiding.

Loop IV

Neurons in this circuit take origin in the motor cortex of the frontal lobes and traverse the pyramidal tracts in the lateral columns of the spinal cord, synapsing on the pudendal sphincter nucleus. This circuit provides voluntary control over the striated muscle of the urethral sphincter during bladder storage and voiding.

Peripheral Innervation of the Lower Urinary Tract

The hypogastric and pelvic nerves supply the bladder and urethra with sympathetic and parasympathetic efferent innervation, respectively. They also conduct sensory afferent nerves to the spinal cord. The extrinsic component of the striated sphincter receives somatic innervation via the pudendal nerve.

The parasympathetic efferent nerves arise from sacral spinal cord segments S2, S3, and S4 and travel in the pelvic nerves to synapse on ganglia in the vesical plexus around the urethrovesical junction and also on ganglia within the interstices of the detrusor muscle. These ganglia are the final common pathways for integration of motor impulses in the lower urinary tract. Some respond exclusively to parasympathetic innervation, some are exclusively sympathetic, and a third group will respond to stimulation by either autonomic input. Neuronal transmission at this level utilizes acetylcholine. The sympathetic nervous supply originates at the T11 to L2 level of the spinal cord, and traverses the sympathetic ganglion chain and hypogastric nerves en route to the bladder and urethra.

Sensory afferent nerves from the bladder conducting proprioceptive (fullness) and enteroceptive (thermal, tactile, and pain) impulses are carried by both the pelvic and hypogastric nerves to the spinal cord where some will synapse on the pudendal nuclei. Enteroceptive afferents travel in the contralateral spinothalamic tract to the thalamus and ultimately to the sensory cortex, and proprioceptive afferents ascend in the posterior columns to the pontomesencephalic reticular formation and thence to the thalamus and sensory cortex.

Interruption of the peripheral nerve supply to the bladder and urethra may result from a variety of lesions. Trauma due to extensive pelvic surgery (such as abdominoperineal resection for carcinoma of the rectum and radical hysterectomy) is a frequent cause. Autonomic neuropathy may result from diabetes, other metabolic lesions, infectious agents, and toxins including alcohol and heavy metals. Herpes zoster, sacral agenesis, and cauda equina tumor and injury also may interrupt the peripheral innervation.

The Intrinsic Innervation of the Vesicourethral Unit

Within the detrusor a single nerve innervates a number of muscle cells, excitation spreading to adjacent muscle cells by low-resistance extrasynaptic pathways, thereby producing a coordinated contraction of the entire detrusor muscle. Cholinergic and adrenergic nerves ramify in the adventitia of the organ, mainly in association with blood vessels. Cholinergic receptors at the termination of the postganglionic parasympathetic fibers predominate in the body of the bladder, and they mediate a contractile response. The sympathetic innervation of the bladder and urethra is mediated by both alpha-adrenergic receptors (producing contraction) and beta-adrenergic receptors (producing relaxation). There is a regional distribution of these receptors, with a predominance of beta receptors in the body of the bladder and alpha receptors in the bladder base and proximal urethra. The differing effects of alpha and beta activity on the bladder and urethral musculature and the regional distribution of these receptors allows for the pharmacologic manipulation of detrusor and sphincter function.[2]

The Neuromechanics of Lower Urinary Tract Function

The lower urinary tract basically serves two functions, those of urine storage and urine expulsion. Storage requires that the bladder accommodate increasing volumes of urine at low intravesical pressure, that there be no inappropriate (uninhibited) bladder contractions until voiding occurs, and that the bladder outlet be closed and functionally competent. During urine expulsion a bladder contraction of adequate magnitude must be established together with coordinated relaxation of both proximal and distal sphincter mechanisms.

During the storage phase as filling progresses, bladder wall tension and volume receptor stimulation occurs and afferent impulses carried by the pelvic and hypogastric nerves are routed to the spinal and bulbar centers. The efferent

limb of this storage reflex is predominantly sympathetic and mediated by the hypogastric nerve, and it results in detrusor relaxation due to a beta-adrenergic response and contraction of the outlet as the result of an alpha-adrenergic effect. In addition the alpha-adrenergic receptors synapsing on parasympathetic ganglia exert an inhibitory effect on parasympathetic ganglion transmission. When the bladder is full and there is maximum afferent stimulation, the involuntary suppression of the detrusor by the higher centers is removed, and contraction occurs in response to activation of parasympathetic motor fibers to the bladder. There is simultaneous inhibition of sympathetic alpha- and beta-adrenergic discharge, thereby further facilitating detrusor contraction and allowing for relaxation of the smooth musculature of the proximal urethra. Striated muscle sphincter relaxation is mediated by the pudendal nerve.

Obviously, successful and efficient storage and voiding requires highly coordinated integration of activity at all levels of the central and peripheral nervous system, and the complexity of this system accounts for the susceptibility of the lower urinary tract to neurogenic dysfunction in the face of even subtle neurological lesions.

The Physiology of Male Sexual Function

Normal sexual function depends on the interaction of a variety of factors, including those of endocrine, vascular, psychological, and neurogenic origin. All levels of the central and peripheral nervous system are involved, and even the most subtle lesions can adversely affect either libido, erectile function, ejaculatory function, or orgasm. Penile erection is a hemodynamic event in which the corpora cavernosa and corpus spongiosum undergo vascular engorgement, the actual mechanics of which are poorly understood.[16] It is undoubtedly a neurologically mediated vasomotor event in which both the pelvic nerves from the sacral cord and the hypogastric nerve from the lumbar sympathetics are involved.

In the male, penile erection may be induced by psychogenic or reflex stimulation. Psychic erections originating from the brain in response to erotic stimuli are mediated by the thoracolumbar sympathetic outflow. Reflex erections, which are stronger than the psychic variety, arise in response to sensory stimuli in the S2 to S4 dermatome, and they are mediated via the parasympathetic centers and pelvic nerves. Spinal cord lesions at or above the sympathetic outflow will hence interfere with psychic erectile function; injuries of the parasympathetic centers or its outflow will interfere with reflex erections while preserving psychic function; and injuries between the two levels may preserve psychic and reflex erectile ability. Incomplete spinal cord lesions may not effect erectile pathways, and this accounts for the exceptions to this schema.

Ejaculation is even more sensitive to neurological injury than is erection. It is ordinarily a two-part process involving emission of semen into the posterior urethra (regulated by sympathetic activity), followed by true ejaculation, which is achieved by contraction of the bulbocavernosus and ischiocavernosus muscles (mediated by pudendal nerve afferents).

Classification of Neurourologic Disorders

Neurourology is bedeviled by a profusion of classifications of bladder dysfunction based on, among other things, descriptive, anatomical, and etiologic terminology, none of which has been entirely satisfactory. More recently, the introduction of urodynamic evaluation has allowed for the accurate identification of the functional deficit at both the urethral and detrusor levels, and this has facilitated a logical approach to classification, diagnosis, and therapy.

Bors and Comarr introduced a classification with 15 different pathological categories, divided essentially according to whether the neurological lesion was an upper motor neuron (suprasacral) or a lower motor neuron (sacral or infrasacral) variety.[3] This classification included comment on the completeness of the neurological lesion and also on whether the sphincter acted in a coordinated fashion with the detrusor. However, urodynamic studies have shown that the bladder does not always act in the predictable upper or lower motor neuron fashion after neurological injury, and, in addition, the classification is unwieldy and not entirely satisfactory for daily clinical use and communication. Lapides popularized a currently widely used, descriptive classification that identifies five categories of neurogenic bladder dysfunction, two being due to upper motor neuron lesions (the uninhibited and reflex neurogenic bladder) and the remaining three being due to lower motor neuron lesions (the autonomous, the sensory paralytic, and the motor paralytic neurogenic bladders).[10] The term *uninhibited bladder* describes a hyper-reflexic detrusor with a normal or balanced sphincter, whereas the *reflex bladder* describes detrusor hyper-reflexia with imbalance (dys-synergia) at the striated external sphincter level. The *autonomous neurogenic bladder,* resulting from a lesion of both sensory and motor limbs of the voiding reflex arc, results in an areflexic bladder incapable of contraction and a sphincter mechanism that is also inactive. The *motor paralytic bladder* also results in an areflexic detrusor, and in the *sensory paralytic bladder* the primary problem is one of sensory denervation of the bladder, although ultimately bladder overdistension causes myogenic damage and contractile failure. This classification is attractive and often is clinically applicable. However, difficulty arises in the many cases that do not fit into one of the five categories, as may result from incomplete neurological lesions, and those cases in which the associated sphincter dysfunction does not fit the customary pattern.

Urodynamics offers a tool for identifying the functional deficit at the four levels that may be altered by neurological disease: the detrusor, the smooth muscle urethral sphincter, the striated muscle urethral sphincter, and sensation. Among others, Krane has developed a classification in which the detrusor muscle activity is classified according to whether it is functionally normal, hyper-reflexic, or areflexic.[8] Hyper-reflexic detrusor activity is defined as the occurrence of involuntary detrusor contractions, and detrusor areflexia is the inability to generate a voiding contraction. Urethral sphincter function at both the proximal and distal sphincter levels can likewise be identified and described as being either normal, hyperactive, or hypoactive. Normal sphincter activity implies normal continence tone during the storage phase of bladder activity and synergistic relaxation during voiding. A hyperactive sphincter, which may synonymously be called uncoordinated, imbalanced, or dys-synergic, may either relax inappropriately during storage or may contract inappropriately during voiding. The hypoactive sphincter has lost the ability to relax or contract appropriately and is generally a result of denervation; it may result in incontinence, or in some circumstances may be obstructive because it fails to relax during voiding. Bladder sensation is categorized during cystometry as being either normal, hyposensitive, or hypersensitive.

A more simplistic classification was introduced by Wein, who divided neurogenic bladders into those that fail to store adequately and those that fail to empty adequately (Table 34-4).[20] This is an excellent classification when it comes to planning treatment, but it too relies upon the urodynamic identification of detrusor and sphincter function. In essence, no single classification of neurogenic bladder dysfunction is ideal, and the neurourologist should have an understanding of each.

Evaluation of the Patient with Neurogenic Vesicourethral Dysfunction

Neurourologic History

The degree of neurological impairment will determine the patient's urologic symptomatology, and those with gross neurological deficits may only recognize their inability to remain continent or their inability to void. However, those with more subtle neurological lesions may present with symptoms that are not immediately identifiable as of neurogenic etiology, and they may mimic bladder irritative or obstructive problems.

Neurogenic disease may lead to any of the various forms of urinary incontinence. Stress incontinence may occur as a result of sphincter incompetence due to sacral cord or peripheral nerve lesions. Urgency incontinence is a manifestation of hyper-reflexic bladder dysfunction. The patient with intact bladder sensation will recognize the urge to void but will not reach the bathroom in time before forceful involuntary urine loss occurs; however, in more complete lesions, when sensation is lost, unconscious reflex incontinence occurs. Overflow incontinence occurs in an areflexic bladder when the bladder fills to the point where intravesical pressure exceeds the urethral closing pressure and continuous dribbling loss of urine results. Total urinary incontinence where the bladder and urethra are converted into a virtual open conduit rarely occurs because of neurogenic dysfunction, and it is more often a result of sphincter compromise by surgery or trauma.

Neurogenic voiding problems may relate to control of the voiding event and to its frequency and its efficiency. The patient should be able to voluntarily initiate voiding, and once established the urinary stream should be continuous and forceful without straining, and the bladder should empty to completion. Each of these factors may be altered in both structural bladder outlet obstruction and neurogenic vesicourethral dysfunction.

Pain is a frequent warning symptom of urological disease. Inflammatory changes in the bladder and urethra usually manifest by dysuria, pyelonephritis by flank pain, and upper urinary tract obstruction by lateralized colicky abdominal discomfort. Depending on the level and completeness of the neurological lesion, such pain may or may not be perceived by the patient.

Hematuria may be the first sign of serious complication in neurogenic bladder disease, and its presence demands further investigation. The causes are numerous, but in the patient with neurogenic bladder disease the most common are urinary infection and calculus disease. In patients on intermittent catheterization, however, catheter trauma may be responsible, and good clinical judgment is necessary to avoid overinvestigation of this group. It is important to note that microscopic and gross hematuria are of equal importance.

Bowel dysfunction frequently accompanies neurogenic vesicourethral disease, and there is considerable incentive to achieve bowel training to avoid soiling. One should document whether the patient has the sensation of desire to defecate, whether the fecal mass can be differentiated from flatus, whether bowel movements can be initiated and interrupted, how often bowel movements occur, and whether diarrhea or soiling are frequent.

Neurourologic Examination

The patient with neurogenic bladder dysfunction should undergo a general physical, a specific urological, and a thorough neurological examination. The neurological examination is designed to ascertain the nature and extent of the neurological impairment so as to predict the likely nature of the resultant bladder dysfunction, and also to determine the patient's ability to accomplish planned urologic management. In most cases the identification of the neurological deficit is a simple matter; however, it is not uncommon for occult neurological lesions to result in neurogenic bladder dysfunction before any other obvious manifestations occur.

The urologic examination should include inspection and palpation of the abdomen, inguinal regions, and external genitalia and a rectal examination. It should also include a pelvic examination in the female. This examination is often rendered difficult in the neurologically impaired patient who is immobile or confined to a wheelchair, making placement on the examining table time-consuming and difficult. For this reason there is a tendency to examine these patients incompletely.

Laboratory Procedures

Urinalysis and Urine Culture

Because the neurologically impaired patient may not experience the usual warning symptoms of urologic disease, urinalysis takes on a greater significance. Many patients with neurogenic bladder disease cannot volitionally void, and specimen collection may be difficult. A voiding reflex may be triggered by suprapubic stimulation or the Credé maneuver; however, it is rarely possible, particularly in the

neurologically impaired female, to obtain an uncontaminated specimen by this method, and sterile catheterization is justified.

In the catheter-free patient the finding of pyuria, microscopic hematuria, bacteriuria, etc., takes on the same significance as it would in the normal urologic patient, and it demands further investigation. However, in the patient managed by intermittent catheterization and the patient with an ileal loop urinary diversion, minimal pyuria and occasional microscopic hematuria and asymptomatic bacteriuria are not infrequent findings. In this group the occurrence is a matter for careful consideration and clinical judgment. The patient with neurogenic bladder dysfunction is more susceptible to urinary tract infection and to stone disease, both of which may manifest as changes in the urinary sediment on microscopy; so it is advisable that these studies be completed at least every 3 to 4 months even in the uncomplicated patient.

Blood Chemistries and Hematologic Studies

Because of the risk of renal impairment in patients with neurogenic bladder dysfunction, an assessment of renal function by serum creatinine and electrolyte levels is customary. Automated clinical chemistry and hematologic profiles have greatly simplified these determinations, making their performance a matter of routine. Baseline studies should be obtained on all patients presenting with neurogenic bladder disease, and thereafter may be repeated on a timely basis, with annual repetition in the uncomplicated patient.

Radiological Procedures

In the normal urologic patient, routine screening radiological studies are rarely justified. However, it is a matter of common practice in the patient with neurogenic vesicourethral dysfunction. This is because of the patient's frequent inability to perceive symptoms, so that surreptitious changes may occur in the upper and lower urinary tract, defying recognition by any means other than x-ray studies.

Plain Abdominal Film

A plain film of the abdomen, including the areas of the kidneys ureters, and the bladder (also called scout film or KUB) is generally performed as an initial study prior to subsequent radiographic examination. This is also valuable as an isolated study for the identification of opaque urinary calculi.

Excretory Urography

This study should be performed as a baseline in all patients with neurogenic vesicourethral dysfunction to look for the changes arising from chronic infection, obstruction, reflux, and stone disease. In the uncomplicated case, it is repeated every 3 years. In patients in whom other urologic parameters are abnormal or in whom prior excretory urograms have shown renal changes, more frequent study may be necessary. Interim examination of the upper tracts may be safely accomplished by a KUB to exclude stone disease and by renal ultrasound to exclude changes in renal size or hydronephrosis.

In the child with myelodysplasia with neurogenic bladder dysfunction, an excretory urogram is obtained during the first month of life to identify the morphological characteristics of the kidneys. Should this study be normal it is customary to follow the child's upper tracts with renal ultrasound or radioisotope renal scans so as to avoid the potential dangers of repeated x-ray exposure. This is discussed later.

Voiding Cystourethrography (VCUG)

This study identifies the morphological characteristics of the bladder and the presence of vesicoureteral reflux, and hints at the functional status of the urethral sphincters. The indications for VCUG in neurogenic bladder dysfunction are controversial. Because there is a high risk of vesicoureteral reflux in these patients, some clinicians routinely perform it for screening purposes at the time of excretory urography. Alternatively, because significant reflux will usually manifest by upper tract changes identifiable on excretory urography or ultrasound, the VCUG may be reserved for such occasions or for patients with recurrent urinary infections. The nuclear cystogram may be used in pediatric practice to avoid excessive radiation exposure.

The iced cystogram may be of value in differentiating neurogenic internal from neurogenic external sphincter obstruction. Refrigerated radiographic contrast material is used for this study for it accentuates the pathophysiological response of the detrusor and sphincter, making radiographic identification of the level of obstruction more easily discernible on the voiding films.

Renal Ultrasound

Because of the need for frequent upper urinary tract re-evaluation in the neurogenic bladder patient, there is a danger of exposure to dangerous levels of radiation. Ultrasonography presents an alternative that is particularly applicable to the pediatric age group. These studies will adequately demonstrate even minor changes in upper tract dilatation, can accurately identify renal size, will demonstrate opaque and nonopaque calculi, and are indispensable in the evaluation of renal masses.

Endoscopic Procedures

Neurogenic bladder disease is a disorder of function, and cystoscopy has little to offer in its identification. However, endoscopy is indicated for the evaluation of other abnormal parameters in the neurogenic bladder patient, such as hematuria, recurrent urinary tract infection or unexplained pyuria, and voiding dysfunction unexplained by urodynamic study.

In most patients, general anesthesia is unnecessary for cystourethroscopy. Bacteremic episodes are common following instrumentation in patients with neurogenic bladder dysfunction, and endoscopy should not be performed in the presence of acute urinary infection.

Autonomic dysreflexia is a syndrome seen in patients with spinal cord lesions above the midthoracic level, and it may be triggered by urologic stimulation such as endoscopy.[9] It is a potentially dangerous condition characterized by headache, sweating, nasal obstruction, and flushing, and it results in bradycardia and severe paroxysmal hypertension that may precipitate cerebral hemorrhage, convulsions, and even death. In the event that it occurs, the endoscopic procedure should be immediately terminated, and if this does not resolve the problem, immediate parenteral administration of either pentolinium, hexamethonium, nitroprusside, hydralazine, trimethaphan, or diazoxide has been recommended. Spinal or general anesthesia will also prevent this condition and is resorted to for endoscopic studies in patients who have a history of dysreflexia.

Urodynamic Evaluation

Urodynamics is the discipline concerned with the identification and measurement of physiological and pathological factors involved in the storage, transportation, and evacuation of urine. I believe that these studies are mandatory in the evaluation of neurogenic bladder disease, for it is only by identification of the functional deficit that logical therapy, be it pharmacologic or surgical, may be selected. A variety of urodynamic studies of varying sophistication are available; however, cystometry and sphincter electromyography are the mainstays in the evaluation of the neurogenic patient (Table 34-1).[18]

The most important questions that urodynamic studies should answer for us in neurourologic dysfunction include:

1. Is the bladder hyper-reflexic during filling?
2. What is the compliance of the bladder during filling?
3. Is sensation of filling events and the need to void present?
4. Can the patient generate a voluntary voiding contraction?
5. Is the contraction of sufficient magnitude and duration to complete emptying?
6. Can a voiding contraction be triggered by stimulation (e.g., suprapubic percussion)?
7. If voiding is incomplete, is it due to detrusor, bladder neck, or external sphincter dysfunction?
8. Is external sphincter activity coordinated—that is, does the sphincter relax appropriately during voiding?
9. What is the nature of the motor unit potentials on the oscilloscopic recording of the electromyogram (EMG)?
10. What is the latency of impulse transmission in the sacral reflex arc?

Answers to these questions will not only dictate the most logical therapy but will also help characterize the neurogenic bladder in terms of its potential for jeopardy to the upper urinary tract.

TABLE 34-1   Urodynamic Armamentarium

Cystometry
Uroflowmetry
Sphincter electromyography
Urethral pressure studies
Multifunction micturition studies
Video urodynamics
Pharmacologic urodynamic testing

The Hyper-reflexic Detrusor

As I have noted in the earlier discussion of the physiology of micturition, detrusor hyper-reflexia generally results from suprasacral neurological lesions. It manifests as loss of control of the detrusor reflex with resultant uninhibited bladder contractions. These contractions are demonstrated by filling cystometry. Depending on the nature of the neurological lesion, the sphincters may be either coordinated or dys-synergic.

Hyper-reflexic Detrusor with Coordinated Urethral Sphincters

This is the uninhibited neurogenic bladder of the Lapides classification. Depending on the completeness of the neurological lesion, the patient may or may not have intact bladder sensation. If it is intact, the onset of the uninhibited contraction will be perceived as an urgency to void. If the long tracts controlling the pelvic floor musculature are also intact, the voluntary sphincter is contracted until the uninhibited detrusor contraction is lost, or leakage occurs, or the patient finds a bathroom. In patients who lack bladder sensation, the uninhibited contraction will cause unconscious loss of urine, or reflex incontinence. A frequent characteristic of the hyper-reflexic detrusor is the inability to generate a voluntary contraction prior to the trigger capacity of the bladder being reached, but contractions may be stimulated by extrinsic triggering mechanisms such as posture change and suprapubic percussion. Because this is an unobstructed system by virtue of the coordinated sphincters, it tends to portend less hazard to the upper urinary tracts.

Hyper-reflexic Detrusor with a Dys-synergic Voluntary Striated Sphincter

This is the reflex bladder of the Lapides classification. Although various types of dys-synergic activity in the striated sphincter are described, the most usual is the occurrence of crescendo contraction of the striated pelvic floor each time the detrusor contracts. This effectively produces obstructed voiding, and it is seen predominantly in patients with suprasacral spinal cord lesions involving both detrusor and sphincter long tracts; generally these patients have no sensation of bladder events. It is a potentially serious variety of neurogenic bladder dysfunction as a high-pressure obstructed system develops. This patient will exhibit both in-

continence and inefficient voiding. Urodynamic evaluation again rests on cystometry to demonstrate the uninhibited contractions and simultaneous sphincter electromyography to show the sphincter dys-synergia.

Hyper-reflexic Detrusor with Dys-synergia at the Proximal Smooth Muscle Sphincter

Identification of this entity requires both cystometry, striated sphincter electromyography, and simultaneous voiding cystourethrography to demonstrate a failure of funneling of the bladder neck (proximal smooth muscle sphincter). This type of neurogenic bladder dysfunction may occur in isolation, but it more commonly occurs in conjunction with dys-synergism at the striated sphincter level, particularly in quadriplegic patients with spinal cord lesions above the level of sympathetic outflow.

The Areflexic Detrusor

This variety of neurogenic bladder dysfunction manifests as a failure to void because of the inability to generate a micturition contraction. There are other causes for detrusor areflexia in the absence of neurological disease, including bladder outlet obstruction, psychogenic inhibition, pharmacologic effects, and myogenic failure due to detrusor overdistension. The neurogenic variety results from lesions of the detrusor sensory afferent nerves (sensory paralytic bladder), the afferent motor nerves to the detrusor (motor paralytic bladder), or both (autonomous bladder). From a functional point of view, however, it is artificial to separate these entities. In patients with suprasacral spinal cord injuries, a period of spinal shock with detrusor areflexia precedes the development of hyper-reflexia.

Urodynamic evaluation should include cystometry, sphincter electromyography, micturition study, and pharmacologic testing using the bethanechol denervation supersensitivity test to confirm that the areflexia is neurogenic and not due to one of the other etiologies mentioned earlier. Disease in the sacral reflex can also be identified by electromyographic sacral latency studies.

Although on many occasions the areflexic bladder may be of large capacity and "flaccid," it may on occasion be hypertonic with a steep rising curve on cystometry, indicating poor bladder compliance (distensibility). This is thought to be due to unopposed alpha-adrenergic activity causing an increase in bladder muscle tone.

As in the case of the hyper-reflexic detrusor, the sphincters may be variably affected by the neurological lesion. In the event the innervation of the sphincters remains intact or partially intact, urethral closing pressure will be good, and continence will be assured providing the bladder is not allowed to fill to the point of overflow. If the sphincter mechanism is denervated, as may occur in spinal cord infarction and in extensive myelomeningocele lesions, the urethral closing pressure may be low, the urethra may be totally incompetent, and continuous incontinence results. Urethral pressure profilometry and striated sphincter electromyography will help identify this disturbance in the outflow tract.

In some cases, the innervation of the proximal muscle and the distal striated muscle sphincters are differentially affected.

Management of the Patient with Neurogenic Vesicourethral Dysfunction

There is no single schema for managing patients with neurogenic genitourinary disease, and a variety of factors will determine treatment selection (Table 34-2). In many cases the underlying neurological disease will predict the type of bladder and sphincter dysfunction to be anticipated; however, urodynamic studies discussed earlier should be used to identify accurately the functional deficit and so allow for logical treatment selection. Conservative management is indicated in patients with potentially fatal neurological disease and for those with potentially changeable problems such as multiple sclerosis. The use of clean, intermittent, self-catheterization is now widespread, but it does require the patient to be able to use his or her hands, and also requires the intelligence, motivation, and reliability to conduct such a program. Age is also an important consideration, and in those children with a congenital neurogenic bladder, intervention is deferred until the child is of school age, providing the bladder dysfunction is of a safe variety.

The goals of management will vary from patient to patient but will usually involve four aims (Table 34-3).[22] To most patients the primary consideration is continence, but achievement of this must be tempered with concern about changes in the upper urinary tracts and the avoidance of urinary infections. These two factors require that the bladder be emptied completely on a cyclical basis with avoidance of any periods of overdistension.

Wein's functional classification of neurogenic bladder presents us with a logical guide for planning treatment (Table 34-4). Therapy is aimed at facilitating either storage or emptying using a variety of conservative and surgical methods depending on whether urodynamic studies have shown the bladder or the outlet to be at fault (Tables 34-5

TABLE 34-2 Factors Determining Treatment Selection in Patients with Neurogenic Vesicourethral Dysfunction

Type of vesicourethral dysfunction
Underlying disease prognosis
Ability to use the hands
Patient age
Patient intelligence, motivation
 and reliability

TABLE 34-3 Goals of Management in Neurogenic Vesicourethral Dysfunction

Preserve normal upper tracts
Control urinary infection
Facilitate complete bladder emptying
Achieve urinary continence

TABLE 34-4 A Functional Classification of Neurogenic Vesicourethral Dysfunction

Failure to store
 Because of the bladder
 Because of the outlet
Failure to empty
 Because of the bladder
 Because of the outlet

TABLE 34-5 Therapy to Facilitate Urine Storage*

Inhibition of bladder contractility
 Pharmacologic manipulation
 Electrical stimulation
 Bladder overdistension
 Detrusor denervation
 Augmentation cystoplasty
Increase in outlet resistance
 Pharmacologic manipulation
 Artificial sphincter prostheses
 Bladder neck surgery
 Pelvic floor electrical stimulation

*Each of these therapies may require intermittent catheterization for emptying.

and 34-6). It has always been my philosophy that the achievement of continence without the use of external devices is optimal. For this reason the treatment route involving augmentation of bladder storage potential with intermittent emptying by clean catheterization has become the mainstay of management, and the treatment options offered in Table 34-5 are systematically explored seeking the least invasive method of achieving this end. This is particularly true for females for whom there is no external collecting device available to control uninhibited urine loss. The alternative route of therapy facilitating bladder emptying is often at the expense of continence, in which case it is only appropriate for male patients able to wear an external collecting device successfully. It is also appropriate for those patients deemed untrustworthy to perform self-catheterization in the optimal fashion, and for those unable to catheterize themselves because of upper extremity dysfunction or because of urethral anomalies.

In the past, and largely responsible for the poor prognosis of many patients with neurogenic bladder, indwelling Foley catheterization or supravesical urinary diversion using the ileal conduit were commonly used. There are few indica-

TABLE 34-6 Therapy to Facilitate Bladder Emptying*

Increase bladder contractility
 Pharmacologic manipulation
 Credé or Valsalva maneuver
 Triggering reflex bladder contractions
 Electrical stimulation
Decrease outlet resistance
 Pharmacologic
 Outlet surgery (sphincterotomy)
 Pudendal nerve interruption

*These methods frequently improve emptying at the expense of continence.

tions for such treatment in this modern medical era; however, the Foley catheter does occasionally find a place in the management of the elderly.

Therapy to Facilitate Urine Storage

In some patients, storage may be improved leaving volitional voiding intact. However, therapy to improve storage generally compromises emptying such that residual urine with the potential for infection results. In this event, a clean intermittent catheterization must be added.

Clean Intermittent Catheterization

The pioneering work in this field was by Guttmann, who with Frankel in 1966 reported aseptic intermittent catheterization for the management of spinal cord injury patients during the period of spinal shock and until balanced bladder function could be achieved by a noncatheter technique.[6] In the hospital environment and particularly during the immediate postinjury period, aseptic catheterization by the nurse or catheterization team is still the rule. However, in the rehabilitation center a clean self-catheterization technique is taught, a concept introduced (in 1971) and popularized by Lapides et al.[11]

Technique The female patient is initially taught to self-catheterize in the recumbent position. She is instructed to wash her hands with soap and water, lie in the recumbent position with the hips abducted, spread the labia with the fingers of the left hand, and visualize the urethra in a mirror stationed on the bed between the legs. She must then insert a lubricated no. 14 French catheter using the right hand, and completely empty the bladder. Once she has learned to catheterize in the recumbent position, the ambulatory patient graduates to where she may perform the procedure seated on the toilet or standing, with one foot on the toilet seat. After the initial period of learning, the patient does not need to use a mirror and learns to locate the meatus by touch. Patients who are confined to a wheelchair who find transfer to the toilet difficult may generally be taught to catheterize in the wheelchair seat. The technique is far easier in males, who should make similar attempts at cleanliness and catheterize the urethra either standing or in the seated position, making certain to thoroughly lubricate the catheter. In the male the catheter may "hang up" at the site of a stricture, a false passage, at the level of the distal sphincter mechanism, particularly if it is dys-synergic, or at the bladder neck. These difficulties may make the program impossible; however, in most instances they can be overcome.

Commercially made disposable plastic catheters are available at reasonable cost. When expense is a consideration, however, the same catheter may be simply reused by thorough washing in soap and water after use and wrapping in a clean towel until the next use.

Bacteria are obviously introduced into the bladder during clean catheterization, but providing that complete emptying is achieved, these organisms are neutralized by the host defense mechanisms and infection is usually avoided. Overdistension of the bladder must be avoided, for it compromises the blood supply to the bladder wall and impairs the host resistance. Using clean intermittent catheterization, sterile urine is achieved in from 39 to 65 percent of cases.[7] Those patients who do not have sterile urine generally have asymptomatic bacteriuria. Most go untreated unless recurrent symptomatic infective episodes occur or anatomical reasons such as reflux make treatment advisable. However, many physicians, uncertain of the long-term adverse effects of chronic bacteriuria, advocate adjunctive prophylactic antimicrobial treatment for all patients on a clean intermittent catheterization program.

Inhibition of Bladder Contractility

In a patient with detrusor areflexia and a competent outlet, intermittent catheterization alone will suffice. However, in many cases one or more of the adjunctive procedures noted in Table 34-5 will be necessary to promote bladder storage.

Pharmacologic Manipulation The agents most often used to inhibit bladder contractility are the anticholinergic drugs and agents with a direct inhibitory effect on smooth muscle.[19] Oxybutynin (Ditropan, Marion Laboratories, Inc., Kansas City, Mo.) is the most widely used agent for this purpose. In addition to its anticholinergic activity it has an independent musculotropic effect and also some moderate local anesthetic effect on the bladder. It is customarily used in adults in a dosage of 5 mg four times daily and is also available in a pediatric suspension. Its antimuscarinic side effects include drying of salivary secretions, mydriasis, blurred vision, tachycardia, drowsiness, and constipation. Alternative agents with the same effect include propantheline, methantheline, flavoxate hydrochloride, dicyclomine hydrochloride, and imipramine hydrochloride.

Use of these agents requires careful follow-up. In some cases, symptomatic improvement with increase in bladder capacity and a decrease in incontinence is rapid, without compromising voiding efficiency. In others, however, the dosage required to reduce continence abolishes the micturition contraction and makes the use of the clean intermittent catheterization program necessary. All of these agents are contraindicated in patients who have glaucoma, and they must be used with great care in patients with obstructive gastrointestinal disease, bladder outlet obstruction, or tachycardia.

Electrical Stimulation Devices designed to stimulate the afferent limb of the pudendal reflex arc have been used for some years to treat urinary incontinence. They were originally designed to improve the urethral closing function by stimulation of the pelvic floor musculature. However, it appears that there is a sacral pathway for the inhibition of detrusor reflex activity, and electrical stimulation of the pudendal afferents has been used clinically to achieve this end. The technology for this therapy is rapidly improving, and should be tried prior to the use of invasive methods to control uninhibited detrusor activity.[12]

Bladder Overdistension This is performed under epidural anesthesia using a specially constructed balloon catheter that is filled within the bladder until the pressure within it approximates systolic blood pressure.[14] This pressure is maintained for four 30-min periods, the bladder being emptied at the end of each period. The procedure results in degeneration in the unmyelinated nerve fibers in the bladder wall with a resultant peripheral denervation and alteration of both sensory and motor function. However, it is not without risk, and rupture of the bladder can result.

Detrusor Denervation These procedures are reserved for patients with intractable detrusor hyper-reflexia unresponsive to other conservative modalities. Central denervation involves interruption of either S2, S3, or S4 nerve roots, the particular roots selected depending on either preliminary diagnostic nerve blocks using local anesthesia, or intraoperative testing by nerve stimulation and the monitoring of the bladder's contractile response. Such selective sacral neurectomy may be performed surgically or by percutaneous radiofrequency coagulation of the nerve. In the patient with an incomplete neurological lesion it is important that denervation procedures do not compromise other functions, nor cause significant somatic sensory loss. Following denervation the bladder becomes areflexic and may be managed by clean intermittent catheterization. Torrens and Hald have summarized the results of sacral neurectomy for the paraplegic bladder from 10 series and report good results.[17]

Augmentation Cystoplasty Enterocystoplasty is a major operative procedure used to augment the capacity of the abnormal neurogenic bladder, and it should be used only as a last resort. In patients with marked bladder hyper-reflexia or poor bladder compliance (distensibility) unresponsive to the previously mentioned procedures, augmentation procedures with or without excision of part of the viscus may result in a continent storage organ that may be emptied by intermittent catheterization or in some cases by the Credé or Valsalva maneuver.

Increase in Outlet Resistance

Pharmacologic Manipulation The innervation of the bladder outlet, detailed earlier, tells us that alpha-adrenergic drugs will have a facilitatory effect on the smooth muscle sphincter mechanism. These agents find their major clinical use in the treatment of pediatric neurogenic incontinence in the myelodysplastic child, in the treatment of the patient with postprostatectomy urinary incontinence, and in the treatment of very mild stress urinary incontinence in the female. The agents most commonly used are ephedrine, pseudoephedrine hydrochloride, and phenylpropanolamine hydrochloride.[19] These agents have limited capacity to improve the urethral closing pressure and only mild incontinence will be corrected.

Artificial Sphincter Prostheses The Brantley Scott genitourinary sphincter prosthesis has undergone remarkable development during the past 10 years, and providing that stringent implantation criteria are met, its success rate in controlling urinary incontinence is approximately 85 percent.[15] It is an implantable hydraulically operated device composed of a silicone constructed cuff for occlusion of the urethra or bladder neck, a pressure balloon that controls the amount of compression, a pump implanted in the scrotum or labia (the squeezing of which activates the device), and a

control assembly that is made up of resistors that control fluid flow within the system. The device finds particular use in the myelodysplastic child who has an incompetent outlet due to sphincter denervation. Devices have also been implanted in adults with acquired neurogenic bladder dysfunction.

Most failures following implantation are due to sphincter erosion due to ischemia of the urethral tissue beneath the occlusive cuff or to prosthesis infection or mechanical malfunction. A prerequisite is that the patient be able to efficiently empty the bladder when the device is activated, and this frequently requires the performance of sphincterotomy or other outlet procedures prior to sphincter implantation.

Bladder Neck Surgery Reconstructive procedures at the level of the bladder neck have been used to improve the competence of the bladder outlet in a variety of congenital and acquired conditions. Inconsistent results have dulled the enthusiasm of most urologists for these operations; however, the fascial sling cystourethropexy does find a role in the myelodysplastic girl with outlet incompetence. The procedure can produce urinary retention, allowing the child to perform clean intermittent catheterization to empty the bladder.

Therapy to Facilitate Bladder Emptying

Bladder emptying may be facilitated either by methods designed to increase bladder contractility or by procedures designed to decrease the outlet resistance (Table 34-6). These procedures often achieve their end only at the expense of continence, in which event they are only appropriate for use in males who can wear an external collecting device.

Urodynamic studies will identify whether the bladder emptying failure is due to problems of bladder contractility, failure of sphincter relaxation, or structural outlet obstruction. The voiding cystourethrogram is also invaluable in this regard.

Maneuvers to Increase Bladder Contractility

Pharmacologic Manipulation The most widely used drug for this purpose is bethanechol hydrochloride (Duvoid, Norwich Eaton Pharmaceuticals, Inc., Norwich, N.Y.; or Urecholine, Merck Sharp & Dohme, West Point, Pa.). It has acetylcholine-like activity and may be administered either subcutaneously or orally. Although it is widely used, there is a considerable body of evidence to suspect the clinical efficacy of the drug, and it is my belief that it probably does not appreciably improve voiding in the oral doses currently used. In patients with detrusor areflexia the medication will not produce a voiding contraction, although the tone of the detrusor muscle may be increased.

Credé or Valsalva Maneuvers An increase in abdominal pressure by the Valsalva maneuver or direct extrinsic bladder compression by the Credé maneuver will improve emptying efficiency in patients with low outflow resistance. In patients with detrusor areflexia due to a sacral or infrasacral spinal cord lesion, this maneuver is rarely successful, for the sphincter mechanisms remain competent and no amount of extrinsic bladder compression will effect complete emptying. In fact, under such circumstances, the procedure may be hazardous. It is also contraindicated in patients with reflux. In effect, it finds its main use in a select group of women with detrusor areflexia and in males who have previously undergone sphincterotomy.

Triggering Reflex Bladder Contractions The areflexic bladder due to sacral or infrasacral spinal cord lesions cannot be triggered to contract by this method; however, suprapubic percussion, pubic hair stimulation, etc., may trigger contractions in the hyper-reflexic neurogenic bladder, helping to complete emptying. One must be certain that there is no striated sphincter dys-synergia because this could result in high-pressure obstructed voiding contractions with potentially damaging effects on the upper urinary tracts.

Electrical Stimulation A variety of electrical implants have been tried to augment bladder emptying, including electrodes implanted in the bladder wall, on the sacral nerves, or in the conus medullaris. Direct bladder stimulation has been largely supplanted by the latter two procedures, and the technology in each continues to improve but cannot yet be considered a therapeutic alternative except in specialized centers.[5,13]

Maneuvers to Decrease Outlet Resistance

Pharmacologic Manipulation Drugs with alpha-adrenergic blocking activity tend to inhibit the proximal smooth muscle sphincter, and striated muscle relaxants may inhibit pelvic floor striated muscle sphincter activity. The most widely used alpha blocking agent is phenoxybenzamine and the striated muscle relaxants used include dantrolene sodium, baclofen, and diazepam.[19] None of these agents acts specifically on the urinary sphincter mechanisms, and other muscular functions are also affected. Although there are some enthusiastic reports of their use, we have not achieved any dramatic improvement in emptying efficiency.

Bladder Outlet Surgery Procedures that have been advocated to surgically decrease outlet resistance include bladder neck incision or resection, radical transurethral prostatectomy, and external sphincterotomy. Each of these procedures may be performed endoscopically, and selection of the appropriate operation is based upon urodynamic features and voiding cystourethrography. These operations frequently compromise continence and are only appropriate in the male. In the patient for whom bladder emptying into an external collecting device is deemed more appropriate than a clean intermittent catheterization program, these procedures are the optimal way to facilitate bladder emptying and thereby reduce the incidence of infection and risk of upper tract deterioration.[23]

Pudendal Nerve Interruption Dys-synergic obstruction to urine flow by the striated muscle of the pelvic floor may be blocked by pudendal nerve interruption. The main disadvantage of this procedure is its invariable adverse effect on erectile potency in the male. In addition, it does not always improve bladder emptying, and before the nerve is surgically or chemically interrupted, the likelihood of success should be checked by a local anesthetic nerve block. This procedure has been largely abandoned in most centers.

Specific Neurourologic Problems

Spinal Cord Injury

Detrusor areflexia due to spinal shock persists for a variable period after injury. During this period, the bladder will be managed by an intermittent catheterization program, usually conducted in the rehabilitation unit.[1] The return of spontaneous reflex bladder activity will depend on the level and completeness of the neurological lesion, and will be heralded by spontaneous voiding occurring between catheterizations. Urodynamic evaluation is delayed until this time, and future urologic therapy is based on the results of these studies and on factors discussed earlier, which dictate whether the patient will follow the route of facilitation of bladder storage with clean intermittent catheterization or facilitation of bladder emptying with the use of an external collecting device. It is important to recognize the potential for rapid renal deterioration that accompanies the neurogenic bladder from spinal cord injury, and careful objective follow-up is mandatory.

Multiple Sclerosis

Although this disease is characterized by a clinical course of remissions and exacerbations, the accompanying micturition dysfunction is often progressive. It may present to the urologist as urinary retention, urinary incontinence, urinary frequency and urgency, or voiding inefficiency with incomplete emptying and urinary infections. We have found the majority of patients to have detrusor hyper-reflexia, which accounts for the frequency, urgency, and incontinence. Inappropriate striated sphincter activity (detrusor sphincter dys-synergia) is not uncommon, and it will result in emptying inefficiency and will increase the potential for complications such as infection and upper tract deterioration.

Because of the variable nature of this disease, aggressive surgical urologic intervention is unjustified, and sphincterotomies, etc., are rarely performed. Because of the frequent cerebellar involvement and upper extremity dysfunction, clean intermittent self-catheterization programs are often impossible. Specific treatment intervention will be dependent largely on the urodynamic features of the disease, the patient's predominant symptoms, the potential for urologic hazard of the neurogenic bladder, and the patient's own ability to perform the specific therapeutic regimens.

Cerebrovascular Disease

Urinary retention is common during the initial period following a cerebrovascular accident (CVA), and a short period of indwelling Foley catheter drainage is often appropriate, after which aseptic intermittent catheterization should be substituted until the bladder regains spontaneous reflex activity. The most common neurogenic bladder dysfunction to result from CVA is detrusor hyper-reflexia with coordinated sphincter function. Detrusor dys-synergia is uncommon, and if bladder emptying is inefficient one suspects outlet obstruction due to structural problems (for example, prostate enlargement) and endoscopic and urodynamic studies are performed for clarification.

Urinary frequency, urgency, and incontinence due to hyper-reflexia may be controlled using anticholinergic medications, but often these maneuvers are unsuccessful until the patient's rehabilitation progresses to the point where he or she recognizes the bladder's cues and is mobile enough to get to the bathroom in time. In patients in whom mental status is also severely compromised, and in the very elderly, an indwelling Foley catheter may be appropriate.

Parkinson's Disease

Neurogenic bladder dysfunction in these patients is among the most difficult to treat. Both detrusor hyper-reflexia and hyporeflexia may result, and in addition, the picture is confused by the fact that males with Parkinson's disease are frequently elderly and have concomitant prostate outlet obstruction, and the fact that antiparkinsonian medications frequently cause urinary retention. Because of motor dysfunction, these patients cannot perform self-catheterization, which would ordinarily be the most appropriate management for such complex dysfunction. Transurethral prostatectomy in the prostate-obstructed group often gives unsatisfactory results with persistent incomplete bladder emptying and frequently with urinary incontinence. Many patients severely incapacitated by their disease may be managed by an intermittent catheterization program performed by a family member, or reluctantly the indwelling Foley catheter may find a role.

Diabetes Mellitus

Diabetic peripheral neuropathy may result in bladder dysfunction. Sensory neuropathy causes a lack of awareness of bladder filling events, and the urge to void is lost. The resulting insidious progressive bladder overdistension will cause myogenic damage and poor bladder contractility. A large capacity hyporeflexic bladder is produced with resultant voiding difficulties, residual urine, and urinary infections. Cholinergic agents have been used to try to improve bladder contractility, but are rarely successful. Alpha-adrenergic blocking agents to lower outlet resistance may be added, and in some cases transurethral incision of the bladder neck or prostate resection are used to decrease the outlet resistance and facilitate emptying. These maneuvers are not always successful, and should the residual urine be excessive and should infections be problematic, intermittent catheterization is required.

Neurourologic Problems in Children

In children, disorders of voiding and continence may be due to structural, functional, or neurogenic etiologies. Functional causes predominate, but in many instances these are difficult to differentiate from neurogenic disease, and the terms *non-neurogenic neurogenic bladder* and *occult neuropathic*

bladder have been coined. Pediatric neurogenic bladder dysfunction may be congenital or acquired in variety. Most cases are due to myelodysplasia, but sacral agenesis, spinal dysraphic states, and cerebral palsy also contribute. Acquired etiologies include trauma, malignancy, and inflammation. Invariably the type of neurogenic bladder dysfunction that results will depend on the level and completeness of the neurological lesion.

In the myelodysplastic child, evaluation of the lower urinary tract dysfunction is generally delayed until just before school age, at which time it becomes important to achieve continence. During the first years of life, the aim is to maintain a sterile urine and to ensure preservation of normal upper urinary tracts. This is achieved by the timely performance of urinalysis and culture, excretory urography, renal ultrasound, radioisotope renal scanning, voiding cystourethrography, and urodynamics. Until school age approaches, the child may be managed for incontinence by the use of diapers, and at 3 to 5 years of age or earlier, should recurrent urinary tract or upper tract changes dictate, a urodynamic study is performed to identify the nature of the dysfunction. In my practice approximately 30 percent of these children have detrusor hyper-reflexia and 70 percent have detrusor areflexia. In the areflexic group, rather than having flaccid bladders, many have poor compliance of the bladder wall with steep cystometrogram curves indicating the poor distensibility. Striated sphincter electromyography shows some degree of denervation in 80 percent of cases. This may not only compromise continence but may result in inefficient bladder emptying due to the sphincter's failure to relax appropriately during voiding attempts.

Few myelodysplastic children will retain voluntary control of micturition and be continent and void to completion. An initial attempt may be made to achieve this end with the help of appropriate pharmacologic manipulation of detrusor and sphincter function as dictated by the urodynamic study. However, currently the majority are managed by a clean intermittent catheterization program, again with appropriate pharmacologic manipulation. A small percentage, in particular those with a low urethral closing pressure due to sphincter denervation, will not achieve continence by this means, and surgical intervention to increase outlet resistance will be necessary. The Brantley-Scott inflatable sphincter prosthesis enjoys excellent success in these patients, providing that all criteria for successful implantation are met. In the past, many myelodysplastic children underwent supravesical urinary diversion, and because of advances in our management of the lower urinary tract, most of these children are now candidates for reversal of diversion and institution of either intermittent catheterization or implantation of the artificial sphincter.

Children with sacral agenesis or an occult spinal dysraphic state and those who develop acquired neurological lesions should be evaluated and managed by the same protocol as described above. Those children who present with apparent neurogenic bladder dysfunction in the absence of an identifiable neurological lesion are diagnosed as the non-neurogenic neurogenic bladder, and it is likely that this is to some degree a learned phenomenon. The potential for upper tract damage is just as great as with true neurogenic bladder dysfunction, and these children generally have continence and voiding problems and recurrent urinary infections.

Their management is by the eradication of infection and pharmacologic manipulation of detrusor and sphincter dysfunction; also, some advocate attempting to retrain a normal micturition pattern using biofeedback.

Evaluation and Therapy of Neurogenic Impotence

The term *impotence* describes not only loss of erectile function but also changes in libido, failure of ejaculation, and loss of orgasm. In the neurologically impaired these may occur individually or together. In the male, sexual potency is generally equated with erectile ability, failure of which may be either organic or psychogenic in origin. Psychogenic cases far outnumber organic, and often both etiologies are active.

The sexual history should explore all aspects of the problem and should be conducted in a frank manner using understandable language. In examining for a possible organic cause, a variety of etiologies must be considered, including anatomical, pharmacologic, endocrine, hematologic, vasculogenic, metabolic, toxic, and postsurgical, as well as neurogenic dysfunction.

Laboratory investigations include screening automated chemistry and hematologic studies; many advocate a routine glucose tolerance test for all impotent males. More detailed endocrine studies may be dictated by the findings of physical examination, and screening serum testosterone levels are suggested.

A specialized psychological interview may identify the cause for the impotence. It is also useful to identify those who are motivated for surgery and those in whom surgery may cause emotional problems. It may also prepare the patient and his wife for the adjustments after surgical intervention. The Minnesota Multiphasic Personality Inventory (MMPI) is one of the tools most often used in this evaluation. Nocturnal penile tumescence monitoring is also a useful tool to differentiate organic from psychogenic impotence. It is believed that patients unable to have nocturnal erections (which occur in association with REM sleep) probably have organic impotence, whereas those who do have nocturnal erections have a psychogenic etiology. Electromyographic studies to measure the latency of the evoked response in the sacral reflex arc may be useful to identify those with subtle neurogenic causes for impotence.

After the initial neurological insult, be it due to spinal cord injury, cerebrovascular accident, or multiple sclerosis, the full extent of the sexual deficit will not be apparent. The patient should be counseled using a positive attitude and indicating all of the possible alternatives, which are many and varied. The patient must be helped to recognize his physical limitations, and if traditional sexual performance (erection, orgasm, ejaculation) is not possible, the psychological rewards of the relationship such as love, companionship, sharing, and warmth should be emphasized. The patient and his partner must be encouraged to experiment, but should not be forced into activities contrary to their moralities.

Some patients will develop satisfactory psychogenic or reflex erections, and in these patients traditional intercourse may be possible with modification only of positioning or other aspect. With time the patient will learn the technique most satisfactory to help him develop good reflex or psychogenic erections, but usually prolonged digital or oral stimulation of the genitalia are necessary.

If vaginal penetration is strongly desired but not possible because of poor erections, then a variety of artificial aids are available. External support of the phallus may be appropriate in some cases; however, the development and perfection of the internally implanted penile prostheses presents a far more satisfactory alternative. These prostheses are basically of two varieties, the semirigid rod and the inflatable prosthesis, and their insertion should be delayed until it is certain that there will be no further recovery. The latter is aesthetically more pleasing to the patient, but mechanical problems lead to a need for surgical revision in a significant percentage. Paraplegic patients unfortunately suffer a significant complication rate from penile prosthetic surgery, and diligent selection criteria must be used. It is important that the neurogenic bladder dysfunction be resolved or properly managed and that the urine be sterile before implantation because infection of the silastic implants will inevitably lead to failure. It is possible to practice intermittent self-catheterization following insertion of the prosthesis, and in addition, the added penile turgidity and bulk will make it easier for a male to wear an external collecting device.

References

1. Barkin M, Dolfin D, Herschorn S, Bharatwal N, Comisarow R: The urologic care of spinal cord injury patient. J Urol 129:335–339, 1983.
2. Bissada NK, Finkbeiner AE: Neuropharmacology of the lower urinary tract, in Finkbeiner AE, Barbour GL, Bissada NK (eds): *Pharmacology of the Urinary Tract and the Male Reproductive System*. New York, Appleton-Century-Crofts, 1982, pp 199–216.
3. Bors E, Comarr AE: *Neurological Urology*. New York, Karger, 1971, p 129.
4. Bradley WE, Timm GW, Scott FB: Innervation of the detrusor muscle and urethra. Urol Clin North Am 1:3–27, 1974.
5. Brindley GS, Polkey CE, Rushton DN: Sacral anterior root stimulators for bladder control in paraplegia. Paraplegia 20:365–381, 1982.
6. Guttmann L, Frankel H: The value of intermittent catheterization in the early management of traumatic paraplegia and tetraplegia. Paraplegia 4:63–84, 1966.
7. Khanna OP: Nonsurgical therapeutic modalities, in Krane RJ, Siroky MB (eds): *Clinical Neuro-Urology*. Boston, Little, Brown and Company, 1979, pp 159–196.
8. Krane RJ, Siroky MB: *Clinical Neuro-Urology*. Boston, Little, Brown, 1979, p 143.
9. Kursh ED, Freehafer A, Persky L: Complications of autonomic dysreflexia. J Urol 118:70–72, 1977.
10. Lapides J: Neuromuscular vesical and ureteral dysfunction, in Campbell MF, Harrison JH (eds): *Urology*, 6th ed. Philadelphia, Saunders, 1976, pp 1343–1370.
11. Lapides J, Diokno AC, Silber SJ, Lowe BS: Clean, intermittent self-catheterization in the treatment of urinary tract disease. Trans Am Assoc Genitourin Surg 63:92–96, 1971.
12. McGuire EJ, Shi-Chun Z, Horwinski ER, Lytton B: Treatment of motor and sensory detrusor instability by electrical stimulation. J Urol 129:78–79, 1983.
13. Nashold BS: Electrical stimulation of the neurogenic bladder from the spinal cord. Presented at the International Symposium

on Electrical Stimulation of the Neurogenic Bladder, Frankfurt, Germany, 1976.

14. Ramsden PD, Smith JC, Dunn M, Ardran GM: Distension therapy for the unstable bladder: Later results including an assessment of repeat distensions. Br J Urol 48:623–629, 1976.

15. Scott FB, Light JK, Fishman IF, West JE: Implantation of an artificial sphincter for urinary incontinence. Contemp Surg 18:11–35, 1981.

16. Siroky MB, Krane RJ: Physiology of male sexual function, in Krane RJ, Siroky MB (eds): *Clinical Neuro-Urology*. Boston, Little, Brown, 1979, pp 45–62.

17. Torrens M, Hald T: Bladder denervation procedures. Urol Clin North Am 6:283–293, 1979.

18. Webster GD: Urodynamic studies, in Resnick MI, Older RA (eds): *Diagnosis of Genitourinary Disease*. New York, Thieme-Stratton, 1982, pp 173–204.

19. Webster GD: Pharmacologic management of lower urinary tract dysfunction. Drug Ther 15:113–135, 1983.

20. Wein AJ: Classification of neurogenic voiding dysfunction. J Urol 125:605–609, 1981.

21. Wein AJ, Raezer DM: Physiology of micturition, in Krane RJ, Siroky MB (eds): *Clinical Neuro-Urology*. Boston, Little, Brown, 1979, pp 1–33.

22. Wein AJ, Raezer DM, Benson GS: Management of neurogenic bladder dysfunction in the adult. Urology 8:432–443, 1976.

23. Yalla SV, Fam BA, Gabilondo FB, Jacobs S, DiBenedetto M, Rossier AB, Gittes RF: Anteromedian external urethral sphincterotomy: Technique, rationale and complications. J Urol 117:489–493, 1977.

35

Preoperative Evaluation of a Neurosurgical Patient

Ted S. Keller

A multifaceted appraisal of patients who are to undergo neurosurgical procedures is often required since the nervous system and its operative manipulation may effect widespread physiologic and metabolic changes in the body. Therefore, a thorough preoperative medical evaluation and optimization of the patient's medical condition may make for a smoother postoperative course or may prevent some postoperative complications. Also, the surgeon and the anesthesiologist must consider how pre-existing disease or malfunction of other body systems will affect the functional integrity of the central nervous system before, during, and following the operation.

Once an indication for a specific operation has been established by the surgeon and surgical consultants, a general assessment of operative risk is necessary, not only to plan the perioperative management but also to inform the patient and/or the patient's family in a rational and honest way of the potential benefits of surgical intervention as well as the risks.

The most prominent consideration in risk assessment for elective neurosurgical procedures is the danger of functional loss related to the primary neurosurgical disease and its direct surgical attack. The primary neurosurgical risks are of two major types: (1) location-specific and (2) disease-specific. Each neural structure, its location, and its function should be appraised in relation to the pathologic lesion to be approached surgically and the susceptibility of each structure to functional damage during surgery should be considered. For instance, when operation on an aneurysm of the circle of Willis or operation for a tumor located in or near the tentorial notch is contemplated, risks of extraocular muscle palsies due to injury of the third, fourth, and sixth cranial nerves should be discussed. Likewise, when a subfrontal intracranial approach is to be employed for surgical attack on aneurysms, cerebrospinal fluid fistulas, or suprasellar masses, the chances of postoperative anosmia due to olfactory nerve injury should be thoroughly discussed with the patient so that he or she will be fully prepared to deal with the possibility of this deficit following operation. Disease-specific considerations would comprise operative complications unique to attack of a particular type of central nervous system pathology. For instance, the risks of significant intraoperative hemorrhage would be higher in a patient with an intracranial aneurysm than in one undergoing surgery for biopsy of an intracerebral neoplasm. However, a patient with a large amount of pre-existing cerebral edema from an intracerebral neoplasm would be at considerably higher risk for significant postoperative brain swelling and intracranial hypertension than would a patient with an unruptured intracranial aneurysm. Other risk considerations may depend on matters other than actual pathology, being related rather to matters such as intraoperative patient positioning, e.g., the risk of air embolism in the sitting position.

Pre-existing cardiac disease is a well-known contributor to operative morbidity and mortality in neurosurgical patients. While this is often a problem from an intraoperative anesthetic standpoint, medical complications from such cardiac problems may also arise in the postoperative course. The patients at highest risk from a cardiac standpoint are those with (1) a history suggestive of myocardial ischemia and (2) those with clinical or diagnostic evidence of left ventricular dysfunction. Preoperative 12-lead EKG, rhythm strip, or even stress testing can be of assistance in revealing the presence of and the severity of potential myocardial ischemia. However the most reliable indicator of the presence of significant ischemic myocardial disease is the patient's history. This may also be true in regard to assessment of left ventricular function. A history of dyspnea on exertion and of peripheral edema may precede any definitive diagnostic evidence of such. Cardiac conduction disturbance and arrhythmias, as well as hypertensive cardiovascular disease, are also powerful contributing risk factors in all operative patients, especially those patients with serious or life-threatening neurosurgical disease entities who require emergent operative treatment before meticulous preoperative stabilization of these conditions can be done. In the patient with severe cardiovascular disease preoperative placement of a pulmonary artery catheter may be advisable for intraoperative monitoring of left ventricular function by way of pulmonary wedge pressure and cardiac output determinations.

The presence of significant pulmonary dysfunction can also affect operative risk. Again, one of the more sensitive indicators of this is the patient's history. A history of dyspnea, either on exertion or at rest, is important in preoperative assessment, as is a history of chronic cough or sputum production, recent respiratory infection, wheezing, or tobacco smoking. If there is a significant history of pulmonary symptomatology, preoperative assessment by pulmonary consultants may be advisable. In addition to the routine chest x-ray, pulmonary function tests and arterial blood gas sampling may be of assistance in determining the degree of pulmonary impairment. Preoperative chest percussion, intermittent positive pressure breathing treatments, and bronchodilator therapy may improve the patient's pulmonary status prior to the anticipated operation. Cessation of tobacco smoking several days prior to operation may also aid in maximal preoperative pulmonary care.

Renal function can affect the perioperative management of the neurosurgical patient. Routine screening of patients with serum electrolytes, blood urea nitrogen, and serum creatinine levels (as well as routine urinalysis) will sort out most patients with significant renal dysfunction so that appropriate management adjustments can be made. These tests may also aid the surgeon in assessing the state of hydration and any water and electrolyte imbalances.

Hepatic dysfunction is rarely a source of significant neurosurgical morbidity and mortality but may affect primary anesthetic management. The one not infrequent exception is coagulopathy secondary to hepatic disease, which may require vigorous correction preoperatively. However, the patient with a history of significant hepatic disease or with laboratory evidence of mild hepatic dysfunction may not be a candidate for intraoperative use of halogenated anesthetic agents that could further disrupt hepatic physiology.

The patient's hematologic status is usually screened adequately by performance of a complete blood count and of a coagulation profile that includes prothrombin time, partial thromboplastin time, and platelet count. Serious anemia and polycythemia can present additional operative risk and should be corrected prior to any elective neurosurgical procedure. Leukocytosis may indicate systemic infection, and leukopenia may pose a risk in terms of *increased* susceptibility to infection. Abnormalities of coagulation can be assessed from the patient's history (e.g., hemophilia) or from appropriate tests of coagulation, and most often preoperative correction of these coagulation deficits is desirable. For elective surgery, preoperative evaluation of the patient by a hematologist may be advisable. The patient with neoplastic disease who has been on chemotherapeutic agents may also be strongly suspected of harboring a significant coagulopathy.

Evidence of an active infectious process, either local (e.g., urinary tract infection) or systemic (e.g., subacute bacterial endocarditis), can also alter operative risk, and appropriate treatment of infections should be considered prior to surgery.

Following complete preoperative assessment, a thorough and frank discussion should take place between the surgeon and the patient (and/or family) regarding the primary neurosurgical disease, the techniques of operation deemed necessary for treatment, indications for operation, optional methods of treatment, risks of surgery, postoperative care, and potential postoperative complications. Chances of success should also be discussed, and the possibility of an unsatisfactory result or failure of surgery to alleviate the pathology or to relieve symptoms should also be presented as potential outcomes. Since the prospect of surgery in itself is often frightening to the patient, a frank discussion of these potential neurosurgical or anesthetic complications, many of which can be quite serious, can further heighten the patient's anxieties. An empathetic approach on the part of the surgeon can often do much to allay the anxieties provoked by the "informed consent" process by making the patient feel comfortable with asking questions about the surgery, which the surgeon answers as honestly as possible without feeling threatened by the patient's fears. If the question of a second opinion arises prior to surgery, it is best to honor or even to encourage the patient's wishes unless the presence of a true surgical emergency makes taking the time for such an opinion inadvisable. In short, an honest and knowledgeable approach will often enhance the surgeon-patient relationship and provide both parties with an optimal psychological advantage for a major neurosurgical operation. Such sensitivity and honesty will usually carry over into the period of postoperative care and outpatient follow-up as long as that attitude is maintained.

After operative indications and risks have been plotted and after any systemic disturbances have been identified, thorough consideration should be given to correction of or optimization of metabolic, hematologic, respiratory, and cardiovascular status. Patients with intraspinal or intracranial disease may also require special premedication with steroid agents to reduce or minimize edema of central nervous system structures or medication to prevent complications such as infection or convulsions.

Common metabolic derangements that may require preoperative treatment include disorders of glucose metabolism (diabetes mellitus) and of electrolyte and water imbalance. The patient with known diabetes should have this condition optimally stabilized by treatment with parenteral or oral hypoglycemic agents before elective surgery is performed, especially intracranial or spinal surgery. The stresses brought about by the surgical procedure itself, by anesthesia, or by the use of high-dose corticosteroid agents will often worsen such patients' hyperglycemia, which could prove detrimental in the postoperative course. Diabetic patients may also be at higher risk for poor wound healing. Patients with intracranial disease of many kinds will either have or develop the syndrome of inappropriate antidiuretic hormone secretion, in which the patient tends to retain water, leading to severe hyponatremia and relative water intoxication.[5] The presence of this syndrome implies the presence of a normal or elevated intravascular volume and should be treated by preoperative fluid restriction until serum sodium approaches a more normal level. If this metabolic aberration is not managed properly, injudicious crystalloid administration during or following operation may worsen the hyponatremia. Water intoxication of itself can cause cerebral edema and convulsions. Disorders of potassium balance may also be present. Hypokalemia (potassium deficiency) can cause dangerous intraoperative or postoperative cardiac arrhythmias, this condition being especially common in patients on chronic diuretic treatment for hypertension or heart failure. Hyperkalemia may be seen in patients with renal failure or in those with massive tissue trauma. This aberration should also be corrected prior to surgery and anesthesia either with enteral ion-exchange resins or with parenteral glucose and insulin infusions.

The state of nutrition may also be an important consideration in the preoperative neurosurgical patient. Chronic alcoholism is well known to affect both metabolic and nutritional factors so that the alcoholic may suffer from malnutrition on the basis of vitamin deficiencies (especially thiamine) or of poor foodstuff intake or poor caloric intake. All alcoholic patients should routinely be given oral or parenteral thiamine both preoperatively and postoperatively. A history of large alcohol intake just prior to hospitalization should also raise the question of acute dehydration.

The chronically obese patient with neurosurgical problems may also pose a unique dilemma. Though the obese patient's nutrition may be more than adequate, systemic problems such as diabetes, hypertension, and pulmonary insufficiency may be more frequent. Mechanical factors relating to the obesity may also present potential perioperative problems. These patients may be more difficult to mobilize physically in the postoperative course, which can predispose to pulmonary and thromboembolic complications. Obesity in patients with spinal disease, especially those with lumbar disc disease, can lead to a suboptimal postoperative result. For these reasons, strong consideration should be given to a strict weight reduction program before elective surgery is performed.

Hematologic disorders should be treated and corrected preoperatively in most patients. Severe anemia may require blood transfusions before surgery. If polycythemia is present, the etiology of this should be determined. "Relative polycythemia" may be seen in acute dehydration, and appropriate treatment may only require intravenous crystalloid administration. If polycythemia rubra vera or polycythemia due to chronic hypoxic lung disease is confirmed, then preoperative phlebotomy may be advisable. If a coagulopathy is identified, the cause of this disorder should be elucidated in the preoperative assessment. The most appropriate treatment, either with parenteral coagulation factors (fresh frozen plasma, factor VIII, platelet concentrate) or with parenteral vitamin K, can then be selected. If the patient has been

anticoagulated with intravenous heparin, discontinuation of the heparin at an appropriate time prior to surgery or medical reversal of heparin with protamine sulfate at the time of surgery may be advisable.

Cardiovascular factors can also play a powerful role in outcome from both the surgical procedure itself and anesthesia. As discussed previously, the pre-existence of symptomatic coronary artery disease, hypertension, or congestive heart failure figures strongly in assessment of preoperative risk, and cardiovascular function should definitely be made optimal by specific medical treatment of each disease entity. Other more subtle cardiovascular deficits may also be present and may be a source of intraoperative or postoperative problems. These subtle but powerful factors include: (1) dehydration, or systemic hypovolemia; and (2) relative hypotension (in the medically treated hypertensive patient).

The primary consequences of dehydration from a cardiovascular standpoint are lowered blood volume and subsequent reduction in cardiac output. The chronically hypertensive patient whose blood pressure is being lowered by medical treatment with diuretics and with arterial vasodilators may also have a low cardiac output because of such treatment. It is known that in chronic hypertensive patients the cerebrovascular autoregulatory curve is "shifted to the right," so that cerebral blood flow will begin to fall during systemic hypotension at a higher blood pressure than in patients without hypertension.[7] Therefore, overly vigorous lowering of blood pressure in the hypertensive patient may cause greater susceptibility to cerebral ischemia in the event that significant cerebrovascular occlusive disease is already present and/or that a major intracranial procedure involving brain retraction or brain manipulation is performed.

Although fluid restriction may be a necessary and advisable preoperative measure in patients with an intracranial neoplasm, patients with cerebrovascular occlusive disease and with ruptured intracranial aneurysms (who are at high risk for ischemic complications in the perioperative course) should have their intravascular volume closely maintained with intravenous crystalloid and colloid since recent experiments and clinical data have revealed a strong relationship between cerebral blood flow to marginally supplied brain regions and the cardiac output.[3,4]

Postoperative infectious complications can often be reduced by appropriate preoperative measures. Thorough preoperative cleansing of the site of proposed surgery is usually advisable. Screening of patients with active infections of the respiratory tract and of the urinary tract by history and physical examination and by routine preoperative testing is often beneficial.

The role of perioperative antibiotic administration remains controversial, but the strongest evidence at present is that intraoperative antibiotic administration only for elective "clean" neurosurgical cases seems to be the most beneficial and rational method for prophylaxis against postoperative neurosurgical infection.[6] The management of "contaminated" cases involving primary infections of the central nervous system varies, but it is often advisable to maintain multidrug therapy in these patients both preoperatively and postoperatively.

Any neurosurgical patient who will require open intraoperative manipulation of the brain or of the spinal cord should be premedicated with moderate to large doses of corticosteroids. This is done in order to minimize postoperative edema formation, and the usual drug of choice is dexamethasone, 10 mg given parenterally or orally the night before surgery and 4 to 10 mg given on call to the operating room. Patients who have been on steroid medications for antiedema therapy, e.g., brain tumor patients, should continue on these medications in the perioperative period. Patients undergoing surgical procedures for masses near or in the pituitary fossa, either by a trans-sphenoidal or a transcranial approach, should be prophylactically premedicated with hydrocortisone, 100 mg, to prevent the possibility of addisonian crisis in the perioperative period.

Some surgeons think that patients undergoing supratentorial intracranial surgery should be treated with prophylactic anticonvulsant therapy although if the patient has not had clinical seizures, it is usually unnecessary to begin these until after the surgery has been completed. The occurrence of intraoperative or immediate postoperative convulsions is rare; therefore it is usually unnecessary to give therapeutic "loading" doses of phenobarbital or phenytoin preoperatively. Patients undergoing routine ventricular shunt procedures for hydrocephalus and patients undergoing surgery of the posterior fossa usually do not require prophylactic anticonvulsant administration.

Vigorous preoperative treatment of serious intracranial hypertension has been recommended in recent years for selected patients with intracerebral hematomas, either traumatic[2] or spontaneous[1] in origin. Though the emergency management of these intracranial clots remains debatable, it is believed that many of these lesions can be managed nonoperatively if intracranial pressure can be controlled by the use of hyperventilation, osmotic agents, and ventricular drainage. If pressure is difficult to control with such conservative measures, then direct surgical evacuation of the

hematoma may then be considered advisable. Such preoperative control of intracranial hypertension may make the surgical procedure safer for the patient.

Preoperative assessment and treatment should therefore be tailored to optimize the patient's clinical condition in regard to both the neurosurgical disease and to any pre-existing disorder of other organ systems in such manner that the operative risks are minimized and postoperative care is facilitated.

References

1. Duff TA, Ayeni S, Levin AB, Javid M: Nonsurgical management of spontaneous intracerebral hematoma. Neurosurgery 9:387–393, 1981.
2. Galbraith S, Teasdale G: Predicting the need for operation in the patient with an occult traumatic intracranial hematoma. J Neurosurg 55:75–81, 1981.
3. Keller TS, McGillicuddy JE, LaBond VA, Kindt GW: Volume expansion in focal cerebral ischemia: The effect of cardiac output on local cerebral blood flow. Clin Neurosurg 29:40–50, 1982.
4. Keller TS, McGillicuddy JE, LaBond VA, Kindt GW: Cardiac output–mediated responses of local cerebral blood flow in monkeys with focal cerebral ischemia: Therapeutic effects of intravascular volume expansion. In press, 1983.
5. Lester MC, Nelson PB: Neurological aspects of vasopressin release and the syndrome of inappropriate secretion of antidiuretic hormone. Neurosurgery 8:735–740, 1981.
6. Malis LI: Prevention of neurosurgical infection by intraoperative antibiotics. Neurosurgery 5:339–343, 1979.
7. Strandgaard S, Olesen J, Skinhoj E, Lassen NA: Autoregulation of brain circulation in severe arterial hypertension. Br Med J 1:507–510, 1973.

36
Blood Coagulation
Salvatore V. Pizzo

Blood coagulation is initiated as a result of vascular injury. This injury may be as subtle as retraction of endothelial cells, creating small gaps that expose the underlying basement membrane, or as gross as the transection of a blood vessel. When an artery or arteriole is injured, neural mecha-

nisms trigger vasoconstriction, which is the most nonspecific means of achieving hemostasis. Capillaries lack a muscular wall, but they constrict in response to humoral and local factors. These local controls involve release by platelets of a number of vasoactive substances. The importance of vasoconstriction in hemostasis is exemplified by the bleeding that follows transection of the middle meningeal artery. This vessel tends to be fixed to the skull and cannot readily constrict.

Vasoconstriction is generally not sufficient to prevent bleeding, and specific mechanisms of coagulation have evolved. This process involves the interaction of platelets, blood coagulation proteins, and various plasma protease inhibitors. The intact, endothelial-lined vessel wall tends to be a nonthrombogenic surface for at least two reasons: (1) the intact wall synthesizes a potent inhibitor of platelet aggregation, prostacyclin; and (2) the endothelium is covered by a glycocalyx containing heparinlike substances (heparinoids). Heparinoids activate the plasma protease inhibitor, antithrombin III, a potent anticoagulant. When the vessel wall is disrupted, prostacyclin synthesis decreases and the heparinoid coating is lost, which favors coagulation. Loss of the endothelium, moreover, exposes the underlying tissue, containing collagen and other substances that trigger platelet adhesion and aggregation. The collagen also serves as a site for factor XII activation, initiating blood coagulation via the intrinsic system. Damaged endothelium around the injury site releases "tissue factor" (thromboplastin), which activates factor VII and initiates the extrinsic system of coagulation.

Platelets are present in the blood at a concentration of 200,000 to 400,000 per mm^3. They circulate as smooth, disc-shaped cells with a diameter of about 2 μm. Platelets adhere to the collagen exposed after endothelial damage and undergo a number of secretory reactions, releasing adenosine diphosphate (ADP), epinephrine, serotonin, and various prostaglandins. The prostaglandin thromboxane A_2 is the most potent platelet aggregation agent yet described. ADP, however, is the most important aggregating agent under physiological conditions. It is released not only by the platelets but also by anoxic red blood cells trapped within the developing clot.

Platelet aggregation also involves various coagulation proteins, including thrombin, factor VIII/von Willebrand factor, and fibrinogen. In the absence of fibrinogen, platelets show little response to ADP. A specific platelet receptor for fibrinogen has been described and characterized, but it is uncertain why this receptor must be occupied before platelets will aggregate in the presence of ADP. Thrombin and factor VIII/von Willebrand factor bind to distinct and specific receptors on the platelets. Occupancy of these receptors directly stimulates platelet aggregation.

The platelet release reactions are accompanied by a dramatic change in platelet shape from smooth discs to spiny spheres. These spiny spheres are quite sticky and aggregate rapidly. The aggregates are capable of establishing hemostasis in small vessels but are unstable and cannot seal a major bleeding site. The activation of the plasma coagulation proteins, along with platelet aggregation, ultimately results in the formation of a hemostatic plug at the site of a vascular injury. The hemostatic plug consists of tangled masses of fibrin and platelet aggregates with variable amounts of other blood cells trapped within the mass.

Blood coagulation involves a cascade of reactions in which an enzyme is generated at each step, and this enzyme then activates the next factor in the cascade. This mechanism offers unique potential for amplification of the initial response to injury. Table 36-1 lists the coagulation proteins. Of these proteins, factors II, VII, IX, X, XI, and XII and prekallikrein are all zymogens, which become converted to proteases during coagulation. Factor V, factor VIII/von Willebrand protein, and high molecular weight kininogen are cofactors required to speed up several of the activation reactions.

The coagulation system is divided into the so-called intrinsic and extrinsic pathways. The sequence of reactions is diagramed in Fig. 36-1. Ultimately, both pathways generate the activated form of factor X (Xa). Factor Xa is then responsible for the activation of prothrombin to thrombin. This latter enzyme cleaves fibrinopeptides A and B from the fibrinogen molecule, generating fibrin. Thrombin also activates the crosslinking enzyme, factor XIII. The resultant factor XIIIa crosslinks fibrin, stabilizing the developing network from attack by the fibrinolytic system.

TABLE 36-1   The Blood Coagulation Proteins

Factor	Synonyms
I	Fibrinogen
II	Prothrombin
III	Tissue thromboplastin, tissue factor
IV	Calcium
V	Accelerator globulin, proaccelerin, labile factor
VI*	———
VII	Proconvertin, stable factor
VIII†	Antihemophilic factor or globulin
IX	Christmas factor, plasma thromboplastin component
X	Stuart factor, Stuart-Prower factor
XI	Plasma thromboplastin antecedent
XII	Hageman factor
XIII	Fibrin-stabilizing factor, fibrinoligase
——	Prekallikrein (Fletcher factor)
——	High molecular weight kininogen (Fitzgerald factor)

*Factor VI was at one time used to designate activated factor V.
†Also designated as factor VIII/von Willebrand factor.

The synthesis in the liver of factors II, VII, IX, and X in activatable form requires vitamin K for the conversion of a number of glutamic acid residues to dicarboxylic acids. These γ-carboxyglutamic acid residues are the binding sites for Ca^{+2} and phospholipid and are essential for the function of the vitamin K–dependent factors. Without the interaction of Ca^{+2} and phospholipid, the reactions involving factors II, VII, IX, and X occur very slowly, if at all. Dicumarol is an anticoagulant because it is an antimetabolite of vitamin K. When patients are treated with this drug, immunologically reactive variants of factors II, VII, IX, and X are produced. These proteins, however, lack the γ-carboxyglutamic acid residues and are inactive. The reversal of the anticoagulant effect of dicumarol depends on the catabolic turnover of the modified forms of factors II, VII, IX, and X. This turnover takes hours to days, depending on the protein.

Division of the coagulation system into intrinsic and extrinsic pathways reflects the traditional belief that the former system functions to produce intravascular thrombi while the latter system is involved in coagulation after major tissue injury. This concept is incorrect since "tissue factor," required for activation of the extrinsic pathway, is produced and released by endothelium as described earlier. Conceptually, it is useful to think of the two pathways separately. In addition, the two most common tests of coagulation, the prothrombin time and partial thromboplastin time, are based on separating the reactions of these two pathways. A brief review of each pathway follows.

Injury of the blood vessel wall exposes collagen, which serves as the initiation site for platelet aggregation. Collagen also binds factor XII, which then undergoes autoactivation to factor XIIa. This process is comparatively slow but the resultant factor XIIa converts prekallikrein to kallikrein. This enzyme, in the presence of a protein cofactor, high molecular weight kininogen, rapidly activates more factor XII. These reactions provide an early amplification of the coagulation cascade. The activation of factor XI occurs on

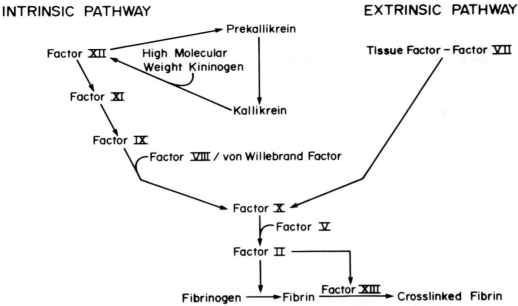

INTRINSIC PATHWAY

Prekallikrein

Factor XII

High Molecular Weight Kininogen

Factor XI

Kallikrein

Factor IX

Factor VIII / von Willebrand Factor

EXTRINSIC PATHWAY

Tissue Factor – Factor VII

Factor X

Factor V

Factor II

Fibrinogen ⟶ Fibrin ⟶ Factor XIII ⟶ Crosslinked Fibrin

Figure 36-1 Diagram of normal blood coagulation indicating the order of the activation reactions. The scheme is read as: "Factor XII activates factor XI, which activates factor IX, . . ." and so on down the cascade.

the same surface at which factor XIIa is bound. This activation also requires high molecular weight kininogen. Factor XIa remains bound to the vessel wall, where it activates factor IX. This reaction requires the presence of Ca^{+2}. Factor IXa is responsible for the activation of factor X. This reaction requires the presence of factor VIII/von Willebrand factor, Ca^{+2}, and phospholipid.

The activation of factor X also occurs as a result of the extrinsic pathway. In these reactions, tissue factor (thromboplastin) released from damaged endothelium reacts with factor VII in the blood. The resultant complex in the presence of Ca^{+2} activates factor X. Activation of factor X, therefore, is the common endpoint of both the intrinsic and extrinsic pathways. Factor Xa in the presence of factor V, Ca^{+2}, and phospholipid will convert prothrombin to thrombin. This enzyme then cleaves fibrinogen, yielding fibrin. The brain is the richest known source of tissue factor. After head injury a considerable amount of this substance may be released, triggering abnormal coagulation.

Fibrinogen consists of three pairs of polypeptide chains, designated $A\alpha$, $B\beta$, and γ. These chains are held together by disulfide bonds. Thrombin cleaves the A and B peptides, yielding fibrin monomer. Fibrin monomers rapidly align to form fibrin polymers. Thrombin also activates factor XIII, which then cross-links the fibrin strands. These cross-links are of several types. Dimers of γ chains form rapidly and the process is completed in several minutes. Subsequently, high molecular weight polymers are formed by the α chains over a period of several hours. These polymers were believed to consist entirely of α chains, but recent amino acid sequence studies indicate that as much as 30 percent of the polymer may consist of mixed polymers of the γ and α chains. The formation of these cross-links is critical because they protect the chains from fibrinolysis.

Hemostasis is achieved by a delicate balance between the coagulation reactions and activation of the fibrinolytic system. The fibrinolytic system consists of plasminogen, plasminogen activator, and α_2-antiplasmin. Plasminogen circulates in the blood in an inactive form. Coagulation triggers release of plasminogen activator from the vessel wall and this substance converts plasminogen to plasmin. Plasmin then digests the clot to yield "fibrin split products." Plasminogen activator is present in only small amounts in vessel walls, preventing massive generation of plasmin. Both plasmin and plasminogen activator bind to fibrin, localizing the fibrinolytic response at the site of thrombosis. Plasma contains a low concentration of α_2-antiplasmin, a potent inhibitor, which will inactivate any plasmin diffusing away from the clot. The fibrinolytic system, therefore, is highly regulated to prevent systemic release of plasmin. This is important because plasmin will digest fibrinogen as well as fibrin.

The fibrinolytic system is subject to a number of therapeutic manipulations. Both urokinase and streptokinase are plasminogen activators that have been used to treat pulmonary emboli and other thrombotic disorders. By contrast, inhibitors of plasminogen activation and plasmin have been used to prevent excess bleeding, such as that occurring in association with ruptured berry aneurysms. The best known of these inhibitors is ϵ-aminocaproic acid, which inhibits plasminogen activation as well as the fibrinolytic activity of plasmin.

The regulation of the hemostatic balance involves not only the coagulation proteins and fibrinolytic system but also a number of plasma proteins that inhibit coagulation. Of these, α_2-macroglobulin, antithrombin III, and α_1-proteinase inhibitor (formerly α_1-antitrypsin) are present in the highest concentration. Antithrombin III (AT III) is a plasma antiprotease and inhibits factors XIIa, XIa, Xa, IXa, and thrombin. The activity of AT III is increased 1000- to 10,000-fold in the presence of heparin, and the efficacy of this anticoagulant is proportional to the level of AT III. Patients with congenital deficiency of AT III therefore have a serious thrombotic disorder responding poorly to heparin, which is itself a very poor thrombin inhibitor.

The coagulation system can be monitored by a number of tests. Of these, the prothrombin time (PT) and partial thromboplastin time (PTT) are the most commonly employed. In both tests, plasma is anticoagulated by addition of a substance which binds Ca^{+2}, preventing activation of the coagulation system. Since all formed elements are removed from the plasma before performing the PT and PTT, neither test is sensitive to platelet defects. The PT is used to monitor the extrinsic system. The test is performed by addition of Ca^{+2} and tissue factor (thromboplastin) to the plasma. This results in rapid activation of factor VII and formation of a clot. The PTT is a test of the intrinsic system. The test is initiated by addition of Ca^{+2} and a source of phospholipid to the plasma.

Defects in coagulation proteins may cause a prolongation of either or both of these tests. A deficiency of factor VII will prolong only the PT. If factors VIII/von Willebrand, IX, XI, and/or XII are deficient, only the PTT is abnormal. Deficiencies of the common pathway components, i.e., factors II, X, and/or V, will result in a prolonged PT and PTT. Moreover, anticoagulant therapy will also prolong these tests. Generally, both tests are prolonged when the patient receives either dicumarol or heparin. However, the PT is most sensitive to dicumarol levels. This follows from the fact that dicumarol tends to suppress the vitamin K–dependent factors in an order that is the inverse of their plasma half-lives. Factor VII has the shortest half-life and is the first factor suppressed, followed by factors IX and X and prothrombin in that order. If a patient is withdrawn from dicumarol, factor VII levels begin returning to normal within several hours because of its 4- to 6-h half-life. This is reflected in a shortening of the PT.

Heparin is best monitored by the PTT since this drug suppresses the coagulation factors by its action on AT III. As described above, AT III inhibits activated factors XII, XI, X, and IX and thrombin. Factor VIIa of the extrinsic pathway, however, is not inhibited. Thus, the PTT is more sensitive to heparin than the PT.

References

1. Murano G: A basic outline of blood coagulation. Semin Thromb Hemostas 6: 140–162, 1980.
2. Pizzo SV: Overview of coagulation, in Koepke JA (ed): *Laboratory Hematology*. New York, Churchill Livingstone, in press, 1984.
3. Pizzo SV: Venous thrombosis, in Koepke JA (ed): *Laboratory Hematology*. New York, Churchill Livingstone, in press, 1984.
4. Weiss HJ: Platelet physiology and abnormalities of platelet function (First of two parts). N Engl J Med 293:531–541, 1975.
5. Wessler, S, Gitel SN: Thrombosis: The relationship of hemostatic mechanisms to drug therapy. J Neurosurg 54:1–11, 1981.

37

Blood Transfusion

Fred V. Plapp
William L. Bayer

Introduction

Several advances in recent years have greatly expanded the capabilities of transfusion therapy. The introduction of a closed system of multiple plastic bags allows a single unit of blood to be collected into a primary bag and then separated into its essential components. In this way a single unit of whole blood can be separated into red blood cells, platelets, plasma, and cryoprecipitated factor VIII:C concentrates, which can be stored and administered individually. Also, the development of hemapheresis techniques has facilitated collection of larger numbers of particular cell types, such as granulocytes and/or platelets, from a single donor since the unused components are simultaneously returned to the donor. Finally, advances in fractionation and chemical processing of larger volumes of pooled plasma have provided several blood derivatives, such as albumin, immune serum globulin, antihemophilic factor, and factor IX (prothrombin) complex.

These advances have made numerous blood components and derivatives available today for transfusion. Physicians need to be well informed about the composition of each of these blood products and the medical indications for their use in order to treat patients safely and effectively. Generally, transfusion is required to improve one or more of the following medical conditions: restoration of blood volume, improvement of oxygen transport, correction of bleeding tendencies, treatment of sepsis in neutropenic patients, and enhancement of immunity. Thorough knowledge of blood component therapy will allow selection of the proper component to treat each of these disorders. Also, the practice of prudent blood component therapy will help to ensure that adequate blood supplies are maintained in the future, since the separation of a single donated unit of blood into multiple components allows each donor to serve the needs of more than one patient.

Blood Components

Whole Blood

Whole blood contains 450 ± 45 ml of blood collected from a single donor, which is mixed with 63 ml of an anticoagulant-preservative. CPDA-1, the most widely used anticoagulant-preservative today, contains citrate, phosphate, dextrose, and adenine. Sufficient citrate is present to chelate the ionized calcium present in a unit of whole blood throughout storage (0.31 g citrate ion per 100 ml blood), thereby inhibiting the calcium-dependent steps of the coagulation cascade. Phosphate, dextrose, and adenine are added so that red cells can continue to synthesize ATP via the glycolytic pathway. These additives allow whole blood and red blood cells to be stored for 35 days at 4°C. Even after 35 days of storage at least 70 percent of the red blood cells will survive and function normally in vivo following transfusion. Whole blood must undergo compatibility testing before transfusion.

Whole blood should not be considered the equivalent of the blood that a patient loses during bleeding since it undergoes several changes during storage. Platelet viability is rapidly lost during storage at 4°C so that by 48 h inadequate numbers of platelets remain for hemostasis. There also is a gradual decline in the activities of factors V and VIII:C, the labile coagulation factors. Factor VIII:C (antihemophilic globulin) levels remain above 80 percent for 1 to 2 days. Factor V (proaccelerin) remains at normal levels for at least 5 days. At 35 days the factor VIII:C level is on the average 40 percent (20 to 100 percent) and the factor V level 30 percent (5 to 55 percent). Factors I, II, VII, IX, X, XI, and XII are stable. All these plasma coagulation factor levels are sufficient to maintain hemostasis.

The pH of the whole blood–CPDA-1 mixture is 7.1 immediately after venipuncture and gradually declines to 6.9 at day 35 owing to accumulation of lactic acid during RBC glycolysis. The concentration of potassium in plasma is 3.5 to 5.0 meq per liter in normal plasma and 100 meq per liter inside red blood cells. During storage there is a slow but constant leakage of potassium from RBCs into the plasma so that by the 35th day the plasma concentration is 13 to 20 meq per liter. Plasma SGOT, LDH, hemoglobin, and whole blood ammonia also gradually increase with storage but present no problems during transfusion.

Whole blood transfusion is indicated for conditions in which there is a need to simultaneously replace blood volume in order to prevent or treat shock and to improve the oxygen-carrying capacity of the blood in order to prevent acute hypoxia. The loss of 500 ml of blood within 5 min is well tolerated by the average adult blood donor, and it is therefore usually inappropriate to transfuse patients with a single unit of whole blood since the recipient probably needs the blood no more than does the donor. Patients who have lost more than 20 percent of their blood volume are more critical and have signs such as tachycardia and decreased systolic blood pressure in spite of compensatory mechanisms such as peripheral vasoconstriction and a shift in fluid from the extravascular to the intravascular space. Hemodilution begins almost immediately after the onset of hemorrhage and continues up to 72 h after cessation of bleeding. Although this influx of fluid does not improve oxygen-carrying capacity, it does help to maintain blood volume and stabilize circulation. In this situation, a single-unit transfusion of blood along with crystalloid or colloid solutions is justifiable since the patient has lost the equivalent of three units of blood.

Adult patients in hemorrhagic shock have usually lost 35 to 40 percent of their blood volume, or approximately 2 liters of blood. These patients will be pale, restless, or unconscious and have hypotension, tachycardia, air hunger, and cold, clammy perspiration. Rapid replacement of fluid volume is more important than blood replacement in shock patients. Blood volume should be immediately replaced with crystalloid solutions such as lactated Ringer's solution or normal saline. Colloids are no more advantageous physiologically than crystalloids during early resuscitation and are more expensive. The early administration of fluids allows sufficient time for ABO typing of the recipient, which takes only a few minutes. In this way, ABO type-specific blood can be given instead of empirically giving units of O negative blood, which often is in short supply. Determination of the patient's Rh type is less important in an emergency since administering Rh-positive blood to an Rh-negative person will not cause significant hemolysis, unlike a transfusion of ABO-incompatible blood. Determination of Rh type is more important when transfusing female patients of childbearing potential, since administration of Rh-positive blood to an Rh-negative female could stimulate the synthesis of anti-D IgG. Anti-D could cause hemolytic disease of the newborn during a subsequent pregnancy. In the event that Rh-positive blood is given to an Rh-negative woman of childbearing potential, anti-D formation can be suppressed by giving one vial of Rh-immune globulin per 30 ml of transfused Rh-positive blood within 72 h after transfusion.

Transfusion of a large quantity of whole blood approaching or exceeding the recipient's blood volume within a 24-h period is considered a massive transfusion. Following transfusions equivalent to one blood volume, approximately 60 percent of the patient's own cells and plasma will be replaced. In our region, 50 to 60 percent of all blood units are transfused before they have been stored 1 week. Patients who are massively transfused receive even a larger proportion of blood that has a shorter storage time. If such patients have not developed shock, bleeding due to depletion of coagulation factors is seldom a problem. If these patients continue to bleed, a platelet count, a prothrombin time, and an activated partial thromboplastin time should be obtained to determine corrective therapy. Massive transfusion with stored red blood cells that are depleted of 2,3-DPG should theoretically interfere with oxygen release to tissues. However, this rarely appears to be clinically significant. Citrate toxicity is also a potential but rarely seen problem, since citrate is rapidly metabolized to bicarbonate and then to carbon dioxide and water. Hypocalcemia is almost never seen, while ionized calcium may be slightly depressed. An adult patient with normal liver function should be able to tolerate a unit of blood every 5 min without receiving supplemental calcium.

Metabolic acidosis is often seen early in patients receiving massive transfusion owing to the cumulative effects of shock and the citric and lactic acids present in stored blood. These acids are readily metabolized to bicarbonate, leading eventu-

TABLE 37-1 Comparison of a Unit of Whole Blood and a Unit of Red Blood Cells

Parameter	Whole Blood	RBCs
Total volume	500–550 ml	250 ml
Red cell mass	200 ml	200 ml
Plasma volume	250 ml	75–100 ml
Hematocrit	40%	70%
Total protein	49 g	36 g
Anticoagulant (citrate)	67 ml	22 ml

ally to metabolic alkalosis and hypokalemia. Blood is stored at 4°C and usually warms up to 10°C by the time it is transfused. Rapid transfusion of large volumes of cold blood can cause hypothermia in a patient, with ensuing cardiac arrhythmias. Infusion of cold blood directly into central veins has even been associated with cardiac arrest. These complications can be prevented by warming blood to 37°C during transfusion by using a blood warmer. Patients receiving larger volumes of blood should always receive blood in this manner.

Red Blood Cells

Red blood cells (RBCs), commonly referred to as packed red cells, are the cells that remain following separation of plasma from whole blood at any time during the dating period. Approximately 225 to 250 ml of plasma and CPDA-1 mixture is removed, resulting in a unit containing about 200 ml of red blood cells and 100 ml of plasma and CPDA-1 with a packed cell volume of 70 percent. A unit of RBCs has the same red cell mass as a unit of whole blood and therefore provides the same oxygen-carrying capacity in half the volume (Table 37-1). RBCs can also be stored for 35 days at 4°C and should undergo compatibility testing prior to transfusion.

Transfusion of RBCs is indicated in clinical situations in which there is a deficit in RBC mass not associated with decreased blood volume or colloid osmotic pressure. A surgical operation or asymptomatic anemia are not, in themselves, indications for transfusion. RBCs, and not whole blood, should be used when transfusion is required for patients with chronic anemia that does not respond to specific therapy, such as iron, vitamin B_{12}, or folic acid. These patients usually have normal or slightly increased total blood volume in spite of their reduced red cell mass. The decision to transfuse these patients should be based on clinical judgment and not an attempt to elevate the patient's hemoglobin or hematocrit to some arbitrary value since most patients with chronic anemia can tolerate hemoglobin levels of 7 to 8 g/dl. One unit of red blood cells should raise a patient's hemoglobin by 1 g/dl or the hematocrit by 3 percent.

RBCs accompanied by crystalloid solutions appear to be as beneficial as whole blood in replacing blood loss during surgery unless there is significant hypovolemia. An operative blood loss of 1000 ml can usually be replaced by crystalloid and/or colloid solutions alone. Greater blood loss should be supplemented by RBC transfusions.

The reduced volume of plasma in a unit of red blood cells compared with whole blood offers several other advantages.

The 50 percent reduction in volume minimizes the possibility of hypervolemia. RBC transfusion is less likely to contribute to congestive heart failure in patients with cardiac problems. Also the removal of plasma reduces the electrolyte, citrate, and organic acid load transfused. Citrate, pyruvate, lactic acid, and ammonia are metabolized by the liver. The use of packed red cells for transfusion of patients with compromised hepatic function will minimize the adverse effects of these substances. Furthermore, a unit of red blood cells contains fewer plasma proteins, cellular fragments, and other potential plasma allergens and such transfusions are associated with a lower incidence of febrile and allergic transfusion reactions.

RBCs also have reduced amounts of the isoagglutinins, anti-A and anti-B, which becomes an important consideration when blood of the same ABO group as the recipient's is not available. When ABO-specific blood is not available, it is important to use RBCs that are still compatible with the recipient's serum, that is, compatibility in the major crossmatch. The donor's RBCs must not contain A or B antigens that react with the anti-A or anti-B present in the recipient's serum. In this situation the large amount of anti-A or anti-B in the recipient's 3 liters of plasma would bind to transfused ABO-incompatible RBCs and possibly cause hemolysis. The reverse situation, in which the donor's red blood cells do not have an antigen that reacts with a recipient's antibody but the recipient's RBCs have an antigen that reacts with an antibody in the donor's plasma, is not as important. In this case, the small amount of antibody present in the 100 ml of plasma remaining in a RBC unit is rapidly diluted about 30-fold in the recipient's plasma before the antibody can injure enough RBCs to be clinically apparent. Whole blood should not be used when switching ABO blood groups since each unit contains 250 ml of plasma and therefore 2 to 3 times more isoagglutinins. Table 37-2 summarizes the proper selection of RBCs for Rh-positive recipients when ABO group-specific blood is unavailable.

Although group O packed red cells can be given to any ABO group recipient and have been designated as universal donor blood, large volumes could possibly give a recipient enough anti-A or anti-B to cause a positive direct antiglobulin test and hemolysis. Therefore, there really is no such thing as universal donor blood.

TABLE 37-2 Selection of Donor Blood When Type-Specific Blood Is Unavailable

Recipient's ABO Group	1st Choice	2d Choice	3d Choice
O+	O+	O−	None
A+	A+	O+ RBCs	O− RBCs
B+	B+	O+ RBCs	O− RBCs
AB+	AB+	A+ or B+ RBCs	O+ RBCs

For Rh-negative recipients the order of choices is the same as far as ABO groups are concerned. Rh-negative patients can be given Rh-positive blood if they lack anti-D antibody. This alternative may be used in emergency or in elective situations when the likelihood of transfusions in the future is low. Rh-positive blood should not be given to patients who have had anti-D antibody and is best not given to Rh-negative women of childbearing potential or to Rh-negative women who have had mutiple pregnancies. Multiparous patients may no longer have detectable anti-D antibody but such a transfusion may lead to an anamnestic response and a delayed hemolytic reaction.

Recently general guidelines have been established regarding the number of red blood cell units that need to be ordered and crossmatched for routine neurosurgical cases[4] (Table 37-3).

Most elective neurosurgery cases require only that one or two units of RBCs be crossmatched before surgery. A type and screen instead of a crossmatch is recommended for those procedures in which a transfusion is seldom required. In the unlikely event that blood is needed on an emergency basis during one of these operations, type-specific blood could be given without any adverse affects 99.9 percent of the time since the antibody screen would have detected any alloantibodies of clinical importance. Furthermore, a crossmatch could be completed within 1 h if necessary since the results of the recipient's blood type and antibody screen would already be known. In most cases the patient could be supported by crystalloid or colloid solutions until then.

Close adherence to this guideline for transfusion will decrease unnecessary crossmatching of blood, which in turn will improve each hospital's available blood supplies, decrease outdating of blood, and decrease the patient's laboratory and transfusion fees.

TABLE 37-3 Need for RBC Units in Neurosurgery

Elective Surgical Procedure	Number of Units Crossmatched
Carotid endarterectomy	1
Carpal tunnel release	Type and screen*
Cordotomy	Type and screen
Craniectomy	1
Cranioplasty	1
Craniosynostosis	1
Craniotomy	
Aneurysm	2
Fistula	1
Pituitary tumor	1
Posterior fossa	1
Tumor	2
Laminectomy	
Cervical	1
Lumbar	Type and screen
Lumbar tumor	3
Thoracic	1
Multiple rhizotomies	Type and screen
Nerve repair (median, ulnar, peroneal)	Type and screen
Trans-sphenoidal hypophysectomy	2
Ventriculoperitoneal shunt	Type and screen

*Type and screen means that an ABO and Rh type and an antibody screen are performed.

Leukocyte-Poor Red Blood Cells

A unit of RBCs can be further modified by removing the bulk of the leukocytes present in the buffy coat. The extent of leukocyte removal depends on the method used. Generally 80 percent of the leukocytes are removed along with some plasma. The resulting unit has a hematocrit of 90 percent and contains less than 10^9 leukocytes. These units can be stored for 35 days and should be compatible before use.

Leukocyte-poor RBCs are primarily indicated for patients with repeated febrile transfusion reactions. Febrile episodes are the most common adverse reaction to blood transfusion, accompanying up to 1 percent of the units of blood transfused. They usually occur in multiparous or multiply transfused patients. These reactions are thought to be caused by cytotoxic antileukocyte antibodies. Most patients who have a single febrile reaction after receiving a unit of RBCs will not have a subsequent second reaction. Approximately 15 percent of all patients will have a second febrile reaction during future transfusions of RBCs.[9] Therefore, it is suggested that an additional unit of RBCs be given to any patient experiencing a single febrile transfusion reaction. If a second reaction occurs, it is reasonable to switch to leukocyte-poor RBCs for future transfusions. Leukocyte-poor red blood cells that have been irradiated with 1500 to 3000 rad to kill lymphocytes are also indicated for children with immunodeficiency disorders to prevent graft versus host disease.

Saline-Washed Red Blood Cells

Saline-washed RBCs are units of whole blood or RBCs that have been washed with saline, either manually or with an automated cell washer. They have a hematocrit of 70 percent and have been depleted of 99 percent of the plasma proteins and 85 percent of the leukocytes. Other RBC metabolites are also removed. Saline washed RBCs must be used within 24 h after washing since the original blood bag has been entered, which breaks the hermetic seal and increases the possibility of bacterial contamination. These units are recommended for patients who continue to experience allergic or febrile transfusion reactions due to plasma proteins, since plasma proteins are almost totally removed in the washing. Patients with IgA deficiencies should receive saline washed RBCs since they often have developed anti-IgA antibodies, which can cause anaphylaxis if the patient receives any blood product containing IgA. RBCs can also be frozen in the presence of glycerol and then washed after thawing to remove glycerol. These RBCs are used for the same purpose as saline washed cells. Additionally, they are used to stockpile rare blood types.

Platelet Concentrates

A *platelet concentrate* is defined as the platelets obtained from a single unit of platelet-rich plasma separated within 6 h after whole blood has been collected. At least 5.5×10^{10} platelets are present, which are suspended in 30 to 50 ml of plasma to maintain the pH greater than 6.3. Immediately after preparation, platelet concentrates are continuously agitated at 20 to 24°C. Previously all platelet concentrates had an expiration date of 72 h after the time of processing. Recently a new polyolefin plastic bag has been developed. Polyolefin has increased permeability to oxygen and carbon dioxide, thereby retarding the accumulation of lactic acid and preventing the fall in pH. Platelets collected in these bags can be stored for 5 days. Platelets can be transfused without compatibility testing and ABO-incompatible platelets can be given unless they contain excessive numbers of red blood cells. Rh-negative units should be used for Rh-negative women of childbearing potential. However, as many of the patients who receive frequent platelet transfusions have terminal illnesses or are in an emergency bleeding situation, Rh-positive platelets may have to be given. One vial of Rh immune globulin may be given to those women who are likely to become pregnant in the future.

Platelets serve at least two major functions in the prevention and stoppage of bleeding. They form the primary hemostatic plug by adhering to injured blood vessels and aggregating to each other. Also, they contribute to the coagulation cascade by supplying platelet factor 3, which enhances the conversion of prothrombin to thrombin. Qualitative or quantitative defects in platelets impair these functions and predispose to bleeding. Normal people have platelet counts between 150,000 and 300,000 per microliter, which appears to be more than adequate to prevent bleeding. Although a correlation exists between the platelet count and the risk of hemorrhage, no absolute threshold has been defined below which bleeding always occurs. Each patient must be evaluated individually. Usually patients have little risk of spontaneously hemorrhaging if the platelet count is greater than 50,000 per μl. However, this level may not be sufficient to prevent bleeding during surgery or trauma. A platelet count between 10,000 to 50,000 per μl is associated with a moderate risk of spontaneous hemorrhage while a platelet count less than 10,000 per μl is associated with higher risk (Table 37-4). Determination of platelet size may also be of value in predicting bleeding tendencies since larger platelets apparently provide better hemostasis.[5]

Transfusion of platelet concentrates is indicated for the treatment of hemorrhage in patients with platelet counts of less than 50,000 per microliter. This includes patients with overt bleeding, such as epistaxis or hematuria, or suspected or proven internal bleeding from intracranial, intracutaneous, intramuscular, abdominal, or thoracic sites. Prophylactic platelet transfusions are indicated for surgical patients if they have thrombocytopenia (<100,000 platelets per microliter) or platelet dysfunction (thrombopathia) to prevent serious intraoperative hemorrhage. In the latter case, patients will have a normal platelet count but a prolonged bleeding time of greater than 9.5 min. As mentioned earlier, patients should also be given platelets after massive transfusion if they have platelet counts of less than 50,000 per microliter and continue to have nonmechanical bleeding.

Platelet concentrates are also indicated prophylactically for the prevention of bleeding in patients with platelet counts below 10,000 per microliter because of the higher risk of spontaneous hemorrhage. This latter category usually applies to patients with malignancies who are receiving chemotherapy. In contrast, patients with aplastic anemia who are likely to remain thrombocytopenic for many months should probably receive platelet concentrates only in

TABLE 37-4 Platelet Count and Risk of Spontaneous Hemorrhage

Risk	Platelet Count, per μl
Low	50,000–100,000
Moderate	10,000–50,000
High	0–10,000

the event of bleeding. These patients are more likely to form alloantibodies to platelets, which would make them refractory to platelet transfusions in the future.

Patients who have thrombocytopenia due to accelerated destruction of platelets, such as occurs in idiopathic thrombocytopenic purpura (ITP) and disseminated intravascular coagulation, seldom benefit from platelet concentrates since the transfused platelets are rapidly destroyed. If neurosurgery is necessary for an ITP patient, the platelets should be infused slowly during the procedure and throughout the recovery period rather than given as a bolus. Correction of the bleeding time should be used to guide therapy.

Uremic patients develop a functional platelet defect, which results from a plasma abnormality. This defect is corrected transiently following dialysis. Transfused platelets will not correct the platelet dysfunction since they are rapidly inactivated by this plasma abnormality.

The total dosage, frequency, and duration of platelet concentrates given to patients varies with the patient's body size, platelet count, clinical condition, and underlying illness. Generally, 4 to 6 platelet concentrates are sufficient to correct or prevent bleeding in an adult patient. More recently, physicians have tended to order 10 platelet concentrates per transfusion, probably in the belief that stored platelets have decreased viability. However, in most cases sufficient numbers of functionally active platelets are present in 4 to 6 platelet concentrates to provide hemostasis. Infants should receive one platelet concentrate per 6 kg of body weight. One platelet concentrate is expected to elevate the platelet count by 5000 to 15,000 per microliter per square meter of body surface. The effectiveness of the platelet transfusion can be monitored by performing a bleeding time or a platelet count 1 to 4 h post-transfusion to see if this increment is obtained.

Following multiple platelet transfusions from random donors, patients may develop alloantibodies to either HLA or platelet-specific antigens. When refractoriness to platelets occurs, further transfusion with random donor platelets will be unsuccessful. Refractory patients often do respond to large numbers of platelets obtained by thrombocytapheresis, especially if the donors are family members, since they are more likely to be HLA-compatible. A single-donor platelet concentrate contains the equivalent number of platelets present in five to seven random donor platelet concentrates.

Granulocytes

Granulocyte concentrates are prepared from a single donor by either continuous- or intermittent-flow centrifugal leukapheresis. Each unit contains 1 to 4×10^{10} granulocytes, 0.2 to 1.5×10^{10} lymphocytes, 1 to 10×10^{11} platelets, and 25 to 50 ml of red blood cells suspended in 200 to

500 ml of plasma. Because of the significant hematocrit, the donor's red cells must be compatible with the recipient's plasma. The transfused granulocytes have normal chemotactic and phagocytic functions, and transfused monocytes retain the ability to differentiate into macrophages.

Granulocyte transfusions are indicated for the support of neutropenic patients who have a granulocyte count of less than 500 per microliter and evidence of infection not responsive to antibiotics.

The optimal dosage of granulocytes is different to determine, but most authorities advocate a dose of 10^{10} granulocytes per day. This dose represents about 10 to 25 percent of the granulocytes produced by a healthy person each day $(1.3 \times 10^{11}$ granulocytes per day) and therefore probably represents a minimal beneficial dose. This dose should be continued daily until the infection resolves, as documented by defervescence or negative blood cultures, or the patient's bone marrow recovers so that the granulocyte count remains elevated about 1000 per microliter. The decision as to how long granulocyte transfusions should be continued is an individual one, which must take into account the patient's clinical response, the status of the underlying disease, and a realistic appraisal of the patient's prognosis.

Single-Donor Plasma, Fresh Frozen

Fresh frozen plasma is the plasma separated from a unit of whole blood and frozen within 6 h. Each unit contains 225 to 275 ml of plasma and CPDA-1 mixture, including about 25 meq of citric acid. Prompt freezing prevents the deterioration of the labile coagulation factors V and VIII:C so that fresh frozen plasma is a good source of all coagulation factors except platelets. We have determined that even after 2 years of storage hemostatic levels of factor V and VIII:C remain (Fig. 37-1).

The wide range of factor levels observed predominantly reflects the normal variability of factors V and VIII:C present in individual donors (50 to 150 percent of the mean) and not random deterioration of factors during storage. Fresh frozen plasma should be ABO-compatible and must be administered within 6 h after thawing. Single-donor fresh frozen plasma is indicated for the control of bleeding in patients with clotting deficiencies when specific concentrates are not available or when a single-factor deficiency has not been identified. Patients with multiple coagulation factor deficiencies, such as occur in liver disease, intravascular coagulation, or massive transfusion, may require fresh frozen plasma to control bleeding. The number of units required will depend on the severity of each case but can be readily evaluated by following routine coagulation tests, including the prothrombin time and the partial thromboplastin time, which should be prolonged at least 4 and 15 s, respectively, above the control. Usually two units of fresh frozen plasma are given initially to an adult and the response is determined by coagulation assays before any more is given.

Patients with severely prolonged prothrombin times due to coumarin therapy, who because of their clinical status may be at high risk for intracranial hemorrhage, should also be given fresh frozen plasma concomitantly with vitamin K therapy.

Fresh frozen plasma is used to treat the rare congenital deficiencies of factors II, V, VII, and X and the more common congenital deficiency of factor XI. All these factors except VII, which has a very short half-life, have half-lives greater than 12 h, and generally these patients can be treated with fresh frozen plasma without immediate concern for fluid overload since the levels necessary for hemostasis are quite low. A practical approach to dosage for an average adult would be to give four units of fresh frozen plasma prior to surgery followed by one unit every 12 h. This dosage schedule should be readjusted after 24 h according to the results of the specific factor assays. Congenital factor VII–deficient patients, particularly infants, are at high risk for central nervous system bleeding.[10] Volume overload can be an overwhelming problem and factor IX complex might be a better choice for their therapy.

Fresh frozen plasma can also be used for patients with mild, infrequently treated hemophilia B. However, during surgical procedures and treatment of head trauma, when factor IX levels should be maintained above 25 percent, factor IX concentrates are preferable, despite their risk of hepatitis.

Cryoprecipitated Antihemophilic Factor

Cryoprecipitate refers to those plasma proteins that precipitate out of solution when a unit of fresh frozen plasma is slowly thawed at 4°C. Each bag contains about 80 to 100

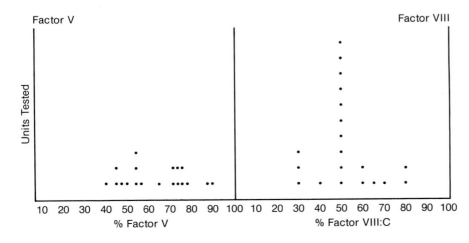

Figure 37-1 The distribution of factors V and VIII in individual units of fresh frozen plasma after 2 years of storage.

units of factor VIII:C, 200 to 250 mg of fibrinogen (factor I), 30 percent of the factor XIII level of the original fresh plasma, and 40 to 50 percent of the original plasma's von Willebrand's factor, suspended in 10 to 15 ml of residual plasma. Cryoprecipitate is stored frozen for up to 1 year and is thawed at 30 to 38°C before use. Since several bags are transfused at a time, they are usually pooled in a sterile plastic transfer pack or syringe and kept at room temperature until administration. ABO-compatible cryoprecipitate is not necessary but is desirable if the patient is expected to receive large doses. Rh comptability is unimportant. Cryoprecipitate must be transfused intravenously through a filter within 6 h after thawing and 4 h after pooling.

Cryoprecipitate is indicated for the treatment of bleeding in patients with mild hemophilia A (factor VIII:C deficiency), von Willebrand's disease, hypofibrinogenemia, dysfibrinogenemia, and factor XIII deficiency. More recently, cryoprecipitate has been found to be beneficial in correcting the thrombopathia associated with uremia.[8] Cryoprecipitate can be used to treat mild to moderate hemophilia A, as an alternative to antihemophilic factor (AHF) concentrates. Since cryoprecipitate is obtained from volunteer single donors, it carries less risk of hepatitis transmission than AHF concentrates, which are prepared from large pools of plasma. The dosage of cryoprecipitate varies according to the severity of factor VIII:C deficiency. Sufficient cryoprecipitate should be given to raise the patient's factor VIII:C level to approximately 50 percent prior to surgery. Initially two bags of cryoprecipitate should be given per 6 kg of body weight since each bag will raise the factor VIII:C level by about 2.5 percent in a 70-kg adult. Maintenance doses should be given at 8 to 12-h intervals to assure that the VIII:C level does not fall below 25 percent since the plasma half-life of factor VIII:C is 8 to 12 h. Therapy should be continued for 1 week to 10 days to maintain hemostasis after major surgery. Actual dosage should be monitored with factor VIII:C assays. Cryoprecipitate (cryo.) dosage may be calculated by the following formula:

$$\text{No. bags cryo.} = \frac{\text{desired change in factor VIII:C} \times \text{plasma volume (ml)}}{80 \text{ units of factor VIII:C per bag}}$$

In this formula,
plasma volume = weight (kg) × 80 × plasmacrit.

Example: This illustrates the number of bags necessary to raise the level of VIII:C from 25 percent to 50 percent in a 40 kg patient with a red cell hematocrit of 38 percent.

$$6.2 \text{ bags cryo.} = \frac{0.25 \times 1984 \,(40 \times 80 \times 0.62)}{80}$$

Since these calculations are approximations, six bags would be transfused.

Hemophilia A patients who have any head injury should be given cryoprecipitate or AHF concentrate immediately to prevent intracerebral hemorrhage. The dosage should be sufficient to raise the patient's level to 25 percent.

Patients with von Willebrand's disease should be treated with cryoprecipitate instead of AHF concentrates since cryoprecipitate more reliably corrects the bleeding time abnormality in this disease. Von Willebrand's patients undergoing surgery may be given cryoprecipitate 30 min prior to the operation, during the procedure, and then every 8 to 12 h depending on their response, which varies within individuals as well as among family members. In addition to watching the clinical response, it is reasonable to measure VIII:C levels and bleeding times, as the duration of the effect on them may vary. In many von Willebrand's patients, the VIII:C level will reach a level far higher than expected and remain sustained for 12 to 24 h while the bleeding time may only remain corrected for 8 to 12 h. (Fig. 37-2). A practical transfusion regimen for von Willebrand's patients undergoing surgery or intracranial bleeding would be to initiate therapy with six to eight bags of cryoprecipitate followed by two bags every 8 to 12 h, depending on the patient's test results.

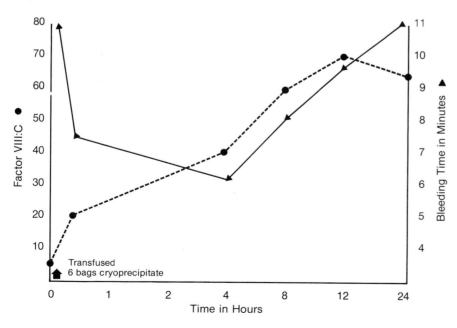

Figure 37-2 Transfusion response in an adult von Willebrand's patient to six bags of cryoprecipitate.

Cryoprecipitate is the only component available today that has a high enough concentration of fibrinogen to treat severe hypofibrinogenemia (<70 mg/dl). Fibrinogen levels need to be greater than 100 mg/dl, which is the minimal hemostatic level. Since each bag of cryoprecipitate contains 200 to 250 mg of fibrinogen, it will increase a 70-kg adult's fibrinogen level by 6 to 8 mg/dl. The number of cryoprecipitate bags needed to correct a fibrinogen deficiency can be calculated by the following formula:

No. bags cryo.
$$= \frac{\text{desired level} - \text{patient's level} \times \text{plasma volume}}{20}$$

Again, plasma volume = weight (kg) × 80 × plasmacrit. Levels are measured in miligrams per deciliter and plasma volume in liters.

Example: A 90-kg patient with an RBC hematocrit of 25 percent has a fibrinogen level of 50 mg/dl. To assure hemostasis, levels greater than 100 mg/dl are needed. This example will illustrate the amount necessary to raise the level to 150 mg/dl.

$$27 \text{ bags} = \frac{150 - 50 \times 5.4 \text{ liters } (90 \times 80 \times 0.75)}{20}$$

In head injuries due to gunshot wounds or blunt trauma, it is not uncommon to detect falling fibrinogen levels and platelet counts. In most incidents this is a self-limited form of disseminated intravascular coagulation.[6] In such cases, eight to ten cryoprecipitate bags can be given.

Recently, cryoprecipitate has been found to correct the prolonged bleeding time associated with uremia.[8] The infusion of 10 bags of cryoprecipitate is indicated in uremic adult patients who are acutely bleeding or are undergoing surgery. The maximum effect of the cryoprecipitate takes at least 4 h to develop. By 24 h after infusion, the bleeding time will return to the preinfusion levels. Thus, cryoprecipitate provides only short-term improvement in hemostasis so that life-threatening hemorrhage can be controlled or surgery can be performed.

Antihemophilic Factor Concentrates

AHF concentrates are lyophilized, partially purified factor VIII:C concentrates prepared from large pools of human plasma. Since they are prepared from large pools, the risk of hepatitis transmission is greater and they should be generally reserved for severe hemophilia A patients. Most vials contain 200 to 400 VIII:C units; however, vials containing 1000 or more units are available and offer some advantages where larger doses are anticipated during intracranial surgery or in the treatment of factor VIII:C inhibitors. These products contain isoagglutinins to red cell antigens and can occasionally cause a hemolytic reaction. For cases in which extremely large amounts are used for patients who are not blood group O, products with lower levels of isoagglutinins are available.

Patients with VIII:C levels greater than 5 percent usually do not have spontaneous bleeding, but they, too, should be treated immediately after any head trauma to obtain a level of 25 percent while they are being evaluated for neurological changes. The dosage of AHF concentrates can be estimated by the following formula:

Units of VIII:C
= desired change in factor VIII:C × plasma volume

As before, plasma volume = weight (kg) × 80 × plasmacrit.

Example: This illustrates the amount of VIII:C necessary to raise the level from <1 to 25 percent in a 70-kg adult with a red cell hematocrit of 43 percent:

798 units of VIII:C = 0.25 × 3192 ml (70 × 80 × 0.57)

If the vials contain more factor VIII:C than necessary to achieve the desired increase, the remaining material should be administered to the patient and not discarded. On the other hand, these calculations are just estimates and if a combination of vials contains slightly less than the estimated need, an additional vial need not be reconstituted. The vials should be reconstituted according to each manufacturer's instructions. For surgical procedures the factor VIII:C level of the patient should be raised to approximately 50 percent and kept above 25 percent. In cases of intracranial surgery, factor VIII:C levels close to 100 percent are sought initially and the goal is to maintain the level above 50 percent for 5 to 7 days; thereafter, levels should be maintained between 50 and 25 percent for another week.

Factor VIII:C half-life is 8 to 12 h, and obviously better control, using less material, can be attained with a more frequent or even continuous dosage schedule, but practicality more often requires scheduling at 8- or 12-h intervals. Factor assays should be done on samples drawn after the loading dose, after surgery, and on a daily basis just prior to another dose so that concentrate dosage can be properly adjusted to maintain the necessary VIII:C levels in the patient.

Factor IX Complex

Factor IX complexes are also known as *prothrombin complexes* and are lyophilized concentrates of coagulation factors II, VII, IX, and X prepared from large pools of human plasma. The number of units of factor IX are listed on each vial. These concentrates are also reconstituted with diluent and administered intravenously with a plastic syringe within 3 h. They should be kept at room temperature during the interim between reconstitution and administration.

Factor IX complex is indicated for the treatment of patients with hemophilia B (Christmas disease, factor IX deficiency). Just as in hemophilia A, head trauma should be treated immediately. For surgical procedures the same guidelines for dosage as were used in hemophilia A can be applied, although the dosage schedule can be adjusted to a longer interval since the half-life of factor IX is 12 to 24 h.

Patients with primary amyloidosis uncommonly have a factor X deficiency and hemostasis can only be maintained with frequent infusions of factor IX concentrates. These concentrates are also used preferentially in the treatment of the rare congenital, severe factor VII–deficient patient. In the above conditions, the vials have to be assayed for potency of the specific factor and the patient's plasma factor levels followed carefully by specific assay.

A summary of coagulation factor deficiencies and their treatment is presented in Table 37-5.

Plasma Protein Fraction and Normal Serum Albumin

Plasma protein fraction consists of about 88 percent serum albumin and 12 percent alpha-and beta-globulins, which are obtained from large pools of human plasma by a process known as Cohn fractionation. The total protein concentration is approximately 5 g/dl. The final product is heat-treated to inactivate hepatitis viruses. Since no isoagglutinins are present, plasma protein fraction can be given to recipients of any ABO blood group. No coagulation factors are present so this product cannot be used to treat coagulopathies. It is administered intravenously through a filter. Hypotensive reactions have been occasionally observed when plasma protein fraction is administered too rapidly, possibly owing to the presence of prekallikrein activator.[1] Because of this potential side effect, it should be administered at less than 10 ml per min.

Normal serum albumin is prepared by the same fractionation method as plasma protein fraction but undergoes several more purification steps, so that the final product consists of 95% albumin. The sodium content ranges from 130 to 160 meq/per liter. Albumin is available as a 5% or a 25% solution. The 5% solution is iso-oncotic with plasma while the 25% solution exerts an oncotic pressure five times greater than that of plasma. Albumin is associated with a lower incidence of hypotensive episodes than is plasma protein fraction.

Because of their oncotic effects, both plasma protein fraction and 5% albumin are indicated for the replacement of lost plasma volume in patients with acute traumatic shock.[11,12] Large volumes of crystalloid solutions can also be used in this situation in younger, previously healthly individuals. However, older patients with other underlying medical illnesses may respond better to volume replacement by albumin than by crystalloid.

The adult respiratory distress syndrome sometimes occurs during shock or following surgery. The syndrome is characterized by inadequate oxygenation due to interstitial pulmonary edema. In addition to the usual treatment with diuretics and careful balancing of fluid intake and output, albumin replacement may be beneficial to prevent a decrease in effective plasma volume following diuresis.[11] Use of 25% albumin is preferable in this situation. The dosage is dependent on the response of the patient's vital signs. The intravenous administration of 20 ml of 25% albumin will draw approximately 70 ml of extravascular fluid into the circulation.

Immune Serum Globulin

Immune serum globulin consists of the immunoglobulin fraction of plasma, which is prepared by Cohn fractionation of very large pools of plasma. It consists of about 95% IgG suspended at a concentration of 16.5% (165 mg/ml). It should be given intramuscularly since it contains aggregates of IgG, which can fix complement and cause anaphylaxis if given intravenously. Since it is prepared from large pools of human plasma, it contains antibodies against common bacteria and viruses.

Immune serum globulin is recommended for IgG replacement in patients with hypogammaglobulinemia due to primary or secondary immunodeficiency disorders. The therapeutic goal is to raise the serum IgG level above 250 mg/dl.[2] This goal can be achieved by administering an initial loading dose of 200 to 250 mg/kg followed by regular doses at 1 to 3 week intervals, depending on the severity of hypogammaglobulinemia. The minimal effective maintenance dose averages 25 mg/kg per week. A 7 to 10 day incubation period is required for development of peak antibody titers. The half-life is 22 days.

More recently, a 5% (50 mg/ml) solution of IgG has been licensed in the United States for intravenous administration. This product has been specially processed to eliminate IgG polymers so that it is safe for intravenous use. This product is intended for use in persons who cannot tolerate repeated intramuscular injections of large volumes of immune serum

TABLE 37-5   Treatment of Coagulopathies

Congenital Factor Deficiency	Plasma Concentration Needed for Surgical Hemostasis	Half-life of Infused Factor	Component Used	
			Mild Deficiency	Severe Deficiency
I (fibrinogen)	100 mg/dl	4–6 days	Cryo	Cryo
II	40%	60 h	FFP	IX
V	10–15%	24 h	FFP	FFP
VII	5–10%	1–7 h	FFP	IX
VIII	25%	8–12 h	Cryo or AHF	AHF
IX	25%	12–24 h	FFP	IX
X	10–20%	48–72 h	FFP	FFP
XI		40–80 h	FFP	FFP
XII	Does not require component therapy			
XIII	1–5%	3–5 days	Cryo	Cryo
von Willebrand's	Variable	Variable	Cryo	Cryo

Abbreviations: FFP = fresh frozen plasma; Cryo = cryoprecipitated antihemophilic factor concentrate; IX = factor IX (prothrombin) complex; AHF = antihemophilic factor concentrate.

globulin at monthly intervals. In contrast to intramuscular IgG, peak serum antibody titers are achieved immediately with the intravenous IgG. The recommended dose is 100 to 200 mg/kg per month. Since this product contains traces of IgA, it should not be administered to patients with combined IgG-IgA deficiencies accompanied by anti-IgA antibodies since anaphylaxis could occur.

Immune serum globulin fractions prepared from patients with high titers of certain antibodies are used as hyperimmune gamma-globulin for treating selected disorders. Their indications and dosages are listed in Table 37-6.

Adverse Reactions to Transfusion

Adverse reactions to transfusion of blood components can be due to the cellular and fluid portions of blood, anticoagulant-preservative solutions, metabolic by-products, or microorganisms. These adverse effects may occur either during the transfusion or much later.

Immediate Reactions

Immediate adverse reactions can be mediated by both immunologic and nonimmunologic mechanisms. Immunologic reactions can occur in two ways: an antibody in the recipi-

ent's plasma may react with an antigen in the donor's blood or an antibody in the donor's plasma may react with an antigen in the recipient's blood. Antibodies that react against plasma protein antigens usually cause allergic reactions ranging from urticaria to anaphylaxis. Antibodies that react with leukocyte or platelet antigens generally cause febrile transfusion reactions, while antibodies directed against red blood cells occasionally cause hemolytic transfusion reactions.

Allergic reactions are usually manifested by hives and may occur in 0.5 to 3.0 percent of recipients. They occur less commonly when red blood cells are transfused instead of whole blood. More rarely, allergic reactions may be more severe and cause glottal edema or asthma. Rare individuals who are IgA-deficient may develop anti-IgA antibodies, which cause anaphylactoid reactions consisting of bronchospasm, dyspnea, and shock if the patient receives blood components containing IgA.

In mild cases, urticaria and pruritus should be managed by slowing the rate of transfusion and administering antihistamines, such as 50 mg diphenhydramine, intravenously or intramuscularly. In more severe reactions the urticaria may be accompanied by anxiety, dyspnea, palpitations, fever, and chills. In these cases the transfusion should be discontinued and the intravenous line should be kept open with normal saline. The patient should be treated with intravenous antihistamines and oral antipyretics. In severe cases intravenous corticosteroids or adrenalin may also be needed.

TABLE 37-6   Uses of Human Immunoglobulin

Disease or Condition	Transmission Conditions	Product	Dose
Hepatitis A	Family contacts Institutional outbreaks	ISG	3.2 mg/kg BW
	Exposure to unhygienic conditions in tropical or developing countries	ISG	3.2–8.0 mg/kg BW every 4 months
Hepatitis B	Percutaneous or mucosal exposure	HBIG	8–11 mg/kg BW; repeat in 1 month
	Newborns of mothers with HBsAg	HBIG	48 mg at birth, 3, and 6 months
	Sexual contacts of acute hepatitis B patients	HBIG	48 mg/kg BW; repeat after 1 month
Rubella	Women exposed during early pregnancy	ISG	20 ml
Varicella-zoster	Immunosuppressed contacts of acute cases or newborn contacts	VZIG	15–25 units/kg BW; minimum of 125 units
Measles (rubeola)	In infants less than 1 year old; or immunosuppressed contacts of acute cases exposed within 6 days	ISG	0.25 ml/kg BW; or 0.5 ml/kg BW if immunosuppressed
Rabies	Subjects exposed to rabid animals	RIG	20 IU/kg BW
Tetanus	Following significant exposure of unimmunized or incompletely immunized person or immediately on diagnosis of disease	TIG	250 units for prophylaxis; 3000–6000 units for therapy
Rh iso-immunization	In Rh(D)-mother on delivery of Rh+ infant, or after abortion (RH+ father), or after transfusion of Rh+ blood	RhIG	One vial (200–300 μg) per 30 ml of Rh(+) blood

Abbreviations: ISG = immune serum globulin (human); HBIG = hepatitis B immune globulin; VZIG = varicella zoster immune globulin; RIG = rabies immune globulin; TIG = tetanus immune globulin; RhIG = Rh immune globulin; BW = body weight.

The donor unit accompanied with the attached administration set should be returned to the blood bank along with a post-transfusion sample of the patient's blood. The blood bank will perform a transfusion reaction workup to rule out a hemolytic transfusion reaction.

Febrile reactions are characterized by fever and chills and occur in 0.5 to 1.0 percent of transfusions. Fever usually occurs 1 h after the transfusion begins and may persist for 8 to 12 h. In some cases fever and chills may be accompanied by headache, flushing, and tachycardia. In severe cases the transfusion should be discontinued and aspirin or acetaminophen can be given if necessary. Antihistamines are not effective in febrile transfusion reactions. If a patient has experienced two or more febrile reactions, leukocyte-poor or saline-washed red blood cells can subsequently be given. Since these reactions mimic the early stages of a hemolytic transfusion reaction, the patient should be monitored carefully and the transfusion service informed so that the appropriate evaluation can be performed.

Hemolytic transfusion reactions may occur when there is an incompatibility between donor red blood cells and recipient plasma. Most immediate hemolytic reactions are due to an ABO mismatch, which most often occurs because of identification errors. Initial symptoms may include fever, chills, tightness in the chest, flank pain, and anxiety. Clinical signs will include tachycardia, fever, and hypotension. Anesthetized patients may exhibit only hemoglobinuria, hemoglobinemia, or oozing of blood from cut surfaces. Renal failure may subsequently occur. Treatment includes discontinuing the transfusion as soon as hemolysis is suspected and supporting the patient's blood pressure and blood volume so that adequate renal blood flow is maintained. This can be achieved by rapidly infusing 20 g mannitol along with other intravenous fluids. Alternatively, 20 to 80 mg furosemide can be given intravenously to induce diuresis. The patient should be observed closely for complications such as acute renal failure and disseminated intravascular coagulation. The blood bank should be immediately notified and clotted and anticoagulated blood specimens should be sent to the laboratory, along with the unit of blood and the attached administration set. A clerical check of all the transfusion records should be made. The blood bank will recheck the unit's compatibility.

Other causes of hemolysis that may mimic a hemolytic transfusion reaction include bacterial contamination of the donor unit. Some bacteria, such as gram-negative bacilli, can grow rapidly in blood at 4°C and produce endotoxins. Transfusion of the contaminated unit would cause septic shock. Transfusion must be begun as soon as the units are set up to prevent possible bacterial proliferation. The administration of hypotonic solutions with whole blood or red blood cells can cause hemolysis. Five or 10% dextrose in water or in 0.45 or 0.225% saline causes red blood cells to swell, resulting in decreased in vivo survival. Therefore, only isotonic saline solutions should be given with red blood cells or whole blood. Overheating or freezing of blood before or during transfusion can also mimic an acute hemolytic reaction. Only blood warmers designed specifically for that purpose should be used.

Several nonimmunologic mechanisms can cause immediate adverse transfusion reactions. Circulatory overload may result when excessive volumes of blood or blood components are administered. This complication occurs most frequently in patients with severe chronic anemia who have a decreased red mass but an increased plasma volume. Patients with incipient heart failure are also at higher risk. These patients will experience tightness in the chest and a dry cough, which could evolve into pulmonary edema. Treatment consists of decreasing the rate of transfusion and sitting the patient upright. Red blood cells, instead of whole blood, should be transfused.

Air embolism is a very rare complication today since the introduction of plastic blood bags, but can occur if air enters the bag during the changing of an infusion set in the middle of a transfusion. If air embolism occurs, the patient will become cyanotic and dyspneic. Cardiac arrest could occur. Patients should be treated by lowering their head and laying them on their side so that air will collect in the right atrium, away from the pulmonary valve.

Metabolic complications, including hypothermia, citrate toxicity, acidosis, and clotting deficiencies may also occur during transfusion. They have already been discussed in the section on massive transfusion.

Delayed Reactions

Delayed Hemolytic Reactions

At the time of transfusion, a patient may have an antibody with a titer too low to be detected by compatibility testing. Transfusion of donor blood possessing the corresponding antigen may provoke an anamnestic response. After several days the antibody titer may become high enough to hemolyze transfused red blood cells. This type of reaction makes it necessary to provide new blood samples for compatibility testing at 48-h intervals for patients receiving multiple transfusions. The clinical signs and symptoms are usually milder than those seen during acute hemolytic episodes. These patients typically become icteric and may have hemoglobinemia and hemoglobinuria. They should be monitored closely for the complications of hemolysis.

Infectious Diseases

Improved testing for hepatitis B surface antigen (HBsAg) and the change in the donor base to volunteers has greatly reduced the incidence of clinical hepatitis associated with transfusion in the United States. Viral hepatitis due to hepatitis B is now infrequently seen in transfusion recipients. Hepatitis A has only been documented on a few occasions. Non-A, non-B hepatitis is the predominant cause of transfusion-related hepatitis.[3] The vast majority of patients with non-A, non-B hepatitis are only diagnosed by elevated transaminases and are anicteric. The incidence of hepatitis transmission varies according to geographic area, socioeconomic status, sex, and ethnic subgroup of donors. The blood components and derivatives with a potential of transmitting hepatitis are listed in Table 37-7.

Blood derivatives such as antihemophilic factor and factor IX (prothrombin) complexes, which are prepared from large pools of human plasma, are associated with a higher

TABLE 37-7 Hepatitis Transmission Risk of Blood Components

Possible	None
Whole blood	Albumin
Red blood cells	Plasma protein fraction (Plasmanate, Protenate, Plasma-plex)
Fresh frozen plasma	
Platelets	Immune serum globulin
Cryoprecipitate	
Factor VIII:C	
Factor IX	

incidence of post-transfusion hepatitis. Albumin, plasma protein fraction, and immune serum globulin are heat treated during processing and do not transmit hepatitis. Overall, transfusion accounts for only a small portion of the exposure risk to infectious agents in the environment that might lead to illness.

The Future

Red blood cells will continue to be the mainstay of transfusion therapy in the future. However, current research is underway to develop substitutes for red blood cell transfusions, such as hemoglobin derivatives and perfluorocarbons. Controlled clinical trials are already in progress to evaluate the safety and efficacy of Fluosol-DA, a 70% perfluorocarbon emulsion.[7] Perfluorocarbons may prove to be most useful as replacements of blood volume and oxygen-carrying capacity during acute hemorrhagic shock. Their usefulness in anemic patients who require multiple transfusions over long periods of time will require further study since these emulsions only circulate about 24 h before they become unstable and are deposited in the liver and spleen.

Both the Fluosol-DA and hemoglobin solutions have oncotic properties and may gain use as plasma expanders. Other artificial plasma expanders presently in use in the United States are prepared from dextrans and starches. These macromolecules are gaining increasing use but only limited volumes can be infused since they can cause bleeding diatheses. Also, starch products may remain associated with cells for long periods of time.

Genetic engineering should also have an impact on blood derivative therapy. Recombinant DNA techniques may provide alternative sources of albumin and coagulation factors. New protein factors may become clinically available. The future possibilities will only be limited by our imagination, perseverance, and knowledge of the function of the body's numerous proteins, which is presently very limited.

For today, it still remains of utmost importance for people to give blood voluntarily to meet the ever-increasing needs of patients and for clinicians to use the materials derived from these donations only for appropriate reasons.

References

1. Alving BM, Hojima Y, Pisano JJ, Mason BL, Buckingham RE Jr, Mozen MM, Finlayson JS: Hypotension associated with prekallikrein activator (Hageman-factor fragments) in plasma protein fraction. N Engl J Med 299:66–70, 1978.
2. Appropriate uses of human immunoglobulin in clinical practice: Memorandum from an IUIS/WHO meeting. Bull WHO 60:43–47, 1982.
3. Bayer WL: Based on your analysis of the benefits and costs of routine donor screening for ALT-GPT to reduce the incidence of posttransfusion non-A, non-B hepatitis in your blood services region, what action would you recommend on this matter? Vox Sang (in press).
4. Boral LI, Dannemiller FJ, Stanford W, Hill, SS, Cornell TA: A guideline for anticipated blood usage during elective surgical procedures. Am J Clin Pathol 71:680–684, 1979.
5. Eldor A, Avitzour M, Or R, Hanna R, Penchas S: Prediction of haemorrhagic diathesis in thrombocytopenia by mean platelet volume. Br Med J 285:397–400, 1982.
6. Feinstein DI: Diagnosis and management of disseminated intravascular coagulation: The role of heparin therapy. Blood 60:284–287, 1982.
7. Geyer RP: Oxygen transport in vivo by means of perfluorochemical preparations. N Engl J Med 307:304–306, 1982.
8. Janson PA, Jubelirer SJ, Weinstein MJ, Deykin D: Treatment of the bleeding tendency in uremia with cryoprecipitate. N Engl J Med 303:1318–1322, 1980.
9. Menitove JE, McElligott MC, Aster RH: Febrile transfusion reaction: What blood component should be given next? Vox Sang 42:318–321, 1982.
10. Ragni MV, Lewis JH, Spero JA, Hasiba U: Factor VII deficiency: Report of three cases and literature review with emphasis on CNS hemorrhage. Am J Hematol 10:79–88, 1981.
11. Shoemaker WC, Hauser CJ: Critique of crystalloid versus colloid therapy in shock and shock lung. Crit Care Med 7:117–124, 1979.
12. Skillman JJ: The role of albumin and oncotically active fluids in shock. Crit Care Med 4:55–61, 1976.

38

Neuroanesthesia

Maurice S. Albin

Prevention is the daughter of intelligence.
(Sir Walter Raleigh, 1593)

The management of neurosurgical cases has changed remarkably since the beginning of the twentieth century, and it would not be unfair to note that many of the quantum jumps have been due in no small part to the concomitant advances in anesthesiology.

A chapter on neuroanesthesia would be incomplete without pausing to mention or paying homage to one of the founders of modern neurosurgery whose contributions are inextricably entwined with the development of modern anesthesia—Harvey Cushing. In a historical sense, we in anesthesia can stake out a prior "claim" on Cushing because he started giving anesthesia (as an "etherizer") while a second-year medical student at Harvard Medical School in 1892. A letter from a fellow medical student, E. A. (Avery) Codman, to Dr. Cushing notes " . . . I also spoke of the case which stopped breathing under ether and interested you in Brain Surgery."[43]

The origins of today's anesthetic record can be traced directly to the "etherization" chart developed by E. A. Codman and Harvey Cushing while medical students.[15,36,43,49,86] The record consisted of two sides: one giving the demographic information, including age, name, diagnosis, drugs, preoperative pulse rate, temperature, and respiration as well as the status of the patient in the recovery room, including rectal temperature, vomiting, and "Remarks (please note shock, apnea, intermittent pulse, etc.)"; and the other showing the time frame at 5-min intervals on the horizontal axis and pulse and respiratory rate and temperature numeration on the vertical axis, also indicating the name of the surgeon, time for anesthesia and surgery, amount of anesthesia, condition of the heart, and presence of mucus during the surgery.[43]

Cushing's classic experimental paper on the relationship of intracranial pressure to blood pressure regulation was published in 1901.[33] This work was done in Kocher's laboratory in Bern, Switzerland, and completed in the spring of 1901 in Turin, Italy. After leaving Turin, Cushing visited Pavia, Italy and met Dr. Orlandi, who gave him a model of Scarpione Riva-Rocci's device for measuring blood pressure noninvasively.[43] At that time the apparatus was being used for routine bedside use by Orlandi, and Cushing immediately realized the practicality and importance of this type of unit during surgical procedures. Interestingly enough, another great pioneer of modern surgery, George Crile, was also interested in blood pressure monitoring, using a Gaertner tonometer.[43] On January 19, 1903 both Crile and Cushing spoke at a special meeting of the Boston Medical Society giving their findings on the importance of blood pressure measurements for surgical procedures. One month later a committee composed of members of the Department of Surgery of Harvard Medical School was formed " . . . in order to determine, so far as the opportunities in this community will allow, the extent to which blood pressure observations in surgical cases may be of value from a clinical point of view."[35] After numerous meetings the committee voted that "the adoption of blood pressure observations in surgical patients does not at present appear to be necessary as a routine measure." In spite of this, blood pressure monitoring survived, owing for the most part to the intensive efforts of Cushing. Blood pressure (in millimeters of mercury) was incorporated into the anesthesia records with Cushing's first chart introduced at the Johns Hopkins Hospital early in 1902.[34]

While an assistant resident on Halsted's service at Johns Hopkins in 1898, Cushing experimented with regional anesthesia, using cocaine infiltration for nerve blocks. It is to be remembered that Halsted was one of the pioneers in defining the use of cocaine for regional anesthesia and by 1885 he had reported its use in more than 1000 procedures.[46] Cushing published a short preliminary note in 1898 on the use of cocaine as a local anesthetic for inguinal hernia repair and in thyroid tumor surgery.[28] Cushing's paper in 1900 on the use of cocaine for hernia repair represents a minor unheralded classic, with important overtones for modern anesthesia.[31] In this document Cushing delineated the criteria of physical status, age, and anesthesia risk; insisted on monitoring the vital signs of high risk patients during surgery; defined the advantages of local anesthesia over general anesthesia; and noted the importance of premedication. Interestingly, Cushing described 200 operations under cocaine in the 18 months prior to publication of the paper, including major operative procedures such as laparotomies, exploratory section, gastrotomies, cholecystotomies, appendectomies, pyloric resection for carcinoma, and gastroenterostomy.[29,30]

Fluid balance and volume replacement are important surgical and anesthesia considerations. In 1901 Cushing reported on the dangers of infusion of plain sodium chloride in a simple but elegant experiment.[32] He noted that ionically balanced low-salt solutions are needed for adequate muscular contraction. Years were to elapse before the importance of this problem was noted by other investigators.[49]

While Gardner was the first to actively utilize induced hypotension, Cushing was the first to voice the concept of hypotension as an adjunct to neurosurgery by observing that hemorrhage was followed by vasoconstriction, which led to a dry operating field.[37]

Cushing's physiological approach to the neurosurgical patient heralded the need to develop similar methodological considerations in anesthetic management and many decades were to elapse before this was to come to pass. The neuroanesthesiologist today must have an understanding of the physiopathological responses to neurological dysfunction; of the effects of pharmacologic agents on cerebral blood flow and metabolism; of the nature and relationships of intracranial pressure (ICP), compliance, and cerebral blood volume;

and of how to utilize invasive and noninvasive monitoring systems to minimize morbidity and mortality. Similarly, surgical therapeutics has been intensely influenced by advances in neuroradiological imaging techniques; microneurosurgical methods and instrumentation; development of specialized neurosurgical nursing and critical care units; understanding of how to achieve reductions in brain volume; ability to reduce blood pressure while operating on vascular lesions during neurovascular surgery; and realization of the physiological restraints during brain retraction.

The interaction between the anesthesiologist and the neurosurgeon is critical and both must have an understanding of each other's problems and limitations. The anesthesiologist should have an adequate knowledge of neuropathology and the therapeutic aims of the neurosurgical procedure. Conversely, the neurosurgeon should understand the physiopathological responses to anesthetic agents and neuroanesthesia techniques. This cooperative approach should not merely focus on the intraoperative period but should include the preoperative and postoperative phases as well.

The Preoperative Period

Evaluation

Evaluation[1] is concerned with a knowledge of the patient's pulmonary, cardiovascular, and renal function; with determination that there are no bleeding or coagulation abnormalities; and with determinations that the patient is not hypovolemic because of hemorrhage, restricted activity, or extended periods of parenteral therapy. A thorough medical history and physical examination are critical, along with knowledge of medications, allergies, and past surgical procedures and anesthetics. Routine evaluation should include x-ray films of the chest, hematocrit and hemoglobin, complete blood and platelet counts, differential blood smear, prothrombin time and partial thromboplastin regeneration time, 12-lead electrocardiogram (ECG), and urinalysis. In anticipation of the possible use of intraoperative diuretics and hyperosmotic agents, screening tests should include serum electrolytes, blood urea nitrogen, creatinine, and glucose. Liver function tests and enzymes are valuable for baseline data.

Preoperative estimation of plasma and red cell volume may be of aid in management of patients with intracranial aneurysms, arteriovenous malformations (AVMs), or other situations in which significant blood loss might occur. Maroon and Nelson[58] have already reported the plasma volume–red cell mass deficits in the patient with a subarachnoid hemorrhage secondary to an aneurysmal bleed. It must also be remembered that the patient at bed rest for many days because of an intracranial bleed, mass lesion, or increased intracranial pressure, whose fluid intake has been restricted and who is on a regimen of hyperosmotic agents and loop diuretics, becomes a potential anesthetic risk. In this type of individual with a contracted blood volume, one may anticipate a marked decrease in total peripheral resistance, with accompanying arterial hypotension upon anes-

thetic induction. This may be exacerbated by age and accompanying cardiopulmonary or renal problems.

Pulmonary function studies, including arterial blood gases before and after 100% oxygen inhalation, should be carried out if there is any suspicion of ventilatory dysfunction or a history of heavy smoking.

Monitoring

Any neurosurgical patient manifesting signs of increased intracranial pressure (ICP), altered level of consciousness, cardiopulmonary instability, or the need for control of hemodynamic variables (as in the aneurysm patient) should be placed in a specialized care unit, kept under constant observation, and monitored for ECG, arterial blood pressure (indwelling catheter), central venous pressure (CVP) and/or pulmonary artery and pulmonary capillary wedge pressures, urinary output, and chemistries and blood gases of samples from the arterial line. If elevated ICP is suspected, monitoring may be accomplished from an intraventricular, subarachnoid, or epidural transducer. Inadequate or periodic ventilation in these patients should be evaluated both clinically and with blood gases. If necessary, the patient should be intubated carefully and ventilated with a volume-controlled ventilator so that the Pa_{O_2} is above 80 mmHg and the Pa_{CO_2} is between 25 and 30 mmHg.

Premedication

Premedication can be of critical importance if the patient has ICP. In this type of patient, we must aim not to increase cerebral blood volume and ICP, especially if we are dealing with an individual who is near the portion of the intracranial compliance curve at which a small increase in cerebral blood volume will give a marked increase in ICP.[76] Any drug or agent which will in any way cause any type of respiratory embarrassment should be avoided. Conversely, the proper use of benzodiazepine derivatives to tranquilize the patient and to attenuate seizure activity is also important. This has special validity in the patient with an intracranial aneurysm,[47] who might develop a serious bleed prior to surgery because of apprehension and an increase of blood pressure. When a surgical procedure is to take place in the morning, it is common practice to withhold food and drink after midnight but to allow the full supper meal. It has been demonstrated that postoperative solid food emesis can take place as long as 48 h after withdrawal of oral food.[8] Therefore, it is suggested that patients have a clear liquid lunch and supper, whenever possible, the day before surgery. It is our practice to give all patients entering the operating room 15.0 ml of 0.3 M sodium citrate orally. The use of glycopyrrolate for premedication combined with oral sodium citrate prior to surgery has been shown to keep gastric contents above a pH of 3.0 during induction of anesthesia.

The ability of the histamine antagonist cimetadine, given at least 1 h prior to surgery, to suppress gastric secretion and raise gastric pH, will probably help to eliminate the problem of chemical pneumonitis during the preoperative and postoperative periods should emesis occur.

Intraoperative Management

Monitoring

The use of monitoring methods makes it possible to profile both rapidly and slowly changing physiological responses. The application of computer techniques for rapid handling of large quantities of intraoperative physiological and biochemical data will enable us to eventually develop predictability curves that will enhance patient safety.

Arterial Blood Pressure

Accurate determination of arterial blood pressure is important because of positional changes, the use of induced hypotension, and the need to know moment-to-moment changes during operative procedures. Although indirect methods are useful, intravascular monitoring is more reliable and sensitive, with the radial artery most commonly used. To ensure adequate collateral flow from the ulnar artery in case of radial artery occlusion, both radial and ulnar arteries should be digitally occluded after fist clenching and the ulnar pressure should then be released. If an adequate flush does not cover the entire hand, insufficient collateral flow is indicated, and the radial artery of that hand should not be used (Allen test). Also, indwelling catheters larger than 20 gauge should not be employed. The arterial line can be kept open by intermittent flushing with heparinized crystalloid solution or by using a pressure infusor. To calculate cerebral perfusion pressure (CPP), the intravascular arterial pressure transducer should be aligned to the superior margin of the surgical incision. CPP calculations, based on mean arterial blood pressure minus central venous pressure or intracranial pressure, whichever is higher, can be critical since even small decreases below the threshold for cerebral blood flow (CBF) autoregulation may be deleterious. The intravascular catheter also serves as a source of arterial blood for blood gases and other biochemical and hematological determinations.

CVP, Right Atrial, and Swan-Ganz Catheters

CVP monitoring has been used as an indication of acute circulatory changes, for evaluating volume status, and for aspiration in case of venous air embolism. Unfortunately, the CVP basically reflects the functional state of the right ventricle, which quite often does not indicate the status of the left heart. One can note a normal CVP in the face of marked changes in functional characteristics of the left heart. An important advance has been the relatively recent development of balloon flotation catheter techniques (Swan-Ganz), allowing for measurements of pulmonary capillary wedge pressure (PCWP) that closely reflect left atrial pressure and serve as an index of left ventricular filling pressure.[20,55]

The PCWP also can denote shifts in fluid from the pulmonary capillaries into the interstitial tissue and alveoli, indicating pulmonary congestion and/or the development of pulmonary edema. The triple lumen Swan-Ganz catheter can also give pulmonary artery (PA) and right atrial (RA) pressures, as well as having the ability to do repeated cardiac output measurements by the thermodilution technique. With the knowledge of flow and pressure, vascular resistances can be easily calculated and the addition of hematocrit, hemoglobin, and blood gases monitoring enables us to calculate a complete cardiopulmonary physiological profile including shunting, stroke volume, and oxygen transport. We have used this technique in difficult cases involving aneurysms and arteriovenous malformations with the catheter often introduced preoperatively. This is an excellent method in controlling volume replacement and continued monitoring in the intraoperative and postoperative periods. The ability to monitor plasma colloid oncotic pressure (COP) is important since a marked decrease in COP can produce pulmonary edema even in the face of normal or slightly elevated pulmonary capillary pressure (hypoproteinemia or large volume of crystalloids).

In terms of air aspiration, the proper positioning of the catheter in the right atrium can be accomplished by radiographic placement; by ECG verification (P-wave changes); and by inserting a 24-in. catheter its maximal length (via the antecubital fossa), attaching it to a strain gauge transducer, looking for a ventricular pulse contour, and then withdrawing until the wave form changes to an atrial pulse. The actual venous pressures may be measured with a strain gauge or water manometer zeroed to the level of the right atrium. For RA catheter placement, the basilic, cephalic, internal jugular, external jugular, or subclavian vein may be used. Because of the many reported complications (pneumothorax, hemothorax, etc.), we have abandoned using the subclavian vein for catheter placement. Recent experimental information has indicated that the optimal placement of the RA catheter tip in terms of maximal venous air aspiration is at the junction of the SVC and right atrium,[22] with use of a multiorifice (5-hole) 14-gauge Bunegin-Albin venous air aspiration set (Cook, Inc., Burlington, Indiana).

For conventional cardiovascular recording, mean arterial pressure (MAP) is measured at the right atrial level and also is referenced at the level of the cranial vertex to determine CPP. The latter figure becomes critical during induced hypotension, in which situation using the right atrium as the reference point for MAP would be misleading. Because of the gradient between the right side of the heart and the elevated incisional area, the MAP would naturally be higher than if the reference point were at the vertex, especially when the patient is in the sitting position and/or when the gradient between right atrium and vertex is greater.

Venous Air Embolism (VAE)

It is difficult to believe that by 1885 the physiopathology, diagnostic criteria, and treatment of VAE had been thoroughly elucidated by scientist-physicians from three different countries and two continents.[2] In 1839 Amussat, of France, published a book on "Research on the Accidental Introduction of Air into the Veins".[9] At the 13th meeting of the British Association for the Advancement of Science in 1843, Erichsen presented a communication "On the proximate cause of death after the spontaneous introduction of air into the veins, with some remarks on the treatment of the accident," which was published in 1844.[41] Finally, in 1885 the *Annals of Surgery* contained a 115-page dissertation by Senn on "An Experimental and Clinical Study of Air Embolism".[75] These three investigators described, collected, and reviewed hundreds of clinical cases of VAE and a host of experiments using a variety of animal species. This trio described the heart tone changes we now call "mill wheel," the gasping respirations, cyanosis, and cardiovascular collapse. They spoke about mechanical distension of the right side of the heart due to air bubble accumulation and about asphyxia from obstruction to the pulmonary circulation, often producing acute "anemia of the brain" and causing "acute cerebral ischemia." They also were familiar with the different responses to venous air and arterial air embolism and experimentally described and clinically documented that the development of gradients between the incisional area and the right heart area was critical in promoting the movement of air ("the force of gravitation"). Amussat, Erichsen, and Senn identified VAE in cases involving internal jugular, external jugular, facial, axillary, anterior thoracic, superficial cervical, femoral, internal saphenous, uterine, pulmonary, and diploic veins, as well as the superior longitudinal and uterine sinuses. They also advocated the prophylactic approach of painstaking hemostasis by compression, flooding the operative field, and vein ligation. In a number of elegant experimental studies they demonstrated that air in the right side of the heart could be removed by needle aspiration or by the introduction of a cannula or catheter via the jugular vein into the atrium and subsequent aspiration.

If one scans the surgical literature published during the 1800s, one can identify more than 150 articles, reports, reviews, and books on VAE. It is to be remembered that VAE was a much feared complication during the nineteenth century in the spontaneously ventilating (anesthetized or non-anesthetized) patient and that many surgical procedures were carried out in the sitting or semisitting position. Recent case reports have indicated the occurrence of VAE in non-neurosurgical cases and it appears that the lessons of history have to be relearned continuously.[61,66]

In terms of its potential side effects relating to VAE, the use of the sitting position is today as controversial as it was when it was first introduced. In 1913 DeMartel in Paris adopted the sitting position for brain tumor surgery under local anesthesia. Frazier in 1928 was the first in the United States to use this position for operations on the gasserian ganglion, and it has been popular ever since. In neurosurgery gradients between the right heart and the incisional area in the head or neck (as seen in the sitting position) enhance the subatmospheric pressures in the open venous channels, thereby enhancing the possibility of developing venous air embolism. Our neuroanesthesia group has noted that significant quantities of air can enter the venous system, even with gradients of not more than 5 cm in the lateral, supine, and prone positions.[7] Similarly, a death was reported in 1969 from venous air embolism in the prone position in which the head was elevated 10 cm above the heart level.[77] The neurosurgical practice of elevating the head above the heart level to allow for adequate venous drainage creates a gradient and potential source of VAE should the veins or dural sinuses be entered. This gravitational gradient can be enhanced by decreasing the mean intrathoracic pressure as well as by increasing the distance of the entrance point above the right side of the heart. A contracted blood volume and low central venous pressure will also enhance the effects of a small gradient. The right heart reference point can be considered to be on a transverse plane running through the fourth intercostal space.[73] For these reasons it is possible for VAE to occur during laminectomies using the Hastings frame, since there is a reduction in the intrathoracic and intra-abdominal pressures, which favors the development of a negative pressure and hence an increased gradient. With patients in the Hastings frame, caval pressures ranging from −2.0 to −6.6 cmH$_2$O have been reported.[39]

Incidence rates of VAE have changed since the introduction of the Doppler ultrasonic air bubble detector by Maroon and colleagues in 1968.[57] Prior to this date VAE was reported to occur in 0.98 to 15 percent[59,62] of the neurosurgical operations performed in the sitting position, while with Doppler monitoring the reported incidence rate has ranged from 21 to 60%.[3] We are concerned with VAE because the entrance of a large quantity of air can produce an air lock, which can block adequate filling of the right heart, and if not evacuated can lead to cardiac arrest. Because of solubility factors, the bubble volume is markedly increased in the presence of nitrous oxide, and at a 1:1 N$_2$O–O$_2$ concentration the bubble size is doubled.[64] Another danger of the entrance of a large volume of air into the right heart arises from the fact that if the right atrial pressure becomes greater than the left atrial pressure and a probe patent foramen ovale exists, the air could enter the left side of the heart and be deposited into the coronary sinuses and/or cerebral vessels. The entrance of air into the pulmonary vasculature can produce severe pulmonary perfusion deficits in humans, as noted by the use of technetium-macroaggregated albumin scans.[7] It is also possible that the passage of air in large quantities might so overwhelm the pulmonary vasculature[71] that passage across the capillary bed might occur, resulting in cerebral air embolism.

Signs of VAE may include spontaneous (gasping) respiration, increases in CVP, dysrhythmias, ECG changes, hypotension, changes in heart sounds, and cyanosis. Unfortunately, the appearance of the mill wheel murmur is a late occurrence and indicates that a substantial quantity of air has already been aspirated into the venous system.

The employment of ultrasonic Doppler techniques for air bubble detection has opened a new era in rapid, sensitive monitoring that now allows for detection of as little as 0.1 ml of air. Criteria for optimal Doppler transducer design involve adequate depth of field, beam coverage across the whole right atrium, and competent squelching circuitry to eliminate radiofrequency interference during electrocoagulation. Calibration for correct transducer localization is easily accomplished by rapid injection of a bolus (10 ml) of a crystalloid solution[87] through the RA catheter, the resultant turbulence giving a sound similar to that of air inflow.

Capnographic techniques for measuring levels of CO$_2$ in the expired air (ET$_{CO_2}$) have been used successfully for VAE detection.[59] Similarly, a rise in pulmonary artery pressure (PAP) occurs in the presence of small quantities of air.[65] The overall sensitivity ranking for detecting VAE is: Doppler >PAP > ET$_{CO_2}$ >MAP >esophageal stethoscope.[23]

Two new devices have recently been reported that may further improve our ability to diagnose VAE. The first is a transesophageal Doppler probe[60] that has a 360-degree arc and the capability to look at both the right and the left side of the heart. The second device[44] is a transesophageal echocardiographic unit with excellent sensitivity to air which also has the capability to monitor both sides of the heart simultaneously. The advantages of these devices are apparent, especially in terms of monitoring the occurrence of paradoxical VAE (movement of air across a patent foramen ovale).

Because of the possibility that VAE will occur, it is customary in some institutions to monitor for VAE with a Doppler monitor and right atrial catheter during any intracranial procedures regardless of the patient's position.

Other methods used to decrease the gravitational gradient have included jugular compression, the Valsalva maneuver, a neck tourniquet, movement of the entrance site to the heart level, controlled ventilation without a negative pressure phase, the antigravity suit (G-suit), and positive-end expiratory pressure (PEEP). The use of the G-suit has not been found to be an adequate preventive measure against VAE,[88] as the initial rise in CVP is soon dissipated to the upper extremities and the highly distensible splanchnic system. It has been thought for many years that the institution of PEEP during neurosurgical procedures in the sitting position might be effective in increasing the CVP enough to eliminate the gradient. I have also thought that 10 cm H_2O PEEP (used with skull closed when there was no increase in ICP or mass lesion or with skull open) might be beneficial in treating VAE in the presence of a small gradient. Bedford and Perkins-Pearson[13] have recently shown that 10 cm H_2O PEEP in the sitting position not only is ineffective in increasing venous pressure high enough to stop VAE but impairs cardiovascular function and also increases right atrial pressure more than left atrial pressure, allowing for the possibility of driving air across a patent foramen ovale into the left side of the heart, where coronary or cerebral air embolism might be formed.[27] For these reasons PEEP should not be instituted as therapy for VAE. When VAE is detected, the surgeon is alerted to look for the site of entrance of air, and the air is aspirated through the right atrial catheter. The N_2O is discontinued, the patient is placed on 100% O_2, and attention is paid to changes in the ECG and end-expiratory CO_2. If vital signs change as a result of large quantities of air, symptomatic treatment is used to combat the possible hypotension, arrhythmias, or cyanosis that may occur. The esophageal stethoscope may resound with a mill wheel murmur, usually a late occurrence, which indicates the uptake of a large volume of air into the right heart. With massive air embolism or inability to deal with steady entrainment of air, it may be necessary to place the head at or below heart level and to abort the operative procedure.

The hallmarks of VAE treatment appear to be early detection and aspiration with a previously inserted SVC-RA catheter. Over the years, neurosurgeons and anesthesiologists have become impatient and annoyed with the difficulties involved in placement of the right atrial catheter. Recently, Bunegin et al,[22] have indicated the precise location for placement of the catheter to obtain maximal air aspiration should VAE occur, and a multiorificed catheter with wire guide is now available, making the antecubital route

simple and successful. That the problem associated with VAE can still plague us can be noted by the reports of Cucchiara and Bowers[27] and Smith et al.[81] which indicate the relatively high incidence of VAE in the pediatric age group.

Electrocardiography

The electrocardiogram (ECG) is important for all neurosurgical cases, and a full complement of arm, limb, and some chest lead electrodes can be placed to help define any ECG abnormalities that may develop. It has been found that changes in rate and wave forms are a sensitive indicator of brain stem compression. Similarly, ECG (ST-T segment) changes have been reported from subarachnoid hemorrhage,[69] and continuous ECG monitoring should be carried out through the intraoperative period and postoperatively. New methods for evaluating myocardial function, in which ECG and arterial wave components are utilized, allow noninvasive evaluation of cardiac performance during neurosurgical procedures.

Urinary Output

An indwelling urinary tract catheter is extremely important in being able to follow the patient's response to the use of loop diuretics and/or hyperosmotic agents, as well as in gauging renal function during prolonged and/or profound hypotension. Similarly, estimates of urinary electrolytes and osmolality can be easily made.

Blood Chemistries, Blood Gases, Ventilation Measurements

The development of rapid microchemical and polarographic techniques has made it relatively simple to obtain a moment-to-moment metabolic profile. A blood sample (from arterial line) for hematocrit, blood gases, (Pa_{CO_2}, Pa_{O_2}, pH, bicarbonate, calculated base excess or deficit, colloid oncotic pressure, and serum osmolality can be reported within 10 min after receipt of a sample, with the addition of serum K^+, Na^+, Ca^{2+}, ionized calcium, and glucose adding another 10 min to the required time. Thus, intraoperative metabolic corrections can be made rapidly in acid-base balance and ventilatory requirements. Control of Pa_{CO_2} levels is critical in the management of CBF and ICP. Similarly, tidal volume, minute volume, and airway pressure should be easily obtained from the anesthesia machine ventilator.

EEG and Evoked Potentials

The clinical use of electroencephalography (EEG) for monitoring anesthesia depth with both inhalational and intravenous agents was pioneered by Faulconer et al.,[42] Bickford,[17] and Courtin et al.[26] These authors were also able to correlate electrophysiological responses and anesthetic depths[42] with blood levels of the inhalational agents. Unfortunately, the administration of premedications and other drugs also having electrophysiological effects makes it extremely difficult to use the EEG as a means of determining depth of anesthesia.

Because of its correlation with CBF,[85] the EEG has been used as an indicator of changes in brain state during hypotension, hypocarbia, and hypercarbia and in monitoring cerebral electrical activity during carotid endarterectomy and other neurovascular procedures.[84] The EEG is also used to monitor brain perfusion during open-heart surgery,[74] when either nonexistent or low-level EEG activity correlates well with serious postoperative neurological deficits.

Such new methods as spectral compression EEG techniques using Fourier processing eliminate the bulky EEG tracing, allow for the display of three-dimensional vertically compressed power spectra, and reduce data to an easily readable small area of paper display.[83] Changes in cerebral perfusion have been easily identified by this means during carotid endarterectomy and open-heart surgery.

The past decade has seen an extraordinary maturation in the development and employment of sensory evoked potential (SEP) measurement in clinical areas.[45] The SEP measurement can give indications of the physiological (and often functional) integrity of the central nervous system areas subserved as the pathways for these responses.[11] In terms of experience, somatosensory evoked potential (SSEP) measurement has been with us for the longest time, being utilized during surgery on the spine and spinal cord.[70] Brain stem auditory evoked potential (BAEP)[50] monitoring is used during posterior fossa explorations, and recording of visual evoked potential (VEP) responses[82] is used during procedures about the optic chiasm or nerves. SEP monitoring has been used as both a diagnostic and prognostic modality; in patients with spinal cord injuries and during spinal cord and spine procedures; in the comatose patient; for determinations of brain death; for delineating neoplasms, vascular abnormalities, infarcts, and other lesions; for evaluating ischemia, hypoxia, limits of induced hypotension,[21] and anesthesia levels; as an indicator of excessive brain retraction[16]; and as a monitor of auditory pathways.

Intraoperatively, better reliability and clinical correlation has been noted with the SSEP and BAEP than with the VEP. The more general use of the SEP as an intraoperative clinical monitoring tool has been limited because of the level of equipment sophistication, expense, technical utilization, and methodology and a lack of understanding and agreement concerning correlative significance. On the other hand, the studies that have already been made indicate that SEP monitoring during neurosurgical procedures will become an important standardized tool in the near future.

Brain Retraction Pressure

"It is evident the oedema is directly proportioned to the amount of insult to the brain during the operation. Gentleness in touching the brain, in traction, in sponging, the use of sharp incisions instead of blunt force in cleavage are all important in lowering the amount of cerebral oedema" (Walter E. Dandy 1932).

During intracranial procedures it is important to assure the brain of an adequate CPP,[12] and in general we would like to have a CPP at or above 50 torr.[76] It is to be remembered that under normal conditions, autoregulation of the intracranial circulation occurs at a mean arterial blood pressure (MAP) between 50 and 150 torr.

In the closed skull: $CPP = MAP - ICP$

While this is a global expression of overall perfusion for the whole brain, it does not indicate the status of regional perfusion pressure with the skull open and in the area where brain retraction is taking place.[53,72] We can make this calculation using

$$rCPP = MAP - BRP$$

where rCPP is the regional cerebral perfusion pressure (in mmHg) and BRP is the measured brain retraction pressure (in mmHg).

During the past decade our research group has been active in looking at many of the problems associated with the use of the brain retractor during neurosurgical procedures.[5] This work was stimulated in part by the findings of Numoto, Donaghy,[68] and Donaghy et al.[40] and the challenges in designing adequate instrumentation for monitoring the BRP.

Our animal data (dogs and subhuman primates) have indicated that the threshold for retraction injury[4,6] is related to the MAP, and thus a BRP of 20 torr is better tolerated at an MAP of 80 torr than at an MAP of 50 torr. Additional factors influencing lesion formation as a result of brain retraction may be due to the intrinsic pharmacologic properties of some of the agents used for induced hypotension[21] (trimethaphan and nitroprusside) and the halogenated anesthetics (halothane, enflurane). The BRP was monitored with a counterpressure pneumoelectronic switch built into a thin plastic sleeve into which the retractor was placed. This unit (Codman Pressure Monitor and Albin-Bunegin Pressure Sensor) cycles at least 20 times a minute and on a hard copy or CRT trace one may even be able to note respiratory fluctuations and vascular pulsations intermixed with the BRP recording.

Our animal data indicate that the BRP threshold for the development of histological changes after 1 h of retraction at normotensive levels was greater than 20 torr; at induced hypotensive levels (to MAP of 50 torr) the threshold dropped to greater than 10 torr.[6] At these threshold levels changes in blood-brain barrier permeability, neurological status, and somatosensory evoked responses (SER) also occurred.[4] A correlation was also seen between the SER and CPP when the BRP lesion threshold was reached. Similarly, a correlation was found between the cortical blood flow and SER at BRP lesion threshold levels.[16]

Our findings concerning the BRP reflection to the contralateral hemisphere are of interest. We noted that application of 20 torr BRP to one hemisphere produced an immediate rise in ICP of almost the same order of magnitude on the contralateral side.[6] Under these conditions, decreases in CBF (measured by microspheres) occurred bilaterally and were considerably greater under induced hypotension, with loss of autoregulation occurring when nitroprusside or trimethaphan was used. Although trimethaphan is a ganglionic blocker and theoretically does not directly affect resistance vessels, one of our studies has indicated that autoregulation is lost initially as the MAP starts to decrease to our endpoint of 50 torr.[21] This may be a dose-related function, for about 10 min after an MAP of 50 torr is reached, autoregulation appears to become reestablished. This may have clinical relevance, indicating the need to avoid retracting for a 10-min period after reaching a hypotensive level near 50 torr MAP. It is to be remembered that BRP pressures greater than 20 torr for 1 h (with an MAP at 50 torr) will produce a defined infarct in both subhuman primates and dogs.

Our studies of BRP in humans have indicated the importance of this monitoring tool in the education of the neurosurgical resident. As a rule, a number of initiates in neurosurgery have no idea as to the "feel" for specific BRP levels and are amazed to discover how easy it is to approach pressures of 50 torr or higher. Within a short time after using the BRP monitor, they are able to retract adequately using a BRP not greater than 20 torr.

While the danger of excessive BRP is obvious with the hand-held retractor, there are also potential problems associated with the use of mechanical retractor holders that may not be evident. We have followed the application of one or more $\frac{5}{16}$ in. De Martel retractors secured in place by retractor holders during initial exposure of the operative field. In some of these cases the brain falls away from the retractor, moving its bulk against the lateral or opposing portion of the inner table. At this time the retractors are repositioned, with a resulting BRP less than 20 torr. The retractors are left in place as the operation proceeds and ignored because the focus of the surgeon is not directly related to the area of mechanical retractors. While the repositioned BRP is less than 20 torr, a "rebound" often occurs, since the brain has no more room to move into the cranial vault, and within 10 to 15 min the BRP can be elevated to above 30 torr as the brain expands against the retractor. Under these conditions, the retractor should be loosened and if possible repositioned at a lower BRP.

Because of the difficulties involved in ensuring the equal distribution of retraction forces on the brain, tremendous shear stresses can be generated on the retractor edges. During neurosurgical procedures it is important not to use ridged or deformed retractor blades or those with sharp edges. Edge pressures can be attenuated by the use of energy-absorbing material and by better retractor design. Brain retraction pressure should be monitored, and whenever possible the retractor should be released periodically. Induced hypotension should be employed as sparingly as possible. Our aim should always be to encourage as adequate a regional cerebral perfusion pressure as possible which is compatible with surgical exposure and hemostasis.

Temperature

A temperature probe at midesophagus or a tympanic temperature probe is essential for monitoring this critical parameter. Esophageal temperature is closely related to intracardiac blood temperature and is within 1.0°C of brain temperature. Rectal temperature reflects that of the body core and may not change as rapidly as esophageal or tympanic measurements. Prompt recognition of such syndromes as malignant hyperpyrexia cannot be accomplished without this aid. Patients lose energy and heat under anesthesia, and body temperatures may fall to levels that increase cardiac irritability. Keeping a thermal blanket under the patient to control body temperature during operation is a worthwhile precaution.

Monitoring the Patient with a Ruptured Aneurysm

Patients with an aneurysmal bleed who are disoriented, comatose, or manifesting signs of cerebral vasospasm should be observed closely. Routine monitoring usually includes the ECG, arterial blood pressure (radial artery), urinary output, blood electrolytes, and blood gases from the arterial line. Elevated ICP, if suspected, can be monitored by one of several methods: an intraventricular catheter, Richmond bolt, or extradural transducer. Adequate ICP monitoring can be used for the monitoring of hyperosmolar therapy, and measurements of intracranial compliance can be obtained by injecting small aliquots of saline either intraventricularly or subdurally, and measuring the accompanying pressure rise and consequent time slope. In this manner one can note ICP changes initiated by changes in Pa_{CO_2}, Pa_{O_2}, acid-base balance, and hyperosmotic agents.

The adequacy of ventilation in these patients should be evaluated both clinically and by blood gas determinations. In the face of inadequate ventilation and an increased ICP, the patient should be intubated and ventilated so that the Pa_{O_2} is above 80 torr and the Pa_{CO_2} between 25 and 30 torr.

Strenuous pharmacological regimens are often instituted in this type of patient in order to avoid rebleeding, to control ICP, and to lower the mean arterial blood pressure from hypertensive levels.[89] Epsilon-aminocaproic acid is given in an attempt to retard fibrinolysis, isoproterenol to maintain adequate cerebral perfusion, aminophylline to dilate the cerebral vessels, kanamycin to block vasospasm by decreasing catecholamines, nitroprusside to lower MAP and enhance CBF, and agents ranging from reserpine to guanethidine to hydralazine to reduced high blood pressure. Calcium channel blockers have also been advocated recently for treatment of vasospasm.

This pharmacologic cornucopia necessitates a high level of vigilance in a special patient care unit, since most of the agents mentioned above are not without their side effects, including drug interactions. The inotropic drugs (isoproterenol) require ECG monitoring because of the arrhythmias they may produce and also require a nursing and professional staff capable of instituting adequate therapy should ventricular dysrhythmias occur; fibrinolytic drugs necessitate clot lysis studies as well as the availability of coagulation profiles in case bleeding problems develop; antihypertensive drugs necessitate the moment-to-moment evaluation of MAP; and the combination of many of these agents involves the potentiality of marked changes in serum osmolality, oncotic pressure, electrolytes, and blood volumes. The old concept of keeping the aneurysm patient "dry as a bone," resulting in decreases in circulating plasma and red blood cell volumes and increases in the levels of circulating antidiuretic hormone (ADH) and catecholamines, has changed to the concept of maintaining an adequate circulating blood volume that will maximize cerebral perfusion (of the microvasculature as well) and hence aid in the problem of cerebral vasospasm. This signifies being able to monitor blood volumes (directly or indirectly) in order to achieve our therapeutic goals and to prepare the patient adequately for the operative and anesthetic stresses encountered during the definitive surgical procedure. Plasma volume and red cell mass (RCM) can be determined by the radioimmunosorbent test with the hematocrit included in the equation. The RCM can also be measured with a radiolabeling technique using ^{59}Cr estimations of blood volume, and replacement therapy can be appreciated by understanding the cardiovascular dynamics involved in the right and left side of the heart, for which the Swan-Ganz triple lumen balloon catheter has been designed.

Anesthesia, Cerebral Blood Flow, and Metabolism

In neuroanesthesia our aims are to maintain optimal CPP while minimally challenging the autoregulatory capacity of the brain. Either primarily or because of associated secondary effects, anesthetic agents influence CBF, metabolic rate of cerebral oxygen consumption (CMRO$_2$), CPP, and cerebrovascular resistance (CVR). The secondary effects can relate to changes in body temperature, blood CO$_2$ and O$_2$ concentrations, and arterial and venous pressures. In general, the volatile inhalation anesthetics are cerebrovascular dilators[76]; they increase CBF and blood volume and can increase ICP although the last two effects may be modified by induced hypocapnia. The relationships between CBF and CMRO$_2$ are extremely important. Anesthetic agents that increase CBF achieve this by uncoupling the relationship of activity and flow and "steal" blood from an area of high function to an area of low function.

Halothane has been shown to be a vasodilator, increasing CBF and decreasing CMRO$_2$. Patients with moderate intracranial hypertension have evidenced further transient increases in ICP that can often but not always be minimized or eliminated by pretreatment to induce hypocapnia. ICP changes can develop after halothane also because of alterations in CPP secondary to hypotension caused by this anesthetic agent.

Methoxyflurane is similar to halothane in its cerebrovascular effects, except that it is very difficult to reduce the increased ICP response by moderate hyperventilation.

Enflurane is capable of increasing CBF and in the presence of intracranial hypertension may increase ICP even with pretreatment by hyperventilation to induce hypocapnia. This increase in ICP and a resultant drop in MAP because of the effect of enflurane on myocardial contractility may cause a decrease in CPP. Enflurane has the added liability of seizure activity at reduced CO$_2$ tensions.

Isoflurane is a new, potent halogenated agent that may be extremely useful in neuroanesthesia since CBF does not increase at anesthetic concentrations that produce surgical anesthesia (0.6 to 1.1 maximum allowable concentration).[10,67]

Nitrous oxide causes ICP elevation at normocapnic levels in patients with intracranial hypertension; this response may be attenuated by hyperventilation.

Of the intravenous anesthetics, ketamine increases CBF, CMRO$_2$, and ICP. Althesin and neuroleptic combinations (e.g., fentanyl-droperidol) decrease CBF, CMRO$_2$, and ICP.[76] The barbiturates have been shown to cause dose-dependent cerebrovascular constriction, with the CBF and CMRO$_2$ consistently decreasing.[78] The increased CVR found after narcotic and barbiturate administration may tend to lower ICP and hence minimize this response to ischemia or hypoxia by decreasing the accompanying cerebral edema. Barbiturates may also act as scavengers for the free radicals that develop during hypoxia-ischemia and may activate the pentose shunt cycle, thus allowing more effective carbohydrate metabolism. The edema response to cold-induced lesions is much less under thiopental and fentanyl-droperidol than under halothane.[79] Halothane has also been shown to cause blood-brain barrier permeability changes.

Recent information from Mann et al.[56] has indicated that anesthetic agents may elicit central nervous system responses other than those affecting CBF and CMRO$_2$. They noted that enflurane and ketamine increase both cerebral spinal fluid (CSF) outflow resistance and CSF resting pressures while enflurane also increases CSF formation. Conversely, pentobarbital has no effect on these CSF dynamics.

Induction of Anesthesia

We prefer to place the monitoring catheters before anesthetizing the patient. The exception may be the patient with an aneurysm, AVM, or elevated ICP in whom stress or anxiety would be dangerous. Quite often patients come to the operating room from the intensive care unit with the lines in place. Sedation with a benzodiazepine may be important in the apprehensive and/or hypertensive patient with a vascular lesion in order to avoid a rebleed.

The induction technique we use consists of preoxygenation with 100% O$_2$ by face mask for at least 5 min followed by 0.1 mg/kg of diazepam and 0.250 mg of fentanyl delivered intravenously. This is followed by the slow intravenous injection of 6.0 mg/kg of thiopental or thiamylal, the injected dose of barbiturate being titrated to changes in arterial blood pressure. In the aneurysm patient, metocurine iodide, a nondepolarizing muscle relaxant that has minimal effect on MAP or heart rate, is used for intubation at an intravenous dose of 0.3 mg/kg. Otherwise, we use pancuronium bromide for intubation and maintenance relaxation, starting with 0.15 mg/kg. A peripheral nerve stimulator is used with the electrodes placed over the ulnar nerve distribution at the wrist; the complete absence of twitch after tetanic stimulation indicates neuromuscular blockade. At this time 1.5 mg/kg of cardiac lidocaine (no preservative) is injected intravenously to attenuate coughing and bucking on endotracheal intubation. Lidocaine also has an effect of transiently decreasing CBF.[14,54] An armored (wire spiral) endotracheal tube with a low-pressure cuff is inserted under laryngoscopy and the patient is placed on a volume-cycled anesthesia ventilator, with the ventilation controlled to obtain a Pa$_{O_2}$ above 100 torr and a Pa$_{CO_2}$ of about 30 torr. Decreases in PCWP and/or pulmonary artery pressure as well as MAP generally indicate a hypovolemic state, which we treat by the infusion of 5% plasma protein. At about the same time that the muscle relaxant is administered for intubation, fentanyl or a fentanyl-droperidol combination is given. Anesthesia is maintained with a fentanyl-O$_2$-N$_2$O-curare combination, with the addition of a continuous infusion of 4.0 mg/kg per hour of thiopental or thiamylal. Because of head elevation above the right heart level, the ultrasonic Doppler air bubble detector is placed on the left sternal area, and an indwelling urinary catheter is inserted.

If deemed necessary, a lumbar subarachnoid malleable needle or catheter is placed for spinal drainage and attached to an appropriate collection system. To anticipate hypertensive surges and to be prepared to maintain MAP at a normotensive or hypotensive level during anesthesia induction and throughout the operative procedure, one must keep at hand a solution of trimethaphan, sodium nitroprusside, or nitroglycerin for intravenous infusion.

The patient is then moved or turned to the appropriate position, the monitoring instruments and anesthesia equipment are checked, and the patient is prepped and draped. Blood gases should be measured, and the patient's ventilatory needs should be estimated during positional changes. Alterations in pulmonary perfusion can occur with the patient in the lateral position. If the sitting position is selected by the neurosurgeon, the patient should be moved into this position slowly, with frequent observations of arterial and CVP, ECG, and adequacy of ventilation and breath sounds.

Control of Brain Volume

Hyperosmotic agents, including urea, mannitol, and glycerol, may be used to raise plasma osmolality so that intracellular water moves from the brain into the vascular system and thence to the kidneys. Urea, first used in 1956, causes local tissue irritation if it infiltrates and also produces a moderate rebound phenomenon. Mannitol, a larger molecule, has less rebound and can be used in the patient with renal disease, but during its active phase it has been noted to produced a transitory increase in $CMRO_2$. All three agents bring about hypervolemia with increase in blood pressure before diuresis, increased blood viscosity after diuresis, and some hemolysis. Glycerol is metabolized to CO_2 and H_2O and no rebound effect of consequence has been demonstrated. It can be used in the presence of diabetic ketoacidosis because insulin is not required for its metabolism. A 20% solution causes marked hemolysis but with a 10% solution hemolysis is minimal, and it may be an acceptable hyperosmotic agent. Loop diuretics (furosemide and ethacrynic acid) seem to be effective in reducing ICP, owing not only to their diuretic action but also to a central effect related to decreased cerebrospinal fluid production by central inhibition of chloride transport.[18]

Induced Hypotension

The successful use of certain microneurovascular surgical techniques depends mainly upon an operative field in which intravascular tension is markedly reduced. Use of the operating microscope and induced hypotension have been partly responsible for the marked decline in utilization of induced hypothermia during these operations. In many neurosurgical procedures in which vessel rupture is a hazard, it is now common practice to induce hypotension.

The concept of hypotension as an adjunct to neurosurgery was first voiced in 1917 by Harvey Cushing,[36] who observed that hemorrhage was followed by vasoconstriction, which led to a dry operating field. Others subsequently attempted to induce hypotension through arteriotomy, but

this technique was abandoned because "controlled shock" affects far more than blood pressure (e.g., pumping ability of the heart, peripheral vascular resistance, microcirculatory mechanisms, blood volume regulation, and blood rheology and coagulability) and produces tissue hypoxia. The production of vasomotor paralysis by blocking preganglionic sympathetic fibers through the use of subarachnoid drugs, reported in 1948, is not without hazard, is time-consuming, and is difficult to control. The selection of high spinal anesthesia merely as a means to produce hypotension has been questioned.

Another method of decreasing peripheral resistance and inducing hypotension is ganglionic blockade, first used by Enderby. Up to the mid-1970s the most common ganglionic blocking agent in use was trimethaphan. Probably owing to its rapid destruction by pseudocholinesterase, this drug has the advantage that its action can be maintained under precise control. Certain side effects, namely tachycardia, tachyphylaxis, inactivation of the pupillary reflex, curarelike action, and histamine release, are drawbacks to its use. The last of these has the potential for increasing ICP by causing cerebral vasodilation, either directly or indirectly by inducing bronchospasm, thus raising Pa_{CO_2}. Recent investigations have shown that trimethaphan can be as deleterious to cerebral metabolism as is acute hemorrhage. Deep halothane anesthesia will also produce hypotension, primarily by direct myocardial depression, with a subsequent fall in cardiac output. This agent has also been shown to cause the loss of cerebrovascular autoregulation, to raise ICP, to augment experimentally induced edema of the cerebral cortex, and at concentrations above 2.3 percent to produce cerebral lactic acidosis even when oxygenation is adequate. Other pharmacologic agents that have been used to decrease peripheral resistance include those that depress the midbrain autonomic centers (hydralazine) and the medullary vasomotor centers (narcotics, hypnotics), those that stimulate the brain stem vasodilator centers (veratrum alkaloids), those that block the postganglionic sympathetic fibers (chlorpromazine, guanethidine, phentolamine), and those that directly affect the vessel walls.

Sodium nitroprusside, acting directly on the vessel wall, is considered by many to be the agent of choice for induction of controlled hypotension because of its ability to easily affect blood pressure moment to moment and its apparent lack of tachyphylaxis. However, one must be cognizant of its potential for harm when considering its use in the neurosurgical patient.[48] The chemical structure of sodium nitroprusside includes five cyanide groups; this structure is rapidly broken down by both free and intracellular hemoglobin to release all five cyanide ions.[80] The majority of the released ions undergo detoxification by liver and kidney rhodanase systems, reacting with thiosulfate and vitamin B_{12} to produce thiocyanate. This end product of cyanide detoxification is not innocuous, however, and can produce toxic psychosis, hyperreflexia, and convulsions. The cause of three deaths after the intraoperative use of sodium nitroprusside was thought to be an inability of the patients to detoxify cyanide.[38] Michenfelder and Theye recommend a maximum acute dose not to exceed 1.5 mg/kg over 1 to 3 h, with a maximum chronic dose of 0.5 mg/kg per hour.[63] Cyanide exerts its toxic effect by interference with cytochrome oxidase, thus blocking the energy flow through the electron transport chain and inhibiting adenosine triphosphate production. Because the brain consumes energy at a constant rate in a variety of states, this metabolic blockade can have serious consequences. Apart from the toxicity inherent in its metabolites, sodium nitroprusside has been shown to increase ICP and to produce wide fluctuations of blood pressure which makes it potentially harmful, especially to patients with loss of autoregulation.[19]

Nitroglycerin (glyceryl trinitrate or GTN) has been part of the medical armamentarium for over 100 years. Its intravenous use was first reported by Christensson et al.[25], who intimated its possible application to obtaining steady vasodilatory effects in "certain clinical conditions." The present use of GTN intravenously is mainly aimed at the treatment of myocardial infarction. Studies have demonstrated that the action of this drug is primarily exerted on the capacitance vessels; it increases flow to ischemic myocardium, in contradistinction to sodium nitroprusside, and improves left ventricular function, all without significantly accelerating the heart rate. Kaplan et al.[51] used intravenous GTN intraoperatively and reported that the drug is easily regulated, produces little overshoot in controlled hypotension, and has no known toxicity.

Intravenous GTN[24] has been used to control blood pressure during such elective neurosurgical procedures as clipping of intracranial aneurysms, resections of AVMs, and microneurovascular decompression of cranial nerves. Recent studies have indicated that, like nitroprusside, GTN affects autoregulation and produces ICP elevations in humans. Because of its low toxicity and positive effect on the coronary circulation, we first use GTN for induced hypotension with the skull open and, in the event of tolerance, then go to nitroprusside.

Since rebound arterial hypertension has been reported after the abrupt termination of nitroprusside infusion and found to be due to activation of the renin-angiotensin system, propranolol[52] (as a renin antagonist) has been used prophylactically prior to initiation of induced hypotension.

Induced hypotension should not be attempted without an arterial line, ECG, and the capability to monitor urinary output continuously. The use of a CVP or Swan-Ganz catheter is also of aid in delineating the cardiovascular responses.

During aneurysm or AVM surgery, an adequate number of transfusion units should be available in a polystyrene cooler in the operating room. At least two large-bore intravenous catheters should be at hand for transfusion routes and they should be kept open.

Regardless of the hypotensive agent used, the drug should be delivered by means of a calibrated system, whether a microdrip infusion set or an infusion pump. The timing and depth of induced hypotension depend on surgical factors and the general condition of the patient. Because the purpose of hypotension is to reduce the arterial transmural pressure, it may be reasonable in many instances to start dropping the intra-arterial pressure by 15 or 20 torr with the opening of the dura. Many neurosurgeons ask that controlled hypotension begin as soon as aneurysm is brought into view and continue until after clipping. Some surgeons ask that the mean arterial pressure be brought to a certain level (e.g., 40 to 50 torr MAP at cranial level) and kept there

until after clipping. A physiological approach seems to be to bring the MAP down to a level at which intravascular pressure is reduced within the aneurysm itself, with the physiological constraints of the patient's condition always kept in mind.

After the need for induced hypotension has passed, the arterial pressure should be restored gradually, without administration of vasopressors, especially in those patients whose autoregulation is compromised. In these individuals CBF passively follows arterial pressure surges, and ICP may increase.

Induced hypotension involves risk in cases of brain stem compression by giant aneurysms, high ICP, vasospasm, chronic hypertension, and glaucoma. Indeed, the BP may even have to be raised temporarily during a short interruption of blood flow in a cerebral vessel.

Conclusion of Anesthesia

After termination of the surgical procedure, the patient should be evaluated, the muscle relaxant should be reversed, and if ventilation is adequate, the endotracheal tube should be removed, possibly after an intravenous injection of lidocaine to suppress the cough reflex momentarily. If any question arises related to ventilatory status, the patient should be sent to a special unit (recovery room, intensive care unit, continuous care unit) and extubated there later.

References

1. Albin MS: The neurosurgical patient. Excerpta Med Int Congr Ser 399:214–216, 1976.
2. Albin, MS: The sights and sounds of air. Anesthesiology 58:113–114, 1983.
3. Albin MS, Babinski M, Maroon JC, Jannetta PJ: Anesthetic management of posterior fossa surgery in the sitting position. Acta Anaesthesiol Scand, 20:117–128, 1976.
4. Albin M, Bunegin L, Bennett MH, Dujovny M, Jannetta PJ: Clinical and experimental brain retraction pressure monitoring. Acta Neurol Scand 56:Suppl 64:522–523, 1977.
5. Albin MS, Bunegin L, Dujovny M, Bennett MH, Jannetta PJ, Wisotzkey H: Brain retraction pressures during intracranial procedures. Surg Forum 26:199–200, 1975.
6. Albin MS, Bunegin L, Helsel P, Marlin A, Babinski M: Intracranial pressure and regional cerebral blood flow responses to experimental brain retraction pressure, in Shulman K, Marmarou A, Miller JD, Becker DP, Hochwold GM, Brock M (eds): Intracranial Pressure IV. Heidelberg, Springer, 1980, pp 131–135.
7. Albin MS, Carroll RG, Maroon JC: Clinical considerations concerning detection of venous air embolism. Neurosurgery 3:380–384, 1978.
8. Albin MS, Figallo E: Delayed postprandial solid food emesis in the postoperative patient. Excerpta Med Int Congr Ser 399:546–548, 1976.
9. Amussat JZ: Recherches sur l'Introduction Accidentelle de L'Air dans les Veins. Paris, Germer Baillière, 1839, p 255.
10. Artu AA: A comparison of the effects of isoflurane, enflurane, halothane, and fentanyl on cerebral blood volume and ICP. Proc Soc Neurosurg Anesth Neurol Supportive Care, Las Vegas, Oct 21, 1982, pp 98–102.
11. Astrup J, Symon L, Branston N, Lassen NA: Cortical evoked

potential and extracellular K$^+$ and H$^+$ at critical levels of brain ischemia. Stroke 8:51–57, 1977.

12. Becker DP, Vries JK, Young HF, Ward JD: Controlled cerebral perfusion pressure and ventilation in human mechanical brain injury: Prevention of progressive brain swelling, in Lundberg N, Ponten U, Brock M (eds): *Intracranial Pressure II*. Berlin, Springer, 1975, pp 440–484.

13. Bedford RF, Perkins-Pearson NAK: PEEP for treatment of venous air embolism. Proc Soc Neurosurg Anesth Neurol Supportive Care, Las Vegas, Oct 21, 1982, pp 94–97.

14. Bedford RF, Winn HR, Tyson G, Park TS, Jane JA: Lidocaine prevents increased ICP after endoctracheal intubation. In Shulman K, Marmarou A, Miller JD, Becker DP, Hochwold GM, Brock M (eds): *Intracranial Pressure IV*. Heidelberg, Springer, 1980, pp 595–598.

15. Beecher, HK: The first anesthesia records (Codman, Cushing). Surg Gynecol Obstet 71:689–993, 1940.

16. Bennett MH, Bunegin L, Albin M, Dujovny M, Hellstrom HR, Jannetta PJ: Evoked potential correlates of graded brain retraction pressure. Stroke 8:487–492, 1977.

17. Bickford RG: Use of frequency discrimination in the automatic electroencephalographic control of anesthesia (servo-anesthesia). Electroencephalogr Clin Neurophysiol 3:83–86, 1951.

18. Bourke RS, Kimelberg HK, Dazé MA, Popp AJ: Studies on the formation of astroglial swelling and its inhibition by clinically useful agents, in Popp AJ, Nelson LR, Bourke RS, Kimelberg HK (eds): *Seminars in Neurological Surgery: Neural Trauma*. New York, Raven Press, 1979, pp 95–113.

19. Brown DF, Hanlon K, Crockard HA, Mullan S: Effect of sodium nitroprusside on cerebral blood flow in conscious human beings. Surg Neurol 7:67–70, 1977.

20. Buchbinder N, Ganz W: Hemodynamic monitoring: Invasive techniques. Anesthesiology 45:146–155, 1976.

21. Bunegin L, Albin MS, Helsel PE, Hoffman A, Hung TK: Positioning the right atrial catheter: A model for reappraisal. Anesthesiology 55:343–348, 1981.

22. Bunegin L, Albin MS, Helsel P, Bell RD: Changes in somatosensory evoked responses and cerebral blood flow following induced hypotension. Anesthesiology 53:S46, 1980.

23. Chang JL, Albin MS, Bunegin L, Hung TK: Analysis and comparison of venous air embolism detection methods. Neurosurgery 7:135–141, 1980.

24. Chestnut JS, Albin MS, Newfield P, Maroon JC, Gonzalez-Abola E: Clinical evaluation of intravenous nitroglycerin for neurosurgery. J Neurosurg 48:704–711, 1978.

25. Christensson B, Nordenfelt I, Westling H, White T: Intravenous infusion of nitroglycerin in normal subjects. Scand J Clin Lab Invest 23:49–53, 1969.

26. Courtin RF, Bickford RG, Faulconer A Jr: The classification and significance of electro-encephalographic patterns produced by nitrous oxide–ether anesthesia during surgical operations. Proc Mayo Clin 25:197–206, 1950.

27. Cucchiara RF, Bowers B: Air embolism in children undergoing suboccipital craniotomy. Anesthesiology 57:338–339, 1982.

28. Cushing HW: Cocaine anesthesia in the treatment of certain cases of hernia and in operations for thyroid tumors. Johns Hopkins Hosp Bull 9:192–193, 1898.

29. Cushing H: Exploratory laparotomy under local anesthesia for acute abdominal symptoms occurring in the course of typhoid fever. Philadelphia Med J 5:501–508, 1900.

30. Cushing H: Observations on the neural anatomy of the inguinal region relative to the performance of herniotomy under local anaesthesia. Johns Hopkins Hosp Bull 11:58–64, 1900.

31. Cushing H: The employment of local anaesthesia in the radical cure of certain cases of hernia, with a note upon the nervous anatomy of the inguinal region. Ann Surg 31:1–34, 1900.

32. Cushing H: Concerning the poisonous effects of pure sodium chloride solutions upon the nerve-muscle preparation. Am J Physiol 6:77–90, 1901.

33. Cushing H: Concerning a definite regulatory mechanism of the vaso-motor center which controls blood pressure during cerebral compression. Johns Hopkins Hosp Bull 12:290–292, 1901.

34. Cushing H: On the avoidance of shock in major amputations by cocainization of large nerve-trunks preliminary to their division: With observations on blood-pressure changes in surgical cases. Ann Surg 36:321–345, 1902.

35. Cushing H: On routine determinations of arterial tension in operating room and clinic. Boston Med Surg J 148:250–256, 1903.

36. Cushing H: *Selected Papers on Neurosurgery*, Matson DD, Germen W (eds). New Haven, Yale University Press, 1969, p 669.

37. Cushing H: *Tumors of the Nervus Acusticus and the Syndrome of the Cerebellopontine Angle*. Philadelphia, W B Saunders, 1917, p 296.

38. Davies DW, Kadar D, Steward DJ, Munro IR: A sudden death associated with the use of sodium nitroprusside for induction of hypotension during anaesthesia. Can Anaesth Soc J 22:547–552, 1975.

39. DiStefano VJ, Klein KS, Nixon JE, Andrews ET: Intraoperative analysis of the effects of position and body habitus on surgery of the low back. Clin Orthop 99:51–54, 1974.

40. Donaghy RMP, Numoto M, Wallman LJ, Flanagan ME: Pressure measurement beneath retractors for protection of delicate tissues. Am J Surg 123:429–431, 1974.

41. Erichsen JE: On the proximate cause of death after the spontaneous introduction of air into the veins, with some remarks on the treatment of the accident. Edinburgh Med Surg J 61:1–24, 1844.

42. Faulconer A, Pender JW, Bickford RG: The influence of partial pressure of nitrous oxide on the depth of anesthesia and the electroencephalogram in man. Anesthesiology 10:601–609, 1949.

43. Fulton JF: *Harvey Cushing: A Biography*. Springfield, Ill, Charles C Thomas, 1946, p 754.

44. Furuya H, Suzuki T, Okumura F, Kishi Y, Uefuji T: Detection of air embolism by transesophageal echocardiography. Anesthesiology 58:124–129, 1983.

45. Grundy, BL: Intraoperative monitoring of sensory-evoked potentials. Anesthesiology 58:72–87, 1983.

46. Halsted, WS: Practical comments on the use and abuse of cocaine. Suggested by its invariably successful employment in more than a thousand minor surgical operations. NY Med J 42:294–295, 1885.

47. Heros RC, Zervas NT: Intracranial aneurysms, in *Recent Advances in Current Neurology*. Boston, Houghton Mifflin, 1978, pp 233–242.

48. Jack RD: Toxicity of sodium nitroprusside (letter). Br J Anaesth 46:952, 1974.

49. Jefferson, G: Harvey Cushing. Manch Univ Med Sch Gaz 22:37–45, 1943.

50. Jewett, DL, Romano, MN, Williston JS: Human auditory evoked potentials: Possible brain stem components detected on the scalp. Science 167:1517–1518, 1970.

51. Kaplan JA, Dunbar RW, Jones LE: Nitroglycerin infusion during coronary-artery surgery. Anesthesiology 45:14–21, 1976.

52. Khambatta HJ, Stone JG, Khan E: Propranolol abates nitroprusside-induced renin release. Anesthesiology 51:574, 1979 (Abstr.).

53. Laha RK, Dujovny M, Rao S, Barrionuevo PJ, Bunegin L, Hellstrom HR, Albin MS, Taylor FH: Cerebellar retraction: Significance and sequelae. Surg Neurol 12:209–214, 1979.

54. Lescanic ML, Miller ED Jr, DiFazio CA, Beckman JJ, Moscicki J: The effects of lidocaine on the whole body distribution

of radioactively labeled microspheres in the conscious rat. Anesthesiology 55:269–273, 1981.

55. Mangano DT: Monitoring pulmonary arterial pressure in coronary-artery disease. Anesthesiology 53:364–370, 1980.

56. Mann JD, Cookson SL, Mann ES: Differential effects of pentobarbital, ketamine hydrochloride, and enflurane anesthesia on CSF formation rate and outflow resistance in the rat, in Shulman K, Marmaru A, Miller JD, Becker DP, Hochwald GM, Brock M (eds): *Intracranial Pressure IV*. Heidelberg, Springer, 1980, pp 466–470.

57. Maroon, JC, Goodman, JM, Horner, TG, Cambell, RL: Detection of minute venous air emboli with ultrasound. Surg Gynecol Obstet, 127:1236–1238, 1968.

58. Maroon JC, Nelson PB: Hypovolemia in patients with subarachnoid hemorrhage: Therapeutic implications. Neurosurgery 4:223–226, 1979.

59. Marshall, BM: Air embolus in neurosurgical anaesthesia, its diagnosis and treatment. Can Anaesth Soc J, 12:255–261, 1965.

60. Martin RW, Colley PS: Evaluation of transesophageal Doppler detection air embolism in dogs. Anesthesiology 58:117–123, 1983.

61. Michel R: Air embolism in hip surgery. Anaesthesia 35:858–862, 1980.

62. Michenfelder JD, Terry HR Jr, Daw EF, Miller RH: Air embolism during neurosurgery: A new method of treatment. Anesth Analg (Cleve) 45:390–395, 1966.

63. Michenfelder JD, Theye R: Canine systemic and cerebral effects of hypotension induced by hemorrhage, trimethaphan, halothane, or nitroprusside. Anesthesiology 46:188–195, 1977.

64. Munson ES, Merrick HC: Effect of nitrous oxide on venous air embolism. Anesthesiology 27:783–787, 1966.

65. Munson ES, Paul WL, Petty JC, DePadua CB, Rhoton AL: Early detection of venous air embolism using a Swan-Ganz catheter. Anesthesiology 42:223–226, 1975.

66. Naulty SJ, Melsel LB, Datta S, Ostheimer GW: Air embolism during radical hysterectomy. Anesthesiology 57:420–422, 1982.

67. Newberg LA: The cerebral metabolic and protective effect of isoflurane. Proc Soc Neurosurg Anesth Neurol Supportive Care. Las Vegas, Oct. 21, 1982, pp 66–88.

68. Numoto M, Donaghy RMP: Effects of local pressure on cortical electrical activity and cortical vessels in the dog. J Neurosurg 33:381–387, 1970.

69. Parizel G: Life-threatening arrhythmias in subarachnoid hemorrhage. Angiology 24:17–21, 1973.

70. Perot PL Jr: Somatosensory evoked potentials in the evaluation of patients with spinal cord injury, in Morley, TP (ed): *Current Controversies in Neurosurgery*. Philadelphia, Saunders, 1976, pp 160–167.

71. Perschau RA, Munson ES, Chapin JC: Pulmonary interstitial edema after multiple venous air emboli. Anesthesiology 45:364–368, 1976.

72. Rosenorn J, Diemer NH: Reduction of regional cerebral blood flow during brain retraction pressure in the rat. J Neurosurg 56:826–829, 1982.

73. Rushmer RF: *Cardiovascular Dynamics*, 3d ed. Philadelphia, Saunders, 1970, p 559.

74. Schwartz MS, Colvin MP, Prior PF, Strunin L, Simpson BR, Weaver EJM, Scott DF: The cerebral function monitor: Its value in predicting the neurological outcome in patients undergoing cardiopulmonary by-pass. Anaesthesia 28:611–618, 1973.

75. Senn N: An experimental and clinical study of air embolism. Ann Surg 2:198–214, 1885.

76. Shapiro H: Intracranial hypertension: Therapeutic and anesthetic considerations. Anesthesiology 43:445–471, 1975.

77. Shenkin HN, Goldfedder P: Air embolism from exposure of posterior cranial fossa in prone position. (Letter to the editor). JAMA 210:726, 1969.

78. Smith AL, Hoff JT, Nielsen SL, Larson CP: Barbiturate protection against cerebral infarction, in Langfitt TW, McHenry LC Jr, Reivich M, Wollman H (eds): *Cerebral Circulation & Metabolism*. New York, Springer, 1975, pp 347–348.

79. Smith AL, Marque JJ: Anesthetics and cerebral edema. Anesthesiology 45:64–72, 1976.

80. Smith RP, Kruszyna H: Nitroprusside produces cyanide poisoning via a reaction with hemoglobin. J Pharmacol Exp Ther 191:557–563, 1974.

81. Smith S, Albin, MS, Boyd R: In press, 1984, Canad Anesth Soc J.

82. Sokol S: Visual evoked potentials, in Aminoff MJ: *Electrodiagnosis in Clinical Neurology*. New York, Churchill Livingstone, 1980, pp 348–369.

83. Stockard J, Bickford RG: The neurophysiology of anaesthesia, in Gordon E (ed): *A Basis and Practice of Neuroanesthesia*. Amsterdam, Excerpta Medica, 1975, pp 3–46.

84. Sundt T: Blood flow regulation in normal and ischemic brain, in *Current Concepts*. Kalamazoo, Michigan, Upjohn, 1979, p 32.

85. Sundt TM Jr, Sharbrough FW, Piepgras DG, Keoms TP, Messick JM Jr, O'Fallon, WM: Correlation of cerebral blood flow and electroencephalographic changes during carotid endarterectomy: With results of surgery and hemodynamics of cerebral ischemia. Mayo Clin Proc 56:533–543, 1981.

86. Thomson, EH: *Harvey Cushing: Surgeon, Author, Artist*. New York, Neale Watson Academic Publications, 1981, p 347.

87. Tinker JH, Gronert GA, Messick JM Jr, Michenfelder JD: Detection of air embolism, a test for positioning of right atrial catheter and Doppler probe. Anesthesiology 43:104–106, 1975.

88. Tinker, JH, Vandam LD: How effective is the G suit in neurosurgical operations? Anesthesiology 36:609–611, 1972.

89. Wilkins RH: Attempted prevention or treatment of intracranial arterial spasm: A survey. Neurosurgery 6:198–208, 1980.

39
Intensive Care
Allan B. Levin

The practice of modern neurosurgery requires the use in most instances of an intensive care unit (ICU). There seems to be a general consensus in recent years that patients with acute neurological disorders, such as head injury, subarachnoid hemorrhage, or rapidly expanding intracranial lesions, as well as postoperative patients who have undergone intracranial and in some cases even spinal surgery, require constant monitoring. This constant monitoring lasts for more than just the few hours available in a recovery room and may extend for several weeks. Certainly as our therapeutic measures and techniques improve, the need for this constant intensive care will continue to grow.

A Neurosurgical Intensive Care Unit

The question of the actual design of a neurosurgical ICU can be a matter of preference or a matter of what has been regulated by hospital planners and administrators. If we consider that major neurosurgical trauma and acute intracranial disorders require intensive care, then some form of an ICU must be available to the neurosurgeon. A general medical ICU used occasionally for neurosurgical patients cannot be considered to qualify as a neurosurgical ICU. The nurses usually have no experience in monitoring the neurosurgical patient. Therefore, the physician may find that he receives frequent calls regarding arrhythmias or significant changes in blood pressure, but if the patient developed pupillary dilatation it might not be reported to the physician. Although this is not a criticism of the nursing staff per se, it does point out the fact that nursing has become as specialized as other fields of medicine. We should not expect cardiovascular critical care nurses to be able to handle neurosurgical patients efficiently unless they take an interest in neurosurgical care and participate in continuing education. Further, these medical ICUs are rarely equipped to monitor the neurosurgical patient.

Although in many instances it would be ideal to have a separate isolated neurosurgical ICU, this is rarely feasible at present. But there are advantages to combined or adjacent ICUs in which the neurosurgical ICU is a portion of, or a satellite of, a larger ICU. This type of setup has the benefit of the presence of nurses trained for neurological-neurosurgical care and also of the constant presence of ancillary medical personnel and medical expertise, specifically that of pulmonary medicine, infectious disease, and respiratory care with their ability to offer ideas and aid in the management of secondary problems and complications.

To develop a neurosurgical ICU two requirements are very important. The first and most important is a nursing staff that has been trained and has developed an interest in the care of neurological and neurosurgical patients. This nursing staff must be aware of what the different symptoms and signs of neurological disorders are, what they mean, and, most importantly, how to treat them effectively in the temporary absence of a neurologically trained physician. Not only must these nurses be trained in this field but to keep abreast of changes they must have some form of continuing education and, even more importantly, they must be continually exposed to neurosurgical problems. Only occasional use of an ICU will lend itself to a gradual deterioration of care in that unit. The second item that is important in a neurosurgical ICU is the monitoring techniques available to the patient. Monitoring should consist not only of standard cardiovascular monitors but also of respiratory monitors, intracranial pressure (ICP) monitors, and in some cases, even more sophisticated equipment such as that used to measure evoked potentials and regional blood flow. Another extremely important item in the monitoring of the neurosurgical patient is the data form that is used. It must be able to connote changes in the patient's neurologic status as well as in temperature and other vital signs. These forms should provide ease of information input, easy visualization of progress (or deterioration), and easy conversion to computer data base input if and when this is available in the ICU.

The use of computers in ICUs has already begun. They have been used for nearly a decade in cardiac ICUs. The advantage of computers in the neurosurgical ICU presently consists of on-line data acquisition of monitored parameters, with the ability to signal an alarm with the development of such abnormalities as intracranial hypertension, cerebral perfusion pressure changes, or the presence of abnormal intracranial pressure wave patterns. It will also allow the physician to review patient status in a fairly condensed report form. Any data that are available on a computer can be transmitted across telephone lines which allows the physician to view patient status from either office or home. Certainly, the future will also allow for feedback mechanisms within the ICU, whereby treatment will be begun by the computer as it detects abnormalities.

It is our experience that the majority of neurosurgical patients in our ICU for longer than 5 days develop pulmonary infections as they are intubated over a prolonged time. It would be ideal to have separate rooms in the ICU to keep cross-contamination to a minimum. Another more expensive option is laminar air-flow rooms.

Last, the design of a neurosurgical ICU should allow for the easy access of patients to support equipment, including monitoring apparatus and respirators. There should be free movement of patients and equipment to and from the emergency area, the neurosurgical operating room area, CT scanning, and any other diagnostic facility. These should all be designed to allow for movement on the same floor so personnel do not have to be squeezed into an elevator while attempting to manage a critically ill patient.

Intensive Monitoring and Care

The neurosurgical model frequently used for intensive monitoring and for acute care is that of the head-injured patient.[10] Although much of the discussion here will refer to such patients, it must be remembered that with very minor modifications the model can be carried over to the acute patient with subarachnoid hemorrhage and vasospasm, the patient with an acute intracerebral hematoma, and even the postcraniotomy patient. When intensive monitoring was utilized, only 11 percent of our patients with post-traumatic mass lesions required surgical decompression, the overall mortality being less than 20 percent[6] Likewise, our group of patients with spontaneous intracerebral hematomas of non-aneurysmal origin could be treated throughout their acute course without requiring surgery and with zero mortality.[3] Certainly some of the improvements in mortality and outcome could be attributed to newer therapy, but overall I think the major factors have been advances in physiological monitoring and more aggressive therapy of derangements in these physiological parameters. This brief chapter does not allow me to discuss in detail all the modalities of monitoring; therefore, many of the references will have to be consulted for more detail.

Intracranial Pressure Monitoring

As neurosurgeons one of our primary concerns is the status of the intracranial contents. High-resolution CT scanning of the head is an absolute necessity in diagnosing and following structural intracranial changes. Major intracranial surgery should not be performed without the availability of such CT scanning. However, CT scanning cannot evaluate the physiological status of the intracranial contents and it cannot tell us the status of the ICP. It is therefore very important to monitor the ICP of all patients who have the potential of developing intracranial hypertension.[6] Certainly any head-injured patient who is comatose on arrival in the emergency room and remains so should have an ICP monitor. Likewise, patients with spontaneous intracerebral hematomas who are comatose or severely lethargic deserve ICP monitoring. Patients with subarachnoid hemorrhage may not require routine monitoring unless there is evidence of either neurologic deterioration or the onset of vasospasm. Postoperative ICP monitoring is usually a matter of preference, but certainly in large intracranial lesions, which entail the potential for severe postoperative edema, delayed hematoma formation, or hydrocephalus, the use of ICP monitoring should be routine. In acute problems monitors should be placed as soon as possible to allow for the early management of intracranial hypertension.

The duration of placement of an ICP monitor is determined by the presence of increased ICP. With normal pressure and improving neurological status, the monitor may be left in place for 3 to 5 days. Among head-injured patients we have found that only 10 percent had returned to normal ICP by 48 h and delayed intracranial hypertension can be seen in the severely contused patient with an onset as late as 5 to 7 days. Increased ICP can also be seen this late in patients with spontaneous intracerebral hematomas and patients who develop vasospasm from a subarachnoid hemorrhage. In view of this, it is our policy to leave the ICP monitor in place either until the patient has returned to an awake status or until the ICP has returned to normal and remained there without therapy for at least 48 h. In our experience the average duration of ICP monitoring in the head-injured patient is approximately 2 weeks, with the same duration in patients with spontaneous cerebral hematomas.

The type of ICP monitor used in the management of clinical problems is usually dictated by ease of use as well as duration of use. Also important is the complication rate of a particular mode of ICP monitoring. The first clinical measurements of ICP were done with an intraventricular catheter and today ventricular catheters remain a popular method for measuring ICP. The catheter is attached via a fluid pathway to either a fluid-filled manometer or a strain gauge. The readings of ICP are accurate as long as a free fluid pathway is maintained. However, because a ventricular catheter uses a fluid pathway means as easily as there is an egress of fluid, there can be an ingress of contamination and subsequent infection. Even when attempts were made to use buried ventricular reservoirs, which were intermittently or continuously punctured by needles, the infection rate remained fairly high. Our personal experience shows that by 10 days an infection rate with ventriculostomy approaches 100 percent. An additional problem that can exist is that of placement of the ventricular catheter in patients with large intracerebral hematomas and compressed or displaced ventricles. Also, as the brain begins to swell, the ventricles can collapse. If there is accidental or purposeful loss of fluid through the ventricular cannula, there will be a loss of monitoring capability at a point where the need for monitoring is the greatest. ICP monitoring from the subarachnoid space, utilizing either subarachnoid bolts or catheters, also requires fluid pathways to strain gauges, and the potential for infection is really unchanged from that of ventricular catheters. A specific drawback with the bolt system is that when there is significant increased pressure, the brain begins to herniate into the bolt and plug the fluid pathway. To overcome some of the problems of fluid pathway as well as cannula placement, miniaturized transducers have been developed, which can be implanted into the epidural space. The electrical ones are fragile and when patients do a fair amount of moving, they are easily broken. There is also the problem of zero drift and temperature instability, which can make them unreliable after a few days. More recently developed sensors that work on a nonelectrical basis in the epidural space have proved to be much more effective and accurate in the long run. It is these systems that we have been using for the past several years, with excellent results. In using epidural sensors it is important to remember to strip the dura from the bone around the area of implantation to prevent a wedge effect, which could artificially elevate the ICP value. There appears to be no problem from epidural scarring or loss of dural compliance throughout the duration of ICP monitoring. The fact that only the epidural space is entered means that the brain and subarachnoid space are protected from potential infections.

Consistent attempts have been made to develop telemetric monitoring. Problems with drift mean that there is a question of reliability of most telemetric systems once this system has been implanted for more than a few days. To date, none of the systems has proved practical in clinical practice. Further, it has not been shown that there is a need for long-term ICP monitoring in acute neurosurgical intensive care that would require the use of expensive and implantable devices. Considering the zero infection rate with the use of epidurally placed sensors with external leads, the potential for infection certainly cannot be said to warrant the additional expense and system complexities of telemetric devices.

Treatment of Intracranial Pressure

Although the treatment of increased ICP is discussed in detail elsewhere, it is important to at least outline it briefly at this point in the discussion of intensive care. The question always arises as to what abnormalities of ICP should be treated. We have long felt that the absolute value of ICP has little relevance per se; we tend rather to treat low perfusion pressure or the appearance of pressure waves. The perfusion pressure is the mean arterial pressure minus the ICP in millimeters of mercury. In patients who have a rapid increase in ICP, it is reasonable to consider a minimal perfusion pressure of 60 torr. If, however, the metabolic rate has been decreased either by hypothermia or by the use of high-dose barbiturates, the additional protective effect allows us to meet metabolic demand with a perfusion pressure as low as 40 torr and sometimes lower. We also have an absolute ICP level, which in our experience usually runs around 40 torr, above which we prefer to treat the patient. Above this level, despite adequate perfusion there most likely is some structural damage caused by compression itself. Another way of setting ICP limits is based upon clinical symptoms. Occasionally there can be a dampening effect of the local pressure, and the pressure actually being measured either through the subarachnoid or the epidural space will be somewhat lower than local pressure. The local pressure can then manifest itself as a change in neurological status or the appearance of a new neurological abnormality such as the dilation of a pupil.

We also treat the appearance of pressure waves. There are two basic wave patterns that are presently of clinical importance, A waves and B waves (Fig. 39-1). These were originally described by Lundberg.[9] A waves are periods of increased ICP with peak values of 50 torr or more lasting 5 to 20 min and usually superimposed on an already elevated baseline. These waves are always pathological, indicating vascular volume changes within the intracranial compartment that are beginning to compromise cerebral perfusion. They should be treated aggressively to prevent appearance of plateau waves, which are longer periods of markedly elevated ICP that may occur after a series of A waves. A terminal plateau wave may develop in which the ICP reaches the level of arterial pressure and cerebral blood flow ceases. B waves are short-term oscillations lower in amplitude than A waves and occurring at a rate of ½ to 2 waves per minute. These may or may not be pathological. Although B waves are clinically less significant than A waves, we sometimes find them in runs associated with pathological depression of consciousness and they can precede the appearance of A waves.

The therapy of ICP abnormalities should follow a logical sequence (Table 39-1). The question of the use of high-dose glucocorticoids always arises. Certainly glucocorticoids are indicated in increased ICP secondary to the cerebral edema of primary and metastatic brain tumors as well as extra-axial intracranial tumors. Their effects have been well documented. A standard dose has been an initial 10 mg dexamethasone followed by 4 mg every 4 to 6 h, but these doses can be raised dramatically with continuing beneficial results. The question of steroids in trauma and spontaneous intracerebral hematomas has been much more controversial. Numerous studies of routine-dose and high-dose glucocorticoids in head injuries have yielded variable results.[1,4] Our own studies have shown no change in the course of the head-injured patient regardless of the dose of steroids and no significant difference in complications with or without the use of glucocorticoids. Our present practice is to use one large dose of glucocorticoids (up to 60 mg per kilogram of dexamethasone) if there is a question of aspiration but otherwise not to persist with the use of steroids. Glucocorticoids are rarely used in our practice in patients with spontaneous intracerebral hematomas or in patients with subarachnoid hemorrhage.

To continue the sequence of increased ICP treatment, all comatose patients are routinely intubated and hyperventilation is instituted to drop the Pa_{CO_2}. We continue to lower the Pa_{CO_2} until the ICP is under control. In children we are not infrequently able to drive the Pa_{CO_2} into the high teens, although we prefer to hold it in the range of the low twenties. In adults this is extremely difficult. At best we can usually get the Pa_{CO_2} down into the low twenties but not much lower. Routine preference is to hold the Pa_{CO_2} in the area between 25 and 28 torr. The CO_2 reactivity of the cerebral vasculature appears to remain intact until brain function ac-

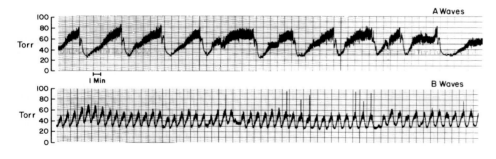

Figure 39-1 Appearance of A waves (upper trace) and B waves (lower trace) as measured by a rapid-response epidural intracranial ICP monitor. The form of these waves may vary with the type of monitor used.

TABLE 39-1 Flow Diagram of Treatment of Increased ICP

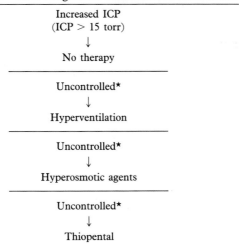

Increased ICP
(ICP > 15 torr)
↓
No therapy
_____
Uncontrolled*
↓
Hyperventilation
_____
Uncontrolled*
↓
Hyperosmotic agents
_____
Uncontrolled*
↓
Thiopental

*See text for definition.

Cerebral Blood Flow

The purpose of evaluating regional cerebral blood flow (rCBF) in the acute neurosurgical patient is to determine whether or not cerebral perfusion is adequate to meet the brain's metabolic demands and also to evaluate the effect of therapy used to control intracranial hypertension and other systemic pathological states. In addition, cerebral blood flow studies may be used in predicting outcome. The presence of global or focal ischemia and its duration may give us an indication of the amount of neural damage; a complete lack of flow can give us a diagnosis of cerebral death. Another parameter that can sometimes be developed from cerebral blood flow studies is the cerebral metabolic rate for oxygen (CMR_{O_2}). This, however, requires measuring the arterial venous difference in the oxygen content across the brain. Obtaining the venous sample requires catheterization of the jugular bulb; because of unequal drainage from the hemispheres it is very likely that the blood flow is not measured simultaneously from the region of the brain where the oxygen is being extracted. This means that the CMR_{O_2} derived is, at best, a rough estimate of brain metabolism.

tually ceases, and continued lowering of the CO_2 can continue to lower ICP. There is no evidence in humans that hyperventilation will lead to cerebral infarction. The major problem that can arise from hyperventilation is a change in pH, which will be discussed later in this chapter.

If patients cannot be treated adequately with hyperventilation, our next step is to use hyperosmotic agents. We have studied various agents including intravenous urea, oral urea, intravenous mannitol, glycerol, and intravenous furosemide[7]. We found that the only consistent effects were from urea and mannitol, and we use these agents exclusively. We initially start with a dose of 0.5 to 1 g per kilogram body weight of urea or 2 to 4 g per kilogram of body weight of mannitol. Recurrent pressure rises are then treated with smaller doses, usually half the initial dose; if a good response is obtained at that dose, then even smaller doses may be given with each ensuing rise. For an adult male weighing somewhere in the neighborhood of 75 to 80 kg we will start out with 40 to 80 g of urea. The second dose would be 40 g of urea and, providing good responses are obtained, recurrent doses would be 20 g of urea. Equivalent doses of mannitol would be 2 to 4 times that of urea in grams per kilogram. We consider continued therapy of a patient with 20 g of urea every 4 to 6 h to be quite reasonable for maintaining the ICP over several days, and in our experience this has been effective for as long as a few weeks. If, however, the dosage and frequency of hyperosmotic therapy continue to climb and the patient either requires hyperosmotic therapy more frequently than every 4 h or requires more than 2 g per kilogram body weight of urea or 6 g per kilogram body weight of mannitol in a 24-h period, we consider placing the patient on high-dose barbiturate therapy.

We have used thiopental as our barbiturate of choice. The advantage is that of a rapid onset because of lipid solubility and the potential of this barbiturate to act as a free-radical scavenger. Thiopental does, however, also appear to have the potential disadvantage of increased inhibition of the immune responses.

Electrophysiological Monitoring

Recording of electrical activity from the brain, whether spontaneous or evoked, has been used as an index of functional activity of the central nervous system and has also been used to demonstrate the integrity of central nervous system pathways. Measurement of electrical activity from the scalp requires appropriate placement of an electrode array, and since the signals being acquired are relatively small, the use of high gain amplifiers. The presence of a great deal of instrumentation in an ICU requires the filtering out of unwanted signals, mainly 60-Hz and very high frequency signals from television and radio. In developing evoked potentials, input stimuli are necessary. Because of the low amplitude of cortical or brain stem evoked responses, signal-averaging computers are necessary. Attempts have been made to utilize evoked potentials for correlation with neurological status after a central nervous system injury as well as for prognosis of outcome.[5] These can also be important in the evaluation and follow-up of the spinal cord–injured patient.

Respiratory System

In our ICU all acute neurosurgical patients who are comatose are intubated and placed on respirators. The use of the soft endotracheal tube allows for prolonged intubation (in excess of one month) without the necessity of tracheostomy. The frequent use of ventilators requires respiratory therapists to manage the technical aspect of the equipment and physicians to have a knowledge of gas exchange and the use of specific physiological measurements. There are many pulmonary factors that can be monitored in patients on respirators. As soon as one suspects any change in pulmonary status, blood gases and a chest x-ray film should be obtained.

Arterial Blood Gases

The most important measurement to determine respiratory status is that of arterial blood gases and the most important single factor is arterial oxygen tension (Pa_{O_2}). A Pa_{O_2} does not represent the absolute amount of oxygen being carried by the blood. Other factors, including both anemia and cardiac output, must be considered before one moves from a diagnosis of a low Pa_{O_2} to one of inadequate oxygenation. There is a nonlinear relationship between Pa_{O_2} and the percent saturation of hemoglobin (Fig. 39-2). This relationship must be kept in mind for two reasons. First, at the far right portion of the curve, very little added oxygen is carried by the hemoglobin with increasing Pa_{O_2}; therefore, little is gained by increases in Pa_{O_2} above 70 or 80 torr. Second, when Pa_{O_2} is at 55 torr, it lies at the beginning of a rapidly descending limb of the curve. Therefore, any decrease in Pa_{O_2} would cause a rapid drop in actual oxygen saturation, leading directly to a marked decrease in oxygen delivered. If adequate oxygen delivery can be provided and the flow of inspiratory oxygen kept under 50 percent, the additional insult of oxygen toxicity will not be added to any underlying pulmonary damage.[2] Keeping the Pa_{CO_2} within a normal range ensures that adequate ventilation of alveoli is occurring. This is of crucial importance in the comatose patient on mechanical ventilation. In neurosurgical patients a low Pa_{CO_2} is usually present and/or desired. However, this can lead to severe respiratory alkalosis. This major toxic effect of low Pa_{CO_2} can be avoided, however, by following the third parameter obtained by blood gases, the pH. Levels lower than 7.5 are relatively safe, but it is best to keep the level between 7.35 and 7.44. Another use of pH is to assess whether the pulmonary system is adequately adjusting for metabolic acidosis. The respiratory response to metabolic pH alterations is very rapid and in most cases very adequate. The pH should be approximately 7.35 in mild to moderate metabolic acidosis.

Gas Measurements

Several measurements of the fraction of gas concentrations have clinical relevance. Measurements of gas concentrations are expressed as either the fraction of the total (F) or, when that fraction is multiplied by the barometric pressure, as the partial pressure (P). The first clinically useful measurement is a routine analysis of the fraction of inspiratory oxygen concentration (FI_{O_2}). This monitoring parameter is a safeguard against inappropriate inspiratory gas concentrations. End tidal gas concentrations can be helpful if the gas analyzer used has a rapid response time. During expiratory flow out of the lung, the first gas expired has a low CO_2 fraction (F_{CO_2}). As more and more alveoli empty, F_{CO_2} rises. Finally, at the end of expiration, flow ceases (end expiration) and there is a plateau of the highest F_{CO_2}. This is thought to be a collection of alveolar gas in equilibrium with the arterialized capillary bed. Because the normal gradient between the arterial P_{CO_2} and the alveolar P_{CO_2} (PA_{CO_2}) is less than 4 torr, the end tidal CO_2 may be used effectively as a rough estimate of the Pa_{CO_2} to assess alveolar ventilation between blood gas determinations. A widening gradient between the arterial and alveolar P_{CO_2} is a very sensitive indicator of pulmonary emboli.[11] Anything that causes a loss of blood flow to alveolar capillary units can cause a widening of the gradient. Following the arterial difference in oxygen allows for overall evaluation of gas exchange.

Dead Space Determination

Another use of gas measurements is to estimate dead space. The *dead space* is the ventilation brought into the lungs that does not match up with perfused alveolar capillaries; thus, it is wasted ventilation. The trachea and major bronchi represent anatomic dead space. Normally about one-third of each tidal breath is dead space. Dead space is calculated by using the arterial P_{CO_2} and the P_{CO_2} in a mixed

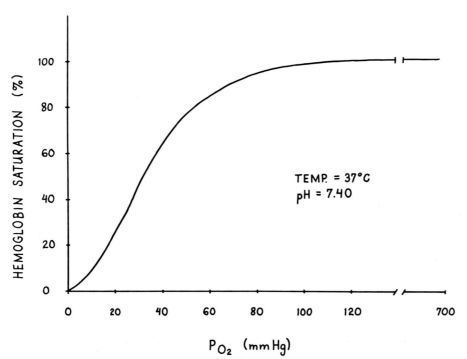

Figure 39-2 Oxyhemoglobin dissociation curve.

expired gas collection. In certain intensive care situations there is a marked increase in dead space. This becomes important when changing volume parameters to improve alveolar ventilation.

Oxygen Consumption

By using both inspiratory and expiratory gas concentrations and the measurement of minute volume, the volumes of O_2 (V_{O_2}) and CO_2 (V_{CO_2}) can be calculated. The ratio V_{CO_2}/V_{O_2} produces an estimate of the respiratory quotient. The V_{O_2} is an important number as it gives some idea of how many calories of energy are needed so that caloric intake can be adjusted properly. The V_{CO_2} is also of value if a patient is constantly having problems of weaning from the respirator because Pa_{CO_2} is elevated. If there is a high V_{CO_2}, one should carefully examine how many calories are being given. Excess calories will produce extra CO_2. In a patient with a borderline pulmonary status the extra work required to move the extra CO_2 may make weaning impossible or at least difficult.

Pressure Measurements

In normal respiration the mechanical act of inspiration involves action of the external intercostals and the diaphragm to make the pleural pressure more negative than the pressure within the lung. The intrapulmonary pressure is less than the atmospheric pressure and this pressure gradient causes movement of air into the lungs. During quiet expiration there is no requirement of muscle action because the rib cage and elastic fibers of the lung are stretched during inspiration and then move the air out of the lung as they return to the resting position.

The work required for ventilation to occur is the work needed to overcome the elastic forces stretching the lung and chest wall as well as the resistance to air flow in the airways. If the lungs have fibrosis or increased fluid within the interstitium, the pressure needed to expand the lungs to a given volume is increased. If the airways are narrowed, as with secretions or bronchial spasm, it takes more pressure to move air through the bronchi.

For the patient on the ventilator, the work of breathing is done by the ventilator. There is an elastic component, but instead of negative intrathoracic pressure pulling air in there is a positive pressure pushing air into the lungs. In addition, pressure is needed to overcome the resistance of the airways. The same conditions that cause stiffness of the lung, such as congestive heart failure or fibrosis, will require more pressure to get a given volume. With secretions or bronchial spasms it takes more pressure from the ventilator to move air into the lung. The measurement used to describe the elastic properties is the compliance (C). The change of volume (ΔV) over the resulting change of pressure (ΔP) is equal to the compliance. Resistance is a measurement that can be described as the pressure required to obtain a given flow through the airway.

The use of positive end-expiratory pressure (PEEP) is helpful in maintaining airway and alveolar patency, thereby improving oxygenation. Although PEEP has the potential for increasing ICP, we have found no significant difficulty when the pressure is kept below 10 cmH_2O. We prefer to keep PEEP below 7.5 cmH_2O and, if needed, add an inflation hold (usually 10 percent). This gives a higher but briefer temporary increase in airway pressure. The added advantage is that an inflation hold will open closed airway passages, whereas PEEP only maintains the airway passages that are already open.

Cardiovascular System

The cornerstone of hemodynamic monitoring is arterial pressure monitoring. This should be done with pressure transducers. This is especially necessary in those patients receiving intravenous infusions of vasoactive drugs, either vasodilators or vasopressors. Continuous monitoring of mean arterial pressure is imperative for calculating cerebral perfusion. An accurate mean arterial pressure is also necessary for calculation of peripheral vascular resistance. Since cardiac output, blood pressure, and peripheral resistance are related by the equation

Blood pressure = cardiac output × peripheral resistance

blood pressure can be maintained in a low output state by an increase in peripheral vascular resistance. In these cases, attempts at measuring blood pressure by cuff may result in gross underestimation of the pressure.

Monitoring Central Pressure and Cardiac Output

Basic goals for the hemodynamic management of critically ill patients are: (1) the optimization of oxygen delivery (the product of cardiac output and arterial oxygen content); and (2) the minimization of extravascular lung water accumulation, that is, pulmonary edema. The introduction of the flow-directed balloon-flotation pulmonary artery catheter (Swan-Ganz catheter) has greatly facilitated the achievement of these goals.[14]

The Swan-Ganz catheter has four lumina. The largest is the distal lumen, which terminates in an opening at the tip of the catheter. A second lumen ends in a latex balloon. The third lumen opens 30 cm from the tip and is used to measure the central venous pressure as well as to inject iced saline for the thermodilution output measurements. The fourth lumen carries the thermistor wires from the tip of the catheter.

As for placement of the Swan-Ganz Catheter, access to the central venous circulation can be gained from a peripheral or central approach. The peripheral approach has fallen into disfavor in most institutions because of difficulty of insertion as well as high risk of sepsis and peripheral vein thrombosis. The anatomical options for central placement include the internal jugular vein and the subclavian vein.

Swan-Ganz catheterization (Fig. 39-3) is performed with continuous monitoring of both pressure and waveforms from the catheter tip and of the ECG. Following introduction of the catheter through the introducer, the catheter is advanced until respiratory fluctuation in the pressure tracing confirms that the catheter tip is in the thorax. At that time the balloon is inflated and the catheter advanced with constant observation of waveform and pressure. The low-

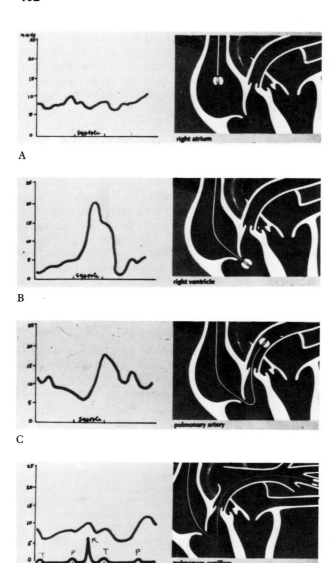

Figure 39-3 Pressure tracing of the Swan-Ganz catheter as it is advanced. *A.* Right atrial placement. *B.* Right ventricular placement. *C.* Pulmonary artery placement. *D.* Pulmonary capillary wedge placement. (American Edwards Laboratories.)

amplitude excursion of the right atrial pressure tracing changes to a high-amplitude excursion of the cone-shaped right ventricular tracing as the catheter tip crosses the tricuspid valve. Normal right ventricular pressures are in the range of 15 to 25 torr systolic and 0 to 8 torr diastolic. The highest risk of arrhythmia exists when the catheter tip is in the right ventricle. When the catheter tip crosses the pulmonic valve, both waveforms and pressure will change. A typical pulmonary artery tracing has a down slope, which is less steep than the up slope and which displays a prominent dicrotic notch. Normal pulmonary artery pressures are 15 to 25 torr systolic and 8 to 15 torr diastolic with a mean of 10 to 20 torr. As the catheter with the balloon still inflated is advanced, it will wedge in a branch of the pulmonary artery

and occlude it. At this point, the pressure present in the central pulmonary artery is effectively blocked off and the catheter tip senses the pressure transmitted retrograde from the left atrium through the pulmonary veins and capillaries. The pulmonary capillary wedge pressure (PCWP) thus approximates the left atrial pressure tracing and has the same configuration as the right atrial pressure tracing.

In the absence of significant lung disease, the mean PCWP is normally 1 to 4 torr less than the pulmonary artery diastolic pressure. After the catheter has been wedged and the pressure recorded, the balloon is deflated and the catheter tip will recoil into a more central pulmonary artery position with the return of the more typical pulmonary artery tracing. Slow reinflation of the balloon will again move the catheter tip into a wedge position. To avoid the possibility of pulmonary artery infarction, the catheter should never be left in the wedge position. Pressure and waveform monitoring is required to ensure that the spontaneous migration of the catheter tip into the wedge position will immediately be detected. Unexplained sepsis in the critically ill patient requires removal and culture of the catheter, as well as other vascular catheters, unless another source of sepsis can be identified.

The cardiac output determined with the Swan-Ganz catheter is obtained by a thermodilution technique. Recording of temperature change at the thermistor tip results in a temperature versus time curve. The area under the curve is inversely proportional to the cardiac output. The thermodilution technique itself most commonly utilizes a cardiac output computer linked to the thermistor.

Clinical Applications of Hemodynamic Measurements

Measurements obtained by the Swan-Ganz catheter combined with several derived hemodynamic parameters can provide important diagnostic information and facilitate therapeutic decision making. The PCWP, as well as being a measurement of the left atrial pressure, is also a reflection of the hydrostatic pressure exerted on the pulmonary capillary bed. Increased hydrostatic pressure and decreased plasma oncotic pressure promote the movement of water across the pulmonary capillary membrane. In a patient with normal pulmonary capillary permeability, an elevated PCWP can be quite predictive of the accumulation of pulmonary edema fluid. While evidence of pulmonary edema on chest x-ray films and by physical examination may persist for 24 to 48 h after the accumulation of edema fluid has ceased, the PCWP will instantaneously reflect responses to therapy. The interpretation of the PCWP must be tempered with the knowledge that oncotic pressure and permeability also play a role in accumulation of edema fluid. The patients with increased permeability or decreased plasma oncotic pressure are at increased risk for edema formation at any given PCWP. Increased permeability is the sine qua non of adult respiratory arrest syndrome, including neurogenic pulmonary edema. A decreased plasma oncotic pressure is common in catabolic, volume-restricted patients.

The patient's left atrial pressure approximates the left ventricular end-diastolic pressure and the PCWP is an indirect measurement of left ventricular end diastolic pressure.

The importance of this relationship lies in the fact that left ventricular end diastolic pressure (or ventricular preload) is one of the important determinants of left ventricular function, the others being afterload and myocardial contractility. The Frank-Starling curves (Fig. 39-4) show the relationship between the PCWP and the cardiac index. The cardiac index is the cardiac output divided by the body surface. The curves are depicted for hearts with decreased and normal contractility. In hearts with decreased contractility large increments in PCWP are attendant, with little or no change in cardiac output. The cardiac function of the patient who responds to a volume challenge with an increase in PCWP but not an increase in cardiac output is represented somewhere in the flat part of the Starling curve. Further volume increments in such a patient will not increase the cardiac output and will only increase the risk of pulmonary edema formation. Conversely, such a patient may respond to diuresis with a decrease in the PCWP and little or no decrements in cardiac output. The construction of the Starling curves is also useful in following drug interventions. Positive inotropic agents such as digoxin or dopamine, which increase contractility, and vasodilating agents, which decrease afterload, will move the curve of a failing heart upward and to the left. Drugs may thus be titrated to obtain an optimal point on the curve in order to maximize cardiac output while minimizing PCWP. These relationships have particular importance in neurosurgical patients with underlying cardiovascular disease, multisystem organ failure, or neurogenic pulmonary edema. They are also important in patients who are being treated with cardiodepressant drugs such as high-dose barbiturates or large doses of osmotic diuretics.

Total peripheral vascular resistance is one of the hemodynamic parameters that can be derived from Swan-Ganz catheter measurements. Total peripheral resistance contributes to afterload, the force the ventricle must overcome to produce a flow of blood, and can be calculated from this formula. Clearly, the Swan-Ganz catheter has replaced the central venous line as the optimum hemodynamic monitoring device for critically ill patients.

Electrical Cardiac Monitoring

Electrocardiographic (ECG) monitoring is the most routine of the intensive care monitors used. Normal electrical cardiac impulses are generated at the sinoatrial node. With a normal sinus rhythm these occur at a rate of 60 to 100 per minute, allowing for proper conduction throughout the remainder of the heart. The heart rate varies somewhat from moment to moment with respiration and venous return. If this moment-to-moment variation increases so that the interval is greater than 0.12 s, there is a sinus arrhythmia.

Sinus bradycardias of less than 45 beats per minute can significantly reduce cardiac output. If the slowing is of vagal origin, it can be blocked with atropine; if not, transvenous cardiac pacing is required. When the cardiac rate exceeds 100 beats per minute, a sinus tachycardia exists. In adults this seldom exceeds 160 beats per minute, or in children 200 beats per minute. Treatment of tachycardias, other than a paroxysmal atrial tachycardia, which can often be stopped with carotid massage, requires treatment of the underlying cause, which can be pain, fever, or shock. Any electrical impulse that arises outside of the sinoatrial node but within the atrium is referred to as an *ectopic atrial beat*. Ectopic beats may cause premature atrial contraction. This can be seen in cardiac ischemia as well as in fluid overloading. The ectopic beats are seldom of hemodynamic significance.

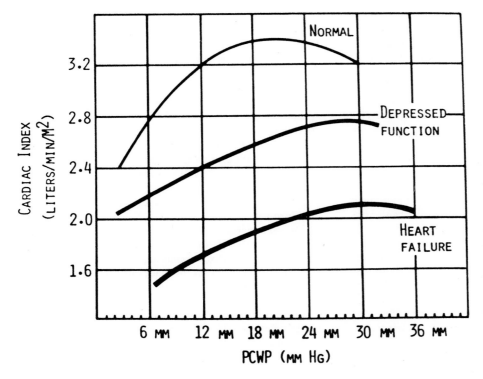

Figure 39-4 Frank-Starling curves of cardiac function: cardiac index vs. pulmonary capillary wedge pressure (PCWP). In the heart with normal function, an increase in PCWP gives an increase in cardiac index. In the heart with depressed function, very little augmentation of cardiac index is obtained by increasing the PCWP. (American Edwards Laboratories.)

Cardiac activity that arises primarily from the atrial-ventricular (AV) node is usually referred to as a *nodal rhythm*. The AV node will usually pace the heart at a rate of 40 to 70 beats per minute. Patients with nodal rhythm may be asymptomatic. Excessive slowing in the nodal rhythm, due to an excess of vagal tone, can be treated with atropine. Electrolyte abnormality or evidence of congestive heart failure should be corrected. There is also a nodal tachycardia. These can be of two types: (1) the paroxysmal type, which is hemodynamically similar to a paroxysmal auricular tachycardia and can usually be corrected with carotid massage; and (2) the nonparoxysmal type, which has a more gradual onset and can be caused by either digitalis toxicity or myocardial infarction.

Paroxysmal atrial tachycardia has a rate of 160 to 240 beats per minute and is characterized by regular P waves and an identical ventricular rate. The onset is usually sudden. Paroxysmal atrial tachycardia usually responds well to carotid massage. Despite the tachycardia there is usually only mild hemodynamic impairment. If, however, the patient has a marginal cardiopulmonary function, this tachycardia can cause a serious decrease in cardiac output. Atrial flutter is not a frequently seen arrhythmia and only occurs with an underlying heart disease. Atrial fibrillation is more frequently seen, with atrial contractions occurring at 400 to 800 beats per minute. There is a variable block so that the ventricular response is only 60 to 180 beats per minute. The ventricular response is grossly irregular in intensity and rhythm. With atrial fibrillation, cardiac function may be reduced by as much as 40 percent. In patients with some degree of heart failure, there is also an increased incidence of systemic emboli from clot formation. The significance of arrhythmias varies with the hemodynamic status of the patient. In any situation in which arrhythmia precipitates or causes shock or severe heart failure, cardioversion is indicated. Propranolol or verapamil are also effective in terminating supraventricular tachycardias.

Cardiac electrical activity that arises from the ventricle and is not the result of a conducted impulse is considered to be an ectopic ventricular beat. If such a beat occurs with sinus beats, then these are premature ventricular contractions (PVCs). PVCs that occur in short succession, are multifocal, or are present in the face of a tachycardia can be extremely dangerous and should be treated aggressively. These PVCs can occur in response to ischemia, hypoxia, or heart failure. They can also occur as an escape phenomena if the atrial impulse is conductive at less than 60 beats per minute. In this case no suppression of the ventricular contractions is indicated. PVCs otherwise should be treated with lidocaine. If the premature ventricular contractions become more regular, a ventricular tachycardia can ensue and may rapidly lead to a ventricular fibrillation, especially if there is underlying heart disease, ischemia, hypoxia, or acidosis. Patients with underlying heart disease will frequently develop heart failure and shock. If the rhythm is irregular and there is a suggestion of multiple ectopic foci, the condition becomes much more dangerous and should be treated immediately. Again, treatment is with lidocaine bolus and drip. If this fails to control the ventricular tachycardia, cardioversion should be performed. The ventricular tachycardia can progress into a ventricular flutter and

then, usually within a few seconds, to a ventricular fibrillation. In ventricular fibrillation there is total disorganization of ventricular contraction and the blood flow ceases. This is an indication for immediate cardiac massage and full-scale cardiac resuscitation, including electrical defibrillation.

Acute Care of the Critically Ill Neurosurgical Patient

Fluid and Electrolyte Therapy

It has been common practice among neurosurgeons to limit the fluid intake in patients with acute intracranial lesions and associated cerebral edema to approximately two-thirds that of normal maintenance. This is reasonable when considering the use of intravenous solutions in patients who are being treated in the early phases of increased ICP or in the early postoperative phases. If high-dose barbiturate therapy is to be used, normal daily fluid maintenance should be instituted. From most studies it appears that a 5% aqueous dextrose solution should not be used in patients with cerebral edema as it tends to enhance the edema process. A certain amount of saline should be utilized per day; we find it easiest to use a 5% dextrose in 0.5 N saline solution with added potassium if needed. Patients who are carried with fluid restriction and the use of hyperosmotic agents may, with time, get into difficulty with serum hyperosmolality and hypernatremia. On occasion we will allow patients to develop a serum sodium value in the range of 160 meq per liter and serum osmolalities around 360 mosm per liter. We try to maintain these values as the upper limits when treating patients with osmotic diuretics. The attempt to rapidly reverse these serum electrolyte abnormalities with dextrose in water solutions can be disastrous. We prefer to rehydrate the patient gradually, utilizing colloid solutions. Although these solutions still have salt, there is a gradual dilution effect, which will lower the serum osmolality and decrease the hypernatremia.

Occasionally diabetes insipidus may develop in head-injured patients and postoperative patients with lesions around the pituitary or hypothalamus. Initially it is best to control the diabetes insipidus with fluid replacement, as many times it will be self-limiting. If, however, the diabetes insipidus should continue, the use of 1-desamino-9-D-arginine vasopressin (DDAVP) as a nasal spray once or twice a day is indicated.[12] Its effects are shorter-acting than those of Pitressin tannate in oil and it has less side effects than aqueous Pitressin.

Directly opposite to diabetes insipidus is the syndrome of inappropriate ADH secretion, which is not infrequently seen in acute neurological conditions. This syndrome is diagnosed by the presence of inappropriate water retention with hyponatremia in the presence of normal kidney function and normal sodium excretion from the kidney. The treatment for this syndrome consists of fluid restriction and, in extremely severe cases, intravenous infusion of hypertonic saline solution. For the most part this syndrome is self-limiting; following several days of fluid restriction, there is a tendency for correction of the electrolyte disturbances.

Alimentation

The protein or crystalloid amino acid requirement for the well-nourished, nonstressed patient is about 1 g/kg per day. This increases 1.5- to 2.5-fold in the stressed patient. These stresses can be craniocerebral trauma, sepsis, or even elective surgery.[8] The stressed patient tends to have an increased protein turnover and protein not used for anabolism is used for fuel. Likewise, stressed patients tend to have an increase in resting metabolism, anywhere up to 1.5 times that of the normal, nonstressed resting patient.[8] The most commonly used source of carbohydrates, dextrose, yields about 3.4 kcal per gram. Nitrogen utilization from protein anabolism increases with increasing carbohydrate calories. The excess calories are stored as glycogen and fat. It is obvious that we cannot maintain the patients in either a neutral or positive metabolism balance utilizing 5% dextrose. Therefore, it becomes necessary in the early phase of intensive therapy to hyperaliment these patients. The most desirable route of alimentation is enteral. This gives the best uptake of the appropriate metabolic needs with the least complications. It also tends to maintain the integrity of the gut mucosa, which atrophies in the face of starvation. Many acute neurosurgical patients will have return of alimentary tract functions within a few days of the acute episode and are therefore good candidates for enteral alimentation. This is most frequently done with a nasogastric tube, although in the comatose patient one must watch for aspiration. It is important to use small, frequent feedings and to keep the patient's head up. Postural drainage should not be done immediately following tube feedings. It is preferable to have the patient intubated and to have the cuff inflated at the time of feeding. In the case of aspiration, feedings should stop temporarily and appropriate measures for aspiration should be taken. In patients who lack alimentary tract function, consideration of parenteral hyperalimentation should begin within the first few days following the acute episode.

Hyperalimentation is begun with 10% dextrose. The patient is then changed to standardized parenteral nutritional solutions with 25% glucose to which are added amino acids and standard electrolytes, i.e., sodium, potassium, chloride, calcium, magnesium, phosphorus, and acetate. To increase caloric content, lipids are added, as the caloric density of fat is about 9 kcal per gram. Hyperalimentation should be administered through a separate central line. Eventually one should plan on giving the average adult approximately 3000 kcal per day. In addition, parenteral vitamins should be added. Standard preparations of multivitamins plus folic acid and cyanocobalamin are placed within the parenteral solution. Trace elements should also include zinc, copper, chromium, and manganese. Phytonadione should be given once a week intramuscularly. Standard hyperalimentation solutions are now available commercially.[13]

When using hyperalimentation one must begin the hyperalimentation slowly, monitoring the serum glucose initially twice a day and then daily, as well as monitoring urine glucose every 8 h. Insulin should be used to control hyperglycemia but one must be careful to avoid hypokalemia. One must carefully observe the patient for sepsis and change the hyperalimentation line periodically in addition to maintaining good catheter care. Electrolytes must also be monitored carefully. Liver enzymes should be checked weekly to avoid complications from excess calories and to document adequate essential fatty acid intake.

Additional Comments

An additional problem that can arise in an immobilized patient, especially one without any active motion in the lower extremities, is the potential for blood clots.[15] Low-dose heparinization is one alternative, but one must be careful in trauma patients of the potential for hemorrhage. In the use of low-dose heparin therapy one should also include the concentration of heparin that is being utilized to keep the intraarterial lines open as well as heparin that might be placed into hyperalimentation lines. These should be totaled up before additional heparin is given. Pneumatic boots constitute another mode of therapy for patients with immobilized lower extremities.

References

1. Cooper PR, Moody S, Clark WK, Kirkpatrick J, Maravilla K, Gould AL, Drane W: Dexamethasone and severe head injury: A prospective double-blind study. J Neurosurg 51:307–316, 1979.
2. Deneke SM, Fanburg BL: Normobaric oxygen toxicity of the lung. N Engl J Med 303:76–86, 1980.
3. Duff TA, Ayeni S, Levin AB, Javid M: Nonsurgical management of spontaneous intracerebral hematoma. Neurosurgery 9:387–393, 1981.
4. Faupel G, Reulen HJ, Müller D, Schürmann K: Double-blind study on the effects of steroids on severe closed head injury, in Pappius HM, Feindel W (eds): *Dynamics of Brain Edema*. Berlin, Springer, 1976, pp 337–343.
5. Greenberg RP, Mayer DJ, Becker DP, Miller JD: Evaluation of brain function in severe human head trauma with multimodality evoked potentials. Part 1: Evoked brain-injury potentials, methods, and analysis. J Neurosurg 47:150–162, 1977.
6. Levin AB, Braun SR, Grossman JE: Physiological monitoring of the head-injured patient. Clin Neurosurg 29:240–287, 1982.
7. Levin AB, Duff TA, Javid MJ: Treatment of increased intracranial pressure: A comparison of different hyperosmotic agents and the use of thiopental. Neurosurgery 5:570–575, 1979.
8. Long CL: Metabolic response to injury and illness: Estimation of energy and protein needs from indirect calorimetry and nitrogen balance. JPEN 3:452–456, 1979.
9. Lundberg N: Continuous recording and control of ventricular fluid pressure in neurosurgical practice. Acta Psychiatr Scand 36 [Suppl 149]:1–193, 1960.
10. Marshall LF, Smith RW, Shapiro HM: The outcome with aggressive treatment in severe head injuries. Part 1: The significance of intracranial pressure monitoring. J Neurosurg 50:20–25, 1979.
11. Robin ED, Forkner CE Jr, Bromberg PA, Croteau JR, Travis DM: Alveolar gas exchange in clinical pulmonary embolism. N Engl J Med 262:283–287, 1960.

12. Robinson AG: DDAVP in the treatment of central diabetes insipidus. N Engl J Med 294:507–511, 1976.
13. Sorkness R: Parenteral fundamentals: Total parenteral nutrition. J Parent Drug Assoc 34:80–89, 1980.
14. Swan HJC, Ganz W, Forrester J, Marcus H, Diamond G,

Chonette D: Catheterization of the heart in man with use of a flow-directed balloon-tipped catheter. N Engl J Med 283:447–451, 1970.
15. Wessler S, Gitel SN: Thrombosis: The relationship of hemostatic mechanisms to drug therapy. J Neurosurg 54:1–11, 1981.

40

Prevention and Treatment of Thromboembolic Complications in a Neurosurgical Patient

Stephen K. Powers
Michael S. B. Edwards

Clinical studies have shown that 29 to 43 percent of neurosurgical patients will develop deep vein thrombosis (DVT) during the acute postoperative recovery period.[1,2,4,8,9] Anticoagulant treatment of these complications increases the inherent risk of hemorrhage into the operative site. Thus, prophylactic measures to prevent DVT appear to be the only logical approach to the problem of preventing postoperative thromboembolism in neurosurgical patients. Without thromboembolism prophylaxis, 1 percent of the patients develop fatal pulmonary embolism at our institution.

Incidence of DVT and Pulmonary Embolism

Without prophylaxis, DVT develops in one out of every three patients older than 40 years of age undergoing an elective general surgical procedure. Approximately 50 percent of orthopedic patients develop DVT. Pulmonary embolism (PE) is known to occur in 1.8 percent of surgical patients; it has been estimated that the incidence of undetected clinical PE ranges from 14 to 45 percent in the general surgical population. The incidence of PE in neurosurgical patients is not known, but in four series with over 1200 acutely paraplegic patients, the incidence of fatal PE was 2 percent.

Predisposing Factors

It has been suggested that a number of factors may increase the risk of developing DVT and PE, but only a few have been documented statistically. Age seems to be the most important factor in the development of DVT in the general surgical population. In particular, prolonged immobilization of patients more than 40 years of age is associated with an increased incidence of thromboembolic complications. In neurosurgical patients, however, age by itself has not been shown to increase risk, although factors that put the patient at risk are more prevalent with increasing age. Previous thromboembolic complications, leg weakness, varicose veins, cardiac disease (particularly congestive heart failure), malignancy, use of oral contraceptives, pregnancy, and myeloproliferative disorders have been associated with an increase in thromboembolism. In neurosurgical patients, a twofold increase in the risk of DVT has been associated with operations that last longer than 4 h. However, the risk of developing DVT after either spinal or intracranial operations is the same. Thus, any condition resulting in venous stasis of the lower extremities or a hypercoagulable state should lead the physician to suspect a greater risk of thromboembolic complications in the postoperative period.

Mechanism of Venous Thrombosis

Figure 40-1 illustrates the mechanisms of the coagulation system. Platelets, the first line of defense in the normal hemostatic mechanism, are activated only after the vascular endothelial lining has been damaged. The adhesiveness (ability to stick to nonplatelet surfaces) and aggregation (ability to stick to one another) of platelets assist in this hemostatic function. The second line of normal hemostatic defense is the fibrin plug. This system is activated by either the intrinsic pathway, which requires only blood components, or the extrinsic pathway, which requires thromboplastins released from tissue for activation.[7]

Clot formation in the intrinsic pathway begins with the sequential activation of four "hemophilioid factors" (so called because of the hemophilic states that exist with decreased activity of factors VIII, IX, and XI) caused by phos-

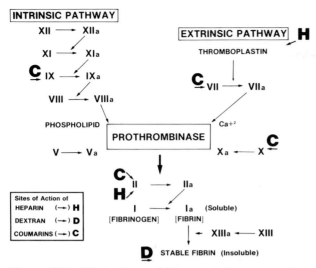

Figure 40-1 Mechanisms of the coagulation system that lead to the formation of a clot. Arrows indicate the points in the pathways at which anticoagulation agents act. (From Powers and Edwards.[8])

pholipids that probably come from platelets. Each step in the clotting cascade begins when an inactive plasma protein factor is changed into an enzymatically active form, which activates the next factor in the sequence. Calcium is involved in these reactions. Activated factor VIII activates factors V and X; with platelet phospholipids and calcium, factors V and X form a fourway complex that has prothrombinase activity and converts prothrombin (II) to thrombin (IIa), the latter of which then converts fibrinogen (I) to fibrin. However, at this point the fibrin clot is soft and fragile, and without the presence of activated factor XIII it would disintegrate rapidly in plasma. The extrinsic clotting pathway is initiated by the activation of factor VII by either tissue phospholipids or thromboplastin. Factor VII in turn activates the formation of the prothrombinase complex (factor Va–factor Xa–phospholipid–calcium) that converts prothrombin to thrombin and then forms fibrin, which is finally stabilized by factor XIIIa.

Blood clots that form in the veins of the pelvis and lower extremities (DVT) consist primarily of fibrin, erythrocytes, a few white blood cells, and some platelets that are randomly distributed throughout the venous plug. In contrast to the products of arterial thrombosis, platelets and platelet debris are rarely found in venous thrombi; activation of platelets by vascular endothelial injury that takes place in arterial thrombosis is not important in this sequence.

The brain contains the highest concentration of tissue thromboplastin in the body. It is therefore not surprising that intracranial surgery or trauma to the brain activates the coagulation mechanism through the release of tissue thromboplastin. Thus, the activation of the coagulation system along with venous stasis of the anesthetized patient initiates the formation of venous thrombosis in neurosurgical cases. The intrinsic and extrinsic pathways converge at clotting factor X, which, as will be discussed later, is the point in the mechanism at which low-dose heparin prevents the formation of thrombi.

Clinical Features

DVT often develops with symptoms or signs that may not be apparent to either the patient or physician. Not uncommonly, the first signs and symptoms that may signal the presence of DVT are those observed with pulmonary embolism. Although edema, increased calf girth, and local deep tenderness (Pratt's sign) are the most reliable physical findings, their absence does not indicate the absence of venous thrombosis.

Likewise, the majority of patients with PE are known to have symptoms and signs that are relatively nonspecific and may mimic any number of cardiopulmonary abnormalities. The sudden onset of dyspnea in a postoperative patient should suggest the diagnosis of PE. Dyspnea is seen in 81 percent of the patients with PE, and the intensity of this complaint by patients tends to be out of proportion to the degree of the objective abnormal findings. Pleuritic chest pain occurs in approximately three-fourths of patients but is not often associated with hemoptysis. In fact, hemoptysis occurs in approximately one-third of all patients with PE and its presence is indicative of infarction. Other symptoms commonly seen with PE are apprehension, a cough that is usually dry and hacking, diaphoresis, and occasionally syncope with massive PE.

The most frequent physical finding in PE is a tachypnea with a respiratory rate of greater than 16 per minute. Tachycardia is also often seen, with a heart rate greater than 100 beats per minute; there tends to be direct relationship between the size of the embolic process and the increase in the heart rate. When rales are present they indicate congestive heart failure. Almost half the patients are febrile, but temperature is usually only modestly elevated (100 to 102°F) and does not have the "spiking" nature of systemic infectious processes. A temperature above 103°F should suggest an etiology other than thromboembolism. Gallop heart sounds (S_3 and S_4) occur in one-third of patients with extensive embolic obstruction. Their presence reflects abnormal right ventricular hemodynamics. Cyanosis is uncommon and occurs only in patients with severe hypoxemia from extensive embolic obstruction.

Although DVT is associated with PE, it is asymptomatic in approximately 50 percent of patients. Only by the application of objective diagnostic tests can DVT be detected with any degree of accuracy. In most patients, DVT will not be recognized before the development of a PE. In fact, only 10 to 17 percent of neurosurgical patients who develop DVT have clinical symptoms or signs of venous thrombosis. One-third of patients with clinically recognized PE die, and half of these patients die within minutes of the onset of symptoms, before therapy can be started.

Assessment of Diagnostic Tests for DVT and PE

The objective of a diagnostic evaluation for PE is to confirm either the physician's clinical suspicion or to exclude the presence of disease as expeditiously as possible. Mortality of untreated PE is three to four times as high as the incidence in patients treated with conventional anticoagulation (8 percent mortality) or thrombolytic therapy. Therefore, early diagnosis and treatment are necessary to reduce mortality.

The importance of early diagnosis of DVT in neurosurgical patients raises several questions. First, the incidence of DVT is much greater than that of PE, and DVT that develops will not necessarily embolize the pulmonary circulation. Second, the risk of treating DVT with either anticoagulant or thrombolytic therapy in postoperative neurosurgical patients is forbiddingly high. Third, the clinical diagnosis of DVT (as has been mentioned previously) is infrequently made so that to make the diagnosis requires screening of all susceptible patients. The questions, then, in neurosurgical patients are whether the cost-benefit and risk-benefit ratios of aggressive diagnosis and management of DVT are acceptable. Because of the limited therapeutic alternatives available to treat the patient after diagnosis, we think that it is unjustified to perform multiple tests to diagnose DVT. We suggest that methods aimed primarily at the prophylaxis of DVT would offer the most benefit to the neurosurgical patient in the postoperative period.

Routine laboratory studies offer little in the diagnosis of PE. There is often a nonspecific elevation of lactate dehydrogenase and serum bilirubin in the presence of normal serum glutamic oxalacetic transaminase. The electrocardiogram may be abnormal, but the findings are often nonspecific, aside from the pattern of acute cor pulmonale or the S_1-Q_3-T_3 pattern. QRS abnormalities are noted in two-thirds of the patients. More commonly, nonspecific ST-T wave changes are seen, along with various ventricular and atrial arrythmias.

Chest x-rays may demonstrate pulmonary infiltration and evidence of pleural effusion if infarction has occurred; however, the chest x-ray is usually normal until 12 to 36 h after infarction. Massive emboli are often associated with arterial hypoxemia, hypocapnia, and respiratory alkalosis. An inverse relationship exists between the size of the embolic obstruction and the Pa_{O_2} in patients without previous cardiopulmonary disease. The perfusion lung scan has been most valuable in the diagnosis of PE and demonstrates abnormalities in the distribution of pulmonary blood flow. Perfusion scans are interpreted as showing lesions of high probability of being caused by PE when there are multiple defects or lesions having configurations compatible with vascular lesions. Medium and low probability scans are those in which there are either singular or multiple filling defects generally corresponding to some abnormality seen on the plain chest x-ray. The performance of ventilation scans before or shortly after perfusion scanning adds specificity to the test. Characteristically, a normal ventilation scan in an area of perfusion abnormality is highly specific for PE. Selective pulmonary angiography is the only means by which anatomical information about the pulmonary vasculature can be obtained. Angiography is most helpful in demonstrating embolism in patients with underlying heart or lung disease whose clinical presentation may be nonspecific and compatible with exacerbation of an underlying disease or whose ventilation-perfusion scans may be less specific. Pulmonary angiography is an invasive procedure and carries an overall mortality of 1 percent when performed by experienced personnel.

Most patients who die from PE will have evidence of DVT of the legs at autopsy. Because of this observation, the assessment of the deep venous system with various noninvasive techniques has recently become a great aid in the indirect diagnosis of PE. The ^{125}I-fibrinogen uptake test is the most sensitive technique for detecting active thrombosis in calf veins. It is the most useful clinical test for establishing the activity of thrombosis in patients in whom recurrence of active venous thrombosis is suspected. However, the technique is insensitive to thrombi that are not actively forming. This technique cannot be used in patients who have leg wounds, hematomas, or inflammatory conditions involving the areas to be examined because of the overlying uptake of ^{125}I-fibrinogen. The technique is also insensitive to proximal thigh-vein thrombosis and particularly to thrombi in the iliac veins.

Doppler ultrasound, which involves a sound pattern recognition, requires considerable experience with the method to achieve maximal accuracy. This method has a 95 percent accuracy for either the identification or exclusion of DVT as compared with contrast phlebography. The technique detects alterations in the normal phasic flow characteristics of the extremities and because of this is quite nonspecific. Therefore, conditions that affect venous outflow will result in Doppler venous abnormalities. Other noninvasive techniques include plethysmography and radionuclide phlebography, which in selected patients have been shown to be effective for the diagnosis of DVT of the lower extremities.

Treatment of DVT and PE

Anticoagulant therapy is the mainstay of management for thromboembolism. Unfortunately, patients who have undergone either intracranial or intraspinal operations are at high risk for major hemorrhage into the operative site and subsequent neurological catastrophe from anticoagulant therapy. The risks from an untreated thromboembolic process must be weighed against the risks of hemorrhagic complications from the anticoagulant therapy. Trials conducted at the National Institutes of Health (NIH) have shown that absolute contraindications for the use of thrombolytic therapy (streptokinase and urokinase) include active internal bleeding states and a recent (within 2 months) cerebral vascular process or procedure.[6] A more remote (greater than 2 months) cerebral vascular process should be considered a very strong but relative contraindication and the decision to use lytic agents must be based on an assessment of the risk-benefit status. The NIH guidelines list as a relative contraindication any recent invasive procedure involving a body cavity (for example, the spinal cord) or vessel that cannot be compressed for a long period unless the risk of the thromboembolic process overrides the risk of bleeding.

Streptokinase and urokinase, which are plasminogen activators that lyse thromboemboli, have been shown to be more effective in the treatment of PE and DVT than high doses of heparin for the dissolution of pulmonary emboli. This is reflected in better improvement in the abnormal hemodynamics of the right heart and pulmonary circulation than is seen with heparin. However, there has been no difference in the mortality rate between patients treated with fibrinolytic agents and heparin. Significant bleeding occurs in 5 to 9 percent of unoperated patients who receive either urokinase or streptokinase. The incidence of bleeding complications is somewhat higher (4 percent) than that for high-dose heparin in unoperated patients. However, the risk of catastrophic hemorrhage from either of these agents for documented thromboembolism in the postoperative neurosurgical patient is substantially increased.

Because the treatments available for a potentially fatal thromboembolic complication are severely limited and because of our experience with hemorrhagic catastrophes in patients who were treated with anticoagulation or thrombolysis, we have relied on vena caval ligation or the placement of a caval "umbrella" in some of our patients who demonstrated pulmonary embolization from a thrombus arising in the pelvis or lower extremities postoperatively. This procedure is not without risk and does not avert half the deaths from sudden PE.

Methods of Prophylaxis

The most widely used prophylactic measures against thromboembolic complications are either mechanical or pharmacological. Mechanical methods are popular because the devices used do not cause hemorrhagic complications, being used primarily to improve venous blood flow to extremities by eliminating the effect of venous stasis on the production of DVT. Operative intervention by caval ligation or the placement of a caval "umbrella" can be considered a subgroup of this category. However, operative procedures are used only to prevent pulmonary embolizations from documented pelvic or lower extremity DVT and are used only when other means of preventing PE have failed or when their use is contraindicated in a given patient.

Standard prophylactic methods, which include ambulation soon after operation, leg elevation, and physiotherapy, have no effect on the incidence of DVT. Elastic stockings do not decrease the risk, but graduated compression stockings effectively decrease DVT. There is no evidence that the latter lower the incidence of postoperative pulmonary embolism.

For general surgical and neurosurgical patients, intraoperative intermittent pneumatic compression of the calf is probably the best available mechanical means for the prophylaxis of postoperative DVT.[10] Although it has not been proved that this technique prevents PE, it should be considered when prophylactic drug therapy is contraindicated. Intraoperative electrical stimulation of the calf lowers the incidence of DVT by 50 percent in general surgical patients, but its effect on PE is not known. Other mechanical methods of prophylaxis that have been used include the intraoperative foot mover and intermittent-pulse graduated pressure stockings; there are no reports of their efficacy. Generally, pharmacological prophylaxis is more effective than mechanical methods for prevention of DVT or PE.

Antiplatelet agents such as aspirin, dipyridamole, and sulfinpyrazone may reduce the incidence of DVT in certain patient groups, but none reduces the incidence of fatal PE. However, the coumarins (warfarin), heparin, and dextran reduce the incidence of PE.

Coumarins have been used primarily in orthopedic patients to lower the incidence of postoperative DVT. Coumarins are vitamin K antagonists and therefore inhibit the production of factors II, VII, IX, and X by the liver (Figure 40-1). However, because of the high incidence of side effects and the interaction of coumarins with many drugs, they are not widely used to prevent thromboembolism. The prophylactic use of coumarins has not been studied extensively in other patient groups.

The prophylactic effect of low-dose heparin has been studied extensively in the past decade and has been shown to diminish effectively the risk of both DVT and PE after operation. In 1975 the first international multicenter trial, carried out with over 2000 patients, showed that treatment with 5000 IU of calcium heparin administered subcutaneously 2 h before operation and continued every 8 h for 7 days or longer (until the patient was ambulatory) reduced the incidence of DVT from 24.6 percent in the control group to 7.7 percent in the treated group and reduced the incidence of fatal PE by 87.5 percent.[5] Recently, it has been shown that 5000 IU of heparin administered subcutaneously twice a day prevents DVT as effectively as the same dose given three times a day. Heparin prophylaxis should begin before surgery and continue until the patient is ambulatory. Although there is a higher frequency of wound hematomas in patients receiving low-dose heparin, the incidence of major bleeding complications is not increased by its use. Barnett et al. have shown that low-dose heparin can be used safely in neurosurgical patients who received a dose of 5000 IU administered subcutaneously preoperatively and twice daily after operation for at least three days.[1] None of 50 patients undergoing a number of neurosurgical procedures developed a major hemorrhagic complication. Among the complications reported were four wound seromas, two wound hematomas, and one nonfatal PE. Barnett et al. concluded that there was no increased risk of either intraspinal or intracranial hemorrhage with low-dose heparin given on this schedule.[1] Cerrato et al. did not find a difference in transfusion requirements, postoperative hemoglobin concentrations, or the occurrence of postoperative hematomas in neurosurgical patients who received low-dose (5000 IU) heparin subcutaneously 2 h before surgery and every 8 h thereafter for at least 7 days.[2] A lower heparin dose (3750 IU) was given to four patients who had abnormal prothrombin and partial thromboplastin times with a normal dose.

Current interest in avoiding the risk of minor bleeding complications with heparin therapy has led to the use of ultralow-dose heparin. A statistically significant decrease in DVT, comparable with the decrease produced by standard low-dose heparin therapy, has been noted on using 1 IU of intravenous heparin per kilogram body weight per hour for 3 to 5 days after major abdominal surgery. This dose is probably equivalent to the amount of heparin used to flush arterial catheters in an intensive care unit. Continuous administration avoids the peaks of hypocoagulability that may occur with periodic heparin administration and theoretically should not create as high an incidence of minor bleeding complications as does low-dose heparin.

Several theories have been proposed to explain why low-dose heparin therapy prevents thromboembolism. Heparin increases the activity of plasma antithrombin III, which acts to inhibit activated factor X and thereby affects both the intrinsic and extrinsic clotting mechanisms (Fig. 40-1). If administered before factor X is activated by tissue thromboplastins released in a surgical operation, lower doses of heparin can effectively prevent clot formation by inhibiting factor X. However, if factor X has been activated by thromboplastins, higher prophylactic doses are necessary to inhibit clot formation. Plasma concentrations of 0.25 to 0.5 IU of heparin per milliliter destroy thromboplastin that has formed, and the formation of intrinsic plasma thromboplastin is prevented by as little as 0.05 to 0.033 IU of heparin per milliliter. Thus, the action of heparin may be mediated both through its effect on thromboplastins and through its effect on antithrombin III. Negus, who was the first to propose the use of ultralow-dose heparin, has shown that the normal postoperative increase in platelet adhesion is reduced by 1 IU of heparin per kilogram body weight given intravenously. Other possible mechanisms of action might include the release of factor IV by vascular endothelium or an increase in plasma thromboxane B_2, which is thought to affect platelet activation by either thromboxane A_2 or thrombin. Irrespective of which mechanism(s) is operative, very small doses of heparin produce antithrombogenicity; at the same plasma concentrations, anticoagulation does not occur.

Several other regimens that either improve DVT and PE prophylaxis or lower the incidence of heparin-associated postoperative wound hematomas are being studied. Semisynthetic heparin analogues and synthetic heparoids are of interest because they reduce the incidence of bleeding complications. The combination of 5000 IU heparin and 0.5 IU of dihydroergotamine subcutaneously twice daily effectively prevents DVT and limits a number of postoperative bleeding complications seen with higher doses of heparin. Dihydroergotamine can increase the velocity of venous blood flow in the leg up to threefold, which potentiates the antithrombogenic effect of heparin by lowering venous stasis.

In a recent Swiss-Scandinavian multicenter trial, infusions of dextran were as effective as heparin in preventing fatal PE in general, orthopedic, gynecological, and neurological surgical patients.[3] Dextran acts by interfering with factor XIII antigen and the von Willebrand cofactor, both of which are related to normal platelet function. Because it increases the activity of the fibrinolytic system, dextran increases the dissolution of formed thrombus. Dextran also reduces blood viscosity and, because it is a colloid volume-expanding agent, it increases blood flow. However, dextran does not prevent DVT although it significantly decreases the risk of PE. The usual method of administration is to give 100 ml of either Dextran 40 or Dextran 70—there is no difference in their antithrombogenic effects—before operation, 400 ml during operation, 500 ml during the evening after operation, and 500 ml during the next morning. The major

side effect is anaphylaxis. That is caused by the presence of serum dextran–reactive antibodies that combine with dextran to form immune complexes, which release vasoactive mediators. In institutions where dextran is routinely used for antithrombogenesis, patients routinely receive monovalent hapten dextran 15% (Dextran 1) as a 20-ml intravenous injection that, because of the hapten inhibition principle, avoids all serious immune reactions. Dextran is, however, a plasma volume expander and may produce congestive failure in patients with borderline cardiac function. In neurosurgical patients with blood-brain barrier defects, this effect may cause increased intracranial pressure; cerebral edema is aggravated by dextran that leaks into the extracellular space of the involved brain and because of its colloid osmotic effect causes the transfer of obligate water. Therefore, dextran would probably not be well tolerated in head-injured patients or in neurosurgical patients harboring intracranial tumors.

References

1. Barnett HG, Clifford JE, Llewllyn RC: Safety of mini-dose heparin administration for neurosurgical patients. J Neurosurg 47:27–30, 1977.
2. Cerrato D, Ariano C, Fiacchino F: Deep vein thrombosis and low-dose heparin prophylaxis in neurosurgical patients. J Neurosurg 49:378–381, 1978.
3. Gruber UF, Saldeen T, Brokop T, Eklöf B, Eriksson I, Goldie I, Gran L, Hohl M, Jonsson T, Kristersson S, Ljungström KG, Lund T, Moe MH, Svensjö E, Thomson D, Torhorst J, Trippestad A, Ulstein M: Incidences of fatal postoperative pulmonary embolism after prophylaxis with dextran 70 and low-dose heparin: An international multicentre study. Br Med J 280:69–72, 1980.
4. Joffe SN: Incidence of postoperative deep vein thrombosis in neurosurgical patients. J Neurosurg 42:201–203, 1975.
5. Kakkar VV, Corrigan TP, Fossard DP: Prevention of fatal postoperative pulmonary embolism by low doses of heparin: An international multicentre trial. Lancet 2:45–51, 1975.
6. National Institutes of Health: Thrombolytic therapy in thrombosis. Stroke 12:17–21, 1981.
7. Owen CA Jr, Bowie EJW: Surgical hemostasis. J Neurosurg 51:137–146, 1979.
8. Powers SK, Edwards MSB: Prophylaxis of thromboembolism in the neurosurgical patient: A review. Neurosurgery 10:509–513, 1982.
9. Valladares JB, Hankinson J: Incidence of lower extremity deep vein thrombosis in neurosurgical patients. Neurosurgery 6:138–141, 1980.
10. Zelikovski A, Zucker G, Eliashiv A, Reiss R, Shalit M: A new sequential pneumatic device for the prevention of deep vein thrombosis. J Neurosurg 54:652–654, 1981.

41

Spasticity and Spasm

Wesley A. Cook, Jr.

Much of the confusion and apparent inconsistency regarding the pathophysiology and therapy of spasticity reflects our failure to adhere to a precise definition of the term. Diverse conditions such as cerebral palsy, decerebrate rigidity, the flexor or extensor spasms associated with paraplegia, and the events following a capsular stroke have all been labeled *spasticity*. While elements of spasticity can be found in each of these conditions, there are also, in the Jacksonian sense, other positive and negative symptoms that do not represent spasticity. Very often it is a negative symptom, such as the lack of strength or coordination, that is the most disabling event for the patient.[11]

From a neurophysiological viewpoint, spasticity is an exaggerated reflex response to stretch of a muscle. With this restricted definition, the clinical abnormalities associated with spasticity include hyperactive deep tendon reflexes (phasic stretch reflex), resistance to passive stretch of a muscle (tonic stretch reflex), clonus, and the clasp-knife phenomenon. Mass reflexes, flexor and extensor spasms, and the dystonic movements of cerebral palsy do not represent spasticity and there are reasons to believe that the pathophysiology of these latter conditions differs from that of simple spasticity.

Physiology

The pathophysiology of spasticity can be approached by a review of the current concepts of the stretch reflex.[12] The neural loop consists of afferent and efferent limbs, the peripheral muscle, and the central spinal cord. The receptors in muscle and adjacent tissue contributing to the afferent fibers in muscle nerves include free nerve endings, pacinian corpuscles, joint receptors, Golgi tendon organs, and muscle spindles. There may also be stretch-sensitive receptors which have not been identified. Present evidence indicates a definite role for Golgi tendon organs and muscle spindles in the stretch reflex.

Golgi tendon organs are found in tendons close to the musculotendinous junction and, more often, in the portions of muscle that attach to aponeuroses. Initially the view was held that tendon organs were placed "in series" between muscle and tendon, so that the receptor would be equally responsive to the tensions generated by passive stretch and by active contraction of the muscle. However, tendon organs are relatively insensitive to stretch, primarily owing to the low elastic compliance of tendon compared with that of muscle. Furthermore, each tendon organ is in series only with the relatively few muscle fibers supplied by its tendinous slip and is "in parallel" with other muscle fibers. In contrast to muscle spindles, which signal muscle length, tendon organs signal tension and especially the tension generated by muscle contraction. Studies of single fiber discharges in humans confirm the above observations, which were obtained from experimental animals.[19] In summary, tendon organs provide continuous feedback to the central nervous system regarding the static and dynamic contraction state of a muscle.

The large afferent fiber arising from a Golgi tendon organ falls into the group Ib muscle afferent classification. The central spinal action of group Ib afferents is inhibitory to motoneurons supplying the muscle of origin and excitatory to antagonistic motoneurons.

The muscle spindle is a specialized receptor composed of a group of intrafusal muscle fibers surrounded by a connective tissue capsule with a central expansion. The intrafusal fibers, in contrast to skeletal muscle fibers or extrafusal fibers, are of two types, nuclear chain and nuclear bag. The latter fibers have their nuclei clustered in the equatorial region and are longer and fatter. In contrast to tendon organs, muscle spindles are in parallel with extrafusal fibers and thus monitor muscle length and not muscle tension.

The muscle spindle is supplied with two different afferent fibers. The larger of the two (annulospiral or primary ending) is distributed to both nuclear chain and nuclear bag fibers, where it wraps about the equatorial region. The smaller afferent fiber (secondary ending or flower spray) terminates on either side of the primary ending and is mainly distributed to the nuclear chain fibers.

Muscle spindles also receive motor fibers (fusimotor or gamma fibers) that terminate on the striated poles of each intrafusal muscle fiber. Activation of these efferent fibers results in shortening of the contractile poles of the intrafusal fibers and produces distortion of the centrally placed afferent terminal. In other words, muscle spindle afferents can be activated either by passive stretch of the muscle or by activation of the gamma system with resultant shortening of the intrafusal fibers. In the latter case spindle discharge will continue even though the muscle as a whole may shorten with contraction.

The primary endings contribute to the group Ia afferents and the secondary endings to the group II afferents. Group Ia afferents are excitatory to motoneurons supplying the muscle of origin and its synergists. This synaptic connection is monosynaptic, whereas the inhibitory connection to antagonistic motoneurons is disynaptic. It has long been held that group II afferents are excitatory to flexor motoneurons and inhibitory to extensor motoneurons irrespective of the muscle or origin. This concept now appears to be an oversimplification since some group II afferents are known to excite extensor motoneurons by both monosynaptic and polysynaptic routes.[12]

In addition to the difference in size and in distribution to

411

intrafusal fibers, primary and secondary endings differ in their response to stretch. The stretch threshold of secondary endings is higher than that of primary endings, and secondary endings signal only the magnitude of the stretch whereas primary endings signal both the magnitude and the velocity of the stretch. A final difference, based on the dynamic properties of primary endings, is that primary endings are responsive to vibration whereas secondary endings are not (Table 41-1).

The motoneurons contributing to the efferent limb of the stretch reflex are of two types: the large alpha motoneurons with large-diameter axons, which are directed to extrafusal muscle fibers, and the smaller gamma motoneurons, which supply the intrafusal fibers of muscle spindles. In addition, some of the smaller alpha axons branch to supply both extrafusal and intrafusal muscle fibers. These are referred to as beta fibers. Their occurrence in humans is unknown, but in the cat the number of beta fibers is believed to be significant.

Stretch Reflexes and Spasticity

The above information can be summarized from the clinical perspective. The group Ia afferents with their primary endings on muscle spindles and their monosynaptic excitatory connection to alpha motoneurons is the reflex arc responsible for the phasic stretch, or in other words, the deep tendon reflex. The magnitude of the response to a tap of a tendon is determined by the excitability of the alpha motoneuron, the amount of gamma drive which sets the responsiveness of the muscle spindle, and the amount of excitatory transmitter agent released by the terminals of the group Ia afferents, which reflects, among other things, the level of presynaptic inhibition. The balance of the evidence from single nerve studies in the human suggests that the excitability level of the alpha motoneuron is the more important factor and that the gamma system does not play the major role once envisioned for it.[19]

The same monosynaptic reflex arc is responsible for clonus. The abrupt dorsiflexion of the foot by the hand stretches the gastrocnemius-soleus muscle, with resultant activation of the primary endings. The relatively synchronous burst of activity in the Ia afferents fires the alpha motoneurons to the gastrocnemius-soleus muscle, which con-

tracts and silences spindle discharge; however, the contraction is resisted by the hand, which restretches the muscle and the next cycle is thereby initiated. Antagonistic muscles, the dorsiflexors of the foot in this case, do not play an active role in clonus.[2]

It is important to realize that hyperactive deep tendon reflexes and sustained clonus, although a manifestation of spasticity, can be elicited in normal individuals. Recall the clonus of one's foot on the brake after a near miss automobile accident or of test-anxious medical students prior to a major examination. All that is required for this expression of spasticity is a general increase in the excitability of the loop mediating the stretch reflex.

The understanding of the tonic stretch reflex is incomplete. As noted before, it was once believed that group II muscle spindle afferents were excitatory to flexor motoneurons and inhibitory to extensor motoneurons. If this were the case, there would be little role for these fibers in the tonic stretch reflex that is usually present in extensor or antigravity muscles. However, with the demonstration that some group II afferents are excitatory to extensor motoneurons, this concept is no longer tenable. This does not mean that group Ia afferents do not contribute to the tonic stretch reflex. Indeed, a selective block of group Ia afferent input abolishes both phasic and tonic stretch reflexes.[3]

Decerebrate Rigidity

Charles Sherrington's description and imaginative analysis of decerebrate rigidity has not been surpassed.[5] The experimental animal used in his tests was prepared by transection of the brain stem at an intercollicular level following bilateral carotid ligation. The resulting rigidity was noted to involve antigravity muscles, that is, extensor or physiological extensor muscle groups. Sherrington further discovered that posterior rhizotomy abolished the rigidity, which laid the groundwork for his investigations of the stretch reflex. He also noted that hemisection of the midbrain cephalad to the pyramidal decussation produced only ipsilateral rigidity and that the rigidity occurred as long as the transection of the brain stem remained cephalad to the level of the auditory nerve. Subsequent investigations have shown that the red nucleus is not critical for the appearance of decerebrate rigidity.

TABLE 41-1 Stretch Receptors

Receptor	Afferent Fiber	Segmental Action	Information Supplied to CNS
Tendon organ	Group Ib	Inhibitory to muscle of origin (disynaptic). Excitatory to antagonists.	Static and dynamic contraction state (tension) of muscle.
Muscle spindle, primary ending	Group Ia	Excitatory to muscle of origin (monosynaptic) and synergists. Inhibitory to antagonists.	Static and dynamic length of muscle.
Muscle spindle, secondary ending	Group II	Inhibitory to extensor muscles. Excitatory to flexor (and some extensor) muscles.	Static length of muscle.

In contrast to the intercollicular decerebrate preparation of Sherrington, the anemic decerebrate animal is produced by ligation of the carotid and basilar arteries. The resulting infarction involves both the midbrain and the anterior cerebellum. The rigidity in this case is not abolished by posterior rhizotomy, which indicates that the persistent discharge of alpha motoneurons is independent of the stretch reflex. The anemic decerebrate is an example of alpha rigidity, and single fiber recordings have shown a decrease in gamma discharge. This is in contrast to the intercollicular decerebrate, in which there is an increase in both static and dynamic gamma discharge to extensor muscles.

In humans, decerebrate rigidity is most commonly caused by trauma and the associated mortality is quite high.[5] The posture of decerebrate rigidity is extensor rigidity of all extremities with pronation of the arms and adduction of the legs. In some patients the extensor rigidity is transient and will intensify with noxious stimuli; in others, the extensor rigidity persists in a continuous state. Decorticate rigidity in humans is characterized by extensor rigidity of the legs and flexion of the adducted upper extremities. Most often bilateral lesions are associated with decorticate rigidity; however, in many patients the clinical distinction between decerebrate and decorticate rigidity is blurred owing to diffuse multiple lesions.

Spasm

In contrast to lesions of the midbrain with the immediate appearance of rigidity, the changes following injury to the spinal cord take days to weeks for their expression. Following a period of spinal shock, spasticity may gradually appear—however, this is usually of less concern to the patient than the development of spasms and mass reflexes, which greatly interfere with rehabilitative efforts. The pathophysiological mechanisms responsible for these responses are poorly understood, although a variety of possibilities have been considered. Denervation hypersensitivity of interneurons or of alpha motoneurons, similar to that occurring after denervation of a muscle, remains an unproven explanation. Sprouting of intraspinal afferent terminals, with subsequent synaptic contact with interneurons or motoneurons, is another possibility of unknown significance. In recent years attention has shifted to changes in synaptic transmitter concentrations and the suppression of normal presynaptic and postsynaptic inhibitory mechanisms to account for these exaggerated reflex responses to often trivial stimuli.[17] It should be clearly understood that spasticity as defined earlier and spasms or mass reflexes are entirely different entities, whether considered physiologically or clinically.

Therapy

Drug Therapy

Before initiating a therapeutic program, the relative role of the positive and negative symptoms for the individual patient should be evaluated. If a positive symptom, for example, flexor spasms, is the most troublesome, therapy may be helpful; however, if it is weakness or the lack of coordination that is the major concern, therapy may be a disappointment to patient and physician alike.

If therapy appears to be indicated, consideration of the available forms of treatment should be undertaken. In most instances the patient's interests are best served if we are not wedded to a single therapeutic maneuver. For example, a patient may most benefit from a combination of drug therapy and a peripheral nerve block with phenol for spasticity of the lower extremities coupled with painful adductor spasms. And finally, there should be no confusion between contracture and the persistent contraction secondary to repetitive firing of motoneurons. In a few cases, this distinction will require differential spinal anesthesia for clarification.

At the present time the three drugs useful in the clinical setting include dantrolene (Dantrium, Norwich-Eaton Laboratories, Norwich, N.Y.), baclofen (Lioresal, Geigy Pharmaceuticals, Summit, N.J.), and diazepam (Valium, Roche Laboratories, Nutley, N.J.). Dantrolene acts peripherally on skeletal muscle whereas the latter two drugs have a central action. Each of these drugs has potentially serious side effects and therapy with these agents should be monitored and then discontinued if there are not substantial clinical benefits.[22]

Dantrolene

In the course of normal excitation-contraction of skeletal muscle, the muscle action potential results in the efflux of calcium from the sarcoplasmic reticulum into the sarcoplasm, where the calcium ions bind to protein and activate the contraction process. Dantrolene acts to reduce this calcium efflux and thus produces muscle weakness in the true sense. The effect of dantrolene is differential in that the fast, phasic motor units are weakened considerably more than the slow tonic units.

Dantrolene is generally most useful when muscle strength is not of primary concern, for example, when the patient is confined to bed. While it is of value to some ambulatory patients, other patients note significant muscle weakness before blood levels of the drug are sufficiently high to reduce spasticity or spasms.

The starting dosage is 25 mg per day and this should be increased by one tablet twice a week to a maximum of 100 mg four times a day or until muscle weakness or diarrhea occurs. If beneficial effects are not apparent within 2 weeks after reaching the maximum tolerated dose, the drug should be discontinued.

Dantrolene is metabolized in the liver although its metabolism is not influenced by concurrent use of diazepam or barbiturates. Hepatitis, as an idiosyncratic reaction, has been reported and the risk of dantrolene hepatic toxicity is greatest in women, older patients, and patients receiving estrogen. Liver function tests should precede dantrolene therapy and be repeated throughout the course of therapy.

Baclofen

This drug is an analog of gamma-aminobutyric acid and acts to depress neuronal function on a widespread basis. It is not known if the drug depresses excitatory transmitter release or has direct postsynaptic actions but the bulk of evidence favors a presynaptic mechanism. The spinal site of action is proven since the drug will reduce flexor spasms equally well in patients with complete or incomplete spinal cord lesions.

In our studies and according to the reports of others, baclofen is most beneficial in those patients with painful flexor or extensor spasms. These patients as a group are the quadriplegics and paraplegics whose conditions are secondary in most instances to trauma or multiple sclerosis.

It is advisable to gradually increase the dosage, beginning with 5 mg twice daily and increasing this twice weekly to 20 mg four times a day. Baclofen is less likely than dantrolene to produce sedation or muscle weakness as a side effect and thus appears to be the preferred initial agent for painful spasms.

In the dose range described there are few major side effects. Sedation is the most common but most patients soon adjust to this. Rapid withdrawal of the drug should be avoided.

Diazepam

This agent is believed to enhance presynaptic inhibition by facilitating the postsynaptic actions of gamma-aminobutyric acid. Although diazepam acts at many levels of the neuraxis, it is effective in reducing spasms in patients with spinal cord transections, which implies a spinal site for this action.

Based on studies to date there appears to be no major difference in the effectiveness of diazepam and baclofen. Patients are more likely to be troubled with sedation and muscle weakness with the former agent. The drug should be started slowly, 2 mg twice a day, and then gradually increased to 60 to 80 mg per day. These high levels can be tolerated by some patients when the dosage is slowly increased over a period of time.

The drug must be used very cautiously in the elderly or when other centrally acting medications or alcohol is being used. It should not be used in the presence of narrow-angle glaucoma or liver, renal, or blood disorders.

Surgical Therapy

In addition to drug therapy, a variety of operative procedures have been utilized in an attempt to alleviate spasticity and spasms. A partial list includes tenotomy, peripheral neurotomy, subarachnoid phenol injection, open or percutaneous rhizotomy, myelotomy, cordectomy, vascular embolization of the spinal cord, and implantation of a neurostimulation device. While the very number of procedures may suggest that any one is not optimal, many carefully selected patients will benefit from one or more of these maneuvers.

Phenol Injection

A major advantage of the subarachnoid injection of phenol is the ease of the procedure and that it can be repeated as needed should there be a recurrence of painful spasms.

However, it is not possible to be highly selective and a number of roots may be involved, including the sacral outflow to bowel and bladder. In the experience at Duke University Medical Center one patient expired from his underlying disease some 6 months following the subarachnoid injection of phenol. Microscopic examination revealed widespread but patchy destruction of anterior and posterior rootlets, with both large- and small-diameter fibers equally affected.

Rhizotomy

The first open rhizotomy was carried out by Foerster following Sherrington's demonstration that dorsal rhizotomy would abolish decerebrate rigidity. Ventral rhizotomy is totally effective but must be reserved for patients without useful motor function. Dorsal rhizotomy can be utilized in patients with retained motor function; however, complete deafferentation renders the limb useless from a functional standpoint. Partial dorsal rhizotomy in which the rootlets to be sectioned are selected on the basis of stimulation and recording patterns will effectively decrease spasticity and spasms while avoiding many of the complications of complete deafferentation.[8]

Percutaneous rhizotomy is a popular procedure at present owing to the ease of the procedure and the high degree of selectivity that can be achieved.[10] The nerve roots to be coagulated can be selected on the basis of the clinical distribution of the spasms and whether interference with motor function or bowel and bladder function can be avoided. Furthermore, lumbar lesions in quadriplegics will often decrease spasticity in the trunk and upper extremities. However, the procedure is not free of complications. Excessive coagulation of nerve roots will produce motor weakness, and coagulation and thrombosis of the artery of Adamkiewicz can produce paraplegia. This artery usually enters the spinal canal from the left side in the lower thoracic or upper lumbar region. Variations do occur and must be kept in mind when performing this procedure, especially when the patient has useful motor function.

Another condition that open or percutaneous rhizotomy will aid is that of the reflex-contracted bladder that imposes frequent voiding patterns on the patient. These patients must first be evaluated urodynamically. The reflex nature of the contracted bladder is proven on two separate occasions by selective nerve root blocks. Only then is the involved root, usually S3, cut or coagulated. At Duke this procedure has been successful in enlarging bladder capacity in all patients who met the criteria noted above.

Myelotomy

The purpose of myelotomy is to destroy the reflex arcs within the gray matter of the spinal cord. Bischof's original procedure consisted of a lateral, longitudinal myelotomy, which divided the spinal cord into dorsal and ventral halves. This procedure abolishes mass reflexes and spasms but also eliminates any useful motor function. In an attempt to avoid destruction of the corticospinal and other motor tracts, a number of surgeons have turned to "inverted T" myelotomies, which are accomplished either freehand or with a myelotome.[21] In these procedures a dorsal midline incision is carried ventrally to the central canal and then extended laterally into the gray matter on each side to complete the inverted T. The results of these procedures have been satisfactory in eliminating spasticity and spasms while preserving useful motor function.

Embolization and Cordectomy

Embolization of the artery of Adamkiewicz is reported to reduce spasticity and spasms without influencing autonomic bladder function.[15] This approach was based on the observation that the arteriographic arterial supply to the spinal cord was deficient in paraplegics who remained flaccid in contrast to those who developed spasticity and spasms. It would appear that neither this procedure nor selective cordectomy[7] should be undertaken as an initial mode of therapy.

Neurostimulation

Chronic stimulation of the central nervous system has been reported to alleviate spasticity and spasm. A major advantage of this approach is the nondestructive nature of the procedure. Arrays of stimulating electrodes are placed on the cerebellum or the posterior columns of the spinal cord. In the latter case, percutaneous placement of the electrodes in the epidural space further refines and simplifies the procedure.[20]

Appropriate stimulation of the anterior lobe of the cerebellum will produce an immediate "melting" of decerebrate rigidity in the cat. Unfortunately, cerebellar stimulation in humans does not evoke such a dramatic response. Although more than 1000 stimulators have been implanted, the results remain controversial.[13] The majority of these patients represent cases of cerebral palsy, which is an example of a very complex dysfunction of the central nervous system of which only a portion is secondary to spasticity. While some investigators have reported a decrease in muscle tone and improvement in daily activities with cerebellar stimulation, double blind evaluations have not demonstrated any consistent beneficial response for the patient. Examples of the controversy regarding this procedure are the back-to-back reports by two groups of investigators at a recent symposium. One group concluded that cerebellar stimulation is a proven valuable aid whereas the other group has abandoned the procedure because of lack of efficacy.[4,9]

Percutaneous epidural neurostimulation has been reported as a successful therapy for paraplegic spasticity,[16] the ataxia and spasticity of multiple sclerosis,[1] peripheral vascular disease, and the autonomic hyper-reflexia associated with spinal cord injury.[14] Although there is less controversy regarding the efficacy of posterior column stimulation as compared with cerebellar stimulation, there is still an immediate need for well-controlled clinical trials to document what benefits this form of therapy holds for the spastic patient.

The mechanism of posterior column stimulation is poorly understood. Antidromic, orthodromic, and long-loop circuit activation all occur with posterior column stimulation but the relative role of each is obscure. Since the effects of the stimulation far outlast the duration of the stimulation, the release of chemical substances such as endorphins has been suggested.[18]

References

1. Cook AW, Taylor JK, Nidzgorski F: Results of spinal cord stimulation in multiple sclerosis. Appl Neurophysiol 44:55–61, 1981.
2. Cook WA Jr: Antagonistic muscles in the production of clonus in man. Neurology (Minneap) 17:779–781, 796, 1967.
3. Cook WA Jr, Duncan CC Jr: Contribution of group I afferents to the tonic stretch reflex of the decerebrate cat. Brain Res 33:509–513, 1971.
4. Davis R, Engle H, Kudzma J, Gray E, Ryan T, Dusnak A: Update of chronic cerebellar stimulation for spasticity and epilepsy. Appl Neurophysiol 45:44–50, 1982.
5. Davis RA, Davis L: Decerebrate rigidity in animals. Neurosurgery 9:79–89, 1981.
6. Davis RA, Davis L: Decerebrate rigidity in humans. Neurosurgery 10:635–642, 1982.
7. Durwood QJ, Rice GP, Ball MJ, Gilbert JJ, Kaufman JCE: Selective spinal cordectomy: Clinicopathological correlation. J Neurosurg 56:359–367, 1982.
8. Fasano VA, Barolat-Romana G, Zeme S, Squazzi A: Electrophysiological assessment of spinal circuits in spasticity by direct dorsal root stimulation. Neurosurgery 4:146–151, 1979.
9. Ivan LP, Ventureyra ECG: Chronic cerebellar stimulation in cerebral palsy. Appl Neurophysiol 45:51–54, 1982.
10. Kennemore D: Radiofrequency neurotomy for peripheral pain and spasticity syndromes. Contemp Neurosurg 5(4):1–6, 1983.
11. Landau WM: Spasticity: The fable of a neurological demon and the emperor's new therapy. Arch Neurol 31:217–219, 1974.
12. Patton HD: Reflex regulation of movement and posture, in Ruch T, Patton HD (eds): Physiology and Biophysics, vol 4. Philadelphia, Saunders, 1982, pp 303–342.
13. Penn RD: Chronic cerebellar stimulation for cerebral palsy: A review. Neurosurgery 10:116–121, 1982.
14. Richardson RR, Cerullo LJ, Meyer PR: Autonomic hyper-reflexia modulated by percutaneous epidural neurostimulation: A preliminary report. Neurosurgery 4:517–520, 1979.
15. Shibasaki K, Nakai S, Higuchi M: Percutaneous embolisation of major spinal cord artery as a treatment for intractable spasticity. Paraplegia 20:158–168, 1982.
16. Siegfried J, Lazorthes Y, Broggi G: Electrical spinal cord stimulation for spastic movement disorders. Appl Neurophysiol 44:77–92, 1981.
17. Smith JE, Hall PV, Galvin MR, Jones AR, Campbell RL: Effects of glycine administration on canine experimental spinal spasticity and the levels of glycine, glutamate and asparate in the lumbar spinal cord. Neurosurgery 4:152–156, 1979.
18. Spiegel E: Relief of pain and spasticity by posterior column stimulation: A proposed mechanism. Arch Neurol 39:184–185, 1982.
19. Vallbo AB, Hagbarth KE, Torebjörk HE, Wallin BG: Somatosensory, proprioceptive and sympathetic activity in human peripheral nerves. Physiol Rev 59:919–957, 1979.
20. Waltz J: Computerized percutaneous multi-level spinal cord stimulation in motor disorders. Appl Neurophysiol 45:73–92, 1982.
21. Yamada S, Perot PL Jr, Ducker TB, Lockard I: Myelotomy for control of mass spasms in paraplegia. J Neurosurg 45:683–691, 1976.
22. Young RR, Delwaide PJ: Spasticity. N Engl J Med 304:28–33, 96–99, 1981.

42

Principles of Rehabilitation of the Disabled Patient

E. Wayne Massey

Rehabilitation of disabled persons re-establishes their capacity to participate in their surroundings and fully utilize their abilities physically, socially, vocationally, and intellectually. The goal of rehabilitation for each individual is to provide optimal physical, psychological, physiological, and social adaptation, with restoration and maintenance of health. After inpatient rehabilitation, maintenance is concerned with continued management of the patient over months or years to preserve optimal performance. Social and psychological adjustments concerned with the personality of the patient as well as family problems may be manifested at the onset of the disability or may develop subsequent to it; therefore, dependency, loss of self-esteem, absence of family support, and economic concerns may negate efforts to restore functional status.

Not every patient needs rehabilitation. The goal of inpatient rehabilitation is primarily to aid patients with self-care and to train them in activities of daily living. With the help of occupational therapy, physical therapy, nursing and medical management, the patient should obtain optimal function.[9] Patients are to be as independent as possible, physically and socially. If they are not physically independent, they can teach others how best to care for them. It is important to establish the limitations of the level of rehabilitation to be expected as early as possible. Comprehensive planned medical management based on the total person, even if the disabled individual has only one disability, is essential for prognostic reasons. This will require a multidisciplinary approach through skilled professional personnel involved with the evaluation and program planning.[9]

The physician in charge must be knowledgeable about the functions and responsibility of all the allied health personnel who contribute to the management. Each professional working with the patient should recognize the patient's entire need for therapy. This is best accomplished on a continuous verbal communication level with interchange of information about progress.

In the rehabilitation setting, optimal care is delivered by a physician, nurse, occupational therapist, physical therapist, speech therapist, recreational therapist, social service counselor and a vocational rehabilitation therapist. Additionally, psychiatric counseling is ideal for the majority of patients. In this chapter we will discuss general areas of management of the neurosurgical patient with a neurological deficit, as well as specific disease entities which require special situations. We will discuss the basic requirements for various forms of neurological disability including hemiplegia, paraplegia or quadriplegia, peripheral neuropathy, multiple sclerosis, Parkinson's disease, peripheral nerve injury, head injury, and cerebral palsy.

Hemiplegia

Hemiplegia is the most frequent of the neurological disabilities requiring rehabilitation. Although usually subsequent to a stroke,[2] in the neurosurgical setting it is seen following operative procedures such as brain tumor resection. The term *hemiplegia* may range from minimal paresis and sensory loss to a complete unilateral paralysis and sensory loss. Therefore rehabilitative treatment of each patient must be individualized, since there can be no one standard treatment for all forms of hemiplegia. For some mild involvement, outpatient therapy may be required for only short periods. Other patients may require a complex, comprehensive rehabilitation program involving highly skilled personnel.[7]

Initial Management

Rehabilitation begins when the patient is admitted to the hospital even though his level of consciousness may not allow initial responsiveness. A neurological examination for precise localization of the cerebral lesion and determination of sensory motor deficits is essential. This may not be possible to complete on the initial assessment. Additionally, a complete medical assessment can determine if any medical problems such as cardiac disease, peripheral vascular disease, hypertension, diabetes mellitus, or urinary dysfunction will impede rehabilitation. Social and psychological evaluation should be done to be aware of patients' previous education, mode of life, goals, and the family and community resources available to them. Before active rehabilitation can begin, the mental status of all patients must be evaluated so that their learning ability, intelligence, memory, orientation, perception, and adaptation to stressful situations can be assessed.

Initially, simple measures to prevent development of decubitus ulcers or contractures may be easily accomplished. A board below a firm mattress is usually helpful and the patient should be placed to prevent heel pressure and external rotation of the hip, as well as upper extremity contractures in the shoulder adductors and rotators and the wrist and finger flexors. Patients who are comatose and unable to move themselves should be turned from supine to one side or the other every 2 h. Each joint of the affected extremity should be moved to a full range of motion three times, at least once daily. Early mobilization is an obtainable goal.

Active rehabilitation begins with a mobilization program consisting of range-of-motion exercises for all joints of the involved side, which may be initially carried out by nursing or physical therapy personnel but subsequently by the patient. Early development of independence in transferring is extremely important in hemiplegic rehabilitation. A patient who is able to come to a sitting position with adequate and safe balance is ready for training from a bed to chair (wheelchair). After coming to the sitting or standing position beside the bed, the patient uses the normal lower extremity for support and pushes up with the normal upper extremity. This is initially done for transfer from bed to chair and subsequently from chair to toilet. A standing pivot transfer with the normal or noninvolved side closest to the toilet may be facilitated by support rails (grab bars) fastened to the wall.

Physical Therapy

Initial physical therapy is a strengthening exercise program consisting of progressive, resistive exercises for the noninvolved extremities, particularly for the muscles required for standing and transfers. On the involved side, strengthening exercises for functional paretic muscles are instituted. A mat exercise program consists of rolling from side to side and from supine to prone and balancing activities that assist in the development of skills necessary to perform elevation and transfers. The use of a stationary bicycle to provide reciprocal motion of lower extremities and to increase endurance is another useful adjunctive preparation for ambulation. Muscle re-education is given to major paralyzed groups to reinforce or assist the spontaneous return. This may be initially to the proximal muscle groups and later to the distal groups as the functional recovery returns.

Occupational Therapy

Occupational therapy emphasizes function to the upper extremity by manual activities, which are used to assist in developing the coordinate control motions of the shoulder and elbow. Obviously the extent of return in the upper extremity is usually what determines the exact form of therapy and how much dependence the patient must place on the noninvolved extremity. The occupational therapy complements the physical therapy in standing and balancing practice and aids the nursing staff in teaching activities of daily living. In addition, they teach compensation training for perceptual deficits, e.g., "neglect."

Ambulation

The majority of hemiplegic patients will learn to walk. After they have learned a safe sitting balance, training with the parallel bars is initiated. Training progresses with walking in these bars as the patients pull themselves forward with their unaffected arms. Ambulation subsequently progresses. Patients change from hemiwalker to four-point cane to single-point cane as they are able to show safety and maintain balance. Ambulation training should be provided twice a day except in older patients with limited endurance, for whom training must be limited. When the best walking pattern is obtained on level ground, the patient is trained in climbing stairs and descending ramps and curbs.

Activities of Daily Living

Independence in essential activities, such as bed activities, hygiene, feeding, dressing, elevation, transfers, and other manipulative activities, is important for the hemiplegic patient. Bed activities and rolling can be accomplished by hooking the unaffected leg under the involved leg and using the unaffected arm with a trapeze or bed rail, which will subsequently allow the patient to develop rolling techniques and to sit up. Hygiene may be taught by having the patient perform all necessary activities such as washing, shaving, grooming, and brushing the teeth and the hair with the uninvolved side. Cooperation must be obtained from the family and friends as these patients must be encouraged to do such activities. Feeding may be done by the patient in some cases in a relatively short period after the stroke. Special cutting and assistance utensils may be of aid. Dressing independence will require considerable training by nursing and therapy personnel. Initially the patients learn to dress while in the bed and subsequently while in a wheelchair. All patients should dress themselves or be assisted in dressing as soon as possible which dispenses with the wearing of hospital gowns except at night.

Bowel and Bladder Management

Initially a hemiplegic patient may require an indwelling catheter to prevent distension of a flaccid bladder. As bladder tone returns and level of consciousness is recovered, intermittent catheterization for retention or, more commonly, for incontinence management is required until control returns. With few exceptions hemiplegic patients are capable of urinary continence. Persistence of bowel and bladder incontinence is an indication of poor rehabilitation potential.

Speech Therapy

Communication difficulties often accompany a right hemiplegia with fluent or nonfluent aphasia presenting additional problems for the patient. In addition to the difficulty with anomia, loss of production of speech sounds, decreased understanding of word meaning, and decreased recall or retention of learned experiences, the patient may have a verbal apraxia with impairment of the ability to coordinately perform articulation. This may occur even without receptive language difficulty. A speech therapist is essential in the complete evaluation of the pathology of these patients.

Although some controversy exists over the value of speech therapy, detailed evaluation of the speech disturbance and the institution of a program will provide patients and their families with understanding of the meaning of a communication disorder. All personnel working with the patient are involved in providing stimulation and reinforcement for the patient to communicate verbally and to write. This is important even in right hemisphere lesions, which may entail severe writing, reading, and spatial problems even with no aphasia.

An evaluation by speech therapy may lead to a prediction of the extent of anticipated recovery from the communicative disorder. Patients with hemiplegia secondary to neurosurgical procedure do better in general than the patients with cerebrovascular infarction. Patients with a minimal receptive component with adequate retention and recall do better than those without.

The right hemiplegic patient often has a dysphasia, with difficulty in comprehension and expression, both verbal and written. Even without language dysfunction there is frequently impairment of recall, auditory retention, and abstract language function. Therefore, utilization of nonverbal correction such as visual demonstrations and gestures is indicated. In the left hemiplegic patient perceptual loss frequently involves spatial concepts and visuomotor relationships. There is often impaired integration and judgment of sensory input along with failure to recognize errors in performance. Patients may ignore their left feet and bump into objects on their left; therefore step-by-step verbal correction is important in development by the patient of symbolic reminders for the performance of motor function. Occupational therapy aids in this area as well.

Psychological Adjustments

Hemiplegic patients will have a severe emotional reaction to the loss of body function. Grief is appropriate while they concentrate on their loss. Gradually, with the perception that they do have significant functional abilities, their self-devaluation may recede. Some studies in stroke however, have indicated that maximum depression may be delayed and not be prominent for several months.

Positive reinforcement is provided by knowledgeable personnel who can establish realistic and achievable goals. Some patients have a large amount of denial or failure to accept the disability, which requires more skillful appraisal and management with psychiatric assistance.

Orthoses

Orthotic aids can be very helpful in patients with hemiplegia. In order to ambulate well, bracing with a polypropylene orthosis (ankle foot device, AFO) of the coil-spring type or a Klenzak ankle-joint short leg brace may be required to correct foot drop. Also, subluxation of the shoulder joint of the paralyzed upper extremity may occur in a flaccid upper extremity, causing pain, which interferes with rehabilitation. Various forms of slings or supports to the elbow help to maintain the head of the humerus in the socket. Upper extremity splinting is of increasing value to aid flexor synergy. Active and passive range of motion may help to prevent contractures in the adducted position.

Complications

A patient who does not initially receive a full passive range of motion may develop a "shoulder hand syndrome" or reflex sympathetic dystrophy on the involved side. The disabling symptom is severe pain, which restricts participation in the program. The patient has pain on minimal motion of the shoulder, which results in contractures, limiting the shoulder motion and causing further pain on motion. The hand may become cold and cyanotic and have accompanying edema, which interferes with the normal range of motion. Relief of the pain and edema and restoration of a full range of motion may be aided by short-term oral steroids and hot packs to the shoulder followed by manual active stretching exercises. In severe cases stellate ganglion block may be indicated.[3]

Social Aspects

The majority of hemiplegic patients can achieve complete independence and return to their homes.[2] Substitution of mechanisms for individual deficits may assist them with adjustment to their disabilities. The family usually requires some counseling and some participation in the rehabilitation activities. Rehabilitation includes evaluation of the home for needed modification, such as wheelchair accessibility. It is important that the physical restoration activities not be terminated abruptly at discharge so that a maintenance program can be continued by the patient after returning home. Active and passive range of motion exercises, ambulation, and independent performance of activities of daily living contribute to the adjustment of the patient and family. Follow-up evaluation should support this as well. In the aphasic patient the family must be involved in the therapy early and subsequent outpatient speech therapy may be continued. Occupational therapy teaches homemaking and community skills.

Vocational rehabilitation of the hemiplegic stroke patient is difficult since the majority of the patients are elderly. Postsurgical vocational status depends on the course of the hemiplegia. Impairment of judgment, comprehension, retention, and recall interferes with job performance and makes vocational rehabilitation less successful. However, successful placement is possible for selected neurosurgical patients.[8]

Paraplegia or Quadriplegia

The initial management of spinal cord injury from trauma, congenital defect, or an infectious process begins with the emergency care of the incomplete or complete cord lesion.[1,5] The care of the acute injury will be discussed in another chapter.

For the paraplegic or quadriplegic, the prevention of skin breakdown is of major importance. Decubitus ulcers develop as a result of pressure and friction and are more likely to occur in the presence of inadequate nutrition, particularly protein intake. From the outset the patient must be turned every 2 h during the entire 24-h day. The patient is turned from side to side and whenever possible from prone to supine without any sliding, which would produce friction or shearing forces. Special beds have been developed to facilitate good preventive skin care. The use of a foam egg crate or alternating-pressure mattress, sheepskin, or flotation mattress is helpful in preventing development of decubiti but does not eliminate the need for turning. The skin, particularly over bony prominences, should be inspected by the nurses every time the patient is turned. When reddened areas develop that do not abate when the pressure is off the area, further pressure must be avoided. As soon as patients are able, they should be taught to turn themselves every 2 h, taking care to avoid sliding and thus friction. Patients may inspect the skin themselves with the use of a hand mirror at some stage in rehabilitation.

Skin cleanliness is essential for paraplegics or quadriplegics. They are bathed with soap and water and the skin is thoroughly dried. Emphasis on keeping the skin dry is to prevent the maceration effects of moisture, which also predisposes to development of decubitus ulcers. When excessive perspiration is a complication of the spinal cord injury, an anticholinergic medication may be beneficial.[4,6]

Mobilization

An exercise program is begun consisting of passive exercises of all joints of the paralyzed or paretic extremities, which carry the joint through the maximum range of motion, and active exercises of all joints in which there is sufficient functional muscle power. When the patient stabilizes, an exercise program of resistive exercises for the functional muscles is begun. Essential muscle groups in this regimen should be shoulder depressors, elbow extensors, and wrist flexors and extensors, which are necessary in transferring and in crutch ambulation.

The patient should be placed in a standing position as soon as possible, although the timing of this step must be individualized. The standing position reduces the development of osteoporosis in the lower extremities, with increased urinary calcium excretion, and aids in the re-establishment of vascular tone to prevent postural hypotension. A tilt table may be used to progress the patient from an angle of 20 to 30 degrees to one of 70 degrees for periods of 30 min to 1 h. Pressure-gradient elastic stockings or elastic bandages on the lower extremities may aid the effectiveness, and on rare occasions, a "G suit" is required. When a spinal injury is due to unstable vertebrae, spinal bracing is desirable prior to the use of a tilt table. A brace may be obtained for wheelchair and ambulation activities, which will vary depending upon whether the injury is in the cervical, thoracic, or lumbar location.

The patient, when able to get out of bed, will require a wheelchair with swinging detachable footrests and removable armrests. Preventive skin care continues when the patient is able to be in a wheelchair since unavoidable pressure over the ischial tuberosities occurs. A foam rubber wheelchair cushion helps to distribute some of the weight to the buttocks and thighs, but no cushion alone is adequate in reducing ischial pressure to a level sufficient to prevent de-

cubiti. Therefore, patients must shift their weight off the tuberosities at least every 15 min. Paraplegics can do this by push-ups on the arms of their chairs and quadriplegics by rocking their trunks sideways.

Development of independence in bed activities and in transferring is provided by nursing and physical therapy personnel. Turning from side to side, rolling over from the supine to the prone position, sitting erect, and reaching and handling objects on the bedside can be learned. A paraplegic patient usually has little difficulty in developing independence whereas a quadriplegic, who has lost grasp and elbow extension, has considerable difficulty.

The erect long sitting position is a prerequisite for independent bed transfer. The bed should be at the same level as the wheelchair seat. A sliding transfer board is required initially for high paraplegics and quadriplegics and for some is always necessary. However, many paraplegics may learn to transfer to an obliquely placed wheelchair from a sitting position by boosting themselves with their upper extremities and swinging into the locked chair. An alternative method for paraplegics to transfer is by boosting the hips across the bed until both hands can be placed upon the armrests of the wheelchair, which is adjusted to the bed. In transferring from the wheelchair to the bed, the reverse process is used.

Transferring from the wheelchair to the toilet is essential. The toilet seat should be at the same height as the wheelchair if possible, and raised seats can be attached to regular toilets. Before transferring patients wearing trousers, these are to be lowered to midthigh, and the patients use the knee armrest and one hand on the far side of the toilet to lift their bodies and swing over onto the toilet seat. Grab bars or overhead trapeze facilities may aid in transfer. Similarly, wheelchair-to-bathtub and chair-to-car transfers must be learned. Patients may learn to transfer from the chair to the floor by extending their legs to the floor and using their arms to lift their hips; they then slide forward and lower themselves to the footrest. These maneuvers must be repeated and practiced to be done safely and adequately.

Exercises

Exercises should be gradually advanced from those confined to the bed area to those that can be done in a physical therapy setting. Stretching exercises can be manual or can be assisted by gradual stretching with use of weights for a 30-min period. A mat exercise program consisting of rolling from side to side and from prone to supine, push-ups, knee stands, and crawling and balancing in the long sitting position aids in balance training. Progressive resistance exercises are instituted in order to develop maximal strength in the muscles necessary for crutch ambulation and transferring. Weighted blocks and looms increase endurance and strength and assist in re-education for nonfunctioning muscles.

Although it is technically possible to train low quadriplegics to ambulate, from a practical standpoint their locomotion is limited to a wheelchair. High thoracic paraplegics are usually more functional from a wheelchair. But functional ambulation for a paraplegic is feasible from the tenth thoracic segment or below, although there are exceptions. Paraplegics with involvement above the tenth thoracic level require so much energy for ambulation that they often prefer the wheelchair and use their skill in ambulation only when there is a barrier to the wheelchair.

Orthoses

Before ambulation, the paraplegic patient will need brace fitting. When the paralysis involves the hip musculature, long leg braces are prescribed. The preferred bracing consists of double-bar steel long leg braces, a bail or a Swiss knee lock, leather cuffs with a buckle or a velcro closure, decor or Klenzak spring ankle joints with a stirrup in the heel, and firm shoes with leather soles and rubber heels. The braces should fit as high as possible without causing pressure on the gluteal crease, on the ischial tuberosity, or in the groin. The use of the pelvic band is usually unnecessary. Paraplegics with residual muscle power sufficient to lock their knees may require only drop foot braces of the ankle.

Braces are prescribed for almost all paraplegics except those with high thoracic involvement, even though it is known that those with lesions above the tenth thoracic segment will likely not use them for functional walking. Ambulation is an important goal for paraplegics, and they must experience for themselves the difficulties of ambulation before accepting the wheelchair for functional use.

Ambulation training begins with parallel bars. The patient is taught balancing and weight shifting and progresses to a swing-through tripod gait. When the gait pattern in parallel bars is perfected, the training can proceed to the use of underarm or forearm crutches, starting with balance and weight shifting and progressing to the swing-through gait. For certain patients, the use of a stable four-point cane is helpful. In addition to the gait pattern, the paraplegic must learn the technique of rising from sitting in a chair, climbing stairs, and descending stairs and curbs, as well as walking on ramps and rough ground.

Activities of Daily Living

Adjunctive therapy to gait training is provided by occupational therapists to help patients learn activities of daily living. Independent performance of some routine hygienic activities, such as brushing the teeth, washing the face, arms, and upper trunk, combing the hair, and shaving, are required of the paraplegic patient. For the quadriplegic patient this may be delayed until more extension can be provided. Because of the loss of grasp in the quadriplegic patient, an elastic palm cuff with a pocket may be used to hold a toothbrush or an electric shaver. When sufficient wrist extensor power is present, a flexor-hinged splint may be used, which may provide a three-finger pinch and significantly increase the manual activities of the patient.

Bowel and Bladder Control

During spinal shock fecal incontinence will be present. Prevention of fecal impaction or diarrhea by means of diet, enema, and digital removal of impactions must be done until the anal reflex returns and bowel training can be started. At this time the patient should be able to transfer to the toilet or be placed on the toilet or bedside commode. Since the upright position facilitates bowel evacuation, the gastrocolic reflex is utilized by placing the patient on the toilet approximately 30 min after eating and requiring that the patient's schedule be adjusted to allow digital stimulation of the anorectal reflex. A suppository (e.g., bisacodyl) 30 min before a bowel movement is frequently beneficial. Stool softeners, mild laxatives, or bulk agents are used when necessary.

Initially the bladder is atonic, so control is obtained by an indwelling catheter. To avoid pressure within the urethra the catheter should be of the smallest size possible. If the urine remains clear, the catheter may be changed every 2 weeks. A fluid intake of $3\frac{1}{2}$ to 4 liters a day will minimize complications from the indwelling catheter. Prophylactic antibacterial therapy may be used in some cases with methenamine mandelate or Septra (Burroughs Wellcome Co., Research Triangle Park, N.C.), but controlled studies suggest that this need not be routine.

As soon as possible, the patient and family are taught the entire program of bladder management (self-catheterization, fluid management). Generally, C6 and lower quadriplegics are capable of independent bladder care.

Diet

The diet should be high in calories and high in protein, with the paraplegic soon feeding himself. The quadriplegic will need to be in a sitting or semireclining position and will require adaptations such as the palm cuff to allow holding of an eating utensil.

Independence

Once paraplegics are able to sit, they are able to dress themselves, including the application of braces. Quadriplegics have limited ability because of loss of hand function. Pull-on straps, button hooks, zippers, and velcro closures permit quadriplegics to have independence.

In occupational therapy, quadriplegics may be taught how to type, write, dial a phone, operate light switches, handle money, address envelopes, open and close doors, etc. Several wrists splints and orthotic devices are available to aid in this function.

Many patients (C6 level and below) are able to drive with the use of automatic shift and power devices for steering, brakes, and window controls. A manual control, usually on the left hand, is installed for the accelerator, brakes, and dimmer switch. Steering is usually by the right hand by use of a swivel knob attached to the steering wheel.

Psychosocial Problems

Paraplegic and quadriplegic patients undergo a high degree of stress when they become aware of the loss of function. A reactive depression will result from grief at the loss (which indicates the patient's acceptance of reality). If this does not occur, it may imply unrealistic denial of the disability and inappropriate hope of restoration of the loss. During this grief, patients will concentrate on the loss but should begin to appreciate the things that they are able to do. Reinforcement by hospital personnel and the family is required. The success of rehabilitation depends a great deal on how patients can resume and participate in the activities they value. The methods used and success in dealing with previous stress prior to the injury will determine how a patient approaches the stress after the injury.

Nursing, occupational therapy, and physical therapy personnel need to be involved on a daily basis to reinforce the patient's positive behavior. Since interruption of social function occurs, a program must be provided that will result in solving the social problems. A social worker may be very important in communication with the family and community resources. Knowledge of the patient's living arrangements, family situation, financial resources, education, and employment will enhance the planning of optimal rehabilitation and goals. This will allow the patient to cope with the social problems to be faced. The social worker may aid the family in seeking out financial and community assistance. Recreation therapy is valuable in getting the patient involved with activities outside of self-care.

Vocational Rehabilitation

A vocational counselor will utilize counseling interviews, vocational psychological testing, and work evaluation to determine the individual patient's needs. The previous level of education, work history, attitude regarding work, sense of responsibility, assets, response to disability, and level of independency must be ascertained.

Following discharge, job placement may be sought, often with a previous employer, or the patient may be referred to a rehabilitation center or sheltered workshop for a training program in a job more suitable for the disability and an educational program directed toward a profession or semiprofession. State divisions of vocational rehabilitation provide a number of services to assist the patient in employment.[8]

Complications

Pain

The paraplegic often complains of a severe, constant pain in the lower extremities, accompanied by paresthesias and aggravated by coughing and sneezing. Patients with spinal cord injury also develop pain sensation and paresthesias at various periods following the injury. This pain may be sharp, dull, burning, or tingling and may be intermittent or constant. Mild analgesics or tranquilizers or even antidepressant medication may aid in adjustments. Various forms of surgical treatment are discussed elsewhere in this textbook.

Spasticity

Following the initial flaccidity, spasticity occurs in the involved extremities and is often beneficial for function; however, in some patients the spasticity is incapacitating

and interferes with mobilization and activities of daily living. Increased spasticity predisposes to urinary tract and skin problems and to development of contractures. It may be exacerbated by infection, decubitus ulcers, yawning, and other external stimuli. The treatment of spasticity is discussed in Chap. 41.

Decubitus Ulcers

Development of such ulcers requires prompt management. All pressure or friction in the area must be eliminated and infection prevented. All dead tissue must be removed and any nutritional defect or anemia corrected. Strict attention to bed position eliminates pressure on these areas. A water bed may be beneficial with large ulcers, but with most patients simply keeping them off the area helps with the healing process. Debridement of the necrotic tissue may be mechanical or enzymatic. The ulcer should be kept dry, with massage of the surrounding skin to increase circulation and decrease edema, allowing healthy granulation tissue to develop. Large ulcers sometimes require closure with flaps.

Urinary Tract Complications

Urinary tract infection requires immediate treatment with high fluid intake, straight catheter drainage, and, after culture, a broad-spectrum antibiotic. Acute pyelonephritis must be considered in cases involving sudden onset of chills and fever. Urinary calculi result from increased urine excretion of calcium and phosphorus together with limited intake. Preventive measures include early mobilization and acidification of the urine. Vesicoureteral reflux is a major cause of upper urinary tract infection; satisfactory bladder drainage prevents reflux.

Autonomic Dysfunction

Alteration in body temperature, sweating abnormalities, and autonomic dysreflexia may occur. These usually only cause discomfort but occasionally produce severe symptoms.

Respiratory Complications

In high quadriplegics respiratory care must be an ongoing part of rehabilitation.

Sexual Function

Sexual adequacy is as important in the paraplegic and quadriplegic as it is in the normal individual. Because of the paralysis, there may have to be a role change between the male and the female. Although orgasm may not be possible for the female, conception is feasible and sexual adjustment is somewhat less of a problem than for the male. Approximately 75 percent of males with spinal cord injury may maintain an erection although ejaculation is either intermittent or not present, so that artificial insemination by donor or adoption may be necessary if a family is desired.[10] In patients who are impotent, recourse to sexual stimulation for the partner by means other than intercourse may be necessary. It is most important that the physician provide an opportunity for discussion of this area, as many patients are hesitant to discuss the problem.

Cerebral Palsy and Myelodysplasia

Any program of cerebral palsy rehabilitation must be flexible since symptoms and findings are not constant and depend on the state of maturation of the child. An approach and a program based upon periodic assessments as the child changes during growth are essential. The therapeutic regimen of the cerebral palsy child must be carried out by the family within the home situation using a program carefully designed within the family's capabilities. There must be continued education and instruction as the child develops.

The neuromuscular symptoms are classified as spasticity, athetosis, rigidity, ataxia, tremor, flaccidity, and combinations of these major neuromuscular symptoms. Training must include sitting balance, hand control, locomotion and ambulation (training will include bracing in many patients), and communication. In addition to neuromuscular development, the program must also provide aids for sensory and perceptual impairments, hearing and visual problems, speech impairments, emotional disturbances, social problems, and intellectual impairment. Parental counseling is important, as is vocational training.

Myelodysplastic children represent a special area of paraplegia for neurosurgeons. With these patients, as with cerebral palsy patients, a knowledge of child development is required, and therapy varies with the patient's age and growth. For example, functional bracing may be practical for T1 paraplegic children whereas it would not be for similarly afflicted adults. Vocational planning for the child should be considered at an early age with the goal of self-sufficiency.[3]

Head Injury

Head injuries cause mental changes but are often accompanied by motor and sensory deficits. Rehabilitation must be continued in a manner similar to that used in the care of the paraplegic and hemiplegic patient. However, the patient's level of consciousness, emotional stability, and intellectual ability may be greatly altered after a head injury. Sometimes, even in relatively minor head injuries, there is marked alteration in personality that affects the patient in every area of rehabilitation.

Patients may show marked apathy or extreme hostility. Obviously each of these areas must be approached in a very different manner. Hostility may be reduced by the use of antipsychotic medications. Family cooperation is essential in both of these extremes to assist in the rehabilitation.[3,5]

Since alteration in cerebral function may significantly affect the outcome of physical therapy, occupational therapy, and nursing care, psychological evaluation as early as possible may aid in the approach of the rehabilitation personnel. Cognitive remediation by therapists with specific training in techniques to improve mental deficits is important.

Polyneuropathy

The patient with the Guillain-Barré syndrome requires rest and other supportive measures initially; the prevention of contractures is essential. Footboards, posterior drop-foot splints, trochanter rolls, and volar or dorsal splints for the wrists and fingers will aid the paretic muscles. A passive range of motion will also prevent contractures and muscle tightness.

In the chronic stage any muscle tightness can be corrected by manual or prolonged stretching preceded by heat in the form of hot packs or whirlpool baths. The program must be carefully graduated, as fatigue or overuse must be avoided.

Prior to ambulation, the tilt table is valuable. If a foot drop is present, a leg brace is usually required. Maintenance of measures directed toward associated hypertensive, renal, and autonomic dysfunctions and sometimes painful paresthesias is an essential part of the rehabilitation program.

Multiple Sclerosis

Rehabilitation management of multiple sclerosis (MS) varies with the clinical course. The patient with paraplegia from transverse myelitis requires different care from the patient with marked ataxia.

Most patients with MS are susceptible to fatigue. Supervised endurance exercises are valuable, and short but frequent periods of activity should be interspersed with rest. Many patients have apparent intolerance to heat so that generalized thermotherapy is avoided, although local application of hot packs is usually tolerated. Severe spasticity may be a problem but its management is not different from that in other paraplegic patients. Cerebellar ataxia is difficult to treat effectively but the use of weighted wristlets or anklets, broad-based canes, or walkers may be helpful. Loss of urinary and bowel control will require training in any paraplegic patient to improve function.

Psychological adjustment must not be forgotten. Some patients have altered affect, with depression and/or euphoria that may be due to structural involvement; however, many times depressive reaction is expected. Therapy may include medical management in addition to psychiatric or group therapy.[3]

Parkinsonism

Rehabilitation is directed at correcting contractures and initiation of a reconditioning active program consisting of mat exercises, calisthenics, and endurance and strengthening programs. Insistence upon the performance of all activities of daily living of which the patient is capable is important. In ambulation training, walking with a wide-base support may aid in the redevelopment of reciprocal arm movements. All rehabilitation measures should be correlated with the proper medical therapy involving use of L-dopa and other medications. Orthostatic hypotension may complicate active therapy.

Many patients with parkinsonism have altered autonomic function or altered sleep patterns (often sleep pattern reversal), and some have an altered mental status. However, those who appear "dull" and markedly depressed owing to a masked facies may improve significantly with the institution of medical therapy.

Peripheral Nerve Lesion

Rehabilitation of a peripheral nerve lesion is done to maximize restoration of muscle function with reinnervation or with substitution of function if reinnervation does not occur. Edema may be kept at a minimum by the use of bandages or stockings, limb elevation, or an arm sling. Braces often maintain functional alignment and prevent overstretching of the paralyzed muscle. An active and a passive range of motion exercises involving the joints should be carried out daily. Electrical stimulation may aid in preventing atrophy and tissue fibrosis.

If reinnervation takes place, muscle re-education is required to establish voluntary control. When reinnervation does not occur, substitution for the loss of function may be accomplished by the use of braces or splints or by means of reconstructive surgery consisting of joint fusions or tendon transfers. Obviously, each patient must be treated individually since different nerve injuries require specific functional assessment and management.

References

1. Boshes B: Traumatic paralysis: Diagnosis and nonsurgical treatment. Med Clin North Am 47:1629–1646, 1963.
2. Feigenson JS: Stroke rehabilitation. Stroke 12:372–375, 1981.
3. Gullickson G Jr: Neurologic rehabilitation, in Baker AB, Baker LH (eds): *Clinical Neurology*, vol 3. Philadelphia, Harper & Row, 1981, pp 1–25.
4. Guttmann L: Discussion on the treatment and prognosis of traumatic paraplegia. Proc R Soc Med 40:219–229, 1947.
5. Guttmann L: Initial management of the paraplegic patient. Practitioner 176:157–170, 1956.
6. Guttmann L: *Spinal Cord Injuries: A Comprehensive Management and Research*, 2d ed. Oxford, Blackwell Scientific, 1976.
7. Knapp ME: Practical physical medicine and rehabilitation. Lecture 2: The hemiplegic patient—rehabilitation. Postgrad Med 39:A143–A149, 1966.
8. Meine E: On after-care of paralysed patients in their homes. Paraplegia 8:154–157, 1970.
9. Roberts DW: Evolution of the rehabilitation center concept in the planning of rehabilitation centers. *Rehabilitation Service Series* 420, US Dept of Health, Education and Welfare, 1957, p 10.
10. Tarabulcy E: Sexual function in the normal and in paraplegia. Paraplegia 10:201–208, 1972.

Part V

Neurosurgical and Related Techniques

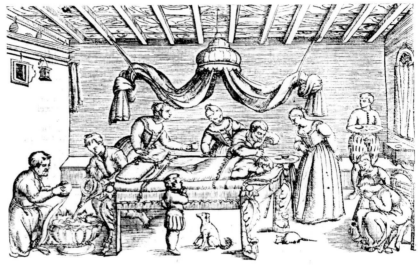

della Croce GA. *Chirurgiae Libri Septem*. Venice, J Zillettus, 1573. An early illustration of a neurosurgical operation.

43

Principles of Neurosurgical Operative Technique

Robert H. Wilkins

Many atlases describe the specific techniques used in various neurosurgical operations, and it is not the intent of this chapter to present such information. Rather, it outlines the principles that underlie all neurosurgical operations.[63] The reader who wants the details about a particular procedure is referred to the appropriate segment of this textbook and to the atlases and textbooks listed at the end of this chapter.

Preparation

Many factors contribute to the successful management of a neurosurgical case, including a prompt and accurate diagnosis and excellent pre- and postoperative care. Regarding the operation itself, the decision about whether and when to operate and the choice of operations are certainly as significant as the specific instruments and methods used during the chosen operation.

However, even considering that it is only one of many factors contributing to a successful outcome, operative technique is important, and the neurosurgeon can improve the results by paying attention to the details of each operation. An approach of this sort begins with the steps taken in advance of the actual surgical procedure.

First and foremost, the neurosurgeon should have an operative "game plan," based on the patient's history, physical findings, and test results, that not only includes the specific steps that will be taken if all goes as it should but also includes contingency plans to deal with unexpected findings or events that might be encountered during the operation. A surgeon who is learning to perform a particular procedure or one whose memory needs refreshing should read about the operation and discuss it with a more experienced surgeon who can give advice and help. In addition, surgeons at any level of expertise should review the patient's record for any previous surgical treatment that might influence how the proposed operation is carried out.

Once the surgeon has a plan in mind, it should be discussed with the patient and the appropriate members of the patient's family. Occasionally this will not be possible because of unusual circumstances; for example, the patient may be unconscious and may require immediate treatment before the next of kin can be contacted. However, usually there is time for this important conversation. The surgeon should discuss the nature of the condition for which the patient is being treated and the nature of the proposed operation as well as the chance of success, the major risks,[24] and the alternative methods of treatment. The surgeon should indicate that the treatment given will be in accordance with customary and usual medical standards but that there is no guarantee of a successful outcome.

Once informed consent has been obtained, specific plans for the proposed operation begin. The procedure in the operating room must be scheduled, and information must be given about patient positioning and about any unusual instruments needed. The surgeon must also write the appropriate preoperative orders. Generally the patient is restricted from eating or drinking after a certain time, the blood bank is requested to prepare a certain number of units of blood for possible transfusion, and the orders for premedications are written. The surgeon needs to consider whether to order one or more analgesic, barbiturate, neuroleptic, anticholinergic, steroid, or antibiotic medications. Elastic stockings may be ordered for use during the operation and in the initial postoperative period. Both the surgeon and the anesthesiologist should review the patient's history, physical findings, and laboratory data to identify any conditions that might affect the outcome of the operation adversely. If such a condition is found, the surgeon and anesthesiologist must then decide how best to deal with it to reduce the operative risk.

In the operating room, just before the procedure is to begin, the surgeon should check with the patient and chart regarding the disease process and exact anatomical localization (side, level, etc.). The surgeon should also review the pertinent radiographic films and should put up the key films on the view boxes in the operating room.

Elastic stockings should be placed on the patient's lower extremities or elastic bandages wrapped around the legs to prevent venous stagnation. After the induction of anesthesia, the ground plate of the cautery should be applied, with plenty of gel for good contact, to a flat surface of the patient's body, away from the external genitalia. The patient's eyes should be protected by instilling ointment into them, taping the lids shut, or both. A urinary catheter should be inserted into the bladder if the operation is expected to last more than two or three hours, if hyperosmotic agents are to be given, or if urinary output is to be monitored during the procedure. During some operations, lumbar drainage of cerebrospinal fluid will facilitate surgical exposure; if this is anticipated, the lumbar needle or catheter should be inserted at this time, and the patency of the system should be tested after final patient positioning by allowing a small amount of CSF to exit.

The surgeon and the anesthesiologist will need to decide in each case which parameters are to be monitored during the operation and to insert or apply the appropriate equipment for these monitors. In addition to arterial blood pressure, pulse, temperature, and ECG measurements, the surgeon and anesthesiologist might wish to monitor arterial blood gas levels, gas concentrations in the exhaled air, central venous pressure, urine output, intracranial pressure, evoked potential patterns, electroencephalographic wave forms, cerebral blood flow measurements, etc. If the patient is to be operated upon in a position in which the area of operation will be significantly higher than the right atrium, a Doppler monitor should be attached to the chest and a venous catheter passed into the right atrium so that any venous air embolism may be detected and treated by aspiration of air from the right atrium.[1,36] If significant bleeding is likely to occur during the operation, at least two intravenous lines should be established. If spinal traction will be needed during the operation, the traction apparatus should be applied before the operative area is prepared and draped.

The patient should be positioned in such a way that the operative area is stabilized and maximum exposure is achieved. However, the person responsible for positioning the patient should minimize the distortion of normal anatomical relationships and should be careful not to put undue pressure on peripheral nerves,[41] eyes, jugular veins, and other sensitive structures. If the patient is to be operated upon in the prone position, the trunk should be supported laterally, allowing room for thoracic and abdominal excursions centrally and avoiding secondary distention of the spinal veins. If the patient's head is to be immobilized by a pin-type head holder, sterile pins should be used, the appropriate regions of the scalp should be prepared with an antiseptic solution, and the force of application of pins should be sufficient to immobilize the skull but not so great as to penetrate the inner table. For posterior fossa surgery, head flexion should not be excessive, especially in a patient with cervical spondylosis, in order to avoid a possible acute compressive myelopathy.

Final preparations for the operation include shaving the operative area. In the case of an unusual or infrequently performed operation, the surgeon may wish to consult an anatomical atlas or some similar source of information and have it available in the operating room for reference during the procedure. The operating table is placed in the optimal position in the operating room, the anesthesia team and their equipment are situated, and any other necessary equipment, such as a C-arm x-ray machine, is also positioned about the patient. The surgeon or assistant, after scrubbing hands and forearms and donning sterile gloves, cleanses the operative area and marks out the proposed incision.

In planning the incision, the surgeon should aim for maximum exposure of the lesion or target and minimum exposure of adjacent normal tissues. In spinal operations, guidance may be provided by palpation of the spinous processes or other bony landmarks or by noting a cutaneous scratch made at the time of myelography to mark the level of the lesion. However, if there is any question about the accuracy of spinal localization, it is best to verify the exact level with a lateral or posteroanterior roentgenogram made in the operating room after the dissection has been started and some anatomical structure has been tagged by a removable metallic marker. For example, the tip of a Penfield dissector or a metal suction tip can be placed against the ligamentum flavum at an interlaminar space or a needle can be inserted into the anterior aspect of an intervertebral disc.

In planning a scalp incision, the surgeon may wish to view the key radiographic films and perhaps even have the circulating nurse hold the lateral angiogram adjacent to the patient's head as a direct guide. In addition, the surgeon should be able to visualize the location of key intracranial structures while looking at the external surface of the patient's head. Studies of craniocerebral topography have provided guidelines for determining the locations of the sylvian and the rolandic fissures, and the surgeon would do well to remember these in planning the surgical approach (Fig. 43-1). The sylvian fissure lies along a line connecting the external angular process of the frontal bone and a point along the sagittal midline three-quarters of the distance from the nasion to the inion. The fissure of Rolando lies along a line connecting the midpoint of the zygomatic arch and a point along the sagittal midline 2 cm posterior to the midpoint between the nasion and the inion.

Scalp flaps should have a broad base and an adequate blood supply. If the base is narrower than the distal end of the flap and if the flap is not based on a good arterial supply, its edges may become gangrenous. Perpendicular or crossing scalp incisions should not be used because of possible ischemia of the pointed flap tip or tips. The scalp incision should be made within a hair-containing portion of the scalp, if feasible, so that it will be hidden after the patient's hair regrows. Any portion of the scalp to be excised should be restricted as much as possible so that the edges of the scalp can be reapproximated at the end of the operation without having to use a rotation flap or some other major maneuver.

The incision should be outlined before the operative area is draped, so that no important landmarks are hidden from the surgeon's view. It may also be of value to make other lines on the skin to mark the sagittal midline, key bony landmarks, alternative or accessory incisions, etc., for the purpose of orienting the surgeon during the period when everything but the operative field is obscured by the drapes.

The main purpose of draping is to isolate the sterile operative field from the surrounding unsterile areas. The first layer should therefore be applied tightly around the edges of the operative field to avoid direct gaps to the outside. An

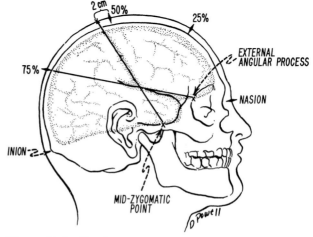

Figure 43-1 Craniocerebral topography, showing the approximate locations of the sylvian and rolandic fissures. (From Wilkins and Odom.[63])

adhesive sterile translucent sheet of plastic is an excellent method of achieving such a barrier while also covering all of the exposed skin and thus reducing the possibility of wound contamination by bacteria remaining on the skin after antiseptic cleansing. Further draping not only serves to protect against infection but also reduces possible visual distractions for the surgical team. The draping and lighting focus their attention on the operative field.

After draping has been completed, the scrub nurse moves the instrument tables into position, and any lines from sterile to unsterile areas (e.g., suction tubes, cautery cords, the energy source for an automatic drill) are attached. If a microscope is to be used, it should already have been draped and should be in a standby position. The surgeon should be sure that illumination, magnification, and suction are adequate for the job at hand and should choose and load the aneurysm clips or set up any other special equipment or instruments that might be needed quickly during the operation, when time might not permit a careful selection.

Wound Healing

The surgeon needs to understand the basics of wound healing, which are so important to the outcome of an operation.[6,9,11,12,14,25–27,49,51] Wound healing is therefore considered at this point, before continuing the discussion of operative technique.

Phases of Healing

There are three phases of wound healing. The first phase, also called the inflammatory, exudative, substrate, or lag phase, lasts for the first four or five days after a wound occurs. This phase involves both a vascular-hemostatic response and a cellular response. Immediately after a tissue is wounded, blood exits from any severed vessels and fills the gap between the wound edges. This blood then clots. Within the tissue at the edges of the wound, vasoconstriction and vessel retraction start within a few seconds and last a few minutes. Platelets aggregate within small vessels. Blood flow in these vessels slows, and white blood cells adhere to the vessel walls. Then vasodilatation begins, reaching a maximum in about 10 min. The small blood vessels become more permeable, and white blood cells (and, to a lesser extent, red blood cells) escape into the tissue. Plasma also escapes, resulting in tissue edema. The fibrin formed by the blood coagulation within the gap unites the wound margins and provides a scaffold for cell migration.

Mast cells in the tissue release histamine and other substances soon after injury. These cells decrease in number within 1 day and then gradually return to normal over 8 days.

Other cells arrive through the bloodstream. Neutrophils appear in the wounded tissue in maximum numbers during the first 2 days, taking 2 to 8 min to emigrate through the vessel wall. Their numbers decrease after the third day. Neutrophils disintegrate, releasing hydrolytic enzymes from their lysosomes, which lyse fibrin and debris and aid in phagocytosis. Neutrophils also phagocytize bacteria and small foreign material.

Monocytes also arrive mainly via the bloodstream, reaching a maximum concentration within a few days. They are the dominant cells in the wound by the fifth day. These monocytes become macrophages, having the main function of phagocytosis, but they also become epithelioid cells and multinucleated giant cells in the presence of materials that cannot be degraded, phagocytized, and removed.

Lymphocytes reach maximum numbers in the wound at about 6 days. These cells are important in the immune response. They are not phagocytic and are not precursors of macrophages.

By the end of the first phase of wound healing, new capillaries and lymphatic channels are beginning to extend out into the coagulum within the gap of the wound. Fibroblasts are also beginning to appear, having originated in the adjacent connective tissue. This first phase, which involves a transient inflammatory response, is necessary for optimal fibroblast proliferation and connective tissue formation during the second phase. If the inflammatory response is reduced, as by steroid administration, fibroplasia is delayed and reduced. If it is unusually prolonged or severe, as by bacterial infection, fibroplasia will also be altered detrimentally.

The second phase of wound healing is also called the proliferative, connective tissue, or fibroblastic phase. It lasts from about the fifth day to the twentieth day, and during this period there is marked physical and biochemical activity involving cells, glycoproteins, mucopolysaccharides, and collagen. Epithelial cells and fibroblasts proliferate and migrate, with cell movement being away from other cells. Contact guidance occurs along structures such as fibrin strands and along planes of tension or compression. Epithelial proliferation occurs at the wound edges, and epithelial cells begin to migrate early in the course of wound healing. Such cell movement is more rapid in moist than in dry wounds. The fibroblasts, which are derived mainly from adjacent connective tissue, start appearing in the wound from the second to the fourth day and reach a maximum on about the eighth day. Early x-ray irradiation of the wound will reduce the numbers of these important cells.

The fibroblasts form collagen, the protein that binds the wound edges together. Within the fibroblast, three polypeptide chains (alpha chains) are synthesized. These chains are bonded together in helical fashion to form a single molecule, which is extruded from the fibroblast as procollagen. Terminal peptides are removed to form tropocollagen, and the tropocollagen molecules aggregate into collagen filaments, being held together by intermolecular bonds. These filaments (about 200 Å in diameter) in turn join other filaments to form collagen fibrils (about 2000 Å in diameter), primitive collagen fibers (about 20,000 Å in diameter), and collagen fibers (about 100,000 to 200,000 Å in diameter). As the number and size of the collagen fibers increase over weeks, there is a progressive increase in tensile strength, which outlasts the period of fibroplasia (Fig. 43-2).

In addition to fibroblasts, new capillaries also extend into the wound during the second phase of wound healing. These begin as solid sprouts from existing capillaries that later canalize. They are quite fragile, and most eventually regress.

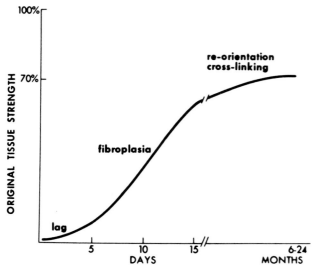

Figure 43-2 Tensile strength–time curve for incised wounds. (From Heughan C, Hunt TK: Some aspects of wound healing research: A review. Can J Surg 18:118–126, 1975.)

In the ground substance of the wound, the mucopolysaccharide content increases to a maximum between the third and sixth days and then diminishes as the amount of collagen in the wound increases.

The third phase of wound healing is the reorganization, or remodeling, phase. This begins at about 21 days and lasts for 2 years or more.

Wound contraction occurs and is most pronounced at around 3 weeks. There is a decrease in the number of cells and vessels within the wound, and the vascular network differentiates. Collagen fibers align in a direction parallel to the direction of tension and stretch forces. Aggregation, cross-linking, and organization of collagen fibers continue, resulting in a further increase in the tensile strength of the wound (though at a progressively diminishing rate) until a plateau is reached (Fig. 43-2).

Healing of Dura Mater and Bone

The dura mater heals in the same fashion as does connective tissue in other parts of the body. However, in addition an encapsulating neomembrane forms on both sides of a healing dural flap or a dural graft of periosteum or fascia. There is little effect on the underlying brain unless it has been injured, in which case adhesions form between the cortex and the dura or dural graft. Dural substitutes elicit a variable foreign body reaction, with an early cellular response (including in the leptomeninges) and eventual encapsulation.[28]

The bone of the skull and spine heals in a predictable fashion. The fracture of any bone is followed by acute inflammation, then debridement and the formation of a reparative blastema. The connective tissue cells in and around the bone (in large part derived from the proliferation of medullary and periosteal cells, including dural cells in the case of cranial bone) constitute a labile pool of interconverti-

ble osteoblasts, chondroblasts, fibroblasts, osteoclasts, and undifferentiated cells. These form a callus of new bone, cartilage, and fibrous tissue that serves as a temporary splint.

Bryant points out that the connective tissue cells

form bone in areas of high oxygen tension and form cartilage in areas of low oxygen tension. As new capillary growth proceeds, new bone replaces cartilaginous callus. . . . The osteogenic cells nearest the bone surface appear to transform directly into osteoblasts and lay down a collagen matrix which calcifies directly into bone. In less well vascularized areas of the wound, the osteogenic cells form cartilage. Whether a given undifferentiated cell manufactures cartilage or bone appears to depend on several factors in its microenvironment, including oxygen tension, pH, and the stresses of compression and tension.[6]

Remodeling of the old and new bone occurs next. Osteoclasts resorb the callus, and new haversian systems are formed as concentric layers of bone are laid down around the new blood vessels.

Following a craniotomy with immediate replacement of the bone flap, there will be slight movement of the bone edges with each heartbeat, as modified by respiration. As a result, the patient may experience a clicking at the operative site until enough fibrous tissue or callus has formed to prevent such movement. The skull flaps will be totally remodeled in the course of healing, and the edges of the flap may reunite with the adjacent skull through bony bridges, especially in infants and children. If the skull flap is removed aseptically at craniotomy and is replaced at a later date, having been stored in frozen condition in the interim, the sequential dynamics of skull revitalization have been found to be revascularization, resorption, and accretion.[43,44] Occasionally the accretion is incomplete, and portions of the skull flap will not be reformed after having been resorbed. If a free bone flap is replaced in a craniotomy defect after it has been autoclaved, resorption is usually more marked and there is an increased risk of subsequent osteomyelitis, especially if the flap has been autoclaved and stored in a frozen state for a period of time before being replaced.

Factors Affecting Healing

Many factors affect wound healing. Local factors of importance include blood supply, mechanical stress, the surgical technique used to treat the wound, suture materials, infection, and radiotherapy. Among important systemic factors are patient age and nutrition, trauma to other parts of the body, hypovolemia, hypoxia, anemia, uremia, malignant disease, jaundice, and the administration of corticosteroid, cytotoxic, or antimetabolite drugs.

Wounds should be closed, if possible, by approximating the sides of the wound closely after removing all foreign matter and devitalized tissue. This approximation should not be so tight that it interferes with the blood supply, but it should be tight enough to prevent dead spaces that retard fibroplasia. During the first 7 to 10 days, immobilization of the wound prevents shearing and rupture of the new capillaries in the granulation tissue, fluid accumulation, and

TABLE 43-1   General Properties of Common Suture Materials

Suture Material	Absorbable (A) or Nonabsorbable (NA)	Breaking Strength	Knot Security	Tensile Strength in Tissues	Tissue Reaction
Plain catgut	A	Variable	Poor	Nil at 3 days	Gross
Chromic catgut	A	Good	Fair	Nil after 10 days	Moderate
Extruded collagen	A	Good	Fair	Nil after 10 days	Moderate
Polyglycolic acid	A	Good	Good	40% at 14 days	Less than catgut
Polyglactin	A	Good	Good	40% at 14 days	Less than catgut
Silk thread	NA	Fair	Good	None at 6 months	Moderate
Linen thread	NA	Fair	Good	None at 6 months	Moderate
Braided polyamide (nylon)	NA	Good	Good	Variable loss at 6 months	Less than silk or linen
Monofilament polyamide (nylon)	NA	Good	Poor	Little loss	Minimal
Braided polyester (Dacron, Orlon, Teflon)	NA	Very good	Good	Retained	Minimal
Polypropylene (monofilament)	NA	Good	Fair	Retained	Minimal
Steel wire (monofilament)	NA	Very good	Good	Retained	Minimal

SOURCE: Irvin, p. 38.[27]

hemorrhage. After 2 to 3 weeks, when tensile strength is improving, a graded increase in activity aids collagen deposition and wound strength.

Any retained foreign material, including a surgical implant, is rejected by the wound. If it is small enough, it is phagocytized. If not, it is "exteriorized" by fibrocollagenous encapsulation within the wound or by inflammatory extrusion from the wound.

Various suture materials have different physical properties, as outlined in Table 43-1. Nonabsorbable sutures supply only 40 to 70 percent of the natural tensile strength of tissue (Fig. 43-3). Ideally, absorbable sutures should be able to hold tissues together long enough until the forming collagen unites the wound at the 40 percent strength level, which may require 2 to 4 weeks.

The catguts are variably tanned condensations of longitudinal muscle fibers of sheep intestine. These and other heterologous proteins, such as reconstituted bovine collagen, evoke a local immune rejection response and provide a maximal stimulus for fibroplasia. The synthetic absorbable sutures formed from polyglycolic acid or polyglactin have certain advantages over catgut.[33] They have a more predictable rate of absorption; they are more dependable in tensile strength, strength retention, and knot security; they cause less tissue reactivity; and they retain their integrity and strength better in the face of infection.

Various tissue adhesives have been introduced to hold tissues together in addition to or instead of sutures.[20,22,39] In general, these have proved to be toxic to neural structures and to incite an inflammatory response in adjacent tissues. For this reason they have been of limited value in neurosurgical practice; they have been used primarily in sealing CSF leaks that cannot be sutured shut, in coating aneurysms that

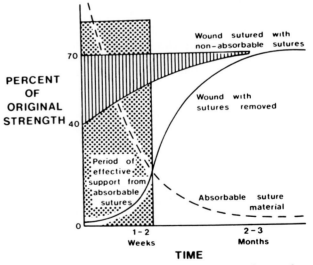

Figure 43-3   Strength is recovered in a sutured wound as a function of the strength achieved by the sutures and the progressive recovery of strength during the three phases of wound healing. As soon as a wound is sutured with a nonabsorbable suture material, it has between 40 and 70 percent of the original tissue strength, and this will last until fibroplasia brings the wound strength to 70 percent. A wound sutured with an absorbable material will lose strength rapidly from the 40 to 70 percent level over the first 2 weeks; at that point fibroplasia has still not supplied 40 percent of the original strength, and the wound is the weakest. (From Forrester JC: Sutures and wound repair, in Hunt, pp. 194–206.[25])

cannot be treated by other means, and for intravascular obliteration of arteriovenous malformations and carotid-cavernous fistulas.

As mentioned previously, the initial transient inflammatory response during the first few days after wounding prepares the wound for the second stage of wound healing. However, bacterial infection of a wound destroys young fibroblasts and interferes with fibroplasia. Bacteria compete with fibroblasts and other host cells for available oxygen within the wound. Furthermore, massive infection with pus formation physically disrupts the wound.

The rate of wound infection after clean neurosurgical operations should be no higher than 4 percent and is usually in the range of 1 to 2 percent. Dunphy has stated unequivocally that tissue injury is a more important factor in wound infection than simple bacterial contamination and that most wound infections after clean operations are the result of poor surgical technique.[11] The rate of wound infection in neurosurgical operations is higher in longer operations and re-explorations, and when external drains are used or the patient has diabetes mellitus.[64,65] It has been reported that the infection rate in clean operations can be reduced by the use of ultraviolet lights in the operating room.[65]

Can the administration of antibiotics also reduce the incidence of wound infection after neurosurgical operations? Theoretically, effective prophylaxis of infection can be achieved if the appropriate antibacterial agent is given in such a way that there is an adequate concentration in the appropriate tissues at the time of bacterial contamination or shortly thereafter but with limitation of the period of antibiotic administration to avoid superinfection by resistant organisms.[8] Despite evidence to the contrary from other investigations, some recent studies have seemed to indicate that prophylactic antibiotics do reduce the incidence of neurosurgical wound infections. Most of these studies have not been randomized or well controlled, but they have been provocative.

In 1975 Horwitz and Curtin reported a series of consecutive operations for lumbar disc herniation by one neurosurgeon.[23] In 128 operations the patient had no antibiotics; there were 11 major infections and one minor infection. In 402 operations the patient was given antibiotics, and there were only four minor infections. During the 5 years prior to 1975 lincomycin was given pre- and postoperatively in 238 cases, and there was only one minor infection, for an infection rate of 0.4 percent.

In 1976 Venes presented a study of 150 consecutive CSF shunting procedures.[62] During the induction of anesthesia, oxacillin at 50 mg/kg was given as an intravenous bolus, and two further intravenous doses of 25 mg/kg were given 6 and 12 h later. There was also a rigid operative protocol, including antiseptic cleansing and draping. In this series there was only one primary infection and two secondary infections.

Then in 1979, Malis reported that the use of an intraoperative prophylactic antibiotic regime consisting of intramuscular gentamicin or tobramycin, intravenous vancomycin, and streptomycin irrigating solution, over a 5-year period at Mount Sinai Hospital in New York, had provided complete protection against neurosurgical operative infections, with no instance of an infection among 1732 clean operative cases and no complication due to the antibiotics.[35]

This startling report prompted other neurosurgeons to adopt this same regimen, with varying degrees of success.

As a result of his review of existing studies, published in 1980, Haines[17] noted the lack of truly scientific randomized clinical evaluations of prophylactic antibiotics in neurosurgery, and he concluded:

> There are no unequivocal indications for the use of prophylactic antibiotics in neurological surgery. If one fact can be gleaned from this review, it is that there is a need for carefully designed, large scale, randomized clinical trials to settle some of these issues. This is not a minor undertaking, for appropriately designed studies will require the cooperation of several large clinical services and the entry of thousands of patients to satisfy statistical requirements.

Reasonable recommendations based on the incomplete data available follow:

1. Final recommendations regarding antibiotic prophylaxis in clean neurosurgical procedures must await the replication of Malis' results. Until then there is support in the literature for either using or not using antibiotics prophylactically.

2. A reasonable case can be made for either using or not using antibiotics when a foreign body is implanted into a clean wound.

3. Surgical entry into a noninfected sinus or the oral or nasal cavities has not been studied sufficiently to allow comment.

4. A reasonable case can be made either way for the use of prophylactic antibiotics in external ventriculostomy.

5. Antibiotics are not necessary in basilar skull fracture without overt CSF leakage, but a reasonable case in either direction can be made for patients in whom CSF leakage is documented.

6. Compound skull fractures may be treated with or without antibiotics unless contamination is so evident as to make antibiotic use therapeutic rather than prophylactic.

Two recent studies of the efficacy of prophylactic antibiotics in preventing hydrocephalus shunt infections have been carried out in prospective, double-blind, randomized fashion. Epstein and his associates found that the administration of cephalothin sodium neutral from 1 h preoperatively through 3 days postoperatively reduced the postoperative infection rate significantly, from 21.1 percent in the 38 control patients to 2.6 percent in the 39 patients receiving cephalothin.[13] Haines and Taylor carried out a study of 74 children, giving the experimental group of 35 patients methicillin at 12.5 mg/kg every 6 h for 72 h beginning 6 h before a ventriculoperitoneal shunting operation, with an additional 12.5 mg/kg of methicillin given intravenously at the time of anesthesia induction. The 39 control patients received saline on the same schedule. There were five infections in the placebo group (12.8 percent) and two in the methicillin group (5.7 percent); however, the difference was not statistically significant.[18] These two studies represent the beginning of a scientific investigative approach to neurosurgical wound infections that should eventually provide important guidelines for the use of prophylactic antibiotics in neurosurgical practice.

As stated above, depending on timing and dosage, radiation therapy, like infection, may impair fibroplasia and wound contraction. Similarly, alkylating agents such as nitrogen mustard may reduce the amount of granulation tissue and collagen concentration and may delay wound contraction.

Although advanced patient age is supposed to retard wound healing, patient age does not seem to be an important factor in the development of a postoperative infection after a clean craniotomy.[64] Likewise, although cortisone in large doses given preoperatively and immediately postoperatively inhibits the inflammatory phase of wound healing and hence inhibits subsequent fibroplasia (it also inhibits wound contraction), steroid administration does not seem to be an important determinant of wound infection after a clean craniotomy.[64] (As an aside, the adverse effects of cortisone on wound healing can be counteracted to some extent with the topical or systemic administration of vitamin A.)

Nutrition plays an important role in wound healing. If the patient has a deficiency of proteins, amino acids, ascorbic acid and other vitamins, or trace minerals such as zinc, fibroblast activity and collagen formation will be retarded. Hypoxia will also affect wound healing adversely. In contrast, if a normal wounded person breathes 40% oxygen at atmospheric pressure, there is a 15 percent increase in the rate of wound healing. This observation, and the success in healing radionecrosis of the mandible with hyperbaric oxygen treatments, provide a clue to better wound healing that should be investigated further.

The reopening of a craniotomy or laminectomy is associated with a higher incidence of wound infection, especially when the operation is repeated more than once or is repeated within a short time.[64,65] However, any wound that is reopened within a few weeks and is then resutured heals more rapidly than a fresh primary wound, probably because the fibroplasia phase is already in progress.

Neurosurgical Materials and Devices

In the United States, tissue adhesives, sutures, and other neurosurgical devices have come under the regulatory control of the Food and Drug Administration (FDA).[7] The Federal Food, Drug, and Cosmetic Act of 1906, as amended in 1938 and 1962, gave the FDA the authority to regulate medical drugs. In addition, the 1938 amendment gave the FDA the power to restrain the sale of unsafe or unproven medical devices. However, until 1976 the FDA had no right to impose pre-marketing clearance restraints on medical devices, and it usually required lengthy court action to stop the manufacture and distribution of fraudulent or harmful devices. The 1976 medical device amendments gave the Food and Drug Administration direct legal authority to control medical devices (and by doing so, to potentially regulate those professionals using such devices).

The 1976 amendments were actually initiated by President Nixon in 1969, who requested the Secretary of Health, Education and Welfare to determine what legislative controls were necessary to protect the public against risk of injury or illness from medical devices. As a consequence, a study group on medical devices was formed under the chairmanship of Dr. Theodore Cooper, Director of the National Heart and Lung Institute. As Burton and McFadden[7] reported:

> The Cooper Committee report recommended a review of the existing medical devices, and the classification of these devices into three categories: 1) those requiring pre-marketing clearance; 2) those for which standards would be appropriate; and 3) those which should be exempt from pre-marketing review and standards.

> At the request of the Secretary of Health, Education and Welfare, the FDA undertook an inventory and classification of existing medical devices from the 1100 manufacturers identified as suppliers in the USA. This task was expedited by the formation of federal advisory panels to assist the FDA.

> By the end of 1974, 14 panels, including a Neurological Panel, had been established.

These panels did their work well, and by 1976 the FDA Panel on Neurologic Devices had finished its classification of neurological devices. The panel was kept intact to review and recommend neurological device standards and to otherwise advise the FDA on device-related affairs.

In addition to interacting with the FDA, neurosurgeons in the United States became involved with other aspects of device development and safety. For many years, numerous organizations around the world have been involved with writing up standards for various types of devices on a voluntary basis. The American Society for Testing and Materials (ASTM), founded in 1898, is the world's largest source of voluntary consensus standards. As of 1976, the ASTM Committee on Surgical Materials and Devices included a neurosurgical subcommittee with 11 sections (materials, aneurysm and blood vessel clips, cranioplasty materials, carotid clamps, shunts, aneurysmorrhaphy and tissue adhesives, electrodes, suture materials, cranial tongs for skeletal traction, stereotaxic instruments, and operating microscopes). Neurosurgeons have taken an active part in the activities of the American Society for Testing and Materials since 1967.

The Association for the Advancement of Medical Instrumentation (AAMI) was organized in 1966. A Neurostimulation Subcommittee was formed in 1972 and the Committee on Neurosurgical Devices in 1975. The third major organization in the United States, the American National Standards Institute (ANSI), began in 1918 as the American Engineering Standards Committee. Internationally, the two main nongovernmental organizations that coordinate and approve voluntary international standards are the International Standards Organization (ISO), which started in 1926 as the International Federation of National Standardization Associations, and the International Electrotechnical Commission.

A specific interest in neurosurgical materials and devices has also grown among members of neurosurgical organizations. In the 1950s an Instrument Committee was formed by members of the Harvey Cushing Society. Subsequently a Committee on Materials and Devices was formed in the Congress of Neurological Surgeons in 1972 and in the American Association of Neurological Surgeons in 1973; the two separate committees fused to form a joint committee in 1974.

Thus for more than a decade there has been an organized group of neurosurgeons in the United States who have been able to advise the FDA about neurosurgical devices and who have been involved with writing standards for such devices. Their activities have become an important part of the continuing effort to improve the technical aspects of neurosurgical care.

Intraoperative Technique

During an operation, the surgeon and the rest of the operative team should be in a proper state of mind—attentive to the task at hand but not so tense as to interfere with their smooth functioning. Elective cases should be scheduled when the operative team is fresh. There is a definite advantage to having the same personnel involved in all the neurosurgical cases; they come to know the equipment and procedures and work together in a progressively more efficient fashion with time. Surgeons and their assistants should operate from a comfortable position. Surgeons should not only continually sharpen their own technical abilities but should learn to use their assistants and other personnel to best advantage. Personnel movement should be limited during an operation. Incoming pages, telephone calls, sudden loud noises, and other distractions should be kept to a minimum.

Any operation consists of a series of steps, such as the division of tissue; achievement of hemostasis; protection and retraction of normal tissue; control of untoward pathophysiological events such as increased intracranial pressure with brain herniation; recognition of pathological tissue and distortions of normal tissue; management of unsterile, contaminated, or infected areas; removal of tissue; insertion of materials or devices; replacement and reapproximation of tissue; insertion and removal of drains; and application of dressings, splints, and braces. In the following paragraphs, some of these steps are considered in relation to neurosurgical operations.

Division of Tissue and Hemostasis

Tissue may be divided in a number of ways, with instruments ranging from the standard scalpel to the latest laser and plasma scalpel (gas jet) techniques. The division and removal of tissue by automated cutting and suction, by ultrasonic emulsification and aspiration, and by laser energy are discussed in subsequent chapters and are not considered here.

The pressure of the assistant's fingers against the skin on either side of a skin incision is usually sufficient to control

bleeding until hemostatic clamps or clips can be applied. The surgeon using Raney clips on the scalp edges must be aware of the degree of compression they are exerting, which will vary according to the thickness of the scalp. If such clips are tightly compressive, are left in place for several hours, and have been applied to a scalp flap that has other impairments to its circulation (e.g., diabetes mellitus, narrow flap base, flap folded sharply at its base during the operation, etc.), ischemia may result. Such ischemia may interfere with the regrowth of hair adjacent to the scalp incision or may impair the healing of the incision.

Electrical energy in the range of 250,000 to 2 million Hz can be used to divide tissue and also to stop bleeding.

> The ability of high-frequency current to damage tissue depends on its concentration or density. As the current density increases, its heating effect becomes more pronounced. The size of the active monopolar electrode is deliberately kept small so that concentrated heating will occur at its point of contact with tissue. The ground, or return electrode, must have a large area of contact to ensure low current density and low tissue heating.[12]

If the ground plate has only a small point of proper contact with the patient, the skin at that point may be burned. Also, the surgeon must keep in mind that the current tends to flow in a direct line from a monopolar electrode to the ground plate and may alter the normal electrical activity of intervening tissue.

If current of correct wave form (Fig. 43-4), voltage, amperage, and continuity of energy is applied to tissue through a suitable electrode, a small, intense arc will form between the electrode and the tissue. A small zone of tissue cells will be vaporized, and the tissues will part. A shallow zone of tissue dehydration (coagulation) is created on the edges of the severed tissue. More dehydration occurs with more electrical power, a slower cutting stroke, and a thicker entering electrode edge. This dehydration has a hemostatic effect to some extent, but it interferes with wound healing. There is more serum accumulation than after a scalpel cut. Healing is

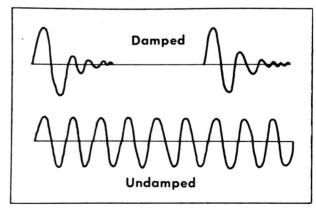

Figure 43-4 Schematic representation of damped and undamped electrical currents. Damped current has primarily hemostatic effects, whereas undamped current will divide tissue well. (From Edlich et al.[12])

about 2 days slower than after a corresponding scalpel incision, the wound has slightly less tensile strength, and the resulting scar is larger. The use of a cutting electrical current also makes the wound more susceptible to infection. "The increased susceptibility of such wounds to infection mitigates against the use of electrosurgery for cutting skin and subcutaneous tissue."[12]

If the current oscillations are damped (Fig. 43-4), the current can be used to achieve hemostasis without cutting the tissue. However, when the wound is closed, all the coagulated tissue must be absorbed in the process of wound healing. By using bipolar coagulation, the surgeon can achieve hemostasis with more precision and less tissue damage. In the bipolar technique, current flows into the tissue through one arm of a forceps and out of the tissue through the other. The effects of the current energy are essentially confined to the space between the two tips of the forceps. Less heat is produced in the adjacent tissues than with the monopolar technique. There is no ground plate and therefore no worry about altering the electrical activity of distant tissue or of causing a burn in the skin under the ground plate. Furthermore, bipolar current is more effective for coagulating tissue under a layer of fluid, such as CSF, than is monopolar current, which will leak off through the fluid.

Bone may be divided in a number of ways. Ordinarily a drill of some type is used first to establish an opening through the bone and then a saw or drill to outline a larger area, or rongeurs are used to remove more bone in piecemeal fashion. Many instruments are available, from hand-held trephines similar to those used in antiquity to high-powered machines with drill points turning as fast as 73,000 revolutions per minute that can cut rapidly through the skull or spine and yet not damage the underlying dura mater. However, the dura may be tightly adherent to the inner surface of the skull, especially across the cranial sutures and especially in elderly patients, and it may be breached accidentally during a craniotomy unless it is stripped from the bone well as the bone is opened. If a Gigli wire saw is used to connect burr holes in the creation of a bone flap, the cut is narrow and can be beveled so that the flap will sit well (and will not tend to sink in) when it is replaced at the end of the operation. The cut made with a power drill is wider, and beveling may not be possible.

Bleeding from bone edges can be stopped by the application of bone wax, which has been used in neurosurgical operations for almost a century. Commercially available bone wax may be too firm to spread easily, especially when it is at room temperature, but a softer bone wax can be prepared by neurosurgeons for their own use in the following way: Olive oil (200 g) is placed in a stainless steel container, and beeswax (700 g) is broken into small pieces and added to it. The oil mixture is heated to dissolve the wax and then cooled a little; to it is added 100 g phenol. The resulting mixture is stirred well with a glass rod, perhaps with some heating so that the phenol blends in well, and poured into clean, dry screw-top jars in about 25-g portions. (This recipe makes approximately 40 jars.) The jars are closed and are sterilized in a hot air oven at 150°C for 90 min.

Recently other hemostatic bone sealants have been developed, but they have not yet replaced bone wax in routine neurosurgical practice. These include Absele—a paste of stabilized fibrin and soluble collagen that absorbs totally with minimal tissue reaction in about 3 weeks—and a paste of absorbable gelatin.

Similar materials have been used for controlling bleeding from other tissues in neurosurgical operations. Chief among these have been absorbable gelatin sponge (Gelfoam, The Upjohn Company, Kalamazoo, Mich.), oxidized cellulose (Oxycel, Parke, Davis & Company, Morris Plains, N.J.), oxidized regenerated cellulose (Surgicel, Surgikos, New Brunswick, N.J.), and microfibrillar collagen hemostat (Avitene, Avicon, Inc., Fort Worth, Tex.). In addition, simple temporary tamponade for a period of time, with or without the application of a small piece of tissue such as muscle and the use of a warm (105 to 115°F) irrigating solution, has been a valuable hemostatic technique that has been used in neurosurgery since its inception.[34]

Metallic clips can be used to advantage to control bleeding from the margins of a dural incision or from intracranial vessels, especially arteries. However, these clips may interfere with the quality of subsequent CT scans, and for this reason should be used sparingly.

Protection and Retraction of Tissue

Exposed tissues may be injured unintentionally during an operation. Even the simple exposure of the brain to air may cause damage to the cortical surface. Surgical exposure should therefore be confined, if possible, to the specific area of the abnormality to be treated, and neural tissue should be kept moist with a physiological irrigating solution to protect against the detrimental effects of drying.

When tissue is retracted, the force of the retraction must always be kept in mind. If possible, retraction should be directed against tissue to be removed (such as a brain tumor) rather than against normal neural tissue. In either case the retractor should be padded in some way to prevent accidental cutting of the neural tissue by the edge of the retractor blade.

Albin and associates studied brain retraction in some detail and found in dogs that cerebral infarction occurred regularly in a portion of the brain retracted for 1 h if the difference between the perfusion pressure in the brain and the retractor pressure was less than 40 mmHg.[2] In other words, if the effective perfusion pressure of the brain beneath the retractor remains below 40 torr for 1 h, infarction results. These studies are pertinent, because brain retraction pressures in human brain surgery may exceed 25 torr, and if the cerebral perfusion pressure happens to fall below 65 torr at the same time, the area of brain being retracted might become ischemic (provided the canine data can be applied directly to humans). During induced arterial hypotension, as during the clipping of an intracranial aneurysm, the threat of retraction-induced cerebral infarction is particularly worrisome.

Self-retaining retraction systems have been used with increasing frequency in neurosurgical operations[15] and are discussed in another chapter. They have been especially helpful in microneurosurgical procedures, in which they give the surgeon better control of a more stable operative field.

Control of Increased Intracranial Pressure

Key studies of intracranial pressure (ICP) alterations during neurosurgical operations were performed by Becker and associates, who pointed out that

> The patient who comes to the operating room with elevated ICP, or with limited remaining compensatory space, is in a precarious situation. Major increases in ICP to levels close to arterial blood pressure can occur at induction or during surgery before dural opening. This ischemic event may go unrecognized and may account for the severely brain damaged patient seen after an otherwise technically perfect operation.[5]

Many factors may elevate the intracranial pressure of a patient undergoing brain surgery, including the condition for which the patient is being treated, insufficient ventilation with resulting hypercarbia (Fig. 43-5), dependent head position, interference with venous drainage from the head, the Valsalva maneuver, the use of halothane (which may reduce the cerebral perfusion pressure not only by elevating the intracranial pressure but also by lowering the systemic arterial blood pressure simultaneously; Fig. 43-6), etc. Special attention should be given to these factors in the perioperative and operative period, especially if the intracranial pressure is not being monitored.

Insertion of Metallic Materials

McFadden, Dujovny, and others have performed important investigations of the behavior of metallic devices such as aneurysm clips that are left in the human body at the end of

neurosurgical operations.[37,38] McFadden points out that all metallic implants corrode with time. Of the commonly used metals, sterling silver is the most corrodible and tantalum the least. Corrosion of metals can be minimized by avoiding the use of different metals near each other (such as clips made of different metals on or near the same aneurysm); by not covering implanted stainless steel with nonviable material; by not burying tied or twisted stainless steel wire in tissue; by not shaping, drilling or otherwise altering stainless steel wire in tissue; by not shaping, drilling or otherwise altering stainless steel plates or mesh at operation; and by not implanting silver clips.[37]

Replacement and Reapproximation of Tissue

The principles of replacing and reapproximating tissues so that they will heal well have been discussed above. Current adaptations of technique by some surgeons include the performance of a posterior fossa craniotomy with bone flap replacement rather than a piecemeal craniectomy with no bone flap replacement and the revival of interest in performing a laminotomy rather than a laminectomy at one or more levels (especially in children), with replacement of the posterior arches at the end of the operation.

The recent development of a well-controlled, low-energy carbon dioxide laser system by Morris and Neblett have enabled them to bond animal tissues together with their laser. They have tested this device in rats and have found that they can make an immediate bond between the divided ends or edges of various tissues such as the walls of small arteries and the epineurium of nerves. In neurosurgery, this technique holds promise as a relatively quick way of sealing together such tubular structures.

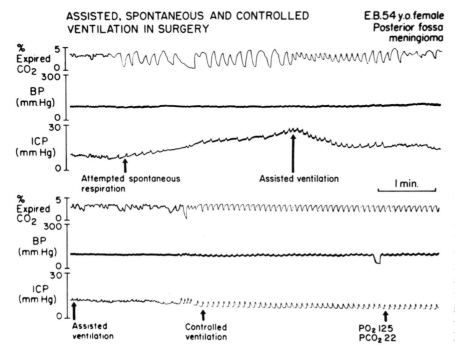

Figure 43-5 Intraoperative measurements of intracranial pressure (ICP), systemic blood pressure (BP), and percentage of expired CO_2 of a 54-year-old woman with a posterior fossa meningioma. She was unable to breathe adequately spontaneously, and the resulting retention of CO_2 was associated with a rise in intracranial pressure. These measurements show the value of assisted and controlled ventilation in maintaining the intracranial pressure at an acceptable level during an operation for a brain tumor. (From Becker et al.[5])

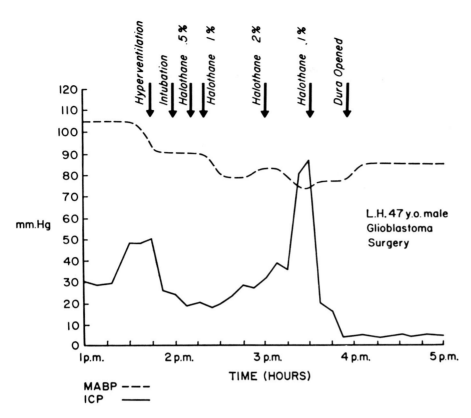

Figure 43-6 Intraoperative measurements of mean arterial blood pressure (*dashed line*) and intracranial pressure (*solid line*) of a 47-year-old man undergoing an operation for a glioblastoma. The use of halothane was associated with a fall in blood pressure and an elevation of intracranial pressure to the point where there was no cerebral perfusion for a short period. The patient was worse after a technically satisfactory frontal lobectomy and internal decompression. (From Becker et al.[5])

References

1. Albin MS, Babinski M, Maroon JC, Jannetta PJ: Anesthetic management of posterior fossa surgery in the sitting position. Acta Anaesthesiol Scand 20:117–128, 1976.
2. Albin MS, Bunegin L, Heisel P, Marlin A, Babinski M: Intracranial pressure and regional cerebral blood flow responses to experimental brain retraction pressure, in Shulman K, Marmarou A, Miller JD, Becker DP, Hochwald GM, Brock M: *Intracranial Pressure IV*. Berlin, Springer-Verlag, 1980, pp 131–135.
3. Alexander E Jr: Neurosurgical techniques. J Neurosurg 24:818–819, 1966 et seq.
4. Asenjo A: *Neurosurgical Techniques*. Springfield, Ill., Charles C Thomas, 1963.
5. Becker DP, Young HF, Vries JK, Sakalas R: Monitoring in patients with brain tumors. Clin Neurosurg 22:364–388, 1975.
6. Bryant WM: Wound healing. Ciba Clin Symp 29(3):1–36, 1977.
7. Burton CV, McFadden JT: Neurosurgical materials and devices: Report on regulatory agencies and advisory groups. J Neurosurg 45:251–258, 1976.
8. Committee on Control of Surgical Infections of the Committee on Pre- and Postoperative Care, American College of Surgeons: *Manual on Control of Infection in Surgical Patients*. Philadelphia, Lippincott, 1976.
9. Dineen P, Hildick-Smith G: *The Surgical Wound*. Philadelphia, Lea & Febiger, 1981.
10. Donaghy RMP, Yasargil MG: *Microvascular Surgery. Report of First Conference, October 1–7, 1966, Mary Fletcher Hospital, Burlington, Vermont*. St Louis, Mosby, 1967.
11. Dunphy JE: *Wound Healing*. New York, Medcom Press, 1974.
12. Edlich RF, Rodeheaver G, Thacker JG, Edgerton MT: Technical factors in wound management, in Hunt TK, Dunphy JE: *Fundamentals of Wound Management*, New York, Appleton Century Crofts, 1979, pp 364–454.
13. Epstein MH, Kumor K, Hughes W, Lietman P: The use of prophylactic antibiotics in pediatric shunting operations—a double blind prospective randomized study. Presented at the 51st Annual Meeting of The American Association of Neurological Surgeons, Honolulu, Hawaii, April 26, 1982.
14. Glynn LE: *Tissue Repair and Regeneration (Handbook of Inflammation, vol 3)*. Amsterdam, Elsevier/North-Holland, 1981.
15. Greenberg IM: Staircase concept of instrument placement in microsurgery. Neurosurgery 9:696–702, 1981.
16. Gurdjian ES, Thomas LM: *Operative Neurosurgery*, 3d ed. Baltimore, Williams & Wilkins, 1970.
17. Haines SJ: Systemic antibiotic prophylaxis in neurological surgery. Neurosurgery 6:355–361, 1980.
18. Haines SJ, Taylor F: Prophylactic methicillin for shunt operations: Effects on incidence of shunt malfunction and infection. Childs Brain 9:10–22, 1982.
19. Handa H: *Microneurosurgery*. Baltimore, University Park Press, 1973.
20. Handa H, Ohta T, Kamijyo Y: Encasement of intracranial aneurysms with plastic compounds. Prog Neurol Surg 3:149–192, 1969.
21. Hoff JT: *Neurosurgery* (from Goldsmith HS: *Practice of Surgery*). Philadelphia, Harper & Row, 1982.
22. Hood TW, Mastri AR, Chou SN: Neural and vascular tissue reaction to cyanoacrylate adhesives: A further report. Neurosurgery 11:363–366, 1982.
23. Horwitz NH, Curtin JA: Prophylactic antibiotics and wound infections following laminectomy for lumbar disc herniation: A retrospective study. J Neurosurg 43:727–731, 1975.

24. Horwitz NH, Rizzoli HV: *Postoperative Complications of Intracranial Neurological Surgery.* Baltimore, Williams & Wilkins, 1982.
25. Hunt TK: *Wound Healing and Wound Infection: Theory and Surgical Practice.* New York, Appleton Century Crofts, 1980.
26. Hunt TK, Dunphy JE: *Fundamentals of Wound Management.* New York, Appleton Century Crofts, 1979.
27. Irvin TT: *Wound Healing: Principles and Practice.* London, Chapman & Hall, 1981.
28. Keener EB: Regeneration of dural defects: A review. J Neurosurg 16:415–423, 1959.
29. Kempe LG: *Operative Neurosurgery,* vol 1: *Cranial, Cerebral, and Intracranial Vascular Disease,* 1968, vol 2: *Posterior Fossa, Spinal Cord, and Peripheral Nerve Disease,* 1970. New York, Springer-Verlag.
30. Koos WT, Böck FW, Spetzler RF: *Clinical Microneurosurgery.* Stuttgart, Thieme, 1976.
31. Krayenbühl H: *Advances and Technical Standards in Neurosurgery.* New York, Springer-Verlag, 1974 et seq.
32. Kurze T: Approaches to the incisura. Clin Neurosurg 25:700–716, 1978.
33. Laufman H, Rubel T: Synthetic absorbable sutures. Surg Gynecol Obstet 145:597–608, 1977.
34. Light RU: Hemostasis in neurosurgery. J Neurosurg 2:414–434, 1945.
35. Malis LI: Prevention of neurosurgical infection by intraoperative antibiotics. Neurosurgery 5:339–343, 1979.
36. Maroon JC, Edmonds-Seal J, Campbell RL: An ultrasonic method for detecting air embolism. J Neurosurg 31:196–201, 1969.
37. McFadden, JT: Metallurgical principles in neurosurgery. J Neurosurg 31:373–385, 1969.
38. McFadden JT: Tissue reactions to standard neurosurgical metallic implants. J Neurosurg 36:598–603, 1972.
39. Mickey BE, Samson D: Neurosurgical applications of the cyanoacrylate adhesives. Clin Neurosurg 28:429–444, 1981.
40. Omer GE Jr, Spinner M: *Management of Peripheral Nerve Problems.* Philadelphia, Saunders, 1980.
41. Parks BJ: Postoperative peripheral neuropathies. Surgery 74:348–357, 1973.
42. Poppen JL: *An Atlas of Neurosurgical Techniques.* Philadelphia, Saunders, 1960.
43. Prolo DJ: The use of transplantable tissue in neurosurgery. Clin Neurosurg 28:407–417, 1981.
44. Prolo DJ, Burres KP, McLaughlin WT, Christensen AH: Autogenous skull cranioplasty: Fresh and preserved (frozen), with consideration of the cellular response. Neurosurgery 4:18–29, 1979.
45. Rand RW: *Microneurosurgery,* 2d ed, St Louis, Mosby, 1978.
46. Ransohoff J: *Modern Technics in Surgery—Neurosurgery.* Mount Kisco, N.Y., Futura, 1979–1981.
47. Rhoton AL Jr: Micro-operative technique, in Youmans JR: *Neurological Surgery: A Comprehensive Reference Guide to the Diagnosis and Management of Neurosurgical Problems,* 2d ed. Philadelphia, Saunders, 1982, pp 1160–1193.
48. Rhoton AL Jr, Yamamoto I, Peace DA: Microsurgery of the third ventricle, part 2: Operative approaches. Neurosurgery 8:357–373, 1981.
49. Ross R: The fibroblast and wound repair. Biol Rev 43:51–96, 1968.
50. Rothman RH, Simeone FA: *The Spine,* 2d ed. Philadelphia, Saunders, 1982.
51. Schilling JA: Wound healing. Physiol Rev 48:374–423, 1968.
52. Schmidek HH, Sweet WH: *Current Techniques in Operative Neurosurgery.* New York, Grune & Stratton 1977.
53. Schmidek HH, Sweet WH: *Operative Neurosurgical Techniques: Indications, Methods, and Results.* New York, Grune & Stratton, 1982.
54. Schneider RC, Kahn EA, Crosby EC, Taren JA: *Correlative Neurosurgery,* 3d ed. Springfield, Ill. Charles C Thomas, 1982.
55. Section of Pediatric Neurosurgery, American Association of Neurological Surgeons: *Pediatric Neurosurgery: Surgery of the Developing Nervous System.* New York, Grune & Stratton, 1982.
56. Seeger W: *Microsurgery of the Brain: Anatomical and Technical Principles.* Vienna, Springer-Verlag, 1980.
57. Seeger W: *Microsurgery of the Spinal Cord and Surrounding Structures.* Vienna, Springer-Verlag, 1982.
58. Seletz E: *Surgery of Peripheral Nerves.* Springfield, Ill. Charles C Thomas, 1951.
59. Shillito J Jr, Matson DD: *An Atlas of Pediatric Neurosurgical Operations.* Philadelphia, Saunders, 1982.
60. Symon L: Neurosurgery (from Rob C, Smith R: *Operative Surgery: Fundamental International Techniques*), 3d ed. London, Butterworth, 1979.
61. Tindall GT, Long DM: *Contemporary Neurosurgery.* Baltimore, Williams & Wilkins, 1979 et seq.
62. Venes JL: Control of shunt infection; Report of 150 consecutive cases. J Neurosurg 45:311–314, 1976.
63. Wilkins RH, Odom GL: General operative technique, in Youmans JR: *Neurological Surgery: A Comprehensive Reference Guide to the Diagnosis and Management of Neurosurgical Problems,* 2d ed. Philadelphia, Saunders, 1982, pp 1136–1159.
64. Wright RL: *Postoperative Craniotomy Infections.* Springfield, Ill. Charles C Thomas, 1966.
65. Wright RL: *Septic Complications of Neurosurgical Spinal Procedures.* Springfield, Ill. Charles C Thomas, 1970.
66. Yasargil MG: *Microsurgery, Applied to Neurosurgery.* Stuttgart, Thieme, 1969.
67. Youmans JR: *Neurological Surgery: A Comprehensive Reference Guide to the Diagnosis and Management of Neurosurgical Problems,* 2d ed. Philadelphia, Saunders, 1982.

44

Instrumentation for Microneurosurgery

John M. Tew, Jr.
Hans Jacob Steiger

During the last decade the value of the surgical microscope has become widely accepted among neurological surgeons. Most hospitals, even in smaller communities, offer the basic equipment and necessary personnel for microsurgery. Magnified vision has improved many procedures, brought about new ones, and caused the major revision of older surgical techniques.[1,3] Less retraction of the brain is needed for microsurgical approaches to lesions at the base of the brain. Delineation of neural and vascular structures is more precise. Perforating arteries arising close to an aneurysm can be identified and spared. Tumors can be separated from brain, spinal cord, and nerves less traumatically. Maintenance of the integrity of the facial nerve during removal of acoustic neuromas is now expected, and hearing function can be preserved in some patients. Even cervical or lumbar discectomies may be performed more safely with the aid of the surgical microscope. Further, the advantages of microsurgical technique have opened new horizons to neurosurgery, such as arterial bypass procedures, pituitary microadenomectomy, vascular decompression of cranial nerves, laser ablation, and reconstructive surgery.

However, microtechnique may lengthen the duration of the operative procedure. Sterility of the operative field may be compromised. More personnel and special training are required to maintain and operate the complicated equipment. Furthermore, the microscope, microinstruments, cameras, and personnel add a financial burden for the hospital.

The improvement of microsurgical techniques and equipment is an evolving process. Refinements of microscope design and accessories, as well as of microsurgical instruments, appear continuously and many are of substantial value. The following description is based on the 1983 state of the art and is recommended for most active neurosurgical centers.

The Neurosurgical Microscope

A surgical microscope should provide the surgeon with detailed visual information without imposing a significant amount of extra effort to manipulate the instrument. The magnification factor and the optical axis of the microscope should be easily adjustable. The image should be free of aberration and the depth of field optimal to reduce operator fatigue. The microscope should not interfere with freedom of motion of the surgeon's hands and instruments. The operative view must be visible for assistants and displayed for operating room personnel; documentation with still cameras and dynamic cameras should be accessible. There are several surgical microscopes with adequate accessories available today. The optical designs are similar, but the Zeiss operating microscope has been more widely used for neurosurgical procedures. Our experience has been limited to Zeiss equipment (Carl Zeiss, Inc., Thornwood, New York) so the following descriptions are specifically related to that line of equipment unless otherwise indicated[2] (Fig. 44-1).

Optical Principles

The primary image from the surgical field enters the microscope body through a large objective lens at the front end. The light rays leaving the front objective are parallel to each other. Exchangeable miniature telescopes or a zoom system, the magnification changer, increase or decrease the magnification very much like a binocular telescope. The system is dual, separated for each eye. The light rays continue in parallel through the magnification changer to the binocular telescope tube for the final magnification step (Fig. 44-2).

The magnification of the microscope can be calculated by the following formula:

$$VM = \frac{f_{\text{tub}}}{f_{\text{obj}}} \times Y \times V_{\text{oc}}$$

where VM is the total magnification, V_{oc} is the magnification factor of the eye pieces, and f_{tub} and f_{obj} refer to the focal length of the binocular tubes and the main objective lens, respectively. Y is the magnification factor of the magnification changer and is displayed on the front window of the microscope body of a zoom microscope or on the manual knob of the drum-type magnification changer of a mechanical microscope. For example, with a tube length of 160 mm (standard tube length of the inclinable binocular head), the objective focal length of 300 mm and a 12.5X eyepiece, the total magnification can be changed between 2.6- and 16.6-fold.

Another important optical quality of the microscope is the depth of field. The exact definition is difficult because in certain microscopes specific parameters are involved and some assumptions regarding the physiology of the observer's eye are necessary. However, it is important to know that the depth of field increases with the square of the focal length of the main objective lens and decreases in a more than linear fashion with increasing magnification. For example, with an objective lens focal length of 200 mm, a binocular tube focal

439

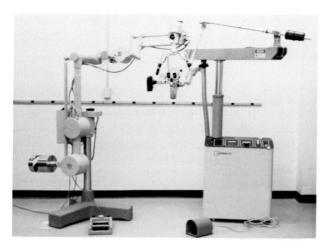

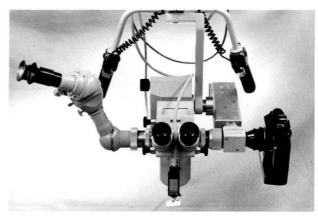

A   B

Figure 44-1 *A*. The Zeiss zoom operating microscope mounted on a Contraves stand. Note the laser and television camera attached to the microscope. *B*. Close-up photograph of the microscope with the attached still and television cameras (*right*) and binocular eyepieces for the assistant (*left*).

length of 125 mm, and a 12.5X eyepiece magnification factor, the depth of field is approximately 15 mm with the minimal magnification setting of the changer and less than 1 mm with the maximal magnification factor.

Essential Modules of the Neurosurgical Microscope

Main Objective Lens

Objectives with focal lengths between 200 and 400 mm are commonly used in neurological surgery. The choice of the objective length (which is identical with the working distance) depends on the required magnification and brightness of the image and the minimum working distance, which is dictated by the depth of the surgical cavity and lengths of the instruments: 250 mm is the ideal focal length for superficial operations such as an extracranial-intracranial bypass graft which requires high magnification and good stereoscopic vision; a 300-mm focal length is optimal for aneurysm surgery or most procedures at the base of the brain; a 400-mm lens may be chosen for trans-sphenoidal operations. The choice of the correct focal length is of primary importance to permit hours in a comfortable surgical position.

An important alternative to the exchangeable objective lens used on the earlier microscopes is the variable length motorized system, which permits continuous adjustment of the focal length. The Siemens-Moeller microscope uses this system for focusing instead of using vertical movement of the microscope body (Siemens Corp., Iselin, N.J.).

Magnification Changer

There are two basic types of magnification changers available, the dual rotating drum type of exchangeable Galilean telescopes and the motorized zoom system. The manual

type consists of two Galilean telescopes mounted on a rotatable drum with one free path. Each telescope can be used in either direction, thus increasing or decreasing magnification. The drum is rotated by a dial knob on the outside of the microscope body. Although this system has been basically unchanged since 1953, many surgeons still prefer its simple design because of the light weight, ease of operation, and excellent optical quality. The motorized system, in contrast, consists of dual moveable lenses within the microscope body controlled by a motor actuated by a mechanical switch. The earlier models allowed less flexibility of magnification than the drum type magnification changer because the zoom lens cannot be used bidirectionally. In addition, the microscope body of the earlier system was exceedingly long. Zeiss' new type 6C body is compact, and the magnification changer works from 0.4 to 2.4 and provides optical quality equal to that of the manual type magnification changer. The advantage of easy adjustment of magnification during suturing and dissection provides freedom of action and improves visual orientation and operative speed. The depth of field at higher magnification has been improved by the addition of a variable shutter which mechanically alters the radius of the lens.

Binocular Tubes

Binocular tubes are available in either a straight configuration or a 45° inclination between the axis of the microscope body and the optical access of the surgeon. The binocular tubes are available also with focal lengths between 125 mm and 160 mm. The choice of appropriate inclination and tube length is determined by the preference of the surgeon for posture and working distance. Most surgeons prefer a new tiltable binocular tube with a variable inclination between 0 and 60°. The system is available with a focal length of 160 mm which does not increase the working distance unduly because the reflected light path permits a more com-

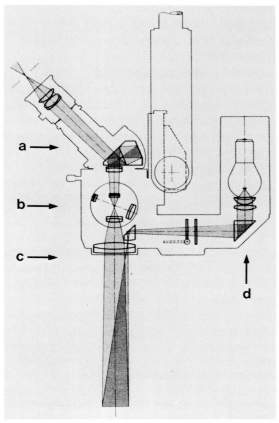

Figure 44-2 Diagram of the optical principles of the operating microscope. (*a*) Inclined binocular tube; (*b*) manual drum magnification changer; (*c*) objective lens; (*d*) illumination bulb. Zoom microscopes differ only by a motorized dual zoom system instead of the manual drum type magnification changer shown. (Courtesy of Carl Zeiss, Inc.)

pact design. The variable inclination is facilitated by a system of prisms and rotary mirrors. Some surgeons may experience difficulty in their initial use of the tiltable binocular tube because of the lack of a constant relation between the ocular access and the axis of the microscope body. However, after an initial adjustment period this design offers a considerable advantage by permitting the surgeon to retain a comfortable position independent of the patient or table position. All binocular tubes provide adjustment for each eyepiece for the individual interpupillary distance and refractive correction.

Illumination

There are two primary sources of illumination for neurosurgical microscopes. One may choose between an integral source or a remote light source with fiberoptic transfer to the microscope housing. The latter design requires less space and permits bulb exchange with minimal disturbance. The integral system requires a 30-watt tungsten bulb, or a 100-watt halogen bulb, which produces approximately 7,000 to 10,000 footcandles of light. The coaxial illumination re-

quired for homogeneous illumination of deep spaces is achieved by two sets of reflecting prisms which align the light beam with the optical axis of the microscope. The light leaves the microscope through the main objective lens, which facilitates final collimation. The 30-watt filament bulb is often insufficient at higher magnifications, especially when a beam splitter divides the available light in half to accommodate cameras and observer tubes. The halogen bulb has the additional advantages of a whiter light, which is preferred for a true color television picture and for photographs. The Wild surgical microscope (E. Leitz, Inc., Rockleigh, N.J.) provides for automatic adjustment of light collimation according to the magnification. This system permits constant brightness of the working field, independent of magnification.

Microscope Suspension

A microscope stand for neurosurgery should provide adequate stability for the microscope in a fixed position, but should permit easy and repeated adjustment of the position and axis of the microscope. There are several different movable floor stands and ceiling-mounted units available. One of these, the Contraves stand (represented by Carl Zeiss, Inc.), is designed for the mobility and stability required for neurosurgery. This heavily built microscope support consists of an assembly of counterbalance arms which in the unlocked mode releases the mechanism for free-floating translational and rotational movement in all directions (Fig. 44-3). The arms are firmly locked by electromagnetic clutches at the arm joints. A hand switch releases all six brakes and permits coarse adjustment of the microscope. Translational movements are possible during surgery by means of a mouth-operated switch, which also guides the microscope through fine adjustments. Time analysis demonstrates that the Contraves stand leads to a considerable reduction in operating time because the conventional mechanical systems require time and effort for frequent adjustments of the microscope. More important, the ease of adjustment allows the surgeon to work at a consistently comfortable position. The microscope stand can be balanced precisely to compensate for the weight of an array of different accessories including laser attachments.

Operative Setup

The preoperative setup of the microscope begins with the attachment of the desired accessories: the assistant's observation tube, cameras, laser micromanipulator and articulated arm, or the quartz fiberoptic cable. The Contraves stand provides sufficient mobility that it is best to position the microscope stand to the left of the head of the patient for supratentorial cranial surgery or for posterior fossa surgery in the sitting position. Therefore, the assistant's binocular tube is attached to the right side of the beam splitter and the cameras are attached to the left side. For posterior fossa procedures in the decubitus position and for trans-sphenoidal operations, the microscope is placed at the cranial end of the operating table. The assistant is positioned between the surgeon and the microscope so the accessories should be

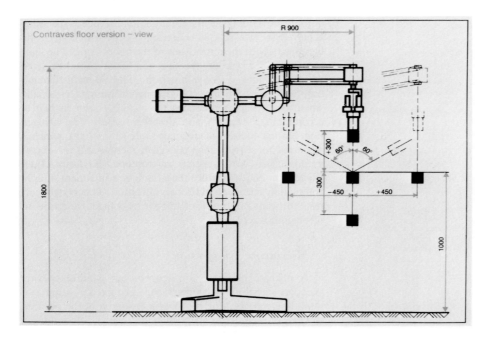

Figure 44-3 Sketch illustrating the degree of freedom provided by the Contraves microscope suspension. The microscope can be moved freely in all three directions by means of a mouth switch. In addition, rotation of the microscope around all three axes is possible. (Courtesy of Carl Zeiss, Inc.)

mounted appropriately. Following the attachment of the microscope observer tube, the laser, and the other attachments, the microscope stand must be balanced. This procedure is very important and the responsible operating room personnel must be thoroughly familiar with the Contraves stand operation manual. The selection and attachment of the objective lens (250, 300 or 400 mm) and the eyepieces for the surgeon and assistant, and the individual adjustment of the eyepieces, must be completed before the draping of the microscope. If this point is neglected, the image may be out of focus for the cameras and assistants. The surgeon's correction can be dialed on the diopter scale of the eyepieces. If the surgeon's spherical ametropia is unknown, the following procedure is recommended:

1. Remove the binocular tube with the eyepieces from the microscope body and use it as a magnification lens for a distant object.
2. Rotate both diopter scales all the way counterclockwise.
3. Adjust each eyepiece separately by rotating the diopter scale clockwise until the image is in focus. Do not go beyond this point.
4. Repeat the procedure several times and take the average correction.

The draping of the microscope is the final step of the preoperative preparation. Disposable polyethylene bags provided by different manufacturers are preferred to cotton drapes or gas sterilization of the microscope. The disposable bags have the advantage that, during the procedure, attachment of additional equipment or adjustment of camera equipment is easily accomplished by cutting holes in the drape and patching with a sterile adhesive drape. Visibility of the equipment is also provided. Attention must be paid to air circulation for cooling of the light bulb for assurance of longer bulb life.

Maintenance of the Microscope

Proper care of the microscope optics is critical for optimal performance. A blurred view is most commonly due to a dirty objective lens. The lens surfaces of the microscope are adversely affected by dust, blood, irrigation solutions and finger prints. Removal of loose particles is best accomplished by a small rubber blowing bulb. This tactic cleans the lens without touching it. Dust particles can also be removed with a special soft brush. To remove finger prints or blood contamination from the objective or eyepieces, small cotton applicators moistened with distilled water may be used. If there is residual dirt, the procedure should be repeated with a cleansing solvent consisting of 25% alcohol, 10% ether, and 65% acetone. Cleaning fluids should be used sparingly because excessive fluid may damage the cemented surfaces of the objective if it enters the space between the lens and the lens mount. The microscope should be covered at all times and stored in a safe place when it is not in use. A ceiling mount pedestal or a track for mounting the microscope is advisable for designated neurosurgery operating rooms. Ceiling mounting of the scope eliminates cords and wires on the floor, frees valuable space, and improves access to the patient. Moreover, care is facilitated and the durability of the microscope is insured. The disadvantage of limiting the microscope to a single room is more than offset by the advantages just listed.

The illumination device also needs attention for trouble-free function. A new tungsten bulb is recommended for a long operation, eliminating the need for replacement during a critical part of the operation. The bulb should not be handled with bare hands but gripped with a cloth to prevent contamination. The correct seating of the bulb is important for shadow-free illumination. A fiberoptic system permits the easy exchange of the bulb outside the sterile field and preventive exchange is not necessary. The fiberoptic cable is a delicate device; it should never be bent or the tiny glass fibers inside the cable will be disrupted.

Microneurosurgical Instruments

In collaboration with many inventive surgeons, surgical instrument companies have developed a great variety of microsurgical instruments. Most products meet the rigorous criteria necessary for microsurgery. The tolerance limits observed in production may be in the range of microns in the case of tools that allow manipulation of microsutures less than 20 μm thick. Knowledge of the critical needs for each instrument will enable the surgeon to make the best selection for each surgical procedure. The final choice of microsurgical tools is greatly influenced by personal preference. Different analogous pieces of equipment should be compared in the animal laboratory or in practice at another neurosurgical center.

In contrast to gross surgical instruments which are guided and manipulated under direct visual control, microsurgery requires a thorough familiarity with the instruments for satisfactory performance because the instruments must be guided blindly into the operative field. During manipulation, only the tip of the instrument is in direct view. The critical properties and performance limitations of an instrument must be known. The surgeon must be confident that a dissector is not so sharp that it may lacerate a fragile neural or vascular structure. Frequent practice in the microsurgical laboratory insures the needed familiarity with new tools prior to performance and sharpens the skills needed for highly technical procedures.

All surgeons should work with a limited number of basic instruments. The set can be extended as one gains more experience. Several companies offer sets of basic instruments consisting of scissors, forceps, needle holders, and dissectors in a matching storage case. Many surgeons prefer to choose a set of instruments that suit their particular needs and place them in a suitable instrument case. We have designed a set of instruments that work effectively for each procedure that is performed with reasonable frequency. Many surgeons have designed important instruments that are likely to satisfy the most discriminating surgeon's requirements.

Microsurgical instruments are delicate tools which demand meticulous care. Damage occurs easily if instruments are dropped, abused, improperly cleaned, or sterilized by autoclave. One person in the operating room should be responsible for the care of microsurgical instruments. A special washing basket should be used and should be designed to separate the delicate instruments from one another. Cleaning should be by ultrasound or a soft brush, with thorough drying afterward. Instruments with moving parts must be periodically oiled with a surgical lubricant and inspected under the microscope for abrasion, chips, and malalignments of scissor blades and forceps tips. During operations microsurgical instruments should be kept in their own tray. Microsurgical instruments should be used only for the procedure for which they are designed. A needle holder for 10-0

sutures will be damaged by use with larger needles. With proper care, microsurgical instruments can last for hundreds of operations.

Microsurgical instruments were originally made of stainless steel. During recent years, titanium instruments have become popular. Titanium is much lighter and the instruments handle differently, do not corrode, and are free of ferromagnetism, important for needle holders and forceps. However, the blades of titanium scissors and the jaws of needle holders are not as resistant to deformation as are instruments made of steel. Because of its higher cost and lower durability, titanium has not gained general acceptance.

Most microsurgical instruments are adaptations of already proven surgical tools. However, there are ergonomic principles which dictate different concepts for microsurgical instruments. For example, they should allow the ulnar aspects of the forearm, wrist, and hand to be balanced on a special arm rest or the border of the wound (Fig. 44-4). Furthermore, they must be designed so that they can be held like a pencil, with the handle long enough to rest on the web between the thumb and index finger. Traditional ring scissors cannot be manipulated with a hand resting on the hypothenar eminence because the main movements are performed with the wrist. The ring handle therefore has limited use in microsurgery. Alligator type forceps and scissors with ring handles are used only for trans-sphenoidal operations.

The design of the instruments must be appropriate for the depth of the surgical cavity. For a superficial operation such as an extracranial-intracranial arterial anastomosis,

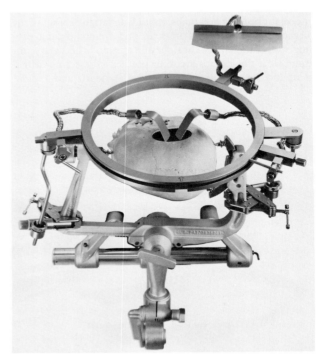

Figure 44-4 The Budde-Halo retractor system attached to the standard Mayfield skull clamp. The base ring allows attachment of a variety of retractors and trays and also serves as a hand rest. (Courtesy of Ohio Medical Instrument Company, Inc., Cincinnati.)

straight instruments provide maximum precision and freedom of motion. If the instruments are equipped with rounded handles, rotation is enhanced by rolling the handles between the thumb and forefinger. For a procedure confined to a deep cavity, longer bayonet type instruments must be used (Fig. 44-5). In these instances, rotation of the tip of the instrument is limited and is substituted by alternating instruments with varied angles and curved tips. Bayonet instruments are offered with a parallel shaft and handle, or with an angulation (Fig. 44-6). Angled instruments allow the hand to be rested more comfortably, but rotation about the shaft of the instrument is less easy. Use of a bayonet instrument requires the ultimate in surgical skill. However, this configuration is essential to avoid blocking of vision through a narrow microscopic channel.

Forceps

Simple jewelers' forceps are suitable instruments for handling tissue and suture material for superficial operations. A no. 5 forceps is delicate and its tips approximate precisely to permit handling of microsuture material, but the instrument is too short for most situations. Longer straight microforceps, scissors, and bipolar forceps have been developed. The ideal length is 7 in., which provides excellent balance and permits the instrument to be used for a variety of procedures. Most designs have a pin alignment guide which eliminates scissoring or malalignment. Ring and platform points on microforceps are designed for microvascular anastomoses.

The tension of the forceps, the resistance to closure, is important because great tension leads to fatigue spasm of the surgeon's intrinsic hand muscles and tremor during prolonged operations, yet considerable tension is necessary, for example, if the forceps are to be used as a dissecting instrument for developing tissue planes. Standard and bipolar

bayonet forceps with 8- or 10-cm shaft lengths and different tips ranging from 0.3 to 1.5 mm are needed for operations at the base of the brain. Upward or downward angled tips may be necessary in special situations such as dissection around the neck of an aneurysm.

Scissors and Knives

Superficial microvascular procedures require a set of straight handled scissors with straight and curved blades of different sizes. The finest scissors should be used for preparation of the cortical artery and for arteriotomy. The larger scissors may be used for preparation of the donor vessel with its tenacious surrounding fascia. The initial step of the cortical arteriotomy is performed with a knife. A disposable small blade is ideal for this purpose. Diamond blades have the sharpest cutting edge, but the cost is prohibitively expensive. Straight and curved bayonet scissors are the basic dissecting instruments for aneurysm surgery. The tips should open approximately 3 mm and cutting should be done with the distal third of the blade to insure accuracy. It is often impossible to align the straight and curved scissor blades properly for the desired line of action in deep cavities. In these situations, the use of scissors with angle blades may be helpful.

Long alligator type scissors are used for trans-sphenoidal operations and for some operations deep in the cranial cavity. These scissors are equipped with blades with various angulations which permit cutting in all directions.

Needle Holders

Most microsurgical firms offer needle holders and scissors of the same design. During recent years an array of sophisticated needle holders have been designed for microanas-

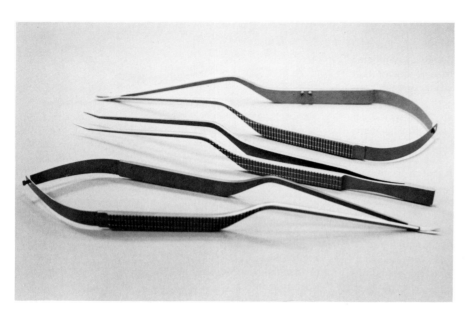

Figure 44-5 Bayonet-type scissors, forceps, and needle holder designed for operations in deep surgical cavities.

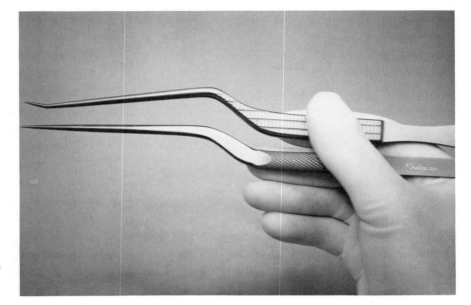

Figure 44-6 Comparison of two different bayonet designs. The Malis instruments (*upper*) with an angle between the shaft and handle prevent the hand of the surgeon obscuring the surgical field. The Rhoton design (*lower*) permits greater rotational freedom because of the rounded handles.

tomotic procedures. The tips of the needle holder should open only 1 mm. The needle holder must be able to hold and direct a needle firmly in any direction, and the jaws must be sufficiently delicate to tie a 10-0 suture without damaging the suture material. Curved needles can be seated in the needle holder perpendicular to the jaw. Some instruments have a groove in the jaw to fix the direction of the needle automatically. Wedge-shaped jaws allow the needle to be seated at an angle and be gripped firmly. Wedge-shaped jaws can also be used for handling suture material almost as accurately as forceps tips. The jaws of micro needle holders should be curved for optimal directional maneuverability of the needle. Straight-handled needle holders are used for superficial intracranial bypass oper-

ations. For operations in deeper cavities, such as suturing the middle cerebral artery or facial nerve, a bayonet type needle holder with round handles and curved jaws should be used. The limited freedom of motion imposed by suturing in deep cavities can be overcome by well-designed instruments and frequent practice in the laboratory.

Dissectors

Spatula and ball tip dissectors are frequently used in microneurosurgery (Figs. 44-7 and 44-8). Developing cleavage planes with spatula dissectors should only be attempted if there are few and fragile adhesions. Sharp dissection with

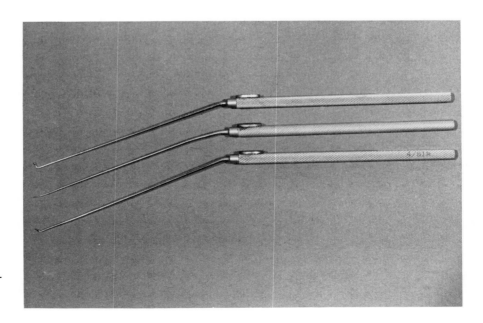

Figure 44-7 Angled microdissectors as used for operations at the base of the brain.

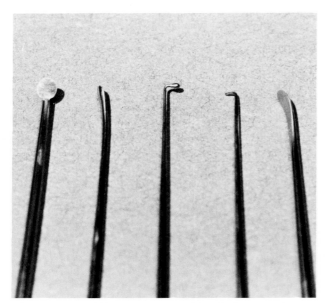

Figure 44-8 Different spatula and hook dissector tips.

scissors or specially designed knives is preferred in order to prevent tearing nerves and vessels. Delicate dissectors with straight or angled shafts are available for use in aneurysm, tumor, and tissue dissection. A Krayenbühl ball dissector is an excellent tool to manipulate healthy vessels and nerves. Angled flat dissectors are excellent for separation of tumor from bone in narrow canals or for developing a plane between a tumor and its capsule. The spatula dissectors for microsurgery should have tips 1 to 2 mm wide. Most surgeons prefer straight handles because of greater rotational ability, but angled instruments are essential in deep cavities to avoid blocking the view. Hook dissectors should have a flat surface or other palpable mark on the handle to indicate

which way the point is directed. A fine hook under a network of perforating vessels or behind an aneurysm cannot be seen.

Suction Tubes

Microsurgical suction tubes are multipurpose instruments (Fig. 44-9). They must serve to clear the operative field of fluid but may function as a retractor for tissue and as a blunt dissector. The tip must be smooth to prevent damage to fragile vascular and neural structures, and suction force must be easily controlled by a thumb plate air vent. The central vacuum system must have a variable control mechanism to allow gentle suction in critical circumstances. A flat angle between the handle and the shaft allows the suction tube to be held in a pencil-like fashion, which frees the ulnar aspect of the hand and allows it to be comfortably rested on the border of the wound. Tip diameters of nos. 3 to 12 French are used in neurosurgery and different shaft lengths of 8 to 15 cm are necessary to accommodate the depth of various operative cavities. The French designation refers to the outer tip diameter: no. 3 French is 1 mm. A no. 3 French tip is too small to remove blood but is superb for removing cerebrospinal fluid and irrigation fluid. A highly flexible tubing should be attached to the suction tip to avoid excessive resistance and provide unencumbered motion.

Bone Instruments

High-speed drills and small punches are necessary for bone removal in restricted areas contiguous to arteries and nerves. Electric and air-powered drills are available. Electric drills are lighter, their speed can be adjusted readily, and the rotation of the drill can be reversed. Rotation should be directed away from important structures. Air-powered drills may achieve higher speed and create less torque. Therefore,

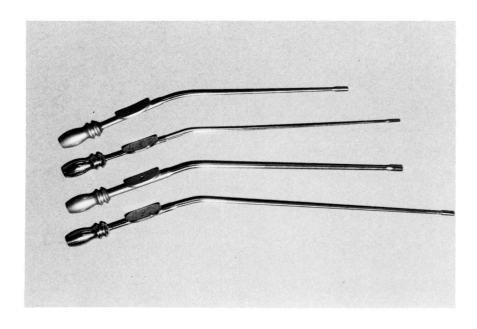

Figure 44-9 Suction tubes designed for microsurgery. Note the obtuse angle between the shaft and handle as well as the blunt tips.

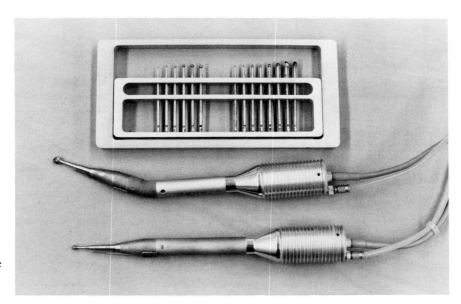

Figure 44-10 Electrical high-speed drill designed for microsurgery. The design shown has an integrated irrigation system.

safety may be enhanced. Continuous irrigation is necessary to cool the drill point and the adjacent bone. Some drills have an integrated irrigation system which is activated simultaneously with the burr (Fig. 44-10). A cutting drill can be used for gross bone removal, but diamond drills are preferred for final bone removal near a critical anatomical structure. The largest drill bit should be chosen for a more even removal of bone. Minute punches and curettes should be used for delicate removal of bone. The tips of a micropunch should be 1 mm wide and possess a very fine foot plate. Obviously, such instruments can only be used for the most delicate maneuvers or they will be broken or damaged.

References

1. Fox JL, Albin MS, Bader DCH, Davis DO, Korczynski SL, Malis LI, Reichman OH, Rhoton AL, Wilson CB: Microsurgical treatment of neurovascular disease. Neurosurgery 3:285–320, 1978.
2. Lang WH, Muchel F: *Zeiss Microscopes for Microsurgery*. New York, Springer-Verlag, 1981.
3. Yasargil MG (ed): *Microsurgery Applied to Neurosurgery*. New York, Academic Press, 1969.

45

Prophylactic Antibiotics

Stephen J. Haines

In the future, systemic penicillin will doubtless become a 48-hour routine treatment after intracranial operations and will close all the doors to bacterial invasion.

A. Dickson Wright, 1950[18]

Wright was wrong.

In the decades since antibiotics came into clinical use, this infection-free promised land has failed to materialize. Both physicians and bacteria have become more sophisticated in their knowledge of antibiotics, and the struggle to control infection continues. There is no doubt that antibiotics play a dominant role in the treatment of infection. It has seemed logical since their first clinical use that antibiotics should also be useful in preventing infection.

Early enthusiasm for the prophylactic use of antibiotics was dampened by lack of evidence of efficacy and by the realization that such use could contribute to serious infection problems. Clarification of the principles governing appropriate prophylactic use of antibiotics has led to a recent resurgence of interest in this subject.

Principles of Prophylactic Antibiotic Use

Antibiotics should be present in the tissues before contamination occurs. This was first demonstrated experimentally and confirmed when review of clinical regimens of postoperative prophylaxis showed them to be ineffective.

Antibiotics should be administered for a short period of time. Serious complications of prophylactic antibiotic administration, such as superinfection and development of resistant organisms, have been associated with administration for more than a few days. In recent years, many studies of surgical antibiotic prophylaxis have shown that very short regimens (one to four doses for a total duration of less than 24 h) are as effective as longer courses.

The antibiotic chosen should be effective against the most likely infecting organisms. In general, the use of wide spectrum antibiotics in an attempt to prevent all conceivable infections has been unsuccessful and more likely to be associated with superinfection than regimens using relatively narrow spectrum drugs.

The higher the risk of infection, the more clearly beneficial are prophylactic antibiotics. In fact, with the exception of infection complicating total hip arthroplasty, prophylactic antibiotics have not been shown to be effective in preventing infections in operations where the expected infection rate is less than 15 percent.

Prophylactic antibiotics will not compensate for sloppiness in other techniques of infection control. Wartime experience has made this clear. Early debridement of war wounds is much more effective in controlling infection than is antibiotic treatment followed by delayed debridement. Many surgeons have had very low infection rates without the use of prophylactic antibiotics.

Using these principles, proposed prophylactic antibiotic regimens can be evaluated, and, where empirical data do not exist, logical recommendations can be made.

Prophylactic Antibiotics for Surgical Procedures

Because the efficacy of prophylactic antibiotics is related to the risk of infection, surgical procedures are here classified on the basis of infection, as outlined by the National Research Council[12] (Table 45-1). Dirty and contaminated wounds have a sufficiently high risk of infection that the use of antibiotics should be considered therapeutic rather than prophylactic. In recent years, scientifically designed clinical research has gradually defined a place for prophylactic antibiotics in some surgical procedures.[4] Those procedures for which prophylactic antibiotics have been shown to be of benefit generally fall into the clean-contaminated category, for instance, hysterectomy, cesarean section, and pharyngeal and laryngeal operations. The only "clean" operation for which prophylactic antibiotics have an established benefit is total hip arthroplasty, and the implantation of a large foreign body in this procedure is an important consideration that will be discussed later.

Dirty Wounds

Such wounds are fortunately rare in neurosurgery. Contamination is present in the wound before operation. Antibiotic use in these wounds is considered therapeutic.

Contaminated Wounds

Here again, contamination is present before antibiotics are considered. The source of contamination is not the airborne or skin organisms usually considered to be the source of wound infection in clean surgical procedures. In grossly contaminated wounds, the indication for therapeutic antibiotic is clear. Many patients with contaminated neurosurgical wounds are the victims of multiple trauma and will be receiving therapeutic antibiotics because of wounds of other organ systems.

All authors emphasize the primary importance of thorough surgical debridement in the treatment of contaminated

TABLE 45-1 Classification of Surgical Wounds

Clean wounds: Nontraumatic, uninfected operative wounds in which neither the bronchi, the gastrointestinal tract, nor the genitourinary tract was entered

Clean-contamined wounds: Operative wounds in which the bronchus, gastrointestinal tract, or oral-pharyngeal cavity was entered but without unusual contamination

Contaminated wounds: Open, fresh traumatic wounds, operations with a major break in sterile technique (e.g., for open cardiac massage), and incisions encountering acute, nonpurulent inflammation

Dirty wounds: Old traumatic wounds and those involving abscesses or perforated viscera

SOURCE: Based on classification of National Academy of Sciences–National Research Council.[12]

wounds. There is less certainty that antibiotic administration is necessary after a wound has been thoroughly debrided. There is acceptable scientific evidence that simple lacerations do not benefit from penicillin prophylaxis. The most commonly encountered neurosurgical contaminated wound is the compound skull fracture, and here there does not appear to be uniformity of opinion regarding the use of antibiotics. A judgment as to whether or not to treat a compound fracture with antibiotics must, at this time, be left to the individual surgeon. The decision should consider the degree of contamination, the state of the patient's immunologic defenses, the adequacy of surgical debridement, the integrity of the dura, and the possible contaminating organisms. Such use should be considered therapeutic, not prophylactic, as contamination is present before antibiotics are started. Those surgeons who have elected to replace free bone fragments in cranial defects have uniformly recommended the use of antibiotics.

Clean-Contaminated Wounds

According to the strict definition of this category, the only neurosurgical procedures that qualify as clean-contaminated are those performed through the oral and nasal cavities. Transoral approaches to the clivus and odontoid and transsphenoidal approaches to the pituitary fossa would be the most common. There is no controlled information available regarding the benefit of prophylactic antibiotics for these procedures. Most neurosurgeons performing them appear to use prophylactic antibiotics. In view of existing studies supporting the use of prophylactic antibiotics in clean-contaminated procedures in other specialties, especially those in pharyngeal and laryngeal surgery, a reasonable case can be made for their use. The antibiotics should be chosen to be effective against the usual resident flora. Some have advocated obtaining preoperative cultures and adjusting the antibiotics on the basis of these results. As with all prophylactic regimens, the antibiotics should be begun prior to surgery and administration continued for only a few doses. The relative efficacy of topical and systemic antibiotics has not been studied.

The paranasal sinuses are generally considered to be sterile.[16] It is not uncommon to enter the frontal sinus or the mastoid air cells during certain surgical procedures. Unless there is prior indication of infection in these sinuses or acute inflammation is encountered, procedures involving entry into these areas need not be considered contaminated and should be treated as clean surgical wounds.

Clean Wounds

It is the use of prophylactic antibiotics in clean neurosurgical procedures that has caused the greatest controversy. Clean neurosurgical wound infection rates have traditionally been low. There are several reports in the literature of infection rates in the range of 1 percent without the use of prophylactic antibiotics. More typical infection rates were in the range of 4 to 5 percent 20 years ago and 2 to 3 percent in recent times. However, the effects of neurosurgical wound infection can be devastating. In addition to pain and discomfort, hospitalization is prolonged and reoperation may be necessary in some cases. Superficial wound infection may lead to infection of the deeper tissues and to the devastating complications of meningitis and brain abscess. It is for this reason that neurosurgeons have continued to work hard to eliminate wound infection despite having an infection rate considered enviably low by other surgical specialists.

Clean procedures must be divided into two groups, those involving implantation of a large foreign body being considered separately. The implantation of a large foreign body generally increases the risk of infection, and removal of the foreign body is generally required if the infection is to be cured. The prototype of such operations is the cerebrospinal fluid shunt. Shunt infection rates have progressively declined in recent years coincident with improvements in shunt design, change from ventriculoatrial to ventriculoperitoneal shunts, and the use of prophylactic antibiotic regimens. Recent reports suggest that shunt infection rates should be less than 5 percent. The controlled studies of the value of prophylactic antibiotics in shunt surgery are all flawed—based on too few infections for conclusions to be drawn. Haines and Taylor's study was prematurely terminated before a sufficient number of patients had been entered for clinically important results to be statistically significant,[8] and Epstein's control group has an infection rate that must be considered exceptionally high by current standards.[3] However, it has been well demonstrated that antibiotics are effective in reducing infection rates in total hip arthroplasty. For this reason, and because Epstein's study has demonstrated its value when the baseline infection rate is quite high, systemic antibiotic prophylaxis is recommended for cerebrospinal fluid shunting procedures. Adhering to the principles outlined initially, the antibiotics should be effective against the staphylococci that are the most common infecting organism in shunt surgery. A semisynthetic penicillin or cephalosporin would seem a logical choice. Antibiotics should be administered with the induction of anesthesia and possibly for one to two doses postoperatively. There is no evidence that a longer course is more effective.

Using the same arguments, a similar regimen would be recommended for cranioplasty, although no direct scientific evidence exists to support this practice.

For clean neurosurgical procedures without implantation of a foreign body, the literature prior to 1979 was reviewed by Haines.[5] The results are equivocal. One cannot argue by analogy from other surgical specialties, for there is no definitive demonstration of the value of prophylactic antibiotics for any operation where the expected infection rate is 5 percent or less. The current controversy arises from Malis's 1979 report of 1732 operations without an infection.[11] He attributes this admirable record to a combination of systemic and topical antibiotic prophylaxis. Others using this regimen have reported infection rates in the range of 1 percent.[7,15] A series of 1000 clean operations without an infection has been reported using a somewhat different systemic antibiotic regimen.[17] These results have led many to believe that prophylactic antibiotics should be used for all neurosurgical procedures. Is this belief justified?

The difficulty in interpreting these data arises from several facts. The baseline infection rate without antibiotics is quite low. Infection rates are known to vary by several percentage points from year to year for reasons that are often not easily discernible. Many services will go for periods of a year or more with infection rates in the 1 percent range. Brief flurries of infection frequently lead to increased attention to details of sterile technique and rapid reduction of the infection rate. The natural variation of the infection rate thus covers a range of several percent. This amount of "noise" in the data makes it impossible to detect changes in infection rates of a few percentage points without a carefully designed controlled trial. We must therefore conclude that the infection rates obtained with prophylactic antibiotics overlap with those obtained without their use and that the value of prophylactic antibiotics for clean neurosurgical procedures has not been demonstrated.

Current scientific information does not support or refute the routine use of prophylactic antibiotics for clean neurosurgical procedures. Neurosurgeons whose infection rate in such procedures exceeds 3 percent would be well advised to reassess their routine aseptic technique. If the infection rate continues to be unacceptably high, the empirical use of prophylactic antibiotics might be justifiable.

Some would argue that the cost and risk of a short course of prophylactic antibiotics is so low that rigid scientific documentation of benefit should not be required. While the costs are relatively low per patient, when this procedure is applied as a general policy to all neurosurgical operations, the total cost may run into the millions of dollars per year. The known risks are small, consisting of a few anaphylactic reactions and occasional aplastic anemia, hemolysis, renal failure, or jaundice. However, there may be unknown risks. Superinfection and the development of resistant organisms in patients with prolonged exposure to antibiotics were unknown risks when antibiotics were first used. Recent experimental work has shown adverse effects on reticuloendothelial system function in rats given short courses of prophylactic antibiotics.[1] It is possible that the widespread use of prophylactic antibiotics could result in development of resistant organisms, not only in single patients but in institutions. Such a selective pressure might take a number of years to manifest itself. The absolute safety of short courses of antibiotics cannot be proved—it can only be disproved, and the history of antibiotic use suggests that it will be.

This is likely to continue to be an area of controversy.

Although surgical wound infections are a relatively small problem as a percentage of surgical procedures, the consequences are serious enough to warrant a careful clinical trial to assess the value of prophylactic antibiotics.

Nonsurgical Uses of Prophylactic Antibiotics

Cerebrospinal Fluid Fistula

There are a number of situations other than surgical procedures in which neurosurgeons would like to prevent the development of infection. When the normal cerebrospinal fluid pathway is violated and there is continuity between the subarachnoid space and the skin or mucous membranes, there is risk of retrograde infection of the central nervous system. Naturally, it has been proposed that when there is a spinal fluid leak, antibiotics should be administered before infection develops, to prevent the development of such infection. The existing data in this regard are contradictory and mostly retrospective in nature. One difficulty in the prophylactic treatment of CSF leaks is that one cannot predict when contamination will take place. This means that antibiotics may have to be continued for many days, weeks, or even months, and past experience suggests that such prolonged prophylactic antibiotic courses are likely to be ineffective and predispose to the development of resistant organisms. Therefore, while many neurosurgeons routinely administer antibiotics prophylactically to patients with cerebrospinal fluid fistulae, the author and many other neurosurgeons do not use prophylactic antibiotics in such patients. Obviously, the development of meningitis must be identified at its earliest stages and treated vigorously.

It has also been recommended that prophylactic antibiotics be used in all patients with basilar skull fracture, on the grounds that there may be an occult CSF leak. Studies of this policy, although too small to allow definite conclusions to be drawn, do not support this use of prophylactic antibiotics.

In special situations, for example, where a CSF otorrhea is complicated by a bacterial otitis externa, a clear case for antibiotic use can be made. In general this will be therapeutic rather than prophylactic antibiotic administration.

Intracranial Pressure Monitoring and Ventriculostomy

Intracranial pressure monitoring, whether through a subarachnoid bolt or an epidural or ventricular catheter, has become a common practice in modern neurosurgery. At the present time, all such devices in some way establish a continuity between the skin and the intracranial space. In some ways they may be viewed as CSF fistulae created under carefully controlled circumstance. As such, they should be at lower risk of infection than traumatic or spontaneous CSF fistulae. In several reported series, the infection rate seems to be about 5 percent, with the risk of infection increasing markedly after the fourth day of monitoring. It seems to be common practice to cover patients with prophylactic antibiotics while a monitoring device is in place. This is based on retrospective reviews which have suggested lower infection rates in patients who received antibiotics. There is no controlled scientific evidence to support the practice.

The theoretical objections are the same as for traumatic CSF leaks. Analogous situations, such as the maintenance of long-term central vein catheters for total parenteral nutrition and long-term urethral catheterization are managed without prophylactic systemic antibiotics. Once again, the key to controlling the infection rate of intracranial pressure monitors and ventriculostomies appears to be meticulous local care of the device and perhaps changing its site periodically. Antibiotics should be reserved for treating infections once they are established. Exceptions to this policy could rationally be made where the patient appears to be at unusual risk of infection—e.g., an immunosuppressed patient, the presence of an infection in some other organ system, or an institutional risk of infection known to be higher than a few percent.

Urinary Tract Infection

Urinary tract infection is common in catheterized patients, and many neurosurgical patients require catheterization at some time during hospitalization. It is clear that sterile, closed drainage catheter systems are superior to open drainage systems. Catheters should be inserted with meticulous aseptic technique. Except in short-term situations or when catheter irrigation must be done frequently, antibiotic or antiseptic irrigation does not appear to be beneficial. Systemic antibiotic prophylaxis in patients with long-term catheterization is counterproductive, leading to infection with resistant organisms. Again, it seems that meticulous care of the catheter is of paramount importance in infection protection, although the specifics of the local care regimen remain controversial.[10] For long-term management of incontinence, intermittent catheterization programs may be superior to indwelling catheterization in terms of infection and other complications.

Pneumonia

Schemes for the prevention of postoperative pneumonia with systemic antibiotics have generally failed. Indeed, in Petersdorf's study of unconscious patients[13] and Price and Sleigh's experience with neurosurgical patients,[14] broad spectrum prophylactic regimens created more trouble than they prevented. Prophylactic aerosol antibiotic treatment of intubated patients has not been proved effective and may be harmful.[2] Again, prevention of infection relies more on good physical care than on antibiotic therapy.

Miscellaneous Indications for Prophylaxis

Patients with structural abnormalities of the heart and great vessels, prior history of infective endocarditis, or intravascular prosthetic devices are at risk for developing serious infec-

tions related to bacteremia caused by dental and surgical procedures. Although there are no controlled trials and the efficacy of prophylaxis for endocarditis has been called into question by some, current recommendations are that patients in the above categories receive prophylaxis with all dental procedures, surgical procedures on the upper respiratory tract, and surgical procedures and instrumentation (including urethral catheterization) of the gastrointestinal and genitourinary tracts.[9] It is logical to include patients with ventriculoatrial shunts in this category and to recommend routine prophylaxis for these patients in these situations. It does not seem necessary to extend prophylaxis to patients with ventriculoperitoneal shunts, as the shunts lie outside the vascular system.

Topical Antibiotic Prophylaxis

Many neurosurgeons have routinely irrigated surgical wounds with antibiotic solutions, bacitracin being the most common. There has been little systematic study of this practice, and there is little information to suggest that it is of value. This literature has recently been reviewed.[6]

References

1. Altura BM, Gebrewold A: Prophylactic administration of antibiotics compromises reticuloendothelial system function and exacerbates shock mortality in rats. Br J Pharmacol 68:19–21, 1980.
2. Eickhoff TC: Pulmonary infections in surgical patients. Surg Clin North Am 60:175–183, 1980.
3. Epstein MM, Kumor K, Hughes W, Lietman P: The use of prophylactic antibiotics in pediatric shunting operations—A double-blind prospective randomized study. Presented at the Annual Meeting of the American Association of Neurological Surgeons, Honolulu, Hawaii, April 26, 1982.
4. Flynn NM, Lawrence RM: Antimicrobial prophylaxis. Med Clin North Am 63: 1225–1244, 1979.
5. Haines SJ: Systemic antibiotic prophylaxis in neurological surgery. Neurosurgery 6:355–361, 1980.
6. Haines SJ: Topical antibiotic prophylaxis in neurosurgery. Neurosurgery 11:250–253, 1982.
7. Haines SJ, Goodman ML: Antibiotic prophylaxis of postoperative neurosurgical wound infection. J Neurosurg 56:103–105, 1982.
8. Haines SJ, Taylor F: Prophylactic methicillin for shunt operations: Effects on incidence of shunt malfunction and infection. Childs Brain 9:10–22, 1982.
9. Kaplan EL, Anthony BF, Bisno A, Durack D, Houser H, Millard HD, Sanford J, Shulman ST, Stillerman M, Taranta A, Wenger N: Prevention of bacterial endocarditis. Circulation 56:139A–143A, 1977.
10. Kunin CM: Urinary tract infections. Surg Clin North Am 60:223–231, 1980.
11. Malis LI: Prevention of neurosurgical infection by intraoperative antibiotics. Neurosurgery 5:339–343, 1979.
12. National Academy of Sciences–National Research Council: Postoperative wound infections: The influence of ultraviolet irradiation of the operating room and of various other factors. Ann Surg 160 (suppl):23, 1964.
13. Petersdorf RG, Curtin JA, Hoeprich PD, Peeler RN, Bennett

IL Jr: A study of antibiotic prophylaxis in unconscious patients. N Engl J Med 257:1001–1009, 1957.

14. Price DJE, Sleigh JD: Control of infection due to *Klebsiella aerogenes* in a neurosurgical unit by withdrawal of all antibiotics. Lancet 2:1213–1215, 1970.

15. Quartey GRC, Polyzoidis K: Intraoperative antibiotic prophylaxis in neurosurgery: A clinical study. Neurosurgery 8:669–671, 1981.

16. Rosebury T. *Microorganisms Indigenous to Man*. New York, McGraw Hill, 1962, pp 310–311.

17. Savitz MH, Katz SS: Rationale for prophylactic antibiotics in neurosurgery. Neurosurgery 9:142–144, 1981.

18. Wright AD: Brain and meningeal infections, in Fleming A: *Penicillin: Its Practical Application*, 2d ed. London, Butterworth, 1950, p 287.

46
Patient Positioning

Donald H. Stewart, Jr.
John Krawchenko

Patient positioning is an integral and important aspect of any operative procedure and can be the most crucial factor in the successful outcome of an operation. Proper positioning should be planned and carried out to achieve the following essential goals:

1. To provide complete and appropriate exposure for the neurosurgical procedure
2. To ensure and maintain adequate cardiovascular and respiratory function during surgery
3. To prevent or minimize unnecessary pressure or traction on important structures such as spinal roots, peripheral nerves, skin, blood vessels, eyes, ears, and extremities
4. To provide a comfortable position for the patient during the procedure
5. To provide a comfortable position for the neurosurgeon during the procedure.

To ensure these goals, positioning should be managed primarily by the operating surgeon and coordinated with the anesthesiologist and operating room personnel. Several important aspects of patient positioning should be considered before the patient enters the operating room. The operating table must be situated to achieve optimal illumination of the operative field and easy access to anesthetic lines, respirator, and outlets for power-driven instruments. Attention should be given to the optimal placement of the surgical technician, neurosurgical instruments, operative assistants, and operating microscope. The actions performed during anesthesia induction must be observed by the surgeon. Extension of

the neck for intubation must be avoided in patients with spondylotic myelopathy or cervical fractures. A smooth induction must be achieved, especially in patients with high intracranial pressure or a cerebral vascular lesion.

As positioning progresses and draping is carried out, the surgeon should remain fully aware of the relationship of the proposed operative site to the surrounding anatomical structures which will be obscured by the drapes. To be adequate, the final position should be matched to the anticipated surgical exposure and peculiarities of the patient as dictated by age, skeletal deformity, and anticipated cardiorespiratory events. The surgeon should always complete the positioning process by personally marking the planned incision, as an inadequate exposure may compromise the intended surgical goal. Some surgeons may even wish to place themselves in the planned position to determine potential beneficial or harmful effects. Positions that would be uncomfortable or compromise neurologic or cardiovascular-respiratory function in the awake patient must also be avoided for the anesthetized patient.

Supine Position

The supine position is utilized for various craniotomies, anterior cervical procedures, and carotid endarterectomies (Fig. 46-1). The patient is placed supine on the operating table with the arms secured at the sides in a supinated position to protect the ulnar nerves. The elbows may be pro-

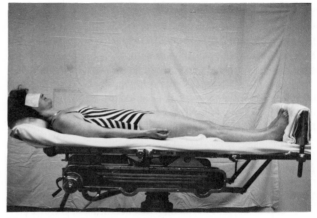

Figure 46-1 Supine position.

tected with padding. The patient's feet should firmly abut on a padded footboard to prevent migration of the body on the operating table. The eyelids should be taped shut after lubricant is inserted to prevent dryness and irritation of the cornea. The surgeon should ascertain that ventilation is satisfactory.

For cranial operations, the head is supported on a doughnut-shaped pad and elevated slightly above the level of the heart to reduce venous engorgement of the brain. However, the surgeon must be alert to the potential risk of air emboli in this position. In all cranial operations the head should be positioned so that the normal brain will fall away by gravity from the route of access to the lesion, reducing the necessity for brain retraction. The head may be rotated in either direction as dictated by the operative procedure. If significant rotation is needed, a padded sandbag is placed under the shoulder to minimize kinking of neck veins and undue strain on the cervical muscles. The neck should not be twisted into an uncomfortable position or one that obstructs the venous outflow. Tape used by the anesthesiologist should not compress the cervical veins. The vertex of the skull should protrude slightly beyond the edge of the table to avoid mechanical interference by the edge of the operating table with the surgeon's hands. This will also allow the drapes to fall directly downward. The dependent ear is positioned in the hollow portion of a doughnut-shaped pad to avoid pressure injury.

Many surgeons prefer to use the head clamp to rigidly immobilize the head for cranial operations in the supine as well as the prone, lateral, or sitting position. This will allow the anatomical structures, as perceived prior to draping, to remain in constant relationship to the operative incision. However, a clamp may significantly limit intraoperative repositioning of the head. The connecting frame for the head clamp is placed underneath the head of the table and should be positioned so as not to press against the legs of a surgeon who will be sitting. The head clamp should be secured to the skull after a final positioning of the head and neck. The pins of the head clamp should enter the skull just below the curve of the parietal boss and frontal boss to prevent upward migration of the pins on the curved portion of the skull during the operative procedure. The pins should be positioned to avoid puncture of the thin temporal squamosa. Care must be taken to avoid pressure on the forehead or occiput by the head clamp bar. Vaseline ointment should be placed around the pins to minimize the risk of air emboli. Vaseline gauze forced between the scalp and the head clamp pins can cause scalp necrosis. The position and function of the endotracheal tube must be rechecked. If the head clamp is used in a pediatric patient, the pins should have a longer base projection and smaller points to accommodate the smaller head diameter and thinner scalp and skull.

For anterior cervical spine and carotid artery procedures, the anesthesiologist is placed at the head of the table and the surgeons at either side of the patient. The head is slightly extended and slightly rotated away from the side of the proposed incision. A small pad is placed between the shoulder blades which will slightly extend the neck and provide a better exposure. In the case of anterior cervical fusions, a halter cervical traction apparatus for intraoperative traction is applied after the induction of anesthesia. The iliac crest is elevated slightly with a small pillow under the buttock to allow better access to the graft donor site. The iliac crest incision should be marked prior to draping to avoid an incision near the anterior superior iliac spine that might injure the lateral femoral cutaneous nerve. In cases of cervical spine fractures requiring open reduction, fusion, or laminectomy, the patient is operated upon while remaining on the fracture frame, and any turning from the supine to the prone position is carefully done while traction is maintained. Some neurosurgeons who employ a halo-type apparatus for the initial management of cervical fractures leave it in place during the cervical procedure, taking off either the back or front portion to gain the necessary exposure and reconnecting it postoperatively to secure adequate long-term immobilization.

Prone Position

The prone position may be used for various spinal and cranial procedures. Most thoracolumbar spine operations are done in the prone position. This requires that the pelvis and lateral chest wall be supported on either a special frame or large rolls. There should be minimal abdominal pressure, thereby permitting unrestricted diaphragmatic movement and a reduction of pressure on the vena cava to reduce possible extradural venous bleeding. Care must be taken to avoid pressure on the lateral femoral cutaneous nerve at the lateral end of the inguinal ligament to reduce the incidence of postoperative meralgia paresthetica. The authors recommend a Wilson frame (Zimmer Docherty Associates, Warsaw, Ind.), as it is adjustable in width and height and can be elevated during lumbar procedures to reverse the lumbar lordosis, thereby placing the lumbar spine in a horizontal position and opening the interlaminar spaces. Such a frame is easily used and obviates the need for supplying various sized cushions and rolls which may shift in position during the operation. The frame can be lowered to allow a lordotic posture, which may assist in the management of troublesome extradural bleeding. The sternum must be protected and the breasts and genitalia comfortably placed.

For lumbar procedures, the arms can be placed on armboards at the head of the table (Fig. 46-2). The neurovascular structures in the axillae must not be compressed by the lateral frame pad. The ulnar nerves must be protected and free of pressure. The position of the shoulders and arms should look comfortable. The authors prefer to have the patient's hips and knees flexed and the feet elevated on pillows to the level of the back, thereby reducing stretch on the sciatic nerve components. The head and neck must rest in a comfortable position supported on pillows to minimize any cervical muscle strain, periorbital edema, or facial venous congestion. There should not be pressure on either eye, which could result in blindness. The surgeon should ascertain that ventilation is satisfactory and should not leave the patient's head and neck positioning solely to the anesthesiologist.

Occasionally the knee-chest position is used for lumbar spine operations.[1] This affords an unencumbered abdomen but in the authors' opinion is not as desirable as the prone or

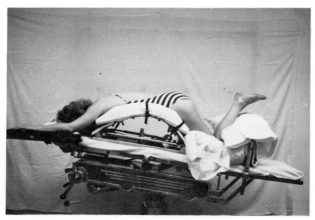

Figure 46-2 Prone position: lumbar procedures.

lateral position, because the height of the surgical field renders the use of some types of microscopes impossible. Additionally, postoperative knee pain is likely should the patient have any pre-existing knee pathology.

For thoracic operations in the prone position, the authors prefer to have the patient's legs straight and the knees supported on pillows, with the feet resting securely on a footboard. The Wilson frame need not be elevated in such circumstances, since a reversal of the lumbar lordosis is not needed (Fig. 46-3).

For midthoracic to low thoracic lesions, the patient's arms may conveniently be placed on armrests at the head of the table, easily accessible to the anesthesiologist. For high thoracic procedures, it is more comfortable for the surgeon to place the patient's arms alongside the body. The position of the head and neck is as described for lumbar procedures.

For procedures extending to or involving the posterior cervical spine, the head is stabilized in a head clamp and flexed on the neck so that the chin is tucked in. Depending on the exposure required in the cervical spine procedure, the spine may be maintained in a neutral or slightly flexed position to expose the interlaminar spaces. The arms are secured at the patient's sides, with care to avoid pressure on the peripheral nerves. Occasionally, access to the cervical-dorsal junction is facilitated by tape placed laterally over the shoulders to pull them dorsally and downward.

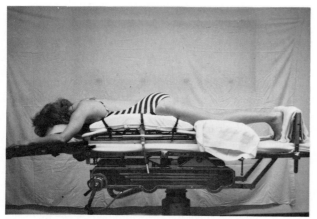

Figure 46-3 Prone position: thoracic procedures.

For spinal operations on large children and small adults, the above principles and techniques apply. For small children and babies, the Wilson frame is not usable, and foam or cloth cushions must provide the necessary support for the body. Prevention of heat loss is a prime consideration in infants. Heat lamps and warming blankets are employed for this purpose.

For posterior cranial procedures, the head is secured in the head clamp. In an infant or child, the cerebellar headrest may be used but must be well padded, and meticulous attention must be given to protecting the eyes from pressure. For posterior supratentorial cranial procedures in the prone position, the head and neck may be maintained in a neutral position. For posterior infratentorial procedures, the head is flexed on the neck, and the neck itself may be slightly flexed to provide maximal exposure of this area (Fig. 46-4).

Whenever the patient's head or neck is flexed after insertion of the endotracheal tube, it is imperative to ascertain the adequacy of ventilation, since in this circumstance the endotracheal tube extends farther down the trachea and may occasionally enter the right main stem bronchus and ventilate only the right lung. With extreme flexion, the tube itself may kink, making ventilation difficult or impossible. Also, with head flexion in the prone position, there should be no pressure on the chin, which may be quite closely approximated to the edge of the operating table. Dependent edema of the tongue is prevented by proper positioning of the tongue relative to the teeth, oropharyngeal tube, and endotracheal tube.

For all the posterior cervical and cranial procedures in the prone position, it is imperative that the feet be firmly supported on a foot plate with the legs extended passively, to prevent the body from sliding as the table is tilted into the reverse Trendelenberg position to bring the neck and head into a horizontal plane. The arms are secured at the patient's sides.

Sitting Position

The sitting position, used for cranial and posterior cervical procedures, requires meticulous attention to details (Fig. 46-5A). A major concern in this position is the occurrence of air emboli or hypotension. A central venous pressure catheter is used to remove possible air emboli. It must be inserted preoperatively into the region of the right atrium under fluoroscopic control and its final position checked with a chest film with the patient in the proposed sitting position. Displacement of the catheter tip by abduction or elevation of the arm, which may occur during positioning of the patient, can be readily checked with the fluoroscope preoperatively in the x-ray suite. Cardiac arrhythmias may occur if the catheter tip abuts the myocardial wall. The catheter should be removed or pulled back into the superior vena cava shortly after the operation to prevent myocardial perforation and cardiac tamponade, which occurred in one of the authors' cases. A small test bolus of fluid or air detectable by the Doppler monitor should be introduced by the anesthesiologist, and the surgeon's ears should be attuned to these formidable sounds, which will necessitate quick remedial action on the part of the entire surgical team.

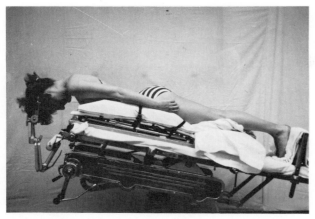

Figure 46-4 Prone position: craniocervical procedures.

As the patient is progressively elevated into the sitting position, the blood pressure and pulse must be carefully monitored by the anesthesiologist. If hypotension occurs, the patient should be returned to the supine position and appropriate remedial action taken. To place the patient in a sitting position, the surgeon must carry out several coordinated maneuvers with the operating table. The back of the table is elevated, while simultaneously the table is flexed at the hips. The knees are then flexed and the table placed in Trendelenberg position. If an arched bar is attached to the table to which the head clamp support bar is attached, care must be taken to avoid pressure on the patient's knees by this device. For cervical procedures, the head is flexed on the neck and the neck itself is maintained in a neutral position. For posterior supratentorial approaches, the head and neck may be maintained also in a neutral position. For posterior infratentorial approaches, full flexion of the head and neck is desirable. The head is flexed on the neck with the chin tucked in, and the neck itself is flexed so that the chin almost touches the sternum, allowing room, however, for insertion of at least one or two fingers. At times, the flexed head and neck may need to be pushed forward to provide optimal exposure of the supracerebellar and tentorial region. For more lateral lesions, especially at the cerebellopontine angle, the head should be rotated sufficiently toward the side of the lesion to allow direct visualization and access to the lesion. As flexion of the head and neck is carried out, the endotracheal tube position and function must be rechecked

as the final positioning point is reached. The head clamp should be secured to the skull after the final position is attained.

A microscope stand that is short may not allow the microscope to be raised up to the surgical field with the patient in the sitting position. Occasionally this can be overcome by further flexion of the neck and forward displacement of the skull, which may allow additional Trendelenberg positioning of the table, bringing the operative site to a position nearer the floor and thus making it possible to use the microscope (Fig. 46-5B). When the final patient and microscope position is achieved, the posture of the surgeon's neck should be comfortable, not in extension, nor should the hands be above eye level.

The patient's arms should be supported in a comfortable position by padded armrests to avoid drooping of the shoulders and passive downward traction on the cervical roots, especially in patients with cervical spondylosis. The ulnar nerves should be well protected. It is advisable to ask the patient, while awake, to assume the anticipated position of the neck and head flexion, and head rotation if that is to be used, to ascertain that the position will be comfortable and easily assumed. If the position cannot be attained in the awake patient, it cannot be used under anesthesia. For some small adults and children, it may be necessary to place a cushion under the buttocks to raise the cervical or cranial area sufficiently above the back of the operating table.

Lateral Position

The lateral position may be used for lumbar and certain thoracic spinal procedures and cranial procedures (Fig. 46-6A). It is especially useful in severely obese or kyphotic patients. If a unilateral spinal approach is planned, it is best to place the symptomatic side uppermost, with the body rolled slightly away from the surgeon. A pad must be placed beneath the dependent chest to elevate it slightly, reducing any pressure on the adjacent dependent axillary neurovascular structures. The head should be in a neutral, comfortable position. For thoracic procedures done in the lateral position, both legs should be extended, with the feet against a fixed, padded foot plate and with care to avoid pressure on the peroneal nerve adjacent to the table. A pillow between the knees is comfortable. For lumbar procedures, the lordo-

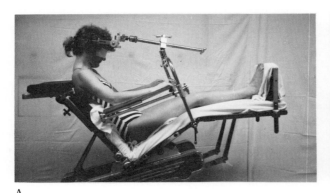

A

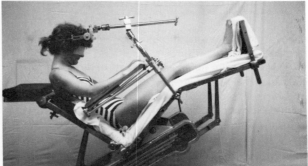

B

Figure 46-5 Sitting position.

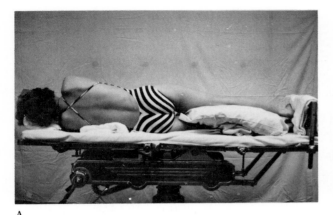

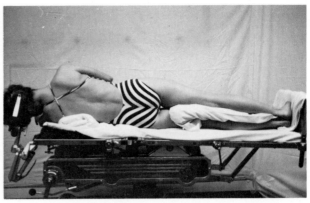

A

B

Figure 46-6 Lateral position.

sis may be reduced by flexion of the dependent hip and knee. In unilateral procedures for disc removal, elevation of the kidney rest will induce an upward convex spine and open to some degree the interlaminar space. The abdomen is free in this position, making ventilation easy and venous pressure elevation minimal. The uppermost arm may be held in a soft, elevated arm sling or taped to the side of the body. Body motion is minimized by straps or tape securing the body to the operating table. This position gives excellent visualization for the surgeon and the assistant for unilateral small-incision procedures and is also satisfactory for extensive thoracolumbar procedures. It is not so satisfactory for combined cervical-thoracic procedures. One advantage is that the surgical technician and the instrument tray can be placed directly opposite the surgeon.

The lateral position may also be used for posterior cranial and cervical procedures (Fig. 46-6B). The head is best supported and fixed in a head clamp. Depending on the operative procedure, head and neck flexion is carried out as discussed for the sitting position. For posterior fossa approaches, the shoulders should be retracted with tape and the neck laterally bent to allow better exposure for the surgeon.

The lateral position is also satisfactory for a retroperitoneal approach to the lumbar bodies, insertion of lumboperitoneal shunts, transthoracic operations on the spine, and unilateral dorsal sympathectomies.

Semiprone, or Tonsillar, Position

The semiprone, or tonsillar, position may be used for posterior cranial operations with or without a head clamp (Fig. 46-7). It is also useful for emergency operations on the posterior fossa. The patient is placed semiprone, in a position much like that assumed when one is sleeping with the dependent arm behind the body and the uppermost arm flexed at the elbow with the hand near the chin. A pillow or sandbag may be placed in front of the chest for support. The head should protrude slightly beyond the end of the table. The dependent eye should be well protected from pressure injury. The head and neck may be flexed. The dependent

leg is extended and the foot firmly fixed against a padded footboard. The dependent knee is padded to protect the peroneal nerve. The uppermost leg is flexed at the hip and knee. The endotracheal tube should be rechecked for any possible kinking. This position affords easy ventilation, as the abdomen is quite free.

Peripheral Nerves

The most frequently performed peripheral nerve operations by neurosurgeons today relate to the median and ulnar nerves. For median nerve compression syndromes at the wrist, the patient is best placed in the supine position, with one or both arms abducted and supinated on a laterally placed armboard. A small pad is placed beneath the distal forearm to allow dorsiflexion of the wrist. The surgeon sits on that side of the arm which allows easiest use of the surgeon's dominant hand. This position is also satisfactory for ulnar nerve exploration at the wrist and hand.

Patients with nerve lesions at the elbow may be positioned similarly. A convenient alternative for good exposure is to secure the hand and forearm of the supine patient to an ether screen directly over the face of the patient in the "sa-

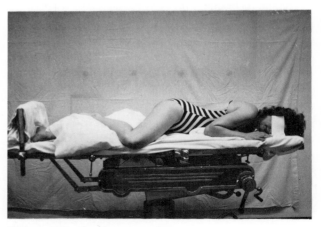

Figure 46-7 Semiprone position.

lute" position, so that the elbow is flexed and protrudes just beyond the operating table.

Lesions of the sciatic nerve at or below the popliteal fossa are best pursued with the patient prone or with the affected side slightly elevated to allow access to the fibular neck. For lesions of the sciatic nerve above the popliteal fossa, the patient is positioned prone, with steps taken during draping to assure mobility of the extremity below the operative site.

For a discussion of patient positioning for more complicated peripheral nerve procedures and exploration of the brachial and lumbosacral plexus, the reader is referred to Omer and Spinner[3] and Pollock and Davis.[4]

In many other specific operations, positioning is dictated by the peculiarity of the procedure itself—e.g., trans-sphenoidal hypophysectomy, stereotactic operations, cordotomy, etc. For specific information concerning patient positioning for these procedures, the surgeon should review articles on the individual procedure.[2,5-8] However, the basic principles are the same as those described in this chapter.

References

1. Cook AW, Siddiqi TS, Nidzgorski F, Clare HA: Sitting prone position for the posterior surgical approach to the spine and posterior fossa. Neurosurgery 10:232–235, 1982.
2. Kempe LG: *Operative Neurosurgery*, vol 1, 1968, vol 2, 1970. New York, Springer-Verlag.
3. Omer GE Jr, Spinner M: *Management of Peripheral Nerve Problems*. Philadelphia, Saunders, 1980.
4. Pollock LJ, Davis L: *Peripheral Nerve Injuries*. New York, Hoeber-Harper, 1933.
5. Rob C, Smith R: Operative Surgery: Fundamental international tecniques, in Symon L: *Neurosurgery*, 3d ed. London, Butterworth, 1979.
6. Schmidek HH, Sweet WH: *Current Techniques in Operative Neurosurgery*. New York, Grune & Stratton, 1977.
7. Shillito J Jr, Matson DD: *An Atlas of Pediatric Neurosurgical Operations*. Philadelphia, Saunders, 1982.
8. Youmans JR: *Neurological Surgery*, 2d ed. Philadelphia, Saunders, 1982.

47

Intraoperative Diagnostic Ultrasound

George J. Dohrmann
Jonathan M. Rubin

Ultrasound has been utilized sporadically in the neurosurgical operating room for over 25 years.[1,2,7,13,15] The need to accurately localize and characterize lesions in the brain is a recurring and important problem for neurosurgeons; this has stimulated a revival in intraoperative ultrasonography as a means for solving some of these problems.

Physical Principles and Historical Development of Ultrasound Scanning

All diagnostic ultrasound scanners work on the same principles. Within their scanheads they contain transducers that convert electrical energy to mechanical or sound energy and vice versa. These transducers contain crystals having the property of changing abruptly in shape when an electrical voltage is placed across them. If they are in contact with a surface, this abrupt change in shape is analogous to sharply hitting the contact surface. A sound wave is then propagated into the surface, much as an impulse is sent into a wall if someone hits it with a fist. This wave will travel continuously into the medium until it contacts another surface or encounters a change in what is termed *acoustic impedance*. Acoustic impedance is a physical property that is a function not only of density but also of the actual composition and internal structure of a substance. Therefore normal biological substances such as muscle and collagen may have quite different acoustic impedances, even though they are both composed of the same elements in about the same proportions.

Once the sound wave strikes a surface, some of the energy is reflected back to the transducer and some continues to propagate forward. This fact is important, since substances that reflect most, if not all, of the sound energy impinging upon them, most notably air and bone, prevent the imaging of structures behind them. Thus structures behind air or bone are invisible by ultrasound. This fact alone makes ultrasonography basically useless as a preoperative diagnostic tool for the central nervous system, since it is encased within bone.

The reflected sound wave returns to the scanhead and hits the transducer. This collision has the reverse effect of changing the shape of the crystal in the transducer, inducing a voltage across it. This induced voltage is recorded by a computer in modern equipment or is directly displayed as an amplitude on an oscilloscope trace in older machines (Fig. 47-1). The displayed amplitude is dependent on the strength of the reflection manifested by the amount of energy that contacts the transducer face. The location within the tissue from which the reflection came can easily be calculated once the speed of sound in the organ being scanned and the inter-

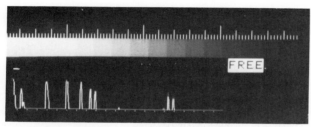

Figure 47-1 The early ultrasound image was unidimensional. The height of the peaks along the bottom of the figure corresponds to the amplitude of an ultrasound beam. Early ultrasound machines could only display these amplitude plots, hence no image could be produced.

val of time between the generation of the impulse by the ultrasound transducer and the reception of the reflected wave are known. This period corresponds to the time it takes the sound wave to travel down and back, or twice the distance from the transducer to any particular reflecting surface. Knowing these facts, it is a simple matter to determine the position of any reflection using the following equation:

Distance = speed of sound × 1/2(time of flight)

Ultrasonography has the additional interesting property that it not only determines the depth of these reflections but also quantifies the position of reflections relative to the scanhead and transducer. This is because all ultrasound transducers are focused, making the ultrasound beam directional. Rather than propagating out in all directions like waves emanating from a stone thrown into a pool of water, the sound waves coming from diagnostic ultrasound transducers move only in the direction in which the transducer is pointing. Therefore a surgeon holding an ultrasound scanhead knows immediately where a reflection has come from, since the reflection's depth is known by its position on an oscilloscope or television screen and its location from the direction in which the scanhead is pointed at the time when the reflection was produced. Ultrasonography is therefore in some sense "inherently stereotactic," since structures are defined in three dimensions relative to the ultrasound scanhead independent of stereotactic frames or grids.[1]

Given these facts, it is not surprising that certain types of ultrasonography have been tried in the neurosurgical operating room over the years. Once the overlying bone has been removed during an operation, a sterilized or sterilely draped scanhead can be applied directly to the dural surface or to the brain for scanning. Since there is normally no bone or air within the brain, the sound easily propagates into the organ. It has been repeatedly demonstrated that normal brain tissue has a markedly different echogenicity than tumors or hemorrhages.[7] Using ultrasonic probes, surgeons have been able to localize and characterize various types of intracranial lesions.[3,5,8,9,12]

Yet intraoperative ultrasonography has had a checkered history over the years, despite its obvious advantages. Further, its limited preoperative intracranial diagnostic applications, except in young infants, have been almost entirely replaced by computed tomography (CT) for several reasons. First, the older scanners did not generate images. As mentioned above, all ultrasound scanners operate by pulsing out sound waves and then recording the positions of reflections in the returning wave. The direction from which the information is recorded depends on the orientation of the scanhead. This direction is a line, and therefore all the information gathered in any particular scan was one-dimensional. Further, the information was displayed as a trace on an oscilloscope, much like an electrocardiogram, with stronger echoes producing higher peaks. Hence all ultrasound scans were simply plots of the reflection amplitudes along the direction of scanning; no image was produced (Fig. 47-1). These facts made interpretation difficult and frequently unreliable. The subjectivity involved in reading these scans impaired the usefulness of the information they contained. Preoperative CT and angiograms were just as valuable and were much less subjective to interpret.

These problems have all but disappeared in the last few years with the development of two-dimensional, real-time ultrasound sector scanners.[5,6,9,10] These machines make two-dimensional slices through the object being scanned, much as do CT scanners. Yet, since they rely on reflected information rather than using a transmitted signal to mathematically reconstruct an image, as does CT, they can scan objects at very rapid rates. If these rates are much more rapid than physiological motion, on the order of 10 to 100 ms per slice, this motion can be represented in the image. Thus the operator can see arterial pulsations and scan across an object much as one does when sweeping a flashlight through a darkened room. The term *real time* has been applied to these ultrasound scanners because their rapid frame rates permit the visualization of physiological motion.

As mentioned earlier, all ultrasound information starts out being one-dimensional. However, there is a modification in the way the information is recorded. Rather than an oscilloscope trace, each reflection is assigned a dot. The brightness of each dot is directly related to the strength of the reflection. Thus, in the usual display mode of white-on-black, structures like bone or air that strongly reflect sound are white, while those that have no reflecting surfaces within them at all, such as cerebrospinal fluid (CSF), are black. This gives a line of dots rather than a graph on an oscilloscope. This line of dots and its orientation relative to the center of the scanhead are stored in a computer memory associated with the ultrasound scanner. If the orientation of the transducer within the scanhead is changed so that it points in a new direction, or if the scanhead contains many transducers and a new one pointing along a different line is employed, a second unique scan line is produced with a new row of dots. These lines, in their relative positions, are then displayed together on a video screen. Eventually, if a single transducer sweeps through enough positions or if a scanhead has enough different transducer elements in it, many lines of dots are generated. If these lines are closely spaced, the entire ensemble produces a two-dimensional slice, which the scanner displays on the video screen (Fig. 47-2).

These slices characteristically have a pie shape, because real-time sector scanners sweep out an angle within the object being scanned, with the scanhead at the apex of the angle. (Rectangular slices can be produced, but these require scanheads with larger contact surfaces and are there-

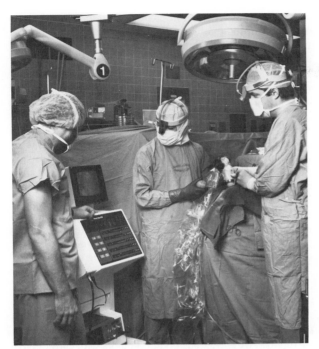

Figure 47-2 Operating room set-up for intraoperative real-time ultrasound imaging of the brain. The ultrasound scanner is at the left, with a video screen at the top. The scanhead is covered by a sterile transparent plastic drape and is held against the dura by the surgeon (*right*). Dynamic imaging of the brain is seen on the videoscreen, and in this case, the surgeon is advancing a biopsy probe toward a deep lesion under continuous ultrasound guidance.

fore not very useful intraoperatively.) These slices can be updated rapidly—more rapidly than the eye can perceive—thus giving the illusion of motion described above.

By holding the scanhead stationary, a continuous representation of one slice can be maintained. Moving the scanhead produces slices through different parts of the object being scanned. Thus it is possible to examine a brain intraoperatively in a matter of seconds. Finally, since the slices are oriented relative to the scanhead, a different slice orientation can be obtained by merely rotating the scanhead 90 degrees. Hence a coronal scan can be converted to a sagittal slice by a twist of the wrist. This great speed and flexibility lets the neurosurgeon evaluate the operative field quickly and accurately immediately after exposing the dura and during the operation.

Some real-time sector scanners allow even more flexibility, in that they permit the operator to rapidly change the frequency of the transducer being used. This is important, since the spatial resolution is directly dependent on the frequency of the transducer employed.[4] The theoretical limit of axial resolution of an ultrasound beam is one-half the wavelength of the beam. Therefore, since the wavelength is inversely proportional to the frequency, the higher the frequency the shorter the wavelength and hence the higher the spatial resolution. However, higher frequency transducers cannot always be used, since the higher frequency waves are

attenuated to a much greater extent by the tissues through which they pass than are lower frequency waves.[4] Hence a higher frequency wave rapidly loses its energy upon entering a tissue, with associated poor depth penetration, while lower frequency waves can penetrate to much greater depths before dissipating their energy; higher resolution is achieved at the expense of decreased penetration. Thus only superficial structures or thin objects such as the spinal cord can be scanned with transducers of relatively high frequency, such as 7.5 megahertz (MHz), whereas a 3-MHz beam can easily traverse both cerebral hemispheres in a coronal section or from anterior to posterior in a sagittal section. Yet fine structural detail such as the central canal in the spinal cord can be imaged only at the higher frequencies. In most ultrasound scanners it is necessary to attach an entire new scanhead assembly each time a different transducer frequency is desired. However, machines are now available that contain multifrequency scanheads, so that transducers of different frequency can be employed merely by pushing a button on the console of the scanner.

Finally, ultrasonography is completely safe. There has never been any proven detrimental effect of ultrasound on human tissue at the energies employed in present-day equipment. The technique can therefore be repeatedly used during an operation without fear of harm to either the patient or the operating room staff.

Intraoperative Ultrasound Scanning

Intracranial

Precise localization and characterization of lesions within the brain have been significant problems in neurosurgery. Static studies such as CT scans of the head and cerebral angiography have served as "road maps," as the information was often displayed in an orientation different from that of the neurosurgeon in the operating room. As the majority of intracranial lesions occur under the surface of the brain or beneath the brain itself, a method of visualizing these in the operating room would be most useful. With accurate localization would come little need for exploration of the brain or "blind" procedures such as biopsy of deep lesions or placement of ventricular catheters. Any unnecessary trauma to the brain should be avoided, so the real-time ultrasound scanner, as described above, offers an enormous advantage in the operating room in allowing the neurosurgeon to explore the brain without opening the dura.[3,5,8,11,14] At the time of exposure of the dura by a burr hole, craniectomy, or craniotomy, the ultrasound scanhead is covered by a sterile plastic bag and touched to the surface of the dura; sterile saline is dripped onto the dura to serve as a coupling agent. Using a low-frequency (3 MHz) transducer, the entire brain may be visualized on the video screen (Fig. 47-2). Orientation is available by determining the position of the ventricles and the interhemispheric fissure. Coronal, transaxial, or sagittal sections can be made, depending upon the location of the exposed dura and the orientation of the scanhead (Fig. 47-3). If less penetration but greater resolution is needed, higher frequencies of 5 or 7.5 MHz are used.

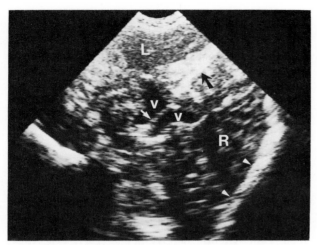

Figure 47-3 Photograph of a dynamic coronal ultrasound image of the brain. The scanhead has been applied to the dura (at top of pie-shaped sector) over the left cerebral hemisphere (L). At 3 MHz, both sides of the brain are imaged. Right cerebral hemisphere (R); falx (*black arrow*); lateral ventricles (V); septum pellucidum (*small arrow*); bone of skull on right side (*arrowheads*).

Real-time ultrasound gives a dynamic image (physiological motion such as pulsation of blood vessels can be seen); however, this image may be frozen on the video screen and the computer can calculate the distance from the surface of the scanhead to a lesion as well as the diameter of the lesion. Because ultrasound images depend upon differences in tissue character rather than the amount of attenuation of x-rays or the permeability of contrast material, as in CT scanning, the ultrasound image can accurately define the size of lesions as well as characterize them (e.g., solid tissue vs. necrosis vs. cyst). Once a lesion within the brain is imaged, the best angle of approach to it may be planned. The dura is opened at this point for either resection or biopsy of the lesion. If a lesion is to be resected, a topectomy is performed and dissection is carried down to the lesion. To check the accuracy of the approach, the wound may be filled with saline and the ultrasound scanhead touched to the saline. The approach to the lesion and the lesion itself can be visualized and midcourse corrections made in the approach. If a lesion is to be biopsied, the probe may be advanced to the lesion through a small dural incision under direct, continuous ultrasound guidance (Fig. 47-4). It can be determined what part of the lesion has been biopsied and whether there is any intracerebral hemorrhage at any time during the procedure.

Tumors

Intraoperative ultrasound is useful in localizing small subcortical tumors, particularly small metastatic neoplasms surrounded by edematous brain.[5] Tumors with considerable mass effect can be scanned prior to opening the dura, and cysts, often not defined by CT scans, can be localized and drained transdurally.[9,10] With the resulting decrease in the mass, the dura then becomes less tense, and an open approach with tumor resection becomes possible with less risk to the surrounding or overlying brain. Deep tumors can be biopsied (Fig. 47-4) as described above.[5,9] Specimens may

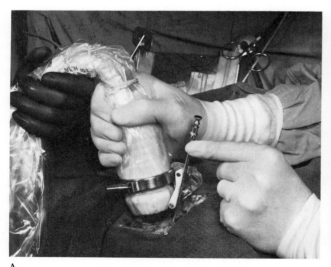

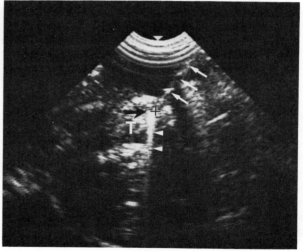

A   B

Figure 47-4 *A.* Biopsy of a deep intracranial tumor, using continuous ultrasound guidance and an instrument guide attached to the draped scanhead by a metal ring. The scanhead is in contact with the surface of the dura, and a thin layer of saline is used as a coupling agent. *B.* Static image of the real-time ultrasound scan of the brain, showing a deep tumor (T) with a plus sign marking the target area (the center of the tumor). Using the instrument guide, a biopsy probe (*white arrows*) was advanced to the target under continuous ultrasound guidance. The area of increased echogenicity corresponds to the tip of the probe (*large black arrow*), with reverberation beneath it (*arrowheads*).

be taken from various areas of the tumor; in the case of low-grade gliomas, this is most helpful in interpreting a pathologist's reading of the frozen section as "low-grade glioma vs. area of gliosis near a tumor," as the exact position of the biopsy probe is known. Following resection of a tumor, the area of resection can be filled with saline and any residual tumor visualized.[10] A portion of a tumor, such as a meningioma, could remain behind a normal structure just out of the neurosurgeon's view; this can be imaged and then resected.

Abscesses

A brain abscess may be localized and drained under continuous ultrasound guidance; the abscess cavity can be seen to decrease in size as the pus is aspirated. Multiple brain abscesses can now be localized and drained. This additional exploration was previously thought to be too traumatic to the brain. Certain abscesses are loculated, and each of these separate areas of the abscess can be identified by real-time ultrasound and drained.

Trauma

Intracerebral hematomas can be visualized with ultrasound and the best approach to them planned. Often the hematoma appears larger on CT scan than with ultrasound because of areas of contusion that may surround the hematoma. Multiple hematomas, depending on their age, may be aspirated under ultrasound guidance. With such aspiration, fresh hemorrhage may be induced, and this can be seen immediately on the video screen of the ultrasound scanner.

In patients with penetrating head injuries, indriven bone fragments can be visualized within the brain by ultrasound. Foreign bodies such as bullet fragments, as well as nonradiopaque foreign bodies such as plastic or some types of glass, can be seen with ultrasound.

Placement of Ventricular Catheters

Ventricular catheters can be placed in optimal position in hydrocephalic patients with the use of intraoperative ultrasound (Fig. 47-5).[9] In infants with an open anterior fontanelle, the placement of the ventricular catheter can easily be monitored by placement of the scanhead on the anterior fontanelle.[12] In patients with normal-sized or small lateral ventricles (e.g., patients with cerebral edema for intracranial pressure monitoring; patients requiring placement of an Ommaya reservoir and ventricular catheter for chemotherapy), the ventricular catheter can be placed accurately.[9] Even if there is no free flow of CSF out of the catheter, some air may be injected via the catheter, and this can be seen by ultrasound to bubble into the ventricle, thereby confirming the intraventricular location of the catheter.

Vascular Lesions

The role of intraoperative ultrasound in patients with vascular lesions is still unclear. The authors have on several occasions found small vascular malformations (5 mm diame-

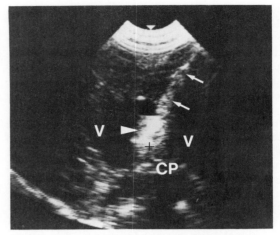

Figure 47-5 Static image of a real-time ultrasound scan of the brain in the sagittal plane in a patient with hydrocephalus. The target area is marked on the screen with a plus sign. Using the instrument guide, a finned ventricular catheter (*arrows*) was advanced into position; the tip of the catheter can be seen (*arrowhead*) as more echogenic than the rest of the catheter. Lateral ventricle (V); choroid plexus (CP).

ter) in a patient with recurrent cerebral hemorrhages and normal cerebral angiograms. It may be of use in finding feeding arteries in patients with large arteriovenous malformations. The role of ultrasound is as yet not clear in the detection of thrombosis of aneurysms or in determination of the thickness of the wall of the aneurysmal sac in the debulking of giant intracranial aneurysms.

Other Uses

During an operative procedure, should there be swelling of the brain, the source of the swelling may be visualized. Hemorrhage has been demonstrated in areas near resected vascular malformations (but not necessarily at the site of the resection) or from bleeding beneath the brain. In a patient with an aneurysm at the junction of the internal carotid and posterior communicating arteries, sudden swelling of the brain was noted by the authors. Ultrasound scanning showed that there was no hemorrhage in the region of the aneurysm but that there had been hemorrhage into the interhemispheric fissure from a bridging vein.

Intraspinal

Exploration of the spinal cord is hazardous; the intraoperative localization of intramedullary lesions has included aspiration of the enlarged portion of the spinal cord and/or posterior myelotomy with microsurgical exploration. The dural sac cannot be explored in the operating room without opening it, and the portion of the spinal canal beneath the spinal cord cannot be visualized by the surgeon. With the development of intraoperative real-time ultrasound scanning in patients with intraspinal lesions, these problems have been solved.[6]

With the patient in a prone position, a laminectomy is performed. The wound is then filled with saline and the scanhead is touched to the saline. This gives a "water path" from the scanhead to the dural sac and its contents. As the scanhead does not touch the dural surface, there is no injury to the spinal cord. Using a frequency of 7.5 MHz, a high-resolution image of the spinal cord and its coverings may be obtained. The lateral and anterior aspects of the spinal cord can be visualized also. Depending upon the orientation of the scanhead, transaxial or sagittal planes may be imaged. In transaxial sections the dural sac and subarachnoid space can be seen, as well as the spinal cord with associated pulsating arteries, the central canal, and nerve roots and dentate ligaments (Fig. 47-6). The central canal is best imaged in sagittal cuts, as are the disc spaces and surfaces of the vertebral bodies.

Intramedullary Lesions

Intraoperative ultrasound is very helpful in delineating intramedullary lesions.[6] Tumors are more echogenic and thus appear on the video screen as whiter than the normal spinal cord (Fig. 47-7). Prior to opening the dura, it can be determined at what point there is tumor and where it comes closest to the posterior aspect of the spinal cord, apropos of biopsy or resection. Cysts, including those within tumors, may be visualized (Fig. 47-7) and aspirated under ultrasound guidance prior to manipulating the spinal cord. Multiple fluid-filled channels are noted in syringomyelia; the largest and most accessible of these can be found by ultrasound and a shunting procedure done. Following drainage, all the fluid-filled cavities may collapse, or the ultrasound scan may show that certain of them are not interconnected, necessitating shunting of those also. Before ultrasound, operative results in syringomyelia were poor, perhaps because, the condition was only partially treated by shunting only one of several syrinx systems.[6]

Intradural Extramedullary Tumors

Prior to opening the dura, the exact location and dimensions of an intradural extramedullary tumor can be imaged. The displacement of the spinal cord can be seen and the operative approach planned accordingly. The complete anterior extent of a tumor can be determined.

Extradural-Intradural Tumors

Intraspinal tumors such as schwannomas often have an intradural and an extradural component (Fig. 47-8). The extent of each of these can be determined by ultrasound, as can the completeness of the resection.

Spondylosis and Disc Herniation

In patients with cervical spondylosis following a multi-level decompressive cervical laminectomy, the dural sac was noted to pulsate and it was the impression of the authors that

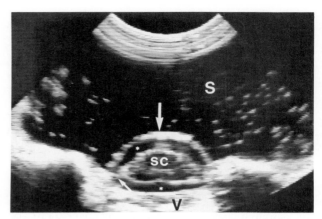

Figure 47-6 Transaxial ultrasound scan of the spinal cord. A laminectomy has been performed, and the wound is filled with saline (S). The white dots within the saline are air bubbles; the white concentric rings seen at the top of the image are the near-field artifact, caused by reverberations within the cap of the scanhead. Posterior surface of dural sac (*large arrow*); spinal cord (SC); nerve root and dentate ligament (*small arrow*); subarachnoid space (*asterisks*); vertebral body (V).

the spinal cord was well decompressed; however, ultrasound scanning showed that, although there was a good posterior subarachnoid space, the spinal cord was still compressed anteriorly by one or more bony bars. Indeed, the spinal cord rocked back and forth over an anterior bar much like a teeter-totter. With this information at hand after the patient had recovered from the laminectomy, the bony bar was resected via an anterior approach.

Herniated lumbar discs have been visualized by ultrasound following laminectomy; after discectomy and evacuation of free disc fragments, the extent of removal of the anterior encroachment on the dural sac and nerve roots could be assessed. Residual displacement of the dural sac and roots was corrected by further removal of more disc material or of an unsuspected disc fragment.

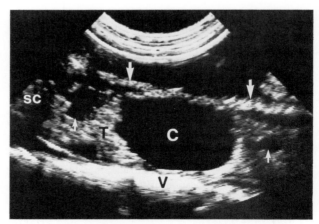

Figure 47-7 Sagittal ultrasound scan showing a cystic low-grade glioma of the spinal cord. Posterior dura (*large arrows*); large cyst (C); smaller cysts (*small arrows*); tumor (T); normal spinal cord (SC); vertebral body (V).

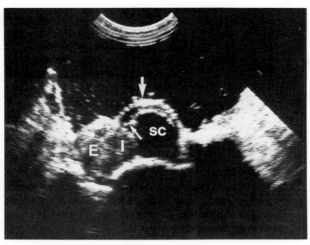

Figure 47-8 Transaxial ultrasound scan showing an extradural-intradural tumor (schwannoma) displacing and rotating the spinal cord (SC) to the contralateral side. Extradural portion of tumor (E); intradural portion of tumor (I); dura (*large arrow*); nerve root and dentate ligament (*small arrow*).

References

1. Backlund EO, Levander B, Greitz T: Stereotactic exploration of brain tumours by ultrasound. Acta Radiol [Diagn] (Stockh) 16: 117–122, 1975.
2. Brownbill D: The clinical value of echoencephalography. Aust NZ J Surg 40: 74–78, 1970.
3. Chandler WF, Knake JE, McGillicuddy JE, Lillehei KO, Sil-ver TM: Intraoperative use of real-time ultrasonography in neurosurgery. J Neurosurg 57: 157–163, 1982.
4. Christensen EE, Curry TS III, Dowdey JE: *An Introduction to the Physics of Diagnostic Radiology*, 2d ed. Philadelphia, Lea & Febiger, 1978, pp 361–394.
5. Dohrmann GJ, Rubin JM: Use of ultrasound in neurosurgical operations: A preliminary report. Surg Neurol 16: 362–366, 1981.
6. Dohrmann GJ, Rubin JM: Intraoperative ultrasound imaging of the spinal cord: Syringomyelia, cysts, and tumors. A preliminary report. Surg Neurol 18: 395–399, 1982.
7. Glasauer FE, Schlagenhauff RE: The use of intraoperative echoencephalography. Neurology (Minneap) 20: 1103–1107, 1970.
8. Masuzawa H, Kamitani H, Sato J, Inoya H, Hachiya J, Sakai F: Intraoperative application of sector scanning electronic ultrasound in neurosurgery. Neurol Med Chir (Tokyo) 21: 277–285, 1981.
9. Rubin JM, Dohrmann GJ: Use of ultrasonically guided probes and catheters in neurosurgery. Surg Neurol 18: 143–148, 1982.
10. Rubin JM, Dohrmann GJ: Intraoperative neurosurgical ultrasound in the localization and characterization of intracranial masses. Radiology 148:519–524, 1983.
11. Rubin JM, Mirfakhraee M, Duda EE, Dohrmann GJ, Brown F: Intraoperative ultrasound examination of the brain. Radiology 137: 831–832, 1980.
12. Shkolnik A, McLone DG: Intraoperative real-time ultrasonic guidance of ventricular shunt placement in infants. Radiology 141: 515–517, 1981.
13. Tanaka K, Ito K, Wagai T: The localization of brain tumors by ultrasonic techniques: A clinical view of 111 cases. J Neurosurg 23: 135–147, 1965.
14. Voorhies RM, Engel I, Gamache FW Jr, Patterson RH Jr, Fraser RAR, Lavyne MH, Schneider M: Intraoperative localization of subcortical brain tumors: Further experience with B-mode real-time sector scanning. Neurosurgery 12: 189–194, 1983.
15. Wild JJ, Reid JM: The effects of biological tissues on 15-mc pulsed ultrasound. J Acoust Soc Am 25: 270–280, 1953.

48

Self-Retaining Retractors

I. M. Greenberg

The evolution of instruments for specialized purposes in surgery is not often given attention, yet mechanical improvements in instrument design and functioning have afforded surgeons opportunities to develop new techniques and greater overall flexibility. For example, self-retaining retractors, particularly those designed for use in neurosurgery, have given surgeons many obvious benefits. These include the reduction of instances of inadvertent suction of tissue; prevention of sudden and unexpected stress to tissue; controlled, precise retraction for long periods of time; and the ability of the surgeon to work with both hands free. Some of these devices are now designed to assist the neurosurgeon with many other tasks in addition to retraction. Interestingly, many of the modifications made to these instruments have come about directly because of the needs (and frustrations) of individual surgeons.

Types of Self-Retaining Retractors

In general there are two categories of self-retaining retractors: some are mounted on the skull, with either direct contact to bone or tissue or indirect contact via a skull clamp; others are mounted on the operating table.

One variety of skull-mounted self-retaining retractor consists of those which are secured directly into an extra drill hole in the skull, e.g., the DeMartel retractor. This instrument, one of the first such devices employed in neurosurgery, was quite simple, consisting only of a post mounted in a drill hole in which a single retractor blade could be mounted. Its limitations were apparent, however, since each retractor could hold only one blade; an additional drill hole was required for each additional blade, and the locations of these holes had to be geometrically precise. Further, the thickness and strength of the skull are simply not consistent enough overall to permit placement of the post in all locations. Thus, while this type of self-retaining retractor was used in some procedures, there was a need to improve upon it.

Hamby, criticizing the DeMartel self-retaining retractor as "clumsy and unstable" (Hamby WB: Personal communication, 1981), modified the device so that it would no longer be necessary to mount the retractor blade on a post secured in a drill hole. Instead, Hamby's self-retaining retractor could be mounted on the edge of the craniotomy wound.[8] Consequently several Hamby self-retaining retractors could be used at the same time and with much greater ease than was possible with the DeMartel retractor. Differences in skull strength and exposure of anchoring bone according to anatomical location, however, were still problems which limited the use of this device.

Other surgeons also sought to improve the capabilities of self-retaining retractors by adapting them so that one instrument could hold several retractor blades simultaneously and could be mounted either on the edge of the skull or in a drill hole. Both the Malis[13] and the Heifetz[19] self-retaining retractors were examples of this, as both could be mounted in either fashion. Instead of attaching the retractor blade directly to the mounting device, however, both these retractors included rods of various lengths which were secured to the mounting point. Retractor blades were then affixed at various positions along the rod. Thus the surgeon had a choice of rod length and blade position, as well as the manner of mounting and the location of these self-retaining retractors. The Dott-Gillingham retractor (sometimes referred to as the Edinburgh retractor) is similar in its use of a rod for multiple retractors, although it can be mounted only in a drill hole.[19]

Another group of skull-mounted self-retaining retractors are those secured by tension against muscle and soft tissue rather than by a connection directly to bone. An immediately obvious limitation is the relative lack of stability of these devices, although Jannetta et al.[10] compensated for this by clamping the retractor to the drapes.

One uniquely designed self-retaining retractor in this group was developed by House and Urban.[2,9] Their mechanically geared retractor blade holder is attached to an Adson retractor and allows finely controlled retraction. One limitation, however, is that only one retractor blade can be used on each device. The House-Urban self-retaining retractor has most often been used for procedures in and about the auditory canal.

The most commonly used self-retaining retractors of this group, however, are modified Weitlaner retractors. The most usual adaptation of the Weitlaner retractor is the attachment of posts to its retractor arms, the so-called pillar and post design. Jannetta et al., for example, use a Weitlaner retractor with two posts on each arm, to which are attached rods on which retractor blades can be secured. They state that this arrangement is both stable and effective.[10] The Kennerdell-Maroon retractor is another similarly modified Weitlaner retractor, which has most often been used in procedures about the orbit. The addition of posts and rods results in self-retaining retractors which are similar in concept to the skull-mounted Malis, Dott-Gillingham, and Heifetz self-retaining retractors mentioned above. All these devices provide options for positioning the retractor blades through the articulations of the posts, rods, and blades. This feature, however, underscores a limitation common to all these devices: the support system for retraction is very close to the operative site. At such close proximity, the articulations provided by the retractor arms, rods, and blades are too few to give flexibility for retraction from all directions about the operative site.

The introduction of a flexible retractor-holding rod whose position could easily be controlled by the surgeon created a completely new concept in self-retaining retractors, offering an alternative to skull-mounted self-retaining retractors. This flexible, ball-jointed device was developed approximately 20 years ago in the Netherlands, where it was known as the Easycheck. Its original function was to hold test indicators in machine shops where precise adjustments had to be made quickly in order to measure concentricity and out-of-round conditions to fine tolerances. After its importation to the United States, the name was changed to Flexbar (Flexbar Machine Corp., Farmingdale, N.Y.), and the device was re-engineered for greater stability and longevity in medical and industrial uses (Adler D: Personal communication, 1982). Two physicians saw the potential advantages in use of the Flexbar as a retractor holder. Dohn and Carton mounted a flexible retractor-holding arm on the edge of a craniotomy wound with a clamp and secured a retractor blade at the other end of the arm (Dohn DF: Personal communication, 1981). The tension, and therefore the position, of the Flexbar arm and its retractor blade could then be adjusted by means of an eccentric cam. In contrast, Apfelbaum chose to mount a flexible arm on a Weitlaner retractor. This combination proved quite practical, particularly in posterior fossa surgery (Apfelbaum R: Personal communication, 1981).

Currently a popular flexible self-retaining retractor is the Leyla retractor (Aesculap, Tuttlingen, Germany), introduced by Yasargil.[24] This device consists of a long flexible arm which is secured by a clamp to the edge of the cranial opening. Another clamp permits two Leyla arms to be mounted at one location, further increasing the versatility of this instrument. An additional advantage of this retractor is that it will accept a variety of retractor blades, with or without handles.

At the same time, the Leyla retractor presented surgeons with a number of mechanical difficulties. Primary among these were problems relating to adjustment. At times it proved difficult to tighten the arm sufficiently to prevent drifting of the retractor blade[3] or to secure the mounting device so as to prevent twisting of the mounting platform.[1,21] Sugita et al.[21] reported that both the adjustment knob and the extreme length of the flexible arm tended to protrude and interfere with the surgeon's hands. In addition, the dura and adjacent tissues beneath the clamp used to secure the Leyla retractor sometimes bled, seemingly as a result of both the size of the clamp and the pressure required to stabilize the instrument.[1,11,21]

One alternative proposed by Yasargil and Fox[25] is to mount the Leyla retractor on the operating table. They utilize an Aesculap retractor-holding bar (Aesculap, Tuttlingen, Germany) for this purpose. Similarly, Kanshepolsky reported the use of a U-shaped bar on which the Leyla arms can be mounted.[11] In both instances the bar is fixed to the operating table and the Leyla arms then secured to the bar. Sugita et al.[21] pointed out, however that these modifications of the Leyla retractor do not completely solve the problems described above. Sugita et al. and Malis[13] have both expressed concern that mounting the retractor arm on the operating table (instead of on either the head or a pin headrest) would appear to allow the possibility of head or retractor-arm movements occurring independently of each other, resulting in movement of the retractor blades against the brain. Further, the length of the Leyla arms would tend to amplify any movements over the distance of the arm, exacerbating this problem.[21]

Thus, while all the self-retaining retractors mentioned above have found acceptance and proved themselves to be valuable tools for the neurosurgeon, each also has limitations. This is particularly true for those which require an additional hole to be drilled in the skull. In some locations, e.g., in the posterior fossa area, it is difficult to provide a mounting post with sufficient stability to provide a base for retraction. In addition, consideration of the variables involved and the drilling of the hole is time-consuming, and the surgeon may not obtain a good mounting in any event. Securing the retractor on the edge of the craniotomy wound is not a great improvement, since here too, bleeding may occur or the skull may simply be unable to bear the strain of the retractor holder. Unseen underlying anatomical structures (e.g., the sagittal sinus, sigmoid sinus, and motor cortex) make it difficult to mount retractor holders supported by either posts or clamps in certain locations. In addition, when the self-retaining retractor is mounted at the edge of the skull, it tends either to further reduce the size of the opening available to the surgeon or to compel enlargement of the craniotomy wound to accommodate it. Pillars, posts, and rods increase the surgeon's options for the positioning of retractors but are capable of only a finite degree of adjustment. Self-retaining retractors mounted via tension on muscle and soft tissue avoid the problem of bone consistency and strength but are inherently less stable. In addition, their location near the operative site presents the same difficulties in terms of crowding.

Flexible retractor holders overcome many of the limitations of adjustment, since their range of movement is far greater than other types of self-retaining retractors. Unfortunately, when they are mounted on the skull or Weitlaner retractors they are subject to the same limitations noted above. Mounting them on the operating table reduces these difficulties but adds the additional risk of retractor-blade movement. Also, many of the self-retaining retractors mentioned thus far suffer from lack of attention to human factors engineering, or ergonomics.

The term *ergonomics* was first used by K. F. H. Murrell almost 20 years ago in discussions of the interface between humans and machines.[14] Referred to as *human factors engineering* in the United States, this science has infrequently been applied to neurosurgery. Pearce and Shackel[17] have stated that "neglect of human factors in the design of instruments can lead to inefficiency by causing the user unnecessary mental and physical strain. The whole job takes longer to do, and the risk of error increases." Michael Patkin[15,16] has written extensively on the application of ergonomics to microsurgery, and the author of this chapter has frequently discussed the importance of applying the principles of work efficiency to neurosurgery.[3-7] The relevance of these principles to self-retaining retractors lies chiefly in the need to improve the design and performance of these instruments as well as the goals of reducing tremor and fatigue and improving surgical techniques.

One approach used to remedy the difficulties mentioned above was to use a flexible arm without mounting it on either the operating table or the skull. Since pin headrests such as the Mayfield or Gardner headrest (Codman and Shurtleff, Inc. Randolph, Mass.) are mounted on the table and then firmly secured to the skull, they have become the base of support for some self-retaining retractors. Greenberg,[3-7] Sugita et al.,[21-23] and Fukushima and Sano[1] have used flexible retractor-holding arms mounted on skull clamps instead. Fukushima and Sano have mounted up to four Leyla retractor arms on a specially developed clamp which is secured to a Mayfield headrest. Both Greenberg and Sugita and his teams, however, have independently designed retractor systems which provide the surgeon with other options in addition to holding retractor blades. Both these systems include the concept of supporting flexible arms with headrests, eliminating the difficulties associated with mounting a retractor holder in a drill hole or at the edge of the cranial wound. The Greenberg Retractor and Handrest, A Universal System (Codman and Shurtleff), described in greater detail below, can be used with either the widely available Mayfield or the Gardner skull clamps, while the Sugita system requires a specially designed skull clamp to which is attached a special multipurpose frame attached to the headrest. Both systems permit several flexible retractor holders to be used simultaneously, regardless of the location of the surgery or the size of the skull opening.

The Sugita system includes small (2, 4 and 6 mm wide) tapered retractors. Because of the length of the Leyla flexible arms used with the Sugita system, Sugita et al.[23] report that there is sometimes difficulty in positioning them so that they do not interfere with the surgeon's hands. They have found that either by placing the Leyla arms under their multipurpose frame and below the surgeon's hands or by positioning the arms above the surgeon's hands and attaching them to a handrest attached to the frame, they can prevent the arms from interfering with the surgeon's movements. Securing the Leyla arm to the handrest also provides increased opportunities for retractor placement.

The inclusion of handrests in a self-retaining retraction and dissection system is unique to the Greenberg and Sugita systems and is a direct result of consideration of human factors when principles of engineering are applied to surgery. Patkin[15] has stated that support for the surgeon's limbs is vital for improving the accuracy of fine movements in microsurgical procedures. The support (or fulcrum), when placed as close to the operative site as possible, reduces the arc of movement of the tip of the surgical instruments as they are used. This has the effect of increasing the surgeon's control and thus improving the accuracy of instrument movements. In addition, muscle tremor and fatigue are reduced, since the arm, shoulder, and back no longer have to bear the full weight of the arm, hand and instrument. This has been accomplished in several ways. Malis,[13] who states that support is required at the forearm, uses a modified Mayo stand. Patkin[16] and Lim[12] prefer that support should be provided to the length of the forearm as well as the hand and even the tips of the fingers. Although Sugita et al.[21] note that handrests can be a hindrance to rapid movements of the hands, they have designed an L-shaped bar which screws into their multipurpose frame and serves as a handrest. The Greenberg system includes a handrest which is mounted via a Flexbar. Both these systems enable the surgeon to support other instruments mechanically as well—e.g., a fiberoptic light source, patty storage tray, suction tube, and microretractors. These two systems differ primarily in their components and the additional options of adjustment of the instruments in the Greenberg system.

The Greenberg System

Conceptually the Greenberg system combines the ball-and-cable design flexible retractor holder with the additional articulations and support provided by metal rods peripheral to the surgical field. Originally its design was similar to Yasargil's Leyla retractor in that the flexible arms were clamped to the edge of the craniotomy wound. The intent, however, was to increase the number of retractor blades which could be used at one time, so the mounting clamp was redesigned to hold a hexagonal bar ¼ in. in diameter and 6 to 10 in. in length). Up to six Flexbars could be mounted on this bar at any one time. The bar itself could be moved laterally within the mounting clamp, further increasing opportunities for retractor placement. Despite the success of this system, it nevertheless limited retraction to a line of 180 degrees from one side of the craniotomy wound. The desire to have a self-retaining retractor which would permit the surgeon to retract from 360 degrees about the operative field led to the development of the Greenberg system as it currently exists. Instead of the long Leyla arms, the Greenberg retractor includes shorter Flexbars. The system also includes versatile vises in which a variety of other instruments can be held. Thus while the number of components may initially seem imposing, the Greenberg system was designed on the basis of human factors and is the product of a deliberate effort to provide surgeons with as many options as possible.

Assembly

The Greenberg system provides a variety of components with which the surgeon creates a supporting framework for the mechanical support of retractor blades, suction tube, patty tray, microdissectors, handrests,[3] fiberoptic illuminator (Bookwalter JR: Personal communication, 1982), scissors,[5–7] a pneumatic drill,[5] and other instruments. The discussion which follows outlines the most popular methods of assembling and using the system, which was designed to provide for alternative techniques as required.

The first component used in the Greenberg system is the primary clamp. As with the flexible arm, industry's machine shops again supplied an important part of this instrument. The Kant-Twist clamp, an invention of Paul Saurenman of the California Institute of Technology in the early 1920s used for clamping setups for machining, was selected as best able to mount securely on a pin headrest (Adler D: Personal communication, 1982). A steel rod 6 in. long and ½ in. in diameter extends from this clamp. Next, longer (12 in.) rods were attached to specially designed vises; these were designated secondary clamps. These new vises were constructed so as to be capable of a high degree of mechanical advantage and gripping surface for secure mounting on both the primary and other secondary bars.

The flexible arms which are the core of the Greenberg system are Flexbars, 9 in. in length and ⅜ in. in diameter. A major difference from the Leyla arms (apart from the shorter length) is the development of an improved device for constantly adjusting the tension of the cable inside the Flexbar. Previously, flexible arms were adjusted by means of an eccentric cam attached to the cable. With use, however, the cable eventually stretched, accounting for the drifting of the arm noted earlier. While it is possible to readjust the cam mechanism to compensate for the longer cable, this can be an awkward, time-consuming, and ineffective procedure. A screw adjustment mechanism attached to a self-compensating drawbar developed by the Flexbar engineers virtually eliminates these problems and ensures that the flexible arms of the Greenberg system will not drift.

The Flexbars of the Greenberg retractor differ from other flexible self-retaining retractor holders in another important respect: the design of the vises which are used with them. At one end is a vise which holds the Flexbar firmly to the secondary bars. At the other end of the Flexbar is a specially designed minivise in which the handles of retractor blades and other instruments (up to ¼ in. in diameter) can be secured. Another newly developed vise, the maxivise, can hold larger instrument handles (up to ½ in. in diameter), while it is, in turn, held by the minivise. A third vise holds handles of up to 1 in. in diameter.

The retractor blades used with this system are 4 in. long and range in ⅛ in. intervals from ¼ to ¾ in. in width. The retractors are attached to shafts which are 2 in. long by ⅛ in. in diameter and fit into the minivises. In addition, microdissectors of from 1 to 7 mm in width can be mounted in maxivises for more precise retraction.[3]

The inclusion of the primary and secondary bars in this self-retaining retraction system enables the surgeon to construct a box around the perimeter of the operative field. The Flexbars holding retractors can be attached at any point around the field, so the surgeon has 360 degrees of opportunity for retraction. Several benefits derive from the fact that the Greenberg system is mounted via primary and secondary bars to the pin headrest. First, there is no need for extra drill holes or stress upon the edge of the skull. The craniotomy wound can, in fact, be smaller, since the mounting clamps are not in immediate proximity. Finally, it is possible to retract less tissue, since smaller retractor blades can be used at exactly the positions required.

The Greenberg self-retaining retractor system also includes handrests. These 1 ½-in.-diameter, 10-in.-long hollow steel tubes are attached to Flexbars which can be clamped by means of a vise grip to either the primary or secondary bars as needed. The handrests may be used singly or in pairs to support the surgeon's forearms and/or hands. The handrests provide stability for the hands of a surgeon in either a standing or a sitting position when the patient is either sitting or prone. Since the handrests of the Greenberg system are attached with Flexbars, they can be adjusted as required by the surgeon, permitting complete freedom of movement.

Experience with the system and consideration of the principles of ergonomics mentioned above has led to incorporation of another feature, that is, continuous suctioning in the microsurgical field by means of a "sump pump." This has been achieved in several ways. Spetzler developed a plastic suctioning device, the Spetzler MicroVac (PMT Inc., Hopkins, Minn.), made malleable by a wire running through its length which can be placed in the operative site without being held by an assistant (Spetzler RL: Personal communication, 1981).[20] Reichman modified a Frazier suction tube (size 12) (V. Mueller, Linden, N.J.) by attaching the shield from a Sherwood Medicut cannula (18 gauge, 2 in. long) (Sherwood Medical Industries, St. Louis, Mo.) (Reichman OH: Personal communication). A Deseret Angiocath (18 gauge, 2 in. long) (Deseret Co., Sandy, Utah) is an acceptable substitute for the cannula shield. Both the Spetzler MicroVac and the Reichman-modified suction tube can be attached to a Flexbar and inserted into the deepest part of the wound to provide continuous stationary suctioning. (It is necessary, however, to fill the thumbhole of the Frazier suction tube with bone wax.) If desired, this sump pump can remain in the microsurgical field throughout the procedure, precisely positioned and repositioned by the surgeon as necessary.

Although the Greenberg system can be used with either the Gardner or the Mayfield pin headrests, differences in the physical designs of these instruments require slightly different protocols when assembling the system (Fig. 48-1). Similarly, the assembly procedures vary slightly depending upon whether the patient is prone or sitting (Figs. 48-1, 48-2). When using either of these headrests, and with the patient either prone or sitting, it is advisable to first rotate, flex and/or extend the patient's head into the position required for surgery. The pin headrest should then be applied so that its base is parallel with the floor of the operating room. This is done in order to provide a perspective and a sense of symmetry, so that the surgeon can more easily assemble the foundation of the Greenberg system, i.e., a boxlike frame around the surgical field. Assembly of the system is initiated only after the pin headrest is in place and the patient draped; sterile conditions are then maintained, with the primary clamps applied over the sterile drapes covering the headrest. The primary clamps are the supporting foundation for the rest of the system; once the secondaries forming the box have been set up, the use of the system is the same with either the Mayfield or the Gardner headrests and with the patient either lying or sitting.

Use of the System

The peripheral box of secondary bars supporting the Greenberg system has sufficient rigidity to assist in the retraction of scalp or skin. Instead of the usual practice of attaching the retracted scalp to the drapes (with the accompanying instability), small towel clips may be attached to the scalp; rubber bands are then secured to the handles of these clips and are twisted around the secondary bars. This arrangement exerts sufficient force for effective, stable retraction. This technique also permits a smaller incision with the rolling back of scalp and the underlying muscle.

After the brain has been retracted, the suction tube (sump pump) should be moved into the field from the periphery where it was placed earlier. Generally, the sump pump should be positioned between the two handrests (which are almost parallel to each other) at either the top or the bottom of the surgical field. The tip is inserted as deep into the field as the surgeon requires. If the tip is placed at the deepest point of the operative site, the field will remain dry; if the tip is elevated slightly, the field will be filled with saline so that coagulation of structures can take place with less charring and adhesion of tissues to the bipolar coagulator.

When dissecting an aneurysm, all surgeons are faced with occasions when the aneurysm ruptures during dissection. The problem is normally handled as originally described by J. L. Poppen.[18] Using his technique, however, it is necessary for the surgeon to hold the suction tube in one hand to keep the field dry while applying the aneurysm clip with the other hand. The author has experienced this problem of rupture and hemorrhage of an aneurysm during dissection on a few occasions. Since the Greenberg system was in place and the sump pump was in the field at the time (secured by a Flexbar), it was possible to modify Poppen's technique by supporting the suction tube mechanically instead of by hand. The plastic tip on the end of the Frazier suction tube can be removed quickly and the large suction tip brought to the rupture site. The aneurysm sac can be maneuvered into the tip of the suction tube; the tube is secured in its position by tightening (if necessary) the Flexbar. This has two benefits: first, the field is clear and dry (as Poppen intended), thus the neck of the aneurysm is sufficiently exposed to facilitate the application of an aneurysm clip while maintaining patency of the parent vessel; second, the surgeon is able to apply the clip with both hands free. Thus the procedure is completed more quickly and efficiently and with far less emotional tension than is usual in such circumstances. After the clip has been applied, the plastic tip can easily be returned to the suction tube as the procedure continues.

The use of mechanically supported microdissectors has been found an especially useful option possible with the Greenberg system. One instance of this is in the dissection of aneurysms, where the instability of the tissues creates difficulty in visualization of the neck and application of the clip. By using the microdissector to give direct support to the aneurysm, the surgeon can more easily dissect to its neck, facilitating application of the clip.

The precision possible with these narrow (1- to 7-mm) blades allows the surgeon to reduce the area of brain tissue

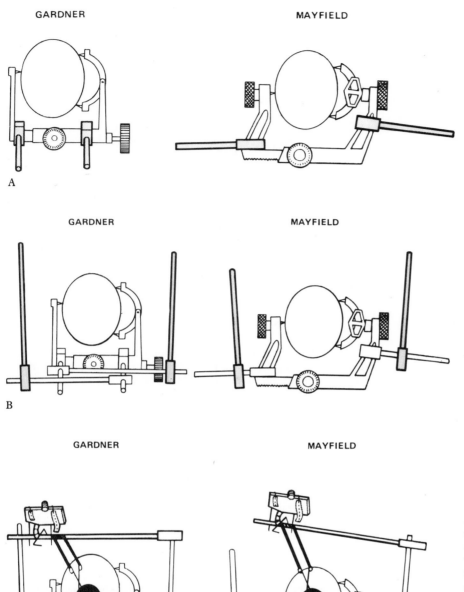

Figure 48-1 *A.* The first step in assembling the Greenberg system is the attachment of the primary bars to the pin headrest. Note the differences in the positions of these bars when using the Gardner or Mayfield pin headrests. *B.* The next step in assembling the Greenberg system with the Gardner headrest requires that two secondary bars be attached as shown. Then, with either headrest, secondary bars are added to each side, angled so that they are below the operative site. *C.* Additional secondaries are added to construct a box around the field. The plane is to be positioned below the operative field. The author has developed a special patty storage tray that can be mounted on the Greenberg system near the operative site. (Note: Although the surgery has not begun at this point in assembly of the system, the craniotomy wound and other instruments are included from here on in order to illustrate various options in the use of the system.)

which is manipulated. Their relatively narrow shaft gives them an advantage over tapered retractors, since the field is not obscured by the shaft. Mechanically supported microinstruments can be used for retraction, sharp and blunt dissection, support, and compression. In addition, the small size of the microdissectors permits their use in retracting small portions of tissue, even in areas crowded with vital structures. As a result, there is a reduced risk of swelling and neurological deficit postoperatively. When they are used as mechanically supported retractors, they create a degree of

stability among the small structures in the field which cannot be achieved with hand-held instruments.

Since the Greenberg system allows retraction from any direction around the target area, the larger Greenberg retractors create a circle of retraction within which the sump pump and microdissectors are used while being supported mechanically. When used in the posterior fossa, microdissectors supported by the system will, for example, hold an acoustic neuroma away from the brain stem for long periods of time, preventing the necessity for redissection from the

GARDNER   MAYFIELD

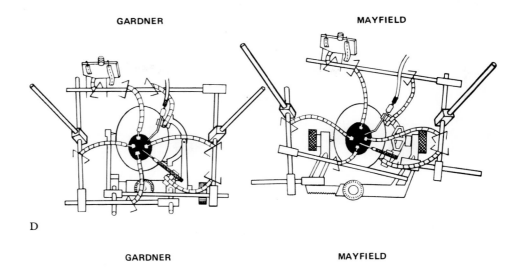

D

GARDNER   MAYFIELD

E

Figure 48-1 (*Continued*)

D. In preparation for mounting handrests, two more secondaries are mounted on either side of the box as shown. *E.* Two handrests are applied directly over the operative field and above the movements of retraction of brain, sump pump, and microdissector(s).

F. During surgery the sump pump is best placed in the deepest part of the operative field. Microdissector(s) should be attached at a point which will permit them to be used anywhere within the field. (Note: The handrest has been omitted from this drawing to better illustrate the other instruments. The profile of the instruments at this level should be low enough so as not to interfere with the dynamic movement of the handrests above and at level 2.)

GARDNER   MAYFIELD

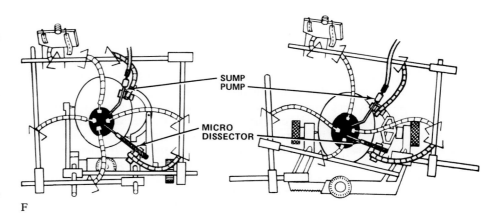

SUMP
PUMP

MICRO
DISSECTOR

F

brain stem or the repeat mobilization of the tumor. Similarly, in microvascular surgery for a cross-compression syndrome, a microdissector can hold a cranial nerve away from the blood vessel while a nonreactive substance is placed between the nerve and the blood vessel.

The mechanical support of other instruments in addition to self-retaining retractors presents the surgeon with many options when performing microsurgery. The techniques described above have facilitated the routine use of multiple instruments in the field at the same time. In addition to

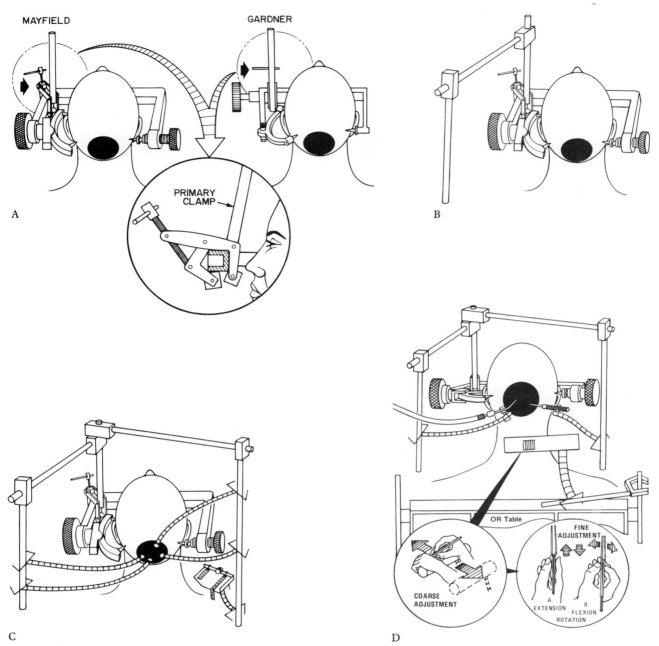

Figure 48-2 *A.* The assembly of the Greenberg system with the patient in a sitting position begins with the attachment of only one primary clamp to the pin headrest. The inset shows the correct position for securing the clamp for maximum stability. *B.* Secondary bars are added to the primary bar as shown. *C.* Flexbars are applied to the secondary bars with a unilateral exposure. For a bilateral exposure, additional secondary bars are added to allow retraction from the opposite side. Instruments can be affixed to any of these bars as required. *D.* When the patient is sitting, the sump pump and microdissector are attached and used in the same manner as when the patient is prone. The handrest is attached as shown. Positioning of the handrest itself (*inset*) executes coarse adjustment, while the surgeon's hand movements control fine adjustment of instruments directly (*inset*).

multiple retractors (three to six), the system provides support for instruments such as the sump pump and a microdissector, leaving the surgeon free to manipulate other instruments, such as a suction irrigator and a bipolar coagulator, by hand (Fig. 48-3).

The simultaneous presence of four instruments in a mi-

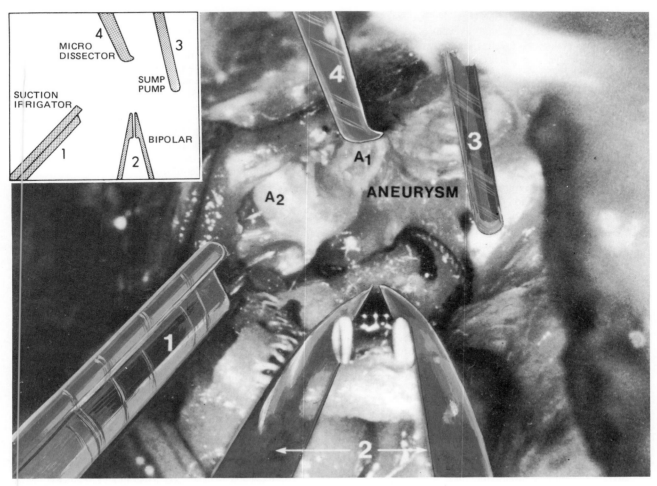

Figure 48-3 Retouched photograph showing four instruments in a microsurgical field. The microdissector (4), and the sump pump (3) are supported by the system. The bipolar forceps (2) is in the surgeon's right hand and the suction irrigator (1) in the left hand.

crosurgical field represents the type of evolution now taking place in microsurgery as a direct result of advances in biomedical engineering. While the surgeon continues to rely on basic hand-held instruments, a systems approach toward instrument use and support within the microsurgical field via mechanical aids increases the options and improves overall efficiency.

Levels of Instrument Performance

The routine use of four or more instruments in the field (in addition to retractor blades) created a need to bring more order to the system. This was accomplished with the development of the concept of levels of instrument placement in the system based on instrument performance.[5] Level 1 consists of the framework of secondary bars around the field and the retractor blades attached to it with Flexbars. Instrument performance at this level includes retraction and mechanical support of the sump pump and microdissector(s). The handrests are at level 2. Thus many of the functions

provided by the system are supported at level 1, while the surgeon's hand-held instruments are supported at level 2 via the handrests. When the patient is prone, the handrests are above the field. When the patient is sitting, the handrests are slightly below the operative field.

Developments and Trends

In assessing the effects of progress in instrument design, it seems clear that the practice of neurosurgery is the beneficiary of collaboration between surgeons and engineers. Advances in instrument design, particularly when influenced by the principles of ergonomics, have produced a vast armamentarium. The trend toward dependence upon instruments which function with some independence from the surgeon is clearly demonstrated by the development of self-retaining retractor systems like the Sugita and Greenberg systems, which provide mechanical support for a variety of instruments. Continuing developments of biomedical engineering are currently expanding these techniques. For example, recently a third performance level has been added to the Greenberg system. At level 3 mechanical support is provided for such dynamic instruments as microscissors and pneumatic drills, allowing the surgeon to use them without having to support their weight and thus giving these instruments stability and preciseness of movement during their use. This technique also reduces the number of entries to and exits from the field.[3,6,7]

The frustration and inventiveness of professionals seeking excellence in performance have been responsible for developments thus far, and the refinement of both instruments and techniques requires these same elements. The benefits of the collaboration discussed above between neurosurgeons, biomedical engineers, and engineers concerned with human factors represent only a sample of the potential gain which can be realized in the near future.

References

1. Fukushima T, Sano K: Simple retractor holder for the Mayfield skull clamp. Surg Neurol 13:320, 1980.
2. Glassock ME III: Surgical techniques for the removal of acoustic tumors: A system of operations. Arch Otolaryngol 88:618–627, 1968.
3. Greenberg IM: Self-retaining retractor and handrest system for neurosurgery. Neurosurgery 8:205–208, 1981.
4. Greenberg IM: New options for the microsurgeon: Multiple instrumentation in a single microsurgical field. Neurosurgery 9:566–572, 1981.
5. Greenberg IM: Staircase concept of instrument placement in microsurgery. Neurosurgery 9:696–702, 1981.
6. Greenberg IM: Proximity storage of instruments during microsurgery. Unpublished manuscript, 1982.
7. Greenberg IM: Rotation of scissors while fixed in the microsurgical field: A technique for increasing the surgeon's efficiency. Unpublished manuscript, 1982.
8. Hamby WB: Mechanical holder for retractors in neurosurgery. Am J Surg 36:732–733, 1937.
9. House WF: Surgical exposure of the internal auditory canal and its contents through the middle cranial fossa. Laryngoscope 71:1363–1385, 1961.
10. Jannetta PJ, Abbasy M, Maroon JC, Ramos FM, Albin MS: Etiology and definitive microsurgical treatment of hemifacial spasm: Operative techniques and results in 47 patients. J Neurosurg 47:321–328, 1977.
11. Kanshepolsky J: Extracranial holder for brain retractors: Technical note. J Neurosurg 46:835–836, 1977.
12. Lim ASM, Khoo CY, Ang BC: Practical microsurgery. Adv Ophthalmol 37:64–70, 1978.
13. Malis LI: Instrumentation and techniques in microsurgery. Clin Neurosurg 26:626–636, 1979.
14. Murrell KFH: Ergonomics: Man in His Working Environment. London, Chapman & Hall, 1965.
15. Patkin M: Ergonomics applied to the practice of microsurgery. Aust NZ J Surg 47:320–329, 1977.
16. Patkin M: Ergonomics and the operating microscope. Adv Ophthalmol 37:53–63, 1978.
17. Pearce BG, Shackel B: The ergonomics of scientific instrument design. J Phys E: Sci Instrum 12(6):447–454, 1979.
18. Poppen JL: An Atlas of Neurosurgical Techniques. Philadelphia, Saunders, 1960.
19. Rhoton AL: Instruments for removal of acoustic neuromas, in Silverstein H, Norrell H (eds): Neurological Surgery of the Ear. Birmingham, Alabama, Aesculapius, 1977, pp 291–302.
20. Spetzler RF, Iversen AA: Malleable microsurgical suction device: Technical note. J Neurosurg 54:704–705, 1981.
21. Sugita K, Hirota T, Mizutani T, Mutsuga N, Shibuya M, Tsugane R: A newly designed multipurpose microneurosurgical head frame: Technical note. J Neurosurg 48:656–657, 1978.
22. Sugita K, Kobayashi S, Shintani A, Mutsuga N: Microneurosurgery for aneurysms of the basilar artery. J Neurosurg 51:615–620, 1979.
23. Sugita K, Kobayashi S, Takemae T, Matsuo K, Yokoo A: Direct retraction method in aneurysm surgery: Technical note. J Neurosurg 53:417–419, 1980.
24. Yasargil MG: Microsurgery Applied to Neurosurgery. New York, Academic, 1969.
25. Yasargil MG, Fox JL: The microsurgical approach to acoustic neurinomas. Surg Neurol 2:393–398, 1974.

49

Automated Cutting and Suction

Martin L. Lazar

Neurosurgical advances in the treatment of mass lesions of the nervous system have occurred in a progressive fashion as a result of a combination of developments in several related fields. The improved diagnostic accuracy offered by neuro-imaging techniques coupled with neuropharmacologic and neuroanaesthetic management has permitted the neurosurgeon to intervene earlier in the course of nervous system diseases, in a more accurate fashion. One of the primary aspirations of neurosurgeons has been to remove these lesions while doing little or preferably no injury to contiguous vital structures. The advent of microneurosurgical techniques, instrumentation, and methods of approaching various regions of the brain while limiting the amount of retraction of the brain has heralded a new era for neurosurgery. Nevertheless, tumors of the nervous system are invariably physically situated in intimate contiguous relationship to vital sensitive centers or structures such as cerebral arteries and cranial nerves. For tumors which do not readily respond to suction removal by virtue of their firmer consistency, our neurosurgical predecessors were faced with the unenviable task of incising, curetting, or pulling these lesions, which added the obvious risks of extending injury to these contiguous or adjacent vital structures. The use of the cutting cautery loop has long been recognized for its potential hazards as well.

Surgical techniques have been developed to specifically address these issues. Among the early advances in instruments were suction devices with a cutting edge on the distal end. A later and significant advance in the attempt to remove tumors more safely by applying a greater physical force in a more controlled limited area and fashion was born from the experience of a neurotologist (Dr. William House) and the engineering laboratories of Urban Engineering Company in Burbank, California: the House-Urban vacuum rotary dissector. This unit is electrically powered by a compact motor. An impressive experience was developed with this unit by neurotologists as well as neurosurgeons, particularly in the treatment of acoustic neuromas. In recent years, other neurosurgeons and engineers have attempted to utilize more modern technology to improve upon the speed and

accuracy of tumor resection while diminishing some of the disadvantages of previously developed instruments. A significant advance occurred with the development of an ultrasonic aspiration device by Flamm et al.[1] called the CUSA (Cavitron ultrasonic surgical aspirator, Cooper Medical Devices, Mountain View, Calif.).

An alternative approach resulted in the development of the Biotome neurosurgical resection device (Cooper Medical Devices).[2] The system consists of a pneumatically activated probe (Fig. 49-1) and a control unit that provides the sources of suction and pressure to operate the cutting probe. The probe consists of slender concentric tubes, one reciprocating inside the other. The tip of the razor-sharp inner tube moves past a specially designed port on one side near the tip of the outer tube (Fig. 49-2). The control unit provides the pneumatic power which drives a sealed bellows housed in the body of the cutting probe and results in the reciprocating motion of the inner tube. The adjustable port at the probe tip can be rotated 360 degrees without changing the position of the surgeon's hand. The position of the cutting port is controlled by a rotatable knob at the posterior part of the probe.

The Biotome was specifically developed for neurosurgical procedures. The probe is well balanced, lightweight, and bayonet-shaped; it is connected to the power source by lightweight pneumatic tubing. It is designed to be used in only one hand. The two probe functions of either suction alone or cutting and suction are activated by depressing the appropriate foot-switch control. The port is always in the open position before the switch is used. When the foot switch is released (Fig. 49-3), the cutting and suction action stops immediately with the probe port in the open position. This will also occur automatically should the system lose power. Controls for the pressure, vacuum, and adjustment of the cutting rate are housed on the control console. A debris collection bottle is located on the top cover panel of the control unit (Fig. 49-3). A disposable tissue trap serves as a tissue collector.

The maximum amount of vacuum is present at the probe port when the surgeon's thumb fully covers the holes on the side of the probe body. When the thumb is removed, air bleeds into the vacuum to reduce the amount of suction at the probe's distal port to a minimum level. This control mechanism, familiar to all neurosurgeons, permits one to control the amount of suction at the tip by varying the degree to which one covers these air bleed holes.

The probe, when in use, sucks a piece of tumor into the distal port, permitting the guillotine action of the inner blade to cut this tumor piece. The tumor fragment is removed through the vacuum tubing to the collection bottle. The surgeon is advised to activate the cutting and suction mode only when the probe's cutting port is visible. The rotatable cutting port is situated on the side, close to the distal tip of the probe. This offers the neurosurgeon the major advantage of directly visualizing whatever tissue is being resected, an advantage which is not available in end-cutting devices. When resecting tumors, the Biotome is most efficient with a technique which allows an initial internal decompression of the mass. In situations where vital vulnerable structures are adjacent to the tumor, one is best advised to interpose a cottonoid or similar substance between the

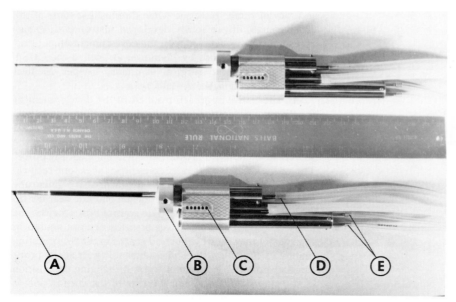

Figure 49-1 Cutting probes of two different dimensions. *A.* The cutting port is part of the outer stationary tube. *B.* The control knob (index wheel) permits the cutting port to be turned 360 degrees. *C.* Fingertip vacuum control. The suction force at the cutting port is directly and instantaneously controlled by covering part or all of the vacuum control ports on this handle. *D.* Reciprocating inner tube attached to the suction hose; small pieces of tumor debris are evacuated through this tubing to a collection bottle. *E.* Air pressure inlets control the reciprocating inner tube. (From Lazar et al.[2] Reproduced with permission.)

vital center or structure and the Biotome in order to limit the risk of injury from inadvertent snaring.

The instrument, of course, is not capable of determining which tissues to preserve and which to resect; the ultimate decision rests with the surgeon, as does the responsibility. However, the instrument has the ability to inflict severe injury in an instant.

On occasion, particularly when insufficient irrigation has been used during tumor resection, the probe may become plugged with debris. Should this occur, the suction force will be reduced. It will not interfere with the reciprocating

action of the inner blade; however, the efficiency of tumor cutting will be lessened, since the diminished suction will not attract the tumor into the cutting port. Several maneuvers are available to "clear the line."

The Biotome is not capable of resecting bone, and attempts to use it for this purpose will damage the blade. The probe is capable of removing material of the consistency of intervertebral disc and substances of somewhat greater density without apparent difficulty. However, the inner blade may become dull more quickly with prolonged use on tough, fibrous tissue. Replacement blades or sharpening

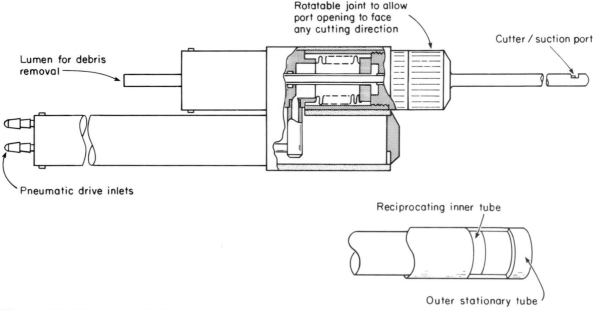

Figure 49-2 Cross-sectional diagram of a cutting probe. The bellows is housed in the body of the probe. The outer tube is stationary and the inner tube reciprocates. (From Lazar et al.[2] Reproduced with permission.)

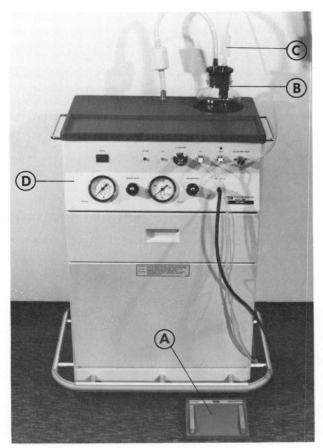

Figure 49-3 Control panel and foot switch. *A.* Dual foot switch that activates suction only or cutting with suction. *B.* Debris collection bottle. *C.* Disposable tissue trap. *D.* Control panel housing on-off power switch, pressure and vacuum adjustment control and gauges, and cutting rate control. (From Lazar et al.[2] Reproduced with permission.)

Among the advantages of this system is its relative cost compared with other devices designed to perform similar functions. Comparing the Biotome and the Cavitron ultrasonic aspirator, the efficiency of removal of diseased tissue is similar for most tissue densities, except for hard consistency lesions, where the ultrasonic aspirator is superior. The Biotome is incapable of removing bone, whereas the ultrasonic aspirator can perform this function.

Like the ultrasonic aspirator and laser resection devices, the Biotome has been utilized to remove almost every kind of tumor of the nervous system in virtually all locations. Intramedullary lesions of the spinal cord and brain stem; tumors of the anterior and posterior third ventricle, orbit, cerebral and cerebellar hemispheres, cerebellopontine angle, and perichiasmatic region; and other lesions have all been successfully removed by experienced surgeons with all these instruments. The success they enjoy and their long-term acceptance will depend upon a number of factors, including not only instrument reliability, cost, ease of handling, and adaptability to a particular surgeon's technical preference but also the integrity and reliability of the manufacturer. The frequency of repairs and the availability of spare parts are potential problems for any device. The clinical experience with the Biotome at our institution extends from May 1977. The prototype units as well as production probes are still being utilized on a regular and frequent basis. In the author's department these devices are regarded as an adjunct to a variety of techniques used to remove nervous system lesions, primarily tumors. The Biotome has proved to be the most useful in deep lesions situated adjacent to vital structures such as firm consistency intraventricular (lateral, anterior and posterior third, and fourth ventricle) tumors, cerebellopontine angle tumors, intraparenchymal firm consistency cerebellar or cerebral hemisphere lesions, and perichiasmatic firm tumors (meningiomas, craniopharyngiomas).

References

1. Flamm ES, Ransohoff J, Wuchinich D, Broadwin A: Preliminary experience with ultrasonic aspiration in neurosurgery. Neurosurgery 2:240–245, 1978.
2. Lazar ML, Wang C, Bland JE: An automated tumor resection device for neurological surgery. Neurosurgery 3:392–395, 1978.

services are available. Two different sizes of probe are manufactured (Fig. 49-1). The more slender probe is better suited for microsurgical techniques, while the larger is well adapted to macrosurgical procedures and is more efficient in removing a tumor with a dense fibrotic consistency.

50

Ultrasonic Dissection

Fred Epstein

In 1928, Cushing and Bovie recorded the use of radiofrequency electric current to facilitate the removal of intracranial tumors.[1] Although the "cutting loop" remains an important surgical adjunct to the removal of firm tumors that cannot be removed by suction, it carries significant hazards as the result of unavoidable heating of surrounding tissue, the danger of hemorrhage from damage to large blood vessels, and the absence of visibility and tactile feedback to the operating surgeon.

The successful application of the Cavitron emulsifier aspirator (Cavitron Ultrasonics, Long Island City N.Y.) to the extraction of cataracts suggested that the same principles of mechanical emulsification and aspiration might be applicable to the removal of firm tumors of the central nervous system, and it was on this conceptual basis that the Cavitron ultrasonic surgical aspirator (CUSA) was designed.[5,6]

The CUSA system (Cooper Medical Devices, Mountain View, Calif.) is self-contained and consists of a control console, flip switch, and handpiece (Fig. 50-1A and B). The vibrating suction device, which is constructed from hollow titanium and activated by a foot plate, oscillates longitudinally along its axis, fragmenting and simultaneously aspirating tissue within a 1- to 2-mm radius of the tip. The console regulates the amount of variable irrigation and suction to the handpiece and vibration to the cutting tip. The surgeon activates the system with a foot switch, while the aspiration and irrigation are regulated at the console. The fragmented and aspirated tissue is deposited in a reservoir on the console.

Indications for and Benefits of Ultrasonic Dissection

The ultrasonic dissecting system is capable of removing a broad range of tissue. When set at maximum stroke, it has the ability to fragment firm tumors such as meningiomas, acoustic neuromas, and firm gliomas. It is not effective in removing heavily calcified craniopharyngiomas or tumors of similar density, although calcified gliomas lend themselves to aspiration by this device.

The CUSA system is also applicable to tumors within the spinal column, including neurofibromas and meningiomas. It is effective in removing intramedullary tumors such as astrocytomas and ependymomas.

With the CUSA, it is possible to debulk the center of a tumor, following which it is technically easier to dissect the capsule from adjacent neural structures and carry out a gross total removal.

The ultrasonic dissector does not obtain hemostasis. The host vessels may bleed profusely, and it is necessary to obtain hemostasis in a conventional way following utilization of the dissector. Therefore it is usually most practical to remove a large volume of tumor with the CUSA and then obtain hemostasis, following which more tumor is removed. If the tip of the dissector is inadvertently applied to a major vascular structure such as the carotid artery, it may cause a laceration of the vessel.

Laboratory investigation has disclosed that normal electrical conduction in neural tissue more than 1 mm from the vibratory tip remains intact. CUSA dissection may thus be carried out immediately adjacent to vital structures with little attendant risk.[5]

Specific Application of the CUSA System

Meningiomas

The CUSA rapidly debulks the center of all but the most heavily calcified meningiomas. The need for the electrocautery cutting loop, with all its inherent hazards, is eliminated by the utilization of ultrasonic dissection. It is possible to rapidly debulk the neoplasm, after which the capsule may be extracted with relatively little manipulation of adjacent normal structures. The CUSA does not seal blood vessels, and these are cauterized by conventional techniques.

Acoustic Neuromas

The CUSA rapidly removes the bulk of the neoplasm, after which the capsule may be more easily separated from adjacent normal structures. Great caution is mandatory to avoid perforating the anterior capsule with the vibrating tip, as the facial nerve may be quickly destroyed.

Gliomas

The majority of glial tumors are easily removed by conventional suction and cautery techniques. The CUSA facilitates the removal of firm or calcified gliomas. These neoplasms are commonly relatively avascular and therefore ideal for ultrasonic dissection. The entire neoplasm may be quickly removed, after which hemostasis is easily obtained in adjacent normal structures.

Craniopharyngiomas

The heavily calcified portion of the craniopharyngioma often does not aspirate readily. However, the firm though less calcified regions of the tumor may be removed by ultrasonic dissection. Following the debulking, the capsule may be more readily dissected from the optic nerves and chiasm.

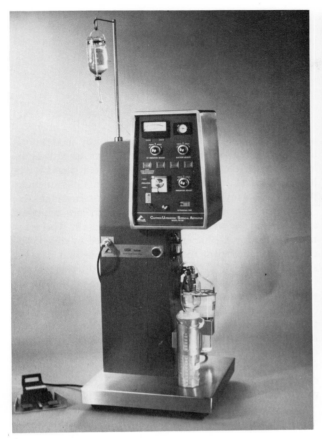

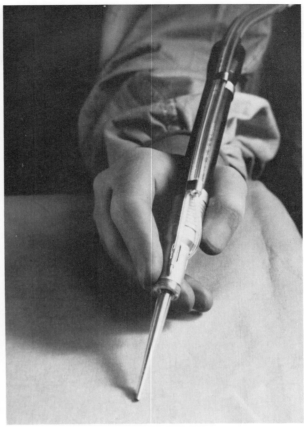

A   B

Figure 50-1 *A.* Console. *B.* Handpiece.

Spinal Neoplasms

Intradural extramedullary tumors such as meningiomas and neurofibromas are easily debulked by ultrasonic dissection. As with similar supratentorial tumors, the dissection of the capsule from the spinal cord is greatly facilitated.

Intramedullary spinal cord neoplasms such as ependymomas and astrocytomas are readily removed with ultrasonic dissection. In ependymomas, debulking the center of the tumor facilitates identification of the cleavage plane that so often exists between the capsule of the tumor and adjacent neural structures. In this way the tumor may be totally excised with little or no retraction on adjacent tissues.

The Cavitron ultrasonic aspirator has been indispensable in the removal of intramedullary spinal cord astroctyomas. Because these tumors are generally firm and do not have a plane of cleavage, the ultrasonic dissector permits the removal of the tumor from "inside out" (2–4). In this way the tumor is debulked until the glial-tumor interface is identified, and it is often possible to obtain gross total tumor resection.

Posterior Fossa Tumors

The CUSA facilitates the excision of relatively firm intra-axial tumors of the cerebellum, as well as exophytic brain stem neoplasms. Whereas conventional suction techniques frequently cause brain stem dysfunction as manifested by bradycardia or arrhythmia, the ultrasonic dissector does not cause movement or traction on adjacent structures more distant than 1 mm from the vibrating tip. Therefore these neoplasms may be relatively quickly removed despite extensive dissection adjacent to, or even within the substance of, the brain stem. In these specific situations, it is an indispensable surgical adjunct.

The author's department has utilized ultrasonic dissection to remove intramedullary spinal cord lipomas. These fatty tumors are traversed by fibrous septa, but the CUSA will remove the bulk of the lesions. Although it is not advisable to attempt a total removal of the intramedullary portion of the tumor, the tumors may be more completely excised than with previous conventional techniques.

References

1. Cushing H, Bovie WT: Electro-surgery as an aid to the removal of intracranial tumors. Surg Gynecol Obstet 47:751–784, 1928.
2. Epstein F, Epstein N: Surgical management of holocord intramedullary spinal cord astroctyomas in children: Report of three cases. J Neurosurg 54:829–832, 1981.
3. Epstein F, Epstein N: Surgical treatment of spinal cord astrocytomas of childhood: A series of 19 patients. J Neurosurg 57:685–689, 1982.
4. Epstein F, Epstein N: Surgical management of extensive intra-

medullary spinal cord astroctyomas in children, in American
Society of Pediatric Neurosurgery: *Concepts in Pediatric Neurosurgery*, vol 2. Basel, S Karger, 1982 pp 29–44.
5. Flamm ES, Ransohoff J, Wuchinich D, Broadwin A: Prelimi-

nary experience with ultrasonic aspiration in neurosurgery.
Neurosurgery 2:240–245, 1978.
6. Kelman CD: Phaco-emulsification and aspiration: A progress
report. Am J Ophthalmol 67:464–477, 1969.

51
Application of the Laser to Neurological Surgery

Leonard J. Cerullo

Physical Basis and Biological Effect

The possibility of *l*ight *a*mplification by the *s*timulated *e*mission of *r*adiation (laser) was originally hypothesized by Einstein[18] but was not realized until 1960 when the first pulsed ruby laser was assembled. The concept of stimulated emission can be understood if one considers a population of atoms that absorb (excited state) and emit (resting state) energy. The energy released when an atom falls from the excited to the resting state is called fluorescence. If, however, an excited atom is further stimulated by a quantum of energy identical to that which brought it from the resting to the excited state, stimulated emission occurs. The energy released is equal to the energy initially absorbed plus the stimulating energy. The waves of electromagnetic energy released are identical in length (monochromatic) and synchronous in space and time (coherent). By containing this system in a tubular structure, the ends of which are closed by partially reflective mirrors, the light waves are bounced back and forth, and the energy is used to restimulate the system over and over again. Eventually, the atoms contained within the tube (plasma tube) are in a generally excited state (population inversion), and the system is self-propagating. Those waves that are not parallel to the long axis of the tube are lost to the environment. Those that are parallel can be released by making one of the mirrors semitransparent or opening it as a shutter. The light that escapes the tube is, therefore, collimated. Because the light is monochromatic

and collimated, it can be efficiently focused by an appropriate lens to a fine point, theoretically one wavelength in diameter. Since the lens can be specific for a single wavelength, essentially all the light is collected. Consequently, the power density (power per unit area) is tremendous.

Each substance that can be so stimulated emits energy of a wavelength (or wavelengths) specific to itself. The spectrum of electromagnetic energy encompassed by this physical phenomenon spans the ultraviolet, visible, and infrared spectra.

When light energy impacts on biological tissues, one of three energy transformations (to chemical energy, to mechanical energy, or to heat) may occur. In photochemical transformation, the energy is converted from electromagnetic to chemical energy, and alterations in the biochemistry of the tissue, cell, or organelle result. An example of this is the use of monochromatic light to activate hematoporphyrin derivative, located within the cell, to produce singlet oxygen, which is toxic to the system and effects cell death.[25]

The mechanical effect of laser light may be seen as an acoustical wave that is generated when laser energy is transformed to mechanical energy. The frequency and amplitude of the acoustical wave are influenced by the power and pulse duration of the laser beam. The end result is tissue shearing. Although generally considered an undesired side effect of laser-tissue interaction, the phenomenon has been used to advantage in the disruption of the opacified posterior lens capsule using the Q-switched (nanosecond pulse duration) YAG laser.[24]

The biophysical interaction that is most often desired at the laser-tissue interface is the transformation of light to heat energy. The practically instantaneous elevation of the intracellular water temperature to the boiling point produces vaporization and explosion of the cell, with obliteration of the extracellular space. The speed of the process protects adjacent cells by a water jacket effect. Experimentally, it has been demonstrated in a variety of tissues that the intense thermal reaction produces three concentric zones of change at the impact site.[1] The central zone (ground zero) is devoid of all but scattered combusted debris. Adjacent to this is a zone of vacuolated cells, which are nonviable but which physically bear some resemblance to an intact biological system. Lateral to the vacuolated area is a zone of edema, in which the thermal effects have been significant enough to result in the accumulation of intracellular water but not in the demise of the functioning unit. A fourth zone, previously hypothesized, has been identified as producing no visible alterations at the light microscopic level but producing reversible histochemical changes.[11] In time, the fourth zone and the edematous zone return to normal, but the combusted and vacuolated zones remain nonviable.

Experimentally, it has been shown that the degree of

thermal trauma, in terms of cell viability, is less with laser than with conventional methods of hemostatic tissue incision such as monopolar and bipolar cautery.[15] Similarly, the degree of mechanical disruption using highly focused laser for incision has been shown to be less than with conventional means of tissue incision using a steel blade.[1] It appears, therefore, that the laser offers a more contained and containable method for incision and coagulation of biological tissues than has heretofore been available.

The Laser As a Tool

The use of the instrument in surgical practice capitalizes on its precision with minimization of trauma, both thermal and mechanical, to surrounding structures. In no surgical specialty is this more highly desired than in the incision, coagulation, and removal of tissue in and around the central nervous system. Precision of incision is exploited in those situations in which nervous tissue must be violated in order to effect a physiological result (myelotomy, cordotomy)[27] or to arrive at deeper pathological structures (tumor, cyst).[9] Precision of vaporization is desirable when removing tissue adjacent to sensitive neural or vascular structures with minimization of thermal or mechanical damage to those elements. Precision of coagulation is essential in directing the thermal energy to those areas in which it is required while protecting the adjacent micro- and macrovasculature.

Characteristics of Laser Media

The energy conversion just described occurs at a specific interface that is dependent on absorption by the cell or a subcellular particle. Each laser medium emits a specific wavelength or wavelengths, and each wavelength has specific coefficients of absorption, penetration, and scatter. Light in the visible spectrum will be absorbed by those structures that are closest in compatible color to that particular wavelength. Argon blue, at 488 nm, is highly absorbed by melanin, whereas the light from a neodymium:yttrium aluminum garnet (Nd:YAG) laser at 1060 nm is most heavily absorbed by the red color of hemoglobin. The energy of the carbon dioxide laser, with a wavelength of 10.6 μm (in the far infrared spectrum), is intensely absorbed by fluids, independent of color. Conversely, the amount of scatter is minimal with the latter, while especially with the argon laser and also the Nd:YAG laser, forward, backward, and side scatter are more prominent. The effects of subcellular particles and blood flow on the continuum of change of tissue being irradiated with laser energy add variables to the eventual degree of absorption and scatter.[8] In general, however, specific biophysical effects have been attributed to each of the main medical laser sources.

The shortest commonly used wavelength is that of argon. Initially the affinity for the argon wavelength by the melanin pigment in the retinal epithelium of the eye allowed ophthalmologists to produce thermal lesions to coagulate retinal vessels and halt the progress of such vasculoproliferative disorders as macular degeneration and diabetic retinopathy.

Argon light can be delivered through an optical fiber with negligible loss of energy, allowing great flexibility. Because of minimal diversion at the fiber tip, a tightly collimated beam is maintained. This can be focused to a fine point to allow high power density and great precision at the target. In addition, because the argon beam is in the visible spectrum, a separate aiming laser is not necessary. The degree of scatter and the nonhomogeneous absorption by tissue, however, effectively increase the volume of tissue destruction at the target.[6] In certain biological systems, the short wavelength of argon appears to have certain ionizing properties, which may result in continued biological effects for some period of time after the application of the energy.[22] This is exploited in retinal and dermatologic surgery, but may be undesirable in nervous tissue. Currently available equipment in the medium power ranges (10 to 20 W output) is bulky and requires specialized electrical (three phase, 80 A) and water supplies because of the relative inefficiency of the laser generation. Lower-power units are of little value in vaporizing tissue, though they may be effective in coagulation.

The Nd:YAG laser emits light in the near infrared spectrum that can also be passed through an optical fiber. The degree of divergence at the fiber tip, however, and the sizable area of scatter upon impact with tissue make this wavelength less suitable for precision than for bulk coagulation. On the other hand, the specific affinity of the Nd:YAG laser for the red color of blood allows a high degree of specificity of coagulation in nonhomogeneous tissue.[28] The ability to coagulate at the distal end of an optical fiber allows the Nd:YAG laser to be used effectively in endoscopic surgery in the upper and lower GI tract and in the GU tract.[17] Recently, increasing use of this instrument for endobronchial coagulation and vaporization has been seen. As a neurosurgical tool, the Nd:YAG laser seems particularly suited for coagulation of the center of a vascular tumor, denaturation of a neoplasm behind structures less absorptive of Nd:YAG energy (e.g., a sinus wall),[4] and endoscopic applications.[2] Present equipment design requires similar electrical and cooling requirements to those of the argon units.

The energy emitted from a carbon dioxide laser is immediately absorbed by fluid and, conversely, has the lowest degree of scatter of the present surgical lasers. At present, there is no readily available fiber that will allow transmission of the carbon dioxide laser without unacceptable loss of energy. Articulating arm systems, using a series of deflecting mirrors, allow the energy to be transmitted from the plasma tube to the target. Most available systems suffer from some degree of vulnerability to trauma, loss of energy, and change of mode (beam pattern). Instruments delivering from less than 1 to over 100 W of output power are activated by house current and do not require external cooling systems. The beam is invisible and must be identified by a coincident pilot laser, in many cases a helium-neon miniwatt laser. If these are not absolutely coaxial, error may result. The minimal spot size of the carbon dioxide laser is larger than that of the argon laser. However, the effect on tissue is more contained and less subject to local variations in color, subcellular particles, and scatter. The carbon dioxide laser has become the most widely used laser instrument in most of the surgical specialities, including neurosurgery, because of its versatility, safety, and predictability.

Safety Considerations

The major safety hazards of the surgical lasers can be grouped into two categories: surface and ocular (retinal). In the former group are thermal burns to the skin of the patient, the surgeon, and other members of the operative team as well as surface burns to the eye involving the cornea and sclera. In addition, untoward effects on tissue in the operative field from reflections of laser energy and the ignition of the endotracheal tube in the oxygen-rich environment of the upper respiratory tract are major sources of concern.[30] Extreme caution should be taken when using the laser in neurosurgery to avoid unanticipated movement of the laser instrument or the target, as either will result in delivery of laser energy to nontarget tissue with potentially disastrous results. When operating on the spinal cord, respiratory excursions and pulse-related movement of neural tissue can be significant and can result in an increased area of tissue destruction.[14] Accordingly, appropriate measures should be taken when performing fine manipulations of the spinal cord.

Because carbon dioxide laser energy is immediately absorbed upon impact and cannot pass a fluid medium, its effects are limited to the surface. The light of the argon and Nd:YAG lasers, however, can pass through clear media such as the cornea and lens of the eye, and therefore these laser sources pose an additional hazard. Energy presented to the globe can be collected by the lens and focused on the retina. This will concentrate even seemingly negligible amounts of energy and may result in severe thermal effects on the retina. Accordingly, protective lenses that are color-specific for the wavelength involved must be worn by the operator, the patient, and all operating room personnel. National safety standards mandate that the operating room in which the laser is being used be clearly identified with signs and/or blinking lights in order to prevent those entering from being inadvertently harmed. Since most lasers are activated by foot switches, it is prudent to limit the use of the laser foot switch to the operating surgeon, while assistants may activate other equipment (e.g., bipolar and monopolar cautery machines) requiring pedal control switches.

The vaporized tissue can generally be removed through routine suction systems. Higher-power vacuum systems are available commercially and may be considered a wise investment. There has not been shown to be active, replicating, material in the laser vapor.[7] Similarly, experimental attempts at tissue culture growth of particles from the vapor, whether from normal or tumorous systems, have been unsuccessful. It appears, then, that aside from its disagreeable odor, the smoke is no health hazard. In a series of over 500 laser operations, we have not experienced untoward effects on surgeon, patient, or operating room personnel.

Advantages and Drawbacks of Laser Use

Each surgical specialty that has come to appreciate the benefits of laser surgery has concentrated on one or another facet of the tool that it considers singularly important. Although all specialties appreciate the precision of tissue destruction offered by the instrument, in neurosurgery the limitation of mechanical and thermal trauma, with minimization of surrounding edema, appears to be the single most important feature. In addition, however, the ability to continually record neurophysiological parameters such as somatosensory and brain stem evoked responses during tissue removal without electrical interference is of major importance.[27] When working in a limited field, the ability to remove or incise tissue without visual impediment by intervening instrumentation is of some consequence. The hemostatic properties of laser are more a function of the wavelength involved than an overall statement, but even the carbon dioxide laser, the least hemostatic because of its immediate energy absorption by fluid, offers a greater degree of hemostatic control when compared with conventional means of tissue incision. This is far more readily appreciated in dealing with bleeding from a tumor bed than with bleeding from the incised edges of normal tissue, including skin, muscle, and central nervous tissue. The sealing effect of laser on tissue has been touted as being responsible on the one hand for a lower rate of recurrence of undesirable phenomena (such as neuroma formation, seroma formation, and recurrence of malignant neoplasm)[3] and on the other hand as being responsible for weakened and delayed wound healing. Probably, neither is of significant validity in neurological surgery.

The basic laser actions of incision, coagulation, and vaporization are a function of the amount of energy delivered to the tissue (radiant exposure) measured in terms of watts over surface area times time, and the reaction of that particular tissue to this quantum of energy of a certain wavelength. While in normal tissues such as skin, muscle, dura, and central nervous tissue, the response is fairly predictable, in tumor the tremendous range of variation in consistency, water content, and vascularity make each experience unique. The corollary is that, while standard tissues can be approached in a relatively stereotyped fashion, the removal of a tumor must proceed on a more empiric basis, beginning with attenuated energy and continuing to more concentrated energy as the situation indicates. In any event, the radiant energy is manipulated by altering the variables of power output, length of exposure, and surface area at impact site.

Power output is a direct function of the laser-generating device. Power output should be considered at the site of tissue impact, rather than at the site of laser generation. There is a significant amount of loss associated with a delivery system, whether it be an optical cable or an articulated arm. In addition, the mode (pattern of energy) at the impact site must be considered. The fundamental mode, or TEM00, is a gaussian distribution of energy with central intensity that gradually diminishes power toward the periphery. Other modes offer different patterns of energy distribution within the limitations of the spot size. It is not uncommon for the mode to vary as a function of the delivery system, particularly fiberoptic ones. With articulated arm systems, the coincidence of laser energy and pilot light should be ascertained, by trial ignition, in each position of use. This prevents accidental maldistribution of energy.

When the pilot light and treating light are the same, this potential error is obviated. As a general rule, it is best to begin with low power and proceed higher as the situation dictates in order to prevent excessive depth of penetration and damage to deep structures. It should be remembered that there is no fail-safe mechanism preventing deeper structures from injury by excessive penetration of laser energy, as this is in the purview of the technical ability of the surgeon. The power density at the impact site is a function not only of power but of the surface area of exposure (power density = power area).

Surface area can be minimized by using an appropriate lens to focus the laser energy to a fine point. The size of the spot is a function of the wavelength of the laser as well as the focal length of the lens. Theoretical physical considerations are generally overshadowed by practical considerations, which dictate the degree of focusing that can be achieved. The area of cross-sectional beam diameter is increased by defocusing either toward (prefocus) or away from (defocus) the focal spot of the lens-laser system. The latter offers the advantage of being continually larger (more attenuated) beyond the plane of laser-tissue interaction. This is a more theoretical than practical concept. As surface area is increased, power density is diminished, resulting in more uniform spread of heat with less depth of penetration. The protection of nontarget tissues that may be located within the radius of the impact site is crucial. When using a carbon dioxide laser, this merely requires a wet substance, such as cotton soaked with saline, to allow the water to completely absorb the energy and protect the underlying structure. With Nd:YAG and argon, the degree of scatter within the tissue makes this less feasible, and consequently these effects must be considered when an attempt is made to attenuate power by increasing the surface area while operating near sensitive neural or vascular structures. Although the power density can be effectively regulated by the two previously mentioned maneuvers, heat buildup at the impact site is more a function of length of exposure.[21]

The time of exposure is a critical factor in promoting or discouraging thermal effects adjacent to the target. With very short exposure times (picosecond, nanosecond) the acoustical effects of the laser are maximized while the thermal effects are practically nonexistent. On the other hand, in using continuous laser energy, local heat buildup may negatively influence the precision of incision and vaporization. By moving the beam rapidly or slowly over the tissue, the thermal effects are altered. The heat sink phenomenon of blood flowing through a tumor or vessel is a third variable that influences the degree of thermal buildup, but this is not generally at the discretion of or under the control of the operating surgeon. In tumorous tissues, the heat sink effect can usually be appreciated only empirically. On the other hand, in dealing with major vessels and sinuses, the heat sink effect can be capitalized on, allowing the surgeon to deliver energy to the wall of the structure while minimizing thermal effects on the circulating fluid within.[5]

The major disadvantage to the use of the laser in neurosurgery is the loss of tactile input from tissue to the surgeon through the intermediary of instrumentation. The ability to manipulate power, surface area, and exposure time enables the competent surgeon to overcome this handicap and, in fact, enjoy a previously unheard of degree of precision and gentleness of surgery of the central nervous system.

Specific Applications

By far, the most commonly used laser in neurosurgery is the carbon dioxide laser. This is because of the relative safety offered by its immediate absorption in fluid with minimal scatter and no demonstrated late effects.[10] In addition, commercially available surgical systems are relatively inexpensive, portable, and versatile. The carbon dioxide laser can be used freehand (with or without optical magnification) or linked to the operating microscope by means of a direct mechanical or electromechanical micromanipulator. A further refinement on the latter allows the surgeon to program an area to be scanned by laser energy, allowing a preset raster to cover the area in uniform sweeps, resulting in a homogenous depth of penetration throughout the surface being treated. However, the use of this refinement has yet to be demonstrated to be effective in neurological surgery.

It appears and is generally accepted that the major use of the carbon dioxide laser is in the removal of extra-axial tumors that are located in neurologically sensitive areas, the resection of which tumors may result in mechanical or thermal damage to surrounding intact structures.[13] Notable in this regard are meningiomas and neuromas at the base of the skull, craniopharyngiomas, intraspinal extramedullary neoplasms, lipomas of the central nervous system, and fibrous tumors located dorsally or ventrally along the midline. In these situations, the atraumatic nature, immediate absorption, and relatively high power of currently available carbon dioxide instruments offer the ability to remove fairly large amounts of tissue in relatively short periods of time, with minimal blood loss, and negligible trauma.

The precision of incision offered by laser, both argon and carbon dioxide, makes neuroablative procedures a second area of major indication. Here, again, the ability to destroy tissue immediately adjacent to that tissue that must be protected, both anatomically and physiologically, allows the laser to demonstrate an unprecedented degree of containment of trauma while offering absolute obliteration (by removal or vaporization) of certain tracts and/or structures. Myelotomy, cordotomy, dorsal root entry zone lesions, and fenestration are notable in this regard. Here, the ability to finely focus the laser with minimal scatter and extreme precision is best done with the argon and carbon dioxide instruments. An extension of a theoretical benefit of this application is the use of the laser for cortical incisions in cerebrotomy and lobectomy. Here, the minimization of thermal and mechanical damage to surrounding intact structures may translate to reduced postoperative morbidity and edema formation. Whether this will be of electrophysiological benefit in reducing postoperative epilepsy remains to be determined.

Nd:YAG and argon lasers appear to have great promise in the treatment of certain vascular tumors and vascular diseases of the central nervous system.[19] The ability to pass these wavelengths through optical cables and their penetrance through fluid (such as CSF) allow for their use in flexible endoscopic and intraventricular surgery.

When considering the use of a laser for a particular application, the benefit/risk ratio must be determined. The use of the laser for treating vascular diseases of the brain and spinal cord is in its infancy. Most likely, Nd:YAG and argon lasers, because of their affinity for hemoglobin-containing structures, will be more applicable than the carbon dioxide laser. Although it is generally stated that the carbon dioxide laser is ineffective for coagulating vessels greater than 1 mm in diameter, the proper application of energy to the vessel wall, prior to its transgression, can allow much larger vessels to be coagulated, particularly if the blood flow through the vessel is temporarily reduced or halted.[29] Preliminary studies have indicated that there is a selective difference in the principal area of the vessel wall affected by different wavelengths, specifically argon and Nd:YAG.[20] The use of the laser, regardless of wavelength, has not been demonstrated to be effective in the treatment or prevention of recurrence of malignant brain tumors, primary or metastatic, except insofar as minimization of trauma to surrounding normal brain is concerned.[31]

The allegation that the use of the carbon dioxide laser as a cutting instrument minimizes postoperative scar tissue formation has not been substantiated. However, the use of the instrument for dissection of muscle results in diminished blood loss and freedom from tetanic muscular contraction coincident with the electric knife.[12] This may translate to reduced postoperative pain. The use of the laser in limited field surgery, such as trans-sphenoidal operations on the pituitary gland and lumbar microdiscectomy, may offer the advantage of freedom from obstruction of the visual field by instrumentation. In addition, the shrinking effect on the pituitary dura and the vaporization of discal material in situ, without mechanical disruption of surrounding discal tissue, may be advantageous. Certainly, neither application would be considered at this time an "absolute" indication for the laser in neurological surgery.

There appear to be certain distinct disadvantages to the use of the laser in cutting tissue. Scalp incision, for instance, is unaided by the laser because of the extreme vascularity of the structure. In fact, the prolongation of operative time and the risk for thermal burn seem to contraindicate the sharp (argon and carbon dioxide) lasers, and certainly the devascularization of the tissue contraindicates the use of the Nd:YAG laser. Bone cutting is slow, and there is a considerable heat buildup because of the relatively dry nature of the tissue on the surface and the heat sink phenomenon within the cancellous portions. In addition, the nonhomogeneous nature of bone renders prediction of degree of penetration impossible. Therefore, underlying structures must be protected against overpenetration of laser energy. Laser incision of dura results in shrinkage of the structure and, therefore, should be limited to those situations in which this effect is desirable (trans-sphenoidal surgery; the dural attachment of a meningioma) and there is no need to directly reclose the structure. Arachnoidal incision can be performed with the carbon dioxide laser, the underlying micro- and macrovasculature being protected by the CSF barrier. The use of the argon or Nd:YAG laser, however, is contraindicated because the light energy would penetrate the arachnoid and CSF to

impact on the underlying central nervous tissue. As the use of laser of several wavelengths becomes more routine, it is anticipated that indications and contraindications will continue to develop and become refined. At present, it appears premature to be dogmatic, except in the most obvious circumstances.

The relatively high cost of laser instrumentation requires judicious planning on the part of medical institutions with sage input from practicing surgeons. Time-sharing by multiple specialties is a method of increasing usage and, thereby, amortizing cost.[16] This is currently not possible with the carbon dioxide laser because of difficulty in beam delivery from a central source. However the easy transportability of the latter in general obviates this necessity. Since the laser is used during only a part of certain operations, there is no need to monopolize an instrument for the entire case. Nevertheless, the high cost may be a deterrent to smaller institutions or, at least, may limit the investment to a single wavelength. The most practical, at this time, is the carbon dioxide laser because of its general usefulness in neurosurgery, otolaryngology, and gynecology. Similarly, the Nd:YAG laser appears to be useful in gastroenterology, urology, and bronchoesophagology. The use of the Nd:YAG laser in neurosurgery is currently experimental but is rapidly gaining popularity.

A major concern is the potential for obsolescence of the various instruments. Potential improvements include sealed-tube systems (eliminating the need for disposable gas tanks), optical fibers to replace cumbersome articulating arms, radiofrequency-excited systems (to replace arc tube devices), multiple-wavelength units, and miniaturization. The basic concept of stimulated emission, however, remains constant. The various proposals for improvement in generating or delivering the beam may change, but these changes, however desirable, will not affect the final result of the laser-tissue interaction. Accordingly, it seems impractical to wait for "next year's model."

The use of the laser is by no means a call for the elimination of other surgical tools. It is, in fact, complimentary rather than competitive with such instruments as ultrasonic fragmentation and aspiration. Similarly, the laser is not a replacement for accepted microsurgical practices. Rather, it is an extension of microsurgical technique. The concepts of gentle tissue handling, minimization of trauma, and elimination of heat buildup are brought to theoretical culmination with this development. Certainly, the instrument is no replacement for surgical judgment and skill. On the other hand, it appears that certain frontiers of neurosurgery may be extended by the use of laser instrumentation and technique.

The future of the laser in neurosurgery is difficult to predict without appearing overly optimistic. The present use of laser and computer systems, coupled to stereotactic devices, makes futuristic predictions appear modest.[23] Certainly the increasing endoscopic use of the instrument with optical cables capable of transmitting laser energy as well as conventional light and channels for mechanical manipulation offers promise for intraspinal, subarachnoid, and intraventricular as well as intravascular navigation and treatment. Likewise, the use of the laser for welding tissues, heretofore considered impossible, has been clearly demonstrated to be effective for anastomosis of small vessels and nerves.[26] Perhaps expansion will include larger structures as well.

At present, it seems safe to predict that the future of the laser in neurosurgery is limited only by the imaginations of surgeons.

References

1. Ascher PW: Newest ultrastructural findings after the use of CO_2-laser on CNS tissue. Acta Neurochir (Wien) [Suppl] 28:572–581, 1979.
2. Ascher PW: Horizons in neurosurgery. Presented at a meeting of the Laser Association of Neurological Surgery International, Houston, Tex, May 1, 1983.
3. Ascher PW, Cerullo LJ: Laser use in neurosurgery, in Dixon J (ed): *Surgical Applications of Lasers*. Chicago, Year Book, 1983.
4. Beck OJ: The use of the Nd-YAG and the CO_2 laser in neurosurgery. Neurosurg Rev 3:261–266, 1980.
5. Beck OJ, Ascher PW: Different lasers in neurosurgery. Presented at the 3rd Annual Meeting of the American Society of Laser Medicine and Surgery, New Orleans, La, January 10–12, 1983.
6. Bellina J: Connective tissue effects of CO_2 and argon lasers. Presented at the Congress on Laser Neurosurgery, II, Chicago, Ill, September 23–25, 1982.
7. Bellina JH, Sterjnoiholm RL, Kurpel JE: Biochemical analysis of carbon dioxide plume emission from irradiated tumors, in Bellina JH (ed): *Gynecologic Laser Surgery*. New York, Plenum, 1981, pp 17–25.
8. Boggan JE, Edwards MSB, Davis RL, Bolger CA, Martin N: Comparison of the brain tissue response in rats to injury by argon and carbon dioxide lasers. Neurosurgery 11:609–616, 1982.
9. Brown JT: Laser fenestration for syringohydromyelia. Presented at the Congress on Laser Neurosurgery, II, Chicago, Ill, September 23–25, 1982.
10. Brown TE, True C, McLaurin RL, Rockwell RJ Jr, Hornby P: Laser radiation: II. Long-term effects of laser radiation on certain intracranial structures. Neurology 17:789–796, 1967.
11. Burke L, Rovin RA, Cerullo LJ, Brown JT, Petronio J: Nd:YAG laser in neurosurgery, in Joffee SN (ed): *Nd:YAG Laser in Medicine and Surgery*. New York, Elsevier, 1983.
12. Cerullo LJ: CO_2 laser surgery in acute spinal cord injury. Presented at the 6th Annual Scientific Meeting of the American Spinal Injury Association, Anaheim, Calif, May 8–11, 1980.
13. Cerullo LJ: Acoustic nerve tumor removal with CO_2 laser: Technique and results. Presented at the Congress on Laser Neurosurgery, II, Chicago, Ill, September 23–25, 1982.
14. Cerullo L, Koht A: Anesthesiologic considerations in laser neurosurgery. Lasers Surg Med 3:35–38, 1983.
15. Cozzens J: Evans blue brain edema model for comparison of CO_2 and bipolar lesions. Presented at the First American Congress on Laser Neurosurgery, Chicago, Ill, October 1–3, 1981.
16. Dixon JA: General surgical and endoscopic applications of lasers, in Dixon J (ed): *Surgical Applications of Lasers*, Chicago, Year Book, 1983.
17. Dwyer RM, Haverback BJ, Bass M, Cherlow J: Laser-induced hemostasis in the canine stomach: Use of a flexible fiberoptic delivery system. JAMA 231:486–489, 1975.
18. Einstein A: Zur quantum Theorie des Strahlung. Phys Z 18:121–128, 1917.
19. Fasano VA: The treatment of vascular malformation of the brain with laser surgery. Presented at the Congress on Laser Neurosurgery, II, Chicago, Ill, September 23–25, 1982.
20. Fasano VA: Effect of different laser sources on vessel wall. Presented at a meeting of the Laser Association of Neurological Surgery International, Houston, Tex, May 1, 1983.
21. Fuller TA: The physics of surgical lasers. Lasers Surg Med 1:5–14, 1980.
22. Goldman L: The argon laser and the port wine stain. Plast Reconstr Surg 65:137–139, 1980.
23. Kelly PJ, Alker GJ Jr, Goerss S: Computer-assisted stereotactic laser microsurgery for the treatment of intracranial neoplasms. Neurosurgery 10:324–331, 1982.
24. Krasnov MM: Q-switched laser iridectomy and Q-switched laser goniopuncture. Adv Ophthalmol 34:192–196, 1977.
25. Laws ER Jr, Cortese DA, Kinsey JH, Eagan RT, Anderson RE: Photoradiation therapy in the treatment of malignant brain tumors: A phase I (feasibility) study. Neurosurgery 9:672–678, 1981.
26. Neblett CR: Reconstructive vascular surgery with use of the CO_2 laser. Presented at the Congress on Laser Neurosurgery, II, Chicago, Ill, September 23–25, 1982.
27. Saunders ML, Young HF, Becker DP, Greenberg RP, Newlon PG, Corales RL, Ham WT, Povlishock JT: The use of the laser in neurological surgery. Surg Neurol 14:1–10, 1980.
28. Taki W, Takeuchi J, Yonekawa Y, Yamagami T, Handa M: Advance in laser microsurgery in neurosurgical operation with special reference to Nd-YAG laser. Presented at the Fourth Congress of the International Society for Laser Surgery, Tokyo, Japan, 1981.
29. Takizawa T: History: Medilaser-S Model MEL-442, in: *Illustrated Laser Surgery, Fundamentals No. 2*. Tokyo, Mochida Pharmaceutical Co, Ltd, 1982.
30. Treyve E, Yarrington CT Jr, Thompson GE: Incendiary characteristics of endotracheal tubes with the carbon dioxide laser: An experimental study. Ann Otol Rhinol Laryngol 90:328–330, 1981.
31. Yokota H, Hara M, Okada J, Ogashiwa M, Motsumoto M, Takeuchi K: Malignant glioma laser surgery. Presented at the Fifth International Congress of Laser Medicine and Surgery, Detroit, Mich, October 7–9, 1983.

52

Interventional Neuroradiology

Fernando Viñuela
Allan J. Fox

The development of techniques of radiological intravascular navigation with particles and balloons has opened a new therapeutic field to some neurological diseases such as intracranial arteriovenous malformations (AVMs) and fistulae. This endovascular approach has received increasing interest from neuroradiologists and neurosurgeons, whether used alone or in conjunction with neurosurgical procedures.

These therapeutic tools require detailed diagnostic angiography to accurately assess the morphology, topography, and hemodynamics of the lesion to be treated. X-ray films showing the cerebral vasculature well are the end product of a complex interaction of many factors: choice of film and screen combination, film processor chemistry, x-ray tubes, radiographic voltage and amperage, filters, grids and collimation, magnification and subtraction. This information is used by the therapist to choose the best delivery system and the best embolic material for each individual vascular lesion.

Intravascular occlusive techniques also require optimal equipment to minimize serious neurological complications from the embolization of normal arteries. It is necessary to have high quality fluoroscopy, either biplane or C-arm type, a good selection of catheters and coaxial systems, and high quality videotape and subtraction capabilities.[23]

The vascular techniques of interventional neuroradiology are predominantly occlusive in nature. The aim of the procedure is to obliterate the congenital or acquired vascular disease, sparing the surrounding normal vascular structures. Thus techniques of superselective vascular catheterization have been developed to position the delivery system as close as possible to the vascular lesion to be treated. These vascular occlusive techniques include embolization with particles, balloons, and fluids (silicone and isobutyl-2-cyanoacrylate).[32] These techniques must be performed by an experienced team of x-ray technicians, neuroradiologists and neurosurgeons, because they have an intrinsic risk of producing a transient or permanent neurological deficit if they are not handled appropriately.

The natural history of the disease, and the advantages and potential iatrogenic complications of therapy, must be discussed thoroughly with the patient and the patient's family as the first step directed to treatment.

Cerebral Arteriovenous Malformations

Cerebral arteriovenous malformations (AVMs) are a conglomerate of abnormal vessels supplied by enlarged arterial feeders and drained by serpiginous dilated veins. They are said to be vascular hamartomas in which there is an arteriovenous shunt of variable degree.[57,59] They occur in the brain more frequently than elsewhere in the body and in addition are the most common of all the vascular anomalies of the central nervous system.[62] In the Cooperative Study, arteriovenous malformations accounted for 6 percent of the subarachnoid hemorrhages studied.[54]

AVMs may be located in the brain parenchyma (pial AVMs), may involve the dura (dural AVMs), or may have dural and pial components (mixed AVMs).[50] They may be supra- or infratentorial and usually receive their blood supply from the internal carotid artery, external carotid artery, and/or vertebrobasilar system, depending on their topography. The middle cerebral artery is the most frequent site of AVMs and the location of the most extensive lesions.[54] AVMs are not infrequently accompanied by aneurysms, located in the same or a different vascular territory.[49]

Histologically, AVMs consist of many enlarged vessels of variable diameter and wall thickness. Vascular thrombosis and/or calcifications are not infrequent findings. The intervening brain tissue shows varying degrees of edema, gliosis, demyelination, and calcification. The brain remote from the lesion may exhibit some gliosis and sometimes loss of neurons.[57]

Patients with brain AVMs may be asymptomatic (unexpected CT finding) or may present with subarachnoid hemorrhage, seizures, progressive neurological deficit, or headaches. The natural history of this disease is not well known. Some authors believe it has a relatively benign natural history,[63] while others stress the point that 10 to 17 percent of patients will die from hemorrhage and 40 to 50 percent will have some deterioration of their working capacity or will become invalids within 20 to 40 years.[25,43]

Treatment

Treatment of brain AVMs is based on the patient's clinical presentation and on the size and topography of the lesion. Patients may be treated by surgery alone if the size and location of the lesion allows safe surgical resection. Endovascular occlusive techniques are indicated mainly in the treatment of large AVMs or those involving the eloquent areas of the brain. They may be used alone or in conjunction with surgery. In some instances embolization of the AVM may result in its complete occlusion.[14] In other cases presurgical embolization can reduce the size of the AVM or obliterate that part of it that poses difficult technical problems for the neurosurgeon.[14]

The goal of endovascular embolization of AVMs is occlusion of the nidus. Proximal surgical or particulate occlusion of feeders has proved to be not only useless but disadvantageous, because of elimination of the natural route for occlusion of the nidus by the uses of transfemoral or intraoperative endovascular embolization with isobutyl-2-cyanoacrylate (IBC or IBCA).[22]

In 1960, Luessenhop and Spence introduced the use of methyl methacrylate spheres for the embolization of brain AVMs.[44] Later, radiopaque Silastic spheres of different sizes were used in a similar fashion.[71] After catheterization of the parent artery via femoral or direct puncture, the spheres are injected into the circulation of the brain, one at a time. The spheres are located radiographically, and the neurological status of the patient is evaluated before more spheres are introduced (Fig. 52-1). The spheres are flow-dependent and are used mainly in angiomas with high flow as determined by the presence of large arterial feeders, taking advantage of the sump effect of the AVM.[71] The pre-embolization angiogram is used to select the sphere size to be used. The smallest sphere possible for the specific AVM should be used, in order to try to reach the core of the AVM without passing into its venous outlet. Wolpert and Stein have stressed the importance of using spheres slightly larger than the nondilated brain vessels but still small enough to occlude smaller feeding vessels close to the nidus.[71] Embolization is discontinued when the flow in the arterial feeders decreases, when a neurological deficit occurs, or when an embolic sphere is seen in a normal artery. Transient postembolization neurological deficits using this technique are frequent, though a complete functional recovery is obtained in most cases. Short-term follow-up angiograms after bead embolization may show a decrease in size and flow of the AVM, although development of collaterals and recanalization of the nidus is frequently seen on long-term follow-up. Patronas et al. believed that they could predict the efficacy of small-silicone-particle embolization of brain AVMs by analyzing the pre-embolization cerebral angiograms.[53] They noted that when the number and caliber of arterial feeders were greater than the number and caliber of draining veins, there was a real possibility of obtaining successful embolization. Wolpert et al. have stated that embolization of brain AVMs with spheres may be helpful to patients complaining of intractable headaches but has no beneficial effect on the frequency of seizures or the development of neurological deficit.[70]

Balloon Occlusion

Several types of latex and silicone detachable balloons are now available. Serbinenko[61] and Romodanov et al.[58] have used the detachable balloon technique to occlude arterial feeders of brain AVMs. This technique may be compared to proximal surgical or particulate obliteration of the feeders of the AVM without occlusion of the nidus. It must be stated that despite good results claimed by the Russian school, long-term follow-up experience demonstrates that in many cases the nidus of the AVM remains patent because of rapid development of collaterals.[22]

Isobutyl-2-cyanoacrylate

Isobutyl-2-cyanoacrylate is one of a group of homologous organic monomers which undergo fast polymerization in the presence of weak bases, including water.[8] This intrinsic property of hardening by polymerization has made it useful in neurosurgery as an adhesive,[42] for reinforcing aneurysms,[24] or for embolizing vascular lesions.[60] The local histotoxicity of IBCA was accurately assessed by Lehman and Hayes in

1966. They noted that this monomer is significantly less toxic to neural and vascular tissue than methyl and ethyl monomers.[41] IBCA also has a fast polymerization time, optimal for clinical use. Further experimental and clinical findings show that IBCA produces a mild to moderate inflammatory reaction, with predominant lymphocyte and monocyte participation, involving the wall of the occluded vessel and nearby brain parenchyma.[26,72] The butyl-cyanoacrylate monomers and polymers have not proved carcinogenic in animals.[41]

The Food and Drug Administration of the United States has approved use of IBCA for investigational use only. The use of commercial cyanoacrylate adhesives which contain the more toxic methyl and ethyl monomers, in addition to unknown additives, should be avoided.[48]

IBCA appears to be an embolizing agent suitable for reaching the nidus of an AVM and permanently obliterating it. In order to use this material it is mandatory to superselectively catheterize the individual feeders of an AVM. Kerber[34] and Pevsner[55] developed a delivery system capable of being positioned in arterial feeders of brain AVMs. A small Silastic calibrated-leak balloon is bonded to a thin, flexible, single-lumen silicone catheter capable of negotiating the curves of the cortical arteries of the brain. When inflated with contrast medium, the balloon is carried by the dominant flow to the AVM's largest feeder. Using continuous fluoroscopic control, the balloon is positioned close to the nidus of the AVM.

Debrun et al.[15] described their experience with a latex calibrated-leak balloon and stated that the physical properties of this material make this balloon safer for cannulation and embolization of cortical arterial feeders.

The procedure is performed in the radiology department, using the transfemoral route, with the patient under neuroleptic analgesia. A no. 6 Cordis sheath (Cordis Corporation, Miami Fl.) is positioned in the femoral artery and a no. 5.8 introducer is positioned either in the internal carotid artery or in the vertebral artery, depending on the topography of the AVM. A latex calibrated-leak balloon bonded to Silastic tubing is coiled in a BD chamber (Becton Dickinson & Co., Rutherford, N.J.) (Fig. 52-2). This chamber is used to inject the balloon through the introducer and into the intracranial vasculature. The balloon's movement is flow-directed, although it may be controlled by inflation and deflation maneuvers with contrast medium under fluoroscopic control. When the balloon is suitably situated for embolization, a pre-embolization superselective angiogram is *always* performed (Fig. 52-3). This angiogram is done safely, and the information obtained may decrease potential technical or clinical complications. Information from this angiogram is classified as anatomical (documentation of the position of the balloon, visualization of normal cortical branches distal to the balloon, and percentage of nidus supplied by the feeder), dynamic (measurement of arteriovenous transit time), and functional (appearance of neurological symptoms during or immediately after injection of pure contrast medium into the feeder).[66]

The superselective angiogram is followed by a slow injection of 10 to 20 mg of sodium amytal.[66] Dubois et al.[23] also recommend temporary reversible balloon occlusion of leptomeningeal arteries for 10 min as a provocative test before permanent occlusion.

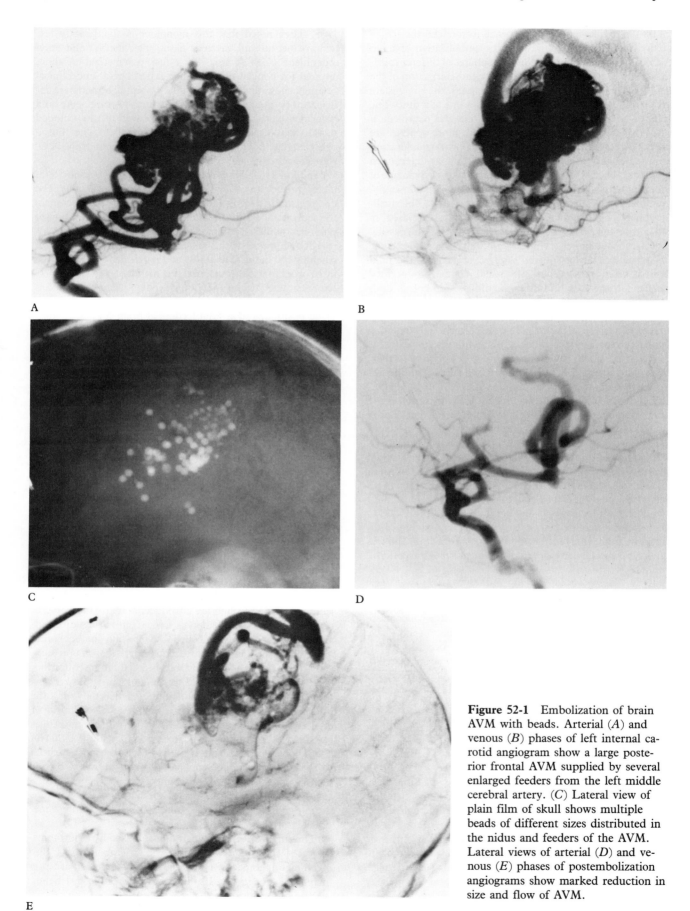

A

B

C

D

Figure 52-1 Embolization of brain AVM with beads. Arterial (*A*) and venous (*B*) phases of left internal carotid angiogram show a large posterior frontal AVM supplied by several enlarged feeders from the left middle cerebral artery. (*C*) Lateral view of plain film of skull shows multiple beads of different sizes distributed in the nidus and feeders of the AVM. Lateral views of arterial (*D*) and venous (*E*) phases of postembolization angiograms show marked reduction in size and flow of AVM.

E

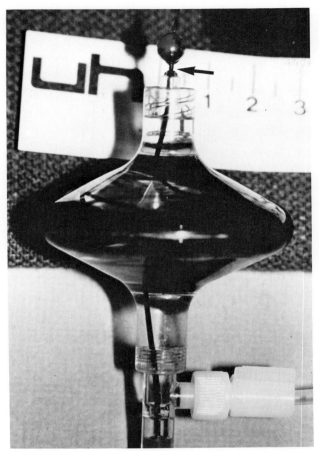

Figure 52-2 Transfemoral embolization of brain AVMs with IBCA. The latex calibrated-leak balloon is bonded to a flexible Silastic tubing (*arrow*). The Silastic tubing has been coiled in a chamber and is ready to be injected through the introducer.

The balloon-catheter system is flushed with a dextrose solution prior to embolization with IBCA. This is followed by manual injection of IBCA under fluoroscopic control. The IBCA is rendered opaque by the addition of 1 g of tantalum powder. The polymerization time of the IBCA is chosen to correspond to the arteriovenous transit time which was measured on the pre-embolization superselective angiogram. The polymerization time may be changed by the addition of iophendylate.[10]

Usually 0.2 to 0.9 cm^2 of IBCA is delivered through the balloon. This amount is regulated by the progression of the radiopaque IBCA column observed by fluoroscopy. When the column stops progressing and starts getting closer to the balloon, the balloon is rapidly deflated by aspiration and withdrawn to avoid gluing it in place.[14] After embolization, the vital signs and neurological status of the patient are checked and an angiogram is performed. When the AVM has several feeders, they may be embolized at the same sitting or on different days, depending on postembolization morphological results and the patient's clinical status. Some authors strongly recommend a sequential approach in order to minimize postembolization cerebral vasogenic edema, produced by sudden postembolization flow changes in the AVM and surrounding brain parenchyma.[22]

Animal and recent clinical experience[30,65] confirms that permanent occlusion is obtained in vessels embolized with IBCA as a result of a foreign body reaction and fibroblastic proliferation within the vessel walls.

Embolization with Isobutyl-2-cyanoacrylate in the Operating Room

This mode of treatment is useful for embolizing distal AVMs or those involving such areas of the brain as the motor or speech cortex. The technique was first described by Allcock et al.,[2] using Pantopaque-impregnated Gelfoam particles (absorbable gelatin sponge, The Upjohn Company, Kalamazoo, Mich.) as the embolic agent. Cromwell and Harris[9] described intraoperative embolization of AVMs with IBCA with the patient asleep. Girvin et al.[29] introduced the technique of intraoperative embolization of AVMs with IBCA with the patient awake.

Individual cortical arterial feeders are dissected and cannulated with a no. 3 French catheter (Fig. 52-4). Pre-embolization videoangiography and a sodium amytal test are performed, using a technique similar to that described in the transfemoral approach. IBCA is injected under fluoroscopic control, and the amount delivered in each injection is again marked by fluoroscopic progression of the radiopaque IBCA column. At the end of the embolization the neurosurgeon may or may not remove the AVM, depending on its topography.

Follow-up CT scans and angiograms are performed 4 to 6 days after therapy. If the AVM has not been completely embolized, a 6-month check angiogram is arranged.

The therapeutic method allows the neurosurgeon to map the functionally important areas of the cortex and to monitor the function of these areas clinically during the procedure. Temporary clipping of multiple vessels allows a more controlled injection of IBCA into the nidus, avoiding the washout effect of the remaining feeders. Continuous functional monitoring of the patient decreases the possibility of an unexpected neurological deficit appearing. The technique also allows a much greater volume of IBCA to be injected through the cannula and embolization of several feeders at the same sitting.[29]

The procedure has some disadvantages. It is associated with more discomfort for both the patient and the operator than the more traditional methods of treating AVMs. Raised intracranial pressure may occur in the awake patient, and this can lead to extremely unpleasant herniation of the brain through the craniotomy. In case of lack of cooperation by the patient, or repeated seizures or vomiting, or shock in the case of hemorrhage, an intubation must be performed immediately, which is unpleasant for the anesthetist in particular. Finally, if one believes that obliteration of AVMs by embolization should be staged, as has been the traditional mode, then, of course, repeated open operations are definitely a disadvantage.[29]

Progressive Thrombosis in Incompletely Embolized Arteriovenous Malformations

This phenomenon has been observed in brain AVMs in which IBCA occluded a substantial portion of the nidus, producing a decrease in flow and marked increase in blood

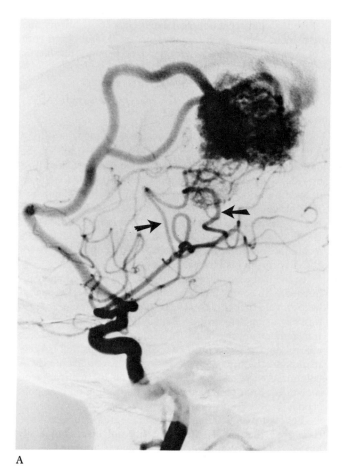

A

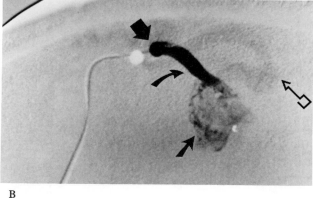

B

Figure 52-3 Pre-embolization superselective angiography. *A.* Internal carotid angiogram shows a mesiofrontal AVM mainly supplied by pericallosal and callosomarginal arteries, with less participation of MCA feeders (*arrows*). *B.* Superselective angiogram of pericallosal artery shows good visualization of the calibrated-leak balloon (*thick arrow*), arterial feeder (*curved arrow*), and AVM nidus (*straight arrow*). Faint visualization of draining vein (*square open arrow*).

stagnation in the AVM's venous outlet. Progressive thrombosis of the AVM may completely obliterate it[14] (Fig. 52-5). This phenomenon may be explained by postembolization hemodynamic changes observed on angiograms and by the active inflammatory process observed in the vessels occluded by IBCA and also in the surrounding brain parenchyma. There is a predominance of lymphocyte and mast cell infiltration in the local inflammatory process, and the infiltration may promote further occlusion of surrounding small vessels.[65] Discovery of this progressive postembolization vascular thrombosis has encouraged IBCA embolization of large AVMs without immediate surgical resection.

Results

Transfemoral and intraoperative embolization of brain AVMs with IBCA offers a promising technique for vascular occlusion in the central nervous system.[14,48] This therapy can substantially decrease or completely obliterate large AVMs or AVMs involving expressive areas of the brain.[14] Several technical modifications have improved its safety.[15,66] A long-term follow-up is now needed to compare morphological with clinical results. It is important to discover whether there is a change in the incidence and/or quality of headaches, seizures, progressive neurological deficit, or subarachnoid hemorrhage in patients with partially embolized

AVMs and to document hemodynamic changes observed after embolization (changes in pressure, flow, and peripheral resistance). These functional parameters may help us to understand the pathophysiology of brain AVMs and to control their therapeutic embolization.

The techniques of embolizing brain AVMs with IBCA need to be handled with great care by an experienced team, because the complexity of this procedure and the delicate brain territory to be embolized carry an intrinsic risk of producing a postembolization transient or permanent neurological deficit. Complications include gluing of the calibrated-leak balloon in place,[4,14] subarachnoid hemorrhage produced by the balloon bursting in a small arterial feeder,[14] dissection of the internal carotid or vertebral artery in the neck by manipulation with large coaxial catheters,[14] transient neurological deficit produced by postembolization vasogenic edema,[14,22] permanent neurological deficit produced by occlusion of normal cortical arteries,[14] and death.[14]

Between August 1978 and September 1982, 64 patients with cerebral arteriovenous malformations were treated by IBCA embolization at University Hospital, London, Ont., Canada; in 113 of the embolizations the transfemoral technique was used and in 45 the intraoperative catheterization technique. All patients had a follow-up angiogram, but there has not been a long enough interval for long-term angiographic and clinical follow-up. The follow-up angiogram al-

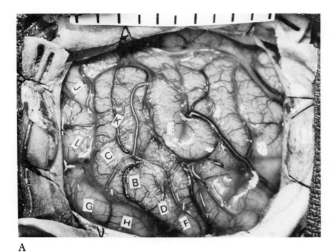

A

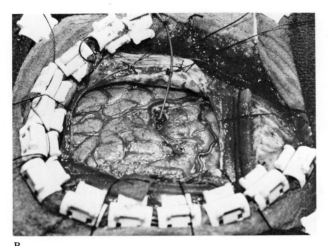

B

Figure 52-4 Intraoperative technique of AVM emboliza-tion. *A.* Functional mapping of the brain cortex by elec-trical stimulation. *B.* Cannulation of a cortical arterial feeder with a no. 3 French catheter through a small arte-riotomy. The cannula is secured in place with a ligature through the dura.

lows an assessment of the degree of obliteration of the AVM (Table 52-1), and 100 percent obliteration was achieved in eight cases by embolization alone (Fig. 52-6). These eight represent close to 20 percent of the 45 patients who had IBCA injected but who did not have resection (from the total of 64 patients). An additional 19, or more than 45 percent of the 45 patients who had embolization and no resection, had

more than two-thirds of the nidus of the AVM obliterated. Considering that the majority of the AVMs embolized with IBCA were considered to be either inoperable or operable only with great risk and difficulty, complete or near com-plete obliteration of these AVMs in the majority of cases is a significant achievement for a new methodology in evolution.

The results were accompanied by some complications (Table 52-2). The series of 64 patients includes three deaths due to hemorrhage that took place during the embolization. Two of these were technique-related, with rupture of a feed-ing vessel in one and the nidus of the AVM in the other caused mechanically by the balloon catheter. Technical ad-justments can be made to avoid this. The third death was caused by a hemorrhage about ½ h after IBCA injection into an arterial feeder in the left thalamus, presumably due to some perfusion change initiated by the embolization, since no arterial rupture could be identified at autopsy. In two cases the balloon catheter was glued in place without neuro-logical deficit. Permanent neurological complications in-cluded seven cases of hemianopsia or quadranopsia, pre-dicted prior to embolization and agreed to in advance by the patient as an expected complication of treatment. Of the five patients with some residual motor weakness, two were con-sidered to have moderate or severe weakness. Both had large malformations in expressive areas. Given the success in ob-literating AVMs by this evolving technique, and comparing it with surgical excision in the same areas, the complications listed do not seem excessive.

Spinal Arteriovenous Malformations

Several articles delineate the anatomical and angiographic details of the blood supply to the spinal cord.[16,28]

Most authors agree on the regional nature of the blood supply to the spinal cord and on its division into three major arterial territories; superior, or cervicodorsal (cervical cord and the first two dorsal segments); middle, or mid-dorsal region (first seven dorsal spine segments) and inferior, or dorsolumbosacral region (from D8 to the conus termi-nalis).[40]

The arterial supply of the spinal cord is generally de-scribed as being derived from the vertebral and subclavian arteries and the thoracolumbar aorta, and occasionally from the iliac and sacral arteries as well.[64] The spinal cord has three longitudinal arterial trunks: the anterior spinal artery and two posterolateral arteries. The anterior spinal artery terminates at the lower end of the spinal cord, 1.5 cm from the end of the conus terminalis, where it anastomoses with

TABLE 52-1 Proportion of AVM Obliteration, Number of Cases

Location	No Embolization	Less Than 70% Oblit.	70–99% Oblit.	100% Obliteration		Total
				Emb. Alone	Emb. + Resection	
Right hemisphere	5	11	7	4	6	33
Left hemisphere	2	6	13	2	4	27
Deep or posterior fossa		2		2		4
Total	7	19	20	8	10	64

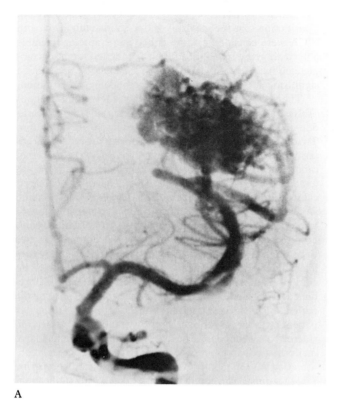

A

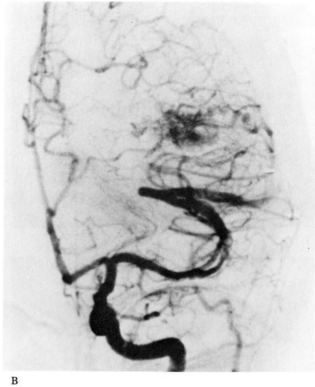

B

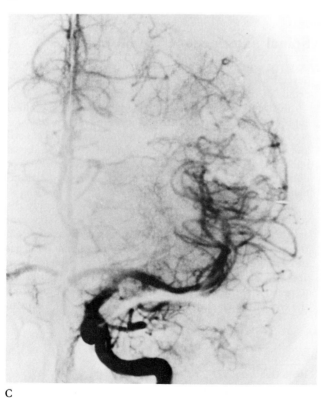

C

Figure 52-5   Postembolization progressive AVM thrombosis. *A*. Pre-embolization left common carotid angiogram shows a left frontal rolandic arteriovenous malformation. *B*. Check angiogram 1 week after IBCA embolization shows some residual AVM and depression of the sylvian point by mass effect. *C*. Check angiogram 6 months after embolization shows complete occlusion of the AVM. The mass effect on the surrounding vessels is no longer seen.

the two posterolateral trunks to form part of the cruciate vascular arch.[31,64] Djinjian et al.[18] played an essential role in the development of superselective angiography of spinal cord feeders and the methodology of embolization of spinal cord AVMs. A combination of standard selective spinal angiography, angiotomography, and angiomyelography is essential in mapping spinal AVMs and assessing their relation to the spinal cord.[17]

A

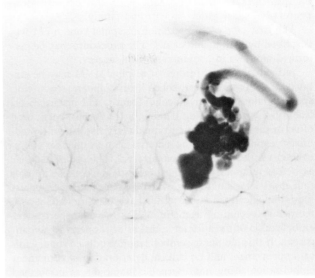

B

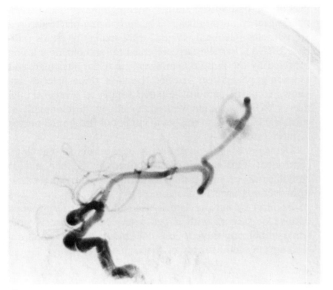

C

Figure 52-6 Complete embolization of brain AVM. Pre-embolization arterial (*A*) and venous (*B*) phases of left carotid angiogram show a parietal AVM supplied by a single left middle cerebral artery feeder. *C.* Check angiogram 1 week after IBCA intraoperative embolization shows complete occlusion of the AVM.

On the basis of the angiographic findings, spinal AVMs may be classified as (1) retromedullary AVMs (blood supply from posterior spinal arteries), (2) intramedullary AVMs (main blood supply from the anterior spinal artery, and (3) extramedullary AVMs with medullary venous drainage.[18]

Treatment

As in brain AVMs, endovascular or surgical treatment of spinal AVMs needs to be preceded by a thorough discussion of the natural history of the disease and the advantages and

TABLE 52-2 Permanent Complications of AVM Embolization

Location	Total Cases	Death	Balloon Glued	Motor Weakness		Visual Field Defect
				Mild	Moderate/Severe	
Right hemisphere	33	1	1	2		4
Left hemisphere	27	2	1		1	3
Deep or posterior fossa	4			1	1	
Total	64	3	2	3	2	7

disadvantages of the treatment with the neurosurgical-neuroradiological team, patient, and family.

The first case of embolization of spinal cord AVM was described by Doppmann et al.[21] The procedure may be performed alone or in conjunction with surgery.[17]

Individual arterial feeders of a spinal AVM may be embolized with particulate solids (dura mater, fresh clot, sponge Ivalon (polyvinyl alcohol foam)), and in rare cases, isobutyl-2-cyanoacrylate. Although IBCA has been used often in the treatment of extramedullary fistulae with medullary venous drainage, the material is rarely used for embolization via the anterior spinal artery.[56] The use of balloons as well as temporary embolization with clot are useful tools to identify lateral networks which are not otherwise detectable radiologically.[56] Riché et al. have used fresh clot as a temporary occluding agent in AVMs in which permanent embolization of the anterior spinal artery appears to be dangerous. If this temporary embolization produced some clinical improvement and no clinical deterioration, a permanent embolization using nonresorbable material was performed later.[56]

Riché et al.[56] reported their results in embolizing spinal AVMs mainly supplied by the anterior spinal artery. They reported 33 patients treated by embolization and/or surgery: of these, 21 were treated by embolization alone, 6 were treated by a combination of embolization and surgery, and 6 had only the surgical procedure (Fig. 52-7). Of the 33 patients, 18 were treated in several sessions separated by intervals of 3 weeks to 3 months. Excellent angiographic and clinical results were reported in the cervical and dorsolumbar regions but less satisfactory results in the middorsal region. The authors postulated that the relatively poor results in the thoracic region could be mainly related to lack of well developed collateral pathways in the thoracic spinal cord.

Berenstein et al.[5] used somatosensory evoked potentials as a guideline to assess the response of the spinal cord when one of the AVM's arterial feeders is temporarily occluded.

Embolization of the External Carotid Artery

The external carotid artery is the dominant blood supply of highly vascularized tumors of the head and neck (hemangiomas of bone and soft tissue, tumors of the cranial nerves, chemodectomas) and dural AVMs.

The development of the technique of superselective catheterization of distal branches of the external carotid artery with standard catheters[20,37] or calibrated-leak balloons[15] allows a safer embolization of lesions supplied by the external carotid artery.

Superselective angiography accurately locates the lesion and also shows the relation between the vascular territory and the several potential nutrient vessels (hemodynamic balance)[37] (Fig. 52-8). It is essential to recognize different collateral pathways between external and internal carotid arteries and their functional balance, because these pathways may be used to embolize lesions otherwise inaccessible or they may be the source of disastrous iatrogenic complications.[1,37]

Embolization of lesions supplied by the external carotid artery is performed alone or in combination with postembolization surgical resection. The combination treatment is used mainly in hypervascular tumors such as chemodecto-

mas of the base of the skull,[36] meningiomas,[6,47] and nasopharyngeal angiofibromas.[39] The embolizing materials used are particles (Gelfoam, Ivalon, dura mater) or fluids (silicone, IBCA). Particles are preferred for embolizing a lesion supplied by the middle meningeal, posterior auricular, and ascending pharyngeal arteries, because these arteries are known to participate in the blood supply to several cranial nerves.[38] Embolization with them allows development of collateral pathways to the blood supply of the cranial nerves in most cases.

Delivery of the embolizing agent should be flow-controlled. This technique, described by Kerber, avoids embolization of intracranial structures by opening extra- to intracranial arterial anastomoses.[35]

Isobutyl-2-cyanoacrylate is used in dural arteriovenous fistulae or tumors with a fast arteriovenous transit time when embolizing these lesions does not carry the risk of occluding the blood supply of the cranial nerves.[15]

Arteriovenous Fistulae

An arteriovenous (AV) fistula is an abnormal direct communication between an artery and a vein, bypassing the capillary system. AV fistulae may be congenital or acquired, with trauma being the most common cause of the latter.

The most common arteriovenous fistulae observed in the head and neck are the carotid-cavernous (CC), the vertebrovertebral (VV), and those involving branches of the external carotid artery.

An AV fistula can be obliterated by surgery or by endovascular occlusion using a Fogarty catheter[7] or a detachable balloon. Occlusion of an AV fistula with a detachable balloon was originally described by Serbinenko[61] and subsequently by Debrun et al.[12] They used latex detachable balloons; Silastic and silicone detachable balloons are now available as well.[69]

In treating a CC fistula, the balloon may be introduced into the cavernous sinus via the arterial route. In some CC fistulae with a predominantly posterior venous outflow, the cavernous sinus may be reached via an enlarged inferior petrosal sinus.[12,46] In selected cases of AV fistula in which treatment by the endovascular or venous route has failed, introduction of the balloon intraoperatively into the cavernous sinus may succeed in obliterating the fistula.[12]

Bank et al.[3] have also described occlusion of CC fistulae by injection of IBCA directly into the cavernous sinus while preserving blood flow in the internal carotid artery.

Traumatic CC Fistulae

The precise location of the fistula is identified in most cases by the technique of vertebral artery injection with concomitant compression of the involved internal carotid artery in the neck, as described by Debrun et al.[12] (Fig. 52-9). The horizontal intracavernous portion of the internal carotid artery is the most common location for a traumatic CC fistula.[12] The external carotid artery rarely participates in the blood supply of a traumatic CC fistula.[12] The cavernous sinus outflow may vary from one patient to another and is

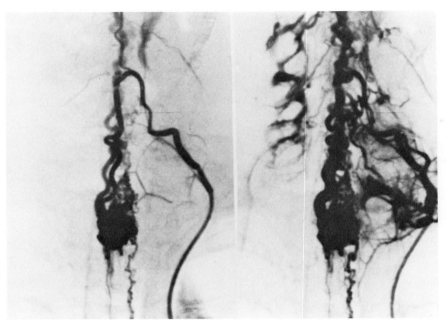

A

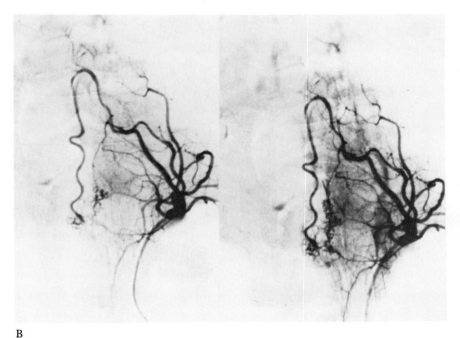

B

Figure 52-7 Embolization of spinal AVM. *A*. Arterial and venous phases of spinal angiogram show a thoracic AVM supplied by the anterior spinal artery. *B*. Check angiogram after embolization with dura shows obliteration of most of the AVM nidus. (Courtesy of Dr. M.C. Riché.)

related to anatomical variation and to possible thrombosis of the cavernous sinus. The venous outflow most commonly observed in traumatic CC fistulae is through the superior ophthalmic vein, the pterygoid plexus, the superior and inferior petrosal sinuses, and the superior sylvian veins, and contralaterally through the coronal veins.

Transarterial Approach to Traumatic CC Fistulae

A no. 8 French introducer is positioned in the internal carotid artery via the transfemoral technique or by direct puncture in the neck. A latex detachable balloon–Teflon catheter system, described by Debrun et al.,[11] is advanced through the introducer into the internal carotid artery. A balloon of appropriate size is selected after estimation from the pre-embolization angiogram of the size of the fistula. Once the balloon enters the cavernous sinus through the fistula, it is slowly inflated under fluoroscopic control until the fistula is occluded. When it is occluded satisfactorily, detachment is effected by sliding a tightly fitting polyethylene catheter over the Teflon catheter until its tip meets the resistance of the latex ligature. At this point, forward pressure on the coaxial polyethylene catheter and traction on the Teflon catheter force the Teflon catheter to withdraw from the balloon without exerting traction on the surrounding

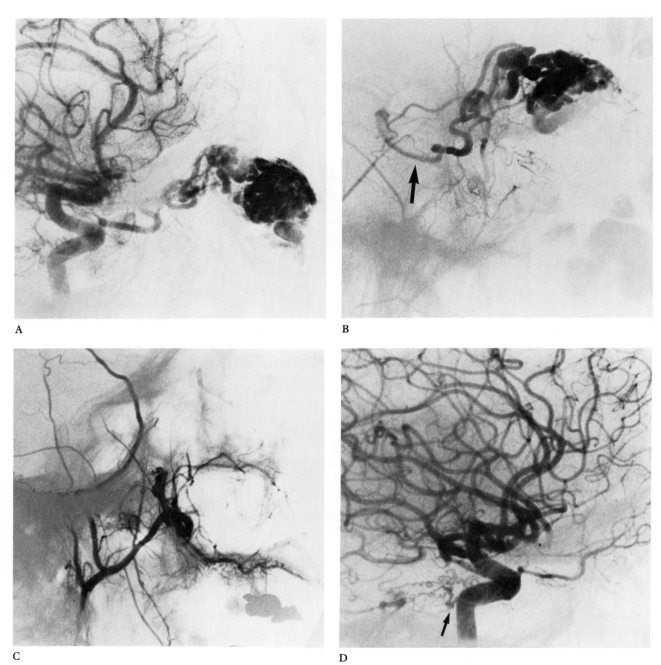

Figure 52-8 Functional embolization of orbital AVM. *A.* Selective internal carotid angiogram shows an orbital AVM supplied by the ophthalmic artery. *B.* Selective injection of the anterior deep temporal artery shows filling of part of the AVM and retrograde visualization of the ophthalmic artery (*arrow*). *C.* Postembolization external carotid angiogram showing complete obliteration of orbital AVM. The AVM was embolized with 0.5 ml of IBCA through the anterior deep temporal artery. *D.* Post-embolization internal carotid angiogram shows complete occlusion of the orbital AVM. Note a small dural AVM supplied by the meningohypophyseal trunk (*arrow*). (Courtesy of Dr. P. Lasjaunias.)

vascular structures.[23] The latex ligature seals the proximal end of the balloon. A confirmatory angiogram is always performed before the balloon is detached in the cavernous sinus. In most cases a single balloon is enough to occlude the

fistula (Fig. 52-10). In some patients with a large cavernous sinus, more than one balloon needs to be detached to achieve occlusion of the AV shunt (Fig. 52-11).

The contrast-filled balloon slowly deflates over a period

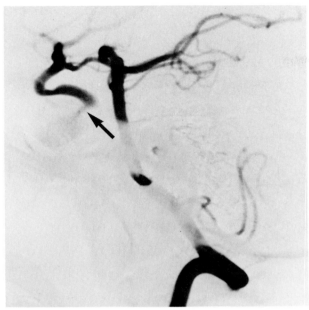

Figure 52-9 Visualization of carotid-cavernous fistula site. Vertebral angiogram with concomitant carotid compression in the neck shows retrograde filling of the carotid siphon and fistula site (*arrow*).

of weeks without recurrence of the already thrombosed fistula. Alternatively, the balloon may be filled with a silicone polymer to achieve permanent inflation.[12]

Debrun et al.[12] were able to occlude 53 of 54 traumatic CC fistulae with this technique. The carotid flow was preserved in 32 of the 54 cases (59 percent). Concomitant occlusion of the fistula and the internal carotid artery was performed in 22 patients. A postembolization intracavernous pseudoaneurysm occurred in 24 of the 54 cases (44 percent) (Fig. 52-12). Pseudoaneurysms that induced severe retro-orbital pain or oculomotor nerve palsy were treated by occlusion of the intracavernous internal carotid artery.

Detachment of more than one balloon in a CC fistula with a large cavernous sinus may produce postembolization nerve palsy and/or severe retro-orbital pain caused by excessive compression by the inflated balloons. Sixth nerve palsy occurred more often than third nerve palsy, and patients recovered faster.[12] Full recovery from this iatrogenic complication was observed in most of Debrun's patients.

Transvenous Approach to Traumatic CC Fistulae

The transvenous approach is another way of reaching the cavernous sinus and fistula when there is predominant posterior venous outflow through an enlarged inferior petrosal sinus. This route appears to be more difficult than the transarterial one, because the detachable balloon must be advanced against the venous outflow and negotiate the often numerous partitions of the cavernous sinus. Debrun et al. used the venous route in 12 patients and obtained complete obliteration of the traumatic CC fistula in only one.[12]

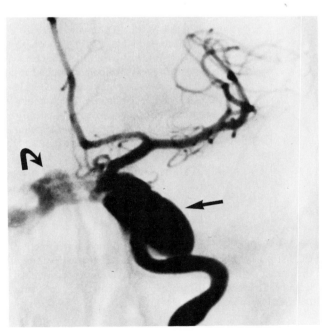

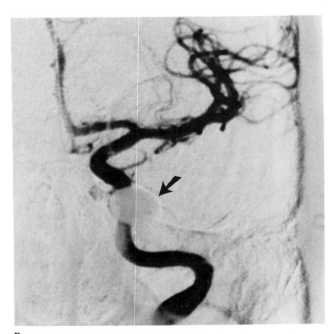

A   B

Figure 52-10 Detachable balloon occlusion of carotid-cavernous fistula. *A.* AP view of left internal carotid angiogram shows abnormal early visualization of ipsilateral cavernous sinus (*straight arrow*). There is also opacification of the contralateral cavernous sinus (*curved arrow*). *B.* Left internal carotid angiogram shows occlusion of the CC fistula by a detachable balloon (*arrow*), with preservation of the internal carotid artery lumen.

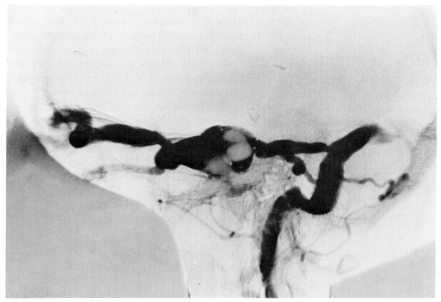

A

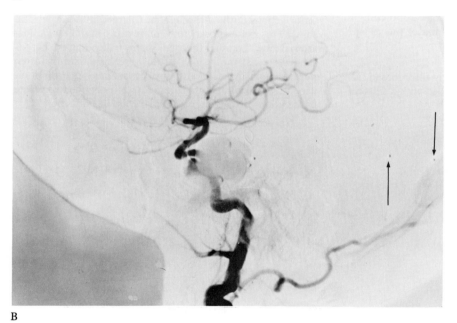

B

Figure 52-11 Traumatic carotid-cavernous fistula. *A.* Venous phase of left internal carotid angiogram shows several balloons detached in a huge cavernous sinus without occlusion of the fistula. *B.* Check angiograms after detachment of several balloons shows successful occlusion of the fistula with preservation of the internal carotid artery lumen. Two balloons burst, and their silver clips are lodged in the ipsilateral lateral sinus (*arrows*).

Surgical Approach to Traumatic CC Fistulae

A combined neurosurgical-neuroradiological approach may be used in those patients in whom the transarterial and venous approaches have failed.[12] The cavernous sinus is exposed, using the approach described by Parkinson.[52] A no. 8 introducer is positioned in the cavernous sinus, and a detachable balloon is introduced through the introducer and slowly inflated until the retro-orbital bruit disappears on Doppler probe, the instrument being positioned over the ipsilateral eye. A postoperative angiogram is then performed after 48 to 72 h.

The three different approaches used for the treatment of CC fistulae with a detachable balloon aim at preservation of the lumen of the internal carotid artery. The experience collected at University Hospital, London, Ont. Canada is summarized in Table 52-3.

Vertebrovertebral Fistulae

In principle, the same technical approach applies to the treatment of VV fistulae. Current neuroradiological experience is mainly based on the transarterial approach.[13] Iso-

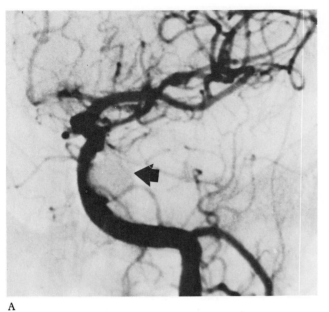

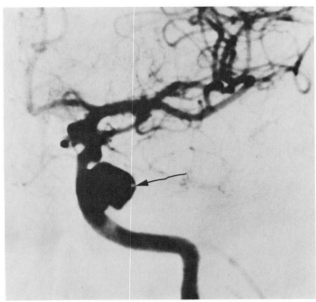

A

B

Figure 52-12   Traumatic carotid-cavernous fistula. *A.* Left common carotid angiogram. AP view shows successful obliteration of a traumatic CC fistula by a single balloon detached in the cavernous sinus (*arrow*). *B.* Pseudoaneurysm formation produced by early deflation of the balloon in the cavernous sinus. The silver clip positioned in the balloon's tip is well visualized (*arrow*).

lated reports on the transvenous and intraoperative approaches have also appeared.[27,33]

The experience at University Hospital is confined to treatment of eight cases of VV fistulae (Table 52-4). All eight were completely obliterated by a Debrun detachable balloon, with preservation of the vertebral artery in six (Fig. 52-13). Two additional cases with a fistula associated with dysplasia of the vertebral artery due to neurofibromatosis were also treated. Both of these were approached to obliterate the vertebral artery along with the fistula, but in one the treatment was incomplete and there was need for further surgical intervention. No neurological complication due to treatment arose in any of these cases.

Spontaneous CC Fistulae

Spontaneous CC fistula and traumatic CC fistula have an entirely different clinical presentation and radiographic appearance.[19] From the clinical viewpoint, spontaneous CC fistulae are seen most frequently in middle-aged women with no history of previous trauma. They have a prolonged clinical course and may sometimes resolve spontaneously. Angiographically they have an external carotid-internal carotid blood supply, with a vascular nidus often being identified and with relatively slow AV shunting [51] (Fig. 52-14).

Spontaneous CC fistulae are infrequently produced by spontaneous rupture of an intracavernous aneurysm.[67] Dif-

TABLE 52-3   Treatment of Traumatic Carotid-Cavernous Fistulae

	Number of Cases	Preservation of Carotid Artery	Temporary Cranial Nerve Dysfunction (III,IV,V,VI)	Other
Complete obliteration	37	25	10	1 transient ischemic attack
Partial obliteration followed by surgery	7	3	3	1 brain abscess
Embolization at surgery	1	1		
Total	45	29	13	2

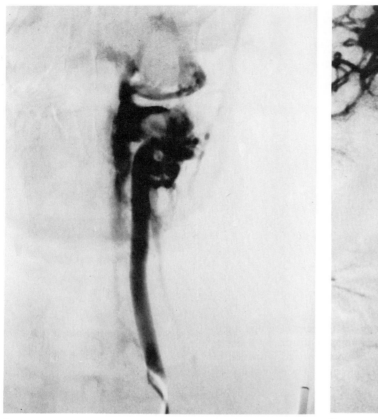

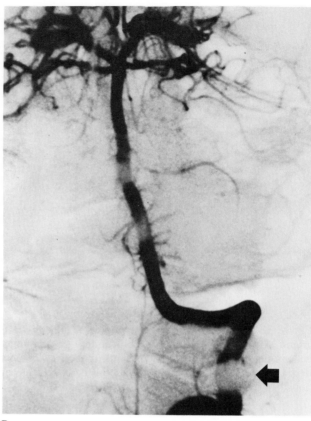

A   B

Figure 52-13   Traumatic vertebrovertebral fistula. *A.* AP view of left vertebral angiogram shows a VV fistula with early filling of paravertebral veins. *B.* Check angiogram after detachment of balloon at the fistula site (*arrow*) shows occlusion of the fistula with preservation of the lumen of the vertebral artery.

ferent therapeutic approaches are used for the treatment of this disease, depending on the angiographic findings. A cavernous dural AVM is treated by embolization of the feeders arising from the external carotid artery with particles, spheres, or isobutyl 2-cyanoacrylate.[45,67] In most cases an incomplete occlusion of the nidus of the AVM is sufficient to obtain substantial clinical improvement, and sometimes this may progress to complete occlusion of the AVM.[67] In cases of spontaneous CC fistula produced by rupture of an aneurysm, it may be necessary to occlude the aneurysm and the internal carotid artery at the same sitting.[67]

Caution must be exercised in approaching treatment of a spontaneous CC fistula, because it may thrombose spontaneously,[51,68] and sometimes partial embolization of the external carotid artery territory alone may be sufficient to obtain a substantial clinical improvement or cure.[67]

Table 52-5 shows the experience in this field at University Hospital, London, Ont. Canada. By far the vast majority of these cases are AVMs involving the dura of the cavernous sinuses or superior orbital fissure region. In seven of ten cases of dural AVMs treated, embolization of the external carotid portion with small particles or liquid acrylic yielded complete obliteration of lesion despite associated feeding from meningeal branches of the cavernous carotid artery (Fig. 52-15). In one case, feeding was from the internal carotid meningeal branches alone, and this was treated by ob-

TABLE 52-4   Treatment of Vertebrovertebral Fistulae

	Number of Cases	Preservation of Vertebral Artery	Complete Obliteration
Spontaneous or traumatic	8	6	8
Neurofibromatosis	2		1

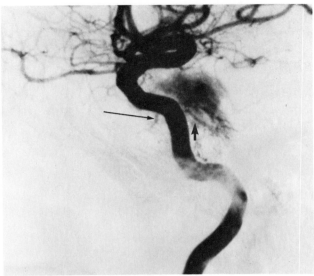

A

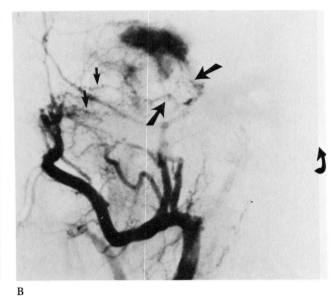

B

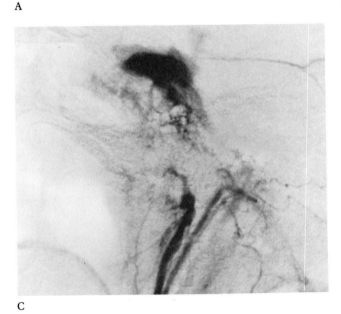

C

Figure 52-14 Spontaneous carotid-cavernous fistula.
A. Selective left internal carotid angiogram shows a cavernous sinus dural AVM supplied by the meningohypophyseal trunk (*short arrow*), and inferolateral trunk (*long arrow*).
B. Selective internal maxillary angiogram shows blood supply also from radicals arising from internal maxillary artery (*small arrows*) and middle meningeal artery (*large arrows*).
C. Selective ascending pharyngeal artery angiogram again shows multiple radicals feeding the cavernous sinus dural AVM.

literation of the carotid by a detachable balloon. Two patients with incomplete obliteration of the AVM had surgery to complete the treatment. In only two cases was a large hole demonstrated in the carotid artery, which was presumed to have been caused by the rupture of an aneurysm. Both these patients were treated by a detachable balloon, and one had

subsequent obliteration of the carotid artery due to filling of the giant aneurysm following obliteration of the fistula. One patient with dural AVM treated with liquid acrylic had an ischemic complication due to retrograde filling of the internal carotid artery through external carotid collaterals.

TABLE 52-5 Treatment of Spontaneous Carotid-Cavernous Fistulae

	Number of Cases	Preservation of Carotid Artery	Complete Obliteration	Partial Obliteration Followed by Surgery
Dural AVM	10	9	8	2
Aneurysm	2	1	2	

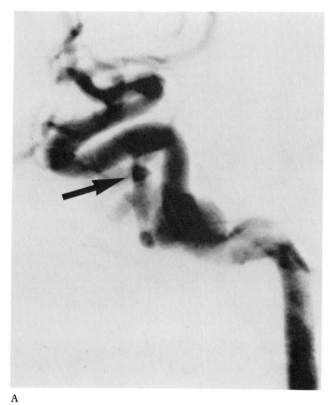

A

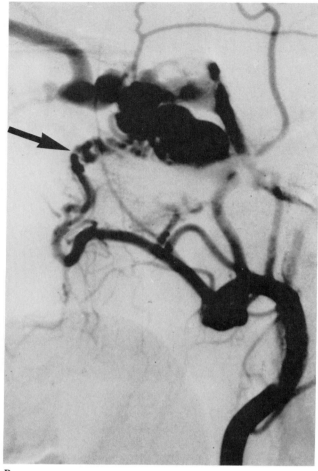

B

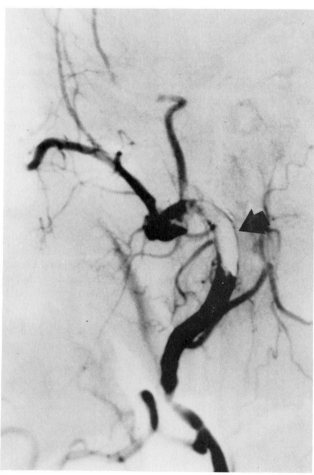

C

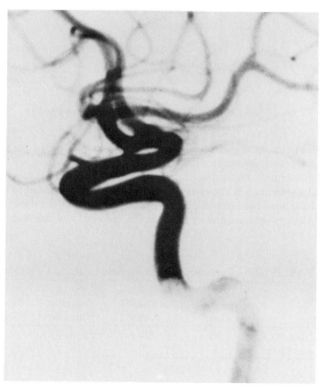

D

References

1. Ahn HS, Kerber CW, Deeb ZL: Extra-to-intracranial arterial anastomoses in therapeutic embolization: Recognition and role. AJNR, 1:71–75, 1980.
2. Allcock J, Drake CG, Fox A, Peerless SJ: Treatment of cerebral arteriovenous malformation by direct embolization into the feeding vessels at craniotomy. Neuroradiology 15:117, 1978 (abstr).
3. Bank WO, Kerber CW, Drayer BP, Troost BT, Maroon JC: Carotid cavernous fistula: Endarterial cyanoacrylate occlusion with preservation of carotid flow. J Neuroradiol 5:279–285, 1978.
4. Bank WO, Tranier FG, Edwards MS, Newton TH: Arterial injury during manipulation of intracerebral microcatheters. Neuroradiology 22:274, 1982.
5. Berenstein A, Young W, Ransohoff J: Somatosensory evoked potentials (SEP) monitoring during spinal angiography and its use during therapeutic transvascular embolization. AJNR 3:96 1982 (abstr).
6. Brismar J, Cronqvist S: Therapeutic embolization in the external carotid artery region. Acta Radiol [Diagn] (Stockh) 19:715–731, 1978.
7. Chowdhary UM: Treatment of carotid-cavernous fistula using a balloon-tipped intra-arterial catheter. J Neurol Neurosurg Psychiatry 41:996–1000, 1978.
8. Collins JA, Pani KC, Lehman RA, Leonard F: Biological substrates and cure rates of cyanoacrylate tissue adhesives. Arch Surg 93:428–432, 1966.
9. Cromwell LD, Harris AB: Treatment of cerebral arteriovenous malformations: A combined neurosurgical and neuroradiological approach. J Neurosurg 52:705–708, 1980.
10. Cromwell LD, Kerber CW: Modification of cyanoacrylate for therapeutic embolization: Preliminary experience. AJR 132:799–801, 1979.
11. Debrun G, Lacour P, Caron J, Hurth M, Comox J, Keravel Y: Detachable balloon and calibrated-leak balloon techniques in the treatment of cerebral vascular lesions. J Neurosurg 49:635–649, 1978.
12. Debrun G, Lacour P, Viñuela F, Fox A, Drake CG, Caron JP: Treatment of 54 traumatic carotid-cavernous fistulas. J Neurosurg 55:678–692, 1981.
13. Debrun G, Legre J, Kasbarian M, Tapias PL, Caron JP: Endovascular occlusion of vertebral fistulae by detachable balloons with conservation of the vertebral blood flow. Radiology 130:141–147, 1979.
14. Debrun G, Viñuela F, Fox A, Drake CG: Embolization of cerebral arteriovenous malformations with Bucrylate: Experience in 46 cases. J Neurosurg 56:615–627, 1982.
15. Debrun GM, Viñuela FV, Fox AJ, Kan S: Two different calibrated-leak balloons: Experimental work and application in humans. AJNR 3:407–414, 1982.

Figure 52-15 Spontaneous carotid-cavernous fistula. *A.* Internal carotid angiogram shows a dural cavernous sinus AVM supplied by the inferolateral trunk (*arrow*). *B.* Internal maxillary artery angiogram shows participation of the artery of the foramen rotundum (*arrow*) in the blood supply to this dural AVM. Abnormal filling of the cavernous sinus, superior ophthalmic vein, and inferior petrosal sinus. *C.* External carotid angiogram after embolization with IBCA shows a cast of IBCA producing partial occlusion of the internal maxillary artery trunk (*arrow*). Nonvisualization of the dural CC fistula. *D.* Postembolization internal carotid angiogram shows no evidence of CC fistula.

16. Djindjian R: Arteriography of the spinal cord. AJR 107:461–478, 1969.
17. Djindjian R, Houdart R, Hurth M: Embolisation dans les angiomes de la moelle. J Neuroradiol 2:73–172, 1975.
18. Djindjian R, Houdart R, Lefebvre J, Fauré C, LeBesnerais Y, Hurth M: L'arteriographie des angiomes de la moelle. Rev Neurol (Paris) 109:640–645, 1963.
19. Djindjian R, Manelfe C, Picard L: Fistules arterioveineuses carotide externe-sinus caverneux: Etude angiographique à propos de 6 observations et revue de la litérature. Neurochirurgie 19:91–110, 1973.
20. Djindjian R, Merland JJ: *Super-selective Arteriography of the External Carotid Artery.* Berlin, Springer-Verlag, 1978.
21. Doppman JL, Di Chiro G, Ommaya AK: Percutaneous embolization of spinal cord arteriovenous malformations. J Neurosurg 34:48–55, 1971.
22. Drake CG: Cerebral arteriovenous malformations: Considerations for and experience with surgical treatment in 166 cases. Clin Neurosurg 26:145–208, 1979.
23. Dubois PJ, Kerber CW, Heinz ER: Interventional techniques in neuroradiology. Radiol Clin North Am 17:515–542, 1979.
24. Dutton J: Acrylic investment of intracranial aneurysms: A report of 12 years experience. J Neurosurg 31:652–657, 1969.
25. Forster DMC, Steiner L, Hakanson S: Arteriovenous malformations of the brain: A long-term clinical study. J Neurosurg 37:562–570, 1972.
26. Freeny PC, Mennemeyer R, Kidd CR, Bush WH: Long-term radiographic-pathologic follow-up of patients treated with visceral transcatheter occlusion using isobutyl-2-cyanoacrylate (Bucrylate). Radiology 132:51–60, 1979.
27. George B, Laurian C: Surgical approach to the whole length of the vertebral artery with special reference to the third portion. Acta Neurochir (Wien) 51:259–272, 1980.
28. Gillilan LA: The arterial blood supply of the human spinal cord. J Comp Neurol 110:75–103, 1958.
29. Girvin JP, Fox AJ, Viñuela F, Drake CG: Intraoperative embolization (IBC) of cerebral arteriovenous malformations in the awake patient. Can J Neurol Sci 9:229, 1982.
30. Goldman ML, Freeny PC, Tallman JM, Galambos JT, Bradley EL III, Salam A, Oen K, Gordon IJ, Mennemeyer R: Transcatheter vascular occlusion therapy with isobutyl-2-cyanoacrylate (Bucrylate) for control of massive upper-gastrointestinal bleeding. Radiology 129:41–49, 1978.
31. Hassler O: Blood supply to human spinal cord: A microangiographic study. Arch Neurol 15:302–307, 1966.
32. Hieshima GB, Mehringer CM, Grinnell VS, Hasso AN, Siegel NH, Pribram HF: Emergency occlusive techniques. Surg Neurol 9:293–302, 1978.
33. Kendall B, Hodare R: Percutaneous transvenous balloon occlusion of arteriovenous fistula. Neuroradiology 20:203–205, 1980.
34. Kerber CW: Intracranial cyanoacrylate: A new catheter therapy for arteriovenous malformation. Invest Radiol 10:536–538, 1975.
35. Kerber CW: Flow-controlled therapeutic embolization: A physiologic and safe technique. AJNR 1:77–81, 1980.
36. Lacour P, Doyon D, Manelfe C, Picard L, Salisacks P, Schwaab G: L'embolisation artérielle thérapeutique dans les chémodectomes (tumeurs glomiques). J Neuroradiol 2:275–287, 1975.
37. Lasjuanias PL: *Craniofacial and Upper Cervical Arteries: Functional, Clinical and Angiographic Aspects.* Baltimore, Williams & Wilkins, 1981.
38. Lasjuanias P, Manelfe C: Arterial supply for the upper cervical nerves and the cervicocarotid anastomotic channels. Neuroradiology 18:125–131, 1979.
39. Lasjuanias P, Picard L, Manelfe C, Moret J, Doyon D: Angio-

fibroma of the nasopharynx: A review of 53 cases treated by embolization: The role of pretherapeutic angiogaphy: Pathophysiological hypotheses. J Neuroradiol 7:73–95, 1980.

40. Lazorthes G, Gouaze A, Zadeh JO, Santini JJ, Lazorthes Y, Bardin P: Arterial vascularization of the spinal cord: Recent studies of the anastomotic substitution pathways. J Neurosurg 35:253–262, 1971.

41. Lehman RA, Hayes GJ: The toxicity of alkyl 2-cyanoacrylate tissue adhesives: Brain and blood vessels. Surgery 61:915–922, 1967.

42. Lehman RAW, Hayes BJ, Martins AN: The use of adhesive and lyophilized dura in the treatment of cerebrospinal rhinorrhea: Technical note. J Neurosurg 26:92–95, 1967.

43. Locksley HB: Report on the Cooperative Study of Intracranial Aneurysms and Subarachnoid Hemorrhage. Section V, Part 1: Natural history of subarachnoid hemorrhage, intracranial aneurysms and arteriovenous malformations. Based on 6368 cases in the cooperative study. J Neurosurg 25:219–239, 1966.

44. Luessenhop AJ, Spence WT: Artificial embolization of cerebral arteries: Report of use in a case of arteriovenous malformation. JAMA 172:1153–1155, 1960.

45. Mahaley MS Jr, Boone SC: External carotid-cavernous fistula treated by arterial embolization: Case report. J Neurosurg 40:110–114, 1974.

46. Manelfe C, Berenstein A: Traitement des fistules carotidocaverneuses par voie veineuse: A propos d'un cas. J Neuroradiol 7:13–19, 1980.

47. Manelfe C, Djindjian R: Techniques de l'embolisation thérapeutique per catheterisme percutané. J Neuroradiol 2:11–27, 1975.

48. Mickey BE, Samson D: Neurosurgical applications of the cyanoacrylate adhesives. Clin Neurosurg 28:429–444, 1981.

49. Miyasaka K, Wolpert SM, Prager RJ: The association of cerebral aneurysms, infundibula and intracranial arteriovenous malformations. Stroke 13:196–203, 1982.

50. Newton TH, Cronqvist S: Involvement of dural arteries in intracranial arteriovenous malformations. Radiology 93:1071–1078, 1969.

51. Newton TH, Hoyt WF: Dural arteriovenous shunts in the region of the cavernous sinus. Neuroradiology 1:71–81, 1970.

52. Parkinson D: Carotid cavernous fistula: Direct repair with preservation of the carotid artery. Technical note. J Neurosurg 38:99–106, 1973.

53. Patronas NJ, Marx WJ, Duda EE, Mullan JJ: Microvascular embolization of arteriovenous malformations: Predicting success by cerebral angiography. AJNR 1:459–462, 1980.

54. Perret G, Nishioka H: Report on the Cooperative Study of Intracranial Aneurysms and Subarachnoid Hemorrhage, Section VI: Arteriovenous malformations: An analysis of 545 cases of cranio-cerebral arteriovenous malformations and fistulae reported to the cooperative study. J Neurosurg 25:467–490, 1966.

55. Pevsner PH: Micro-balloon catheter for superselective angiography and therapeutic occlusion. AJR 128:225–230, 1977.

56. Riché MC, Melki JP, Merland JJ: The current state of embolization of spinal cord vascular malformations via the anterior spinal artery. Presented at the XII Symposium Neuroradiologicum, Washington, D.C., October 10–16, 1982.

57. Rodda RA, Calvert GD: Post-mortem arteriography of cerebral arteriovenous malformations. J Neurol Neurosurg Psychiatry 32:432–439, 1969.

58. Romodanov AP, Zozulia YA, Shcheglov VI: Balloon catheter occlusion of the feeding vessels of arteriovenous malformations of the brain. Zentralbl Neurochir 40:21–25, 1979.

59. Russell DS: The pathology of spontaneous intracranial haemorrhage. Proc R Soc Med 47:689–693, 1954.

60. Samson D, Ditmore QM, Beyer CW Jr: Intravascular use of isobutyl 2-cyanoacrylate: Part 2. Treatment of carotid-cavernous fistulas. Neurosurgery 8:52–55, 1981.

61. Serbinenko FA: Six hundred endovascular neurosurgical procedures in vascular pathology: A ten-year experience. Acta Neurochir [Suppl] (Wien) 28:310–311, 1979.

62. Stehbens WE: *Pathology of the Cerebral Blood Vessels.* St. Louis, Mosby, 1972.

63. Svien HJ, McRae JA: Arteriovenous anomalies of the brain: Fate of patients not having definitive surgery. J Neurosurg 23:23–28, 1965.

64. Tveten L: Spinal cord vascularity: I. Extraspinal sources of spinal cord arteries in man. Acta Radiol [Diagn] (Stockh) 17:1–16, 1976.

65. Vinters HV, Debrun G, Kaufmann JCE, Drake CG: Pathology of arteriovenous malformations embolized with isobutyl-2-cyanoacrylate (Bucrylate): Report of two cases. J Neurosurg 55:819–825, 1981.

66. Viñuela F, Debrun GM, Fox AJ: The role of the pre-embolization superselective angiogram in the treatment of brain arteriovenous malformations with isobutyl-2-cyanoacrylate (IBC). Presented at the XII Symposium Neuroradiologicum, Washington, D.C., October 10–16, 1982.

67. Viñuela F, Fox AJ, Debrun GM, et al: Spontaneous carotidcavernous fistula: A dural AVM. Presented at the XVII Canadian Congress of Neurological Sciences, Toronto, Ontario, June 23–26, 1982.

68. Voigt K, Sauer M, Dichgans J: Spontaneous occlusion of a bilateral caroticocavernous fistula studied by serial angiography. Neuroradiology 2:207–211, 1971.

69. White RJ, Kaufman SL, Barth KH, DeCaprio V, Strandberg JD: Therapeutic embolization with detachable silicone balloons: Early clinical experience. JAMA 241:1257–1260, 1979.

70. Wolpert SM, Barnett FJ, Prager RJ: Benefits of embolization without surgery for cerebral arteriovenous malformations. AJNR 2:535–538, 1981.

71. Wolpert SM, Stein BM: Factors governing the course of emboli in the therapeutic embolization of cerebral arteriovenous malformations. Radiology 131:125–131, 1979.

72. Zanetti PH, Sherman FE: Experimental evaluation of a tissue adhesive as an agent for the treatment of aneurysms and arteriovenous anomalies. J Neurosurg 36:72–79, 1972.

Part VI

Neuro-oncology

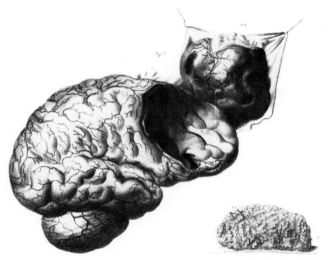

Cruveilhier J. *Anatomie Pathologique du Corps Humain*. Paris, 1829–1842. A convexity meningioma.

SECTION A

Neuro-oncology: An Overview

53

Genetic Factors in Brain Tumors

Robert L. Martuza

Recent developments in genetic research suggest that most tumors may be caused by an abnormality in the structure or function of one or more genes. This is true not only for tumors associated with inherited syndromes but also for the much more common tumors which are sporadic, solitary, and nonhereditary. Such gene abnormalities have been identified in tumors from both animals and humans. In some cases such genes are similar in structure to genes found in normal tissues, suggesting that tumor development may be due to a small abnormality in the structure or function of a gene normally present in all cells.[2] The function of such genes in the normal state is not known, but it has been suggested that they may be involved in embryogenesis or normal cellular differentation. Other studies have suggested that this mutation from normal gene(s) to abnormal tumor gene(s) may in some instances occur in more than one step.[9,11,12] The eventual effect of several mutations at one or more loci is the development of a tumor.

This accumulating body of evidence is gradually developing into a concept of oncogenesis that unifies prior theories of viral, chemical, radiation, and "natural" mechanisms of tumor induction. A virus carrying an abnormal "oncogene" or an abnormal gene segment that regulates another gene can integrate this DNA into a cell and, in one step, cause tumor development. Various chemical carcinogens may cause DNA base pair abnormalities that lead to tumor development. However, since these mutations are generally more random than those of viruses, carcinogenesis may in some cases be caused by a single exposure to the chemical but in other instances may require multiple exposures. Similarly, radiation-induced tumors are dose-dependent and

may, in some instances, represent an accumulation of several mutations leading to tumor formation. The same mechanism may be responsible for the naturally developing tumors. A single large mutation such as a partial chromosomal deletion may lead to tumor formation in one step; however, most naturally occurring mutations involve small segments of DNA, often a single base pair. Tumor development in the natural setting may require several small mutations developing over a period of time during the life of the animal or human being. Ingestion or inhalation of carcinogens or exposure to ionizing radiation may accelerate such mutational events.

Some people may be born with one or more abnormal genes acquired through inheritance or through a spontaneous mutation in early embryogenesis. Such germ cell mutations have been grouped as hereditary tumor syndromes. Patients carrying these genes have a higher incidence of certain tumors than the rest of the population. The development of these tumors is not simply due to the inherited gene(s), since the gene(s) is present in all cells of the body, and clearly, all cells do not develop into tumors. Some additional event is usually necessary. Whether this event is an additional mutation or simply modulation ("turning on") of the existing gene is not known. However, the pathology of the lesions that form in these hereditary tumor syndromes is usually similar to the pathology of analogous tumors that develop sporadically in other patients in a nonhereditary fashion. This fact underscores the importance of studies of the hereditary tumor syndromes. An understanding of the genes that cause these hereditary syndromes is important not only to the families harboring these mutations but also to the rest of the population and to all who are interested in neuro-oncology.

The hereditary tumor syndromes provide a window into the genetic causes of most of the tumors seen by neurosurgeons. In this chapter such syndromes are subdivided according to the type of cell primarily affected: (1) neuronal tumors (retinoblastoma, neuroblastoma, pheochromocytoma, multiple endocrine neoplasia, other paragangliomas); (2) meningiomas; (3) gliomas. The phakomatoses (neurofibromatosis, tuberous sclerosis, von Hippel-Lindau disease, and the neurocutaneous angiomatoses) are of such importance that they are covered in detail in a separate chapter.

Many of these tumors are of neural crest origin, and the term *neurocristopathy* has been applied to them.[3] Studies of normal neural crest differentiation have documented the many tissues that derive from this important embryologic structure, and Table 53-1 shows these normal derivatives as well as the abnormalities noted in these syndromes. It is

TABLE 53-1 Normal Tissues and Tumor Syndromes Derived from Neural Crest

Tumor syndrome	Neural crest derivative	Tumor syndrome
	Carotid body	
	Glomus jugulare	Paragangliomas
	Nodose ganglion	
Neuroblastoma	Sympathetic neurons	
	Anterior pituitary	
	Pancreatic islets	MEN I
	Parathyroids	
MEN II	Thyroid C cells	
	Adrenal medulla	MEN III
	Schwann cells	
Neurofibromatosis	Arachnoid cells	
	Melanocytes	

possible that a family of genes is responsible for the orderly sequence of development of the normal neural crest. Small mutations in these genes could account for each of these syndromes. Larger mutations could account for the overlap between the syndromes.

Neuronal Tumors

Retinoblastoma

Retinoblastoma is a rare, highly malignant tumor of the retina seen mostly in young children.[1] Although the retina is anatomically a part of the central nervous system and involvement of the brain by retinoblastoma has been reported, this type of tumor usually is seen by ophthalmologists and only rarely treated by neurosurgeons. Yet the genetics of this neural tumor have been more extensively and productively studied than those of most other tumors, and therefore retinoblastoma forms a useful model for neurosurgeons to use in understanding the possible genetic factors operative in other nervous system tumors.

Retinoblastoma occurs in approximately one in 20,000 live births and is usually detected within the first 4 years of life. It shows no preference for sex or race, and the incidence is fairly constant worldwide. There is no predilection for the right or the left eye. The tumor occurs unilaterally in about 70 percent of patients and bilaterally in approximately 30 percent. In patients with bilateral retinoblastoma, multiple retinal tumors are the norm. In patients with unilateral retinoblastoma, the lesions are solitary in about 85 percent and multiple in 15 percent. Therefore multifocal retinoblastoma occurs overall in 40 percent of affected patients. It is suggested that the multifocal disease, whether unilateral or bilateral, is due to a germ cell mutation, whereas a truly solitary lesion is more likely due to a somatic cell mutation. A patient with multifocal retinoblastoma, whether unilateral or bilateral, will transmit the disorder to 50 percent of offspring in an autosomal dominant fashion. Patients with lesions that are either unifocal or of undetermined focality generally have a somatic mutation and will not transmit the disorder; however, transmission occurs in up to 15 percent of the offspring of this group. This suggests that some may have a germ cell mutation with only partial or local expres-

sion of the tumor. Nonexpression (the carrier state) may also be seen in about 1 percent of phenotypically normal children born to parents with multifocal retinoblastoma.

Retinoblastomas have been subjected to extensive chromosomal analyses. Most studies have used peripheral leukocytes and have revealed that a small subset of patients (5 percent) with retinoblastoma plus other associated abnormalities (abnormal facies, psychomotor and growth retardation) have a deletion of part of the long arm of chromosome 13 (13q-). Studies of a number of patients harboring slightly different chromosomal deletions have suggested that the deletion of band 14 on the long arm of chromosome 13, probably in its proximal or middle segment, is the common feature in this group of patients.[7,20] Such studies suggest that the gene responsible for retinoblastoma may be at this locus.

Although localization of a gene responsible for oncogenesis is of obvious importance, two major concerns have been raised: (1) since this deletion (13q14) is found in only 5 percent of all retinoblastoma patients, perhaps it is the cause of only a small portion of retinoblastomas; and (2) retinoblastoma has been reported in only 14 percent of patients with deletions of the long arm of chromosome 13, suggesting that other factors may also be involved. In answer to the first concern, one should recognize that chromosome banding techniques are useful only for detecting deletions or additions of large chromosomal segments consisting of many genes. Mutations of a single gene are beyond the resolution of such techniques. Therefore it might be hypothesized that the only patients who show abnormalities of chromosome banding are those with large chromosomal abnormalities. For the remaining group—namely, those with retinoblastoma but without the mental, facial, or psychomotor abnormalities—it is possible that a much smaller mutation at the same locus is responsible for the disorder. Such mutations will become evident as the techniques for detecting them grow more sophisticated.

It must be remembered that mutations at other loci or on other chromosomes have not been excluded as possible causes of some retinoblastomas. This point addresses the second concern mentioned above, that not all patients with deletions of the long arm of chromosome 13 develop retinoblastoma. In addition, it is possible that other factors modulate this gene and are necessary to produce the tumor.

Strong and coworkers advanced one possible explanation

for the carrier state.[20] They have described a family in which band 13q14 is not deleted but rather is translocated to chromosome 3 in some persons. Such an arrangement leads to an unbalanced distribution of this chromosomal material in their offspring. Those with a balanced translocation do not have retinoblastomas. However, this group transmits the translocated chromosomal material to their offspring, with an unbalanced translocation in some children. This latter group develops retinoblastoma.

The study of retinoblastoma has been important not only because it advances our knowledge of this specific heritable tumor but also because it provides insight into the genetic causes of other tumors as well. After studying hereditary patterns in populations of patients with unifocal and multifocal retinoblastoma, Knudson and coworkers suggested that the development of a retinoblastoma requires two mutational events.[11] In nonhereditary situations, the chance of both events occurring in a single cell is exceedingly small, thus accounting for the rarity of multifocal lesions and the later age of presentation in this group of patients. In contrast, hereditary cases have one of these two mutations already present in every cell before birth. Later, a second mutation randomly occurs in one or more cells during embryogenesis or early neonatal life, causing multifocal lesions. While others have argued about some of the details of Knudson's theory, this "multihit" hypothesis of several mutations has gained increasing acceptance in explaining oncogenesis.

Esterase D is an enzyme whose production has been linked to a gene in the chromosome 13q14 region. Therefore, Benedict and coworkers studied chromosomal patterns and esterase D levels in one patient with retinoblastoma and demonstrated decreased levels of esterase D in peripheral tissues (fibroblasts, leukocytes) without a demonstrable chromosomal deletion in these tissues.[1a] However, tissue taken directly from the tumor showed absent esterase D activity and the karyotype showed a missing chromosome 13 (monosomy 13). Taken together, these data suggested that one mutation which was present at the 13q14 locus in all cells of the body accounted for diminished esterase D levels throughout the body but was not by itself sufficient to cause a tumor. A second genetic abnormality, in this case loss of the normal chromosome 13, was associated with the development of a retinoblastoma with no detectable esterase D. This study is important for two reasons. First, it provides direct evidence for a "two-hit" theory of tumor development as initially suggested by Knudson. Second, it suggests that although the disorder of inherited retinoblastoma acts in an autosomal dominant fashion at the level of the organism, the transmitted gene acts in a recessive fashion at the level of the cell and, in this case, it is only expressed as a tumor when the remaining normal gene at that locus is deleted through a second genetic event. Thus, a recessive gene may be related to a dominant disorder if a second event necessary for expression is frequent enough to ensure its occurring within the lifetime of the organism.

This "multihit" hypothesis has also recently been demonstrated in other systems, such as bladder cancer.[13a,17a] The oncogene isolated from the EJ bladder cancer routinely transformed a mouse fibroblast cell line (3T3) but not cells from primary cultures. Transformation of the latter re-

quired a "second hit" in the form of an additional mutation and this is thought to be more representative of the in vivo situation.

The importance of this concept of multiple mutation in explaining bilateral (hereditary) retinoblastoma vs. unilateral (nonhereditary) retinoblastoma becomes obvious to the neurosurgeon when analogous tumors of the central nervous system are considered, e.g., bilateral (hereditary) acoustic neuromas vs. unilateral (nonhereditary) acoustic neuromas, or multiple (hereditary) meningiomas vs. solitary (nonhereditary) meningiomas. Therefore, retinoblastoma has become a well-studied model system of the genetic aspects of neuro-oncology and the concepts learned from retinoblastoma can be applied to a number of other nervous system tumors.

Neuroblastoma

Neuroblastoma, the most common extracranial solid tumor of childhood, arises from elements of the sympathetic nervous system.[10] Despite advances in surgery, chemotherapy, and radiotherapy, neuroblastoma still carries a 50 percent mortality during the first 6 months after diagnosis. Two features of this tumor that have piqued the interest of neurobiologists are the regression and maturation of tumor cells. Autopsies of children who have died of other diseases show an incidence of neuroblastoma that is higher than the incidence of clinically evident neuroblastoma developing later in life. This suggests that some neuroblastomas regress. Indeed, it has been suggested that neuroblastoma has the highest rate of spontaneous remission of any tumor found in human beings. In those tumors that do not regress, remission is at times due to maturation of the malignant neuroblastoma cells into more differentiated, and fortunately benign, ganglioneuroma cells.

In contrast to most other tumors, 60 to 70 percent of neuroblastomas produce substances that can be detected in the serum or urine and are helpful both in tumor detection and in follow-up studies. These catabolites of catecholamines include vanillylmandelic acid, or 3-methoxy-4-hydroxy-mandelic acid (VMA); homovanillic acid (HVA); and 3-methoxy-4-hydroxy-phenyl ethylene glycol (MHPG). The synthesis of these compounds, as well as the unique morphology of neurons and the occasional identification of specific cell surface markers, has allowed growth, identification, and study of this tumor in tissue culture.

Although most neuroblastomas are sporadic, some familial cases have been identified, and these offer insight into the genetic mechanisms responsible for the tumor. A study of such cases led Knudson and Meadows[12] to postulate a two-mutation model for the development of neuroblastoma. As in retinoblastoma, a familial tendency toward neuroblastoma implies the inheritance of one of these mutations. The second mutation then occurs later during embryogenesis or early life and induces the tumor.

Recent studies have demonstrated that human neuroblastomas contain double minute chromosomes and homogeneously staining regions of chromosomes. This abnormal chromosomal material has been shown to contain amplified copies of DNA which is related to the myc oncogene.[18a]

This genetic material is amplified up to 140-fold in some neuroblastoma cells, raising the possibility that one or more genes within this amplified region are responsible for tumorigenesis. A possible association between neuroblastoma and colonic aganglionosis (Hirschsprung's disease) in several patients raises the possibility that the gene responsible for neuroblastoma may be related to a gene responsible for normal autonomic development. Of further interest is the rare coincidence of neuroblastoma and von Recklinghausen's neurofibromatosis. In addition, ganglioneuromas may be found in patients with neurofibromatosis. Also, disseminated neuroblastomas occasionally mature or differentiate into tumors indistinguishable from neurofibromas.

Although some neuroblastomas occur in the cerebrum, most arise in the thorax or abdomen, and are therefore usually treated by the pediatrician and the pediatric surgeon. Nonetheless, these are truly nervous system tumors, and such observations suggest that the biological importance of neuroblastoma to the neurosurgeon and neuro-oncologist far outweighs their current clinical importance for these specialties.

Pheochromocytoma and Multiple Endocrine Neoplastic Syndromes

The multiple endocrine neoplastic syndromes can be subdivided into three categories. All three demonstrate an autosomal dominant pattern of inheritance with variable expression.[18] Family members in each group may have one, a few, or all of the possible tumors of that particular syndrome.

Multiple endocrine neoplasia, type I (also called MEN I, or Wermer's syndrome), is familiar to the neurosurgeon because of the presence of pituitary adenomas. The incidence of pituitary adenoma was previously estimated to be 65 percent, but the current availability of more sensitive hormonal and radiological tests may prove this to be an underestimation. Most of the tumors are chromophobe adenomas of either the nonsecretory or the prolactin-secreting type. In others, growth hormone hypersecretion and acromegaly have been described. Although adrenocorticotropic hormone (ACTH)–secreting pituitary tumors may occur, other causes of Cushing's syndrome must also be considered in patients with MEN I. Overproduction of ACTH may be due to an adrenal adenoma, a carcinoid tumor, an islet cell tumor, or a thymoma.

The treatment of a pituitary tumor in a patient with MEN I is similar to that of a patient with a nonhereditary pituitary tumor. The trans-sphenoidal route is usually the preferred surgical approach. Of course, care must be taken to evaluate other abnormalities that could affect anesthestic management. In particular, one should ensure adequate control of blood pressure as well as normal levels of calcium and glucose. Patients with a pituitary tumor who are thought to have MEN I should be carefully evaluated for other possible lesions.

Patients with hyperparathyroidism may be asymptomatic or may exhibit severe manifestations, including renal, skeletal, and neuromuscular disorders. The parathyroids are involved in up to 90 percent of patients with MEN I. Of these, half have multiple adenomas, another third have a solitary adenoma, and the rest show diffuse parathyroid hyperplasia.

Significant hyperparathyroidism usually requires surgery.

Pancreatic islet cell tumors are present in over 80 percent of patients with MEN I and may secrete gastrin, insulin, or glucagon. Ulcers occur in 58 percent of patients with MEN I because of the Zollinger-Ellison syndrome of gastric hyperacidity secondary to overproduction of gastrin. Mild cases can be controlled with cimetidine, but many require total gastrectomy. Insulinomas are the second most common islet cell tumor and are usually multiple. Because of this, total or near total pancreatectomy is often required. In contrast, glucagon-secreting tumors are rare. When present, they may be associated with weight loss, skin rash, anemia, stomatitis, and mild glucose intolerance.

Multiple endocrine neoplasia, type II (also called MEN II, or Sipple's syndrome) is associated with medullary thyroid carcinoma, pheochromocytoma, and hyperparathyroidism. Medullary thyroid carcinoma derives from thyroid C cells, which are of neural crest origin, and is present in 95 percent of patients with MEN II. These cancers develop any time after age 7 and may be asymptomatic. Calcitonin radioimmunoassay makes possible screening and early diagnosis as well as proper timing of surgical intervention.

Pheochromocytoma occurs in over 50 percent of patients with MEN II and is bilateral in more than half. Symptoms such as headache, hypertension, sweating, and palpitations are due to hypersecretion of catecholamines. As with neuroblastoma, measurement of catecholamine catabolites in serum and urine can be useful in the diagnosis and management of these patients. Proper preoperative management must be undertaken to preclude a possible intraoperative hypersecretory crisis.

Hyperparathroidism, present in 40 percent of patients with MEN II, is usually due to diffuse parathyroid hyperplasia. Diagnosis and treatment are similar to those described for MEN I.

Multiple endocrine neoplasia, type III (also called MEN III or MEN IIb) is a syndrome of multiple mucosal neuromas, medullary thyroid carcinomas, and pheochromocytoma. Medullary thyroid carcinoma is present in 95 percent and pheochromocytoma in 50 percent of patients with MEN III. Their diagnosis and treatment are similar to those discussed for MEN II. Mucosal neuromas are present in virtually all patients with MEN III and can be present on the lips, tongue, buccal mucosa, eyelids, conjunctiva, skin, or gastrointestinal tract. Examination with a slit lamp may show hypertrophied corneal nerve fibers. Since such lesions may also be present in patients with neurofibromatosis, the overlap is obvious. However, patients with MEN III lack café au lait spots, skin neurofibromas, and other stigmata of neurofibromatosis. Nonetheless, the possibility that both these autosomal dominant syndromes may be due to abnormalities of related genes underscores their importance to the neurosurgeon.

Paragangliomas of the Cervical Region

Paragangliomas, also called *chemodectomas* or *glomus tumors*, are relatively rare, highly vascular tumors. The most common locations are the carotid body, the nodose ganglion of the vagus nerve, and the jugulotympanic region. Less commonly, a similar tumor may occur in the nose, orbit, larynx, or other location.[13] The histology of these tumors is similar regardless of location, so only the carotid body tumor is here considered in detail.

Carotid body paragangliomas can occur as solitary, sporadic, nonhereditary lesions or in a hereditary fashion. Like retinoblastoma and pheochromocytoma, bilateral tumors occur more commonly in the familial cases (33 percent) than in the sporadic cases (5 percent).[8] Familial cases are thought to transmit in an autosomal dominant fashion with variable expression. Moreover, the expression of the gene causing this tumor may be modulated by other factors. For example, the normal role of the carotid body is to function as a chemoreceptor for blood pH and oxygen tension. Therefore it is noteworthy that enlarged carotid bodies have been reported in patients subjected to chronic hypoxemia and that there is an increased incidence of carotid body paragangliomas in persons dwelling at high altitudes. This modulation of a tumor gene by other factors is reminiscent of the modulation of normal breast tissue in some cases of breast cancer by estrogen and becomes an additional consideration in von Recklinghausen's neurofibromatosis, where hormonal modulation must also be considered.

Carotid body tumors usually present as a painless mass in the neck but may be associated with tenderness, carotid sinus syndrome, dysphagia, or Horner's syndrome. Malignant degeneration occurs in about 2 to 12 percent of the cases. Other tumors, both benign and malignant, have been reported in 6 to 19 percent of these patients. In those patients with familial carotid body tumors, half of these other tumors are paragangliomas at other sites.

Radiation may not be effective in the treatment of carotid body tumors, and surgical resection is usually required. Because of the highly vascular nature of the tumor, angiography is essential. Blood supply to the tumor is often from the external carotid artery, allowing preoperative embolization of the tumor. This procedure can significantly facilitate surgery. Carotid body tumors and other paragangliomas represent a formidable technical challenge and should not be undertaken by the inexperienced surgeon.

Meningiomas

Standard metaphase banding techniques have been used to study both tumor cells and nontumor cells (usually leukocytes) in patients harboring various types of neoplasms.[15] For most malignant tumors, multiple chromosomal abnormalities are found, and no particular pattern is seen from one patient's tumor to the next. A noteworthy exception is the abnormality of chromosome 22 (termed the *Philadelphia chromosome*) which is typical of chronic myelogenous leukemia. The chromosomal patterns of the meningiomas have been studied more extensively than those of any other solid tumor.[23] To date, more than 267 meningiomas have been examined. Most studies of meningioma have been done early in tissue culture, within a week of explantation. However, studies done directly from biopsy material have produced similar results. Metaphase banding of such tumors shows a reduced number of chromosomes (hypoploidia) in about 70 percent of meningiomas. The most common abnormality is the loss of one chromosome 22 (monosomy 22).

This is true in about half the arachnothelial, fibromatous, and benign angiomatous subtypes. An isolated loss of chromosome 22 is found in only 10 percent of syncytial meningiomas, whereas a loss of chromosome 22 plus one or more other chromosomes is found in 83 percent. Additional chromosomal abnormalities may also be associated with more aggressive meningiomas, in that 75 percent of invasive tumors and 70 percent of recurrences show loss of several chromosomes or atypical chromosomal aberrations.

A correlation has been noted between the karyotype and the sex of the patient. Overall, meningiomas are three times more common in females than in males. This female preponderance holds true for those meningiomas with either 46 chromosomes (normal karyotype) or with 45 chromosomes (monosomy 22). In contrast, meningiomas with more marked chromosomal aberrancy—less than 45 chromosomes or more than 46 chromosomes—show no female predilection. Since hormonal modulation of these tumors has been postulated as a possible reason for the usual female preponderance, one must wonder if the additional loss of genetic material in some way alters this modulating factor.

Of additional interest is that meningiomas with marked hypoploidia show a spontaneous rate of chromosomal breakage and rearrangement of about 20 percent as compared with a rate of 2 percent for normal fibroblasts. The cause of this increased chromosomal fragility is not known, but increased rates of chromosomal breakage are well known for another group of genetic tumor-related syndromes (clastogenic syndromes) such as Bloom's syndrome, Fanconi's anemia, and possibly ataxia telangiectasia.

Using immunofluorescent techniques, Zang and coworkers have detected SV40 virus–related antigens in about one-third of meningiomas and have suggested that this virus may, in some way, be related to the chromosomal abnormalities that have been detected.[23] To date, however, the role of SV40 or related viruses has not been conclusively shown.

In summary, meningiomas are a rather common neoplasm of the central nervous system and are associated with a relatively uniform karyotypic abnormality, namely, loss of chromosome 22. Recently, prophase banding techniques have increased the ability to detect smaller chromosomal abnormalities. In meningiomas, such techniques may allow the detection of smaller deletions of chromosome 22 that are still compatible with tumorigenesis. Hormonal modulation has been postulated, but the interaction of the proposed hormones with cultured chromosomally aberrant meningioma cells has not been tested to date.

Most meningiomas occur as solitary, sporadic lesions, but familial meningiomas, often multiple, have been described. In addition, meningiomas can be associated with neurofibromatosis, in particular with bilateral acoustic neurofibromatosis. However, chromosomal studies of meningiomas occurring in these hereditary settings have not yet been reported.

Gliomas

Gliomas are more common and are associated with a higher morbidity and mortality than any of the previously discussed tumors, yet genetic studies of gliomas have thus far been less rewarding. Such studies fall into three categories: (1) defined genetic syndromes associated with gliomas, (2) familial aggregations of gliomas, and (3) analysis of chromosomes or DNA from sporadic gliomas.

Familial polyposis of the colon may be associated with other abnormalities. In Gardner's syndrome, it is associated with bone and skin lesions. In Turcot's syndrome, colonic polyps are associated with adenocarcinomas and with brain tumors.[21] This is a rare disorder, and only a few affected families have been reported. The pattern of inheritance is autosomal. Most studies suggest that the gene is recessive, although too few reports exist to exclude the possibility of dominant inheritance with variable expression. In most cases the central nervous system lesion is either a glioblastoma or a medulloblastoma. Only an occasional patient shows café au lait marks, hairy nevi, or other stigmata that would implicate other genetic mechanisms. One family with hepatic focal nodular hyperplasia, polyposis, café au lait marks, and glioblastoma has been reported,[6] and other sporadic cases of intestinal polyposis with glioblastoma have been noted. However, these associations are rare, genetic transmission is uncertain, and environmental causes cannot be excluded.

Multiple nevoid basal cell carcinoma syndrome may also be associated with gliomas.[17] This autosomal dominant disorder usually becomes evident in childhood with the development of multiple small, lightly colored papular lesions having the pathological features of basal cell carcinoma. Cerebellar tumors may develop, usually in infancy or early childhood. Most cases have proved to be medulloblastoma. Only rarely has a cerebellar astrocytoma been noted.

Gliomas may be associated with other defined genetic syndromes such as tuberous sclerosis (subependymal astrocytoma, gliomatosis cerebri) or neurofibromatosis (optic glioma, cerebral or spinal astrocytoma or glioblastoma). These are covered in more detail in the chapter on the phakomatoses.

Familial aggregations of gliomas in the absence of other common stigmata have also been noted. Van der Weil studied 5262 relatives of 100 glioma patients and found that the mortality from glioma was four times greater in this group than in controls.[22] He also noted a higher incidence of spinal dysraphism in this glioma-prone population. However, studies by other groups have presented conflicting data concerning the incidence of glioma in families of glioma patients, and as yet, no firm conclusions can be drawn. Nonetheless, a number of well documented familial aggregations of gliomas have been noted by several authors in different parts of the world. In some cases more than one generation is involved, and genetic transmission is suggested. To date, no specific chromosomal abnormality has been identified,[4] nor has the role of an environmental agent been excluded.

Chromosomal patterns of sporadic gliomas have been extensively studied, using standard metaphase banding techniques.[14] Studies of established glioma lines have shown numerous complex karyotypic abnormalities.[16] An excess of chromosomes (hyperploidy) is common, but no marker chromosome or specific pattern has been identified; however, an excess of part or all of chromosome 7 seems to be the most common aberrancy.

References

1. Abramson DH: Retinoblastoma: Diagnosis and management. CA 32:130–140, 1982.
1a. Benedict WF, Murphee AL, Banerjee A, Spina CA, Sparkes MC, Sparkes RS: Patient with chromosome 13 deletion: Evidence that the retinoblastoma is a recessive cancer gene. Science 219:973–975, 1983.
2. Bishop JM: Oncogenes. Sci Am 246:80–92, 1982.
3. Bolande RP: The neurocristopathies: A unifying concept of disease arising in neural crest maldevelopment. Hum Pathol 5:409–429, 1974.
4. Chadduck WM, Netsky MG: Familial gliomas; Report of four families, with chromosome studies. Neurosurgery 10:445–449, 1982.
5. Cuatico W: Characterization of tumor-specific DNA sequences: Molecular grading of astrocytomas. Cancer 46:303–307, 1980.
6. Everson RB, Fraumeni JF Jr: Familial glioblastoma with hepatic focal nodular hyperplasia. Cancer 38:310–313, 1976.
7. Francke U, Kung F: Sporadic bilateral retinoblastoma and 13q chromosomal deletion. Med Pediatr Oncol 2:379–385, 1976.
8. Grufferman S, Gillman MW, Pasternak LR, Peterson CL, Young WG: Familial carotid body tumors: Case report and epidemiologic review. Cancer 46:2116–2122, 1980.
9. Kakati S, Sandberg AA: Chromosomes in solid tumors. Virchows Arch [Zellpathol] 29:129–137, 1978.
10. Kemshead JT, Black J: Developments in the biology of neuroblastoma: Implications for diagnosis and treatment. Dev Med Child Neurol 22:816–829, 1980.
11. Knudson AG Jr, Hethcote HW, Brown BW: Mutation and childhood cancer: A probabalistic model for the incidence of retinoblastoma. Proc Natl Acad Sci USA 72:5116–5120, 1975.
12. Knudson AG Jr, Meadows AT: Developmental genetics of neuroblastoma. J Natl Cancer Inst 57:675–682, 1976.
13. Lack EE, Cubilla AL, Woodruff JM, Farr HW: Paragangliomas of the head and neck region. Cancer 39:397–409, 1977.
13a. Land H, Parada LF, Weinberg RA: Tumorigenic conversion of primary embryo fibroblasts requires at least two cooperating oncogenes. Nature 304:596–602, 1983.
14. Mark J: Chromosome patterns in benign and malignant tumors in the human nervous system, in German J (ed): *Chromosomes and Cancer*. New York, Wiley, 1974, pp 481–495.
15. Mark J: Chromosomal abnormalities and their specificity in human neoplasms: An assessment of recent observations by banding techniques. Adv Cancer Res 24:165–222, 1977.
16. Mark J, Westermark B, Ponten J, Hugosson R: Banding patterns in human glioma cell lines. Hereditas 87:243–260, 1977.
17. Naguib MG, Sung JH, Erickson DL, Gold LHA, Seljeskog EL: Central nervous system involvement in the nevoid basal cell carcinoma syndrome: Case report and review of the literature. Neurosurgery 11:52–56, 1982.
17a. Newbold RF, Overell RW: Fibroblast immortality is a prerequisite for transformation by EJ c-Ha-ras oncogene. Nature 304:648–651, 1983.
18. Pont A: Multiple endocrine neoplasia syndromes. West J Med 132:301–312, 1980.
18a. Schwab M, Alitalok, Klempnauer KH, Varmus HE, Bishop JM, Gilbert F, Brodeur G, Goldstein M, Trent J: Amplified DNA with limited homology to myc cellular oncogene is shared by human neuroblastoma cell lines and a neuroblastoma tumor. Nature 305:245–248, 1983.
19. Shih C, Weinberg RA: Isolation of a transforming sequence from a human bladder carcinoma cell line. Cell 29:161–169, 1982.
20. Strong LC, Riccardi VM, Ferrell RE, Sparkes RS: Familial retinoblastoma and chromosome 13 deletion transmitted

via an insertional translocation. Science 213:1501–1503, 1981.

21. Todd DW, Christoferson LA, Leech RW, Rudolf L: A family affected with intestinal polyposis and gliomas. Ann Neurol 10:390–392, 1981.

22. Van der Wiel HJ: *Inheritance of Glioma*. New York, Elsevier, 1960.

23. Zang KD: Cytological and cytogenetical studies on human meningioma. Cancer Genet Cytogenet 6:249–274, 1982.

54

Neuro-fibromatosis and Other Phakomatoses

Robert L. Martuza

The term *phakomatosis* was coined by van der Hoeve in 1920 and has been used to describe a group of disorders that have cutaneous, ocular, and neurological manifestations, show hereditary features, and often demonstrate progression. Four general groups are recognized: neurofibromatosis, tuberous sclerosis, von Hippel-Lindau disease, and neurocutaneous angiomatoses. With time, subgroups have been recognized. Neurofibromatosis exists in two genetically distinct forms: (1) classic von Recklinghausen's neurofibromatosis, or peripheral neurofibromatosis; and (2) bilateral acoustic neurofibromatosis, also called central neurofibromatosis. Tuberous sclerosis and von Hippel-Lindau disease, or retinocerebellar angiomatosis, have not been subdivided. The neurocutaneous angiomatoses have several subdivisions: (1) ataxia-telangiectasia (Louis-Bar disease); (2) Sturge-Weber syndrome (encephalotrigeminal angiomatosis); (3) Klippel-Trénaunay-Weber syndrome (spinal-cutaneous angiomatosis); (4) Osler-Rendu-Weber syndrome (familial telangiectasia); (5) Wyburn-Mason syndrome (bulbar-facial angiomatosis), and (6) Fabry's disease (angiokeratoma corporis diffusum).

An understanding of the phakomatoses is important to neurosurgeons for several reasons. First, as a group, the phakomatoses account for significant neurological disability. Moreover, the recognition of one of these disorders in a patient suggests genetic screening of other family members for the purpose of providing genetic counseling as well as early treatment for manifestations of the disease. Second, the

presence of disseminated hamartomas or angiomas both in the central nervous system (CNS) and in the skin makes possible ready observation as well as skin biopsy for research into these disorders. Using the skin as a window into the nervous system provides a unique opportunity to study the mechanisms of cellular growth in both normal and abnormal, or neoplastic, tissues. Third, although each of these syndromes is a distinct entity, enough patients have overlapping stigmata to suggest the possibility that all of them may be caused by various mutations among a small family of related genes. Finally, since the CNS abnormalities associated with the phakomatoses (arteriovenous malformation, glioma, schwannoma, meningioma) are also seen as solitary abnormalities in patients without these disorders, identification of the gene(s) involved in causing the phakomatoses may also identify the abnormal gene(s) responsible for the tumors and vascular malformations that make up a large part of most neurosurgical practices. As such, the phakomatoses may be conceptualized as a neurological Rosetta stone which, if understood, can provide a key to the genetic hieroglyphics responsible for neurological tumors and malformations.

Neurofibromatosis

Neurofibromatosis (NF) is a relatively common autosomal dominant disorder (one in 3000 births) that has high penetrance but variable expression.[13,14] Prior reports have not always distinguished the two forms of NF—classic von Recklinghausen's (VRNF) and bilateral acoustic (BANF)—as separate genetic entities, and this has led to some confusion. It is now believed that these two syndromes are distinct genetic abnormalities caused either by different genes or by different alleles of the same gene. Both syndromes show autosomal dominant transmission and are highly penetrant (90 percent or over), suggesting that when the NF gene is present, it is usually expressed. A corollary is that an asymptomatic carrier state (where the gene is present but not expressed) is uncommon in NF.

Von Recklinghausen's Neurofibromatosis

While the penetrance of the VRNF gene is nearly 100 percent, the expression is variable, and therefore the diagnosis can be difficult. The most common manifestations of VRNF are seen in the skin. Multiple cutaneous or subcutaneous neurofibromas (Fig. 54-1) are pathognomonic of this disorder. Patients may have no tumors, a few, or thousands,

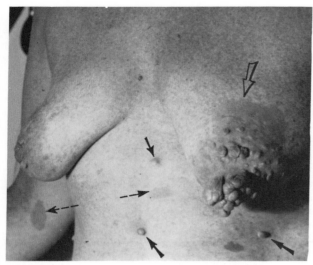

Figure 54-1 Café au lait marks (*broken arrows*), cutaneous neurofibromas (*solid arrows*) and areolar neurofibromas (*open arrow*) are seen in this patient with von Recklinghausen's neurofibromatosis.

usually located in the dermis. These may vary in size from millimeters to a few centimeters and usually invaginate when pressed. Histological study of these lesions shows Schwann cells, often with nuclear palisading, admixed with fibroblasts, neurons, mast cells, and vascular and connective tissue. It is thought that Schwann cells deriving from the neural crest are the essential tumor-forming cell, with the fibroblasts a reactive component; however, conclusive evidence for this concept is lacking. The role of the mast cell also is unclear: some believe it to be reactive, others suggest that its function is to inhibit tumor growth, while recent studies have implicated it in neurofibroma production. Additional studies in this area are needed.

While cutaneous neurofibromas can occur anywhere on the body, they are often most numerous in the thoracic-abdominal area. On many women and some men, neurofibromas are present on the nipple or areolar area of the breast (Fig. 54-1). Whether this is related to the pigmented nature of the area or to possible hormonal factors is not clear.

Abnormal patches of skin pigmentation are another diagnostic feature of NF. Café au lait (CAL) spots usually appear soon after birth and can vary in size from a millimeter to many centimeters (Fig. 54-1). Crowe et al.[3] noted that 95 percent of adult NF patients had one or more CAL spots and 78 percent had six or more, each 15 mm in size or larger. Therefore, for adult patients, the presence of six such spots is a useful diagnostic criterion. It is not a *sufficient* criterion, however, because 22 percent of NF patients have five or fewer CAL spots and 10 percent of the normal population have one CAL spot. In addition, some families have been noted to have multiple CAL spots but no other evidence of NF. Moreover, the pediatric patient has a smaller skin surface and hence smaller CAL spots. Whitehouse has recommended that five CAL spots 5 mm or larger be used as the diagnostic criterion in the pediatric population.[18] It is recommended that all examinations be performed with a

Wood's lamp, since CAL spots can be overlooked in room light.

An additional confounding feature can be the differential diagnosis of NF versus Albright's syndrome, since both may present with precocious puberty and multiple CAL spots. While prior teaching emphasized the importance of the shape of the CAL spot in these two disorders ("coast of California" vs. "coast of Maine"), this has not proved to be a consistently useful feature. Biopsies of the CAL spot can be studied for melanin. Abnormally large melanosomes (macromelanosomes) are seen in NF but not in Albright's syndrome.[2] Whether similar techniques can be used to distinguish the CAL spot associated with NF from the CAL spot seen in 10 percent of the normal population has not yet been conclusively determined, but studies of this are currently under way.

Freckling of areas exposed to the sun is common in many fair-skinned persons. However, the freckles of NF are also seen in hidden areas such as the axilla, groin crease, submammary area, and buttocks. Whereas CAL spots typically appear in early infancy, this intertriginous freckling may not appear until late childhood or early puberty (Fig. 54-2).

Lisch nodules are pigmented, raised hamartomas of the iris. Examination with a slit lamp is necessary to distinguish them from other abnormalities of the iris. In early childhood they are usually absent; from age 6 to puberty they are variably present; after puberty they are present in more than 94 percent of patients with von Recklinghausen's neurofibromatosis (Fig. 54-3).

Plexiform neurofibromas are usually associated with peripheral nerves or with the sympathetic chain. If asymptomatic, they are best left untreated. If they are small and cause significant pain, they often can be resected with the use of the operating microscope without motor dysfunction. However, large lesions may encase sizable neural bundles, and total removal can involve significant removal of functioning axons. This is particularly a problem in brachial plexus neurofibromas. Such large neurofibromas also may be associated with generalized enlargement of the limb (hemihypertrophy; Fig. 54-4). In some of these cases, the final results of surgery may be less than optimal. Realistic goals must be outlined, and appropriate treatment may re-

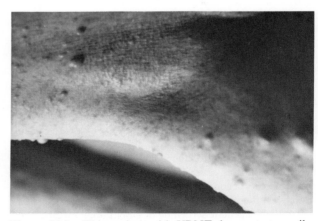

Figure 54-2 This patient with VRNF demonstrates axillary freckling.

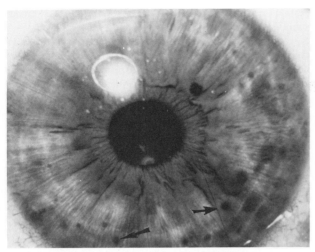

Figure 54-3 Iris hamartomas or Lisch nodules (*arrows*) are found in over 94 percent of patients with VRNF. (Courtesy of Dr. Johan Zwaan.)

quire a combination of partial tumor removal and tendon transfers.

Rapid growth of a plexiform neurofibroma usually suggests the development of a neurofibrosarcoma. It has been suggested that the appearance of a neurofibrosarcoma in a patient with NF may be due to a second local mutation in addition to the already present genetic defect of NF. Because of the life-threatening aspects of this tumor, immediate surgery is necessary to confirm the diagnosis. Amputation of a limb may be required, and radiotherapy and sometimes chemotherapy are necessary. The overall 5-year survival is approximately 23 percent, but location, size, and

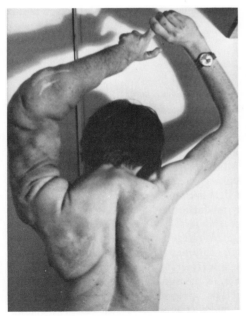

Figure 54-4 Extensive plexiform neurofibromas may be associated with hemihypertrophy of an extremity.

invasiveness are important factors in determining individual results.

Other features, while not diagnostic of NF, may be associated with the disorder. These include pseudoarthrosis in less than 1 percent of patients, pheochromocytoma in less than 1 percent, and kyphoscoliosis in 2 percent. This latter condition is usually a rotatory scoliosis involving a relatively short spinal segment and is often progressive. In many cases bracing can be helpful, but for some, surgery is necessary.

Bilateral Acoustic Neurofibromatosis

Bilateral acoustic neuromas (Fig. 54-5) are the hallmark of a form of NF termed central NF, or bilateral acoustic neurofibromatosis, which is genetically distinct from peripheral NF, or classic von Recklinghausen's disease.[7] Families with bilateral acoustic neurofibromatosis transmit this disorder in an autosomal dominant fashion, and all affected members have bilateral acoustic neuromas. In contrast, families with VRNF exhibit more variable expression. For example, a mother with numerous cutaneous neurofibromas and CAL spots may have a son with a unilateral plexiform neurofibroma and a hemihypertrophied limb but virtually no CAL spots or cutaneous neurofibromas. It has been suggested that there are differences in nerve growth factor between these two disorders, but this remains to be confirmed and, to date, has not proved clinically useful.

While patients with bilateral acoustic neuromas may have some of the cutaneous stigmata typical of VRNF, they usually have fewer or more subtle lesions. Of 15 patients with bilateral acoustic neurofibromatosis, only 2 had six or more CAL spots. Similarly, cutaneous neurofibromas were noted in only 7 of these 15 patients, and they were few in number and often difficult to detect.[9] Oblique lighting may be necessary to detect minimally raised skin plaques in these patients. Nevertheless, biopsy shows these lesions to have the typical histology of a neurofibroma. It is noteworthy that we have not seen Lisch nodules in any patient with bilateral acoustic neuromas; however, congenital cataracts may be associated with this disorder. Macromelanosomes are uncommon in biopsies of CAL spots in these patients (unpublished studies).

While patients with nonhereditary unilateral acoustic neuromas usually become symptomatic in their forties or fifties, patients with bilateral acoustic neuromas usually develop symptoms in their teens. The growth rate of these lesions is variable, and sequential computed tomography (CT) may be necessary to document growth and to plan appropriate treatment. Because bilateral deafness and/or facial dysfunction is significantly more debilitating than unilateral loss, attempts should always be made to preserve both cochlear and facial function whenever surgery is necessary.

As with all hereditary disorders, the identification of a patient with BANF requires the examination of other family members. However, since skin stigmata may be absent in BANF, identification of the disorder has been problematic. Currently, testing of brain stem auditory evoked response has proved useful for detecting small acoustic neuromas. An abnormal test should be confirmed by a CT scan with intravenous contrast or with subarachnoid air contrast. In se-

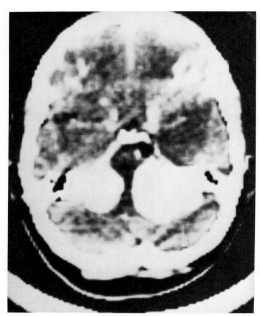

Figure 54-5 Significant brain stem compression already was present when these large bilateral acoustic neuromas were detected. In such advanced cases, sparing of facial nerve and cochlear nerve function may not be possible during complete tumor removal. (From Martuza and Ojemann.[9])

lected cases, surgery on small asymptomatic lesions should be considered in order to have the best possible chance of removing the tumor while sparing hearing and facial function (Fig. 54-6).

Central Nervous System Abnormalities In NF

Although BANF and VRNF are transmitted as distinct genetic entities, both are associated with multiple spinal neurofibromas. In one series, symptomatic spinal neurofibromas developed in 6 of 15 patients with bilateral acoustic neuromas. These tumors are most common on the dorsal roots or their ganglia. Similar lesions also occur with peripheral neurofibromatosis. There is no way to predict the growth characteristics of any of these lesions, and surgery is recommended only for lesions that become symptomatic or show significant growth. Again, because the patient may face multiple operations, preservation of all possible neurological function is essential. In this regard, intraoperative monitoring of somatosensory evoked potentials has proved useful in many instances. Surgical techniques such as ultrasonic aspiration or use of the CO_2 laser facilitate gentle tumor resection and minimize retraction but do not interfere with the evoked response recordings.

Meningiomas are thought to arise from arachnoidal cells, and multiple spinal or intracranial meningiomas can occur with either form of NF. Pathologically, these lesions are identical to meningiomas not associated with NF. Some meningiomas remain dormant for long periods of time, so removal of all such lesions is not necessary. Surgery is rec-

ommended for symptomatic lesions or for those showing significant growth.

Optic gliomas are most common in infancy and early childhood and in many cases may develop prenatally. There has been significant controversy surrounding the appropriate treatment of optic gliomas. Some investigators have noted a histological difference between the optic gliomas found in patients with other stigmata of NF and those in patients without NF stigmata.[15] Some have suggested that optic gliomas are benign hamartomas that do not require surgery or radiotherapy, whereas others contend that there are histological and clinical differences between optic gliomas arising in the anterior chiasm and optic nerves and those arising in the posterior chiasm, hypothalamus, and optic tracts. Currently, there is no hard evidence upon which to base decisions for an individual patient.

Non-neoplastic abnormalities involving the nervous system include macrocephaly, sphenoid wing dysplasia, speech impediments, low IQ, decreased attention span, poor fine motor skills, and seizures. Many patients with NF have a larger than average head size, and the mean head size of all NF patients is in the 70th percentile. Such macrocephaly appears to develop postnatally and is not necessarily associated with neurological dysfunction. A CT scan may show ventriculomegaly or even ventricular asymmetry. Although hydrocephalus can occur in a patient with NF, the presence of relative macrocephaly with moderate ventricular enlargement is not, in itself, proof of hydrocephalus nor is it adequate justification for a ventricular shunt.

In the absence of a tumor, the incidence of seizures in patients with NF is approximately 3 percent. Frank retardation affects only a small percentage of NF patients, but speech impediments, intellectual handicaps, or poor fine motor skills may be present in 30 to 40 percent of these patients. A disorder in cerebral cytoarchitecture has been documented in some patients with frank retardation and has been postulated as a cause of the more subtle cerebral disturbances as well.

Pathogenesis

To date, neither the gene nor the chromosome harboring the NF mutation has been identified. Karyotypes of cells from NF patients are normal, suggesting that the mutation is small, perhaps a point mutation. Studies are under way to locate this gene. Yet even if the gene were identified, genetic engineering has not progressed to the point where it can be applied to the clinical care of the patient with NF. However, the possibility that hormones or other growth-controlling substances may modulate the NF gene is suggested by the following observations: (1) cutaneous neurofibromas may first appear or may enlarge with puberty or pregnancy; (2) bilateral acoustic neuromas appear earlier in patients inheriting the disease from their mother than in those inheriting it from their father; (3) neurofibromas are often most prominent on the areola or nipple of the breast; (4) both meningiomas and Schwann cell tumors have been noted to contain hormonal receptors. Additional research on the factors that modulate the NF gene may allow beneficial therapeutic intervention without requiring direct manipulation of the genome.

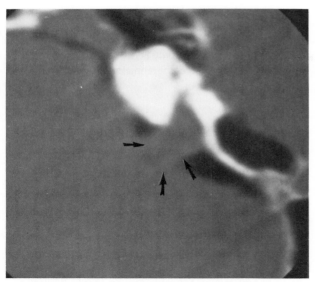

Figure 54-6 Bilateral acoustic neurofibromatosis was detected in this 23-year-old female by abnormal brain stem evoked response testing as part of a genetic screening program. This cisternal air-contrast CT scan shows a 1.5-cm acoustic neuroma. It was completely removed surgically with preservation of hearing. (Courtesy of Dr. Robert Ojemann.)

While it is clear that the NF gene is present in every cell of the body of the NF patient and that hormones or other systemic factors may play a role in the expression of the NF gene, local factors are also important. For example, it is thought that all Schwann cells develop from the neural crest, yet Schwann cell tumors commonly occur only on the sensory or sympathetic nerve roots or ganglia. Schwann cell tumors of the ventral spinal roots or motor cranial nerves are much rarer. Indeed the abundant cutaneous neurofibromas

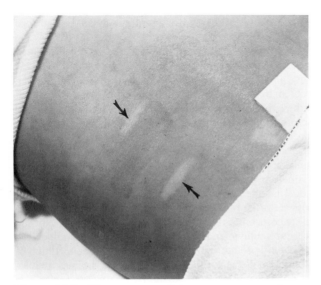

Figure 54-7 The presence of three or more macules (ash-leaf spots) makes it possible to diagnose tuberous sclerosis in a newborn when other stigmata are absent. (Courtesy of Dr. Thomas B. Fitzpatrick.)

associated with VRNF are probably Schwann cell tumors associated with sensory or sympathetic nerve endings. In contrast, neurofibromas at motor end plates, i.e., intramuscular neurofibromas, are virtually nonexistent. These observations suggest that the nerve itself may play a role in controlling Schwann cell growth and hence tumor formation. Studies demonstrating that the membrane of sensory neurons contains a factor mitogenic for Schwann cells lends support to this possibility. Recently developed tissue culture techniques allow the study of the interaction of neurons (and other cells) with human Schwann cells taken from normal persons and from patients with NF. With the development of such techniques, our understanding of NF is expected to evolve from the current level of gross clinical description to a level involving identification of specific cellular pathology. It is hoped that this will make diagnosis more accurate and make treatment finally possible.

Tuberous Sclerosis

Tuberous sclerosis is an autosomal dominant disorder with an incidence of one in 6000 to one in 15,000 births, or about half that of NF.[5] The earliest diagnostic feature is a depigmented, ash-leaf-shaped (one end round, the other end pointed) area on the skin (Fig. 54-7). As with the CAL spots of NF, a Wood's lamp is useful in searching for the ash-leaf spots of tuberous sclerosis. In about 85 percent of cases in which three or more lesions are present, it allows the diagnosis to be made in the neonatal period when other stigmata are often absent. Within 2 to 4 years, patients develop angiofibromas of the face (adenoma sebaceum; Fig. 54-8), subepidermal fibrosis (sharkskin or shagreen skin patch; Fig. 54-9), and subungual angiofibromas of the fingers and toes (Fig. 54-10). Hamartomas may also be found in the retina, kidneys, and lungs. About half of all cardiac rhabdomyomas are due to tuberous sclerosis. Pitting of the tooth enamel is also noted. In the CNS, giant cell subependymal astrocytomas of the third and lateral ventricles are typical of this disorder and are rarely found in the absence of tuberous sclerosis. When numerous but small, these hamartomas resemble candle drippings. On CT scan, they may take on the appearance of multiple periventricular calcifications, usually in the striothalamic zones (Fig. 54-11). Occasionally one of these lesions may show more aggressive growth characteristics or even malignant degeneration with hemorrhage (Fig. 54-12).[17] When a biopsy is needed, CT-directed stereotactic techniques can be utilized. When resection is necessary, a transcortical, intraventricular route has been used.

Gliotic cortical plaques are common central nervous system features and give this syndrome, first described by Bourneville, its name. Only rarely do significant cortical tumors develop, but in some cases diffuse gliomatosis may extend through the hemisphere. The neonate with tuberous sclerosis is often neurologically normal. Later, delayed milestones may be noted, and within 2 or 3 years, seizures and mental retardation may become evident. Initially the seizures take the form of flexion myoclonus with hypsarrhythmia on the electroencephalogram but later evolve into psychomotor or grand mal seizures. In general, mental function continues to deteriorate slowly. However, with increased

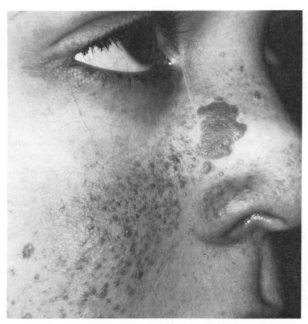

Figure 54-8 Adenoma sebaceum in tuberous sclerosis. (Courtesy of Dr. Thomas B. Fitzpatrick.)

recognition of mild forms of tuberous sclerosis, several recent reports have documented patients with preserved mentation and without seizures.

Tuberous sclerosis is transmitted as a single-gene defect in an autosomal dominant fashion with a penetrance of approximately 80 percent. As with neurofibromatosis, tuberous sclerosis shows variable genetic expression, making detailed family screening by knowledgeable physicians essential. The causative gene has not yet been identified, nor

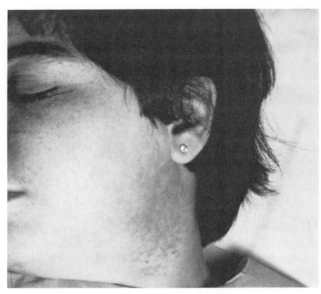

Figure 54-9 Shagreen skin patch of tuberous sclerosis. The posterior lumbosacral area is the more common site. This patient's CT scan is shown as Fig. 54-12. (Courtesy of Dr. Thomas B. Fitzpatrick.)

has a way been devised to halt symptomatic progression. Treatment is aimed at genetic counseling, control of seizures, psychiatric and social assistance, facial dermabrasion for selected patients, and only occasional neurosurgical intervention for progressive symptomatic tumors or for hydrocephalus.

Von Hippel-Lindau Disease

Like the previously described phakomatoses, von Hippel-Lindau disease (VHL) is an autosomal dominant disorder with variable expression.[6] The penetrance is approximately 70 percent. This disorder has been called Lindau's disease when retinal angiomas are absent and von Hippel-Lindau's disease when the retinal defect is present. It is doubtful that it is worth classifying these as separate genetic entities, and since variable genetic expression is common, the all-inclusive term von Hippel-Lindau's disease should be used for this disorder.

The characteristic lesion of VHL is the capillary hemangioblastoma, which is usually a benign tumor. Retinal angiomas are present in over 50 percent of patients with this disorder and are symptomatic in 20 percent. On ocular examination, these pink, vascular tumors with tortuous arteriovenous pairs are a characteristic feature of VHL and are important in the diagnosis and in family screening (Fig. 54-13). In questionable cases, fluorescein retinal angiography is useful to detect small lesions.

Within the cranial and spinal cavities, cerebellar hemangioblastomas predominate, being found in 60 percent of cases of VHL coming to autopsy (Fig. 54-14). They are often multiple and may be in similar locations in members of the same family. Substantial erythropoietic activity may be associated with an elevated hematocrit reading caused by cysts of cystic cerebellar hemangioblastomas in VHL. Less commonly, spinal cord (28 percent) or brain stem (14 percent) lesions are found. Syringomyelia occurs in 24 percent and is usually associated with an intramedullary spinal cord hemangioblastoma.

Although the first symptoms of VHL are usually related to the posterior fossa (55 percent) or to visual loss (18 percent), a renal tumor or pheochromocytoma is the presenting problem in 10 percent. Less commonly, angiomas are found in the liver, spleen, epididymis, or other tissues. The renal tumor is usually a hypernephroma, and malignant degeneration with the development of vascular renal cell carcinoma poses a serious threat to this population and is the cause of death in 14 percent.

Pheochromocytomas can occur in VHL, NF, or multiple endocrine adenomatosis. In each genetic syndrome the tumors are often bilateral; this is in contrast to the spontaneous pheochromocytoma, which is usually solitary. Normal levels of vanillylmandelic acid (VMA) do not eliminate the need of a thorough evaluation, and the close cooperation of an endocrinologist is vital. During surgery, the anesthesiologist must be aware of the possibility of a massive release of catecholamines during manipulation of the tumor, and proper preoperative preparation is essential.

Evaluation of patients with VHL is aimed initially at de-

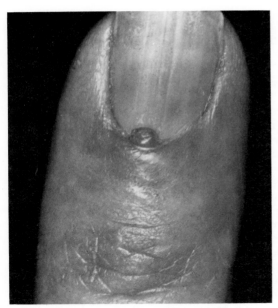

Figure 54-10 Subungual fibroma of tuberous sclerosis. (Courtesy of Dr. Thomas B. Fitzpatrick.)

termining which family members are affected. An affected member should have the extent of the disorder delineated. Such an evaluation should include a fundoscopic examination and measurement of intraocular pressure. Cerebral involvement is best determined by a contrast-enhanced CT scan. Renal and adrenal involvement are evaluated with a hematocrit determination, urinalysis (including VMA, calcium, and phosphate measurements) and plasma catecholamine levels. Radiological testing may include abdominal CT scanning, ultrasonography, and intravenous pyelography,

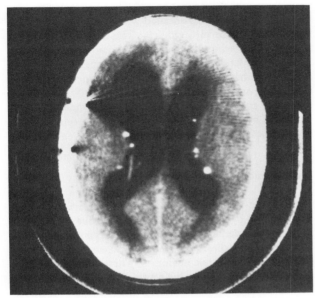

Figure 54-11 This CT scan demonstrates the typical periventricular calcifications seen in tuberous sclerosis. Hydrocephalus is also present.

with tomograms when indicated. Negative results do not exclude the possible later development of lesions, and periodic examination is necessary.

Early recognition of retinal lesions is important, since laser photocoagulation and cryotherapy are safe, effective means of treatment in the early stages. Failure to recognize and treat these lesions may lead to retinal hemorrhage and exudate, total retinal detachment, glaucoma, and visual loss. Symptomatic cerebellar or spinal lesions are usually surgically removed. Lesions may be solitary or multiple and can be either solid or cystic, with a mural nodule. In all cases they are quite vascular. Some lesions may be deeply located, making them subject to substantial surgical risk. In selected cases, stereotactic Bragg peak proton beam therapy may be useful.

Neurocutaneous Angiomatoses

Whereas the most common CNS abnormality of NF is in the Schwann cell and that of tuberous sclerosis is in the astrocyte, the most common abnormality of the neurocutaneous angiomatoses is in the blood vessels. Angiomas are seen in association with cutaneous stigmata that are typical for each of these disorders.

Ataxia-Telangiectasia

Ataxia-telangiectasia (AT) is a syndrome characterized by progressive ataxia, multiple cutaneous telangiectases, and specific immunologic abnormalities.[10] In the neonatal period the patient may be asymptomatic. In the toddler stage, walking is clumsy and unsteady. By 3 years of age and later, cutaneous telangiectases appear and are most prominent over the ears, nose, cheeks, conjuctivae, the exposed parts of the neck, and the flexion creases of the forearm. The disorder is progressive, and by school age, ataxia, choreoathetosis, and dysarthria may be noted. By age 10 or so, intellectual impairment and a mild polyneuropathy may appear.

Patients with ataxia-telangiectasia may have significant immunologic abnormalities, manifested by recurrent respiratory infections, a high incidence of leukemia or lymphoma (10 percent), IgA deficiency, and a low response to phytohemagglutinin. Death usually occurs in the second decade from recurrent infection or neoplasia (lymphoma, glioma).

Lymphocytes from patients with AT have been shown to have increased sensitivity to radiation as manifested by an increased number of chromosomal breaks after irradiation. Some studies suggest that AT cells show deficient excision repair after exposure to hypoxic x-radiation. However, other investigators have demonstrated that DNA synthesis is radioresistant in AT but the mitotic delay seen in irradiated normal cells is absent in AT cells. Therefore it has been suggested that AT cells divide before repair can occur, leading to an increased number of observed chromosomal breaks. AT may thus be classified as an inherited syndrome of chromosomal breakage, or clastogenic syndrome. Other clastogenic disorders include Fanconi's anemia, Bloom's syndrome, and xeroderma pigmentosum. All four show au-

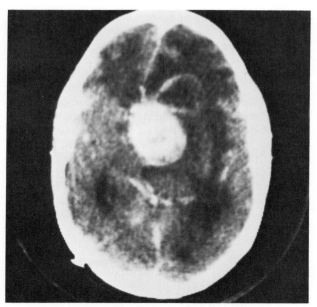

Figure 54-12 This 22-year-old female with tuberous sclerosis and prior radiation had a rapid neurological deterioration. CT scan and surgery revealed a malignant astrocytoma with hemorrhage into the tumor and into the ventricle.

tosomal recessive transmission and are associated with an increased risk of malignant tumors.

Since AT is a recessive disorder, the heterozygous state without overt genetic expression (carrier state) exists. Heterozygous relatives of patients with AT are at higher risk of malignant disease than the normal population. The gene for AT is reasonably common, and it has been estimated that heterozygotes for AT could make up nearly 1 percent of the population of the United States and could account for up to 5 percent of cancer deaths prior to age 45.[12] To date, the autosomal recessive gene responsible for AT has not been identified. In the nervous system, AT causes degeneration of the cerebellar cortex; loss of myelinated fibers in the pe-

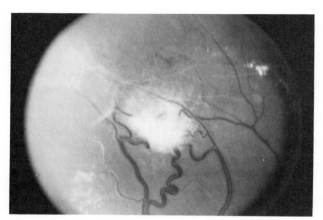

Figure 54-13 A pinkish-white retinal tumor associated with an enlarged arteriovenous pair is typical of von Hippel-Lindau disease. (Courtesy of Dr. Johan Zwaan.)

ripheral nerves, posterior columns, and cerebellospinal tracts; and degenerative changes of the posterior roots and sympathetic ganglia. No treatment is known.

Sturge-Weber Syndrome

Sturge-Weber syndrome can be considered among the phakomatoses because both the skin and the nervous system are involved. Most cases, however, appear to be due to a somatic mutation rather than to a germ cell mutation in that they are sporadic rather than inherited.[4,19] Patients with Sturge-Weber syndrome usually demonstrate a unilateral facial angioma (port-wine stain) in the dermatomes of the first or second division of the trigeminal nerve, associated with ipsilateral parieto-occipital leptomeningeal venous angiomatosis. The cortex underlying the meningeal abnormality demonstrates cortical atrophy, with calcifications in the second and third cortical layers. Angiomas occasionally may be seen in the eye as well as in other parts of the body along the distribution of sensory nerves. Resistance to outflow of aqueous humor due to increased scleral venous pressure can lead to glaucoma and visual loss.

Neurological abnormalities may include seizures or deficits such as a spastic hemiparesis or hemianopia contralateral to the angiomatosis. Fortunately, subarachnoid hemorrhage is uncommon. Successful treatment of the skin lesion with the argon laser has been noted, but similar attempts to treat the brain lesion have not been reported to date.

Klippel-Trénaunay-Weber Syndrome

Klippel-Trénaunay-Weber syndrome is an uncommon neurocutaneous disorder characterized by extensive skin hemangiomas that often appear in a dermatomal pattern and are associated with hemangiomas of the spinal cord in the same dermatomal distribution.[4,19] The lesions are usually unilateral and may be associated with osseous or muscular hypertrophy of the involved area. The disease is similar to Sturge-Weber syndrome and may be considered a spinal variant of the latter. Although some cases suggest autosomal dominant inheritance with incomplete penetrance, most hereditary patterns are not obvious, and both Sturge-Weber syndrome and Klippel-Trénaunay-Weber syndrome could be caused by a similar somatic mutation affecting different dermatomes during development.

Osler-Rendu-Weber Syndrome

Osler-Rendu-Weber syndrome is an uncommon disorder characterized by angiomas of the skin, mucous membranes, and nervous system.[4,8,19] In childhood, this autosomal dominant disorder is diagnosed from the development of multiple small red or purple angiomas. These generally enlarge and in later years may be the cause of recurrent epistaxis or gastrointestinal or genitourinary hemorrhages. Scattered angiomas may develop in the brain or spinal cord, producing hemorrhage or localized cerebral or spinal dysfunction.

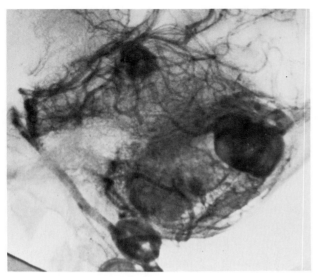

Figure 54-14 This vertebral arteriogram shows three cerebellar hemangioblastomas in a patient with von Hippel-Lindau disease.

Wyburn-Mason Syndrome

Wyburn-Mason syndrome is an uncommon disorder characterized by an arteriovenous aneurysm of the midbrain associated with a unilateral retinal arteriovenous malformation, facial nevi, and mental changes. The hereditary aspects of this uncommon problem are uncertain.

Fabry's Disease

Although not usually considered among the phakomatoses, Fabry's disease (angiokeratoma corporis diffusum) is a genetic abnormality with nervous system, skin, and systemic manifestations which should be considered with the other angiomatoses. Fabry's disease is the only one of the phakomatoses with a known biochemical abnormality.[1,11] It is characterized by multiple small, flat, or slightly raised telangiectases on the abdomen and lower extremities, which are caused by a deficit in α-galactosidase, leading to an accumulation of ceramide trihexoside in the endothelium and media of blood vessels. Although the skin lesions are diagnostic, the vascular involvement is usually more diffuse and can lead to impaired renal function, hypertension, and myocardial infarction.

Neurological involvement includes a painful polyneuropathy caused by ceramide trihexoside deposition both perineurally and intraneurally. In addition, cerebrovascular involvement may lead to cerebral thromboembolic lesions during the teens or early adulthood.

Fabry's disease is an X-linked recessive disorder, so symptoms are found mostly in males. The presence of occasional symptomatic heterozygous females has been explained by hypothesizing the presence of a gene that causes preferential inactivation of the X chromosome carrying the normal allele. For the most part, heterozygous females are

asymptomatic carriers who can be diagnosed by assaying α-galactosidase activity. At present, Fabry's disease is the only phakomatosis that can be diagnosed prenatally.

Diagnostic Considerations

The phakomatoses are syndromes with specific associations between cutaneous, ocular, and neurological abnormalities. However, since the Greek word *phakos* may have more than one meaning and since the "phakoma" of each disorder may show a different histology, it has been suggested that this nondescriptive term be abandoned. Yet, to date, no satisfactory alternative exists. Table 54-1 presents a summary of the major findings and modes of inheritance. Because of the variable expression of many of these disorders, diagnosis can be difficult. Evaluation of multiple systems and of multiple family members is best accomplished by an interdisciplinary group including a geneticist, an ophthalmologist, a dermatologist, a neurologist, and a neurosurgeon. Diagnosis and treatment should be designed for the affected patient and his family in a way that avoids fragmentation of medical care.

Only in Fabry's disease has the genetic defect been identified. For each of the other syndromes, it is not known whether the variable nature of the clinical presentation is due to variable expression of one gene or to an abnormality that can occur in any of several genes leading to the development of similar stigmata.

While the historical tendency has been to divide the phakomatoses into smaller and smaller subcategories, it should be recognized that similarities exist between these groups. Spinal neurofibromas, café au lait spots, and cutaneous and plexiform neurofibromas occur both in classic von Recklinghausen's neurofibromatosis and in bilateral acoustic neurofibromatosis. Pheochromocytoma, often bilateral, may occur in neurofibromatosis or in von Hippel-Lindau disease. Several families have been reported with overlapping manifestations of two phakomatoses. In one family, the retinal angiomas of von Hippel-Lindau disease were associated with the lesions of neurofibromatosis including iris nodules and café au lait spots containing macromelanosomes. One member had cerebellar hemangioblastoma, pheochromocytoma, and renal cell carcinoma.[16] Other reported familial groupings have included tuberous sclerosis associated with Klippel-Trénaunay-Weber syndrome[5], a father and son with adenoma sebaceum and Sturge-Weber syndrome, and tuberous sclerosis associated with visceral lesions of von Hippel-Lindau disease.

One possible explanation for these associations is that common genetic defects may occasionally occur together, or, to put it another way, the presence of one genetic defect does not prevent a person from having a second genetic defect. A second possible explanation is that the phakomatoses are caused by small genetic mutations in a family of genes responsible for the proper embryologic development and organization of the neuroectoderm and mesoderm. Under this concept, neurofibromatosis and tuberous sclerosis may be seen as generalized abnormalities of neuroectodermal growth control due to a gene defect in a germ cell. Von

TABLE 54-1 Clinical Features of the Phakomatoses

Disorder	Transmission	Clinical Findings		
		Nervous System	**Skin**	**Other**
Neurofibromatosis: VRNF	Autosomal dominant	Spinal neurofibroma, plexiform neurofibroma, optic glioma, meningioma, other gliomas, learning disorders, macrocephaly, seizures	Neurofibromas, café au lait spots, intertriginous freckles	Iris hamartomas, scoliosis, pheochromocytoma, hemihypertrophy
BANF	Autosomal dominant	Bilateral acoustic neuroma, meningioma, spinal neurofibroma, gliomas, seizures	Few neurofibromas and café au lait spots	Congenital cataracts but no iris hamartomas
Tuberous sclerosis	Autosomal dominant	Subependymal astrocytoma, cortical nodules, malignant glioma, seizures, retardation	Ash-leaf spots, shagreen patches, adenoma sebaceum, subungual fibromas	Tooth pitting, cardiac rhabdomyomas
von Hippel-Lindau	Autosomal dominant	Hemangioblastoma of cerebellum, spinal cord, or brain stem		Retinal angioma, renal hypernephroma, visceral angioma, pheochromocytoma
Neurocutaneous angiomatoses: Ataxia-telangiectasia	Autosomal dominant	Ataxia, dysarthria, choreoathetosis, polyneuropathy, spinal degeneration, intellectual impairment	Telangiectases	Leukemia, lymphoma, IgA deficiency
Sturge-Weber	Usually a somatic mutation	Parieto-occipital angioma, seizures	Facial hemangioma	Glaucoma
Klippel-Trénaunay-Weber	Uncertain	Spinal hemangioma	Dermatomal hemangioma	
Osler-Rendu-Weber	Autosomal dominant	CNS angiomas and hemorrhage	Hemangiomas	Epistaxis, gastric hemorrhage
Wyburn-Mason	Uncertain	AV aneurysm of midbrain, mental changes	Facial nevi	Unilateral retinal AVM
Fabry's disease	X-linked recessive defect in α-galactosidase	Painful polyneuropathy, stroke	Telangiectases of leg and abdomen	Renal failure, hypertension, myocardial infarction

Hippel-Lindau disease, ataxia-telangiectasia, Osler-Rendu-Weber syndrome, and Fabry's disease might be caused by germ cell defects primarily affecting the control of mesodermal growth. In contrast, the sporadic angiomatoses such as those of Sturge-Weber, Klippel-Trénaunay-Weber, and Wyburn-Mason may represent similar mutations in the genes of somatic cells occurring in early embryogenesis, which may account for their localized dermatomal patterns and lack of transmission. This unifying concept allows one to consider specific genetic defects leading to specific abnormalities of cell growth and organization and, thus, to the development of benign or hamartomatous lesions.

The next decade will see an abundance of genetic research. Genetic studies of the phakomatoses should not only increase our understanding of these disorders, but also broaden our knowledge of the genetic control of the developing nervous system and its vasculature as well as provide an insight into the genes responsible for lesions such as gliomas, schwannomas, acoustic neuromas, meningiomas, and arteriovenous malformations, which occur in the absence of the phakomatoses. Could it be that these solitary lesions, which represent a major portion of neurosurgical problems, are caused by mutations similar to those causing the phakomatoses, but occurring in a somatic cell later in life? We all await the answers to such important questions.

References

1. Beaudet AL, Caskey CT: Detection of Fabry's disease heterozygotes by hair root analysis. Clin Genet 13:251–258, 1978.
2. Benedict PH, Szabó G, Fitzpatrick TB, Sinesi SJ: Melanotic macules in Albright's syndrome and in neurofibromatosis. JAMA 205:618–626, 1968.
3. Crowe FW, Schull WJ, Neel JV: *A Clinical, Pathological and Genetic Study of Multiple Neurofibromatosis*. Springfield, Ill. Charles C Thomas, 1956.
4. Edgerton MT, Hiebert JM: Vascular and lymphatic tumors in infancy, childhood, and adulthood: Challenge of diagnosis and treatment. Curr Probl Cancer 2:1–44, 1978.
5. Gomez MR (ed): *Tuberous Sclerosis*, New York, Raven, 1979.
6. Horton WA, Wong V, Eldridge R: Von Hippel-Lindau disease. Arch Intern Med 136:769–777, 1976.
7. Kanter WR, Eldridge R, Fabricant R, Allen JC, Koerber T: Central neurofibromatosis with bilateral acoustic neuroma: Genetic, clinical and biochemical distinctions from peripheral neurofibromatosis. Neurology (NY) 30:851–859, 1980.
8. King CR, Lovrien EW, Reiss J: Central nervous system arteriovenous malformations in multiple generations of a family with hereditary hemorrhageic telangiectasia. Clin Genet 12:372–381, 1977.
9. Martuza RL, Ojemann RG: Bilateral acoustic neuromas: Clinical aspects, pathogenesis and treatment. Neurosurgery 10:1–12, 1982.
10. Patterson MC, Smith PJ: Ataxia telangiectasia: An inherited human disorder involving hypersensitivity to ionizing radiation and related DNA-damaging chemicals. Ann Rev Genet 13:291–318, 1979.
11. Pilz H, Heipertz R, Seidel D: Basic findings and current developments in sphingolipidoses. Hum Genet 47:113–134, 1979.
12. Purtillo, DT, Paquin L, Gindhart T: Genetics of neoplasia: Impact of ecogenetics on oncogenesis. Am J Pathol 91:607–687, 1978.
13. Riccardi VM: Von Recklinghausen neurofibromatosis. N Engl J Med 305:1617–1627, 1981.
14. Riccardi VM, Mulvihill JJ (eds): *Neurofibromatosis (von Recklinghausen disease): Genetics, Cell Biology, and Biochemistry*. New York, Raven, 1981.
15. Stern J, Jakobiec FA, Housepian EM: The architecture of optic nerve gliomas with and without neurofibromatosis. Arch Ophthalmol 98:505–511, 1980.
16. Thomas JV, Schwartz PL, Gragoudas ES: Von Hippel's disease in association with von Recklinghausen's neurofibromatosis. Brit J Ophthalmol 62:604–608, 1978.
17. Waga S, Yamamoto Y, Kojima T, Sakakura M: Massive hemorrhage in tumor of tuberous sclerosis. Surg Neurol 8:99–101, 1977.
18. Whitehouse D: Diagnostic value of the café-au-lait spot in children. Arch Dis Child 41:316–319, 1966.
19. Williams HB: Hemangiomas and lymphangiomas. Adv Surg 15:317–349, 1981.

55

Virus-Induced Brain Tumors

Jeffrey S. Walker
Darell D. Bigner

Viruses have been known to be oncogenic agents since the discovery of the Rous sarcoma virus in 1912. The first intracranial tumors were induced by Vasquez-Lopez in 1936.[1] He inoculated 3- to 5-month-old chickens intracranially with avian sarcoma virus (ASV). Perivascular sarcomas developed in 75 percent of the infected birds. Vigier et al., in 1957, repeated this experiment using neonatal rather than adult Leghorn chickens. All the inoculated chicks developed meningeal and perivascular sarcomas. In 1964, Rabotti and Raine virally induced intracerebral gliomas in mammals. The Schmidt-Ruppin strain of ASV was injected intracerebrally in newborn Syrian hamsters, resulting in a combination of gliomas and sarcomas. Gliomas will occur in 89 to 100 percent of intracerebrally inoculated animals when the Schmidt-Ruppin strain is used. Following this experiment, an explosion in the recognition of CNS oncogenic viruses

and susceptible animal models occurred (Table 55-1). The major experimental viruses used in neuro-oncology and the type of neoplasm induced by each are reviewed in this chapter.

DNA Tumor Viruses

Two important families of DNA tumor-producing viruses are papovavirus and adenovirus. Papovaviruses are subdivided into the papilloma, or wart viruses and the oncogenic polyomaviruses. From the polyomaviruses are derived the experimentally useful classes of DNA neuro-oncogenic viruses. Each virus strain produces certain tumor types, depending upon the animal model used. As a general rule, neonatal animals produce the highest tumor yield, with the Syrian hamster being the most susceptible animal. Most viruses require intracerebral inoculation in order to produce CNS tumors. Following intracerebral injection, the virus particles are distributed widely within the CNS, especially throughout the ventricular system.

Papovaviruses

Bovine papilloma virus, human JC virus, simian vacuolating virus (SV40) and polyomavirus are the important oncogenic viruses in the papovavirus family. Bovine papilloma virus will induce meningiomas, fibromas, and fibrosarcomas following intracerebral inoculation in calves and hamsters. A latent period of less than 1 year is commonly observed.

One of the most interesting recently discovered tumorigenic virus strains is the human JC papovavirus. Approximately 10 years ago the virus was isolated from the brain of a

TABLE 55-1 Specificity of Virus-Induced Experimental Brain Tumors

Tumor Type	Inducing Virus	
	Group	Type
Anaplastic astrocytoma or	RNA oncornavirus	ASV, MSV, SSV
glioblastoma multiforme	DNA papovavirus	Human JC
	DNA adenovirus	SA7
Pilocytic astrocytoma	RNA oncornavirus	ASV
Gemistocytic astrocytoma	RNA oncornavirus	MSV
Medulloblastoma	DNA papovavirus	Human JC (Mad-1,-2 strains)
	DNA adenovirus	SA7, HA12
Neuroblastoma or	DNA adenovirus	HA12
retinoblastoma	DNA papovavirus	Human JC
Ependymoma	DNA adenovirus	SA7
	RNA oncornavirus	ASV
	DNA papovavirus	SV40, human JC
Choroid plexus papilloma	DNA papovavirus	SV40, human BK
	DNA adenovirus	CELO
Meningioma	DNA papovavirus	Human JC, Bovine papilloma
	RNA oncornavirus	ASV, MSV
Sarcoma	DNA papovavirus	Human JC, murine polyoma, bovine papilloma
	DNA adenoviruses	SA7, HA12, HA18
	RNA oncornavirus	ASV, MSV
Pineocytoma	DNA papovavirus	Human JC (Mad-1,-4 strains)

patient with progressive multifocal leukoencephalopathy (PML). It is named JC virus after the initials of the first patient from whom the virus was cultured. Five different strains have proved to induce neoplastic transformation: Mad-1, -2, -3, and -4 and the SV40 PML isolates from Johns Hopkins University. Mad-1 and -2 strains produce the highest incidence of medulloblastomas. Intracerebral injection of the JC virus into newborn Syrian hamsters produces medulloblastomas near or within the internal granular layer of the cerebellum. Meningiomas, pineocytomas, meningeal sarcomas, intraventricular ependymomas, and thalamic gliomas are also produced. A lack of tumor specificity hinders most of the virally induced tumor models. However, 85 to 95 percent of the animals infected with this virus will produce CNS tumors. The latent period in neonatal animals is generally 3 to 7 months. Increases in the latent period and a lower incidence of tumor production occur in non-neonatal animals. Tumor development preferentially occurs in the cerebellum, followed by the thalamus, piriform lobes, olfactory-frontal regions, ventricles, and occasionally the spinal cord. Neuroblastomas are common peripheral nervous system tumors induced by the JC virus following intracerebral inoculation, indicating the systemic distribution of a virus injected intracranially. Intraocular administration will increase the incidence of neuroblastoma formation and will also induce retinoblastomas. Pineocytomas are exclusively produced by the JC papovavirus. Mad-1 and -4 strains are the most effective strains in producing pineocytomas, with a latent period between 5 and 8 months.

In two primate species the JC virus has induced glioblastomas with the typical features present in the human tumor. The owl monkey (*Aotus trivirgatus*) and squirrel monkey (*Saimiri sciureus*) are susceptible to tumor formation. Rhesus monkeys have been resistant to tumor production with this virus. A glioblastoma and a mixed glial neuronal tumor developed in two of four adult owl monkeys at 16 months and 2 years after inoculation.[3] Four of ten squirrel monkeys developed astrocytomas (graded III to IV) with a latency between 14 and 29 months.

Another related virus, which was isolated from a human, is the BK virus, discovered in the urine of a renal transplant patient who had received immunosuppressive drugs. When it was inoculated intracerebrally into newborn hamsters, choroid plexus papillomas were formed. SV40 will also produce choroid plexus papillomas, along with meningeal sarcomas, in the same experimental animal model. A viral dose of more than 10^6 TCID$_{50}$ is required for tumor production. At this dose a tumor incidence of 15 to 80 percent, with a latent period between 80 and 238 days, is achieved. From these tumors the SV40 genome has been recovered, using hybrid fusion techniques. No evidence of viral particles is found on electron microscopy. Tumors derived from this virus are transplantable.

Using the polyomavirus, CNS anaplastic fibrosarcomas have been produced in the rabbit following intracerebral or subcutaneous viral inoculation. Depending upon the route of administration, a tumor incidence of 33 to 46 percent is achieved, with a latent period of 44 to 228 days. Syrian hamsters and rats are also susceptible animals. The highest incidence of tumor formation, with the shortest latency, occurs in the rat.

Adenoviruses

The major adenovirus strains used in experimental neuro-oncology are the human adenovirus strains 12 (HA12) and 18(HA18), simian adenovirus strains 7 (SA7) and 20 (SA20), and the avian adenovirus strain, CELO. Adenovirus 12 is used for producing neuroblastomas, medulloepitheliomas, and retinoblastomas. Neuroblastomas occur following intracranial and intraperitoneal virus administration. Retinoblastomas result from intraocular virus administration. A wide latent period of 31 to 235 days occurs in susceptible animals (hamsters, mice, rats, and mastomys). An inoculum of $10^{4.5}$ TCID$_{50}$ in 0.1 ml will usually cause tumor formation in 100 percent of susceptible animals.

Simian adenovirus 20 produces undifferentiated tumors of unclear histology. Simian adenovirus 7 induces a wide variety of tumors in the rat and hamster, including fibrosarcomas, malignant ependymomas, choroid plexus carcinomas and sarcomas, medulloblastomas, glioblastomas, and other highly undifferentiated tumors.

The avian adenovirus CELO provides an experimental model for the production of intraventricular choroid plexus papillomas in hamsters. Of 17 animals inoculated, 15 developed tumors, with a latent period between 44 and 228 days. The virus has not been recovered from these tumors, even though viral antigens are expressed. The most common virus-specific antigen is the T antigen.

RNA Tumor Viruses

All neuro-oncogenic RNA viruses are members of the retrovirus family, subfamily oncornavirus. These viruses contain high molecular weight RNA and the enzyme reverse transcriptase. Unlike DNA viruses, they reproduce by budding instead of by cell lysis. Reverse transcriptase transcribes the viral RNA into a DNA strand, which can then be incorporated into the host cell's genome. This results in neoplastic transformation of the host cell without causing cell death. Only one virus particle is necessary to obtain such a transformation. The major oncogenic RNA viruses which have been used in neuro-oncology are the avian sarcoma virus (ASV), murine sarcoma virus (MSV), and simian sarcoma virus (SSV). Oncornaviruses have experimentally produced tumors in a wide variety of animals. The type of tumor produced varies with the site of inoculation and the animal used.

ASV is a commonly used and reliable glioma tumor model. Four different strains are known to induce neoplastic transformation following intracerebral inoculation: Bryan, Schmidt-Ruppin (subgroup D) (Fig. 55-1), CT559, and Bratislava 77 (subgroup C). Introduction of ASV into the cortex or subependymal plate of a dog or rat will produce anaplastic astrocytomas in 100 percent of inoculated animals. Experimentally the viral genome can be recovered from the tumors. Astrocytomas induced with ASV have virus-specific antigens. ASV is not known to have produced any human brain tumors.

The ASV model was refined by Bigner et al. in 1975. Neonatal rats inoculated intracerebrally with 2 μl of ASV

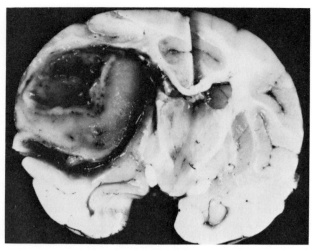

Figure 55-1 A reticulum cell sarcoma of the meninges induced by an intracranial inoculation of Schmidt-Ruppin strain ASV into a rhesus monkey. (From Bigner and Swenberg, p. 35.[1])

(10^7 FFU per milliliter) develop tumors in 1 month. Animal death occurs in approximately 3 months. Uniform mortality distributions make possible experimental evaluation of various therapeutic protocols for efficacy. The ASV-induced tumor model is used extensively for chemotherapy research. It has been shown to be responsive to carmustine (BCNU), lomustine (CCNU), methyl-CCNU, and 5-azacytidine, but not to procarbazine or mithramycin. According to Swenberg's studies, BCNU is more effective than CCNU. BCNU and radiation, in combination therapy, significantly prolongs animal survival.[5] There are conflicting reports of the efficacy of immunotherapy against ASV-induced tumors. Mahaley et al.,[4] were able to prevent ASV glioma induction by intracerebral inoculation of a combination of ASV and bacillus Calmette-Guérin (BCG) wall preparation. The mechanism of this inhibition remains undefined. One advantage of using the ASV model is that a virus pool of uniform dose can be produced and stored for up to 10 years. This assures consistency and reproducibility within an experimental protocol over time.

MSV produces malignant gliomas in rats after intracerebral administration. The Maloney strain induces glioblastomas, oligodendrogliomas, gemistocytic astrocytomas, and hemangioendotheliomas, while the Harvey strain produces only sarcomas. Malignant gliomas, consistent with glioblastomas, have been induced in Wistar-Furth rats using the Kirsten strain. Marked vascular proliferation is present within these tumors. No virus has been detected by electron microscopy. These tumors generally appear 16 days after injection, with death occurring in 4 to 5 weeks in 90 percent of the animals. A question of whether this tumor has true vascular proliferation or neoplastic vascular endothelial transformation makes it a controversial model.

The SSV strain was isolated in 1975 from a fibrosarcoma of a woolly monkey. Intracerebral inoculation of neonatal marmosets produced glioblastomas in 6 of 10 animals. A maximum latent period of 26 months followed the administration of 2×10^3 FFU. SSV was isolated from both the brain and the CSF of the tumor-bearing primates. No such virus particles have been recovered from the CSF in human brain tumor patients.

Newer generation CT scanners have been able to visualize intracranial tumors in experimental animals. Groothuis et al. examined the primary ASV canine tumor model by CT scan. They reported the ability to detect all tumors more than 5 mm in diameter, with a tumor size estimate accurate within 3 mm on contrast-enhanced scans. The owl monkey and squirrel monkey glioma models have also been examined by CT. Transplanted intracranial tumors have been detected by CT in many mammalian species, the smallest of which is the rat. Better resolution CT scanners should help neuro-oncologists identify tumor-bearing animals. This would make possible a direct, noninvasive, in vivo assessment of a tumor's responsiveness to various therapeutic regimens.

Evidence of Viral Induction of Human Brain Tumors

Currently, no conclusive evidence links viral infections to the production of human brain tumors. There are reports of viral inclusion bodies, antigens, and genomes in experimental and human brain tumors. A BK virus from an intracerebral reticulum cell sarcoma and an SV40-type virus from a glioblastoma have been recovered from patients, using cell fusion techniques. Unfortunately, there is no way to determine whether the isolated virus caused the tumor to occur. Alternatively, the virus could be a contaminant or a latent benign infection. Many of the reports of viral nucleic acids detected by nucleic acid hybridization techniques may be artifactual because of contaminated probes.

A papovavirus, SV40, has been suggestively associated with an increased incidence of childhood intracranial tumors. An SV40-contaminated Rhesus monkey kidney cell line was used in preparing the Salk vaccine from 1954 through 1960; the virus was not discovered until 1960. Estimates place the number of people who received the contaminated vaccine as high as 30 million.[6] Intracerebral inoculation of this virus into newborn hamsters results in malignant ependymomas and choroid plexus papillomas. Epidemiologic studies of children exposed to the virus-contaminated vaccine suggest an increased incidence of medulloblastomas in those who were exposed to the virus transplacentally, but no conclusive evidence has been found to support this hypothesis.

PML has been directly associated with the JC virus, which has caused medulloblastomas in newborn hamsters but no proven human tumors. Castaigne et al. reported multiple small gliomas arising within demyelinated areas in a patient with PML. Reports of gliomatous transformation in other demyelinating diseases, such as multiple sclerosis, are rare.

Using viral-specific DNA or DNA hybridization techniques, BK viral DNA homology has been found in more than 10 human intracranial tumors. SV40 viral homologues were found in one of seven glioblastomas by Meinke et al. and also in an oligodendroglioma by Krieg et al.[2] The tumors which experimental data suggest might be related to a viral etiology—medulloblastomas, choroid plexus papillomas, ependymomas, and ependymoblastomas—need to be examined more thoroughly. Krieg et al. did detect an SV40 genome in one of two medulloblastomas tested. No BK or JC viral genomes were found in the one positive medulloblastoma, nor had the patient been exposed to the contaminated Salk vaccine. These investigators found 8 tumors (5 of them meningiomas) with viral genome homology out of 35 human intracranial tumors examined. No cause and effect relationship was proved; however, the study of human viral oncogenesis is still in its infancy.

References

1. Bigner DD, Swenberg JA (eds): *Jänisch and Schreiber's Experimental Tumors of the Central Nervous System*, 1st Engl ed, Kalamazoo, Mich., The Upjohn Co., 1977.

2. Johnson RT: *Viral Infections of the Nervous System*, New York, Raven, 1982, chap 12, pp 295–310.
3. London WT, Houff SA, Madden DL, Fuccillo DA, Gravell M, Wallen WC, Palmer AE, Sever JL, Padgett BL, Walker DL, ZuRhein GM, Ohashi T: Brain tumors in owl monkeys inoculated with a human polyomavirus (JC virus). Science 201:1246–1249, 1978.
4. Mahaley MS Jr, Aronin PA, Michaels A, Bigner DD: Prevention of glioma induction in rats by simultaneous intra-cerebral inoculation of avian sarcoma virus plus BCG cell wall preparation. Submitted for publication, 1982.
5. Steinbok P, Mahaley MS Jr, U R, Zinn DC, Lipper S, Mahaley JL, Bigner DD: Synergism between BCNU and irradiation in the treatment of anaplastic gliomas. J Neurosurg 51:581–586, 1979.
6. Walsh JW, Zimmer SG, Perdue ML: Role of viruses in the induction of primary intracranial tumors. Neurosurgery 10: 643–662, 1982.

56
Radiation-Induced Brain Tumors

Jeffrey S. Walker
Darell D. Bigner

Radiation has been implicated in the induction of human intracranial neoplasms for over thirty years. Numerous articles have reported development of various intracranial tumors in patients following radiation therapy, but obstacles arise in determining whether these tumors were directly caused by radiation. Currently no definitive biochemical abnormalities are linked to radiation-induced tumors, and they exhibit no distinguishing morphological characteristics. Cytogenetic alterations are under investigation, but to date no specific genetic or chromosomal changes can be attributed to radiation. The inability to scientifically link neoplastic cellular alterations to previous radiation makes this area extremely controversial. This chapter reviews the pertinent animal experiments and human case reports of central nervous system tumors associated with radiation that may have played a role in tumor induction.

Animal Experiments

Lacassagne and Vinzent, in 1933, were the first to induce a radiation-related neoplasm.[11] They injected bacteria subcutaneously into a rabbit's leg in order to cause an inflammatory reaction. The animal's legs were then irradiated, using the noninjected leg as a control. A fibrosarcoma developed 18 months after irradiation within the area of inflammation. The experiment was repeated using diatomaceous earth as the inflaming agent, and two rabbits developed fibrosarcomas. These experiments demonstrated the possibility that radiation could induce a tumor. Inflammation was believed to be the prerequisite for radiation induction of a neoplasm.

In another experiment, by Kent and Pickering, focal gamma radiation to the right orbit induced fibrosarcomas within the irradiated area in two of twelve monkeys (*Macaca mulatta*).[8] The radiation dose was 2000 rad, with a latent period of 853 days in the first animal. A latent period of 474 days occurred in the animal that received 3000 rads, indicating a probable relationship between the total dose of radiation and the length of the latent period. Fibrosarcomas developed only in the animals receiving ^{60}Co gamma (1.2 MeV) radiation, whereas monkeys subjected to thermal and fast neutron irradiation developed no such lesions.

Numerous animal experiments have attempted to prove a causal relationship between radiation and primary CNS neoplasms. Haymaker et al. reported on 21 rhesus monkeys (*Macaca mulatta*) who survived 2 years or longer after receiving 200 to 800 rad of whole body proton or x-ray radiation.[5] A glioblastoma multiforme developed in three of ten monkeys who survived 3 to 5 years following the radiation treatment. These three monkeys received 600 to 800 rad of 55-MeV proton whole body irradiation. Two of the monkeys with tumors also had significant areas of radionecrosis. The third animal with a glioblastoma had radiation-induced vascular changes and scattered areas of white and gray matter calcification. The incidence of brain tumor in this group of animals was 14 percent, as compared to known control groups, where the spontaneous development of glial tumors is less than 0.1 percent. One should still recognize that radiation played an ill-defined role in the development of these three tumors.

McDonald et al.,[13] in 1973, also implicated radiation as a cause of glial tumors. They implanted intracerebral pellets of 60 μCi of ^{60}Co into 26- to 30-day-old rats, and 19 of 27 animals developed glioblastomas. The latent period was between 365 and 410 days. When the dose of radiation was increased to 350 μCi of ^{60}Co, all the animals died within 192 days without developing any tumors. It is assumed that more time was needed for tumor development.

Negative results were reported by Jänisch and Kirsch[7] in 1967. They implanted radioactive gold seeds (0.135 to 37 mCi) above the cerebral convexity in 88 different experimental animals without producing a CNS tumor. Daels and Biltris,[4] were also unsuccessful in producing a glial tumor after implanting epidural radium in over 100 guinea pigs.

Some experiments do support the premise that high-dose radiation can cause primary CNS tumors if the animals survive long enough. How to extrapolate these data to a human population is still unclear.

Criteria for Radiation-Induced Neoplasia

In order to incriminate radiation therapy in the development of a human CNS tumor, one must demonstrate that (1) the tumor occurs within the ports of radiation; (2) an adequate latent period exists following radiation, commensurate with the dose of radiation given; (3) no factors predisposing to tumor development exist, such as neurofibromatosis or multiple endocrine neoplastic syndromes; (4) there is a definitive tumor diagnosis, and (5) the tumor would rarely occur spontaneously in a control group of nonirradiated patients. This must be individualized for each patient according to age and sex, in conjunction with tumor type and location. For example, a cerebellar astrocytoma in an adult is unusual, as is a bitemporal glioblastoma. Another interesting phenomenon would be the simultaneous development of a glial tumor in association with a meningioma within the irradiated area. The inability to differentiate spontaneously occurring tumors from radiation-induced ones restricts the ability to prove that radiation induces human brain tumors.

Molecular Basis of Radiation-Induced Neoplasia

The molecular events preceding radiation-induced neoplasia remain obscure. Many authors think that radiation-induced inflammation causes a faulty regeneration in inflamed tissue, leading to tumor formation—an old theory that sheds no light on the causation of the tumors. Radiation is most damaging when given during the mitotic phases of the cell cycle. The production of DNA seems to be diminished in irradiated cells, but whether this is due to an alteration in the DNA structure or in the replicating enzyme systems is un-

known. According to Kleihues and Bigner, a genetic mutation leading to a quasi-permanent yet inheritable change in DNA sequence may be the initiating event in neoplastic transformation.[9] It is unknown whether single or multiple mutations are required for transformation of a normal cell into a neoplastic one. The probability of a radiation-induced mutation leading to a neoplasm remains a popular but unproven theory. Cellular changes following radiation have been reported, but it is unclear how this could result in neoplastic transformation.

Radiation-Induced Tumors in Humans

Fibrosarcomas are the most common tumor type to develop after radiation therapy. Intracranial fibrosarcomas have usually been reported following radiation therapy for pituitary tumors. Waltz and Brownell,[16] in 1966, reported two cases of fibrosarcoma developing after radiation therapy and reviewed 13 previously reported cases. Only a few cases have been reported since 1966. All the patients cited received over 3500 rad. The latent period was generally between 5 and 12 years. To judge from the small number of reported cases, development of a fibrosarcoma after radiation therapy must be a rare occurrence. Unfortunately, no large group of high-dose-irradiated patients surviving over 10 years has been reported, so the incidence of intracranial tumor development following irradiation in humans is still unknown.

Meningiomas have been reported following radiation therapy for pituitary tumors, glial tumors, and scalp abnormalities. Mann et al.,[12] in 1953, first reported a malignant meningioma 6 years after radiation to an optic nerve glioma. Approximately 40 cases have since been reported. These cases were recently reviewed by Iacono et al.,[6] who noted that the latent period for meningioma development in patients receiving less than 800 rad was 31.3 years, while in the high-dose-irradiated group (more than 2300 rad) the average latent period was 20.8 years. These data again suggest that the higher the dose of irradiation the shorter the latent period. The most convincing evidence that radiation was associated with an increased incidence of meningiomas was presented by Modan et al.[14] in 1974. They reviewed almost 11,000 children with tinea capitis who received radiation treatments to the scalp upon immigrating to Israel before 1960. The children received 350 to 400 rad to each of five scalp fields, with a calculated brain dose of 140 rad. Compared with a well-matched control group, a fourfold increase in the incidence of meningiomas occurred in the irradiated group. A latent period of 16 years elapsed before tumor discovery in most of those cases. Some of the children in the study received multiple courses of radiation because of recurrent fungal infection, and most of the patients who developed meningiomas had associated scalp changes and alopecia. It seems logical that these meningiomas were in some way related to the low-dose radiation, but conclusive proof is lacking.

Approximately 16 glial tumors have been reported following radiation to the head. Chung et al.[2] reviewed these cases in 1981 (Table 56-1). Not all the cases cited, however, meet the stringent criteria outlined earlier in this chapter.

TABLE 56-1 Patients with Glioma following Irradiation

First Author, Year, and Reference	Reason for Therapy	Age,* Years	Sex	Radiation Dosage, rad	Latent Period,† Years	Radiation-Induced Glioma
Jones (1960)[2]	Meningioma (left frontal)	33	M	4000	10	Astrocytoma (right hemisphere)
Saenger (1960)[2]	Cervical adenitis	11	M	400	11	Glioblastoma multiforme
Albert (1966)[2]	Tinea capitis	4	M	500–800	4	Astrocytoma (optic chiasm)
Albert (1966)[2]	Tinea capitis	10	M	500–800	1	Astrocytoma (cerebrum)
Kosmaki (1977)[2]	Craniopharyngioma	28	M	5400	6	Glioblastoma multiforme (temporal lobe)
Sogg (1978)[2]	Craniopharyngioma	9	F	6007	5	Malignant astrocytoma (right temporal lobe)
Robinson (1978)[2]	Teratoma (pineal)	10	M	4000	26	Astrocytoma, grade 4 (right frontal lobe)
Robinson (1978)[2]	Meningioma	36	M	2750	21	Astrocytoma, grade 3 (right temporal lobe)
Preissig (1979)[2]	Glomus jugulare tumor (right middle ear)	43	M	4480	8	Anaplastic astrocytoma (right cerebellum)
Chung (1981)[2]	CNS prophylaxis for acute lymphocytic leukemia	2	M	2400	5	Glioblastoma multiforme (left parietal lobe)
Klériga (1978)[10]	Medulloblastoma (left cerebellum)	1	M	5000 cranial 2500 spinal	11	Astrocytoma (left cerebellum)
Bachman (1978)[1]	Papillary ependymoma (left lateral ventricle)	1	F	3960 cranial 2300 spinal	5	Glioblastoma multiforme (left occipital lobe)
Cohen (1981)[3]	Medulloblastoma	4	F	4500 post. fossa 3500 whole brain 3500 spinal	14	Astrocytoma (left frontal lobe)
Pearl (1980)[15]	Medulloblastoma	5	M	4000 post. fossa 3000 whole brain 2000 spinal	13	Glioblastoma multiforme (left occipital lobe)
Piatt‡	Pituitary tumor causing acromegaly	39	M	6000	13	Glioblastoma multiforme (bitemporal)
Walker‡	Hemangioblastoma (left cerebellum)	44	M	3075	24	Glioblastoma multiforme (right occipital lobe); right parasagittal occipital meningioma

*Age at time of therapy.
†Interval between irradiation and diagnosis.
‡In preparation for publication.

From the relatively few reported cases it is impossible to make a definite statement on the role that radiation plays in the development of glial tumors. Could there be some underlying or predisposing factor to cause tumor formation in this small number of patients?

References

1. Bachman DS, Ostrow PT: Fatal long-term sequela following radiation "cure" for ependymoma. Ann Neurol 4:319–321, 1978.
2. Chung CK, Stryker JA, Cruse R, Vannuci R, Towfighi J: Glioblastoma multiforme following prophylactic cranial irradiation and intrathecal methotrexate in a child with acute lymphocytic leukemia. Cancer 47:2563–2566, 1981.
3. Cohen MS, Kushner MJ, Dell S: Frontal lobe astrocytoma following radiotherapy for medulloblastoma. Neurology (NY) 31:616–619, 1981.
4. Daels F, Biltris R: Contribution à l'étude de la provocation de tumeurs malignes expérminentales au moyen de substances radio-actives. Bull Assoc Fr Cancer 20:32–77, 1931.
5. Haymaker W, Rubinstein LJ, Miquel J: Brain tumors in irradiated monkeys. Acta Neuropathol (Berl) 20:267–277, 1972.
6. Iacono RP, Apuzzo MLJ, Davis RL, Tsai FY: Multiple meningiomas following radiation therapy for medulloblastoma: Case report. J Neurosurg 55:282–286, 1981.
7. Jänisch W, Kirsch M: Tierversuche zur Induktion von intrakraniellen Geschwülsten durch ionisierende Strahlen. Exp Pathol 1:226–233, 1967.
8. Kent SP, Pickering JE: Neoplasms in monkeys (*Macaca mulatta*): Spontaneous and irradiation induced. Cancer 11:138–147, 1958.
9. Kleihues P, Bigner DD: Tumours of the nervous system, in Davison AN, Thompson RHS (eds): *The Molecular Basis of Neuropathology*. London, E. Arnold, 1981, pp 81–103.
10. Klériga E, Sher JH, Nallainathan SK, Stein SC, Sacher M: Development of cerebellar malignant astrocytoma at site of a medulloblastoma treated 11 years earlier. J Neurosurg 49:445–449, 1978.

11. Lacassagne A: Conditions dans lesquelles ont été obtenus, chez le lapin, des cancers par action des rayons X sur des foyers inflammatoires. C R Soc Biol (Paris) 112:562–564, 1933.
12. Mann I, Yates PC, Ainslie JP: Unusual case of double primary orbital tumour. Br J Ophthalmol 37:758–762, 1953.
13. McDonald LW, Lippert W, Brownson RH, McDougal HD: Induction of neuroglial tumors by implanted ^{60}Co radiation sources, in Sanders CL, Busch RH, Ballou JE, Mahlum DD (eds): *Radionuclide Carcinogenesis: Proceedings of the Twelfth Annual Hanford Biology Symposium of Richland, Washington,* May 10–12, 1972. Oak Ridge, US Atomic Energy Commission Office of Information Services, No. 720505, 1973, pp 391–405.
14. Modan B, Baidatz D, Mart H, Steinitz R, Levin SG: Radiation-induced head and neck tumours. Lancet 1:277–279, 1974.
15. Pearl GS, Mirra SS, Miles ML: Glioblastoma multiforme occurring 13 years after treatment of a medulloblastoma. Neurosurgery 6:546–551, 1980.
16. Waltz TA, Brownell B: Sarcoma: A possible late result of effective radiation therapy for pituitary adenoma: Report of 2 cases. J Neurosurg 24:901–907, 1966.

57

Chemically Induced Brain Tumors, Primary and Transplanted

Jeffrey S. Walker
Darell D. Bigner

Primary Brain Tumors

The chemical induction of neural tumors has supplied neuro-oncologists and neuroscientists with an inexpensive, reliable, and easily producible supply of experimental glial neoplasms. The first attempt at CNS chemical carcinogenesis was made by Roussy et al. in 1930.[7] They applied coal-tar-soaked gauze to exposed rabbit cortex but failed to produce any tumors. Seligman and Shear, in 1939, first successfully induced brain tumors in mice by implanting methylcholanthrene pellets 1 to 4 mm into the brain substance.[9] Two general types of compounds have subsequently been found to reliably produce experimental CNS tumors: polycyclic hydrocarbons (PCHs) and alkylating agents. They have induced brain tumors in a wide spectrum of experimental animals. Administration of chemical compounds intravenously, intraperitoneally, subcutaneously, intracranially, transplacentally, and into the carotid artery has resulted in the production of nervous system tumors. Because of wide variability in available animal models,

forms of chemical application, and route of administration, the chemical induction of neural tumors has broad experimental versatility. Chemically derived tumors make possible experimental investigations into CNS tumor kinetics, biochemistry, genetics, immunology, pharmacokinetics, histogenesis, and the efficacy of radiation therapy and chemotherapy. This chapter concentrates on the major classes of compounds used to experimentally induce CNS tumors, the types of tumors produced, and transplantation models which have been derived from them.

Factors Influencing Tumor Production

Various factors can affect the incidence of chemically mediated tumor production. Dimant et al.[1] demonstrated a statistically significant increase in the number of intravenous methylnitrosourea (MNU)-induced tumors in female rats castrated by irradiation. Gonadectomy in male rats, however, had little effect. No evidence to date supports the production of human CNS neoplasms from iatrogenic hormone administration. In experimental animals the pH of the carcinogen vehicle, age of the animal, species and strain of the animal, method of administration, chemical solubility, and dosage all affect the number of CNS tumors formed. Hormonal promotion as a mechanism has not been demonstrated for CNS tumors.

Polycyclic Hydrocarbons

The major experimental PCH used for tumor induction is 3- or 20-methylcholanthrene. Other experimentally useful PCHs are 1,2- or 3,4-benzpyrene; dibenzpyrene; 1,2,5,6- or 1,2,6-dibenzanthracene; 9,10-dimethyl-1,2-benzanthracene; and trimethylbenzanthracene. All these compounds must be placed in direct contact with the brain in order to induce tumors. Dimethylbenzanthracene and two derivatives of PCHs, N-2-fluorenylacetamide and N, N'-2,7-fluorenylenebisacetamide, have caused tumors without direct intracranial application. Dimethylbenzanthracene induces tumors when administered to neonatal rats orally or when injected into pregnant rats on the 21st day of gestation. The fluorenylacetamide compounds can also be given orally to rats in a 0.025 to 0.07 percent concentration; the animals develop various gliomas between 7 and 14 months after exposure. Direct surgical application of PCHs within the brain is experimentally disadvantageous, as it creates a traumatic disruption of the surrounding neural tissue, which may alter the vascular supply to the region. The PCH tumor model has another disadvantage in that the average tumor production is 40 to 60 percent and can range from 10 to 100 percent. The incidence of tumors induced is dependent upon many factors, such as species and strain, type of chemical, route of administration, and the animal's age at exposure. Mice, frogs, hamsters, and dogs are most susceptible to tumor production by these substances, while birds, guinea pigs, rabbits, cats, and monkeys are much more resistant.

There are some advantages to the PCH tumor model. Direct implantation enables the experimenter to precisely place the chemical pellet so that a single easily localized neoplasm is formed. Placing the pellet in contact with the dura will produce meningiomas and sarcomas, while ependymomas are more common from intraventricular placement. Oligodendrogliomas occur from frontal lobe white matter placement, but if the pellets are implanted in the subcortical parietal white matter, astrocytomas are commonly formed. Placement of the pellet within the cerebellum generally results in medulloblastomas.

The exact mechanism of PCH carcinogenesis is unknown. It is presumed that one or several metabolites are involved; diolepoxides are commonly incriminated. Benzpyrene's proposed active metabolite is a 9,10 epoxide, which experimentally binds stereoselectively to guanine in DNA.[6] As research continues with this class of compounds the role of carcinogenesis should become clearer. PCHs have not been implicated in human CNS tumors, probably because of the obvious lack of direct brain exposure.

Alkylating Agents

Alkylating agents, or N-nitroso compounds, are the most frequently used agents to experimentally induce nervous system tumors. In the mid-1950s these chemicals were shown to induce hepatocarcinoma in laboratory animals. Druckrey et al., in 1965, demonstrated that N-methyl-N-nitrosourea (MNU) selectively induced CNS tumors.[2] This is accomplished by weekly intravenous injections, in inbred rats, of 5 mg/kg per week of MNU for 8 to 9 months. Malignant gliomas of the CNS develop in 90 to 100 percent of animals. Direct application of the carcinogen to the brain, as needed with the PCHs, is therefore avoided. Besides intravenous administration, MNU may be given orally, subcutaneously, or intraperitoneally, but with fewer neural tumors resulting. As the dose of MNU is increased more mesenchymal tumors are formed, indicating a dose dependency of neural tumor induction. Anaplastic and mixed gliomas, along with oligodendrogliomas, are the predominant MNU-produced CNS tumors. They occur preferentially in the subcortical white matter, hippocampus, and periventricular regions. Dogs, rats, and rabbits are the most susceptible species, while mice, monkeys, cats, swine, guinea pigs, and sheep are more resistant to MNU-induced tumor devel-

opment. In Fischer 344 rats, peripheral nervous system neoplasms are more common than CNS tumors.

Ethylnitrosourea (ENU) is another, more commonly used alkylating agent in neuro-oncology. Ivanković et al. found that a single ENU dose of at least 20 mg per kg given in the third trimester of pregnancy induced neural tumors in 100 percent of the offspring.[5] Injection of ENU on the 15th day of gestation results mainly in brain tumors, while exposure to ENU on the 21st day of gestation leads primarily to spinal cord tumor formation. Mixed gliomas, oligodendrogliomas, anaplastic neuromas, and an occasional anaplastic spinal cord ependymoma are the tumors commonly formed. A latency period of 211 days was noted for the 50 mg/kg dosage. Lower ENU dosages increase the latency period. Rats are the most susceptible species to CNS tumor production, although intracranial tumors in the patas monkey have been induced with ENU. Repeated transplacental exposure to ENU induced ganglioglioma, embryonal sarcoma, angiosarcoma, fibroblastic meningioma, and astrocytoma in these monkeys. A latency period of 2 months to 4 years from birth was observed (Rice JM: Personal communication, 1982). Hamsters, on the other hand, develop tumors confined to the peripheral nervous system. ENU has the advantage that a single injection results in almost 100 percent tumor formation, low systemic toxicity, and tumors that are very similar to human gliomas.

The disadvantage of using alkylating agents is the variability of tumor type and the formation of multiple scattered tumors with variable latencies. Many other nitrosourea compounds have been used experimentally to induce glial tumors, but these have no advantage over ENU and MNU and are not discussed. No evidence of human brain tumor resulting from exposure to these alkylating agents has been reported.

The metabolism and mutagenesis of the nitrosoureas has been fairly well described. After injection, the compounds are widely distributed in the body and cross the blood-brain barrier easily. They are rapidly hydrolyzed and generally have a serum half-life of less than 10 minutes. According to Kleihues and Bigner, the alkylating agents cause the formation of O-alkylated bases, especially O^6-alkylguanine.[6] This molecular alteration results in mispairing of the DNA bases and presumed initiation of neoplastic transformation. They note that the DNA repair systems are much less effective in the brain than in the liver.

Hydrazines

Druckrey et al.,[4] in 1966, used an intravenous injection of 1,2-diethylhydrazine on the 15th day of rat gestation to induce glial and mesenchymal tumors in 93 percent of the offspring. All but two of those animals died of a malignant tumor. Using the same compound but administering it subcutaneously once a week, they induced eight intracranial tumors—gliomas, mixed glial-mesenchymal tumors, and sarcomas—among 45 animals. Hydrazines must be activated by microsomal enzymes; mixed function oxidases hydroxylate one of the alkyl groups. This leads to the formation of alkyldiazonium hydroxide, the proposed active carcinogen.

Triazenes

Triazenes were found to be neurotropic carcinogens by Druckry et al. in 1967.[3] They induced both central and peripheral nervous system tumors in 20 of 33 rats given 3,3-dimethyl-1-phenyltriazene. This compound may be given orally, subcutaneously, or intravenously. Transplacental administration increases the incidence of tumor production to over 90 percent of exposed offspring. Peripheral tumors, especially of the kidney, are commonly found. Methylated triazenes seem to be the most effective carcinogens. Triazenes are bioactivated by the liver and kidneys to 3-methyl-1-phenyltriazene. According to Kleihues and Bigner, hydrolytic fission results in unstable metabolites which are thought to methylate nucleophilic groups in cellular macromolecules.[6]

Human Exposure to Chemical Carcinogens

Two industrial chemicals have been implicated in the production of nervous system tumors in experimental animals and possibly humans. Rats exposed to high levels of vinyl chloride developed brain tumors in no more than 10 percent of exposed animals. Eight epidemiologic evaluations of vinyl chloride workers suggest a small increased risk of developing a brain tumor. These studies, however, have multiple technical problems, and the role of vinyl chloride as a human neurocarcinogen remains tenuous and speculative.

Acrylonitrile (ACN) is another plastic monomer implicated in experimental neural carcinogenesis. It is well established that ACN is mutagenic in bacteria. No chromosomal abnormalities, however, have been discovered in workers exposed to ACN. Rats chronically exposed to ACN have been reported to develop microgliomas, although definitive tumor classification has not been made. Oral ingestion or inhalation of this chemical will induce neoplastic transformation. No evidence exists to relate ACN to the induction of human brain tumors. Better prospective epidemiologic studies, it is hoped, will answer the question of ACN's carcinogenic potential in humans.

Transplantable Brain Tumors

Tumors induced with methylcholanthrene were first transplanted intracerebrally in mice by Zimmerman and Arnold in 1941.[11] They transplanted a murine ependymoblastoma tumor line and obtained 90 to 100 percent tumor production. Two basic types of transplantable tumor models have since been derived: in the syngeneic model, tumors are transplanted into animals with the same genetic background; in the heterotransplant model, tumors derived from another species or strain are transplanted into an animal of different genetic makeup. This may be accomplished by using an immunoincompetent animal or by introducing the tumor into an immunologically privileged site. Neural tumors have been successfully transplanted into the anterior chamber of the eye, muscle, and cheek pouch of a hamster and the subcutaneous region of nude mice, and various metastatic brain tumors have been produced by introducing non-neural tumors into the immunologically privileged brain.

The most commonly used PCH-induced transplantable cell lines are murine ependymoma, ependymoblastoma A, glioma 26, and glioma 261. Intracerebral injection of a brei of cells or implantion of a 1-mm³ piece of tumor in syngeneic mice usually results in death within 2.5 to 3.5 weeks in nearly all animals. Using transplantation models, various treatment modalities may be evaluated for effectiveness. The ependymoblastoma A tumor has been the basis of chemotherapeutic agent testing by the Drug Evaluation Branch of the National Cancer Institute. Good correlation between the response of human glial tumors and the experimental effectiveness of carmustine (BCNU) and lomustine (CCNU) has been demonstrated in these models. Mithramycin proved to be effective against the experimentally produced tumors but not against human brain tumors. These transplantable systems provide short latencies, predictable location, uniformity of growth, morphological tumor uniformity, and a high rate of tumor production at a relatively low cost. Disadvantages of these models are traumatic brain disruption for tumor inoculation, sarcomatous degeneration of tumor lines over time, inability to exactly duplicate the chemotherapeutic sensitivities of human CNS tumors, and possible viral or mycoplasmal contamination on serial passage.

Nitrosourea-induced tumors are commonly used for drug pharmacokinetic and cell kinetic studies in the rat. The methylnitrosourea-induced rat tumor lines commonly used are C-6 (a glioma), and 9L (a gliosarcoma). The C-6 rat glioma was originally induced with methylnitrosourea. It provides a commonly used glial cell line for in vitro studies. Unfortunately, it can be transplanted only into irradiated or neonatal rats, because noninbred rats were used for the initial induction. MNU also induced the 9L gliosarcoma line in Fischer 344 rats. This line was considered an anaplastic astrocytoma, but through successive generations it evolved into a gliosarcoma or sarcoma. Though a somewhat unstable line, its ability to be frozen and successfully thawed has resulted in widespread distribution. Other chemically induced, virally induced, and endogenous animal tumors have been transplanted, each with its own characteristics, advantages, and disadvantages.

Transplantable Human Brain Tumors

Heterotransplant models are the most recently developed and hold great potential for scientific advancement. Nude or athymic mice provide an immunologically incompetent host for transplantable tumors. Serial transplantation of various human tumors intracranially or into the subcutaneous tissue of the flank is easily performed. These tumors include glioblastomas, astrocytomas, medulloblastomas, craniopharyngiomas, gliosarcomas, and meningiomas. Following initial transplantation, a latent period of months to almost a year occurs before the exponential growth phase is reached. Constant tumor growth rates are reliable once this rapid growth phase occurs. Through serial transplantations, tumor lines can change morphologically and in regard to growth kinetics. It has been proposed that with serial passage highly malignant cell populations are preferentially selected, which decreases the latent period and increases the growth rate. Schold and Bigner successfully transplanted 16 of 17 anaplastic human gliomas subcutaneously into the nude mouse flank.[8] They noted tumor doubling times between 4 and 19 days as determined from direct tumor measurements. Tumor volume can be calculated from direct measurement of these flank tumors, permitting an accurate assessment of the efficacy of any treatment modality. Human glioma implantation into the nude mouse flank directly after surgical extirpation has been successful in 50 to 100 percent of tumors tested,[10] depending upon the type of tumor transplanted. Highly malignant glioblastomas have the highest success rate. In the near future, this technique may be used to evaluate in vivo a battery of chemotherapeutic agents for each individual human brain tumor, making possible treatment with agents proven effective against each patient's brain tumor.

References

1. Dimant IN, Loktionov GM, Sataev MM, Israilyan AA: Further study of induction of brain tumors in rats by methylnitrosourea. Bull Exp Biol Med 69:566–568, 1970.
2. Druckrey H, Ivanković S, Preussman R: Selektive Erzeugung maligner Tumoren im Gehirn und Rückenmark von Ratten durch N-methyl-N-nitrosoharnstoff. Z Krebsforsch 66:389–408, 1965.
3. Druckrey H, Ivanković S, Preussmann R: Neurotrope carcinogene Wirkung von Phenyl-dimethyl-triazen an Ratten. Naturwissenschaften 54:171, 1967.
4. Druckrey H, Preussman R, Matzkies F, Ivanković S: Carcinogene Wirkung von 1,2 diäthylhydrazin an Ratten. Naturwissenschaften 53:557–558, 1966.
5. Ivanković S, Druckrey H, Preussman R: Erzeugung neurogener Tumoren bei den Nachkommen nach einmaliger Injektion von Äthylnitrosoharnstoff an schwangere Ratten. Naturwissenschaften 53:410, 1966.
6. Kleihues P, Bigner DD: Tumours of the nervous system, in Davison AN, Thompson RHS (eds): The Molecular Basis of Neuropathology. London, E. Arnold, 1981, pp 81–103.
7. Roussy G, Oberling C, Raileanu C: Lésions expérimentales des centres nerveux provoquées par application locale de goudron. C R Soc Biol (Paris) 104:762–764, 1930.
8. Schold SC Jr, Bigner DD: A review of experimental brain tumor models that have been used for therapeutic studies, in Walker MD (ed): Oncology of the Nervous System. Boston, Martinus Nijhof, 1983, pp 31–63.
9. Seligman AM, Shear MJ: Studies in carcinogenesis: VIII. Experimental production of brain tumors in mice with methylcholanthrene. Am J Cancer 37:364–395, 1939.
10. Shapiro WR, Basler GA, Chernik NL, Posner JB: Human brain tumor transplantation into nude mice. JNCI 62:447–453, 1979.
11. Zimmerman HM, Arnold H: Experimental brain tumors: I. Tumors produced with methylcholanthrene. Cancer Res 1:919–938, 1941.

58

Cell Kinetics of Brain Tumors

Takao Hoshino

The brain is a unique organ from a kinetic point of view, since unlike cells in other tissues, neurons become incapable of cell division shortly after birth. The glial cells in the supportive tissue of the brain retain their proliferative capacity, as shown by reactive and reparative gliosis;[1] but so far there has been no evidence that they proliferate at the rapid rate observed in cells in other tissues. Several reports suggest that there is continually a low level of mitotic activity in the glial population of the adult rat brain[5] and that this slow production of new cells is enough to balance glial cell loss. This proliferation rate is too slow for cell cycle time to be measured by current methods.

The kinetic state of normal brain clearly contrasts with that of brain tumors, in which there is an obviously proliferating cell population.

Glioma is a unique type of brain tumor. As it rarely metastasizes, even in its most malignant form (glioblastoma multiforme), the cause of death of patients with gliomas is usually cerebral or cerebellar herniation resulting from increased intracranial pressure and thus depends on the size of the tumor. Knowledge about tumor growth, therefore, may be of value in predicting the survival of patients with brain tumors, as well as in providing information for improvement in multimodality treatments.

Labeling Index and Survival

Most tumors contain two major cell types: (1) cells in the nonproliferating pool (G_0) and (2) cells in the proliferating pool. The latter, which are the main source of increase in the cell population of the tumor, can be classified in four groups according to their phase in the mitotic cycle: postmitosis (G_1), DNA synthesis (S), premitosis (G_2), and mitosis (M).

The cells in mitosis can be identified by routine microscopic study of the tissue; but cells in the other phases of the cycle, including those in the G_0 pool, cannot be distinguished. When, however, ^{3}H-thymidine or ^{14}C-thymidine is administered intravenously, the cells in S phase, which are synthesizing DNA in preparation for mitosis, take up the labeled thymidine while the thymidine is present in the blood and can thus be identified readily by autoradiography. The S-phase cells of a glioblastoma labeled with thymidine can be recognized easily on an autoradiograph by the black grains on their nuclei. The ratio of the labeled cells to the total tumor cell population, called the *labeling index* (LI), provides a rough idea of the proliferative activity of that tissue, as the proportion of labeled cells indicates the proportion of cells actually in proliferation cycles.

The first in vivo study of this sort in a human glioblastoma was carried out in 1960 by Johnson et al.,[9] who injected multiple doses of ^{3}H-thymidine intravenously into a patient who was in the terminal stage of disease; they calculated an LI of 0.6 percent. Chigasaki[2] studied the in vitro uptake of ^{3}H-thymidine in biopsy specimens of a glioblastoma, an astrocytoma, and an oligodendroglioma, obtaining LIs of 0.94, 0.44, and 0.33 percent, respectively. He estimated the generation time of glioblastoma to be 45 to 60 days. A few years later, Kury and Carter[11] examined the LI of several gliomas in vitro, using a method almost identical to Chigasaki's. They reported that two glioblastomas had LIs of 3.6 and 6.0 percent and five astrocytomas (grade 2 or 3) had LIs of 2, 2, 2.6, 5.5, and 7.4 percent—all considerably higher than the indices reported by Johnson et al.[9] and by Chigasaki.[2] Kury and Carter[11] estimated generation times (approximating potential doubling time, in our terms) of glioblastomas and malignant astrocytomas to be 3 to 5 days and 2 to 10 days, respectively, assuming an S phase of 6 h. Fukuma et al.,[4] using local injection of ^{3}H-thymidine into glioma tissue at the time of craniotomy, reported LIs similar to those obtained by Kury and Carter.[11]

The LIs derived from 28 gliomas[8] by the author are summarized in Table 58-1: the average LIs for medulloblastomas and glioblastomas were 13.2 percent and 9.3 percent, respectively; benign gliomas had an average of 1 percent, and the average for anaplastic astrocytomas was 4 percent, varying from 2 percent to 8 percent according to the extent of anaplasia. In order to determine how this difference in LIs correlates with the growth rate of each tumor, the 28 patients with gliomas were classified into two groups: (1) patients, except those with medulloblastoma, whose tumor had an LI of 5 percent or more (almost all were glioblastomas); and (2) patients whose tumor had an LI of less than 5

percent. A Kaplan-Meier analysis of the survival times of these two groups of patients, from the date of biopsy (when the LI was determined) to the date of death (Fig. 58-1), clearly indicated the significance of the LI: whereas all 14 patients with an LI of more than 5 percent died within 6 months after surgery, patients who presented with an LI of less than 5 percent survived—with few exceptions, more than 1 year, and usually 5 years, after diagnosis (including the preoperative and/or postoperative interval). This difference was statistically significant ($p < 0.001$) according to the Gehan test. These striking results imply that an LI of more than 5 percent may indicate distinct growth characteristics—specifically, malignant behavior.

Cell Cycle Time and Growth Fraction

While the LI represents some of the proliferative activity of gliomas, the characteristics of brain tumor growth cannot be understood without determining several additional factors: (1) the cell cycle, or generalization, time (Tc); (2) the growth fraction (GF), or ratio of proliferating to nonproliferating cells; (3) the cell loss factor; and (4) the tumor doubling time, or time required for approximate doubling of the existing volume of the tumor, which can be measured by serial radiological studies. Although the last two parameters are important in predicting the patient's prognosis, the most significant, both for understanding the basic proliferative activity of tumors and for planning treatment, are GF and Tc.

Tym[12] introduced the stathmokinetic method, adding to the flash-labeling technique the use of vinblastine sulfate. Vinblastine, like colchicine, facilitates kinetic analysis by arresting and holding cells in metaphase. Studying a single glioblastoma, Tym obtained an LI of 1.6 percent and calculated a cell cycle time of 125 h (5.4 days) to 242 h (10 days).

Table 58-2 presents the GFs and Tcs, determined by autoradiography with the aid of a stathmokinetic method,[8] for nine malignant gliomas studied in the author's laboratory. The mean GF was calculated to be approximately 30 percent and the Tc to be 2 to 3 days. These results were based on examination of only those parts of the tumor that showed no microscopic necrosis and fairly homogeneous labeling; the GF would be less if the entire tumor, which includes a large nonviable portion, were considered. Although there was considerable variability among the Tcs calculated from different samples of the same tumor, the average values were

TABLE 58-1 Average Labeling Index (LI) and Mean Survival of Glioma

Tumor Type	No. of Cases	LI (Range),* %	Mean Survival†, Months
Medulloblastoma	3	13.2 (11.2–14.4)	NA
Glioblastoma	13	9.3 (4.5–15.9)	8
Anaplastic astrocytoma	7	4.0 (2.2–8.3)	60
Astrocytoma	3	0.8 (0.3–0.9)	99
Ependymoma	1	1.9	109

*Range of the average LI for each tumor.
†From time of onset to death of patient.

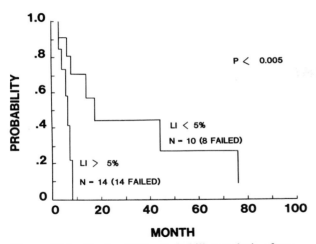

Figure 58-1 Kaplan-Meier probability analysis of survival times (months from date of biopsy) of glioma patients correlated with labeling index (LI). (From Hoshino T: The cell kinetics of gliomas: Its prognostic value and therapeutic implications, in Paoletti P, Walker MD, Butti G, Knerich R (eds): *Multidisciplinary Aspects of Brain Tumor Therapy.* Amsterdam, Elsevier/North Holland, 1979, pp 105–112.)

similar for all tumors except in the first two cases shown in Table 58-2. For the nine tumors, the mean Tc was 3 days. In contrast, the GFs were variable, that for case 2 of the anaplastic astrocytoma series being markedly lower than the others. The fact that the pretreatment interval for this patient was much longer than that interval in the other patients appears to indicate a good correlation between a lower GF and slower growth of the neoplasm.

From the foregoing data it appears that the low LIs found in slow-growing brain tumors may be a function of a low GF rather than a reflection of a prolonged Tc.

Flow Cytometry and DNA Distribution

The heterogeneous nature of the cellular components of human gliomas and their morphological complexity are well documented. This heterogeneity encompasses chromosomal abnormalities, variability in proliferation kinetics, and variations in DNA content. Together, these characteristics suggest that human gliomas may consist of multiple cell populations that are distinct in terms of DNA content, biological behavior, or both.

Until now, it has been difficult to study individual cell populations in a tumor because there have been no satisfactory sorting techniques. Recent developments in flow cytometry (FCM), however, have made it possible to quantitate populations efficiently and accurately on any substrate at the rate of up to 10,000 cells per second, once the substrate has been stained with fluorescent dye. Besides affording this cytometric ability, FCM makes it feasible to sort out any specific cell group(s) on the basis of its characteristics as seen under fluorescence.[13]

Hoshino et al.,[7] Frederiksen et al.,[3] and Kawamoto et al.,[10] all of whom have analyzed the DNA content of human glioma cells by means of FCM, have reported that malignant gliomas, including glioblastoma multiforme, have a highly variable distribution of cell populations as reflected by DNA content. These gliomas consist of cell populations containing not only a diploid (2C) and/or aneuploid amount of DNA but also greater amounts of DNA.

According to the author's observations, benign brain tumors such as meningiomas, pituitary adenomas, and well-differentiated gliomas, all of which grow slowly, have characteristics in common: (1) there are few cells in DNA synthesis; (2) the greater part of the tumor is composed of a single karyotype (the term *karyotype* is used here to denote cells that have identical amounts of DNA in their nuclei rather than the same number of chromosomes); and (3) there is little variability within a tumor. In contrast to these findings, malignant gliomas, including glioblastoma multiforme, exhibit the following characteristics: (1) there is a substantial population of cells in DNA synthesis; (2) there is a wide distribution of nuclear DNA complement, ranging from 2C to 8C (assuming that the initial peak represents diploid nuclei); and (3) different regions of the same tumor vary greatly with respect to the distribution of the predominant ploidy—for example, in some areas, the nuclear population seems to be primarily diploid (2C), whereas in other regions the nuclei are mainly tetraploid (4C).

Thus malignant gliomas are heterogeneous not only with respect to ploidy but also with respect to the populations within different areas of the same tumor. In addition, these multiple populations in terms of DNA content are found to be similarly clonogenic[6] and may respond differently to different chemotherapeutic agents.

General Strategy of Chemotherapy for Gliomas

It is essential to know the Tc in order to plan effective treatment with chemotherapeutic agents, such as vinca alkaloids and purine or pyrimidine analogues, that are specific to cer-

TABLE 58-2 Growth Fraction (GF) and Cell Cycle Time (Tc)

Case No.	LI (SD), %		GF (SD)		Tc (SD), h	
Glioblastoma						
1	15.9	(3.4)	0.44	(0.13)	145.0	(63.4)
2	11.0	(1.4)	0.40	(0.14)	151.7	(63.4)
3	8.6	(3.1)	0.39	(0.10)	64.1	(12.9)
4	15.5	(4.6)	0.35	(0.11)	55.8	(11.6)
5	9.8	(2.6)	0.32	(0.10)	55.4	(11.5)
6	13.0	(3.2)	0.29	(0.07)		
7	5.1	(1.2)	0.21	(0.06)	36.4	(16.6)
Anaplastic Astrocytoma						
1	2.3	(3.7)	0.25	(0.03)	43.9	(7.1)
2	3.4	(1.0)	0.14	(0.06)	52.3	(26.5)

LI = labeling index.
SD = one standard deviation.
SOURCE: Hoshino T, Wilson CB.[8]

tain phases of the cell cycle. Single doses of these agents will kill only cells that are in the sensitive phase of the cycle at the time of drug administration. The maximal effect of the agent can be achieved by maintaining effective drug levels long enough for all cells in cycle to pass through the sensitive phase. However, cell cycle–specific drugs affect only a part of a population, corresponding to the GF, and cannot be expected to achieve a cell kill of more than 30 percent. It is important to note, moreover, that the continued administration of drugs—either by frequent injections or by continuous infusion—for periods significantly longer than the Tc of the tumor may increase drug toxicity by affecting normal regenerating systems, such as the bone marrow and intestinal epithelium, without actually increasing tumor cell kill, assuming that these drugs do not perturb cellular proliferation.

It should be noted that even a drug achieving an exponential cell kill of several logs may not produce an immediate clinical improvement; for, as recent studies show, treated cells usually complete the division process before they die, and actual decrease of the mass is slowed by retarded removal of dead cells from the brain, swelling of dead cells, and repopulation by surviving cells. In order to obtain a sequential decrease in tumor size with drugs, it is necessary to administer repeated courses of therapy with cell kill sufficient to prohibit repopulation of the tumor.

The feasibility of repeated courses of chemotherapy depends on the recovery of normal cell populations during the retreatment interval, during which selective treatment modalities may play an important role. The clinical benefit can also be enhanced by accelerating the cell kill and the removal of dead cells by facilitating phagocytic activities, autolytic processes, or both. Chemotherapeutic agents that provide 2-log to 3-log cell kill are available on an experimental basis. Sophisticated combinations of these drugs in chemotherapy schedules based on these data from cell kinetics studies should improve the treatment of malignant gliomas.

References

1. Cavanagh JB: The proliferation of astrocytes around a needle wound in the rat brain. J Anat 106:471–487, 1970.
2. Chigasaki H: [Studies on the DNA synthesis function of glial cells by means of H-3-thymidine microradioautography.] Brain Nerve (Tokyo) 15:767–781, 1963.
3. Frederiksen P, Reske-Nielsen E, Bichel P: Flow cytometry in tumours of the brain. Acta Neuropathol 41:179–183, 1978.
4. Fukuma S, Taketomo S, Ueda S, Tohyama M, Kitamura T, Yoshida S, Maeka va J, Nakajima K, Fujita T: [Autoradiographic studies of the growth of brain tumors using local labeling with ^{3}H-thymidine in vivo.] Brain Nerve (Tokyo) 21:1029–1035, 1969.
5. Hommes OR, Leblond CP: Mitotic division of neuroglia in the normal adult rat. J Comp Neurol 129:269–278, 1967.
6. Hoshino T, Knebel KD, Rosenblum ML, Dougherty DV, Wilson CB: Clonogenicity of multiple populations of human glioma cells in vitro sorted by DNA content. Cancer 50:997–1002, 1982.
7. Hoshino T, Nomura K, Wilson CB, Knebel KD, Gray JW: The distribution of nuclear DNA from human brain-tumor cells: Flow cytometric studies. J Neurosurg 49:13–21, 1978.
8. Hoshino T, Wilson CB: Cell kinetic analyses of human malignant brain tumors (gliomas). Cancer 44:956–962, 1979.
9. Johnson HA, Haymaker WE, Rubini JR, Fliedner TM, Bond VP, Chronkite EP, Hughes WL: A radioautographic study of a human brain and glioblastoma multiforme after the in vivo uptake of tritiated thymidine. Cancer 13:636–642, 1960.
10. Kawamoto K, Herz F, Wolley RC, Hirano A, Kajikawa H, Koss LG: Flow cytometric analysis of the DNA distribution in human brain tumors. Acta Neuropathol 46:39–44, 1979.
11. Kury G, Carter HW: Autoradiographic study of human nervous system tumors. Arch Pathol 80:38–42, 1965.
12. Tym R: Distribution of cell doubling times in in vivo human cerebral tumors. Surg Forum 20:445–447, 1969.
13. Van Dilla MA, Steinmetz LL, Davis DT, Calvert RN, Gray JW: High-speed cell analysis and sorting with flow systems: Biological applications and new approaches. IEEE Nucl Sci 21:714–720, 1974.

59

Biochemistry of Brain Tumors

C. J. Cummins
B. H. Smith
P. L. Kornblith

The complexity of brain tumor biochemistry, like that of other neoplastic growths, has been increasingly appreciated. The search for a single critical cellular defect responsible for the development of neoplasia has led instead to the finding of a diversity of biochemical phenomena indicative of a wide range of abnormalities of the genetic regulation of phenotypic expression. Also appreciated has been the importance of the interactions between the tumor cells themselves and between the primary tumor cells and the vascular cells, as well as other normal cell types. Substances such as sarcoma growth factor have been shown to be released by tumor cells and are capable of altering the growth of normal cell populations in a reversible fashion.[24] Thus released factors, as well as circulating hormones, have a role in the ultimate pattern of growth shown by neoplastic cell populations.

Brain tumors, the majority of which are of glial origin, have special characteristics, as well as features typical of solid tumors. Special characteristics include their location in the brain or spinal cord; their interaction with the vasculature of the central nervous system (CNS) and its blood-brain barrier; a relatively low potential for metastasis but a high degree of local infiltration and invasion; and a poor prognosis despite combined surgery, radiation, and chemotherapy. The location of these tumors in the CNS leads to problems of increased intracranial pressure and brain shift or herniation, as well as local interference with or destruction of critical brain functions. The margin of clinical and physiological safety with these tumors is small.

In common with other solid and lymphoid malignant diseases, brain tumor cell populations are heterogeneous with respect to a variety of their cell biological properties, ranging from karyotypic patterns and growth rates to metabolic, immunologic, and chemotherapeutic sensitivity properties. This heterogeneity is found not only from one tumor grade to another but also within tumors of the same pathological grade and even in the cell populations of a single tumor.[2,14,19,20] These facts have important implications for understanding and utilizing the range of biochemical properties described for CNS tumors. While the "average" properties of whole tumors continue to be essential and use-

ful, caution in interpreting their therapeutic implications is indicated.

Beyond heterogeneity, brain tumors also share many other biochemical properties with other solid tumors. Although somewhat dated, the most complete review of brain tumor biochemistry is that of Wollemann.[30] Increased glycolytic activity; decreased respiratory rate; increased glycogen and mucopolysaccharide content; decreased phospholipids and glycolipids; increased proteinase, peptidase, and lysosomal activity; and increased nucleic acid metabolism are among the abnormalities documented. More recently, various specialized aspects of the biochemistry of brain tumors, such as cyclic nucleotide regulation,[8] polyamine production,[9,17] cell surface antigens and humoral immunology,[13] and glycolysis[23] have been reviewed. Altered glycolysis is a property shared by brain tumors with other solid neoplasms and has long been of interest in cancer research. The development of 2-deoxyglucose methodology by Sokoloff et al.[21] for the determination of in situ CNS glucose metabolic rates and the further addition of ^{18}F-2-deoxyglucose (FDG) positron emission tomography (PET) for evaluation of tumor glucose metabolic rates in intact patients has made the study of glucose metabolism a rapidly developing area of brain tumor biochemistry. This is the focus of this chapter, both because it is an important topic in its own right and because it illustrates the problems and prospects of brain tumor biochemistry.

Characteristic of tumor cells generally is an increased glycolytic capacity and a high rate of lactate formation from glucose in the presence of oxygen. Early in this century, Otto Warburg observed this accumulation of lactate, as well as pyruvate, and a decreased respiratory rate, even in the presence of excess glucose and oxygen, in tumor tissue.[27] He coined the term *aerobic glycolysis* for the production of lactate and pyruvate in the presence of adequate carbon sources and oxygen. Today, from Weber's work with hepatomas,[28] it is known that aerobic glycolysis is not a necessary or invariant feature of all neoplastic cells but is seen primarily in tumors with a rapid growth rate and high degree of dedifferentiation. Furthermore, aerobic glycolysis is not a unique feature of neoplastic cells, since intestinal mucosa, renal medulla, and normal cells stimulated to proliferate by hormones also show it.[4,15]

As a general rule, better differentiated, slower growing tumor cells have a lower rate of glycolysis, and faster growing, more poorly differentiated cells exhibit higher rates of glycolysis. With the availability of positron emission tomography (as mentioned above), it has become possible to evaluate this relationship directly in patients with CNS tumors, utilizing FDG as a measure of glucose uptake to define local cerebral metabolic rate of glucose ($LCMR_{glc}$). The authors have recently reported the use of the FDG-PET scanning technique for determining the $LCMR_{glc}$ of 60 in situ gliomas.[5] The data from this study demonstrate that elevated glucose uptake is a common feature of high-grade gliomas. Grade I or II gliomas show an $LCMR_{glc}$ that is somewhat lower than that of contralateral normal brain structures. Grade III gliomas have an $LCMR_{glc}$ that is slightly greater; and grade IV gliomas have an $LCMR_{glc}$ that is 1.6-fold greater than that of contralateral normal brain structures (Fig. 59-1). Making the critical (and very likely true) as-

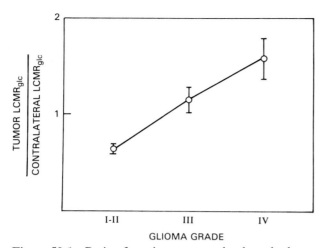

Figure 59-1 Ratio of maximum tumor local cerebral metabolic rate for glucose (LCMR$_{glc}$) to the metabolic rate of normal-appearing contralateral brain structure, measured by ^{18}F-2-deoxyglucose. Metabolic rates for low-grade gliomas appear somewhat less than normal brain and are increased in high-grade gliomas. (From data of DiChiro et al.[5])

sumption that the glucose uptake is driven solely by glycolytic rate, one can conclude that the glycolytic rate is altered in gliomas and increases with increasing grade of malignancy.

Such in situ data correlate well with several lines of evidence collected from previous and current biochemical studies. Beginning with the studies of Victor and Wolf in 1937[26] and continuing on through the data of Heller and Elliot (1955),[10] Kirsch and Leitner (1967),[12] Allen (1972),[1] and Lowry et al. (1977),[16] a consistent picture of a high rate of aerobic glycolysis with a low respiratory rate has been characteristic of gliomas, with a direct correlation to the grade of the tumor. In normal brain, the respiratory quotient (RQ), or ratio of CO_2 evolved to O_2 consumed, is close to 1.0, indicating that carbohydrates are the major energy source for the brain and that they are completely oxidized to CO_2 and H_2O. Both the rate of oxygen consumption and the RQ are depressed in brain tumors of glial origin. The O_2 consumption of gliomas is approximately 10 to 25 percent and the RQ 70 to 80 percent of that of normal brain (see Allen[1] for a more complete discussion). When measured directly in ethylnitrosourea-induced rat tumors, the rates of glucose oxidation via the Krebs cycle and the hexose monophosphate pathway are reduced 33 and 78 percent, respectively. Such tumor RQ values are compatible with either altered glycolysis or the metabolism of alternative fuels. In addition, these data are consistent with Warburg's model of tumor metabolism[27] The only significant exception has been in oligodendrogliomas, where a higher oxygen uptake and respiratory rate seem to persist.

What is the basis of the changes in glycolytic metabolism seen in malignant tumors? Weber, working with hepatomas, provided the first insights into this problem with his hypothesis that the regulatory enzymes of glycolysis are increased and that enzymes involved in the removal of carbon from the glycolytic pathway are reduced in malignant

cells.[28] Because gliomas, like hepatomas, exhibit a continuum of growth rates, invasiveness, and anaplastic characteristics, it is not surprising that their neoplastic features parallel the pattern observed in hepatomas. The activities of hexokinase and phosphofructokinase, which regulate glycolysis by limiting flux at the second and fourth steps in the glycolytic chain, are increased in high-grade gliomas[23,30] and in cultures derived from high-grade gliomas.[3] Glucose-6-phosphatase, which catalyzes the reverse reaction to hexokinase, has been reported to be almost totally absent in the more undifferentiated neuroectodermal tumors,[30] possibly conserving glucose-6-phosphate for energy production via glycolysis or for nucleic acid synthesis via the pentose phosphate shunt. Several other enzymes of glycolysis, including phosphohexose isomerase, aldolase, glyceraldehyde-3-phosphate dehydrogenase, and lactic dehydrogenase, have been reported to have increased activity (see Timperley[23] for review). It is not clear, though, how important they are in determining glycolytic flux, since they are "downstream" from the key regulatory steps of hexokinase and phosphofructokinase.

Glucose not only serves as an energy source in tumors and other proliferating cells but also is converted to ribose sugar, the precursor of nucleic acids, via the pentose phosphate pathway. High concentrations of the intermediates of this pathway, such as 5-phosphoribosyl-1-pyrophosphate (PRPP), are found in tumors (but not the adult brain), suggesting that the pentose phosphate pathway is very active in tumor tissues. On the basis of this fact, one might expect increased enzymatic rates for the two enzymes which regulate this pathway, glucose-6-phosphate dehydrogenase (G6PD) and 6-phosphogluconate dehydrogenase (6PGD). Increased activities of G6PD have been reported by Timperley[23], although the authors of this chapter were unable to confirm this finding in tissue-cultured astrocytomas.[3]

Ribose sugar can be synthesized from glucose carbon in another manner. In the normal course of glycolysis, glucose is metabolized to fructose and then cleared to two three-carbon fragments, glyceraldehyde-3-phosphate (GA3P) and dihydroxyacetone phosphate (DHAP), by aldolase. These molecules, in turn, can enter the pentose phosphate pathway, and their carbon can be recovered as ribose sugar (specifically, as PRPP). If glycolysis is blocked "downstream" from aldolase and a heavy demand for ribonucleotides exists, it is possible that GA3P and DHAP could be removed from glycolysis and shunted into the synthesis of ribose sugars.

Eigenbrodt and Glossmann argue that the terminal step in glycolysis, pyruvate kinase, is predominantly found as the fetal isoenzyme (M2) in tumor tissues.[6] This isoenzyme is regulated somewhat differently from the adult isoenzyme and can be inactivated by phosphorylation by the enzyme cyclic AMP (cAMP)–independent protein kinase. Inactivation would thus slow the flux of glucose carbon into the Krebs cycle and make glucose carbon available for the pentose pathway.

The scheme outlined in the preceding paragraph takes on further plausibility from studies of pyruvate kinase in 101 human brain tumors by van Veelen et al.[25] These investigators found a shift to fetal isoenzymes of pyruvate kinase that correlated with the degree of tumor malignancy. Importantly, the abnormal pyruvate kinase is much more susceptible to alanine inhibition than the normal adult isoenzyme, so that brain tumors appear to fit the general paradigm.

What is the significance of the glycolysis story for understanding brain tumors? As pointed out earlier, aerobic glycolysis is not unique to tumor cells, being found in a variety of proliferating normal cells as well. Thus the glycolysis of tumor cells may or may not be truly unique for the tumor cells. It may instead be secondary to other primary changes in genetic regulation, such as increased nucleic acid synthesis supporting rapid cell division and population growth. Although many of these theories deserve to be experimentally tested for brain tumors, it is clear that in brain tumors (1) the glycolytic capacity is increased because of elevated activities in the main regulatory enzymes and altered activity of hexokinases; (2) the oxidation of glucose is incomplete, since lactate and pyruvate accumulate; (3) considerable glucose carbon flows into the pentose pathway; and (4) pyruvate kinase is altered in some fundamental way. Taken together, the glycolytic metabolism of brain tumors more closely resembles that of the fetal or neonatal brain. Such changes in the glycolytic pathway may also help to account for the relative resistance of gliomas to ischemia and anoxia suggested by Kirsch and Leitner.[12]

Consideration of the mechanism of glycolysis in brain tumors, however, has a broader significance for understanding such tumors. It serves to illustrate the wide-ranging abnormalities of gene regulation and resultant misprogramming of protein synthesis that, as Weinhouse has pointed out,[29] are the essence of the neoplastic cell, whatever the initiating event (oncogene derepression, insertion of viral DNA, etc.). In neoplasia, then, isoenzymes characteristic of adult, differentiated glial cells under tight host control are replaced by abnormal enzymes, perhaps of a fetal type that were inactivated during normal development, which are not tightly controlled and lead to processes critical to initiating and maintaining neoplastic growth. Additional protein products may disrupt normal membrane-cytoplasmic-nuclear regulatory coupling and further advance the abnormal process. The net effects are a complex of abnormalities that are seen in the laboratory end-product analysis as heterogeneity of sensitivity or resistance to chemotherapy agents, to cellular or humoral immunological reagents, or to the normal differentiating signals of the biological microenvironment of the host.

Weinhouse utilizes the term *disordered differentiation* to characterize the cancer cell.[29] This is a particularly apt expression, because it fits with increasing data that it is possible to drive a tumor cell in the direction of producing normal, terminally differentiated progeny (see, for example, Illmensee and Mintz,[11] Sachs,[18] and Stenzel et al.[22]), and human tumors are known to spontaneously regress.[7] If disordered differentiation can be turned to redifferentiation, then safe, effective anticancer therapy is likely to be available. The achievement of redifferentiation may not be simple to achieve or near at hand.

Along the way, some of the other facts of glycolysis, as well as other aspects of brain tumor biochemistry, may provide clues to useful anticancer agents. For example, the fact that malignant brain tumors are dependent on increased membrane-bound mitochondrial hexokinase activity makes the antimitochondrial toxicity of aziridinylbenzoquinone (AZQ), a drug now in phase II clinical trials, more interesting. Perhaps another agent can be found to disinhibit the tumor-type pyruvate kinase and thus inhibit nucleic acid synthesis in the neoplastic cells, while leaving normal pyruvate kinase unmolested. These and other potential therapeutic avenues seem worthy of exploration.

References

1. Allen N: Oxidative metabolism of brain tumors. Prog Exp Tumor Res 17:192–209, 1972.
2. Bigner DD, Bigner SH, Pontén J, Westermark B, Mahaley MS, Jr., Ruoslahti E, Herschman H, Eng LF, Wikstrand CJ: Heterogeneity of genotypic and phenotypic characteristics of fifteen permanent cell lines derived from human gliomas. J Neuropathol Exp Neurol 40:201–229, 1981.
3. Cummins CJ, Graham JF, Galarraga J, Smith BH, Kornblith PL: Alteration in glycolytic enzymes in cultured human brain tumors. In press, 1983.
4. Diamond I, Legg A, Schneider JA, Rozengurt E: Glycolysis in quiescent cultures of 3T3 cells: Stimulation by serum, epidermal growth factor, and insulin in intact cells and persistence of the stimulation after cell homogenization. J Biol Chem 253:866–871, 1978.
5. DiChiro G, DeLaPaz RL, Brooks RA, Sokoloff L, Kornblith PL, Smith BH, Patronas NJ, Kufta CV, Kessler RM, Johnston GS, Manning RG, Wolf AP: Glucose utilization of cerebral gliomas measured by [^{18}F] fluorodeoxyglucose and positron emission tomography. Neurology (NY) 32:1323–1329, 1982.
6. Eigenbrodt E, Glossmann H: Glycolysis—one of the keys to cancer? Trends Pharmacol Sci 1:240–245, 1980.
7. Everson TC, Cole WH: *Spontaneous Regression of Cancer.* Philadelphia, Saunders, 1966.
8. Frattola L, Cerri C, Villani R, Trabucchi M: On the role of cyclic nucleotides in tumor of human nervous tissue: An overview. J Neurosurg Sci 23:257–263, 1979.
9. Fulton DS, Levin VA, Lubich WP, Wilson CB, Marton LJ: Cerebrospinal fluid polyamines in patients with glioblastoma multiforme and anaplastic astrocytoma. Cancer Res 40:3293–3296, 1980.
10. Heller IH, Elliot KAC: The metabolism of normal brain and human gliomas in relation to cell type and density. Can J Biochem 33:395–403, 1955.
11. Illmensee K, Mintz B: Totipotency and normal differentiation of single teratocarcinoma cells cloned by injection into blastocysts. Proc Natl Acad Sci USA 73:549–553, 1976.
12. Kirsch WM, Leitner JW: A comparison of the anaerobic glycolysis of human brain and glioblastoma. J Neurosurg 27:45–51, 1967.
13. Kornblith PL: Humoral immunity, in Thomas DGT, Graham DI (eds): *Brain Tumours: Scientific Basis, Clinical Investigation and Current Therapy.* Boston, Butterworth, 1980, pp 133–144.
14. Kornblith PL, Smith BH, Gately MK: Tumor cell and host response parameters in designing brain tumor therapy, in Walker M (ed): *Oncology of the Nervous System.* Boston, Mass., Martinus Nijhoff, in press, 1983.
15. Krebs HA: The Pasteur effect and the relations between respiration and fermentation. Essays Biochem 8:1–34, 1972.
16. Lowry OH, Berger SJ, Chi MM-Y, Carter JG, Blackshaw A, Outlaw W: Diversity of metabolic pattens in human brain tumors: I. High energy phosphate compounds and basic composition. J Neurochem 29:959–977, 1977.
17. Marton LJ: Polyamines and brain tumors. Natl Cancer Inst Monogr 46:127–131, 1977.
18. Sachs L: Control of normal cell differentiation and the phenotypic reversion of malignancy in myeloid leukaemia. Nature 274:535–539, 1978.

19. Shapiro JR, Yung W-KA, Shapiro WR: Isolation, karyotype, and clonal growth of heterogeneous subpopulations of human malignant gliomas. Cancer Res 41:2349–2359, 1981.

20. Shitara N, McKeever P, Whang Peng J, Smith BH, Schmidt S, Kornblith PL: Cytofluorometric-DNA determination and cytogenetic analysis in human cultured cell line derived from brain tumors. Acta Neuropathol (Berl): In press, 1983.

21. Sokoloff L, Reivich M, Kennedy C, Des Rosiers MH, Patlak CS, Pettigrew KD, Sakurada O, Shinohara M: The [^{14}C] deoxyglucose method for the measurement of local cerebral glucose utilization: Theory, procedure, and normal values in the conscious and anesthetized albino rat. J Neurochem 28:897–916, 1977.

22. Stenzel KH, Schwartz R, Rubin AL, Novogrodsky A: Chemical inducers of differentiation in Friend leukaemia cells inhibit lymphocyte mitogenesis. Nature 285:106–108, 1980.

23. Timperley WR: Glycolysis in neuroectodermal tumours, in Thomas DGT, Graham DI (eds): Brain Tumours: Scientific Basis, Clinical Investigation and Current Therapy. Boston, Butterworth, 1980, pp 145–167.

24. Todaro GJ, Fryling C, De Larco JE: Transforming growth factors produced by certain human tumor cells: Polypeptides that interact with epidermal growth factor receptors. Proc Natl Acad Sci USA 77:5258–5262, 1980.

25. van Veelen CWM, Verbiest H, Zülch KJ, van Ketel B, van der Vlist MJM, Vlug AMC, Rijksen G, Staal GEJ: Pyruvate kinase in human brain tumours: Its significance in the treatment of gliomas. Acta Neurochir (Wien) 61:145–159, 1982.

26. Victor J, Wolf A: Metabolism of brain tumors. Res Publ Assoc Res Nerv Ment Dis 16:44–58, 1937.

27. Warburg O: The Metabolism of Tumours. London, Constable, 1930.

28. Weber G: Enzymology of cancer cells. N Engl J Med 296:486–493, 541–551, 1977.

29. Weinhouse S: New dimensions in the biology of cancer. Cancer 45:2975–2980, 1980.

30. Wollemann M: Biochemistry of brain tumors, in Lajtha A (ed): Handbook of Neurochemistry, vol VII: Pathological Chemistry of the Nervous System. New York, Plenum Press, 1972, pp 503–542.

60

Immunology of Brain Tumors

Michael L. J. Apuzzo

General Concepts

All normal cells express antigenic determinants which make them recognizable to the host as self. In the event that transformation occurs, as in a neoplastic process, determinants may emerge that are recognized as being foreign. These so-called tumor associated or tumor-specific antigens are recognized as such by the host's immune system and initiate an immune response. Such a response represents a dynamic interaction between the neoplasm and the multiple biological elements that constitute the immune system.[1]

Tumor Antigens

Tumors exhibit transplantation antigens. Therefore the development of genetically identical inbred strains of animals possessing identical antigenic substrates was necessary before evidence of the specific antigenicity of experimental tumors could be verified. These studies indicated that all experimentally induced tumors possess tumor-specific transplantation antigens (TSTA), but that immunity to these determinants could protect the host against only relatively small numbers (10^6) of tumor cells. Within the experimental animal setting, transplantation antigens, tumor-specific antigens, viral antigens, and fetal antigens were all found to be tumor-associated.

In humans, it is obviously not possible to demonstrate tumor-specific antigens by transplantation techniques. Methodology has relied on demonstration of cell-mediated immunity or humoral responses against tumor cells or cell extracts. In addition, preparation of heteroantisera has been employed. Since such antisera are obtained by immunization of animals with tumor tissue, it might well be that the animals do not possess the genetic repertoire to detect and respond to the human neoantigens used as immunogens. Also, relatively weak antigens may be hidden on the cell membrane by their close proximity to strong antigens (i.e., histocompatability antigens) or might be present in low concentration. Immunogenicity has been detected in Burkitt's lymphoma, neuroblastoma, malignant melanoma, osteosarcoma, Wilms' tumor, testicular tumors, carcinomas of the breast, lung, endometrium, and ovary, leukemia and central nervous system neoplasms.

Elements of the Immune Mechanism

The immune mechanism represents a dynamic interplay between cellular systems, antibodies, and antigenic mediators. The response has three distinct phases:

1. *Recognition,* in which the antigen is appreciated by the basic elements of response
2. *Proliferation,* in which the multiplication of specific elements ensues prior to immune impact
3. *Effector,* in which the immune system exerts its cytoreductive capacity

In the most simplistic of senses, the immune response may be considered to be composed of two major elements: cellular (cell-mediated), or that response which may be transferred by cells alone; and humoral, which may be transferred by serum or soluble factors alone. While their activities are separable, it should be emphasized that in the rejection of foreign cells, including cancer, these two components must act in concert. Often the two collaborate in a multifaceted process of killing in which antibodies serve to prepare the tumor cells for destruction by leukocytes.

Cellular Immunity

Lymphocytes and macrophages constitute the major elements of cellular immunity. Primary in this group is the T cell, or thymus-derived lymphocyte. Several subclasses or subsets of T cells have been recognized that interact in a dynamic balance. The cytotoxic effector cell, the inducer or helper cell, and the suppressor cell are the components of the cell populations. The balance between helper and suppressor cells is critical in the emergence of an immune response capable of reducing tumor burden. It is the balance between effector and regulator subsets that governs the outcome of antigen triggering. The helper-inducer subset is critical for the activation of many effector elements of the immune response. This inductive influence is regulated by the presence of suppressor T cells that function to govern the inducer subsets, or alternatively, the effector population itself. Loss or activation of these subsets may result in a variety of imunologic states characterized by immunodepression or autoimmunity.

Stimulation of T cells leads to the secretion of lymphokines. One of these, macrophage-activating factor (MAF), nonspecifically activates macrophages and recruits previously unstimulated mononuclear cells. They become cytotoxic effector cells and secrete monokines, which augment the pool of activated lymphocytes.

Natural killer (NK) cells have been described and in the animal setting have been considered an early defense against neoplastic emergence. They are not under genetic control and may provide the host with immunoreactivity without prior immunization or sensitization. Morphologically these appear to be large, granular lymphocytes. Immunologically they share characteristics of both T cells and macrophages. They appear to serve in an immunosurveillance role.

Macrophages are involved in almost every phase of the immune response.[12] This cellular population is made up of subgroups which act in antigen recognition, mediation, and effector toxicity, as well as suppressor feedback into the entire immune mechanism. Effector (killer) macrophages destroy tumor cells by inhibiting their growth rather than by cytolysis. Superoxide radicals, exoenzymes, and transfer of lysosomes are some of the proposed mechanisms of action. Afferent (recognition) macrophages initiate virtually every immune response by attaching antigenic materials to their cell membranes and presenting them to helper T lymphocytes. Antigens not bound to macrophages are usually poorly immunogenic and induce only a weak or transient immune response. Another service of macrophages is to concentrate antigens on their surface and thus present a large number to the T cell. This presentation and release of soluble mediators leads to clonal proliferation of T-cell subsets. The process is amplified by lymphokines from activated T cells, which in turn activate effector macrophages to participate in the specific immune response.

Humoral Immunity

Antibodies (immunoglobulin), alone or in concert with complement, are the major components of the humoral response. The constituents are produced after recognition of antigen by B lymphocytes. There is no distinct lymphoid organ in mammalian development responsible for B-lymphocyte maturation; rather, they are generated in sites of general hematopoiesis. Following recognition, B cells proliferate and differentiate into plasma cells, which secrete the antibodies. Helper (inducer) T cells are important components for facilitation of this response. Antigen alone will not induce B-cell proliferation and antibody production. Most antigens are known to be thymus-dependent, i.e., T cells recognize the larger part of the molecule and B cells produce antibodies against a few antigenic determinants (hapten) within the molecule. Initiation of a humoral response is recognized as a multi-stage event in which antigens must be bound by macrophages and then presented to helper T cells. Proliferation of this T-cell subset occurs, helper cell factors are released, clonal expansion of the corresponding B lymphocyte is induced, and finally antibody production occurs.

The complement system represents the principal effector mechanism of the extracellular fluid; activation of a cascade of responses is triggered by an appropriate antigen-antibody complex. Such a cascade has cell lysis as an end point.

Although a number of immunoglobulins are elaborated, IgG and IgM are considered the most pertinent mediators in immune neoplastic events. Both these antibodies are cytotoxic in vitro in the presence of complement. IgG may assist in cell-mediated cytotoxic responses by arming such cells as macrophages, K cells, and effector cells, thus increasing their effector capacity. IgG is the principal cytophilic antibody binding not only target cells but also effector cells.

Of considerable importance is the consideration of issues attendant on "immune escape," or blocking of effector systems.

In thymus leukemia systems, transient or complete loss of surface tumor antigen has been observed after exposure of the antigen-bearing cells to specific antibodies. This is termed antigenic modulation and is one recognized method of immune escape.

Usually, during a time of rapid tumor growth, large amounts of tumor antigen are present in the host's circulation, while tumor-specific antibodies occur after tumor debulking. The presence of free tumor antibody has been shown to be concurrent with restored immunity. It is well established that soluble tumor antigens or specific immune complexes consisting of specific tumor antigens and tumor antibody are the blocking and tumor-enhancing elements in the immune suppressive tumor sera. The precise mechanisms of effecting suppression are still a major question.

Although the mechanism is not clearly defined, it is believed that free tumor antigen or antigen-antibody complexes induce the emergence of suppressor T-cell predominance. These elements produce glycoproteins which impair the emergence and efficiency of effector subsets. Macrophage subsets of suppressor influence also elaborate prostaglandin-type mediators which reduce effector cell development, especially during the proliferation phase of the immune response. Lymphocytes without identifiable markers (null cells) likewise may have suppressor activity.

Immunology of Glial Tumors

Is the Brain an Immunologically Privileged Site?

Initial perspectives regarding immune responses in brain neoplasia seemed to imply minimum activity; the concept of the brain as an immunologically privileged site arose from the knowledge of the absence of lymphatic channels and presence of the blood-brain barrier. Work sixty years ago indicated rapid tumor growth with intracerebral heterologous transplants with no evidence of rejection. Allogeneic skin grafts in rabbit brains were not rejected. Therefore the issue of immune privilege seemed well established.

However, studies over the past twenty years have effectively refuted the concept by demonstration of clear-cut and reproducible intracerebral graft rejection, induction of immune responses secondary to intracerebral implants, and entry of systemic effector cells to brain parenchyma.

The premise of partial privilege seems more tenable and assumes an alteration in barrier integrity which is attendant on various pathological processes, including neoplasia.[1]

Organ- and Tumor-Related Antigens

Extensive study has disclosed a well-defined antigenic substrate of the intracellular compartment of brain tissue. These include S-100 protein, 14-3-2 protein, glial fibrillary acidic protein (GFAP), alpha-2 glycoprotein, and myelin basic protein (MBP). Because of cross reactivity with microorganisms and other vertebrate tissues, individual cell-surface glial antigens are less satisfactorily defined.

Glial tumors share their antigenic substrate with normal brain, but as anaplastic changes evolve there is an observed trend toward reduction in the expression of this similarity.

Efforts to define precisely the antigenic substrate of intrinsic gliomas have been unsuccessful to date. Initial efforts focused on the study of antigenic determinants through the preparation of antisera in laboratory animals. As already noted, interspecies preparation of antisera is problematic in terms of clearly establishing specificity of response; the technique requires exhaustive absorption studies and strict consideration of potential contamination with cross-reacting microorganisms. Available data indicate that, besides sharing antigenic substrates with normal brain, gliomas also express constituents found in fetal tissues and other tumor systems as well, particularly those derived from tissues of ectodermal origin. No consistent virally coded neoantigen has been reported.

Hybridoma methodology has emerged as a potent probe in the immunologic laboratory which renders the need for standard preparations of heteroantisera virtually obsolete. Monoclonal antibody produced by hybridoma progeny of a

normal B cell and myeloma tumor cell has been utilized as a precise marker for cell-surface determinants related to naturally occurring cells and neoplastic tissues.[5] It appears that this technology will be applied to gliomas to lend further definition to the antigenic substrate.[14]

Cellular and General Immune Responses

Peripheral Cell Pool

The ability of the cellular component of the immune system to respond to antigen has classically been assessed by delayed hypersensitivity responses to skin-test antigens and by quantitative studies of circulating lymphocytes. In vitro assays of the functional responses of lymphocytes have also been commonly employed.

Early major contributions in the evaluation of patients harboring glial tumors were made by Mahaley et al.,[10] Brooks et al.,[4] and Young et al.[19] On the basis of their work, it is clear that patients with malignant gliomas preoperatively exhibit (1) decreased responses to common skin-test antigens, (2) depressed peripheral lymphocyte counts, characterized by decreased percentage of T cells; and (3) impairment of the ability of lymphocytes to respond in vitro. These findings are apparent in spite of the demonstrated sensitivity of peripheral blood leukocytes to extracts of tumor cells.[2]

Assays devised to demonstrate cytotoxic responses are complex in design and require meticulous attention to variables and controls. Results regarding in vitro cytotoxicity are contradictory.[18] More specifically, no clear, reproducible evidence of in vivo cytotoxicity in humans in available.[1]

Recent study of the peripheral blood leukocyte compartment has focused on definition of T-cell subsets.[8] Utilization of monoclonal antibodies specific for cell-surface determinants and fluorescence-activated cell sorting devices have indicated relative suppressor cell predominance in the preoperative period. This suppressor influence has been observed concurrently in patients whose lymphocytes respond poorly in assays of antigenic stimulation.

Tumor Matrix Cellular Constituents

Histologic assessment of glial tumors indicates round cell infiltration in the perivascular regions in approximately 35 to 65 percent of cases. These infiltrations, characterized by various techniques, are composed of combinations of lymphocytes, monocytes, and macrophages.[16] Recently, employing monoclonal antibody immunoperoxidase technique, populations of T-cell subgroups of helper-inducer and suppressor cytotoxic phenotypes have been defined within the tumor matrix and perivascular regions.[15]

Clinical assessment in association with round cell infiltration and its extent has correlated these findings with prolongation of the patient's overall course and survival.[13]

Humoral Response

Quantitative levels of immunoglobulins have been observed to be well within normal ranges, with some studies observing higher mean preoperative levels of IgM in patients with glioblastoma.[10]

Indirect immunofluorescence has indicated the presence of circulating antibodies to glioma cells in 50 percent of cases.[2] In well-designed complement-mediated cytotoxic assays, Kornblith et al. have shown that 82 percent of glioma patients give positive responses indicative of the presence of cytotoxic antibody.[7] However, variable numbers of neuroectodermally derived neoplasms also give positive responses. Studies have indicated that IgM antibodies were more effective than IgG in their ability to fix complement on cultured glioma target cells.

Antibody-dependent cytotoxic assays have yielded no consistent evidence of cytotoxicity.

Mechanisms of Suppression and Blocking

Of singular importance in the study of the immune response to neoplasia is the precise comprehension of mechanisms mediating natural suppression of immune activity and elements of blocking. Insight into pathways and components involved in these events would appear to be essential for rational embarkation on any immunotherapeutic endeavor.

Glioma patients manifest blocking factors in their serum. Brooks et al.[4] demonstrated suppression of lymphocyte proliferation responses to antigenic stimuli with both patient and normal cells in the presence of the patient's serum. This effect was enhanced with increasing serum concentrations and appeared to be related to the tumor burden, as reduction of the effect was observed with postoperative sera following major decompression and tumor debulking.

Kumar and Taylor's cytotoxicity studies[9] indicated that impairment of responsiveness was evident in 80 percent of cases with the addition of autologous patient serum; such a response was not evident with serum from persons who were tumor-free or normal donors.

In a complementary study, Young et al.[19] likewise confirmed the presence of inhibitory factors in the serum of glioblastoma patients, but this autologous serum response was not observed with serum from patients with benign astrocytomas.

As immune complexes are currently seen as the primary instigators of suppressor cell emergence, the study by Martin-Achard et al.[11] of the sera of 208 patients with intracranial neoplasms is especially pertinent to this discussion. Some 28 percent of patients with malignant gliomas manifested immune complexes in their sera as detected by complement fraction C1 binding assays. The mean survival in those patients demonstrating complexes was half of that observed in those who did not manifest such findings. Only 14 percent of benign gliomas were positive in this assay.

Brook's group initially considered that the blocking or suppressor factor was related to the IgG serum fraction.[4] More recent work by Wood and Morantz[17] has supported the validity of this concept.

Garson et al.[6] have demonstrated cell-bound IgG-antigen complexes which impair the emergence of complement-mediated cytoxic responses that are more effectively mediated by IgM. In this cytotoxic mechanism, duplicate IgG binding at the antigen site is required to initiate the complement-mediated response. The presence of one IgG molecule blocks the binding of IgM, which is the more effective initiator.

At the cellular level, monoclonal antibodies detecting the phenotype expression of cell-surface determinants have been employed to define peripheral blood T-cell subsets in patients with both benign and malignant intracranial tumors. Suppressor subsets have been shown to predominate in anaplastic intrinsic neoplasms, while inducer-helper influence is primary in histologically and biologically benign lesions.[8] Similar suppressor T cells have been identified in the matrix of malignant tumors by monoclonal antibody conjugated to immunoperoxidase markers.[15] The suppressor cellular predominance has been concurrently associated with depression of lymphocytic response to antigenic stimulation in vitro.[3]

References

1. Apuzzo MLJ, Mitchell MS: Immunological aspect of intrinsic glial tumors. J Neurosurg 55:1–18, 1981.
2. Apuzzo MLJ, Sheikh KMA, Weiss MH, Heiden JS, Kurze T: The utilization of native glioma antigens in the assessment of cellular and humoral immune responses in malignant glioma patients. Acta Neurochir (Wien) 55:181–200, 1981.
3. Braun DP, Penn RD, Flannery AM, Harris JE: Immunoregulatory cell function in peripheral blood leukocytes of patients with intracranial gliomas. Neurosurgery 10:203–209, 1982.
4. Brooks WH, Netsky MG, Normansell DE, Horwitz DA: Depressed cell-mediated immunity in patients with primary intracranial tumors. J Exp Med 136:1631–1647, 1972.
5. Diamond BA, Yelton DE, Scharff MD: Monoclonal antibodies: A new technology for producing serologic reagents. N Engl J Med 304:1344–1349, 1981.
6. Garson JA, Quindlen EA, Kornblith PL: Complement fixation by IgM and IgG autoantibodies on cultured human glial cells. J Neurosurg 55:19–26, 1981.
7. Kornblith PL, Pollock LA, Coakham HB, Quindlen EA, Wood WC: Cytotoxic antibody responses in astrocytoma patients: An improved allogeneic assay. J Neurosurg 51:47–52, 1979.
8. Kril MP, Apuzzo MLJ, Sheikh KMA: Definition of lymphocyte subsets by monoclonal antibodies and fluorescent activated cell sorting in intracranial neoplastic disorders. Clin Neurosurg 30:125–136, 1983.
9. Kumar S, Taylor G: specific lymphocytotoxicity and blocking factors in tumours of the central nervous system. Br J Cancer [Suppl] 28:135–141, 1973.
10. Mahaley MS, Brooks WH, Roszman TL, Bigner DD, Dudka L, Richardson S: Immunobiology of primary intracranial tumors: Part 1. Studies of the cellular and humoral general immune competence of brain-tumor patients. J Neurosurg 46:467–476, 1977.
11. Martin-Achard A, de Tribolet N, Louis JA, Zander E: Immune complexes associated with brain tumors: Correlation with prognosis. Surg Neurol 13:161–163, 1980.
12. Oehler JR, Herberman RB, Holden HT: Modulation of immunity by macrophages. Pharmacol Ther A 2:551–593, 1978.
13. Palma L, Di Lorenzo N, Guidetti B: Lymphocytic infiltrates in primary glioblastomas and recidivous gliomas: Incidence, fate, and relevance to prognosis in 228 operated cases. J Neurosurg 49:854–861, 1978.
14. Schnegg JF, Diserens AC, Carrel S, Accolla RS, de Tribolet N: Human glioma-associated antigens detected by monoclonal antibodies. Cancer Res 41:1209–1213, 1981.
15. von Hahnwehr R, Hofman F, Taylor CR, Apuzzo MLJ: Mononuclear lymphoid populations infiltrating primary intrinsic central nervous system gliomas: Characterization of cellular subsets with monoclonal antibodies. In press, 1984.
16. Wood GW, Morantz RA: Immunohistologic evaluation of the

lymphoreticular infiltrate of human central nervous system tumors. JNCI 62:485–491, 1979.

17. Wood GW, Morantz RA: In vitro reversal of depressed T-lymphocyte function in the peripheral blood of brain tumor patients. JNCI 68:27–33, 1982.

18. Woosley RE, Mahaley MS, Mahaley JL, Miller GM, Brooks

WH: Immunobiology of primary intracranial tumors: Part 3. Microcytotoxicity assays of specific immune responses of brain tumor patients. J Neurosurg 47:871–885, 1977.

19. Young HF, Sakalas R, Kaplan AM: Inhibition of cell-mediated immunity in patients with brain tumors. Surg Neurol 5:19–23, 1976.

61

Tissue Culture Techniques in the Study of Human Gliomas

Joseph Bressler
Barry H. Smith
Paul L. Kornblith

The value of culturing human glial tumors has long been recognized. Theoretically both diagnostic (prognostic) information and the ability to plan individualized therapy would be increased by employing culture techniques to study their biological characteristics, chemotherapeutic sensitivity, and immunologic properties. It should be possible to design more rational therapeutic agents or modalities, based on combinations of cytotoxicity, differentiation control, and improved immunologic detectability or cytolytic sensitivity of the target cells.

The first attempts to culture human gliomas were made in the laboratories of Fischer[15] and Cushing.[4] Cushing's purpose in culturing tumors was to relate the in vitro growth rate to the in vivo growth rate, as well as to determine the embryonic origin of some intracranial tumors.[37]

This early work was fraught with technical difficulties. Russell's group seemed to have more success in the number of tumors they were able to culture, and they were also the first to use tissue culture studies to verify the histological origin.[55,56]

It is difficult to imagine working in a tissue culture laboratory without an inverted phase contrast microscope or a ready supply of nutrient mixtures and serum, but such were the conditions in these early studies. Workers planted pieces of tumors on plasma clots and fixed and stained these clots

to monitor growth. After World War II, as a result of technical advances, more and more success in culturing central nervous system (CNS) tumors has been achieved. In fact, almost every type of CNS-derived tumor has now been cultured for at least short periods of time. It is not surprising that the more malignant tumors, such as astrocytomas grades III and IV or glioblastomas, have been the easiest to establish in culture.

Many of the early accounts of brain tumor tissue culture have been summarized and appear in Lumsden's chapter in Russell and Rubinstein's *Pathology of Tumours of the Nervous System*.[43] Much of this work continued the study of cellular growth from tissue explants. In many cases, primary cell cultures exhibited distinct morphological patterns which were characteristic for the particular tumor. Lumsden argued that culture studies might help the pathologist verify the classification of a tumor and might add to prognostic information, since the vigor of growth in culture could be related to the degree of malignancy.

More recent efforts have continued the basic studies of morphology and growth kinetics and have also added assessments of chromosomal patterns,[59] differentiated properties,[2] chemotherapeutic agent sensitivities,[35,36,53,54,63,69] and immunologic properties.[16,17,31–34] It appears that tissue culture is now at the point where it can be applied to learning more about the cell biology of brain tumors. This work will encompass genetic and biochemical analyses, thus making it necessary to grow well-characterized cell lines in large quantities. This understanding of brain tumor cell biology may suggest new diagnostic treatment modes.

Definition of Key Terms

The following terms are used frequently in this chapter:

Primary culture: a culture derived directly from the tissue without any prior culturing.

Cell line: derived from the first subculture of a primary culture; the term *line* suggests that cells present in the cell line were also present in the primary culture.

Established cell line: a line maintained in culture for many passages with defined, stable biological characteristics.

Clonal cell line: a cell line derived from a single cell.

Organ culture: in vitro maintenance and/or growth of an organ or piece of tissue allowing the expression of differentiated characteristics and preservation of tissue architecture.

Tissue culture: the in vitro growth and/or maintenance of tissue in a manner allowing the expression of one or more properties which were also expressed in vivo.

Basic Tissue Culture Techniques

Basic references on standard tissue culture techniques abound.[38] Emphasis is needed for the following points.

After excision, the tumor tissue should be placed in a container with a nutrient medium at 4°C and immediately sent to the tissue culture laboratory. The more quickly the tumor is placed in culture, the greater is the likelihood of success in achieving a viable cell line. Under a vertical laminar flow hood, the necrotic areas, macroscopic blood vessels, and any encapsulating material should be cut away, so that only the most homogeneous, healthy tumor tissue is used for culture. This remaining tissue should then be cut into approximately 1-mm pieces, using two scalpels in a scissorslike motion. This cutting motion is important, since a clean edge, rather than a jagged one, ensures better cell growth. At this point the experimenter has a choice of two different methods of culturing the tumor cells: the use of explants or of single-cell suspensions.

In the authors' laboratory explant cultures have been used, because the process involves the least amount of manipulation, decreasing the chance of damaging the cells. The 1-mm pieces of tumor are placed in a tissue culture flask (approximately nine pieces per 25-cm² flask). To ensure adhesion of the explants, the flask is then inverted and placed in a well-humidified incubator at 37°C. After 30 min, medium is added to the flask so that the explants are barely covered. The next day more medium is added (10 ml per 75-cm² flask, 3 ml per 25-cm² flask). The flasks are put back into the incubator and not disturbed for a least 1 week. If explants float off the surface, they can be replanted in another flask, using the same procedure.

A tumor can also be cultured by creating a single-cell suspension. Dispersion can be achieved by either of two methods: mechanical or enzymatic. For mechanical dispersion, 1-mm pieces of tumor are withdrawn through a sequential series of needles ranging from 18-gauge through 25-gauge. It is recommended that this be done in the presence of 30 percent fetal calf serum (FCS). The high protein concentration absorbs shock generated during dispersion. Mechanical dispersion is especially applicable to soft tumors. In fact, as the tumor is cut into 1-mm pieces, cells will be dispersed. Enzymatic dispersion can be accomplished with trypsin, diaspase collagenase or a combination of these. Many procedures have been devised;[23,49,66] the goal of all such procedures is to maximize single-cell yield and viability.

It is important to realize that the method chosen for initial establishment of the culture may determine the predominant cell type ultimately grown. Although the explant method involves the least manipulation of the tumor cells, only those tumor cells that migrate out of the explant will be found in the line or lines established in culture.[59] Not all cell types migrate out at the same time or with the same success. For the single-cell dispersion methods other selection factors may be operative and may affect the extent to which the original tumor cell population is represented.

Also critical is the type of medium used. Many types of medium (varying in both the complexity and the concentration of their nutrients) have been devised in the past thirty years. Many of these media require supplementation with serum in order to provide sources of growth factors and additional nutrients. Investigators have found the use of conditioned media (media derived from an established cell line) or feeder layers to be of benefit in the establishment of primary cell cultures. A detailed study of the nutrient requirements of human glioma cells has not, to the authors' knowledge, been undertaken. It is recommended that human glioma cell lines be grown in one of Ham's formulated media, since these contain the greatest range of nutrients.[22] The authors' laboratory uses Ham's F-10 medium, but Ham's F-12 medium or media with the designation MCDB may be equally satisfactory. Barnes and Sato have found that Ham's F-12 medium mixed with Dulbecco's modified essential medium (DMEM) is also quite good.[1] The addition of fetal calf serum and/or human AB serum (5 to 30 percent) is required for successful growth. Although it would be desirable to grow glioma cultures in chemically defined media (i.e., without serum), this is not yet practical. Finally, it should be noted that no one medium or combination of media will be optimal for all cell lines.

Contamination

A potentially serious problem in tissue culture is contamination. There are four types of contamination: bacterial, fungal, mycoplasmal, and that by cells from other lines. Bacterial and fungal contamination can usually be observed macroscopically, although on occasion a slowly growing organism will be hard to detect. Because of this it is important to examine the cultures at least twice each week by light microscopy. If contamination is observed, the culture should be destroyed. If contamination is recurrent or appears to be spreading, it is advisable to send samples of the contaminated medium to the bacteriology laboratory for culture and sensitivity testing. Additionally, all reagents should be checked in order to trace the source of the contamination. Incubators and their water supplies should also be cleaned and cultured if necessary.

Contamination by mycoplasmas (pleuropneumonia-like organisms, or PPLO) is more difficult to detect, since it is not evident with a light microscope. Sometimes a slower growth rate of an otherwise healthy culture may provide a clue to the presence of mycoplasmas. Since mycoplasmal contamination can render any data obtained on a cell line uninterpretable, it is worthwhile to perform routine checks (every 3 months, for example) on a representative sampling of the cell lines being carried. Mycoplasmal contamination can be detected by various means, including growth in *Mycoplasma* agar,[24] uridine incorporation,[57] or the fluorochrome method of Del Guidice and Hopps.[10] Certain commercial tissue culture supply laboratories offer *Mycoplasma* testing.

Two precautions can be taken to avoid mycoplasmal contamination: (1) use of a propipette or pipette aid instead of a mouth pipette and (2) avoidance of the use of antibiotics in normal culture maintenance (antibiotics mask both bacterial and mycoplasmal contamination). Bacterial infection indicates a breakdown in sterile technique. If antibiotics are used, this indicator is lost, making it possible for another type of infection, such as a *Mycoplasma* infection, to be established.

The contamination of one cell line with one or more cells from another line is more common than might be supposed. Such contamination may render all the laboratory cultures useless or may invalidate months of research. Contamination of human with animal cell lines is a special problem because of the aggressive growth characteristics of certain animal lines. Even if the laboratory has only human lines, it is still possible to cross-contaminate the various lines from different tumors.

Morphology alone is not a guarantee that the line is not contaminated; karyotyping and LDH isoenzyme analysis are necessary. Simple preventive measures include using a different pipette and medium bottle for each line and never touching any flask with a pipette. Scrupulous cleanliness of all hoods and other culture work surfaces will also help.

Methods of Characterizing Glioma Cultures

Glial tumors are made up of heterogeneous cell populations. Besides the vascular elements (endothelial cells, pericytes) and other mesenchyme-derived cells (fibroblasts), the tumor contains glial cell subpopulations varying in both karyotype and phenotype.[2,58] Since all these cell types have the potential to grow in vitro, the cultures must be characterized to ascertain the cell subpopulations which have been selected by the culture process. Morphological characterization is not sufficient, since it can vary with the culture conditions; therefore biochemical markers must be utilized. Unfortunately, cells may lose the ability to express one or more of these markers (usually markers of differentiation) as they adapt to the tissue culture conditions. Thus a panel of markers may be required to define the populations present.

Glial Markers

Glial Fibrillary Acidic Protein (GFAP)

GFAP is a protein with a molecular weight of 50,000 which constitutes the intermediary filaments of and is restricted to mature astrocytes. Antibody prepared in a number of laboratories has been used in immunocytochemical studies to identify cells expressing GFAP.[12,48] More quantitative assays are also available.[13,52] The specificity of the antibody and the particular preparation to be used should be carefully ascertained, since other intermediary filaments (desmin, epithelial cells; vimentin, fibroblasts) share antigenic determinants with GFAP.[51]

The absence of GFAP does not necessarily mean that a cell is of nonglial origin. If the hypothesis that glial tumors are derived from stem cells is accepted and if those stem cells have not yet expressed GFAP (see Dahl[8]), then tumors derived from these cells may not express GFAP. Some apparently neoplastic cells in the intact glial tumors do not, in fact, stain for GFAP. In addition, glial cells lose the ability

to synthesize GFAP after adaptation to culture conditions. In primary culture, glial cells may express GFAP; but most cell lines, except for U-251[12] and a few others, lose this property with increasing time in culture. This loss is not necessarily irreversible. For example, a transformed rat glial cell line grown in monolayer will not express GFAP, but GFAP expression can be induced by growing the cells on cellulose sponges.[3] This suggests that a chemically defined three-dimensional matrix is important in GFAP expression.

S-100 Protein

The name of this protein is derived from its solubility in 100% ammonium sulfate, a property which is utilized in its purification.[47] In the CNS, the protein is localized in the membrane and cytoplasm of astrocytes and in the plasma membrane of oligodendrocytes and possibly neurons.[28] Other cell types of neuroectodermal origin also express S-100 protein.[18] The greatest S-100 synthesis occurs after the cells reach confluency, suggesting that cell density is an important regulator.[40] The function of this protein is probably related to Ca^{2+} regulation, since it binds Ca^{2+}.[62] To detect S-100, microcomplement fixation[43] and immunoelectrophoresis[41] have been used.

S-100 content has been determined both in biopsies of glial tumors and in the cell lines established from them.[2,11,21,29] Although virtually all the tumors examined were positive for S-100, a 19-fold range of levels was detected.[11] In cultures, detection has been more variable, which may suggest changes with time in culture similar to those for GFAP.

CNPase

This enzyme, which is myelin-associated,[39] catalyzes the conversion of 2′,3′-cyclic nucleotides to 3′-cyclic nucleotides. In the rat, the CNPase enzyme is associated with oligodendroglia-derived cells.[46] Its distribution in solid tumor gliomas and glioma-derived cell lines has been studied.[11] CNPase is found in all tumors derived from CNS tissue, although its levels vary over an 835-fold range. No clear correlation of CNPase level with tumor type is evident.

It is clear that more and better markers are needed. Monoclonal antibodies are the subject of active current investigation and may ultimately be the most useful.[5,6,68]

Determination of Neoplastic State

Tumorigenicity

Besides determining the glial origin of cell lines in culture, it is imperative that the tumorigenicity of the cells be established. Cells can lose their tumorigenic potential. Cultured cells may revert to a nontransformed state as they adapt to culture conditions. The ultimate criterion for determining tumorigenicity is the ability of the cells to form a tumor in nude mice.[19] The nude mouse is thought to be a mutant lacking T-cell immunity. This immunodeficiency allows the growth of allografts, such as human tumors, that would normally be rejected in an immunologically competent host. Non-neoplastic cells do not grow. (It should be pointed out that nude mice are expensive and require a specific protocol for maintenance, especially if they are housed in an environment containing other rodents.)

Chromosome Analysis

Chromosome analysis is another method by which to determine whether cells are neoplastic. Neoplastic cells vary widely in ploidy, from hypodiploid to octaploid, while human non-neoplastic cells remain diploid. From the data of Shapiro et al.,[58] it appears that there are 3 to 21 subpopulations of chromosomal patterns in individual glial tumors, thus emphasizing the heterogeneity of these tumors. In addition, these investigators have shown that the cell lines established from these tumors undergo further chromosomal changes with time in culture, consistent with the genetic instability that seems to characterize malignant solid tumors generally.

Anchorage-Independent Growth

Anchorage-independent growth is yet another method by which to distinguish neoplastic from non-neoplastic cells. In this assay, cells are grown in or on a substrate (agarose, agar, or methylcellulose) which does not allow the cell to adhere.[44] The cell body therefore remains spheroidal. Although this technique is useful, there is not a perfect correlation between anchorage-independent growth and tumorigenicity. Cell lines have been established which grow in soft agar but cannot form tumors in vivo, and tumorigenic cell lines have been established which do not exhibit anchorage-independent growth.

Tissue Culture and Glioma Cell Biology

What has been learned from human glioma-derived cell lines in culture? Data have been gathered with respect to such features as growth kinetics;[25,26] morphology at both the light and electron microscopic levels,[2,30] karyotypic and chromosomal analysis, including flow cytometry;[27,58,60] metabolic properties (anaerobic glycolysis) (see Chap. 59); glycolytic and other enzyme isoenzymes;[65] plasminogen activator;[64,70] secreted proteins and/or peptides, including TAF-like activity;[46] DNA methylation repair;[9] response to cAMP, bromodeoxyuridine, and dimethylformamide;[20,50] surface receptors;[59] and surface antigens.[7,34] These findings are in addition to those found for the glial markers described above (i.e., GFAP, S-100, CNPase).

No information as to the cause of these tumors has been gained to date from culture studies. Efforts to find evidence of viral transformation have been negative, although both viral and chemical glial transformations are known for animal systems.

The picture of glial tumors that has emerged from tissue culture studies is much like that for other solid tumors.[19]

Dysregulation of genetic programming, with a tendency for increased expression of certain properties, is a clear pattern. Two major characteristics which have substantial experimental and clinical therapeutic implications are (1) heterogeneity with respect to multiple intrinsic and "response" properties and (2) genetic and phenotypic instability. Two practical areas affected by these features are chemotherapeutic sensitivity or resistance and immunologic properties of human glioma-derived cells.

Glioma Cell Sensitivity to Chemotherapeutic Agents: In Vitro Studies

Several in vitro systems have been employed in the study of the sensitivity of human glioma-derived cells to chemotherapeutic agents. These include the colony formation assay,[54] the microcytotoxicity assay,[35] the surface plating assay,[61] the radioisotope-based microcytotoxicity assay,[67] and the DNA alkaline elution assay.[14] Drugs tested have included carmustine (BCNU), PCNU, chloroethylnitrosourea (CNU), aziridinylbenzoquinone (AZQ), procarbazine, cis-platinum, and spirohydantoin. Common to all these tests except the alkaline elution assay has been a determination of rate of cell killing or growth inhibition. In the DNA alkaline elution assay, the critical measure is the rate of formation of interstrand cross-links and strand breaks, which in turn correlates with cytotoxicity as measured by the colony formation assay or, in certain cases, with data derived from the microcytotoxicity assay.[14]

Without commenting on the significant differences between the assays, one can state that the common theme is heterogeneity of response from tumor to tumor and from clone to clone of cells derived from a single tumor.[69]

The biological characteristics of gliomas, as well as their chemotherapeutic sensitivity, suggest that individualization of antiglioma chemotherapy will be needed to improve therapeutic response in the clinic. Can the in vitro assays described above provide a means to achieve optimization of therapeutic planning despite that fact that the in vitro systems bypass the problems of drug delivery in intact tumors? There is some preliminary evidence that in vitro response does have predictive value, especially for resistance,[35,53] but much more data will have to be gathered before the limits of the in vitro assays are known. Since the various assays may evaluate different aspects of sensitivity, the use of more than one assay may ultimately improve predictive accuracy.

Whether or not the in vitro chemotherapy assays have value for the preselection of one antiglioma drug or a combination of them for individual patients, they will continue to be of use in examining the basis of sensitivity or resistance to both available and new agents. For example, it has been shown that resistance to BCNU is (at least in part) based on the capacity of a given glioma cell for alkylation repair.[14] Furthermore, the cytotoxicity of cis-platinum, also an alkylating agent, is unaffected by the alkylation repair mechanisms that render BCNU ineffective. Thus the in vitro methods are capable of suggesting new, rational approaches to clinical therapy trials and to the design of new, more effective agents.

In Vitro Immunologic Assays in Glioma Patients

The availability of glioma-derived cell lines also provides the opportunity to study tumor cell immunologic properties, as well as host cellular and humoral immune responses. In autologous humoral microcytotoxicity testing, 44 percent of glioma patients have shown positive cytotoxic response to their own tumor cells in culture,[7] with the highest proportion of responders (67 percent) in grades I to III astrocytomas. Among the glioblastomas, the response rate was only 10 percent. These data appear to correlate with patient survival.[32]

With respect to cellular immune response to glial tumors, Gately et al., in a mixed lymphocyte-tumor culture system, have shown that there are three mechanisms by which glioma cells can evade cellular immune attack.[16] In the first, the glioma cells are defective as immunogens, thus provoking no cellular immune attack. This deficiency can be overcome by supplying helper T cells derived from an allogeneic mixed lymphocyte reaction. A second glioma cell defense mechanism is the production of a lymphocyte-suppressor factor. Third, at least some glioma cells produce a protective, extracellular mucopolysaccharide coat that prevents cytotoxic lymphocytes from approaching. Until the coat is removed by hyaluronidase, the sensitized lymphocytes are unable to approach the tumor cells to kill them.

References

1. Barnes D, Sato G: Methods for growth of cultured cells in serum-free medium. Anal Biochem 102:255–270, 1980.
2. Bigner DD, Bigner SH, Pontén J, Westermark B, Mahaley MS Jr, Rouslahti E, Herschman H, Eng LF, Wikstrand CJ: Heterogeneity of genotypic and phenotypic characteristics of fifteen permanent cell lines derived from human gliomas. J Neuropathol Exp Neurol 40:201–229, 1981.
3. Bissel MG, Rubinstein LJ, Bignami A, Herman MM: Characteristics of the rat C-6 glioma maintained in organ culture systems: Production of glial fibrillary acidic protein in the absence of gliofibrillogeneis. Brain Res 82:77–89, 1974.
4. Buckley RC: Tissue culture studies of the glioblastoma multiforme. Am J Pathol 5:467–472, 1929.
5. Cairncross JG, Mattes MJ, Beresford HR, Albino AP, Houghton AN, Lloyd KO, Old LJ: Cell surface antigens of human astrocytoma defined by mouse monoclonal antibodies: Identification of astrocytoma subsets. Proc Natl Acad Sci USA 79:5641–5645, 1982.
6. Carrel S, De Tribolet N, Mach JP: Expression of neuroectodermal antigens common to melanomas, gliomas, and neuroblastomas: I. Identification by monoclonal anti-melanoma and anti-glioma antibodies. Acta Neuropathol (Berl) 57:158–164, 1982.
7. Coakham HB, Kornblith PL: The humoral immune response of patients to their gliomas. Acta Neurochir [Suppl] (Wien) 28:475–479, 1979.
8. Dahl D: The vimentin-GFA protein transition in rat neuroglia cytoskeleton occurs at the time of myelination. J Neurosci Res 6:741–748, 1981.
9. Day RS III, Ziolkowski CHJ: Human brain tumour cell strains with deficient host-cell reactivation of N-methyl-N'-nitro-N-nitrosoguanidine-damaged adenovirus 5. Nature 279:797–799, 1979.
10. Del Guidice RA, Hopps HE: Microbiological methods and fluorescent microscopy for the direct demonstration of mycoplasma infection of cell cultures in McGarrity GJ, Murphy DG, Nichols WW (eds): Mycoplasma Infection of Cell Cultures. New York, Plenum, 1978, pp 57–69.
11. Dohan FC Jr, Kornblith PL, Wellum GR, Pfeiffer SE, Levine L: S-100 protein and 2', 3'-cyclic nucleotide 3'-phosphohydrolase in human brain tumors. Acta Neuropathol (Berl) 40:123–128, 1977.
12. Eng LF, DeArmond SJ: Glial fibrillary acidic (GFA) protein immunocytochemistry in development and neuropathology, in Vidrio EA, Fedoroff S (eds): Eleventh International Congress of Anatomy: Glial and Neuronal Cell Biology (Progress in Clinical and Biological Research, vol 59A). New York, Alan R Liss Inc, 1981, pp 65–79.
13. Eng LF, Lee YL, Miles LEM: Measurement of glial fibrillary acidic protein by a two-site immunoradiometric assay. Anal Biochem 71:243–259, 1976.
14. Erickson LC, Zlotogorski E, Sariban E, Laurent G, Kohn K, Day R III, Ziolkowski C, Smith BH, Pepin C, Kornblith PL: Differences in chloroethylnitrosourea-induced DNA cross-linking in cell lines derived from human malignant gliomas. In press.
15. Fischer A: Observations on the division of sarcoma cells in vitro. J Cancer Res Clin Oncol 9:71–84, 1925.
16. Gately MK, Glaser M, Dick SJ, Mettetal RW Jr, Kornblith PL: In vitro studies on the cell-mediated immune response to human brain tumors: I. Requirement for third-party stimulator lymphocytes in the induction of cell-mediated cytotoxic responses to allogeneic cultured gliomas. JNCI 69:1245–1254, 1982.
17. Gately MK, Glaser M, McCarron RM, Dick SJ, Dick MD, Mettetal RW Jr, Kornblith PL: Mechanisms by which human gliomas may escape cellular immune attack. Acta Neurochir (Wien) 64:175–197, 1982.
18. Gaynor R, Irie R, Morton D, Herschman HR: S100 protein is present in cultured human malignant melanomas. Nature 286:400–401, 1980.
19. Giard DJ, Aaronson SA, Todaro GJ, Arnstein P, Kersey JH, Dosik H, Parks WP: In vitro cultivation of human tumors: Establishment of cell lines derived from a series of solid tumors. JNCI 51:1417–1423, 1973.
20. Gumerlock MK, Smith BH, Pollock LA, Kornblith PL: Chemical differentiation of cultured human glioma cells: Morphologic and immunologic effects. Surg Forum 32:475–477, 1981.
21. Haglid KG, Stavrou D, Rönnbäck L, Carlsson CA, Weidenbach W: The S-100 protein in water-soluble and pentanol-extractable form in normal human brain and tumours of the human nervous system: A quantitative study. J Neurol Sci 20:103–111, 1973.
22. Ham RG: Importance of the basal nutrient medium in the design of hormonally defined media, in Sato GH, Pardee AB, Sirbasku DA (eds): Growth of Cells in Hormonally Defined Media: Book A (Cold Spring Harbor Conferences on Cell Proliferation, vol 9). New York, Cold Spring Harbor Laboratory, 1982, pp 39–60.
23. Hamburger AW, White CP, Tencer K: Effect of enzymatic disaggregation on proliferation of human tumor cells in soft agar. JNCI 68:945–949, 1982.
24. Hayflick L: Screening tissue cultures for mycoplasma infections, in Kruse PF Jr, Patterson MK Jr (eds): Tissue Culture: Methods and Applications. New York, Academic, 1973, pp 722–728.
25. Hoshino T, Barker M, Wilson CB: The kinetics of cultured human glioma cells: Autoradiographic studies. Acta Neuropathol (Berl) 32:235–244, 1975.

26. Hoshino T, Barker M, Wilson CB, Boldrey EB, Fewer D: Cell kinetics of human gliomas. J Neurosurg 37:15–26, 1972.

27. Hoshino T, Nomura K, Wilson CB, Knebel KD, Gray JW: The distribution of nuclear DNA from human tumor cells: Flow cytometric studies. J Neurosurg 49:13–21, 1978.

28. Hyden H, McEwen B: A glial protein specific for the nervous system. Proc Natl Acad Sci USA 55:354–358, 1966.

29. Jacque CM, Kujas M, Poreau A, Raoul M, Collier P, Racadot J, Baumann N: GFA and S100 protein levels as an index for malignancy in human gliomas and neurinomas. JNCI 62:479–483, 1979.

30. Kornblith PL: Role of tissue culture in prediction of malignancy. Clin Neurosurg 25:346–376, 1978.

31. Kornblith PL: Humoral immunity, in Thomas DGT, Graham DI (eds): *Brain Tumours: Scientific Basis, Clinical Investigation and Current Therapy*. London, Butterworth, 1980, pp 133–144.

32. Kornblith PL, Coakham HB, Pollock LA, Wood WC, Green SB, Smith BH: Autologous serological responses in glioma patients: Correlation with tumor grade and survival. In press.

33. Kornblith PL, Dohan FC Jr, Wood WC, Whitman BO: Human astrocytoma: Serum-mediated immunologic response. Cancer 33:1512–1519, 1974.

34. Kornblith PL, Pollock LA, Coakham HB, Quindlen EA, Wood WC: Cytotoxic antibody responses in astrocytoma patients: An improved allogenic assay. J Neurosurg 51:47–52, 1979.

35. Kornblith PL, Smith BH, Leonard LA: Response of cultured human brain tumors to nitosoureas: Correlation with clinical data. Cancer 47:255–265, 1981.

36. Kornblith PL, Szypko PE: Variations in response of human brain tumors to BCNU in vitro. J Neurosurg 48:580–586, 1978.

37. Kredel FE: Tissue culture of intracranial tumors: With a note on the meningiomas. Am J Pathol 4:337–340, 1928.

38. Kruse PF Jr, Patterson MK Jr (eds): *Tissue Culture: Methods and Applications*. New York, Academic, 1973.

39. Kurihara T, Tsukada Y: The regional and subcellular distribution of 2', 3'-cyclic nucleotide 3'-phosphohydrolase in the central nervous system. J Neurochem 14:1167–1174, 1967.

40. Labourdette G, Mahony JB, Brown IR, Marks A: Regulation of synthesis of a brain-specific protein in monolayer cultures of clonal rat glial cells. Eur J Biochem 81:591–597, 1977.

41. Laurell CB: Quantitative estimation of proteins by electrophoresis in agarose gel containing antibodies. Anal Biochem 15:45–52, 1966.

42. Levine L: Micro-complement fixation, Weir DM (eds): *Handbook of Experimental Immunology*, 3d ed. Oxford, Blackwell Scientific Publications, 1978, pp 5B.1–5B.8.

43. Lumsden CE: Tissue culture in relation to tumours of the nervous system, in Russell DS, Rubinstein LJ (eds): *Pathology of Tumours of the Nervous System*, 3d ed. London, E. Arnold, 1963, pp 281–334.

44. Macpherson I: Agar suspension culture for quantitation of transformed cells, in Habel K, Salzman NP (eds): *Fundamental Techniques in Virology*. New York, Academic, 1969, pp 214–219.

45. McCarthy KD, de Vellis J: Preparation of separate astroglial and oligodendroglial cell cultures from rat cerebral tissue. J Cell Biol 85:890–902, 1980.

46. McKeever PE, Quindlen E, Bans MA, Williams U, Kornblith PL, Laverson S, Greenwood MA, Smith B: Biosynthesized products of cultured neuroglial cells: I. Selective release of proteins by cells from human astrocytomas. Neurology (NY) 31:1445–1452, 1981.

47. Moore BW: A soluble protein characteristic of the nervous system. Biochem Biophys Res Commun 19:739–744, 1965.

48. Paetau A, Mellström K, Westermark B, Dahl P, Haltia M, Vaheri A: Mutually exclusive expression of fibronectin and glial fibrillary acidic protein in cultured brain cells. Exp Cell Res 129:337–344, 1980.

49. Penning JJ, LeVan JH: A modified enzymatic technique for production of cell suspensions of a murine fibrosarcoma. JNCI 66:85–87, 1981.

50. Prasad KN, Sahu SK, Sinha PK: Cyclic nucleotides in the regulation of expression of differentiated functions in neuroblastoma cells. JNCI 57:619–631, 1976.

51. Pruss RM, Mirsky R, Raff MC, Thorpe R, Dowding AJ, Anderton BH: All classes of intermediate filaments share a common antigenic determination defined by a monoclonal antibody. Cell 27:419–428, 1981.

52. Rasmussen S, Bock E, Warecka K, Althage G: Quantitation of glial fibrillary acidic protein in human brain tumours. Br J Cancer 41:113–116, 1980.

53. Rosenblum ML, Gerosa MA, Wilson CB, Barger GR, Pertuiset BF, deTribolet N, Dougherty DV: Stem cell studies of human malignant brain tumors: 1. Development of the stem cell assay and its potential. J Neurosurg 58:170–176, 1983.

54. Rosenblum ML, Vasquez DA, Hoshino T, Wilson CB: Development of a clonogenic cell assay for human brain tumors. Cancer 41:2305–2314, 1978.

55. Russell DS, Bland JOW: A study of gliomas by the method of tissue culture. J Pathol Bacteriol 36:273–283, 1933.

56. Russell DS, Bland JOW: Further notes on the tissue culture of gliomas with special reference to Bailey's spongioblastoma. J Pathol Bacteriol 39:375–380, 1934.

57. Schneider EL, Stanbridge EJ: Comparison of methods for the detection of mycoplasmal contamination of cell cultures: A review. In Vitro 11:20–34, 1975.

58. Shapiro JR, Yung W-KA, Shapiro WR: Isolation, karyotype, and clonal growth of heterogeneous subpopulations of human malignant gliomas. Cancer Res 41:2349–2359, 1981.

59. Shitara N, McKeever PE, Cummins C, Smith BH, Kornblith PL, Hirata F: β-adrenergic receptor desensitization stimulates glucose uptake in C$_6$ rat glioma cells. Biochem Biophys Res Commun 109:753–761, 1982.

60. Shitara N, McKeever PE, Whang-Peng J, Knutsen T, Smith BH, Kornblith PL: Flowcytometric and cytogenetic analysis of human cultured cell lines derived from high- and low-grade astrocytomas. In press.

61. Smith BH, Cooke C, Pepin C, Hawkins C, Kornblith PL: Surface plating of chemotherapy agents: A new in vitro assay. In press.

62. Starostina MV, Malup TK, Sviridov SM: Studies on the interaction of Ca^{2+} ions with some fractions of the neurospecific S-100 protein. J Neurochem 36:1904–1915, 1981.

63. Thomas DGT, Darling JL, Freshney RI, Morgan D: In vitro chemosensitivity assay of human glioma by scintillation autofluorography, in Paoletti P, Walker MD, Butti G, Knerich R (eds): *Multidisciplinary Aspects of Brain Tumor Therapy*. Amsterdam, North-Holland, 1979, pp 19–34.

64. Tucker WS, Kirsch WM, Martinez-Hernandez A, Fink LM: In vitro plasminogen activator activity in human brain tumors. Cancer Res 38:297–302, 1978.

65. van Veelen CWM, Verbiest H, Zülch KJ, van Ketel B, van der Vlist MJM, Vlug AMC, Rijksen G, Staal GEJ: Pyruvate kinase in human brain tumours: Its significance in the treatment of gliomas. Acta Neurochir (Wien) 61:145–159, 1982.

66. Waymouth C: To disaggregate or not to disaggregate: Injury and cell disaggregation, transient or permament? In Vitro 10:97–111, 1974.

67. Weller RO: Perspectives in neuro-oncology, in Thomas DGT, Graham DI (eds): *Brain Tumours: Scientific Basis, Clinical In-*

vestigation and Current Therapy. London, Butterworth, 1980, pp 1–9.

68. Wikstrand CJ, Bigner DD: Expression of human fetal brain antigens by human tumors of neuroectodermal origin as defined by monoclonal antibodies. Cancer Res 42:267–275, 1982.
69. Yung WK, Shapiro JR, Shapiro WR: Heterogeneous chemosensitivities of subpopulations of human glioma cells in culture. Cancer Res 42:992–998, 1982.
70. Zänker KS, Stavrou D, Blümel G: Fibrin degradation products, produced by glioma cell–associated fibrinolysis and the partial inhibition of cell growth and migration in tissue culture. Cell Mol Biol 25:387–394, 1979.

62
Tumor Markers

Dennis E. Bullard
S. Clifford Schold, Jr.

A tumor marker is any substance that makes possible either a qualitative diagnosis of neoplasia or a quantitative estimate of tumor burden. The ideal tumor marker should be produced only by neoplastic tissue and should be released into an easily accessible fluid compartment in measurable quantities during an early stage of tumor development. As a screening tool, markers should allow early detection of malignant disease, with the potential for improving prognosis. As a staging instrument, they should provide a reliable estimate of tumor extent, prognosis, and location. As a reflection of tumor burden, they should allow evaluation of response to therapy and detection of early tumor recurrence. The value of tumor markers would be substantial with substances that even approximate this ideal. In most cases, however, this has not been realized, although promising putative tumor markers do exist. Biochemically these are usually proteins or glycoproteins circulating in any of the body fluids, functionally representing either excessive amounts of normally occurring hormones, enzymes, or antigens or substances such as oncofetal antigens and placental hormones, which are not normally found in most patient populations. With systemic malignant disease, a considerable amount of information has been generated, primarily with the oncofetal antigens, the placental proteins, and ectopic polypeptides.

Oncofetal Proteins

The first oncofetal antigen to be evaluated was carcinoembryonic antigen (CEA), a glycoprotein with a molecular weight of approximately 200,000.[14] This antigen is normally found in fetal endodermal cells and repressed during differentiation. CEA was initially described with adenocarcinoma of the rectum, and early reports seemed to indicate a specificity for colonic and rectal tumors, with high serum levels being found in almost all cases. Subsequent work, however, has shown elevated serum CEA levels in a wide spectrum of both malignant and nonmalignant conditions, including endodermally derived lung tumors, hepatic involvement from any malignant lesion, inflammatory bowel disease, pancreatitis, cirrhosis, rectal polyps, ethanol abuse, and cigarette smoking.[12,17] With many types of terminal malignant disease, especially with hepatic involvement, elevated CEA levels are seen in 50 to 90 percent of patients. Also, while a value of more than 2.5 ng/ml is abnormal, patients with nonmalignant disease may have serum values as high as 20 ng/ml, presenting a considerable degree of overlap with those patients having smaller tumor burdens.[12] This lack of specificity prevents CEA from being a definitive diagnostic test but does not preclude its use to follow tumor burden after initial diagnosis and treatment. In this respect, serum CEA provides a valuable indicator of early tumor recurrence or metastases and allows an estimation of the completeness of tumor resection, since in patients with persistently elevated CEA levels more than 1 month after surgery, the chances of residual or metastatic tumor being present are quite high. In patients who later develop elevated CEA levels, the biochemical diagnosis of recurrent tumor can often be made long before the clinical diagnosis.

Cerebrospinal fluid (CSF) CEA values above 1 ng/ml have been reported with leptomeningeal spread of lung cancer (89 percent), breast cancer (60 to 67 percent), malignant melanoma (25 to 33 percent), and carcinoma of the bladder.[13–16] It is unclear why elevation of CSF CEA values has been seen with tumors not usually associated with elevated serum levels. In general, CEA levels have paralleled the CNS tumor burden, although a direct relationship between cytology and CEA level has not been established. With intraparenchymal metastases, CEA determination has not proved consistently reliable even with CEA-positive primary tumors, unless the tumors are in approximation to the subarachnoid space or concomitant carcinomatous meningitis exists. This has been thought to be due to the combined high molecular weight of CEA and lack of direct subarachnoid space access of these intraparenchymal tumors; but no firm data exist to substantiate these speculations. Cerebrospinal fluid (CSF) CEA in patients with primary intracranial tumors is also usually nondetectable, although in approximately 10 percent of cases mild elevations in CSF CEA have been reported. Only carcinomatous meningitis from lung or breast carcinoma consistently elevates the CSF CEA levels in a majority of patients, and most of these patients will also have positive cytological tests.

A second oncofetal protein, alpha fetoprotein (AFP), has also proved useful in the evaluation of certain diseases.[2,12] Like all oncofetal proteins, AFP is a gene product expressed during a certain phase of fetal development—in this case, one which peaks at the third through fourth months of gestation, then gradually declines to normal serum levels by the end of the first year of life. AFP is a glycoprotein with a molecular weight of approximately 70,000 and has the electrophoretic mobility of an α_1-globulin. Like CEA, AFP is synthesized by fetal gastrointestinal tissue, and expression in adults is related most commonly to gastrointestinal and testicular malignant disease. Elevated serum AFP levels have also been seen in patients with carcinoma of the ovary, stomach, pancreas, colon, or lung; in patients with hepatitis or cirrhosis; in patients with ataxia telangiectasia; and in patients from areas of endemic liver disease. While serum levels greater than 500 ng/ml are usually associated with primary hepatic tumors, AFP lacks absolute specificity, and its usefulness is largely to monitor tumor burden following therapy in patients with embryonal and hepatic carcinomas.

Testicular tumors have been reported to metastasize to the CNS in 16 to 25 percent of patients, and elevated CSF levels of AFP have been reported with CNS involvement in a small number of patients.[14–16] Certain primary germ cell CNS tumors, specifically primary intracranial yolk sac tumors, endodermal sinus tumors, and embryonal carcinomas, have been reported to have elevated CSF AFP with normal serum levels or to have abnormal CSF-to-serum gradients. The presence of elevated CSF AFP appears to be a more reliable and sensitive marker for these tumors than cytological findings. Utilizing a panel of markers, such as the beta chain of human chorionic gonadotropin (hCG), in addition to AFP and cytological studies, both the diagnosis and the response to therapy may be evaluated. Given the relative difficulty of surgically biopsying these tumors in their location around the pineal region and their variable radiosensitivity, the use of CSF AFP and other markers should be a primary step in the diagnostic evaluation of all patients with pineal region tumors.

Another important use of AFP has been as a marker for neural tube defects.[2] The elevation of AFP in the amniotic fluid of pregnant women has been consistently seen with open meningomyeloceles, anencephaly, and other severe midline neural tube anomalies. Elevated amniotic fluid AFP levels, however, are not specific for neural tube defects and may rarely be elevated in other conditions. Moreover, with certain midline fusion anomalies, specifically skin-covered myelomeningoceles, which may represent up to 20 percent of neural tube lesions, the amniotic AFP may not be elevated. While not as sensitive, maternal serum elevations of AFP have also proved useful as a general screening procedure. Since neural tube anomalies occur most frequently without a prior family history, serum AFP monitoring selects those women who may benefit from the more invasive amniocentesis.

A third oncofetal protein, pancreatic oncofetal antigen (POA), has been demonstrated in the serum of patients with pancreatic cancers.[12] Somewhat lower levels, however, have also been found in patients with cancers of the lung, colon, stomach, and breast. The role of this protein in the CSF has not been assessed.

Placental Proteins

The placental proteins are substances normally elaborated by the placenta and found in the serum of pregnant and postpartum women.[1,9] Human chorionic gonadotropin, a glycoprotein with a molecular weight of 45,000, is structurally related in its alpha subunit to the anterior pituitary hormone, human luteinizing hormone (hLH), and is secreted by the placental trophoblastic epithelium. The immunologically specific beta chain fraction, hCG-β, is found normally only in fetal blood and in the serum of pregnant and immediately postpartum females. Its presence in other situations is a sensitive marker for disease. Classically an elevated hCG level is diagnostic of uterine choriocarcinoma, most specifically the syncytiotrophoblastic elements of that tumor. However, elevated hCG levels have also been found in patients with choriocarcinomas, embryonal cell tumors, and teratocarcinomas of the testis, primary and metastatic ovarian tumors, and cancers of the pancreas, stomach, liver, and breast.

The CSF hCG usually is 0.5 to 2 percent of the serum level in non-CNS tumors. The presence of a significantly higher CSF level is usually a reliable diagnostic sign of metastatic CNS involvement by choriocarcinoma of the uterus or testis or of primary choriocarcinoma or embryonal cell carcinoma in the pineal region or suprasellar region.[14–16] With metastatic tumors, the level of CSF hCG appears to accurately reflect the tumor burden, although a definitive study to establish this has not been performed. The use of hCG in conjunction with other germ cell tumor markers, such as AFP, also appears to be helpful in establishing the histological diagnosis among posterior third ventricular tumors. The sensitivity and specificity of CSF hCG as an indicator for the presence of these tumors appears quite good.

Two other placental proteins, human placental lactogen (hPL) and placental alkaline phosphatase (PAP), are secreted by trophoblastic tissue and found normally in the serum of pregnant women. Both proteins are also found in the serum of women with trophoblastic tumors and in a small percentage of patients with nontrophoblastic tumors. Neither of these proteins has been evaluated in the CSF.

Ectopic Hormones

An extremely wide variety of tumors are also associated with hormone and prohormone production.[1,3,7,11,12] These tumors may be endocrine or nonendocrine in nature and are frequently ectopic in location. The substances produced by them are virtually all peptides, and most are similar to peptides normally found in the anterior pituitary gland, the remainder of the CNS, or the gastrointestinal tract and its embryologic derivatives. These cells are classified as amine precursor uptake and decarboxylation (APUD) cells. They are widely distributed in the body and include melanocytes, adrenomedullary cells, pancreatic cells, thyroid C cells, and epithelial cells found in the thymus, respiratory tract, and genitourinary system. APUD cells were originally thought to be derived solely from the neural crest, but more recent evidence suggests that they are derived from primitive epithelial neuroendocrine cells. Although almost any type of neoplasm may be involved, certain types are more prevalent. Presently, more than twenty hormones or prohormones are reportedly secreted by tumors. The most common is the ectopic production of ACTH by oat cell carcinoma of the lung. The lung tumors which secrete ACTH, however, may be of several histological types, not all of which have APUD features. In fact, the overall APUD functions of the tumor cells has not been demonstrated to be linked to the hormone production.

Detection and identification of ectopic hormone product, while not tumor-specific, has often proved useful in early diagnosis and evaluation of tumor response to therapy. The widespread nature of these cells and the fluctuations in hormone production with tumor differentiation, however, have precluded consistent reliability for tumor localization or as a monitor of tumor burden. Their role in estimating CNS involvement has not been addressed.

Enzymatic Markers

Other substances utilized as tumor markers have consisted primarily of enzymatic markers, polyamines, sterol metabolites, and immunochemically defined proteins. Each of these types of marker has been evaluated in relation to CNS tumors, primarily by quantitating levels in the CSF. Because of the diversity of these substances and the scope of this section, only the relation of these markers to CNS tumors is here addressed.[4,12–15] Of these substances, the enzymatic markers have received the most attention, and over twenty have been evaluated. Several of these deserve detailed discussion.

β-Glucuronidase, which hydrolyzes the β-glycoside bond between glucuronic acid and other moieties, is found in many body tissues and tends to increase in concentration with malignant change, levels in the CSF being normally below 45 mU per liter. With meningeal carcinomatosis, especially from carcinoma of the breast or lung, or malignant melanoma, these levels can be markedly elevated. With leukemic meningeal involvement, intraparenchymal metastases, and primary intracranial tumors, the results have not been so reliable.

Similarly, lactic dehydrogenase (LDH), which is involved in anaerobic glycolysis, is widely distributed in the body, especially in the CNS. With malignant transformation, the isoenzyme distribution of the five fractions of LDH changes; specifically, there is a shift from the normally dominant fractions 1 and 2 to fractions 4 and 5. With carcinomatous meningitis this abnormality is usually present, while with metastatic intraparenchymal tumors and primary tumors, no significant difference from controls has been consistently noted. Unfortunately, similar shifts have also been seen with granulocytic meningitis, and the sensitivity and specificity for LDH is rather poor when measured in CSF rather than directly from brain homogenates.

The remainder of the enzymatic markers have had only limited investigation. They include isocitrate dehydrogenase, aspartate aminotransferase, creatine phosphokinase, acid phosphatase, glucose phosphate isomerase, leucine aminopeptidase, adenylate kinase, lysozyme, glycerol phosphate dehydrogenase, enolase, aldolase C, carbonic anhydrase, and glutamine synthetase.

Polyamines

The polyamines appear to be produced as side products by cells undergoing RNA synthesis during the growth phase, and increased intracellular concentrations of the polyamines have been reported in neoplastic cells.[15] The original studies with these substances reported increased urine levels of three of the polyamines—spermidine, spermine, and putrescine—in patients with solid tumors, including patients with CNS tumors. Subsequent work with the polyamines has closely linked levels of CSF polyamines with cell metabolism and proliferation, without demonstrating a relationship to CSF protein levels.[7,15] Present data suggest that the polyamines may have value in detecting tumor recurrence in patients with malignant primary tumors. However, technical difficulties have prevented wide use of this assay. With glioblastomas, CSF putrescine has been uniformly elevated while elevated spermidine levels have been reported less consistently. In medulloblastoma patients, CSF putrescine and spermidine levels are also elevated in the CSF, appearing to correlate well with response to therapy and serving as an early indicator of tumor recurrence. Tissue homogenates of astrocytomas have shown elevations of putrescine, which increase with the degree of anaplasia, while benign CNS tumors have lower levels than normal brain. The spermidine and spermine levels, however, vary widely without a clear pattern. With large tumors, the sensitivity of the combined polyamines for medulloblastomas and malignant gliomas has been reported to be more than 95 percent. With medulloblastomas, the total CSF polyamine level has been demonstrated to be predictive of recurrence in the majority of patients,[7] but the value of this assay with smaller or less malignant tumors is not clear. Blood levels of polyamines, although less sensitive than CSF levels, have also been reported to be elevated in patients with primary intracranial tumors and to parallel the degree of anaplasia. These substances have not been well analyzed in metastatic tumors or with carcinomatous meningitis.

Desmosterol

Desmosterol (24-dehydrocholesterol), the precursor of cholesterol, is known to be found in high concentrations in the developing brain and to be related to the high degree of brain sterol biosynthesis.[15,16] In the adult, desmosterol is usually undetectable in the CSF even with the administration of triparanol, an agent which blocks the conversion of desmosterol to cholesterol. When given to patients with a wide spectrum of primary and metastatic tumors, however, triparanol usually induces a significant elevation in CSF levels of desmosterol. In two limited studies, CSF levels of desmosterol have correlated reasonably well with recurrence of glioblastomas, ependymomas, medulloblastomas, meningiomas, and pituitary adenomas. Triparanol, however, has a known degree of toxicity, and detection of desmosterol in the CSF of patients without prior administration of triparanol has not been consistently noted. Controversy has also surrounded the techniques utilized by various investigators to measure the desmosterol levels. While present data suggest a relation between desmosterol levels in the CSF and the presence of tumor, the problems associated with induction and measurement of the sterols have prevented this test from being widely used diagnostically.

Beta-2-Microglobulin

Beta-2-microglobulin (β_2m) is a component of cell membrane that is closely related to HLA antigen expression. Serum levels are frequently elevated in patients with hematologic neoplasms. Cerebrospinal fluid β_2m levels have been reported elevated in patients with leukemia or lymphoma involving the leptomeninges,[8] as well as in patients with leptomeningeal metastases from solid tumors.[10] Like other markers, this peptide appears to be less useful in the diagnosis of parenchymal metastases or primary brain tumors, although in the report from Memorial Hospital Sloan Kettering Institute, two of three patients with primary CNS lymphomas had elevated CSF β_2m levels.[10] A commercial kit is now available for the radioimmunoassay of β_2m, and its value as a CNS tumor marker should be determined in the near future.

Immunochemically Defined Markers

This group of markers is broadly defined and consists of those substances which have been discovered or characterized by immunochemical means. Several of the previously discussed markers, most notably AFP, would also fall into this group by definition. For this section, however, the common thread is that these substances were immunochemically identified during attempts to characterize the cell populations present in the CNS.[4] As such, they often bridge the gap between brain tissue markers and brain tumor markers.

The first of these substances studied was S-100 protein, which consists of two acid proteins that are soluble in saturated ammonium sulfate at pH 7.1. Initial work demonstrated this substance to be associated with astrocytes and to a lesser extent with oligodendroglia and neurons. Recent work, however, has shown S-100 to be present also in neural crest–derived tumors. Studies of human brain tumors have shown varying levels of S-100 with glioblastomas, anaplastic astrocytomas, oligodendrogliomas, and acoustic neuromas. The levels of S-100 have not been found useful in either diagnostic or prognostic studies. The potential exists, though, that S-100 may be beneficial in evaluating the cell of origin for certain highly undifferentiated tumors.

The second protein, glial fibrillary acidic protein (GFAP), was first isolated in 1968 from brain tissue of patients with Tay-Sachs disease and was believed to be specific for fibrillary astrocytes. A similar protein was identified several years later by a second laboratory in association with multiple sclerosis plaques and postleukotomy scars. Subsequent immunochemical studies have demonstrated identical specificities for these two substances, and it is now known that GFAP is an acidic intracellular protein found in association with morphologically astroglial cells. Evaluation of GFAP with normal brain and glioblastomas has demonstrated a two- to sixfold increase of GFAP in non-necrotic brain tumors. Some equivocal evidence exists, however, that correlates the degree of differentiation of the glial tumor directly with the level of GFAP, demonstrating higher levels of GFAP with cellular differentiation.

As with S-100, GFAP has also been used to investigate the cellular origin for certain tumors. GFAP has been found in small amounts in metastatic tumors, meningiomas, and craniopharyngiomas, where it has most frequently been postulated to be a contaminant, and in higher levels in a few hemangioblastomas, ependymomas, and medulloblastomas, where it has been used to question the nature of the cellular subpopulations and the origins of these tumors. Presently, GFAP is often used clinically in the diagnosis of highly primitive or anaplastic tumors to support or refute an astrocytic origin for the lesion.

Attempts to use CSF GFAP levels as a marker for glial tumors have not been consistently successful. While the highest CSF levels to date have been from patients with malignant gliomas, a wide spectrum of nonglial tumors and non-neoplastic neurological diseases have also shown consistently elevated CSF GFAP levels. The diagnostic usefulness of GFAP still needs to be defined, although it appears that its histopathological value may outweigh its value as a CSF tumor marker.

Recent Developments

With the development of monoclonal antibodies by the fusion of mouse spleen and myeloma cells, a new frontier in immunochemistry has evolved.[4–6] Utilizing this method, the specificity, sensitivity, and reproducibility of immunologically defining substances has improved immensely. It is now possible to produce large amounts of single-class antibodies to a specific antigenic determinant. Monoclonal antibodies have already been produced against several normal CNS antigens, including nicotinic acetylcholine receptors and substance P, and against a panel of human glioma–derived cell line antigens.[4] It appears likely that this technological advance will allow greater specificity and sensitivity in defining all cell populations and therefore in the evaluation of tumor antigenic expression.

References

1. Baylin SB, Mendelsohn G: Ectopic (inappropriate) hormone production by tumors: Mechanisms involved and the biological and clinical implications. Endocr Rev 1:45–77, 1980.
2. Brock DJH: Alphafetoprotein and the prenatal diagnosis of neural tube defects. JR Coll Surg Edinb 23:184–192, 1978.

3. Frohman LA: Ectopic hormone production. Am J Med 70:995–997, 1981.

4. Jones TR, Bigner DD: Distribution of cell and tissue-associated markers in normal brain and central nervous system neoplasia, in Sell S: (ed): *Cancer Markers: Diagnostic and Developmental Significance.* Clifton, N.J., Humana Press, 1980, pp 381–422.

5. Kennett RH, Jonak ZL, Bechtol KB: Monoclonal antibodies against human tumor-associated antigens, in Kennett RH, McKearn TJ, Bechtol KB (eds): *Monoclonal Antibodies: Hybridomas: A New Dimension in Biological Analysis.* New York, Plenum, 1980, pp 155–168.

6. Köhler G, Milstein C: Continuous cultures of fused cells secreting antibody of predefined specificity. Nature 256:495–497, 1975.

7. Marton LJ, Edwards MS, Levin VA, Lubich WP, Wilson CB: CSF polyamines: A new and important means of monitoring patients with medulloblastoma. Cancer 47:757–760, 1981.

8. Mavligit GM, Stuckey SE, Cabanillas FF, Keating MJ, Tourtelotte WW, Schold SC, Freireich EJ: Diagnosis of leukemia or lymphoma in the central nervous system by beta-2-microglobulin determination. N Engl J Med 303:718–722, 1980.

9. Odell, WD: Endocrine manifestations of tumors: Ectopic hormone production, in Wyngaarden JB, Smith LH Jr (eds): *Textbook of Medicine.* Philadelphia, Saunders, 1982, pp 1022–1026.

10. Rogers LO, Fleisher MD, Schold SC, Schwartz MK, Posner JB: CSF beta-2-microglobulin in patients with systemic cancer and primary brain tumors. Neurology (NY) In press.

11. Rosen SW, Weintraub BD, Vaitukaitus JL, Sussman HH, Hershman JM, Muggia FM: Placental proteins and their subunits as tumor markers. Ann Intern Med 82:71–83, 1975.

12. Schein PS: Tumor markers, in Wyngaarden JB, Smith LH Jr (eds): *Textbook of Medicine.* Philadelphia, Saunders, 1982, pp 1020–1022.

13. Schold SC, Bullard DE: Cerebrospinal fluid analysis in central nervous system cancer, in Wood JH (ed): *Neurobiology of Cerebrospinal Fluid*, vol I. New York, Plenum, 1980, pp 549–559.

14. Schold SC, Wasserstrom WR, Fleisher M, Schwartz MK, Posner JB: Cerebrospinal fluid biochemical markers of central nervous system metastases. Ann Neurol 8:597–604, 1980.

15. Seldenfeld J, Marton LJ: Biochemical markers of central nervous system tumors measured in cerebrospinal fluid and their potential use in diagnosis and patient management: A review. JNCI 63:919–931, 1979.

16. Wasserstrom WR, Schwartz MK, Fleisher M, Posner JB: Cerebrospinal fluid biochemical markers in central nervous system tumors: A review. Ann Clin Lab Sci 11:239–251, 1981.

17. Zamcheck N: The present status of carcinoembryonic antigen (CEA) in diagnosis, detection of recurrence, prognosis and evaluation of therapy of colonic and pancreatic cancer. Clin Gastroenterol 5:625–638, 1976.

Gliomas

63

Gliomas: Pathology

Peter C. Burger

Gliomas are exceptionally diverse in location, morphology, differentiation, ease of excision, and response to postoperative therapy.[5,17,18,23–25] Knowledge of their pathology is a great practical aid, since it provides a conceptual framework in which to place specific lesions, defines reasonable expectations of surgery for each neoplasm, and clarifies the significance of histological diagnoses as formulated according to current classifications.

Astrocytic Neoplasms

Neoplasms derived from astrocytes make up an extremely large and heterogeneous group. However, since some oversimplification is appropriate in this limited discussion, astrocytic neoplasms are divided here into two large categories: (1) fibrillary astrocytic neoplasms (including glioblastoma multiforme), and (2) a group of childhood tumors encompassing optic nerve astrocytoma, juvenile pilocytic astrocytoma of the hypothalamus, and cerebellar astrocytoma.

Fibrillary Astrocytic Neoplasms

Fibrillary, or fibrous, astrocytes diffusely populate the brain and are especially prominent in the white matter, where their stellate processes can be identified with the historically significant but technically capricious gold impregnation of Cajal. Antibodies to glial fibrillary acidic protein (GFAP) and the immunoperoxidase method have been combined to bring a more specific and predictable technique to bear on the identification of this protein.[8] Fibrillary astrocytes are readily seen, since their processes are rich in the "glial" filaments which are the predominant site of this protein.

When neoplastically transformed, the fibrillary astrocyte produces over 80 percent of all astrocytic neoplasms and the majority of all gliomas. Like other gliomas, these astrocytic neoplasms extend as a continuum from well-differentiated lesions to anaplastic tumors. Several grading systems have been formulated for therapeutic and prognostic purposes. The first to be widely used in this country was that of Bailey and Cushing, who likened the morphology of the neoplastic cells in these lesions to astrocytes in three stages of embryologic development, namely, the astrocyte, the astroblast, and the spongioblast. Accordingly, the neoplasms which resembled these cells were named, in increasing order of malignancy, astrocytoma, astroblastoma, and spongioblastoma (later glioblastoma) multiforme (Table 63-1).[1] At the Mayo Clinic, meanwhile, surgical pathologists were refining a four-tiered grading system for carcinomas, and from this environment emerged the Kernohan system dividing this same group of neoplasms into four grades (astrocytoma grades I, II, III, and IV) (Table 63-1).[12]

TABLE 63-1 Classification of Fibrillary Astrocytic Neoplasms

Bailey & Cushing[1]	Kernohan[12]	Others	WHO[25]
Astrocytoma	Astrocytoma grade 1	Astrocytoma	Astrocytoma (grade 2)*
Astroblastoma	Astrocytoma grade 2	Anaplastic astrocytoma	Anaplastic astrocytoma (grade 3)
Spongioblastoma multiforme	Astrocytoma grade 3 Astrocytoma grade 4	Glioblastoma multiforme	Glioblastoma multiforme (poorly differentiated glioma, grade 4)†

*Lesions considered grade 1 include the optic nerve glioma, pilocytic astrocytoma, and cerebellar astrocytoma.
†Not classified as an astrocytic neoplasm.

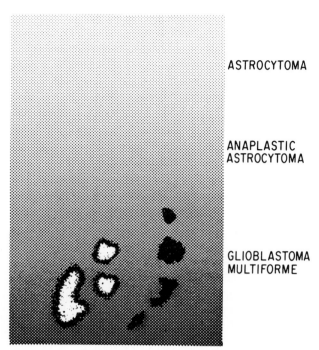

Figure 63-1 Fibrillary astrocytic neoplasms. The classification utilized in this chapter divides fibrillary astrocytic neoplasms into three lesions on the basis of increasing cellularity and cytologic abnormality. As is apparent from this illustration depicting the gradations of cellularity, there is no precise division between astrocytoma, anaplastic astrocytoma, and glioblastoma on the basis of these criteria alone. The glioblastoma is readily recognized when necrosis with pseudopalisading (*bottom left*) and abundant vascular proliferation (*bottom right*) are present, although this diagnosis may not be possible in small specimens when these two features are not observed.

In recent years there has been a general, although not universal, reluctance to subdivide glioblastoma multiforme into the two grades required by the Kernohan classification, and the fibrillary astrocytic neoplasms are now often classified into three subdivisions as originally suggested by Bailey and Cushing. At present, however, there is little effort to seek similarities between neoplastic and embryologic cells, and the three lesions are often referred to as the astrocytoma, the anaplastic (malignant) astrocytoma, and glioblastoma multiforme. The following discussion employs this latter classification (Fig. 63-1), although it is not ideal, since the term *anaplastic* astrocytoma suggests a fully malignant lesion rather than the intermediate neoplasm it denotes. Abroad, it is used in this most malignant sense and is often synonomous with glioblastoma multiforme. Furthermore, the use of the three-tiered system by some pathologists and the Kernohan classification by others is an obvious source of confusion that is most apparent in the interpretation of lesions designated as grade III. In the Kernohan system, such a neoplasm is a glioblastoma, while to many pathologists it now refers to a tumor of intermediate malignancy—the anaplastic astrocytoma. Unfortunately, some authors do not define the

meaning of grade III, although it is often apparent from survival statistics that the anaplastic astrocytoma is intended.

Astrocytoma

The lower and "benign" end of the spectrum of fibrillary astrocytic neoplasms begins with the astrocytoma (Fig. 63-1). In adults, most of these lesions arise in the cerebral hemispheres where the symptoms, especially seizures, may be of long standing. In children, the brain stem, particularly the pons, is favored.[13] The spinal cord is affected in both age groups. In the cerebral hemispheres, the well-differentiated astrocytoma is less common than the glioblastoma, whereas the opposite is true in the spinal cord. In any location, the neoplasm alters the color and texture of the parent tissue, but this is most obvious in the cerebral hemispheres, where the imparted yellow stringiness of the white matter is most readily seen and felt (Fig. 63-2).[21,24] Cysts filled with clear yellow fluid may be seen, and gritty grains of calcium may be encountered in a minority of cases. The ill-defined borders of these lesions are reminders that complete surgical excision is an elusive goal. The brain stem lesions are similarly ill defined and may lobulate the external surface of the pons and partially surround the basilar artery. Some well-differentiated solid or cystic brain stem astrocytomas protrude far into the fourth ventricle.

Microscopically, the nuclei of neoplastic well-differenti-

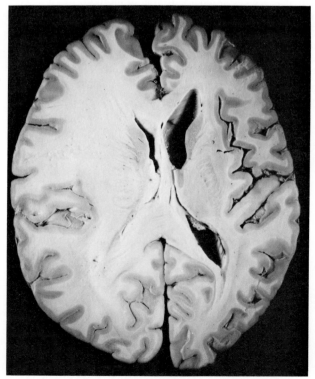

Figure 63-2 Astrocytoma. As in this 45-year-old man with weakness and signs of increased intracranial pressure, the well-differentiated astrocytoma produces a diffuse, ill-defined expansion of the white matter.

ated astrocytes are round and generally uniform. They congregate in a density not markedly different from that of normal white matter. Mitoses are rare, and the vascular proliferation and necrosis which characterize the glioblastoma are not observed. A helpful diagnostic feature is a vacuolated state produced by small pools of eosinophilic fluid and known as *microcystic change*. This is not usually found either in reactive astrocytosis or in markedly anaplastic neoplasms. The pink cytoplasm with the multiple filament-rich processes characteristic of astrocytes may or may not be seen in standard histological sections but are visualized by electron microscopy or staining for GFAP (Figs. 63-3 and 63-4). These astrocytic characteristics are exaggerated in the process-laden astrocytes which predominate in the subcategory of astrocytomas known as *gemistocytic astrocytomas*. Some think that gemistocytic lesions behave aggressively and are more likely to evolve into glioblastomas.[17,18]

The ease of histological diagnosis of the well-differentiated astrocytoma depends on the extent to which the lesion differs from normal or gliotic brain. This difference may not be great, and a firm diagnosis may not always be possible, especially in small specimens such as those from the brain stem, spinal cord, or edge of a cerebral lesion. As much tissue as possible should be submitted for histological studies, especially from the macroscopically most abnormal area. Frozen section examination should also be directed at this latter site to minimize the likelihood of a "consistent with" or "I think this is" diagnosis that can be the pathologist's way of hedging when there is uncertainty about the nature of the lesion.

Anaplastic (Malignant) Astrocytoma

The anaplastic astrocytoma is intermediate in anaplasia between astrocytoma and glioblastoma multiforme. In its common location in the cerebral hemispheres of adults, it is

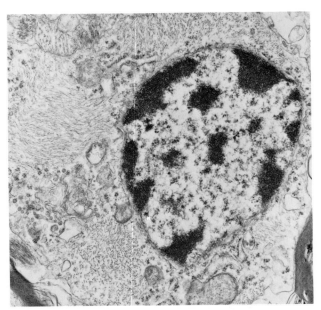

Figure 63-4 Astrocytoma. Intracytoplasmic intermediate filaments are largely the ultrastructural correlate of GFAP positivity in the well-differentiated astrocyte. (×25,500.)

also intermediate in the age of highest incidence (40 to 50 years), duration of preoperative symptoms, and degree of macroscopic abnormality. The lesion also occurs in the brain stem and spinal cord.

The increment of cellularity over the well-differentiated astrocytoma makes macroscopic abnormality more apparent, so that the anaplastic astrocytoma is better defined from the surrounding brain. Microscopically it is also more abnormal, as the cells are more populous, more pleomorphic, and more often present in mitotic division (Fig. 63-1). The cells may invade the cerebral cortex to satellite neurons and mass within the subpial position.[21] Cells with cytoplasmic features of astrocytes are often prominent, but less well differentiated cells may also be seen. Absent is the necrosis which characterizes glioblastoma multiforme, although vascular proliferation may be seen in limited degrees (Fig. 63-1).

The diagnosis of anaplastic astrocytoma depends on the histological distinction between well-differentiated astrocytoma on one hand and glioblastoma multiforme on the other. The better differentiated varieties of the anaplastic astrocytoma are separated from the well-differentiated astrocytoma by imprecise and subjective differences in cellularity and pleomorphism. The criteria for distinguishing these two lesions may therefore vary among observers, and the dividing line may wander even in the same microscopist from observation to observation. At the other extreme the anaplasia of this lesion overlaps with that of glioblastoma, and there is no well-established criterion to separate these two lesions on the basis of cellularity or anaplasia alone. As discussed below, the glioblastoma is often diagnosed only when necrosis and/or vascular proliferation are present. If one holds rigorously to this rule, many glioblastomas will be underdiagnosed as anaplastic astrocytomas in small specimens, such as needle biopsies, that do not happen to include

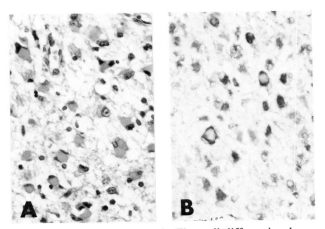

Figure 63-3 Astrocytoma. *A.* The well-differentiated astrocytoma is frequently composed of cells with copious pink cytoplasm and prominent cytoplasmic processes. (Hematoxylin and eosin, ×300.) *B.* The immunoperoxidase method for the identification of glial fibrillary acidic protein (GFAP) discloses the cytoplasmic positivity in these well-differentiated astrocytes. (×300.)

necrosis or vascular proliferation. It is not surprising, therefore, that some patients with "anaplastic astrocytomas" in the cerebral hemispheres do not survive for the 2 years expected for such patients.

Glioblastoma Multiforme

The graded anaplasia of the glioma group reaches its extreme in glioblastoma multiforme. The author considers this lesion to be a neoplasm of astrocytes because (1) the glioblastoma merges as a clinical entity with the two better differentiated lesions just discussed, (2) pathologically the glioblastoma sometimes evolves out of a better differentiated astrocytic tumor, and (3) it often contains neoplastic astrocytes. It is recognized, however, that many glioblastomas appear to arise *de novo*, some are totally undifferentiated; and a rare glioblastoma evolves out of another glioma such as an oligodendroglioma. Accordingly, some classifications such as that of the World Health Organization assign glioblastoma multiforme (along with a strange bedfellow—medulloblastoma) to a group of grade IV poorly differentiated lesions and do not classify it as an astrocytic neoplasm (Table 63-1).[25]

In any site, the glioblastoma expresses its outright anaplasia as the induration and sometimes fleshy grayness of high cellularity and the hemorrhagic necrosis of rapid growth (Fig. 63-5). These features are most apparent in the cerebral hemispheres of adults, where the characteristically deep-seated lesion is most common, but can also be observed in the brain stem or in the rare lesion of the spinal cord. The gray fleshiness is typical of any markedly cellular lesion and is often most apparent in areas of invaded cortical gray matter. The necrotic regions are usually more centrally placed and are known for distinctive variegation by reds, browns, and yellows. Unlike the well-differentiated astrocytoma, the mass often appears well defined, and any cysts are filled with dirty brown, rather than clear yellow, fluid. The neoplastic cells diffuse freely through the white matter and can funnel into fiber pathways such as the corpus callosum, internal capsule, or anterior commissure. Expansion into the opposite cerebral hemisphere then produces the classic butterfly lesion.

At surgery, the circumscription of the glioblastoma can be sufficiently pronounced, especially in the giant cell variant, to suggest a metastatic carcinoma. The deposition of collagen, either as a reactive process or as part of a neoplastic proliferation of fibroblasts ("gliosarcoma"), can enhance this definition and produce a discrete, firm mass. In general, however, the glioblastoma's infiltrating border, large size, and prominent central area of necrosis are distinguishing features. The soft necrotic character of some glioblastomas can be simulated by the primary cerebral lymphoma or the occasional infarct that comes to surgery. The latter shows prominent softening of the cerebral cortex and lacks the fleshy grayness of the glioma. A rare patient with a glioblastoma has the acute effects of a large intratumoral hemor-

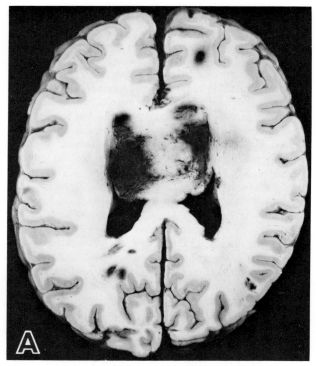
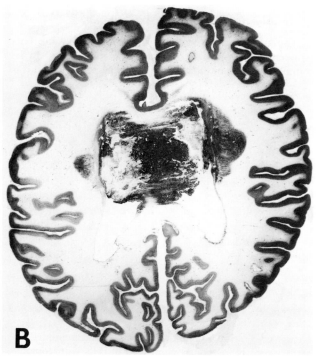

Figure 63-5 Glioblastoma multiforme. *A.* In contrast to the well-differentiated astrocytoma, the glioblastoma is hemorrhagic, necrotic, and sometimes macroscopically well defined. *B.* A whole-mount histologic section of the lesion in *A* emphasizes marked cellularity, necrosis, and apparent but misleading discreteness of the glioblastoma. (Cresyl fast violet.)

rhage, although the incidence of this event in this neoplasm is much lower than in metastatic neoplasms such as malignant melanoma and choriocarcinoma. The incidence is high enough, however, to justify pathological study of tissue fragments adherent to intracranial hematomas.

Microscopically, most of the viable neoplastic cells in the glioblastoma are concentrated in a region of high cellularity which circumscribes a central area of necrosis. In less advanced neoplasms, only scattered smaller areas of necrosis may be seen. The cellular areas are apparent macroscopically as the fleshy rim and radiographically as the ring of contrast enhancement.[4] Peripherally, the neoplastic cells diffuse away into the surrounding edematous brain for distances which must be considerable in light of the failure of large *en bloc* resections to cure the lesion. In contrast to the well-differentiated astrocytoma, calcification is rare.

The cytological composition of the glioblastoma includes a remarkably heterogeneous array of cell types such as fibrillary astrocytes, gemistocytes, larger and more pleomorphic astrocytes, and large bizarre cells with extreme pleomorphism (Fig. 63-6). For the most part these elements have characteristics generally attributed to astrocytes; that is, they have stellate processes as in the fibrillary and gemistocytic astrocytes and a prominent glassy cytoplasm as in the more bizarre astrocytes and giant cells. With immunoperoxidase staining, the fibrillary and gemistocytic astrocytes are often positive, whereas the pink cytoplasm of the other cells shows a variable positivity. By electron microscopy, the positivity with immunoperoxidase is correlated with the presence of the cytoplasmic "glial" filaments. These are numerous in the fibrillary astrocytes and unpredictably present in the large glassy cytoplasm of the remaining cell types.

A cell which often predominates in the glioblastoma but is present also in limited numbers in the anaplastic astrocytoma is a small anaplastic form with a round to elongated nucleus. These cells proliferate to a remarkably high density and are usually responsible for gray, fleshy areas. They also are extremely mobile and diffuse freely through the corpus callosum or other fiber tracts, invade the cortex to satellite neurons, and aggregate in the subpial position. In addition, they often are prominent about areas of necrosis, suggesting that this distinctive peripheral concentration of cells could be a consequence of their motility by which they accumulate at the edge because they are unable to pass through the necrotic center.

Some glioblastomas contain many large, bizarre cells, and such neoplasms have been variously referred to as giant cell glioblastoma, giant cell fibrosarcoma, or a type of gliosarcoma. The author would classify most of these lesions as gliomas and has noted that, in spite of their alarming microscopic appearance, the survival rate for patients with these lesions is somewhat more favorable than for those with the typical glioblastoma.[6] This may relate to their well-circumscribed nature and ease of surgical excision and/or to the reduced biological aggressiveness of bizarre giant cells.

Reactive fibroblasts populate some glioblastomas, whereas neoplastic fibroblasts proliferate in others. In either setting, mesenchymal cells are distinguished from the glial component by the former's polarity, association with reticulin and collagen, and absence of GFAP. A higher incidence in the temporal lobes has been suggested for the mixed neo-

plastic lesions known as gliosarcomas. It is worth noting that the distinction between reactive and neoplastic fibroblasts is often quite subjective: what is a gliosarcoma to one observer may be a glioblastoma with reactive fibrosis to another. The distinction appears largely academic, however, since the presence of a sarcomatous component does not appear to modify the prognosis.[15]

For diagnostic purposes, the histological diagnosis of glioblastoma is usually made as much on the basis of two distinctive secondary features as on cytological characteristics.[20,21] The first of these is vascular proliferation, by which vascular cells divide to produce coiled masses resembling renal glomeruli (Fig. 63-7). These new vessels often have a directional orientation, as the coils point toward a common site such as an area of high cellularity or necrosis. A response to an angiogenic factor liberated by the neoplasm has been suggested. The phenomenon is commonly called endothelial proliferation, although a recent study has noted that only part of the proliferating cells express the endothelial cell–specific factor VIII (von Willebrand's factor).[14]

As discussed below, vascular proliferation is an important feature differentiating glioblastoma multiforme from the well-differentiated fibrillary astrocytoma and the anaplastic astrocytoma, although a small amount of this proliferation is acceptable within the latter lesion. Although characteristic of the glioblastoma, vascular proliferation is found also in limited extent in other neoplasms, such as pilocytic astrocytoma, cerebellar astrocytoma, oligodendroglioma, and medulloblastoma.

The second diagnostically helpful feature in glioblastoma is necrosis (Fig. 63-7). The author believes that this feature, with or without associated pseudopalisading, is a firm differential point distinguishing glioblastoma from anaplastic astrocytoma. In lesions which have been previously treated with radiation therapy, of course, necrosis may not have this diagnostic value. A distinctive feature of necrotic areas in glioblastoma multiforme, especially the smaller foci, is a concentration of neoplastic cells that jostle with one another at the periphery. Because these cells are often elongated and oriented perpendicularly to their tangents with the necrotic area, the term *palisade* or *pseudopalisade* is applied. In a cerebral hemispheric glioma, this pseudopalisading is virtually diagnostic of glioblastoma. Neither the presence nor the absence of pseudopalisading, however, affects the prognostic or diagnostic value of necrosis.[6]

The pathological diagnosis of the glioblastoma is usually not difficult in generous specimens but can be problematic in small ones. The pathologist's need for an adequate specimen cannot be overemphasized. More diagnostic problems can be resolved by larger specimens than by application of special stains, including available immunologic techniques. Although purists contend that glioblastoma should be diagnosed only in the presence of necrosis and/or endothelial proliferation, in practice there is a justifiable temptation in surgical material to diagnose glioblastoma multiforme on the basis of extreme cellularity or pleomorphism alone, especially in the face of typical clinical and radiographic findings. This is not condoned in the less cellular lesions, however. The size of some small specimens also makes it difficult to exclude other malignant neoplasms such as a metastatic carcinoma. For this reason it is desirable to sub-

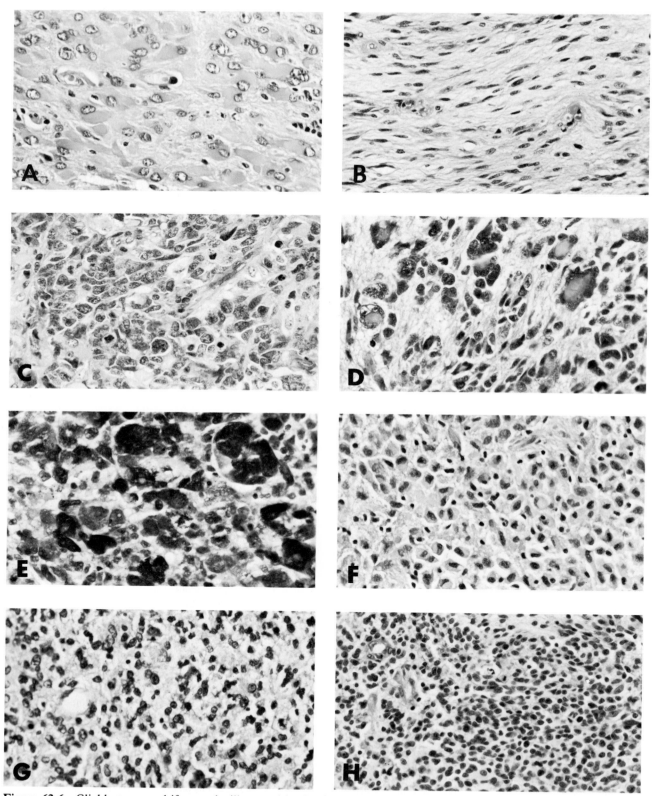

Figure 63-6 Glioblastoma multiforme. As illustrated in these panels from eight neoplasms, the predominant cell types in the glioblastoma are extremely varied. (Hematoxylin and eosin, ×250.)

mit to the pathologist specimens from the edge of the most cellular areas. Such tissues define the relationship of the neoplasm to the surrounding brain—a relationship that in the case of glioblastoma is one of diffuse infiltration and in metastatic carcinoma is the expansion of a cohesive mass. The diagnostically helpful endothelial proliferation and necrosis with pseudopalisading are also often prominent in this peripheral region. A positive GFAP stain indicates a glial, rather than an epithelial, neoplasm, but, like other special stains, it is often negative in the anaplastic lesion where its diagnostic value is most needed.

Radio- and chemotherapy produce marked changes in the glioblastoma that may be encountered at reoperation. Radiotherapy destroys small cells, leaving better differentiated astrocytes behind, and induces pleomorphism in residual neoplastic or reactive glia. Macroscopically, such treated lesions in remission are discrete, fibrotic, necrotic, and sometimes calcified.[4] The author's experience suggests that the subsequent phenomenon of recurrence relates largely to the regrowth of the small anaplastic cells discussed above. At this point, such cells are widely invasive and frequently extend down, or in the case of brain stem lesions up, the cerebral peduncles. Perhaps 10 percent of the lesions seed the ventricular and subarachnoid spaces. In such cases, CSF cytological study can be an effective diagnostic tool.[3]

Optic Nerve Astrocytoma, Hypothalamic Glioma, and Cerebellar Astrocytoma

The common gliomas in these three positions share incidence in childhood, a number of similar pathological features, and a slow rate of growth. These three neoplasms are grouped together at this point to emphasize these similarities, not to imply that they are necessarily the same histopathological entity, although this view has been expressed and the three lesions united under the term *spongioblastoma*.[23,24] The World Health Organization considers these neoplasms grade I.

Optic Nerve Astrocytoma (Optic Nerve Glioma)

The optic nerve is a cylindrical extrusion of the central nervous system partially compartmentalized along its long axis by fibrovascular septa. The proliferation of cells within the nerve enlarges these compartments and, as a consequence, the nerve itself. Additional expansion is produced by the cells' extension into the subarachnoid space, where they proliferate into a circumferential mass made firm by a secondary collagenous reaction. This is sometimes referred to as hyperplasia of the optic nerve sheath. At surgery, the well-developed lesion is therefore a fusiform swelling which, in cross section, contains a central or eccentrically placed hypertrophic nerve surrounded by a firmer and whiter corona of leptomeningeal neoplasm and collagen (Fig. 63-8). The neoplasm may occur anywhere along the nerve, from the optic chiasm to the globe. Multicentricity is common in neurofibromatosis.

Microscopically, the uniformity of the nuclei of the optic nerve glioma is commensurate with the lesion's leisurely growth. The cells are either elongated forms or stellate cells

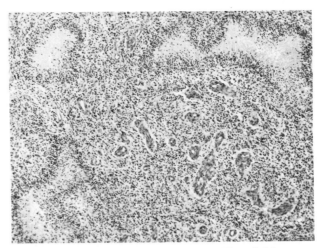

Figure 63-7 Glioblastoma multiforme. The glioblastoma multiforme is characterized by two diagnostically important features—necrosis with pseudopalisading and (*bottom right*) vascular proliferation. (Hematoxylin and eosin, ×100.)

producing a spongy tissue rich in mucopolysaccharide. The latter substance often lends a gelatinous quality to the macroscopic lesion, particularly the centrally placed enlarged nerve (Fig. 63-8). The elongated cells often contain Rosenthal fibers, whose structure and function are discussed in more detail in the following section on hypothalamic astrocytoma.

Although the neoplastic cells in the lesions are astrocytic in morphology, their cell of origin is unknown, since similar cells are not recognized components of the normal nerve.

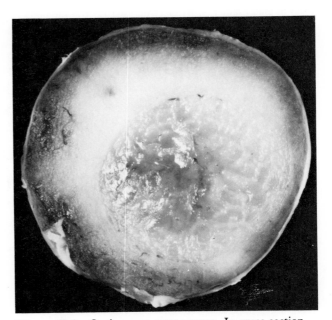

Figure 63-8 Optic nerve astrocytoma. In cross-section, the optic nerve astrocytoma produces a gelatinous enlargement of the nerve and a firmer surrounding halo of dense collagen and infiltrating neoplastic cells. (From Burger and Vogel.[5])

The normal fibrillary astrocytes of the optic nerve produce only rare neoplasms. These occur predominantly in adults and are similar in their invasiveness and aggressiveness to the fibrillary astrocytic neoplasms.

The treatment of optic nerve gliomas has been controversial because of the long post-treatment intervals required to compare different therapies.[9] From the point of view of a pathologist, the lesion has the expansile and invasive qualities of a neoplasm, albeit one well differentiated and slowly growing.

Hypothalamic Astrocytoma

The hypothalamic glioma is a soft, lobular, gray-tan lesion that, because of its slow growth, can attain considerable size. Positioned in the walls of the third ventricle, it is sometimes cystic and calcified. The lesion is often referred to as the *juvenile form of pilocytic astrocytoma*, but the term *spongioblastoma* is also sometimes used. Anteriorly, the lesions merge clinically and pathologically with the optic nerve glioma. The distinction between a large chiasmal glioma and a hypothalamic glioma may be arbitrary, depending only on the predominant position of the lesion. A neoplasm similar to the hypothalamic glioma occasionally occurs in the brain stem, especially in neurofibromatosis.

Microscopically, hypothalamic glioma is formed of bland cells in solid sheets and lobules and a curious juxtaposition of elongated cells in fascicles about attentuated areas of microcysts (Fig. 63-9A). The elongated cells are especially likely to contain a structure of considerable diagnostic importance, the Rosenthal fiber (Fig. 63-9B). This intracytoplasmic hyaline eosinophilic body stains bright red with Masson's stain and dense blue with PTAH. Tinctorially, the Rosenthal fiber therefore is consistent with an aggregated mass of glial filaments. By electron microscopy, the body is a dense amorphous structure anchored to the cytoplasmic glial filaments which are abundant in such cells. The body is negative, or only weakly positive, for GFAP. The Rosenthal

fiber is an extremely helpful histological feature, although it is not a diagnostic one, since it can occur also in periventricular gliosis—that secondary to craniopharyngioma being a notable and germane example. Vascular proliferation is sometimes noted in hypothalamic glioma, but it lacks the malignant connotation it has in fibrillary astrocytic neoplasms of the cerebral hemispheres, brain stem, or spinal cord.

The hypothalamic glioma of the juvenile type is histologically benign, and in only extremely rare cases has histological malignancy ensued. Because of the anatomical location, however, it cannot be completely excised.

Cerebellar Astrocytoma

The cerebellar astrocytoma is a well-circumscribed, often cystic, mass in the hemisphere or, less commonly, the vermis. Like the hypothalamic glioma, the neoplasm is remarkable microscopically for elongated areas of cellular polarity alternating with large or small areas of spongy microcystic change. The nuclei are characteristically uniform and euchromatic. Rosenthal fibers, calcium, and endothelial proliferation are frequently found. In common with the optic nerve and hypothalamic astrocytomas, cells closely resembling oligodendrocytes are often seen.

This classic lesion grows slowly and is amenable to total resection because of its location and circumscribed nature. Long survivals have followed even subtotal resections.[10]

Oligodendroglioma

Oligodendrocytes maintain myelin and hover obediently about large neurons in the cerebral cortex. They occur, therefore, in both gray matter and white matter but are much more numerous in the latter, where they are regimented along axis cylinders. Neoplasms derived from these cells are found principally in adults and primarily in the cerebral hemispheres, where the frontal lobes are greatly favored. Only rarely does an oligodendroglioma appear in the cerebellum, brain stem, or spinal cord. Radiographic calcification is common, and seizures may be present for many years preoperatively.[7]

At surgery, the lesions are infiltrating tumors and therefore can resemble the well-differentiated astrocytoma. Focally, however, the neoplasm is often extremely cellular, gray, and fleshy, so it can simulate an anaplastic neoplasm. Heavy calcification in a cerebral neoplasm in an adult should alert the surgeon and the pathologist to the possibility of this entity.

The oligodendroglioma has a number of distinctive histological features which usually permit a ready and unequivocal diagnosis in permanent sections, although the neoplasm can be difficult to recognize in frozen tissues. The nuclei are monotonously round and uniform, and are packed into cellular sheets that abut rather abruptly on the adjacent brain. In zones of cortical infiltration, perinuclear satellitosis is often more pronounced than in astrocytomas. Calcium is common as freestanding laminated bodies (calcospherites) or mineralization of blood vessel walls (Fig. 63-10). The presence of delicate angulated segments of capillaries that

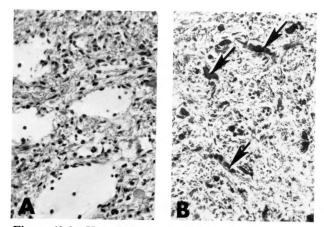

Figure 63-9 Hypothalamic pilocytic astrocytoma. *A.* The hypothalamic glioma of childhood contains well-differentiated glia surrounding microcysts. (Hematoxylin and eosin, ×100.) *B.* Intracytoplasmic eosinophilic bodies, or Rosenthal fibers (*arrows*), are a helpful diagnostic feature, although these structures may be found also in reactive astrocytes. (Hematoxylin and eosin, ×40.)

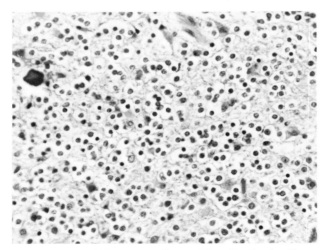

Figure 63-10 Oligodendroglioma. The oligodendroglioma is usually recognized by the perinuclear clear zones that produce the appearance of fried eggs. Calcification (*top left*) is common. (Hematoxylin and eosin, ×197.)

parenthesize focal areas of the parenchyma is an additional vascular change. Vascular cells commonly proliferate in the oligodendroglioma, although not usually in the marked glomeruloid formation as noted in glioblastoma. These cells may be present in even the well-differentiated lesion, where it does not necessarily have malignant connotations.

The most distinctive and diagnostic feature of the oligodendroglioma is an artifact due to its propensity for imbibing water during ischemia or autolysis (Fig. 63-10). When this fluid distends the cytoplasm, the bloated cells contain lucent perinuclear halos resembling the whites of fried eggs about their yolks. As diagnostically helpful as it is esthetically pleasing, this artifact is, unfortunately, not present in tissues which are fixed rapidly, particularly those used for frozen sections. The presence of this artifact constitutes the one, and probably the only, occasion when a pathologist is pleased that tissues are transported in the physiological but autolysis-promoting warm saline to which neurosurgeons entrust even excised tissue.

The classic oligodendroglioma is readily recognized in permanent section, although the absence of the characteristic halos in frozen sections may make recognition of this neoplasm difficult during surgery. Such a lesion may be interpreted as an astrocytoma or, because of its high cellularity, an anaplastic astrocytoma. The presence of sheets of high cellularity, monotonous nuclear roundness, calcium, and the typical vascular formations at this point are all suggestive features. If difficulty persists in permanent sections, the GFAP method can be extremely helpful, since oligodendroglia contain microtubules rather than glial filaments. The oligodendrocyte is therefore negative with this technique. The possibility of an astrocytic subpopulation in oligodendrogliomas is frequently raised, however, because of cells with the pink GFAP-positive cytoplasm typical of astrocytes. Some of these cells have the density and cytological appearance of reactive cells, whereas others have cytoplasmic and nuclear features suggesting neoplasia. The prognostic significance of the latter mixed lesions remains to be defined.

The typical oligodendroglioma described above merges with a continuum of increasingly cellular and pleomorphic lesions; the most anaplastic have nuclear or nucleolar enlargement, frequent mitoses, foci of necrosis, and abundant vascular proliferation. A detailed four-tiered grading system is not generally used for oligodendroglioma, but the term *oligodendroblastoma* is sometimes applied to these histologically malignant lesions. Although one would anticipate a considerable difference in survival between patients with the best differentiated and those with the most anaplastic lesions, this is not as striking as has been noted for astrocytic tumors. Recent studies, however, identify histological findings indicating a poorer prognosis, such as necrosis, mitotic figures, and abundant vascular proliferation.[22] A rare lesion has features of both anaplastic oligodendroglioma and glioblastoma multiforme. For prognostic purposes the author would consider such a neoplasm a glioblastoma multiforme.

Ependymoma

In common with their cell of origin, ependymomas are found throughout the central nervous system—from frontal horns to filum terminale. Intracranially, most occur in the fourth ventricle of children, although supratentorial neoplasms appear in both children and adults (Fig. 63-11).[2,16] The spinal lesions, especially those of the filum terminale, are usually seen in adults. A rare neoplasm arises as a primary tumefaction in sacral soft tissues or bone.

The intracranial lesions meet little resistance to intraventricular expansion and can become sizable exophytic masses before the onset of obstructive symptoms (Fig. 63-11). Such neoplasms are lobular, well circumscribed, and broadly attached to the ventricular floor from which they arise. Secondary adhesions to other ventricular surfaces may also

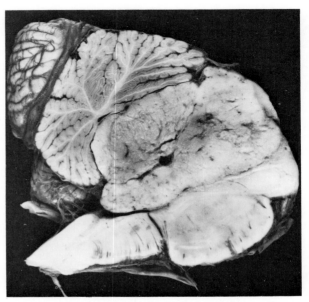

Figure 63-11 Ependymoma. Posterior fossa ependymomas are lobulated, discrete masses that arise from the fourth ventricular floor.

form. Characteristically, in the fourth ventricle, there is little invasion of the ventricular wall, and but for their origin from the brain stem, the neoplasms could be excised in toto. The larger ependymomas in any site may be cystic. Calcification may be present.

Intraoperatively, the fourth ventricular ependymoma can resemble a medulloblastoma pendent from the vermis, although it is not usually as soft and necrotic as the medulloblastoma in its typical form or as firm as the cerebellar neoplasm in its desmoplastic variety. In the spinal cord, an ependymoma's discreteness helps differentiate it from the infiltrating astrocytoma (Fig. 63-12). It can, however, be mimicked by the similarly discrete but more vascular and much less common spinal hemangioblastoma. Caudally, the filum terminale can be confused with a nerve root and an ependymoma be mistaken for a schwannoma.

Microscopically, there are two classes of ependymoma: (1) the classic lesion of the brain and spinal cord and (2) the distinctive myxopapillary ependymoma of the filum terminale. The classic ependymoma is a cellular neoplasm formed of cells with small, dark nuclei. Cytoplasmic differentiation produces two basic patterns. The first is the cells' expression of their glial heritage in cell processes packed with filaments (Fig. 63-13A).[8] When the ependymal cells are present in low density and these processes are abundant, the lesion can resemble the well-differentiated astrocytoma, and it may be difficult to distinguish the two lesions in small specimens. One helpful differential feature characteristic of ependymomas in such fibrillar areas, as well as in more cellular regions, is the orientation of cell processes to the wall of blood vessels. This produces a perivascular eosinophilic anuclear zone that, together with the perivascular nuclei, is known as a *perivascular pseudorosette.*

The second distinctive feature of the classic ependymoma is the epithelial differentiation by which cuboidal cells form

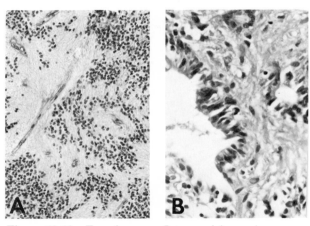

Figure 63-13   Ependymoma. Intracranial ependymomas often demonstrate both glial and epithelial features. *A.* The typical cellular ependymoma has perivascular clear zones filled with cytoplasmic glial processes. (Hematoxylin and eosin, ×40). *B.* Epithelia are present as ependymal rosettes and canals. (Hematoxylin and eosin, ×400).

epithelial surfaces (Fig. 63-13B). These include small canals known as *true ependymal rosettes,* large, flat epithelial surfaces, and crude papillations. In contrast to the choroid plexus papilloma, the epithelial features are never exclusive, and cells with more glial features are found within the interstices between rosettes and canals. As is also true of astrocytomas of the hypothalamus, optic nerve, and cerebellum, clusters of cells resembling oligodendrocytes are occasionally seen.

The structure of the myxopapillary ependymoma is quite different and may reflect the differences in embryology and anatomy between the caudal nervous system, derived from the caudal cell mass, and the principal portion of the nervous system, derived by neurulation. This lesion is extensively vacuolated by microcysts, whose expansion forces the nuclei into intravacuolar interstices. The mucosubstance also swells the walls of the blood vessels to which the neoplastic cells cling as the papillae that give this distinctive lesion its name (Fig. 63-14).

As in the other gliomas, there is a spectrum of histological anaplasia in the classic ependymoma from the well-differentiated lesion to the markedly cellular neoplasm. Anaplastic lesions are not recognized in the myxopapillary group, although the lesion is capable of wide dissemination though CSF pathways in rare instances. The Kernohan group developed a grading system of four tiers similar to that used for the astrocytomas, but this is not widely used, since it has been difficult to establish precise correlations between histological grade and biological behavior, because of the overriding importance of location and extent of excision in the length of postoperative survival. It appears, however, that the more anaplastic lesions behave more aggressively.[16] The term *ependymoblastoma* has sometimes been used for these more anaplastic lesions, although others reserve this term for a separate, extremely rare, neoplasm of childhood with epithelial surfaces similar to that of the primitive neuroepithelium.[17,18]

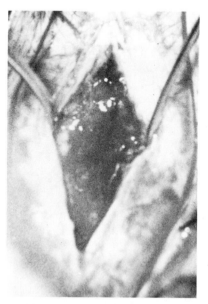

Figure 63-12   Ependymoma. In contrast to the spinal astrocytoma, the intramedullary ependymoma is a discrete mass.

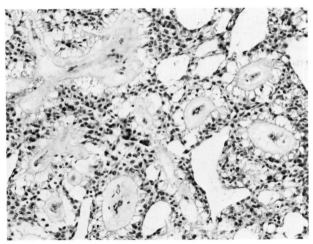

Figure 63-14 Myxopapillary ependymoma. The myxo-papillary ependymoma of the conus medullaris and filum terminale is characterized by mucoid substance that distends the walls of blood vessels and fills cystic spaces. The lesion is histologically distinct from the intracerebral and intramedullary ependymomas as illustrated in Fig. 63-13. (Hematoxylin and eosin, ×100.)

A neoplasm related to the ependymoma is the subependymoma. This discrete lobulated lesion occurs in either the anterior lateral ventricle or the posterior fourth ventricle.[19] In either, it is a reasonably common incidental necropsy finding but a rare surgical entity. Histologically, subependymomas are remarkable for the clustering of uniform nuclei in a highly fibrillar background. Some lesions in the lateral ventricles can be totally excised, but attachment to the medulla precludes this possibility in the fourth ventricle.

Mixed Gliomas

Although the preceding gliomas are often portrayed as pure entities, many contain other cell types or hybrid cells with partial expressions of more than one type. Thus the oligodendroglioma can contain cells with astrocytic characteristics, or an ependymoma or cerebellar astrocytoma may include dozens of "fried eggs." The term *mixed glioma* is applied when a second cell type is present in quantity,[11] but when present in limited numbers, a second cell type can be noted but not included in the diagnosis. At present, the significance of these mixed lesions is not known. Presumably, the application of markers for specific glia will continue to define the incidence and character of mixed gliomas, and careful correlative clinical studies will establish their prognostic significance.

References

1. Bailey P, Cushing HA: *A Classification of the Tumors of the Glioma Group on a Histogenetic Basis with a Correlated Study of Prognosis.* Philadelphia, Lippincott, 1926.
2. Barone BM, Elvidge AR: Ependymomas: A clinical survey. J Neurosurg 33:428–438, 1970.
3. Bigner SH, Johnston WW: The cytopathology of cerebrospinal fluid: II. Metastatic cancer, meningeal carcinomatosis and primary central nervous system neoplasms. Acta Cytol (Baltimore) 25:461–479, 1981.
4. Burger PC, Dubois PJ, Schold SC, Smith KR Jr., Odom GL, Crafts DC, Giangaspero F: Computerized tomographic and pathologic studies of the untreated, quiescent, and recurrent glioblastoma multiforme. J Neurosurg 58:159–169, 1983.
5. Burger PC, Vogel FS: *Surgical Pathology of the Nervous System and Its Coverings,* 2d ed. New York, Wiley, 1982.
6. Burger PC, Vollmer RT: Histologic factors of prognostic significance in the glioblastoma multiforme. Cancer 46:1179–1186, 1980.
7. Chin HW, Hazel JJ, Kim TH, Webster JH: Oligodendrogliomas: I. A clinical study of cerebral oligodendrogliomas. Cancer 45:1458–1466, 1980.
8. Deck JHN, Eng LF, Bigbee J, Woodcock SM: The role of glial fibrillary acidic protein in the diagnosis of central nervous system tumors. Acta Neuropathol (Berl) 42:183–190, 1978.
9. Dosoretz DE, Blitzer PH, Wang CC, Linggood RM: Management of glioma of the optic nerve and/or chiasm: An analysis of 20 cases. Cancer 45:1467–1471, 1980.
10. Gjerris F, Klinken L: Long-term prognosis in children with benign cerebellar astrocytoma. J Neurosurg 49:179–184, 1978.
11. Hart MN, Petito CK, Earle KM: Mixed gliomas. Cancer 33:134–140, 1974.
12. Kernohan JW, Mabon RF, Svien HJ, Adson AW: A simplified classification of the gliomas. Proc Staff Mtg Mayo Clin 24:71–75, 1949.
13. Littman P, Jarrett P, Bilaniuk LT, Rorke LB, Zimmerman RA, Bruce DA, Carabell SC, Schut L: Pediatric brain stem gliomas. Cancer 45:2787–2792, 1980.
14. McComb, RD, Jones TR, Pizzo SV, Bigner DD: Immunohistochemical detection of factor VIII/von Willebrand factor in hyperplastic endothelial cells in glioblastoma multiforme and mixed glioma-sarcoma. J Neuropathol Exp Neurol 41:479–489, 1982.
15. Morantz RA, Feigin I, Ransohoff J II: Clinical and pathological study of 24 cases of gliosarcoma. J Neurosurg 45:398–408, 1976.
16. Mørk SJ, Løken AC: Ependymoma: A follow-up study of 101 cases. Cancer 40:907–915, 1977.
17. Rubinstein LJ: *Tumors of the Central Nervous System,* Atlas of Tumor Pathology, fasc. 6, 2d ser., Washington, DC, Armed Forces Institute of Pathology, 1972.
18. Russell DS, Rubinstein LJ: *Pathology of Tumours of the Nervous System,* 4th ed. Baltimore, Williams & Wilkins, 1977.
19. Scheithauer BW: Symptomatic subependymoma. J Neurosurg 49:689–696, 1978.
20. Scherer HJ: Structural development in gliomas. Am J Cancer 34:333–351, 1938.
21. Scherer HJ: Cerebral astrocytomas and their derivatives. Am J Cancer 40:159–198, 1940.
22. Smith MT, Ludwig CL, Godfrey AD, Armbrustmacher VW: Grading of oligodendrogliomas. Cancer 52:2107–2114, 1983.
23. Zülch KJ: *Atlas of the Histology of Brain Tumors.* New York, Springer, 1971.
24. Zülch KJ: *Atlas of Gross Neurosurgical Pathology.* New York, Springer 1975.
25. Zülch KJ: *Histological Typing of Tumours of the Central Nervous System.* Geneva, World Health Organization, 1979.

64

Supratentorial Gliomas: Radiology

Kenneth R. Maravilla

The neuroradiological evaluation of the patient suspected of harboring a central nervous system neoplasm has been greatly enhanced since the introduction of computed tomography (CT). Prior to CT, the presence of an intracranial mass could be detected only by indirect radiographic findings such as abnormal intracranial calcification, demineralization of the dorsum sellae secondary to increased intracranial pressure, or hyperostosis along the cranial vault. Even specialized, invasive studies, including arteriography and pneumoencephalography, relied on indirect signs such as distortion of the normal cerebral vascular architecture or displacement and deformity of the cerebral ventricles or the subarachnoid space to suggest the diagnosis of an intracranial neoplasm.

For the first time computed tomography enables us to see, more or less directly, the brain tissue in a living patient, and exquisitely defines both normal and pathological intracranial anatomy. This has led to increased sensitivity and, in the majority of cases, increased specificity of diagnosis. For instance, one can detect subtle masses deep within the cerebral hemispheres or small midline tumors that previously would have been difficult or even impossible to diagnose. Through detailed analysis of the morphology of a mass as seen on CT scans and by correlating this with our knowledge of the gross pathological appearance of cases seen at the autopsy table, one can often arrive at a very specific preoperative diagnosis. Certain physiological changes that often accompany intracranial neoplasms can also be evaluated with CT and can help to establish the correct diagnosis. These include compromise of the blood-brain barrier and the presence of surrounding intracerebral edema.

The CT technique is not without its limitations, however. Despite the exquisite detail obtained with CT images of the head, it should be realized that this diagnostic modality still does not provide a histological diagnosis, and there is considerable overlap among the characteristic morphological changes associated with various intracranial abnormalities. Furthermore, the CT image is basically a map outlining the distribution of relative differences in tissue electron density throughout the brain. Significant pathological abnormalities

may occur, but because the density of the abnormality in some cases is not significantly different from that of normal brain tissue, the lesion may go undetected. This phenomenon is best illustrated by the isodense, subacute subdural hematoma. Finally, computed tomography presents a static picture of the brain, and evaluation of dynamic and physiological changes within the brain is extremely limited at best.

Traditional radiographic methods of diagnostic evaluation often add critical information in the diagnosis of tumors. Plain x-ray films of the skull, for instance, may show hyperostosis in the presence of a meningioma or erosion of the internal auditory canal with a neurinoma involving the eighth cranial nerve. Similarly, the differentiation between a low density infiltrating glioma and a cerebral infarct, when unclear from CT criteria alone, may be influenced by changes on the skull film of increased intracranial pressure which would indicate a mass lesion of some duration and of progressive onset, rather than an acute cerebral infarction. Angiography may be particularly helpful in the diagnosis of brain tumors by defining tumor vascularity and early draining veins in the presence of a glioblastoma. In contrast, abscess formation or an arteriovenous malformation may show characteristic changes that are very different and that allow for the proper preoperative diagnosis of these lesions.

Recent advances in neuroradiology, in addition to providing more accurate and more efficient diagnosis, have also been of great benefit to the patient undergoing a diagnostic evaluation. Many such patients are now spared the risk and the discomfort of invasive angiographic or myelographic procedures when the CT scan has provided sufficient information. Pneumoencephalography, which was once the most uncomfortable diagnostic neuroradiological procedure, is now rarely, if ever, indicated.

The subsequent sections provide an overview of the neuroradiological approach to the diagnosis of cerebral gliomas. The emphasis on computed tomographic findings is in direct proportion to the relative importance of these techniques in modern neuroradiology.

Skull Films

The plain x-ray film of the skull was once the initial diagnostic study performed in the evaluation of all patients presenting with CNS symptoms. Skull films have declined markedly in importance and have now been relegated to a secondary position in the workup of patients with intracranial tumors. The reasons for this change in philosophy are many. First, reviews in the literature show that skull films in large series of patients presenting with symptoms suggestive of an intracranial abnormality demonstrate findings related to intracranial lesions in only a very small percentage of cases. Even in a selected series of 136 patients with proven intracerebral tumor reviewed by Stenhouse, the incidence of positive findings on x-ray films of the skull was a disappointing 17.6 percent.[14] Second, most of the findings seen on

564

skull films, including demineralization of the dorsum sellae secondary to increased intracranial pressure, intracranial hyperostosis, bone erosion, abnormal intracranial calcification, and shift of the pineal gland are all nonspecific findings and provide little or no information for localization and characterization of the lesion. Third, in the presence of symptoms suggesting an intracerebral neoplasm, the patient will still require CT evaluation whether or not changes are seen on the skull films. Finally, in most cases bony changes within the calvarium, the presence and location of intracranial calcification, and the degree of midline shift are all better evaluated on a properly performed CT exam.

This is not to say, however, that skull films are totally without merit. They can add much valuable information in selected cases. For instance, in the presence of mass lesions at the base of the brain, plain x-ray films may show the presence or absence of bony erosion or hyperostosis at the base of the skull (Fig. 64-1). The presence of these findings would greatly aid in narrowing the differential diagnostic possibilities. Similarly, in the patient presenting with severe or atypical headaches but with no abnormality seen on CT scans, plain films may provide evidence of disease within the sinuses that may account for the patient's symptoms since visualization of most of the paranasal sinuses is usually excluded on routine CT scanning of the brain. In other patients with a similar presentation, demineralization of the dorsum sellae secondary to chronically increased intracranial pressure but no abnormality on CT scans suggests pseudotumor cerebri as the cause (Fig. 64-2).

In nearly all instances, it can be strongly argued that a CT scan of the brain should be the first radiographic procedure obtained in patients suspected of harboring an intracranial neoplasm. Skull films should be reserved for secondary evaluation and obtained only in those instances where they may be needed to answer specific questions. This has been the approach in the author's institution. It should be emphasized, however, that a very different approach is used in patients suspected of harboring extracerebral tumors (i.e., bony metastases or nasopharyngeal tumors) and in patients suffering acute head trauma.

Computed Tomography

As indicated from the foregoing discussion, computed tomography is the primary diagnostic technique for patients with a suspected intracranial glioma. Optimal study includes scans obtained both prior to and following the intravenous injection of an iodinated contrast material. The precontrast scan provides a baseline density of the lesion to determine if the lesion is of increased density (hyperdense), decreased density (hypodense), or similar density (isodense) relative to normal brain. This baseline density measurement is also used for comparison to determine the degree of contrast enhancement which may occur. When a lesion is hyperdense following IV contrast, the precontrast study is necessary to

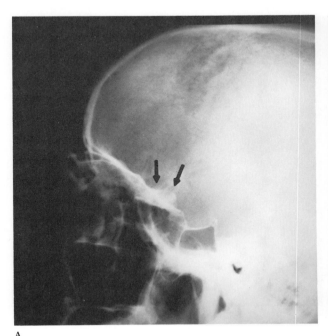
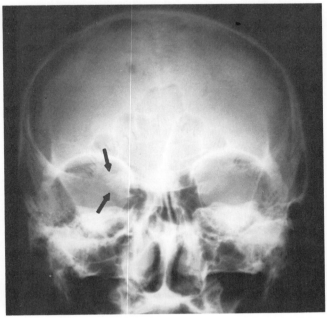

A   B

Figure 64-1 *A.* Lateral view of the skull clearly shows hyperostosis or "blistering" of the planum sphenoidale (*arrows*). *B.* Anteroposterior view of the skull shows that the hyperostosis also involves the lesser wing of the sphenoid and the anterior clinoid on the right (*arrows*). These abnormal findings on the plain skull films are highly specific and indicate the presence of a meningioma that was proved surgically.

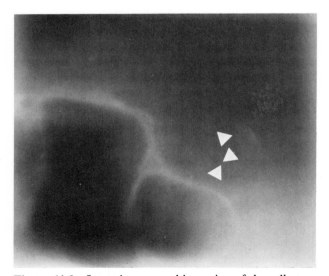

Figure 64-2 Lateral tomographic section of the sella turcica shows marked demineralization of the dorsum sellae secondary to increased intracranial pressure. This pattern can be distinguished from direct erosion of the dorsum sellae by a mass lesion since the dorsum remains intact although barely visible (*arrowheads*). In this patient, who had a normal CT scan, the findings on the skull film indicate the diagnosis of benign intracranial hypertension or pseudotumor cerebri.

evaluate for the presence of intralesional calcification or the presence of associated hemorrhage. In some cases, additional anatomical projections may be necessary for complete evaluation of a lesion. Such images may be obtained either by direct coronal scanning of the patient with the neck hyperextended (Fig. 64-3) or through computer reformatting of the routine axial images into sagittal and coronal displays (Fig. 64-4).

The diagnosis of an intracranial neoplasm is usually made by the combination of an area of abnormal intracerebral density together with anatomical deformity of regional cerebral structures due to compression and displacement by the mass effect of the tumor. However, in many cases of very slow-growing lesions or predominantly infiltrating gliomas, such mass effects may be minimal or absent. One needs to be especially observant of subtle anatomical deformities in the presence of isodense lesions, where a subtle midline shift and slight deformity of the white matter structures and ventricles may be the only clues to the presence and location of a tumor.

Abnormal density on the CT scan can be divided into lesions of increased density, those of decreased density, and those with mixed or inhomogeneous density. The density abnormality on the CT scan serves to localize the lesion and will usually provide information regarding the size and extent of the lesion. An exception to this, however, is a low density tumor with associated surrounding edema. Intracer-

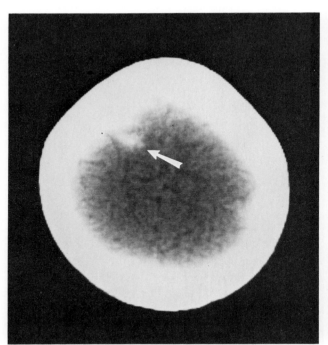

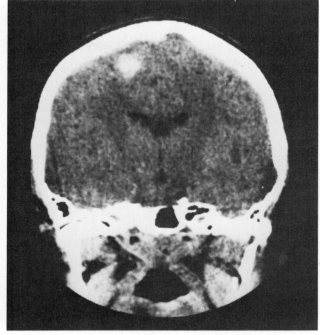

A   B

Figure 64-3 *A.* An axial CT scan near the top of the brain shows a high-density parasagittal lesion on the right side (*arrow*). This single view does not reveal whether the lesion arises extra-axially from the dura at the top of the skull or represents an intraparenchymal mass lesion. *B.* A direct coronal CT scan with the patient's head in hyperextension shows that the lesion is an intraparenchymal mass unattached to the cranial vault. It proved to be grade II astrocytoma.

ebral edema is also seen as a low density change on the CT scan, and in the case of a hypodense mass, the tumor cannot be distinguished from the surrounding edema on the noncontrast CT scan.

Many of the lesions will increase in attenuation or be enhanced following the intravenous injection of an iodinated contrast material. This provides valuable information. Most importantly, lesions that are isodense on the nonenhanced scan but that exhibit increased density following enhancement are much more readily detected and their margins are precisely defined. Contrast enhancement is also of great value in the presence of a low density tumor surrounded by edema. In such a case, if the tumor can be enhanced, its precise extent is easily defined, and the tumor is readily separated from the surrounding edema (Fig. 64-5). The ability of brain lesions to exhibit contrast enhancement is most directly related to increased permeability of the blood-brain barrier, which results in interstitial extravasation of the contrast material.[7,8] Hypervascularity within the lesion may also play a minor role in contrast enhancement in hypervascular tumors, but it plays a much greater role in vascular

lesions such as arteriovenous malformations (AVMs). Conversely, nonenhancement of the tumor implies a hypovascular lesion with an intact blood-brain barrier. This pattern is seen in many low grade gliomas or cystic abnormalities.

Morphological characteristics associated with an intracranial mass lesion are also very important in formulating a differential diagnosis. Characteristic CT findings are associated with the various gliomas, and the CT changes associated with benignancy or malignancy roughly correlate with the histological grading of the tumors.[2,15,16] In general, masses that are sharply marginated, are homogeneous in density, and that show little or no contrast enhancement tend to be benign. On the other hand, masses that show poor margination, are inhomogeneous in density, and demonstrate considerable contrast enhancement, especially when this enhancement is irregular in pattern and outline, tend to be malignant lesions. These are general characteristics, and all of the morphological findings of a lesion must be considered together. Individual changes may differ from the norm. For instance, some histologically benign, low grade astrocytomas that are primarily infiltrating may demonstrate poor margination with the surrounding brain, while, by contrast, some rapidly growing, malignant glioblastomas and many metastases may show relatively sharp demarcation from the surrounding normal brain.

Nonenhancing zones within an enhanced mass suggest areas of necrosis and indicate rapid tumoral growth and ma-

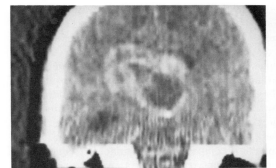

A

Figure 64-4 *A*. Axial CT scan image shows a glioblastoma multiforme involving the body and splenium of the corpus callosum. Coronal (*B*) and sagittal (*C*) reformatted images of the same patient clearly show the true extent of the lesion in multiple projections together with its precise anatomical relationships. Unlike the image in Fig. 64-3*B*, these do not represent rescans of the patient, but rather computer reformatting of the axial image data to display pictures in the sagittal and coronal projections. This technique is helpful when the patient cannot tolerate the direct coronal view or when the sagittal view is desired.

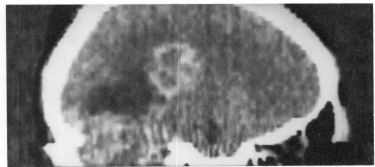

B   C

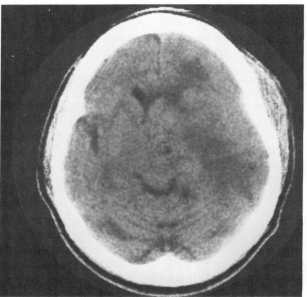 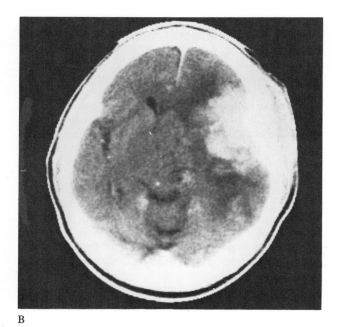

A   B

Figure 64-5 *A*. An axial CT scan section shows an obvious mass effect with compression of the lateral ventricles and displacement to the right. An abnormal area of low density can be seen within the left hemisphere. With this noncontrast view a question remains as to the exact location and extent of the mass lesion. *B*. A CT scan section taken at approximately the same level following the intravenous injection of a contrast agent now clearly shows the location and extent of a large, irregular enhancing mass. The lesion lies peripheral to the low-density zone that represents surrounding cerebral edema. This mass was not clearly defined on the precontrast scan since it was isodense with the adjacent brain parenchyma.

lignant behavior. Similarly, areas of hemorrhage within a mass favor a malignant lesion and are most often seen with glioblastomas and metastases.

Large amounts of surrounding edema also favor the diagnosis of a malignant lesion. Benign astrocytomas and ependymomas tend to exhibit little or no surrounding edema. A prominent exception to this rule is the meningioma, which, although a benign lesion, may nonetheless be associated with very large amounts of edema out of proportion to the size of the mass.[4]

The presence of calcification within the tumor is usually an indication of a slow-growing mass. Calcification is very often detected in oligodendrogliomas[10,11] and may also be seen with astrocytomas and ependymomas. However, if an adjacent area of the tumor shows intense contrast enhancement, this may indicate a lesion that started out as a benign glioma but has undergone degeneration with areas exhibiting CT and histological characteristics of glioblastoma multiforme.

Low Grade Astrocytoma (Astrocytoma Grades 1 and 2)

This is the so-called benign astrocytoma. This terminology may be misleading for, although the lesion exhibits the histological characteristics of a benign lesion, it nonetheless is

an infiltrating lesion, which may grow extensively throughout the brain and is not completely resectable. The most typical CT presentation is that of a low density mass that is poorly marginated from the surrounding brain tissue (Fig. 64-6). These astrocytomas usually infiltrate along white matter tracts and may even cross the midline via the corpus callosum (Fig. 64-7). They usually exhibit a mild to moderate mass effect due to their slow growth, and calcium may be present in a minority of these tumors. The texture of these masses is rather homogeneous in character. Most often they are nonenhancing or show only minimal contrast enhancement.

In some cases these lesions may show a homogeneous pattern of moderate contrast enhancement (Fig. 64-8). This pattern is more often seen in children. They may also occasionally show a large cystic component which is represented by a round, sharply circumscribed area of further decreased density that may or may not be surrounded by a rim of enhancement, i.e., a "ring lesion" (Fig. 64-9). An enhancing tumor nodule is sometimes present within the wall of the cyst. These lesions are most often seen in children and young patients, and are usually found in the posterior fossa. However, they may be seen in adult patients in the cerebral hemisphere, especially in the periventricular region. Drainage of the cystic component of the tumor is frequently accompanied by striking relief of symptoms and a marked decrease in the mass effect seen on CT scans. These lesions are discussed further elsewhere in this textbook.

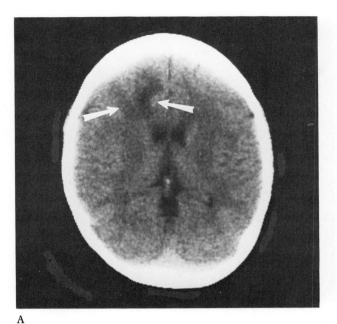

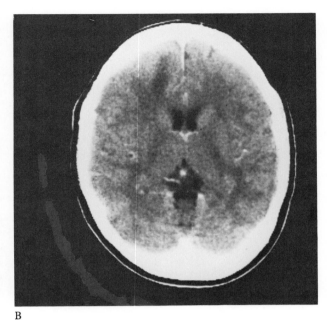

A   B

Figure 64-6   Precontrast (*A*) and postcontrast (*B*) CT scans show an ill-defined, nonenhancing low-density region in the forceps minor on the right side (*arrows*). This represents a low-grade astrocytoma. Note the ill-defined nature of the margins surrounding this lesion and the almost total absence of mass effect. This is due to the slow growth and infiltrating nature of low-grade astrocytomas.

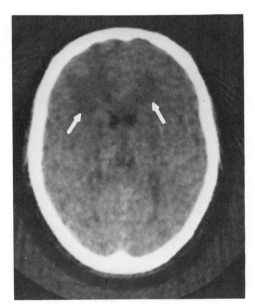

Figure 64-7   A low-grade astrocytoma with infiltration through the corpus callosum and involvement of both frontal lobes (*arrows*). The appearance of this lesion with the bulk of the mass on the right side suggests that the tumor arose primarily on the right and subsequently infiltrated to involve the left hemisphere as well. This pattern of involvement has been referred to as a "butterfly" glioma.

The differential diagnosis of a low grade astrocytoma may include a cerebral infarct. The latter can usually be distinguished by a characteristic clinical history of an abrupt onset of symptoms together with a typical CT pattern of an infarct. The CT scans of a patient with an infarct usually show an area of low density that conforms to the distribution of a vascular territory. This is characterized by a wedge-shaped lesion that is broad-based against the surface of the brain and that tapers medially. Also, unlike the astrocytoma which tends to infiltrate throughout the white matter and shows relative sparing of the cerebral cortex, the infarct usually shows nondiscriminatory involvement of both the gray and white matter (Fig. 64-10). In the case of small, deep infarcts, the CT characteristics may overlap. If distinction between the two is not clear-cut, a follow-up CT scan in approximately 5 to 10 days will show typical evolutionary changes within a cerebral infarct.[5,13] These include a decreasing mass effect together with a characteristic peripheral rim of contrast enhancement along the edge of the infarct and along the cerebral gyri. By contrast, a tumor will show no change in appearance in this short period of time.

Additional diagnostic consideration must be given to an area of demyelination that also presents as a low density lesion conforming to the white matter. These changes are usually more widely distributed, showing either diffuse involvement of the cerebral white matter bilaterally, or a patchy distribution of multiple widely-separated zones of demyelination. Furthermore, demyelinating processes are usually accompanied by changes of parenchymal loss and atrophy, whereas infiltrating gliomas are usually accompanied by a mass effect.

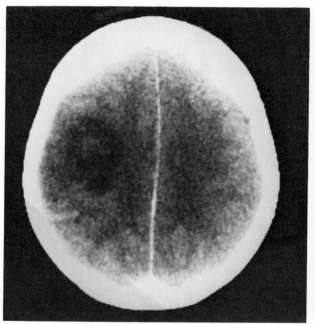
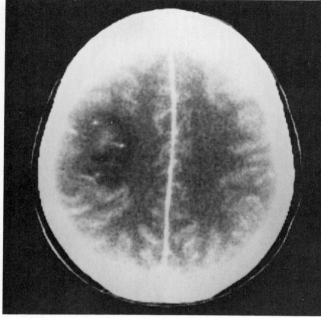

A   B

Figure 64-8 *A.* A precontrast CT scan of a low-grade astrocytoma shows a nearly isodense tumor nodule surrounded by low-density cerebral edema deep within the right hemisphere. *B.* Following the intravenous administration of a contrast agent, there is a mild to moderate degree of homogeneous enhancement within the tumor nodule. The low-density edematous zone does not enhance. Compare this pattern of enhancement with that seen with malignant astrocytomas, as illustrated in Figs. 64-4 and 64-11.

High Grade Astrocytoma (Astrocytoma Grades 3 and 4)

This is the malignant astrocytoma or glioblastoma multiforme. The characteristic CT pattern is that of an irregular mass lesion showing poor margination from the surrounding brain tissue. The texture of the mass is inhomogeneous on the nonenhanced scan, and following contrast enhancement there is intense contrast enhancement that is irregular in outline and often shows a swirl-like pattern surrounding multiple areas of low density (Fig. 64-4). The low density zones correspond to areas of necrosis within the tumor mass, indicating the rapid growth and malignant behavior of the tumor. Occasionally, glioblastomas may show a paradoxically sharp margination from the surrounding brain tissue as a result of the destruction and displacement of the surrounding parenchyma. This should not dissuade one from the diagnosis of a malignant glioma since the other changes are usually overwhelmingly characteristic. Glioblastomas are often accompanied by moderate to severe associated surrounding edema and a large mass effect (Fig. 64-11). Areas of hemorrhage within the lesion are not infrequent and even when not obvious are often contributing factors to the inhomogeneous nature of the lesion. Calcium is not an accompanying feature of glioblastoma.

The differential diagnosis in the case of a glioblastoma includes a metastasis, which also may present as an enhanc-ing mass with a necrotic center. Metastatic lesions are round or oval and are relatively sharply marginated from the surrounding brain.[3] Multiple lesions strongly favor the diagnosis of metastases. Furthermore, metastases usually are not irregular in outline as are most glioblastomas (Fig. 64-12). Metastases are often accompanied by an amount of edema which is excessive relative to the size of the mass. In some cases when confronted with a solitary lesion, a distinction between the two cannot be made by CT criteria alone.

Abscess formation may also mimic changes seen in some glioblastomas. Abscesses are usually round, smoothly-outlined, thin-walled, enhancing masses with a low density center. The wall, however, unlike the rim of most glioblastomas, is thin, is uniform in thickness, and shows a regular outline[17] that is round or oval in shape (Fig. 64-13). Abscesses may also show surrounding edema, although oftentimes it is less in degree than that seen with a glioblastoma or a metastasis. When an abscess is multiloculated, it presents changes on a CT scan that can easily be confused with the irregular, swirl-like pattern of a glioblastoma. Similarly, some glioblastomas may present as a solitary round mass with a central lucency. However, in these cases almost invariably the wall is not of uniform thickness and will show some areas with a shaggy margin or with nodule formation along the inner margin (see Fig. 64-19*B*).

In some cases, the CT scan shows a low density infiltrating mass with either no contrast enhancement or with a

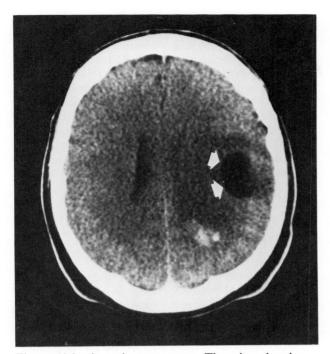

Figure 64-9 A cystic astrocytoma. There is a sharply defined low-density mass on the left (*arrows*). Unlike the infiltrating low-grade gliomas, the margins of this mass are sharply defined and the density more closely approaches that of CSF. These characteristics indicate the presence of an astrocytoma with a cystic component. An area of calcification that lies more posteriorly in the left hemisphere probably represents tumor calcification in a posteriorly infiltrating component of the astrocytoma. This case also illustrates the fact that these lesions are oftentimes inhomogeneous in character with both infiltrating as well as cystic components.

small area of contrast enhancement. All of the characteristics may be those of a benign astrocytoma, as cited previously. However, following biopsy, a histological diagnosis of glioblastoma is obtained. In these cases, the apparent discrepancy between CT presentation and histology is most likely due to the fact that the tumor contains areas of different histological grading. In such cases the tumor is graded pathologically according to the most malignant section even though it may represent only a small portion of the mass. The CT changes, however, will be characterized by the bulk of the mass, which, in the example cited above, is that of a low grade glioma. The pathological grading of glioblastoma is justified since the tumor will usually behave clinically and will follow the natural history of the most malignant portion of the mass.

Oligodendroglioma

Oligodendrogliomas are slow-growing tumors which account for approximately 5 percent of gliomas. They occur most frequently in the centrum semiovale of the cerebral

hemispheres and are found predominantly in adult patients. The most characteristic radiographic finding associated with these tumors is the frequent occurrence of prominent, irregular clumps of calcification within the tumor mass (Fig. 64-14). Such calcification has been shown to be detectable on plain x-ray films of the skull in approximately 40 to 60 percent of patients with an oligodendroglioma.[6,11] The percentage is probably even higher using CT as the method of diagnosis, although no large series of CT cases has been reported thus far to confirm this observation. The tumor surrounding the calcification has a CT appearance similar to that of a benign astrocytoma; it is often of low density and shows little or no contrast enhancement (Fig. 64-15). Oligodendrogliomas may occur within the cerebral ventricles, in which case they may be easily confused with ependymomas or intraventricular meningiomas, both of which may also show the presence of intratumoral calcification (Fig. 64-16). An oligodendroglioma may also undergo malignant degeneration to a glioblastoma. In such cases malignant transformation may be seen as adjacent areas of intense, irregular contrast enhancement and necrosis.

Ependymoma

Ependymomas arise from the ependymal cells lining the ventricles and are most often found in childhood, usually originating from the fourth ventricle. Less commonly, they occur in adults, and in this age group they are more often

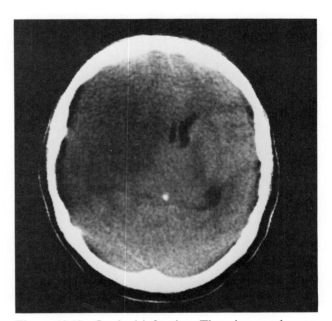

Figure 64-10 Cerebral infarction. There is a poorly marginated low-density area in the distribution of the right middle cerebral artery. Note the wedge-shaped character of the low density and, most importantly, the fact that both the gray and the white matter of the brain are involved. This is in direct contrast to the low-grade astrocytomas, which tend to infiltrate through the white matter tracts.

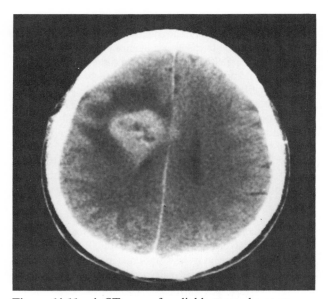

Figure 64-11 A CT scan of a glioblastoma shows an inhomogeneously enhancing mass with irregular areas of low density, which represent tumor necrosis. Note the large amount of surrounding edema peripheral to the tumor, and compression of the right lateral ventricle.

seen in the cerebral hemispheres associated with the lateral ventricles or the third ventricle. Despite their histologically benign nature, the adult form of ependymoma may invade the cerebral parenchyma rather than grow predominantly within the ventricle. They are reported to show calcification but in our experience the incidence is uncommon. Ependymomas frequently exhibit a low density mass, often accompanied by a moderate homogeneous contrast enhancement within the tumor mass, and little surrounding edema (Fig. 64-17). In addition to the ability of these tumors to extend and invade locally, they may also show seeding or drop metastases throughout the cerebrospinal fluid pathways.

Angiography

Cerebral angiography is an important diagnostic modality that provides additional information in the diagnosis and evaluation of central nervous system (CNS) tumors. The angiogram is usually done in the presence of a known mass lesion already detected on the CT scan, and the type of angiographic evaluation is tailored to provide additional infor-

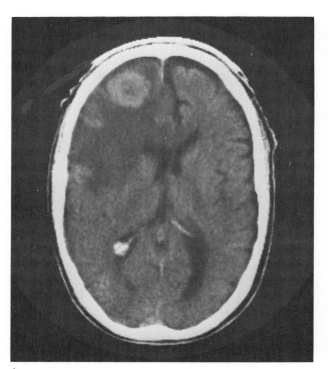

A

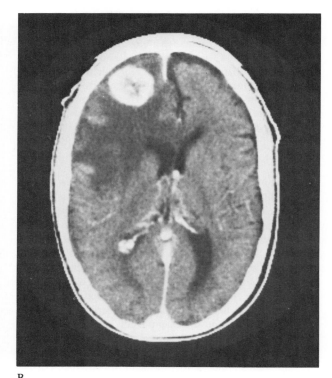

B

Figure 64-12 A metastatic nodule in the right frontal region without (A) and with (B) contrast enhancement; this lesion shows as a well-marginated round mass that enhances markedly. The thick wall of enhancement surrounding a relatively low density center has often been referred to as the "donut" sign of a metastatic lesion. The low-density center represents a central zone of relative avascularity or necrosis. Also note the disproportionate amount of cerebral edema that extends far back into the cerebral hemisphere. This amount of edema is greater than that seen with astrocytomas and is highly characteristic of metastatic tumors.

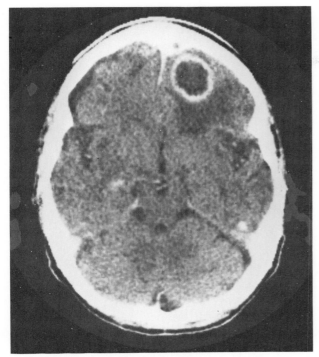

Figure 64-13 A brain abscess in the left frontal lobe. A mature brain abscess shows a low-density central area of liquefaction with a smooth, round, thin-walled capsule, which is best seen following intravenous contrast enhancement. Such lesions are usually surrounded, as in this case, by a mild to moderate amount of cerebral edema. Contrast this picture with the marked irregularity of the tumor walls seen with glioblastomas and with the thick-walled donut sign of a metastasis.

mation about the CT abnormality. The indications for cerebral angiography in the presence of a mass lesion include the following:

1. to aid in narrowing the differential diagnosis of a mass lesion;
2. to eliminate the possibility of a giant aneurysm or vascular malformation as the cause of the CT abnormality;
3. to determine the involvement or lack of involvement of key anatomical structures;
4. to distinguish between an intra-axial versus an extra-axial mass; and
5. to assist in preoperative planning by providing detailed localization of the mass relative to regional vascular anatomy.

Angiography is particularly useful in those lesions that show contrast enhancement and are located at the base of the brain or adjacent to dural surfaces. A giant aneurysm must be considered in the differential diagnosis, and this can be easily diagnosed by angiography (Fig. 64-18). A meningioma also has a characteristic angiographic appearance and may be distinguished from an intra-axial glioma. As evidence of their extra-axial nature, meningiomas receive all or the bulk of their vascular supply from dural arteries. Meningiomas also exhibit a characteristic pattern within the mass that has been described as a sunburst or spoke wheel distribution of feeding vessels. They also show an intense stain that occurs late in the arterial phase and persists well into the venous phase. Usually early draining veins are not an accompanying feature of meningiomas.

Similarly, vascular lesions such as a giant aneurysm may simulate a tumor at the base of the brain on the CT scan.

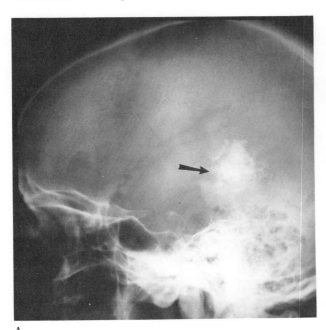

A

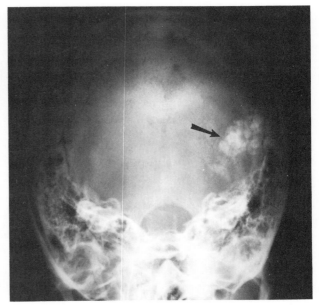

B

Figure 64-14 Lateral (A) and Towne's (B) views of the skull show large, irregular clumps of calcification in the left posterior temporal region (arrows), which represents intratumoral calcification in a large oligodendroglioma. This pattern of calcification is highly characteristic of these lesions.

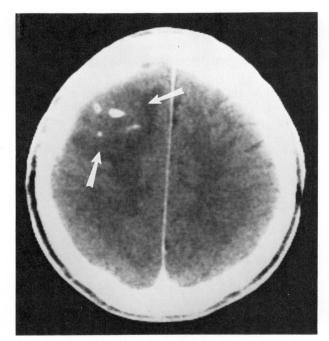

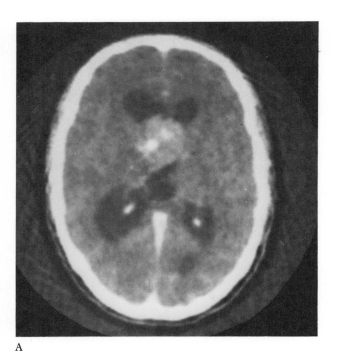

A

Figure 64-15 An oliogodendroglioma with clumps of intratumoral calcification is shown on an axial CT scan. The mass lesion in this case is nearly isodense with the surrounding brain tissue (*arrows*) and shows no contrast enhancement. There is a minimal amount of surrounding low-density edema also noted.

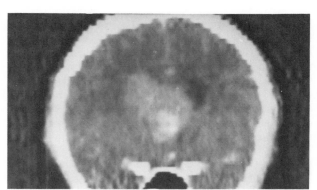

B

Figure 64-16 An intraventricular oligodendroglioma. Axial (*A*) and reformatted coronal (*B*) and sagittal (*C*) views show the three-dimensional relationships. Note the clumps of calcification and moderate, homogeneous contrast enhancement, characteristics indistinguishable from those of a meningioma or ependymoma. Cerebral angiography showed increased vascularity to the lesion, further suggesting a meningioma, but at operation the lesion proved to be an oligodendroglioma.

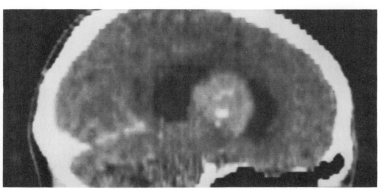

C

Occasionally, an arteriovenous malformation can also mimic an intra-axial tumor, but the correct nature of the lesion is easily diagnosed by angiography.

Of all the intracranial gliomas, glioblastoma has the most characteristic angiographic pattern. These lesions exhibit an intracerebral mass effect with displacement of the regional vessels. Glioblastomas tend to be hypervascular and show intense neovascularity with many small vessels within the tumor. These exhibit a disorganized pattern and the fine vessels are irregular in caliber. There is often a prominent tumor blush that occurs in the midarterial phase. This tumor blush may be associated with nonstaining areas

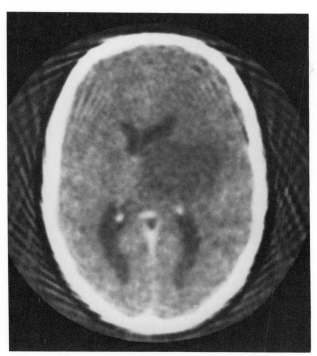

Figure 64-17 A cerebral ependymoma. A low-density, nonenhancing mass lesion is seen in the left paraventricular region. Despite the fact that these tumors arise from the ependymal cells lining the ventricular system, they may often show parenchymal invasion, as in this case, rather than primary intraventricular growth.

within the mass that correspond to areas of necrosis within the tumor. Early draining veins are a frequent accompaniment, and oftentimes these veins may fill very quickly in the midarterial or late arterial phase, indicating a degree of arteriovenous (AV) shunting within the tumor mass (Fig. 64-19).

Due to the intense proliferation of small vessels within the tumor mass and the AV shunting, the changes can sometimes be confused with those of an arteriovenous malformation. The latter is distinguished by several characteristics. AVMs produce little or no mass effect, and vessels within the arteriovenous malformation appear more closely packed, are more organized in appearance, and exhibit a more uniform caliber. This characteristic appearance of an AVM has been described as a "bag of worms" appearance. Furthermore, due to the congenital nature of AVMs and because of the high degree of arteriovenous shunting, the arterial feeders are markedly dilated. This is in contrast to the arterial feeders accompanying glioblastomas, which tend to be normal in caliber or minimally dilated. Similarly, the draining veins accompanying an arteriovenous malformation are larger and appear more redundant than the early draining veins of a glioblastoma, which again tend to be normal in caliber or mildly dilated.[9] Finally, arteriovenous malformations generally show more rapid arteriovenous shunting than is seen with glioblastomas.

Low-grade astrocytomas and oligodendrogliomas tend to be hypovascular or avascular masses at angiography. No

characteristic findings are present to distinguish these lesions. Ependymomas may show an increase in small vessels within the mass, but not to the extent of a glioblastoma. The vessels are also more regular in character and less disorganized in appearance. There is a tumor stain often present at angiography which is usually homogeneous in character. Early draining veins are often seen, but no AV shunting is present.

Differentiation between intraventricular ependymoma, oligodendroglioma, or an intraventricular meningioma may be difficult or impossible by angiographic criteria. Solitary metastases may also be difficult to distinguish from vascular gliomas by angiography alone.

Radionuclide Scanning

Conventional radionuclide brain scanning is not very useful when high-quality CT techniques are available. The mechanisms of detection of cerebral lesions are similar for both radionuclide scans and enhanced CT scans. Both techniques are based upon the abnormal extravasation of material (radionuclide or iodinated contrast material, respectively) across an abnormally permeable blood-brain barrier to enter the interstitial tissues of the brain or tumor. In addition to merely detecting the presence of an abnormality, CT has the added advantage of showing detailed morphology of the lesion together with an accurate demonstration of the surrounding anatomy. Furthermore, CT is better at detecting small lesions that lie deep within the cerebral hemispheres, near the midline, or near the base of the skull. These are all areas of difficulty for diagnosis by radionuclide scanning. Thus, CT has the advantages of increased sensitivity and far better specificity than radionuclide scanning.

Two types of radionuclide studies, however, may prove to be valuable techniques for obtaining unique information in patients with CNS abnormalities. The first is positron emission tomography, or PET scanning, and the second is single photon emission CT, or SPECT scanning. Both of these techniques are currently used as research modalities and provide dynamic and physiological information about the brain which is not obtainable with x-ray transmission CT. These techniques supply information regarding brain function and regional cerebral perfusion that may someday prove to be clinically valuable in the evaluation and treatment of CNS tumors. There is further discussion of these important modalities in other chapters of this book.

Postoperative Evaluation

The relative noninvasiveness of computed tomography has improved our ability to monitor the course of tumor patients following treatment by surgery, radiation, or chemotherapy. Postoperative changes can be grouped into two categories: immediate postoperative changes, which occur during the period of hospitalization following surgery, and delayed

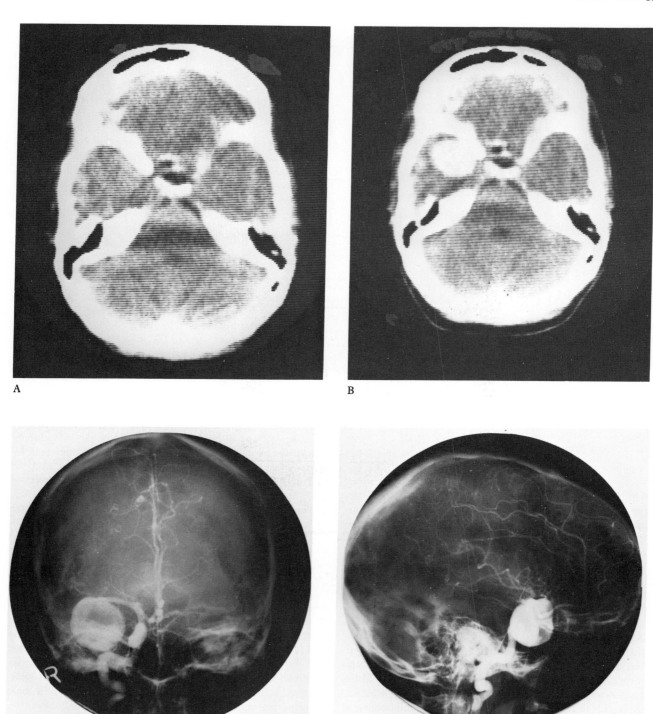

A

B

C

D

Figure 64-18 A giant aneurysm. Precontrast (*A*) and postcontrast (*B*) CT scans show a markedly enhancing mass within the right anterior temporal region. The CT picture suggests a neoplastic mass as the cause, but because of the location near the base of the skull, a giant aneurysm must be considered in the differential diagnosis. Anteroposterior (*C*) and lateral (*D*) views of the cerebral arteriogram establish the correct diagnosis of a giant intracranial aneurysm. This case indicates the critical necessity of arteriography prior to surgical intervention in lesions with this type of appearance.

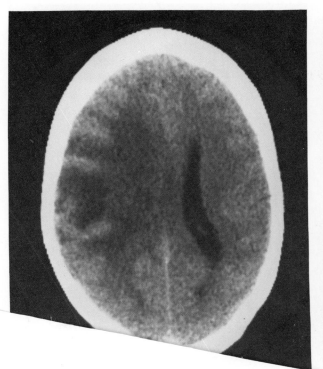

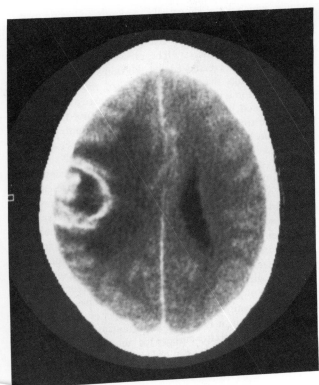

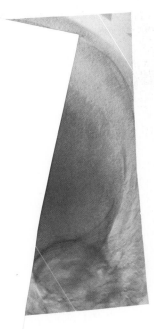

Computed tomography
of calcified brain tumor.

cation in intracranial gliomata.

Kricheff II, Wiggli U: Computed
erative care of neurosurgical patients.
-189, 1977.
a B, Rubino FA: Evaluation of recent cere-
computerized tomography. Arch Neurol

Plain radiography of the skull in the diagnosis of
tumours. Br J Radiol 21:287–300, 1948.
Scotti G, Terbrugge K, Melançon D, Bélanger G,
C, Ethier R: Computerized tomography as a possible aid
stological grading of supratentorial gliomas. J Neurosurg
:735–739, 1977.
Thomson JLG: Computerized axial tomography and the diagnosis of glioma: A possible aid
proven cases. Clin Radiol 27:431–441, 1976.
17. Whelan MA, Hilal SK: Computed tomography as a guide in the
diagnosis and follow-up of brain abscesses. Radiology 135:663–
671, 1980.

changes, which occur some weeks to months following treatment.

Immediate postoperative changes include primarily the complications of surgery.[12] The presence of postoperative hemorrhage or increased edema following surgery are the primary findings that are sought. Also, the adequacy of tumor resection is evaluated. In the case where only a biopsy was attempted, the question of whether or not the proper area of the tumor was biopsied to provide a representative sample can be answered with the use of postoperative CT scanning.

Delayed evaluation of tumor treatment is designed to answer questions predominantly related to the presence or absence of recurrent tumor, or to the shrinkage or growth of residual tumor following radiotherapy or chemotherapy. In these cases it must be remembered that radiation necrosis may often mimic recurrent tumor[1] and is an important pitfall that one must be constantly aware of in the evaluation of the post-treatment patient (Fig. 64-20). It is important for the radiologist to know whether or not the patient has had a full course of radiation therapy or merely has undergone surgical extirpation of the tumor. In proper evaluation of the delayed CT scan, it is usually important to have a baseline CT scan done soon after surgery for comparison with subsequent follow-up CT scans in order to properly evaluate the delayed changes.

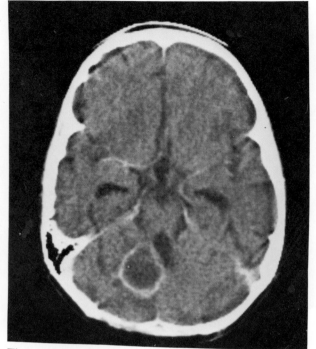

Figure 64-20 Radiation necrosis. A CT scan of a patient who had prior removal of an ependymoma of the fourth ventricle. The CT scan done some months following surgery and radiation therapy shows a thin-walled, ring-enhancing mass in the inferior cerebellum and cerebellar vermis. The appearance of this lesion suggests either a recurrent tumor or a brain abscess. However surgical exploration this proved to be an area of necrosis.

References

1. Brismar J, Roberson GH, Davis KR: Radiation necrosis of the brain: Neuroradiological considerations with computed tomography. Neuroradiology 12:109–113, 1976.
2. Butler AR, Horii SC, Kricheff II, Shannon MB, Budzilovich GN: Computed tomography in astrocytomas. Radiology 129:433–439, 1978.
3. Constant P, Renou AM, Caille AM, Dop A: Cerebral metastasis—A study of computerized tomography. Comput Tomogr 1:87–94, 1977.
4. Davis DO: CT in the diagnosis of supratentorial tumors. Semin Roentgenol 12:97–108, 1977.
5. Davis KR, Ackerman RH, Kistler JP, Mohr JP: Computed tomography of cerebral infarction: Hemorrhagic, contrast enhancement, and time of appearance. Comput Tomogr 1:71–86, 1977.
6. Davis L, Martin J, Padberg F, Anderson RK: A study of 182 patients with verified astrocytoma, astroblastoma and oligodendroglioma of the brain. J Neurosurg 7:299–312, 1950.
7. Gado MH, Phelps ME, Coleman RE: An extravascular component of contrast enhancement in cranial computed tomography. Part I. The tissue-blood ratio of contrast enhancement. Radiology 117:589–593, 1975.
8. Gado MH, Phelps ME, Coleman RE: An extravascular component of contrast enhancement in cranial computed tomography. Part II. Contrast enhancement and the blood-tissue barrier. Radiology 117:595–597, 1975.
9. Goree JA, Dukes HT: The angiographic differential diagnosis between the vascularized malignant glioma and the intracranial arteriovenous malformation. AJR 90:512–521, 1963.

10. Gouliamos AD, Jimenez JP, Goree JA, and skull radiography in the diagnos AJR 130:761–764, 1978.
11. Kalan C, Burrows EH: Calcifi Br J Radiol 35:589–602, 196
12. Lin JP, Pay N, Naidich T tomography in the posto Neuroradiology 12:18
13. Masdeu JC, Azar-K bral infarction b 34:417–421, 19
14. Stenhouse D intracrania
15. Tchang Milne to h 46
16.

65

Supratentorial Gliomas: Clinical Features and Surgical Therapy

Michael Salcman

The most common supratentorial tumors are those of glial origin, hence it is not surprising that the clinical study and surgical treatment of gliomas is virtually coextensive with the historical development of neurological surgery as a specialty. In 1884, Bennett and Godlee performed the first successful removal of a brain tumor that had been localized by neurological examination; the lesion was a low-grade astrocytoma, and the patient succumbed to infection less than 2 weeks after the procedure.[1] Although Sir Victor Horsley was greatly fascinated by this case, he was soon discouraged by his inability to save his own patients with malignant gliomas. During the early years of neurosurgery, periods of enthusiasm and neglect waxed and waned in regard to the surgery of the gliomas, and this fact was reflected in the conflicting recommendations put forward by Cushing, Dandy, and MacKenzie. Indeed, the development of Cushing's own surgical technique often mirrored the evolution of prevailing views concerning the relative merits of active therapy and benign neglect. Initially, Cushing advocated external decompression, with removal of the bone flap and creation of subgaleal and muscular pockets into which the tumor might herniate. Toward the end of his career, he came to accept the concept of radical internal decompression (i.e., tumor resection) with preservation of contiguous brain; his own technical contributions, especially the development of silver clips and electrocautery, were largely responsible for making such procedures possible. From 1901 to 1912, Harvey Cushing's operative mortality for glial tumors was 30.9 percent, but by the end of his career he had reduced this to 11 percent.[3] The technical difficulties of dealing with these tumors remained relatively unchanged until the introduction of corticosteroids and other perioperative aids in the 1960s. Because glial tumors are so common in clinical practice and because successful application of new therapeutic modalities may well depend upon the continued development of surgical technique, the early diagnosis and operative treatment of glial tumors remain a major challenge for every neurosurgeon.

Clinical Features

The symptoms and signs produced by intracranial tumors fall into two general categories, nonspecific findings secondary to elevations in the intracranial pressure (ICP) and site-specific findings secondary to the actual location of the neoplasm. Although the tempo with which symptoms and signs develop may give a clue to the underlying nature of the tumor, their specific character depends on the location of the tumor and not on its histology. The nonspecific symptoms and signs of elevated ICP include headache, drowsiness, visual obscuration, nausea, vomiting, nuchal rigidity, papilledema, and sixth nerve palsy. The headache of brain tumor is usually nonlocalizing but may lateralize to the side of the lesion. The headache is typically worse in the morning and may be relieved after an episode of vomiting or the onset of physical activity. It is thought that morning headaches are secondary to mild CO_2 retention during sleep and concomitant cerebral vasodilatation. Eventually the headache becomes nearly constant, but its intensity is rarely as severe as that of migraine or subarachnoid hemorrhage. Headache is the initial symptom in almost 40 percent of patients with glioblastoma multiforme[5,15] and in more than 35 percent of all patients with cerebral gliomas.[11] It is the most frequent chief complaint and the most prevalent symptom at the time of diagnosis (Table 65-1). Headache is the universal complaint of patients with brain tumors and must be carefully investigated in all likely suspects.

The drowsiness observed in brain tumor patients is caused by mechanical and vascular compromise of the diencephalon, and the neck stiffness is produced by herniation of the cerebellar tonsils through the foramen magnum. Of course, papilledema or choked disc is a direct reflection of an elevated ICP. It is important to remember that the presence of venous pulsations is almost always indicative of an ICP of less than 180 mmH$_2$O. Falsely localizing signs in brain tumor suspects, such as a sixth nerve palsy, are usually caused by compression of the involved cranial nerve against an adjacent structure (e.g., the petrous pyramid) and are usually reflective of brain swelling or hydrocephalus. Nonspecific signs and symptoms secondary to elevated ICP are more commonly observed in high-grade tumors than in relatively more benign low-grade astrocytomas and oligodendrogliomas. Nevertheless, a quarter to a third of all glioma patients complain of drowsiness or lethargy (Table 65-1); at diagnosis, more than one-half of all patients have papilledema, and almost 40 percent of the patients with glioblastoma have a depressed level of consciousness (Table 65-2).

The site-specific findings of supratentorial tumors are either irritative or destructive in nature, but their precise expression always depends upon the location of the tumor in respect to the functional organization of the brain. Lesions within the substance of the temporal lobe or in the vicinity of the motor cortex are far more likely to produce seizures than are similar neoplasms of the occipital pole. Similarly, mental apathy, memory loss, and personality disturbance are more frequently seen with frontotemporal tumors and hemiparesis and sensory loss with frontoparietal lesions. Seizures are the second most common complaint at the time of diagnosis and are more frequently seen with oligoden-

TABLE 65-1 Symptoms at Assessment in Glioma Patients (% of Cases)

Symptom	Tumor Type		
	All Gliomas* N = 653	Glioblastoma Multiforme† N = 870	Oligodendroglioma‡ N = 52
Headache	71.4	76.8	23.1
Seizures	53.9	29.2	86.5
Grand mal	20.4		
Focal	22.8		36.5
Psychomotor	8.6		28.8
Minor absence	2.1		17.3
Mental change	52.2	43.8	38.5
Hemiparesis	43.3	42.8	19.2
Vomiting	31.5	30.7	
Dysphasia	27.0	29.0	3.8
Impaired consciousness	24.8	27.7	
Hemianesthesia	13.6	14.1	5.8
Hemianopsia	8.1	1.0	

*McKeran and Thomas, 1980.[11]
†Compiled from Roth and Elvidge, 1960;[15] Frankel and German, 1958;[5] Jelsma and Bucy, 1967.[8]
‡Chin et al., 1980.[2]

drogliomas and astrocytomas (75 and 65 percent of cases, respectively) than with glioblastoma multiforme.[11] More than a third of all glioma patients suffer from seizures as the initial manifestation of their disease, and the average duration of this symptom prior to diagnosis is about 12 months in patients with glioblastoma[15] and about 3 years in patients with low-grade gliomas. Focal neurological findings are much more common in malignant astrocytomas than in other glial tumors, and this is especially true for motor weakness (Table 65-2). Nevertheless, it must be emphasized that although more than 60 percent of patients with glioblastoma suffer from hemiparesis at the time of diagnosis, only 3 percent complain of weakness as the initial symptom.[5] At the outset of their disease, patients with gliomas have relatively low rates of hemiparesis, dysphasia, hemianesthesia, and hemianopsia, but by the time of diagnosis, some or all of these findings are present in the majority of patients. Tumors in relatively silent areas produce symptoms and signs by virtue of edema that extends into adjacent functional zones, and the symptoms can often be ameliorated through the administration of corticosteroids. Of course, complete loss of function is indicative of direct invasion and is rarely reversed by any form of therapy.

The frequency with which different site-specific findings are encountered in clinical practice (Tables 65-1 and 65-2) depends heavily upon the diagnostic acumen of the physicians in charge of the patient. For example, retrospective studies of patients with malignant astrocytoma have indicated that subtle personality change is often missed on the initial history and physical examination. In patients with glioblastoma, personality change occurs an average of more than 8 months prior to diagnosis[15] and is the second earliest warning signal, next to seizures. At the time of diagnosis, up to 60 percent of patients with gliomas demonstrate some disturbance of orientation, memory, emotion, or judgement; this appears to be especially true for patients with oligodendroglioma.[2,11] Late in the clinical course, it is much more difficult to evaluate personality and mental change in the presence of a depressed sensorium.

Since the benefits of therapy to a certain extent depend upon the functional status of the patient, it is vitally important that the correct diagnosis be made and proper treatment instituted prior to the onset of hemiplegia or stupor. The majority of patients with glioblastoma multiforme, malignant astrocytoma, and oligodendroglioma have tumors in the frontal and temporal lobes or at the frontoparietal junction. Hence it is not surprising that the frequency of site-specific findings in these diseases is roughly similar, although there is some tendency for seizures to be associated with oligodendrogliomas and for personality disturbances to be more common in patients with glioblastoma. Of far greater importance is the tempo with which the site-specific findings appear. A rapid evolution of symptoms and signs is associated with malignancy, while a history of many years' duration is more consistent with a low-grade astrocytoma or oligodendroglioma. Finally, the proper interpretation of symptoms and signs can be made only within the context of the whole patient, especially as certain demographic factors (e.g., age and sex) bear heavily upon the correct diagnosis.

In summary, headache, seizures, mental change, and hemiparesis are the cardinal clinical features of supratentorial gliomas. A first seizure in a patient over 40 years of age should be considered indicative of a brain tumor until proved otherwise. Together with papilledema, mental change and hemiparesis are the most frequent findings on the initial physical examination; they provide important clues as to the location and extent of the tumor. Prior to the advent of computed tomography, underdiagnosis of bilateral spread in cases of glioblastoma was common, but careful neurological assessment often yields insights complementary to those provided by modern imaging techniques. Irrespective of the precise combination of clinical findings, it is the relentless progression of the disease that stamps it as an intracranial tumor. In a series of 615 cases of cerebral glioma, only 1 failed to progress clinically.[11] Since apoplectic onset is rare and radiographic progression usually accompanies clinical deterioration, there should be little difficulty in separating brain tumor suspects from patients with such other intracranial processes as cerebrovascular diseases.

TABLE 65-2　Physical Signs at Assessment in Glioma Patients (% of Cases)

Sign	Tumor Type			
	Astrocytoma* Grade 1 $N = 48$	Astrocytoma* Grade 2/3 $N = 341$	Glioblastoma multiforme† $N = 826$	Oligoden- droglioma $N = 36$
Hemiparesis	45.8	58.6	66.9	58.3
Cranial nerve signs‡	64.6	45.5	63.5	41.7
Papilledema	56.3	47.2	58.2	50.0
Mental change §	39.6	50.4	38.3	52.8
Hemianesthesia ¶	20.5	32.5	37.9	27.8
Depressed sensorium	n.a.	n.a.	37.3	n.a.
Hemianopsia	18.8	32.2	31.7	33.3
Dysphasia	22.9	24.3	29.2	25.0

*McKeran and Thomas[11] (includes some cerebellar tumors).
†Compiled from Roth and Elvidge,[15] Jelsma and Bucy,[8] McKeran and Thomas.[11]
‡Includes facial palsy.
§Includes confusion and disorientation.
¶Includes parietal lobe syndromes, sensory loss, astereognosis.

Surgical Therapy

The successful extirpation of a supratentorial glioma without further increase in the pre-existing neurological deficit of the patient is among the most difficult of all neurosurgical exercises. Significant palliation with good functional recovery cannot be achieved on a routine basis unless the surgeon undertakes such procedures with the same seriousness of purpose and attention to detail more commonly lavished upon less frequent disorders. It is my belief that optimal results are achieved when maximal resection of the tumor has been combined with minimal disturbance of the surrounding brain. Careful preoperative planning, scrupulous surgical technique, and the selective use of such aids as the operating microscope and the carbon dioxide laser all play a role in the gentle removal of the tumor and the fastidious preservation of adjacent nervous tissue. It is now possible to safely remove large glial tumors from virtually any hemispheric location without significant impairment of the patient. Radical removal accomplishes several goals for the oncologist-surgeon: (1) adequate sampling of the tissue for histopathological study and diagnosis; (2) maximal mechanical cytoreduction of the tumor mass prior to the institution of other forms of therapy; (3) immediate relief from elevated ICP, permitting adequate exposure of the patient to other treatments; and (4) the removal of cells known to be insensitive to other treatment modalities. Since the length of survival of patients with gliomas can be correlated with the extent of the surgical resection, it is the policy on our service to offer radical removal to all patients in whom an acceptable level of function can be predicted. As with other operations, the number of such patients tends to increase as the skill, experience, and judgement of the surgeon grow. Nevertheless, there remain some patients for whom a radical resection is an inappropriate procedure, and reasonable alternatives are discussed later in this chapter.

Preoperative planning begins with a careful review of the neurological findings, the functional status of the patient, and the relevant features of the CT scan. The general condition of the patient, the presence or absence of specific neurological deficits, the prospects for useful recovery, and the precise location of the lesion all have considerable bearing upon the selection of a specific operative approach. For example, a tumor located close to a cortical surface is generally attacked through that surface if the associated cortical function is already lost, the prospect for its recovery is small, or the potential loss of function (e.g., quadrantanopsia or weakness restricted to the distal leg) is considered justified by both patient and physician in view of the potential gains of the procedure.

Once the general approach has been chosen, rational design of an appropriate scalp incision and bone flap may proceed; it is highly preferable for these matters to be decided prior to the day of surgery. The surgeon should measure the maximum extent of the lesion in the vertical, transverse, and rostrocaudal directions as it appears on the enhanced CT scan, remembering to use the appropriate conversion factor (usually in the range of 3.0 to 3.5) to obtain the true physical dimensions in centimeters; the resection cavity obtained at the end of the operation will also be measured and should not exceed in any direction the preoperative radiographic estimates. It is important for the surgeon to develop the capacity of forming a mental image of the three-dimensional extent of the lesion in such a way as to be capable of revising the relationship of the lesion to the important anatomical structures that surround it. Among the most critical of these relationships are the location of the tumor vis-à-vis the motor strip, the thalamus, the basal ganglia, the ventricle, the angular gyrus, the superior temporal lobe, the tentorial incisura, the falx, the pterion, the coronal suture, and the external ear. An arteriogram is usually not necessary, but if it is available, the relationship of the tumor to the superficial cortical veins is sometimes useful information. It is all too easy for the unprepared surgeon to become lost within the substance of the brain and to inadvertently wander into areas that preclude the successful recovery of the patient.

A few words are in order concerning the premedication of the patient. It is the practice on our service to place all glioma patients on glucocorticosteroids and prophylactic anticonvulsants. Since transcortical approaches are required in virtually all glial tumors, it is vitally important to minimize the amount of postoperative depression, brain swelling, and seizure activity. A minimum of 2 to 3 days of dexamethasone (4 to 10 mg every 4 to 6 h) or an equivalent dose of methylprednisolone is required to adequately prepare the brain for surgery. Aggressive use of corticosteroids and good neuroanesthesia can avoid unnecessary intraoperative administration of mannitol or ethacrinic acid. Several days should also be allowed for preoperative loading of anticonvulsants; sodium phenytoin is the preferred drug because it does not cause CNS depression at therapeutic levels and because it can be given intravenously during the operation. Patients who have not received adequate amounts of anticonvulsants may suffer a seizure during emergence from anesthesia, and the associated motor activity and systemic hypertension pose serious threats to hemostasis and relaxation at the operative site. Many postoperative problems can be avoided by careful preoperative planning and close communication between the surgeon and the neuroanesthesiologist.

All patients are operated on under general anesthesia. Airway management and intubation must be smooth so as not to produce elevations in the ICP or sudden bleeding within the tumor. Proper positioning of the patient is essential in producing a relaxed brain and a relaxed surgeon. The major axis of the tumor should lie in a plane parallel to the floor of the operating theater. The head of the patient is slightly elevated above the level of the chest so as to promote venous drainage; for similar reasons, extreme rotation of the neck is avoided, as is extreme forward flexion. The majority of glial tumors can be operated upon in the supine position and in an ordinary headrest; this is especially the case for many frontal and temporal and some parietal lesions. When the major axis of the tumor requires that the patient be placed in either full lateral, three-quarter prone, or semisitting position, secure fixation in head pins is always employed; this situation is frequently encountered with high parietal, posterior temporal, true occipital, parapineal, and paramidline tumors. The line of incision is always marked, even for reoperations, because the combination of an iodine preparation and a plastic drape will usually obscure the old incision scar as well as all superficial landmarks.

In general, operations for a tumor require much larger craniotomies than procedures carried out in similar locations for cerebrovascular, infective, or traumatic diseases. Retraction can be quite difficult during tumor surgery, and some provision must be made for swollen brain. In addition, the exposure must be large enough and versatile enough to permit a change in either the angle of attack or the general nature of the procedure (e.g., intratumoral resection as opposed to lobectomy). In other words, although radical intratumoral resection is sufficient in most cases, the incision is planned as if a major lobectomy might have to be carried out. For frontal lobe tumors, the incision must give access to the frontal pole, the pterion, the orbital plate, the sphenoid wing, and the midline (Fig 65-1A). Anterior temporal lobe tumors are best approached through a question mark incision that begins on the zygoma, just anterior to the ear, and curves forward above the superior temporal line until it meets the external orbital angle (Fig. 65-1B). Incisions close to the ear spare the main trunk of the superficial temporal artery and the superior branch of the facial nerve. Posterior temporal lobe and inferior parietal lobe lesions require a formal temporal craniotomy, either through a reverse question mark or through a horseshoe incision. The posterior limb of the incision comes down at or just behind the interaural line (Fig. 65-1C) and should not reach the asterion. The latter is however, the most anterior and inferior point of large occipital horseshoe flaps, the mesial limbs of which may reach the posterior midline. Parietal flaps are almost always made as horseshoe incisions, the apex just touching or crossing the sagittal suture; the base of the flap is at the level of the superior temporal line (Fig. 65-2). All the standard incisions are planned in such a way as to provide access to important anatomical landmarks with preservation of the superficial blood supply as it enters the flap from the inferior margin. Fresh incisions are infiltrated with a mixture of xylocaine and epinephrine to prevent blood loss and undue traumatization of the scalp from clips and cauterization. Since glioma patients are likely to be subjected to radiation, reoperation, and chemotherapy, every attempt must be made to handle all tissue layers with the utmost gentleness. The plastic barrier drape will usually serve to keep the skin towels in place; if it does not, the towels should be sewn and not clipped to the skin. If the incision is made in short segments with firm finger pressure on either side, the use of clips and epinephrine should keep blood loss at a minimum.

It is a common error for the surgeon to progressively reduce the exposure by placing the burr holes well within the margins of the scalp incision and making the dural opening much smaller than the bone flap; this tendency must be avoided at all costs, since it defeats the purpose of designing a generous scalp flap in the first place. Prior to placement of the burr holes, the scalp margins should be retracted so as to take maximum advantage of the skin opening. Saw cuts are made at the outer margin of each burr hole so as to include the entire burr hole within the boundaries of the bone flap. During these maneuvers, tears in the dura must be avoided, since they may lead to strangulation of the brain as it herniates through the laceration. When mannitol is to be used, it should be given as a continuous drip of the 20 percent solution and not as a bolus; the infusion is usually begun with the first burr hole and continued until a total dose of 0.5 to 1.0 mg per kg body weight has been achieved. Osteoplastic bone flaps are preferable in patients likely to be exposed to devitalizing adjuvant treatments, since the bone is hinged on its own blood supply; but free flaps are quicker and are the sole option for parietal lesions. When control of the midline is required and the sagittal sinus must be crossed, burr holes should be placed on either side of the sinus; unilateral parietal flaps require only four holes and are rectangular in shape. Temporal and frontal flaps must sit low enough to expose the skull base, and extra burr holes may be required to cross the coronal and squamosal sutures. It is always useful to place burr holes directly over the pterion and on the external orbital process (the "keyhole"), to achieve control of the sphenoid wing and orbital plate, respectively.

The first point of danger is reached with the dural opening. If the dura feels tight, the head should be elevated and the neck checked for undue rotation. If these maneuvers are unsuccessful, hyperventilation may have to be increased and mannitol administered. The dura is rapidly opened so as to prevent strangulation of the brain in a small incision, and a

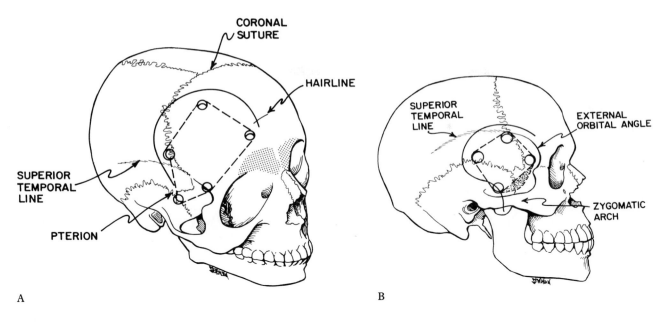

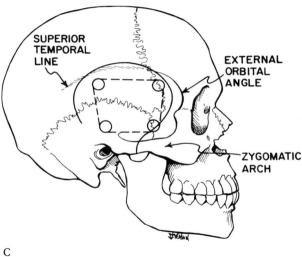

Figure 65-1 Frontal and temporal craniotomies for supratentorial glioma. *A.* In frontal craniotomies, control of the floor must be obtained through burr holes placed at the external orbital angle and at or behind the pterion. *B.* Frontotemporal craniotomies employ a question mark incision and can be used to remove the anterior temporal lobe; the bone flap rests below the superior temporal line. *C.* Temporal craniotomies employ a reverse question mark incision and are used for middle and posterior temporal lobe lesions. Scalp incisions are shown as solid lines, saw cuts as broken lines; the stippled area in *B* must be bitten away with rongeurs. All saw cuts are made at the outer edges of the burr holes.

decision is made as to whether the herniating tissue will be resected. If the dura is slack, it is recommended that it be opened in the following manner. The dural incision is planned to take maximal advantage of the bony opening, and the base of the dural flap is placed in the direction of the structures to be protected. In a frontoparietal exposure, for example, the apex of the incision points forward and the limbs are drawn backward toward the unexposed motor cortex; in a parietal exposure, the base is toward the sagittal sinus; and so forth. A dural stitch is first placed in the longest side of the intended incision, and a no. 11 blade is used to just nick the dura; the knife is employed with its cutting edge up, so that inadvertent laceration of the cortex is nearly impossible, and narrow cottonoid strips (¼-in. width) are immediately inserted to depress the brain from the dura. Advancement of the strip under the dura is much easier if it is floated by intermittent irrigation from a miniature irrigating bulb. The rest of the dura is then opened with small Metzenbaum scissors reserved only for this purpose. Once

adequate control of the midline, the temporal fossa, the orbital plate, and other anatomical landmarks has been obtained, the further and unnecessary exposure of cortex not pertinent to the procedure should be avoided.

The general location of the cortical incision is chosen prior to the design of the scalp incision and the bone flap. Tumors located superficially in the hemisphere are usually approached directly through the overlying cortex (Fig. 65-3), and those deep in the hemisphere are often reached through a paramedian approach (Fig. 65-4). At all times, the approximate location of the motor strip and all language areas must be known. A useful rule is to draw a line from the pterion to a point 2 in behind the coronal suture in the midline and at a 45° angle to the orbital plate (Fig. 65-5); the motor strip can be expected to lie along this line, and Broca's area just posterior to it in the inferior frontal gyrus. The dominant angular gyrus is usually located just above the ear. When the cortical incision must be made in the vicinity of the motor strip, it should be drawn at an acute angle to the

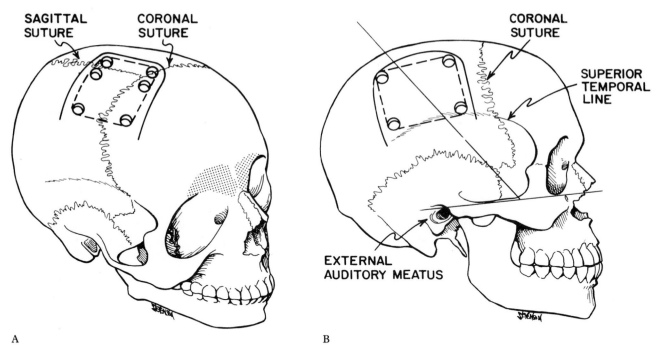

A   B

Figure 65-2 Parietal craniotomy for supratentorial glioma. *A*. Parasagittal exposures require incisions that reach or cross the midline; burr holes are made on either side of the sagittal sinus to provide a safe crossing. *B*. Exposures on the parietal boss are based above the superior temporal line, and most flaps can be located in relation to the ear. It is important to determine the approximate location of the motor strip within the bony exposure; this can be done in a number of ways. (See text and Fig. 65-5.)

45° line, cutting across the motor homunculus at a single point; the incision should always be drawn toward the motor strip and never along its long axis. The approximate location of the motor strip can also be determined through use of the

Taylor-Haughton lines and by noticing that the initial segment of the middle meningeal artery at the pterion usually points in the direction of the 45° line. It is useful to keep eloquent cortex covered by a large cottonoid throughout the

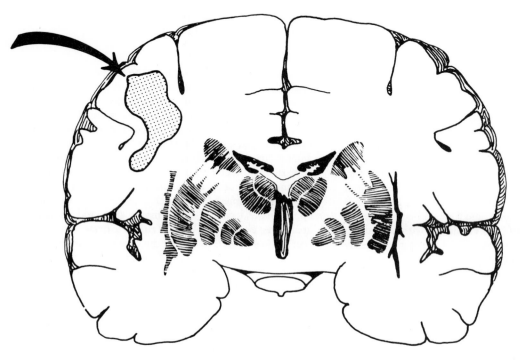

Figure 65-3 Coronal section of brain with superficial tumor in the dominant hemisphere. When a tumor comes to the surface, even in the dominant hemisphere, the safest point of attack (*arrow*) is an incision directly over the lesion.

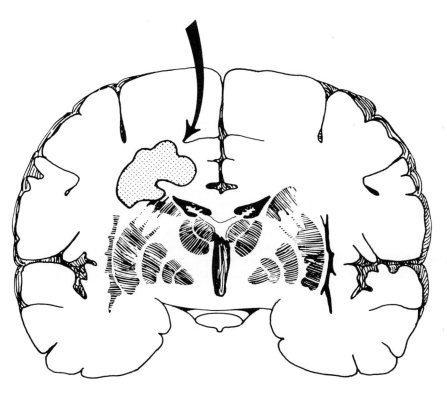

Figure 65-4 Coronal section of brain with deep tumor in dominant hemisphere. When a tumor is deep in an eloquent area, the safest point of attack (*arrow*) is an approach anterior, posterior, or medial to the involved region. In the example illustrated here, it is more acceptable to compromise the functioning of a dominant leg than a dominant hand or arm; the correct approach is the paramedian.

operation and to run the free edge of the cottonoid along the long axis of the motor strip.

The average length of the cortical incision is 2 to 3 cm, and it is made with the aid of a two-point suction cautery; I prefer the Scarff modification of the original Greenwood bipolar forceps. The instrument combines the advantages of restricted bipolar coagulation with suction at the tips of a

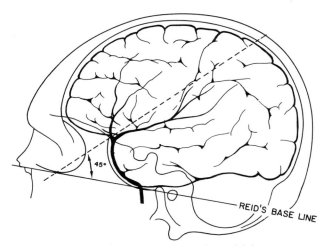

Figure 65-5 Safe resection line for frontal lobectomy. A line drawn at a 45° angle to the plane of the orbital roof and through the lateral edge of the sphenoid wing (pterion) will point in the direction of the motor strip; resections carried out posterior to this line may encroach upon the basal ganglia and Broca's area. The permissible frontal resection area is a wedge-shaped volume that extends further posteriorly along its superior surface than it does along the floor of the skull.

bayonet forceps that also can be used for grasping; as a consequence, the other hand is free to hold another bayonet forceps or a microdissector or microscissors. Although the initial subpial incision for lobectomies is made with the unaided eye, I prefer to use the operating microscope in making the small cortical incisions required for deep hemispheric work in critical areas. The suction of the two-point cautery is pinched off and the cautery used to paint the incision on the pial surface; the incision is opened with the no. 11 blade and large microscissors. The incision is deepened by spreading with the two-point forceps; no cortical plug is resected. Copper blades are attached to a Leyla self-retaining retractor, and the lips of the cortical incision are gently spread apart; the blades are always oriented parallel to the long axis of the incision, since a transverse orientation tends to cut into the brain and produce subpial hemorrhage. At this point, use of the operating microscope is absolutely essential, since a 5- to 8-cm tumor cannot be gently and safely removed through a 2-cm incision without it.

The improved illumination provided by the microscope readily permits exploration of a large space through a narrow aperture and facilitates the delineation of edematous white matter from either a low-grade glioma or the peripheral fringe of a glioblastoma. Resection of the tumor must be restricted to those areas of tissue that are clearly abnormal by virtue of their altered consistency, texture, or color. Most soft tumors can be resected with just the large two-point suction cautery, a large microscissors for cutting coagulated blood vessels, and a large microfreer dissector for establishing planes. Firm areas in fresh oligodendrogliomas, calcified astrocytomas, or previously irradiated glioblastomas are best handled with the carbon dioxide laser. With the two-point suction cautery in one hand and the micromanipulator of the laser in the other, it is possible to gently and efficiently remove large tumors with a minimum loss of blood. Small vessels are coagulated by the laser and large ones by the two-point suction cautery; the laser can be used to transect coagulated vessels as well as to vaporize the tumor on the edges of the resection field. When the low-power laser is used at 30 watts, the suction of the two-point cautery is sufficiently strong to keep the microsurgical field clear of smoke. As soon as edematous white matter is reached, fluid will be seen to glisten under the illumination of the microscope, and in some areas, actual weeping of the tissue will be observed. Throughout the resection, the size of the cavity should be measured along its major axes and these measurements compared with radiographic determinations made by CT; it goes without saying that both the actual scans and the measurements should be immediately available on the viewer of the operating theater.

At the conclusion of the resection, scrupulous hemostasis must be obtained through patient irrigation of the field and liberal use of the two-point suction cautery. The return from the irrigating fluid should be crystal clear prior to the use of oxidized cellulose or microfibrillary collagen to line the walls of the cavity. The oxidized cellulose should be laid down in thin wisps so as not to decrease the size of the resection cavity; because gelatin sponge swells and because it does not provide as satisfactory a surface for platelet adhesion, I tend to avoid leaving it in tumor resection beds. When the self-retaining retractor blades are removed, the two edges of the cortical incision should just come to rest against each another without any obvious holes or bruises in the cortical surface. The dura is always closed in a watertight fashion, and the bone flap is secured with heavy silk sutures. The scalp is closed in multiple layers and a closed drainage system inserted into the subgaleal space. On our service the practice of perioperative antibiotic coverage has recently been adopted, as well as soaking the bone flap in an iodine solution during the operation and the liberal use of iodine irrigation after the dura is closed.

When radical intratumoral resection is not feasible, normal brain may have to be sacrificed in order to achieve decompression; under these unfortunate circumstances, formal lobectomy becomes the procedure of choice. Lobectomies are always carried out as subpial resections in which the pial envelope is circumferentially incised at the point of amputation and every attempt is made to avoid repeated violation of the pial surface at other points. The frontal lobe is removed along a 45° plane with its base at the edge of the sphenoid wing and its superior edge more posteriorly placed along the upper surface of the lobe. In this fashion it is possible to avoid entering the frontal horn and endangering either the thalamus or the basal ganglia. Since the main trunk of the anterior cerebral artery winds tightly around the rostrum of the corpus callosum, this structure is usually not visualized and all major frontal arteries may be sacrificed with impunity. In the temporal lobe, it is always safer to carry out lobectomies in the anterior and inferior portions of the lobe. The inferior and middle temporal gyri, as well as those areas medially located along the edge of the tentorium, are always safe to remove. The dominant superior temporal gyrus should not be removed any farther posteriorly than 6 cm back from the temporal tip; remember that the temporal pole is hidden under the edge of the sphenoid wing and that

the measurement must be made from there. It is sometimes easier to free the tentorial edge under the operating microscope, and every temporal lobectomy should conclude with removal of the most medial aspects of the temporal lobe, a maneuver that is sure to prevent most midnight surprises.

Stereotactic Biopsy and Irradiation

Patients who are too ill for formal craniotomy or those with tumors confined to the basal ganglia and thalamus are candidates for stereotactic biopsy. Such procedures are also useful for patients with recurrent tumors in whom a change in histopathology is anticipated and when the use of interstitial irradiation or hyperthermia is planned. Some patients with cystic recurrences obtain symptomatic relief from stereotactic aspiration of the cyst. The advent of computed tomography and CT-compatible stereotactic frames (e.g., the Leksell instrument) has greatly simplified the performance of stereotactic procedures for both large and small target lesions. Nevertheless, simple biopsy carries a 2 to 3 percent mortality rate and a 3 percent serious complication rate. Although the smear preparations from such procedures yield a correct diagnosis in 95 percent of glial tumors when adequate tissue has been obtained, in 11.8 percent of the cases either the diagnosis is incorrect or the material is inadequate.[14] After stereotactic biopsy, all patients with a confirmed diagnosis of a glial neoplasm should undergo some form of external irradiation. Combined stereotactic biopsy and postoperative irradiation is an especially appropriate method of handling young and neurologically intact patients with large, nonenhancing, low-density lesions on CT. In cases of diffuse spread of a low-grade astrocytoma through large volumes of critical tissue, it is usually impossible at open craniotomy to do more than a biopsy, because the margins of the lesion are totally undefined. Since open biopsy without resection carries a higher complication and mortality rate than either closed biopsy or radical removal, it seems only prudent to subject such patients to stereotactic biopsy instead.

Surgical Results and Complications

The length and quality of postoperative survival are the most important indicators by which one can evaluate the results of any treatment for supratentorial brain tumors. The inherent risk of surgery as a treatment modality requires that some analysis also be made of perioperative morbidity and mortality. As can be seen from Table 65-3, the 30-day operative mortality for glioma surgery remained in the range of 20 to 40 percent until the advent of corticosteroids and modern neuroanesthesia in the early 1960s. Since then there has been a steady decline in surgical risk, and the authors of several published series have achieved mortality rates of less than 3 percent.[8,18] Recent attention to the details of surgical technique have also probably contributed to this steady improvement. It is the general opinion of experienced operators that limited biopsy at open surgery poses a

TABLE 65-3 Operative Mortality Rates for Patients with Glial Tumors

Series	Year	Tumor	No. Cases	Mortality, %[*]
Davis et al.[4]	1949	Glioblastoma	187	41.1
Grant[6]	1956	Astrocytoma	279	20.0
		Glioblastoma	350	38.0
		Oligodendroglioma	48	19.0
Frankel and German[5]	1958	Glioblastoma	183	18.5
Roth and Elvidge[15]	1960	Glioblastoma	399	21.5
Ley et al.[10]	1962	Astrocytoma	37	16.2
		Glioblastoma	207	31.4
		Oligodendroglioma	40	30.0
Hitchcock and Sato[7]	1964	Glioblastoma	222	19.0
Jelsma and Bucy[8‡]	1967	Glioblastoma	122	27.9
		Glioblastoma	35	2.9
Leibel et al.[9]	1975	Astrocytoma[§]	147	17.0
Salcman et al.[17,18]	1982	Glioblastoma	74	0.7

[*]One month mortality except as indicated.
[†]One week mortality.
[‡]The first series is 1948–1961; the second, 1962–1964.
[§]A number of cerebellar astrocytomas are included.

greater risk to the patient than either radical excision or a stereotactic procedure[5,7,8], and this is borne out by a retrospective analysis of the available survival data (Fig. 65-6). The selection bias in these data is quite strong, since there is a tendency for older and sicker patients to receive more limited surgical procedures. Nevertheless, the analysis is based on 603 patients drawn from the literature who did not receive postoperative radiation for glioblastoma, and it is quite unlikely that any better data will ever be accrued on the effects of surgery uncontaminated by the influence of other concomitant therapies. Since the extent of surgical resection for cancers elsewhere in the body can also be correlated with the length of postoperative survival, the general principle that radical excision is preferable to either partial removal or simple biopsy is adequately supported. It is my impression that the operating microscope and the carbon dioxide laser facilitate the performance of a more radical tumor removal

in greater numbers of patients and with correspondingly less operative morbidity and mortality.

Somewhat surprisingly, relatively little attention has been paid to postoperative morbidity, because survival was the prime issue of importance in the early series. Davis and his associates did provide several anecdotal reports of patients retaining the ability to fulfill their economic and social obligations but made no statistical analysis.[4] In 44 patients surviving more than 3 months after surgery for glioblastoma, Hitchcock and Sato found that 76 percent had a "useful" survival of at least 6 months but that only 28 percent were able to return to work.[7] Of course, the failure of patients to return to work is subject to many factors other than the postoperative neurological condition; among these are familial, social, psychological, and economic influences. Up to 40 percent of postoperative survivors are neurologically normal or suffer from such minimal deficits as facial weak-

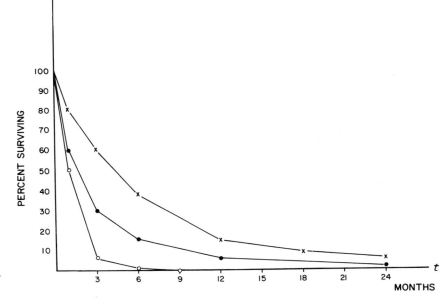

Figure 65-6 Percentage of glioblastoma patients surviving as a function of time and type of surgery. The curves are based on 603 patients drawn from the literature in which extensive surgical resection (X's, 172 cases), partial surgical resection (closed circles, 301 cases), and simple biopsy (open circles, 130 cases) were used *without* subsequent irradiation or chemotherapy.

ness and quadrantanopsia;[5,15] another 26 percent suffer from more severe deficits, including hemiparesis, but remain ambulatory and able to care for themselves.[15] Patients undergoing extensive resections have the greatest likelihood of improving their preoperative condition and achieving some degree of independent existence.[8] It is reasonable to suppose that those procedures with the highest postoperative mortality (i.e., biopsy and partial removal) also result in the greatest degree of functional impairment among the survivors.[8] Only one systematic study has been made comparing the preoperative and postoperative neurological grading of patients with malignant glioma.[20] Eighty-two patients with gliomas were examined for evidence of abnormalities in speech, personality, and visual, sensory, or motor function. Preoperative abnormalities were observed in 191 of the 410 functional areas examined, and 151 of these were improved or unchanged after surgery, in comparison with only 40 that became worse. Overall, patients were helped rather than hurt by the surgical procedure ($p < 0.05$), and Shapiro concluded that the "resection of neuroectodermal tumors is more likely to alleviate existing symptoms than to produce additional ones."[20]

It is common practice to give postoperative irradiation to patients with glioblastoma but it is not equally appreciated that a similar policy should be adopted in regard to all grades of supratentorial astrocytoma.[9,19] The 5-year survival rate for patients with grade 1 and grade 2 astrocytomas is only 19 percent after incomplete resection but is 46 percent when postoperative irradiation is added.[9] In some series, the magnitude of the beneficial effect of irradiation for low-grade tumors has even been independent of the extent of the resection.[19] Patients with oligodendroglioma also appear to benefit from combined-modality therapy. In a series of 35 patients evaluated at more than 5 years after surgery, the 5-year survival rate for surgery alone was 82 percent and the recurrence rate (including deaths) was 36 percent; in contrast, the 5-year survival rate after both surgery and irradiation was 100 percent, and there were no clinical or radiographic recurrences.[2] An important consideration, in this regard, is the theoretical necessity of providing maximal therapy at the earliest possible juncture in the clinical course, since recurrence is almost invariably fatal. Two-thirds of all astrocytomas are of a more malignant grade at the time of first recurrence, with nearly one-third of grade 1 tumors and nearly one-half of grade 2 tumors having become frank glioblastomas.[12] Similarly, 50 percent of recurrent oligodendrogliomas appear to be histologically more malignant at reoperation, and nearly 20 percent recur as glioblastomas.[13] Hence it is my current recommendation that all adult patients with a supratentorial astrocytoma or oligodendroglioma undergo postoperative irradiation.

Without radiation, the median postoperative survival for patients with glioblastoma is only 4 months, even if all cases with limited resections or simple biopsies are excluded.[16] The addition of postoperative irradiation increases this figure to 9.25 months and improves the 2-year survival rate from 3 to 11 percent. Although the use of postoperative irradiation increases the proportion of patients surviving at all intermediate points in the first 18 months following surgery, the natural course of the disease is such that all survival curves, irrespective of the mode of treatment, appear to converge at 18 to 24 months after diagnosis. Nevertheless, the value of irradiation is unequivocal, since virtually all study groups that have reported a zero percent 2-year survival rate also failed to irradiate their patients.[16] Unfortunately, the amount of external irradiation that can be safely delivered is limited by the sensitivity of the brain and its blood vessels to the detrimental effects of ionizing radiation.

Further small increments in the length of postoperative survival can be obtained through the use of nitrosourea chemotherapy; the number of long-term survivors is increased in randomized studies,[21] and the median survival in a retrospective analysis of maximally operated patients rises to almost 10 months.[16] Nevertheless, the beneficial effect of chemotherapy is so modest that it is easily obscured by the impact of such major prognostic variables as age and performance status;[17,21] in addition, chemotherapy does not appear to influence the shape of the survival curve or the likelihood of cure in the majority of patients.[16] It is my impression that some tumors in young patients are inherently more sensitive to nitrosourea than virtually any tumors in older patients, thus contributing to the marked dependency of survival statistics on the patient's age at diagnosis.[17] The end result of this and other biological factors is an inability to extend either the median survival beyond 15 months or the 2-year survival rate beyond 25 percent in patients with malignant astrocytoma, even when they are subjected to an extremely aggressive combination of radical resection, maximum radiation, high-dose chemotherapy, and frequent reoperation.[17] It is conceivable that therapeutic failures are rooted in the cellular heterogeneity of most solid tumors and the tendency to deliver treatments sequentially in isolation rather than in combination.[18]

Indications for Reoperation

Relatively few data exist concerning the efficacy of reoperation in the treatment of recurrent gliomas; for this reason, if for no other, considerable controversy surrounds the proper role of surgery in the context of primary treatment failure. Historically speaking, published reoperation rates have been low, generally in the range of 0 to 10 percent, and the surgical mortality for such procedures has been high, in the range of 10 to 20 percent. Additionally, most surgeons have been highly selective in their choice of patients for reoperation, so the available data are biased by an inordinate number of cases of low-grade astrocytoma and oligodendroglioma. Reoperations are usually carried out in patients who are relatively young and in good neurological condition, in those who have tumors that are favorably situated, and in those in whom recurrence has occurred long after operation. In the case of low-grade tumors, this inconsistent policy has hampered the histological study of recurrent tumors and delayed the understanding of their biological evolution.[12,13] Even fewer patients with glioblastoma have been submitted to reoperation, on the possibly erroneous assumption that surgery has nothing to offer the patient with a malignant glioma. As this chapter has already indicated, there are several good reasons for questioning this assumption: (1) the rough correlation between the length of postoperative survival and the extent of surgical resection in patients with malignant astrocytoma and medulloblastoma; (2) the importance of early and radical surgery in the treatment of solid cancers elsewhere in the body; (3) the existence of cell compartments within malignant gliomas that are inherently resistant to all other treatment modalities; and (4) the possible potentiation of other treatments by mechanical cytoreduction. Therefore the rationale for primary surgery may apply equally well to reoperation, especially if sampling of the tissue is adequate and a fresh evaluation of both the tumor and the effects of previous therapy can be made.

Roth and Elvidge reoperated on only 13 of their 399 patients (3 percent) with glioblastoma and achieved an average additional survival of 4.5 months;[15] it should be noted, however, that the survival of one of these patients after reoperation (17 months) was greater than the interoperative interval of 14 months. Frankel and German reoperated on 28 of their 183 patients (15.3 percent) but did not comment on the effect of these procedures, despite the fact that one patient was subjected to 5 operations.[5] In another series, approximately 10 percent of all patients with intracerebral gliomas were reoperated on, but only 4.4 percent of the patients with glioblastoma;[11] once again, the effectiveness of this policy was not commented on. Young and associates carefully analyzed a series of 24 reoperated cases of glioblastoma accumulated over a 12-year period and found that the length of survival after the second operation correlated significantly with the preoperative neurological status and weakly with the length of the interoperative interval.[22] The patients in this retrospective study were operated on at two separate institutions by a large number of neurosurgeons and represented less than 5 percent of their treated cases. We have recently reported a consecutive series of 74 patients admitted to an aggressive multimodality treatment program, in which reoperation was prospectively offered to all malignant astrocytoma patients prior to the institution of any new therapy, irrespective of the age of the patient, the histologic grade of the tumor, the location of the tumor, or its previous response to treatment.[17] Reoperation was withheld when the performance status or neurological function was so poor that no further therapy of any kind was actively considered. In 36 months, 40 patients had second operations and achieved a median survival of 37 weeks from the time of reoperation (Fig. 65-7). Virtually all the procedures were carried out with the aid of the operating microscope and the carbon dioxide laser in the context of aggressive multimodality treatment. There were no operative deaths in 60 reoperations. There were four serious infections; the total morbidity rate for reoperation was 8.3 percent. In our series, the length of survival after the second operation was not correlated with patient age, performance status, tumor grade, or the interoperative interval, and it was concluded that reoperation for malignant astrocytoma is safe, feasible, and of potential benefit in combination with other therapies. The routine use of reoperation to "set up" other treatment modalities deserves further study.[17,18,20]

It must be emphasized that reoperation requires exquisite attention to the details of surgical technique, since the incidence of postoperative infection is high and the condition of the tissues often poor. The majority of patients pre-

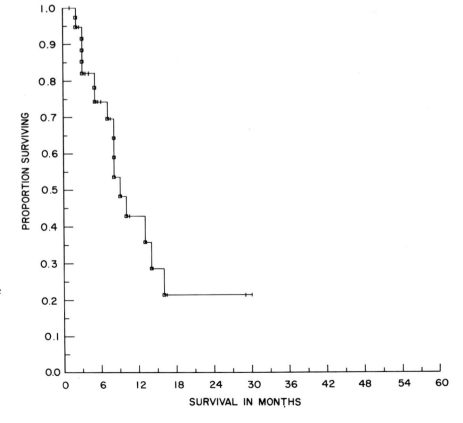

Figure 65-7 Kaplan-Meier survival curve after repeat surgery for malignant astrocytoma. The calculated probability of survival from the time of the *second* operation is plotted for 40 patients reoperated upon in a consecutive series of 74 in which reoperation was prospectively used during aggressive multimodality therapy; the median additional survival time is 37 weeks. (From Salcman et al.[17])

senting for reoperation have already failed some combination of surgery, radiation, and chemotherapy; the scalp is usually devitalized and the dura in poor repair. It is my impression that the operating microscope and the carbon dioxide laser are of great benefit in minimizing the neurological cost to the patient while maximizing the extent of the surgical resection. Parenthetically, it should be mentioned that previously irradiated gliomas are often easier to remove by virtue of their impaired blood supply. Nevertheless, firm areas of radionecrosis and calcification still pose intraoperative risks to the patient if undue manipulation results in the brain being "rocked" around; hence the great advantage of resection techniques such as the laser that do not cause visible movement of the brain.

References

1. Bennett H, Godlee RJ: Excision of a tumor from the brain. Lancet 2:1090–1091, 1884.
2. Chin HW, Hazel JJ, Kim TH, Webster JH: Oligodendrogliomas: I. A clinical study of cerebral oligodendrogliomas. Cancer 45:1458–1466, 1980.
3. Cushing H: *Intracranial Tumours: Notes Upon a Series of Two Thousand Verified Cases with Surgical-Mortality Percentages Pertaining Thereto.* Springfield, Ill., Charles C Thomas, 1932.
4. Davis L, Martin J, Goldstein SL, Ashkenazy M: A study of 211 patients with verified glioblastoma multiforme. J Neurosurg 6:33–44, 1949.
5. Frankel SA, German WJ: Glioblastoma multiforme: Review of 219 cases with regard to natural history, pathology, diagnostic methods, and treatment. J Neurosurg 15:489–503, 1958.
6. Grant FC: A study of the results of surgical treatment in 2,326 consecutive patients with brain tumor. J Neurosurg 13:479–488, 1956.
7. Hitchcock E, Sato F: Treatment of malignant gliomata. J Neurosurg 21:497–505, 1964.
8. Jelsma R, Bucy PC: The treatment of glioblastoma multiforme of the brain. J Neurosurg 27:388–400, 1967.
9. Leibel SA, Sheline GE, Wara WM, Boldrey EB, Nielsen SL: The role of radiation therapy in the treatment of astrocytomas. Cancer 35:1551–1557, 1975.
10. Ley A, Ley A Jr, Guitart JM, Oliveras C: Surgical management of intracranial gliomas. J Neurosurg 19:365–374, 1962.
11. McKeran RO, Thomas DGT: The clinical study of gliomas, in Thomas DGT, Graham DI (eds): *Brain Tumours: Scientific Basis, Clinical Investigation and Current Therapy.* Boston, Butterworth, 1980, pp 194–230.
12. Müller W, Áfra D, Schröder R: Supratentorial recurrences of gliomas: Morphological studies in relation to time intervals with astrocytomas. Acta Neurochir (Wien) 37:75–91, 1977.
13. Müller W, Áfra D, Schröder R: Supratentorial recurrences of gliomas: Morphological studies in relation to time intervals with oligodendrogliomas. Acta Neurochir (Wien) 39:15–25, 1977.
14. Ostertag CB, Mennel HD, Kiessling M: Stereotactic biopsy of brain tumors. Surg Neurol 14:275–283, 1980.
15. Roth JG, Elvidge AR: Glioblastoma multiforme: A clinical survey. J Neurosurg 17:736–750, 1960.
16. Salcman M: Survival in glioblastoma: Historical perspective. Neurosurgery 7:435–439, 1980.
17. Salcman M, Kaplan RS, Ducker TB, Abdo H, Montgomery E: Effect of age and reoperation on survival in the combined modality treatment of malignant astrocytoma. Neurosurgery 10:454–463, 1982.
18. Salcman M, Kaplan RS, Samaras GM, Ducker TB, Broadwell RD: Aggressive multimodality therapy based on a multicompartmental model of glioblastoma. Surgery 92:250–259, 1982.
19. Scanlon PW, Taylor WF: Radiotherapy of intracranial astrocytomas: Analysis of 417 cases treated from 1960 through 1969. Neurosurgery 5:301–308, 1979.
20. Shapiro WR: Treatment of neuroectodermal brain tumors. Ann Neurol 12:231–237, 1982.
21. Walker MD, Green SB, Byar DP, Alexander E Jr, Batzdorf U, Brooks WH, Hunt WE, MacCarty CS, Mahaley MS Jr, Mealey J, Owens G, Ransohoff J II, Robertson JT, Shapiro WR, Smith KR Jr, Wilson CB, Strike TA: Randomized comparisons of radiotherapy and nitrosoureas for the treatment of malignant glioma after surgery. N Engl J Med 303:1323–1329, 1980.
22. Young B, Oldfield EH, Markesbery WR, Haack D, Tibbs PA, McCombs P, Chin HW, Maruyama Y, Meacham WF: Reoperation for glioblastoma. J Neurosurg 55:917–921, 1981.

SECTION C

Metastatic Brain Tumors

66

Factors That Govern the Metastatic Process

Leonard Weiss

The staging of cancer and its treatment are dependent on the presence or absence of metastases. The specific clinical details and the biology of metastases vary with the site and extent of target organ involvement and with the nature of the primary cancer. The picture is complicated by individual variations in host response and anatomy and by the natural history of the metastatic process as modified by treatment. Detailed discussions of basic and clinical aspects of metastasis to the lung,[8] brain,[12] lymphatic system,[11] bones,[9] and liver[10] are given in the References; this chapter provides a brief overview of some of the factors thought to govern various steps of the so-called metastatic cascade.

The metastatic cascade consists of a number of exceptionally complex, overlapping, repetitive steps as outlined in Figure 66-1. The first phase is concerned with invasion and ultimately involves the entry of cancer cells into blood and lymphatic vessels as well as body spaces and cavities. The second phase of dissemination involves the transport of cells that have gained access to the various disseminative channels and their arrest at target sites. Most of the arrested cells are released either before or after being killed. The comparatively few viable cells retained in the target organs develop into micrometastases, which in themselves are relatively harmless. However, as a result of cancer-host interactions, the micrometastases may enter a growth phase and develop into metastases. A major clinical problem is the detection of micrometastases and the prevention of their development. The final step is the metastasis of the metastases.

A major problem in determining the mechanisms involved in metastasis is obtaining suitable animal models. Although the genetics and immunology of mouse tumor systems are well documented, the short life span and hemodynamics of the mouse make it in some respects an unsuitable model. In larger animals, although their life spans and hemodynamics are more relevant to the human situation, the genetic uncertainties, problems in obtaining transplantable cancers, and practical difficulties associated with procuring large animals with spontaneous tumors make it difficult to perform reproducible experiments. In the author's opinion, no experimental system provides a total model for human metastasis, but judicious studies with these systems provide useful information on parts of this disease process. The development of noninvasive techniques will, it may be hoped, permit the ethical study of metastasis in humans.

Cell Detachment from the Primary Cancer

Detachment is an essential part of the metastatic process, since by definition, a metastasis is a cancer which has lost contiguity with the tumor generating it. This topic has been reviewed in detail by Weiss and Ward.[15]

The suggestion that the undeniable tendency of cancer cells to detach from their parent tumors is an inherent part of the malignant phenotype is a misleading simplification, since it focuses exclusively on hypothetical stable cancer-specific properties of the cancer cells themselves. Cell detachment is not cancer-specific, and although normal tissues do not metastasize, it must be emphasized that detachment is not synonymous with metastasis. The relative ease with which cancer cells detach from tumors varies not only with the pathophysiological status of the malignant cells themselves but also with the dynamic properties of the whole tumor, which contains cancer and noncancer cells, both modified by host response.

Factors Affecting Detachment

Many tumors exhibit considerable heterogeneity, not only with respect to the cancer cells which they contain, but also with respect to regions of proliferation and necrosis, host cell infiltration, fibrosis, encapsulation, and blood supply.

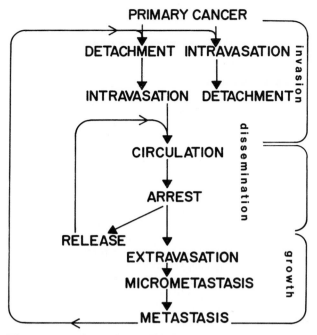

Figure 66-1 A much simplified overview of the various steps in the invasive, disseminative, and growth phases of metastasis.

The effects of some of these variables on cell detachment have been quantitated by various techniques in which cultured cells are detached from their substrata by known hydrodynamic forces or are shaken free of small blocks of tissues under carefully standardized conditions.

Growth Rate

A number of experiments made with cancer and noncancer cells have revealed that the higher the growth rate the more easily the cells are detached from one another and from artificial substrates. As cell detachment is only an initial step in a complex series, it is unlikely that correlations could be demonstrated between tumor growth rate, detachment, and metastasis over the whole range of cancers, where so many other variables come into play. Attempts to correlate growth rate with metastasis reveal many apparent contradictions, such as rapidly growing tumors which do not metastasize and slow-growing tumors which do. However, in a number of palpable human epitheliomas in which growth rate could be assessed by size change measured with calipers, Glücksmann[4] reported a striking correlation between growth coefficient and the incidence of local lymph node metastasis.

Necrosis

Necrosis is a common feature of solid tumors, as a consequence of growth-associated vascular insufficiency, host-defense reactions, and therapeutic intervention. In studies on W256 tumors, regions of central necrosis developed in tumors exceeding 1 cm in diameter. It was shown that viable cancer cells were more readily detached from each other in the juxtanecrotic regions than in the more peripheral regions of tumors. This effect was mimicked by exposing samples from the tumor peripheries to saline extracts of the necrotic core. When W256 tumors grow in the rat liver, the parenchymal cells close to the tumor edges may be more easily separated from each other than those located 0.5 or 1 cm from the tumor periphery. The evidence suggested that the necrotic material acted as a pool of free lysosomal enzymes and other material which acted on the various cells present in the tumors and facilitated their detachment by direct or indirect mechanisms.

Whether the demonstrable necrosis-associated facilitation of detachment actually promotes metastasis depends on whether the released cancer cells are free to disseminate. On the one hand, the facilitated detachment of cells in the tissues surrounding a tumor is reasonably expected to promote its invasion, particularly as necrotic extracts promote the active movements of some types of cancer cells. On the other hand, if necrosis results from vascular insufficiency, immediate dissemination of detached cancer cells may not occur. Depending on the accessibility of cancer cell "escape routes," there is the possibility that by causing necrosis in the absence of a 100 percent kill, local therapy may actually promote dissemination. In this connection it is of interest that exposure of cancer cells to a variety of antimetabolites promotes their detachment in vitro.

Enzymes

Many pathological processes associated with inflammation, immune response, therapy, etc. are ultimately expressed in enzyme release; in events related to metastasis, the enzymes may be derived from the cancer cells themselves, from vascular endothelial cells, from cells of the reticuloendothelial system, and other types of cell. It has been known for many years that viable cells may be liberated from a variety of tissues by the action of enzymes combined with the application of distractive forces generated by muscle movements, surgical trauma, etc. In essence, free enzymes may facilitate cell detachment by lysis of intercellular material. In addition, the release of endogenous enzymes by both cancer cells and nonmalignant "bystanders" also facilitates detachment. The lysosomes constitute an obvious and well-documented nonexclusive source of such enzymes, and a large number of factors activating lysosomes promote detachment, whereas a number of agents stabilizing lysosomes inhibit the process.

Stress

Although the effects of surgical manipulation on cancer cell release are well documented, it is not generally appreciated that the appearance of malignant cells in the bloodstream and the release of cells from tissues can be promoted by anesthesia. These disquieting phenomena are worthy of further study!

Cell Movement

Cell movement may be active or passive. In invasive processes, cancer cells may crawl through tissues and breach basement membranes during intravasation and extravasation. Alternatively, invasion may result from the expansive forces generated by growing tumors (*vis a tergo*), and movement will occur along the paths of least mechanical resistance. Expansion by growth can result in arrested tumor emboli bursting out of blood vessels. Although active movement of cancer cells was recognized by Virchow in 1863, for various technical reasons the relative importance of crawling and growth-associated expansive movements were never quantitatively assessed until recently. A technique has been developed in which, from statistical analyses of cancer cell density counts made on tumor sections, the diffusive density patterns associated with active cell movement may be discriminated from the more abrupt patterns associated with growth. Tests of the technique made on sections of malignant melanomas in human skin confirm the validity of the technique and indicate that actively moving melanoma cells invade the dermis to a depth of up to 500 μm in advance of the main tumor body. Within this zone, it appears that the cancer cells stop migrating and proliferate. The whole process is then repeated.[14]

For active locomotion to occur, cancer cells must first make contact with and adhere to tissues through which they move; locomotor energy generated by the cell acts on these adhesive regions, and finally, localized detachment must occur to permit translatory movements. Therefore, agents promoting initial cell adhesion and cell detachment and stimulating the actin-containing contractile microfilaments in cancer cells are expected to promote active movements and vice versa. Enzymes are expected to have paradoxical effects, because they may inhibit the formation of focal adhesions or destroy them and may also promote detachment. The action of any agent will probably depend on its effects on a rather delicate balance of the three basic components of active movement. In addition to these effects, enzymes, by acting on the noncancerous tissues surrounding a tumor, may facilitate movement by expansion. In contrast, by destroying the substrate through which a cell could move and thus preventing adhesion, enzyme-related tissue lysis could also prevent or inhibit active movements of cancer cells.

Circulating Cancer Cells

Cancer cells may gain direct access to the venous circulation, or alternatively may gain access first to the lymphatic system and then to the bloodstream. There are so many communications between the lymphatic and venous systems that except in the earliest stages of metastatic cancer, it seems unrealistic to consider metastasis as being limited to one system or the other. This view should not be confused with the question of the desirability of lymph node removal in the treatment of early cancers, since this has the double function of staging and the eradication of potential generalizing sites.

The question of why carcinomas disseminate via the lymphatics and sarcomas via the blood should be rephrased. The evidence is that lymphnode metastases are approximately three times as common in carcinomas as in sarcomas, which does not make lymphogenous metastasis of sarcomas rare, and the postregional lymphnode pattern of metastasis from carcinomas is frequently hematogenous. The initial disseminative route is to some extent influenced by the site of cell detachment from the primary lesion. If detachment occurs prior to contact between the tumor and blood channels, as in the case of early cutaneous melanomas, for example, where cancer cells actively locomote through the dermis, they will have the opportunity to gain early access to the lymphatic system. If contact with blood channels occurs prior to detachment, venous dissemination will be the preferred initial route. If parts of an invasive tumor project into lumen of a blood vessel, cells can be detached by a combination of factors described above. An alternative mode of entry takes place in sarcomas, where vascular clefts lined by cancer cells are present and shedding is directly into the bloodstream.

Any quantitative assessment of hematogenous metastasis requires knowledge of the numbers of cancer cells entering the bloodstream. Much of the earlier literature on the occurrence of circulating cancer cells in people is suspect because in a number of papers, megakaryocytes and degenerate cells were erroneously described as cancer cells. However, reports of positive identification of cancer cells in the venous effluents of many tumors clearly indicate that large numbers enter the bloodstream, although quantitation is lacking. Using tumor grafts into the ovarian bed of rats, where the entire venous drainage occurs through a single cannulated ovarian vein, Butler and Gullino[2] estimated that approximately one million cancer cells were liberated into the venous blood per gram of tumor every 24 hours. On the reasonable assumption that millions of viable cancer cells are liberated into the blood of patients with cancer, then as overt metastases usually occur with a frequency which is orders of magnitude less, one is forced to conclude that in terms of the cancer cells involved, metastasis is a remarkably inefficient process. It is paradoxical that an inefficient process should result in the deaths of so many patients! However, even an inefficient process will succeed if repeated often enough.

By all accounts, the circulation is a hostile environment for cancer cells, and unless they can extravasate, the vast majority perish. Part of the circulatory trauma appears to be due to the mechanical deformation imposed on cells in passing through the microcirculation. In some cases at least, the more deformable cancer cells are, the less circulatory trauma they suffer. As with most other properties of cancer cells, their deformability is not a constant property but probably varies with a number of intracellular factors such as stage in the cell cycle and nonlethal digestion of the cancer cell periphery by enzymes released by the cancer cells themselves and/or nearby cancer or noncancer cells.[7] It is of interest that some of the enzymes and enzyme-release mechanisms implicated in cell detachment and the invasive processes associated with intravasation should also apparently enhance the survival of circulating cancer cells. In addition to mechanical trauma, naturally occurring cytotoxic factors in the serum may also contribute to cancer cell death. However, in a review of the literature on experimental work in this area, it was often impossible to discriminate between rather ill-defined humoral immunologic factors which are of doubtful relevance to the human situation and nonimmunologic agents.

Arrest of Circulating Cancer Cells

As noted earlier, without arrest metastasis cannot occur, and continuously circulating cancer cells die.

The surfaces of all types of human cells carry a net negative electric charge. This results in an average electrostatic repulsion between cancer cells and vascular endothelial cells, which tends to prevent their contact and adhesion. The charged groups on a number of cells tend to be arranged in clusters, and in some cells contact is made via fine probes or macromolecules and those surface regions between the clusters, where the charge density is low.[13] The macromolecules which could be involved include the glycoproteins laminin and fibronectin.

Another factor inhibiting contact relates to fluid displacement from between the vascular endothelium and approaching cancer cells. When a cancer cell moves in the blood, hydrodynamic forces are generated which cause pressure changes and plasma movements close to its surface. This hydrodynamic field is significantly perturbed when the distance separating the cancer cell from the vascular endothelium is less than the cancer cell radius, leading to retardation in contact and hence cell arrest. If the cancer cells are deformed in the contact-making process, so that the cancer cell is flattened to match the contours of the opposing endothelium, the average distance between the two surfaces will be decreased and contact and arrest will take longer. Thus, on the one hand, cancer cell deformability increases survival in the circulation and hence promotes metastasis; on the other hand, deformability may serve to keep cancer cells in the circulation longer, thereby decreasing the chances of metastasis. The balance of this paradoxical situation is doubtless variable within the same population of cancer cells and may vary between cancer cells of different types.

Another interaction of cancer cell emboli and the vascular endothelium involves embolic size. Single cancer cells tend to be at least temporarily arrested at the level of capillaries and postcapillary venules, subject to electrostatic and hemodynamic considerations. Multicellular emboli tend to be shunted through larger vessels and to be physically impacted. Not only is the arrest mechanism somewhat different, but arrest is more permanent in the case of multicellular emboli, where, in addition, the outer cells tend to protect the innermost cells. In experimental animals, these and possibly other factors lead to a greater metastatic efficiency of multicellular than of unicellular emboli.

If the microcirculation of an organ is considered in terms of microcirculatory units, the arrest of cancer cells at the precapillary sphincter can cause microinjury in the distal capillary bed. It is argued that as a result of this injury there is increased arrest of cancer cells in this region, and that in association with the increased permeability the extravasation of the arrested cells is facilitated.[6]

Thrombosis and Cancer Cell Arrest

Fibrin and platelet deposition is often seen associated with arrested cancer cells, particularly where there is defect in the vascular endothelium revealing the underlying basement membrane. Studies by the author and his associates in mice[3] revealed no changes in the arrest patterns of several types of intravenously injected cancer cells when the platelet release reaction was depressed by the administration of aspirin. In addition, therapeutic doses of heparin and warfarin, which affect different levels of the coagulation cascade, were also without effect on cancer cell arrest patterns in both normal mice and tumor-bearing animals with the coagulopathies typically associated with cancer. These experiments suggest that coagulation factors do not play a key role in cancer cell arrest, although other studies on different tumor systems have shown that drugs either inhibiting coagulation or promoting fibrinolysis reduce the incidence of lung tumors if given before the intravenous injection of cancer cells, but not if given 24 hours after. The implication is that fibrin provides necessary short-term protection for arrested cancer cells. Both experimental and human cancer cells exhibit differing degrees of plasminogen activation, and the resulting fibrinolysis would thus be expected to reduce their metastatic potential.

In view of the association of platelets and fibrin with the metastatic process, there have been many attempts to utilize anticoagulants in antimetastatic therapy. Although the reports of these attempts are both conflicting and confusing, it appears that under certain conditions anticoagulants can reduce the incidence of metastases.[5,15] However, this antimetastatic effect may not be due to their anticoagulant activity. For example, aspirin interferes with prostaglandin biosynthesis, and warfarin can inhibit cell motility. Another complicating factor is that some agents, for example aspirin, appear to have differential activity on platelets and on vascular endothelial cells.

A physiological role of the vascular endothelium is to maintain vascular integrity by means of self-purging mechanisms. In situations where thrombi involving platelets are concerned, there is a delicate intravascular balance between the activities of thromboxane A_2 (TXA_2), which aggregates platelets as part of host defense, and prostacyclin (PGI_2), which is released by the vascular endothelium and which inhibits TXA_2-induced platelet aggregation. The PGI_2-TXA_2 balance is disturbed in the presence of some cancer cells in favor of TXA_2-induced platelet aggregation, which is thought to promote metastasis. On this basis, Honn and colleagues[5] have administered agents either promoting PGI_2 activity or synthesis or inhibiting TXA_2 synthesis to mice injected with cancer cells or bearing tumors and have demonstrated antimetastatic activity. Regardless of whether this form of therapy proves applicable to humans, the observations serve to illustrate the importance in metastasis of interactions involving the vascular endothelium.

Release of Arrested Cancer Cells

When radiolabeled cancer cells are injected directly into the systemic venous system of experimental animals, counts made within 5 minutes usually indicate that 70 to 100 percent of the labeled cells are arrested within the pulmonary microvasculature. After this time there is a progressive loss of cancer cells, so that by 24 hours the lung counts usually represent less than 5 percent of those injected. As the cells leave the lungs, there is a concomitant increase in counts in other organs; however, the majority of the cells secondarily arrested are nonviable, and most of the radioactivity is excreted by the animals, indicating that the vast majority of injected cancer cells are killed in association with passage through the pulmonary vasculature. The surviving cells form tumors, commonly in the lungs, with few extrapulmonary lesions. In some cases, particularly with cancer cells previously subjected to in vitro or in vivo selection, there may be no overt pulmonary tumors but a predominance of tumors in other specific organs; the relevance of these specific patterns to naturally occuring metastatic patterns is currently receiving much attention. However, the chief phenomenon is that a major cause of metastatic inefficiency in experimental animals appears to be the intravascular transpulmonary passage of cancer cells, and that either prior to release or after release from their temporary arrest sites most of them are killed. Other studies in which cancer cells are widely disseminated following left ventricular injection into mice also demonstrate almost total clearance over 24 hours in the liver, kidneys, brain, pancreas, myocardium, and ileum.

Cell detachment is not in itself a lethal procedure, but assessment of the release of viable cancer cells from secondary target organs in humans is very difficult, because a number of different phenomena may be involved. In experimental animals there is little question that injected cancer cells can rapidly pass through various organs via vascular or lymphatic shunts. However, in assessing the relevance of these observations to humans, it must be borne in mind that in mice, with a blood volume of approximately 2 ml, the rapid intravenous injection of 0.2 ml of cancer cell suspension can modify arrest patterns and may open up "abnormal" vascular pathways. Comparison of circulating cancer cells with leukocytes raises the possibility that at least some of the cancer cells passing through the microcirculation of an organ marginate and make very slow transit without adhering to the vessel walls. In both these cases, lethal interactions with the cells of the vascular endothelium are expected to be minimal, although mechanical damage is expected to increase with shear rate. In some cases, temporary arrest by virtue of cancer cell adhesion to the vascular endothelium does occur; some retained cells survive to form metastases, and in others, cellular contact interactions probably result in cell death. If death is associated with the release of factors such as detachment-active enzymes, for example, living cells close to the dead cells could also be released; but it should be emphasized that the release of such enzymes is not necessarily lethal. Finally, as metastasizing of metastases is probably a common event,[1] the cancer cells leaving an organ need not be the identical cells arriving in it but their descendants and are subject to the same considerations as cells released from the primary cancer.

The mechanisms causing the release of temporarily arrested tumor emboli are not clear. They involve not only the cancer cells but also the vascular endothelium and associated leukocytes. In general, the factors promoting the release of cells from primary cancers are also expected to promote their release from temporary arrest sites at the vascular endothelium.

The retention of cancer cells by the vascular endothelium may be modified by the immune response associated with tumor bearing. It has been shown that following sensitization, retention of injected cancer cells in the lungs is increased in some tumor-host situations; in others it is decreased, and in others not changed at all.

Cancer cell release can also be mediated in part by so-called natural killer (NK) cells, which are part of the nonimmunologic defense system. Vascular clearance is impaired in animals with defective NK function and is increased in animals with increased NK activity. The reticuloendothelial system (RES), which includes the mobile and sessile mononuclear phagocytes, leukocytes, and vascular endothelial cells, also participates in clearance of arrested cancer cells. This is indicated by studies in which stimulation of the RES by glucan, BCG, *Corynebacterium parvum*, endotoxin, and zymosan was associated with increased clearance, whereas inhibition of the RES by silica and trypan blue was associated with reduced clearance.

The final common pathway in many host defense mechanisms, including inflammation and immune response, involves enzyme release over and above background levels. Enhancement of enzyme release may on the one hand favor cell detachment from primary cancers and thereby promote invasion and metastasis, but on the other hand release of cancer cells from their arrest sites at the vascular endothelium may inhibit metastasis and constitute a major contribution to metastatic inefficiency. The extent to which secondary release precedes or follows cancer cell death remains to be determined.

Further Development of Metastases

Cells retained in the vasculature of an organ extravasate at an early stage in metastasis development. Extravasation can occur if cancer cells actively migrate through vessel walls, or alternatively, growing emboli can burst out. Both these processes would presumably be aided by enzyme-mediated lysis of basement membranes and the weakening associated with increases in vascular permeability.

While the developing metastasis is less than approximately 2 mm in diameter, it can obtain its nutrition by diffusion processes. This provides a functional definition of a micrometastasis, since the increase in size of a micrometastasis to a metastasis requires vascularization. This is achieved by diffusion of angiogenic factors from the tumor to local host capillaries; the endothelial cells are stimulated into mitosis and grow toward and invade the tumor, ensuring its nutrition and growth. The role of neovascularization is emphasized by experiments showing that agents such as cartilage inhibit tumor growth by inhibition of angiogenesis. Angiogenic factors are not specific for cancer cells but may also be produced by inflammatory cells and fibroblasts. It appears likely that two components in the neovascularization cascade are prostaglandin E_1 (and other prostaglandins to a lesser extent) and copper utilization.[16] It is therefore of interest that prostaglandin E (PGE) production is one of a number of factors involved in the failure of the immune system to eliminate tumor growth; while immune stimulation results in enhanced PGE production, the prostaglandins produced inhibit function by a negative feedback mechanism.

Failure of micrometastases to grow is associated with the so-called dormant state, which is well recognized by clinicians. In this condition, patients with removed primary cancers survive for long periods with no overt metastases. In apparent response to apparently trivial stimuli they then develop a metastatic "explosion." When recurrence or new cancers are ruled out, the dormant state may represent true dormancy, in which micrometastases behave in an inert manner, with their constituent cancer cells apparently in the nondividing (G_0) state. Alternatively, the situation may represent a pseudodormant state in which cancer cell multiplication is balanced by loss. Either way, if by definition micrometastases are not vascularized, it is not difficult to understand their resistance to systemic chemotherapy.

A final step in the development of the metastatic process is the metastasis of metastases. It appears that most human cancers metastasize to so-called generalizing sites[1] determined by anatomical considerations, the commonest being lymph nodes, lung, and liver. From these secondary sites, tertiary metastases occur. The consequent metastatic patterns depend partially on "mechanical" factors, including target organ blood flow, and partially on as yet undefined "seed and soil" factors. The elucidation of the mechanisms of pattern formation in humans is rendered exceptionally difficult by the perturbations induced by therapy.

The Cell Periphery and Metastasis

From the previous comments it is clear that at least some of the components of the metastatic cascade are dependent on the nature of the cancer cell periphery. Contrary to popular belief, little concrete information emerges from the mass of published biochemical and other anecdotes. As far as the author is aware, no general rules have emerged relating metastasis to specific cancer cell properties with respect to topography, physical chemistry, biochemistry, or in vitro behavior; this is not surprising in view of the complexity of metastasis and the variability of cancer cells. The heterogeneity of "pure" populations of cancer cells is well known even in clonal derivatives. In addition, some peripheral properties of cancer cells also vary with respect to growth, degeneration, organ site, and host response.

Whatever their function, a number of antigenic markers have been described at the peripheries of different types of cancer cells, although individuality at the patient level is common. The development of specific antibodies against such antigens will, it is hoped, permit homing of therapeutic and diagnostic modalities.

References

1. Bross IDJ, Viadana E, Pickren J: Do generalized metastases occur directly from the primary? J Chronic Dis 28:149–159, 1975.
2. Butler TP, Gullino PM: Quantitation of cell shedding into efferent blood of mammary adenocarcinoma. Cancer Res 35:512–516, 1975.
3. Glaves D, Weiss L: Initial tumor cell arrest in animals of defined coagulative status. Int J Cancer 21:741–746, 1978.
4. Glücksmann A: The relation of radiosensitivity and radiocurability to the histology of tumour tissue. Br J Radiol 21:559–566, 1948.
5. Honn KV, Busse WD, Sloane BF: Prostacyclin and thromboxanes: Implications for their role in tumor cell metastasis. Biochem Pharmacol 32:1–11, 1983.
6. Warren BA: Arrest and extravasation of cancer cells with special reference to brain metastases and the microinjury hypothesis, in Weiss L, Gilbert HA, Posner JB (eds): *Brain Metastasis.* Boston, G.K. Hall, 1980, pp 81–99.
7. Weiss L: Cell deformability: Some general considerations, in Weiss L (ed): *Fundamental Aspects of Metastasis.* Amsterdam, North-Holland, 1976, pp 305–310.
8. Weiss L, Gilbert HA (eds): *Pulmonary Metastasis.* Boston, G.K. Hall, 1978.
9. Weiss L, Gilbert HA (eds): *Bone Metastasis.* Boston, G.K. Hall, 1981.
10. Weiss L, Gilbert HA (eds): *Liver Metastasis.* Boston, G.K. Hall, 1982.
11. Weiss L, Gilbert HA, Ballon SC (eds): *Lymphatic System Metastasis.* Boston, G.K. Hall, 1980.
12. Weiss L, Gilbert HA, Posner JB (eds): *Brain Metastasis.* Boston, G.K. Hall, 1980.
13. Weiss L, Harlos JP: Cell contact phenomena and their implication in cell communication, in DeMello WC (ed): *Intercellular Communication.* New York, Plenum, 1977, pp 33–59.
14. Weiss L, Suh OW: A morphometric analysis of invasion in human malignant melanomas. In press, 1983.
15. Weiss L, Ward PM: Cell detachment and metastasis. Cancer Met Rev 2:117–127, 1983.
16. Ziche M, Jones J, Gullino PM: Role of prostaglandin E_1 and copper in angiogenesis. J Natl Cancer Inst 69:475–482, 1982.

67

Metastatic Brain Tumors

Joseph H. Galicich
Narayan Sundaresan

The intracranial compartment is a common site of metastatic cancer. Of the 430,000 patients projected to die of systemic cancer in the United States in 1983, approximately 25 percent, or over 100,000, can be expected to have intracranial metastasis. The magnitude of this problem in neuro-oncology may, perhaps, be better appreciated when this figure is compared with the projected 10,800 deaths from *primary* malignant tumors of the central nervous system. The importance of intracranial metastasis is, however, not due primarily to its frequent occurrence, but to the fact that the large majority of the new foci become symptomatic. Furthermore, as compared with other organs such as the lung and liver, in which the incidence of metastasis is even higher, the manifestations of metastases affecting the brain are usually more overt and disabling, and, if untreated, tend to be rapidly lethal. It is for these reasons that brain metastasis demands prompt attention both diagnostically and therapeutically.

A sense of frustration is justifiably inherent in the treatment of patients suffering from disseminated cancer. With few exceptions, even the eradication of a presumed solitary metastasis is followed sooner or later by the discovery of metastases elsewhere or at the primary site. Nevertheless, treatment of metastases that are associated with a high morbidity and mortality, such as those within the brain, can, and often is, rewarded by meaningful palliation. In this regard, the best results are not achieved by rigidly standardized methods of therapy. Rather, the task of the oncologist is to select the most rational treatment based on, among other criteria such as age and general health, a careful assessment of the extent of the patient's disease and the expected or proven response of that particular neoplasm to various modes of therapy. In some instances, the most appropriate course of action may consist of corticosteroid therapy alone or even no treatment at all, while in others, radical multidisciplinary therapy, including surgery directed at the brain metastasis and primary tumor, may provide the most benefit to the patient and family. The purpose of this chapter is to present some of the data and techniques that we have found useful in caring for patients who have intracranial metastases with an emphasis on criteria for selection of those patients most likely to benefit from surgery.

Incidence and Classification

Autopsy studies of large numbers of cancer patients dying in the hospital, while imperfect, provide useful guides as to the frequency and distribution within the cranium of metastases from various primary neoplasms. The overall frequency of intracranial metastases reported from autopsy series carried out over the past several decades ranges from 12 to 35 percent. These studies differ in respect to the population and time period surveyed and, undoubtedly, the thoroughness of examination of the central nervous system. Series reporting lower figures generally cover earlier time periods and therefore do not reflect the steep rise in deaths from lung cancer, which have doubled in the past 30 years. They also tend not to include leukemia, lymphoma, or dural or pituitary metastases. Taking such factors into consideration, it is reasonable to assume that 25 to 30 percent of cancer patients now develop intracranial metastases in the course of their disease. The two most recent large series both report a frequency of about 25 percent.[20,24] Table 67-1 lists the frequency of intracranial and brain (parenchymal) metastases from various primary sites found at autopsy by Takakura et al. and a corresponding estimate of the number of patients in the United States who will develop these lesions.[21,24]

The propensity of tumors of different primary origin to metastasize to the cranial contents, as well as to the various intracranial compartments, differs widely. Among other factors, ready access to the arterial circulation of the head and an environment necessary to sustain the growth of tumor emboli are of importance. For example, primary tumors of the lung, and tumors that commonly metastasize to the lung early in the disease, such as breast carcinoma and melanoma, have a very high incidence and wide distribution of intracranial metastases. Lymphoma metastasizes almost exclusively to the meninges; and prostatic cancer, which has a much lower frequency of intracranial metastases, has a distinct predilection for the skull and dura.

Anatomical Site

Individual intracranial metastases are conveniently classified as to their probable site of origin within the skull, dura, leptomeninges, or brain. Although the opposing surface of the dura is commonly secondarily invaded by tumors that begin in the skull and not infrequently by those that metastasize to the parenchyma, this structure generally acts as a barrier to further invasion. Occasionally a single tumor (usually originating in the skull or dura) involves all four structures (Fig. 67-1).

Skull and Dura

Although surgically of less importance than parenchymal tumors, those metastatic to the skull or dura occasionally reach considerable proportions within the intracranial space and may warrant excision (Fig. 67-1). Those located at the vertex or in the low occiput may produce neurological dys-

TABLE 67-1 Frequency and Number of Estimated Cases of Intracranial and Brain Metastases (United States)

Type of Malignancy	Number of Expected Deaths (1983)[21]	Intracranial Metastases		Brain Metastases	
		Frequency,%	Number*	Frequency,%	Number*
Lung	117,000	41	48,000	35	41,000
GI tract	81,000	8	6,500	6	5,000
Breast	38,000	51	19,000	21	8,000
Liver, pancreas	33,000	6	2,000	5	1,500
Prostate	24,000	17	4,000	6	1,700
Female genital	24,000	7	4,000	2	500
Urinary tract	19,000	21	4,000	17	3,200
Leukemia	16,000	48	8,000	8	1,000
Lymphoma	14,000	22	4,000	5	700
Head and neck	13,000	18	2,000	7	900
Melanoma	5,000	65	3,250	49	2,500
Sarcoma	4,000	22	900	15	600
Thyroid	1,000	24	240	17	1,700
Others†	41,000	26	11,000	19	8,000
Total‡	430,000	27	117,000	18	76,000

*Derived by multiplying frequency (see text) by corresponding figure in column 1.
†No reliable data on frequency available; mean frequency of other solid tumors used.
‡All totals derived from Table 67-1; figures rounded off.

function by compression of the sagittal or lateral sinuses, and at the skull base, by compression of cranial nerves. Skull or dural metastases are common in the following malignancies: prostate carcinoma, lymphoma, breast carcinoma, melanoma, neuroblastoma, and osteogenic sarcoma.

Pituitary

Although infrequently included in autopsy series, metastases to the pituitary are not rare. In the series of Takakura et al., metastases to the pituitary were present in 6 percent of all cases and in 20 percent of patients dying with breast cancer.[24]

Leptomeninges

Metastases to the leptomeninges and spread within the cerebrospinal pathways (neoplastic meningitis) are discussed in depth elsewhere. Virtually all malignant neoplasms have been reported to have produced this entity, which can result in an extremely variable constellation of neurological symptoms and signs by invasion of the brain, cranial nerves, spinal cord, and spinal nerve roots. Obliteration of the subarachnoid spaces with consequent hydrocephalus is more prevalent in our experience in patients with carcinomatous, as opposed to leukemic meningitis, reflecting, perhaps, the better response to treatment of the latter. Neoplastic meningitis is most common in patients who have leukemia, especially the acute lymphocytic variety, non-Hodgkin's lymphoma, and breast carcinoma; and there is a significant incidence in lung cancer and melanoma. Timely diagnosis requires a high degree of suspicion in patients with these cancers and familiarity with the often subtle symptoms and signs that present early in the disease. Since the neurosur-

geon may be called upon to provide chronic access to the cerebrospinal fluid for delivery of intrathecal chemotherapy, it is important to recognize that these patients often have an abnormally small ventricular system as a result of diffuse cerebral swelling. With few exceptions, safe, accurate placement of an indwelling ventricular cannula requires preoperative pneumoencephalography and the use of fluoroscopy at operation.[9]

Parenchyma

Approximately 16 to 18 percent of cancer patients develop brain metastases, and in about 9 percent they represent the only intracranial site of cancer.[20] Because metastases originate from emboli (most often trapped at the site of acute arterial narrowing near the surface) and grow in a soft, yielding matrix without significant tissue planes, such tumors tend to be peripherally located and roughly spherical. Their distribution among the cerebrum, cerebellum, and brain stem corresponds to the relative weight of subdivision. Overall, 40 to 45 percent of solid parenchymal metastases as determined by current diagnostic techniques are single; of these, roughly 80 percent are located in the cerebrum, 16 percent in the cerebellum, and 3 percent in the brain stem. However, the presence of a truly solitary metastasis in the brain, as borne out by long follow-up after total removal, is rare. Most frequently reported solitary lesions originate from renal cell carcinomas; but others, including metastases from lung carcinomas, certainly occur.

As is the case with metastases to other sites, the interval between the diagnosis of the primary cancer and the diagnosis of brain metastases varies with the tumor type (Table 67-2). The median interval in lung cancer is notably short, and it is protracted in breast cancer. The range for each type of cancer, however, varies considerably. Brain metastases

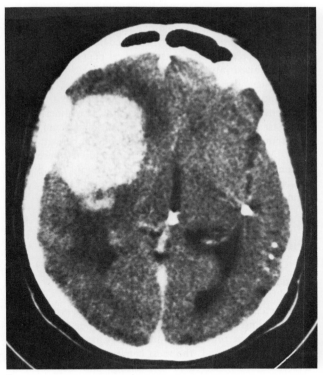
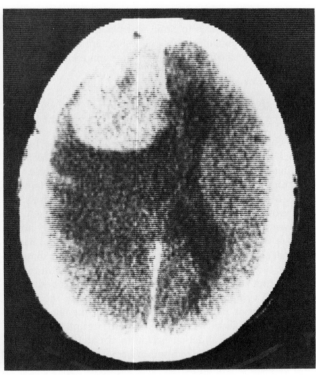

A   B

Figure 67-1 *A.* Carcinoma of the prostate metastatic to the right sphenoid ridge and extending to involve the dura, subdural space (sylvian fissure), and parenchyma. *B.* Lymphoma metastatic to the dura with intracerebral extension. In each case, angiography was consistent with the diagnosis of meningioma. Both lesions were successfully removed.

may be synchronous, i.e., present at the time of the diagnosis of the primary tumor, or, conversely, may occur more than a decade later. Histological verification is necessary to distinguish between metastases from a neoplasm believed to be long-cured, and a new primary tumor. Multiple primary tumors occur in about 15 percent of patients with cancer.

Because of their prevalence or unusual frequency, brain metastases originating from cancer of the lung, breast, colon, and kidney and from melanoma are of special interest. Carcinoma of the lung is presently responsible for approximately 40 percent of all intracranial metastases and 60 percent of brain metastases in the United States (Table 67-1). Of the histological varieties of lung cancer, squamous cell

carcinoma is less likely to metastasize to the brain than is adenocarcinoma or undifferentiated carcinoma. The frequency of brain metastases in patients with small cell carcinoma is extremely high (70 percent). Approximately 40 percent of non-small cell metastases are single and 15 percent are synchronous.[22] Breast carcinoma, while the second most common source of metastatic brain tumor, is also the most widely distributed throughout the intracranial contents and is apt to involve several compartments simultaneously. Fortunately, it is usually moderately radiosensitive. Both colon and kidney metastases have a marked predilection for the brain as compared with other intracranial compartments, tend to be single, and are radioresistant. Of the common

TABLE 67-2 Interval between Diagnosis of Primary Cancer and Cerebral Metastasis*

Type of Malignancy	Total Number	Within 12 Months	After 12 Months	Median Duration, Months	Range, Months
Lung	20	12	8	11	0–74
Testicular	8	2	6	19.5	6–42
Melanoma	13	2	11	36	5–239
Breast	5	1	4	51	11–36
Others	19	7	12	20	2–73

*Data from a series of 65 patients who underwent surgical removal of a single brain metastasis at Memorial Sloan Kettering Cancer Center.

malignant tumors, disseminated melanoma has the highest incidence of metastasis to brain and has the greatest tendency to bleed spontaneously. The lesions are usually multiple and characteristically occur in large numbers.

Clinical Manifestations

The neurological symptoms and signs of metastatic brain tumors are indistinguishable from those of many other expanding intracranial mass lesions and, without the presence or history of cancer, cannot be diagnosed on clinical grounds alone. Most metastatic brain tumors are subcortical in location, grow rapidly, and, even when relatively small, produce extensive edema. Neurological deterioration commonly proceeds at a rapid pace and can be measured in terms of days or weeks. It is the spread of edema through the white matter and not the increase in the size of the tumor per se in most patients that accounts for the relatively rapid onset and progression of symptoms and signs and the fact that the latter are generally of limited value in localizing the site of the metastatic neoplasm with precision. An abrupt strokelike onset of neurological deficit occurs in about 10 percent of patients and may result from tumor hemorrhage or compromise of local blood supply by the neoplasm.

As might be expected, symptoms of increased intracranial pressure are common in patients with metastatic brain tumors. Headache is the initial complaint in 50 to 60 percent of patients. Decrease in cognitive function and nausea and vomiting are less frequent.[24] Papilledema is observed in about 10 percent of patients. Cerebral edema is the usual cause of raised intracranial pressure, but it also may result from ventricular obstruction secondary to cerebellar (Fig. 67-2) and brain stem metastases and occasionally from concomitant carcinomatous meningitis. Focal weakness is the presenting symptom in about 40 percent of patients, but is apparent on the initial examination about 60 percent of the time. Ataxia is the first symptom noted in 20 percent of patients, and seizures (predominantly focal) in approximately 15 to 20 percent. Seizures are predictably more common in patients who have multiple brain metastases.

Differential Diagnosis

Primary Tumors

Most cancer patients who illustrate a full-blown syndrome of an expanding intracranial mass lesion have metastatic brain tumors. Yet at times a second primary neoplasm may be found. Meningioma is the most common primary intracranial tumor encountered in this setting, and may occur in association with breast carcinoma. Presumably because of the high blood flow to these tumors, meningiomas may

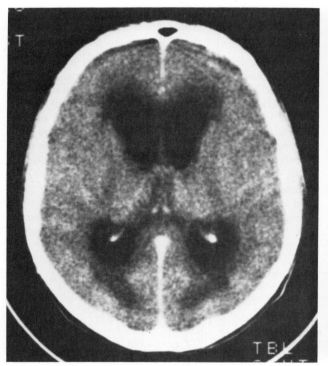
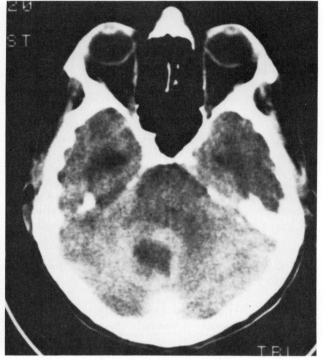

A   B

Figure 67-2 CT scan reveals hydrocephalus with periventricular edema caused by a cerebellar metastasis from lung cancer, as shown in (*B*). The study was prompted by symptoms of increased intracranial pressure. Chest films revealed a right upper lobe mass that proved to be adenocarcinoma on needle biopsy.

themselves be the site of metastases. Malignant gliomas are occasionally present in patients with systemic cancer, but it is uncertain whether or not the association is mere chance.

Abscess

Brain abscesses, while quite uncommon in cancer patients, occur with a greater frequency than in the general population. Patients who have profound depression of the immune system as a result of their disease (e.g., lymphoma) or its treatment are prone to infection by opportunistic organisms and may develop fungous or toxoplasma abscesses or viral encephalitis. Surgically significant bacterial abscesses are probably most common in patients in whom a communication between the intracranial space and the body surface develops following unsuccessful radical surgery and radiation therapy for malignant tumors near the skull base. They may also orginate from septic emboli in patients who have lung abscesses secondary to bronchial obstruction by primary or metastatic tumors.

Infarction and Hemorrhage

Cerebrovascular lesions are common in patients with cancer; they are found at autopsy in about 15 percent of cases.[12] Hemorrhage and infarction occur with equal frequency, and about one-half of each are symptomatic. Both entities, at times, produce clinical symptoms and CT findings that may be confused with metastatic tumors. In addition to their potential for creating diagnostic problems and the fact that they most frequently occur during the end stages of disease, several cerebrovascular lesions, namely intracerebral and subdural hematomas, are of surgical importance. Intracerebral hematoma is encountered in about 4 to 5 percent of cancer patients at autopsy, and subdural hematoma in 1 to 2 percent. The most common cause of hemorrhage is a coagulopathy, usually from thrombocytopenia. In some patients, a transient thrombocytopenia may be responsible for a chronic subdural hematoma. In most instances, acute, coagulopathy-induced hemorrhage into the subdural space or brain is massive and attempts at salvage are futile.

Intra- or peritumoral hemorrhage, usually spontaneous, is responsible for about 25 percent of intracerebral hemorrhages. The majority are associated with melanoma and choriocarcinoma, but can be produced by any metastatic tumor. Bleeding usually emanates from relatively small vessels and dissects along fiber tracts in the centrum, displacing rather than destroying significant amounts of neural tissue. The neurological deficit after surgical removal is, therefore, often insignificant even with very large clots. In a neurologically deteriorating patient, the most effective treatment is prompt, thorough removal of the clot and tumor. This may not only be lifesaving but, in patients with no other intracranial disease and limited or treatable disease elsewhere, can result in prolonged and meaningful survival (Fig. 67-3). Since delay in the removal of large clots usually results in death or profound deficit in such patients, the frequent practice of "watchful waiting" should be condemned.

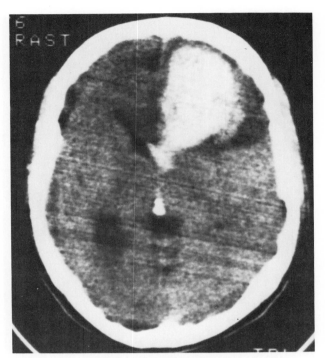

Figure 67-3 A noncontrast CT scan shows a large left frontal hemorrhage in a patient with metastatic lung cancer. The metastasis responsible for the hemorrhage was obscured by the hematoma on the contrast scan. The patient made an uneventful recovery after evacuation.

Radiological Evaluation

Current CT scanners, capable of detecting tumors less than 5 mm in diameter, provide a simple method for early, accurate diagnosis of metastatic brain tumors and meaningful follow-up after treatment. In some instances, however, skull films, tomography, angiography, and radionuclide scans may still be required for optimal diagnosis and treatment.

The typical parenchymal metastasis on CT scans is a discrete, rounded mass with extensive surrounding edema (Fig. 67-4). Multiple lesions are seen in approximately 60 percent of patients. Most metastatic tumors are hypodense, and the majority (90 percent) show enhancement following the administration of a contrast medium. Heterogenous enhancement is common in large tumors (more than 2 cm in diameter) and is usually due to central necrosis. Metastases that are largely cystic show ringlike enhancement with a clear center, a pattern that is also typical of an abscess (Fig. 67-5). Acute hemorrhage within and surrounding a metastatic tumor may obscure the presence of the tumor nodule (Fig. 67-3).

A number of other important pathological entities must be considered in the differential diagnosis when lesions consistent with metastatic tumor are present on CT scans. Especially in patients with breast cancer, if radiotherapy is contemplated, it is wise, but not always possible, to exclude meningioma by cerebral angiography when a juxtadural tumor with dense, homogeneous uptake of contrast is dis-

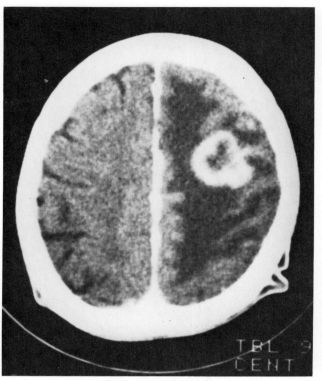
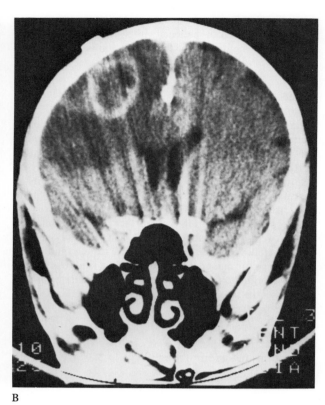

A   B

Figure 67-4   Axial (A) and coronal (B) scans of a patient with a single metastasis from lung cancer in the left posterior frontal lobe. Both scans demonstrate the peripheral location, central necrosis, and extensive edema characteristic of metastases. In B, note the marker applied to the scalp over the tumor (see text).

covered (Fig. 67-1B). In patients with depressed cellular immunity, who have fungous or toxoplasma abscesses, the only radiological clue may be the atypical location of the intracranial mass (e.g., basal ganglia). Malignant gliomas, although usually irregular in shape and uptake of contrast, sometimes appear as single or multiple (10 to 15 percent) discrete, round lesions (Fig. 67-6). If such patients do not have other evidence of cancer, excisional biopsy is usually necessary for a definitive diagnosis, although angiographic findings may sometimes be conclusive. Cerebral infarction may produce discrete areas of enhancement, which, however, resolve on repeat sequential scans. Delayed brain necrosis as a sequela of therapeutic radiation may resemble recurrent metastatic tumor by appearing as a discrete mass, which occasionally shows progressive enlargement on repeat scans.[23]

Patients considered for surgery should undergo scans in both axial and coronal planes to provide a two-dimensional view of the tumor (Fig. 67-7). To plan the surgical approach, localization markers are positioned on the scalp over the point at which the tumor is most superficial (Figs. 67-4 and 67-5). The use of delayed high-dose contrast scans may identify additional tumors not appreciated on routine scans. By this method, Hayman et al. reported finding unsuspected lesions in 15 percent of patients evaluated for brain tumors.[13] We use this technique routinely before surgery.

In the postoperative period, computed tomography is extremely useful in distinguishing between increasing

edema and postoperative clot. Varying degrees of enhancement at the margins of the tumor bed frequently occur in the first few weeks after surgery, presumably from breakdown of the blood-brain barrier and neovascularization. Such abnormal ring enhancement may be difficult to differentiate from residual tumor without sequential scans.

Cerebral angiography is occasionally used preoperatively to determine the magnitude of increased vascularity in such tumors as those of thyroid and kidney origin or to demonstrate the position of a tumor with respect to major blood vessels, such as those in the sylvian fissure. In the latter instances, prior to angiography, a radiopaque marker is placed over the localization point previously established by CT scanning.

Both radionuclide scans and routine radiography are useful in the detection of skull metastases; they often reveal the extent of osseous involvement by tumor more clearly than do CT scans. Polytomography is especially useful in evaluating the presence and extent of metastases involving the skull base.

Treatment

The options for treatment of metastatic intracranial neoplasms include corticosteroids, surgery, radiation therapy, and chemotherapy, either alone or in various combinations.

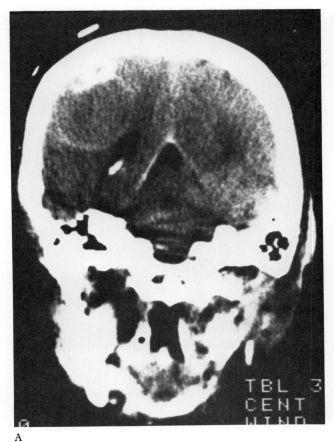
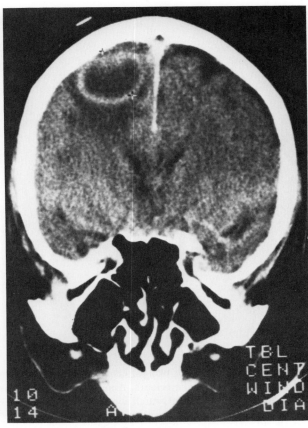

A   B

Figure 67-5 *A.* Large cystic metastasis from a thyroid carcinoma in the left parietal lobe in a patient who had failed whole brain radiation therapy. *B.* The scan of a patient with a brain abscess suspected of having a metastatic tumor prior to craniotomy. Compare with *A.*

At present, therapy in the vast majority of these patients is palliative since most have or will develop widely disseminated disease. There exists, however, a small but significant group of patients with no evidence of cancer elsewhere, perhaps 5 percent of the total, in whom eradication of intracranial disease carries with it the possibility of cure. For this reason, comparison of the effectiveness of various treatment modalities should be made in terms of their potential for eliminating specific intracranial lesions rather than on the basis of survival statistics alone.

Corticosteroids

Corticosteroids are unique in this armamentarium since they may not only effect significant palliation of neurological symptoms and signs when used alone, but also are of immense value when used in conjunction with other treatment modalities. The primary role of these compounds is in the reduction of tumor-induced edema in the white matter, but by decreasing permeability of normal and edematous brain, they also retard edema formation resulting from surgical trauma, ionizing radiation, and chemotherapy. A direct oncolytic action of corticosteroids, while reported for some

tumors, is rare. We have, however, observed shrinkage of metastatic lymphomas with corticosteroid therapy.

Dexamethasone, 10 mg initially and 4 mg q 6 h, or equivalent doses of an analogue, usually results in noticeable clinical improvement within 12 h in most patients.[8] If practical, treatment with corticosteroids should begin 3 to 5 days before surgery (or other specific therapy) to achieve maximal clinical benefit. This not only assures a significant reduction of edema before operation and reduces edema resulting from surgery, but also may provide an indication of whether or not major neurological deficits are fixed or potentially remediable. The success of the surgeon or oncologist in avoiding increased deficit should be gauged in relation to the neurological condition of the patient following a maximum response to corticosteroid therapy and not on the basis of the presenting neurological signs.

Patients with symptomatic brain metastases who are preterminal or in whom specific therapy has failed often receive significant palliation from corticosteroid therapy. Even in the patient who obviously has only days or a few weeks to live, such treatment may bring welcome relief from headache or incapacitating neurological deficit. Although an increase in the median survival of 1 month for patients treated with corticosteroids alone is widely quoted, extension of a

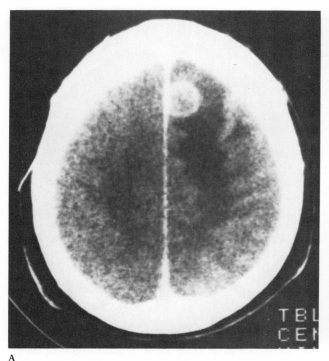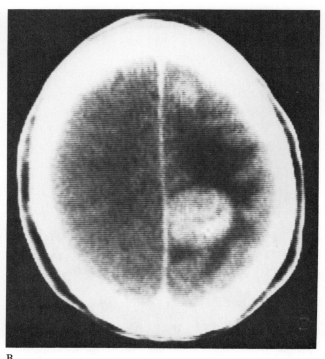

A   B

Figure 67-6   The scans of two patients demonstrating discrete spherical nodules compatible with metastatic tumors. Angiography in both cases revealed avascular lesions. After an unsuccessful search for a primary tumor, the single lesion in the patient shown in A and the larger, posterior, tumor in the patient shown in B were excised. The histological diagnosis in both cases was malignant glioma.

tolerable existence for many months is quite common, especially in those patients in whom radiation therapy has failed to ablate the metastases. Some metastases from relatively radioresistant tumors, such as kidney and colon cancer and melanoma, may respond to radiation therapy by shrinkage and very occasionally by disappearance, but it is from the concomitant use of corticosteroids and not the radiation therapy that the majority of these patients benefit.

Much larger doses of corticosteroids than those noted above may be necessary in some patients to achieve palliation or to control cerebral edema following treatment. However, in order to minimize side effects such as myopathy, diabetes, and immunosuppression associated with the long-term use of corticosteroids, continued efforts should be made to reduce the dosage to the lowest level that prevents recurrence of major neurological symptoms. Prolonged corticosteroid dependency (more than 4 to 6 weeks) following surgery or radiation therapy usually indicates the presence of residual tumor and has been used as a criterion of treatment failure.

Surgery

Scope of Surgery

The primary role of surgery is largely confined to the treatment of patients with a single brain metastasis who do not have widespread or rapidly progressive cancer. This group, unfortunately, represents only about 20 to 25 percent

of patients with parenchymal brain metastases; and ideal candidates for surgery constitute an even smaller percentage.[11] Occasionally, patients with multiple brain metastases may benefit from surgery, for example, those with several radioresistant but surgically accessible tumors who are apparently free of disease elsewhere and those with potentially radiosensitive tumors in whom a single large tumor is life-threatening.

A secondary role of surgery in patients with intracranial metastases includes excision of some metastases to the skull or dura (Fig. 67-1), biopsy of lesions that are clinically and radiologically obscure, removal of subdural and intracerebral hematomas (Fig. 67-3), insertion of indwelling catheters and reservoirs for the delivery of intrathecal chemotherapy, and insertion of cerebrospinal fluid shunts for the treatment of hydrocephalus. Although several of these surgical entities have been discussed briefly, a thorough discourse is beyond the scope of this chapter.

Parenchymal Metastases

The majority of metastatic brain tumors are superficial in location, moderate in size, and relatively avascular, and can be easily and cleanly separated from the surrounding brain by gentle dissection. For these reasons, the risk of increased neurological deficit as a result of extirpation is usually small. In contradistinction to a seemingly widely held belief, we have noted no major differences in this regard in the removal of single lesions from the dominant hemisphere or cerebel-

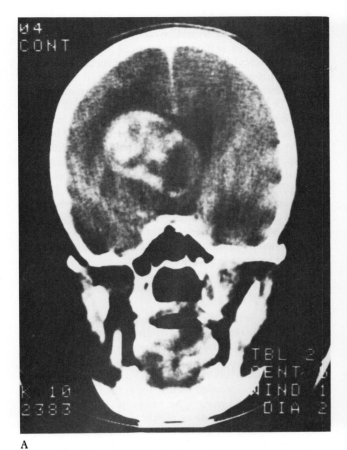

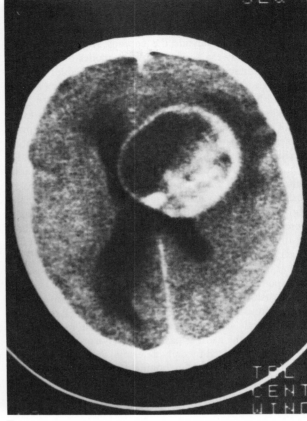

A

B

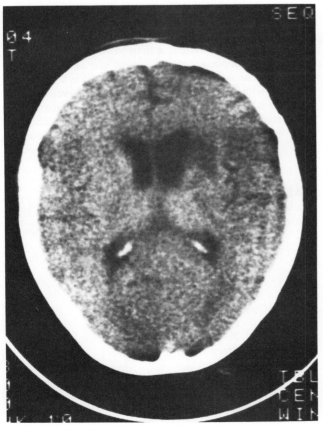

C

Figure 67-7 Preoperative coronal (*A*) and axial (*B*) scans of a 38-year-old woman with a tumor deep in the left hemisphere metastatic from a leiomyosarcoma of the vagina. Scan *C* was carried out 2 months after surgery and radiation therapy. Aside from a slight memory defect, the patient was neurologically intact for 14 months, at which time she died of disseminated systemic cancer.

lum as opposed to those in the nondominant hemisphere (Figs. 67-2 to 67-7). The risk of death within a 30-day period following craniotomy (i.e., standard operative mortality) in these patients is primarily a function of their neurological and general physical condition prior to operation rather than of complications directly related to the operation.[7] Although it is certainly not desirable to restrict the use of surgery to patients who are at least risk, since many others may benefit from operation, analysis of the cause of death in patients undergoing the removal of a brain metastasis reveals that it would be entirely possible to reduce overall operative mortality to considerably under 5 percent by the selection of patients (see below).

In our experience, three major factors influence survival in patients undergoing surgery and radiation therapy for single metastases.[10] These include (1) neurological grade prior to craniotomy, which at the extremes of the scale is predictably reflected in surgical mortality; (2) the interval between the diagnosis of the primary neoplasm and that of the brain metastasis, a rough estimate of the aggressiveness of the cancer; and (3) the extent of systemic disease, perhaps the most important variable, since the major cause of death is progression of cancer outside the nervous system. Any valid comparison between series or various modes of therapy of metastatic brain tumors must take these variables into account, in addition to those usually considered, such as age, sex, and histological diagnosis.

Because cancer or its treatment commonly impairs function of many organs and systems, laboratory evaluation prior to surgery in patients undergoing craniotomy must be especially thorough. Aside from studies routinely used to determine the presence of metastases such as chest roentgenograms and bone and liver-spleen scans, extensive cardiopulmonary evaluation may be required in patients who have received cardiotoxic and pneumotoxic chemotherapy, who have had pulmonary resection, or who have existing primary or metastatic disease of the lung. Elective surgery in patients undergoing chemotherapy must be timed so that the operation and early postoperative phase will not correspond to the nadir in the platelet and white blood cell counts. Although the timing of major depression in bone marrow function can be fairly well predicted for most chemotherapeutic agents, if possible, it is best to carry out the surgery after the nadir is past and a stable or rising platelet count is documented by daily determinations. A count of at least 100,000 normally functioning platelets is necessary to ensure hemostasis in edematous brain. A bleeding time within the normal range with lower platelet counts should not be accepted as safe, since the test is carried out in an organ, i.e., skin, in which the vessels are normal and the physical properties are markedly different from the tumor and brain.

Surgery of all intracranial tumors, including metastatic brain tumors, should be carried out with magnified vision using microsurgical techniques. Even the very large intracerebral tumors can usually be removed via small, well-planned cortical incisions. Sacrifice of large areas of cortex ("uncapping") or lobes of the brain is necessary only if they are involved with tumor.

Although some metastatic tumors present on the surface of the brain, most are entirely subcortical, and, even if quite superficial, rarely produce reliable signs of their location on inspection and palpation of the brain. It is, therefore, often essential to have one or more CT localization points in choosing the most appropriate placement of the cortical incision and the direction of the transparenchymal approach. The ideal cortical incision, and the one oftentimes appropriate, follows the precise center of a single gyrus perpendicular to its transverse diameter. This incision minimizes the risk of major damage to the large arteries in the adjacent sulci as well as to their branches, which run transversely across the surface of the intervening gyrus to end or anastomose at its center. The lack of major deficit following removal of small tumors from immediately beneath primary motor, sensory, and speech cortex at our institution suggests that careful splitting of a gyrus in this manner is compatible with its continued function.

For tumors below the surface of the brain, a small incision to the surface of the tumor is first made, and the wound is thereafter enlarged in the appropriate direction and only to the extent needed for removal of the neoplasm. Incisions through white matter should be carried out by careful blunt dissection parallel to the major tracts. A well-defined plane is usually present between the surface of metastatic tumors and the surrounding brain. In such instances, if the tumor is of a moderately firm consistency, it can and should be removed in one piece if this can be accomplished without major injury to critical areas of the brain. Large and deep tumors, and those with ill-defined margins, should be dealt with by progressively reducing the center and carefully dissecting, folding in, and removing the adjacent margins of the tumor (Fig. 67-7). Surgery of this type of neoplasm is greatly facilitated by use of the ultrasonic aspirator. The relative danger of seeding the wound with viable cells as opposed to incomplete removal of tumor in the margins of the cavity as a source of recurrence is unknown. The use of the laser in attempts at total removal of extremely friable tumors may help to provide such an answer.

Results of Surgery

The treatment of metastatic tumors by surgery followed by radiation therapy is highly effective. In a typical consecutive series of 75 patients who underwent surgery for removal of a single brain metastasis at our institution over a 3-year period beginning July 1977 (Table 67-3), sequential postoperative CT scans revealed recurrence at the operative site in eight patients (11 percent). An additional 10 percent developed intracranial metastases at other sites, despite the fact that the majority (61 patients) had received postoperative radiation therapy. The remaining 14 patients underwent surgery after radiation failure.

Although relapse rate is a more accurate means of evaluating efficacy of therapy directed at a specific complication of cancer (in this instance, a defined metastasis), survival time is more important in gauging the impact of that treatment. Median survival for the entire group was 8.9 months. Patients with disease limited to the central nervous system (Fig. 67-8, Group A) had a 1-year survival of approximately 75 percent. The median survival for patients who had disease in the chest or elsewhere (Group B) was 4.5 months, and less than 10 percent survived 1 year. The 2-year overall

TABLE 67-3 Surgical Treatment of Single Brain Metastases: Site or Type of Primary Tumor In 75 Patients*

Site	Number of Patients
Lung	23
Melanoma	14
Kidney	11
Unknown	6
Sarcoma	6
Colon	4
Testis	4
Breast	3
Others	4
Total	75

*The series included 42 males and 33 females with an age range of 8 to 72 years. Postoperative radiation therapy was given to 61 patients; 14 patients had failed radiation therapy prior to surgery.

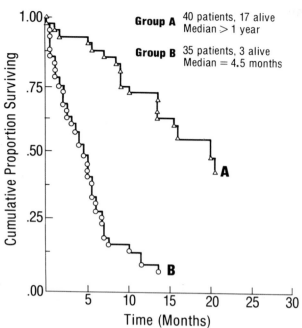

Figure 67-8   Survival curves (Kaplan-Meier product-limit method) of 75 patients undergoing surgery for single brain metastases, 1977–1980 (see text). Group A represents patients in whom metastatic disease was evident only in the brain; group B had radiological evidence of metastases elsewhere.

survival was 18 out of 75 (24 percent). Five patients have lived for 5 years following treatment. "Surgical mortality" is also greatly influenced by the presence of active systemic cancer. The 30-day mortality of the entire series was 9 percent, but it was 2 percent in the 40 patients who had no evidence of disease outside of the brain as determined by preoperative chest films and radionuclide bone and liver-spleen scans.

Carcinoma of the lung is not only the leading cause of death from cancer in the United States but also is responsible for the majority of brain metastases (Table 67-1). An analysis of 50 consecutive patients at our institution operated upon for brain metastases from non-small cell lung cancer serves to emphasize several major determinants of survival, including the treatment directed at the primary lesion. The histology of the primary lesion was adenocarcinoma in 38 patients, epidermoid cancer in 9 patients, and large cell, undifferentiated carcinoma in 3 patients. The discovery of brain metastasis was synchronous with the diagnosis of the primary tumor in 14 patients, occurred within 1 year of treatment of the primary tumor in 21 patients, and after 1 year in 15 patients. In patients with synchronous metastases, thoracotomy was carried out 5 to 10 days following removal of the brain tumor. Fifteen patients had undergone whole brain radiation previously (radiation failures), and 34 patients received radiation therapy after craniotomy.

The overall median survival was 18 months. There was no difference in survival in those patients who presented with a synchronous brain metastasis, as compared with those in whom the diagnosis of metastatic brain tumor was made after that of the primary tumor. Median survival in patients with disease limited to the brain was 24 months, as compared with a median of 6 months for those who had metastases elsewhere or persistent or "recurrent" chest tumors (Fig. 67-9). Patients undergoing curative resection of the primary tumor had a median survival of 28 months, which was significantly different from those undergoing palliative resection or no surgical treatment of the primary lesion (Fig. 67-10). Patients with negative mediastinal nodes (N0 or N1) had a median survival of 28 months, as opposed to a median survival of 18 months in patients with positive nodes.

There was a much higher incidence of local recurrence of the brain tumor at the original site (67 percent) in patients who had previously failed whole brain radiation as compared with those who received radiation therapy following surgery (10 percent). In addition, the patients who had previously failed radiation therapy tended to be corticosteroid-dependent even after the apparent successful surgical removal of the tumor.

Postoperative Radiation Therapy

Important issues in regard to the treatment of single brain metastases are whether radiation therapy should be given following surgery and whether focal or whole brain radiation should be used. The latter question also applies to patients with single lesions treated by radiation therapy alone. The use of postoperative whole brain radiation is predicated on the assumption that even in lesions cleanly removed microscopic foci may be left in the tumor bed and that undetected metastases reside elsewhere in the brain. While seemingly logical, neither assumption is based on extensive evidence. In a small series of 33 patients who underwent resection of single brain metastases, Dosoretz et al. found no difference in survival in patients receiving radiation therapy after surgery as compared with those who underwent surgery alone.[5] However, the markedly increased recurrence rate noted in our series of patients who did not receive postoperative radiation (see section above), while conceivably due to preselection of exceptionally radioresistant tumors, leads us to believe it prudent to give postoperative radiation therapy.

The relative efficacy of whole brain versus focal radiation in patients with apparent single metastases has not been determined. The fact that the incidence of single metastasis observed by CT scanning is essentially the same as that found at autopsy suggests that micrometastases are uncommon in these patients. Apart from preventing the untoward consequences of whole brain radiation such as dementia, the use of focal therapy affords the possibility of radiation of subsequent metastases in long-lived patients.[23]

Radiation Therapy and Chemotherapy

The use of radiation therapy and chemotherapy as a primary treatment modality or for palliation in patients with brain metastases is fully discussed in other chapters. Response to ionizing radiation, of course, varies with tumor type; and reduction of the mass lesion, even in cases in which there is

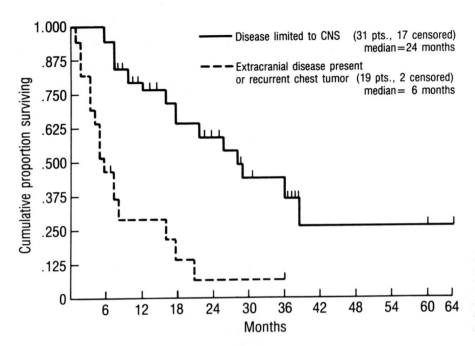

Figure 67-9 Survival curves of 50 patients treated surgically for brain metastases from non-small cell lung cancer, 1978–1982. The median survival of the entire series was 18 months (see text).

complete tumor kill, is relatively slow since it is dependent upon mechanisms such as phagocytosis. Nevertheless, combined with the use of corticosteroids, radiation therapy has been shown to extend survival of significant numbers of patients with multiple brain metastases and should be used in patients who have a life expectancy of more than 2 to 3 months. Demonstration by the Radiation Therapy Oncology Group of the effectiveness of a higher-dose fraction delivered over a shorter period of time (e.g., 2000 rads in 1 week or 3000 rads in 2 weeks) has improved the socioeconomic impact of whole brain radiation.[1]

The role of chemotherapy in patients with brain metastases is limited. However, the concept that it is almost always ineffective is being challenged by recent studies. In some tumors (germ cell neoplasms, small cell lung carcinoma, and possibly some breast carcinomas), the combined use of chemotherapy and radiation therapy may enhance the therapeutic response. Although conventional chemotherapy is generally ineffective, intra-arterial infusions via the carotid or vertebral artery have the theoretical advantage of improving drug delivery to the brain with less systemic toxicity. The most widely used drug is BCNU, although cisplatin and doxorubicin hydrochloride are agents that are being evaluated in Phase II trials. Madajewicz et al., using intra-arterial BCNU, reported response rates of 50 percent in patients with metastatic brain tumors from lung cancer.[17] A similar study by Cascino et al. showed a 20 percent response rate at this center.[3]

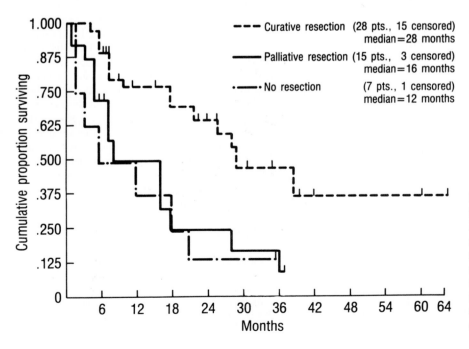

Figure 67-10 Survival curves of the same patients presented in Fig. 67-9 subdivided by the method of treatment of the primary tumor. Palliative resection consisted of removal of the tumor-involved lung and implantation of ^{131}I seeds in adjacent structures manifesting residual disease.

Comparison of Treatment Modalities

At the present time, valid comparison of the two most important treatment modalities of brain metastases (i.e., surgery versus radiation) is difficult. No prospective randomized trials, which would eliminate bias due to patient selection, have been carried out, and even retrospective matched comparisons are rare. The largest reported series of patients treated by radiation and corticosteroid therapy alone does not separate results achieved in patients with single versus multiple metastases, making even a simple comparison with surgery difficult.

Clearly, the longest survivals reported in the literature are patients with single brain metastases who have undergone surgical resection followed by radiation therapy; this is true even for such traditionally radiosensitive tumors as breast carcinoma. In addition, surgery has several obvious advantages when compared with the use of radiation therapy (or chemotherapy) alone. Extirpation of the tumor eliminates the immediate cause of cerebral edema and consequently the necessity for chronic corticosteroid therapy, accomplishes rapid decompression of the brain in acutely deteriorating patients with large tumors or associated intracerebral hemorrhage, and provides accurate histology in patients in whom the diagnosis is uncertain.

Also, surgical excision is currently the only reliable method of eradicating most metastases from malignancies of the colon, thyroid, and kidney and from melanoma as well as many sarcomas and some primary carcinomas of the lung.[7] Although many of us have long held the seemingly logical assumption that treatment of these radioresistant tumors was best carried out by surgery, it has been only recently that confirmation of this premise has appeared in the literature. Retrospective comparison of treatment modalities used in patients with single brain metastases from kidney or colon cancer and from melanoma all overwhelmingly favor surgery.[2,4,6,15,16]

While the role of surgical excision in improving the quality and length of survival is not now generally questioned for radioresistant neoplasms, the management of brain metastases from lung cancer continues to be controversial. During the past decade, Order, Hazra, Montana, and their colleagues had found no difference in outcome between patients who had undergone surgical resection of brain metastases versus those who were treated with whole brain radiation alone.[14,18,19] In view of the overall poor survival, they reported that radiation therapy should be the treatment of choice for these patients because their life expectancy was so limited. In our recent series of 50 patients discussed above, the overall median survival is approximately 18 months, which is clearly superior to survivals achieved by the authors cited above with radiation therapy alone. This figure also compares favorably with the best prognostic subgroup reported by the Radiation Therapy Oncology Group: of 373 ambulatory lung cancer patients with the primary tumor absent and no extracerebral metastases, the median survival was 28 weeks, and less than 50 percent of these patients were neurologically stable until death.[1] In our series, almost 90 percent improved neurologically following surgery, and 65 percent maintained improvement until death. Although a selection bias is undoubtedly involved,

current morbidity and mortality from craniotomy are low enough in experienced hands that no patients should be denied the possible benefits of surgery.

References

1. Borgelt B, Gelber R, Kramer S, Brady LW, Chang CH, Davis LW, Perez CA, Hendrickson FR: The palliation of brain metastases: Final results of the first two studies by the Radiation Therapy Oncology Group. Int J Radiat Oncol Biol Phys 6:1–9, 1980.
2. Byrne TN, Posner JB: Treatment of brain metastases in melanoma. In press.
3. Cascino TL, Byrne TN, Deck MDF, Posner JB: Intrarterial BCNU in the treatment of metastatic brain tumors. In press.
4. Cascino TL, Leavengood JM, Kemeny N, Posner JB: Brain metastasis in colon cancer. Neurology (NY) 32:A74, 1982 (abstr).
5. Dosoretz DE, Blitzer PH, Russell AH, Wang CC: Management of solitary metastasis to the brain: The role of elective brain irradiation following complete surgical resection. Int J Radiat Oncol Biol Phys 6:1727–1730, 1980.
6. Fell DA, Leavens ME, McBride CM: Surgical versus nonsurgical management of metastatic melanoma of the brain. Neurosurgery 7:238–242, 1980.
7. Galicich JH: Surgery of malignant brain tumors, in Vick NA (ed): Seminars in Neurology. New York, Thieme-Stratton, 1981, vol 1, pp 159–168.
8. Galicich JH, French LA, Melby JC: Use of dexamethasone in the treatment of cerebral edema associated with brain tumors. J Lancet 81:46–53, 1961.
9. Galicich JH, Guido LJ: Ommaya device in carcinomatous and leukemic meningitis: Surgical experience in 45 cases. Surg Clin North Am 54:915–922, 1974.
10. Galicich JH, Sundaresan N, Arbit E, Passe S: Surgical treatment of single brain metastasis: Factors associated with survival. Cancer 45:381–386, 1980.
11. Galicich JH, Sundaresan N, Thaler HT: Surgical treatment of single brain metastasis: Evaluation of results by computerized tomography scanning. J Neurosurg 53:63–67, 1980.
12. Graus F, Rogers L, Posner JP: Cerebral vascular complications of systemic cancer. In press.
13. Hayman LA, Evans RA, Hinck VC: Delayed high iodine dose contrast computed tomography. Radiology 136:677–684, 1980.
14. Hazra T, Mullins GM, Lott S: Management of cerebral metastasis from bronchogenic carcinoma. Johns Hopkins Med J 130:377–383, 1972.
15. Katz HR: The relative effectiveness of radiation therapy, corticosteroids, and surgery in the management of melanoma metastatic to the central nervous system. Int J Radiat Oncol Biol Phys 7:897–906, 1981.
16. Macdonald DR, Walker R, Posner JB: Brain metastasis from renal carcinoma. Neurology 33 [Suppl 2]:139, 1983 (abstr).
17. Madajewicz S, West CR, Park HC, Ghoorah J, Avellanosa AM, Takita H, Karakousis C, Vincent R, Caracandas J, Jennings E: Phase II study: Intra-arterial BCNU therapy for metastatic brain tumors. Cancer 47:653–657, 1981.
18. Montana GS, Meacham WF, Caldwell WL: Brain irradiation for metastatic disease of lung origin. Cancer 29:1477–1480, 1972.
19. Order SE, Hellman S, Von Essen CF, Kligerman MM: Improvement in quality of survival following whole-brain irradiation for brain metastasis. Radiology 91:149–153, 1968.
20. Posner JB, Chernik NL: Intracranial metastases from systemic cancer. Adv Neurol 19:579–592, 1978.

21. Silverberg E, Lubera JA: A review of American Cancer Society estimates of cancer cases and deaths. CA 33:2–8, 1983.

22. Sundaresan N, Galicich JH, Beattie EJ: Surgical treatment of brain metastases from lung cancer. J Neurosurg 58:666–671, 1983.

23. Sundaresan N, Galicich JH, Deck MDF, Tomita T: Radiation necrosis after treatment of solitary intracranial metastases. Neurosurgery 8:329–333, 1981.

24. Takakura K, Sano K, Hojo S, Hirano A: *Metastatic Tumors of the Central Nervous System.* Tokyo, Igaku-Shoin, 1982.

68
Meningeal Carcinomatosis

John R. Little
Maurice R. Hanson

The term *meningeal carcinomatosis* refers to diffuse metastasis of the leptomeninges by systemic cancer. Saenger in 1900[9] and Lilienfeld and Benda in 1901[6] were the first to recognize this form of spread of primary malignant tumors from outside the central nervous system. Once thought to be rare, this condition, according to reports appearing during the past ten years, may be present in up to 8 percent of patients with systemic cancer at autopsy.[8,11]

Clinical Features

Symptoms and signs of diffuse leptomeningeal metastases from a primary carcinoma outside the central nervous system may be the first evidence of a malignant disease. In one series,[7] 48 percent of patients with clinical manifestations of leptomeningeal involvement had no previous history of cancer. Many cases have also been identified years after apparently successful treatment of the primary lesion.

The clinical manifestations of meningeal carcinomatosis are similar to those of diffuse meningeal metastases from lymphoma, sarcoma, and leukemia. In some cases a coexistent discrete metastatic tumor produces symptoms and signs in addition to those resulting from the leptomeningeal infiltration.

Widespread involvement of the leptomeninges, present in most cases, results in the simultaneous occurrence of neurological findings in more than one area of the neuraxis. In one report, symptoms and signs indicating involvement of both intracranial and intraspinal structures were found in 90 percent of cases. Usually the neurological signs indicate more widespread involvement than would be expected from the patient's complaints alone.

The clinical findings can be classified according to the level of the neuraxis that is involved: (1) brain, (2) cranial nerve, and (3) spinal nerve and spinal cord. The most frequent symptoms and signs of cerebral and cerebellar involvement include headache, disturbed mentation, lethargy, seizures, and ataxia. These findings have been attributed to communicating hydrocephalus which is occasionally seen with diffuse leptomeningeal metastases or to direct superficial infiltration of the cerebral and/or cerebellar cortex.

Cranial nerve involvement has been reported in up to 94 percent of patients during the course of the disease.[8] Any cranial nerve can be involved, and multiple cranial nerve palsies are the rule during the course of the illness. The cranial nerves most often affected are VII, III, V, and VI, in decreasing order of frequency. Decreased visual acuity from second cranial nerve infiltration appears to be less common than reported earlier.[1,3,4]

Infiltration of the spinal leptomeninges and nerve roots is frequently manifested by pain along the spinal axis or in a radicular distribution in the extremities. Neurological examination frequently shows more widespread involvement of spinal nerve roots than indicated by the patient's symptoms. In one series,[8] 40 percent of patients had spinal root symptoms, whereas 78 percent were found to have signs of root involvement. Meningismus, reported in up to 50 percent of cases, tends to be less severe than that seen with purulent meningitis. Lumbosacral roots are more frequently involved than cervical roots. This predilection for the cauda equina is probably related to the gravitation of malignant cells into the cul-de-sac and to the greater length of the lumbosacral roots within the subarachnoid space. Long tract signs, occasionally found in patients with meningeal carcinomatosis, are thought to be related to superficial infiltration of the spinal cord.

Primary Sites of Carcinoma

The most frequent sites for the primary carcinoma are the breast and lung.[7,8] Malignant melanoma is the third most common primary tumor. Primary tumors of the gastrointestinal tract, initially thought to have a predilection for diffuse metastases to the leptomeninges,[3,4,5] are seen less frequently, perhaps partly because of the declining incidence of gastrointestinal tumors, particularly gastric carcinoma, in the western world. The incidence of lymphomatous meningitis appears to be similar to that of carcinomatous meningitis secondary to primary tumors of the breast or lung.[8]

Pathology

Metastatic carcinoma may gain access to the leptomeninges through a number of routes. Once infiltration has occurred, there is a potential for widespread dissemination throughout the cerebrospinal fluid compartment. Hematogenous metastasis to the choroid plexus has been implicated as the most frequent initiating event. Metastasis to superficial regions of the brain parenchyma, with subsequent infiltration into the subarachnoid or ventricular spaces, is probably an important mechanism in some cases. Infiltration along spinal nerve roots is probably more common in lymphoma than in carcinoma because of its more frequent growth in the paravertebral region.

The most frequent sites of gross involvement are the basal cisterns, anterior sylvian cistern, dorsal aspect of the spinal cord, and lumbosacral cul-de-sac. Predilection for these sites is thought to be related to gravitation of malignant cells into dependent areas. Although certain areas are more commonly affected, macroscopic involvement of any part of the cerebrospinal fluid compartment can occur.

Diffuse or focal opaque thickening of the leptomeninges is the most common gross finding. These changes are sometimes difficult to differentiate from those leptomeningeal changes seen with aging. Discrete tumor nodules or petechial hemorrhages are occasionally seen.

Involved nerve roots usually appear diffusely swollen, although discrete nodules may also be present. The affected nerve roots of the cauda equina or those in other regions are often ensheathed with tumor and firmly stuck together.

Sectioning of the brain occasionally reveals mild to moderate hydrocephalus. In a small number of cases, cerebral swelling results in reduction in the size of the lateral and third ventricles. Examination of the choroid plexus or ventricular walls may demonstrate diffuse or nodular tumor infiltration.

Adenocarcinoma is the most frequent histological type of carcinoma to metastasize diffusely to the leptomeninges and subarachnoid space.[7] Lymphoma, although not a true carcinoma, also appears to have a predilection for leptomeningeal metastasis.[8] Microscopic involvement ranges from one to many cell layers. Associated fibrosis or inflammation is occasionally seen. Infiltration into the parenchyma along the perivascular Virchow-Robin spaces is a common finding. Direct invasion of the brain or spinal cord is less common. Tumor deposits may be seen in the choroid plexus or lining the walls of the ventricular chambers. Diffuse or nodular infiltration of multiple nerve roots is invariably present.

Investigations

Cerebrospinal Fluid Findings

Examination of the cerebrospinal fluid is the most useful diagnostic procedure. Repeated cytological studies, however, are frequently necessary to identify malignant cells. Olson et al.[8] reported the identification of malignant cells in 45 percent of patients on the first examination, whereas 34 percent of patients required repeated studies (i.e., as many as six lumbar punctures) before malignant cells were found. In another report,[7] 81 percent of patients were eventually found to have malignant cells in the cerebrospinal fluid.

The cerebrospinal fluid is abnormal in more than 95 percent of cases.[7,8] Aside from malignant cells, reduced glucose content or increased protein content has been reported in up to 76 percent of cases.[7] Inflammatory cells, either polymorphonuclear leukocytes or lymphocytes, are commonly present, but cultures for bacteria or fungi are always negative.

At the present time there are no biochemical markers to confirm the presence of meningeal carcinomatosis in the absence of malignant cells; however, Shuttleworth and Allen[10] have shown that β-glucuronidase levels can be elevated in the cerebrospinal fluid of patients with this disorder. In a recent report, levels of CSF β-glucuronidase activity above 80 mU per liter were thought to strongly suggest the presence of leptomeningeal metastases.[11]

The diagnostic significance of carcinoembryonic antigen or elevated lactate dehydrogenase isoenzyme levels in the cerebrospinal fluid in patients with leptomeningeal metastases has yet to be determined.

A computed tomography (CT) scan of the head is recommended before a lumbar puncture is performed for CSF examination, to rule out the presence of a significant brain mass or severe hydrocephalus, which would make lumbar puncture hazardous.

Computed Tomography

A CT scan of the head may show ventricular dilatation, usually mild. Studies performed with intravenous contrast have been reported in some cases to show enhancement of the involved basal cisterns or ventricular walls.[2] This is thought to represent disturbed vascular permeability to the contrast medium in the areas of tumor infiltration.

Myelography

Myelographic changes are most commonly seen in the lumbosacral cul-de-sac. Typical findings include irregular granular filling defects and enlargement and adherence of nerve roots. In one study,[8] multiple nodular defects on nerve roots were seen in 7 of 18 patients examined. The abnormalities seen in meningeal carcinomatosis may be difficult to differentiate from those seen in chronic lumbar arachnoiditis.

Meningeal Biopsy

Arachnoid biopsy may be indicated in those cases where the diagnosis of meningeal carcinomatosis is strongly suspected clinically but where other investigations (particularly CSF examination) have failed to provide confirmation. The arachnoid membrane in the region of the cisterna magna can be easily and safely biopsied through a small craniectomy 1 to 2 cm posterior to the foramen magnum. In those few patients with symptoms and signs exclusively at the spinal level, a low lumbar laminectomy with biopsy may be preferable.

Differential Diagnosis

The clinical diagnosis of meningeal carcinomatosis is particularly difficult in patients with no previous history of malignant disease. The correct diagnosis often is not readily appreciated at the time of the initial evaluation. The most frequent incorrect diagnosis is brain metastasis or spinal cord compression. The findings of meningeal irritation, multiple nerve root palsies, and hydrocephalus together with CSF abnormalities such as decreased glucose content, increased protein content, and inflammatory cells in the absence of malignant cells makes it difficult to differentiate meningeal carcinomatosis from chronic meningitis from a tuberculous or fungal origin or sarcoidosis. Misdiagnosis in patients with predominant mental aberrations include metabolic encephalopathy, drug toxicity, or a paraneoplastic syndrome. In these cases the CSF examination usually points to the correct diagnosis.

Therapy

Treatment of meningeal carcinomatosis must be directed toward the entire neuraxis because of the diffuse nature of this condition. Options include irradiation of part or all of the neuraxis and/or chemotherapy. Widespread irradiation, although an effective treatment, carries the risk of bone marrow depression. The likelihood of bone marrow depression is greater in this group of patients, as many will also be receiving systemic chemotherapy for the primary tumor. Consequently, focal radiation is recommended in most cases.

Chemotherapy for meningeal malignant disease appears to be most effective when the chemotherapeutic agent is injected directly into the CSF compartment. The use of an indwelling Ommaya reservoir with the catheter in the right lateral ventricle is preferable to repeated lumbar punctures because of (1) ease of administration of the chemotherapeutic agent, (2) more reliable delivery of the agent to the CSF compartment, (3) more widespread distribution of the agent, and (4) higher chemotherapeutic agent concentration. Methotrexate and/or cytosine arabinoside have been used intrathecally in cases of meningeal carcinomatosis.[11] Methotrexate is given initially at a dose of 7 mg/m^2 biweekly, then monthly, then at 6-week intervals, depending upon clinical response and CSF parameters. Citrovorum factor is given by mouth during treatment with methotrexate (9 mg PO twice daily for 4 days after treatment). Cytosine arabinoside (35 mg/m^2) may be given in a time frame similar to that described for methotrexate. Potential complications of ventricular injection of chemotherapeutic agents include aseptic meningitis and generalized encephalopathy or focal encephalopathy secondary to pooling of the agent or backtracking along the ventricular catheter.

The use of an indwelling shunt for hydrocephalus should be avoided if possible. Hydrocephalus in some cases may resolve with irradiation or chemotherapy. The use of a shunting device carries the risk of further spread of the tumor.

Prognosis

The prognosis in untreated patients is universally poor, with survival being 2 months or less in most instances. Improved prognosis with aggressive therapy is possible, although long-term survival is unlikely. In one large series,[11] treatment with a combination of focal radiation and intrathecal chemotherapy (methotrexate with or without cytosine arabinoside) resulted in periods of neurological stabilization or improvement in 50 percent of patients for more than 1 month. Median survival time was 5.8 months after diagnosis (range: 1 to 29 months). In 18 patients with disease limited to the nervous system, median survival time was 8 months, with four patients surviving 1 year and two patients surviving 2 years. Side effects of this treatment were relatively minor. The CSF findings tended to stabilize or improve with this form of therapy.

References

1. D'Andrea F, Constans JP, De Divitiis E: A propos de la carcinose leptoméningée. Neurochirurgia 8:1–11, 1965.
2. Enzmann DR, Krikorian J, Yorke C, Hayward R: Computed tomography in leptomeningeal spread of tumor. J Comput Assist Tomogr 2:448–455, 1978.
3. Fischer-Williams M, Bosanquet FD, Daniel PM: Carcinomatosis of the meninges: A report of three cases. Brain 78:42–58, 1955.
4. Heathfield KWG, Williams JRB: Carcinomatosis of the meninges: Some clinical and pathological aspects. Br Med J 1:328–330, 1956.
5. Jacobs LL, Richland KJ: Carcinomatosis of the leptomeninges: Review of literature and report of four cases. Bull Los Angeles Neurol Soc 16:335–356, 1951.
6. Lilienfeld F, Benda C: Fall von metastischer Karcinose der Neiven und Hirnhaute. Berl Klin Wochenschr 38:729–730, 1901.
7. Little JR, Dale AJD, Okazaki H: Meningeal carcinomatosis: Clinical manifestations. Arch Neurol 30:138–143, 1974.
8. Olson ME, Chernik NL, Posner JB: Infiltration of the leptomeninges by systemic cancer: A clinical and pathologic study. Arch Neurol 30:122–137, 1974.
9. Saenger A: Ueber Hirnsymptome bei Carcinomatose. Munch Med Wochenschr 47:341–342, 1900.
10. Shuttleworth EC, Allen N: Early differentiation of chronic meningitis by enzyme assay. Neurology 18:534–542, 1968.
11. Wasserstrom WR, Glass JP, Posner JB: Diagnosis and treatment of leptomeningeal metastases from solid tumors. Cancer 49:759–772, 1982.

SECTION D

Meningiomas

69

Meningiomas: Pathology

Venkata R. Challa
William R. Markesbery

Meningiomas, so named by Harvey Cushing in 1922, are common tumors that arise from cells of the meninges. Although others have proposed different names such as fibroma or endothelioma of the meninges, these terms have not found general acceptance. A large amount of information on the biology and clinical features of meningiomas has accumulated in the five decades since Cushing and Eisenhardt published the classification and morphological descriptions of these tumors.[5] Their pathology is so variable as to equal or exceed the morphological complexities associated with glioblastoma multiforme. Controversies over the histogenesis and terminology of these tumors still exist.

Histogenesis

Meningiomas are thought to originate from arachnoidal cap cells (cells forming the outer lining of the arachnoid membrane), related cells such as arachnoidal fibroblasts, and perhaps the precursor cell of meninges as a whole—the so-called meningoblast. Whether the arachnoidal cap cell is derived from the neural crest or the mesoderm is itself still controversial. Rubinstein[17] includes all meningiomas under mesodermal tumors, probably because many of these tumors show fibroblastic differentiation and some show other mesenchymal features such as chondromatous foci, xanthomatous foci, bone formation, etc. Irrespective of this problem, it is accurate to consider the meningiomas as tumors derived from the arachnoidal cells. The similarities in

ultrastructural features between normal meningeal cap cells and the tumor cells of meningiomas, as well as the tendency of both to form whorls are well known. The deeper cells of the arachnoid show some changes from the typical characteristics of the cap cells, especially a decrease in cell junctions and in number of cell processes formed. These cells are mixed with the more typical fibroblasts near the arachnoid space. Two types of meningiomas, the transitional and the fibroblastic types, mimic the features of the fibroblasts at the light microscope level. While the histogenesis of the majority of meningiomas (i.e., the meningothelial, transitional, and fibroblastic types) is thus explained, the origin of some types, especially the angioblastic type, is controversial.[9,11] The histogenetic relationship of the angioblastic meningioma to the capillary hemangioblastoma of the cerebellum, which it mimics histologically, is poorly understood.

Incidence

Meningiomas constitute about 15 percent of primary brain tumors[11] and 25 percent of spinal cord tumors.[17] However, since most meningiomas are benign and completely resectable, the mortality figures are much lower; only about 6 percent of brain tumors causing death are meningiomas. While reports from most countries give similar figures, Froman and Lipschitz[6] reported that in the Bantu population of Transvaal, South Africa, meningiomas form over 30 percent of primary brain tumors.

Meningiomas are tumors of adults, with the age of incidence ranging between 20 and 60. The peak incidence is around the age of 40. A female preponderance is seen, especially in the spinal cord meningiomas. Most meningiomas are solitary, but multiple meningiomas can occur, alone or in association with neurofibromatosis.

Gross Features

Most meningiomas are well-demarcated, round or oval, frequently lobulated tumors attached to the dura (Figs. 69-1, 69-2). However, in a minority of tumors a dural attachment cannot be shown. The benign meningiomas tend to compress the brain but not invade it (Fig. 69-3). An occasional meningioma, called *meningioma-en-plaque*, has a flattened appearance that conforms to the curves of the brain and the

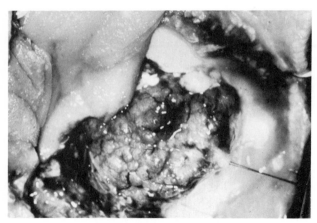

Figure 69-1 A typical meningioma at operation. The tumor surface is finely lobulated and pinkish. Blood vessels on the surface are prominent.

inside of the skull. A delicate compressed layer of arachnoidal cells intervenes between the tumor and the brain, but often this is highly attenuated in places. On cut surfaces the typical meningioma is a grayish pink homogenous tumor with a faint whorled appearance. Occasionally, yellow flecks representing collections of fat-containing (xanthoma) cells may be seen. Grossly visible cystic degeneration and hemorrhage are infrequent.[17] The angioblastic meningiomas are grossly not much different from the ordinary meningothelial and fibroblastic meningiomas, but a deeper pink coloration may be present. Most meningiomas, especially the transitional and fibroblastic types, are firm to hard in consistency. The presence of numerous psammoma bodies and calcification may impart a gritty feeling when the tumor is sliced for frozen section diagnosis. A significant number of meningiomas invade surrounding tissues, including the dura, adjacent bone and extracranial musculature, soft tissue of the orbit, and the paranasal sinuses. This feature suggests increased chance of recurrence after operation. However, most meningiomas are completely resectable.

In the spinal canal, meningiomas are usually round or oval small tumors attached to the dura and compressing the adjacent spinal cord. Sometimes they may be en plaque and partly or totally encircle the spinal cord. Although they may invade epidural soft tissue or intervertebral foramina, they do not show the typical dumbbell shape of the spinal schwannoma. Occasional tumors in this site tend to invade bone and adjacent soft tissues, but the majority of spinal cord meningiomas are slow-growing and well circumscribed.

Histological Types

Except for the less common angioblastic, papillary, and atypical meningiomas, which are aggressive, there is no relationship between the histological type of meningioma and

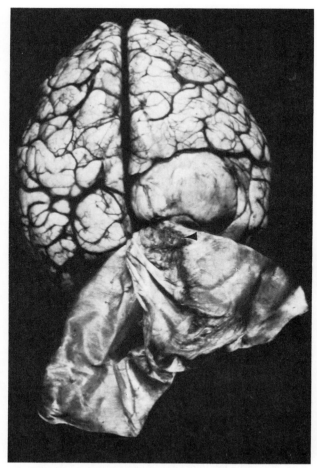

Figure 69-2 A large meningioma over the cerebral convexity. It is attached (*arrowhead*) to the dura, which has been pulled down toward the occipital region. Because of formalin fixation the tumor is more gray than pink.

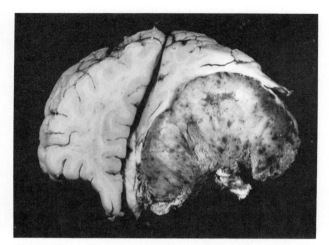

Figure 69-3 Even large meningiomas tend to compress the brain rather than invade it. This example shows the clear demarcation between the tumor and the underlying brain. The dusky color indicates a highly vascular tumor.

prognosis, but it is customary for pathologists to divide meningiomas into several types.

The *meningothelial* (also called syncytial or endothelial) type is characterized by broad sheets or medium-size lobules of fairly uniform cells with round or oval nuclei, ample light pink cytoplasm, and indistinct cytoplasmic borders (Fig. 69-4). It is this indistinctness of the cytoplasmic borders that gave rise to the term *syncytial*. However, as will be shown presently, ultrastructural examination shows that these cells are not truly syncytial like the syncytial trophoblast. A slight to moderate tendency to whorling of the cells may be observed in these tumors, but whorling is more common in the next type, the *transitional* meningioma (Fig. 69-5). The cells in this type are more elongated and separated from one another and thus appear less syncytial. Bundles of several cells sweep in different directions, and a few elongated fascicles can also be seen. The most important feature of this type of meningioma is the propensity of the cells to form small whorls by partly encircling other cells; this whorl formation (Fig. 69-6) is an important feature for frozen section diagnosis of these tumors. The number of whorls formed varies from tumor to tumor and from one place to another in the same tumor. Some whorling is also observed around small blood vessels, but most whorls contain tumor cells in the center. When a whorl in a meningioma undergoes degeneration of the cells in the middle followed by calcium deposition, a rounded, partly or totally calcified structure called the *psammoma body* is formed. The number of psammoma bodies in a meningioma varies from nil to tumors wholly composed of these bodies with a few cells in between—the psammomatous meningiomas (Fig. 69-7). These are basi-

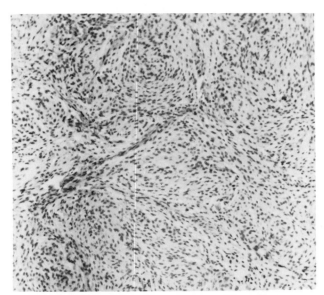

Figure 69-5 Transitional meningioma. The cells are somewhat elongated and tend to flow in different directions. (Hematoxylin-eosin, ×120.)

cally a variant of transitional meningiomas. The presence of psammoma bodies in abundance indicates slow growth and good prognosis. Psammomatous meningiomas are more common in the spinal canal than elsewhere in the nervous system.

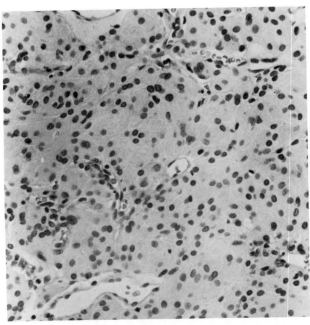

Figure 69-4 Meningothelial meningioma. The cells have indistinct cytoplasmic margins and uniform round or oval nuclei; delicate blood vessels are present. (Hematoxylin-eosin, ×240.)

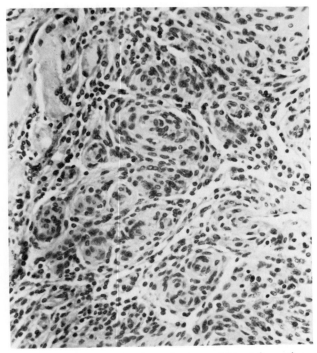

Figure 69-6 Transitional meningioma. Whorl formation is prominent in the center. (Hematoxylin-eosin, ×240.)

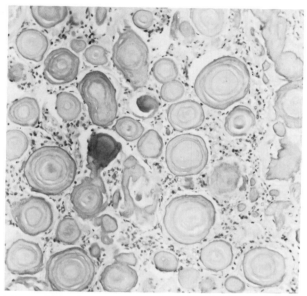

Figure 69-7 Psammoma bodies. When these are this numerous, the tumor may be called a psammomatous meningioma. (Hematoxylin-eosin, ×120.)

Another frequent type of meningioma is called the *fibroblastic* meningioma because the cells mimic fibroblasts in appearance (Fig. 69-8) and also form true reticulin and col-

lagen fibrils (Fig. 69-9). The cells of the fibroblastic meningioma are usually arranged in fascicles crossing other fascicles. The amount of reticulin and collagen fibers formed varies from one place to another. Reticulin fibers are often easily seen with special stains. The pink collagen bundles seen in hematoxylin-eosin-stained sections vary from place to place.

The *angioblastic* meningioma is a less common type that is more aggressive than the preceding types,[9,16] and several documented cases of metastases from these tumors are known.[11] Currently, this type is subdivided into the *hemangioblastic* type, which superficially mimics the cerebellar hemangioblastoma, and the *hemangiopericytic* type, which is histologically similar to hemangiopericytomas elsewhere in the body and is aggressive in its behavior. Some tumors may show a mixture of these patterns and transitions to more regular meningothelial meningiomas.[9] In addition, the term *angiomatous meningioma* has often been used, mainly to denote a richly vascularized meningioma (Fig. 69-10). Since the prognosis of a completely resected, richly vascularized meningioma is the same as that of an ordinary meningothelial meningioma, it may be better not to use this term, to avoid confusion with the angioblastic meningioma.

The hemangioblastic variant of angioblastic meningioma is characterized by a rich network of small blood vessels, with one or a few cells wrapped around the vessel. Occasional fat-laden cells are found between the blood vessels, much like the fat-laden cells found in cerebellar hemangioblastoma (Fig. 69-11). Some authors argue that cerebellar hemangioblastoma and angioblastic meningioma (hemangioblastic type) are one and the same. However, the absence of

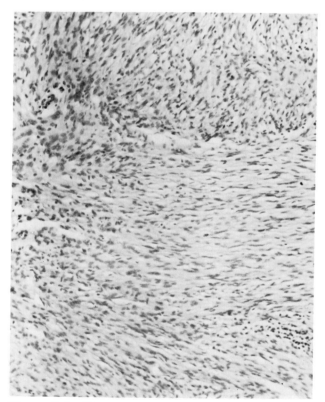

Figure 69-8 Fibroblastic meningioma. Elongated fibroblast-like cells are arranged in fascicles passing in different directions. (Hematoxylin-eosin, ×240.)

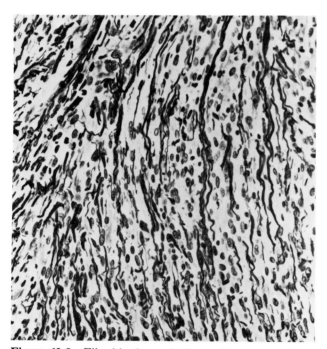

Figure 69-9 Fibroblastic meningioma. Numerous reticulin (fine) and collagen (coarse) fibers are seen between the cells. Only cell nuclei are apparent. (Wilder's reticulin, ×240.)

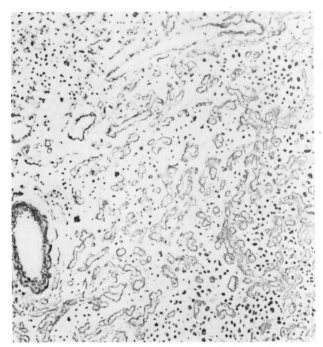

Figure 69-10 Richly vascularized meningioma. Numerous small blood vessels are shown prominently by the reticulin method. (Wilder's reticulin, ×240.)

a cystic component, the attachment to dura, and the presence of recognizable meningothelial cell clusters are features of angioblastic meningioma that are not seen in cerebellar hemangioblastoma.[11] Moreover, other features of von Hippel-Lindau disease, such as retinal hemangiomas and adrenal pheochromocytomas, are associated with capillary hemangioblastoma of the cerebellum but not with angioblastic meningioma.

Histologically, hemangiopericytic meningioma is characterized by closely packed small cells with hyperchromatic nuclei and ill-defined cytoplasmic boundaries between numerous thin-walled vessels (Fig. 69-12). Mitoses are common, and with special stains, reticulin may be demonstrated around individual cells and groups of cells. These tumors are aggressive and prone to recurrence or development of distant metastases.

Less common types of meningiomas are the *xanthomatous* type, with large numbers of fat-laden cells mixed with recognizable meningothelial cell types. More commonly, however, small xanthomatous foci are seen in meningothelial or other types of meningiomas. The fat droplets in these cells are multiple and of various sizes. The *lipoblastic* meningioma is also an uncommon type; it is characterized by numerous cells resembling adult fat cells plus a component of meningothelial cells. The term *chondromatous* meningioma means a transitional or fibroblastic meningioma with prominent focal islands of imperfect but benign cartilage formation. Two rare types of meningiomas are the *papillary* and *atypical* types. In the papillary type, alignment of cells around small

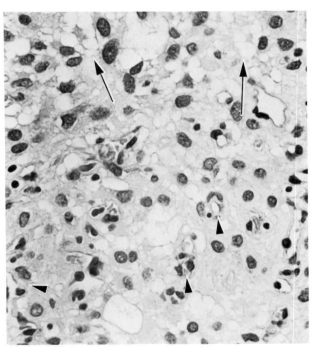

Figure 69-11 Angioblastic meningioma. Capillaries (*arrowheads*) are surrounded by tumor cells. Some of the cells between blood vessels show fat vacuoles in the cytoplasm (*arrows*). (Hematoxylin-eosin, ×240.)

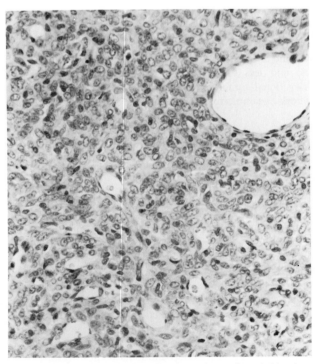

Figure 69-12 Hemangiopericytic variant of angioblastic meningioma. Numerous small empty vessels are surrounded by densely crowded tumor cells. (Hematoxylin-eosin, ×240.)

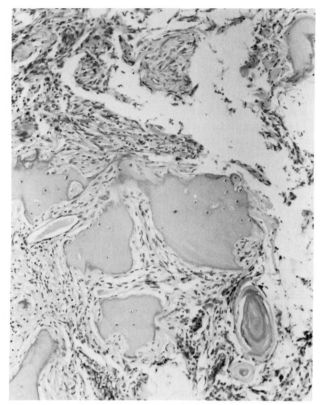

Figure 69-13 Fibroblastic meningioma with bone formation. (Hematoxylin-eosin, ×120.)

blood vessels results in the formation of papillary structures.[13] The second type is a cellular meningioma with atypical and crowded nuclei and mitoses. It appears more epithelial and less easily recognizable as a meningothelial or transitional tumor, especially because it shows few or no whorls, psammoma bodies, and calcifications.

Histological Variation

One is often surprised by the number of histological variations exhibited by meningiomas. These are mainly of interest to pathologists but occasionally have significance for the neurosurgeon. An extensive discussion of the subtle changes in meningiomas can be found in the monograph by Kepes.[11] Calcification other than formation of psammoma bodies can occur in meningiomas; it usually involves fibrous septa between the tumor lobules. Ossification (bone formation) may also occur (Fig. 69-13). Aggregates of hyalinized blood vessels are also commonly seen.

Another peculiar change sometimes seen in meningiomas is the formation of pseudopsammoma bodies (hyaline bodies). These are noncalcified, globular, pink, extracellular blobs of proteinaceous material surrounded by meningothelial cells (Fig. 69-14). The surrounding cells seem to shed

small processes of their cell membranes into the center and contribute to the formation of the pseudopsammoma body. Because of their content of glycoprotein, these bodies stain a bright magenta color with the periodic acid Schiff (PAS) technique. Kepes[11] has described the formation of the pseudopsammoma bodies in detail.

Another change seen in some meningiomas, hyaline droplet degeneration, appears as pink intracytoplasmic droplets of different sizes. Although grossly visible cyst formation in meningiomas is unusual, microcystic degeneration is considerably more common (Fig. 69-15), especially in the well-vascularized meningothelial examples.

Some meningothelial meningiomas and angioblastic meningiomas may show uninucleate or multinucleate giant cells, often with bizarre nuclei; these features do not indicate malignancy. The nuclei of many meningiomas (especially the meningothelial types) show intranuclear vacuoles of two types. One type is formed by invagination of cytoplasm into the nucleus (Fig. 69-16), the other by clearing of chromatin material from the center of the nucleus (Fig. 69-17). The latter type is more common and is of diagnostic help. Some meningiomas contain bloated cells with well-defined cytoplasmic borders, mimicking gemistocytic astrocytes.[11] Some meningiomas (focally at least) may mimic the fried egg pattern of oligodendrogliomas.[2]

In view of such problems arising in frozen section diagnosis, it is imperative that the requisition for frozen section diagnosis be accompanied by information about the exact location of the tumor, i.e., whether intra-axial or extra-axial, and the structures invaded by it. In addition, specimens obtained with the CUSA system (Cavitron ultrasonic surgical aspirator, Cooper Medical, Mountain View, California) show crushing of cells mimicking necrosis (Fig. 69-18). This form of pseudonecrosis does not have the grave implication of true necrosis seen in malignant meningiomas.

A peculiar proliferation of small, dark cells in the walls of

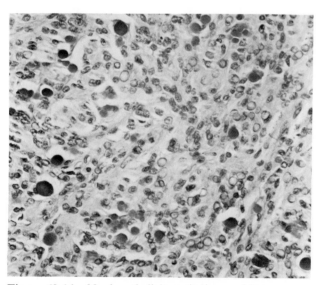

Figure 69-14 Meningothelial meningioma with numerous globular bodies called pseudopsammoma bodies. (Periodic acid Schiff stain, ×240.)

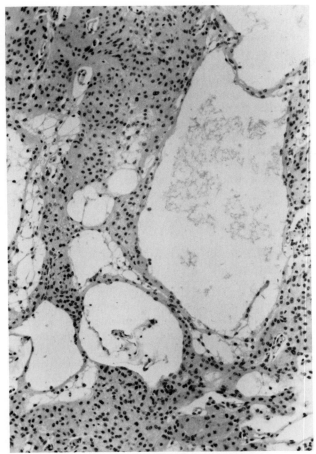

Figure 69-15 Meningothelial meningioma with microscopic cystic degeneration. The cysts are of various sizes. (Hematoxylin-eosin, ×120.)

blood vessels has been observed in some meningiomas. According to Mirra and Miles [15] and Challa et al., [4] these cells have features of proliferating pericytes. The relation of these tumors to true hemangiopericytic meningiomas is unclear. Challa et al. [4] and Smith et al. [18] think that there is a relationship between the occurrence of these vascular proliferative changes and the presence of severe cerebral edema adjacent to the tumor.

Finally, a rare condition called *meningioangiomatosis*, first described by Worster-Drought et al., [20] needs to be considered under the histology of meningiomas, for it can cause confusion. In this rare condition, possibly related to neurofibromatosis, there is invasion of the brain by benign-appearing clusters of meningothelial cells and pial blood vessels. The condition is neither malignant nor is it presently considered to be a form of meningioma.

Ultrastructure

The ultrastructural features of meningiomas are typical and are often helpful in determining the meningiomatous nature of aggressive tumors. However, routine electron microscope examination is not needed in the diagnosis of ordinary meningiomas. As mentioned before, the ultrastructural features of the meningothelial cell are reflected in the tumor cells of meningiomas. The most important of these are (1) formation of complex and intertwining cells processes,[14] (2) formation of variable numbers of intercellular junctional complexes, especially desmosomes,[8] and (3) presence of

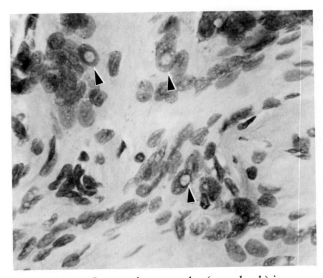

Figure 69-16 Intranuclear vacuoles (*arrowheads*) in a meningioma. This type of vacuole is caused by invagination of the cytoplasm into the nucleus. (Hematoxylin-eosin, ×460.)

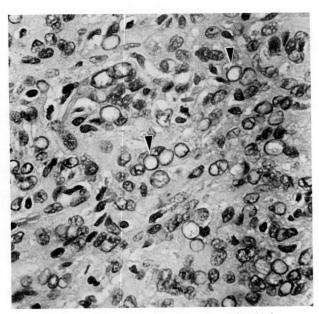

Figure 69-17 Intranuclear vacuoles (*arrowheads*) in a meningioma. Many cells show this feature. This type of vacuole is caused by clearing of chromatin from the center to the periphery. (Hematoxylin-eosin, ×460.)

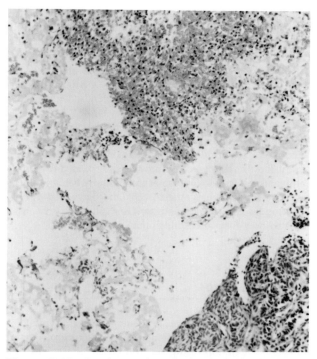

Figure 69-18 Specimen of meningioma obtained with the CUSA unit. An appearance of pseudonecrosis is seen, along with an intact fragment of tumor at the lower right corner. (Hematoxylin-eosin, ×120.)

numerous fine fibrils in the cytoplasm of these cells[10] (Figs. 69-19, 69-20). The nuclei of some tumor cells may show invagination of cytoplasm. A nucleolus is often recognized. Usual cell organelles like mitochondria, as well as rough-surfaced endoplasmic reticulum, are found between the cytoplasmic filaments. An electron-dense granular material is often found between some of the tumor cells (Fig. 69-21). Unusually the meningothelial tumor cells may show formation of basal bodies and cilia.[3] The scanning electron microscopic features of meningiomas are mostly of academic interest and play no part in routine diagnostic studies. The fusion of tumor cells, formation of microvilli, and globular clusters of whorls have all been documented by this method.[1,19]

Other Lesions Associated with Meningiomas

The vast majority of meningiomas are solitary tumors. However, multiple meningiomas can occur in the central form of von Recklinghausen's disease.[17] In this entity meningiomas may be mixed with schwannomas and gliomas. Multiple meningiomas can occur both within the cranial cavity and within the spinal canal. More common are the bone changes associated with meningiomas. Hyperostosis is seen in the

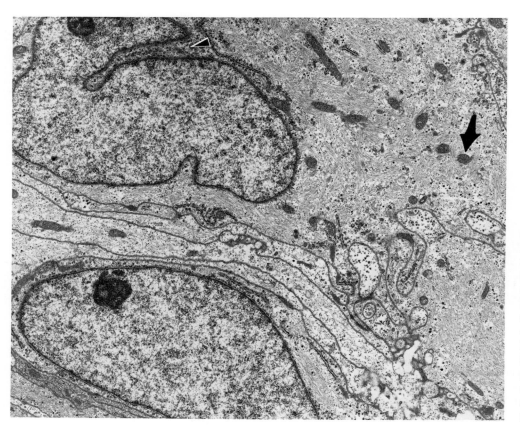

Figure 69-19 Meningioma, showing two nuclei, each with a nucleolus. The upper nucleus shows an invagination of cytoplasm (*arrowhead*) responsible for the appearances shown in Fig. 69-16. The cytoplasm of the cells is filled with fibrils, with mitochondria (*arrow*) dispersed among them. Between the two nuclei are cell processes from other cells. Under the light microscope this intertwining of cell processes suggests a syncytium; in reality the cells are uninucleated. (EM, ×9000.)

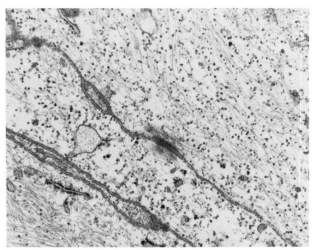

Figure 69-20 Meningioma, showing a desmosome (at center) between adjacent cell processes. Again, fibrils are seen in the cytoplasm. (EM, ×32,000.)

part of the skull overlying the meningioma. This may or may not be related to actual invasion of the bone by the tumor.

Malignant Meningiomas

Meningiomas are mostly benign tumors, and metastasizing malignant meningothelial and fibroblastic meningiomas are not common. Lungs, liver, lymph nodes, bones, and other sites are involved by metastases in that order of frequency. In recent years it has been realized that the hemangioperi-

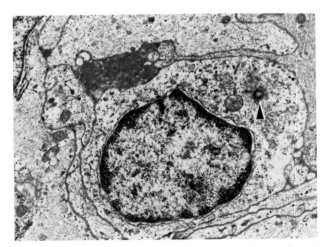

Figure 69-21 Meningioma, showing, above the nucleus, an aggregation of dark granular material between membranes of adjacent cells. Above and to the right of the nucleus is a basal body (*arrowhead*). (EM, ×12,000.)

cytic meningioma is also a dangerous tumor, one that has a high propensity to invade locally, grow quickly, and metastasize.[9,11,16] However, well-documented examples of malignant meningothelial meningiomas also are on record.[11] The features of malignancy are high cellularity, brain invasion, frequent mitoses, and blood vessel invasion. Invasion of dural venous sinuses in itself does not denote malignancy, however; it is seen frequently in benign meningiomas and is unassociated with later metastases. Necrosis is also not common in benign meningiomas and should arouse suspicion of aggressive growth potential. It was Ludwin et al.[13] who first pointed out that tumors of the papillary type were prone to metastasize. Foci of these papillary formations may be seen in aggressive meningothelial or angioblastic meningiomas.[11] Some malignant meningiomas have been known to spread along the CSF pathways.[12] It must be emphasized that local recurrence and local invasion in themselves are not criteria for malignancy, for these properties are shown by many nonmetastasizing meningiomas.

Meningeal Sarcomas

Sarcomas similar to those elsewhere in the body can arise in the meninges. Their histogenetic relationship to malignant meningioma is unclear. It must be pointed out that when a diagnosis of sarcoma is made, the pathologist usually means that no identifiable features of an aggressive or malignant meningothelial meningioma can be found. Sarcomas form less than 1 percent of primary intracranial tumors,[17] and sarcomas of the spinal dura or epidural space are even rarer. The authors have recently observed a patient with a malignant fibrous histiocytoma arising either in the dura or in the epidural space of the lumbar spinal canal with subsequent metastases to the lung.

Primary sarcomas of the central nervous system can occur at any age but are more common in infants, children, and young adults. Grossly they may simulate meningiomas by their location and consistency but are more fleshy and do not show the fine lobulation of the meningiomas. Local invasion is found at the time of operation, and the surface of the brain is often invaded. Sarcoma should be suspected if the duration of presenting complaints is short and the tumor on various radiological examinations appears to be large. The histological features of these sarcomas are quite variable, ranging from the appearance of a well or poorly differentiated fibrosarcoma to polymorphic cell sarcomas and undifferentiated sarcomas. In general, fascicles of plump spindle cells with large hyperchromatic nuclei (Figs. 69-22, 69-23) and formation of extracellular reticulin and/or collagen bundles are observed. Giant cells are uncommon. Uni- or multinucleated giant cells with often foamy cytoplasm suggest the possibility of a malignant fibrous histiocytoma, which has been documented as occurring in the meninges.[7] A rare tumor is the mesenchymal chondrosarcoma, which shows foci of undifferentiated sarcoma as well as recognizable islands of cartilaginous differentiation. The prognosis of these tumors is poor, mainly because they are not amenable to complete resection and their radiosensitivity is only moderate.

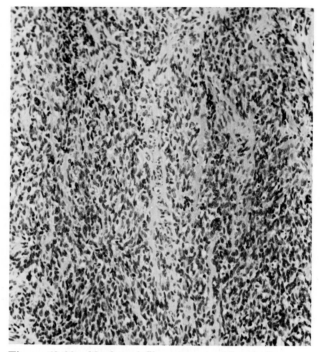

Figure 69-22 Meningeal fibrosarcoma with spindle-shaped tumor cells arranged in fascicles. The tumor is highly cellular. (Hematoxylin-eosin, × 120.)

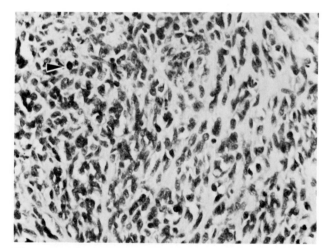

Figure 69-23 Meningeal fibrosarcoma. The cells are elongated and have hyperchromatic, spindle-shaped nuclei. Fine intercellular collagen fibrils are present. A mitosis is seen (*arrowhead*). (Hematoxylin-eosin, × 240.)

References

1. Arnold A, Burrows D: Scanning electron microscopy of cerebral tumors and glial cells. Recent Results Cancer Res 51:52–62, 1975.
2. Burger PC, Vogel FS: *Surgical Pathology of the Nervous System and Its Coverings.* New York, Wiley, 1976, p 93.
3. Cervós-Navarro J, Vazquez J: Elektronmikroskopische Untersuchungen über das Vorkommen von Cilien in Meningiomen. Virchows Arch [Pathol Anat] 341:280–290, 1966.
4. Challa VR, Moody DM, Marshall RB, Kelly DL, Jr: The vascular component in meningiomas associated with severe cerebral edema. Neurosurgery 7:363–368, 1980.
5. Cushing H, Eisenhardt L: *Meningiomas: Their Classification, Regional Behaviour, Life History, and Surgical End Results.* Springfield, Ill., Charles C Thomas, 1938.
6. Froman C, Lipschitz R: Demography of tumors of the central nervous system among the Bantu (African) population of the Transvaal, South Africa. J Neurosurg 32:660–664, 1970.
7. Gonzalez-Vitale JC, Slavin RE, McQueen JD: Radiation-induced intracranial malignant fibrous histiocytoma. Cancer 37:2960–2963, 1976.
8. Gusek W: Submikroskopische Untersuchungen als Beitrag zur Struktur und Onkologie der "Meningiome." Beitr Pathol Anat 127:274–326, 1962.
9. Horten BC, Urich H, Rubinstein LJ, Montague SR: The angioblastic meningioma: A reappraisal of a nosological problem. J Neurol Sci 31:387–410, 1977.
10. Kepes JJ: Electron microscopic studies of meningiomas. Am J Pathol 39:499–510, 1961.
11. Kepes JJ: *Meningiomas: Biology, Pathology & Differential Diagnosis.* New York, Masson, 1982.
12. Ludwin SK, Conley FK: Malignant meningioma metastasizing through the cerebrospinal pathways. J Neurol Neurosurg Psychiatry 38:136–142, 1975.
13. Ludwin SK, Rubinstein LJ, Russell DS: Papillary meningioma: A malignant variant of meningioma. Cancer 36:1363–1373, 1975.
14. Luse SA: Electron microscopic studies of brain tumors. Neurology (Minneap) 10:881–905, 1960.
15. Mirra SS, Miles ML: Unusual pericytic proliferation in a meningotheliomatous meningioma: An ultrastructural study. J Neuropathol Exp Neurol 39:376, 1980 (abstr).
16. Pitkethly DT, Hardman JM, Kempe LG, Earle KM: Angioblastic meningiomas: Clinicopathologic study of 81 cases. J Neurosurg 32:539–544, 1970.
17. Rubinstein LJ: *Tumors of the Central Nervous System,* Atlas of Tumor Pathology, fasc 6 2d ser. Washington, Armed Forces Institute of Pathology, 1972.
18. Smith HP, Challa VR, Moody DM, Kelly DL, Jr: Biological features of meningiomas that determine the production of cerebral edema. Neurosurgery 8:428–433, 1981.
19. Virtanen I, Lehtonen E, Wartiovaara J: Structure of psammoma bodies of a meningioma in scanning electron microscopy. Cancer 38:824–829, 1976.
20. Worster-Drought C, Dickson WEC, McMenemey WH: Multiple meningeal and perineural tumors with analogous changes in the glia and ependyma (neurofibroblastomatosis). Brain 60:85–117, 1937.

70

Meningiomas: Radiology

Dixon M. Moody

The dawn of radiology in the diagnosis of meningioma came in 1902 when Pfahler, on a living patient, achieved

> . . . an exposure of four minutes made with a moderately hard vacuum. I placed the anode of the tube directly opposite to the area in which Dr. Mills had located the tumor and at a distance of eighteen inches from the plate, for the reason that at this distance the shadows in the upper side of the skull would be dissipated by the divergence of the rays, and yet good definitions of the structures on the opposite side of the skull would be obtained."[7]

This tumor was reported at autopsy to be a fibrosarcoma. The term *meningioma* would not be used for over 20 years.[4]

In 1916 Heuer and Dandy reported the radiographic findings in 100 brain tumors, 9 of which were probably meningiomas.[5] It is interesting that a large number of these "endotheliomas" produced "vascular changes in the skull." Of the five cases with local hypertrophy of the skull, three were "dural endotheliomas."

Today, a wide variety of radiographic imaging techniques are available and useful in the diagnosis of meningioma.

Plain Roentgenograms

A local accumulation of calcium in tiny globular bodies over the surface of the brain is direct evidence of meningioma[15] and can be seen in up to 18 percent of cases at initial presentation (Fig. 70-1). Sclerosis of the inner table of the calvarium, a reactive change in the bone, usually does not indicate bone involvement by tumor. The sclerosis can have the appearance of blistering when the tumor is adjacent to a paranasal sinus and represents parallel layers of bone. Spiculation in the area of sclerosis indicates penetration of the bone by tumor, as do lytic skull defects (Fig. 70-2) and sclerosis of the outer table of the calvarium. An increase in number and tortuosity of meningeal vessels grooving the inner table of

the calvarium (Fig. 70-1) and associated enlargement of the foramen spinosum is another indication of meningioma, but this finding can also be seen in arteriovenous malformations and in long-standing carotid occlusive disease.

Indirect signs of meningioma are those of increased intracranial pressure such as demineralization of the sella turcica and a shift of the brain best identified on plain films by displacement of the calcified pineal gland. Olmsted and McGee[10] found a lytic destructive reaction in the adjacent calvarium associated with meningiomas that were likely to recur. With a purely sclerotic calvarial reaction, recurrence following surgery was much less likely, and the predictive value was more accurate than cell type or other histological characteristics.

Radionuclide Scintigraphy

Prior to the advent of computed tomography (CT), radionuclide studies of the brain were very important in the workup of a patient with a possible intracranial mass lesion. If the radionuclide studies did not suggest meningioma, the angiographer could forgo a selective external carotid or common carotid artery injection in favor of a selective internal carotid study. False-negative scintigraphy in meningioma occurs in up to 16 percent of cases.[8,17] When performed on a modern high performance scintillation camera with a high-sensitivity parallel-hole collimator and combined with a dynamic study, the technique was positive in 28 consecutive meningiomas reported by Sheldon et al.[12] In this regard it compares favorably with computed tomography. The increase in radioisotopic activity in the tumor is due to an increased blood volume in the tumor and to leakage of the radionuclide into the extracellular fluid of the tumor. Examinations performed 2 h after injection of the radionuclide proved to be more accurate than scintigraphy done immediately after injection of the agent.

Radionuclide techniques are also available which can predict the patency of the major dural venous sinuses. A helpful diagnostic feature of a convexity meningioma is that it will often exhibit as much radioisotopic activity as the nearest major dural sinus. Radionuclide scintigraphy is useful in the detection of recurrent meningioma, especially when metallic clips are present intracranially, causing artifact on the CT image (see, for instance, Figure 70-17C). Computed tomographic radionuclide studies are now in limited use (Fig. 70-3) and show promise for the future.

Computed Tomography

CT has become the single most important radiographic test in the diagnosis of meningioma. It has eclipsed radionuclide studies because, in addition to identifying the tumor, it will demonstrate brain anatomy, shift, calcification, and edema, as well as bone changes. Classically, the noncalcified areas of

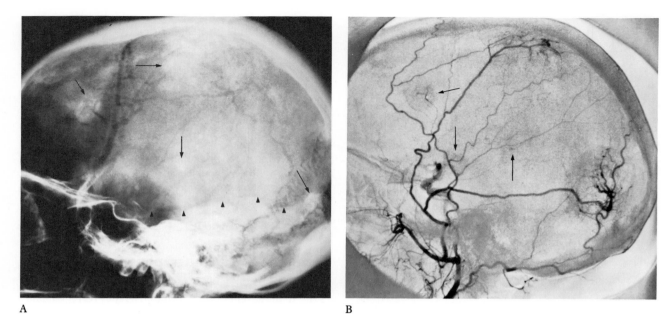

A

B

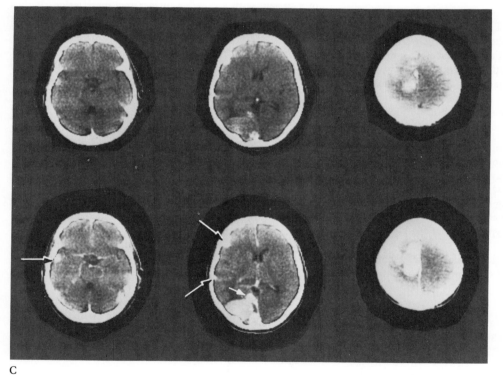

C

Figure 70-1 Multiple meningiomas. *A.* Dilated vascular channels are seen. Note groove for the posterior branch of the middle meningeal artery (*arrowheads*). Several tumors contain calcific densities (*arrows*). *B.* Subtracted selective external carotid arteriogram with minimal spillover into internal carotid system reveals opacification of meningeal feeding arteries to the tumors (arrows on smaller tumors), as well as scalp vessels which perforate the calvarium to contribute supply. From the vascular "hilus" of the tumor radiate small corkscrew tumor vessels. *C.* Uninfused (*top row*) and infused (*bottom*) CT scans demonstrate at least six tumors (arrows indicate smaller lesions). The posterior lesion is actually two tumors, a small one at the free edge of the tentorium and a larger component originating from the occipital squama.

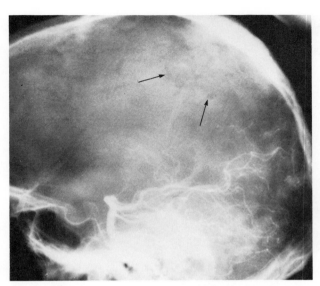

Figure 70-2 Vertex meningioma. Alternating areas of sclerosis and lysis (*arrows*) in the parietal bone. The lytic feature usually indicates direct involvement of the bone by tumor.

the lesion will appear slightly dense (40 to 80 Hounsfield units, or HU) prior to infusion and dura-based, extra-axial, with globular smooth margins and homogeneous dense enhancement following contrast infusion (Fig. 70-4). Rarely, a large tumor will show weak contrast enhancement (Fig. 70-5). Meningiomas may exhibit calcification which can be psammomatous, nodular, or rimlike (Figs. 70-1, 70-6). Calcification is seen in a higher percentage of posterior fossa meningiomas than in meningiomas elsewhere.[8]

Many of the bone changes caused by meningioma and described in the previous section on plain roentgenograms can be seen, sometimes to greater advantage, on CT. Certainly penetration of bone by tumor can be accurately predicted if the soft tissue component of the tumor can be seen on either side of the bone (Fig. 70-7).

Approximately half the meningiomas can impart some vasogenic edema to the brain, and it is striking how much edema can be present in some of the smallest lesions (Figs. 70-8 to 70-10), while often large meningiomas incite little or no radiographically apparent edema in the adjacent brain[13] (Fig. 70-11). The explanation for this has not yet been definitely elucidated. Some theories to explain the phenomenon include direct compression of a draining cerebral vein, direct communication between the tumor's extracellular fluid and the brain's extracellular fluid space, exudation of a humoral agent from the tumor, loss of vascular regulation, transition to hemangiopericytoma cell type, and rapid enlargement of the tumor.[2]

A low-density area is sometimes seen at the margin of a meningioma. This may be a dilated cerebrospinal fluid (CSF) space, an arachnoid cyst (Fig. 70-12), a necrotic portion of the tumor, or brain edema.[1] Vasogenic edema can be identified by its characteristic pattern of cortical sparing and

spread along predictable fiber tract pathways[3] (Figs. 70-8 to 70-10). Posterior fossa meningiomas rarely are associated with brain edema (Fig. 70-6).

If multiple meningiomas or a meningioma in the temporal horn are seen, von Recklinghausen's disease should be considered in the diagnosis. Differential diagnoses of the classic appearance seen on CT include plasmocytoma, chloroma, and fibrous dysplasia (Fig. 70-7). If the lesion is near the internal auditory canal (Fig. 70-6) or sella turcica (Fig. 70-13), acoustic neuroma or pituitary adenoma would enter the differential consideration.

CT without and with contrast is reported to be positive in 96 percent of meningiomas and specific for diagnosis in 90 percent.[8] Of tumors detected by CT, 2 percent will be mistakenly called meningioma and later prove to be another kind of tumor.

The reasons for misdiagnosis are observer error and atypical appearance of the lesion. On uninfused CT, New et al.[8] found the soft tissue component of meningioma isodense with brain in 10 percent (Fig. 70-5) and hypodense in 4 percent. Russell et al.[11] reviewed 131 cases of meningioma and found 8 percent focally atypical and 7 percent generally atypical. The ultimate histological finding of tumor necrosis, cystic change, scarring, lipomatous infiltration, or hemorrhage in these cases correlated excellently with the atypical CT appearance of low density or inhomogeneous enhancement. Recent hemorrhage in the tumor, although rare, was seen in three cases in this series.[11]

Recurrence of meningioma is suspected when any one of three CT features is present: (1) mass, (2) vasogenic edema, (3) contrast enhancement more than 1 year after surgery. The rate of recurrence is reported to be 9 to 13 percent in tumors judged to be completely removed. In another report New et al.[9] attempted to correlate CT findings with malignant histological features. They concluded that (1) indistinct margins, (2) fingers of the tumor penetrating deeply into adjacent brain (Fig. 70-6), (3) vasogenic edema, (4) bone lysis, (5) necrosis, (6) absent calcifications, and (7) "mushrooming" pattern or a large en plaque component all correlated with histological malignancy, the last of these findings being the most specific. It remains to be seen if these CT findings correlate directly with recurrence of tumor.

Small intraventricular meningiomas may cause symptoms due to CSF obstruction if located in the temporal horn (Figs. 70-14, 70-15) or foramen of Monro. Tumors in the atria, however, may attain large size before they become symptomatic (Fig. 70-16).

Water-soluble positive contrast CT cisternography has in many instances replaced pneumoencephalography (PEG) as a diagnostic tool for visualizing small basal extra-axial masses. A PEG may be useful in instances of intraventricular[14] or basal meningioma.

Angiography

The objectives of angiography are to serve as a road map for surgery, to confirm encasement of the carotid artery, to consider and plan a preoperative embolization as an adjunct to

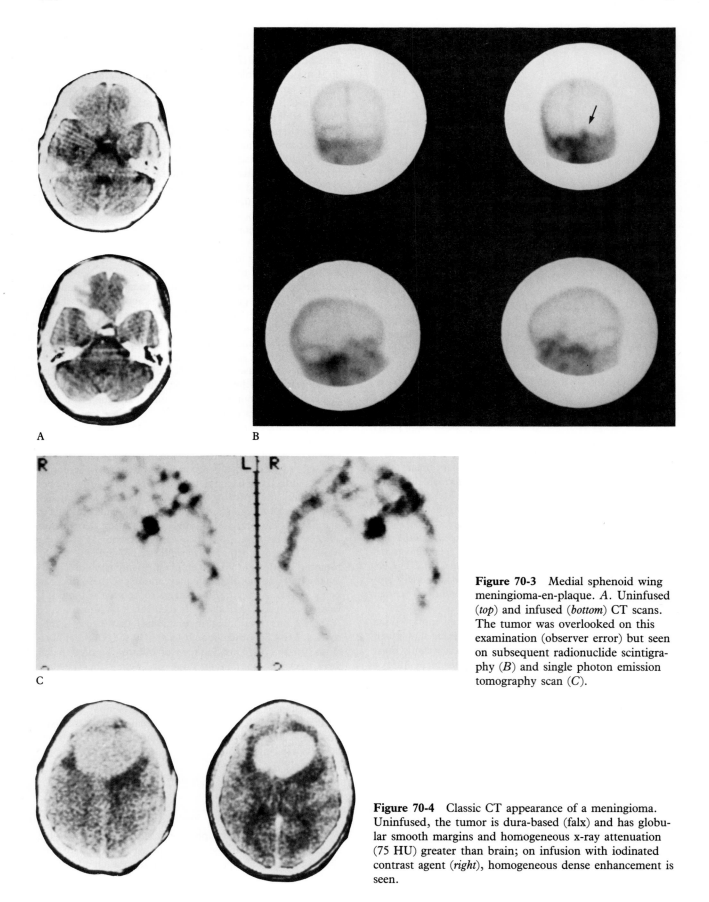

A

B

C

Figure 70-3   Medial sphenoid wing meningioma-en-plaque. *A.* Uninfused (*top*) and infused (*bottom*) CT scans. The tumor was overlooked on this examination (observer error) but seen on subsequent radionuclide scintigraphy (*B*) and single photon emission tomography scan (*C*).

Figure 70-4   Classic CT appearance of a meningioma. Uninfused, the tumor is dura-based (falx) and has globular smooth margins and homogeneous x-ray attenuation (75 HU) greater than brain; on infusion with iodinated contrast agent (*right*), homogeneous dense enhancement is seen.

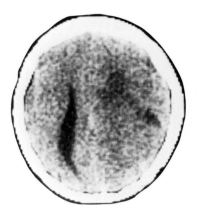
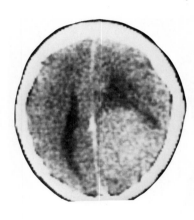

Figure 70-5 Large parieto-occipital meningioma. Prior to infusion (*left*) the tumor is isodense with normal brain, although it has an interface with edematous brain. Twenty minutes after infusion, only faint enhancement is present. This is an unusual CT appearance.

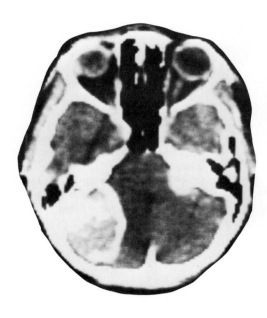

Figure 70-6 Posterior fossa meningioma in a patient with central neurofibromatosis. CT demonstrates both rim and discrete nodular calcification within the tumor. Note the small tumor in the opposite cerebellopontine angle, presumed to be an acoustic neurinoma (unconfirmed).

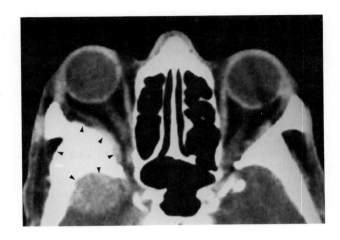

Figure 70-7 Greater sphenoid wing meningioma. The bone is thickened (*arrowheads*), and the soft tissue component extends into the middle fossa and the orbit. The soft tissue component differentiates this tumor from fibrous dysplasia.

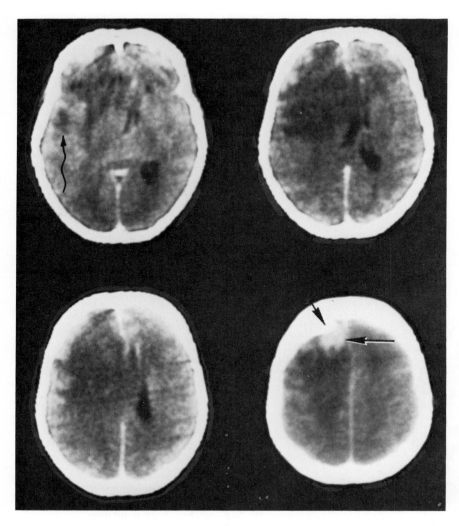

Figure 70-8 Frontal meningioma. Infused CT; small tumor (*arrows*) with indistinct margins which extend like tentacles into the brain incites massive brain edema and herniation. Vasogenic edema extends down the uncinate fasciculus to the temporal lobe (*wavy arrow*). Surgical specimen revealed some hemangiopericytoma elements. (From Challa, et al.[2])

surgery, to establish patency of the major dural sinuses (Fig. 70-17), to identify the length of attachment of the tumor (Fig. 70-18), and in patients with an atypical CT appearance, to confirm the diagnosis. In the study reported by New et al., angiography was found to be equivocal or negative in 6 percent of cases but in 83 percent made the specific diagnosis of meningioma.[8] In 18 percent, angiography increased the level of diagnostic confidence and specificity initially achieved by CT (some of which were uninfused scans). Classic findings include (1) modestly enlarged and tortuous afferent vessels, usually from the external carotid system; (2) abnormal arborization of the afferent arteries, with the distal branches often larger than the parent arteries;[16] (3) sunburst appearance of the arteries at the hilus or attachment of the meningioma to the dura mater, which is the tumor's site of origin; (4) tumor vascularity, or corkscrew appearance of the small arteries in the interstices of the lesion (Fig. 70-18); (5) enlarged draining veins; (6) usually normal circulation time; (7) dense tumor capillary blush in the late venous phase (Fig. 70-18). The primary meningeal vascular supply to the hilus of the tumor is a reasonably constant finding and is derived from the normal meningeal arterial supply (Fig. 70-19) to that area of the dura mater (Table 70-1). Knowledge of the derivation of the normal meningeal arterial supply is imperative in the arteriographic evaluation of meningioma suspected in a particular location (Fig. 70-19).

TABLE 70-1 Parent Meningeal Arterial Supply of Meningiomas by Location

Site	Parent Artery
Cranial convexity	Middle meningeal
Falx cerebri	Ophthalmic–middle meningeal
Olfactory groove	Ophthalmic
Sphenoid wing	Ophthalmic
Diaphragma sellae	Internal carotid
Middle fossa	Internal carotid–middle meningeal
Tentorium	Internal carotid
Posterior fossa:	
Anterior compartment	Internal and external carotid
Posterior compartment	Vertebral
Intraventricular	Anterior or posterior choroidal

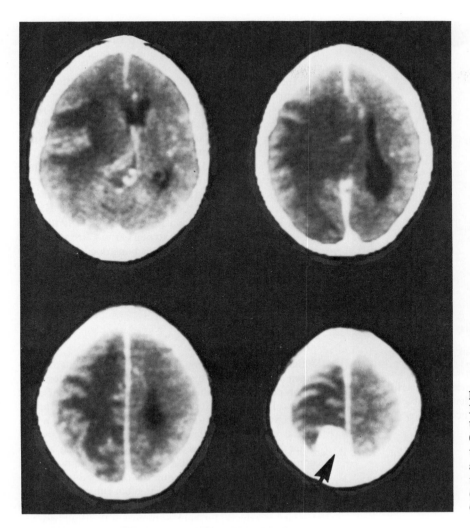

Figure 70-9 Occipital meningioma. Inordinate brain edema and herniation caused by a small tumor (*arrow*). Note the characteristic pattern of vasogenic edema extending along white matter fiber tracts, in this case the subcortical association ("U") fibers, to each gyrus. (From Challa et al.[2])

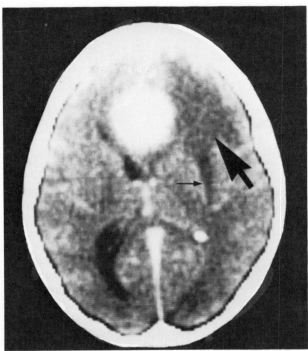

Figure 70-10 Falx meningioma. On infusion CT the tumor extends equally into both frontal lobes, but vasogenic edema (*large arrow*) is present only on right side. Note extension of edema along the inferior fronto-occipital fasciculus (*small arrow*), a characteristic of vasogenic edema. (From Smith et al.[13])

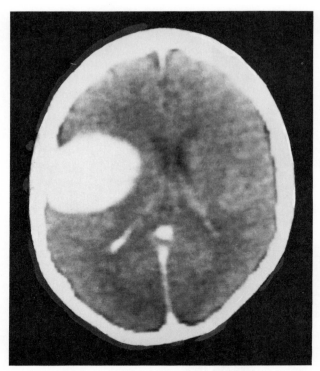

Figure 70-11 Convexity temporal meningioma. Infused CT of a large meningioma with no demonstrable edema. Shift of brain is due solely to space occupied by tumor. (From Smith et al.[13])

With increasing size a meningioma may recruit pial vascularity (brain vessels) to supply the periphery of the tumor. Often, a selective internal carotid arteriogram reveals a doughnut-like tumor stain; a selective external carotid injection then stains the hilus of the lesion. Some meningiomas, particularly those at the skull base and cerebellopontine angle, stain poorly. This may be more apparent than real if on the photographic mask film (used to make the subtraction) there is contrast material trapped in the tumor from earlier test injections or injections into other vessels.

Kieffer et al.[6] found an unusually high incidence (38 percent) of arteriovenous shunting (Fig. 70-17) in the 40 meningiomas they reported, while most others report an incidence of 5 percent for this phenomenon. In the Kieffer series, 11 of 40 did not demonstrate a stain; 22 of 40 received some blood supply from the external carotid artery. All five of the angioblastic meningiomas demonstrated early venous filling. Other angiographic features rarely seen include encasement or entrapment of an artery and subarachnoid hemorrhage with spasm.

Digital Subtraction Angiography

While of lesser resolving capability than standard film-screen arteriography, digital video subtraction angiography has no peer in the evaluation of patency in the major dural sinuses. It can be performed safely as an outpatient procedure. Usually the contrast material is injected into a vein instead of an artery. The technique can nicely show the tumor blush, but the exact nature of the feeding arteries cannot be sorted out on this low-resolution study. Digital subtraction arteriography (using the digital subtraction capability during an arteriogram) can often enhance the tumor blush of those lesions which commonly blush poorly on standard arteriography, such as tumors at the skull base and cerebellopontine angle.

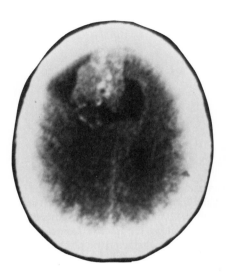
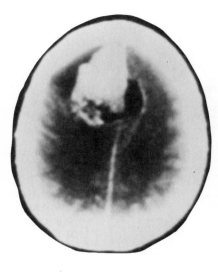

Figure 70-12 Atypical CT appearance of a parasagittal meningioma due to an associated intra-arachnoid cyst. Uninfused scan (*left*) demonstrates globular areas of calcification interspersed in the tumor and low-density areas with sharp margins adjacent to the tumor. These low-density areas proved at surgery to be intra-arachnoid cysts. Infused scan is at right. (Courtesy of Dr. A. R. Cowley, Greenville, S.C.)

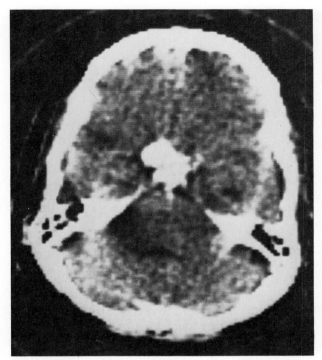

Figure 70-13 Diaphragma sellae meningioma. Infused CT demonstrates tumor extending into the suprasellar cistern.

Nuclear Magnetic Resonance

This imaging technique shows a great deal of promise in many lesions of the brain which heretofore were poorly imaged by other methods. Although meningiomas can be visualized with the technique, it is hard to imagine how diagnostic accuracy could be improved over the procedures now employed. At this early stage no one knows what role in the workup of a meningioma nuclear magnetic resonance (NMR) will play, but our preliminary work suggests that small calcified meningiomas, imaged on CT, are frequently not seen on NMR, especially if the tumor does not incite edema of the adjacent brain. NMR images bone poorly, which is a distinct disadvantage in intracranial meningioma evaluation, but this same characteristic may be used to advantage in the cerebellopontine angle, an area notorious for artifact on CT. It is often impossible to successfully image the brain with CT in patients with a number of areas of high x-ray absorption density such as Pantopaque or metallic clips. NMR may be useful in these instances, provided the metallic objects are not set in motion by the strong magnetic field.

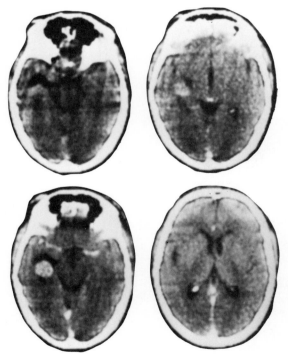

Figure 70-14 Meningioma in temporal horn of lateral ventricle. Uninfused CT (*top row*) reveals "trapped" temporal horn. Infusion (*bottom row*) reveals homogeneous enhancement of tumor.

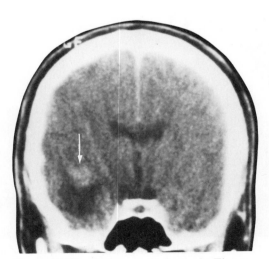

Figure 70-15 Same case as shown in Figure 70-14. Direct coronal CT scan demonstrates trapped horn and tumor (*arrow*) behind it.

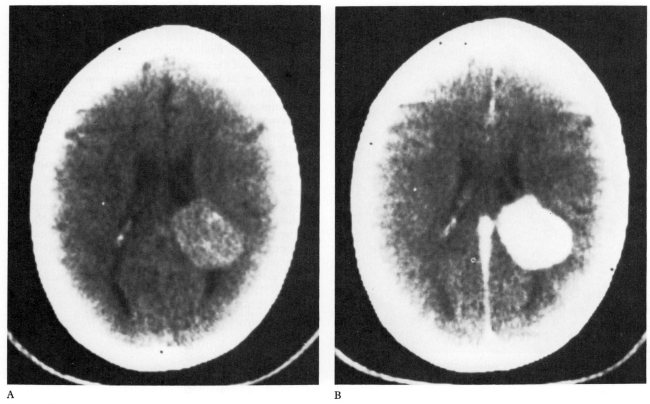

A   B

Figure 70-16   Intraventricular meningioma. Uninfused (*A*) and infused (*B*) CT scans reveal large tumor in atrium without shift of brain, CSF obstruction, or edema.

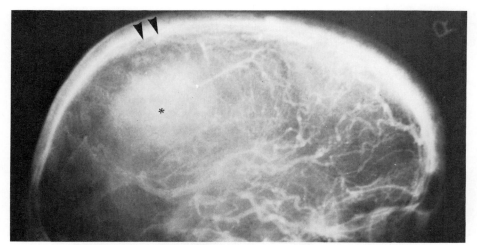

Figure 70-17   Posterior falx meningioma. Venous phase of angiogram demonstrates tumor blush (*asterisk*) and an obstructed superior sagittal sinus (*arrowheads*). Note numerous markedly tortuous collateral venous channels draining downward toward the sphenoparietal sinus and basal vein.

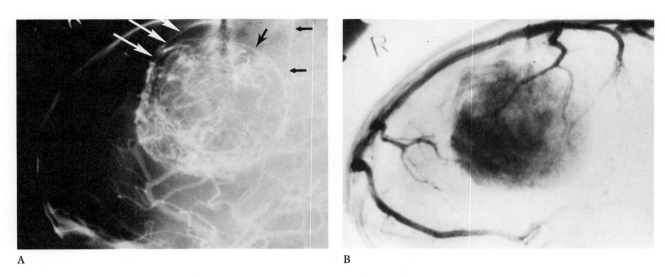

A   B

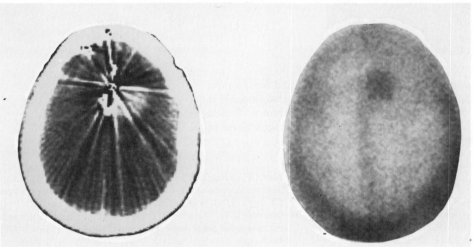

C

Figure 70-18   Falx meningioma, hemangiopericytoma type, in a 15-year-old. *A*. There are corkscrew-like tumor vessels in the lesion, which has recruited pial vascular supply. Early appearance of veins (*arrows*) which have "washed out" by the late venous phase (*B*) is unusual. Note the sustained tumor blush into the late venous phase, which is more characteristic of a meningioma. This tumor, thought to be completely removed, recurred within 2 years. *C*. Infused CT scan is inconclusive for recurrence because artifacts are induced by the metallic clips; radionuclide scintigraphy vertex view (*right*) demonstrates recurrent tumor.

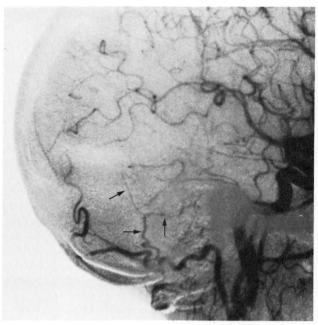

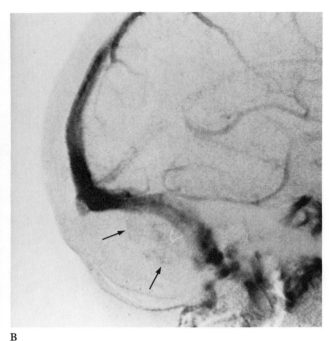

A   B

Figure 70-19 Posterior fossa meningioma. *A*. This tumor, suspected from a prior radionuclide brain scan, was situated laterally just below the transverse sinus. It did not derive vascular supply from the vertebrobasilar circulation but from perforating mastoidal branches of the external carotid artery (*arrows*). *B*. The venous phase reveals the classic persistent tumor blush of meningioma (*arrows*).

References

1. Becker D, Norman D, Wilson CB: Computerized tomography and pathological correlation in cystic meningiomas: Report of two cases. J Neurosurg 50:103–105, 1979.
2. Challa VR, Moody DM, Marshall RB, Kelly DL Jr: The vascular component in meningiomas associated with severe cerebral edema. Neurosurgery 7:363–368, 1980.
3. Cowley AR: The influence of fiber tracts on the CT appearance of cerebral edema: An anatomic-pathological correlation. AJNR 4:915–925, 1983.
4. Cushing H: The meningiomas (dural endotheliomas): Their source, and favoured seats of origin. Brain 45:282–316, 1922.
5. Heuer GJ, Dandy WE: Roentgenography in the localization of brain tumor, based upon a series of one hundred consecutive cases. Bull Johns Hopkins Hosp 27:311–322, 1916.
6. Kieffer SA, Larson DA, Gold LHA, Prentice WB, Stadlan EM, Seyfert S: Rapid circulation in intracranial meningiomas. Radiology 106:575–580, 1973.
7. Mills CK, Pfahler GE: Tumor of the brain localized clinically and by the Roentgen rays: With some observations and investigations relating to the use of the Roentgen rays in the diagnosis of lesions of the brain. Philadelphia Med J 9:268–273, 1902.
8. New PFJ, Aronow S, Hesselink JR: National Cancer Institute study: Evaluation of computed tomography in the diagnosis of intracranial neoplasms: IV. Meningiomas. Radiology 136:665–675, 1980.
9. New PFJ, Hesselink JR, O'Carroll CP, Kleinman GM: Malignant meningiomas: CT and histologic criteria, including a new CT sign. AJNR 3:267–276, 1982.
10. Olmsted WW, McGee TP: Prognosis in meningioma through evaluation of skull bone patterns. Radiology 123:375–377, 1977.
11. Russell EJ, George AE, Kricheff II, Budzilovich G: Atypical computed tomographic features of intracranial meningioma: Radiological-pathological correlation in a series of 131 consecutive cases. Radiology 135:673–682, 1980.
12. Sheldon JJ, Smoak WM, Gargano FP, Watson DD: Dynamic scintigraphy in intracranial meningiomas. Radiology 109:109–115, 1973.
13. Smith HP, Challa VR, Moody DM, Kelly DL Jr: Biological features of meningiomas that determine the production of cerebral edema. Neurosurgery 8:428–433, 1981.
14. Smith H, Moody D, Ball M, Laster W, Kelly DL Jr, Alexander E Jr: The trapped temporal horn: A trap in neuroradiological diagnosis. Neurosurgery 5:245–249, 1979.
15. Taveras JM, Wood EH: *Diagnostic Neuroradiology*, 2d ed. Baltimore, Williams & Wilkins, 1976, pp 159–189.
16. Wickbom I: Tumor circulation, in Newton TH, Potts DG (eds): *Radiology of the Skull and Brain*: vol. 2. *Angiography*. St. Louis, Mosby, 1974, pp 2257–2285.
17. Witcofski RL, Maynard CD, Roper TJ: A comparative analysis of the accuracy of the technetium-99m pertechnetate brain scan: Followup of 1000 patients. J Nucl Med 8:187–196, 1967.

71

Meningiomas: Clinical Features and Surgical Management

Robert G. Ojemann

TABLE 71-1 Locations of Meningiomas in 200 Consecutive Patients Treated Surgically

Parasagittal	20	Anterior fossa	2
Anterior third	3	Floor	1
Middle third	15	No dural attachment	1
Posterior third	2	Middle fossa floor	2
Falx	8	Cerebellopontine angle	27
Convexity	51	Cerebellopontine angle	
Parasagittal	17	and middle fossa	3
Coronal	9	Cerebellar convexity	6
Anterior sylvian	7	Tentorial	8
Other	18	Clivus	3
Olfactory groove	9	Intraventricular	2
Tuberculum sellae	18	Foramen magnum	3
Sphenoid wing	31	Optic sheath	7
Hyperostosing	12		
Middle ridge	3		
Medial	16		

The basis for the surgical management of meningiomas was presented in the classic two-volume work *Meningiomas* by Harvey Cushing and Louise Eisenhardt.[4] Most of these tumors are benign, and the majority are curable. The objective of the operation is total removal of the meningioma, including the involved dura and bone, if at all possible. The completeness of surgical removal of the tumor is the single most important prognostic factor.[4,12] However, this goal must always be tempered by surgical judgment which considers that the first priority is to preserve and improve function. In some patients, in whom total removal carries a significant risk of morbidity, it is better judgment to leave some tumor and plan to follow the patient with clinical evaluation and CT scans, perform a further operation at a later time, or use radiation therapy, as indicated.

The material in this chapter is based on personal experience with a consecutive series of 200 patients with meningiomas operated upon during a 15-year period (1968–1982). Some of the patients reported in a previous publication that covered a different time period are included.[16] The locations of the tumors are recorded in Table 71-1. The overall operative mortality was 1 percent, with two deaths, one due to myocardial infarction and the other to pulmonary embolus. The results are summarized in Table 71-2 and are discussed in more detail in the section on specific sites. The status of the patient was determined as of the last contact or just prior to death or disability from an unrelated illness.

General Aspects of Management

Preoperative Preparation

The patient is given steroids for at least 48 h before surgery and longer if there is considerable edema in the adjacent brain tissue. This is important in helping prevent the problems with cerebral edema that may follow removal of a meningioma.

Preoperative embolization may be indicated in some meningiomas in which there is extensive vascularity from external carotid artery branches which might prove difficult to control early in the course of the operation. However, this procedure must be done with care, since there is the risk that emboli may flow back into the internal carotid artery during the injection. Surgical removal of the tumor should be done within 24 to 48 h of embolization, or collateral blood supply may develop. The different methods of embolization have been reviewed[12] and are also discussed in another chapter of this textbook.

Preoperative radiation was not used in this series. The literature on this subject has been reviewed and is discussed below.[12,25]

Preparation at the Time of Surgery

The neurosurgeon should have available an anesthesiologist who is knowledgeable in the field of neurosurgery. The operating room should be dedicated to neurosurgery and include the availability of trained personnel, operating microscope, bipolar coagulator, laser, and Cavitron ultrasonic surgical aspirator (Cooper Medical, Mountain View, Calif.). The recovery room and intensive care unit should be staffed with personnel familiar with neurosurgical problems.

When the patient arrives in the operating room, a radial artery catheter is inserted for continuous monitoring of blood pressure and evaluation of blood gases. The P_{CO_2} is kept near 30 torr during the operation.

A smooth induction of anesthesia without the patient straining or coughing and careful control of blood pressure are important factors in getting the surgery off to a good start. An indwelling Foley catheter is inserted. As soon as this is done the patient is given 10 to 20 mg of furosemide. During the preparation and exposure, a 20 percent solution of mannitol is given in a dosage of 1 to 1.5 g/kg over 20 to 30 min. Prior to making the skin incision, an antibiotic, usually a cephalosporin, is administered and is continued until 24 h after surgery.

TABLE 71-2 Results of Surgical Treatment Using Microsurgery and Other Adjuncts (1968–1982)

Tumor Location	Removal		Recurrence	Results*			Postoperative Mortality†
	Total	Subtotal		Excellent or Good	Fair	Poor	
Parasagittal	13	7	5‡	14	2	3§	1
Falx	8			7	1		
Cerebral convexity	51		1	48	2		1
Olfactory groove	9			8	1		
Tuberculum sellae	10	8	1	14	2	2¶	
Sphenoid wing:							
Hyperostosing		12	4	12			
Middle	3			3			
Medial		16	5	10	4	2¶	
Cerebellopontine angle:							
<3.0 cm	11	1		12			
>3.0 cm	2	16	5	10	5	3¶	
Cerebellar convexity	6			6			
Tentorial	6	2		8			
Clivus		3		2		1	
Intraventricular	2			1	1		
Foramen magnum	3			3			
Other	11			11			

*Excellent = full recovery with no deficit
 Good = fully functional and able to work but slight neurological deficit
 Fair = able to be active but some limitation because of neurological deficits
 Poor = significant impairment because of neurological deficits
†Death related to operation—one myocardial infarction and one pulmonary embolus.
‡Two patients had subsequent total removal; the other three had malignant meningiomas.
§Two late deaths occurred in patients with malignant meningioma.
¶One late death at each site due to tumor.

After careful positioning, the patient's head is held with the three-point skeletal fixation headrest. Care is taken to keep the head above the heart level and to avoid compression of the jugular veins in the neck. The position must take into account the effects of gravity, the need to minimize brain retraction, and the avoidance of compression of the brain against the edge of the dura. If the head is to be well elevated or a semisitting position is used, a central venous pressure line is placed in the right atrium, using x-ray guidance.

General Principles of Operation

Some type of magnification (either loupes or the operating microscope) is used for the entire operation. The skin incision must allow for full exposure of the tumor. Blood supply to the scalp flap must be adequate, and a wide enough base must be left to provide good vascularization. The cosmetic result of the scar and bone flap should be considered.

A free bone flap will allow wide, expeditious exposure of tumor and can be easily enlarged if necessary. Blood supply coming through the bone is occluded, and the pericranial tissue is kept intact so that it can be used for a dural graft if necessary. At the end of the operation the bone flap is wired solidly in place with several no. 28 wires. If burr holes or bone removal due to tumor will leave a cosmetic deformity or a large bone defect, a cranioplasty is done. For a burr hole or small bone defect, a no. 28 wire is placed across the opening through holes drilled on each side, and the area is filled with acrylic.

Bleeding from the dura is controlled with bipolar coagulation, Surgicel (oxidized cellulose; Johnson and Johnson, New Brunswick, N.J.), or Gelfoam (absorbable gelatin sponge; The Upjohn Co., Kalamazoo, Mich.). The dura is held to the inner table of bone along the craniotomy opening with 4-0 Neurolon (Ethicon, Somerville, N.J.) sutures placed from dura to pericranial tissue or into holes drilled in the bone.

For superficial meningiomas the dura is opened at the margin between brain and tumor. One should always try to expose as little normal brain as possible, especially when the brain is still full because of the presence of a large tumor mass. All dura attached to the tumor is eventually removed, but in convexity and parasagittal meningiomas it is usually wise to leave it attached to help in retraction. At the end of the operation the convexity dura is replaced with a graft of pericranial tissue which is taken from the back of the scalp flap.

Everything is done to avoid retraction or removal of adjacent brain tissue. Gentle pressure is placed against the capsule of the tumor or on the dural attachment to help define the plane with adjacent brain tissue. Brain tissue is gently separated from the capsule of the tumor using fine dissectors. As blood vessels between capsule and brain tissue are encountered, they are coagulated with bipolar coagulation and cut with microscissors. In some patients it is best to carry out an extensive internal decompression of the tumor prior to trying to dissect the capsule. The decompression is facilitated by use of the ultrasonic aspirator, which fragments and aspirates tissue at the tip of the instrument, or the carbon dioxide laser, which vaporizes tissue. The use of the

CO_2 laser in the operative management of intracranial meningioma has been described in detail.[23] Bleeding from within the tumor will often cease spontaneously, but in some cases bipolar coagulation or Surgicel may be needed.

Postoperative Care

Steroids are continued for several days and then gradually tapered. Anticonvulsants are given to patients with supratentorial meningiomas for at least 6 months.

If there is evidence of worsening in the patient's condition postoperatively, a CT scan is done to look for hematoma, cerebral edema, and hydrocephalus. The most frequent cause is cerebral edema, which may require increased steroids or intermittent mannitol administration.

Recurrence

If the meningioma can be totally removed by surgery, the recurrence rate is low.[25] Simpson made a detailed study of the frequency of recurrence of meningiomas after surgery:[21] total removal, including the site of attachment, 9 percent; total removal with dura attachment being cauterized, 19 percent; total removal without full treatment of attachment, 29 percent; partial removal, 40 percent.

Even if total removal is not possible, no further immediate treatment may be indicated. Many sphenoid wing tumors, primarily those involving bone, are so slow-growing that they cause little trouble over many years. Some parasagittal tumors that cannot initially be totally removed because the sagittal sinus is still open can subsequently be cured by surgery when recurrence occludes the sinus.

When recurrence develops, the treatment for most patients is operation. Usually recurrent meningiomas do not change their basic histological characteristics.[19] The role of radiation therapy is discussed below. The demonstration of estradiol binding in some meningiomas suggests that a trial of hormone therapy be considered in some recurrences.[11]

Malignant Meningioma

The pathological diagnosis of malignant meningioma was discussed in a previous chapter. Two types of problems are considered by the neurosurgeon: one is the hemangiopericytoma (a variant of angioblastic meningioma), and the other is the meningioma that has an increased number of mitotic figures.

Treatment of the hemangiopericytoma is total removal if at all possible, followed by radiation therapy. In the Mayo Clinic series the rate of recurrence was 80 percent and the rate of metastasis 23 percent.[10]

The meningioma with an increased number of mitotic figures usually does not have such a poor prognosis. If the tumor can be totally removed, radiation is not given and the patient is followed with CT scans. If the tumor cannot be totally removed and is invasive, or if it is in an area where total removal will not be possible, radiation therapy is considered. If total removal might be feasible in the future, as

with a parasagittal lesion, the patient is followed and reoperation for complete removal is performed when the sagittal sinus becomes occluded.

Radiation Therapy

In the series reported here, radiation therapy was used for some meningiomas involving the cavernous sinus, medial sphenoid wing, or petrous bone and also when total removal of a malignant meningioma could not be assured or when patients had hemangiopericytoma.

Two reports, one of 34 and the other of 68 patients in whom radiation therapy had been used for meningiomas, concluded that this therapy is of benefit for residual or recurrent tumors and should be used in patients with malignant meningioma.[3,25]

The use of preoperative radiation for extremely vascular meningiomas has been reported to be of benefit.[12] Wara et al. recommended 5000 to 5500 rad given over 5½ to 6 weeks, with a 6-month delay between irradiation and surgery.[25] In their series this allowed successful removal of 7 of 12 meningiomas for which surgery had not been considered feasible.

One report has proposed that radiation therapy be considered as a primary treatment in some basilar meningiomas.[3] In that report, all 11 patients treated were alive over a 3- to 6-year follow-up period, and 9 were improved.

Metastases

Distant metastases of meningiomas are rare. In 1974, 56 cases were reviewed.[7] Sites of spread included lung, 60 percent; abdominal viscera, 34 percent; long bones, pelvis, and skull, 11 percent; and vertebrae, 11 percent. In that series, 10 patients had no surgery on the primary tumor or died on the day of operation. There was no correlation with histopathology or with the location of the tumor.

In the series reported here, one patient presented with a seizure. CT scan showed a parasagittal tumor, and chest x-ray showed a peripheral lung nodule. Needle biopsy of the lung lesion disclosed a benign meningioma, and both tumors were completely removed.

Clinical Features and Surgical Management

Parasagittal and Falx Meningiomas

Clinical Features

The term *parasagittal meningioma* applies to those tumors involving the sagittal sinus and the adjacent convexity dura and falx. Only the lateral wall of the sinus may be involved, or the tumor may grow to partially or completely occlude the sinus. Involvement of the overlying bone is common and may occur with or without hyperostosis. Many meningiomas occurring in the parasagittal region arise entirely from the convexity dura, do not involve the sinus, and have a small rim of cerebral tissue between the capsule of the tumor and the falx and sinus. These are grouped with the convexity meningiomas. Falx meningiomas are often bilateral and are completely concealed by the overlying cerebral cortex.

In considering both the symptoms and the surgical aspects of these tumors, it is useful to divide them, according to the area from which they arise, into anterior, middle and posterior thirds of the sagittal sinus, and falx.[4,13,16] The anterior third of the sinus extends from the crista galli to the coronal suture, the middle third from the coronal to the lambdoid sutures, and the posterior third from the lambdoid suture to the torcular. Those tumors arising from the middle third of the sagittal sinus and falx are the most common and present with focal motor or sensory seizures or gradual loss of neurological function, usually beginning in the lower extremity. Meningiomas arising from the anterior third tend to have a more insidious onset and often become large before a diagnosis is made. There may be a gradual change in personality, progressive dementia, and/or apathy. Seizures can occur but are infrequent and nonfocal. Headache is common. Tumor arising from the posterior third often presents with headache or other symptoms and signs of increased intracranial pressure. There may be visual symptoms, often with some type of field defect.[13,19]

The CT scan and angiographic findings have been discussed in Chap. 70. The surgeon must be sure that angiographic views are adequate to determine the status of the sagittal sinus and the relationship of the cortical veins to the tumor. In parasagittal tumors this information is vital, particularly in middle and posterior third lesions, in deciding what to do about the sinus at operation. With a falx meningioma, the location of the cortical veins is important in planning the approach. In some patients only a selective external carotid injection will show the vascular supply to the tumor.

Surgical Management

Positioning of the patient is determined by tumor location. For meningiomas located anterior to the coronal suture, the patient is placed supine with head slightly elevated. A coronal incision is used. For tumors at the coronal suture and in the middle third of the sagittal sinus, the patient is placed in a semilateral position with the head well elevated (Fig. 71-1A). The scalp over the center of the tumor should be the highest point. A horseshoe-shaped incision is used, extending 2 cm across the midline, with the anterior limb at the hairline and the posterior limb well behind the tumor (Fig. 71-1B). For some tumors at the coronal suture, the skin flap may be turned forward rather than laterally. In the posterior third lesions, the same type of position and the horseshoe incision are usually preferred. However, a prone or semisitting position may be indicated for some patients. The use of an S-shaped incision has been suggested by some surgeons.[10,13]

The skin and underlying tissue, including the pericranial tissue, are carefully elevated as one unit. A free bone flap which crosses the midline for 1 to 2 cm is used. Normally eight burr holes are placed, three across the base on the side of the bone flap, one on each side of the sagittal sinus, and one halfway between the holes on the side opposite the

tumor. If there is bone involvement, more burr holes may be placed near the tumor, and occasionally an area of bone is left attached to the tumor while a bone flap is turned around it. As the bone is elevated, bleeding from meningeal vessels is controlled with coagulation and that from the sagittal sinus with Gelfoam or Surgicel.

The dura is opened, usually starting anterior to the tumor, which in parasagittal lesions can usually be seen or palpated through the dura. The incision then curves around the tumor in a circumferential fashion, staying several millimeters from any involved dura. Great care is used, especially with middle third tumors, to avoid injury to the cortical veins. The dura is left attached to the tumor. If the sinus is going to be removed, the dura is then opened on the opposite side and the sinus ligated anterior and posterior to the tumor, as shown in Figure 71-3C. In some patients, the falx is now divided inferior to the tumor; in other patients this step is performed after dissection of the tumor. In anterior third meningiomas the sagittal sinus can and should be excised even if it is still open. If the sinus is open in middle or posterior third tumors, it cannot safely be removed because of the cortical venous infarction that will probably occur in the motor-sensory cortex; a subtotal removal may be indicated. In many patients the tumor involves only the edge or lateral wall of the sinus, and this can be removed. However, at this stage it is often better to make an incision in the tumor a few millimeters away from the sinus and completely free the tumor, coming back after the tumor mass has been removed to deal with the involved sinus.

Attention is now turned to the attachment to the surrounding brain. In many patients the arachnoid and pial attachments are progressively divided in a circumferential fashion and the brain separated, placing traction on the tumor and avoiding as much as possible retraction of the surrounding brain tissue. In some patients the plane between brain and tumor cannot be defined without undue retraction of the brain. In this situation it is useful to use the Cavitron to internally decompress the tumor and then proceed with the dissection. In large tumors one must be aware of the anterior cerebral artery branches, which may be adherent to the deep surface.

After the tumor that is compressing the brain has been removed, attention is turned again to the sinus area. Beginning at one end, the lateral edge of the sinus is opened and the tumor and walls of the sinus excised. After cutting 2 to 3 mm, the two leaves of the sinus are held with a forceps and the edge closed with a running suture of a material such as Prolene (Ethicon) (Fig. 71-1C). This step is repeated until the attachment has been completely divided and the tumor removed. An alternative method is to use fine, curved hemostats.[8,13] The use of various types of grafts to replace or repair a portion of the sagittal sinus has been reported.[1]

The area of brain which was compressed by tumor is lined with Surgicel. Using a graft of pericranial tissue from the back of the scalp flap, the dural defect is closed.

For tumors of the falx the same incision and bone flap are utilized. Often the tumor is bilateral but is much larger on one side. The dura is opened to 1 to 2 cm from the midline, with the exposure planned in relation to the cortical veins draining to the sagittal sinus. Arachnoid and pacchionian granulation attachments are divided. It is only necessary to retract the medial cerebral cortex 1 to 2 cm from the falx to

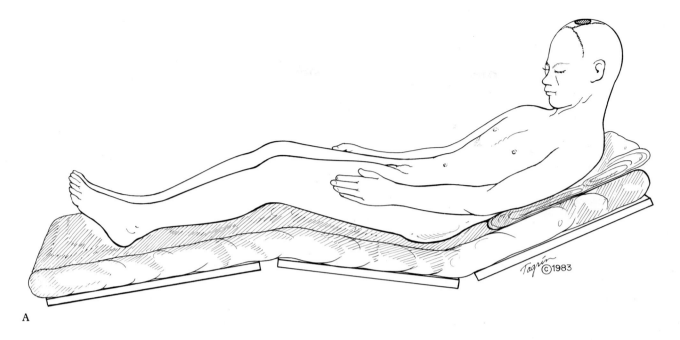

A

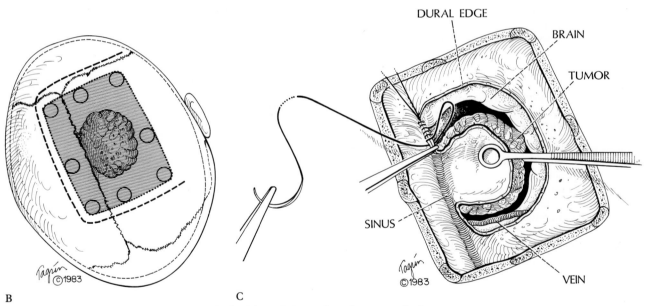

B   C

Figure 71-1 Parasagittal meningioma. *A.* Position of the patient for removal of a tumor involving the middle third of the sagittal sinus. The head is well elevated so that the scalp over the tumor will be the highest point. *B.* The skin incision (*dashed line*) and free bone flap (*dotted line*) are outlined. The exposure crosses the midline. *C.* Complete removal of the tumor may involve entering the lateral edge of the sagittal sinus. As the incision is made, the two sides of the sinus are grasped with a forceps and the opening closed with a continuous suture.

expose the tumor. In some cases a bridging vein can be freed from the cortex for a few millimeters to give the required exposure without sacrificing the vein. A self-retaining retractor is placed.

The key to the operation is to carry out an extensive internal decompression of the tumor with the Cavitron and gradually draw the capsule into the area of decompression.

Sometimes it is easier to work through the falx from the side of lesser involvement; at other times a bilateral exposure is required. At some point in the operation, depending on the size and configuration of the tumor, the falx is divided well away from the tumor attachment. The inferior sagittal sinus can be occluded. Great care must be taken not to injure the pericallosal and callosomarginal arteries.

Results

In the 23 patients in the series tabulated here who had total removal (21 at the initial operation and 2 after surgery for recurrence) there was no evidence of later recurrence (Table 71-2). At the first operation, two patients with middle third parasagittal tumors had tumor left growing into the wall of the sagittal sinus because angiography showed that the sinus was open. With subsequent recurrence the sinus was occluded by tumor and could be totally removed.

Those patients who had large tumors arising from the middle third of the sagittal sinus and falx frequently had an increase in their neurological deficit in the immediate postoperative period, but this gradually cleared over several weeks to a few months, giving a good to excellent result. However, in three patients with total removal of large tumors, there was a significant postoperative neurological deficit with partial recovery which gave only a fair result.

Two other patients had subtotal removal of middle third lesions because the sinus was still open and the involvement too extensive to resect the wall of the sinus. One is well without evidence of recurrence; the other died in the postoperative period from a myocardial infarction. Two patients with subtotal removal of massive malignant meningiomas had severe neurological deficits that did not improve after surgery, and both have had recurrence of the tumor. One patient did well after the initial operation but died several years later from metastatic hemangiopericytoma.

Cerebral Convexity Meningiomas

Clinical Features

Convexity meningiomas may arise from any point on the dura, but the most common sites of occurrence are in the parasagittal region, along the coronal suture, and at the frontal-temporal junction (anterior sylvian or pterional meningioma). Convexity tumors often become quite large before causing symptoms. Headache is a frequent complaint. The presence of a progressive neurological deficit or focal motor or sensory seizure is associated with tumors over the posterior frontoparietal or temporoparietal region.

Surgical Management

Most of these meningiomas can be removed intact and the patient cured. In positioning the patient for the operation, the scalp overlying the central portion of the tumor is placed at the highest level, if this is possible. Usually a horseshoe-shaped incision is used. A free bone flap is elevated, being careful to preserve the pericranial tissue that will be needed for a graft to replace the dural defect. Hyperostosis or involvement of bone with the tumor is handled as discussed in the general section. After dural pericranial sutures are placed, the dura is opened circumferentially around the tumor, occluding the meningeal arteries as these are encountered. The dura is left attached to the tumor and used to apply gentle traction. The removal of tumor from the brain and the closure are the same as described for parasagittal meningiomas.

A special circumstance occurs when the tumor arises over the frontotemporal junction (Fig. 71-2A). Two points should be emphasized. First, the middle cerebral artery branches may be adherent to the medial capsule, and great care must be exercised in removing this tumor (Fig. 71-2B). Second, some of the dural attachment may extend over the floor of the anterior fossa, sphenoid wing, and floor and anterior wall of the middle fossa. This dura must be removed, sometimes even into the lateral edge of the superior orbital fissure. The dural defect can usually be repaired by sewing the graft directly to the edge of the remaining dura, using a small needle. After the intracranial dura is sewn, the graft can be tented along the bone edge and then the convexity margin of dura closed.

Results

All 51 patients in the series reported here had a total removal of the tumor, with most having good to excellent results (Table 71-2). In some patients with tumors compressing the motor-sensory cortex, there was a temporary neurological deficit with recovery leaving little or no disability. Some patients with preoperative disability did not make a full recovery, and some required long-term anticonvulsant therapy. One patient died of a pulmonary embolus 6 weeks after operation.

One patient had a recurrence after what was thought to be total removal. The first specimen was thought to be an atypical meningioma with six mitoses per ten high-power fields. At the second operation 5 years later, total removal was again done and the tumor was a malignant meningioma. The patient is being followed with CT scans.

Olfactory Groove Meningiomas

Clinical Features

These tumors arise from the midline of the anterior fossa between the crista galli and the tuberculum sellae. They are usually bilateral but may be asymmetric and attain a large size before causing symptoms. The most common presenting symptom is a subtle change in mental function or headache alone or in combination with mental function change, but a disturbance in vision or seizure disorder may also be the initial manifestation. Loss of the sense of smell was recorded as "possibly" the primary symptom in only 3 of 28 patients in Cushing's series, and he questioned the reliability of this finding.[1] Only 1 of the 9 patients in the present series had visual symptoms, and none complained of impairment of the sense of smell.

Surgical Management

In planning the operation, it is important to remember that the blood supply comes into the tumor through the bone in the midline of the anterior fossa from branches of the ethmoidal, middle meningeal, and ophthalmic arteries; the posterior capsules may be attached to the optic nerves, chiasm, and anterior cerebral arteries.

A bifrontal craniotomy for removal of these tumors is

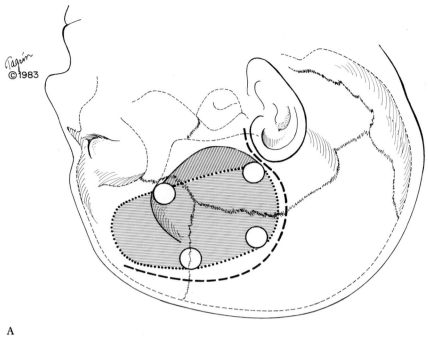

A

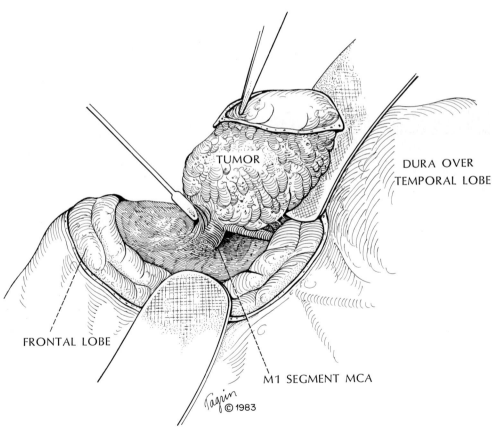

B

Figure 71-2 Anterior sylvian convexity meningioma. *A.* The skin incision (*dashed line*) and free bone flap (*dotted line*) are outlined. The lateral sphenoid wing is removed. *B.* The dura is cut circumferentially and left attached to the tumor to use for traction. Usually the tumor is left intact as it is gradually separated from the surrounding brain tissue. Care must be taken as the medial capsule is dissected, because the middle cerebral artery branches may be attached.

usually preferred. This allows the least amount of traction on the frontal lobes and gives direct access to both sides and the posterior surface of the tumor. MacCarty et al.[10] and Morley[14] also prefer the bifrontal exposure. Kempe[8] described a unilateral right subfrontal approach, and Northfield[16] used a unilateral frontal craniotomy and resected part of the frontal lobe. Logue[9] and Symon[24] use either exposure and also resect part of the frontal lobe.

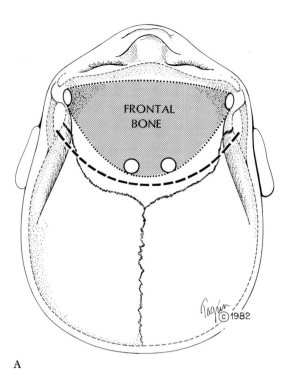

A

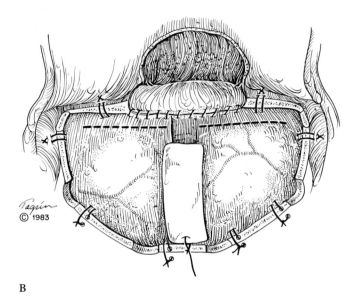

B

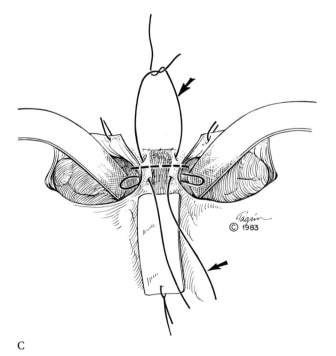

C

Figure 71-3 Olfactory groove meningioma. *A.* The skin incision (*dashed line*) and free bone flap (*dotted line*) are outlined. *B.* The frontal sinuses are almost always entered. The mucosa is removed, the sinuses packed with bacitracin-soaked Gelfoam, and the opening covered with a flap of pericranial tissue. *C.* The anterior sagittal sinus is ligated. *D.* Internal decompression of the tumor has been accomplished. The blood supply coming through the midline of the frontal fossa is being interrupted. *E.* The posterior capsule is being separated from the frontal lobe. The frontal polar artery is often adherent to the tumor and may need to be divided (*arrow*). *F.* The left optic nerve and carotid artery (*arrows*) have been exposed. The tumor is being separated from the arachnoid over the nerve.

The patient is carefully placed in the supine position with the head elevated and slightly extended. Using a coronal incision, the skin flap and underlying tissue, including pericranial tissue, are turned down together. Burr holes are placed just below the end of the anterior temporal line and on each side of the sagittal sinus at the level of the skin incision (Fig. 71-3A). The cut just above the supraorbital ridge is made from each side as far medially as possible. Usually this leaves a centimeter or less of bone in the midline. Because of the irregular bone projecting from the inner table of the skull in this area, it is often not possible to cut completely across the area, but the bone can be broken at this point. The frontal sinuses are almost always entered. The mucosa is removed and the sinuses are packed with bacitracin-soaked Gelfoam. A flap of pericranial tissue from the back of the skin flap is turned down over the sinuses and sewn to the adjacent dura (Fig. 71-3B).

The dural incision is made over each medial inferior frontal lobe just above the edge of the craniotomy opening. While carefully retracting the frontal lobes, the sagittal sinus is divided between two silk sutures and the falx is cut (Fig.

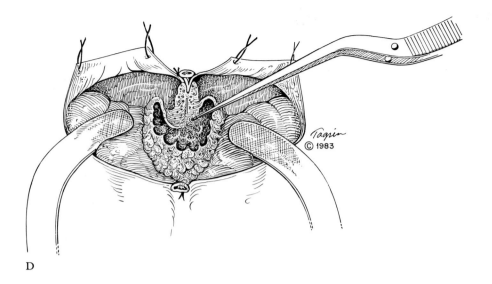

D

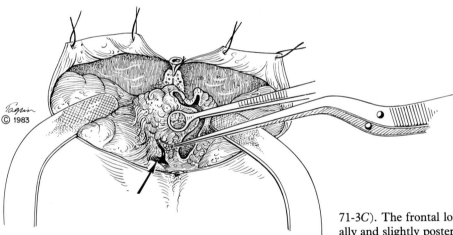

E

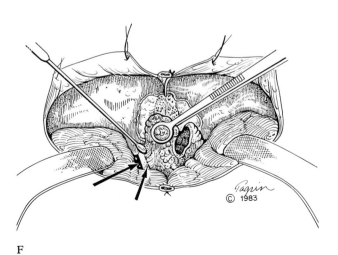

F

71-3C). The frontal lobes are then carefully retracted laterally and slightly posteriorly. The tumor will come into view
in the midline; at times it is found to have grown into the
region of the crista galli and falx. The anterior capsule of the
tumor is exposed, and then an extensive internal decompression is done. The base of the tumor in the midline is
gradually divided, interrupting the blood supply which is
coming in through numerous openings in the bone (Fig.
71-3D). These are occluded with coagulation and bone wax.
The capsule can now be reflected into the area of the decompression without undue pressure on the frontal lobes. Great
care is taken during the dissection of the posterior portion of
the capsule, reflecting it anteriorly and being careful to look
for the pericallosal branch of the anterior cerebral artery
complex, which may be embedded in the tumor. The frontal
polar branch will often be adherent to the tumor and may
need to be divided (Fig. 71-3E). It is usually possible to
follow the capsule back to the sphenoid wing and then,
working medially, to identify the anterior clinoid processes
and the optic nerves (Fig. 71-3F). At times it may be difficult to see the nerves because of the posterior and inferior
compression and the thickened arachnoid. However, under
magnification, the tumor can be reflected off the optic
nerve(s).

Once the bulk of the tumor is removed, the dural attachment is totally excised and any bone hyperostosis removed. The region of the cribriform plate is covered with a graft of pericranial tissue and Gelfoam to prevent a CSF leak.

Results

In this series all nine tumors were totally removed, with restoration of normal mental function and full activity in eight patients (Table 71-2). The postoperative course in one patient was complicated by a subdural hydroma that required a subdural-peritoneal shunt. Another had a postoperative wound infection, and a third had a CSF leak through the ethmoid sinus that required a transethmoidal repair. In the series of MacCarty et al., this type of meningioma patient had the highest long-term survival rate of the major types of meningiomas.[10]

Tuberculum Sellae Meningiomas

Clinical Features

The most common symptom is an asymmetrical visual loss starting with a unilateral decrease in central visual acuity or blurring in the visual field, followed by progression to bilateral involvement. The pattern of visual loss may be acute, gradual, or fluctuating. The onset of headache or a change in a previous headache pattern is seen in two-thirds of these patients.[6]

On examination there is almost always a reduction of visual acuity in at least one eye, and most patients have bilateral field defects. Incongruity and asymmetry of the field defect is the common finding; a symmetrical bitemporal field loss is the exception. Optic atrophy is frequently found and correlates better with the visual acuity loss than with the peripheral field impairment.[6]

Surgical Management

In planning the operation, several important points should be kept in mind:

1. The blood supply usually comes through the tuberculum, and this should be systematically interrupted.
2. Internal decompression of the tumor is essential before trying to dissect the tumor off important visual and arterial structures.
3. When the tumor partially surrounds the A_1 segment of the anterior cerebral artery, it may be possible to remove it by microsurgical techniques.
4. Tumor may grow into the optic foramen and/or involve the dura under the optic nerve.
5. In some patients the internal carotid artery may be located under the medial edge of the nerve just posterior to the optic foramen and be involved with the tumor.
6. The dura over the tuberculum should be removed.
7. The pituitary stalk is behind the tumor and is usually covered by arachnoid.

The operative approach the author prefers in most patients is a right frontotemporal craniotomy with a lateral subfrontal exposure just in front of the sphenoid wing. In many patients at least one olfactory nerve can be saved, and there is minimal trauma to the frontal lobes. Occasionally in large tumors a bifrontal exposure is indicated. A catheter is often placed in the lumbar subarachnoid space to drain cerebrospinal fluid to help reduce brain tension, since drainage from the basal cisterns may not be adequate.

Kempe also approaches tuberculum sellae meningiomas from a right lateral subfrontal exposure.[8] MacCarty et al. use the subfrontal approach but come from the side of greatest visual loss, and they also use a bilateral craniotomy if the tumor is very large.[10] Logue[9] and Symon[24] use a unilateral right subfrontal exposure but approach the tumor along the midline.

The patient is carefully placed in the supine position, with the head elevated, held with the three-point skeletal fixation headrest, and rotated about 60° to the left so that the anterior zygoma is uppermost. An incision is made beginning just above the zygoma a few millimeters anterior to the ear and then, staying behind the hairline, extending medially to end in the midline of the forehead (Fig. 71-4A). The skin, underlying temporalis muscle, and pericranial tissue are turned down together, exposing the inferior lateral frontal and anterior temporal bones.

The most important burr hole is the one placed just below the anterior end of the superior temporal line just behind the zygomatic process of the frontal bone. It is important that this hole be properly placed so that the exposure will be on the floor of the anterior fossa. Two or three other burr holes are placed as shown and the bone flap is cut.

The lateral portion of the sphenoid wing is removed, as is bone over the anterior superior temporal region. The dura is opened over the inferior frontal and anterior temporal regions. Draining veins from the anterior temporal lobe along the sphenoid wing are divided. The frontal lobe is carefully elevated along the sphenoid wing, revealing the posterior part of the olfactory tract. This normally will lead the surgeon to the optic nerve unless there is significant displacement.

The dura anterior to the optic nerve may be reddish and have increased vascularity. Slightly more exposure reveals the anterior clinoid process, the carotid artery, and a varying portion of the right optic nerve, depending on the size of the tumor. In patients with smaller tumors, the arachnoid over the lateral optic nerve and internal carotid artery is opened and CSF is aspirated to give further decompression. In some patients with larger tumors, both the optic nerves and carotid artery may be surrounded by tumor (Fig. 71-4B). The frontal lobe tissue is carefully freed from the surface of the tumor, and self-retaining retractors are placed.

The tumor capsule is opened. Attachments of the tumor along the tuberculum are divided to interrupt the blood supply as it comes into this area. Internal decompression of the tumor is done, using the bipolar coagulator, Cavitron, or laser. The tumor is then carefully reflected from the right optic nerve. A small, straight microdissector has been the most useful instrument in freeing the tumor from the optic and vascular structures (Fig. 71-4C).

When a large tumor projects beneath or surrounds a portion of the right optic nerve, it is usually possible to free the tumor from above and below the nerve, remove it from its loose attachment to the carotid artery, and roll it out from beneath the right optic nerve and carotid artery (Fig. 71-4D).

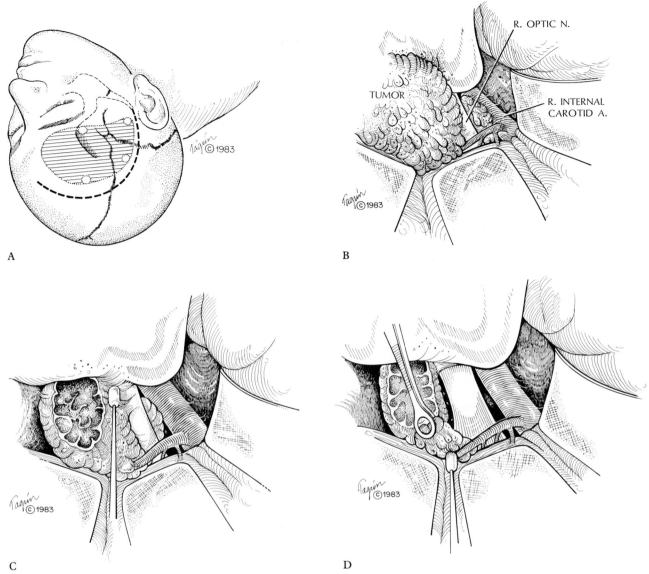

A

B

C

D

Figure 71-4 Tuberculum sellae meningioma. *A*. The skin incision (*dashed line*) and free bone flap (*dotted line*) are outlined. *B*. Tumor surrounds a portion of the right optic nerve and right anterior cerebral artery and displaces the right internal carotid artery. *C*. Internal decompression of the tumor has been accomplished. The attachments to the right optic nerve are being separated. *D*. The tumor surrounding the right anterior cerebral artery is being carefully separated.

In smaller tumors, the left optic nerve may be seen as the anterior capsule is depressed into the area of decompression. In large tumors it is sometimes best to identify the chiasm and the left optic nerve by dissection of the posterior capsule, taking great care to visualize directly any attachment to the anterior cerebral vessels. It is sometimes easier to remove tumor from under the left optic nerve because of direct vision into this area.

The A$_1$ segment of the anterior cerebral artery and the anterior communicating artery complex may be surrounded by tumor. Usually tumor can be removed from these arteries (Fig. 71-4*D*). In some of these patients a small portion of the tumor will need to be left if it is densely adherent. Infre-

quently, some arterial supply to the tumor will come off the A$_1$ or A$_2$ segments of the anterior cerebral artery, and great care must be taken to coagulate and divide this attachment and not avulse it from the artery.

As the tumor is removed from between the optic nerves and in front of the chiasm, arachnoid is encountered which may be thickened. Just beneath this is the pituitary stalk, which may have been displaced by the tumor. This structure can usually be preserved.

After tumor removal has been completed, the dura over the tuberculum and adjacent area is excised. Usually, this is all that is required, but on occasion there may be hyperostosis which needs to be removed with a diamond burr.

Results

Gregorius et al. found that a long history of decreased visual acuity or a severe visual field defect did not preclude postoperative recovery of vision.[6] They noted that improvement occurred most frequently within the first several weeks after operation and that further return of vision did not occur after a year.

The 18 patients in this report often presented a difficult surgical problem because of the extensive growth beneath the optic nerves and posterior to the internal carotid artery and/or the involvement of the anterior cerebral artery complex. Three patients were operated upon for extensive recurrence of tumor who had previously had surgery elsewhere. All had severe involvement of vision which did not improve, and in one the ability to count fingers progressed to no useful vision. One also had evidence of severe frontal lobe impairment which did not improve, and eventually the patient died from the secondary effects of the tumor. One other patient with a massive tumor had both severe visual and frontal lobe dysfunction which did not improve from direct surgery or subsequent placement of a shunt for hydrocephalus. The other 14 patients had good or excellent results. In 10 a total removal was possible, including several in whom tumor was removed from around the anterior cerebral or internal carotid arteries. In the other four patients areas of tumor were left under the optic nerve, around the carotid artery, or on the anterior cerebral artery complex. In 12 of the 14 patients, vision improved. One patient had a temporary worsening in one eye, which recovered to be better than the preoperative status. However, in two the vision was worse in one eye and improved in the other eye.

From the author's experience, it is best to carry out as complete a removal of tumor as possible at the initial operation. The patient should then be carefully followed with CT scans and radiation therapy considered if there is evidence of recurrence.

Sphenoid Wing Meningiomas

It is useful to modify Cushing's classification of these tumors and divide them into three groups because of the different clinical syndromes and operative approaches associated with each.[4,10] These are the hyperostosing meningioma-en-plaque involving the lateral and often a large portion of the sphenoid wing, usually associated with a plaque of tumor on the adjacent dura and in the orbit, and at times associated with a significant intracranial mass. The second group are the globular meningiomas arising from the middle third of the ridge. The final group are the medial, or clinoidal, meningiomas. The globular meningiomas at the pterion are included with the convexity lesions.

Hyperostosing Meningioma-en-Plaque

Clinical Features　There is usually a history of a slowly progressive, painless, unilateral exophthalmos. In some patients there may be a palpable mass in the anterior temporal region. The exophthalmos may be present for many years before there is a change in visual acuity or extraocular movements. Some patients have headache and impairment of sensation in the first or second division of the trigeminal nerve, and in others significant intracranial extension of the tumor may cause a seizure disorder or evidence of impairment of neurological function.

Surgical Management　These tumors are slow-growing, and complete surgical removal is usually not possible by the time the diagnosis is made.[2,19] Surgery is indicated for disfiguring proptosis or decreased visual acuity.

The hyperostosis is due to invasion of bone by meningioma.[2,18] The blood supply is from meningeal branches, but many of these tumors are relatively avascular. The tumor often involves the orbital capsule and the dura around the superior orbital fissure, orbital apex, and cavernous sinus.

The position and the skin incision are essentially the same as are used for tuberculum sellae tumors. If the exposed bone is not involved with tumor, a frontotemporal free bone flap is turned, as illustrated in Fig. 71-4A. If tumor is growing into the bone, the flap is turned around the area.

Using the air drill and appropriate bone instruments, the lateral sphenoid wing is removed and the orbit entered, being careful to keep the orbital capsule intact (Fig. 71-5). Gradually bone is removed to expose both frontal and temporal dura and the orbital fascia. The lateral edge of the superior orbital fissure will be encountered and is marked by a small fold of dura that extends into the orbital fascia. There often is a small arterial vessel at that point. The entire lateral wall and roof of the orbit are removed. If hyperostotic bone extends over the optic canal, this is also removed. The dura is then opened and, if indicated, the intracranial tumor resected and the dura replaced with a graft. In many patients, tumor will be growing into the superior orbital fissure and medial dura and it will not be possible to remove this area. The last step is to open the orbital fascia; if this is done earlier, the orbital fat will be in the way of the intracranial procedure. A localized mass of tumor may involve the orbital capsule. Sometimes this can be removed, but in many patients the lateral rectus muscle and/or orbital apex are involved with tumor, and a judgment will have to be made about the extent of removal. It is not necessary to replace the orbital roof. Pulsations of the eye gradually diminish and usually will not be a bother to the patient.

Results　The experience in this series as well as others indicates that total removal of the tumor is rarely possible.[2,19] Of the 12 patients in this series, none had a total removal. Two had a significant intracranial mass that was removed, and all had en plaque tumor involving the dura along the sphenoid wing and orbital capsule. Four required operation for symptoms due to recurrent tumor several years later. However, all were able to return to normal function, and no death or disability other than the ocular manifestations was due to the tumor or operation. Radiation therapy was not used.

In a report of 21 patients with meningiomas involving the sphenoid ridge, only two of the tumors could be totally removed, and after extensive subtotal removal there was no recurrence within the first 8 years of follow-up.[2] Later recurrence occurred in three of eight who were followed 9 years or more.

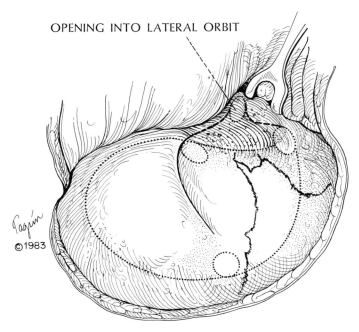

OPENING INTO LATERAL ORBIT

©1983

Figure 71-5 Hyperostosing lateral sphenoid wing meningioma. The bone over the lateral sphenoid wing may be thickened and irregular. In some patients tumor will be growing into the temporal muscle. The bone flap is turned around the involved bone. A separate opening is made through the markedly thickened bone into the lateral orbit.

In some patients improvement of exophthalmos occurs, and in most it is at least stabilized. A more optimistic outlook has been reported following extensive extradural resection of bone and adjacent tumor by Pompili et al.[18] In a series of 30 patients, preoperative exophthalmos regressed completely in 18 and partially in 9. Among 22 patients with bone involvement of the lateral or middle ridge and orbit, there were 13 complete removals with full recovery and 6 subtotal removals with improvement; 3 patients had recurrence of tumor or a permanent deficit due to postoperative complications.

Middle Third Meningiomas

These tumors arise from the edge of the ridge and grow in a globular fashion, compressing the frontal and temporal lobes. In this series one patient presented with increased intracranial pressure, one with headache, and one with a seizure. The approach is the same as described for tuberculum sellae and medial sphenoid wing tumors. If the attachment of the tumor can be divided, most of the blood supply will be interrupted. All three patients had total removal with no neurological complications.

Medial (Clinoidal) Meningiomas

Clinical Features In the series of patients previously reported, the tumors can be divided into two general categories.[17] In one category, the tumor is predominantly a mass arising from the medial sphenoid wing, involving the carotid and middle cerebral arteries to varying degrees, and compressing the optic nerves, optic tract, and/or adjacent frontal and temporal lobes (Fig. 71-6A). These patients usually present with evidence of compression of the optic nerve, but a seizure disorder or progressive hemiparesis may also be the presenting symptom. On the angiogram it is important to look for encasement of the internal carotid and mid-

dle cerebral arteries, which is indicated by segmental narrowing or irregularity of the vessel.

In the second category are those patients in whom the tumor grows diffusely in the region of the anterior clinoid, cavernous sinus, and adjacent medial sphenoid wing, often without a significant intracranial mass (Fig. 71-6B). These patients may present with evidence of optic nerve involvement, third nerve palsy, and/or sensory loss in the first division of the trigeminal nerve. There may be proptosis due to venous congestion, tumor in the orbit, or hyperostosis.

Surgical Management Great care must be taken in the approach to these lesions, since the carotid and middle cerebral arteries may be embedded in the tumor. Usually only a subtotal removal is possible because of the growth of the tumor around these arteries and into the base of the skull.

The operative approach is similar to the frontotemporal exposure outlined in the section on tuberculum sellae meningiomas, with more temporal exposure and with the side being determined by the site of the tumor. A similar subfrontal approach is used by Kempe[8] and by MacCarty et al.[10] Logue[9] does an elective resection of the lateral inferior frontal lobe, and Morley[14] may resect the temporal lobe tip.

After the initial exposure, it may be necessary to open the medial aspect of the sylvian fissure. Internal decompression of the tumor is carried out, and the blood supply along the sphenoid wing, often a hypertrophied branch of the middle meningeal artery, is divided. As the dissection progresses on the lateral aspect of the tumor, it is important to look for the middle cerebral artery branches and to follow these medially to determine whether they or the internal carotid artery are involved with tumor.

When the tumor grows into the optic foramen or involves the bone around the foramen and superior orbital fissure, the dura over this area is excised and the bone is removed under the operating microscope, using an air drill with a diamond burr and then fine curettes.

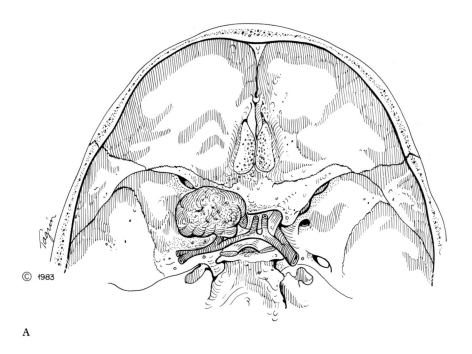

A

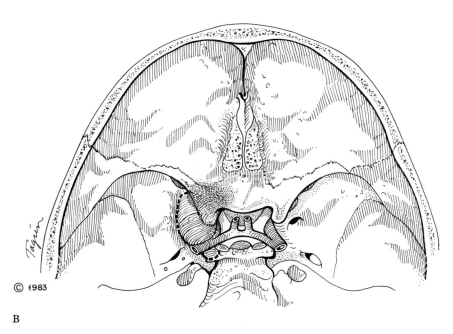

B

Figure 71-6 Medial sphenoid wing meningioma. *A*. Some tumors grow as a mass, involve the optic nerve and carotid and middle cerebral arteries, and compress the frontal and temporal lobes. *B*. Other tumors grow as a plaque involving the anterior clinoid and medial middle fossa, affecting structures within the cavernous sinus.

Results In none of the 16 patients in the series reported here was it possible to be absolutely sure that a total removal had been done (Table 71-2). Ten were able to resume normal activity. Four were improved but had some limitations from residual neurological deficits present prior to surgery. One with a severe preoperative deficit did not improve and subsequently died from the effects of the tumor. In one patient, hemorrhage occurred 5 days postoperatively from a middle cerebral artery branch in the residual tumor capsule, and the patient was left with a serious disability. Improvement in visual function with optic nerve decompression was the exception.

Three patients required reoperation for recurrence of a significant intracranial mass. One of these and two other patients who did not have surgery for recurrence received radiation therapy with arrest of growth of the tumor.

Cerebellopontine Angle Meningiomas

Clinical Features

The most common presenting symptoms are hearing loss, vertigo or imbalance, and tinnitus, typical for any tumor arising in the cerebellopontine angle (CPA).[26] Other symptoms depend on the size of the tumor and the area of dura over the petrous pyramid from which the tumor arises; they include numbness or tingling of the face, facial pain, headache, and difficulty swallowing. Occasionally there are symptoms of hydrocephalus. Examination confirms the cranial nerve deficits and frequently shows ataxic gait.

Unfortunately, many CPA meningiomas reach a significant size before diagnosis. These lesions present a formidable challenge to the neurosurgeon. It is important that all patients have a high-resolution contrast CT scan if they present with a progressive sensorineural hearing loss, symptoms of fifth nerve dysfunction, or other symptoms or signs which raise the slightest suspicion of a CPA lesion. If this study is negative and clinical findings or the brain stem auditory evoked responses suggest a tumor, an air cisternogram with CT is indicated if the patient is under 60 years of age.

Surgical Management

These tumors arise from the dura over the petrous bone. It is useful to divide them into those tumors originating anterior and those originating posterior to the internal auditory meatus (IAM). In this series of 30 patients, 26 tumors were primarily in the CPA, 1 involved the petrous bone, and 3 were in the CPA and middle fossa. Five of the 26 tumors arose posterior to the IAM, compressing the seventh or eighth nerve anteriorly or inferiorly and the cerebellum medially and often extended into the anterior edge of the meatus. In those patients with tumors arising anterior to the IAM, the surgeon is confronted with the seventh and eighth nerves bowed around the posterior inferior surface of tumor, the fifth nerve anterior or superior, and the brain stem compressed medially. Any one of these nerves, as well as the sixth nerve and the anterior inferior cerebellar artery, may be encased in tumor.

Prior to operation it is important to perform angiography that includes selective injection of the vertebral and the external and internal carotid arteries. This will not only define the major arterial supply but will also indicate whether it would be useful to consider preoperative external carotid embolization.

Early in this series the operations were performed with the patient in the semisitting position. A modified supine position is now used. (Fig. 71-7A). This approach has worked well from the standpoint of visualization of important anatomical structures, tumor removal, comfort of the operator and avoidance of any problem with air embolism.

The operating table is turned around so that the surgeon can comfortably sit with the feet under the table. The patient's ipsilateral shoulder is slightly elevated. If there is cervical spondylosis or limitation of neck motion, a lateral position is used. The head is turned parallel to the floor, elevated, and held with the three-point skeletal-fixation headrest. During the operation the line of sight to the brain stem may be altered by rotating the table from side to side.

A vertical incision is centered 1 cm medial to the mastoid process (Fig. 71-7B). A pericranial tissue graft is taken from the bone over the occipital region to be used in closing the dura at the end of the operation. The craniectomy exposes the lateral two-thirds of the dura over the cerebellar hemisphere and is carried over the edge of the transverse sinus

above the sigmoid sinus laterally. If a small opening is made into the mastoid air cells, it is occluded with bone wax, but a large opening is filled with an adipose tissue graft taken from the abdomen.

The dura is opened vertically, usually about 2 cm from the lateral edge of the exposure. The medial dura is kept intact. The lateral dura is cut so that superior, lateral, and inferior dural flaps allow exposure to the edge of the venous sinuses (Fig. 71-7C). The cerebellum is carefully elevated. The arachnoid below and posterior to the ninth, tenth, and eleventh nerves is opened and CSF is allowed to drain (Fig. 71-7D). This will usually relieve whatever tension remains in the cerebellum. In some patients with a large tumor some of the lateral cerebellar hemisphere will need to be resected.

Once the cerebellum is slack, exploration in the CPA will reveal the tumor adherent to the petrous bone. The arachnoid is opened and the cerebellum reflected from the capsule. Stimulation will either confirm the presence of the seventh nerve or locate it if it is not seen.

For tumors arising posterior to the IAM, the seventh and eighth nerves will not be identified initially. The posterior capsule is opened, and gradually the attachment to the petrous bone is divided, using bipolar coagulation to interrupt the blood supply. Internal decompression is carried out with the Cavitron, laser, and/or bipolar coagulator. The capsule is then gradually reflected from the surrounding gliotic cerebellum. As the anterior capsule is reached, the seventh and eighth nerves are identified and separated, using microsurgical techniques. In large tumors the lower cranial nerves may also need to be separated from the capsule. Once the tumor mass is removed, the dural attachment is completely excised. This may require going into or removing a portion of the posterior wall of the IAM.

The tumor arising anterior to the IAM may present a difficult problem (Fig. 71-7E). After the posterior capsule is exposed and self-retaining retractors placed, the lower cranial nerves are visualized and, if possible, carefully separated from the capsule and covered with a small rubber dam for protection. The seventh and eighth nerves will be displaced posteriorly and slightly inferiorly, and the surgeon will need to work around these during the tumor removal. In some patients, tumor grows within the fibers of these nerves. Internal decompression, as described above, is followed by meticulous microsurgical dissection of the capsule. There may be marked adherence to the brain stem. The dural attachment is removed if possible. Some of the attachment may involve the petrosal sinus. In some patients, especially those with large tumors, it will be better to leave some tumor attached to these important structures.

After tumor removal is completed, no attempt is made to suture the original dural opening. Instead, a graft of pericranial tissue is used for this closure.

Results

In this series of 30 patients the results were directly related to the size of the tumor (Table 71-2). In tumors 3 cm or smaller (12 patients) it was usually possible to do a total removal with good to excellent results. The most common disability was reduced or absent hearing, but one patient had difficulty swallowing. Usually facial nerve function can be preserved.

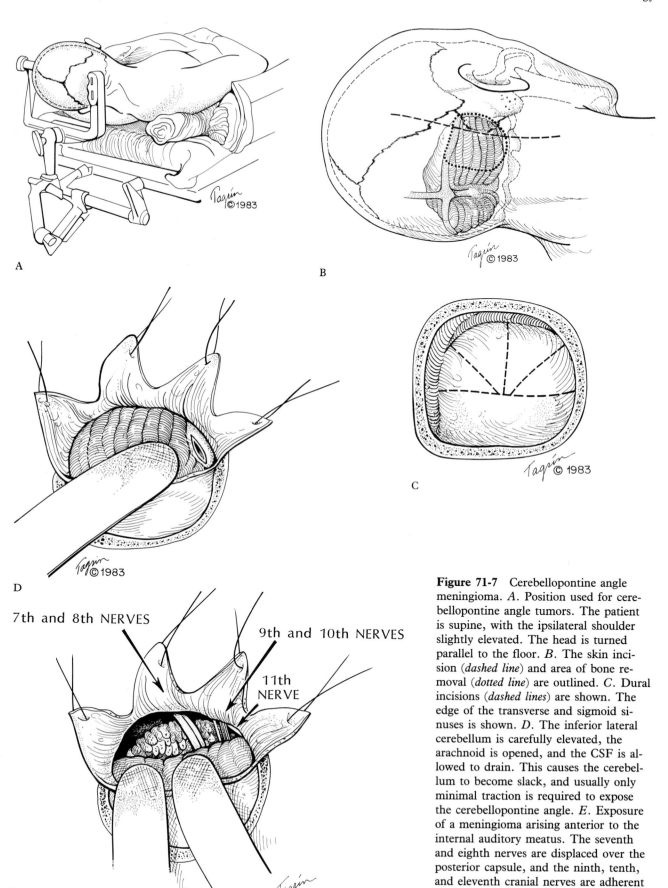

A

B

C

D

7th and 8th NERVES

9th and 10th NERVES

11th NERVE

E

Figure 71-7 Cerebellopontine angle meningioma. *A.* Position used for cerebellopontine angle tumors. The patient is supine, with the ipsilateral shoulder slightly elevated. The head is turned parallel to the floor. *B.* The skin incision (*dashed line*) and area of bone removal (*dotted line*) are outlined. *C.* Dural incisions (*dashed lines*) are shown. The edge of the transverse and sigmoid sinuses is shown. *D.* The inferior lateral cerebellum is carefully elevated, the arachnoid is opened, and the CSF is allowed to drain. This causes the cerebellum to become slack, and usually only minimal traction is required to expose the cerebellopontine angle. *E.* Exposure of a meningioma arising anterior to the internal auditory meatus. The seventh and eighth nerves are displaced over the posterior capsule, and the ninth, tenth, and eleventh cranial nerves are adherent inferiorly.

In patients with large tumors (18 patients) it was usually possible to do only a subtotal removal because of involvement of important structures. Eight patients had a good or excellent outcome; three had a fair and three a poor result. There were a number of serious complications causing the fair or poor results. In one patient the sixth, seventh, and eighth nerves were surrounded by tumor, and postoperative deficits were noted plus a significant ataxia. Three patients did well for several years after a subtotal removal, but with recurrence and reoperation for recurrence, severe impairment of swallowing and other neurological deficits were present which eventually led to one patient's death, after an attempt to remove tumor tissue growing within the fibers of the lower cranial nerves. Three patients required a shunt for hydrocephalus, one had treatment of CSF rhinorrhea by mastoid obliteration with adipose tissue graft, and one had treatment of a wound infection.

When there is facial paralysis, a lateral tarsorrhaphy may be needed to protect the cornea. This should be done as soon as possible, especially if there is loss of fifth nerve function as well. One of the most serious complications is damage to the lower cranial nerves, causing inability to swallow and handle secretions. Recovery from this disability is slow, and a feeding gastrostomy and at times a tracheostomy may be necessary until function improves.

One patient had diffuse involvement of the petrous bone and a plaque of tumor in the dura. She was treated with radiation therapy and has remained stable. Three patients had large tumors involving both the middle fossa and CPA. One is stable after subtotal removal and radiation therapy, but two are only fair, being worse after extensive surgery. One required a shunt and one an operation for recurrence.

In the series of 30 patients reported by Yasargil et al., 19 were free of neurological deficits postoperatively; 9 others were fully employable, and all had total removal.[26]

Cerebellar Convexity Meningiomas

Clinical Features

These tumors typically arise near the junction of the sigmoid, transverse, and petrosal sinuses and involve the petrous and posterior fossa dura and at times the tentorium. Occasionally they come directly off the posterior fossa dura. Frequently they attain a large size before causing symptoms. Usually the patient presents with headache and signs of hydrocephalus or a progressive cerebellar deficit. Occasionally there is a CPA clinical syndrome.

In this series two patients presented with headache, two with a normal pressure hydrocephalus syndrome, one with signs of posterior fossa compression, and one with diplopia. It is important to know from angiography the status of both the right and left transverse and sigmoid sinuses.

Surgical Management

The approach is that for a CPA meningioma and the principles of tumor removal are those for a cerebral convexity meningioma, with internal decompression and careful separation from surrounding cerebellum. The cranial nerves are usually covered by compressed cerebellum.

The major problem is the attachment of the tumor to the region of the sinuses. In some patients the dura, tentorium, and transverse sinus may need to be removed.

Results

In this series of six patients, all had good or excellent results (Table 71-2). All the tumors were large and arose from the junction of the sinuses.

Tentorial Meningiomas

Clinical Features

Meningiomas arising from the tentorium may cause primary cerebral or cerebellar symptoms or both. When the growth is supratentorial, the most common manifestation is a seizure. Infratentorial growth causes evidence of cerebellar dysfunction or hydrocephalus.

Surgical Management

These tumors may occur at any site on the tentorium. Those along the medial tentorial edge receive their main blood supply from the tentorial branch of the internal carotid artery (artery of Bernasconi and Cassinari). For these medial tumors a subtemporal craniotomy is used.[8] During temporal lobe retraction, the vein of Labbé is preserved if at all possible. After the tumor is exposed, self-retaining retractors are placed on the temporal lobe. If the tumor is large, intracapsular decompression is performed. Usually the tentorium can be opened lateral to the tumor and then a cut made around the tumor toward the anterior tentorial edge to divide the blood supply. Care is taken to avoid injury to the fourth nerve and superior cerebellar artery.

In posterior and lateral tentorial meningiomas, the position used for the operation is the same as described for CPA tumors. A paramedian incision is used. A bone flap is turned over the inferior occipital region and crosses the transverse sinus (Fig. 71-8). A suboccipital craniectomy is performed if posterior fossa exposure will be needed. The dura is opened just above and parallel to the lateral sinus. The occipital lobe is carefully elevated. If the tumor does not involve the sinuses, it is carefully freed from the occipital lobe and an incision made in the tentorium. A circumferential cut is made around the tumor, separating it from the underlying cerebellum. Some tumors present primarily below the tentorium, and in these patients a posterior exploration is done first and the tumor decompressed. When the tumor involves the transverse sinus, complete excision of the sinus may be possible if the opposite sinus is open.

Results

Total removal was done in six of eight patients, including two with involvement of the transverse sinus. All had excellent or good results. One patient had a tumor involving the medial tentorium and tentorial edge with a large middle fossa extension. A small ribbon of tumor was left adherent to the brain stem and the superior cerebellar and posterior cerebral arteries. One patient had a tumor arising in the midline

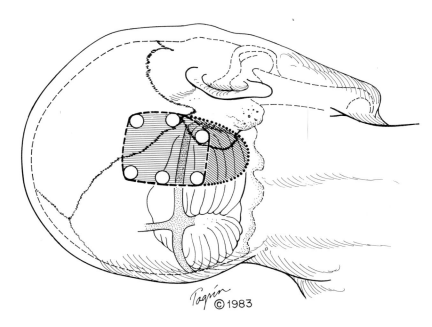

© 1983

Figure 71-8 Tentorial meningioma. The position for the patient is the same as described for cerebellopontine angle meningioma. The skin incision and bone flap depend on the location and size of the tumor. A free bone flap (*dashed line*) and craniectomy (*dotted line*) are outlined for removal of a lateral tentorial tumor.

within the leaves of the medial tentorium and falx, compressing the midbrain, causing hydrocephalus, and obliterating the normal venous anatomy. The patient presented with headache, and the CT scan showed hydrocephalus. A shunt was placed and subtotal removal done.

Clivus Meningiomas

Clinical Features

The most common initial symptoms are facial numbness or paresthesias, decreased hearing, and headache (26). Other initial manifestations have included gait disturbance, third and sixth nerve palsies, vertigo or imbalance and temporal lobe seizures. Frequently, examination reveals a reduced corneal reflex and decreased facial sensation. Decreased hearing and gait and limb ataxia may also be present. In large tumors there are signs of pyramidal tract compression.

Surgical Management

Removal of a clivus meningioma is technically feasible but carries a significant risk, and total removal may not be possible or indicated. Important blood supply to the midbrain and brain stem is often involved by the tumor; the third, fourth, and sixth nerves may be encased; and the tumor capsule may be adherent to the upper brain stem.[8,26] Yasargil has described his approaches in detail;[26] he used a suboccipital, temporal, or frontolateral-temporal exposure, depending on the direction of tumor growth.

The author generally uses a right temporal craniotomy unless there is a predominant left side extension, with provision for a paramedian suboccipital extension from the posterior limb of the incision. The temporal lobe is elevated, keeping as many draining veins intact as possible. The tumor is exposed and the medial tentorium opened, with care to stay behind the entrance of the fourth nerve into the dura. Internal decompression of the tumor is carried out.

Results

Yasargil et al. have reported the results from operation on 20 patients using microsurgical techniques.[26] There were 13 subtotal and 7 total removals. Results were good (fully employable) in 11, fair in 5, and poor in 2; 2 patients died. Only one patient was free of neurological deficits. There were a number of serious postoperative complications and new permanent neurological deficits.

In the series reported here, three patients were treated with subtotal removal. One is well but required a shunt; one is working but has a sixth nerve palsy from injury to this nerve, which was surrounded by tumor; and one has a moderate postoperative disability after an attempt to dissect the tumor from the brain stem.

Intraventricular Meningiomas

Clinical Features

These tumors most commonly are located in the trigone of the lateral ventricle but may be found in the third or rarely the fourth ventricle.[19] There is no diagnostic syndrome for the lateral ventricle meningioma.[5,10] The symptoms are often vague, with headache, mental change, and visual complaints the most frequent. Occasionally there may be a spontaneous hemorrhage.

Surgical Management

The patient is positioned for a temporal craniotomy. The cortical incision is made in the middle temporal gyrus (Fig. 71-9).[8] In the dominant hemisphere it is especially important that damage to the posterior superior temporal gyrus be avoided. This approach allows access to the tumor with the least chance of brain damage. In most patients the blood supply is from the choroidal arteries. The anterior choroidal supply can be picked up, and after internal decompression, the medial vessel can be divided.

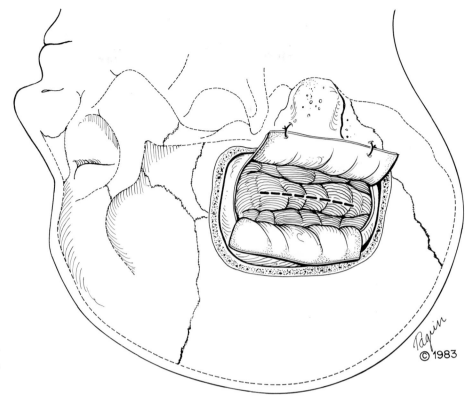

Figure 71-9 Intraventricular meningioma. Cortical incision in the middle temporal gyrus is used to remove a meningioma from the trigone of the right lateral ventricle. The same incision (on the left) may be used for a dominant hemisphere tumor.

MacCarty et al. prefer a posterior parietal approach just above the lambdoidal suture.[10] Fornari et al. use a sagittal paramedian parieto-occipital incision.[5] The advantages and disadvantages of the approaches that have been used for intraventricular tumors are nicely summarized by Spencer and Collins.[22]

Results

One patient made a normal recovery. The other had a significant preoperative disability which did not fully improve, leaving a fair result.

Foramen Magnum Meningiomas

Clinical Features

The earliest symptoms are cervical pain, neck stiffness, and dysesthesias of the hands and fingers followed by clumsiness in the hands.[27] Asymmetrical quadriparesis may develop, with the greatest involvement in the ipsilateral arm. The spinal accessory nerve may be affected, but other cranial nerve abnormalities are rare.

Surgical Management

The tumor usually arises from the anterolateral dura above the entrance of the vertebral artery. The posterior inferior cerebellar artery and spinal accessory nerve overlie the tumor. The ninth and tenth nerves are against the superior capsule, and the dura around the exit of the hypoglossal nerve may be involved.

The prone position is used with a midline skin incision, laminectomy of C1 and C2, and craniectomy over the inferior posterior fossa. The dura is opened laterally on the side of the lesion. The medulla is displaced toward the opposite side and posteriorly and is left covered by dura. In order to safely remove the tumor, internal decompression is required, with careful dissection from the structures noted above. The dural attachment is removed.

Results

The three patients in this series all had a good to excellent result after total removal.

Meningiomas at Other Sites

Meningiomas of the optic sheath are discussed in another chapter. Reports of meningiomas of the pineal region, arising from the velum interposition without dural attachment, have been summarized by Yasargil et al.[19] Other meningiomas without dural attachment were reported by Cushing.[4] There was one in the series reported here, located in the medial anterior frontal lobe.

Rarely, tumors arise from the orbital roof, away from the sphenoid wing, and project into the anterior fossa. Cushing knew of only one such patient.[4] There was one in this series.

Meningiomas may arise from the floor of the middle fossa. Of the two patients in this series, one presented with a seizure disorder and the other with increased intracranial pressure. When the tumor involves the gasserian ganglion, trigeminal neuralgia may be the presenting symptom.[15]

Multiple meningiomas may occur in association with neurofibromatosis but may also be found without any other manifestation of that disease.

References

1. Bonnal J, Brotchi J: Surgery of the superior sagittal sinus in parasagittal meningiomas. J Neurosurg 48: 935–945, 1978.
2. Bonnal J, Thibaut A, Brotchi J, Born J: Invading meningiomas of the sphenoid ridge. J Neurosurg 53:587–599, 1980.
3. Carella RJ, Ransohoff J, Newall J: Role of radiation therapy in the management of meningiomas. Neurosurgery 10:332–339, 1982.
4. Cushing H, Eisenhardt L: *Meningiomas: Their Classification, Regional Behaviour, Life History and Surgical End Results.* Springfield, Ill., Charles C Thomas, 1938.
5. Fornari M, Savoiardo M, Morello G, Solero CL: Meningiomas of the lateral ventricles: Neuroradiological and surgical considerations in 18 cases. J Neurosurg 54:64–74, 1981.
6. Gregorius FK, Hepler RS, Stern WE: Loss and recovery of vision with suprasellar meningiomas. J Neurosurg 42:69–75, 1975.
7. Karasick JL, Mullen S: A survey of metastatic meningiomas. J Neurosurg 40:206–212, 1974.
8. Kempe LG: *Operative Neurosurgery:* vol. 1, *Cranial, Cerebral, and Intracranial Vascular Disease.* New York, Springer, 1968.
9. Logue V: Surgery of meningiomas, in Symon L (ed): *Operative Surgery: Neurosurgery.* London, Butterworth, 1979, pp 128–173.
10. MacCarty CS, Piepgras DG, Ebersold MJ: Meningeal tumors of the brain, in Youmans JR (ed): *Neurological Surgery: A Comprehensive Reference Guide to the Diagnosis and Management of Neurosurgical Problems,* 2d ed. Philadelphia, Saunders, 1982, pp 2936–2966.
11. Martuza RL, MacLaughlin DT, Ojemann RG: Specific estradiol binding in schwannomas, meningiomas, and neurofibromas. Neurosurgery 9:665–671, 1981.
12. Maxwell RE, Chou SN: Preoperative evaluation and management of meningiomas, in Schmidek HH, Sweet WH (eds): *Operative Neurosurgical Techniques: Indications, Methods, and Results.* New York, Grune & Stratton, 1982, pp 481–489.
13. Maxwell RE, Chou SN: Parasagittal and falx meningiomas, in Schmidek HH, Sweet WH (eds): *Operative Neurosurgical Techniques: Indications, Methods, and Results.* New York, Grune & Stratton, 1982, pp 503–515.
14. Morley TP: Tumors of the cranial meninges, in Youmans JR (ed): *Neurological Surgery: A Comprehensive Reference Guide to the Diagnosis and Management of Neurosurgical Problems,* 1st ed. Philadelphia, Saunders, 1973, pp 1388–1411.
15. Nijensohn DE, Araujo JC, MacCarty CS: Meningiomas of Meckel's cave. J Neurosurg 43:197–202, 1975.
16. Northfield DWC: The meningiomas: Hemangioblastoma, in *The Surgery of the Central Nervous System: A Textbook for Postgraduate Students.* Oxford, Blackwell Scientific Publications, 1973, pp 229–262.
17. Ojemann RG: Meningiomas of the basal parapituitary region: Technical considerations. Clin Neurosurg 27:233–262, 1980.
18. Pompili A, Derome PJ, Visot A, Guiot G: Hyperostosing meningiomas of the sphenoid ridge—clinical features, surgical therapy, and long-term observations: Review of 49 cases. Surg Neurol 17:411–416, 1982.
19. Quest DO: Meningiomas: An update. Neurosurgery 3:219–225, 1978.
20. Rozario R, Adelman L, Prager RJ, Stein BM: Meningiomas of the pineal region and third ventricle. Neurosurgery 5:489–495, 1979.
21. Simpson D: The recurrence of intracranial meningiomas after surgical treatment. J Neurol Neurosurg Psychiatry 20:22–39, 1957.
22. Spencer DD, Collins WF: Surgical management of lateral intraventricular tumors, in Schmidek HH, Sweet WH (eds): *Operative Neurosurgical Techniques: Indications, Methods, and Results.* New York, Grune & Stratton, 1982, pp 561–574.
23. Strait TA, Robertson JH, Clark WC: Use of the carbon dioxide laser in the operative management of intracranial meningiomas: A report of twenty cases. Neurosurgery 10:464–467, 1982.
24. Symon L: Olfactory groove and suprasellar meningiomas, in Krayenbühl H (ed): *Advances and Technical Standards in Neurosurgery,* vol 4. Vienna, Springer-Verlag, 1977, pp 67–91.
25. Wara WM, Sheline GE, Newman H, Townsend JJ, Boldrey EB: Radiation therapy of meningiomas. AJR 123:453–458, 1972.
26. Yasargil MG, Mortara RW, Curcic M: Meningiomas of basal posterior cranial fossa, in Krayenbühl H (ed): *Advances and Technical Standards in Neurosurgery,* vol 7. Vienna, Springer-Verlag, 1980, pp 3–115.
27. Yasuoka S, Okazaki H, Daube JR, MacCarty CS: Foramen magnum tumors: Analysis of 57 cases of benign extramedullary tumors. J Neurosurg 49:828–838, 1978.

SECTION E

Epidermoid and Dermoid Tumors

72

Epidermoid and Dermoid Tumors: Pathology

Jere W. Baxter
Martin G. Netsky

Epidermoid and dermoid tumors are uncommon lesions making up roughly 1 percent of all intracranial neoplasms. Epidermoids are about 10 times more frequent than dermoids. These masses most often are not clinically manifest at birth. They are easily recognizable both grossly and microscopically. Histologically, epidermoid tumors are composed only of dermal epithelium and associated connective tissue. Dermoid tumors, in addition, contain dermal appendages such as hair follicles, sweat glands, and sebaceous glands.

The medical literature concerning these tumors consists largely of isolated case reports. Reviews of large series and accounts of advances in knowledge are sparse. Most of these tumors are derived from developmental ectodermal inclusions, a result of imperfect embryogenesis. The pathogenesis of so-called cholesteatomas of the middle ear, however, is still debated; these lesions may be the result of two or more mechanisms discussed later in this chapter. Epidermoids and dermoids are similar in appearance, derivation, pathogenesis, and clinical outcome and may therefore be considered as one entity. The difference in histological appearance is the usual basis of separation, but they may also be considered as separate types because of differences in age of clinical onset, rate of progression, preferential location, and frequency of associated lesions.

Epidermoid tumors occur at all ages, but the peak onset is in the fifth decade. Dermoid tumors more often are found in younger patients in the first and second decades. Epidermoids grow more slowly, mainly by desquamation of epithelial cells and by accumulation of cellular debris. Dermoids enlarge by glandular, largely sebaceous, secretions as well as by desquamation. Epidermoids occur more often in men, although women are said to predominate in some series. Dermoids lack sex predilection.

Sites of preference of epidermoids include the diploe of the skull, pons and cerebellopontine angle, ventricular system (lateral, third and fourth), optic chiasm, parapituitary region, and collicular plate. In the spinal canal, both types occur least often in cervical segments. They increase in frequency in the thoracic region and occur most often in the lumbosacral regions. The reason for spinal caudal predominance is that the lowest part of the spinal cord has a cutaneous attachment in early fetal life.[17] The rise in position of the spinal cord relative to the site of attachment creates a path of potential epithelial inclusions added to the usual mechanism of midline folding. Epidermoids produced by repeated lumbar punctures have caused tumors in the lumbar region. Dermoids, although much less frequent, may occur in any of the various locations but are found most often in the cerebellar midline, the cauda equina, and the scalp, orbit, and paranasal region.

Epidermoids usually occur without associated anomalies or with minimal dimpling of the skin. Dermoids more often are associated with dermal sinuses, tufts of external hair, and focal skin pigmentation, and in the spinal cord, with malformations such as spina bifida.

Histology of Skin and Dermal Appendages

Epidermoid and *dermoid* are terms meaning "skinlike." Both epidermoid and dermoid masses contain structures found in normal skin. The squamous epithelium lining these tumors resembles the keratinizing epidermis of skin. Pilosebaceous units and sweat glands of normal skin also occur in dermoids. The fibrous capsule of both types of tumor is dermal connective tissue.

The squamous epithelium of the skin has four cell layers: the stratum basalis, stratum spinosum, stratum granulosum, and stratum corneum. The basal layer is a single layer of cuboidal germinative cells giving rise to the other strata. Intercellular bridges (prickles, or spines) characterize the multilayered cells of the stratum spinosum. The stratum granulosum is a superficial thin layer of cells with coarse keratohyaline granules in the cytoplasm. The stratum corneum is composed of living and dead flattened cells forming layers of keratin.

Pilosebaceous units, sweat ducts, and sweat glands are the dermal appendages. The proximal deep portions lie in the dermis. The distal parts of hair follicles and glandular ducts traverse the epidermis.

Appearance of Epidermoid and Dermoid Tumors

Solitary lesions, when, rarely, they are removed intact, have a smooth, round, multilobulated external surface. The tumors are almost never multiple. Gross and microscopic recognition of the lesions is generally uncomplicated, even when the surgical specimen consists of multiple fragments of cyst contents and wall. A pearly sheen is characteristic of the external appearance of many epidermoids and dermoids.

A stratified squamous epithelial lining resembling skin is the diagnostic histological finding (Fig. 72-1). This lining produces keratinized squamous cells that accumulate centrally, contributing to the volume of the tumor (Fig. 72-1). As in stratified squamous epithelia elsewhere, the single basal layer of germinative cells gives rise to the other strata. The epithelial cells rest on a basement membrane anchored in a capsule of fibrous connective tissue. Granular and cornified layers are absent in mucosal epithelia, such as those giving rise to craniopharyngioma (see below).

Epidermoids contain solid, cheesy, dry material because of accumulated kerantinized epidermal debris and the absence of sebaceous and sweat gland secretions.

Pilosebaceous units in the cyst wall and frequently hair in the cyst characterize dermoids; adipose tissue and sweat glands may also be present. Dermoids may then be recognized by the presence of sebaceous material and hair in addition to keratinized debris (Fig. 72-2). The contents are fluid and resemble soft butter.[31] Teeth are rarely encountered.

Pathogenesis and Embryology

Epidermoids and dermoids may be formed by congenital, iatrogenic, or inflammatory mechanisms.

Congenital: Epithelial Misplacement during Embryonic Development

During the third to fourth week of embryonic life, the neural plate invaginates in the dorsal midline to form the neural groove and folds.[21] The neural folds approach the midline, then fuse to form the neural tube, which then separates from the overlying ectoderm. Ectopic epithelium may be deposited at sites between the neural canal and skin when the sequence of development is imperfect. The concept of mis-

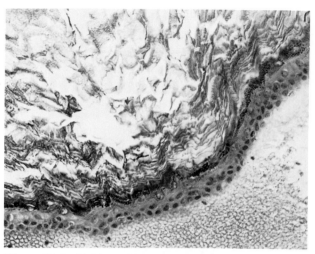

Figure 72-1 Epidermoid tumor. The wall of the cyst contains many layers of accumulated keratin. The stratum corneum and stratum granulosum lie above the thin stratum spinosum. The basal cell layer is moderately disrupted. Hematoxylin-eosin, ×250. (From Toglia et al.[30])

placed epithelium is supported by the identification of epithelial rests in tracts leading to deeply placed lesions. Secondary vesicles formed in development (e.g., otic and optic) may also result in epithelial misplacements, accounting for laterally placed, squamous-lined cysts.[8] The early attach-

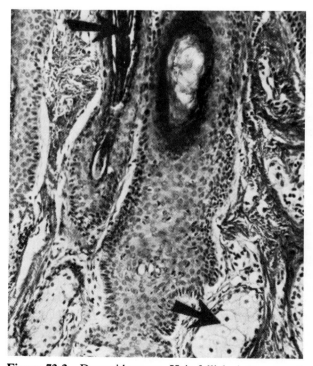

Figure 72-2 Dermoid tumor. Hair follicle (*upper arrow*) and sebaceous glands (*lower arrow*) are present in addition to the dermal epithelium. Hematoxylin-eosin, ×110. (From Toglia et al.[30])

ment of spinal cord to skin and the subsequent upward migration of the cord have already been considered.

This theory explains the frequency of midline lesions, the association of intraspinal tumors with spinal anomalies and dermal sinus tracts, the common occurrence of laterally situated tumors in the cerebellopontine angle and lateral orbit, and the frequence of lesions in the cauda equina. It also suggests these biological correlates: misplaced epithelium alone or epithelium and mesenchyme not yet containing organizer substances, hence early in development, results in a simple squamous-lined cyst (epidermoid); misplaced epithelium and adjacent mesenchyme later in fetal life contains organizer substances and results in a squamous-lined cyst with skin appendages (dermoid). Epidermoids probably form earlier in development, since they lack the organizers.[30]

Iatrogenic: The Physician as a Cause of Epidermoids

Intraspinal epidermoids may be caused by physicians, most often in connection with multiple lumbar punctures for intrathecal administration of drugs.[7] Single lumbar punctures rarely produce epidermoids.[28] Suturing of skin to form a pocket may also result in an epidermoid.[30]

Inflammatory Response: Epidermoids of the Middle Ear

The pathogenesis of so-called cholesteatomas of the middle ear is currently debated, as indicated earlier. Major theories include congenital origin, migration, and metaplasia.[3] The concept of congenital origin suggests derivation from misplaced epithelial cells.[5] The migration and metaplasia theories presume middle ear or mastoid inflammation as a precursor of tumorigenesis. Acute inflammation may result in perforation of the tympanic membrane or adjacent bone. This break provides a portal of entry for epidermis migrating from the external auditory canal. Alternatively, chronic inflammation may cause the formation of retraction pockets. These inward movements of the tympanic membrane may be the result of negative pressure in the middle ear or of adhesive bands.[12] Desquamated cells and secretions accumulate, and the pockets expand to accommodate the squamous epithelium in the middle ear. According to this theory, squamous metaplasia in response to chronic inflammation occurs in the ear as in other organs. This surface process leads to accumulation of cellular debris in the aural cavity. Budding of metaplastic epithelium into surrounding connective tissue results in cyst formation.[26]

It is suggested here that both congenital epithelial rests and acquired inflammatory metaplasia may give rise to epidermoids of the middle ear. This region begins as a collection of mesenchyme giving rise to the auditory ossicles. The ossicles are covered by mucosal epithelium arising from the first pharyngeal pouch. The external ear arises from an ectodermal invagination. Both the mucosal pouch and the ear canal contribute epithelium to the tympanic membrane. This confluence of epithelia derived from multiple invagina-

tions and coverings provides numerous opportunities for epithelial misplacement. It also accurately predicts the high prevalence of epidermoids in this region.[30]

Sadé has recently championed the metaplasia theory.[26] He cites the phenomenon of contact inhibition between mature epithelial cells and the location of most epidermoids in a position medial to the malleus and incus as evidence against invasion (migration) of the middle ear by benign epithelium. He suggests that many epidermoids are actually poorly visualized retraction pockets, and that negative pressure in the "atelectatic" middle ear is insufficient to elevate retraction pockets into the epitympanic space.

Cholesteatomas are said to occur less frequently in affluent communities and among members of higher economic strata.[3] This decreased prevalence may be a result of better access to modern medical treatment, implicating untreated otitis media in the pathogenesis of cholesteatomas. On the other hand, a striking decline in the frequency of otitis media when antibiotics were first introduced did not result in a comparable decline in epidermoid tumors of the middle ear, suggesting lack of a cause-and-effect relationship between inflammation and production of epidermoids.[30]

Location

Epidermoids and dermoids occur throughout the skull, brain, and spinal cord but almost never in the vertebrae. They may occur in subcutaneous, subperiosteal, or intraosseous locations adjacent to the neuraxis, as well as in the substance of the brain and spinal cord, and may be connected by sinuses to the skin. They are here grouped by location: scalp, skull, cranial contents, spine, and middle ear cavity.

Scalp

Pericranial dermoids often occur near the anterior fontanelle. Epidermoids are uncommon in this region. The dermoids may be present at birth, and most become evident clinically in the first few years of life. They are round protuberances, soft and slightly mobile, ranging up to 6 cm in diameter. Characteristically, a sinus tract does not occur, but an overlying dimple of the skin may be present. Radiographs reveal erosion of both bony tables in older children.[9]

Skull

Intraosseous tumors occur in the cranial diploe, paranasal sinuses, orbit, and petrous bone. Epidermoids are more common than dermoids except in the paranasal region. Calvarial lesions are evenly distributed in the calvarium in proportion to the surface area of the various bones.[25] The frontal sinus is frequently involved. A laterally situated dermal sinus and associated frontotemporal intradiploic dermoid occurs rarely.[22] Characteristically, radiography reveals a scalloped, sclerotic margin.[18] This appearance is produced by slow widening of the space between the two tables, causing centrifugal expansion. One or both tables may be destroyed. Headache is common, but the symptoms depend on the location and involvement of intracranial structures.[10] Surgical removal is usually complete, with little operative morbidity.

The petrous bone may contain epithelial rests giving rise to congenital (primary) epidermoids. These deeply situated tumors should be distinguished clinically from the more frequent cholesteatomas of the ear. The usual presenting complaints are gradual onset of facial palsy, hearing loss, and vestibular disturbance. Marginal perforation of the tympanic membrane is absent, but the roof of the petrous bone is usually eroded. Aural cholesteatoma rarely presents with an intact membrane.[4]

Paranasal and orbital tumors exemplify the destructive nature of these histologically innocuous lesions. Paranasal familial dermoids occupy the glabella, bridge and tip of the nose, and deep part of the septum.[24] They may extend into the anterior cranial fossa. Orbital tumors usually arise superolaterally at sites of embryologic fusion; they cause downward deviation of the eye and proptosis, erode the orbit, and also may enter the anterior fossa.

Cranial Contents

Epidermoids are more frequent than dermoids within the cranium, except in the cerebellum. Epidermoids have an affinity for the subarachnoid cisterns at the base of the brain. The suprasellar region and cerebellopontine angle are favored sites. Less frequent locations include the lateral ventricles, optic chiasm, collicular plate, paratrigeminal area, and pineal gland.[14] Symptoms depend upon location; seizures and dementia are frequent.[31] Tumors in the paratrigeminal region present with slowly progressive, unilateral facial anesthesia, paralysis of the muscles of mastication, and occasionally trigeminal pain.[2] Suprasellar lesions produce visual alterations but usually minimal endocrinologic disturbance.

Intracranial epidermoids often are a few centimeters in diameter but may enlarge to involve more than one cranial fossa (Fig. 72-3). They may infiltrate the brain or occur entirely within the substance of the brain.[6,16] The usual reaction of the surrounding brain is a fibrillary gliosis and a thickening of the overlying leptomeninges. The meninges may contain foreign-body giant cells, usually as a reaction to cholesterol from the epidermal cells.[32] Successful removal is difficult when lesions are deeply situated, extensive, and intimately related to vital structures. Lesions recur if not totally excised, although years may elapse between recurrences.

Cerebellar tumors are usually dermoids in the midline in young children, most often in association with dermal sinuses. They are commonly found in the cerebellar parenchyma, but may sometimes be mainly in the meninges. Dermoids occur less frequently at the base of the brain.

Roentgenographic examination is useful in demonstrating intracranial lesions. In the past, tumors within the ventricles were diagnosed by the characteristic cauliflowerlike appearance on pneumoencephalography.[27] Plain skull films may disclose a fluid level of fat in the rare instance when a

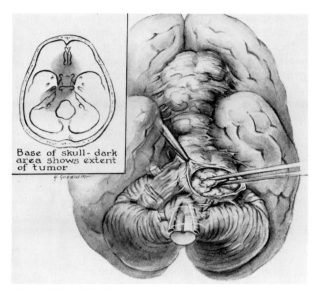

Figure 72-3 Epidermoid tumor at base of brain extends from anterior to posterior fossa. Numerous adhesions bind the mass to the brain. (From Toglia et al.[30])

cyst ruptures into a lateral ventricle.[20] Computed tomography identifies intracranial dermoids or epidermoids as areas of low attenuation. This technique occasionally indicates rupture of a cyst when multiple foci of low attenuation within the cerebrospinal fluid system are identified.[15]

Spine

Both epidermoids and dermoids occur intraspinally. List[17] found fewest in the cervical region and an increasing frequency in the lower portions of the spinal cord. Dermoids were more common than epidermoids, according to List. Other authors state that epidermoids are more common intraspinally or that they predominate in the thoracic region. Two-thirds are in the leptomeninges, one-fifth are intramedullary, and the remainder are in the epidural space.[17] Epidermoids caused by lumbar puncture once accounted for many lumbar tumors;[19] iatrogenic production of epithelial cysts now is uncommon, because serial lumbar punctures are infrequently performed.

Dermoids are more frequently associated with dermal sinus tracts and malformations of the spinal column.[1] They may become large enough to compress the spinal cord severely (Fig. 72-4). Special attention should be given to inspection of the dorsal midline. Patches of pigmentation and tufts of hair may overlie these tumors. Spinal roentgenograms often definitively characterize bony defects.

Middle Ear

Epidermoids of the middle ear usually occupy the epitympanic space (the tympanic attic) and are commonly called *attic cholesteatomas*. These attic epidermoids involve the mastoid antrum and air cells. The masses usually communi-

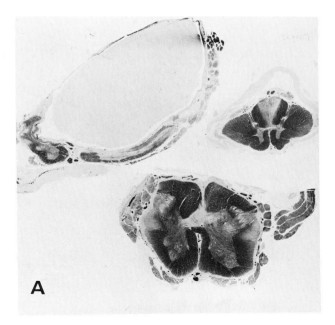

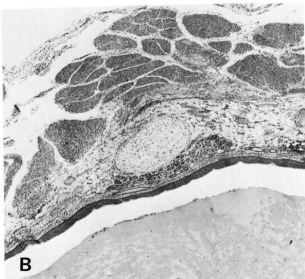

Figure 72-4 *A.* Large dermoid tumor compresses and distorts the lower thoracic region of the spinal cord. Ascending and descending demyelination are present in upper thoracic and lumbar segments, respectively. Weil stain, ×5. *B.* Higher power view of edge of mass shown in *A.* Squamous epithelium and dermal appendages separate the nerve roots (above) from the center of the mass. Island of cartilage suggests relation to teratoma (see text). Hematoxylin-eosin, ×36.

cate with the external ear through a marginal perforation. They characteristically erode bone and encroach upon the superior portions of the malleus and incus to cause conductive loss of hearing. Although it has become increasingly acceptable to identify certain tumors by naming them for specific tumor products (aldosteronoma or insulinoma), cholesteatoma is the only example of a tumor named for a nonspecific product of cellular degeneration. *Attic epider-*

moid is a more acceptable term for both the histological appearance and the derivation from skin, whether the mass is congenital or consequent to inflammation.

Malignancy

Most of these squamous-lined cysts are benign. The extremely rare malignant growths are squamous cell carcinomas, neoplasms that are cytologically malignant and histologically invasive (Fig. 72-5). A recent review cites 13 cases of squamous cell cancer occurring predominantly in the parapontine and cerebellopontine regions.[23] Patients with these malignant growths usually die within a year. Metastases have not been reported. These tumors should be considered in the differential diagnosis of metastatic squamous cell carcinoma in the central nervous system. Dermoids might be expected also to result in other types of carcinoma, but a search of the literature revealed only one report of an invasive atypical hidradenoma.[13]

Complications

Superficial lesions are easily accessible and readily removed, generally with uncomplicated recovery. Deeper lesions are often extensive and close to vital structures, and the capsule may be firmly adherent to brain or spinal cord. These factors frequently preclude total removal of the squamous epithelium, resulting in recurrences. Total removal, when feasible, is the optimal treatment, but lesser procedures may provide long intervals of symptom-free life. The use of an

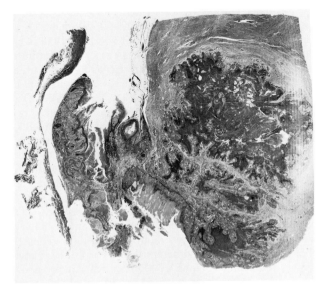

Figure 72-5 Malignant epidermoid tumor (primary squamous cell carcinoma). The neoplasm lies beneath the dura on the left and extends into the pons. Edematous neural tissue is seen at top and right side of the picture. Hematoxylin-eosin, ×3. (From Toglia et al.[30])

Ommaya reservoir for drainage of a recurrent cyst of the conus medullaris is an alternative to repeated surgical exposure.[11]

Complications result from persistence, rupture, or manipulation of the tumors. Chemical meningitis (no organism identified) may accompany rupture of the cyst; repeated episodes are caused by intermittent release of cystic contents into the cerebrospinal fluid. Sterile meningitis may also occur postoperatively, presumably as a result of contamination of the cerebrospinal fluid by lipid and cellular debris. Keratinized squamous cells may be identified cytologically in these circumstances. Brain abscess may result from chronic suppurative otitis media associated with cholesteatoma.[29]

Differential Diagnosis

The characteristic gross and microscopic appearance of these lesions assures a definitive pathological diagnosis in almost all cases. Near the pituitary, craniopharyngioma, pituitary adenoma, teratoma, and meningioma must be considered preoperatively. In the cerebellopontine angle, acoustic neuroma and meningioma are frequent. In the spine, schwannoma, metastatic lesions, and myeloma contribute to the differential diagnosis. Encephaloceles, mucoceles, and arachnoidal cysts may also be mistaken clinically for epidermoids or dermoids.

Microscopically, the distinction of epidermoids and dermoids from most of these other tumors is easily made by finding mature squamous epithelium forming the usual strata. Difficulty is encountered in the rare instances when compression by the cyst eliminates evidence of squamous epithelium. Laminated zones of stratum corneum are, however, more resistant to pressure.

Two other types of tumor containing squamous epithelium should be histologically distinguished: craniopharyngioma and teratoma. Craniopharyngiomas occur in the midline near the sella turcica. A single large cyst or multiple small cavities contain cholesterol crystals and a viscid fluid resembling machine oil. Two histological variants are found: mucosal and adamantinomatous (Figs. 72-6, 72-7). The mucosal type (Fig. 72-6) contains stratum basalis and stratum spinosum, as found in normal skin and in epidermoids, but lacks stratum granulosum and stratum corneum. The adamantinomatous type resembles the primitive tooth bud. Basal columnar cells lie peripherally in islands surrounding a loose connective tissue matrix (Fig. 72-7); squamous cells form anastomosing fine epithelial trabeculae.

Teratomas usually occur in the midline but may be found laterally and in various sites. They often contain mature kerantinizing squamous epithelium, hence must be considered in the microscopic differential diagnosis. Epidermoid tumors containing the four layers of normal skin are not a differential diagnostic problem. Dermoid cysts in most instances also are easily distinguished, as they contain skin and dermal appendages. When hair is present, the physician often considers a gross diagnosis of teratoma, but hair is produced by appendages of skin and occurs in many dermoids. The problem is made more difficult because dermoid

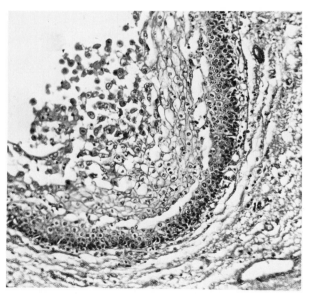

Figure 72-6 Craniopharyngioma. Mucosal epithelium with cells desquamating into central cavity. The epithelium resembles that shown in Figure 72-2, but the stratum corneum and stratum granulosum are absent. Hematoxylin-eosin, ×135.

cysts are often viewed as teratomas. It is contended here that the two lesions are separable on both theoretical and practical grounds in most cases, although borderline cases may occur. The lesion illustrated in Figure 72-4B is an instance of an intermediate type. An otherwise typical dermoid cyst contains a small island of cartilage. If the cartilage has a potential for cellular growth, the lesion is a teratoma.

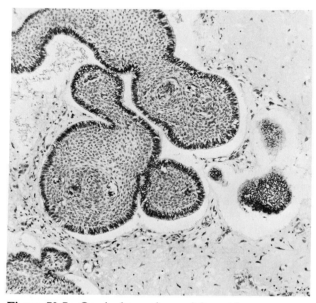

Figure 72-7 Craniopharyngioma. Adamantinomatous type of epithelium is formed by outer layer of basal cells around islands of mesenchymal cells. The appearance is that of primitive tooth buds. Hematoxylin-eosin, ×144.

The modern definition of teratoma no longer relates to a hypothetical derivation from the three germ layers. Willis[33] states that a teratoma is "a true neoplasm composed of multiple (two or more) tissues foreign to the part in which they arise." The teratomas discussed here are thus readily diagnosed by the presence in the tumor of *nondermal* elements such as intestinal epithelium, neural tissue, cartilage, or bone.

The importance of the distinction is that dermoid cysts are developmental in origin. They are not neoplasms, although they may, rarely, become malignant. They enlarge by desquamation of normal cells and by secretion. Teratomas, however, whether benign or malignant, are neoplasms; they grow by progressive mitotic division of the cells.

References

1. Bailey IC: Dermoid tumors of the spinal cord. J Neurosurg 33:676–681, 1970.
2. Baumann CHH, Bucy PC: Paratrigeminal epidermoid tumors. J Neurosurg 13:455–468, 1956.
3. Beales P: Pathogenesis of attic cholesteatomas. J R Soc Med 71:707–708, 1978.
4. Cawthorne T: Congenital cholesteatoma. Arch Otolaryngol 78:248–252, 1963.
5. Cawthorne T, Pickard B: The pathology and treatment of cholesteatoma auris. J Laryngol Otol 79:945–951, 1965.
6. Chandler WF, Farhat SM, Pauli FJ: Intrathalamic epidermoid tumor. J Neurosurg 43:614–617, 1975.
7. Choremis C, Economos D, Papadatos C, Gargoulas A: Intraspinal epidermoid tumours (cholesteatomas) in patients treated for tuberculous meningitis. Lancet 2:437–439, 1956.
8. Fleming JFR, Botterell EH: Cranial dermoid and epidermoid tumors. Surg Gynecol Obstet 109:403–411, 1959.
9. Glasauer FE, Levy LF, Auchterlonie WC: Congenital inclusion dermoid cyst of the anterior fontanel. J Neurosurg 48:274–278, 1978.
10. Grant FC, Austin GM: Epidermoids: Clinical evaluation and surgical results. J Neurosurg 7:190–198, 1950.
11. Hoffman HJ, Holness RO, Flett NR. Long-term control of recurrent cyst of the conus medullaris: Case report. J Neurosurg 47:953–954, 1977.
12. Juers AL: Cholesteatoma genesis. Arch Otolaryngol 81:5–8, 1965.
13. Keogh AJ, Timperley WR: Atypical hidradenoma arising in a dermoid cyst of the spinal canal. J Pathol 117:207–209, 1975.
14. Kirsch WM, Stears JC: Radiographic identification and surgical excision of an epidermoid tumor of the pineal gland. J Neurosurg 33:708–713, 1970.
15. Laster DW, Moody DM, Ball MR: Epidermoid tumors with intraventricular and subarachnoid fat: Report of two cases. Am J Roentgenol 128:504–507, 1977.
16. Leal O, Miles J: Epidermoid cyst in the brain stem: Case report. J Neurosurg 48:811–813, 1978.
17. List CF: Intraspinal epidermoids, dermoids and dermal sinuses. Surg Gynecol Obstet 73:525–538, 1941.
18. MacCarty CS, Leavens ME, Love JG, Kernohan JW: Dermoid and epidermoid tumors in the central nervous system of adults. Surg Gynecol Obstet 108:191–198, 1959.
19. Manno NJ, Uihlein A, Kernohan JW: Intraspinal epidermoids. J Neurosurg 19:754–765, 1962.
20. Maravilla KR: Intraventricular fat-fluid level secondary to rupture of an intracranial dermoid cyst. AJR 128:500–501, 1977.
21. Moore KL: *The Developing Human: Clinically Oriented Embryology*. Philadelphia, Saunders, 1973.
22. Neblett CR, Caram PC, Morris R: Lateral congenital dermal sinus tract associated with an intradiploic dermoid tumor: Case report. J Neurosurg 33:103–105, 1970.
23. Nosaka Y, Nagao S, Tabuchi K, Nishimoto A: Primary intracranial epidermoid carcinoma: Case report. J Neurosurg 50:830–833, 1979.
24. Plewes JL, Jacobson I: Familial frontonasal dermoid cysts: Report of four cases. J Neurosurg 34:683–686, 1971.
25. Rengachary S, Kishore PRS, Watanabe I: Intradiploic epidermoid cyst of the occipital bone with torcular obstruction: Case report. J Neurosurg 48:475–478, 1978.
26. Sadé J: Pathogenesis of attic cholesteatomas. J R Soc Med 71:716–732, 1978.
27. Scott M: Epidermoid tumor (cholesteatoma) of the lateral cerebral ventricle: Case report. J Neurosurg 14:110–113, 1957.
28. Tabaddor K, Lamorgese JR: Lumbar epidermoid cyst following single lumbar puncture. J Bone Joint Surg [Am] 57:1168–1169, 1975.
29. Tarkkanen J, Kohonen A: Otogenic brain abscess: Report of three cases. Arch Otolaryngol 91:91–93, 1970.
30. Toglia JU, Netsky MG, Alexander E Jr: Epithelial (epidermoid) tumors of the cranium: Their common nature and pathogenesis. J Neurosurg 23:384–393, 1965.
31. Tytus JS, Pennybacker J: Pearly tumors in relation to the central nervous system. J Neurol Neurosurg Psychiatry 19:241–259, 1956.
32. Ulrich J: Intracranial epidermoids: A study on their distribution and spread. J Neurosurg 21:1051–1058, 1964.
33. Willis RA: *Teratomas*. Atlas of Tumor Pathology, sect III, fasc 9. Washington, Armed Forces Institute of Pathology, 1951.

73

Epidermoid and Dermoid Tumors: Radiology

Dennis R. Osborne

Scalp

Dermoids and epidermoids of the scalp cannot be distinguished radiologically; however, dermoids have a predilection for the midline or the upper outer quadrant of the orbit, and lesions in these sites are likely to be dermoids rather than epidermoids. Both present as soft tissue masses deep in the dermis which may erode the outer table of the skull and occasionally extend intracranially. The margins of the erosion are typically sclerotic. The lesions of the scalp are best demonstrated radiographically when they are profiled with soft tissue technique (Fig. 73-1). Bone erosion, when it occurs, can usually be detected with conventional skull radiography. It is not possible to differentiate these lesions radiographically from other tumors of the scalp.

Orbital dermoids are usually associated with proptosis. They typically produce a circumscribed erosion elevating the lateral orbital roof and supraorbital ridge.[14,17] They may scallop or trabeculate bone (Fig. 73-2).

Skull

Both dermoid and epidermoid tumors can be found in all the flat bones of the calvarium—paranasal sinuses, maxilla, mandible, tympanum, and petrous bone.[12] Primary epidermoids cannot be radiologically distinguished from those secondary to or associated with chronic infection; the secondary lesions, however, have a predilection for the middle ear and paranasal sinuses.

Cushing gave the first radiological description of an epidermoid in the medical literature.[5] He noted, as have subsequent authors, that the epidermoid produced a discrete area

of bone destruction with margins sharply demarcated by a thin rim of increased density (Fig. 73-3). The destructive area is typically rounded but may appear scalloped or honeycombed and may cause local expansion of the cranial vault. A tangential view of the lesion or a CT scan with bone windows will distinguish pericranial, intradiploic, and intracranial epidural lesions (Fig. 73-4). Both epidermoids and dermoids of the diploe may contain some calcium; dermoids also occasionally contain teeth (Fig. 73-5). If there is an intracranial component, it is best detected by computed tomography and is typically limited by the dura. CT scanning at bone windows will frequently determine the probable site of origin of the lesion (Fig. 73-6). Angiography and radionuclide bone scanning are unhelpful in the evaluation of intradiploic dermoids or epidermoids.

Differential Diagnosis

Other intradiploic lesions share some of the radiological characteristics of epidermoids and dermoids and need to be included in a differential radiological diagnosis. Mucoceles may cause local destruction and expansion of the diploe, but they characteristically extend from a paranasal sinus and produce a more florid hyperostosis than is present with dermoids and epidermoids. The histiocytoses produce a destructive lesion with a less well-defined margin and almost invariably excite no reactive bony sclerosis. Metastases typically produce multiple areas of irregular bony destruction without much reactive marginal sclerosis. Glial rests are usually quite small and usually involve the inner table of the skull; they are not typically associated with much marginal sclerosis. Pacchionian granulations may excavate the inner table of the skull and are typically closely related to a venous sinus but do not produce the sclerotic reaction characteristic of dermoids and epidermoids. Intradiploic hemangiomas, which may be associated with local bony lysis, characteristically produce a spokelike trabeculation of bone and are usually easily recognized. Fibrous dysplasia may cause a radiolucent area in the skull, but this is usually associated with an

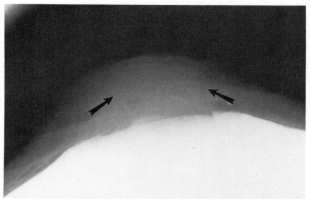

Figure 73-1 Profile view of soft tissue dermoid of scalp (*arrows*) causing erosion of outer table of skull.

adjacent focus of increased density. Osteomyelitis, which can cause extensive irregular bony destruction, typically shows an accompanying florid reactive hyperostosis.

Intracranial Lesions

Intracranial epidermoids are much more frequent than intracranial dermoids (4 to 1). Epidermoids occur in four typical sites: cerebellopontine angle and petrous apex; suprasellar region; cerebral hemisphere, including the lateral ventricle; and cerebellum or fourth ventricle. Dermoids characteristically occur in the midline, usually in the suprasellar region or posterior fossa (the latter may communicate with the skin via a sinus tract).

Radiological Findings

Epidermoid Tumors

CT is the imaging modality of choice in the radiological assessment of epidermoids. The lesions typically present as a mass having a low attenuation value (-22 to $+32$

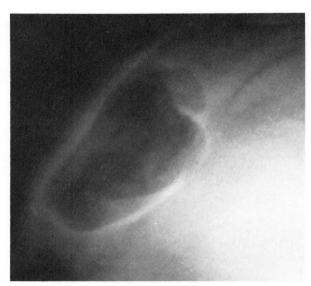

Figure 73-3 Epidermoid of skull vault causing focal bony defect, with margins defined by a thin rim of increased density.

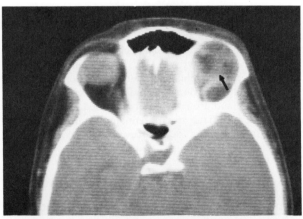

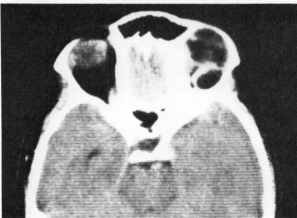

Figure 73-2 CT scan of orbit demonstrating multiloculated dermoid (*arrow*). Note low attenuation values of contents of tumor (similar to orbital fat).

Hounsfield units, or HU) (Fig. 73-7), although lesions of relatively high density (80 to 120 HU) can occur. This range of values reflects the varying amounts of low-density lipid and high-density keratin in the desquamative debris of the tumor. Braun et al.[2] described two cases of epidermoid tumor with attenuation values of 80 to 120 HU and suggested that calcification and saponification of the keratinized debris of the tumor were responsible for the increased attenuation. Fat and fluid can be seen within the tumor.[4] After rupture of the tumor, fat and fluid may be seen in the subarachnoid space or ventricle[10] (Fig. 73-8). Discrete foci of calcification may be noted in the tumor capsule of an epidermoid but are uncommon.

Epidermoid tumors grow slowly, and their shape characteristically conforms to the space in which they are located. This is typically seen with intraventricular and fissural epidermoids. The surface of the lesion often has interstices which can be shown to fill with appropriate contrast agents, producing a characteristic filigree appearance on pneumoencephalography[8]—a feature which can also be demonstrated by intrathecal water-soluble-contrast CT cisternography or ventriculography.[11] The lesions are often present in strategic locations, but because of their slow growth they dilate or distort the ventricular system rather than obstruct it. The gradual accommodation of the ventricular system to a tumor and the presence of interstices within the lesion allow a slow but definite CSF flow even with large tumors. Hydrocephalus is only occasionally seen. This is a useful discriminator in the differential diagnosis of fourth ventricular and cerebellopontine angle tumors, as most other cerebellopontine angle, cerebellar, and fourth ventricular tumors obstruct the ventricular system.

Epidermoid tumors do not enhance after the intravenous injection of a contrast agent.[6,9] This reflects the avascular nature of their contents and their thin, avascular wall. One case of enhancement of the periphery of an epidermoid,

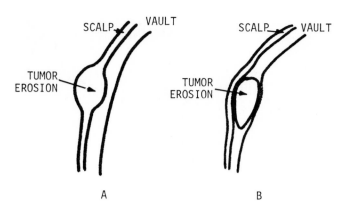

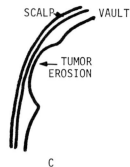

Figure 73-4 Radiological differentiation of epidermoid and dermoid tumors of scalp (*A*), skull vault (*B*), and cranial cavity (*C*).

thought to be due to gliosis and wall thickening, has been reported. Malignant intracranial epidermoids are extremely rare; in three reports of malignancy in the literature, however, contrast enhancement of a portion of the lesion has been noted.[7]

Dermoid Tumors

Dermoid tumors exhibit many of the radiological features of the epidermoid, and the two cannot easily be distinguished. Dermoid tumors are, however, more frequently calcified, are more frequently associated with an external dermal sinus tract, and have a greater range of attenuation values than epidermoids (Fig. 73-9). Associated developmental anomalies of the skeleton are often present.

Ancillary Radiological Techniques

The plain radiographic examination is usually normal, although occasionally the sella may be flattened or deformed by parasellar lesions and intracranial calcification may be demonstrated. Radionuclide examinations of the head are unhelpful. Angiography demonstrates an avascular mass

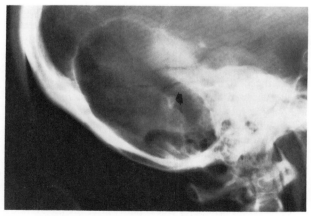

Figure 73-5 Occipital dermoid. A thin margin of sclerosis defines the bony limits of an occipital dermoid. Note intratumoral tooth (*arrow*). The tumor had a large intracranial component.

and occasionally vascular encasement.[16] Pneumoencephalography is rarely necessary, although it can localize the lesion precisely and may demonstrate the interstices of the tumor as a filigree lacework and spongelike, irregular collection of air.

Differential Diagnosis

Cerebellopontine Angle Masses

Arachnoid cysts have discretely defined margins, may insinuate themselves around the brain stem, do not have calcification in their walls, and are characterized by attenuation values of the same range as CSF. Dermoids and epidermoids have a wider range of attenuation values. Acoustic neuromas and meningiomas typically enhance with intravenous contrast and are occasionally calcified. Parasitic cysts are sometimes difficult to differentiate, but their occasional calcified margin and a focal enhancing arachnoid response aid in distinguishing them.

Suprasellar Masses

Craniopharyngiomas characteristically enhance at least in part, and their walls, and occasionally their contents, are partially calcified. Arachnoid cysts can cause a real problem in differentiation in the supra- and parasellar regions, but the absence of calcification, the discreteness of their limits, and the absence of any variation in their attenuation values (CSF density) help. Rathke's pouch cysts can be similarly differentiated. Cystic chromophobe adenomas enhance at least in part after the intravenous administration of an iodinated contrast medium.

Fourth Ventricular and Cerebellar Masses

Arachnoid cysts can usually be distinguished by the absence of any variation in their attenuation values (CSF density) and the absence of calcification in their margins. Hemangioblastomas, cystic astrocytomas, and ependymomas have a density slightly higher than that of CSF (reflecting their proteinacious contents) and an irregularly enhancing margin or mural nodule. All these lesions typically produce an obstructive hydrocephalus. This is an important differen-

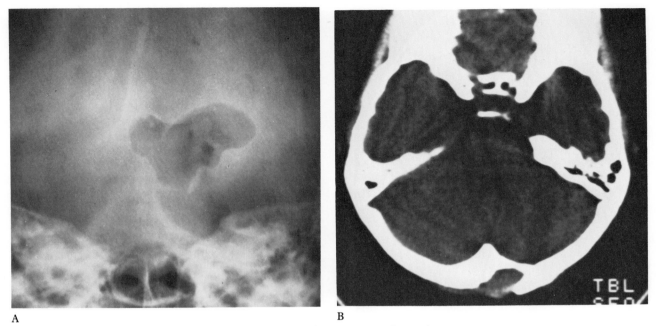

A   B

Figure 73-6 *A*. Dermoid of occipital bone. *B*. CT scan demonstrates primary intra-diploic site and extension of tumor to involve and destroy outer table of skull.

tial point in diagnosis, as dermoid and epidermoid tumors of the fourth ventricle and cerebellum only occasionally produce hydrocephalus. The demonstration of interstices within the tumor by intrathecal metrizamide or air may fur-

ther assist in the differentiation of epidermoids from the other lesions. A large cisterna magna may be differentiated by its characteristic CSF density and the fact that it is transgressed by vessels.

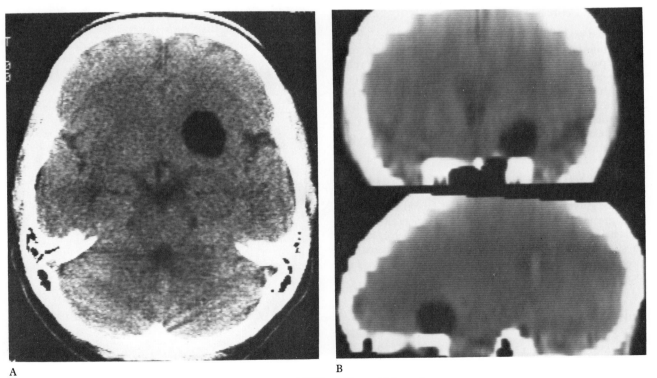

A   B

Figure 73-7 Epidermoid tumor. *A*. Low-density (−15 HU) epidermoid lateral to olfactory gyrus. *B*. Reformatted coronal and sagittal images show relation of lesion to floor of anterior cranial fossa.

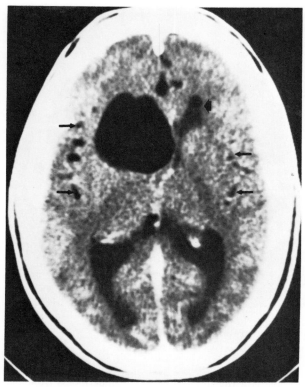

Figure 73-8 Ruptured epidermoid. Note fat-fluid level in left lateral ventricle (*large arrow*) and seeds in subarachnoid cisterns (*small arrows*).

Lateral Ventricular Tumors

Choroid plexus papillomas typically enhance after intravenous injection of a contrast medium, are often small, and may be partially calcified. They characteristically cause ventricular enlargement. Meningiomas have higher attenuation values than dermoids or epidermoids and characteristically enhance. Ependymomas may be cystic but have a higher attenuation value than epidermoids and dermoids and typically enhance, at least in part, after the intravenous injection of an iodine-containing agent.

Cerebral Parenchymal Masses

Cystic gliomas characteristically have a mean attenuation value greater than that of dermoids and epidermoids and characteristically enhance, at least in part. Other cystic lesions of the parenchyma can usually be differentiated by associated intracranial findings such as encephalomalacia or focal ventricular enlargement.

Spinal Lesions

Epidermoid and dermoid tumors of the spinal column are uncommon.[1,15] The lesions are typically intradural and involve the contents of the thecal sac, including the spinal cord.[13] Epidermoid tumors occur over the length of the vertebral canal; in the lumbar region they may be due to im-

plantation of an epidermal seed into the thecal sac by a spinal puncture needle.[3] Both epidermoids and dermoids may involve the spinal cord. Dermoids typically occur in the lumbar region and are often associated with developmental vertebral anomalies and a dermal sinus. It is not possible to distinguish dermoids and epidermoids by their radiographic characteristics.

The plain film findings include local widening of the vertebral canal at the level of the lesion, scalloping of the posterior margins of the vertebrae, and flattening of the pedicles. There may be associated anomalies of the vertebral column, a finding more frequent with dermoids. The tumors are usually quite large when they present, and myelography characteristically demonstrates a block or evidence of a significantly compromised thecal sac (Fig. 73-10). The lesion has a characteristic smooth margin and may be either extra- or intramedullary. Computed tomography demonstrates a low-density lesion obliterating the vertebral canal and failing to enhance after intravenous contrast injection (Fig. 73-10).

Differential Diagnosis

The radiological findings are nonspecific, and the differential diagnosis has to include meningioma and neurofibroma among the extramedullary lesions and ependymoma, gli-

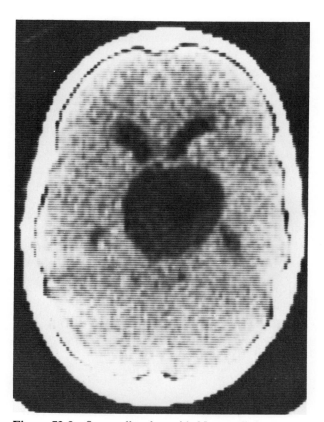

Figure 73-9 Suprasellar dermoid. Note well-demarcated low-density lesion obstructing interventricular foramina and causing hydrocephalus. Attenuation values of the tumor ranged from −10 HU to +20 HU.

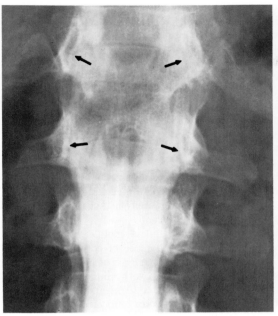 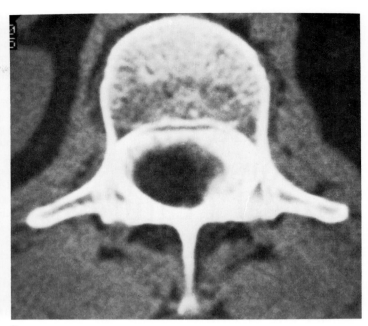

A B

Figure 73-10 Dermoid tumor, conus medullaris. *A*. The interpediculate distance is widened and the pedicles flattened (*arrows*). Myelography demonstrates an intradural intramedullary lesion completely obstructing the thecal sac. *B*. Computed tomography (after myelography) demonstrates the obstructing tumor with characteristically low attenuation values (− 10 HU).

oma, and lipoma among the intramedullary lesions. There is no simple way to differentiate these entities radiographically, although the low attenuation values of epidermoids and dermoids can be a useful aid to diagnosis when CT is used.

References

1. Bailey IC: Dermoid tumors of the spinal cord. J Neurosurg 33:676–681, 1970.
2. Braun IF, Naidich TP, Leeds NE, Koslow M, Zimmerman HM, Chase NE: Dense intracranial epidermoid tumors: Computed tomographic observations. Radiology 122:717–719, 1977.
3. Choremis C, Economos D, Papadatos C, Gargoulas A: Intraspinal epidermoid tumours in patients treated for tuberculous meningitis. Lancet 2:437–439, 1956.
4. Cornell SH, Graf CJ, Dolan KD: Fat-fluid level in intracranial epidermoid cyst. AJR 128:502–503, 1977.
5. Cushing H: A large epidermal cholesteatoma of the parieto-temporal region deforming the left hemisphere without cerebral symptoms. Surg Gynecol Obstet 34:557–566, 1922.
6. Davis KR, Roberson GH, Taveras JM, New PFJ, Trevor R: Diagnosis of epidermoid tumor by computed tomography: Analysis and evaluation of findings. Radiology 119:347–353, 1976.
7. Dubois PJ, Sage M, Luther JS, Burger PC, Heinz ER, Drayer

BP: Malignant change in an intracranial epidermoid cyst. J Comput Assist Tomogr 5:433–435, 1981.
8. Dyke CG, Davidoff LM: Encephalographic appearance of an intraventricular epidermoid. Bull Neurol Inst N Y 6:489–493, 1937.
9. Fawcitt RA, Isherwood I: Radiodiagnosis of intracranial pearly tumours with particular reference to the value of computer tomography. Neuroradiology 11:235–242, 1976.
10. Ford K, Drayer B, Osborne D, Dubois P: Transient cerebral ischemia as a manifestation of ruptured intracranial dermoid cyst. 5:895–897, 1981.
11. Gellad F, Rao KCVG, Arora S, Chiantella N, Salcman M: Epidermoid tumor of the fourth ventricle: Use of metrizamide-computed tomography. J Comput Assist Tomogr 6:231–235, 1982.
12. Haig PV: Primary epidermoids of the skull: Including a case with malignant change. AJR 76:1076–1080, 1956.
13. King AB: Intramedullary epidermoid tumor of the spinal cord. J Neurosurg 14:353–357, 1957.
14. MacCarty CS, Leavens ME, Love JG, Kernohan JW: Dermoid and epidermoid tumors in the central nervous system of adults. Surg Gynecol Obstet 108:191–198, 1959.
15. Manno NJ, Uihlein A, Kernohan JW: Intraspinal epidermoids. J Neurosurg 19:754–765, 1962.
16. Mikhael MA, Mattar AG: Intracranial pearly tumors: The roles of computed tomography, angiography, and pneumoencephalography. J Comput Assist Tomogr 2:421–429, 1978.
17. Tytus JS, Pennybacker J: Pearly tumours in relation to the central nervous system. J Neurol Neurosurg Psychiatry 19:241–259, 1956.

74

Epidermoid and Dermoid Tumors: Clinical Features and Surgical Management

Frances K. Conley

Clinical Features

Epidermoids and dermoids, which are inclusion tumors of the central nervous system, are rare, usually benign, slow-growing, and can cause protean symptoms. Epidermoids are estimated to constitute 0.5 to 1.5 percent of brain tumors; dermoids occur less frequently, constituting approximately 0.3 percent of brain tumors. Dermoid cysts have a greater tendency than epidermoids to occur in a midline location and are most commonly diagnosed and treated in the pediatric age group. By contrast, epidermoid tumors most often become symptomatic between the ages of 20 and 40 and more often occur in a lateral location. The only other important differentiation between dermoids and epidermoids is histological: the cyst lining of the epidermoid is composed of a capsule of stratified squamous epithelium only, while the cyst lining of the dermoid contains, in addition to skin, dermal elements such as hair and sebaceous glands. Both tumors expand slowly by progressive desquamation of capsular components into the interior of the cyst itself, and both can produce clinical symptoms by deformation of, compression of, and insinuation around adjacent neural and vascular structures. Because the breakdown products produced by both tumors are soft and because the pliable capsule wall continues to grow slowly, these tumors can literally flow into any available space, and in the past often have reached a large size before sufficient symptoms developed to warrant invasive neuroradiological diagnostic studies. In the future, these tumors should be diagnosed more frequently (autopsy studies suggest a higher incidence that do clinical studies[18]) and at an earlier stage in their development as CT scanning is applied to more patients who present with nonspecific neurological complaints.

Dermoids and epidermoids produce symptoms by virtue of their location, by interference with spinal fluid or vascular pathways, or by cyst rupture into the subarachnoid space or ventricular system. This latter event releases keratin and cholesterol breakdown products which are irritating and may cause a chemical meningitis or ventriculitis which can be severe and long-lasting. Fascinating features of many of the case reports available in the literature are long duration (up to 53 years) of mild symptoms, a history of waxing and waning symptoms mimicking demyelinating disease, and long-term remission of neurological symptoms in the absence of tumor removal.

Dermoids and epidermoids can occur in the scalp, the calvarium, and the spinal canal, can extend into the epidural space, and can present intradurally in a variety of locations or within the ventricular system.

Scalp cysts are usually painless, mobile, rubbery masses which are important only because of cosmetic deformity (Fig. 74-1). The midline dermal cysts of infancy and childhood are frequently associated with midline fusion defects (spina bifida, failure of vertebral segmentation, cleft palate, etc.) and in 25 percent of cases are connected by a congenital sinus or stalk to intracranial structures or to the spinal canal. The presentation and surgical management of the dermoid with a sinus tract are presented more completely elsewhere in this volume.

Epidermoids or dermoids confined to the diploe of the calvarium usually present as painless masses which by x-ray evaluation have thinned or eroded both inner and outer tables of the skull (Figs. 74-2, 74-3). Cysts which arise in the diploe of the petrous bone can cause a slowly progressive seventh nerve paresis. Orbital tumors usually arise from the lateral orbital roof and gradually displace the eye downward and medially, often without producing a change in visual accuity or causing other neurological symptoms (Fig. 74-4).[17]

Most intracranial cysts arise in the basal cisterns and produce symptoms by slow, progressive, expansive growth from their point of origin. Although the clinical signs and symptoms produced by intracranial cysts do not necessarily reflect the full mass extent of the lesion, the cysts can be roughly divided into four categories describing their anatomical origin and primary location: suprasellar-chiasmatic, parasellar-sylvian fissure, retrosellar-cerebellopontine angle, and basilar-posterior fossa.

Suprasellar cysts most commonly produce symptoms referable to the optic apparatus. Visual impairment, optic atrophy, and bitemporal hemianopsia are common, particularly because the optic nerves are so vulnerable to compression. Pituitary dysfunction may or may not be evident along with the visual symptoms,[4,12,15] and occasionally these patients will develop diabetes insipidus. From a suprasellar location the cyst can expand forward into the anterior fossa, posteriorly over the dorsum in front of the pons, and/or laterally under the temporal lobes.

Because of their close proximity to the temporal lobe, parasellar tumors frequently are associated with a seizure disorder, which may be typical for the temporal lobe involvement or grand mal in type. The tumor may grow into the Sylvian fissure, widely spreading the temporal and frontal lobes, and at the base may extend into the internal cap-

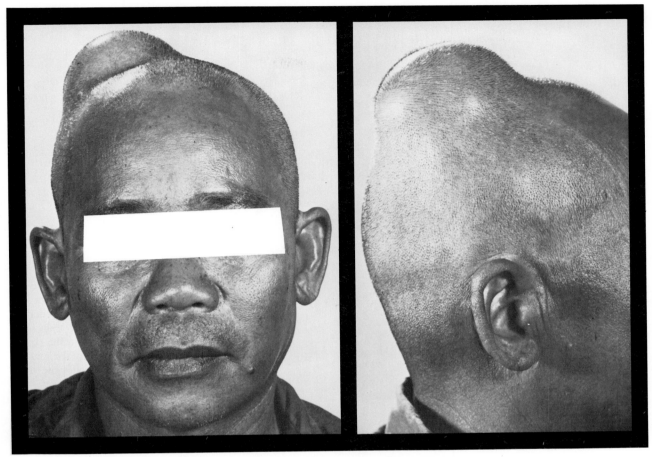

Figure 74-1 Epidermoid cyst of scalp, calvarium, and epidural space. (Courtesy Dr. John W. Hanbery.)

sule and thalamus[3] and involve the postganglionic fibers of the fifth cranial nerve, producing hemiparesis and trigeminal nerve deficits.

Trigeminal neuralgia is a frequently encountered symptom produced by cysts in the retrosellar-cerebellopontine angle. Since the cyst and its contents tend to envelop and enclose adjacent neural structures, rather than displacing them, it is not surprising that the early symptoms produced are irritative rather than dysfunctional in nature. Therefore, any young adult presenting with trigeminal neuralgia or hemifacial spasm should be carefully investigated for evidence of an epidermoid cyst. As the cyst in the cerebellopontine angle enlarges, multiple cranial nerve deficits may develop, most frequently involving nerves V, VII, and VIII, and these cranial nerve deficits often will be accompanied by cerebellar ataxia, nystagmus, and hemiparesis.

Cysts which arise in the basilar region interfere with the function of lower cranial nerves and may produce both cerebellar deficits and pyramidal tract abnormalities. Progressive growth of these lesions may slowly erode through the entire substance of the brain stem.[9]

Intraventricular dermoids and epidermoids can produce a great variety of symptoms; some of the most interesting case reports are those of patients with intraventricular tumors. Cysts occur more frequently in the fourth ventricle than in the rest of the ventricular system (Fig. 74-5), but cysts arising in the third and lateral ventricles are not unknown. Many cases of fourth ventricular inclusion tumors, not unexpectedly, present with signs and symptoms resulting from obstructive hydrocephalus. More surprising, however, are case reports of failure of hydrocephalus to develop despite the fact that the third or fourth ventricular cyst fills the entire ventricle and even extends into the aqueduct.[14] These tumors grow linearly, not exponentially, with time, and their plasticity allows progressive slow deformity of the surrounding neural structures and also allows for maintenance of a percolating type of cerebrospinal fluid pathway. The patients may present with strange combinations of symptoms which are difficult to interpret,[1] may wax and wane, and often are ascribed to demyelinating disease. Symptoms which develop include headache, dementia, psychiatric problems, and local compressive events with cranial nerve palsies, ataxia, and hemiparesis.

Dermoids and epidermoids involving the spinal column have been reported at all levels, but the vast majority occur in the thoracic or upper lumbar areas. Both clinical and experimental evidence suggest that in the past, many reported epidermoid tumors of the lower lumbar region were iatrogenic in origin, following implantation of epidermal tissue by lumbar puncture with a needle lacking a stylet.[15] If these

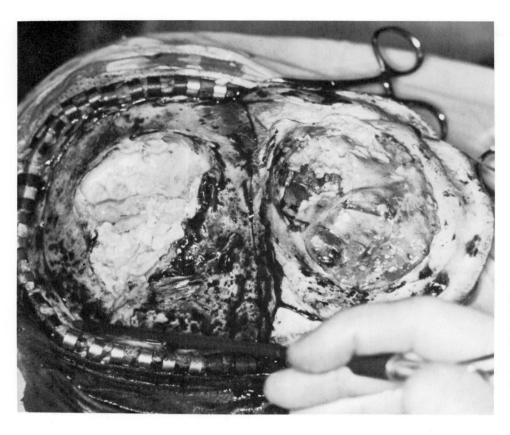

Figure 74-2 Operative photo of patient shown in Figure 74-1. The epidermoid cyst of the scalp has been reflected to the right; the calvarial epidermoid completely erodes the skull on the left. (Courtesy Dr. John W. Hanbery.)

iatrogenic cases are eliminated in order to assess the clinical characteristics of the true congenital lesions, it is obvious that congenital cysts have a predilection for involving the conus and low to midthoracic regions and for an intramedullary location.[11] These tumors are often associated with other abnormalities of the spinal cord and bony vertebral column. Assuming that congenital inclusion cysts have been present since birth, the clinical data suggest that they, like intracranial cysts, are slow-growing lesions which become symptomatic during the second decade of life. The symptoms produced are back and leg pain and/or slowly progressive impairment of spinal cord function with paraparesis, sphincter dysfunction, and sensory disturbance. Dermoids of the spinal canal, which tend to be associated with a clinical history of recurrent meningitis and a congenital dermal sinus, are considered in more detail elsewhere in this volume.

Operative Technique

Regardless of location or histological type, the therapeutic goal in the treatment of epidermoid and dermoid cysts is complete surgical excision of both the cyst lining and its contents; radiation therapy and chemotherapy play no role whatever in the management of these lesions. Whether total excision can be achieved, of course, depends on the location and extent of the individual tumor. Scalp lesions should be excised with sufficient margins to assure that no remnants of cyst lining have been left behind, bearing in mind that cer-

tain of the superficial tumors will be connected by a stalk through bone and/or dura to a second lesion located intracranially or intraspinally.

Intradiploic tumors of the calvarium are most reliably removed by an enbloc excision with a surrounding margin of bone, followed by cranioplasty. These tumors have also been successfully removed by meticulously scraping away the cyst contents and lining from the surrounding bone. Since there can be epidural and/or intracranial extension of the cyst from these diploic sites, the surgeon should have investigated the patient thoroughly preoperatively, (as with scalp lesions), in order to be prepared to handle any demonstrated intracranial extension of the cyst at the time the calvarial lesion is excised. Lesions located over major dural vascular sinuses are of special concern, as there may be involvement of these venous conduits by the cyst,[13] and the surgeon must be prepared to surgically repair them.

Total excision of intracranial tumors can be considerably more difficult than that of scalp and diploic lesions. Preoperatively, the surgeon must be fully cognizant of the exact location and extent of the tumor to be removed.[8,16] Multiple fingers of the cyst may invaginate arachnoid spaces separating neural components or extend from one cranial fossa into another. Since intracranial cysts tend to arise from the basal cisterns, the operating surgeon must be prepared to follow the lining of the cyst capsule to its origin and meticulously dissect the lining from adjacent neural and vascular structures. Thus for many cases the use of an operating microscope is mandatory, and dehydrating agents must be used in those cases in which extensive retraction of the brain is necessary to reach the cyst origin at the base of the brain. Many

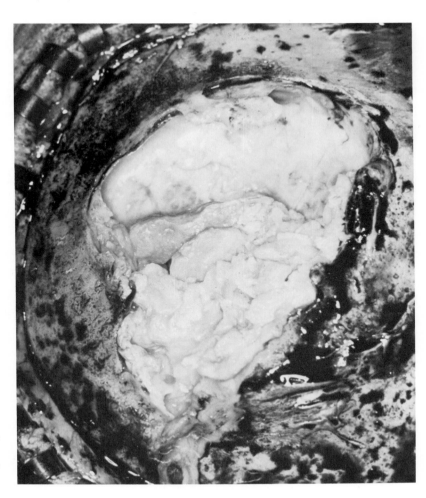

Figure 74-3   Close-up of Figure 74-2 showing the irregular, glistening "mother-of-pearl" epidermoid tumor eroding the outer and inner tables of the skull. (Courtesy Dr. John W. Hanbery.)

cysts or portions of cysts show a clear plane of dissection between the cyst lining and arachnoid layers. However, in others, a chronic granulomatous reaction which may have

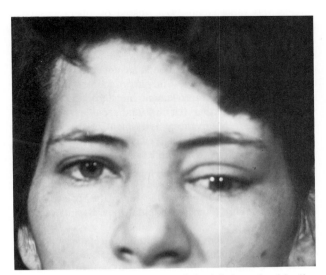

Figure 74-4   Epidermoid cyst of the left lateral orbit displacing the left eye downward. (Courtesy Dr. John W. Hanbery).

been present over many years[18] can make the surgical separation difficult, if not impossible. The lining of these tumors is often remarkably adherent to vascular structures such as the carotid and basilar arteries, as well as to cranial nerves and brain stem substance.[5] In such cases it is preferable to leave small tags of cyst lining rather than attempt a complete removal at the expense of irreparable damage to the involved vascular and neural structures.[6] Complete removal of spinal cysts can also be very difficult in cases in which the cyst lining invaginates the roots of the cauda equina or is densely adherent to the substance of the spinal cord. Use of the operating microscope and great tenacity on the part of the surgeon should allow more of these tumors to be totally removed in the future.

During removal of intradural tumors, either cranial or spinal, it is advisable to avoid, as much as possible, contamination of the surgical field and spillage of the cyst contents into the subarachnoid or ventricular spaces. Seeding of the subarachnoid space with the irritating breakdown products from the interior of the cyst can cause a severe chemical meningitis and/or ventriculitis which can be long-lasting. Some surgeons have reported beneficial results in avoiding this inflammatory response from adding hydrocortisone to the irrigating fluid used during the operation and from the use of systemic steroids perioperatively and postoperatively.[2]

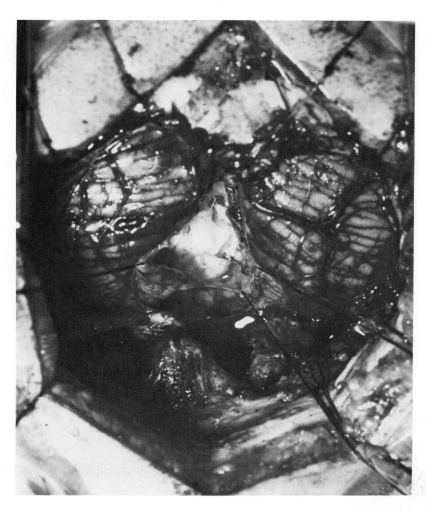

Figure 74-5 Epidermoid cyst of the fourth ventricle.

Surgical removal of intraventricular cysts does not present any special features different from what has been stated above. These cysts may, indeed, be more easily removed than tumors in the cerebellopontine angle or suprasellar regions, where there are more neural and vascular structures which may be trapped by the insinuating fingers of a cyst. The point of attachment of intraventricular tumors may be very adherent to vital neural structures, especially in the floor of the fourth ventricle. An attempt should be made to define the attachment of the cyst lining as closely as possible and to meticulously remove all cyst lining except that which obviously invades the brain stem.[14] Careful operative monitoring of vital signs is essential during the course of this dissection. In the future, operative use of evoked potentials may prove to be a benefit in the surgical management of intraventricular cysts, as well as those cysts in the suprasellar region and in the cerebellopontine angle.

Operative Results

Operative mortality from the attempted removal of these cysts has declined remarkably during the course of this century. Prior to 1936, the operative mortality rate approached

70 percent for removal of intracranial epidermoid and dermoid cysts. This rate dropped to approximately 20 percent in the 1950s, and more recently an operative death rate of 10 percent was reported in 1977,[7] based on operations performed since 1953. A review of case reports from the 1970s suggests an even lower recent operative mortality rate following the removal of these tumors. The improvement in operative results can be ascribed to advances in neuroradiology, neuroanesthesiology, and microneurosurgical technique. The marked improvement in neuroradiological investigation allows earlier diagnosis and provides the surgeon with a complete preoperative assessment of the size, location, and extent of the tumor. Newer techniques of anesthesia permit operations to continue safely for many hours and provide sophisticated monitoring of vital neural functions. The operating microscope provides the neurosurgeon with an invaluable tool for visualizing the planes of separation between cyst lining and arachnoidal, neural, and vascular structures.

Almost 100 percent of scalp and diploic epidermoids and dermoids and 50 to 80 percent of intraspinal and intracranial cysts can be removed completely. Over the past ten years an "incomplete removal" has meant, in the majority of cases, leaving only tiny remnants of cyst lining behind when removal of those final fragments would unduly jeopardize neural or vascular structures. In most of these cases postoperative CT scans have revealed no tumor residual. The recurrence rate for dermoids and especially epidermoids was considerably higher twenty or thirty years ago than it appears in the more recent literature. It is possible that the higher recurrence rate in earlier studies is related more to unrecognized incomplete removal of cysts than to regrowth from small remnants of cyst lining known to have been left behind. Clinical recurrence in more recent cases where only small fragments of cyst lining have been left has not been frequent.

Operative Complications

Operative complications which result from damage to nerves, blood vessels, or brain or spinal cord substance are not unique to the surgical removal of epidermoids and dermoids. Since these tumors may intimately involve neural and vascular structures and be densely adherent to them, such structures are at high risk for both direct and stretch injury during the course of surgery, as they are during the removal of many other types of tumors. Prolonged and often permanent sphincter disturbance is the most common complication in cases where a spinal intramedullary tumor has been excised.[10]

An operative complication which is unique to this type of tumor and which occurs in approximately 40 percent of cases is postoperative aseptic meningitis, which can last for a number of weeks. Case reports from the available literature suggest that this complication occurs far more frequently when removal of the cyst has been incomplete. Even when only a few remnants of the capsule are known to have been left behind there is a higher incidence of aseptic meningitis than when removal has been complete.[7] If the chemical meningitis is severe and long-lasting, it can lead to a "granulomatous" type of arachnoiditis in which nearby nerve roots become encased in a thick layer of reactive arachnoidal tissue. In the cauda equina region and sometimes in cysts involving the cerebellopontine angle, removal of this abnormal arachnoidal tissue from the involved cranial nerves or lumbosacral nerve roots has been of benefit in restoring neural function.

Postoperative hydrocephalus is another not uncommon complication following removal of these tumors. It occurs more frequently in those patients who develop postoperative aseptic meningitis, and it may be concurrent with this inflammatory condition in the postoperative period. Shunting is usually required, and such patients frequently remain shunt-dependent.

References

1. Bailey P: Cruveilhier's "tumeurs perlées." Surg Gynecol Obstet 31:390–401, 1920.
2. Cantu RC, Ojemann RG: Glucosteroid treatment of keratin meningitis following removal of a fourth ventricle epidermoid tumour. J Neurol Neurosurg Psychiatry 31:73–75, 1968.
3. Chandler WF, Farhat SM, Pauli FJ: Intrathalamic epidermoid tumor: Case report. J Neurosurg 43:614–617, 1975.
4. Fawcitt RA, Isherwood I: Radiodiagnosis of intracranial pearly tumours with particular reference to the value of computer tomography. Neuroradiology 11:235–242, 1976.
5. Gagliardi FM, Vagnozzi R, Caruso R, Delfini R: Epidermoids of the cerebellopontine angle (cpa): Usefulness of CT scan. Acta Neurochir (Wien) 54:271–281, 1980.
6. Grant FC, Austin GM: Epidermoids: Clinical evaluation and surgical results. J Neurosurg 7:190–198, 1950.
7. Guidetti B, Gagliardi FM: Epidermoid and dermoid cysts: Clinical evaluation and late surgical results. J Neurosurg 47:12–18, 1977.
8. Hamer J: Diagnosis by computerized tomography of intradural dermoid with spontaneous rupture of the cyst. Acta Neurochir (Wien) 51:219–226, 1980.
9. Leal O, Miles J: Epidermoid cyst in the brain stem: Case report. J Neurosurg 48:811–813, 1978.
10. MacCarty CS, Leavens ME, Love JG, Kernohan JW: Dermoid and epidermoid tumors in the central nervous system of adults. Surg Gynecol Obstet 108:191–198, 1959.
11. Manno NJ, Uihlein A, Kernohan JW: Intraspinal epidermoids. J Neurosurg 19:754–765, 1962.
12. Mohanty S, Bhattacharya RN, Tandon SC, Shukla PK: Intracerebral cystic epidermoid: Report of two cases. Acta Neurochir (Wien) 57:107–113, 1981.
13. Rengachary SS, Kishore PRS, Watanabe I: Intradiploic epidermoid cyst of the occipital bone with torcular obstruction: Case report. J Neurosurg 48:475–478, 1978.
14. Rosario M, Becker DH, Conley FK: Epidermoid tumors involving the fourth ventricle. Neurosurgery 9:9–13, 1981.
15. Tan TI: Epidermoids and dermoids of the central nervous system. Acta Neurochir (Wien) 26:13–24, 1972.
16. Toglia JU, Netsky MG, Alexander E Jr: Epithelial (epidermoid) tumors of the cranium. J Neurosurg 23:384–393, 1965.
17. Tytus JS, Pennybacker J: Pearly tumours in relation to the central nervous system. J Neurol Neurosurg Psychiatry 19:241–259, 1956.
18. Ulrich J: Intracranial epidermoids: A study on their distribution and spread. J Neurosurg 21:1051–1058, 1964.

SECTION F

Tumors in the Region of the Pineal Gland

75

Pineal Tumors: Classification and Pathology

Maie Kaarsoo Herrick

The Normal Pineal Gland

The pineal organ (Latin *pineale*, pine cone), or more appropriately, the pineal gland, first becomes visible in the human during the second fetal month, when a diverticulum and adjacent cellular thickening develop in the roof of the diencephalon. The pineal parenchyma is formed of tubules which are transformed into solid cell masses, separated by connective tissue and nerve twigs. By the middle of the first decade the structure of the pineal approaches that of a mature gland, consisting of pineocytes arranged into lobules separated by delicate connective tissue septa and thin-walled blood vessels (Fig. 75-1).

The pineal cells are a specialized type of neuroepithelial cells, closely related to neurons. They lack axons but have one or more elongated cytoplasmic processes, which end chiefly in the perivascular space around capillaries. Ultrastructurally, besides the usual cellular organelles, mammalian pineocytes have granular (dense-cored) vesicles, generally considered to be of secretory nature. Small numbers of astrocytes are present between the pineal cells. Typical neurons are found rarely in the human pineal, although a ganglion of about 20 nerve cells (Pastori's ganglion) is present in the tissue at the tip of the gland.[5] Foci of mineralization (*acervuli*), largely of hydroxy- or carbonate apatite structure, develop from early infancy and increase with age but do not

become radiologically demonstrable until the second decade. The adult pineal weighs about 140 mg (100 to 800 mg) and measures 8 to 12 mm in length, 5 to 8 mm in width, and 4 to 5 mm in thickness. Its blood supply is derived from the posterior cerebral arteries via their posterior choroidal branches. In humans, at least some of the blood drains into the junction of the great cerebral veins.

During its phylogenetic development, the pineal undergoes remarkable changes.[8] In fishes and amphibians, it is chiefly a neurosensory photoreceptor organ. In reptiles and birds, the photosensory function is gradually lost and replaced by an exclusively secretory function. The concept of direct derivation of the mammalian neurosecretory pineocyte from the pineal photoreceptor cell of the lower vertebrate is reinforced by the finding of similar organelles in both these cells. The mammalian pineal gland has a neurotransmitter secretory function. Photic stimuli from the retina reach the pineal gland by the way of a polysynaptic pathway whose final links are postganglionic sympathetic fibers from the superior cervical ganglia.

Most of the research concerned with the biological behavior of the pineal gland has been performed on animals which show considerable species variation. The major attention has been directed toward melatonin, named for its blanching effect on tadpole skin. Melatonin is synthesized in

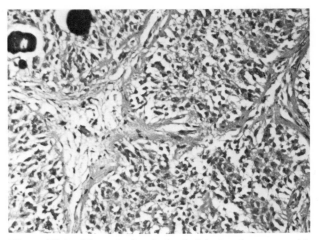

Figure 75-1 Normal pineal gland: lobulated pattern with delicate intersecting connective tissue septa and foci of calcification, left upper corner. (Hematoxylin-eosin, ×120.)

pineocytes from tryptophan through a series of metabolic reactions, of which one is the formation of serotonin. Serotonin is found in the pineal tissue in concentrations higher than in any other area of the brain. It is subsequently converted to melatonin in two steps. The final reaction is catalyzed by an enzyme, hydroxyindole-O-methyl-transferase (HIOMT). This enzyme is capable of producing other related methoxyindoles, such as methoxytryptophol, which may eventually be found to be of importance. The pineal is also rich in noradrenalin and peptides such as arginine vasotocin.

Melatonin in animals is essential in regulating circadian rhythms in endocrine activity, producing an antigonadal effect primarily through the hypothalamic-adenohypophyseal axis. Light inhibits melatonin production. In humans the importance of melatonin is less well defined and alterations in melatonin levels are less closely tied to changes in light. In one study, an abrupt fall in concentration of melatonin and methoxytryptophol in the blood of boys preceded the onset of puberty. Other effects of melatonin reported in humans have been tranquilization, mild euphoria, and induction of sleep.[7]

Masses in the Pineal Region: Histogenesis, Classification, and General Features

About 1 percent of all intracranial tumors arise from the pineal region.[9] Not only are they rare, but neoplasms of a great variety of histological types can occur and have been described.[2,3,9-11] Some of the tumors arise from the pineal parenchymal cells, others from supportive tissues in and around the gland, and the most frequently occurring pineal neoplasm, the germinoma, is derived from presumably misplaced germ cells which are not a normal component of the pineal at all. In the past, the name *pinealoma* was used to designate this most common pineal growth and the term *ectopic pinealoma* was used when it was found at other intracranial sites, such as the suprasellar region. As the histological similarity of the pinealoma to a common testicular neoplasm was recognized, the name *atypical teratoma* was proposed for the pineal tumor, to emphasize its relation to germ cell tumors. Eventually the name *germinoma* supplanted both previous terms as the similarity between this tumor, the testicular seminoma, and the ovarian dysgerminoma became well established. The classification of pineal neoplasms is based on this concept (Table 75-1).

Tumors of Germ Cell Origin

The hypotheses of origin, the classification, and considerations of the pathogenesis of this group of neoplasms in the context of extragonadal germ cell tumors has recently been thoroughly reviewed.[4] The source of these tumors is believed to be primordial germ cells that failed to migrate properly during the first few weeks of embryonic development. This explanation also accounts for the location of such neoplasms at other intracranial sites, most often in the

TABLE 75-1 Classification of Pineal Tumors

Tumors of germ cell origin
    Germinoma (atypical teratoma) and closely related tumors
    Teratoma—typical and teratoid
Tumors of pineal parenchymal cells
    Pineoblastoma
    Pineocytoma
Tumors of glial and other cell origin
Non-neoplastic cysts and masses

suprasellar region and extracranially elsewhere in the midline of the body. The spectrum of tumors arising from the pineal site is similar to that of gonadal tumors of germ cell derivation (Table 75-2). The concept of a common germ cell origin of these neoplasms is reinforced by the frequent finding of more than one histologic pattern in the same tumor.

Tumors of all types of germ cell origin occur predominantly in males and are most frequent in the first three decades, with a peak in the middle of the second decade, although no age group is totally immune. A similar age distribution exists for this group of neoplasms in the suprasellar region, but at the latter site the sexes are more equally affected. The capacity of extracranial endodermal sinus tumors to produce alpha fetoprotein (AFP) and of choriocarcinomas to secrete human chorionic gonadotropin (hCG) has prompted attempts to demonstrate similar activity in pineal neoplasms. In several cases elevated serum, urine, or CSF concentrations of AFP or hCG have been demonstrated in patients with endodermal sinus tumor or choriocarcinoma. The same substances have also been identified with immunofluorescent or immunoperoxidase staining techniques in the corresponding tumor cells. The demonstration of AFP and hCG in an embryonal carcinoma and some suprasellar germinomas implies the presence of some endodermal sinus tumor and choriocarcinomatous elements in these particular tumors.

The potential usefulness of such tumor markers in diagnosis and monitoring of therapy is unquestioned, but further work is required to understand them. The demonstration of the melatonin-synthesizing enzyme HIOMT in a dural extension of a suprasellar germinoma and of melatonin, HIOMT, and serotonin in a soft tissue metastasis of a pineal germinoma does not fit the theory that melatonin and HIOMT are almost exclusively produced by the pineal parenchymal cell, which also contains high concentrations of serotonin.

The *germinoma* is the most common tumor of germ cell

TABLE 75-2 Histological Types of Tumors of Germ Cell Origin and Their Biological Behavior

Germinoma (atypical teratoma, dysgerminoma, seminoma)	Malignant
Embryonal carcinoma—tumor of totipotential cells	Malignant
Endodermal sinus tumor—extraembryonic structures	Malignant
Choriocarcinoma—extraembryonic structures	Malignant
Teratoma—embryonic endo-, meso-, ectoderm	Malignant or benign

origin arising at the pineal site and accounts for more than 50 percent of all neoplasms at this location. An unusually high occurrence of germinomas is seen in Japan, where their incidence is reported to be 5.6 to 9 percent of all intracranial tumors, and 11 percent if only children are considered.[10] The germinoma is extremely malignant and fast-growing but also highly radiosensitive. With therapy, about two-thirds or more of the patients survive more than 5 years. Spinal cord metastases have been reported in 14 percent of patients with biopsy-proven germinoma. Extraneural hematogenous and shunt metastases have been reported rarely.

On gross examination the tumor is usually poorly circumscribed. At times the pineal mass is connected with suprasellar tumor by continuous invasion of the walls of the third ventricle, so that it is not possible to be certain of its site of origin. The cut surface of the tumor is light gray, granular, and usually solid. Hemorrhage, necrosis, grossly visible cysts, and degeneration may be seen but are uncommon.

Microscopically the germinoma is composed of two cell types (Fig. 75-2). There are islands and trabeculae of large round or polyhedral cells with well-defined cytoplasmic membranes. The cytoplasm may be clear or eosinophilic. The nuclei are prominent, round, and rather vesicular, with some coarse peripherally clumped chromatin and one or more prominent nucleoli. Mitoses are variable. The large cells are separated by a fibrovascular stroma which is infiltrated by lymphocytes, the majority of which have in a few cases been identified as T cells. The additional presence of inflammatory granulomas, complete with giant cells in many of these tumors, may represent an immunologic response. Microcysts containing proteinaceous fluid and also liquefaction necrosis have sometimes been described. Other tissue elements such as glands with columnar epithelium, cartilage, squamous epithelium, and trophoblast may be present.

Other closely related tumors of germ cell origin, the embryonal carcinoma, endodermal sinus tumor, and choriocarcinoma, are also highly malignant and tend to invade locally and to seed throughout the spinal fluid pathways. Rarely, extraneural metastases have been described in all the tumor types. Although mixtures of various elements of germ cell origin, including the germinoma, are often seen, purer forms also may occur. Unlike the germinoma, the tumors in this group are not radiosensitive but do respond to some chemotherapeutic agents. On gross inspection, small and large cysts, necrosis, and hemorrhage may be apparent.

The *embryonal carcinoma* is the most primitive of these tumors. It is composed of cells of cuboidal or columnar epithelium growing in a glandular, tubular, or papillary pattern or in solid sheets.

The *endodermal sinus tumor* (Fig. 75-3), which is probably the most frequent of this rare group, is believed to represent extraembryonic differentiation of the totipotential cell. Less than two dozen such pineal tumors have been reported in the literature. This tumor carries a poor prognosis. Several distinctive histological patterns are described, consisting of reticular arrangement of primitive epithelial cells, communicating cavities and channels, papillary structures, solid areas, and so-called Schiller-Duval bodies. The latter are characterized by the presence of delicate blood vessels surrounded by primitive columnar cells, lying in a space lined

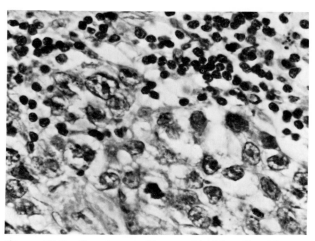

Figure 75-2 Germinoma, 11-year-old girl: cells with large nuclei and prominent nucleoli, below, separated by bands of lymphocytes, above. (Hematoxylin-eosin, ×480.)

by flattened cells. Hyaline intra- and extracellular globules containing alpha fetoprotein are present, and detectable levels of this substance may be measured in the serum, urine, and CSF of affected patients.

The *choriocarcinoma* also is thought to represent extraembryonic differentiation of totipotential cells and most often is a component of another malignant germ cell neoplasm. This tumor is characterized by large, round cytotrophoblastic cells with clear cytoplasm growing with sheets of multinucleated syncytiotrophoblastic cells. Chorionic gonadotropin may be secreted by these cells, and a search for this tumor marker may be of value.

The *teratoma* results from further differentiation of embryonic structures and contains the derivatives of all three germ layers. Like other tumors in this group, the pineal teratomas occur mainly in young males. This is in contrast to the neonatal intracranial teratomas, most of which occur in female infants.[4] These latter are usually massive, and often their precise site of origin cannot be determined, but

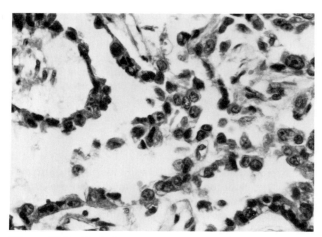

Figure 75-3 Endodermal sinus tumor, 5-year-old boy: channels lined by cuboidal epithelial cells, which also surround delicate blood vessels. (Hematoxylin-eosin, ×480.)

several such tumors arising at the pineal site have been recognized.

Usually teratomas are grossly well-defined and spherical or lobulated, generally remaining localized while compressing surrounding structures. The cut surface is variegated, and areas of cartilage, bone, or even teeth may be recognizable. Cysts are frequently seen and may contain fluid, hair, or keratinous material. Isolated instances of rupture of such cysts have been reported, with discharge of irritating materials into the cerebrospinal fluid compartment.

Microscopically, any combination of tissue elements from the various germ cell layers may be identified. These may be present in the form of mature tissues, frequently including epidermoid or dermoid cysts. Teratomas composed only of fully differentiated tissues are probably the rarest of the group; tumors with immature elements are more common (Fig. 75-4). The presence of immature tissue components does not in itself denote malignancy. The teratomas which behave in an aggressive manner usually contain germ cell elements and less commonly may have a carcinomatous or sarcomatous component such as rhabdomyosarcoma. Intracranial metastases distant from the primary tumor are exceedingly rare. An instance of a pineal tumor with the features of Wilms' tumor probably represents overgrowth of one component of a teratoma.

Tumors of Pineal Parenchyma

Approximately 20 percent of the pineal tumors are derived from the pineal parenchymal cells. About two-thirds of the affected patients are male. The neoplastic cells appear to possess the ability to differentiate along several lines, so that neurons, astrocytes, and retinoblastomatous structures may be identified. The types of pineal parenchymal tumors and their malignant potential are summarized in Table 75-3. The tumors fall into two broad categories: the *pineoblastomas*, in

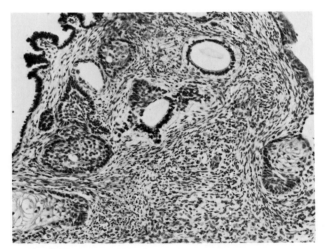

Figure 75-4 Immature teratoma, 11-year-old girl: papillary structures covered by apocrine cells, top left; nests of immature squamous epithelium and small cyst lined by columnar epithelium, middle; respiratory epithelium, far upper right. (Hematoxylin-eosin, ×80.)

TABLE 75-3 Cytological Variants of Tumors of Pineal Parenchymal Cells and Their Biological Behavior

Pineoblastomas:	
With pineocytic differentiation	Malignant
With retinoblastomatous differentiation	Malignant
Pineocytomas:	
With astrocytic differentiation	Malignant or benign
With neuronal differentiation	Benign
With neuronal and astrocytic differentiation ("ganglioglioma of pineal")	Benign

which the predominant component is the undifferentiated immature pineoblastic cell, and the *pineocytomas*, in which cellular differentiation toward the more mature pineocyte has occurred. Combined forms are not infrequent.

In a personally examined series of 28 cases and 12 collected from the literature,[6] it was found that 43 percent (17 patients) of pineal parenchymal tumors were pineoblastomas, 3 of which manifested focal retinoblastomatous differentiation. These tumors occurred primarily in the first two decades, although a few were seen in young adults. They were extremely malignant and disseminated widely throughout the spinal fluid pathways.

In 25 percent (10 patients) the tumors were pineocytomas, which in two instances had an astrocytic component. These tumors occurred at any age, and in about half the cases widespread metastases in the CSF pathway had taken place. The metastases, in both pineoblastomas and pineocytomas, were always of the pineoblastic type. The patients with pineoblastoma or pure pineocytoma did not survive beyond 2 years. Of the two pineocytomas which contained astrocytes, one behaved in a benign, the other in a malignant manner.

The remaining 32 percent (13 patients) were pineocytomas with neuronal or neuronal and astrocytic differentiation. These tumors were seen in the older age groups. They remained localized and grew slowly. The longest survivals, up to 8 years, were recorded in this group. These findings were similar to those of another recently published series.[1]

Accurate histological classification is important and allows prediction of the clinical course as well as selection of the therapeutic approach. Radiotherapy directed not only locally but along the entire neuraxis would be expected to benefit more than two-thirds of the pineal parenchymal tumors, the pineoblastomas, and pure pineocytomas or those with astrocytic differentiation. One-third of the pineal parenchymal tumors which exhibit neuronal or neuronal and astrocytic differentiation, however, are not expected to be radiosensitive. Such neoplasms should be treated by surgical resection.

At the present time only rare attempts have been made to assay HIOMT or melatonin in the serum or tumor tissue from patients with pineal parenchymal neoplasm, so far with inconclusive results. The availability of a radioimmunoassay for melatonin will, it is hoped, encourage future efforts to elucidate the diagnostic usefulness of this substance as a tumor marker.

The gross appearance of tumors of pineal parenchymal origin does not permit them to be distinguished from other

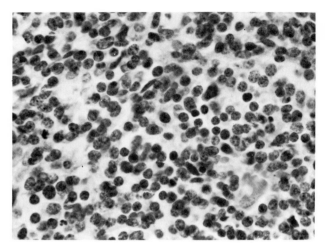

Figure 75-5 Pineoblastoma, 5-year-old boy: closely packed small, round, dark nuclei with scanty cytoplasm and suggestion of neuroblastic (Homer Wright) rosette formation. (Hematoxylin-eosin, ×480.) (Ref. 6, Case 3.)

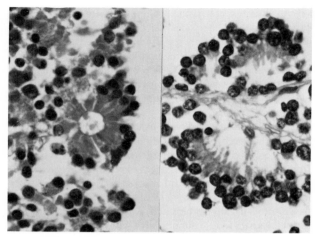

Figure 75-6 Pineoblastoma with retinoblastomatous differentiation, 2¾-year-old boy: left, retinoblastoma (Flexner-Wintersteiner) rosette; right, two fleurettes. (Hematoxylin-eosin, ×480.) (Ref. 6, Case 11.)

pineal neoplasms. Although the benign forms remain circumscribed focal masses, the malignant types will invade locally and disseminate widely. One instance of extracranial metastasis of pineoblastoma has been recorded. Necrosis, cysts, and focal hemorrhages are not uncommon. A special silver carbonate impregnation for pineal parenchyma may help to verify the identity of the tumor cells.

The pineoblastoma is a highly cellular tumor with small, round to oval nuclei, variable numbers of mitoses, and ill-defined, wispy cytoplasm (Fig. 75-5). The tumor resembles .the medulloblastoma, and neuroblastic (Homer Wright) rosettes, characterized by a circular arrangement of nuclei around a fibrillary center, may occasionally be seen. Focal hemorrhages and necrosis are frequent. Areas of pineocytomatous differentiation are not uncommon. Several additional features may be seen. In a small but well-documented number of cases, retinoblastomatous differentiation is recognized in the form of fleurettes and retinoblastoma (Flexner-Wintersteiner) rosettes (Fig. 75-6). These structures represent abortive attempts at photoreceptor development. The fleurettes are believed to be more advanced and consist of a semicircular arrangement of columnar cells with terminal membranes through which project club-shaped processes. The Flexner-Wintersteiner rosettes are more primitive and are characterized by a circular arrangement of columnar cells with a distinct apical membrane. It is not surprising to find such retinoblastomatous differentiation in tumors of pineal origin, in view of the evolution of the pineal gland from a neurosensory photoreceptor organ.

Additional evidence for the close relation between some pineal and retinal neoplasms has accumulated from recent reports of so-called trilateral retinoblastomas. These are bilateral retinoblastomas in young children associated with pineoblastomas and apparently arising from a hereditary genetic abnormality. Isolated cases of pineoblastomas with the mosaic pattern of the developing pineal gland or presence of melanin pigment in pineoblastic cells have also been reported.

The pineocytomas resemble more the normal pineal gland, with a tendency to lobular arrangement (Fig. 75-7) and better defined cellular cytoplasmic processes (Fig. 75-8), which may be directed toward blood vessel walls. Neuronal differentiation may be recognized in pineocytomas and is characterized by two patterns. The first consists of small, dark, round nuclei arranged in groups and sometimes in large rosettes (Fig. 75-9). This picture may predominate or may blend with a more pleomorphic pattern, the second pattern, in which clearly recognizable ganglion cells are identified. A few reports of electron microscopic examination of pineocytomas have verified the neuronal nature of some of the tumor cells. The presence of ganglion cells is usually accompanied by an astrocytic component. In a few instances astrocytic differentiation alone, without neuronal differentiation, has been noted, and in at least one case the astrocytes also appeared malignant.[6]

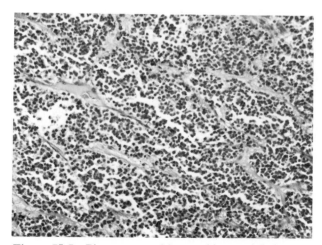

Figure 75-7 Pineocytoma, 26-year-old man: lobular pattern reminiscent of normal pineal gland. (Hematoxylin-eosin, ×120.) (Ref. 6, Case 12.)

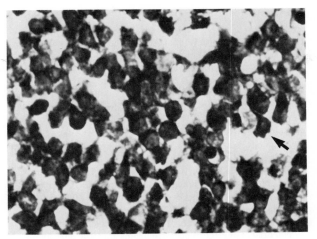

Figure 75-8 Pineocytoma, 69-year-old woman: tumor cells with scant black cytoplasm which is sometimes extended into a single process. (Achucarro-Hortega silver carbonate stain modified by DeGirolami and Zvaigzne, ×960.) (Ref. 6, Case 18.)

Tumors of Glial and Other Cell Origin

The occasional tumors of glial origin which arise at the pineal site are derived either from astrocytes present normally in the gland or from elements of the intimately related surrounding brain tissues. Astroblastoma, astrocytoma, glioblastoma, ependymoma, oligodendroglioma, and choroid plexus papilloma have been identified.[2,9] All histological subtypes of meningiomas have also been described. These are thought to arise from the velum interpositum in the roof of the third ventricle, the junction of the falx and tentorium to which they may be attached, or possibly the connective tissue of the pineal gland itself. Other even rarer findings are a single chemotectoma and craniopharyngioma. Involvement of the pineal gland by metastases from disseminated malignant neoplasms has been reported infrequently. In one series of autopsies of 130 such patients, pineal tumor was present in five, and only in three was the tumor grossly visible.

Non-Neoplastic Cysts and Masses

Small cysts, usually containing gelatinous material, are not infrequent findings in the pineal gland at routine autopsy. Rarely, such cysts become large enough to produce a mass effect. Although usually the result of focal degeneration of the pineal parenchyma, distention of an obliterated portion of the pineal diverticulum has also been postulated as their source. The report of a pineal cyst associated with polycystic kidney disease is intriguing but probably represents coincidence. Epidermoid cysts at the pineal site are usually a part of teratoma, although rare instances without a demonstrable teratomatous component are recognized. Other rare lesions at the pineal site include arachnoid cyst, cysticercus lesions, sarcoid without any systemic manifestations, tuberculoma, and syphilitic gumma.

Behavior and Complications of Pineal Neoplasms

Tumors in the pineal region, like tumors elsewhere, may form a local mass (Fig. 75-10), extend directly to surrounding structures, or metastasize to distal sites. Although in most instances the pineal gland is enlarged or even obliterated by the neoplasm, occasionally there may be only slight change in its size even while the tumor has spread extensively. Sometimes the pineal gland is spared altogether as the tumor arises in the parapineal region. Usually early in the course of the disease the aqueduct of Sylvius is compressed, with consequent increase in intracranial pressure.

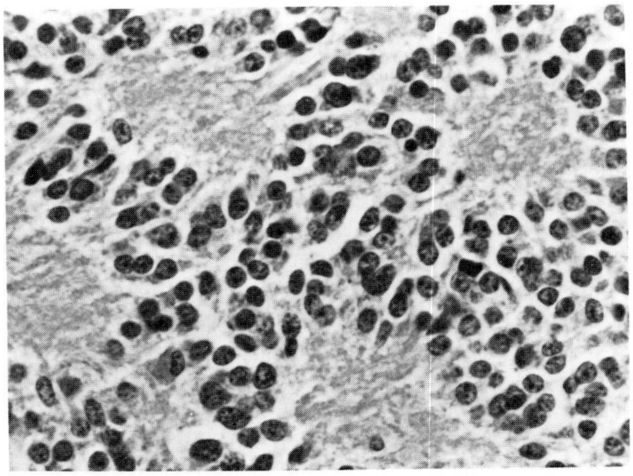

Figure 75-9 Pineocytoma with neuronal differentiation, 78-year-old woman: giant rosettes formed by small, darkly staining nuclei around acellular, faintly fibrillary areas. (Hematoxylin-eosin, ×480.) (Ref. 6, Case 21.)

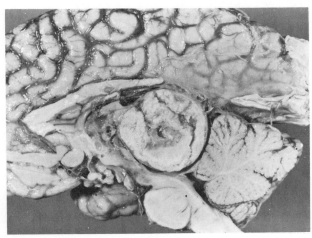

Figure 75-10 Pineal teratoma, 13-year-old boy: circumscribed mass, compressing the midbrain and projecting into the third ventricle. Only mature elements of all germ layers were found.

The neoplasm may compress or infiltrate the tectum of the midbrain, extend into the third ventricle and hypothalamus, and invade infratentorially into the posterior fossa. Dissemination of neoplastic cells throughout the subarachnoid compartment can result in cranial nerve palsies and masses in the distal neuraxis. Extracranial metastases are rare but may occur, usually after surgical intervention. They have been described in tumors of both germ cell and pineal parenchymal cell origin. The tumor disseminates by the hematogenous route, appearing in lungs or other organs. Occasional shunt metastases also have been reported. An uncommon but catastrophic complication is massive hemorrhage into a pineal tumor, which may be accompanied by subarachnoid extension of the blood. Again, several histological tumor types have been involved. In isolated instances hemorrhage into a pineal tumor has also been described with no recognizable predisposing abnormality, as well as hemorrhage into a pineal cyst in a patient receiving anticoagulants.

The importance of arriving at a precise histological diagnosis of each pineal tumor cannot be emphasized enough, since these tumors differ in their biological behavior and response to various modes of therapy.

References

1. Borit A, Blackwood W, Mair WGP: The separation of pineocytoma from pineoblastoma. Cancer 45:1408–1418, 1980.
2. Burger PC, Vogel FS: *Surgical Pathology of the Nervous System and Its Coverings*, 2d ed. New York, Wiley, 1982, pp 398–410.
3. DeGirolami U: Pathology of tumors of the pineal region, in Schmidek HH (ed): *Pineal Tumors*. New York, Masson, 1977, pp 1–19.
4. Gonzalez-Crussi F: *Extragonadal Teratomas*. Atlas of Tumor Pathology, ser 2, fasc 18. Washington, Armed Forces Institute of Pathology, 1982.
5. Haymaker W, Liss L, Vogel FS, Johnson JE Jr, Adams RD, Scharenberg K: The pineal gland, in Haymaker W, Adams RD (eds): *Histology and Histopathology of the Nervous System*. Springfield, Ill, Charles C Thomas, 1982, pp 1801–2023.
6. Herrick MK, Rubinstein LJ: The cytological differentiating potential of pineal parenchymal neoplasms (true pinealomas): A clinicopathological study of 28 tumours. Brain 102:289–320, 1979.
7. Mullen PE, Smith I: The endocrinology of the human pineal. Br J Hosp Med 25:248, 253–256, 1981.
8. Reiter RJ: The mammalian pineal gland: Structure and function. Am J Anat 162:287–313, 1981.
9. Rubinstein LJ: *Tumors of the Central Nervous System*. Atlas of Tumor Pathology, ser 2, fasc 6. Washington, Armed Forces Institute of Pathology, 1972, pp 269–284.
10. Rubinstein LJ: Cytogenesis and differentiation of pineal neoplasms. Hum Pathol 12:441–448, 1981.
11. Russell DS, Rubinstein LJ: *Pathology of Tumors of the Nervous System*, 4th ed. Baltimore, Williams & Wilkins, 1977, pp 283–298.

76

Pineal Region Masses: Radiology

Robert A. Zimmerman

The diagnostic radiographic approach to pineal tumors has changed over the course of the past ten years. Skull radiography, once an important study for a possible pineal neoplasm, has fallen into disuse, because of its low sensitivity in detecting tumor. Unless the neoplasm is calcified, or unless the calcification in the pineal gland is displaced by contigu-

ous tumor or hydrocephalus, or unless changes of increased intracranial pressure are reflected in the sella, sutures, or calvarium, the skull x-ray is not informative. Prior to the advent of computed tomography, the emphasis was on contrast examination of the ventricles and subarachnoid space. In the patient with obstructive hydrocephalus, ventriculography using air or a positive contrast agent was used to define the anatomy of the posterior third ventricle and cerebral aqueduct. In the patient without obstructive hydrocephalus, pneumoencephalography with air introduced by the lumbar route was used to outline the position of the cerebral aqueduct, the configuration of the posterior third ventricle, and the anatomy of the quadrigeminal plate cistern. Carotid arteriography and vertebral arteriography were used to identify the arterial blood supply to the pineal gland, the venous drainage, and vascular displacements due to mass effect and obstructive hydrocephalus. Since the advent of computed tomography, pneumoencephalography and ventriculography are rarely, if ever, done in the diagnostic evaluation of pineal tumors. On occasion a contrast agent such as metrizamide is introduced into the ventricular system or subarachnoid space before computed tomography (CT) of the pineal region is done.[11]

At present, plain and contrast-enhanced CT scans, with or without reconstruction (sagittal or coronal), usually suffice to make the diagnosis of a mass lesion in the region of

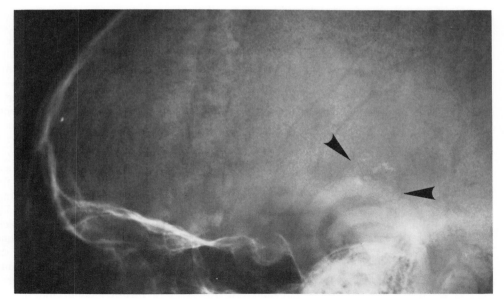

Figure 76-1 Calcified pineocytoma. Lateral skull film of 60-year-old demented male with obstructive hydrocephalus shows a calcified mass (*arrowheads*). There was demineralization of the sella secondary to increased intracranial pressure.

the pineal gland. Cerebral angiography retains a role in the evaluation of pineal neoplasms—that of defining the arterial anatomy, venous drainage, and contiguous critical venous anatomy (position of the internal cerebral veins) when surgical resection is contemplated. Occasionally, blood supply characteristics such as dural tentorial blood supply (tentorial meningioma) may indicate the histological nature of the lesion. The role of nuclear magnetic resonance (NMR), a new imaging modality, in the diagnosis of pineal neoplasms is as yet uncertain. Preliminary evidence, with transverse and sagittal sections, suggests that NMR will be an effective diagnostic modality in identifying abnormalities of the pineal gland. Its histological specificity is at present unknown.

Plain Roentgenograms

A normal pineal gland measures 5 to 9 mm in length and has a height of 3 to 5 mm and a width of up to 6 mm.[8] The calcified pineal gland that is larger than 1 cm in any dimension should be looked upon with suspicion (Figs. 76-1, 76-2). Not only the size of the pineal calcification and its location are important but also the age at which the calcification appears.[17] In the literature on the evaluation of skull roentgenograms it had generally been held that calcification of the pineal gland under the age of 10 was abnormal. However, Schey[14] found that physiological calcification could be seen in persons as young as 6 years. The overall incidence of calcification in childhood has been given by Willich et al.[16] as 0.83 percent and by Peterson and Kieffer[13] as 5.1 percent.

It is clear from the literature on pineal calcification detected on skull roentgenograms that the incidence varies according to the age of the population examined, the quality of the examination, and the genetic makeup of the population.[17] Vastine and Kinney reported an incidence of 47.9 percent[15] in 1927, and Dyke reported an incidence of 51 percent[7] in 1930. The high incidence of pineal calcification

in these series is attributed to the fact that most of their patients were older adults and to their failure to differentiate between pineal calcification and calcification in adjacent structures such as the habenula, choroid plexus, and tento-

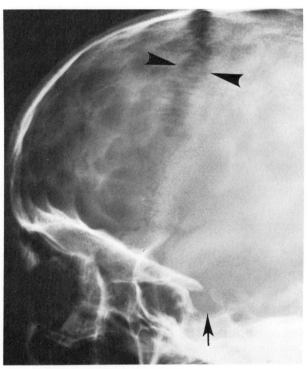

Figure 76-2 Increased intracranial pressure due to pineal tumor. Skull roentgenogram of a child who presented with headaches and paralysis of upward gaze showed splitting of the coronal sutures (*arrowheads*), increased digital markings (so-called beaten copper skull), and demineralization of the floor of the sella (*arrow*).

rium. In the more recent series of Adeloye and Felson,[2] the overall incidence of pineal calcification was 12.2 percent.

Another factor in the incidence of skull radiographic evidence of pineal calcification is genetic. There is a body of literature which gives different rates for pineal calcification according to the country of origin. Thus the incidence for Nigerians has been reported as 5 percent,[6] for Japanese as 9.9 percent,[5] for Fijians as 15 percent,[10] and for Indians as 19 to 24 percent.[10] In contrast to these reports are the similar incidences found for calcification per decade of life by Adeloye and Felson[2] in the American population and by Bhatti and Khan[4] in the Pakistani population. For the first decade of life the incidence was zero in both series, for the second decade it was between 1.5 and 2.3 percent, and for the third decade it was 10.5 percent. The incidence of pineal calcifications in both Americans and Pakistanis rises to 30 percent as the population ages into the middle and later years.

Roentgenograms of the skull may be of diagnostic value in the patient with a pineal tumor if (1) the tumor produces calcification that is visible on the skull films (Fig 76-1); (2) the pineal tumor produces obstructive hydrocephalus with increased intracranial pressure which demineralizes the floor of the sella (Fig. 76-2) or separates the sutures (Fig. 76-2) or the dilated third ventricle amputates the dorsum sellae; or (3) the obstructive hydrocephalus causes inferior and posterior displacement of the pineal calcification(s).

The frequency of positive plain skull films in a series of pineal tumors varies. Abay et al.,[1] in a series of 24 patients with pineal tumors found that in 25 percent the skull roentgenograms were abnormal on the basis of pineal tumor calcification, pineal calcification position, or evidence of increased intracranial pressure. Lin et al. reported a series of 32 pineal neoplasms,[9] with calcifications seen in the region of the pineal in 75 percent. Of those with pineal calcification, the pineal gland was abnormal in size in 21 percent and in an abnormal position in 67 percent. The presence of the pineal calcification was abnormal by age in four of five patients 5 years of age or under (80 percent). The histological classification of the tumors in the patients with abnormally large pineal calcifications was teratoma in two, atypical teratoma in one, and pineoblastoma in two.

Computed Tomograms

Factors that affect the detection of pineal calcification by CT are the thickness of the CT section, the size of the gland, the portion that is calcified, and the density of the calcification.[12] Denser calcifications, thinner sections, and greater calcific portions make identification easier. It has been demonstrated[12] that 8-mm-thick CT sections are eight times more sensitive than skull roentgenograms for the detection of 3-mm calcifications and 22 times more sensitive for 10-mm calcifications.

The youngest patient with a normally calcified pineal gland on CT was age 6½ years in the series of Zimmerman and Bilaniuk.[17] In this series, from ages 8 to 14 years the incidence of pineal calcification ranged between 8 and 11 percent. At age 15 the incidence rose to 30 percent and at

age 17 to 40 percent. Thus the incidence of pineal calcification as detected by CT shows an increase that coincides with the onset of puberty. The presence of a small pineal calcification on CT, in and by itself, from age 6½ up is not evidence for a pineal neoplasm. Calcification under age 6 should be looked upon with suspicion.

Computed tomography has become the primary diagnostic radiographic test for demonstrating the presence or absence of a pineal tumor. In the series of Abay et al.[1] eight of nine CT studies were positive for pineal tumors. In one instance the CT was thought to be normal. In this false-negative study done on a first-generation CT scanner, the image quality was not ideal. In the first 44 pineal neoplasms diagnosed in the author's department since the advent of CT, there were two instances (4.5 percent) in which the pineal tumor was not initially appreciated. In one case, a 12-year-old female presented with abnormal contrast enhancement of the subarachnoid space and a normal pineal region. Several subsequent CT examinations showed the same findings. Eight months after the onset of her headaches, a high-resolution, thin-section CT examination demonstrated the presence of a small pineal tumor. Biopsy revealed pineoblastoma, and examination of the subarachnoid space revealed evidence of tumor seeding. The other patient had previously been treated for bilateral retinoblastomas. She was found to have an "incidental" CT finding of pineal calcification at age 3 (Fig. 76-3A). The patient was followed for a year, during which a soft tissue mass grew around the calcification, producing obstructive hydrocephalus (Fig. 76-3B). Biopsy of this revealed a pineoblastoma. The first case represents a false-negative CT examination due to the small size of the lesion, while the second case represents a failure to appreciate the significance of a too early appearing pineal calcification.

Thirty-one patients with pineal, parapineal, or histologically related tumors were reported by Zimmerman et al.[18] The CT characteristics in that series allowed differentiation between benign (germinal) tumors such as teratomas and epidermoids from malignant germinal tumors such as the germinoma and embryonal cell carcinoma. Primary pineal tumors (pineoblastoma, pineocytoma) could not be differentiated from malignant germinal tumors on the basis of CT criteria alone. Germinomas appeared as a soft tissue mass of slightly greater density than normal brain tissue (Fig. 76-4A). Calcification was not a feature of the tumor matrix in germinomas.[18] Frequently the germinoma surrounded a centrally placed normal-appearing pineal calcification. In the smaller tumors, the germinoma was well defined and did not appear to invade the surrounding brain or subarachnoid spaces. Uniform contrast enhancement was the rule (Fig. 76-4B). With larger germinomas the margins became poorly defined and infiltration into the adjacent brain parenchyma and subarachnoid spaces became common. Cystic changes within the nonoperated tumor were unusual. Embryonal cell carcinomas had similar soft tissue densities to the germinoma, commonly contained tumor calcification (Fig. 76-5), but in contrast to the germinoma more often showed cystic areas. The benign teratomatous tumors showed cystic areas. The benign teratomatous tumors showed evidence of tissue derived from all three germinal layers, such as calcification, ossification, fat, and soft tissue densities (Fig. 76-6).

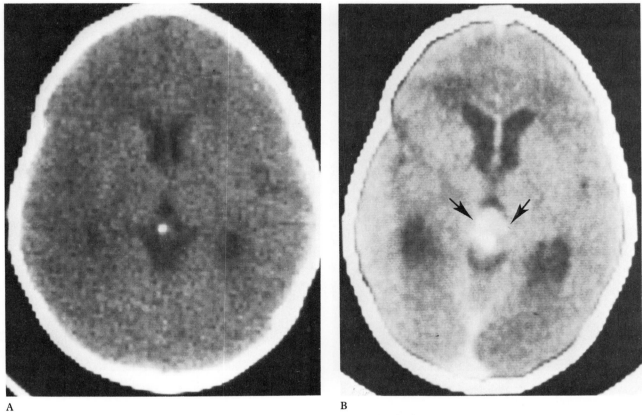

A   B

Figure 76-3 Pineoblastoma. *A*. Pineal calcification without evidence of soft tissue mass is present at age 3. *B*. CT examination 16 months later, following injection of contrast material, shows enhancement of the tumor mass (*arrows*). (From Zimmerman and Bilaniuk.[17])

Epidermoid tumors of the pineal region have a density in the range of CSF and thus may be confused with arachnoid cyst or encysted ventricular structures.

Both the pineocytomas and pineoblastomas show an isodense tumor matrix, contrast enhancement (Figs. 76-3*B*, 76-7), and a tendency toward parenchymal calcifications within the tumor matrix. Two patients with pineoblastomas, when followed by sequential CT examinations prior to treatment, showed rapid tumor growth. All but one of the pineoblastomas presented within the first 12 years of life. The case in which the pineoblastoma presented later, at age 40, occurred in the mother of the child who had presented at age 12 with a pineoblastoma. The increased incidence of pineoblastomas in patients with congenital bilateral retinoblastomas[3] and the occurrence of pineoblastoma in mother and daughter raise the interesting question of genetic predisposition in at least some patients.

Astrocytomas that arise within the pineal gland or adjacent to it either expand the gland, invade it, or displace it. Since a glial stroma supports the pineocytes and is an integral part of the gland, some astrocytomas, presumably a small proportion of those which involve the gland, arise directly from the pineal gland. Most often these tumors are of decreased density relative to brain parenchyma. The contrast enhancement that occurs is usually inhomogeneous.

Calcification infrequently occurs in these tumors, but when it does it may be of such a nature and position that it makes the differential diagnosis between astrocytoma of adjacent structures and nonastrocytic pineal tumor difficult. Because of their location, posterior hypothalamic astrocytomas (Fig. 76-8) and astrocytomas of the tectum of the mesencephalon are also difficult to differentiate from primary pineal tumors on transverse section CT.[18] They frequently abut on the cerebral aqueduct or on the posterior third ventricle, producing obstructive hydrocephalus in a manner similar to that produced by the primary pineal neoplasm. In order to differentiate these tumors by location, careful attention needs to be paid to the size and shape of the tectal region; the radiologist needs to look for forward displacement of the calcified pineal gland by an upper brain stem mass.[18] Sagittally reconstructed sections may be of particular advantage in this situation, as may be the use of subarachnoid metrizamide at the time of sectioning.

In interpreting the computed tomographic findings, attention should be paid to the patient's age and sex. Teratomatous tumors of the pineal region occur almost exclusively in males.[18] Germinomas occur in both males and females, most frequently in the second and third decades. Embryonal cell carcinoma occurs most often in the male in the second decade. Both germinomas and embryonal cell

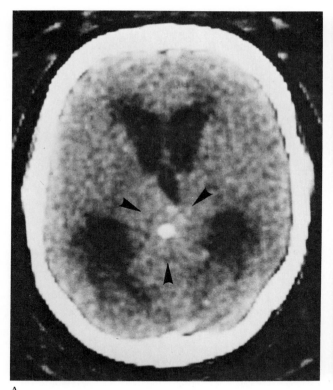

A

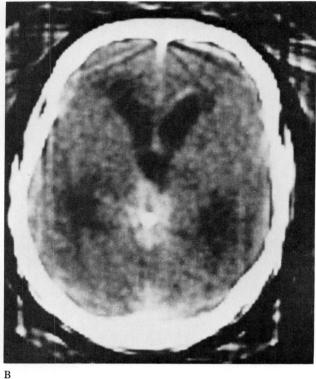

B

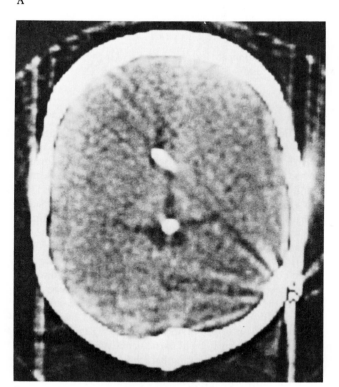

C

Figure 76-4 Pineal germinoma. *A.* Preinjection CT shows a mass (*arrowheads*) of slightly increased density surrounding the calcified pineal gland. The posterior third ventricle is amputated. *B.* CT scan at the same level following contrast injection shows homogeneous enhancement of the mass. (*A* and *B* from Zimmerman et al.[18]) *C.* Computed tomographic study 6 months after radiation therapy shows complete absence of tumor. A shunt is in place.

pineoblastoma group appears equal. In a female patient with a calcified tumor in the pineal region, the most likely diagnosis is primary pineal tumor.

Cerebral Angiograms

The primary blood supply to the pineal gland arises from the posterior medial choroidal artery, a branch of the posterior cerebral artery. This vessel arises from the interpeduncular segment of the posterior cerebral artery, extends superiorly through the cistern of the lamina tecti, and comes to lie on the lateral surface of the pineal gland. The artery continues on past the pineal to supply blood to the choroid plexus in the roof of the third ventricle (Fig. 76-9). The pineal gland is drained by veins that originate from its superior and inferior surfaces. These veins drain into either the internal cerebral

carcinomas are radiosensitive, but only the germinoma (in the author's experience) is radiocurable (Fig. 76-4C). Embryonal cell carcinoma after a period of regression tends to recur promptly. Sex distribution in the pineocytoma-

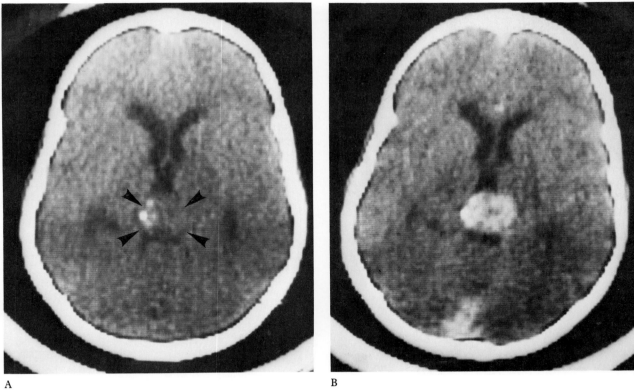

A   B

Figure 76-5 Embryonal cell carcinoma of pineal. *A*. Precontrast CT demonstrates an isodense mass (*arrowheads*) obstructing the posterior third ventricle. Clumps of calcification are present in the tumor. *B*. Postcontrast CT shows dense homogeneous enhancement of the tumor. (From Zimmerman et al.[18])

vein or the great vein of Galen. Superimposed upon the pineal vein anatomy on the lateral vertebral angiogram are the thalamic veins. It is difficult to differentiate pineal from thalamic veins. The internal cerebral vein lies in the roof of the third ventricle, extends posteriorly through the velum interpositum into the cistern of the lamina tecti, where it joins the opposite internal cerebral vein and, with both basilar veins of Rosenthal, forms the vein of Galen. The vein of Galen lies just beneath the splenium of the corpus callosum and extends posteriorly to join with the inferior sagittal sinus, forming the straight sinus which lies at the point of insertion of the falx cerebri onto the tentorium.

In the pathological situation a number of adjacent arterial and venous structures may be displaced or deformed or may provide an abnormal source of blood supply or venous drainage. How often these findings are appreciated angiographically is uncertain. It is probable that the degree to which these findings are appreciated depends upon the quality of the examination. A high-quality examination requires magnification angiography with subtraction, following the deliverance of an adequate volume of contrast agent to the tumor bed in a patient who is able to cooperate. Abay et al.,[1] in a series of 12 pineal tumors studied by angiography, reported the presence of tumor vascularity or stain in 4 (33 percent).

More important than the presence of tumor stain is the recognition of the displacement of adjacent arteries and

veins. Vascular displacements are dependent upon the direction of growth of the neoplasm and upon enlargement of the ventricular system from obstruction of the posterior third ventricle or aqueduct. When the pineal gland is enlarged, the posterior medial choroid artery is displaced posteriorly and laterally (Fig. 76-10*A*), and the superior and inferior pineal veins become more separated. The internal cerebral vein, which lies just above the pineal gland, is impinged on, elevated, and stretched. If the mass effect is sufficient, an angular deformity occurs at the point of juncture between the internal cerebral vein and the vein of Galen (Fig. 76-10*B*). If the tumor is large and extends posterolaterally, the vein of Rosenthal can also be deformed. As the tumor extends back into the cistern of the lamina tecti, down onto the tectum of the mesencephalon, and against the anterior-superior vermis, other changes occur. The superior cerebellar arteries are spread apart within the lamina tecti cistern (Towne projection vertebral arteriogram), the precentral cerebellar veins are flattened and displaced from front to back (lateral vertebral angiogram), and the superior cerebellar artery branches, as they go over the anterior superior vermis, are flattened and deformed from front to back (lateral vertebral arteriogram). If the tumor extends forward (inferiorly), into the floor of the third ventricle, or as the third ventricle dilates from obstructive hydrocephalus, the thalamus-perforating branches that arise from the proximal posterior cerebral arteries and posterior communicating ar-

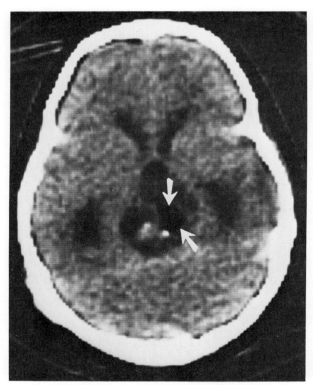

Figure 76-6 Teratoma. Computed tomographic study shows a mass containing fat (*arrows*), ossifications, and soft tissues (two teeth were found at surgical excision). (From Zimmerman et al.[18])

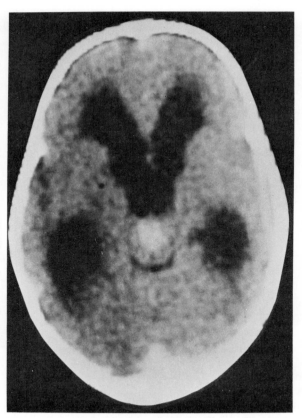

Figure 76-8 Posterior hypothalamic glioma. Postcontrast CT examination shows enhancement of a posterior hypothalamic astrocytoma (surgical biopsy, grade I). (From Zimmerman et al.[18])

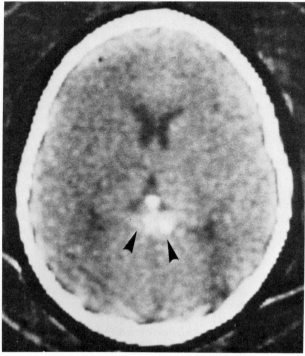

Figure 76-7 Pineocytoma. Postcontrast CT scan shows enhanced tumor filling the quadrigeminal cistern (*arrowheads*). Tumor is contiguous to the posterior aspect of the pineal calcification. (From Zimmerman et al.[18])

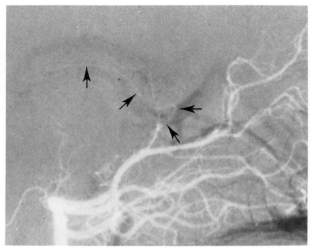

Figure 76-9 Normal vertebral angiogram. Arteries in white, veins in black. Note the normal appearance of the posterior medial choroid artery (*arrows*). The artery terminates in the choroid veins in the roof of the third ventricle.

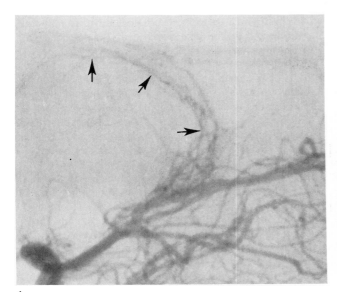
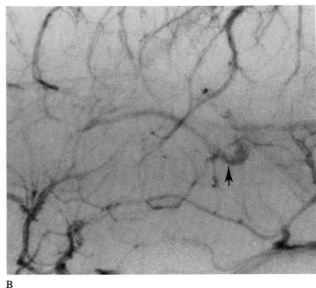

A   B

Figure 76-10   Nine-year-old male with embryonal cell carcinoma of pineal gland. *A.*
Posterior medial choroid artery (*arrows*) is stretched and deformed posteriorly. *B.*
Deformity at the point of juncture of the internal cerebral vein and the vein of Galen
(*arrow*).

teries are displaced and stretched (lateral vertebral arteriogram). With obstructive hydrocephalus, the posterior lateral choroidal arteries (branches of the posterior cerebral artery that supply the choroid plexus in the lateral ventricles) are stretched. In the rare instance of a parapineal tentorial meningioma, selective injection of the internal carotid artery may show its dural blood supply, which arises from the intracavernous portion of the internal carotid artery through the tentorial branch of the meningohypophyseal trunk. Internal carotid arteriography as well as vertebral arteriography are of use in the differential diagnosis of pineal neoplasms when the lesion proves to be a vascular anomaly (such as a vein of Galen aneurysm) that simulates a pineal tumor on CT examination.

References

1. Abay EO II, Laws ER Jr, Grado GL, Brackman JE, Forbes GS, Gomez MR, Scott M: Pineal tumors in children and adolescents; Treatment by CSF shunting and radiotherapy. J Neurosurg 55:889–895, 1981.

2. Adeloye A, Felson B: Incidence of normal pineal gland calcification in skull roentgenograms of black and white Americans. AJR 122:503–507, 1974.

3. Bader JL, Meadows AT, Zimmerman LE, Rorke LB, Voute PA, Champion LAA, Miller RW: Bilateral retinoblastoma with ectopic intracranial retinoblastoma: Trilateral retinoblastoma. Cancer, Genet, Cytogenet 5:203–213, 1982.

4. Bhatti IH, Khan A: Pineal calcifications. JPMA 27:310–312, 1977.

5. Chiba M, Yamanda M: About the calcification of the pineal gland in the Japanese. Folia Psychiatr Neurol [Jpn] 2:301–303, 1948.

6. Daramola GF, Olowu AO: Physiological and radiological implications of a low incidence of pineal calcification in Nigeria. Neuroendocrinology 9:41–57, 1972.

7. Dyke CG: Indirect signs of brain tumor as noted in routine Roentgen examinations: Displacement of the pineal shadow; A survey of 3,000 consecutive skull examinations. AJR 23:598–606, 1930.

8. Harwood-Nash DC, Fitz CR: *Neuroradiology in Infants and Children.* St Louis: Mosby, 1976, vol 2, pp 484–486.

9. Lin S, Crane MD, Lin Z, Bilaniuk L, Plassche WM Jr, Marshall L, Spataro RF: Characteristics of calcification in tumors of the pineal gland. Radiology 126:721–726, 1978.

10. McKay RT: Pineal calcification in Indians and Fijians. Trans R Soc Trop Med Hyg 67:214–216, 1973.

11. Nakstad P, Sortland O, Hovind K: The evaluation of ventriculography as a supplement to computed tomography. Neuroradiology 23:85–88, 1982.

12. Norman D, Diamond C, Boyd D: Relative detectability of intracranial calcifications on computed tomography and skull radiography. J Comput Assist Tomogr 2:61–64, 1978.

13. Peterson HO, Kieffer SA: *Introduction to Neuroradiology.* Hagerstown, Md., Harper & Row, 1972, p 10.

14. Schey WL: Intracranial calcifications in childhood: Frequency of occurrence and significance. AJR 122:495–502, 1974.

15. Vastine JH, Kinney KK: The pineal shadow as an aid in the localization of brain tumors. AJR 17:320–324, 1927.

16. Willich E, Sellier W, Weigel W: Die intrakraniellen Verkalkungen des Kindes alters. Fortschr Geb Roentgenstr Nuklearmed Erganzungsband 116:735–750, 1972.

17. Zimmerman RA, Bilaniuk LT: Age-related incidence of pineal calcification detected by computed tomography. Radiology 142:659–662, 1982.

18. Zimmerman RA, Bilaniuk LT, Wood JH, Bruce DA, Schut L: Computed tomography of pineal, parapineal, and histologically related tumors. Radiology 137:669–677, 1980.

77

Pineal Masses: Clinical Features and Management

Henry H. Schmidek
Alan Waters

Clinical Features

Pineal tumors are a heterogeneous group of mass lesions originating in or located adjacent to the pineal gland. Neoplasms in this region cause symptoms when they compress or invade local structures or are disseminated beyond the confines of the tumor. When these tumors occlude the cerebral aqueduct, obstructive hydrocephalus with intracranial hypertension occurs; if the superior colliculus and pretectal area are involved, characteristic eye signs develop, which may include impairment of upward gaze and abnormalities of the pupil, paralysis or spasm of convergence, and nystagmus retractorius. This sylvian aqueduct syndrome is indicative of a periaqueductal lesion. Parinaud's syndrome, the paralysis of upward gaze alone, is often and incorrectly used as synonymous with sylvian aqueduct syndrome. The anatomical substrate underlying these functions is located just anterior to the aqueduct and below the posterior part of the third ventricle. Downward gaze, which may also be impaired in these patients, has its localization caudal to that of upward gaze in the brain stem. Compression or invasion of the cerebellum results in dysmetria, hypotonia, and intention tremor. There may be altered consciousness due to intracranial hypertension or direct invasion of the brain stem by tumor. Some of these tumors metastasize to the spinal cord or cauda equina or to structures outside the nervous system. These metastases may pass through the shunts inserted to treat intracranial hypertension. Less common symptoms, occurring in less than 10 percent of male patients with pineal tumors, are precocious puberty or delayed onset of sexual maturation. Even less common is the occurrence of pineal apoplexy, in which a patient undergoes sudden neurological deterioration secondary to intratumoral hemorrhage and sudden expansion in the size of the posterior third ventricular tumor.

The lesions in the posterior third ventricle represent a diverse group of tumors; however, the crucial differentiation prognostically is between those lesions which are benign and those which are malignant. Approximately 10 percent of le-

sions in this area are truly benign, including cysts, lipomas, arteriovenous malformations and aneurysms, pineocytomas, and meningiomas. Another 5 to 10 percent of tumors are relatively benign, including the low-grade gliomas and dermoids. The remaining 80 to 85 percent of pineal region neoplasms are highly malignant lesions. These include the germ cell tumors typified by the atypical teratoma (pineal germinoma), also teratocarcinoma, choriocarcinoma, endodermal sinus tumor, pineoblastoma, glioblastoma, metastatic tumor, sarcoma, and mixed tumors with two or more of these components.

The suprasellar germinomas are included in this family of neoplasms. These are a subgroup of tumors, histologically identical to the pineal germinoma, which arise in or beneath the anterior part of the third ventricle. Germinomas represent a distinct pathological entity arising from germ cells that originate from yolk-sac endoderm, migrate widely, and settle in the gonadal ridges of the embryo. Normally, the nongonadal cells disappear from these sites; a failure of these cells to involute in the retroperitoneum, sacrococcygeal region, mediastinum, cerebral hemisphere, or pineal or suprasellar region forms the cellular basis for an identical group of tumors which occasionally arise at these diverse locations. Many suprasellar germinomas represent anterior extension of a pineal germinoma; however, suprasellar germinomas have been shown to exist free of pineal involvement.

Kageyama and Belsky[9] categorized these suprasellar tumors. The type 1 suprasellar germinoma is a metastatic tumor from the pineal which invades the floor of the third ventricle, hypophysis, and optic pathways. The symptoms are those typical of pineal tumor and of hypothalamic and chiasmatic involvement. At the time of diagnosis there is commonly an admixture of these signs and symptoms, indicating involvement of both anterior and posterior third ventricular structures. Type 2 germinomas are those which arise within the third ventricle and produce an obstructive hydrocephalus early in the disease; later findings are indicative of invasion of the hypothalamus, pituitary, and optic pathways. Type 3 germinomas are those which originate in the region of the optic chiasmal region, grow outside the ventricular system, and only late in the disease invade the third ventricle and hypothalamus.

When there is suprasellar involvement, the patient may present with a triad of findings including diabetes insipidus, visual defects, and other evidence of endocrine dysfunction. Diabetes insipidus is the most common manifestation of these tumors and may precede the development of other findings by years. The abnormalities of the visual system encountered include reduction in visual acuity, often in conjunction with optic atrophy. There are isolated reports of extraocular paralysis or severe exophthalmos due to infiltration of the tumor into the optic chiasm, nerves, and orbit. Papilledema may not be evident, even in the presence of severe intracranial hypertension, because of the associated optic atrophy. Visual field studies may demonstrate bitemporal inferior scotomas, indicating a lesion on the dorsum of the chiasm. Macular fiber involvement by tumor growing into the posterior and superior part of the chiasm, associated with a bitemporal inferior scotomatous defect, is particularly characteristic of this tumor. Hypopituitarism is the third most common finding, after diabetes insipidus and visual abnormalities, and is often associated with growth arrest when the tumor occurs before puberty or with hypogonadism and amenorrhea when it occurs in older patients. Pathological obesity, neurogenic hypernatremia, abnormalities in temperature regulation, and excessive somnolence are uncommon manifestations reported in conjunction with these lesions. Elevated intracranial pressure is seen in tumors arising by extension from pineal region neoplasms. Suprasellar germinomas may also metastasize throughout the neuraxis.

The skull roentgenograms are abnormal in approximately 50 percent of patients with pineal region tumors, indicating changes secondary to chronic intracranial hypertension, and there may be abnormalities in the amount and configuration of calcification in the pineal region suggesting the presence of an aneurysm, dermoid, meningioma, low-grade glioma, or germinoma. Subtle abnormal findings are also found on the skull films in about 50 percent of suprasellar germinomas. These may disclose ballooning of the sella or decalcification of the posterior clinoid. Chest radiography is part of the investigation, to exclude a primary malignant disease of the lung or a tumor that may have metastasized to both lung and brain.

Computerized tomography of the head with enhancement indicates the size and position of the lesion; whether there is a calcific, cystic, or hemorrhagic component; the degree of hydrocephalus; and whether there is evidence of subependymal extension or extension into the lateral ventricles or the suprasellar region. The suprasellar extension from a posterior third ventricular mass may be quite subtle and may require serial thin sections for detection, especially of the subependymal enhancement. The suprasellar germinomas may show obliteration of the suprasellar cistern, irregular margins, moderate enhancement by contrast material, and tumor infiltration of the wall of the third ventricle and both lateral ventricles. There may also be extension into the orbit and expansion of the optic nerves or chiasm due to tumor infiltration.

Cytological examination of the cerebrospinal fluid is important, since the presence of malignant cells may establish the nature and extent of the lesion. Seeding of the cerebrospinal fluid is a particularly characteristic feature of the germinomas, although this property is also exhibited by an occasional pineoblastoma. Among brain tumors, the medulloblastomas have the highest incidence of malignant cells in the cerebrospinal fluid, 61.9 percent; however, the incidence of this phenomenon in patients with malignant pineal tumors is not known. There are reports of this occurrence in up to 60 percent of cases serially examined, especially when the sensitivity of the cerebrospinal fluid examination is improved by the use of millipore-filtered CSF tissue culture techniques.

Angiographic examination of both the carotid and the vertebral systems should allow identification of aneurysms of the posterior cerebral artery, arteriovenous malformations, abnormalities of the vein of Galen, and meningiomas, thereby allowing these lesions to be appropriately treated. Although germinomas are vascular, it is unusual for them to contain neovascularity demonstrable by angiography, whereas embryonal carcinoma and teratocarcinoma show tumor vessels, and the presence of such tumor vascularity is suggestive of these malignant tumors. In addition, angiography provides important preoperative information about the relation of the internal cerebral veins, vein of Galen, basal veins of Rosenthal, and precentral cerebellar vein to the mass lesion.

Whether a myelographic examination of the spinal axis should be performed in patients with a posterior third ventricular neoplasm of undefined character is problematic. It is the policy on the authors' service to undertake this examination as part of the investigation both during the initial set of diagnostic studies and often serially in the patient with a malignant tumor, in order to identify asymptomatic spinal metastases or assess the response of these to therapy. The presence of such lesions is of major diagnostic and therapeutic importance, particularly since one cannot determine with a high degree of accuracy the nature of an isolated posterior third ventricular mass on the basis of radiographic studies alone. Currently, one cannot distinguish the benign from the malignant posterior third ventricular tumor on the basis of tumor enhancement, size, and tumor margination alone.

The patient with a posterior third ventricular tumor requires as part of the investigation a careful assessment of endocrine function.[13] Diabetes insipidus is the most common endocrine abnormality associated with pineal tumors; when present, it is probably due to anterior third ventricular extension of the neoplasm. Such cases are often overlooked. The physician should be suspicious and should undertake appropriate provocative tests. Tests of anterior pituitary function are also part of the investigation, to exclude ACTH deficiency and secondary, possibly life-threatening, adrenocortical insufficiency. Abnormalities of sexual maturation require that the levels of LH, FSH, testosterone, prolactin, and growth hormone and the melatonin-forming activity of the cerebrospinal fluid and serum be surveyed.

Neuro-ophthalmologic examination is mandatory in search of the defects seen in conjunction with these lesions and to provide evidence of the extent of the tumor involvement—which may not be apparent from the other studies—as well as a baseline for comparison after treatment.

Immunoassay for alpha fetoprotein (AFP) and the beta chain of human chorionic gonadotropin (hCG) may allow the diagnosis of an intracranial germ cell tumor (i.e., germinoma, teratocarcinoma, choriocarcinoma, or embryonal carcinoma). Forty to fifty percent of germinomas and embryonal carcinomas are hCG-producing tumors, and the embryonal carcinoma can also produce AFP. Cases have been reported in which the tumor produces both AFP and hCG, although no tumor has been reported as producing AFP alone.[7] In addition, the plasma level of these tumor markers correlates with tumor growth and regression and may be used to assess the response to therapy.[6] Plasma melatonin has also been used as a marker of pineal tumors, although there may be significant extrapineal sources of melatonin, so that even when a pineal tumor and raised melatonin levels exist, the value of this test has been questioned.[1]

Since pineal region tumors are among the most dangerous intracranial masses to excise, there has been an ongoing debate for at least the last half-century concerning their surgical management. The debate centers on whether it is in the patient's best interest to explore these lesions at the time of their diagnosis, or whether the obstructive hydrocephalus should be treated with a shunt and the posterior third ventricular tumor irradiated without a tissue diagnosis—maneuvers which can be carried out with a mortality rate of under 5 percent. Until the last decade the high morbidity and mortality associated with attempts to biopsy or excise tumors in this location provided ample reason for this debate. In response to the challenge, the last decade has seen increasingly frequent reports of exploration of these tumors by standard microsurgical techniques, with an ever lessening mortality and morbidity. These reports, by Jamieson,[8] Neuwelt et al.,[11] Chapman and Linggood,[2] Sano and Matsutani,[12] Ventureyra,[20] and Stein,[15] represent an aggregate of 128 cases of posterior third ventricular tumor subjected to direct exploration. In this combined series there were two operative deaths, one from hemorrhage into a glioblastoma occurring 1 week after surgery, the other related to a large infiltrating tumor of the midbrain which had been previously irradiated.[15]

Even though it is now feasible for highly experienced surgeons to operate on lesions in the posterior third ventricle with an acceptable risk, patients in whom cytological examination of the cerebrospinal fluid shows malignant cells, patients with evidence of either spinal or extraneural metastases, and patients in whom both an anterior and a posterior third ventricular tumor are demonstrable (particularly if one of the tumor marker assays is abnormally high) are harboring a germinoma or other malignant germ cell tumor and may not require direct intervention. In contrast to these cases, there is a strong indication for surgical intervention in those tumors which, on the basis of the investigations, have a particularly high likelihood of being benign—e.g., the cyst or dermoid; those cases in which investigations do not allow characterization of the tumor; and those patients previously treated with shunt and radiation without a tissue diagnosis who present with progressive neurological problems in the presence of a functioning shunt. Patients in this latter group have often survived for a period of years, and benign or relatively benign tumors are particularly frequent among this select group of cases, whereas the danger of radionecrosis from further radiotherapy is high. A significant percentage of cases in the surgical series reported since 1971 associated with a favorable outcome include cases of this type.

Surgical Techniques for Biopsy or Excision

Several approaches which do not involve craniotomy can be used to biopsy and treat pineal tumors. A particularly interesting report is that of Moser and Backlund[10] of 19 patients with solid pineal region tumors managed by stereotactic radiosurgery at the Karolinska Hospital, Stockholm, between 1969 and 1981. In 17 of these patients satisfactory biopsy samples were obtained by stereotactic biopsy carried out without complication. Patients with germinoma were then treated with conventional radiotherapy, and those with astrocytoma, pineocytoma and pineoblastoma, ependymoma, and medulloblastoma received a single radionecrotizing dose of 5000 to 7500 rad to the tumor volume, using the gamma radiosurgical instrument. The radiosur-

gical procedure is usually accomplished in 30 to 60 min, and the patients are routinely discharged the following day. With a mean follow-up period of 5.4 years, there is a 69 percent survival rate in this group of patients.

Conway[4] reported an experience with 31 deep-seated intracranial tumors stereotactically biopsied. In 28 of these cases diagnostic specimens were obtained. Six patients in this group had tumors of the posterior third ventricle. There were no deaths and no significant morbidity among this group of 31 patients. This experience was then reaffirmed by Sugita et al.,[16] who performed stereotactic biopsies in 10 patients with pineal masses without complications. In two patients Conway repeated the biopsies when the patients exhibited clinical progression in the absence of intracranial hypertension or shunt malfunction 1.5 and 3 years after radiation. After the biopsies, which in one case yielded residual evidence of tumor and in the second case a fresh blood clot and white matter, a cryoprobe replaced the biopsy instrument and the area was frozen incrementally for a total of 6 min at between −40 and −80°C. The liquefied tissue was aspirated. Subsequently, the patients' brain stem and pupillary signs improved.

There are as yet no reports of biopsy of pineal region masses guided by CT scanning. This technique is now routinely used in dealing with a variety of brain tumors and will undoubtedly allow the pineal area to be biopsied accurately and safely.

Fukushima,[5] using the flexible ventriculoscope, has been able to successfully biopsy pineal region tumors. This instrument, which has an outside diameter of 4 mm and a tip capable of bending 30° in an upward direction and 130° downward, is introduced into the ventricle through a burr hole, and the lesion is then biopsied. Fukushima takes only one biopsy in avascular tumors, using a small cup-type probe. A definitive diagnosis was obtained in 11 of 21 intracranial tumors studied (52.4 percent). The relatively low yield compared with the stereotactic procedure is largely attributable to either too small or too few specimens being taken.

Since the early decades of this century a variety of operations have been devised to allow direct surgical exploration of the pineal region. Dandy's transcallosal approach is performed through a parieto-occipital craniotomy, exposing the posterior half of the cerebral hemisphere (Fig. 77-1). When the hemisphere is retracted laterally, the corpus callosum is exposed and the posterior half of the corpus callosum is incised, exposing the deep cerebral veins and the pineal tumor. In this exposure the veins are usually dorsal and lateral to the tumor. Horrax modified the operation by excising the occipital lobe, to overcome the amount of retraction needed to expose a large tumor.

Both Poppen and Jamieson[8] initially used this approach to the pineal region but subsequently modified it. Poppen modified the operation so that after exposing the occipital lobe, the lateral ventricle is cannulated and the occipital lobe mobilized in an upward direction, exposing the tentorium. A wedge of tentorium is removed, exposing the tumor, which is then aspirated, biopsied, or excised. The corpus callosum is not sectioned. Jamieson experienced difficulty with Poppen's approach and the limited exposure and excessive retraction required in attempting to remove a pineocy-

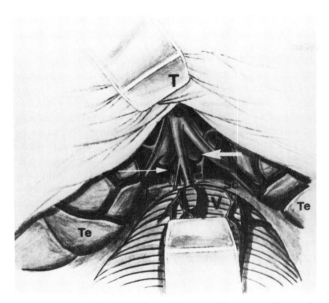

Figure 77-1 Infratentorial-supracerebellar view. Internal cerebral vein (*large white arrow*); pineal gland (*thin white arrow*). G, vein of Galen; Sc, superior colliculi; T, tentorium; Te, medial inferior temporal lobe; V, superior vermis. (From Quest DO, Kleriga E: Microsurgical anatomy of the pineal region. Neurosurgery 6:385–390, 1980.)

toma. Because of the subsequent hemorrhage into the occipital lobe, it was then necessary to perform an occipital lobectomy after the tumor's removal, which resulted in a permanent homonymous hemianopsia. Jamieson's operation is performed with the patient lying on the left side, with the head rotated downward; the surgeon operates from behind the patient's right shoulder. The right lateral ventricle is cannulated and the cerebrospinal fluid aspirated. The occipital pole is then mobilized in a superior and lateral direction, exposing the tentorium. The tentorium is divided to its free edge, and the posterior cerebral artery, superior cerebellar artery, and third and fourth cranial nerves are identified. The tumor is exposed, along with the vein of Galen and its branches draped over the surface of the mass. The tumor is then removed from beneath these venous structures, using standard microsurgical techniques and instrumentation. Clark[3] performs essentially this same operation with the patient in a sitting rather than a recumbent position.

Ten years after Dandy's original report, Van Wagenen[19] reported exploration of a pineal tumor through a right parieto-occipital craniotomy and corticectomy. The corticectomy extends from the superior parietal lobule to the superior temporal gyrus and enters the atrium of the lateral ventricle. After the medial wall of the ventricle is opened, the tumor is exposed, as are the deep veins at its base. Van Wagenen was able to remove all but a small amount of the tumor using this exposure. Postoperatively the patient had a hemiparesis, hemisensory loss, and hemianopsia which cleared within the next year.

In 1971 Stein[14] reintroduced the posterior fossa–supracerebellar approach to the pineal region (Fig. 77-2). This approach was first discussed by Horsley, who in 1910 used it to excise pineal tumors in two patients. In 1926,

Krause formally described the infratentorial–supracerebellar approach to the pineal region. The operation has the specific advantage of avoiding the deep venous structures usually situated dorsal and lateral to these tumors. (Injury to these veins, which drain the diencephalon, basal ganglia, midbrain, and medial part of the hemisphere, results in a venous infarction which is usually fatal.) The approach has the specific disadvantage that the distance between the collicular plate and the tentorial hiatus may be very small, limiting the exposure above the tentorial notch when viewed from an infratentorial position. This may present a problem in exposing a lesion above the tentorial notch in the region of the posterior third ventricle and especially paramedian lesions adjacent to this area. The tentorium may, however, be sectioned through the posterior fossa to provide the necessary exposure. In addition, the amount of retraction of important structures is less than required with the supratentorial operation.

This procedure is performed in the sitting position except in young children. A suboccipital craniectomy extending to the transverse sinus and torcular is performed and extended inferiorly to the foramen magnum. The tentorium is retracted upward, and the bridging veins from the upper surfaces of the cerebellum are sacrificed. Under magnification, the arachnoid of the quadrigeminal region is opened. This tissue is usually thickened and opaque in the presence of a tumor. The deep veins above and lateral to the tumor are apparent. The tumor is aspirated, and if it is not vascular or cystic, the capsule is opened and the tumor decompressed. Only in the encapsulated lesion that dissects easily from the surrounding structures is total excision even at-

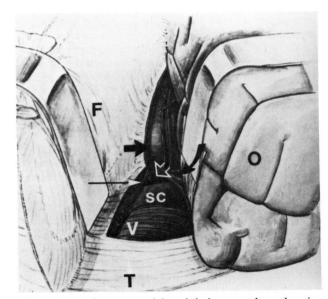

Figure 77-2 Supratentorial-occipital approach to the pineal region. Splenium of the corpus callosum (*straight black arrow*); pineal gland (*open arrow*); basal vein of Rosenthal (*curved black arrow*); superior vermian vein (*white arrowhead*). F, falx; O, occipital lobe; T, tentorium; V, superior vermis; SC, superior colliculus. (From Quest DO, Kleriga E: Microsurgical anatomy of the pineal region. Neurosurgery 6:385–390, 1980.)

tempted. Tumors may begin in the pineal region and expand either superiorly or below the tentorium, and it may then be necessary to divide the overlying splenium when dealing with superior extensions or to split the upper vermis for inferior tumor extensions. Should the obstructive hydrocephalus not have been relieved by a previous operation, a ventriculocisternostomy or another type of shunt can be performed. Alternatively, external ventricular drainage may be continued for several days and a shunt performed subsequently.

There are several alternative surgical approaches to deal with tumors in the pineal region. In the presence of an obstructive hydrocephalus it is often wise to divert the cerebrospinal fluid through a shunt prior to undertaking direct exploration of the tumor. If the area is to be explored via craniotomy, for these lesions within the posterior third ventricle a parietal transcallosal approach may be most suitable, whereas lesions situated within or below the quadrigeminal cistern can be explored by the supracerebellar-infratentorial approach, and lesions above the quadrigeminal cistern and bulging into the posterior third ventricle by the occipital transtentorial approach.

Several surgical options also exist for the exploration of a tumor adjacent to the anterior third ventricle, depending on whether the mass is predominantly intra- or extra-axial. For lesions within the third ventricle, a transfrontal-transcortical approach, a transcallosal approach, or a closed biopsy by one of the techniques described above can be used. The exploration of suprasellar germinomas, unlike that of tumors of the posterior third ventricle, is not controversial. The results of several series show that these tumors can be explored safely at the time they are diagnosed, vital structures can be decompressed, and the pathologic nature of the tumor can be verified prior to radiotherapy. There is little justification for the irradiation of these tumors prior to surgical intervention. In the series of Sano and Matsutani, 20 suprasellar germinomas were operated on without deaths and with 1-year and 5-year survival rates of 100 percent following radiation therapy and a 10-year survival rate of 92 percent.[12]

There is controversy as to whether, in treating malignant pineal tumors, radiation should be confined to the head or extended to include the entire neuraxis. The exquisite responsiveness of the germinoma to radiation, as assessed by serial CT scans performed during treatment in five cases of presumed (i.e., not histologically confirmed) germinoma, has been described by Takaki et al.[18] It was possible to detect evidence of clinical improvement when the patient had received 1200 rad, with a change in the clinical effects preceding the changes to be seen on CT scanning. At 1500 rad a marked decrease in tumor size was detectable, coincident with a decrease in the tumor's contrast enhancement. With further radiation there was gradual normalization of the ventricular system and cisterns, and by 5000 rad the tumor had disappeared entirely. The concern is whether the prophylactic irradiation of the entire neuraxis is necessary in tumors, such as the germinoma and pineoblastoma, which have a propensity to seed throughout the nervous system, since bone marrow suppression, growth arrest of the spine, and radiation effects on the ovaries or testes attend this approach. The other reason for controversy is that reliable figures are not available on the incidence of spinal metastases,

although there are estimates of 15 to 57 percent.[17] Symptomatic spinal metastases occur in approximately 15 percent of cases. On the authors' service, neuraxis radiation is currently reserved for patients with histologically proven germinoma and for patients with a posterior third ventricular neoplasm and cerebrospinal fluid cytology positive for malignant cells or in whom spinal implants are revealed on myelography. The remaining patients are treated on an individualized basis in consultation with the radiotherapist.

The absence of the blood-brain barrier in the pineal gland suggests that lesions located there may have an increased vulnerability to systemic chemotherapy. Objective remission has been reported in a pineal tumor with pulmonary metastases treated with chlorambucil, methotrexate, and dactinomycin. In addition, testicular germinomas, which are histologically identical to pineal germinomas, have shown an 82 percent remission rate when treated with bleomycin, vinblastine, and cis-platinum.[11] These forms of chemotherapy are currently reserved for patients presenting with systemic, extraneural metastases or those with recurrent disease within the neuraxis following full courses of radiation therapy in whom further radiation is not an option.

References

1. Barber SG, Smith JA, Hughes RC: Melatonin as a tumour marker in a patient with pineal tumour. Br Med J 2:328, 1978.
2. Chapman PH, Linggood, RM: The management of pineal area tumors: A recent reappraisal. Cancer 46:1253–1257, 1980.
3. Clark K: The occipital transtentorial approach to the pineal region, in Schmidek HH, Sweet WH (eds): *Operative Neurosurgical Techniques: Indications and Methods*. New York, Grune & Stratton, 1982, pp 595–597.
4. Conway LW: Stereotaxic diagnosis and treatment of intracranial tumors including an initial experience with cryosurgery for pinealomas. J Neurosurg 38:453–460, 1973.
5. Fukushima T: Endoscopic biopsy of intraventricular tumors with the use of a ventriculofiberscope. Neurosurgery 2:110–113, 1978.
6. Gindhart TD, Tsukahara YC: Cytologic diagnosis of pineal germinoma in cerebrospinal fluid and sputum. Acta Cytol (Baltimore) 23:341–346, 1979.
7. Haase J, Nielsen K: Value of tumor markers in the treatment of endodermal sinus tumors and choriocarcinomas in the pineal region. Neurosurgery 5:485–488, 1979.
8. Jamieson KG: Excision of pineal tumors. J Neurosurg 35:550–553, 1971.
9. Kageyama N, Belsky R: Ectopic pinealoma in the chiasma region. Neurology 11:318–327, 1961.
10. Moser RP, Backlund EO: Stereotactic radiosurgery in pineal region tumors. Presented at the 51st Annual Meeting of the American Association of Neurological Surgeons, Honolulu, Hawaii, April 25, 1982.
11. Neuwelt EA, Glasberg M, Frenkel E, Clark WK: Malignant pineal region tumors: A clinico-pathological study. J Neurosurg 51:597–607, 1979.
12. Sano K, Matsutani M: Pinealoma (germinoma) treated by direct surgery and postoperative irradiation: A long-term follow-up. Childs Brain 8:81–97, 1981.
13. Schmidek HH (ed): *Pineal Tumors*. New York, Masson, 1977.
14. Stein BM: The infratentorial supracerebellar approach to pineal lesions. J Neurosurg 35:197–202, 1971.
15. Stein BM: Supracerebellar approach for pineal region neo-

plasms, in Schmidek HH, Sweet WH (eds): *Operative Neurosurgical Techniques: Indications and Methods*. New York, Grune & Stratton, 1982, pp 599–607.

16. Sugita K, Matsuga N, Takaoka Y, Hirota T, Shibuya M, Doi T: Stereotaxic exploration of para-third ventricle tumors. Confin Neurol 37:156–162, 1975.

17. Sung DI, Harisiadis L, Chang CH: Midline pineal tumors and suprasellar germinomas: Highly curable by irradiation. Radiology 128:745–751, 1978.

18. Takaki S, Hikita T, Ishii C, Nakayama K, Aiba H: Serial computed tomographic studies of pineal region tumor treated by irradiation. Kurume Med J 26:163–173, 1979.

19. Van Wagenen WP: A surgical approach for the removal of certain pineal tumors: Report of a case. Surg Gynecol Obstet 53:216–220, 1931.

20. Ventureyra ECG: Pineal region: Surgical management of tumours and vascular malformations. Surg Neurol 16:77–84, 1981.

SECTION G

Cerebellopontine Angle Tumors

78

Tumors of the Cerebellopontine Angle: Pathology

F. Stephen Vogel

An angle is defined geometrically as the intersection of two lines. This definition inadequately depicts the physical union of the cerebellum with the pons. Alternatively, an angle is "a secluded place, a nook." Although this definition characterizes a property of the anatomy, it does not truly portray its configuration, for the ventral aspect of the cerebellum adjoins the pons with the conformation of an elongated cleavage, a furrow, bounded by two hemispheric structures. Cranial nerves V and VII to XI cross this cleavage as strands of a necklace (Fig. 78-1), and the leptomeninges drape it as a diaphanous shawl.

The native structures of the cerebellopontine angle give rise to three categories of neoplasms: schwannomas, meningiomas, and arachnoid cysts. The last two are discussed elsewhere in this textbook, since their frequency is greater in other locations. Epithelial cells are displaced into the posterior fossa during embryonic development and, with the passage of time, evolve dermoid and epidermoid cysts. These are the so-called cholesteotomas, also discussed in other chapters. The anatomical structures that are contiguous to the cerebellopontine angle also spawn a variety of neoplasms which enlarge, impinge upon, disfigure, and occupy the angle. These neoplasms include exophytic pontine gliomas (Fig. 78-2), cerebellar hemangioblastomas, papillomas and carcinomas of the choroid plexus, ependymomas, and a variety of insurgent lesions that penetrate the base of the skull. Among the latter are chemodectomas or glomus jugulare tumors (Fig. 78-3), chordomas, metastatic lesions (Fig. 78-

4), and nasopharyngeal carcinomas (the latter referred to as *Schmincke's tumors*). These lesions also are discussed in other chapters.

Uncertainty of the cell of origin contributed to the multiplicity of names for the schwannoma, notably, perineural fibroblastoma (Penfield), neurilemmoma, schwannoma, and neurinoma. Among these, the term *schwannoma* seems most appropriate, since it designates the constituent cell.

Schwannomas manifest a penchant for involvement of the acoustic nerve. This makes it appropriate to discuss this entity in its anatomical relation to the cerebellopontine angle.

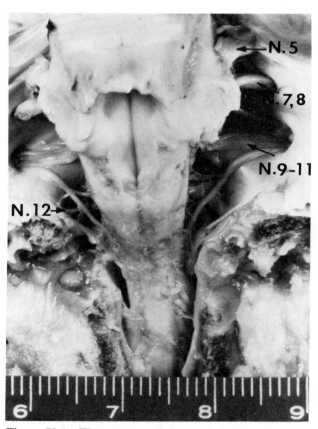

Figure 78-1 The anatomy of the cerebellopontine angle is revealed upon excision of the cerebellar hemispheres. Note the proximity of cranial nerves VII, V, and IX to XI to the porus acusticus.

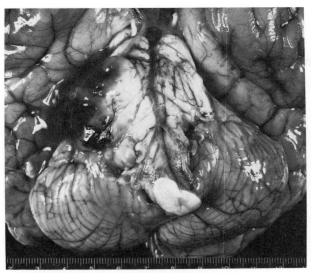

Figure 78-2 An exophytic mass protrudes from a pontine glioma into the right cerebellopontine angle of a 19-year-old girl, who died after a 2-week history of headaches, weakness, ptosis, and coma.

The anatomical peculiarities of the acoustic nerve predispose it to neoplastic transformation, for unlike other cranial and spinal nerves, glia form the matrix of the proximal 8 to 12 mm, and only upon entry through the porus acusticus does the nerve acquire a vestment of Schwann cells and assume the true characteristics of a peripheral nerve. It is at

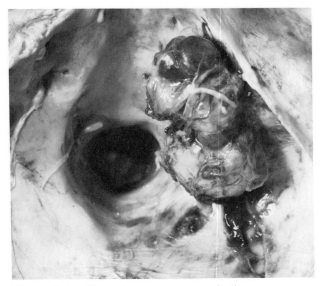

Figure 78-3 Chemodectomas may erode the petrous bone and enter the cerebellopontine angle. This lesion became symptomatic in the auricular area in a 32-year-old man who received irradiation therapy. This protrusion into the cerebellopontine angle is visualized 11 years later. (From Burger and Vogel.[1])

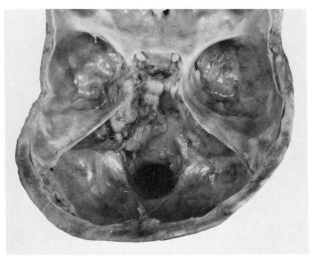

Figure 78-4 Malignant tumors may reach the cerebellopontine angle as blood-borne metastases to the skull or by direct penetration from primary lesions of the nasopharynx, as shown in this illustration. The primary carcinoma of the breast in this 44-year-old woman had been treated by radical mastectomy 5 years prior to symptomatic involvement of the base of the skull. (From Burger and Vogel.[1])

this interface, between the stroma of oligodendroglia and Schwann cells, that neoplastic transformation occurs. Interestingly, a propensity for neoplasia is also evidenced at this same location in fetal rats exposed transplacentally to nitrosourea.[5]

This structural uniqueness of the acoustic nerve and its propensity for neoplasia prompt a brief review of its embryonic development. The eighth nerve is derived from the lateral margin of the primitive rhombencephalon, from a group of cells known as the acousticofacial ganglion, which lies medial and ventral to the auditory vesicle. The cells of the vestibular ganglion are the first to extend fibers toward the auditory vesicle; shortly thereafter there is an outgrowth of fibers from the cochlear ganglion. This egress of fibers is accompanied by primitive Schwann cells; however, the fibers grow rapidly, and glia are drawn from the rhombencephalon into the proximal segment of the nerve. The adult acoustic nerve, in the human, is approximately 18 mm in length; its proximal 8 to 12 mm is endowed with neuroglia. The distal portion elaborates an endoneurium, epineurium, and perineurium from Schwann cells and fibroblasts, after the manner of a true peripheral nerve. The interface of neuroglia and Schwann cells is usually situated more distally in the vestibular than in the cochlear division, and the transition zone in the former is generally marked by a greater degree of intermingling of the two cell types and by a regional overproduction of Schwann cells.

Characteristically, acoustic schwannomas arise in the vestibular division, predictably in that short segment which traverses the porus acusticus or the internal auditory meatus (Fig. 78-5). Early enlargement compresses the cochlear division and may also obstruct the labyrinthine blood vessels

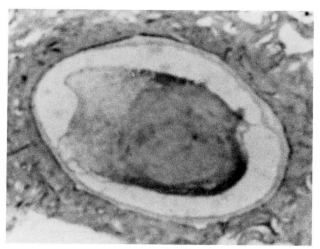

Figure 78-5 Cross section of porus acusticus discloses an incidental acoustic schwannoma in a patient with von Recklinghausen's disease. This early lesion involves approximately two-thirds of the diameter of the acoustic nerve. The porus acusticus was normal in size.

which supply the organ of Corti and the vestibular end organs. Although the neoplasm typically has its origin in the vestibular division, the earliest symptoms generally do not express this localization but rather the compression of the auditory component. Tinnitus is the most common initial symptom, soon accompanied by vertigo, in approximately 25 percent of cases.[2]

The neoplasm expands and erodes the porus acusticus. Thereafter, the mass intrudes from its bony canal into the cerebellopontine angle, where it lies between the petrous pyramid, the tentorium cerebelli, the cerebellum, and the brain stem. The new growth remains closely applied to the petrous pyramid, and its ventral surface thereafter acquires the mosaic irregularities of this bony ridge. By contrast, the vertex of the mass encounters only the soft tissues of the cerebellum and pons and is therefore dome-shaped, smoothly contoured, or slightly bosselated. The color is variegated with gray, yellow, and red, in accordance, respectively, with areas of dense cellularity, regions of xanthomatous degeneration, and degrees of vascularity. The yellow areas are generally soft and reflect their rich content of lipid. They contrast with the firmer gray tissues, which histologically are dense with Schwann cells.

The mass characteristically attains dimensions of 3 to 6 cm before its recognition and surgical excision. As this size is approached, the tumor mass contacts cranial nerves sequentially; first the facial nerve, which even at the time of surgical excision generally remains stretched across the ventral dome of the tumor (Fig. 78-6). The fifth nerve is compressed as it exits from the lateral aspect of the pons. Thereafter, caudal extension of the tumor brings it into contact with the ninth and tenth nerves and, occasionally, the eleventh. Medial growth disfigures and displaces the lateral aspects of the pons and, to a lesser degree, the medulla. The mass may then incorporate major blood vessels, the basilar and vertebral arteries or their branches. This medial exten-

sion brings the mass in contact with the sixth cranial nerve. Cephalad growth carries the edge of the tumor against the sigmoid sinus and, on occasion, directs it into the jugular foramen.

The expanding lesion within the posterior fossa thrusts the cerebellum downward and imprints the bony ridge of the foramen magnum against the inferior aspect of the cerebellum. Herniation of the cerebellar tonsils is imminent. The increased pressure in the posterior fossa and the disfigurement of the foramina of Magendie and of Luschka dispose to obstruction of cerebrospinal fluid flow and the development of hydrocephalus.

As the intruder enters the cerebellopontine angle, it acquires a vestment of arachnoid. This delicate membrane may thicken, but more often it blends with the fibroblastic tumor and imparts an appearance of encapsulation. The relation of the arachnoid and the tumor may also lead to the formation of cul-de-sacs that become filled with clear liquor, presumably cerebrospinal fluid. These cysts may add significantly to the dimensions of the mass and augment its compressive quality.

Acoustic schwannomas also extrude into the internal auditory canal, and later may penetrate into the inner ear.[1] This slender cylindrical extension of tissue is easily fractured and then remains in its bony compartment when the mass in the cerebellopontine angle has been removed bluntly at surgery or at postmortem examination. Thus its presence and

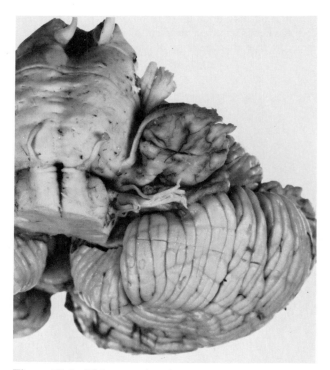

Figure 78-6 This acoustic schwannoma embodies the eighth nerve and deflects the seventh across its vertex. Note the proximity of the mass to the fifth cranial nerve, above, and to the ninth to eleventh nerves caudally, as well as its more distant relation to the sixth nerve in its medial position. (From Burger and Vogel.[1])

significance may be overlooked by both the surgeon and the pathologist.

Upon microscopic examination, the schwannoma presents two distinctive architectural patterns,[1,3,4] designated *Antoni A* and *Antoni B* patterns. Both tissues are formed of spindle cells with elongated nuclei and fibrillated cytoplasm; both are formed predominantly of Schwann cells (Fig. 78-7). The two tissue types differ in their cellular density and weave. Antoni A tissue is compact, with a variable prominence of interwoven fascicles. Antoni B tissue is porous and less structured. Its cells are clustered randomly about blood vessels, microcysts, collections of xanthomatous cells, and sites of antecedent hemorrhage. Lymphocytes also mark these loose reactive and degenerative tissues of the Antoni B type. The degree of nuclear pleomorphism varies considerably among schwannomas and also between different areas within the same tumor. This pleomorphism often includes a random population of large, bizarre nuclei that torment the pathologist with the notion of anaplasia; however, fortunately, malignant transformation is so rare (perhaps even nonexistent) as to completely reassure the pathologist of benignity, even in the presence of marked cellular pleomorphism (Fig. 78-8). Mitotic figures are rarely encountered. The occurrence of necrosis testifies to the meagerness of the native vascular bed rather than to the rapidity of tumor growth.

The differential diagnosis of a neoplasm of the cerebellopontine angle initially embraces the many lesions mentioned above. When histological examination excludes such distinctive entities as ependymoma, chemodectoma, chordoma, and carcinoma and special stains disclose a collagen stroma to distinguish the mesenchymal lesion from the exophytic glioma, the differential diagnosis narrows sharply to schwannoma and meningioma. In turn, the nodular architecture of the meningioma, created by whorls of menin-

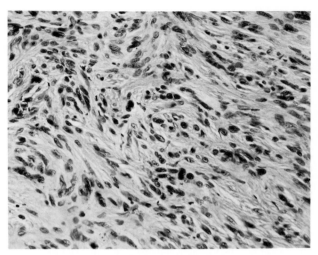

Figure 78-8 A histological preparation of an acoustic schwannoma. Nuclear pleomorphism may be marked in such a tumor but it does not bear malignant connotations. (Hematoxylin-eosin, ×189.)

gothelial cells with their psammoma bodies, individualizes this lesion and distinguishes it from the schwannoma. Generally, even in frozen section, the monotonous, woven appearance of a schwannoma is readily recognized.

Electron microscopy has resolved the issue of the cell of origin. Schwann cells possess a basement membrane that lies external to and closely applied to the plasma membrane (Fig. 78-9). This feature distinguishes the Schwann cell from the fibroblast with full assurance. In addition, the presence of wide-spaced collagen reaffirms this interpretation. Electron microscopy is generally an extravagance of

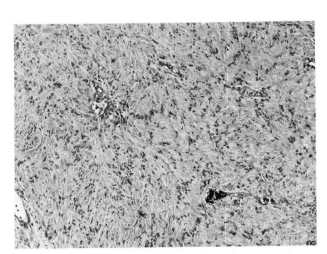

Figure 78-7 A histological preparation of an acoustic schwannoma. The Schwann cells variably align in fascicles and appear in loose, haphazard arrangement. This area depicts Antoni A tissue. (Hematoxylin-eosin, ×79.)

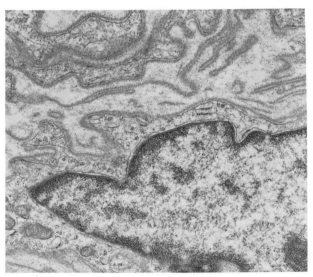

Figure 78-9 An electron micrograph of an acoustic schwannoma. The interdigitating processes of Schwann cells are separated by delicate basement laminae. This distinguishes them from fibroblasts. (×14,000.)

money, effort, and time in the diagnosis of individual case material. The histological features of an acoustic schwannoma are diagnostic, and the assessment of anaplasia or malignancy has already been resolved in favor of benignity by the natural biological behavior of prior lesions.

Acoustic schwannomas occur more often in women than men, in an approximate ratio of 3 to 2. Interestingly, this ratio also obtains with meningiomas. The peak incidence of this neoplasm has been variably cited at between 35 and 55 years of age. These statistics indicate that there is a plateau of high incidence and that this plateau spans the several decades of mid-adult life. Like the spinal, peripheral, and other cranial nerve schwannomas, the acoustic lesions have a heightened incidence in persons with von Recklinghausen's disease. This unfortunate hereditary state also enhances the bilateral tendency of the acoustic schwannoma.

Cure of this lesion calls for complete surgical excision. Continued indolent growth follows subtotal resection, much

in the manner and tempo of the meningioma. Although the possibility of bilaterality may shadow the patient's prognosis, fortunately, malignant transformation is not an issue.

References

1. Burger PC, Vogel FS: *Surgical Pathology of the Nervous System and Its Coverings*, 2d ed. New York, Wiley, 1982.
2. Harner SG, Laws ER: Diagnosis of acoustic neurinoma. Neurosurgery 9:373–379, 1981.
3. Rubinstein LJ: *Tumors of the Central Nervous System.* Atlas of Tumor Pathology, ser 2, fasc 6. Washington, Armed Forces Institute of Pathology, 1972.
4. Russell DS, Rubinstein LJ: *Pathology of Tumours of the Nervous System*, 4th ed. Baltimore, Williams & Wilkins Co, 1977.
5. Swenberg JA, Clendenon N, Denlinger R, Gordon WA: Sequential development of ethylnitrosourea-induced neurinomas: Morphology, biochemistry, and transplantability. JNCI 55:147–152, 1975.

79

Tumors of the Cerebellopontine Angle: Neurotologic Aspects of Diagnosis

Patrick D. Kenan

Acoustic neuromas of the internal auditory canal and other tumors of the cerebellopontine angle (CPA) generate symptoms because of pressure upon or destruction of contiguous neural and vascular structures. As expected, various eighth nerve symptoms are usually the first to be sensed by the patient. These include tinnitus, hearing loss, and vestibular symptoms, usually unsteadiness without true vertigo.

Unfortunately, there is no classic symptom complex or progression of symptoms pathognomonic of the acoustic neuroma, or CPA tumor. Except in rare circumstances, such

as von Recklinghausen's disease with bilateral neurofibromas of the internal auditory canals, the acoustic neuroma is unilateral, therefore the physician should maintain an index of suspicion for the presence of acoustic neuroma in any patient with unilateral tinnitus, hearing loss, and vestibular symptoms. Suspicion is heightened when fifth and seventh nerve symptoms are present, such as unilateral facial numbness or weakness or loss of corneal sensitivity. When there is also impairment of cranial nerves IX, X, and XI, there is a strong possibility of a CPA tumor of significant size. Very large CPA tumors may interfere with CSF flow and reabsorption and result in increased intracranial pressure.

These symptoms and neurological signs of acoustic neuroma may occur and progress in any order. They may be sudden and abrupt in onset, continuous or intermittent, and may begin with purely auditory or purely vestibular symptoms. Despite the close association of the seventh and eighth cranial nerves, facial weakness or paralysis is rarely the presenting complaint. The exception is a primary facial neuroma. Actually, fifth nerve involvement is relatively more common than seventh nerve deficits and is related to growth of the tumor out of the internal auditory canal and porus acusticus into the cerebellopontine angle.

If there is any "classic" presentation of the early acoustic neuroma, it is unilateral tinnitus and mild vestibular disturbance in the form of unsteadiness, with hearing impairment characterized by mild to moderate pure-tone sensorineural loss greater in the higher frequencies and loss of speech discrimination out of proportion to the pure-tone impairment. One must be wary of accepting this "classic" description, though, because acoustic neuromas and CPA tumors are noted for their exceptional behavior.

A comment regarding sudden vascular occlusion is in order before progressing to the primary purpose of this chapter, which is a discussion of testing techniques. A neuroma may be present for a prolonged period of time with minimal auditory or vestibular symptoms yet ultimately reach a size sufficient to produce complete occlusion of the internal auditory artery. This will result in an immediate and permanent loss of labyrinthine function, with resultant total hearing loss and complete loss of end-organ vestibular function on the involved side. This is precisely comparable to intentional surgical destruction of the labyrinth, often used in the treatment of advanced Ménière's disease. This produces sudden and perhaps intense vestibular symptoms coupled with complete loss of hearing, but the remainder of the vestibular system adapts quite readily and spontaneously to the loss, and subsequently the patient may function at close to normal from a vestibular point of view. The diagnosis of "inner ear apoplexy" is sometimes used in such cases, and the patient may be falsely reassured that "the damage is done, there is no treatment, but it isn't serious." One should always proceed with appropriate testing and scanning in this clinical situation to rule out a mass lesion of the internal auditory canal or CPA.

Ruling Out Acoustic Neuroma and Other CPA Tumors

Auditory Evaluation

This chapter does not discuss the diagnostic role of radiographic evaluation or that of brain stem evoked response audiometry, as these are dealt with more specifically in other sections. It focuses primarily on the classic auditory and vestibular tests, with a few general comments regarding fifth and seventh nerve testing and other tests of brain stem, cerebellar, and proprioceptive function.

Historically, behavioral auditory testing in suspected acoustic neuromas gives the most qualitatively and quantitatively accurate data the neurotologist and audiologist can provide. Formerly, the usual battery of tests included pure-tone air and bone thresholds, speech audiometry, tone decay, short-increment sensitivity index (SISI) measure-

ments, alternate binaural loudness balance (ABLB) as a measurement of recruitment, and Békésy audiometry. Through these various audiometric measurements, the audiologist could readily differentiate between conductive and sensorineural hearing loss, and in the case of the latter, between indicators of cochlear and of retrocochlear pathology. For historical reasons and because in some practices these classic behavioral audiometric tests may still be done in the absence of impedance audiometry and brain stem evoked response testing, Table 79-1 is included in this presentation to give the general diagnostic guidelines indicated by these tests. One therefore expected, in the classic presentation of acoustic neuroma, unilateral sensorineural hearing loss with speech discrimination out of proportion to the level of puretone loss, positive tone decay, negative or low SISI scores, negative recruitment as demonstrated by ABLB, and type III or IV Békésy tracings.

In recent years, two forms of nonbehavioral auditory testing have become standard in most neurotologic and audiologic practices: impedance audiometry and brain stem evoked response audiometry. Impedance audiometry is especially valuable in assessing middle ear, eustachian tube, and ossicular disease but is also quite valuable in showing normal versus abnormal acoustic reflex (stapedial reflex) behavior. This measurement is proving to be an extremely sensitive index of retrocochlear disease.

Impedance audiometry consists of three separate measurements: (1) static compliance, or "stiffness" of the eardrum-ossicle-middle ear conducting apparatus; (2) pressure differentials between the outer ear canal and middle ear (tympanometry); and (3) acoustic (stapedial) reflex, an afferent-efferent arc utilizing an intense sound signal delivered to the eighth nerve, producing reflex contraction of the stapedius muscle innervated by the seventh nerve.

Abnormalities of compliance and of pressure differentials are sensitive indicators of middle ear disease. The acoustic reflex is a nonbehavioral audiometric procedure which has proved to be of considerable value in the detection of retrocochlear lesions. Measurement of the acoustic reflex relies on changes in the relative impedance of the middle ear appa-

TABLE 79-1 Previous Auditory Workup for Acoustic Neuroma

Auditory Test	Conductive Loss	Sensorineural Loss Cochlear Origin	Retrocochlear Origin
Pure-tone air conduction	Elevated thresholds	Elevated thresholds	Elevated thresholds
Pure-tone bone conduction	Normal thresholds	Elevated, equal to pure-tone air conduction	Elevated, equal to pure-tone air conduction
Speech reception threshold	Threshold about equal to average air conduction	Threshold about equal to average air conduction	Threshold about equal to average air conduction
Speech discrimination	Normal	Mild to moderate loss	Moderate to severe loss
Tone decay	Negative	Negative	Positive
Short-increment sensitivity index	Negative	Positive	Negative
Alternate binaural loudness balance (recruitment)	Negative	Positive	Negative
Békésy	Type I	Type II, sometimes I	Type III or IV

ratus which occur when the stapedius muscle contracts in response to an intense auditory signal.

To measure the acoustic reflex, a low-frequency probe tone (220 Hz or 660 Hz) is transmitted to the ear through a tight-fitting rubber tip which seals the external auditory canal. The reflex is detected as a marked increase in the amplitude of the sound reflected off the tympanic membrane when the stapedius muscle contracts and stiffens the middle ear mechanism.[9]

The acoustic reflex is bilateral, so it is convenient to place the probe tone in the nontest ear and to present the tone eliciting the reflex through an earphone on the test ear. In addition to this contralateral reflex testing, most reflex-measuring apparatuses also permit ipsilateral testing in which both the probe and the signal tones are presented to the test ear. When it is important to differentiate between eighth nerve and brain stem lesions, ipsilateral and contralateral reflexes are compared.

In the normal hearing population approximately 95 percent of people demonstrate the acoustic reflex at about 85 dB above their behavioral threshold.[3] People with a cochlear hearing impairment with recruitment often show an abnormally small gap (less than about 55 dB) between the acoustic reflex threshold and their behavioral hearing threshold.[6] In contrast, patients with eighth nerve or CPA lesions show elevated or absent acoustic reflex thresholds. For these patients, ipsilateral and contralateral reflexes are abnormal when the high-intensity stimulus is presented to the affected ear and normal when the sound is presented to the unaffected ear.[10]

When a patient demonstrates the acoustic reflex and a retrocochlear lesion is suspected, the audiologist routinely measures rate of adaptation of the reflex (amplitude decay). To measure reflex decay, a sustained tone is presented 10 dB above the patient's reflex threshold for a period of 10 s. If the reflex amplitude reduces more than 50 percent during this time period, the results are suggestive of an eighth nerve lesion. Reflex decay testing is usually conducted at frequencies below 2000 Hz, because normal persons frequently show reflex decay at higher frequencies.

It must be cautioned that one would not expect to elicit an acoustic reflex in a patient with severe to profound hearing loss regardless of cause. Further, a patient with even a slight conductive hearing loss may show no reflex, because the middle ear problem may hide any subtle impedance changes produced by the acoustic reflex.

Acoustic reflex testing is certainly not the definitive test for an eighth nerve lesion, but it takes less than 5 minutes to conduct and provides useful information regarding the need for more extensive diagnostic procedures. Reflex test equipment is available in all complete audiologic facilities. Such testing should be a routine part of the workup of any hearing-impaired patient, and most definitely in any neuroma subject. In a series of 117 neuroma patients from the Otological Medical Group of Los Angeles, more than 80 percent showed decay or absence of the acoustic reflex. After brain stem audiometry, the acoustic reflex is the most highly positive auditory test in neuroma diagnosis.[4]

Brain stem evoked response audiometry (BERA) is described in depth elsewhere in this textbook and is not discussed here except to say that it is probably the single most accurate auditory test in neuroma diagnosis. Selters and Brackmann[8] have reported a series of 414 cases (148 proven tumors and 266 nontumors). There was a 96 percent tumor detection rate by BERA testing, with an 8 percent false-positive rate and a 4 percent false-negative rate. No other test, including x-ray studies, acoustic reflex testing, and electronystagmography, proved as consistent or gave such low false-positive or false-negative rates as BERA.

As a consequence of the routine use of impedance audiometry, which includes acoustic reflex testing, and brain stem audiometry, it now is considered unnecessary to include tone decay, SISI, ABLB, or Békésy testing in the routine workup of the suspected neuroma or CPA tumor. The recommended battery of auditory tests that should be conducted in the neuroma workup, listed in Table 79-2, consists of pure-tone air and bone conduction thresholds, speech audiometry, impedance testing with stapedius reflex, and BERA. The "usual" neuroma would present with the following auditory findings: Unilateral sensorineural hearing loss with discrimination impairment out of proportion to the pure-tone thresholds, normal tympanometry and compliance, absent acoustic reflex or with reflex decay, and positive (delayed) brain stem conduction by BERA.

TABLE 79-2 Current Auditory Workup for Acoustic Neuroma

Auditory Test	Conductive Loss	Sensorineural Loss Cochlear Origin	Sensorineural Loss Retrocochlear Origin
Pure-tone air conduction	Elevated thresholds	Elevated thresholds	Elevated thresholds
Pure-tone bone conduction	Normal thresholds	Elevated, equal to pure-tone air conduction	Elevated, equal to pure-tone air conduction
Speech reception threshold	Threshold about equal to average air conduction	Threshold about equal to average air conduction	Threshold about equal to average air conduction
Speech discrimination	Normal	Mild to moderate loss	Moderate to severe loss
Tympanometry	Usually abnormal	Normal	Normal
Static compliance	Usually abnormal	Normal	Normal
Acoustic reflex	Usually abnormal	Normal	Absent or decayed
Brain stem evoked response audiometry	Normal	Normal	Delayed

A few concluding comments regarding costs of equipping a complete audiologic testing laboratory are in order. Costs are substantial for the equipment alone, not including installation. Four basic units are necessary, at the following approximate price ranges: Sound-treated room, $5000 to $10,000; clinical audiometer, $10,000; impedance bridge, $4000 to $5000; BERA unit $15,000 to $20,000. Total equipment costs would range (at 1982 prices) from $34,000 to $45,000. Cheaper screening units are of course available and are often used for audiologic screening, but a definitive neurotologic workup for the neuroma suspect will justify costly and sophisticated instrumentation.

Vestibular Evaluation

Historically, caloric stimulation and Bárány chair rotation were the earliest methods of producing vestibular symptoms, with an observable and measurable effect, nystagmus. Although the two methods are seemingly disparate, in actuality both create vestibular effects by stimulating a flow of endolymph over the neuroreceptors of the vestibular end organ. In caloric stimulation, the vestibular effects are the result of convection currents in endolymph resulting from the cooling or warming effects of water or other suitable thermal agents in the outer ear. Because of the relatively exposed position of the lateral semicircular canal and its lie of 30° elevation from the horizontal with the head upright, a backward 60° tilt of the head places the canal in a vertical position. Cool water in the outer ear conveys its caloric effects through the tympanic membrane and middle ear, and downward convection currents are produced in the endolymph of the lateral canal. The opposite, or upward, convection currents result from the thermal effects of warm water irrigation. The flow of endolymph across the cupula of the vestibular hair cells of the cristae which lie within the ampulla of the lateral canal stimulates a predictable nystagmoid response with certain expected parameters (delay in onset, duration, and intensity, coupled with subjective vertigo). Cold convection currents produce an endolymph flow away from the ampulla (ampullofugal), with the fast component of nystagmus opposite the ear being stimulated, while warm stimulation produces flow of endolymph toward the ampulla (ampullopetal), with the fast component of nystagmus toward the stimulated ear. The mnemonic, COWS (cold-opposite; warm-same), applies, and the combination of cold stimulation (30°C, 7°C below normal body temperature of 37°C) alternately to each ear followed by warm stimulation (44°C, 7°C above normal body temperature of 37°C), with appropriate measurement of the results, constitutes the classic bithermal Fitzgerald-Hallpike caloric stimulation test.

In his first monograph devoted to acoustic neuromas,[7] House reported on 53 proven neuromas with 96 percent decreased or absent caloric responses. In his second monograph,[5] 82 percent of 200 neuromas were reported to have demonstrated reduced caloric responses, but small tumors showed impaired caloric responses in slightly less than 50 percent. Caloric responses were therefore not considered reliable indicators of neuroma in comparison with other forms of vestibular disease.

Bárány stimulation is actually quite similar to caloric stimulation but depends upon rotation of the subject with the head tilted forward 30° to place the lateral semicircular canals in the horizontal plane. As rotation begins, there is first an inertia of endolymph that is ampullofugal on one side, ampullopetal on the other, with a brief vestibular effect. A constant rotation rate allows the endolymph to "catch up" until such time as rotation ceases, at which point momentum produces a significant endolymph flow, comparable to simultaneous caloric stimulation with cold water in one ear and warm water in the other. Again, certain measurable parameters result from Bárány rotation which allow one to differentiate between normal and abnormal.

A major difference between Bárány and caloric stimulation is that the former is a simultaneous stimulation of both vestibular end organs, whereas the latter attempts to test and quantify individually each end organ.

Additional forms of vestibular evaluation include optokinetic tracking, testing for positional or postural nystagmus, ocular dysmetria and gaze testing, sinusoidal tracking, spontaneous nystagmus, paroxysmal nystagmus, and averaging of bithermal bilateral caloric responses to establish directional preponderance or unilateral weakness. The composite of these vestibular tests constitutes what is traditionally offered by the technique of electronystagmography, or ENG testing.[1,2,11]

ENG recordings are possible because of the difference in electrical potential between the cornea and retina of the eye, the cornea being positive, the retina negative. The small change in potential as the eyes move from side to side in controlled movements or uncontrolled nystagmus is recorded by the ENG. Nystagmus may be suppressed by ocular fixation but will be evident by ENG recording with the eyes closed. This is called *latent nystagmus* and is a subtler form of spontaneous nystagmus.

The ENG is conducted with the patient supine and, except for positional nystagmus testing, with the head elevated 30° (or back 60° from the vertical) to place the lateral semicircular canals in a vertical plane for maximal response to bithermal caloric stimulation. Electrodes are taped near each outer canthus, and a ground electrode is placed in the midline of the forehead. Electrical leads are connected to the two-channel recorder. Sensitivity is adjusted so that 10° of eye shift produces 10 mm of shift on recording paper. The test is calibrated by having the patient look alternately at two lights 10° on either side of center. Overshoots, in which the eyes go significantly beyond, then return to the 10° mark, are termed *ocular dysmetria* and are believed to indicate possible brain stem or cerebellar disease.

To test gaze nystagmus, the patient is observed for significant and sometimes intense nystagmus on lateral gaze, either bilaterally equal or unequal or unilateral only. Minimal end-gaze nystagmus is normal. Otherwise, gaze nystagmus indicates either drug effects (barbiturates, phenytoin, alcohol, etc.) or brain stem dysfunction. Vertical nystagmus is often seen with brain stem, pons, or cerebellar lesions.

Sinusoidal tracking involves having the patient follow the movement of a point or finger across the horizontal. The recording will appear as a sine curve. A breakup in the sine curve may indicate oculomotor or other brain stem lesions and is usually associated with gaze nystagmus.

Spontaneous nystagmus is tested with the patient in a

sitting or neutral position with the eyes closed. Positive findings are nonlocalized and may result from central or peripheral lesions or from medications.

Positional nystagmus testing requires position changes from supine, right or left lateral, and head-hanging positions. Positive nystagmus which fatigues is nonlocalized and may relate to transient neurovascular changes. Nonfatiguing nystagmus is usually indicative of an abnormality of the central or peripheral vestibular system.

Optokinetic (OPK) testing involves having the patient watch a rotating drum with vertical stripes. If bilateral inability to track is not due to poor cooperation, a high brain stem lesion should be considered. An abnormal unilateral response suggests a cerebral hemisphere lesion, with the predominant beating toward the side of the lesion.

The Dix-Hallpike test for paroxysmal nystagmus, like positional nystagmus testing, is done with sudden supination, head-hanging, and right and left positions. A positive test requires a latency of 5 to 25 seconds of no nystagmus, followed by a sudden burst of nystagmus with subjective vertigo, which fatigues with time or with repetition. The positive Dix-Hallpike test suggests peripheral vestibular disease in the downward ear.

Bithermal irrigations, using 30°C water then 44°C water irrigation of the ears, with 30° elevation of the head from horizontal to place the lateral semicircular canal in the vertical plane, are the final ENG test. While the fast component of nystagmus is the most obvious outward sign of response, it is the slow or return nystagmoid movement which is related to vestibular activity. Therefore the speed of the slow component (SSC) is measured for each irrigation and averaged for each ear (cold, then warm) and compared, right to left. Unilateral weakness indicates peripheral disease. Directional preponderance of left versus right nystagmus (fast component), on the other hand, is a nonlocalized finding related to either CNS or peripheral disease.

Basic ENG laboratories require a two-channel recorder, closed-loop caloric bath, optokinetic drum, ENG table, and calculator, all for less than $6000 (1982 prices). More elaborate systems, including computers with printed readouts, are available but probably offer no better interpretation than that provided by a trained and experienced ENG technician. This basic vestibular testing laboratory is within the reach of virtually any neurotologic practice. The training and experience of the ENG technician is important to the reliability of the results. The usual ENG technician can achieve a high degree of proficiency and skill within 6 months to 1 year of training and experience and can be quite as competent in analyzing and interpreting test results as the neurotologist.

Another system for evaluation of vestibular function deserves discussion and indeed support in this presentation. As the ENG was to caloric stimulation, so low-frequency sinusoidal harmonic acceleration may be to ENG testing for vestibular disorders. This new system has greater sensitivities for demonstrating the presence and the locus of vestibular lesions than electronystagmography. It is not really "new," because it utilizes Bárány's rotational stimulation, but in an oscillating (sinusoidal) manner, to stimulate the vestibular system and measure its responses. The system requires substantial instrumentation, including an isolation chamber, a motorized and computerized oscillating rotational chair, optokinetic and sinusoidal tracking units, and a computer for interpretation of results. Equipment and installation costs alone would be in the range of $100,000 to $150,000 for the complete system. Many names apply to such a system, the simplest being the *rotary chair system*; but a more elaborate and technically correct designation would be *low-frequency sinusoidal harmonic acceleration tracking unit*. No matter, cost notwithstanding, the rotary chair system is unquestionably a qualitatively and quantitatively more accurate method for measurement of vestibular dysfunction than the ENG and represents a major step forward in clinical vestibular physiology. Numerous instances of suspected vestibulopathies despite normal ENGs have been proved and the focus pinpointed by rotary chair results.[12]

A number of medical centers now offer harmonic acceleration vestibular testing as a matter of routine in their neurotologic vestibular laboratories. The technique is more than a research tool, it is here to stay and can be a highly sensitive indicator of early vestibular disease. Considering the current great interest in the diagnosis of early intracanalicular acoustic neuromas which may be successfully removed while sparing cochlear and seventh nerve function, perhaps the rotary chair low-frequency sinusoidal acceleration tracking system will be the ultimate diagnostic tool. After all, if a small neuroma produces only minimal and atypical auditory changes and negative radiographic findings but might be diagnosed by exquisitely sensitive vestibular testing, then the costs of the system are probably justified. The next decade should decide clearly what place the rotary chair system has in the neurotologic diagnosis of acoustic neuroma.

ENG testing is warranted in every neuroma suspect and indeed in most vestibular complaints of a continuing nature. The more costly rotary chair testing is presently available in only a limited number of major medical centers. This testing technique has a higher degree of accuracy than caloric or ENG testing but may be open to criticism as to its cost effectiveness. If the equipment and installation costs, cost of training and retaining technicians, and cost of testing can ever be brought within reason, harmonic rotational testing will probably be the best vestibular function test available in the workup of the neuroma suspect. Until such time, ENG will remain the standard, while its limitations in differentiating between neuroma and non-neuroma are recognized.

Order of Workup

In evaluating neuroma suspects, history taking is all important. Suspicion of neuroma should immediately be aroused by presenting complaints of unilateral hearing loss, tinnitus, and vestibular symptoms. Facial weakness or numbness and other signs or symptoms of brain stem or cerebellar disease should further heighten the suspicion of neuroma or CPA tumor. The introductory section of this chapter presents these signs and symptoms, and they need not be dealt with further except to say that a small intracanalicular tumor or a small CPA tumor may be atypical in every aspect of its presentation. It is usually the astuteness of the clinician that accounts for diagnosis of the extremely small eighth nerve or CPA tumor.

After history taking and before any specialized auditory, vestibular, or radiographic evaluation, the neurotologic examination should include routine visual inspection of the ear canals, drums, and middle ear landmarks, preferably using the pneumatic otoscope and operating microscope for optimal visual assessment. The examiner should look for spontaneous nystagmus or differences in lateral gaze nystagmus. Nose, throat, and laryngeal examinations are important, particularly to rule out any impairment of palatal, pharyngeal, or laryngeal innervation. Deficits of ninth, tenth, and eleventh cranial nerves are not uncommon with CPA tumors. Tongue involvement through hypoglossal impairment is uncommon except in massive CPA or brain stem lesions, in which multiple neurological signs would be expected, including possible increased intracranial pressure. Ophthalmoscopic examination should therefore be routine.

The neurotologist should pay particular attention to fifth nerve impairment. Facial hypesthesia, paresthesia, or anesthesia are significant signs of trigeminal nerve involvement, as is loss of strength of the muscles of mastication on the involved side. Impaired corneal sensitivity is the earliest indicator of fifth nerve involvement; the test for this is the easiest and quantitatively the most accurate test to perform in the neurotologic examination of fifth nerve function.

Seventh nerve function is usually unimpaired grossly except in the larger neuromas. Slowed or impaired blink reflexes may be detected by the careful observer. Impaired taste through involvement of the chorda tympani nerve may occasionally be elicited by history taking or even by testing with sweet, sour, or salty substances, but the technique is fraught with error and subjective overlay. The electronic taste tester has been used to some advantage but has never enjoyed widespread use. The Schirmer test for bilateral comparison of lacrimation is of value when gross seventh nerve deficits are present and helps place the lesion proximal or distal to the greater superficial petrosal nerve.

Tests of cerebellar and proprioceptive function are usually conducted by gait and station observation, the Romberg test, finger-to-nose or finger-to-finger testing with eyes closed, rapid alternating hand movements, having the patient hop on one foot with eyes closed, etc.

From a practical point of view, the entire battery of history taking, ear-nose-throat examination, and basic neurological examination can be performed by the neurotologist in a relatively brief time at the initial intake evaluation and should be considered routine in most evaluations of hearing loss and/or vestibular symptoms.

Arrangements are next made for the orderly conduct of auditory and vestibular evaluation. These are frequently conducted the same day but at separate times. The author's preference is to carry out auditory testing first, with routine performance of pure-tone and speech audiometry and impedance audiometry, which includes auditory reflex testing. Because of the greater costs and time associated with brain stem audiometry, this can be scheduled at a second consultation, depending upon the need indicated by initial auditory testing.

Vestibular testing in the form of ENG can be scheduled the same day subsequent to the auditory battery. Because there may be continuing vestibular effects, particularly in the form of nausea that may last some hours following caloric stimulation in some patients, the cooperation and concentration required for accurate auditory evaluation can be impaired if conducted following unpleasant vestibular stimulation; hence the desirability of performing the routine auditory battery before vestibular testing.

Everything described to this point can in most instances be performed in the space of one day, including certain aspects of the radiographic evaluation. If brain stem audiometry is indicated, it is usually done as a separate study after initial auditory and vestibular tests are completed. It is quite feasible for BERA, like the previous components of the workup, to be done on an outpatient basis.

Many neuroma suspects are referred for direct hospital admission, in which case all the foregoing studies are usually done on an inpatient basis, and sometimes in whatever order the consultations and services become available. It is not unusual, therefore, that the auditory and vestibular studies be carried out after a radiographic diagnosis has been established by scanning techniques. The recommendation would be that auditory and vestibular evaluation be performed prior to radiographic scanning. In certain instances a non-neuroma diagnosis may be made and treatment already be under way, which might negate the need for a costly full radiographic evaluation. Obviously, this would not apply to the true neuroma suspect but only to otologic disorders such as otomastoiditis or hearing loss of middle ear origin. Considering that various disorders of the middle ear may also present with unilateral hearing loss, tinnitus, vestibular effects, and even facial nerve paralysis, all of which may strongly suggest neuroma, it should be kept in mind that conventional and impedance audiometry and conventional mastoid roentgenograms may unequivocally diagnose the middle ear origin of the disease and dictate appropriate and immediate otologic treatment, all without the substantial costs and time required for BERA and CT scanning. Discretionary judgment is therefore advised in the order of the tests required for neuroma workup, reserving BERA and CT scanning for the true neuroma suspect and using them only after conventional auditory, vestibular, and radiographic evaluation have confirmed a reasonable concern for acoustic neuroma or CPA tumor.

References

1. Baloh RW, Honrubia V: *Clinical Neurophysiology of the Vestibular System.* Philadelphia, F. A. Davis, 1979.
2. Coats AC: Electronystagmography, in Bradford LJ (ed): *Physiological Measurements of the Audio-Vestibular System.* New York, Academic, 1975, pp 37–85.
3. Jerger J, Jerger S, Mauldin L: Studies in impedance audiometry: I. Normal and sensorineural ears. Arch Otolaryngol 96: 513–523, 1972.
4. Johnson EW: Results of auditory tests in acoustic tumor patients, in House WF, Luetje CM (eds): *Acoustic Tumors: Diagnosis.* Baltimore, University Park Press, 1979, Vol 1, pp 209–224.
5. Linthicum FH Jr, Churchill D: Vestibular test results in acous-

tic tumor cases, in House WF (ed): *Monograph II: Acoustic Neuroma.* Arch Otolaryngol 88:604–607, 1968.

6. Metz O: Threshold of reflex contractions of muscles of middle ear and recruitment of loudness. Arch Otolaryngol 55:536–543, 1952.
7. Pulec JL, House WF, Hughes RL: Vestibular involvement and testing in acoustic neuromas, in House WF (ed): *Monograph: Transtemporal Bone Microsurgical Removal of Acoustic Neuromas.* Arch Otolaryngol 80:677–681, 1964.
8. Selters WA, Brackmann DE: Brainstem electric response audiometry in acoustic tumor detection, in House WF, Luetje CM

(eds): *Acoustic Tumors, vol. I: Diagnosis.* Baltimore, University Park Press, 1979, pp 225–235.

9. Sheehy JL, Hughes RL: The ABC's of impedance audiometry. Laryngoscope 84:1935–1949, 1974.
10. Sheehy JL, Inzer BE: Acoustic reflex test in neuro-otologic diagnosis. Arch Otolaryngol 102:647–653, 1976.
11. Simmons FB, Gillam SF, Mattox DE: *An Atlas of Electronystagmography.* New York, Grune & Stratton, 1979.
12. Wolfe JW, Engelken EJ, Olson JW, Kos CM: Vestibular responses to bithermal caloric and harmonic acceleration. Ann Otol Rhinol Laryngol 87:861–867, 1978.

80

Tumors of the Cerebellopontine Angle: Radiology

Philip Dubois

The most common primary tumors of the cerebellopontine angle are acoustic neurinomas (80 to 90 percent), meningiomas (5 to 10 percent), and epidermoid tumors (5 percent). Many other mass lesions may mimic these neoplasms, and a list of these is given in Table 80-1.

Radiographic Modalities

Plain Roentgenography

When a patient presents with the clinical syndrome of a cerebellopontine angle mass, computed tomography may theoretically provide a complete analysis of the presence, characteristics, and extent of the lesion. However, in practice, plain skull films, including specialized temporal bone views (Fig. 80-1), continue to be useful to detect extensive destruction of the skull base, as may occur in aggressive neoplastic or inflammatory processes, or widening of the internal auditory canals or basal foramina. Where older computed tomographic units that do not have the capability to obtain ultra-thin sections are available, the superior spatial resolution of conventional roentgenograms is essential to

detect bony changes. Additionally, in centers where computed tomography is not readily available, conventional films provide a low-cost screening method with a sensitivity of approximately 50 percent in the detection of acoustic neurinomas.[10]

Polytomography

Thin-section polydirectional tomography enjoyed considerable popularity prior to the advent of high-resolution CT scanning by enhancing the detection of subtle erosions of the internal auditory canal and thereby elevating the sensitivity of the radiographic detection of acoustic neurinomas to approximately 78 percent.[10] However, the development of CT units capable of imaging with thin sections, with a spatial resolution better than 0.8 mm, with a wide window width to depict bone detail, and with the capability to perform direct coronal CT sections has rendered polytomography virtually obsolete.

In centers where a polydirectional tomographic unit is available, there is an occasional utility in mapping the bony contour of cerebellopontine angle mass lesions that have extensive adjacent bony destruction (Fig. 80-2) and in which

TABLE 80-1 Cerebellopontine Angle Masses

Acoustic neurinoma
Meningioma
Epidermoid and dermoid tumors
Metastasis
Trigeminal neurinoma
Arachnoid cyst
Aneurysm
Dolichobasilar ectasia
Extensions of
  Brain stem or cerebellar glioma
  Pituitary adenoma
  Craniopharyngioma
  Chordoma and tumors of the skull base
  Fourth ventricle tumor (ependymoma)
  Choroid plexus papilloma
  Neurinomas of lowest four cranial nerves
  Glomus jugulare tumor
  Primary tumors of the temporal bone

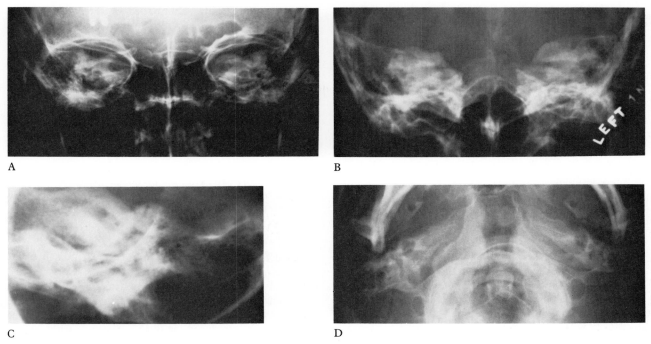

A   B

C   D

Figure 80-1 Specialized roentgenograms of the temporal bone to display the petrous pyramid and internal auditory canal: *A*, frontal view; *B*, Towne's view; *C*, Stenver's view; *D*, submentovertex view.

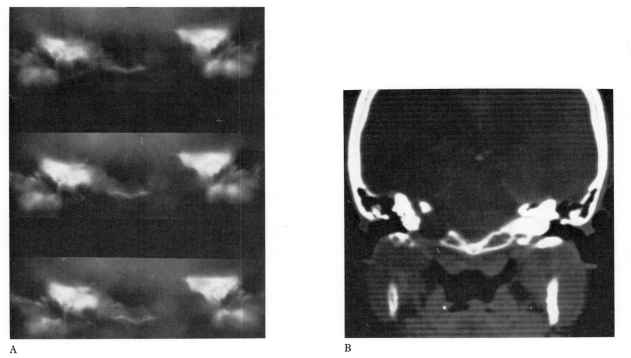

A   B

Figure 80-2 *A*. An epidermoid tumor of the left petrous temporal bone invading the cerebellopontine angle. Coronal polydirectional tomograms demonstrate the intra-osseous extent of the lesion and the characteristic discrete bony margin, but give no information regarding the soft tissue component. *B*. A high-resolution CT scan in another patient with a similar lesion shows the low-density soft tissue component of the epidermoid tumor extending intra- and extracranially, as well as the bony contour.

the coronal plane best displays the anatomical region. Even though polytomography cannot display the soft tissue component of the lesion as can CT, coronal sections are technically much easier to perform with a polydirectional tomographic unit than with computed tomography. In the latter, patients are required to hyperextend the neck, lying prone or supine, to obtain direct coronal sections. On the other hand, similar uncomfortable positioning was necessary to obtain horizontal (axial) sections at polytomography. Thus high-resolution CT, which creates sections in this projection in the comfortable supine position has proven far more useful in analyzing both bony (as well as soft tissue) pathology in this projection.

Posterior Fossa Myelography

This procedure was originally developed using the lumbar intrathecal injection of Pantopaque [ethyl 10-(p-iodophenyl) undecylate; Picker Corporation, Cleveland, Ohio] instilled into the cerebellopontine angle using a conventional tilting myelographic table and spot filming.[8] Originally, a relatively large volume of Pantopaque was used to detect extra-axial mass lesions in the posterior fossa (Fig. 80-3A). This procedure has been rendered totally obsolete with the advent of computed tomography.

Small-volume Pantopaque studies in which 1 to 2 ml of Pantopaque is positioned in the cerebellopontine angle cistern and internal auditory canal (Fig. 80-3) have been used as the "gold standard" for the detection of small intracanalicular neurinomas for over a decade.[3] This technique, using specialized horizontal beam films or polytomography, remains useful when a thin-section CT examination reveals no extracanalicular component of an acoustic neurinoma, despite strongly positive clinical or audiometric signs.

Enthusiasm for water-soluble contrast media led to the development of the technique of a C1-C2 level subarachnoid injection of 5 ml of hypertonic metrizamide, positioned into the cerebellopontine angle and internal auditory canal for plain radiographic and tomographic filming,[1] but this technique has largely been superseded by gas CT cisternography.

Computed Tomography

High-resolution computed tomography is the mainstay of the diagnostic evaluation of cerebellopontine angle mass lesions.[7] Technically adequate computed tomographic studies require sections no thicker than 5 mm to be obtained through the posterior fossa, and in most instances the study should be performed before and after enhancement by the intravenous infusion of a contrast agent (Fig. 80-4). Studies obtained only after contrast enhancement may lead to an equivocal interpretation since the variable prominence of the jugular tubercle may mimic an enhancing cerebellopontine angle mass lesion (Fig. 80-5A), unless an unenhanced image is available for comparison. The unenhanced study will, of course, reveal the high-density bony tubercle in a position in which the "tumor" is seen on the enhanced study (Fig.

80-5B). Alternatively, reformatted or direct coronal CT sections will clarify the bony nature of the "lesion" (Fig. 80-5C).

Axial CT sections usually suffice for a complete analysis, and these may be in the plane of the anatomical baseline or at 15 degrees to the anatomical baseline, depending on the preference of the examining radiologist. Reformatted images in sagittal, coronal, or oblique projections are sometimes helpful in the analysis of the spatial relationships of large tumors (Fig. 80-6A). Direct coronal CT examinations offer higher spatial resolution than reformatted coronal images and are sometimes useful for both small and large mass lesions. (Fig. 80-6B). They are particularly helpful in analyzing the relationships of tumor masses to the fourth ventricle and the foramen magnum.

Gas CT Cisternography

In this technique, which is used to detect or exclude small intracanalicular acoustic neurinomas that are beyond the resolution of conventional CT scans, approximately 5 ml of sterile gas is introduced via lumbar puncture with the patient on a tilting fluoroscopic table or tilting gurney.[6,9] The patient is positioned on the side, with the side to be examined uppermost, and with a head-up tilt of between 45 and 75 degrees, gas is slowly bubbled into the lumbar subarachnoid space via a 22-gauge needle until the patient experiences a "popping" sensation in the uppermost ear. The patient is transported to the CT scanner in the decubitus position, and CT sections are obtained through the internal auditory canal (Fig. 80-7). If the capability of imaging with ultra-thin sections is not available, 5-mm sections overlapped 2 mm between sections are adequate to visualize the neurovascular bundle and the contents of the internal auditory canal. The procedure is usually performed on inpatients with at least an overnight hospital admission following the procedure, but in several centers radiologists have had considerable experience with performing this procedure on an outpatient basis, with no significant side effects.

Metrizamide CT Cisternography

The intrinsically high contrast resolution capability of computed tomography can be utilized to visualize a very low concentration of intrathecal metrizamide. In this technique, 5 ml of metrizamide in isotonic concentration (170 mg of iodine per milliliter) is instilled into the lumbar subarachnoid space via a 22-gauge needle and with 60 s of steep head-down tilt. The metrizamide opacifies the subarachnoid cisterns and fourth ventricle. Adequate visualization of the contents of the cerebellopontine angle cisterns is provided with 5-mm CT sections performed in the supine position, but intracanalicular detail is only resolved if the patient has relatively large internal auditory canals. In average or small-size internal auditory canals, gas CT cisternography is still necessary and is preferable if there is a clinical suspicion of a small intracanalicular tumor.

Metrizamide CT cisternography is most useful in analyz-

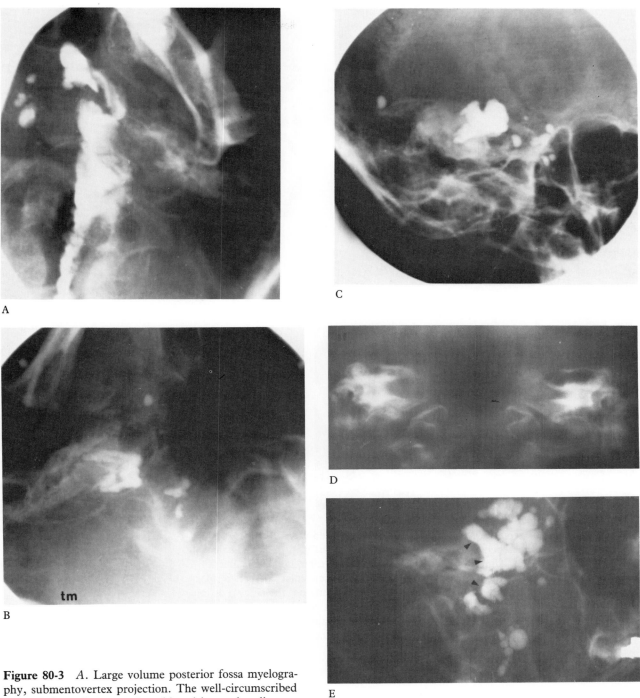

Figure 80-3 *A.* Large volume posterior fossa myelography, submentovertex projection. The well-circumscribed filling defect adjacent to the widened internal auditory canal is caused by a 2.5-cm acoustic neurinoma. *B.* A small-volume Pantopaque study in the same projection shows filling of the internal auditory canal in this normal patient. *C.* In the same patient, Stenver's projection again shows the intracanalicular extension of the Pantopaque. *D.* A frontal tomogram in a patient with a 1.5-cm right acoustic neurinoma shows characteristic flaring of the internal auditory canal. *E.* A small-volume Pantopaque study in the same patient shows the extracanalicular tumor component displacing the Pantopaque (*arrowheads*) away from the internal auditory canal.

ing the relationships of relatively large cerebellopontine angle mass lesions to the brain stem, that is, in determining whether a mass lesion in the angle arises intra- or extra-axially (Fig. 80-8).

These procedures are usually performed on inpatients since there is a significant incidence of headache, nausea, and vomiting following the intracranial instillation of metrizamide. The epileptogenic side effects of metrizamide are not considered a significant problem at the low doses and con-

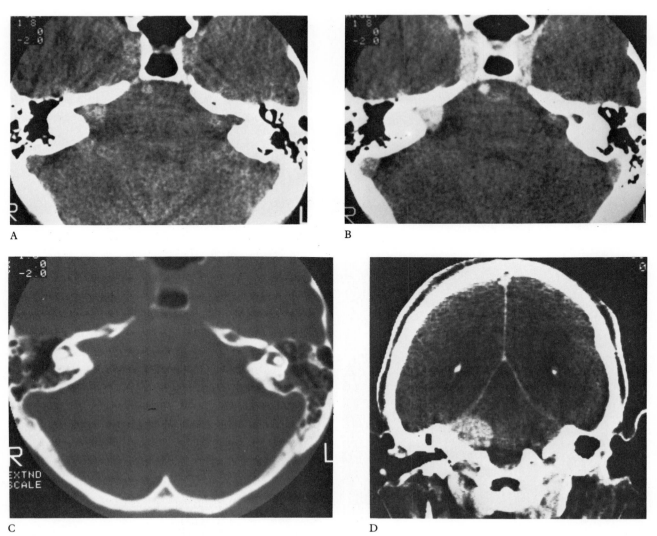

Figure 80-4 A right acoustic neurinoma: *A.* The unenhanced CT in this case shows a slightly higher than cerebellar-density soft tissue mass in the right porus acusticus. *B.* After the intravenous administration of a contrast agent, there is prominent enhancement and the well-circumscribed margin of the extracanalicular component of the tumor is well demonstrated. *C.* Using bone window technique, the erosion of the right internal auditory canal and the intraosseous details are well demonstrated. *D.* The CT scan of another patient with a larger acoustic neurinoma; the tumor shows characteristic homogeneous enhancement and a well-circumscribed margin.

centrations that are used, unless the patient has a previous history of a seizure disorder, or alcoholism, or is receiving neuroleptic medications.

Angiography

Prior to the advent of computed tomography, angiography was useful in assessing patients with a raised intracranial pressure and a suspected posterior fossa tumor, but its role has diminished considerably in recent years. Angiography is now reserved for patients in whom a vascular neoplasm (for

example, a hemangioblastoma or glomus jugulare tumor) is suspected, for embolization therapy of glomus jugulare and other hypervascular tumors, to rule out the possibility of an aneurysm mimicking a neoplasm in the cerebellopontine angle, and to provide a preoperative "road map" of the arteries adjacent to a detected neoplasm.

Selective vertebral angiography with subtraction technique displays the vertebral, basilar, posterior inferior cerebellar, anterior inferior cerebellar, and superior cerebellar arteries. Cerebellopontine angle mass lesions characteristically elevate (less often, depress) the anterior inferior cerebellar artery and efface the characteristic loop that lies adja-

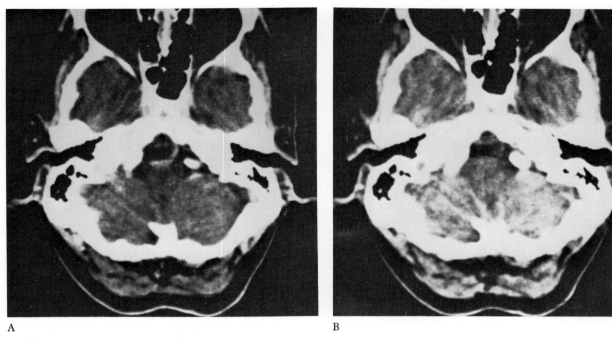

A   B

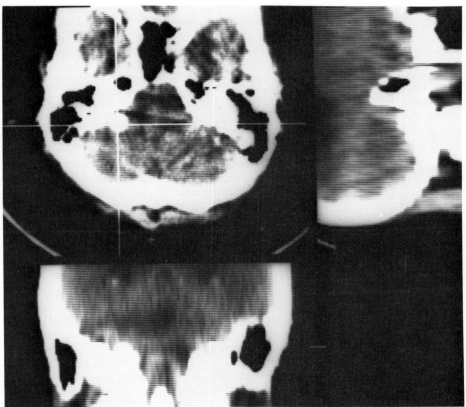

C

Figure 80-5 Normal CT studies using 10-mm-thick sections and without high-resolution reconstruction: *A*. After contrast enhancement, bilateral high-density "lesions" in the cerebellopontine angles mimic acoustic neurinomas. *B*. Twenty-four hours later the study was repeated, and this unenhanced section at the same level shows that the "lesions" are in fact prominent jugular tubercles. *C*. In another normal patient with a unilateral high jugular tubercle, sagittal and coronal reformatting of 5-mm CT sections clarifies the nature of the high-density structure in the cerebellopontine angle.

cent to the internal auditory canal (Fig. 80-9*A*). Large mass lesions will displace the basilar artery to the contralateral side, elevate the superior cerebellar artery, and depress and displace posteriorly the choroidal point of the posterior infe-

rior cerebellar artery (Fig. 80-9*C*). In the venous phase of vertebral angiography, the petrosal vein is usually obliterated in the presence of a cerebellopontine angle mass lesion (Fig. 80-9*B* and *D*).

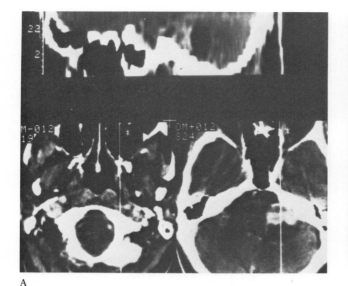

A

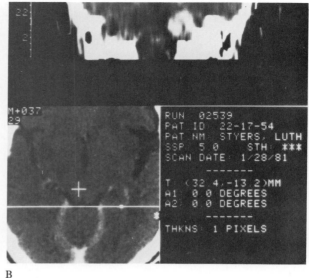

B

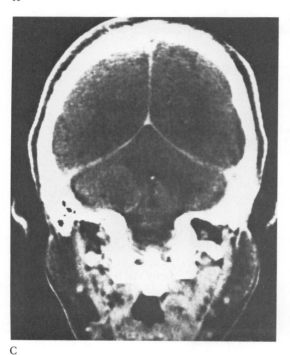

C

Figure 80-6 An acoustic neurinoma with an unusual large cystic component: sagittal (*A*) and coronal (*B*) reformatting define the tumor relationship to the temporal bone and cerebellum, but spatial resolution is inferior. *C*. In another patient, a direct coronal CT scan more clearly defines the tumor margins and the relationship to the displaced fourth ventricle, vallecula, and tentorium.

Digital subtraction angiography by computer technique simplifies arterial studies technically, and additionally may permit the characterization of the vascularity of a cerebellopontine angle mass lesion following a venous injection of a contrast agent (Fig. 80-11). The increased contrast resolution of this technique compared with conventional subtraction angiography offers the potential for a more complete, relatively noninvasive preoperative analysis of these lesions. However, there is some sacrifice of spatial resolution at this time in evolution of computer subtraction units in comparison with conventional angiography.

Jugular Venography

Jugular venography is uncommonly required when high-quality subtraction angiography is available. This procedure is employed when the extent of a demonstrated glomus jugulare tumor invading the jugular vein needs to be defined accurately. It may also occasionally be useful to confirm the suspected diagnosis of an anomalous high position of the jugular bulb in a patient who usually presents with pulsatile tinnitus and who has a demonstrated, smoothly marginated enlargement of the jugular fossa on films of the petrous bone (Fig. 80-12). In this technique, a retrograde high-volume

Selective external carotid angiography is most useful in analyzing glomus jugulare tumors, and most commonly these tumors are markedly hypervascular, deriving their blood supply from the ascending pharyngeal branch or other branches of the external carotid artery (Fig. 80-10). Embolization of these feeding arteries using particles of Gelfoam (absorbable gelatin sponge, The Upjohn Company, Kalamazoo, Mich.), polyvinyl alcohol, or polymerizing liquids may aid the surgeon by devascularizing such a tumor prior to its resection. In inoperable tumors, palliation or even ablation may be achieved by multiple arterial embolizations.

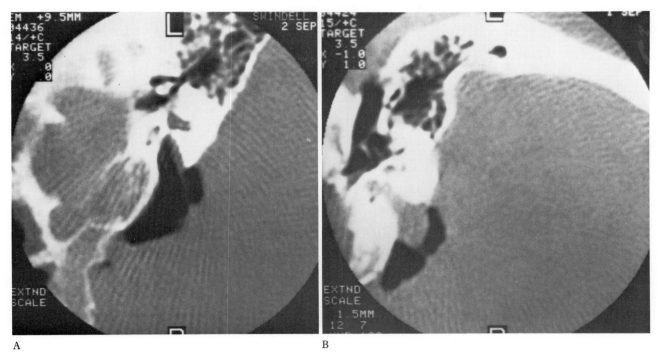

Figure 80-7 Gas CT cisternography in detecting small acoustic neurinomas: *A*. In this normal patient, gas enters the internal auditory canal and clearly defines the neurovascular bundle. *B*. In this patient with a small acoustic neurinoma, widening of the porus acusticus and a well-circumscribed tumor margin preventing entrance of gas into the canal are seen.

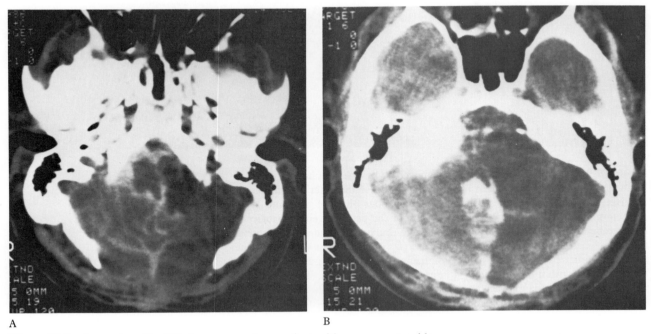

Figure 80-8 A metrizamide CT cisternogram in a patient with a recurrent epidermoid tumor of the left cerebellopontine angle. Displacement of the medulla (*A*) and fourth ventricle (*B*) away from the tumor mass distinguishes a recurrent epidermoid tumor from a surgical defect filled with cerebrospinal fluid. The subarachnoid and intraventricular metrizamide outlines the lesion with a precision unachievable by conventional computed tomography.

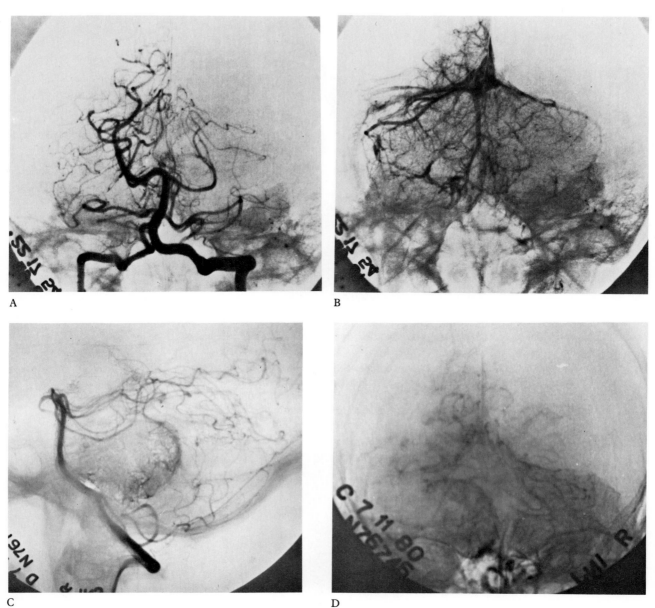

A

B

C

D

Figure 80-9 A large left acoustic neurinoma: *A.* The arterial phase of a left vertebral angiogram shows effacement of the normal loop of the anterior inferior cerebellar artery opposite the porus acusticus. *B.* The venous phase of the same Towne's
projection angiographic run shows obliteration of the petrosal vein, a paucity of surface cerebellar veins, and a subtle capsular vein draped over the superior surface of
the tumor mass. The lateral (*C*) and Towne's (*D*) projections of a vertebral angiogram in another patient shows more prominent capsular vessels and subtle stippled
neovascularity within the margin of a large acoustic neurinoma. The posterior inferior cerebellar artery is displaced posteriorly and inferiorly while the basilar artery
preserves its normal position in the lateral projection.

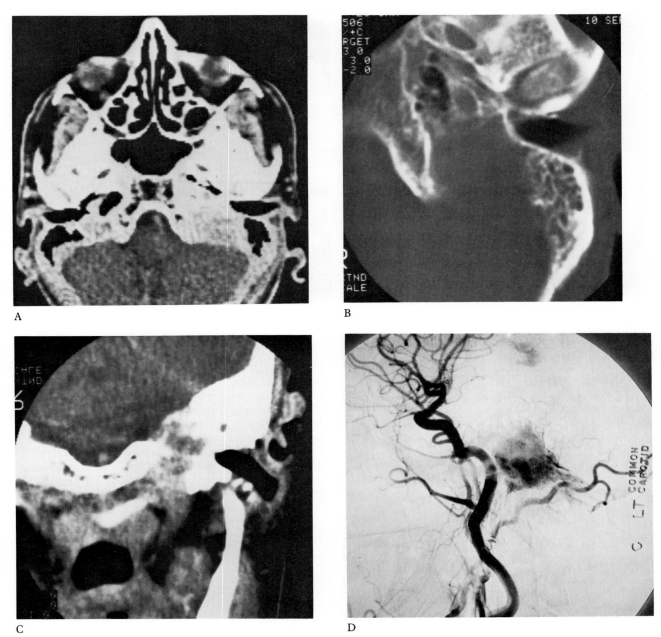

A

B

C

D

Figure 80-10 A glomus jugulare tumor: *A*. A contrast enhanced axial CT scan with conventional technique shows fairly well circumscribed enhancing pathological tissue in the region of the right jugular foramen, with possible bony invasion. *B*. Small field of view imaging with bone window reconstruction technique shows the extensive bony destruction involving the mastoid air cells and bony labyrinth as well as the margin of the soft tissue mass. *C*. A direct coronal high-resolution CT scan with an intermediate window setting shows the enhancing tumor tissue, bony destruction, and extension of the tumor into the jugular vein beneath the jugular foramen. *D*. A common carotid arteriogram following partial embolization (note the wire coil in an external carotid branch) reveals extensive tumor hypervascularity in the arterial phase. The feeding vessels were chiefly the ascending pharyngeal artery and un-named branches of the external carotid artery.

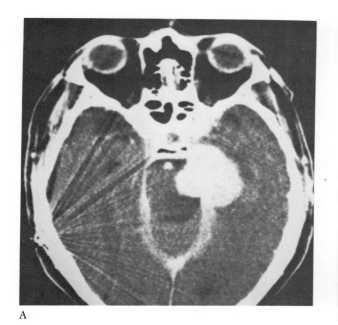

A

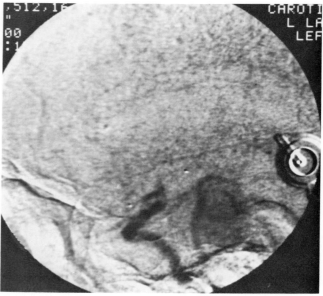

B

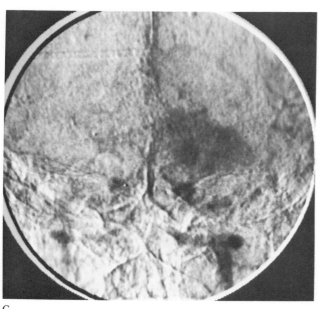

C

Figure 80-11   A meningioma of the tentorial edge with extension to the cerebellopontine angle: *A.* An intravenously enhanced CT examination reveals a typical well-circumscribed tumor mass arising from the tentorial edge. The brain stem is displaced to the contralateral side. Artifacts are induced by a metal ventricular shunt apparatus. *B,C.* Digital subtraction angiography (venous injection) shows a typical meningioma blush and defines the relationship of the tumor to the posterior cerebral and basilar arteries.

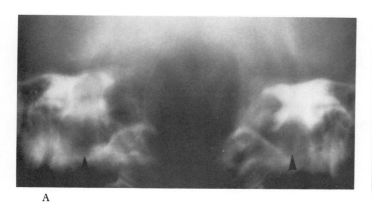

A

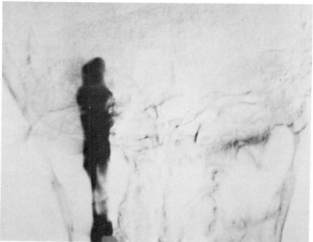

B

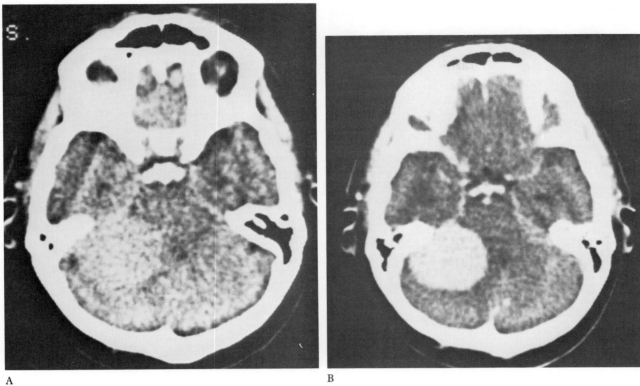

A   B

Figure 80-13 A meningioma of the cerebellopontine angle: *A*. An unenhanced CT scan shows a well-circumscribed lesion of greater than cerebellar tissue density arising in the angle and displacing the fourth ventricle and brain stem. *B*. After intravenous contrast agent administration, there is marked homogeneous enhancement, and a well-circumscribed margin is better defined.

injection of a contrast agent into the jugular vein is performed using either a transfemoral venous catheterization or a percutaneous puncture of the jugular vein.

Individual Tumors

Acoustic Neurinoma

Computed tomography performed correctly readily detects all acoustic neurinomas provided their extracanalicular component has a diameter greater than 1.5 cm. This is assuming that an intravenous contrast agent is administered, since a noncontrast CT scan will often fail to show acoustic neurinomas. In noncontrast CT scans, large lesions cause effacement of the cerebellopontine angle cistern and displacement

Figure 80-12 An anomalous high right jugular bulb: *A*. Frontal polydirectional tomogram shows a well-circumscribed defect immediately posterior to the internal auditory canal in the right petrous temporal bone. *B*. A retrograde jugular venogram shows the anomalous high jugular bulb responsible for the patient's pulsatile tinnitus.

of the fourth ventricle, but the tumor is usually almost isodense with the adjacent cerebellar tissue. Calcification is exceedingly rare and, if demonstrated, should raise the suspicion of a meningioma or a "collision tumor" composed of a meningioma as well as a neurinoma. After the intravenous infusion of a contrast agent, almost all acoustic neurinomas exhibit contrast enhancement. Two-thirds of them enhance homogeneously and have well-defined margins (80-4). About one-third of tumors exhibit ring enhancement,[7] and in such cases, delayed CT scanning at 30 to 90 min will usually show diffusion of the contrast agent into the center of the tumor. Uncommonly, cysts are demonstrated in association with acoustic neurinomas; these are usually small and contiguous with the surface of the tumor (Fig. 80-6).

Computed tomography using bone window techniques and appropriate thin sections (5, 2, or 1.5 mm) will reveal the characteristic widening of the porus acusticus and internal auditory canal in the vast majority of patients with acoustic neurinomas. This bony change aids in differentiating this lesion from meningiomas and neurinomas of other cranial nerves. Occasionally, large tumors will be purely extracanalicular and there will be no bony erosion. In such cases, obviously, plain film and polytomographic findings correlate very poorly with the size of the tumor present. Rarely, acoustic neurinomas have lobulated contours and a less spherical contour than the typical tumor, and in such

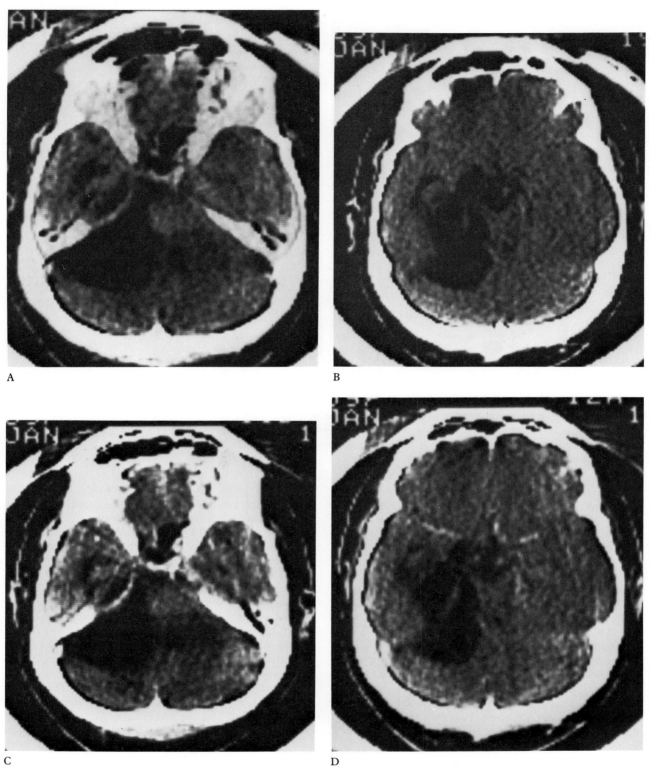

A

B

C

D

Figure 80-14   An epidermoid cyst of the cerebellopontine angle with supratentorial
extension: *A,B*. Before contrast enhancement, the lower than CSF density lesion
with relatively little mass effect for its size is detected infratentorially, in the ambient
cistern, and above the tentorial hiatus. *C,D*. Following intravenous contrast agent
administration, there is no change in the attenuation value of the cyst.

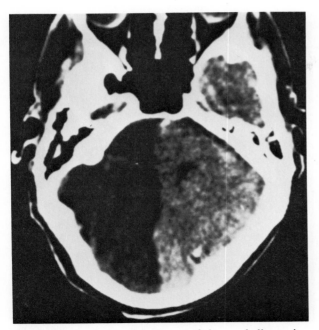

Figure 80-15 An arachnoid cyst of the cerebellopontine angle. This unusually large lesion in a 48-year-old male has a density approximately equal to that of cerebrospinal fluid and demonstrated no increasing density after intravenous contrast agent administration. There is bony remodelling of the petrous temporal bone and marked displacement of the fourth ventricle to the contralateral side.

cases, differentiation from an intra-axial tumor with an exophytic component is difficult. Characteristic widening of the porus acusticus is a useful differentiating feature.

Metrizamide CT cisternography may be valuable, and the use of a low-volume technique and a small-gauge spinal needle has significantly reduced the risk of tonsillar herniation, which exists with any large posterior fossa tumor.[5] However, this procedure should not be performed if there is demonstrated enlargement of the lateral and third ventricles at CT, or if there is a large posterior fossa mass lesion and no precautions are taken for emergency ventriculostomy. The enhanced depiction of the cerebrospinal fluid spaces by metrizamide will usually enable differentiation between intra-axial and extra-axial tumors (Fig. 80-8).

Angiography is rarely necessary in patients with typical clinical, audiometric, and computed tomographic findings. Typically, acoustic neurinomas are hypovascular, with tiny irregular tumor vessels demonstrated in the periphery of the tumor on selective external carotid angiography. The lesions are usually avascular at vertebral angiography, where a defect in the capillary phase, displacement of the anterior inferior cerebellar artery, and obliteration of the petrosal vein by pressure effect are usually seen (Fig. 80-9).

Gas CT cisternography using overlapped 5-mm sections or contiguous 1.5- to 2.0-mm sections is the "gold standard" today for detecting or excluding small intracanalicular tumors that are beyond the resolution of intravenous enhanced CT. If the internal auditory canal of the clinically symptomatic side fills completely to the area cribrosa and no spherical filling defect is present in the porus or canal, the diagnosis of a small acoustic neurinoma is confidently excluded (Fig. 80-7A). In centers where only thick-section low-resolution CT scanners are available, posterior fossa myelography using low-volume technique and polydirectional tomography is still useful in the detection of small intracanalicular lesions (Fig. 80-3).

Meningioma

Computed tomography of meningiomas in the cerebellopontine angle usually reveals a well-circumscribed spherical mass lesion with higher than brain density on the noncontrast CT scan (Fig. 80-13A). Occasionally, calcification is demonstrated within the tumor mass. After intravenous contrast administration, prominent contrast enhancement is the rule (Fig. 80-13B). Bony erosion of the porus acusticus or of the temporal bone surface is uncommon. Reactive hyperostosis is also uncommon with meningiomas in this location.

Because these tumors have usually obtained a diameter of at least 1 cm before presentation with symptoms, there is rarely any need to perform CT gas cisternography or other cerebrospinal fluid enhancing techniques. Angiography is occasionally performed to aid in the differentiation from a calcified aneurysm or other neoplasm; the characteristic homogeneous late blush of a meningioma is usually demonstrable (Fig. 80-11).

Epidermoid Tumor

Epidermoid tumors constitute the third most common lesion of the cerebellopontine angle, and CT scanning characteristically reveals a low-density, irregularly contoured lesion with less mass effect than would be expected with a meningioma or acoustic neurinoma of equivalent size. The low-density center reflects a high lipid content, and attenuation values below those of CSF may be seen.[4] The tumor usually exhibits no change in CT attenuation after intravenous contrast agent administration (Fig. 80-14). Calcification is occasionally encountered in the rim of the cyst, and this usually indicates a lesion of considerable age. Rarely, high-density epidermoids are encountered on unenhanced CT scans, but again, pathological enhancement is absent.[2] These tumors tend to extend along cleavage planes between cerebral and cerebellar structures, may extend supratentorially, and may reach quite a large size before becoming symptomatic because of their minimal mass effect.

Glomus Jugulare Tumor

When this tumor is large enough to extend into the cerebellopontine angle, there is always extensive irregular bony destruction in the region of the jugular foramen (Fig. 80-10). CT scanning reveals slightly higher than cerebellar at-

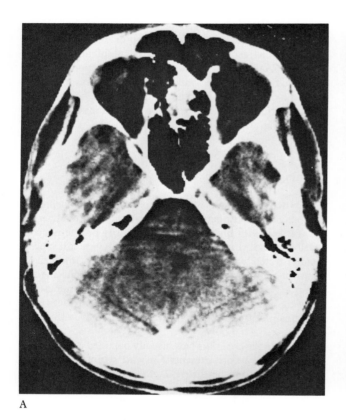

A

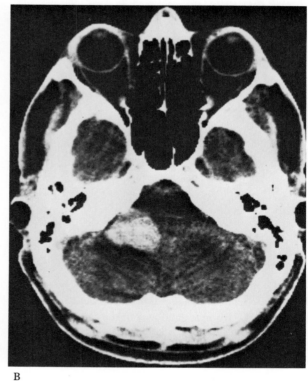

B

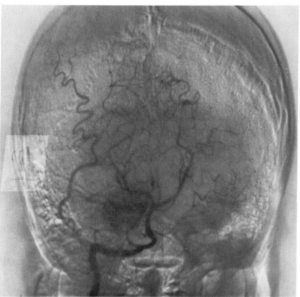

C

Figure 80-16 A cerebellar hemangioblastoma, shown in unenhanced (*A*) and enhanced (*B*) CT scans, and by angiography (*C*). This solid lesion extended into the cerebellopontine angle.

Other Tumors

Arachnoid cysts (Fig. 80-15) mimic epidermoid tumors in the cerebellopontine angle, but their CSF density usually enables characterization. Neurinomas of the lower cranial nerves (IX to XII) may extend to the cerebellopontine angle. The location and CT features (similar to those of acoustic neurinoma) of these uncommon lesions challenge the radiological investigator, and metrizamide CT studies and angiography may be indicated. Large pituitary adenomas occasionally extend caudally through the tentorial hiatus to present in the cerebellopontine angle; high-resolution CT scanning usually makes the diagnosis clear. Hemangioblastomas (Fig. 80-16) and choroid plexus papillomas may present atypically in the cerebellopontine angle; angiography is usually sufficiently characteristic to separate these vascular tumors from meningiomas and neurinomas. Primary intrapetrous neoplasms (Fig. 80-17) and nasopharyngeal and clival tumors may extend into the cerebellopontine angle; to

tenuation values on the noncontrast study, and after intravenous contrast enhancement, there is a marked increase in attenuation values reflecting hypervascularity. Angiography always produces a prominent early arterial and capillary phase blush, usually with large feeding vessels from the external carotid artery.

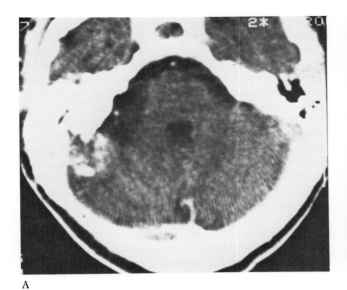
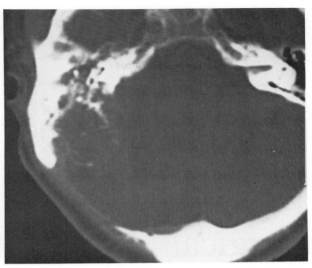

A   B

Figure 80-17 A ceruminoma. This rare, locally invasive tumor arising from the external auditory canal has recurred following partial resection. *A*. The enhancing intracranial component is well demonstrated with small field of view, narrow window technique. *B*. With wider window technique, the origin of this invasive tumor from the middle ear and mastoid, and marginal calcifications, are displayed.

correctly analyze their origin and extent requires careful technique in CT examinations with specialized projections, intravenous contrast enhancement, and bone window widths.

References

1. Anke IM: Metrizamide cisternography of the cerebello-pontine angle by lateral C1-C2 puncture. Neuroradiology 25:81–83, 1983.

2. Braun IF, Naidich TP, Leeds NE, Koslow M, Zimmerman HM, Chase NE: Dense intracranial epidermoid tumors. Radiology 122:717–719, 1977.

3. Britton BH Jr, Hitselberger WE: Iophendylate examination of posterior fossa in diagnosis of cerebellopontine angle tumors. Arch Otolaryngol 88:608–617, 1968.

4. Davis KR, Roberson GH, Taveras JM, New PJ, Trevor R: Diagnosis of epidermoid tumor by computed tomography: Analysis and evaluation of findings. Radiology 119:347–353, 1976.

5. Dubois PJ, Drayer BP, Bank WO, Deeb ZL, Rosenbaum AE: An evaluation of current diagnostic radiologic modalities in the investigation of acoustic neurilemmomas. Radiology 126:173–179, 1978.

6. Kricheff I, Pinto RS, Bergeron RT, Cohen N: Air-CT cisternography and canalography in the diagnosis of small acoustic neuromas. AJNR 1:57–63, 1980.

7. Naidich TP, Lin JP, Leeds NE, Kricheff II, George AE, Chase NE, Pudlowski RM, Passalaqua A: Computed tomography in the diagnosis of extra-axial posterior fossa masses. Radiology 120:333–339, 1976.

8. Scanlan RL: Positive contrast medium (iophendylate) in diagnosis of acoustic neuroma. Arch Otolaryngol 80:698–707, 1964.

9. Sortland O: Computed tomography combined with gas cisternography for the diagnosis of expanding lesions in the cerebellopontine angle. Neuroradiology 18:19–22, 1979.

10. Valvassori GE: The diagnosis of acoustic neuromas. Otolaryngol Clin North Am 6:391–400, 1973.

81

Tumors of the Cerebellopontine Angle: Clinical Features and Surgical Management

William A. Buchheit
Tomas E. Delgado

The history of surgery of the posterior fossa is reflected in the history of acoustic neuromas. Prior to the twentieth century, occasional attempts at surgery within the cerebellopontine angle (CPA) were carried out. These were associated with extremely high mortality, and most people, including surgeons, considered the operations suicidal. After the turn of the century, improvements in anesthesia and surgical technique led to a dramatic reduction in mortality and morbidity of neurosurgery in general and surgery of the posterior fossa in particular. The mortality dropped from 85 percent in Henschen's cases reported in 1910[4] to 4 percent by Cushing[2] 22 years later. Progressive improvement in diagnostic and surgical techniques has led to the modern era. It is now possible, with computed tomograms, to identify tumors in an early stage and, with microneurosurgery, to remove them with a consistently low mortality. An operation which was once believed to be impossible is now performed daily. Nowhere has the progress of neurosurgery been so dramatically demonstrated as in the history of posterior fossa surgery.

Clinical Features

The clinical features of cerebellopontine angle lesions are uniquely specific. The close proximity of a number of important structures permits the clinical diagnosis of cerebellopontine angle masses with great certainty. On the other hand, the uniformly slow growth rates of these lesions make a clinical histological diagnosis practically impossible. Fortunately, diagnostic aids (discussed elsewhere) permit the differentiation of tumor types with a high degree of reliability. Thus a combination of clinical examination and specific neuroradiological, audiologic, and neurophysiological evaluation allows the neurosurgeon to come to the operating room with a fairly accurate preoperative diagnosis.

The acoustic neuroma is the most common cerebellopontine angle tumor and may serve as a prototype for lesions in this area. A history of progressive unilateral hearing loss, usually over many months and sometimes years, is a hallmark of this tumor. It is associated with tinnitus in most cases, and as the tumor enlarges the patient complains of unsteadiness and loss of balance. True rotational vertigo is rare.

The resistance of the facial nerve to stretching and distortion is a curiosity which has been observed consistently. The nerve usually functions normally until the tumor reaches a large size. When a problem with the nerve does develop, it is usually mild. Total facial paralysis is rare and is usually seen only with the largest tumors.

Involvement of the trigeminal nerve likewise occurs late and is seen primarily in tumors more than 3 cm in diameter. As the tumor grows upward into the superior aspect of the cerebellopontine angle, it encroaches upon the trigeminal nerve, producing the diminution, and later loss, of the corneal reflex. Facial analgesia and anesthesia follow progressively as the tumor enlarges. Anesthesia of the face, like seventh nerve palsy, is usually associated with a large tumor. Tic-like pain occurs rarely.

Cerebellar signs and symptoms occur late in the growth of these lesions and are often associated with dysfunction of the trigeminal and facial nerves. Papilledema and hydrocephalus occur, usually in the late stages of the development of these tumors.

Hearing loss is the most consistent symptom in patients with acoustic lesions. Details of the audiologic manifestations are discussed in another chapter.

Meningiomas are the second most frequent tumor of the angle. These tumors have the same general signs and symptoms as acoustic tumors, with several exceptions. Often these lesions originate from the superior anterior lip of the porus acusticus[9] and are associated with early involvement of the seventh nerve. Hearing loss, on the other hand, occurs later. In terms of the facial and auditory function, meningiomas are the exact opposite of acoustic tumors. Involvement of the posterior root of the fifth nerve may lead to numbness of the face and tic-like symptoms. These symptoms, preceding hearing loss, tip the scales in favor of a meningioma or, less likely, a tumor of the trigeminal nerve.

The growth downward of any of these lesions leads to hoarseness, numbness of the throat, difficulty swallowing, etc., as the ninth, tenth, and eleventh nerves are compromised. Ataxia becomes prominent when the lesions compromise the cerebellum and its peduncle. Exceptionally large tumors lead to brain stem compression and pyramidal tract signs.

Those meningiomas that arise far up in the cerebellopontine angle ultimately produce similar signs, but they are preceded by the fifth nerve symptoms. When the tumor growth is in the direction of the incisura, early signs and symptoms of hydrocephalus and increased intracranial pressure may occur. Associated with this are, ultimately, upper pontine and midbrain signs, including involvement of the third, fourth, and sixth cranial nerves.

Metastatic tumors of the angle occur less frequently than either meningiomas or acoustic tumors. Differentiation between these lesions is practically impossible without knowledge of the primary tumor.

Headaches occur in these patients and are generally of two types. The more common is secondary to hydrocephalus and intracranial pressure; the less common is related to involvement of the trigeminal fibers in the adjacent dura.

Anatomy

The cerebellopontine angle is an inverted triangular cistern in which the fifth, seventh, and eighth cranial nerves, along with the anterior inferior cerebellar artery (AICA) and the superior petrosal vein, are located (Fig. 81-1). From a surgeon's viewpoint, the cistern is bounded laterally by the back wall of the petrous bone, medially by the pons, and cephalad by the tentorium which forms the base of the triangle. This cistern communicates freely with the other cerebrospinal fluid spaces within the posterior fossa, including a small diverticulum which extends down into the porus acusticus.[11]

At the upper aspect of the cistern, the fifth nerve is a broad white band, extending from the lateral aspect of the pons into Meckel's cavity. At the upper posterior edge of this nerve is the petrosal vein, which drains from the superior aspect of the cerebellum to the superior petrosal sinus. This vein is usually 1 to 2 mm in diameter and at times may be made up of a cluster of veins.[5,15]

The seventh and eighth nerves course laterally from the pontomedullary junction to the internal auditory canal. They cross the cistern in what appears to be a single nerve, which is composed of four discrete nerves—the superior and inferior vestibular nerves, the cochlear nerve, and the facial nerve. When viewed from the suboccipital approach, the vestibular nerves form the posterior aspect, or the portion closest to the surgeon. The facial nerve makes up the anterior superior portion within this bundle, and the cochlear division of the eighth nerve makes up the anterior inferior portion.[12] When one looks into the posterior fossa from the extreme lateral aspect of a suboccipital approach, the sixth nerve is occasionally seen coursing from its origin at the pontomedullary junction to its entrance into the dura of the clivus. In situations where the tumor has rotated and displaced the brain stem, this nerve may be confused with the seventh nerve, inasmuch as it exits on the same plane as the seventh nerve and enters the dura at the same level as the internal auditory canal.

The ninth, tenth, and eleventh nerves, although not specifically within the cerebellopontine angle cistern, are found immediately below its inferior margin. The most superior of these nerves, the ninth, is round and shiny and made up of a single filament. The tenth nerve consists of multiple filaments which are flat, and the eleventh nerve is unique in having a spinal root traversing the foramen magnum.

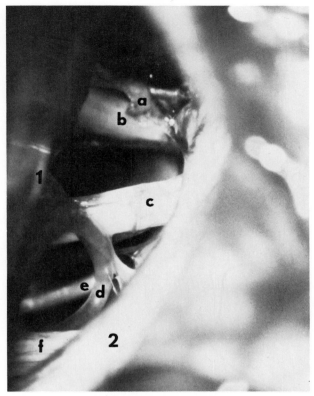

Figure 81-1 Normal microsurgical anatomy of the right cerebellopontine angle. (1) Cerebellar retractor; (2) petrous bone; (a) petrosal vein; (b) trigeminal nerve; (c) VII-VIII nerve complex; (d) anterior inferior cerebellar artery; (e) VI nerve; (f) IX-X-XI nerve complex.

The anterior inferior cerebellar artery has a variable location within the cistern. In acoustic tumors, this vessel is usually located in the arachnoid over the cleft between the cerebellum and the dome of the tumor.

Operative Approaches to the Cerebellopontine Angle

Middle Fossa Approach

The middle fossa approach, as described by House in 1961,[6] involves an extradural subtemporal approach with microsurgical unroofing of the internal auditory canal. This approach is limited to the excision of small intracanalicular tumors that have not escaped the confines of the internal auditory canal. It is usually performed in patients in whom audition remains at a functional level, providing a chance of hearing preservation.

The procedure is performed with the patient in the lateral position. A linear temporal incision is made from the zygomatic arch to the insertion of the temporalis fascia (Fig. 81-2). A bone flap is constructed as a square, two-thirds anterior and one-third posterior to the external auditory canal. Once the dura is elevated from the floor of the tempo-

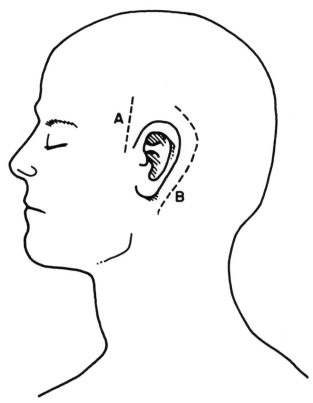

Figure 81-2 Surgical incisions used for A, middle fossa approach and B, translabyrinthine approach to acoustic tumors.

ral fossa, the House-Urban retractor is secured in place. Several anatomical structures come into view as the dural dissection continues. First is the middle meningeal artery, exiting the foramen spinosum. This landmark is used as the anterior limit of the dural elevation. Next, the petrous ridge is identified, at the point where it has been grooved by the superior petrosal sinus. Care must be taken not to injure the geniculate ganglion or the greater superficial petrosal nerve, both of which lie unprotected by bone in about 5 percent of cases. The greater superficial petrosal nerve, when followed posteriorly, leads to the facial nerve. At this point in the operation, it is usually possible to identify the middle meningeal artery, the arcuate eminence, the greater superficial petrosal nerve, and the facial hiatus. Bone removal over the auditory canal follows. It is easier to identify the internal auditory canal by following the facial nerve. The entire superior wall of the canal is exposed and removed (Fig. 81-3). The lateral end of the internal auditory canal is dissected, and the vertical crest of bone separating the facial from the superior vestibular nerve (Bill's bar) is identified. The dura is opened along the posterior aspect of the internal auditory canal. The tumor is removed by first freeing it from the facial nerve and internal auditory canal, posterior to and beneath the facial nerve.

The search for the anterior inferior cerebellar artery is begun after a plane has been developed between the facial and cochlear nerves and the tumor. This artery is most likely

to be spared from injury if it is identified early and dissected free from the tumor capsule.

A temporalis muscle graft is used to obliterate the defect in the internal auditory canal. The craniotomy and skin flap are then closed in the usual fashion.

Translabyrinthine Approach

The microsurgical translabyrinthine approach was developed by House in 1964.[7] It exposes the posterior fossa dura in the retromeatal trigone (Trautmann's triangle) formed by the sigmoid sinus, jugular bulb, and superior petrosal sinus. This approach is usually reserved for patients with moderate-sized tumors (1.0 to 2.5 cm in diameter). Unfortunately, any preoperative auditory function is lost as a result of this approach.

The mastoid is exposed through an incision approximately 2 cm behind the ear (Fig. 81-2). The mastoidectomy and labyrinthectomy are performed with a high-speed drill with a diamond burr, under the operative microscope. The facial nerve is exposed and freed from the tumor in the vicinity of the porus acusticus.

Following bone removal (Fig. 81-4), the dura in front of the sigmoid sinus is opened, and this opening is carried forward to the porus acusticus, exposing the tumor. Dissection around the tumor is carried superiorly and medially to free the cerebellum and then continued in the direction of the superior petrosal sinus and the anterior inferior cerebellar artery. Care must be taken to visualize the ninth, tenth, and eleventh nerves and to dissect them away from the lower pole of the tumor capsule. The tumor is then incised and removed in a piecemeal fashion (Fig. 81-5). Further dissection is carried out between these neurovascular structures and the capsule as tumor removal continues.

After the tumor has been removed, the dural defect is covered with a temporalis muscle graft or fat. The soft tissues are closed in layers in the usual fashion.

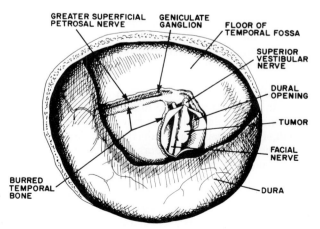

Figure 81-3 Middle fossa approach. Schematic overall view of an intracanalicular acoustic neuroma.

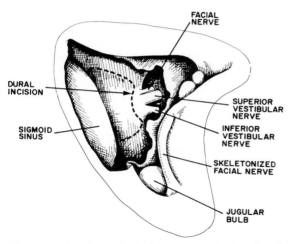

Figure 81-4 Translabyrinthine approach. Landmarks and exposure seen during microscopic dissection.

Posterior Fossa Transmeatal Approach

The authors prefer to have the patient in the sitting position for surgery of lesions in the angle (Fig. 81-6). The patient is placed on the operating table with the neck in the neutral position and the head turned gently toward the side of the lesion. Then, to avoid flexing the cervical spine, access up into the cerebellar pontine angle is gained by forward rotation of the entire operating table. This maneuver is particularly important in patients with cervical spondylosis. An alternative is the lateral position, with the patient's head extended off the foot of the table to give more room for the surgeon's legs (Fig. 81-7).

With the patient appropriately prepared and draped, a modified "hockey stick" incision is made (Fig. 81-8). No preliminary burr hole is made. In patients with hydrocephalus, shunting is done at an earlier operation, and those with

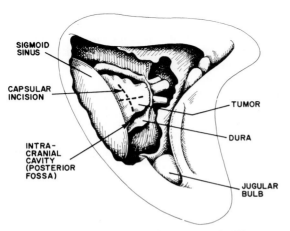

Figure 81-5 Translabyrinthine approach. The dura has been entered and the tumor exposed. Tumor removal is begun by debulking the center of the tumor, as illustrated.

normal ventricles are monitored with a pressure bolt following the operation.

The horizontal limb of the skin incision is made 2 cm above and parallel to the nuchal line, avoiding transection of the suboccipital muscles. The lateral vertical limb of the incision is made over the mastoid process and quite far lateral. The skin and muscle flap is turned down in the standard way. In doing this, care must be taken in the region of C1 and the foramen magnum to avoid injury to an aberrant vertebral artery, which may loop unexpectedly up into the cervical muscles.

The craniectomy should extend up to the edge of the sigmoid sinus, which corresponds roughly to the medial border of the petrous bone. If necessary, the mastoid air cells are opened and sealed with bone wax. With completion of the craniectomy, furosemide or mannitol is given to relax the dura. Once slack, the dura is opened at the midpoint of the craniectomy and then further opened to the edges of the transverse and sigmoid sinuses. The final 1 to 2 mm of the dural incision is made with the aid of fiberoptic transillumination, the light being inserted into the subdural space and the dura transilluminated (Fig. 81-9). The dural flaps are sewn back to the fascial edges. The cerebellum is elevated to expose the cisterna magna, which is then opened. With the cerebrospinal fluid drained, a self-retaining retractor is inserted and the cerebellar hemisphere elevated superiorly and medially. Most angle neoplasms arise outside the cerebrospinal fluid space, and their continued growth is associated with the involution or infolding of the arachnoid back into the cistern. As the tumor grows, this involuted lateral arachnoid comes into contact with the more medial arachnoid, forming a distinct double-layered cap (Fig. 81-10). This arachnoid cap contains the important vessels and nerves of the cerebellopontine angle and serves as a cleavage plane and barrier between the tumor and brain stem. This cleavage plane facilitates the dissection of tumors and should be preserved. With sharp dissection, the arachnoid overlying the tumor is removed, setting the stage for the tumor's removal (Fig. 81-11).

The site of origin of the tumor determines the direction in which the lower cranial nerves will be displaced. In acoustic tumors, for example, the seventh nerve is usually displaced anteriorly around the tumor on the side away from the surgeon. On the other hand, in meningiomas arising from the anterior lip of the porus acusticus, the seventh nerve will be displaced posteriorly toward the surgeon. In meningiomas of the clivus, the nerves are displaced laterally over the tumor. In all circumstances, the location of the nerve may be confirmed by stimulation.

Once the landmarks have been identified, the tumor is reduced in size by internal decompression (Fig. 81-12). Many of these tumors are soft, and it is possible to remove them by aspiration. In others it is necessary to use ultrasonic aspiration or the laser. The decompression process allows the walls of the tumor to cave in and eventually converts a large tumor to a small one. As the walls of the tumor collapse, it may be necessary to return to arachnoid dissection to mobilize the cranial nerves, the anterior inferior cerebellar artery, and brain stem. It is the authors' preference to dissect the medial aspect of the tumor from the brain stem

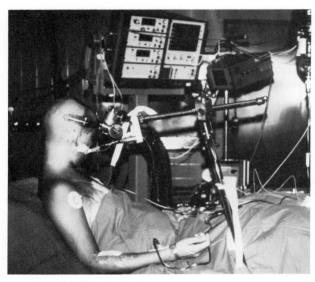

Figure 81-6 Sitting position.

first. In general, tumors are dissected with microscissors and an absolute minimum of traction. No attempt is made to remove the lesion in one piece. Once the medial portion of the tumor is free, the lateral part is removed. It is usually necessary to drill off the posterior wall of the porus in order to expose the intracanalicular portion. This is done by removing the dura over the posterior aspect of the porus and drilling off the bone. Once exposed, the dural lining of the porus is opened and the contents dissected.

In the large tumors it is at times necessary to remove the lateral third of the cerebellar hemisphere in order to gain exposure. The authors prefer resection to forcible retraction of the cerebellar hemisphere. With smaller tumors, furosemide, mannitol, and judicious elevation of the hemisphere are usually adequate to gain exposure. Once the tumor has been removed, hemostasis is obtained by the usual means. Bilateral jugular compression and a normal systemic blood pressure confirm hemostasis. Prior to closure, the integrity

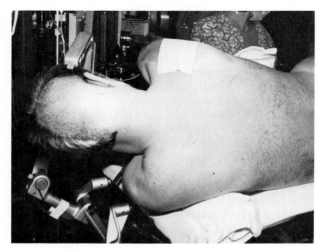

Figure 81-7 Lateral position.

of the seventh nerve is demonstrated by electrical nerve stimulation and facial muscle recordings.[3] In the event that the nerve has been severed, intracranial anastamosis is attempted. Following this, the dura is closed along with the scalp flap. A nondominant frontal Richmond screw is inserted to monitor intracranial pressure and provide a site for ventricular catheterization if it becomes necessary.

Operative Complications

Complications related to surgery within the cerebellopontine angle may be divided into three distinct groups: those occurring during surgery, those occurring during the early postoperative period, and those occurring during the late postoperative period. The complications that occur during surgery may be further subdivided into anesthetic, surgical, and positional.

With the patient in the sitting position, the most common anesthetic complication is air embolization. Although usually not a serious problem, it has the potential to become one. Careful maintenance of hemostasis, beginning with the skin incision and continuing right through to wound closure, minimizes the risk. A Doppler precordial stethoscope and an expiratory CO_2 monitor alert the anesthesiologist and the surgeon to the presence of emboli. When evidence of embolization occurs, if nitrous oxide is being used it must immediately be discontinued and an attempt made to aspirate air from the atrial catheter.[13] Occasionally the site of the embolus is not apparent, and it may be necessary to pack the wound and discontinue surgery until the problem is under control. In extreme cases it is necessary to move the patient from the sitting position.

The most serious complication related to the sitting position is quadriplegia. Although the mechanisms are not clear, certain steps may be taken to minimize the risk of its occurrence. The most obvious precautionary measure is careful positioning of the head and neck in skeletal fixation, as described in the operative procedure. Cervical spine films, including flexion-extension views, may be taken to identify occult subluxation and cervical stenosis that could contribute to cord compression. It is possible that spinal cord infarction secondary to ischemia accounts for this complication; therefore maintenance of blood volume and pressure appear to be particularly important.

Two other complications of the sitting position are stretch injuries of the sciatic nerve and of the brachial plexus.[1] The sciatic nerve may be injured if the patient's legs are straight on the operating table, with hips flexed and knees extended. This position, over a period of several hours, may lead to neuropathy. This is easily avoided by flexing the knees to release the tension on the sciatic nerve. The arms should not be allowed to hang at the patient's side, producing drag on the brachial plexus. This is avoided by securing the arms comfortably across the abdomen.

Hemorrhage during surgery in the angle is usually not a major problem. Occasionally the petrosal vein is torn, and this can usually be managed with gentle packing. Laceration of an artery may lead to hemorrhage, but more importantly,

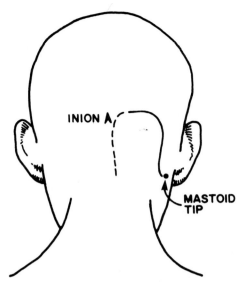

Figure 81-8 Surgical incision. Standard incision used for cerebellopontine angle tumor (*solid line*). Extension of the incision for large tumors (*dotted line*).

an injury of the anterior inferior cerebellar artery may lead to pontine infarction and death.

An unpleasant intraoperative complication is cerebellar swelling. There are two major causes for this. The most frequent is CO_2 retention, and this may be dealt with by the anesthesiologist. The other common source of cerebellar swelling is occult hemorrhage, above or anterior to the cerebellum. The bleeding must be controlled directly, and often this is not easy.

During the early postoperative period, monitoring of intracranial pressure aids in the detection of complications. The most serious of these complications is bleeding into the tumor bed, which, if not properly diagnosed and treated,

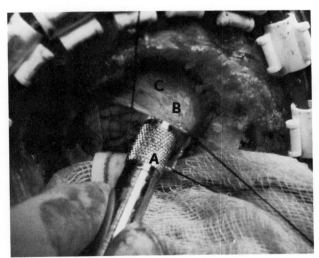

Figure 81-9 Dural transillumination. (A) Fiberoptic light; (B) dura; (C) transverse sinus.

may lead to catastrophe. The diagnosis is usually not difficult in the patient who has awakened from anesthesia and then becomes stuporous or comatose. If the deterioration is slow, there may be time for a CT scan. If, on the other hand, the deterioration is rapid, the patient is best taken to the operating room for re-exploration. This is a difficult decision to make, after a long operation, but experience leads the authors to believe that if a postoperative hemorrhage is suspected, re-exploration is best. Postoperative subdural hematomas are not common, and they usually develop more insidiously than do clots within the tumor bed.

Acute hydrocephalus may occur during the early postoperative period and may be difficult to differentiate from postoperative hemorrhage or may occur along with it. A CT scan is helpful, if time permits. If it does not, ventriculostomy prior to re-exploration of the surgical site will settle the issue. During the late postoperative period a more chronic form of hydrocephalus may develop; this may be managed in a routine way.

Postoperative bacterial meningitis most commonly occurs on the fifth to seventh day. The occurrence of fever, leukocytosis, and nuchal rigidity suggest this complication. The diagnosis may be made only with a spinal fluid analysis and culture. A sterile meningitis may also occur and can be differentiated by the spinal fluid analysis and culture.

Cerebrospinal fluid leakage results from poor wound healing, increased intracranial pressure, or wound infection. The treatment of the leak actually begins at the time of the initial incision. A clean, sharp incision and careful handling of the wound edges is most important in preventing its occurrence. Meticulous anatomical closure of the wound edges, including the dura, follows as a logical second step. In spite of good wound care, cerebrospinal fluid leak may still occur if intracranial pressure is elevated or if wound infection develops. Unfortunately, a few simple wound stitches seldom control a leak unless the underlying increased intracranial pressure is managed. In patients with hydrocephalus, a ventriculoperitoneal shunt will usually control the pressure and stop the drainage. The difficult problems occur in patients with meningitis and hydrocephalus; the authors are unwilling to insert a ventriculoperitoneal shunt in these patients and prefer a ventriculostomy with instillation of intraventricular antibiotics. When the culture is normal, a shunt is inserted.

The surgeon must be alert for occult cerebrospinal fluid leakage through the mastoid air cells that were opened either during the craniectomy or while drilling the porus acusticus. The fluid drains from the mastoid cells into the middle ear and then through the eustachian tube down the pharynx or out the nose. When this occurs, the authors usually insert a lumbar external drain for a few days. If the leak does not stop, the wound is re-explored.

Fifth nerve injury may follow removal of any size tumor. Within several days, the resultant corneal anesthesia may lead to corneal ulceration if proper eye care is not given. The fifth nerve function should be evaluated as soon as the patient awakens from anesthesia, even if there is no suspicion of injury to the nerve. When the corneal reflex is diminished, the eye should be covered with a protective shield and artificial tears inserted every 4 h. If the reflex is absent or if

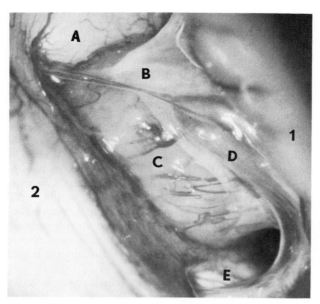

Figure 81-10 Acoustic tumor. (1) Cerebellar retractor; (2) temporal bone; (A) tentorium; (B) CPA arachnoid. (C) acoustic tumor; (D) AICA; (E) IX-X-XI nerve complex.

there is an associated facial palsy, a tarsorrhaphy is performed (Table 81-1).

Postoperative facial nerve paralysis is of two types—one that occurs immediately following surgery and a second that occurs within 3 to 4 days after surgery. The immediate type is the result of either anatomical disruption of the nerve or, more frequently, contusion and axonotmesis. With the immediate type, a curious phenomenon of spurious facial function may occur for 24 to 48 hours. During this period the eye closes and the face moves, but within several days the functions disappear. The reasons for this are not clear.

The delayed type of facial palsy develops between the third and fifth postoperative days and presumably is a consequence of edema or ischemia of the nerve. Regardless of the time frame, postoperative facial nerve palsy is a problem, because it impairs the blink reflex.

Immediately upon the patient's awakening from surgery, the seventh nerve function should be evaluated. If the face is paralyzed, the eye should be covered with a protective shield and artificial tears inserted every 4 h, and a tarsorrhaphy should soon be performed.

If the facial nerve has been totally disrupted during surgery, plans should be made for reinnervation of the face with nerve anastomosis, or reanimation by plastic surgery (Table 81-2). Generally, the authors delay both these procedures for 3 to 4 months, sometimes longer, giving the patient time to recover completely from the posterior fossa surgery. Details of the nerve anastomosis are presented elsewhere in this chapter.

TABLE 81-1 Management of Trigeminal Lesions

Facial nerve intact	:	Observation
Facial nerve paralyzed	:	Immediate tarsorrhaphy

TABLE 81-2 Management of Facial Paralysis

Facial nerve intact:
1. Tarsorrhaphy
2. Biofeedback
3. Physical therapy

Facial nerve not intact:
1. Tarsorrhaphy
2. Cranial nerve anastomosis
3. Static facial support (plastic surgery)

Bilateral Acoustic Tumors

Bilateral acoustic tumors are pathognomonic of central neurofibromatosis and often are associated with intracranial and intraspinal meningiomas. Deafness is a strong possibility in these patients, so prior to surgery they should be encouraged to learn lip reading; when this skill has been mastered, surgery can proceed.

The authors do not remove both tumors during one operation, although initially a bilateral skin incision is made that will be suitable for both operations. In general, the larger tumor is operated on first. Removal of the tumor is carried out with the technique outlined earlier in this chapter. The patient returns to the hospital for surgery on the second side only after there has been complete recovery from the first operation. This includes wound healing and facial nerve function. In the event of facial nerve paralysis following the first operation, the second one is delayed until the nerve recovers or the face is reanimated by other means. In gen-

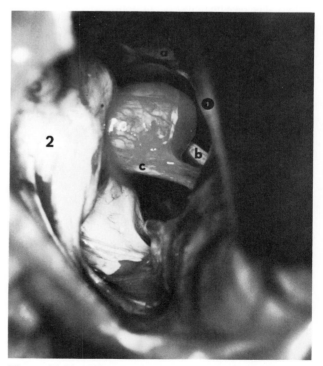

Figure 81-11 Microscopic view of small acoustic tumor. (1) Cerebellar retractor; (2) temporal bone; (a) nerve V; (b) nerve VII; (c) nerve VIII and acoustic tumor.

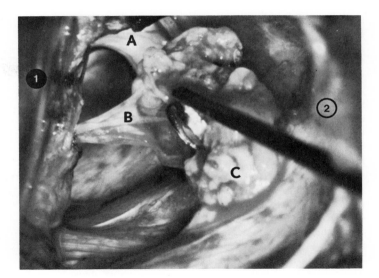

Figure 81-12 Tumor excision. (1) Cerebellar retractor; (2) temporal bone; (A) nerve V; (B) VII–VIII nerve complex; (C) acoustic tumor.

eral, the smaller tumor is removed before the patient becomes deaf, as there is a possibility that some degree of existing hearing may be preserved.

Facial Paralysis

Several procedures have been developed to improve facial tone and motor function in patients with postoperative facial nerve paralysis. The choice of procedure is tailored to the individual case. The ideal treatment is intracranial end-to-end anastomosis of the facial nerve during the initial operation. Unfortunately, most often the nerve has been attenuated or destroyed, making this impossible. The alternatives then are hypoglossal-facial, spinal accessory–facial, or phrenic-facial anastomosis. The authors prefer the hypoglossal-facial anastomosis, particularly for patients who are not dependent upon speech for their livelihood.

Timing of Surgery

The timing of surgery depends on the state of integrity of the facial nerve. If it is anatomically severed and cannot be repaired intracranially, it is the author's practice to wait 3 to 4 weeks, then readmit the patient for hypoglossal-facial anastomosis. If the nerve is anatomically and physiologically preserved during surgery but is without postoperative function, the anastomosis is generally not done for at least 2 years, since 90 percent of the patients on the authors' service seem to have adequate, although delayed, functional facial nerve recovery.

Surgical Technique

Hypoglossal-Facial Anastomosis

This procedure is performed under general anesthesia, with the patient supine on the operating table, head turned to the contralateral side. The earlobe is stitched up anteri-

orly, out of the operative field. A postauricular incision is made, from half an inch above the tip of the mastoid down in front of the sternocleidomastoid muscle, for a length of approximately 10 cm (Fig. 81-13). The skin and subcutaneous tissue are opened, and the fascia and platysmal muscles are then divided in a longitudinal fashion. The sternocleidomastoid muscle is identified and retracted laterally. Dissection continues superiorly and medially, and the cervical fascia is identified and opened. The posterior belly of the digastric muscle is identified and dissection is carried

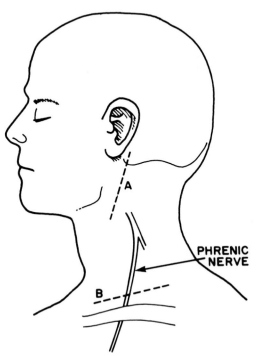

Figure 81-13 Surgical incisions for A, hypoglossal-facial and spinal accessory–facial nerve anastomoses; B, second incision used for the phrenic-facial anastomosis.

around it until the anteromedial tendinous portion is identified. The hypoglossal nerve is located underneath the posterior belly of the digastric muscle. It may be identified by following the descending ansa hypoglossi up until it meets with the hypoglossal nerve.

Attention is turned to the area of the mastoid tip. Using the periosteal elevator, the digastric muscle is partially separated from the periosteum of the mastoid process. The tip of the mastoid process is rongeured away, improving visualization of the area of the styloid process and the stylomastoid foramen. The authors prefer sharp dissection for the exposure of the facial nerve at its exit from the stylomastoid foramen (Fig. 81-14). Occasionally one must go through the posterior portion of the parotid gland to identify this nerve. Once both the facial and hypoglossal nerves have been identified, the hypoglossal nerve is sectioned at the point where it begins to branch.

The facial nerve is sectioned at the stylomastoid foramen. The proximal end of the hypoglossal nerve is swung upward posteriorly, in contact with the distal end of the facial nerve, adjacent to the posterior belly of the digastric muscle. Using microsurgical technique, the two ends are joined, using 8-0 Prolene (Ethicon, Inc., Somerville, N.J.). Care must be taken to ensure that the nerve is not angulated or under tension. After the anastomosis is complete, the wound is closed in standard fashion.

Spinal Accessory–Facial Anastomosis

The incision is identical to the one used for the hypoglossal-facial anastomosis. The sternocleidomastoid muscle is identified and retracted laterally and inferiorly, exposing the posterior belly of the digastric muscle. The spinal accessory nerve may be identified entering the posterior aspect of the sternocleidomastoid muscle (Fig. 81-14). To expose the distal end of the facial nerve, the technique described above is used. Once the facial nerve has been dissected at the stylomastoid foramen, the spinal accessory nerve is sectioned in its most distal portion, roughly where it enters the sternocleidomastoid muscle. The proximal spinal accessory nerve is swung around superiorly and posteriorly and anastomosed to the distal facial nerve.

Phrenic-Facial Anastomosis

Two incisions are used, one similar to the one described for the hypoglossal-facial and the spinal accessory-facial anastomoses, in order to expose the distal facial nerve right at the stylomastoid foramen, and another which is placed approximately two fingerbreadths above the clavicle in the supraclavicular fossa (Fig. 81-13). The sternocleidomastoid muscle is retracted medially and superiorly, and the anterior scalene muscle will then come into view. The phrenic nerve is in front of the anterior scalene muscle, underneath the fascia. Once it is identified, it is cut at the lowermost end on the anterior scalenus. The proximal end of the phrenic nerve is brought up underneath the sternocleidomastoid muscle and anastomosed to the facial nerve. It is recommended that the phrenic nerve be cut and brought up first, to help judge the length of facial nerve that will be needed to perform the anastomosis without tension. If there is trouble obtaining

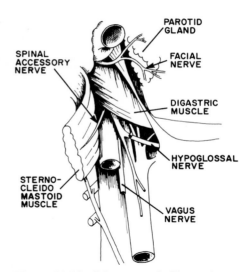

Figure 81-14 Diagrammatic illustration of the anatomy and landmarks used for hypoglossal-facial and spinal accessory–facial anastomoses.

the needed length, it is always possible to perform a mastoidectomy and expose the facial nerve higher up at the stylomastoid foramen (Fig. 81-15).

With these anastomotic procedures, satisfactory functional results are obtained in most cases. Recovery is not expected until at least 4 to 6 months after anastomosis. In some cases it takes a year for the expected surgical results to occur.

Operative Results

The authors' series, reported in Table 81-3, includes only microsurgery of acoustic neuromas. These cases were performed with the patient in the sitting position, with the ex-

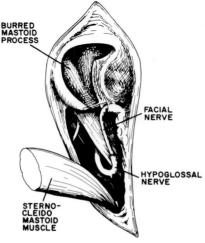

Figure 81-15 Surgical alternative when a further length of facial nerve is required.

TABLE 81-3 Acoustic Neuromas: Preservation of Nerve Function

Size of Tumor	No. of Patients	Function Preserved Postoperatively	
		Nerve VII (%)	Nerve VIII (%)
> 2 cm	85	65 (76)	5 (6)
1–2 cm	36	33 (92)	12 (33)
< 1 cm	14	14 (100)	8 (57)
Total	135		

ception of two that were performed in the lateral position. Two deaths occurred in patients who underwent surgery in the sitting position. The first of these patients had a postoperative hematoma secondary to disseminated intravascular coagulopathy, and the second had a cerebral infarction 6 weeks after operation.

References

1. Buchheit WA, Delgado TE: The surgical removal of acoustic neuromas, in Schmidek HH, Sweet WH (eds): *Operative Neurosurgical Techniques: Indications, Methods and Results.* New York, Grune & Stratton, 1982, vol 1, pp 637–647.
2. Cushing H: The surgical mortality percentages pertaining to a series of two thousand verified intracranial tumors. Arch Neurol Psychiatry 27:1273–1280, 1932.
3. Delgado TE, Buchheit WA, Rosenholtz HR, Chrissian S: Intraoperative monitoring of facial muscle evoked responses obtained by intracranial stimulation of the facial nerve: A more accurate technique for facial nerve dissection. Neurosurgery 4:418–421, 1979.
4. Henschen F: *Ueber Geschwülste der hinteren Schädelgrube, insbesondere des Kleinhirnbruckenwinkels: Klinische und anatomische Studien.* Jena, Gustav Fischer, 1910.
5. Hollinshead WH: *Anatomy for Surgeons,* 2d ed: vol 1. *The Head and Neck.* New York, Harper & Row, 1968.
6. House WF: Surgical exposure of the internal auditory canal and its contents through the middle cranial fossa. Laryngoscope 71:1363–1385, 1961.
7. House WF (ed): Monograph: Transtemporal bone microsurgical removal of acoustic neuromas. Arch Otolaryngol 80:597–756, 1964.
8. Leksell L: A note on the treatment of acoustic tumours. Acta Chir Scand 137:763–765, 1971.
9. Miller R: Meningiomas of the posterior fossa, in Buchheit WA, Truex RC Jr (eds): *Surgery of the Posterior Fossa.* New York, Raven Press, 1979, pp 99–110.
10. Norlén G, Leksell L: Stereotatic treatment of acoustic tumors, in Szikle G (ed): *Stereotactic Cerebral Irradiation.* Amsterdam, Elsevier, 1979, pp 241–244.
11. Portmann M, Sterkers JM, Charachon R, Chouard CH: *The Internal Auditory Meatus: Anatomy, Pathology and Surgery.* Edinburgh, Churchill-Livingstone, 1975.
12. Rhoton AL Jr: Microsurgery of the internal acoustic meatus. Surg Neurol 2:311–318, 1974.
13. Smith WH, Harp JR: Anesthesia for neurosurgery in the sitting position, in Buchheit WA, Truex RC Jr (eds): *Surgery of the Posterior Fossa.* New York, Raven Press, 1979, pp 89–97.
14. Wald SL, Schmidek HH: The laser and ultrasonic aspirator in neurosurgery, in Schmidek HH, Sweet WH (eds): *Operative Neurosurgical Techniques: Indications, Methods and Results.* New York, Grune & Stratton, 1982, vol 2, pp 1541–1550.
15. Wilson M: *The Anatomic Foundation of Neuroradiology of the Brain,* 2d ed. Boston, Little, Brown, 1972.

SECTION H

Posterior Fossa Tumors

82

Radiology of Posterior Fossa Tumors

Shelley B. Rosenbloom
Arthur E. Rosenbaum

The resection and decompression of masses of the posterior fossa have demanded the best of neurosurgical skills and neuroradiological localization. The sloping dorsum sellae and clivus, geometrically complex and usually asymmetrical vasculature, and topographically varied tentorium and calvarium, as well as the surgeon's fear of transtentorial and foramen magnum herniation(s), all affect the interpretation of abnormalities of the posterior fossa.

The methods of radiological investigation include plain skull roentgenography; geometric tomography; ventriculography and pneumoencephalography; direct magnification, selective vertebrobasilar (and internal carotid) angiography; radionuclide brain scanning; x-ray computed tomography (CT), and magnetic computed tomography (or nuclear magnetic resonance, NMR). The predominant current techniques are computed tomography and vertebral angiography. These techniques may be more specifically classified as follows:

I. X-ray computed tomography
   A. Unenhanced
   B. Intravenously enhanced
   C. Intrathecally enhanced
II. Magnetic computed tomography
   A. Unenhanced: spin-echo, inversion recovery sequences, saturation recovery
   B. Paramagnetically enhanced

III. Vertebral angiography
   A. Selective catheterization techniques: transfemoral or transaxillary, usually
   B. Countercurrent brachial arteriography: Unilateral or bilateral; less valuable; may show some resurgence with digital imaging
   C. Digital subtraction intravenous, intra-arterial, or selective intra-arterial angiography

Real-time ultrasound has important applications in infants and children (less than 2 years of age) and, used via a burr hole or craniectomy defect, in the intra- or postoperative patient.

The value of x-ray computed tomography is well appreciated. Unenhanced slices may not be worthwhile in the absence of any abnormality on the intravenously enhanced slices. However, unenhanced slices are necessary at the onset when a hemorrhagic lesion is suspected clinically, or secondarily when a hyperdense lesion is found on the IV-enhanced examination, to determine whether blood or calcification is present. Both pre-enhanced and IV-enhanced studies may be indicated when rescanning later is not convenient, as in the case of sedated children or outpatients.

The use of vertebral angiography is often related to the neurosurgeon's need to better define regional morphology. In the CT era, pediatric neurosurgeons request angiography less frequently in their presurgical planning process than do neurosurgeons dealing with adult patients. When the lesion enhances, angiography may prove useful to evaluate prominence of vessels. Whether angiography is needed also depends on how detailed the CT information is. Additional information may be gained by high-resolution algorithms, multiplanar reconstruction, dynamic scanning, or a 3-D-like display for showing sequential vascular opacification. Intrathecal enhancement usually minimizes x-ray CT artifacts in the posterior fossa; however, when the enhancing medium is introduced by lumbar puncture, the usefulness of enhancement must be balanced against the risk of inducing herniation in patients with posterior fossa tumors.

Cerebellar Tumors: Vermian

Common posterior fossa tumors (medulloblastoma, cerebellar astrocytoma, and ependymoma) may be difficult to differentiate on CT. Absence of cysts and calcifications on CT favors the diagnosis of medulloblastoma (calcification found in only 10 percent of medulloblastomas).[33] Dystrophic calci-

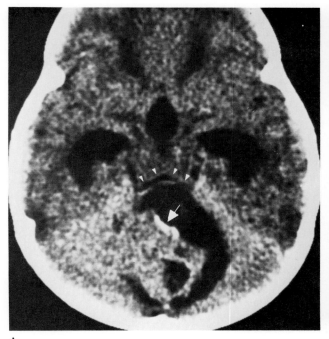

A

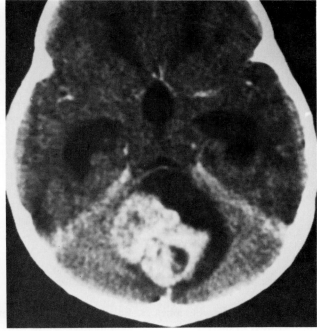

B

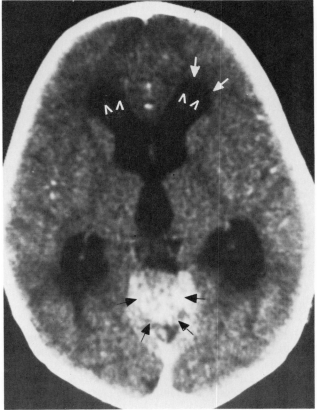

C

Figure 82-1 Medulloblastoma. *A.* Noncontrasted CT scan shows a variegated, nearly isodense mass occupying the posterior and lateral portion of a ballooned fourth ventricle. On the medial surface is a small focus of calcification (*arrow*), an unusual feature in a medulloblastoma. A cystic component is also seen within the mass. The most anterior aspect of the fourth ventricle, which at this level represents the superior medullary velum (*arrowheads*), is bowed forward, and the brain stem is displaced anteriorly. *B.* Contrast-enhanced CT scan demonstrates nonuniform enhancement of the neoplasm. *C.* Enhanced CT scan 12 mm higher demonstrates periventricular hypodensity or "edema," (between white arrows and carets) accompanying the hydrocephalus. Within the tentorial incisura is a densely enhancing mass (*black arrows*), indicating that the tumor extends into the cerebellar vermis.

fication in medulloblastoma after radiotherapy has a higher incidence.[12,48] Homogeneity of appearance has been described as typical of medulloblastomas;[26,48] however, "atyp-

ical" features, including cysts or necrosis (5 of 28 cases), calcification (4 of 28 cases), hemorrhage (1 of 28 cases), failure of enhancement (3 of 28 cases), and eccentricity (2 of 28 cases), have also been described.[44] It is the authors' impression that so-called atypical features are seen frequently with improved imaging techniques.

The most common pediatric vermian tumor is medulloblastoma (Figs. 82-1 to 82-3). On precontrast CT scan, a hyperdense or isodense, partially intraventricular mass,[42] usually surrounded by hypodensity (edema),[20] is characteristic of medulloblastoma.[48] Some tendency for this lesion to

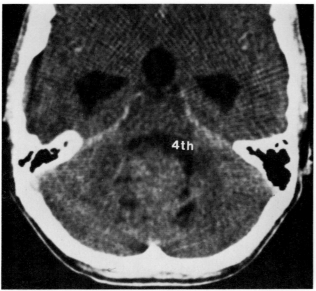
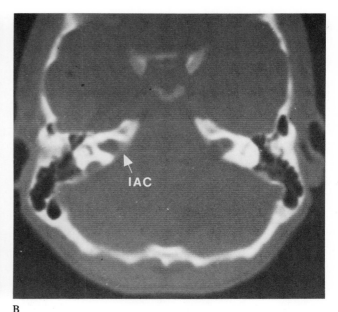

A   B

Figure 82-2 Medulloblastoma. *A*. Enhanced CT scan demonstrates patchy minimal enhancement in the predominantly midline mass which invaginates into the dorsal aspect of the fourth ventricle. The fourth ventricle appears enlarged and ventrally displaced. The brain stem is compressed and displaced anteriorly. Dilatation of the temporal horns and inferior third ventricle signals obstructive hydrocephalus. *B*. A "bone window" (wide window width) image demonstrates a capacious sella turcica and bilaterally wide internal auditory canals (*IAC*) consistent with chronically elevated intracranial pressure.

occur more laterally in older children is reported.[48] Extension from the foramina of Luschka or Magendie through the cerebellum or via the CSF spaces may result in tumor presenting in the cerebellopontine angle, supracerebellar cistern, or other subarachnoid cisterns. Obstructive hydrocephalus is usually present (75 percent in one series[26] and 85 percent in another[48]), and the fourth ventricle may be expanded. IV-enhanced CT scan shows tumor enhancement in most cases, usually well marginated and predominantly homogeneous in character,[25] although patchy and minimal enhancement patterns have been reported.

Angiography is requested uncommonly, since CT sagittal reconstructions generally define the tumor and its relation to other structures. Sagittal reconstructions showing involvement of the region of the superior medullary velum favor a diagnosis of medulloblastoma, whereas involvement of the floor of the fourth ventricle suggests ependymoma. Medulloblastomas are usually avascular on angiography, producing only mass effect (e.g., posterolateral displacement and spreading of posterior inferior cerebellar arteries).[3]

Vermian pseudotumor is the CT depiction of a prominent and generally hyperdense normal vermis (Fig. 82-4).[19] In the context of cerebellar dysfunction, the discrete dense

region may be misinterpreted as a vermian tumor. The normal appearance of the fourth ventricle and symmetry of the vermian blush are diagnostic clues.

Cerebellar Tumors: Hemispheric

Astrocytoma

Cerebellar astrocytoma (Figs. 82-5 and 82-6) is a common cerebellar hemispheric or vermian tumor with equal incidence in the 5-year and under and in the 5- to 10-year age groups.[15] The higher grade lesions tend to be solid or to have a mixed cystic and solid pattern on CT.[48] Midline tumors are predominantly solid and lateral lesions predominantly cystic.[15] Although the origin of these lesions may be in the vermis, extension into the cerebellar peduncles, hemisphere, and recesses of the fourth ventricle usually gives the tumors a lateralized appearance. (The brain stem is generally spared, although is may be displaced by the mass.)

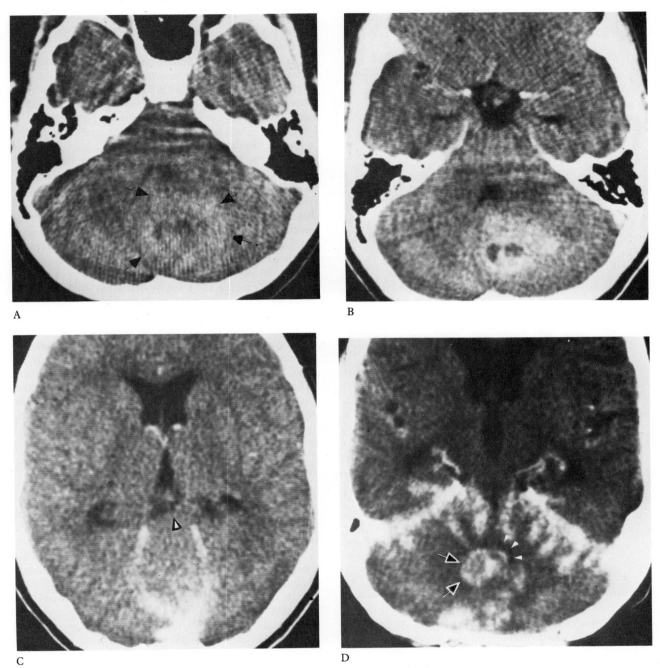

Figure 82-3 Medulloblastoma. *A*. Plain CT scan shows a rounded zone of subtle hyperdensity (*arrows*) posterior to and to the left of the fourth ventricle. The fourth ventricle is displaced ventrally and contralaterally without marked compression. *B*. After the intravenous administration of contrast medium, distinct enhancement occurs and hypodense regions become better defined. *C*. Mild ventriculomegaly accompanies a posterior fossa tumor. Encroachment on the left portion of tentorial hiatus (*arrow*) relates to upward transtentorial herniation. *D*. Meningeal seeding is seen on this contrast-enhanced CT scan 1 year after operation. There is also recurrence of tumor (*arrows*) at the site of the primary lesion. The fourth ventricle is represented by only a thin, left-sided, crescentic hypodensity (*arrowheads*).

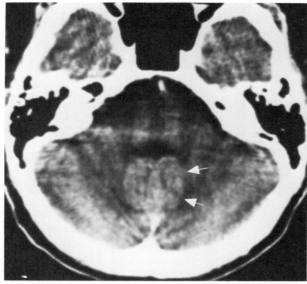

A

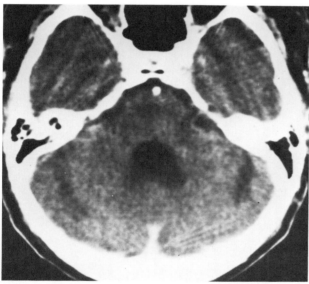

B

Figure 82-4 Vermian pseudotumor (normal). *A.* Just posterior to the fourth ventricle on this intravenously enhanced CT scan is a well-circumscribed, symmetrical midline hyperdensity (*arrows*). Note that there is no distortion or displacement of the ventricle or the basilar artery, so no mass effect is present at this plane. Transversely oriented black streaks posterior to the basilar artery and anterior to the fourth ventricle represent an interpetrous artifact from "beam hardening" and bone/air/tissue interfaces. A fan-shaped artifact emanates from endinion. *B.* On a slice 4 mm higher, an enlarged, uncompressed fourth ventricle is seen. Had the appearance in *A* actually represented a mass, ventricular distortion would have been expected.

The value of the precontrast CT in diagnosis of this tumor is to show calcification; Naidich et al. reported a 22 percent incidence of calcification, usually chunky in character, on CT.[26] The solid tumor component is often of mixed density or hypodense; hyperdense lesions are unusual. The cystic portion contains fluid of variable density and protein content; the wall may contain neoplastic elements. Intratumoral hemorrhage is rare but has been reported.[40]

On IV-enhanced CT scan, the solid cerebellar astrocytoma may show diffuse, focal, or ringlike enhancement.[20] Cystic astrocytomas usually show enhancement of the cyst wall (representing cerebellar margin or tumor) or of a mural nodule. Focal dense enhancement implies a mural nodule. Higher tumor grade correlates with greater cyst wall enhancement and/or nodularity.[47] Layering of the contrast medium in the cystic portion of the tumor may occur.[18] Occasionally, adjacent thinning of the calvarium (better seen on "bone" windows and algorithms) attests to the chronicity of these usually benign tumors.

Sagittal and coronal reconstructions aid in further demonstrating the spatial relationships determined by serial axial sections.

In the study of astrocytomas, angiography is infrequently performed today. When a hyperdense tumor is found on CT, angiography may be used to better characterize its nature; and when the tumor is cystic and shows focal dense enhancement, angiography may aid in differentiating astrocytoma, which is usually avascular, from hemangioblastoma.

Metastatic Deposits

Metastatic deposits are the commonest posterior fossa tumors in adults.[28] The cerebellum is predominantly affected (Fig. 82-7); meningeal and brain stem involvement can also occur (Fig. 82-8).[11,24]

The usual value of the precontrast CT in metastatic disease is its detection of hemorrhage and calcific components. Necrotic or mucin-producing tumors such as those from breast, colon, or ovarian primaries may, rarely, have calcified metastases.[29] Hypervascular lesions such as hypernephroma, choriocarcinoma, and melanoma may present with intratumoral hemorrhage,[10] but intratumoral bleeding is rare.[21] Precontrast CT is usually not indicated in metastatic disease. When it is performed however, if it demonstrates a complete definite ring, self-limited entities such as resolving hematoma or infarct can be excluded.[3]

On the IV-enhanced CT scan, the appearance of these lesions is usually nonspecific (ring, nodule, etc.); multiplicity of lesions is the greatest diagnostic aid, since it is most often seen in neoplasms (rather than circulatory or inflammatory diseases). When a solitary enhancing lesion is discovered, additional lesions are most likely to be demonstrated when high-dose intravenous iodinated contrast (80 g of iodine) is used, with a delay of about an hour before scanning. Almost without exception, metastases will enhance. Enhancement is frequently nodular; when ring enhancement occurs, the margins are characteristically thick-walled,

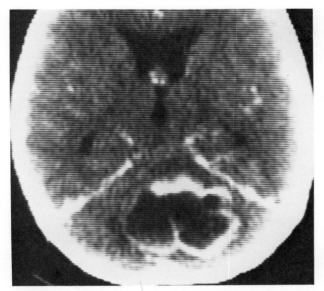

Figure 82-5 Cystic cerebellar astrocytoma (juvenile). An irregularly thick, rim-enhancing large mass nearly centered in the midline compresses the fourth ventricle beyond clear recognition, resulting in mild hydrocephalus in this preteenager. Low density within the mass probably represents cyst contents. Surrounding the lesion is a zone of hypodensity probably composed of edema, portions of the fourth ventricle, and gliosis.

unilocular, and shaggy. Occasionally smooth, thin-walled rings may be seen, making differentiation from abscess difficult.

Hemangioblastoma

Hemangioblastoma of the cerebellum is the commonest *primary* adult intra-axial posterior fossa tumor (Figs. 82-9 to 82-11). Although the cerebellum is the commonest location, lesions may also occur in the brain stem and spinal cord.

The precontrast CT scan characteristically shows an eccentric mass consisting of a usually isodense solid tumor or a mural nodule with a cyst.[14] There is often hypodensity of the surrounding white matter representing edema, gliosis, or necrosis. Calcification is not seen in these lesions. Nodules, which tend to be close to a pial surface, are often associated with cysts, which are very large in comparison with the size of the nodule. Mass effect usually distorts or displaces the fourth ventricle.

On IV-enhanced CT scan, solid tumors and nodules usually enhance markedly, sometimes with central lucencies. Large draining veins may be apparent on CT, a clue to the diagnosis. In cystic lesions, the rim either does not enhance or enhances discontinuously.

Angiography is performed when the diagnosis is uncertain from CT and particularly when multiple hemangioblas-

tomas are suspected (because smaller lesions may be missed on CT scanning). The solid portions of these tumors appear highly vascular, with early appearance of large draining veins. Compared to arteriovenous malformations, hemangioblastomas tend to show more mass effect and fewer draining veins. These highly vascular tumors may also be demonstrable by digital subtraction angiography, even on intravenous injection (Fig. 82-11).[7]

Non-Neoplastic Tumors

Certain non-neoplastic masses may mimic neoplasms of the cerebellum. Among these are cerebellar abscess (Fig. 82-12),[41] parasitic diseases (e.g., cysticercosis[5] and echinococcosis[1]), and granulomatous disease.[42] The CT findings are usually nonspecific, and the diagnosis is based on clinical information.

Cerebellar abscess may appear as an isolated lesion on CT, or may be associated with mastoid air cell opacification or sclerosis (mastoiditis). Noncontrast CT may show focal hypodensity and mass effect; within the hypodensity an isodense rim or nodule is sometimes seen. Obstructive hydrocephalus may be present. Intravenously enhanced scans characteristically show small nodular or ring enhancement. The abscess ring is usually thin-walled but occasionally has thick or irregular walls. In cerebritis, prior to frank abscess formation, the interior of the lesion may enhance on delayed scans. Thin walls and multiloculation favor a diagnosis of abscess rather than neoplasm. The preoperative diagnosis is reached by the usual combination of clinical context and CT findings.[41]

CNS cysticercosis may present with meningitis, parenchymal masses, and intraventricular lesions.[5] Frequently showing calcifications, the nodular components of these lesions vary in density. After IV contrast, rings and nodules (average size 10 to 20 mm) enhance. Hydatid disease involves the CNS in less than 2 percent of cases. CT characteristically shows large, solitary cystic lesions with little or no rim enhancement.[1] The lesions have a predilection for subcortical locations, but their appearance is nonspecific.

The cerebellum is the commonest site for tuberculomas (Fig. 82-13). These lesions may be spherical or multiloculated, with caseated centers and firm rims. Calcifications, edema, and seeding of the meninges may be evident on CT.[42] Angiography, when performed, may demonstrate an avascular mass effect with or without focal or multifocal basal (or peripheral) arterial narrowings.

Two other important non-neoplastic cerebellar tumors are infarction[37] and hematoma.[17] Cerebellar infarctions (Fig. 82-14) often manifest considerable mass effect, resulting in obstructive hydrocephalus. Intravenous enhancement is variable, depending on timing and the magnitude of the ischemic insult. Hypertensive cerebellar hematomas are generally discovered on noncontrast CT scanning in the context of a critically ill patient. They are usually hyperdense lesions but may be lower in density in anemic patients or when they are not acute.[17] Cerebellar hematoma may also be the first sign of initially occult metastatic disease of the cere-

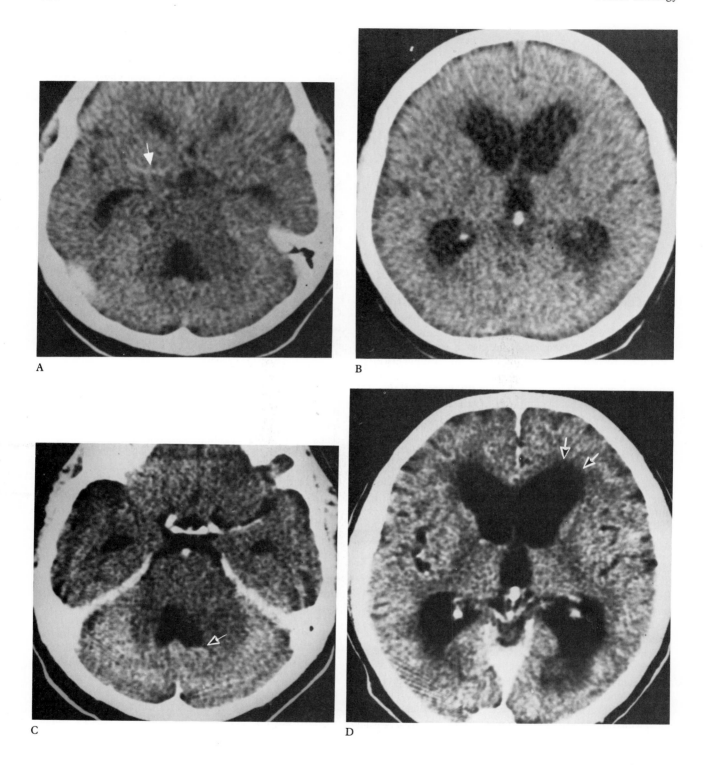

A

B

C

D

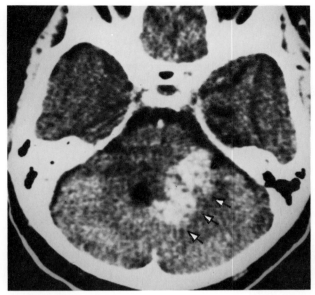

E

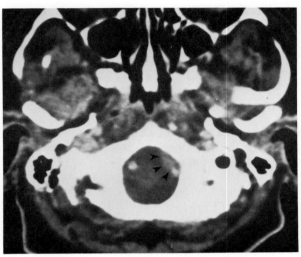

F

Figure 82-6 Cerebellar astrocytoma (adult). *A, B.* Initial intravenously enhanced CT scan: fourth ventricle is subtly shifted without deformity, and ventricular system is dilated. These scans had been interpreted at another institution as showing hydrocephalus (no cause discerned) in this 75-year-old man with progressive ataxia and nausea. Note only faint opacification of the circle of Willis and right middle cerebral artery (*arrow*), indicating unsatisfactory coordination of contrast administration and scanning. *C.* Contrast study 1 month later. Subtle indentation of the back of the left posterolateral recess of the fourth ventricle is caused by nodular hyperdensity (*arrow*). Fourth ventricle dilatation, canting, and shift are unchanged. *D.* Note periventricular hypodensity, i.e., edema (*arrows*), and large third ventricle. *E.* CT scan at the mid posterior fossa level (8 mm below *C*). There is considerable enhancement of an irregularly-shaped mass in the left cerebellar parenchyma. It extends anterolaterally (*arrows*) from behind and beside the fourth ventricle to the cerebellopontine angle, where a lobulated protrusion is seen. *F.* CT slice through the foramen magnum shows enhancing tumor (*arrowheads*) just anterior and medial to the left vertebral artery. Tumor also displaces the spinal cord contralaterally.

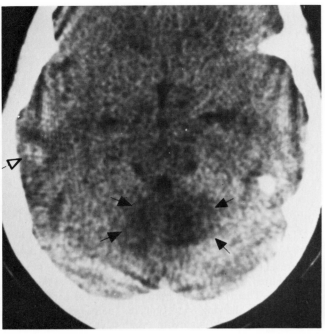

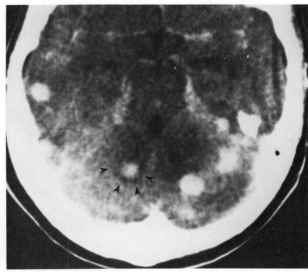

A   B

Figure 82-7 Cerebellar (and cerebral) metastases. *A*. There is asymmetry of the cerebellar medulla (*solid arrows*), but the cause is unclear on this precontrast CT scan. Subtle parenchymal hyperdensity is suggested (*open arrow*). *B*. Enhanced CT scan at same level reveals numerous round enhancing deposits, some with distinct hypodense halos (*arrowheads*).

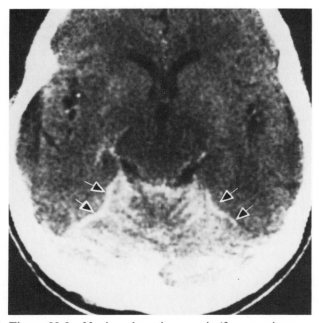

Figure 82-8 Meningeal carcinomatosis (from carcinoma of breast). This 69-year-old woman with positive CSF cytological studies has striking enhancement of the meninges throughout the posterior fossa. The tentorium also enhances excessively (*arrows*). Cerebellar folia stand out in relief against the diffusely diseased, opacifying meninges.

bellum, ruptured aneurysm, cerebellar arteriovenous malformation (AVM), vasculopathy, trauma, or hemorrhagic primary vascular tumor.

Brain Stem Tumors

Brain stem gliomas are among the commonest pediatric posterior fossa tumors (peak incidence at 6 to 8 years of age), and they may also occur in adult life. The usual epicenter of these lesions, the pons, often demonstrates asymmetrical enlargement on CT (Figs. 82-15, 82-16). Exophytic growth into the cerebellopontine angle cistern or interpeduncular cistern may mimic the appearance of a tumor of the cerebellopontine angle (CPA). Of the various x-ray CT techniques, CT cisternography affords the best definition.

Isodensity or hypodensity on a plain CT scan is usual; hyperdensity is uncommon.[2] The hypodense brain stem gliomas are believed to be of higher grade histologically.[2] Asymmetrically narrowed basal cisterns are caused by brain stem expansion and exophytic components. Brain stem gliomas usually displace the fourth ventricle posteriorly and/or extend into it. Unlike fourth ventricular or cerebellar tumors, brain stem neoplasms have been considered unlikely to induce hydrocephalus early.[30] In the authors' experience, however, incipient ventriculomegaly is frequently demonstrated by CT at the time of initial presentation. Calcification is rarely associated (seen in 1 of 24 cases in one series[2]).

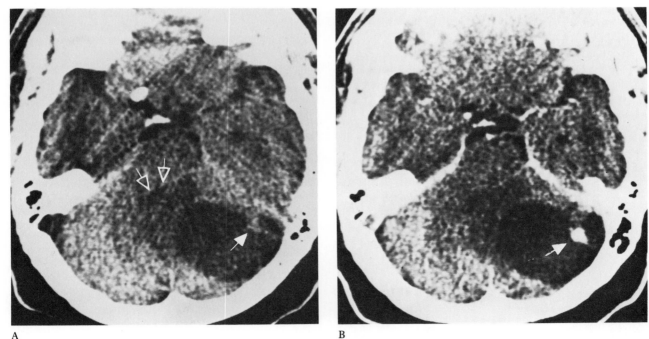

A   B

Figure 82-9 Solitary hemangioblastoma. *A*. Plain CT scan shows a large ellipsoidal, cerebellar hemispheric "cystic" lesion which has shifted, rotated, and compressed the fourth ventricle (*open arrows*). Subtle, brain-isodense excrescence (*arrow*) projects into or is within the cyst. *B*. Enhanced study shows dense opacification of what proved at operation to be the mural nodule (*arrow*) of a hemangioblastoma.

After the administration of an intravenous contrast agent, tumor enhancement may be seen (in about half the cases, especially in exophytic lesions) but is variable and appears to correlate poorly with the histology.[2]

Metrizamide cisternography (CTC) best demonstrates brain stem morphology (size, symmetry) and differentiates exophytic components from other extra-axial masses, defining a site for biopsy. CT cisternography minimizes the artifacts seen in the posterior fossa on standard scans. The plane of section in brain stem CTC should be perpendicular to the long axis of the brain stem, rather than at the conventional angle used in CT of the head, to reduce geometric distortion of the brain stem.

The differential diagnosis of brain stem enlargement must include hematoma (Fig. 82-17),[39] arteriovenous malformation of the brain stem,[43] lymphomatous infiltration, acute multiple sclerosis, brain stem encephalitis, and central pontine myelinolysis (Fig. 82-18), although these are rare lesions, often with characteristic clinical courses, laboratory findings, and CT features. Angiography, when performed, may better characterize lesions by demonstrating vasculature; capillary telangiectasia, cavernous hemangioma, and venous angioma may not be evident, however. Historically, angiography was also used to differentiate intra- from extra-axial lesions.

Fourth Ventricular Tumors

Ependymoma

Fourth ventricular ependymoma accounts for approximately 10 percent of pediatric posterior fossa tumors.[13]

Ependymomas arise from the floor of the fourth ventricle and may extend into the brain stem, cerebellar hemispheres, cerebellopontine angle cisterns, or cisterna magna (Fig. 82-19).[8,26] As seen on plain CT scan, they are usually of variable or mixed density.[26,35] Rare tumoral hemorrhage has been reported.[35,46] Obstructive hydrocephalus is generally present (92 percent in one series[26]). Calcification is present in some 50 percent of ependymomas[33] (vs. 10 percent of medulloblastomas). Small internal lucencies, cysts, or necrosis are also more characteristic of ependymoma than of medulloblastoma.[33]

On IV-enhanced CT scan, solid or ring enhancement is usually noted,[25] but there may be no enhancement.[13] Sagittal reconstructions are more definitive than axial sections for demonstrating involvement of the floor of the fourth ventricle, which suggests the diagnosis of ependymoma rather than medulloblastoma. Recurrences are usually discovered locally or within the ventricular system.[12] Subependymal

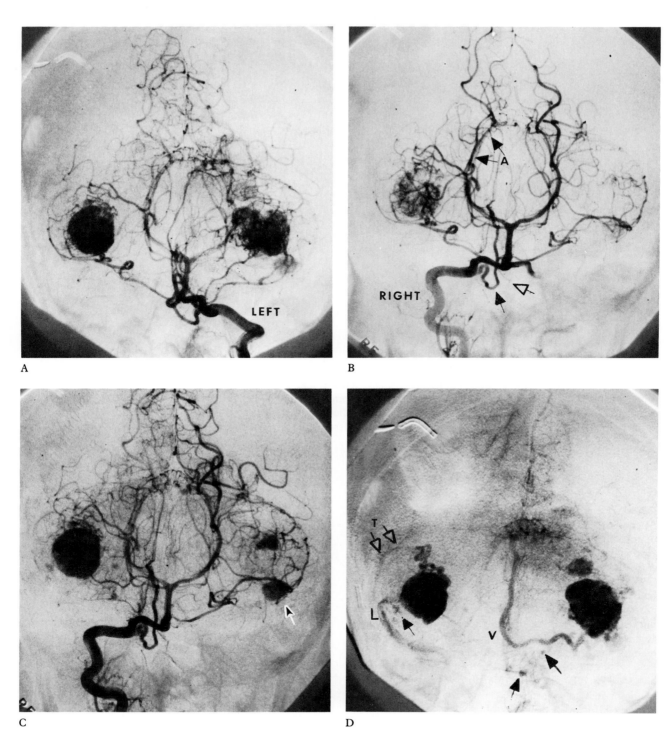

A

B

C

D

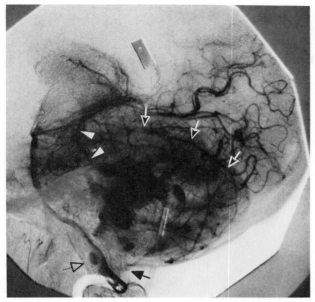

E

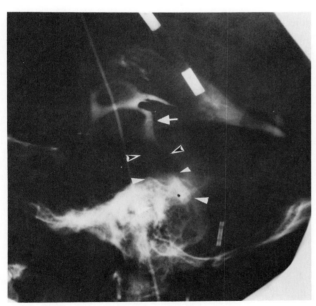

F

Figure 82-10 Hemangioblastomas in von Hippel-Lindau disease. *A.* Selective left vertebral angiogram shows bilateral large, highly vascular cerebellar tumors supplied predominantly by large anterior inferior cerebellar arteries. Subtle additional tumor blushes are suggested. Note the widened midbrain (shown by splaying of the anterior ambient portions of the posterior cerebral and superior cerebellar arteries). This separation of its encircling vessels indicates brain stem compression in upward transtentorial herniation. *B.* Selective right vertebral angiogram (early arterial phase, Towne's projection). Delicate angioarchitecture of the right-sided tumor is well seen in this early phase. Depression of both the caudal loop (*solid arrow*) and hemispheric branch (*open arrow*) of the posterior inferior cerebellar artery (PICA) indicate downward foramen magnum herniation. Inferior vermian branches of the PICA are also shifted toward the right-sided lesion, implying mass effect related to the less opacified left cerebellar lesion(s). *C.* Selective right vertebral angiogram (midarterial phase, Towne's projection). Note differential opacification of tumors between right and left (*A*) vertebral injections (shown, for example, at arrow). In evaluation of hemangioblastoma, examination of both vertebral arteries may uncover additional lesions. *D.* Capillary phase (left vertebral study) shows persistence of dense tumor blush with shunting into a vermian vein (V), transverse sinus (T), and lateral sinus (L). Two (or more) small additional hemangioblastomas are seen (*arrows*). *E.* Selective vertebral angiogram (later arterial phase, lateral projection). Mass effects from these tumors are manifested by the exaggerated curve of cerebellar hemispheric branches (*white arrows with black centers*); forwardly displaced precentral cerebellar artery (*arrowheads*); herniated tonsillohemispheric branches of the AICA-PICA complex (*solid black arrow*) which lie within the foramen magnum; superiorly displaced, taut posterior cerebral arteries; and backward bowing of the vertebral artery (*open arrow*). *F.* Metrizamide ventriculogram via the shunt (lateral projection) shows kinking of the upper cerebral aqueduct (*arrow*), ventricularization of the lower aqueduct (*black-center arrowheads*), and forward displacement of the fourth ventricle (*white arrowheads*), closely paralleling the mass effects visualized on the vertebral angiograms. (Courtesy of Dr. Richard A. Baker.)

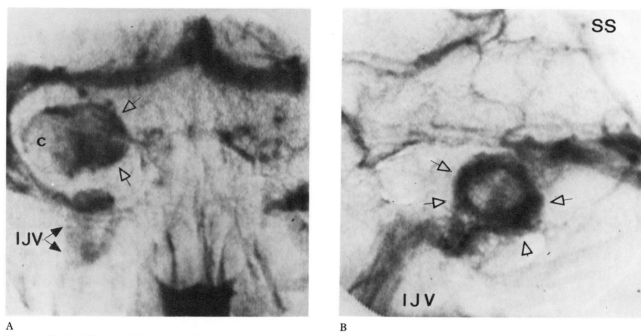

Figure 82-11 Hemangioblastoma. Frontal (*A*) and lateral (*B*) projections of digital intravenous angiogram demonstrate opacification of a rounded cerebellar hemispheric mass (*open arrows*) with a hypervascular rim and a lateral cystic portion (c). Internal jugular vein, IJV; straight sinus, SS. (Courtesy of Dr. Gary J. DeFilipp.)

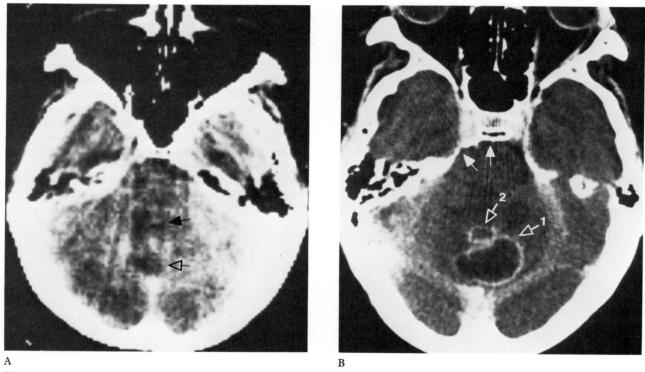

Figure 82-12 Cerebellar abscess. *A.* CT scan submitted for review shows mottling, streaking, and poor anatomical definition. Fourth ventricle is obscured (*arrow*) and could be confused with the midline centrally hypodense lesion (*open arrow*) in this 33-year-old man with history of intravenous drug abuse. *B.* Intravenously enhanced CT scan on high-resolution scanner demonstrates biloculated lesion (*1,2*) in midline (vermis). Pons is displaced anteriorly, as manifested by the fact that the pontine cistern is nearly effaced on the right side (*arrows*).

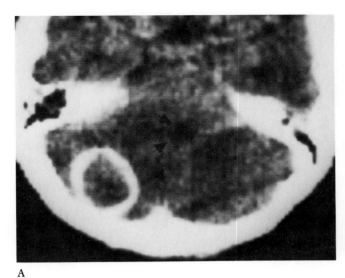

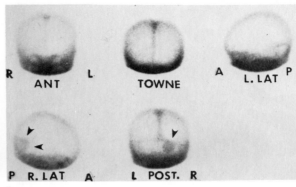

A   B

Figure 82-13 Tuberculoma in a 34-year-old patient with scrofula who presented with subtle neurological findings. *A.* Contrast-enhanced CT scan. A nearly uniformly thick-walled ring-enhancing mass lies in right cerebellar hemisphere. Fourth ventricle (*arrows*) is shifted contralaterally and anteriorly. *B.* Radionuclide scan with ^{99m}Tc. Mass is readily seen on posterior and ipsilateral (right lateral) images (*arrowheads*).

seeding and extension of tumor via the foramina of Luschka and Magendie occurs in ependymoma, as in medulloblastoma.[12] Angiography, now uncommonly performed in children, characteristically shows delicate tumor vessels in the capillary and late venous phases, with some staining.[16] More extensive hypervascularity has also been reported.[27]

Choroid Plexus Papilloma

Although choroid plexus papillomas are commoner in children than in adults, most choroid plexus papillomas in children involve the lateral ventricles, whereas adults have these lesions in the fourth ventricle (Fig. 82-20).[45] On the plain CT scan, hydrocephalus is usually present with a hyperdense, sometimes calcified, intraventricular mass. After administration of contrast medium, marked tumor enhancement occurs. Seeding of the subarachnoid space may be detected rarely. Angiography demonstrates a highly vascular lesion with an early, dense, and prolonged blush. Fourth ventricular choroid plexus papillomas are generally supplied by midline choroid branches of the posterior inferior cerebellar artery (PICA) or arteries. Choroid plexus carcinomas tend to occur in patients of younger age and manifest signs of invasion of the ventricular walls on CT.[20,45]

Other, less common, fourth ventricular tumors include astrocytoma, meningioma (rare in the fourth ventricle[27]), metastasis, epidermoid/dermoid/teratoma,[4] and subependymoma.[32]

Extra-Axial Posterior Fossa Lesions (Excluding Cerebellopontine Angle Tumors)

Extra-axial masses in the posterior fossa include chemodectoma, cranial nerve schwannoma or neurofibroma, aneurysm, meningioma, arachnoid cyst, dermoid and epidermoid, lipoma, chordoma, chondroma, chondrosarcoma, giant cell tumor, lymphoma, plasmacytoma, metastatic lesions, abscess or inflammatory mass, and hematoma.

Chemodectomas of the posterior fossa include glomus jugulare, glomus tympanicum, and glomus vagale lesions. Radiological methods of study have included plain films, geometric tomography, computed tomography, and angiography. CT elegantly assesses the bony involvement and, on intravenous enhancement, the profuse vascularity of these lesions.[22] Jugular bulb involvement can also be assessed by CT.

Glomus tumors are multicentric and bilateral in a minority of cases. CT of the neck and base of the skull in patients with chemodectomas is indicated for evaluation of additional lesions. Occasionally a malignant glomus lesion metastasizes to other intracranial foci or systemically.

Cranial nerve schwannomas, like glomus tumors, may occur in the region of the jugular fossa[38] and present some difficulty in differential diagnosis. These are rare, generally small, firm tumors which may erode bone but preserve smooth bony margins. They may arise sporadically or occur

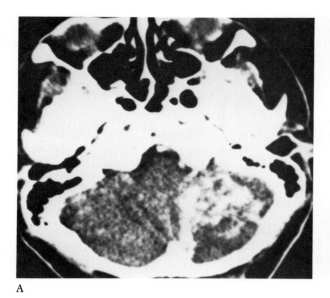

A

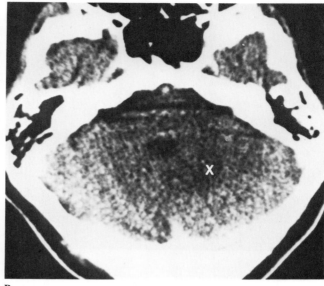

B

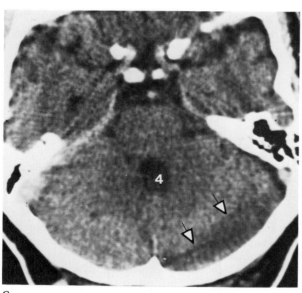

C

Figure 82-14 Evolving cerebellar infarction. *A*. CT scan (early fourth generation scanner) after intravenous injection of contrast medium. Note the broad, convoluted enhancement with long columnar density along its medial aspect. These features are nonspecific and might represent an arteriovenous malformation or an infiltrative tumor. *B*. Contrast-enhanced scan 1 month later. Lack of enhancement at this later time (patient was not taking corticosteroids) excludes neoplasm and large vascular malformation from differential diagnoses. The fourth ventricle is now seen but is shifted contralaterally, indicating some residual mass effect. The cerebellar parenchyma is hypodense (*X*), consistent with edema and/or infarction. *C*. Enhanced CT scan 6 months later, made with higher resolution scanner, shows tissue loss in the left cerebellar hemisphere (posterior surface, *arrows*). The fourth ventricle has shifted to the side of the lesion and is more dilated, particularly ipsilaterally.

Figure 82-15 Brain stem glioma. Intravenously enhanced CT scan demonstrates a lumpy, irregular contour of the grossly enlarged pons. Opacified choroid plexus and vessels about the fourth ventricle (*arrows*) are shifted by the asymmetrically growing tumor. Temporal horns are not visualized and therefore are probably not enlarged.

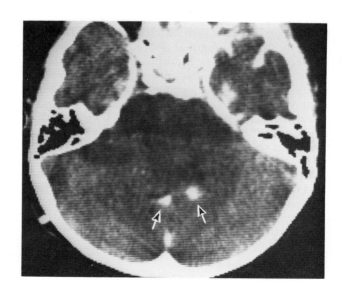

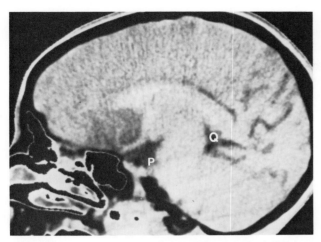

Figure 82-16 Brain stem glioma. Direct sagittal CT scan obtained close to the midline shows forward bulging of the pons and increased distance between the pontine (P) and interpeduncular, and quadrigeminal (Q) cisterns.

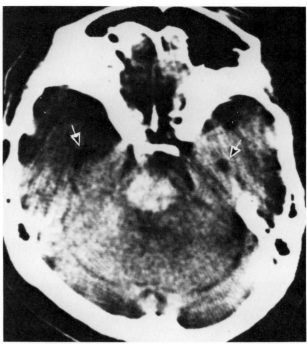

Figure 82-17 Pontine hematoma. Hyperdense, sharply marginated lesion occupies the basis pontis. Thin, hypodense rim (edema) outlines the mass, which is flattening the anterior aspect of the fourth ventricle. Prominence of the temporal horns (*arrows*) in this 40-year-old man indicates obstructive hydrocephalus.

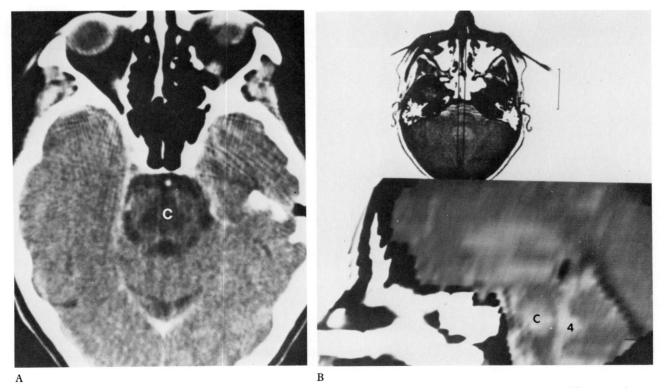

A   B

Figure 82-18 Central pontine myelinolysis. *A.* Axial image of the pons demonstrates a hypodense lesion (C) occupying the bulk of the pons. Pontine and ambient cisterns are capacious, indicating that the lesion has no mass component. *B.* Sagittally reformatted image shows the hypodense defect (C) in the pons anterior to the fourth ventricle (4), which is mildly enlarged.

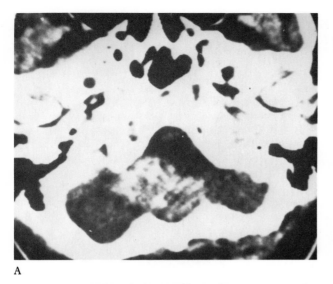

A

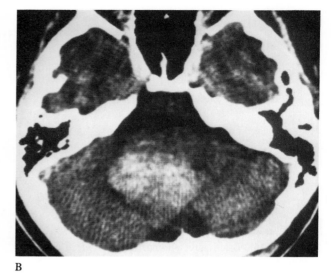

B

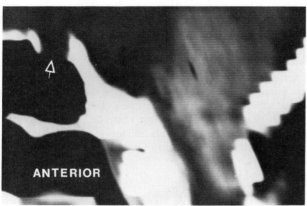

C

Figure 82-19 Malignant ependymoma. *A, B.* Enhancing, somewhat lobulated paramidline mass occupies the region of the fourth ventricle. Hypodense rim in eight o'clock position may represent the residual posterolateral recess of dilated fourth ventricle rather than focal edema. *C.* Indirect sagittal reconstruction demonstrates heterogeneously enhancing tumor in the region of the fourth ventricle; it extends superiorly, as well as inferiorly to the axis vertebra. Floor of sella turcica is not visualized (*arrow*), indicating chronically raised intracranial pressure.

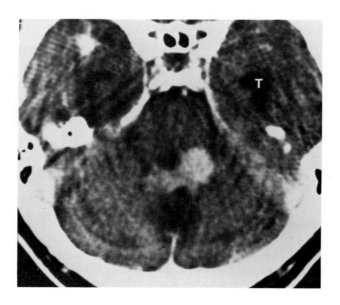

Figure 82-20 Choroid plexus papilloma. Dumbbell-shaped, densely enhancing, transversely oriented mass with hypodensity anterior and posterior to it occupies the region of the fourth ventricle. Moderate prominence of the temporal horns (T) and dilatation of cerebellar sulci are consistent with a cerebrospinal fluid circulation abnormality.

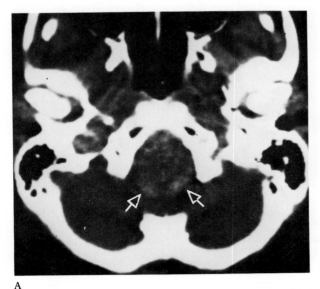

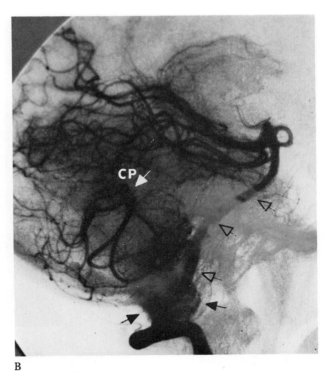

A

B

Figure 82-21 Foramen magnum meningioma. *A.* Postcontrast CT scan of low posterior fossa shows variegated hyperdense lesion (*arrows*) occupying the normal position of the medulla. *B.* Selective vertebral angiogram (arterial phase) shows a tumor blush which extends from the midclivus (*open arrows*) to below the foramen magnum (*solid arrows*). Lateral medullary segment of PICA is stretched and displaced posteriorly, and choroid arch (CP) is elevated.

in association with neurofibromatosis. As with a glomus jugulare tumor, CT demonstrates a soft tissue mass close to the jugular foramen which may manifest bone erosion and contrast enhancement. Calcification does not occur.[23] Angiographic hypervascularity in schwannomas is characteristically less dramatic than in glomus tumors.

Common sites for posterior fossa meningioma, apart from the CPA, include the foramen magnum, torcular, jugular bulb, petrosal sinus areas, and clivus.[13] Hyperostosis and calcification may give a clue to the nature of the lesions. Like meningiomas elsewhere, they appear as dura-based isodense or slightly hyperdense masses which enhance uniformly after administration of intravenous contrast material (Fig. 82-21). Meningiomas in the region of the foramen magnum may be studied by CT of the craniocervical junction, by myelography and CT metrizamide cisternography, and by angiography. They usually originate at the anterolateral aspect of the foramen magnum and may cause displacement and compression of the cervicomedullary junction. At angiography, these lesions usually show meningeal arterial feeders, relatively uniform-size vessels, and a circumscribed, prolonged tumor blush. Patency of dural sinuses may be evaluated by contrast-enhanced CT, cerebral angiography (preferably via bilateral, simultaneous, selec-

tive internal carotid opacification), or digital subtraction angiography.

Dermoid tumors of the posterior fossa generally occur in the midline between the cerebellar hemispheres or in the fourth ventricle, although they may present in the cerebellopontine angle cistern. They may be associated with endodermal transcranial sinus tracts and fistulae. Calcification and fatty components in the capsules of these lesions may be detectable on CT.[25] Enhancement of portions of these lesions is described. Epidermoids in the posterior fossa are most commonly located in the cerebellopontine angle cistern.[4]

Chordomas of the clivus and sella, although histologically benign, are invasive lesions (Fig. 82-22).[6] On CT, marked bone destruction with bony detritus is usually seen, in association with a soft tissue mass which may be relatively large. Enhancement with an intravenous contrast agent has been reported.[6] The lesions are usually in the midline and may be associated with intracranial and/or nasopharyngeal extension. On CT cisternography, the dural margins can be visualized, and dural displacement by the tumor without dural invasion can be seen. Arteriography, when performed, usually demonstrates an avascular extra-axial mass, although vascular tumors have been reported.[34]

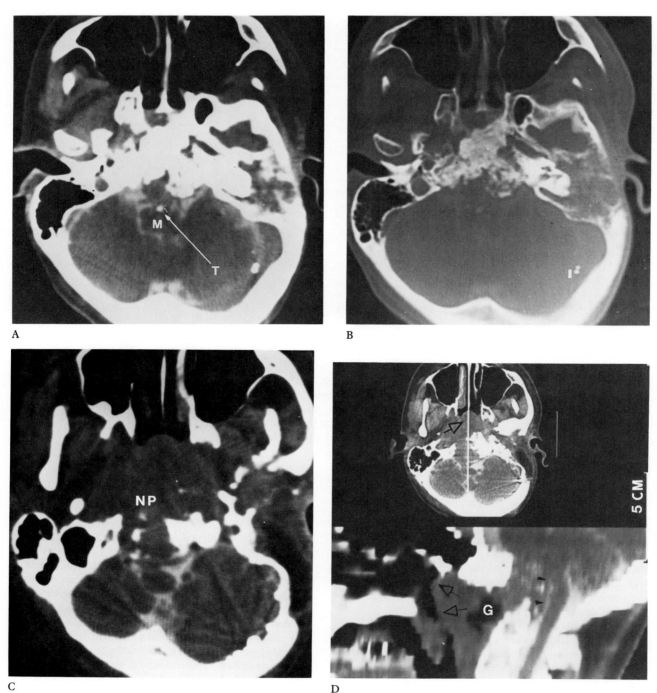

Figure 82-22 Clivus chordoma. CT cisternogram with metrizamide. *A.* The medulla (M) is displaced posteriorly and flattened by larger, lobulated, extra-axial paramidline mass (T). Hyperdensity ventral to the medulla represents either residual iophendylate or bony detritus. Widening of the lateral portion of the medullary cistern bilaterally is caused by the extra-axial tumor. *B.* Computer processing of the same image shows better bone detail. Hyperdense focus ventral to brain stem becomes recognizable at these wide windows as a bone sequestrum. Improved resolution of bone reveals asymmetric permeative destruction of the clivus and bone along the skull base. Bony defects at the right petrous apex and left mastoid region are consequences of surgery. *C.* Slice 12 mm lower shows extension of the tumor into the nasopharynx (NP). *D.* Sagittally reconstructed image. Upper image is axial reference image for the reconstructed sagittal section below. CT cisternogram shows marked posterior displacement of the lower brain stem and cervical spinal cord by patchy hyperdensities (calcifications or bony detritus). The clivus was partially resected surgically in gaining exposure to the tumor. A soft tissue mass (partially composed of Gelfoam) extends through the bed of the clivus, displacing the metrizamide column posteriorly (*arrowheads*) and growing anteriorly (*arrows*) to narrow the nasopharynx. The mass contains pocket of gas (G) in immediate postoperative period.

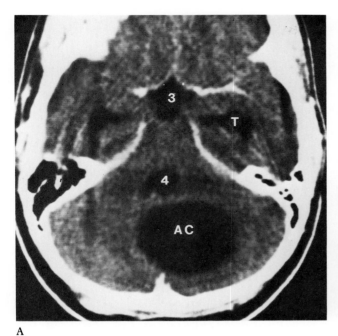

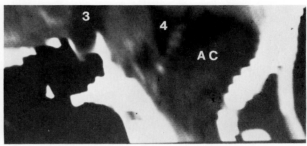

A   B

Figure 82-23 Arachnoid cyst. *A.* Elliptical lesion (AC) matching cerebrospinal fluid in density is visualized posterior to the fourth ventricle and anterior to the torcular. Temporal horns (T), third ventricle (3), and fourth ventricle (4) are enlarged. The fourth ventricle is also displaced slightly anteriorly and ventrally. Cerebellopontine angle cisterns and cerebellar sulci are effaced from compression. *B.* Advanced technology scanner gave this sagittally reconstructed midline image demonstrating extension of the cystic lesion (AC) from the level of the apex of the fourth ventricle to below the foramen magnum. Anterior displacement of the fourth ventricle and brain stem can be appreciated better in the sagittal plane. Protrusion of the cyst through the foramen magnum, once believed to be pathognomonic of Dandy-Walker cyst, is equally characteristic of arachnoid cysts in the region of the cisterna magna. (It is thought not to occur in giant cisterna magna.)

Chondromas are confined to those portions of the skull base which are preformed in cartilage. The densely calcified matrix of these masses can be readily seen. CT characteristically shows less aggressive bone destruction than in chordoma.[31]

Arachnoid cysts of the posterior fossa occur in the CPA, the region of the cisterna magna, the pontine cistern, the quadrigeminal cistern, and the suprasellar cistern, from which they may extend into the posterior fossa (Fig. 82-23). These lesions are hypodense (equivalent to CSF density) and usually well circumscribed. They may cause thinning of the adjacent bone. Whether a hypodense lesion is a cystic intra-axial mass or an extra-axial cyst may be determined by multiplanar reconstruction or intravenously enhanced CT (where the brain's surface vessels lie within the inner margin of the cyst). CT cisternography, however, is the most definitive CT examination; the cyst may be shown to be com-

pletely circumscribed by the nonionic contrast medium, establishing its extra-axial location and its noncommunication with the cisterns.[9] Occasionally an arachnoid cyst opacifies on CT, either early (by direct communication with the subarachnoid space) or several hours later by transmural diffusion.

Large aneurysms may present as extra-axial posterior fossa masses on CT (Fig. 82-24)[36] and thus come into the differential diagnosis of posterior fossa masses. Vertebral angiography has been the definitive method to demonstrate such aneurysms. Dynamic CT scanning, however, may confirm the diagnosis of aneurysm by demonstrating an arterial pattern of transit of the contrast medium through the lumen of the lesion. Digital subtraction angiography may also demonstrate these lesions.

The radiological features discussed in this chapter are summarized in Table 82-1.

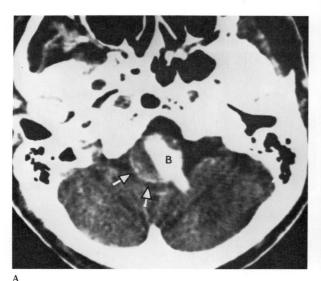

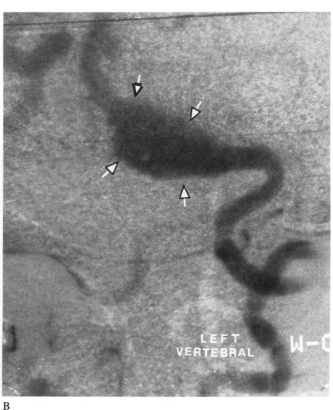

A   B

Figure 82-24 Basilar artery aneurysm. *A.* Intravenously enhanced CT scan demonstrates round, thin-rimmed mass near the midline in the posterior fossa (*arrows*).
Mass contains a broad-based, elongated hyperdensity (B), probably the basilar artery,
which extends obliquely from twelve o'clock position posterolaterally through and
beyond the rim of the mass. *B.* Digital subtraction angiography shows aneurysmal
enlargement of the lumen of the elongated basilar artery.

TABLE 82-1 Posterior Fossa Tumors: Radiological Features

Location	Anatomical Aspects	Computed Tomography Depiction	Depiction by Angiography and Other Techniques
INTRA-AXIAL SITES			
Cerebellar Lesions			
Medulloblastoma	90% originate in vermis, 10% in hemispheres. Fourth ventricle may be filled with tumor, displaced anterolaterally or anterosuperiorly, or (uncommonly) enlarged (suggests ependymoma). Hydrocephalus common. Brain stem anteriorly displaced.	Hyper- or isodense, oval or lobulated, well circumscribed. Nearly all enhance, usually homogeneously. Usually some edema. "Cysts" and calcifications uncommon.	Angiogram: avascular mass. Sagittal and coronal CT reconstructions show relation of tumor and fourth ventricle. Radioisotope scan frequently negative.
Vermian pseudotumor	Limited to vermis. Undistorted ventricles and cisterns.	Vermis hyperdense; some enhancement.	Angiogram normal.
Cerebellar astrocytoma	Commonest primary posterior fossa tumor. Usually grows laterally but originates in vermis. Fourth ventricle contralaterally displaced and compressed, cisterns effaced. Hydrocephalus	Iso- or hypodense solid tumor or nodule. Frequently associated with cysts. Solid tumor, nodule, and cyst wall may enhance, frequently nonhomogeneously. Cyst contents may	Angiogram: avascular mass. Cyst wall and nodule may blush.

TABLE 82-1 Posterior Fossa Tumors: Radiological Features (*continued*)

Location	Anatomical Aspects	Computed Tomography Depiction	Depiction by Angiography and Other Techniques
	common. Brain stem anteriorly displaced.	be denser than CSF. Degree of enhancement correlates with tumor grade. Calcification in about 20%. Calvarial focal thinning.	
Cerebellar metastasis	Commonest adult posterior fossa neoplasm. Vermian or hemispheric. Mass effect on cisterns and fourth ventricle. Solitary or multiple.	Variable density, sometimes with "cysts" of variable wall thickness. Nodular or ring enhancement. May show edema. Rarely hemorrhagic or calcific.	Angiogram: variable vascularity and mass effect. Double-dose delayed CT valuable in identifying a second lesion.
Hemangioblastoma	Commonest in cerebellum, especially hemispheres. May be vermian or medullary. Arises near pial surface, displaces fourth ventricle. May be multiple (von Hippel-Lindau)	Isodense small nodule or solid tumor; very large cyst often associated with nodule. Solid portion enhances intensely; cyst wall may enhance. Not calcified.	Angiogram: solid portion hypervascular with arteriovenous shunting. Large solitary draining veins. Mass effect disproportionate to nodule size (because of cysts). Additional lesions (missed on CT) may be seen angiographically.
Abscess of cerebellum	Unusual in cerebellum. May be related to mastoiditis.	Nodule or ring, usually with thin wall. Central hypodensity within ring. Nodule or ring enhances. May show source (mastoid opacified).	Angiogram: avascular mass. Sometimes ring-shaped blush of capsular vessels.
Cysticercosis	Parenchymal, intraventricular, or meningeal lesions.	Variable density 10- to 20-mm nodules. May show ring enhancement or calcification.	
Tuberculoma	Cerebellum is commonest site. May seed meninges, constricting the basal cisterns.	Pre-enhanced iso- or hyperdense nodules. Solid rim enhancement (after caseation). Single or multiloculated. Edema sometimes present. May be calcified.	Angiogram: avascular mass. Vessel pruning and irregularities.
Infarct	Mass effect on cerebellar hemispheres and CSF pathways may be striking. Hydrocephalus common.	Hypodense, sometimes "cystic," lesion; may enhance dramatically.	Follow-up CT may show gradually resolving mass effect; sometimes enhancement increases as patient improves.
Hematoma	Displacement of regional structures (fourth ventricle and cisterns) common.	Acutely hyperdense lesion; enhancement may be difficult to detect because of clot. Surrounding edema frequent.	Angiogram sometimes helpful in showing AVM or tumoral cause of hemorrhage.
Brain Stem Lesions Glioma	Usual origin is pons, especially if exophytic. Brain stem torsion with widening of ipsilateral CPA cistern. Fourth ventricle displaced and indented; floor may appear convex. Hydrocephalus becomes advanced late in course.	Typically hypodense before contrast; enhancement infrequent and not indicative of grade. Calcification and cysts unusual. Brain stem asymmetrically enlarged.	Metrizamide cisternogram is most sensitive diagnostic modality for subtle abnormalities of brain stem contour. Sagittal reconstructions on CT facilitate assessment of tumor extent rostrocaudally. Angiogram: avascular mass may encase basilar artery. NMR may prove useful.
Vascular malformation	Often pontine.	May present with brain stem enlargement and hemorrhagic foci; may be calcified.	Angiogram: sometimes shows abnormal vessels. Small or thrombosed lesions may escape detection.
Central pontine myelinolysis	Centered in basis pontis. May extend symmetrically rostrocaudally. May be associated with atrophic changes (wide cisterns and fourth ventricle).	Hypodense, well-circumscribed, symmetrical lesion; may be isodense early in clinical course.	NMR may prove useful.

TABLE 82-1 Posterior Fossa Tumors: Radiological Features (*continued*)

Location	Anatomical Aspects	Computed Tomography Depiction	Depiction by Angiography and Other Techniques
Fourth Ventricle Lesions			
Ependymoma	Arising in wall or floor of fourth ventricle, may invaginate into fourth ventricle and/or protrude via outlet of foramina. Hydrocephalus common. May seed via CSF.	Iso- or hyperdense, sometimes with focal lucencies or cysts. Enhancement nearly invariable, may be nodular or ring-shaped and heterogeneous. Most commonly calcified. Edematous rim is common.	Angiogram: sometimes hypervascular. Fourth ventricle enlargement and involvement of fourth ventricle floor seen on sagittal and coronal reformatted images.
Choroid plexus papilloma or carcinoma	Fourth ventricle occupied; tumor may expand via outlet foramina. Hydrocephalus disproportionate to tumor size. May seed via CSF.	Usually hyperdense; sometimes calcified; marked enhancement. Rarely causes subarachnoid hemorrhage.	Angiogram: hypervascular lesion, usually with prolonged blush; supplied by choroid branches of PICA.
Meningioma	Rare in fourth ventricle.	Iso- or hyperdense; rarely cystic; perhaps calcified. Intense "homogeneous" enhancement.	Angiogram: prolonged tumor blush or may be avascular; supplied by meningeal vessels and choroid branches of PICA.
Metastasis	Rare in fourth ventricle.	Variable density; usually circumscribed; enhances as nodule or ring. Sometimes edema (hypodense surround).	
Epidermoid	Unusual in fourth ventricle.	Usually hypodense; may be hyperdense if rich in keratin. Enhancement is unusual.	
Dermoid	Oval lesion may occupy fourth ventricle or vallecula. May have transcalvarial sinus tract.	Usually hypodense but may be hyperdense. May not enhance. calcification unusual, may be present in tumor capsule. Fatty constituents may be evident. Focal bone defect may be present associated with sinus tract.	Plain films may show calcifications.
Subependymoma	Commonest site is fourth ventricle. Occasionally multiple. Usually small and nonobstructive.	Variable density before contrast. May be calcified. Heterogeneous, ill-defined enhancement.	Sagittal and coronal CT reconstructions may be useful in defining relation of lesion to fourth ventricle.
EXTRA-AXIAL SITES			
Chemodectoma	From jugular fossa may extend intra- and extracranially (CPA, incisura, carotid sheath); from middle ear may extend to hypotympanum. May be multicentric, especially in familial cases (25–33%).	Hyperdense before contrast. Marked enhancement. Sometimes calcification.	Angiogram: hypervascular tumor, supplied by external carotid and frequently AICA. "Meniscus" defect in jugular vein is characteristic. Venous collaterals common.
Schwannoma	CPA, jugular fossa, hypoglossal canal, and foramen magnum are common sites.	Density variable. Usually enhances. Smoothly margined bone erosion.	
Meningioma	Jugular fossa, cerebellopontine angle, torcular, petrosal sinuses, and clivus are common locations.	Hyperdense before contrast. May be calcified. Usually dense, homogeneous enhancement. Associated often with hyperostosis. Rarely cystic.	Angiogram: external carotid or meningeal vessel supply. May have dense, prolonged tumor blush.
Epidermoid	Tend to occur off-midline in posterior fossa, especially in CPA.	Usually hypodense but rarely hyperdense. Rarely enhances. May be cystic.	
Dermoid	Usually midline; may lie in fourth ventricle. May be connected via sinus tract to extracranial space.	Usually hypodense but occasionally hyperdense. Enhancement rare. May be partly cystic and may contain fat and calcifications.	

TABLE 82-1 Posterior Fossa Tumors: Radiological Features (*continued*)

Location	Anatomical Aspects	Computed Tomography Depiction	Depiction by Angiography and Other Techniques
Lipoma	May be midline or CPA.	Hypodense compared to CSF. Nonenhancing.	
Chordoma	Destruction of base of skull (clivus, sphenoid) with nasopharyngeal soft tissue mass and intracranial extra-axial mass components.	Variable density, variably enhancing soft tissue mass. Aggressive bone destruction with or without detritus. Does not respect sutures or synchondroses.	Plain films may show clivus destruction, nasopharyngeal mass, and detritus. Metrizamide cisternogram gives best definition of extent of disease and brain stem compromise.
Chondroma or chondrosarcoma	Usual origin in portions of skull base preformed in cartilage; may originate from dura, choroid, brain, or arachnoid.	Hyperdense before contrast enhancement. Destructive lesion which may contain mottled calcification. May cause bone expansion, soft tissue mass. Metastases from chondrosarcoma occur late.	Angiogram: usually avascular (but mesenchymal chondrosarcoma may be vascular).
Aneurysm	Vertebral artery, basilar artery, AICA, PICA.	Hyperdense, rounded. Mural curvilinear calcification may be present. Marked enhancement.	Dynamic CT shows arterial contrast transit pattern. Arteriography is diagnostic.
Arachnoid cyst	Pontine cistern, collicular plate, cisterna magna, and CPA are common sites.	Hypodense, nonenhancing. Bone expansion, if present, indicates chronicity.	Variable communication with subarachnoid space.

References

1. Abbassioun K, Rahmat H, Ameli NO, Tafazoli M: Computerized tomography in hydatid cyst of the brain. J Neurosurg 49:408–411, 1978.
2. Bilaniuk LT, Zimmerman RA, Littman P, Gallo E, Rorke LB, Bruce DA, Schut L: Computed tomography of brain stem gliomas in children. Radiology 134:89–95, 1980.
3. Braun IF, Chambers E, Leeds NE, Zimmerman RD: The value of unenhanced scans in differentiating lesions producing ring enhancement. AJNR 3:643–647, 1982.
4. Braun IF, Naidich TP, Leeds NE, Koslow M, Zimmerman HM, Chase NE: Dense intracranial epidermoid tumors: Computed tomographic observations. Radiology 122:717–719, 1977.
5. Carbajal JR, Palacios E, Azar-Kia B, Churchill R: Radiology of cysticercosis of the central nervous system including computed tomography. Radiology 125:127–131, 1977.
6. Clark WC, Robertson JH, Lara R: Chondroid chordoma: Case report. J Neurosurg 57:842–845, 1982.
7. DeFilipp GJ, Pinto RS, Lin JP, Kricheff II: Intravenous digital subtraction angiography in the investigation of intracranial disease. Radiology 148:129–138, 1983.
8. Dohrmann GJ, Farwell JR, Flannery JT: Ependymomas and ependymoblastomas in children. J Neurosurg 45:273–283, 1976.
9. Drayer BP, Rosenbaum AE, Maroon JC, Bank WO, Woodford JE: Posterior fossa extraaxial cyst: Diagnosis by metrizamide CT cisternography. AJR 128:431–436, 1977.
10. Enzmann DR, Kramer R, Norman D, Pollock J: Malignant melanoma metastatic to the central nervous system. Radiology 127:177–180, 1978.
11. Enzmann DR, Krikorian J, Yorke C, Hayward R: Computed tomography in leptomeningeal spread of tumor. J Comput Assist Tomogr 2:448–455, 1978.
12. Enzmann DR, Norman D, Levin V, Wilson C, Newton TH: Computed tomography in the follow-up of medulloblastomas and ependymomas. Radiology 128:57–63, 1978.
13. Gado M, Huete I, Mikhael M: Computerized tomography of infratentorial tumors. Semin Roentgenol 12:109–120, 1977.
14. Ganti SR, Silver AJ, Hilal SK, Mawad ME, Sane P: Computed tomography of cerebellar hemangioblastomas. J Comput Assist Tomogr 6:912–919. 1982.
15. Gol A: Cerebellar astrocytomas in children. Am J Dis Child 106:21–24, 1963.
16. Harwood-Nash DC, Fitz CR: *Neuroradiology in Infants and Children.* St Louis, Mosby, 1976.
17. Kasdon DL, Scott RM, Adelman LS, Wolpert SM: Cerebellar hemorrhage with decreased absorption values on computed tomography: A case report. Neuroradiology 13:265–266, 1977.
18. Kingsley D, Kendall BE: Dependent layering of contrast medium in cystic astrocytomas. Neuroradiology 14:107–110, 1977.
19. Kramer RA: Vermian pseudotumor: A potential pitfall of CT brain scanning with contrast enhancement. Neuroradiology 13:229–230, 1977.
20. Lee SH, Rao KCVG (eds): *Cranial Computed Tomography.* New York, McGraw-Hill, 1983, pp 241–370.
21. Mandybur TI: Intracranial hemorrhage caused by metastatic tumors. Neurology (Minneap) 27:650–655, 1977.
22. Marsman JWP: Tumors of the glomus jugulare complex (chemodectomas) demonstrated by cranial computed tomography. J Comput Assist Tomogr 3:795–799, 1979.
23. Martin F Jr., Lemmen LJ: Calcification in intracranial neoplasms. Am J Pathol 28:1107–1131, 1952.
24. Naheedy MH, Kido DK, O'Reilly GV: Computed tomographic evaluation of subdural and epidural metastases. J Comput Assist Tomogr 4:311–315, 1980.
25. Naidich TP, Lin JP, Leeds NE, Kricheff II, George AE, Chase

NE, Pudlowski RM, Passalaqua A: Computed tomography in the diagnosis of extra-axial posterior fossa masses. Radiology 120:333–339, 1976.

26. Naidich TP, Lin JP, Leeds NE, Pudlowski RM, Naidich JB: Primary tumors and other masses of the cerebellum and fourth ventricle: Differential diagnosis by computed tomography. Neuroradiology 14:153–174, 1977.

27. Numaguchi Y, Kishikawa T, Fukui M, Komaki S, Russell WJ, Ikeda J, Okudera T, Matsuura K, Kitamura K: Angiographic diagnosis of fourth ventricle tumors. Radiology 128:393–403, 1978.

28. Potts DG, Abbott GF, von Sneidern JV: National Cancer Institute study: Evaluation of computed tomography in the diagnosis of intracranial neoplasms: III. Metastatic tumors. Radiology 136:657–664, 1980.

29. Potts DG, Svare GT: Calcification in intracranial metastases, AJR 92:1249–1251, 1964.

30. Raimondi AJ, Tomita T: Hydrocephalus and infratentorial tumors: Incidence, clinical picture, and treatment. J Neurosurg 55:174–182, 1981.

31. Sarwar M, Swischuk LE, Schecter MM: Intracranial chondromas. AJR 127:973–977, 1976.

32. Scheithauer BW: Symptomatic subependymoma: Report of 21 cases with review of the literature. J Neurosurg 49:689–696, 1978.

33. Segall HD, Zee CS, Naidich TP, Ahmadi J, Becker TS: Computed tomography in neoplasms of the posterior fossa in children. Radiol Clin North Am 20:237–253, 1982.

34. Smink KWF, Hekster REM, Bots GTAM: Clivus chordoma with distinct vascularity demonstrated by angiography. Neuroradiology 13:273–277, 1977.

35. Swartz JD, Zimmerman RA, Bilaniuk LT: Computed tomography of intracranial ependymomas. Radiology 143:97–101, 1982.

36. Thron A, Bockenheimer S: Giant aneurysms of the posterior fossa suspected as neoplasms on computed tomography. Neuroradiology 18:93–97, 1979.

37. Tsai FY, Teal JS, Heishima GB, Zee CS, Grinnell VS, Mehringer CM, Segall HD: Computed tomography in acute posterior fossa infarcts. AJNR 3:149–156, 1982.

38. Uslø C, Sehested P, Overgaard J: Intracranial hypoglossal neurinoma: Diagnosis and postoperative care. Surg Neurol 16:65–68, 1981.

39. Vaquero J, Areitio E, Leunda G, Bravo G: Hematomas of the pons. Surg Neurol 14:115–118, 1980.

40. Vincent FM, Bartone JR, Jones MZ: Cerebellar astrocytoma presenting as a cerebellar hemorrhage in a child. Neurology (NY) 30:91–93, 1980.

41. Whelan MA, Hilal SK: Computed tomography as a guide in the diagnosis and follow-up of brain abscesses. Radiology 135:663–671, 1980.

42. Whelan MA, Stern J: Intracranial tuberculoma. Radiology 138:75–81, 1981.

43. Yeates A, Enzmann D: Cryptic vascular malformations involving the brainstem. Radiology 146:71–75, 1983.

44. Zee CS, Segall HD, Miller C, Ahmadi J, McComb JG, Han JS, Park SH: Less common CT features of medulloblastoma. Radiology 144:97–102, 1982.

45. Zimmerman RA, Bilaniuk LT: Computed tomography of choroid plexus lesions. CT 3:93–103, 1979.

46. Zimmerman RA, Bilaniuk LT: Computed tomography of acute intratumoral hemorrhage. Radiology 135:355–359, 1980.

47. Zimmerman RA, Bilaniuk LT, Bruno L, Rosenstock J: Computed tomography of cerebellar astrocytoma. AJR 130:929–933, 1978.

48. Zimmerman RA, Bilaniuk LT, Pahlajani H: Spectrum of medulloblastomas demonstrated by computed tomography. Radiology 126:137–141, 1978.

83

Cerebellar Astrocytomas

David G. McLone

Cerebellar astrocytomas constitute 10 to 20 percent of childhood brain tumors. They are rare in the first year of life, exhibit peak incidence in the middle of the first decade,[7] and are encountered infrequently in adult life. The tumors occur equally frequently in males and females.[5] Although no obvious race or sex predilection has been reported, in our series of 36 cerebellar astrocytomas, all five black children were females.

Children with cystic astrocytomas of the central nervous system have a generally good prognosis.[1,3,8] Certainly these children fare far better than those with cerebellar medulloblastoma, ependymoma, or brain stem glioma. In children with astrocytoma, long-term survival can follow even incomplete removal of the tumor. Overall, only 5 to 20 percent of their tumors will have histological characteristics which would indicate a malignant course.

History of Illness

The vast majority of children present with morning headaches and vomiting of several weeks' duration. Often these are episodic and are followed by variable periods of apparently good health. Preschool children often present with shorter histories of unexplained vomiting alone. The older children have often already been seen by psychologists because of inferred behavioral problems, and the younger children by gastroenterologists because of the unexplained vomiting. However, close inquiry usually elicits a history of antecedent or coincident clumsiness and headache. Occasionally the onset of deterioration is precipitous or is confused because of association with a minor head injury.

Symptoms and Signs

Mental Status and Cranial Nerves

The typical child is well nourished, has a placid personality, and exhibits an abnormal gait. Diplopia, head tilt, and altered level of consciousness are common. Complaints of pain in the neck, opisthotonic posture, bradycardia, bradypnea, and hypertension indicate impending deterioration and require immediate attention to relieve pressure on the brain stem. Depressed consciousness indicates a poor prognosis.

Papilledema was present in 83 percent of the children in the Children's Memorial series and was most common in the older children with closed sutures. Optic atrophy was occasionally noted. Chronic papilledema reduced one child's visual acuity to 20/200. Obscuration of vision occurred in another patient, but none of the patients was blind at the time of presentation. Cushing reported that 22 of 76 children with cerebellar astrocytoma (29 percent) were blind at admission.[2] Early diagnosis appears to prevent this debilitating consequence.

Abducens palsy was observed in 15 percent of the children in this series and was the second most common cranial nerve finding. Teenage children often complain of dizziness (light-headedness) but rarely have true vertigo. Multiple cranial nerve involvement was seen in only a few of the children.

Cerebellar Function

Truncal ataxia is common. In many of the children, especially the younger ones, this presents as gross gait problems. In older children the ataxia is more subtle and must be brought out by examination of tandem gait or rapid turning. Dysmetria is more common in older children, possibly because of the difficulty of eliciting it in younger children. The ataxia observed may reflect the presence of hydrocephalus more than actual cerebellar involvement, because it frequently resolves completely following ventriculoperitoneal shunting. Nystagmus is far less common than ataxia and dysmetria and tends to be a late sign. The nystagmus is usually worse when gaze is directed toward the side of the lesion. "Cerebellar fits" are uncommon today, because of early diagnosis and treatment.

Management

The biological behavior of this tumor is not well understood. It is consequently impossible to answer precisely parents' common questions about the cause of the tumor and the length of time the tumor has been present. Because not all cystic posterior fossa tumors are benign, it is also impossible to answer parents' questions about prognosis until after pathological verification of tumor histology.

Purely hemispheric astrocytomas and those extending to the midline are mostly cystic (80 to 85 percent).[6] About 50 percent of midline astrocytomas are cystic. Solid tumors occur more frequently in the midline vermian location.[4] The cyst fluid is usually pale yellow and contains 1 to 2 gm per 100 ml of protein. Occasionally the fluid will be thick like motor oil or show evidence of a recent hemorrhage. Hemorrhage into the tumor is one cause of precipitous deterioration in a child.

Preoperative Radiological Evaluation

Skull roentgenograms usually reveal changes consistent with long-standing increased intracranial pressure, including thinning and asymmetric bulging of the occipital squama, chronic splitting of the cranial sutures, and (in those with closed sutures) demineralization or erosion of the sella turcica. It is likely that the tumor itself causes only minor symptoms and signs and that the period of rapid deterioration signifies the onset of secondary hydrocephalus from obstruction of cerebrospinal fluid (CSF) pathways in the posterior fossa. The child's ventricular system then becomes the most rapidly expanding component of the total "tumor" and causes the precipitous clinical decline.

At present, the key step in the radiological evaluation of patients with a possible posterior fossa tumor is computed tomography (CT), without and with intravenous contrast enhancement. Since the advent of CT, the indications for angiography in the evaluation of posterior fossa tumors have decreased. Increasing experience indicates that tumors with typical CT appearance may safely be operated upon without angiography. It is still indicated, however, for (1) lesions without mass effect, which might, therefore, be arteriovenous malformations (AVMs); (2) multiple lesions that might be hemangioblastomas, multifocal AVMs, or other atypical processes; (3) lesions which extend into the cerebellopontine angle; (4) lesions with central enhancement that could be (partially thrombosed) aneurysms; and (5) lesions in patients with stigmata of neurocutaneous or vascular malformation syndromes. Ventriculograms[5] and pneumoencephalograms are now probably of only historical interest in the diagnosis of cerebellar tumors.

Nuclear magnetic resonance (NMR) scanning is highly useful for the diagnosis of posterior fossa lesions, because it can produce sagittal, coronal, and axial images from a single study without exposing the patient to ionizing radiation. It readily identifies tumor extension into the spinal cord, brain stem, and posterior cervical subarachnoid space. Because bone yields no NMR signal, bone artifacts will not obscure the cerebellopontine angles and brain stem as they so commonly now do with CT.

Preoperative Management

The surgeon confronted with a cerebellar astrocytoma needs to determine whether the patient will benefit from preoperative and/or intraoperative corticosteroid therapy and from preoperative decompression of hydrocephalus by shunt diversion of CSF. It must also be determined whether to employ the sitting, prone, or lateral decubitus position for surgery, whether to perform a craniotomy or craniectomy, and whether to attempt gross total resection of the tumor. Postoperatively, it must be determined whether radiation therapy and/or chemotherapy are indicated, and whether reoperation should be considered at any specific time.

Corticosteroid therapy with dexamethasone or an equivalent has proved beneficial in preparing children with posterior fossa tumors for surgery, in performing the actual resection, and in managing them postoperatively. In many of these children, use of steroids alleviates the need for shunting. Complications of such pre- and postoperative steroid use are rare in children.

Emergency preoperative shunting is required in the few cases in which the patient is rapidly deteriorating from high intracranial pressure and is a poor risk for immediate posterior fossa surgery. In the Children's Memorial series, elective ventriculoperitoneal shunting was carried out prior to craniotomy in the majority of patients with secondary hydrocephalus, and tumor resection was delayed until the papilledema had resolved and most of the clinical signs and symptoms had remitted over the 7 to 10 days following shunting. In patients with chronic hydrocephalus and thin cortical mantles, elective shunting is not done, because subdural hematomas may complicate rapid ventricular decompression, especially if surgery is performed with the patient in the sitting position. In such patients, an external ventricular drain may be placed immediately prior to or at the time of surgery, and the surgery should be performed with the patient in the prone or the lateral decubitus position. Because elective shunting carries some risk, including that of upward herniation of posterior fossa structures, some have advocated direct attack on the tumor without shunting. Many pediatric neurosurgeons, in fact, do operate on cerebellar astrocytoma directly, even when hydrocephalus is present, with equally good clinical outcomes.

The patient position selected for approaching posterior fossa tumors depends largely on the prior experience of the neurosurgeon. Each position affords certain advantages and carries certain risks. The sitting position allows drainage of blood and CSF from the surgical site and probably offers better access to the superior vermis. Air embolism is more common in the sitting position, but the actual risk can be reduced by intraoperative fluid expansion and use of positive airway pressure. Patients to be operated upon in the sitting position should have a right atrial central venous catheter placed preoperatively and should be monitored by Doppler ultrasonography and end-expiratory CO_2 in order to detect and treat any air embolism that occurs. In the sitting position, decompression of the ventricles also allows substantial quantities of air to pass into the subdural and subarachnoid spaces during surgery, so these patients are much sicker in the immediate postoperative period.

The prone position reduces the risk of air embolism but subjects the facial structures to increased pressure and potential damage. The lateral decubitus position offers the advantages of good access to the airway and little possibility of air embolism. However, the weight of the cerebellar hemisphere on the superior side makes retraction of the hemisphere and exposure of large cystic tumors a significant problem.

In the author's and other institutions, craniotomy is preferred over craniectomy for opening the posterior fossa. Craniotomy is as easily performed as craniectomy in children and allows anatomical reconstruction at the closure of the posterior fossa. In the occasional patient examined at reoperation, the squamous occiput has healed almost without evidence of prior surgery. The author's service has employed this technique for a number of years with satisfactory results and without significant complications. Whether salvaging the bone flap actually affords any further benefit such as protection from trauma remains to be proved.

Surgical Procedure

A midline skin incision from the external occipital protuberance to the midcervical level is adequate for nearly all cerebellar tumors. This incision is then carried deeply through the relatively avascular ligamentum nuchae to reach periosteum. Cutting cautery is not necessary in this plane. The periosteum deep to the cervical musculature is stripped away to expose the occipital bone from mastoid to mastoid. Osteotomy is performed just inferior to the torcular and the transverse sinuses and is then extended caudad into the foramen magnum on each side. The arch of C1 is always exposed at this time, but the arch is actually resected only when it is necessary to free up impacted cerebellar tonsils.

If the dura is tense, it is important to decompress the posterior fossa by needle aspiration of any cystic component of the astrocytoma prior to opening the dura. It is often helpful to use ultrasonic scanning prior to opening the dura in order (1) to determine the relative positions and sizes of cyst and mural nodule, so that the aspirating needle may be directed away from the mural nodule into the largest diameter of the cyst, and (2) to determine the location of the most superficial portion of the tumor, so that the dural incision and cerebellar incision may be tailored to coincide with the line of optimal surgical attack.

The dura mater is then opened in a U, with the midpoint of the U located just above the annular sinus at the foramen magnum. It is important to open the dura over the cisterna magna before opening the dura overlying the foramen magnum and cervical cord, so that the intact lower dura cradles the cerebellar tonsils until the posterior fossa is partially decompressed. Especially in children, great care must be exercised in carrying the dural incision across the midline falx cerebelli and the annular venous sinus at the foramen magnum, since any inadvertent trauma to these vascular structures may cause rapid blood loss and air embolism.

Early in the operation, soon after the dura mater is opened, the vallecula and fourth ventricle should be identified. A cotton pledget should be placed in the fourth ventricle to identify its location and to protect the vital structures in its floor during subsequent surgery.

It is helpful to employ optical loupes or the operating microscope during surgery to trace the tumor and to avoid injury to vital structures. Loupes afford the surgeon greater mobility but provide less magnification than the operating microscope. Exophytic tumors which extend into the cerebellopontine angle often require the higher magnification of the operating microscope for optimal resection.

Total removal should be the goal of the surgeon. The demarcation between tumor and brain is usually quite distinct, even in those tumors which do not exhibit pseudoencapsulation. The major portion of the astrocytoma, therefore, may usually be removed easily by microdissection, suction, and bipolar cautery. Small residual portions of the tumor in difficult areas may be removed with the CO_2 laser. In patients with cystic astrocytomas, extirpation of the mural tumor nodule may be sufficient to effect cure. However, it is preferable to remove the cyst wall as well, especially if the wall is thick.

In other patients, especially those with solid tumors, tumor growth through the cerebellar peduncles into the brain stem may make complete resection impossible. Despite the surgeon's desire for complete tumor removal, these lesions should not be followed into the brain stem, lest violation of the floor of the fourth ventricle cause additional neurological deficit. Every effort should be made to avoid inflicting cranial nerve palsies and incapacitating ataxia on these children.

At the end of the resection, the dura mater should be closed tightly to prevent postoperative pseudomeningocele. Often intraoperative shrinkage of the dura requires use of a dural substitute or pericranial graft to achieve the dural closure.

Postoperative Management

The postoperative course may be complicated by a meningitis-like syndrome. Clinical evidence of headache and meningeal signs are consistent with the diagnosis of bacterial meningitis. Laboratory evaluation of CSF obtained via lumbar puncture (determined to be safe after precautionary CT scan of the posterior fossa) is also consistent with bacterial meningitis, but all cultures are negative. This postresection syndrome usually resolves over a few days and probably represents chemical meningitis secondary to intraoperative bleeding and residual surgical debris. Seizures may occur in patients with posterior fossa tumors, both prior to and after surgery. A postoperative seizure incidence as high as 12 percent has been reported, leading some to advocate use of prophylactic anticonvulsants. In the author's experience, however, prophylactic anticonvulsants are not necessary, since such seizures are readily controlled and since no child's condition has deteriorated because of such seizures.

Failure of the patient to return to an alert state or progressive neurological deficits in the immediate postoperative period are reasons to obtain a CT scan. If a postoperative hematoma is present, the patient should be returned to the operating room for its evacuation.

Postoperative radiation therapy is indicated for those tumors which are histologically malignant. Those benign tumors in which brain stem invasion has prevented gross total removal can be followed clinically and with CT scanning for evidence of progression. Evidence of progression is an indication for radiation therapy. Only time will demonstrate which agent(s) and which administration protocols are most effective in controlling the growth of cerebellar tumors.

Early reoperation should be undertaken if a large portion of respectable tumor was left behind because of technical problems encountered at the time of the initial resection. Late reoperation should be considered in patients whose tumors recur more than 1 year after the initial resection.

References

1. Bucy PC, Thieman PW: Astrocytomas of the cerebellum: A study of a series of patients operated upon over 28 years ago. Arch Neurol 18:14–19, 1968.
2. Cushing H: Experiences with the cerebellar astrocytomas: A critical review of seventy-six cases. Surg Gynecol Obstet 52:129–204, 1931.
3. Fulchiero A, Winston K, Leviton A, Gilles FH: Secular trends of cerebellar gliomas in children. JNCI 58:839–843, 1977.
4. Gol A, McKissock W: The cerebellar astrocytomas: A report on 98 verified cases. J Neurosurg 16:287–296, 1959.
5. Grant FC, Jones RK: A clinical study of two hundred posterior fossa gliomas in children. Clin Neurosurg 5:1–24, 1957.
6. Ringertz N, Nordenstam H: Cerebellar astrocytoma. J Neuropathol Exp Neurol 10:343–367, 1951.
7. Sayers MP, Hunt WE: Posterior fossa tumors, in Youmans, JR (ed): *Neurological Surgery: A Comprehensive Reference Guide to the Diagnosis and Management of Neurosurgical Problems.* Philadelphia, Saunders, 1973, pp 1466–1489.
8. Winston K, Gilles FH, Leviton A, Fulchiero A: Cerebellar gliomas in children. JNCI 58:833–838, 1977.

84

Medulloblastomas

Luis Schut
Derek A. Bruce
Leslie N. Sutton

The term *medulloblastoma* originated in 1925 when Bailey and Cushing [1] reported clinical and pathological features in 29 patients with "a very cellular tumor of a peculiar kind." Most of these 29 patients were children, and the tumors were usually located in the cerebellar vermis over the roof of the fourth ventricle. They also reported seeing five other patients with similar tumors in the cerebellar hemisphere which they felt were "unquestionably of the same histogenesis." They thought that the tumor represented a subtype of glioma and coined the term *spongioblastoma cerebelli* to describe it. Globus and Strauss,[8] however, used the term for a different type of malignant central nervous system tumor, and a confusion of terms resulted. Bailey and Cushing at first considered changing the name of their reported tumor to *undifferentiated spongioblastoma*, but finally settled on the name *medulloblastoma* to avoid further confusion. Since then, many reports have appeared in the literature describing this tumor, and the name *medulloblastoma* has remained firmly entrenched in the classification of tumors of the central nervous system.

Medulloblastomas have long been recognized as one of the most common tumors in the posterior fossa and account for 4 to 10 percent of primary brain tumors. In patients under the age of 20, they account for between 15 and 20 percent of CNS tumors. Since it is known that the incidence of CNS tumors in children is 2.1 per 100,000 population, it can be roughly estimated that between 300 and 500 new cases of medulloblastoma will occur per year in the United States. Medulloblastoma affects boys more commonly than girls, with a ratio between 4:3 and 2:1. They most commonly occur in the first decade, with 70 percent of tumors occurring in patients less than 8 years of age. However, medulloblastomas have been reported from the newborn period to the seventh decade.

In a recent review of 1350 children with brain tumors reported from the Children's Hospital of Philadelphia, Children's Memorial Hospital in Chicago, and the Hospital for Sick Children in Toronto, the total incidence for tumors in the posterior fossa was reported to be 54.7 percent.[3] While the majority of these masses were astrocytomas, between 12 and 15 percent of all pediatric brain tumors are medulloblastomas.

Gross and Microscopic Pathology

Medulloblastomas are most frequently found in the region of the fourth ventricle, adherent to the posterior medullary velum in the midline, but sometimes they present laterally in the cerebellar hemisphere. The tumor may be visible between the tonsils (Fig. 84-1) or may lie completely within the fourth ventricle. In many cases the tumor is intimately attached to the anterior medullary velum or the region of the aqueduct of Sylvius or the floor of the fourth ventricle. It is usually reddish and friable and often has a pseudocapsule; some tumors are vascular, others are necrotic. In 15 percent of cases there is evidence of recent or old hemorrhage within the tumor.[11] Diffuse thickening of the arachnoid by tumor spread is occasionally seen over the tonsils and cerebellar hemispheres, referred to in the literature as *sugar coating* (Fig. 84-2).

Histologically, the medulloblastoma is a highly cellular tumor, consisting mainly of small pear-shaped or round cells with round to oval hyperchromatic nuclei and little cytoplasm. The cellular borders are poorly defined (Fig. 84-3). A large number of mitoses are commonly observed in the microscopic field along with occasional rosettes of the Homer-Wright type, suggesting neuroblastic differentia-

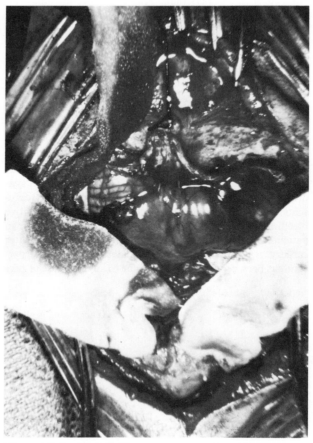

Figure 84-1 Medulloblastoma at operation. The tumor is presenting between the cerebellar tonsils and is readily visible upon opening the dura.

758

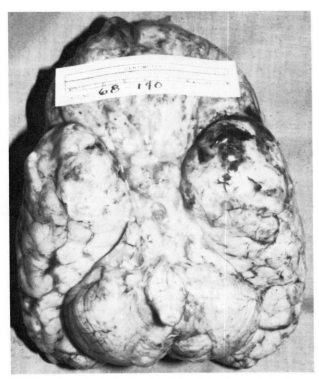

Figure 84-2 Pathology specimen of the base of the brain in medulloblastoma. Diffuse subarachnoid spread of tumor gives the brain surface a "sugar-coated" appearance.

tion. On close examination, the cells forming the rosettes are carrot-shaped, mostly with tapering unipolar processes, but they are occasionally bipolar. Sometimes neurofibrils can be demonstrated with silver stains, and differentiation toward

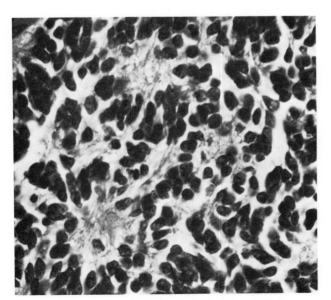

Figure 84-3 Histopathologic section of a medulloblastoma. The tumor is highly cellular, with round to oval cells forming rosettes. (Hematoxylin and eosin.)

ganglion cells, spongioblasts, astrocytes, and even oligodendroglia can be seen. These tumors are not usually very vascular, and blood vessels are not a prominent feature of the histological picture.

A subtype of medulloblastoma is the desmoplastic medulloblastoma, said to be more frequently found in older patients, particularly those over the age of 20.[4] These tumors are located laterally in the cerebellar hemisphere more commonly than in the vermis or fourth ventricle. They are made up of islands of cells surrounded by a network of fibrous and connective tissue. The cells in the islands are small, round to oval, with the nucleolus sometimes visible. Cytoplasm is scant, and there may be distortion of the cells because of compression by the connective tissue element. In a review of 201 cases of medulloblastoma by Chattey and Earle,[4] 42 were believed to comply with this description of desmoplastic medulloblastoma and 159 were of the classic type. The desmoplastic group had an average survival of 51 months, while the classic type had an average survival of 18 months.

Controversy still exists among different schools of neuropathology regarding the cell of origin of medulloblastoma. In 1925, Bailey and Cushing outlined their concept of brain tumor classification based on the cell of origin.[1] They hypothesized a primitive cell, the primitive medullary cell or neuroepithelial cell, which could differentiate into five different cell types: choroidal epithelium, pineal parenchymal cells, primitive spongioblasts, medulloblasts, and polar neuroblasts. According to this idea, the medulloblast was a sort of extraembryonal cell distinct from the spongioblast and neuroblast yet capable of differentiation along both lines. Bailey and Cushing thought this primitive medulloblast was the cell giving rise to the medulloblastoma. However, there is justification for the view that medulloblastoma originates from the germinative cell, which is derived from the external granular layer of the cerebellum and is capable of bipotential differentiation. This view was suggested by Kershman in 1938[10] and by Fujita et al.[7] Another theoretical possibility is that medulloblastomas are really cerebellar neuroblastomas derived from young neuroblasts, a view supported by the work of Tola[15] and others. Because of the well-known tendency of medulloblastoma to differentiate along spongioblastic and glial, rather than neuronal, lines, however, it has been suggested that this tumor is quite separate from neuroblastoma and conceivably not derived from the external granular layer at all. Finally, Rorke[14] recently suggested that medulloblastoma is essentially a primitive neuroectodermal tumor, with or without glial differentiation, neuronal differentiation, or multi- or bipotential differentiation, which is located in the cerebellum.

Clinical Features

Because the fourth ventricle is the preferred site of the medulloblastoma, the most common presenting clinical signs are those referable to increased intracranial pressure secondary to obstruction of the flow of cerebrospinal fluid and secondary hydrocephalus. The typical history is one of lethargy, headaches, and vomiting, at first occurring rarely but as time passes occurring every morning upon awakening. The predominance of morning symptoms is explained by the fact that intracranial pressure rises during the night as a result of position, decrease in the reabsorption of cerebrospinal fluid, and elevation of $PaCO_2$. As the blood volume increases, the intracranial volume increases and raises the intracranial pressure. Upon awakening, the patient complains of severe headache and may vomit, inducing hyperventilation and a decrease in the $PaCO_2$. Also, as the patient assumes an upright position, there is an increase in venous return and a secondary decrease in intracranial pressure. The child feels better and is able to return to normal activities, and because of this the symptoms are dismissed as psychogenic in nature, resulting in delay in diagnosis of the tumor.

If these early symptoms do not lead to a neurological examination and diagnosis of the tumor, they tend to progress to gait ataxia, nystagmus, and, on occasion, cranial nerve palsies, particularly of the sixth and the fourth nerves. When the tumor is located eccentrically and not in the vermis or the fourth ventricle, the patient presents with unilateral cerebellar signs. The duration of the symptoms before a diagnosis is made varies from a few days to as long as 3 to 4 months, with a median duration of 6 to 7 weeks.

On neurological examination, the single most important and most common finding is bilateral papilledema. In many cases papilledema is so severe as to produce marked central scotomas and may progress to severe loss of vision and blindness. In more advanced cases, ataxia, nystagmus, past pointing, and cranial nerve palsies are found. In the younger child, percussion of the skull produces hyperresonance described as the cracked-pot, or Macewen's, sign. Some of these patients present to the pediatrician with an acute ictus suggesting subarachnoid hemorrhage due to spontaneous bleeding within the tumor bed. In the authors' clinic, 15 percent of all nontraumatic spontaneous subarachnoid hemorrhages were due to a tumor, and of these, almost half were tumors in the posterior fossa, most commonly medulloblastoma.[11] Occasionally patients have presented with symptoms of spinal cord compression or hemispheric signs later found to be due to cerebral metastases of a previously undiagnosed fourth ventricle medulloblastoma.

The clinical picture should quickly lead to radiological studies. The plain skull films may show separation of the sutures in the patient under the age of 15, and computed tomography makes the diagnosis of mass lesions with uncanny precision. In the Children's Hospital recent experience, 97 percent of brain tumors were demonstrated by computed tomography, and the indicated histological character of the masses was correct in over 80 percent.

Surgical Therapy

Controversy still exists regarding the initial management of the patient with a medulloblastoma. Some groups advocate routinely shunting the hydrocephalus as the first step, claiming lower morbidity and mortality and a better surgical field after the intracranial pressure is relieved for a period of several days to a few weeks. The proponents of this initial step are divided over the need to insert a filter in the shunting system to prevent the spread of tumor cells to the peritoneal cavity or systemically, since in some studies [9] an incidence of up to 19 percent of extracranial metastases was reported after shunting. Other groups claim that this is an extremely rare occurrence and see no need for filters in the shunting system. Certainly when filters are used, it can be expected that there will be a large incidence of shunt malfunction, since the filters tend to clog rapidly with tissue debris. Because of this, recent efforts have been made to develop a shunt with a bypass system, which can be opened or closed at will. Another problem with early shunting is that decreasing the pressure in the supratentorial system by draining the hydrocephalus can produce an upward herniation of the tumor, necessitating emergency decompression of the posterior fossa and removal of the mass. This complication has been reported in up to 4 percent of all the patients treated initially with shunts. In the authors' experience, shunting for hydrocephalus in patients with medulloblastoma has been necessary in only a relatively small number, roughly one-third. For these reasons, it is the Children's Hospital policy not to shunt initially but to treat the patient presenting with increased intracranial pressure secondary to suspected medulloblastoma with large doses of corticosteroids (dexamethasone once daily in a dosage of 1 mg/kg) for a period of 2 to 3 days prior to surgical intervention. This usually produces a remarkable improvement in the symptoms, and often the neurological examination will revert to normal.

Surgery is usually performed with the patient in the prone position and is preceded by the placement of a posterior parietal burr hole and external ventricular drainage. When there is hydrocephalus, a ventricular catheter is inserted subcutaneously into the lateral ventricle which can, if necessary, be converted to a formal shunting device. The prone position allows good visualization of the region of the cisterna magna, foramen of Magendie, and fourth ventricle and in many cases obviates the necessity of splitting the vermis itself. A posterior fossa craniectomy is commonly performed, including the rim of the foramen magnum, and if necessary, the posterior arch of C1 is easily excised. Frequently the tumor is visible in the cisterna magna upon opening the dura mater (Fig. 84-1). Occasionally, "sugar coating" of the cerebellum and arachnoid can be seen (Fig. 84-2). The surgical goal is to perform total gross removal of the tumor, which can frequently be done in a piecemeal fashion, avoiding traction to the vital structures of the brain stem and cerebellar peduncles. The use of bipolar coagulation, magnification, self-retaining retractors, high-frequency ultrasound aspirators, and the laser beam has greatly improved the chances of obtaining satisfactory removal of the tumor without damage to the surrounding structures. After the tumor is removed, the floor of the fourth ventricle is inspected for infiltration, and cerebrospinal fluid is readily seen draining from the dilated aqueduct of Sylvius. The surgical plan is always to try to perform a gross total removal; there is evidence in the literature [12,13] that this will enhance the likelihood of long-term survival for the patient. By decreasing the amount of manipulation of the structures surrounding the tumor, morbidity such as swallowing difficulties, involvement with speech mechanisms, and other cranial nerve palsies is greatly decreased. The mortality for the operation should certainly be less than 2 percent; it depends greatly on the quality of the team as a whole, including the neuroanesthesiologist and the intensive care specialist.

It has been the policy at Children's Hospital to repeat the CT scan as soon as feasible, and certainly before initiating further therapy. Because of the recent report of a large number of unsuspected spinal cord metastases,[5] myelography with metrizamide has also been performed prior to further therapeutic measures, although few positive studies have been found.

After surgery, early mobilization is encouraged and the steroid dosage is decreased over the course of 2 weeks. The patient is carefully watched for sterile meningitis. When this occurs, an increase in steroid dosage usually produces dramatic improvement in the symptoms.

Adjunctive Therapy and Complications

Since the time of Cushing, it has been clearly demonstrated that the most important single therapeutic procedure after surgery for removal of a medulloblastoma is radiation therapy. The commonly accepted radiotherapeutic regime for the management of medulloblastoma is 5000 to 5500 rad to the posterior fossa, 4000 to 4500 rad to the whole cranial cavity, and 3000 to 3500 rad to the spinal axis. This program is usually started within 3 weeks of surgical removal and is spread over a course of 6 to 7 weeks. The x-rays should be carefully collimated, and it is of utmost importance that there be adequate overlap of the fields. In many recent instances of patients referred because of recurrence of metastatic medulloblastoma, review of the earlier x-ray therapy fields has shown that metastasis occurred in gaps between the fields.

The major problem resulting from this regime is the inability of the young, developing brain to tolerate these large amounts of radiation therapy. Because of this, radiation therapy in the child under the age of 2 is avoided and chemotherapy used instead. Nevertheless, it should be pointed out that the prognosis in the very young child with medulloblastoma is far more pessimistic than in the child over the age of 2, with few of the younger children surviving.

During the past few years, two major studies have been undertaken to try to demonstrate the usefulness of chemotherapy as an adjunctive mode of treatment for patients with medulloblastoma. The Société International Oncologique Pédiatrique (SIOP) examined two groups of patients, one group treated with surgery and radiation therapy and the other with surgery, radiation therapy, and a chemotherapeutic trial of vincristine and lomustine (CCNU).[2] Simultaneously, the Children's Cancer Study Group and the Radiation Therapy Oncology Group joined in a study of children with medulloblastoma in the United States.[6] This study was randomized, with one group receiving vincristine 1.5 mg/cm² for eight injections during the postoperative period and concurrent with radiation therapy. Four weeks after completion of the radiation therapy, vincristine was reinstituted at the same dosage, as well as CCNU, 100 mg/m² by mouth,

and prednisone, 40 mg/m² by mouth, in three divided doses for 14 days. During this 14-day cycle, vincristine was given on days 1, 8, and 15. The cycle was repeated every 6 weeks for a total of eight cycles over a period of 1 year. While these two studies suggested a beneficial effect of chemotherapy in the early stages of the investigation, long-term results have shown little statistical difference between the treated and untreated children, with the European trial suggesting a slightly improved outcome in those treated with chemotherapy.

Results of Therapy

The 5-year survival for this tumor has been reported to vary between 25 and 70 percent. In a hospital specializing in the treatment of children with cancer, a 5-year survival rate of 60 percent or more can be expected following total excision and radiation in patients over the age of 2. In younger patients, an almost 100 percent mortality can be expected within 2 to 3 years. Several attempts have been made to analyze the results of treatment of medulloblastoma. The concept of a period of risk is important. It has been postulated that for tumors of congenital origin, particularly in Wilms' tumor, the period of risk encompasses a time equal to the age of the patient at diagnosis plus 9 months (Collins' law). However, in recent years, with prolonged survival of patients with medulloblastoma and with better record keeping, numerous exceptions to this law have been found, with medulloblastoma recurring after a period far exceeding the predicted term of risk, in some cases by as much as 10 years.

Finally, in discussing the prognosis of this tumor, the complications of combined therapy should be mentioned. Growth hormone deficiency has been reported in as many as 80 percent of the children so treated, and neuropsychological disorders, particularly in performance and short-term memory function, can usually be shown.

References

1. Bailey P, Cushing H: Medulloblastoma cerebelli, a common type of midcerebellar glioma of childhood. Arch Neurol Psychiatry 14:192–224, 1925.
2. Bloom HJG, Thornton H, Schweisguth O: S.I.O.P. medulloblastoma and high grade ependymoma therapeutic clinical trial: Preliminary results. Excerpta Med Int Congr Ser 570:309–322, 1982.
3. Bruno LA, Schut L: Survey of pediatric brain tumors, in Section of Pediatric Neurosurgery, The American Association of Neurological Surgeons: *Pediatric Neurosurgery: Surgery of the Developing Nervous System.* New York, Grune & Stratton, 1982, pp 361–365.
4. Chatty EM, Earle KM: Medulloblastoma: A report of 201 cases with emphasis on the relationship of histologic variants to survival. Cancer 28:977–983, 1971.
5. Deutsch M, Reigel DH: The value of myelography in the management of childhood medulloblastoma. Cancer 45:2194–2197, 1980.
6. Evans AE, Anderson J, Chang C, Jenkin RDT, Kramer S,

Shoenfeld D, Wilson C: Adjuvant chemotherapy for medullo-blastoma and ependymoma, in Paoletti P, Walker MD, Butti G, Knerich R (eds): *Multidisciplinary Aspects of Brain Tumor Therapy*. Amsterdam, Elsevier/North-Holland, 1979, pp 219–222.

7. Fujita S, Shimada M, Nakamura T: H3 thymidine autoradiographic studies on the cell proliferation and differentiation in the external and the internal granular layers of the mouse cerebellum. J Comp Neurol 128:191–207, 1966.

8. Globus JH, Strauss I: Spongioblastoma multiforme, a primary malignant form of brain neoplasm: Its clinical and anatomical features. Arch Neurol Psychiatry 14:139–191, 1925.

9. Hoffman HJ, Hendrick EB, Humphreys RP: Metastasis via ventriculoperitoneal shunt in patients with medulloblastoma. J Neurosurg 44:562–566, 1976.

10. Kershman J: The medulloblast and the medulloblastoma: A study of human embryos. Arch Neurol Psychiatry 40:937–967, 1938.

11. Laurent JP, Bruce DA, Schut L: Hemorrhagic brain tumors in pediatric patients. Childs Brain 8:263–270, 1981.

12. Norris DG, Bruce DA, Byrd RL, Schut L, Littman P, Bilaniuk LT, Zimmerman RA, Capp R: Improved relapse-free survival in medulloblastoma utilizing modern techniques. Neurosurgery 9:661–664, 1981.

13. Raimondi AJ, Tomita T: Medulloblastoma in childhood: Comparative results of partial and total resection. Childs Brain 5:310–328, 1979.

14. Rorke LB: The cerebellar medulloblastoma and its relationship to primitive neuroectodermal tumors. J Neuropathol Exp Neurol 42:1–15, 1983.

15. Tola JS: The histopathological and biological characteristics of the primary neoplasms of the cerebellum and the fourth ventricle, with some aspects of their clinical picture, diagnosis and treatment (on the basis of 71 verified cases). Acta Chir Scand [Suppl] 164:1–112, 1951.

85

Brain Stem Gliomas

Mark S. O'Brien
Mary M. Johnson

The area of the brain between the diencephalon and the cervical spinal cord, derived from the primitive mesencephalon and rhombencephalon and consisting of the midbrain, pons, and medulla oblongata, is generally referred to as the brain stem, and neuroectodermal neoplasms of the astrocytic series occurring in the brain stem are commonly called *brain stem gliomas*.

Previous reports have given the incidence of brain stem gliomas as 10 to 20 percent of all intracranial tumors of childhood and the third most frequently encountered tumor in the posterior fossa of children, trailing the cerebellar astrocytoma and the medulloblastoma.[26,29,33] Recent reviews, however, suggest a higher relative incidence of 25 percent of all intracranial tumors of childhood and an occurrence rate equal to that of cerebellar astrocytoma and medulloblastoma.[2,5] This discrepancy in incidence is probably explained by the more accurate diagnosis afforded by the availability of computed tomography (CT).[2]

This tumor occurs equally in males and females, and there is no race predilection.[26] While it has been reported in all age groups from the newborn[16] to adults,[30] the brain stem glioma is primarily a tumor of childhood, most commonly presenting between the ages of 3 and 9 years.[4,14,17]

Gross Pathology

Of the three divisions of the brain stem, the pons is by far the most frequent site of origin. In time, the tumor usually involves the medulla and midbrain. There have been several reports indicating that malignant tumors tend to arise more commonly in the medulla, whereas the midbrain is more often the site of origin of the benign form.[21,23]

The early growth of this neoplasm is usually characterized by a diffuse proliferation which causes an enlargement, or hypertrophy, often without a discrete neoplastic mass. Such expansion is usually symmetrical bilaterally, but in some instances it is unilateral and halts abruptly at the midline (Fig. 85-1). Spread into the cerebellar peduncles and cerebellum is common. Extension upward into the diencephalon or downward into the cervical spinal cord may occur. Continued growth generally produces bilateral masses which distort the surface of the brain stem (Fig. 85-2), extend into the cerebellopontine angle or interpeduncular fossa, and elevate or rupture through the floor of the fourth ventricle. These exophytic nodules may completely envelop the basilar artery, displacing it posteriorly from the clivus. In the more differentiated lesions the fine architectural detail is obscured but the major landmarks are not effaced. Gelatinous consistency, cystic change, hemorrhage, and necrosis are indexes of poorer differentiation (Fig. 85-3). This neoplasm often either begins as, or degenerates into, the more malignant forms of astrocytoma.[6]

At autopsy, approximately 60 to 70 percent of brain stem gliomas exhibit foci of hemorrhage, necrosis, and pleomorphism that have the microscopic features of glioblastoma multiforme.[18,25] In a small percentage of cases, the tumor

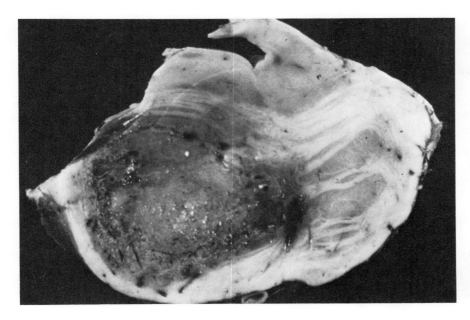

Figure 85-1 Unilateral involvement of the pons by glioblastoma multiforme extending to the midline.

has a wholly benign appearance and contains a large central cyst or multiple microcysts not unlike astrocytomas in the cerebellum and spinal cord.

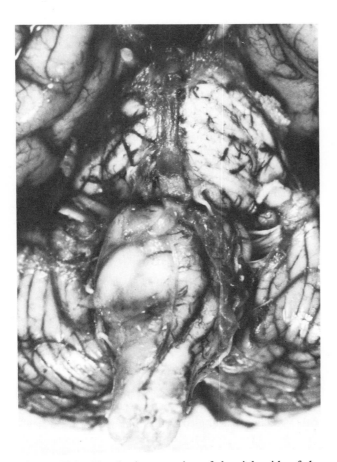

Figure 85-2 Exophytic expansion of the right side of the brain stem displacing the basilar artery dorsolaterally.

Clinical Features

Tumors of the brain stem produce symptoms referable to involvement of the motor and sensory pathways passing through it and particularly to involvement of the nuclei of the cranial nerves which lie within it, so that the frequent combination of cranial nerve plus long-tract signs and cerebellar dysfunction is a natural consequence of the anatomical location of the lesion.

Disturbance of gait is the most common presenting complaint. It is often not clear whether this is the result of weakness or ataxia. The next most common symptom is internal deviation of the eyes. Half the patients are described as having undergone some personality change prior to diagnosis, ranging from apathy, withdrawal, and lethargy to hyperkinesia and aggressive behavior. In school-age children there is a significant deterioration in scholastic ability; in some cases there has been progressive dementia. Swallowing difficulties and speech disturbances are more commonly reported as late symptoms. Headaches and vomiting are reported in one-third of patients and are unrelated in most cases to other evidence of increased intracranial pressure. It is probable that the vomiting is due to direct involvement of the medullary nuclei. Other less common symptoms include focal weakness or ataxia, tinnitus, hearing loss, hiccups, acute hemiplegia, and generalized seizures.[7,24]

Corticospinal tract signs are common in patients with brain stem glioma. Hemiparesis associated with hyperreflexia and an extensor plantar response is the usual finding. Not infrequently, bilateral reflex changes and occasionally quadriparesis are seen.

The most commonly involved cranial nerves are the seventh, sixth, ninth, tenth, and fifth, in that order. Facial diplegia has been reported to occur in up to 25 percent of all patients at some time during the course of their disease.[4] Ocular signs include nystagmus and gaze palsy.[19] Horizontal nystagmus is present in over half the patients and vertical

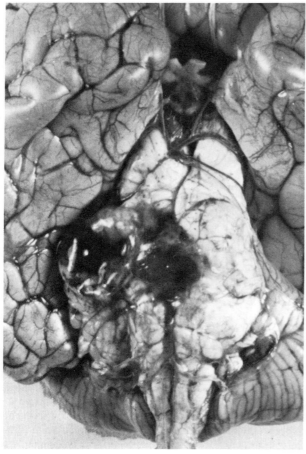

Figure 85-3 Rupture of the exophytic cerebellopontine angle component of a hemorrhagic malignant astrocytoma of the brain stem, causing subarachnoid hemorrhage following an air encephalogram.

nystagmus in less than one-third. Disturbance in lateral gaze can be present, but internuclear ophthalmoplegia is rare.[28] Upward gaze paralysis is less common and indicates upper midbrain involvement.

In general, signs of increased intracranial pressure are not initially present, because of the continued patency of the aqueduct despite the progressive enlargement of the brain stem. However, tumors arising in the midbrain cause hydrocephalus earlier in their clinical course than those arising in the more caudal brain stem. Rapidly growing malignant tumors may also cause obstructive hydrocephalus in the early stage of the disease. Hydrocephalus may develop in the late stages of the disease or with predominantly unilateral lesions, especially those with a significant extrinsic component causing earlier aqueductal distortion. Extension of the tumor into the cerebral peduncle and basal ganglia is often associated with hydrocephalus.[14,20]

The fully developed picture of the patient with corticospinal tract signs, involvement of multiple cranial nerve nuclei, and cerebellar ataxia is usually quickly recognized as a progressive disease of the central nervous system. The patient with insidiously developing symptoms, however, may go unrecognized for some time.

Diagnostic Studies

CSF obtained by lumbar puncture is usually normal in cell count and in protein and sugar content. Rarely, growth of the tumor into the CSF cisterns will produce a low-grade pleocytosis and elevated CSF protein value. Because of these nondiagnostic findings and the risk involved in lumbar puncture in the presence of a posterior fossa mass, there is no place for lumbar puncture, especially before obtaining a CT scan, in the evaluation of a patient suspected of having a brain stem glioma. However, when the diagnosis is in doubt and an infectious lesion is suspected, CSF viral or bacteriologic studies may be of value.[32]

Computed tomography (CT) has replaced pneumoencephalography as the primary radiographic study in the diagnosis of lesions of the brain stem. The CT detection rate for brain stem tumors in children is 96 percent, and its accuracy in diagnosing gliomas is 100 percent.[2] The lowest portion of the medulla and its contiguous cisterns may be poorly visualized because of movement artifact and the overshoot phenomenon from the adjacent petrous bone. Thin sections and the use of metrizamide cisternography are useful adjuncts in delineating small exophytic tumors projecting into the subarachnoid spaces. With the ability of the latest generation of scanners to obtain sagittal and coronal projections, the need for pneumoencephalography has been essentially eliminated.

Information obtained by the CT scan of brain stem gliomas is essential in planning therapy. By indicating the presence and location of an exophytic component, the CT can indicate whether partial resection is possible. The accurate delineation of a large cyst or necrotic area of tumor will help in the surgical decision for internal decompression of the tumor mass and obviate exploratory surgery when these conditions are not present. The presence of obstructive hydrocephalus necessitating a ventricular shunt is easily determined by CT. CT studies are a prerequisite for delineation of the tumor in setting up radiotherapy portals and are useful in postoperative, postradiotherapy, and postchemotherapy evaluations.

Occasionally cerebral angiography is indicated for evaluation of suspected vascular lesions such as an arteriovenous malformation involving the brain stem.

Differential Diagnosis

The differential diagnosis of brain stem glioma includes such non-neoplastic entities as arteriovenous malformation, subacute necrotizing encephalomyelopathy, focal encephalitis, hematoma, tuberculoma, and epidermoid cyst. While these lesions have been reported to mimic brain stem gliomas, they are relatively rare, and most are associated with a specific clinical picture that may suggest the diagnosis. Other tumors, such as chordoma and meningioma, cerebellar astrocytoma, medulloblastoma, and ependymoma can usually be differentiated by CT, metrizamide cisternography, and cerebral angiography.

Therapy

Surgical intervention for brain stem glioma has become a controversial subject, with several recent reports challenging the previously held opinion of radiation treatment without biopsy. Certainly no one would claim that this neoplasm can be extirpated surgically. But no one would reject surgical exploration and biopsy whenever the diagnosis of brain stem glioma is in doubt following thorough evaluation with up-to-date neuroradiological techniques. Patients with brain stem tumors with significant exophytic extension into the extra-axial posterior fossa CSF space or with significant extension of the tumor mass into the fourth ventricle may well benefit from partial tumor removal.[11] Those patients with large intraaxial tumor cysts or large areas of tumor necrosis may benefit from surgical decompression.[13] In these circumstances, the decision for surgical intervention should be based primarily on the patient's clinical condition and prospects for temporary improvement. Follow-up data are insufficient to conclude that surgery for cystic or exophytic lesions is of long-term benefit.

This essentially limits the area of controversy to whether or not all patients with strong clinical and radiological evidence of brain stem glioma should have biopsies. In this case, the major reason for biopsy is specific histopathological correlation with the clinical course and management. Certainly no criticism can be made here. The ability to predict the clinical course can be enhanced when the physician knows whether the patient has a high-grade or low-grade brain stem astrocytoma. This can be helpful not only to the treating physician but also to the patient's parents. When more effective chemotherapeutic agents are available, it might allow for using them adjunctively in the more malignant lesions. Knowledge of the tumor histology might help in evaluating the results of both radiotherapy and chemotherapy and might lead to better therapeutic methods for brain stem gliomas.

The mortality of biopsy is reported to be low with pre- and postoperative use of steroids.[13,23] In one series of biopsied patients there was a worsening of the cranial nerve deficits in 44 percent, of the cerebellar deficit in 40 percent, and of the corticospinal tract deficit in 12 percent.[23]

The problem with biopsy of a brain stem glioma is twofold. One difficulty is the obtaining of tissue suitable for diagnosis. This has improved from 29 percent without the advantage of CT localization[13] to 58 to 75 percent with CT.[15,23] The second is the wide range of histological variation often seen in different areas of the same tumor.[9] Consequently, histological examination of a necessarily limited region by surgical biopsy may not reveal the tumor's true nature. This regional variability points to the limited usefulness of small surgical biopsies.

In view of this heterogeneity of some lesions in degrees of differentiation, the propensity for dedifferentiation following the initial tissue sampling, and the overriding importance of the location of the lesion, it has been difficult to correlate the degree of anaplasia with prognosis. However, it can generally be assumed that the presence of poorly differentiated areas heralds a more rapid course. Patients with such lesions survive on the average for 4 to 10 months after the onset of symptoms. Survival figures for the benign neoplasms are difficult to evaluate, but generally the interval between the onset of symptoms and death in those patients treated with radiation averages 49 months. The benefits of radiation have been debated, but survivals of 5 years or more have been reported.[9,19,22]

Radiotherapy is considered to be generally of benefit in relieving some of the symptoms and signs of brain stem gliomas and in prolonging survival. Various reports indicate that 70 to 90 percent of patients demonstrate some clinical improvement during or after the initial course of radiation.[3,31] However, in histologically verified cases, patients with malignant gliomas usually show little or no improvement and continue to deteriorate. Indeed, this lack of initial response may be used clinically in determining the prognosis, since most long-term survivors initially respond well, while the poor responders succumb quickly.

The 5-year survival rate following the initial course of radiotherapy has varied between 15 and 40 percent,[3,10] with most series reporting 20 to 30 percent.[12,15,19] Again, there is a discrepancy between histologically verified malignant and benign brain stem gliomas. In one series of malignant gliomas, the mean survival time for untreated patients was 2.7 months following diagnosis and for patients who completed the initial course of radiotherapy, 6.3 months.[9]

In a series of adult patients, those with histologically proven glioblastoma or mixed astrocytoma-glioblastoma survived for an average of 8.3 months, while those patients with benign astrocytomas had a mean survival of 30.5 months. Two of the patients in the benign group were still alive 78 and 120 months after the onset of symptoms.[30]

In a series of children, those with benign astrocytomas had symptoms for an average of 17 months before diagnosis and survived for an average of 32.4 months after diagnosis. Children with mixed glioma with anaplasia were diagnosed 3 months after the onset of symptoms and survived on the average an additional 6.4 months. Children with glioblastoma multiforme of the brain stem were diagnosed 3 months after the first symptoms and survived an additional 2.8 months.[19]

It is likely that the discrepancies in survival time in some series and the broad range of survival times in individual cases are, in part, a function of the tumor histology.

While the total dose of radiation seems to play an important role in survival rate, the reported optimum time-dose relationship is not uniform in the literature.[27] The most frequently reported total dose is in the range of 5000 to 6000 rad to the tumor area in 5 to 7 weeks. Particularly in children, total doses in excess of 5500 rad are considered to significantly increase the likelihood of radiation damage to normal brain tissue. Portals should be defined by CT, as this is the best single method for demonstrating the full extent of the lesion. In view of the low incidence of CSF seeding found at autopsy and the fact that progression or recurrence of symptoms is secondary to tumor at the primary site, whole brain and spinal axis radiation is not recommended.

Retreatment by radiation following adequate initial dosage is usually not recommended. One recent paper suggested a significant immediate response rate and a surprisingly high short-term survival with retreatment. However, none of the patients survived more than 3 years.[12] Another report of retreatment in children with recurrent gliomas showed a 37 percent survival for longer than 18 months and a 15 percent long-term survival.[1]

Most recent reports on chemotherapy for brain stem gliomas suggest delaying its use until the time of tumor progression following radiation therapy. Because of the relatively small number of patients in any given study, it is not possible at the present time to evaluate the efficacy of chemotherapy in prolonging survival time in patients with brain stem gliomas. Cooperative trials will be necessary to determine this.[8]

References

1. Abramson N, Raben M, Cavanaugh PJ: Brain tumors in children: Analysis of 136 cases. Radiology 112:669–672, 1974.
2. Bilaniuk LT, Zimmerman RA, Littman P, Gallo E, Rorke LB, Bruce DA, Schut L: Computed tomography of brain stem gliomas in children. Radiology 134:89–95, 1980.
3. Bloom HJG: Recent concepts in the conservative treatment of intracranial tumours in children. Acta Neurochir (Wien) 50:103–116, 1979.
4. Bray PF, Carter S, Taveras JM: Brain stem tumors in children. Neurology 8:1–7, 1958.
5. Bruno L, Schut L: Survey of pediatric brain tumors, in Section of Pediatric Neurosurgery, American Association of Neurological Surgeons: Pediatric Neurosurgery: Surgery of the Developing Nervous System. New York, Grune & Stratton, 1982, pp 361–365.
6. Burger PC, Vogel FS: Surgical Pathology of the Nervous System and Its Coverings. New York, Wiley, 1976, p 246.
7. Fischer AQ, McLean WT Jr: Intractable hiccups as presenting symptoms of brainstem tumor in children. Childs Brain 9:60–63, 1982.
8. Fulton DS, Levin VA, Wara WM, Edwards MS, Wilson CB: Chemotherapy of pediatric brain-stem tumors. J Neurosurg 54:721–725, 1981.
9. Golden GS, Ghatak NR, Hirano A, French JH: Malignant glioma of the brain-stem: A clinicopathological analysis of 13 cases. J Neurol Neurosurg Psychiatry 35:732–738, 1972.
10. Greenberger JS, Cassady JR, Levene MB: Radiation therapy of thalamic, midbrain and brain stem gliomas. Radiology 122:463–468, 1977.
11. Hoffman HJ, Becker L, Craven MA: A clinically and pathologically distinct group of benign brain stem gliomas. Neurosurgery 7:243–247, 1980.
12. Kim TH, Chin HW, Pollan S, Hazel JH, Webster JH: Radiotherapy of primary brain stem tumors. Int J Radiat Oncol Biol Phys 6:51–57, 1980.
13. Lassiter KRL, Alexander E Jr, Davis CH Jr, Kelly DL Jr: Surgical treatment of brain stem gliomas. J Neurosurg 34:719–725, 1971.
14. Lassman LP, Arjona VS: Pontine gliomas of childhood. Lancet 1:913–915, 1967.
15. Littman P, Jarrett P, Bilaniuk LT, Rorke LB, Zimmerman RA, Bruce DA, Carabell SC, Schut L: Pediatric brain stem gliomas. Cancer 45:2787–2792, 1980.
16. Luse SA, Teitelbaum S: Congenital glioma of brain stem. Arch Neurol 18:196–201, 1968.
17. Matson DD: Neurosurgery of Infancy and Childhood, 2d ed. Springfield, Ill., Charles C Thomas, 1969, p 469.
18. Milhorat TH: Pontine glioma. JAMA 232:595–596, 1975.
19. Panitch HS, Berg BO: Brain stem tumors of childhood and adolescence. Am J Dis Child 119:465–472, 1970.
20. Pool JL: Gliomas in the region of the brain stem. J Neurosurg 29:164–167, 1968.
21. Queiroz L de S, Neto JN da C, de Faria JL: Glioblastoma multiforme of the medulla oblongata: A case report. Acta Neuropathol (Berl) 29:355–360, 1974.
22. Redmond JS Jr: The roentgen therapy of pontine gliomas. AJR 86:644–648, 1961.
23. Reigel DH, Scarff TB, Woodford JE: Biopsy of pediatric brain stem tumors. Childs Brain 5:329–340, 1979.
24. Rothman SJ, Olanow CW: Brain stem glioma in childhood: Acute hemiplegic onset. Can J Neurol Sci 8:263–264, 1981.
25. Russell DS, Rubinstein LJ: Pathology of Tumours of the Nervous System. London, Edward Arnold, 1971.
26. Schoenberg BS, Schoenberg DG, Christine BW, Gomez MR: The epidemiology of primary intracranial neoplasms of childhood: A population study. Mayo Clin Proc 51:51–56, 1976.
27. Sheline GE: Radiation therapy of tumors of the central nervous system in childhood. Cancer 35:957–964, 1975.
28. Troost BT, Martinez J, Abel LA, Heros RC: Upbeat nystagmus and internuclear ophthalmoplegia with brainstem glioma. Arch Neurol 37:453–456, 1980.
29. Walker MD: Diagnosis and treatment of brain tumors. Pediatr Clin North Am 23:131–146, 1976.
30. White HH: Brain stem tumors occurring in adults. Neurology (Minneap.) 13:292–300, 1963.
31. Whyte TR, Colby MY Jr, Layton DD Jr: Radiation therapy of brain-stem tumors. Radiology 93:413–416, 1969.
32. Yalaz K, Tinaztepe K: Brain stem encephalitis. Acta Paediatr Scand 63:235–240, 1974.
33. Yates AJ, Becker LE, Sachs LA: Brain tumors in childhood. Childs Brain 5:31—39, 1979.

86

Ependymomas

George J. Dohrmann

This chapter reviews various aspects of ependymal neoplasms (ependymoma and ependymoblastoma) including incidence, age and sex distributions, anatomical location, clinical features, therapy, and prognosis. The pathology and radiology of ependymomas are covered elsewhere in this textbook. Ependymomas are discussed relative to an overall population and then, because they occur most often in the first two decades of life, the aspects of ependymal neoplasms occuring in childhood are discussed separately.

Ependymal Neoplasms in General

Incidence

The incidence of ependymal neoplasms in series of primary intracranial tumors is approximately 5 percent, although it varies from series to series (2 to 9 percent)[1,11,17,18] relative to referral patterns and mean age of patients.

Age and Sex Distributions

Twenty-three years is the mean age of presentation of patients with ependymal neoplasms.[8] At least half the ependymal neoplasms occur during the first two decades of life.[4,7,18] Although there is variation from one series to another, there is a slight male predominance in the occurrence of ependymal tumors.[15,17,18]

Location

The majority of ependymomas occur beneath the tentorium; a good rule of thumb is that one-third occur supratentorially and two-thirds occur infratentorially.[15,17] Approximately half the supratentorial tumors arise from the wall of the ventricle; the remainder arise in an area remote from the ventricular wall, presumably from fetal rests of ependymal cells.[10,17] Almost all the infratentorial ependymomas occur in the midline, often involving the floor of the fourth ventricle; these infratentorial tumors are more solid, while those occurring supratentorially have more cystic components.[17]

Seeding of ependymal neoplasms via cerebrospinal fluid (CSF) pathways has been reported. The evidence of this var-

ies from series to series and varies also as to whether the series was based on autopsy or on clinical data. Svien et al.[17] reported autopsy findings of seeding of the spinal subarachnoid space in over 30 percent of patients with infratentorial ependymal tumors; however, no such seeding was noted in patients with supratentorial ependymal tumors. Of a total of 112 patients with intracranial ependymal neoplasms, only three had clinical evidence of spinal seeding.[7,9] In a review of pooled data on patients with ependymal tumors, 1 of 48 supratentorial tumors had spinal seeding, while 11 of 83 patients with infratentorial tumors had such seeding.[14]

Clinical Features

Symptoms and physical findings are related to the location of the tumor. In general those patients with ependymal tumors involving the cerebral hemispheres present with focal deficits, while those with infratentorial tumors present with nausea and vomiting and ataxia. Most patients present with headache and papilledema, indicative of increased intracranial pressure. Seizures are described in approximately one-third of patients with supratentorial tumors.[6]

Operative and Preoperative Approach

In patients with supratentorial tumors, a craniotomy is performed, and a total gross resection may be done, depending upon the location and the extent of the tumor. The principle here is that of reducing the tumor burden (the number of tumor cells) as much as possible.

Most patients with infratentorial tumors present with hydrocephalus. This should be treated before any other operative procedure is done. In a few patients the hydrocephalus may resolve with the use of steroids preoperatively (see next section); however, almost all patients need diversion of CSF before the posterior fossa is opened so that the brain does not herniate downward. This can be done by placing a shunt (i.e., a ventriculoperitoneal shunt) several days to a week before the tumor resection. Usually the patient improves clinically to the point of reaching a plateau; then the tumor may be operated on. As these tumors can seed via the CSF, incorporation of a filter device into the shunt system is a consideration. Another method of CSF diversion is the placement of a ventricular catheter at the time of the operation or before; the intracranial pressure is monitored via this catheter, and CSF drainage can be used to decrease the pressure.

In operations for infratentorial ependymal tumors, the patient may be operated on in a prone or a sitting position. Because of the increased risk of air embolism with use of the sitting position, Doppler monitoring should be done. A midline incision is used. A suboccipital craniectomy is performed and the posterior arch of C1 is removed. The dura of the posterior fossa is opened with a Y-shaped incision. Most of these lesions occur in the midline; therefore, the vermis is split and the tumor is exposed. As much of the tumor is excised as is possible. Many of these tumors derive their blood supply from the brain stem; therefore total gross removal of tumor is often not possible.

At the time of exposure of the surface of the dura, in patients with supra- or infratentorial ependymomas, real-time ultrasound may be used to dynamically image the tumor. The precise location of the tumor can be obtained from this as well as the tissue characterization (solid tumor vs. necrotic tumor vs. cyst). If a large cystic component is identified, a probe may be advanced with continuous ultrasound guidance and the cyst can be drained. The immediate reduction in the mass of the lesion and the resulting decrease in intracranial pressure lessen the risk of injury to the brain when the dura is opened. Depending upon the circumstances, an operating microscope and microinstruments may be of use with certain ependymomas, as may a laser for vaporization and an ultrasonic aspirator.

In general, the author treats patients with steroids (dexamethasone 4 to 12 mg q 6 h) preoperatively for a minimum of several days but always to the point where they have improved clinically and then have plateaued. The principle is that of improving brain function as much as possible before any operation. At the time of operation, if the dura is tight despite pretreatment with steroids and perhaps a CSF diversion procedure, mannitol (1.5 gm/kg) is given until there is a good urinary response. Usually at that time the dura becomes slack and pulsatile.

Adjunctive Therapy

Ependymal tumors are sensitive to radiation.[13,14] The recommended dose is 4500 rad or more (4500 to 6000 rad over 5 to 6 weeks).[9] As the clinical evidence of spinal seeding of the tumors is slight, many authors do not recommend prophylactic radiation of the spinal cord.[7,9] The role of chemotherapy in the treatment of ependymal neoplasms is uncertain; however, it has been reported to delay recurrence of ependymal tumors for up to several years, although the cure rate is not increased.[3]

Prognosis

Operative mortality for ependymal tumors currently is probably on the order of 10 or 15 percent, but published figures include operative mortalities of over 30 percent.[1] The best survivals are in those patients who have an operation to remove as much of the tumor as possible, followed by radiation therapy. In such patients, Phillips et al.[9] reported a 5-year survival of 80 percent in those with supratentorial tumors and a 5-year survival of 90 percent in those with infratentorial tumors; these figures were for patients who had received 4500 rad or more.

Subependymomas

1945, Scheinker[12] described subependymomas. These indolent tumors occurring just beneath the wall of the tricle and are made up of cells with astrocytic characters and some ependymal features as well. These tumors nble the normal subependymal periventricular glial tissue, hence are quite different from the ependymal neoplasms (ependymomas and ependymoblastomas) discussed here.

Ependymal Neoplasms in Childhood

As half of the ependymal neoplasms (ependymomas and ependymoblastomas) occur in children, these ependymal neoplasms of the first two decades of life are here considered separately.

Incidence

In a review of published series of primary intracranial neoplasms occurring in children, approximately 10 percent were of ependymal origin. The number of intracranial ependymomas is twice that of their more malignant counterparts, ependymoblastomas.[4]

Age and Sex Distributions

The mean age at diagnosis of ependymoma is 5 years, and it is approximately the same for children with ependymoblastoma. Suptratentorial ependymal tumors occur at a younger mean age than infratentorial tumors (Fig. 86-1). Male and female incidence of intracranial ependymal neoplasms is approximately equal; however, a clear male predominance is noted in supratentorial ependymal tumors (1.4:1).[4]

Location

Approximately half the tumors occur above the tentorium and half below, but this varies with the histological type of tumor: 61 percent of ependymomas are infratentorial and 39 percent supratentorial, whereas 81 percent of ependymoblastomas occur supratentorially and 19 percent infratentorially.[4,5]

Clinical Features

Nausea and vomiting, headache, and lethargy are the most common presenting symptoms. The majority of ependymomas occur infratentorially, and the presenting physical findings include ataxia (80 percent), papilledema (40 percent), and dysmetria (40 percent). Ependymoblastomas mainly occur supratentorially, and presenting physical findings are papilledema (62 percent), cranial nerve palsies (46 percent), and paresis (38 percent).[4]

Operative and Preoperative Approach

As discussed above.

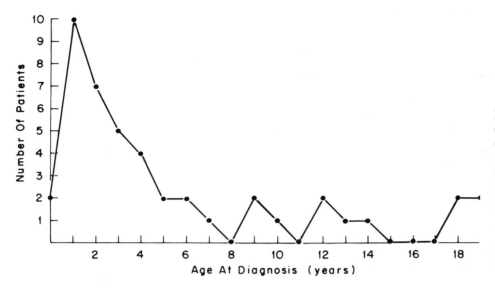

Figure 86-1 Incidence of ependymal neoplasms (ependymoma and ependymoblastoma) in children. The peak incidence was at 1 year, with half the cases occurring before 5 years of age. The distribution was approximately the same for ependymomas as for ependymoblastomas. (From Dohrmann, Farwell, and Flannery.[4])

Adjunctive Therapy

There is no evidence that steroid therapy has had a statistically significant effect on survival.[4] However, the use of steroids probably contributed to the decrease in operative mortality to 17 percent from a value over twice that prior to steroid therapy. Responsiveness of ependymal neoplasms to radiation has been reported to be greater in younger children, and the recurrence rate has been lowest when doses of more than 4500 rad have been used.[16] Nonirradiated ependymal neoplasms have always recurred.[16]

Prognosis

The longest survivals are in children treated initially by operation, followed by radiation. A median survival of 50 months is noted in those children with supratentorial ependymal neoplasms and 31 months in those with infratentorial neoplasms. In children with ependymomas the 1-, 2-, and 5-year survivals are 81 percent, 71 percent, and 21 percent, respectively, while they are 67 percent, 44 percent, and 15 percent for children with ependymoblastomas.[4] It is interesting to note that the survival of adults with ependymal

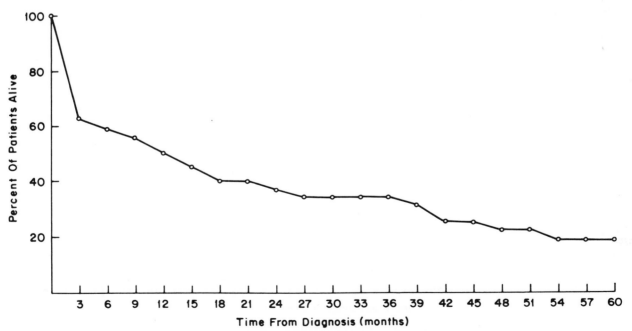

Figure 86-2 Survival of children with intracranial ependymal neoplasms (ependymoma and ependymoblastoma). Approximately half the children died within a year of diagnosis. (From Dohrmann, Farwell, and Flannery.[4])

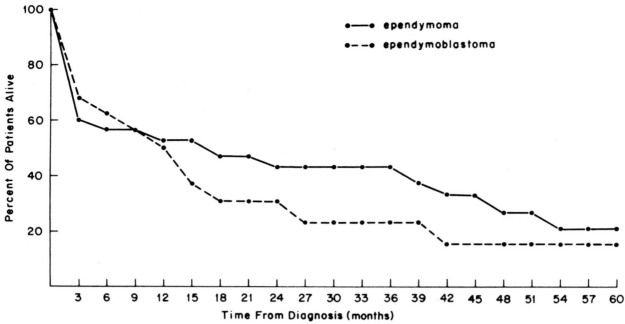

Figure 86-3 Survival time from diagnosis of intracranial ependymal neoplasms in children. Relative survival times are shown for ependymoma and ependymoblastoma. (From Dohrmann, Farwell, and Flannery.[4])

neoplasms is approximately the same as that of children (Table 86-1); the clinical course of ependymal tumor appears to be the same regardless of whether the tumor occurs in an adult or a child. This emphasizes that the biological activity of the tumor is related more to the histological type than to the patient's age (Figs. 86-2 to 86-4).

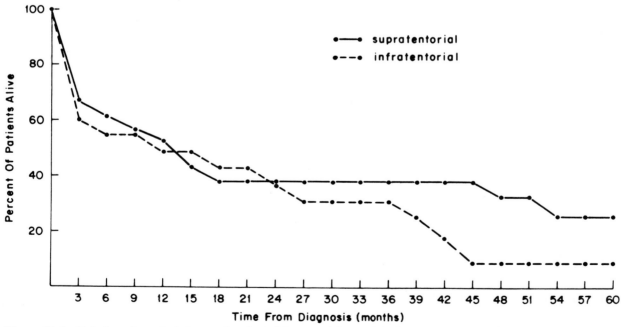

Figure 86-4 Relation of survival time to location of intracranial ependymal neoplasms (ependymomas and ependymoblastomas) in children. Children with supratentorial neoplasms had longer survivals, but the difference became statistically significant ($p < 0.05$) only by 42 months after diagnosis. (From Dohrmann, Farwell, and Flannery.[4])

TABLE 86-1 Survival of Patients with Ependymal Neoplasms in Two Operative Series*

Length of Follow-up, Years	Percent Survival	
	Adults	**Children**
All intracranial		
0.5	54	62
1	50	55
2	38	40
5	32	20
Supratentorial		
0.5	64	64
1	64	54
2	45	39
5	31	27
Infratentorial		
0.5	56	61
1	50	55
2	44	41
5	33	10

*Survival was calculated by an actuarial method.[2] The adult series is that of Ringertz and Reymond,[10] and the series of childhood tumors is that of Dohrmann et al.[4]

References

1. Barone BM, Elvidge AR: Ependymomas: A clinical survey. J Neurosurg 33:428–438, 1970.
2. Berkson J, Gage RP: Calculation of survival rates for cancer. Proc Staff Meet Mayo Clin 25:270–286, 1950.
3. Bloom HJG: Intracranial tumors: Response and resistance to therapeutic endeavors, 1970–1980. Int J Radiat Oncol Biol Phys 8:1083–1113, 1982.
4. Dohrmann GJ, Farwell JR, Flannery JT: Ependymomas and ependymoblastomas in children. J Neurosurg 45:273–283, 1976.
5. Farwell JR, Dohrmann GJ, Flannery JT: Central nervous system tumors in children. Cancer 40:3123–3132, 1977.
6. Haller P, Patzold U: Der diagnostische Wert epileptischer Anfälle für Topik und Morphologie von Hirngeschwülsten: Zugleich ein Beitrag zum Vorzugssitz der häufigsten Grosshirngeschwülste. Z Neurol 203:311–336, 1973.
7. Kricheff II, Becker M Schneck SA, Taveras JM: Intracranial ependymomas: Factors influencing prognosis. J Neurosurg 21:7–14, 1964.
8. Mabon RF, Svien HJ, Kernohan JW, Craig WM: Ependymomas. Proc Staff Meet Mayo Clin 24:65–71, 1949.
9. Phillips TL, Sheline GE, Boldrey E: Therapeutic considerations in tumors affecting the central nervous system: Ependymomas. Radiology 83:98–105, 1964.
10. Ringertz N, Reymond A: Ependymomas and choroid plexus papillomas. J Neuropathol Exp Neurol 8:355–380, 1949.
11. Rubinstein LJ: *Tumors of the Central Nervous System (Atlas of Tumor Pathology*, fasc 6, ser 2). Washington, Armed Forces Institute of Pathology, 1972.
12. Scheinker IM: Subependymoma: A newly recognized tumor of subependymal derivation. J Neurosurg 2:232–240, 1945.
13. Schulz MD, Wang CC, Zinninger GF, Tefft M: Radiotherapy of intracranial neoplasms: With a special section on the radiotherapeutic management of central nervous system tumors in children. Prog Neurol Surg 2:318–370, 1968.
14. Sheline GE, Wara WM: Radiation therapy of brain tumors, in Youmans JR (ed): *Neurological Surgery*, 2d ed. Philadelphia, Saunders, 1982, pp 3096–3106.
15. Shuangshoti S, Panyathanya R: Ependymomas: A study of 45 cases. Dis Nerv Syst 34: 307–314, 1973.
16. Shuman RM, Alvord EC Jr, Leech RW: The biology of childhood ependymomas. Arch Neurol 32:731–739, 1975.
17. Svien HJ, Mabon RF, Kernohan JW, Craig WM: Ependymoma of the brain: Pathologic aspects. Neurology (Minneap) 3:1–15, 1953.
18. Zülch KJ: *Brain Tumors: Their Biology and Pathology*, 2d Am ed. New York, Springer-Verlag, 1965, pp 62–88.

87

Hemangioblastomas

Setti S. Rengachary

Hemangioblastoma of the Cerebellum; Von Hippel-Lindau Complex

Hemangioblastomas are histologically benign tumors occurring exclusively within the neuraxis, most commonly in the posterior fossa. They account for 1.5 to 2.5 percent of all intracranial tumors and 7 to 12 percent of posterior fossa tumors. The term *hemangioblastoma* was originally suggested by Cushing and Bailey to describe these tumors, which were thought to arise from "vasoformative" cells (endothelial cells) of the central nervous system. It stressed the neoplastic nature of the lesion and thereby served to distinguish it from the more common hemangiomas of the nervous system (the latter are not true tumors but hamartomas). Despite the objection that the term *hemangioblastoma* conveyed an erroneous impression of cellular components of primitive nature, implying a malignant potential, it has been widely accepted and is well established in the literature. It is preferred over such synonyms as hemangioma, capillary hemangioendothelioma, Lindau's cyst, Lindau's tumor, or angioreticuloma. Lindau's tumor specifically refers to the tumor of the cerebellum and von Hippel's tumor to hemangioblastoma of the retina. Lindau's disease, or von Hippel-Lindau's (VHL) complex, designates a more diffuse inherited disorder characterized by multiple hemangioblastomas in the neuraxis associated with certain visceral manifestations. The minimal criteria required to justify the diagnosis of VHL complex are debatable, but there is some agreement that if there is more than one hemangioblastoma within the neuraxis (strongly implying multicentricity) or if a solitary hemangioblastoma of the neuraxis is associated with at least one visceral manifestation, a clinical diagnosis of VHL complex is established.

Historical Aspects[3,13,15,23]

Hughlings Jackson reported in the *Medical Times and Gazette* of 1872 the case of a 20-year-old woman who had suffered from failing vision for 3 months. She had a sister who, after two previous "fits," died in the third. Physical examination revealed "double optic neuritis." No ataxia or nystagmus was noted. The patient became totally blind after a period of observation and died suddenly. At autopsy a cyst measuring 1 by 1½ in. was found in the right cerebellar lobe. The cyst contained clear yellow fluid; a tumor described as angiomatous and the size of a shilling was found in the outer wall.

Drs. Vigla, Duchenne, and Dolbeau had a patient with a brain tumor and retinal tumors in the right eye. The patient died in 1864, and a fundus painting of his eye depicting a typical hemangioblastoma appeared in Galezowski's atlas published in 1886.

In a textbook of ocular pathology published in 1879, Panas and Remy illustrated a retinal hemangioblastoma. Their patient had advanced disease, and the basic lesion was not recognized. Instead, these investigators described a complication—"cystic detachment of the retina."

The first accurate description and illustration of the fundus picture was by Fuchs in 1882, who described a case as arteriovenous aneurysm and attributed it to trauma. Lagleyze, in 1884, reported a typical case in the South American literature. In 1885, Pye-Smith presented a case report of a patient who had a cerebellar cyst as well as pancreatic and renal cysts.

In 1892, D. J. Wood of London presented a case of "retinal detachment with unusual dilatation of retinal vessels and other changes." This report is especially significant because Treacher Collins, in 1894, gave the pathological description of the eye from Wood's case as well as the patient's sister's eyes. He observed that the lesions were "made up of plexus of very thin walled blood vessels and there are in them cystic spaces." His conclusions were that this was a new disease, that it was hereditary, and that it was best described as a capillary nevus.

In the American literature, a case described by Millikan from Cleveland, in 1904, probably represents a typical case when one examines the accompanying fundus painting.

Von Hippel's classic paper appeared in 1904; in it he presented two patients with a retinal mass associated with enormously dilated artery and vein and with retinal detachment and exudation. Unaware of Collins' work and lacking tissue for diagnosis, he was unable to assign a cause to this unusual disease. Seven years later, from histologic examination of enucleated eyes from his patients described in previous reports and from becoming aware of Collins' work, he concluded that the primary lesion in the retina was a hemangioblastoma. He thus publicized a new and fascinating clinical entity which soon bore his name as an eponym. After the death of one of von Hippel's patients, Brandt published the autopsy results. In the central nervous system, tumors were found in the cerebellum, in the base of the brain near the petrous bone, and in the cauda equina. In the kidneys, there were cysts and tumors. The pancreas was studded with cysts. The bladder contained papillomas, and the epididymes bore cysts. Brandt also described one other patient with angiomatosis retinae, who had died of brain tumor.

Search of the literature revealed that in at least 10 percent of all cases of angiomatosis retinae, the stigmata of central nervous system neoplasms were also present. Of particular interest was Seidel's report of cerebellar cyst associated with retinal hemangioblastoma in two brothers. Before the onset of cerebellar dysfunction, these men had been earning their living as tightrope walkers!

Thus the time was ripe for Arvid Lindau, a young Swedish pathologist whose monograph in 1926 brought together into one coherent entity the retinal, cerebellar, and visceral components of this disease. Lindau's work had begun as an investigation of cerebellar cysts. Most of these were associated with a mural tumor, and most of the mural tumors were angioblastic. Lindau was particularly impressed by the small size of these mural nodules and emphasized that they could be missed unless meticulous dissection of the cyst wall was carried out. He collected the data on 40 such cases, 24 from the literature and 16 of his own. He found that the hemangioblastomas were not confined to the cerebellum but were present in the medulla and spinal cord as well. The visceral lesions he encountered were pancreatic cysts, renal cysts, renal cell carcinoma, adrenal adenoma, hepatic adenoma, cavernoma of the liver, and tumor of the epididymis.[13,15]

Cushing and Bailey, concurrently with Lindau's work, had begun an attempt to classify gliomas on a clinicopathological basis.[3] In the course of the study they soon found that a number of tumors once regarded as vascular gliomas were indeed blood vessel tumors (hemangioblastomas). They were in the process of assembling these tumors with the intent of publishing these cases when, in reviewing the literature on the subject, they came upon Lindau's monograph. They did not fully appreciate its value because of the misleading title, "Studien über Kleinhirncysten." Further intensive clinicopathological study by Cushing and Bailey confirmed Lindau's meticulous observations. They credited Lindau by attaching his name to the disease.

Genetics[1,6,20]

Hemangioblastomas may occur sporadically as isolated tumors of the cerebellum[1] or may represent a familial disorder as part of VHL complex. In the latter it is transmitted, as an autosomal dominant disorder with varying degrees of penetrance, by either affected or unaffected members of either sex. The clinical syndrome is thus comparable to neurofibroma, which may occur as a solitary lesion involving, say, the acoustic nerve or may be a manifestation of a more diffuse disorder, von Recklinghausen's disease. Both these diseases belong to a group of disorders, the phakamatoses (*phakos*, birthmark), or neurocutaneous syndromes, which are discussed more fully elsewhere in this textbook.

Clinical Features[7,8,16,17]

The cerebellar or retinal tumors are the first to present clinically in patients with the VHL complex. Indeed, cerebellar hemangioblastoma is the most significant manifestation of this disorder and the one that produces the greatest morbidity and mortality. In several reported series there is a slight male preponderance, with a male-to-female ratio of 1.3:1. The average age at onset of symptoms in familial cases is 30 years, with a range of 3 to 83 years. Occurrence of symptoms in children less than 10 years old is distinctly rare. The peak incidence is in the third decade, with a second peak occurring in the fifth decade. The nonfamilial, or sporadic, cerebellar hemangioblastomas tend to present somewhat later, with the mean age at initial presentation being 42 years. The

average duration of symptoms is 13 months, with a range of 3 weeks to 7 years.

The symptoms and signs vary to some extent, depending upon the precise location of the tumor in the posterior fossa. As a general rule, symptoms and signs of increased intracranial pressure with varying expressions of cerebellar or brain stem deficits tend to dominate the picture. Headache is the most common symptom, being present in 95 percent of the cases. It is located in the suboccipital region and tends to be worse in the mornings but becomes relentlessly continuous in later stages. Patients with tumor located in the inferior vermis and tonsils, with chronic impaction of the tumor extending into the foramen magnum, may have continuous occipital pain, neck stiffness, an intermittent shocklike sensation radiating into the occiput, and lapses of consciousness. Vomiting, the next most common symptom, may be due either to obstructive hydrocephalus from a vermian lesion or to irritation of the vagal nucleus from the tumor's origin in the vicinity of this nucleus. In the latter situation vomiting may occur before any other neurological signs appear, leading to a mistaken diagnosis of upper gastrointestinal disorder. Vertigo tends to be a prominent symptom if the tumor is situated directly in the brain stem or in the middle or inferior cerebellar peduncle, with pressure on the vestibular nuclei. Gait disturbance and inability to maintain balance are generally expressions of cerebellar or brain stem hemangioblastoma. Papilledema was recorded in 80 percent of cases in the earlier literature, but this incidence rate is rapidly dropping, thanks to earlier diagnosis of the tumor by universal use of computed tomograms. Diplopia is usually due to sixth nerve paralysis from increased intracranial pressure. Ataxia in the extremities, dysmetria, and intention tremor are observed in cerebellar hemispheric lesions, whereas vermis lesions produce a broad-based gait and truncal ataxia. Nystagmus, especially with a vertical or rotatory component, signifies brain stem involvement. Occasionally in elderly patients, dementia may be the sole or major manifestation of the disease.

Pathology[9,10]

The majority of hemangioblastomas occur in the posterior cranial fossa clustered around the fourth ventricle, generally in the vermis or hemisphere(s) of the cerebellum, medulla oblongata, or pons. Less commonly they are found in the supratentorial compartment or in the spinal cord. Retinal hemangioblastomas occur in 6 percent of patients with cerebellar hemangioblastomas. Structurally, hemangioblastomas occurring at all locations are identical. In familial cases, tumors tend to be multiple. No satisfactory explanation is available for the preponderance of these tumors in the posterior fossa. Lindau suggested that in the twelfth week of intrauterine life, a segment of the primitive choroid plexus was incorporated into the developing cerebellum. Hemangioblastomas were thought to develop from these choroid remnants. This theory is especially attractive in the light of the observation that one of the functions of the primordial choroid plexus is hematopoiesis, but it does not account for the occurrence of hemangioblastomas elsewhere in the neuraxis.

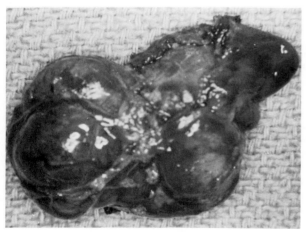

Figure 87-1 Surgically excised specimen of cerebellar hemangioblastoma. The tumor is smooth and multilobulated and has large dilated vessels on the surface. Although it does not have a true capsule, the tumor margin is well defined.

Without any exception, all hemangioblastomas are benign tumors. Occasionally the tumor may spread along the subarachnoid space after a surgical procedure, but it remains histologically benign. Distant metastases have never been reported. Hemangioblastomas do not have a true capsule, but grossly the tumor margin is well circumscribed (Fig. 87-1). The tumors may be either solid or cystic. A higher proportion of cerebellar hemangioblastomas (70 percent) tend to be cystic, compared to supratentorial or brain stem lesions (20 percent). In cystic lesions, the solid component is a small nubbin at some point along the cyst wall, generally close to the pial surface, described commonly as a mural nodule (Fig. 87-2). The cyst contains clear, golden yellow, highly proteinaceous fluid which clots readily after aspiration. The inner surface of the cyst wall is smooth and is made up of glial cells and compressed cerebellar tissue; the tumor itself does not line the cyst wall. The cut surface of the solid tumor appears beefy red from rich vascularity; multiple cysts and cavernous spaces may be seen across the section; in areas the tumor may appear yellow from lipid deposition.

Microscopic Features

Histologically the tumor is composed of three groups of cells: (1) endothelial cells, (2) pericytes, and (3) stromal cells (Fig. 87-3). Whether all three sets of cells participate in the neoplastic process has been the subject of debate; also unresolved is the question of whether these cells interconvert.

The cardinal feature of the tumor is the presence of numerous capillary channels which form an anastamosing plexiform pattern, lined by a single layer of plump endothelial cells (Fig. 87-4). The capillary channels are surrounded by reticulin fibers, best demonstrated by reticulin stains

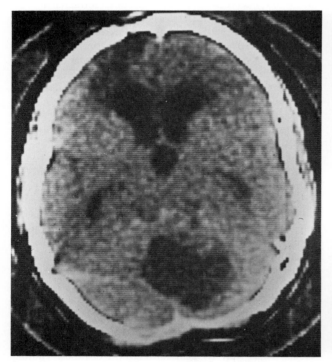

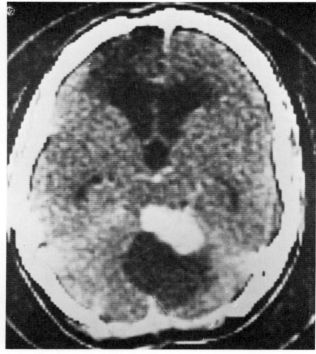

A   B

Figure 87-2 Computed tomograms of cystic cerebellar hemangioblastoma. *A.* In the precontrast scan the mural nodule is isodense and is not readily apparent; the cystic component appears as a low-density lesion. *B.* After contrast injection there is intense staining of the mural nodule.

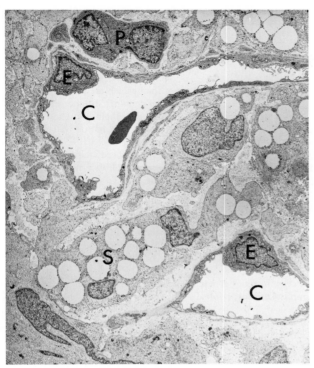

Figure 87-3   Electron micrograph of hemangioblastoma showing the three cell types constituting the tumor: endothelial cell (E), pericyte (P), and lipid-laden stromal cell (S). Capillary lumen (C). (Courtesy of Saing Lee, M.D.)

(Fig. 87-5). The pericytes are difficult to discern with light microscopy and are best visualized with electron microscopy (Fig. 87-4). They lie just outside the periendothelial basement membrane and are themselves completely surrounded by a basement membrane. Between the capillary structures are numerous polygonal cells, the *interstitial*, or *stromal*, *cells*,

with foamy clear cytoplasm. The stromal cells are generally laden with lipid.

Intense research has centered around the question of the origin and nature of the stromal cells ever since Lindau gave an accurate description of the histology of these tumors in 1926. Numerous investigators have, over the years, tried to solve the problem by utilizing a newly introduced histological technique that became available to them. Each investigator or group came up with a fresh hypothesis and believed this was the final word on the subject, only to find a newer technique introduced shortly thereafter which gave rise to different results and to a new, equally firm hypothesis. It is uncertain when the final "final word" will be spoken. In a clinical essay such as this, space does not permit detailed discussion of these hypotheses, but they are briefly summarized in Table 87-1.

Investigations[18]

Computed tomography of the head in the axial and coronal views is the best screening test for patients with hemangioblastomas of the posterior fossa, especially the cystic ones, but is not quite as sensitive as vertebral angiography in detecting small tumor nodules. These two tests provide complementary information and thus should be used together in patients with suspected VHL complex. On computed tomograms, the solid lesions generally appear isodense with cerebellar tissue but stain intensely on contrast injection, with either a homogeneous or a mottled appearance; in some cases there may be a high-density rim with central lucency from an intratumoral cyst. Dilated vessels may be seen in the vicinity of the tumor. The cystic lesions appear as sharply defined low-density lesions with or without a mural nodule. The attenuation values of the cyst may be the same as or slightly higher than those of spinal fluid. The mural nodule, if present, enhances intensely on contrast injection, but the cyst margin itself generally does not enhance. If a cyst is seen alone, without a nodule, in a

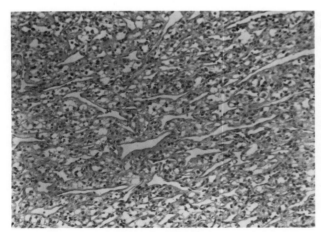

Figure 87-4   Light microscopic appearance of hemangioblastoma. The tumor is composed of numerous capillary channels forming a plexiform pattern and lined by a single layer of endothelial cells.

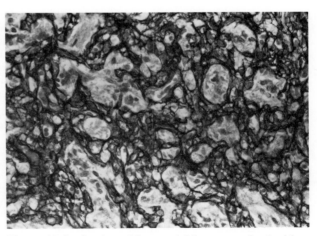

Figure 87-5   Section of hemangioblastoma stained with reticulin stain. The reticulin fibers surrounding the capillary channels are easy to see.

TABLE 87-1 Hypotheses Regarding the Origin and Nature of Stromal Cells in Hemangioblastomas

Author and Year	Technique Used	Findings	Interpretations and Conclusions
Lindau (1926)	Light microscopy	Stromal cells often filled with lipids.	Disturbance of circulation in tumor tissue accompanied by stagnation of lymph rich in lipids which are phagocytized by the endothelial tumor cells, changing them into foam cells.
Various neuropathologists (1930–1940)	Metallic stains for neuroglia and microglia	Stromal cells not stained with metallic stains.	Stromal cells not derived from glial cells.
Cancilla and Zimmerman (1965)	Electron microscopy	Close ultrastructural similarity between endothelial cells and stromal cells.	Hemangioblastomas composed of a single cell type which originates from the endothelium.
Castaigne et al. (1968)	Electron microscopy	Certain ultrastructural observations.	Stromal cells are neoplastic reticulum cells; endothelium and pericytes are nonneoplastic.
Cervós-Navarro (1971) and Kawamura et al. (1973)	Electron microscopy	Overlapping ultrastructural features between endothelial cells, pericytes, and stromal cells.	Stromal cells derived from "vasoformative elements" (endothelium and pericytes).
Jellinger and Denk (1974)	Red-cell adherence technique for blood group isoantigens	Endothelial cells in tumor contain blood group isoantigens, stromal cells do not.	Stromal cells unlikely to be of endothelial origin.
Spence and Rubinstein (1975)	Organ culture and electron microscopy	Endothelial cells, pericytes, and stromal cells maintain their identity in organ culture.	Endothelial cells, pericytes, and stromal cells all neoplastic and replicate in parallel with one another. Interconversion between these cells does not occur.
Jakobiec et al. (1976)	Electron microscopy and lipid analysis	Lipid in stromal cells mostly cholesterol stearate, a plasma lipid; fibrous astrocytes are in different stages of lipidization.	Stromal cells represent lipidized astrocytes; source of lipid is blood plasma; lipidization alters tinctorial properties so that cells no longer stain with metallic stains; occurrence of hemangioblastomas exclusively in nervous system further attests to neuroectodermal origin of tumor rather than angiogenic mesenchymal elements.
Kepes, Rengachary and Lee (1979)[10]	Immunoperoxidase method for detection of glial fibrillary acidic protein (GFAP)	In about half the cases, stromal cells are negative for GFAP; in the remainder, variable amounts of GFAP are demonstrated.	Stromal cells may be of heterogeneous origin; deposition of lipid droplets in cells of diverse origin may make them appear similar.
Jurco et al. (1982)[9]	Immunoperoxidase method for factor VIII–related antigen (VIII R:Ag) and GFAP	All cases show positive staining for VIII R:Ag in stromal cells; astrocytes staining positively for GFAP noted peripherally and centrally in the tumor; but all stromal cells negative for GFAP.	Stromal cells are of endothelial origin; occasional stromal cells other investigators have identified as reacting positively for GFAP may represent stromal cells capable of ingesting extracellular GFAP derived from reactive astrocytes within tumor or may be lipidized astrocytes.

patient with known VHL complex, one has to conclude that the nodule is too small to be defined by CT. In such instances, angiography is mandatory to locate the mural nodule, because the cyst is bound to recur unless the mural nodule is removed.

On vertebral angiography four different vascular patterns may be observed: (1) a vascular mural nodule within an avascular cyst, (2) a doughnut ring of abnormal vessels surrounding an avascular space representing an intratumoral cyst, (3) a large, solid vascular mass (Fig. 87-6), (4) multiple small, widely separated vascular nodules (Fig. 87-7). Since vertebral angiography is highly sensitive in detecting small tumor nodules, it is especially helpful in detecting high spinal lesions as well; thus the neck should be routinely imaged during vertebral angiography in patients with VHL complex. A solid hemangioblastoma in the anterior surface of the cerebellum abutting against the petrous bone may on occasion simulate a cerebellopontine angle tumor on computed tomogram; in such instances the characteristic angiographic pattern will help in their differentiation.

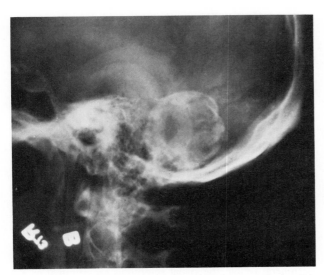

Figure 87-6 Vertebral angiogram showing a typical solid cerebellar hemangioblastoma.

Hemangioblastomas in Other Locations

Supratentorial Hemangioblastomas[4,14,21]

Supratentorial hemangioblastomas are distinctly rare. Sporadic case reports have appeared in the literature; less than 75 cases have been recorded to this date. They may occur in the brain parenchyma of the frontal, parietal, temporal, or occipital lobes, in the corpus callosum or basal ganglia, along the walls of the lateral and third ventricles, in the choroid plexus, and in the leptomeninges. Clinical features are widely variable, depending upon the location of the tumor.

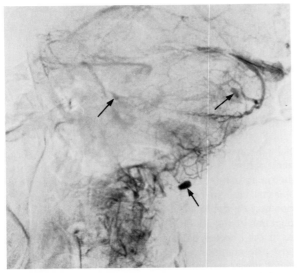

Figure 87-7 Vertebral angiogram showing multiple small vascular nodules in posterior fossa in patient with known VHL complex (*arrows*). Vertebral angiography is more sensitive than computed tomography in detecting nodules of this size.

Association with other features of von Hippel-Lindau complex has been demonstrated in 10 of 63 reported cases. In 7 of the 63 cases, polycythemia was present. Two-thirds of the tumors have been solid, with the remainder having at least some cystic component. Although the radiological features of supratentorial lesions may closely resemble those of hemangioblastoma in the cerebellum, hemangioblastoma is seldom entertained in the differential diagnosis, because of its rarity in the supratentorial compartment, unless the patient has overt signs of von Hippel-Lindau complex.

The relation of angioblastic meningioma to hemangioblastoma, especially with regard to their identity, is controversial. Lee and associates[11] provide a logical classification of highly vascularized meningeal tumors occurring in the supratentorial compartment:

1. Meningiomas with highly vascularized stroma. In these tumors, the basic architecture of the meningioma (meningothelial, fibroblastic, or transitional) can be identified as the principal component of the tumor, and the blood vessels are considered as part of the stroma and not themselves neoplastic.
2. Meningiomas in which meningothelial or fibroplastic components can still be recognized but with a truly neoplastic endothelial component—the "angioblastic" meningiomas.
3. "Angioblastic meningiomas of Cushing and Eisenhardt," which are presently classified as hemangiopericytoma of the meninges, with histological characteristics common to hemangiopericytomas elsewhere in the body. These tumors may not show meningothelial components under light microscopy, but in tissue culture they produce whorls, thus displaying kinship with tumors of meningothelial origin.
4. True hemangioblastoma of the meninges. The histological composition of these tumors is identical to that of hemangioblastomas in other locations, such as the cerebellum or spinal cord. In true hemangioblastomas one does not see meningothelial elements.

The principles of therapy are the same as those described for cerebellar hemangioblastoma.

Hemangioblastomas of the Spinal Cord[2,23]

Hemangioblastomas of the spinal cord represent 1.5 to 2.5 percent of all spinal cord neoplasms. The median age of onset of symptoms is around 35 years. In patients with VHL complex, the spinal symptoms may occur concurrently with or (more often) after the onset of cerebellar or retinal symptoms. Stated differently, the onset of spinal symptoms in a patient with known VHL complex should alert the clinician to the possibility of a spinal hemangioblastoma. Sixty percent of hemangioblastomas are intramedullary and are located in the dorsal half of the spinal cord near the midline. Extramedullary intradural hemangioblastomas tend to be attached to the posterior nerve roots. The thoracic spinal cord is most frequently involved, with the cervical segments next in frequency. Syringomyelia is associated with more than half the cases of spinal hemangioblastoma. The development of syringomyelia is analogous to the development of a cyst in a cerebellar hemangioblastoma, i.e., it arises from transudation of fluid from the tumor capillaries and tubular dissection along the gray matter near the central canal which offers the least resistance. Syringomyelia in patients with VHL complex has never been reported without the accompaniment of a hemangioblastoma within the spinal cord except in the cervical region, where it may be related to a similar tumor in the brain stem.

The clinical presentation is variable. Three common types are described: (1) slow evolution of long tract symptoms and signs (posterior column and corticospinal tracts) with or without radicular symptoms, (2) subarachnoid hemorrhage without focal neurological signs, (3) subarachnoid hemorrhage with abrupt onset of long tract signs.

Roentgenograms of the spine may show erosion of the pedicles and widening of the spinal canal in about half the cases. Myelographic appearances are indicative of an intramedullary mass, and in some cases, serpiginous filling defects may simulate an arteriovenous malformation (in the latter the spinal cord is not usually enlarged). Spinal angiography is most helpful in arriving at the specific diagnosis. A densely staining tumor nodule is visualized, with evidence of rapid circulation through the tumor.

With the use of the operating microscope and bipolar coagulation, total excision of the tumor is possible in the majority of cases. The dura should be opened carefully to avoid damage to the dilated pial vessels. The tumor should be dissected in the plane between the tumor and the parenchyma of the spinal cord, meticulously coagulating all feeding vessels. No attempt should be made to biopsy the tumor or excise it piecemeal.

Angiomatosis Retinae: Von Hippel's Disease[22]

The lesions start as small, discrete foci of dilated capillaries during childhood or adolescence. With time, the angioma appears as a raised or globular reddish mass fed by dilated, tortuous arterioles and drained by engorged serpiginous veins (Fig. 87-8), resulting from low vascular resistance

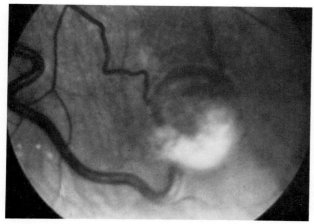

Figure 87-8 Fundus photograph showing retinal hemangioblastoma fed by tortuous artery and drained by engorged draining vein. (Courtesy of Professor A. Lemoine.)

within the tumor. Fluorescein angiography confirms hyperdynamic circulation with intense staining of the nodule and early venous return. Although most commonly located in the peripheral parts of the retina, retinal hemangioblastoma has been observed in the macula, at the border of the optic disc, or on the optic disc. These tumors generally affect both eyes. In long-standing cases a gray-white exudate of variable degree surrounds the mass, the feeding artery, and the draining vein. The exudation is thought to result from increased capillary permeability due to the presence of fenestrations in the lining endothelium. Frequently there is retinal separation, massive gliosis, and retinal edema. On occasion a macular star or papilledema may develop. Recurrent bleeding from the lesion is not infrequent. In late stages, secondary glaucoma with narrowing of the anterior chamber, dilatation of pupil, and extreme congestion may render the eye functionally useless.

In uncomplicated cases of hemangiomas situated in the peripheral retina, the visual symptoms are minimal or absent in the early stages. At this stage the lesion may be diagnosed by diligent fundoscopic examination, especially in patients with a known family history of this condition. Scotomas or a decrease in visual acuity results when there are complicating factors such as exudation, retinal separation, gliosis, or hemorrhage; visual loss may be disproportionately severe when the lesions are located in the macula or on the optic disc.

The histological appearance of the retinal lesions is similar to that of hemangioblastomas occurring in the cerebellum or spinal cord. Hemangioblastoma of the retina should be distinguished clinically from arteriovenous malformations of the retina, Coat's disease, glioma of the retina, melanoma of the choroid, Eales' disease, and multiple retinal aneurysms.

Photocoagulation is the treatment of choice. Despite successful treatment, however, new lesions may develop in other parts of the retina and become apparent with continued follow-up examinations.

Numerous visceral lesions are associated with VHL complex (Table 87-2). The clinically significant ones are described in the following sections.

Related Conditions

Renal Cell Carcinoma

Renal cell carcinoma (Fig. 87-9) is found in one-fourth of patients with VHL complex.[12] The frequency tends to be higher in autopsy series than in clinical series because these neoplasms tend to remain silent in the early stages. The tumor may be the last one to be detected unless computed tomograms of the abdomen are done as a screening procedure in the affected patient or relatives. As more patients survive the common and potentially fatal posterior fossa hemangioblastoma, more cases of renal cell carcinoma will be observed in the respective kindred. The renal cancer differs from its sporadic counterpart in its earlier age of onset, slight male predominence, multicentricity, and synchronous or metachronous bilateral involvement.

TABLE 87-2 Lesions in von Hippel-Lindau Complex

Retinal angiomatosis*	Renal angioma
Cerebellar hemangioblastoma (cystic or solid)*	Renal adenoma
Medullary hemangioblastoma*	Renal cell carcinoma (unilateral or
Spinal hemangioblastoma*	bilateral)*
Supratentorial hemangioblastoma (parenchymal, ventricular wall, choroid plexus, pituitary body, leptomeninges)	Splenic cyst
	Splenic angioma
	Lung cyst
	Lung angioma
Cerebellar ependymoma	Omental cyst
Syringomyelia	Skeletal hemangioma
Pancreatic cyst*	Adrenal cortical angioma
Pancreatic adenoma	Adrenal cortical adenoma
Islet cell carcinoma of the pancreas	Adrenal medullary pheochromocytoma
Adenocarcinoma of the pancreas	Sympathetic paraganglioma
Liver cyst	Epididymal cyst
Liver angioma	Epididymal adenoma
Liver adenoma	Ovarian cyst
Renal cyst*	Ovarian carcinoma

*The more common lesions.

These factors pose special problems in surgical therapy. Some have suggested bilateral nephrectomy, renal dialysis for 5 years, and a renal transplant if the patient survives that long without recurrence of tumor. However, an annual attrition rate of 10 to 12 percent of patients on hemodialysis or after transplantation remains a distressing concern. In addition, a 4 to 6 percent incidence of *de novo* neoplasia and up to 38 percent incidence of recurrent or metastatic carcinoma have been reported in transplant recipients, presumably secondary to immunosuppression. One may expect that these

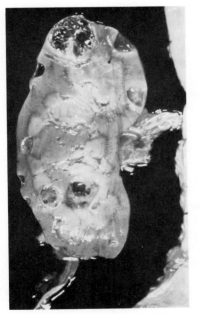

Figure 87-9 Section of a kidney from a patient with von Hippel-Lindau complex, showing multiple renal cysts and a malignant renal tumor at the upper pole of the kidney.

incidence rates will be even higher in patients with VHL complex, who are genetically predisposed to neoplasia. Therefore conservative extirpative surgery with preservation of as much functional renal tissue as possible appears justified in these patients.

Pheochromocytoma

Pheochromocytoma is seen in about 10 percent of patients with VHL complex. A review of reported families with VHL complex suggests that certain families are more prone to the development of this tumor than others. The tumor tends to occur bilaterally, implying that persons with VHL complex with unilateral pheochromocytoma are at risk of developing a second tumor in the opposite adrenal. As a corollary, a patient who presents with bilateral pheochromocytomas should be examined for other evidence of heritable syndromes in which bilateral pheochromocytomas are known to occur: (1) von Recklinghausen's neurofibromatosis, (2) VHL complex, (3) multiple endocrine neoplasia syndrome, (4) simple familial pheochromocytoma. In certain instances adrenal medullary hyperplasia may precede the actual development of tumor.

Pheochromocytomas were so named because of their affinity for chromium salts. As with tumors arising from the anterior pituitary gland, there is imperfect correlation between the functional activity of the tumor and its tinctorial properties with light microscopy. All catecholamine-secreting tumors arising from the adrenal medulla are now designated as pheochromocytomas regardless of whether they stain with chromium salts. Thus the older term *nonchromaffin paraganglioma* for a functioning tumor of the adrenal medulla that fails to stain with chromium salts is unacceptable. Ten percent of pheochromocytomas are malignant, but the malignant variant cannot be distinguished from the benign tumor on histological grounds; the sole criterion is development of metastases, with the malignant tumor at sites where chromaffin tissue does not normally occur.

The cardinal symptoms are episodic headaches, excessive

sweating, palpitation, nervousness and tremor. Headaches in a patient with VHL complex may be due to a cerebellar tumor with increased intracranial pressure or to catecholamine excess from a pheochromocytoma, or both. In the first, the headaches tend to be suboccipital in location, dull, persistent, and often associated with nausea and vomiting. The headaches from catecholamine excess tend to be paroxysmal, pounding or throbbing in character, lasting from a few minutes to several hours; they tend to be associated with other paroxysmal symptoms such as feelings of apprehension, excessive truncal sweating, tremors, tachycardia, palpitations, and anginal pain. There may be paroxysmal or nonparoxysmal elevations in blood pressure. Occasionally the first manifestation of pheochromocytoma may be a dangerous elevation of blood pressure noted during an elective operative procedure in a patient with VHL complex. Impaired glucose tolerance and hypermetabolism with weight loss are often observed.

The best screening test is urinary metanephrine assay in a single voided (spot) specimen. Values ranging from 1.0 to 2.2 μg metanephrine per milligram of creatinine are considered suspicious, and 24-h urine specimens should be examined for metanephrine, vanillylmandelic acid (VMA), and catecholamines. Plasma catecholamine levels are more expensive and technically more difficult to measure and are indeed less reliable because of wide swings in their values even under physiological conditions.

Tumor localization is best determined by an abdominal computed tomogram. Therapy is directed toward resection of the tumor(s) with intensive monitoring and pharmacologic control of blood pressure perioperatively. Ninety percent of these tumors are surgically curable.

Polycythemia

Hemangioblastoma is the only central nervous system tumor to be associated with polycythemia. Polycythemia has been reported in 9 to 20 percent of cases of posterior fossa and supratentorial hemangioblastomas but has not been reported with purely spinal lesions. There is erythrocytosis with no associated splenomegaly or increase in the white cell or platelet count. The red cell volume increases, but the plasma volume remains normal. The red cell life span is within the normal range. There is no evidence of accelerated red cell destruction in the liver or spleen. The rate of red cell synthesis is increased, and the red cell iron turnover is increased proportionately. The bone marrow may show erythroid hyperplasia.

Erythrocytosis in patients with hemangioblastoma is believed to be due to the unregulated secretion of erythropoietin or an erythropoietin-like substance by the neoplastic tissue. Histological sections of a hemangioblastoma may show areas of hematopoietic activity, but this is insufficient to induce polycythemia. Injection of tumor cyst fluid or extracts from solid tumors has induced erythrycytosis in experimental animals. Erythropoietin is known to promote the differentiation, proliferation, and maturation of red cell precursors in the bone marrow. It is a glycoprotein with a molecular weight of approximately 40,000; it migrates as an α-globulin during electrophoresis. Although the kidneys are

TABLE 87-3 Diagnostic Workup of Patient with Suspected VHL Complex

1. Elicitation of family history and clinical examination
2. Detailed fundoscopic examination by an ophthalmologist and possible fluorescein angiography if a lesion is found; fundus photographs for follow-up evaluation; visual acuity and fields
3. Hematocrit and red blood cell count
4. Computed tomography in axial and coronal planes without and with contrast enhancement; upper cervical spine area included
5. Arteriography with subtraction technique; upper cervical area included
6. Urine for metanephrine screen; if positive, 24-h VMA and catecholamine determinations
7. Abdominal computed tomography without and with contrast enhancement; special emphasis on pancreatic, renal, and suprarenal areas
8. Myelography and spinal angiography if spinal lesion suspected

thought to produce erythropoietin under physiological conditions, the exact role the kidneys play in its production remains controversial, in as much as it has not been possible to isolate erythropoietin from kidney extracts. Two alternative roles for the kidneys have been put forward. They may produce an enzyme (erythrogenin) which may act on a substrate in the plasma (erythropoietinogen) which is produced by the liver; or they may synthesize erythropoietin in an active form that may be rapidly inhibited by a complex lipid. The stimulus for secretion of erythropoietin is tissue hypoxia. Erythropoietin levels are increased in patients with anemia, renal artery stenosis, renal cysts, and renal neoplasms. Thus erythrocytosis in a patient with VHL complex may be due to a renal lesion or to a nervous system hemangioblastoma. The erythrocytosis induced by hemangioblastoma may improve after total excision of the tumor or irradiation, only to reappear with recurrence of the tumor. Ultrastructural studies of certain hemangioblastomas have shown granules thought to represent intracellular erythropoietin, but positive proof about their identity is lacking. Table 87-3 summarizes an outline of the diagnostic workup of a patient with suspected VHL complex.

Treatment

Surgery of Posterior Fossa Hemangioblastoma

The operative exposure is through a standard posterior midline or paramedian approach for vermis or cerebellar hemispheric lesions, respectively (Figs. 87-10 and 87-11). A transoccipital transtentorial approach may be desirable for lesions located in the anteroventral surface of the cerebellum abutting against the petrous bone. The patient may be in the sitting, semisitting, prone, or semiprone position, depending on the surgeon's preference. Magnification and bipolar coagulation are mandatory adjuvants. If the dura is extremely tense from a cerebellar cyst, the cyst may be tapped through the dura or through a small durotomy, taking care to avoid striking the mural nodule. The location of the

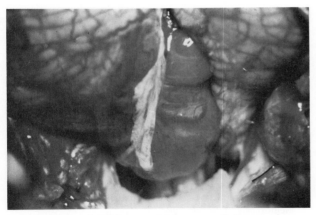

Figure 87-10   Solid hemangioblastoma of the vermis presenting between the cerebellar hemispheres, as exposed through a midline approach to the posterior fossa.

tumor is marked on the surface by dilated pial vessels. The mural nodule is quite small and generally located close to the pial surface. It would suffice to excise the mural nodule and drain the cyst; it is not necessary to excise the cyst wall, since it is not composed of tumor. But drainage of the cyst alone without removal of the mural nodule invites recurrence of the cyst in the immediate postoperative period.

Solid tumors should be dealt with in the same way as vascular malformations. No attempt should be made to biopsy the tumor or to remove it piecemeal. One should recall the histological appearance of the tumor, composed of a meshwork of vascular spaces lined by endothelial cells but no contractile elements. Thus an ill-conceived biopsy may lead to profuse, uncontrollable bleeding, and piecemeal removal of the tumor invites disaster. The surgeon should

cautiously make a cortical incision until the surface of the tumor is reached; at this point the white matter adjacent to the tumor should be dissected all around, coagulating the feeding vessels through the dissection (Fig. 87-11). If the bipolar coagulator is used in the cutting rather than coagulation mode, there is minimal charring at the forceps tips and less stickiness, allowing more rapid dissection around the tumor. The tumor should be excised in toto as a single mass. It is worthy of note that solid tumors tend to involve the brain stem more often than cystic ones.

Tumors arising primarily from the brain stem should be closely scrutinized. Only those with attachment to the floor of the fourth ventricle in the midline are hazardous to remove because of cardiorespiratory complications. Those attached laterally to the inferior cerebellar peduncle may be removed with surprisingly slight morbidity. The author has followed the practice of controlled ventilation with total muscle relaxation until the tumor dissection from the brain stem is started. At this point the patient is allowed to breath spontaneously, with manual assistance if necessary. This permits close monitoring of spontaneous respiratory activity, which is a sensitive indicator of brain stem neuronal activity.

Excision of hemangioblastomas from the brain stem utilizing extracorporeal circulation, profound hypothermia, and elective cardiac arrest has been described. The fact that expertise in the safe use of this technique is available in only a few select centers restricts its general usefulness.

Multiple hemangioblastomas in the posterior fossa pose a special and difficult problem. If the tumors are at least 0.8 to 1 cm in diameter and are easily accessible, they may be removed in the same way as solitary tumors; but if the tumors are smaller and are deep, they may be difficult to find. This is especially so if a prior posterior fossa exploration has led to adhesions and distorted anatomy. In such situations, it may

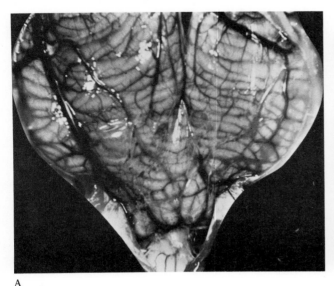

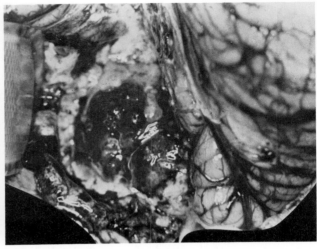

A   B

Figure 87-11   *A.* Left-sided swelling and chronic herniation of the tonsil into the foramen magnum from a hemangioblastoma. *B.* Cortex has been incised and a plane of cleavage developed between the tumor and adjacent cerebellar tissue without disturbing the tumor. No attempt is made at piece-meal removal of this highly vascular tumor.

be prudent to follow these tumors on serial computed tomograms and expose them when they are just large enough to be detected, or better still, when they develop a cyst. With further refinements in CT assisted stereotaxic approaches to deep brain lesions, it may be possible in the near future to approach them with greater certainty and precision and eradicate these lesions either with radiofrequency current or with cryoprobes.

In all instances where the posterior cranial fossa is explored for hemangioblastoma, the dura should be closed in a watertight manner, using grafts if necessary. Given that recurrences of these tumors are common and that the tumor is known to be multicentric, the surgeon should be prepared for re-exploration of the posterior fossa. Re-exploration becomes extremely difficult if there are adhesions due to prior failure to close the dura adequately.

Radiation Therapy

Reliable data on the effects of radiation in hemangioblastomas based on prospective controlled studies on a large series of patients are not available. Recent evidence, however, suggests that high-dose radiation (4500 to 5000 rad given over 4 ½ to 5 weeks) may significantly reduce the size of the tumor or at least retard the rate of growth of the mass, decrease its vascularity, and extend the symptom-free interval and survival time of patients.[5,19] One tangible effect of radiation on the tumor, besides the decrease in size and vascularity seen on angiograms, is the resolution of erythrocytosis. However, it should be emphasized that, unlike surgical resection, radiation treatment is not curative. There is little justification for considering radiation therapy for this benign lesion in the cerebellum, spinal cord, or cerebral hemisphere. For inoperable lesions in the brain stem or for solid lesions of the cerebellum that extend into the brain stem via the cerebellar peduncles, however, radiation therapy may be the only choice.

Prognosis

The long-term prognosis is best for a solitary cystic tumor in the cerebellum. Given that 70 percent of cerebellar hemangioblastomas are cystic and the tumors are always benign, the majority of nonfamilial hemangioblastomas can be resected with minimal morbidity and less than 2 percent mortality. The solid tumors tend to be larger and more vascular and tend to involve the brain stem; for them, the operative mortality is on the order of 15 percent. Lesions with deep midline attachment to the medulla oblongata are invariably lethal. Occurrence of multicentric malignant genitourinary and other visceral tumors in patients with VHL complex becomes a major determinant in assessing expected survival even after successful removal of a cerebellar hemangioblastoma. The multicentric origin of these tumors within the neuraxis in patients with VHL complex further adds to the morbidity and mortality; the recurrence rate is 3 to 10 percent after total excision of the initial tumor, and the symptom-free interval averages 5 years.

References

1. Bonebrake RA, Siqueira EB: The familial occurence of solitary hemangioblastoma of the cerebellum. Neurology 14:733–743, 1964.
2. Browne TR, Adams RD, Roberson GH: Hemangioblastoma of the spinal cord: Review and report of five cases. Arch Neurol 33:435–441, 1976.
3. Cushing H, Bailey P: Hemangiomas of cerebellum and retina (Lindau's disease). Arch Ophthalmol 57:447–463, 1928.
4. Diehl PR, Symon L: Supratentorial intraventricular hemangioblastoma: Case report and review of literature. Surg Neurol 15:435–443, 1981.
5. Helle TL, Conley FK, Britt RH: Effect of radiation therapy on hemangioblastoma: A case report and review of the literature. Neurosurgery 6:82–86, 1980.
6. Horton WA: Genetics of central nervous system tumors. Birth Defects 12:91–97, 1976.
7. Horton WA, Wong V, Eldridge R: Von Hippel-Lindau disease: Clinical and pathological manifestations in nine families with 50 affected members. Arch Intern Med 136:769–777, 1976.
8. Jeffreys R: Clinical and surgical aspects of posterior fossa haemangioblastomata. J Neurol Neurosurg Psychiatry 38:105–111, 1975.
9. Jurco S, Nadji M, Harvey DG, Parker JC, Font RL, Morales AR: Hemangioblastomas: Histogenesis of the stromal cell studied by immunocytochemistry. Hum Pathol 13:13–18, 1982.
10. Kepes JJ, Rengachary SS, Lee SH: Astrocytes in hemangioblastomas of the central nervous system and their relationship to stromal cells. Acta Neuropathol (Berl) 47:99–104, 1979.
11. Lee KR, Kishore PRS, Wulfsberg E, Kepes J: Supratentorial leptomeningeal hemangioblastoma. Neurology 28:727–730, 1978.
12. Levine E, Collins DL, Horton WA, Schimke RN: CT screening of the abdomen in Von Hippel-Lindau disease. AJR 139:505–510, 1982.
13. Lindau A: Discussion on vascular tumours of the brain and spinal cord. Proc R Soc Med 24:363–370, 1930.
14. McDonnell DE, Pollock P: Cerebral cystic hemangioblastoma. Surg Neurol 10:195–199, 1978.
15. Melmon KL, Rosen SW: Lindau's disease: Review of the literature and study of a large kindred. Am J Med 36:595–617, 1964.
16. Obrador S, Martin-Rodriguez JG: Biological factors involved in the clinical features and surgical management of cerebellar hemangioblastomas. Surg Neurol 7:79–85, 1977.
17. Okawara S: Solid cerebellar hemangioblastoma. J Neurosurg 39:514–518, 1973.
18. Seeger JF, Burke DP, Knake JE, Gabrielsen TO: Computed tomographic and angiographic evaluation of hemangioblastomas. Radiology 138:65–73, 1981.
19. Sung DI, Chang CH, Harisiadis L: Cerebellar hemangioblastomas. Cancer 49:553–555, 1982.
20. Tishler PV: A family with coexistent Von Recklinghausen's neurofibromatosis and Von Hippel-Lindau's disease: Diseases possibly derived from a common gene. Neurology 25:840–844, 1975.
21. Tomasello F, Albanese V, Iannotti F, Di Iorio G: Supratentorial hemangioblastoma in a child. J Neurosurg 52:578–583, 1980.
22. Walsh FB, Hoyt WF: Clinical Neuro-Ophthalmology, 3d ed. Baltimore, Williams & Wilkins, 1969.
23. Welch RB: Von Hippel-Lindau disease: The recognition and treatment of early angiomatosis retinae and the use of cryosurgery as an adjunct to therapy. Trans Am Ophthalmol Soc 68:367–424, 1970.

88

Choroid Plexus Papillomas

Hector E. James

Choroid plexus papillomas are benign neoplastic growths that arise from the ventricular choroid plexus and can be considered of ependymal origin.[6] They are slow-growing. They remain asymptomatic for considerable periods, are commonly associated with hydrocephalus, and are liable to hemorrhage spontaneously.[6,7]

Incidence

Considering adults and children together, choroid plexus papillomas are rare, constituting less than 1 percent of all primary intracranial tumors. Although they occur at any age, the majority occur in the first decade; thus in children they constitute 3 percent of intracranial neoplasms.[3] Forty-eight percent of those reported in the literature were in children under 10 years of age and 20 percent in infants under 1 year of age.[3] They are among the more frequent tumors in children under the age of 3 years.[3]

The tumor affects both sexes equally, and genetic factors do not seem to play a role.

Pathology

In adults, the choroid plexus papilloma is most often located in the fourth ventricle, whereas in children it usually arises in the lateral ventricles, the left more commonly than the right.[3,6,7] The third ventricle is seldom involved.

To gross examination the tumor is a dark pink or red meaty mass with an irregular papillary surface. In the lateral ventricle it is accompanied by a considerable enlargement of the ventricle. If it is located in the lateral recess of the fourth ventricle, it can significantly distort surrounding structures. It is characteristically easy to separate from the surrounding brain. Small foci of hemorrhage may be present in its interior.[6,7]

Typical of the choroid plexus papilloma in microscopic examination is its resemblance to the normal choroid plexus. Resting on a slender vascular connective tissue stroma is a delicate arrangement of papillary formations, of usually single layers of cuboidal or columnar epithelium (Fig. 88-1). Cilia and blepharoplasts are found in some infantile tumors.[6] Malignant changes indicate that the tumor is the rare choroid plexus carcinoma, representing an entirely different clinical condition than the choroid plexus papilloma.[3,6,7]

On occasion gross and microscopic spread in the leptomeninges of a benign choroid plexus papilloma is seen at postmortem examination. In these cases there are no malignant histological changes, and such lesions do not cause clinical symptoms.[6]

In the differential histological diagnosis papillary ependymoma and xanthogranuloma of the choroid plexus must be considered. In the former the cells are usually piled up in multiple layers and the stromal support is neuroglial, not connective tissue. The latter consists of small lesions, yellowish and firm, with deposition of cholesterol in their stroma; they are often bilateral.[6]

Pathogenesis of Hydrocephalus

Ventricular enlargement is seen in association with most but not all choroid plexus papillomas. This may be due to a combination of factors: overproduction of CSF, obstruction of CSF pathways by the tumor mass, or subarachnoid scarring due to recurrent bleeding from the tumor.

In those tumors located in the fourth and third ventricles the tumor may reach a size that can obstruct CSF flow. In these cases removal of the tumor mass may resolve the hydrocephalus.

Recurrent occult bleeding is a known complication of these tumors, and the subarachnoid obstruction due to basal meningitis and fibrosis may then lead to hydrocephalus, thus accounting for the lack of resolution of the hydrocephalus despite tumor removal in some cases.[7]

Overproduction of CSF by the tumor mass has long been suspected and was thought to be documented in two

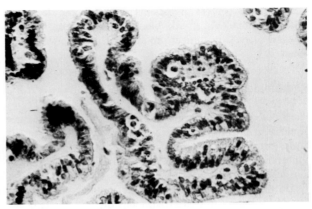

Figure 88-1 Microscopic appearance of a choroid plexus papilloma. Note the delicate papillary structures formed by a single layer of epithelium on a fine connective tissue stroma. Hematoxylin-eosin stain. (Courtesy of Dr. Luis Schut.)

patients.[1,4] In one of these, measurement of CSF production by ventriculolumbar perfusion revealed a formation rate of 1.05 ml/min prior to surgical removal of the tumor; 8 weeks after surgery it was measured at 0.2 ml/min.[4] This may explain the resolution of hydrocephalus in some cases after the removal of a choroid plexus papilloma from the lateral ventricle.[3,5]

Clinical Features

Clinical Presentation

Choroid plexus papillomas may present with overt intracranial hypertension with or without focal neurological signs, with progressively increasing head size, or with insidious hydrocephalus.

As indicated above, obstruction to CSF flow by the tumor mass, subarachnoid fibrosis, or overproduction of CSF will create hydrocephalus. As volume increases, intracranial hypertension follows. Thus, except for headaches, irritability, vomiting, and malaise, there may be no symptoms and a paucity of findings. In the tumor situated in the lateral ventricle, hemiparesis and corticospinal tract findings may be present.

In infancy a common referral is for macrocephaly, and the tumor may then be detected as part of a hydrocephalus workup. In 16 of 23 children in Matson's series,[3] progressive enlargement of the head was one of the important findings. Papilledema was present in over half the patients.[3]

The hydrocephalus may have a slow and progressive course in the adult patient, leading to an insidious presentation. In these cases difficulty with mentation and occasional headaches may be the only symptoms.

CSF Findings

Elevation of CSF protein values is characteristic in choroid plexus papillomas and is found in over two-thirds of patients.[3] In 50 percent of patients there is some degree of xanthochromia, but frank blood is uncommon.[3] When measured, the CSF lumbar pressure has nearly always been elevated.[3]

Radiological Findings

Plain skull roentgenograms will reveal nonspecific changes of elevated intracranial pressure, such as separation of sutures, craniofacial disproportion, and the "beaten silver" appearance of the calvarium.[2] In children, tumor calcification has been reported in 21 percent.

On noncontrast CT scanning the tumor is noted to be similar in density to brain tissue, but there is dramatic enhancement with intravenous injection of a contrast agent.[2] CT provides detail about the outline, extent, and size of the tumor and demonstrates the degree of hydrocephalus.

Cerebral angiography reveals the vascular supply of the tumor, which can aid in surgical removal.[2] The tumor is fed by the corresponding choroid arteries and shows a diffuse blush in the capillary phase. In choroid plexus carcinomas and in ependymomas, the irregular vessels and early venous shunting seen may aid in the differential diagnosis.[2]

Surgical Therapy

The treatment of choroid plexus papilloma is total surgical excision with minimal damage to the surrounding neural elements. Subtotal removal and radiation therapy play no role.

Tumor in the fourth ventricle location is reached through a midline suboccipital approach. Ligation of the vascular plexus coming from the choroid supply aids in removal of the tumor. Those tumors in the fourth ventricle are commonly quite free and easy to remove. Those in the cerebellopontine angle and foramen of Luschka are best treated by piecemeal removal through both the angle and the fourth ventricle.

The rare third ventricle tumors are best approached through a transcallosal incision, although a transfrontal cortical incision and access through an enlargement of the foramen of Monro has been described.[3]

Tumors in the lateral ventricle are most commonly located in the trigone. Two approaches have been advocated for choroid papillomas in this location. One is via a temporoparietal craniotomy, with a linear cortical incision in a convenient thinned gyrus overlying the tumor if the ventricles are enlarged or through an opening of a cone of cerebral tissue to the ventricle if the ventricles are small.[3] Another approach to the trigone is through a linear incision in the superior temporal gyrus which allows access to the choroid supply under the tumor, rather than approaching it superiorly.[4] In both approaches, emphasis is placed on interrupting the vascular supply early in the operation, since this can reduce the tumor size dramatically and minimize bleeding from the highly vascular neoplasm.

Total surgical removal of the neoplasm not only cures the tumor but may lead to complete resolution of the hydrocephalus. However, in 50 percent of cases the hydrocephalus will not resolve and a shunt will be needed.[5] It is imperative, therefore, to follow these patients in the postoperative period and assess the size of their ventricles.

Results and Complications

Total surgical removal of a choroid plexus papilloma cures the disease, and no recurrence following such a procedure has been noted.[3] Although a mortality of 22 percent is noted by Matson,[3] the death of 5 of the 23 patients was not due to the operative intervention itself in 2, and 2 others were moribund upon admission. Present-day anesthesia, microneurosurgery, and pediatric intensive care support should allow for an operative and perioperative mortality of less than 1 percent.

Neurological handicaps vary according to the size of the tumor and the location and degree of transcortical surgery.

Postoperative epilepsy can occur in those patients with supratentorial neoplasms. However, overall the surgeon can
expect a normal outcome in these patients.

References

1. Eisenberg HM, McComb JG, Lorenzo AV: Cerebrospinal fluid
   overproduction and hydrocephalus associated with choroid
   plexus papilloma. J Neurosurg 40:381–385, 1974.
2. Harwood-Nash DC, Fitz CR: *Neuroradiology in Infants and
   Children.* St. Louis, Mosby, 1976, pp. 751–754.
3. Matson DD: *Neurosurgery of Infancy and Childhood,* 2d ed.
   Springfield, Ill., Charles C Thomas, 1969, pp 581–595.
4. Milhorat TH: *Pediatric Neurosurgery* (Contemporary Neurology
   Series, vol 16). Philadelphia, Davis, 1978, pp 95–99.
5. Raimondi AJ, Gutierrez FA: Diagnosis and surgical treatment
   of choroid plexus papillomas. Childs Brain 1:81–115, 1975.
6. Rubinstein LJ: *Tumors of the Central Nervous System* (Atlas of
   Tumor Pathology, 2d ser, fasc. 6). Washington, Armed Forces
   Institute of Pathology, 1972, pp 257–262.
7. Russell DS, Rubinstein LJ: *Pathology of Tumours of the
   Nervous System,* 3d ed. Baltimore, Williams & Wilkins, 1971,
   pp 163–166.

89

Chemodectomas
James T. Robertson

Chemodectoma refers to any tumor of the chemoreceptor system. The tumors of great interest to neurological, head and
neck, and otologic surgeons are those arising from the carotid body, from the adventitia of the jugular bulb, or along
the course of Jacobson's nerve as it crosses the promontory
of the middle ear. The carotid body was first described in
1743 by Van Haller.[5] The first excision of a carotid body
tumor was accomplished by Riegner in 1880.[17] Guild described the glomus jugularis (changed to jugulare) in the
adventitia of the jugular bulb in 1941, and Rosenwasser first
reported the removal of a carotid body–like tumor from the
middle ear and mastoid in 1945.[12,18,27] The origin of the
tumors has been controversial, with various theories giving
rise to synonyms describing the tumors such as paragangliomas, glomus tumors, nonchromaffin paragangliomas, and
chemodectomas.[19,21] Histologically, carotid body tumors
and tumors of the glomus jugulare are similar. In addition to
the carotid body and the glomus jugulare and tympanicum,
cardioaortic bodies, laryngeal bodies, and heterotopic cell
rests have been reported in association with the entire parasympathetic outflow of the autonomic nervous system. Lawson has concluded that the glomus cell, which differentiates
into an epithelioid-type cell, is a modified neuroblast of presumed neural crest origin.[19] This neurogenic nature and its
secretory capacity make it a true neurocrine cell.

Recently, nonchromaffin paragangliomas and carcinoid
tumors have been classified as apudomas.[7,25] The term
APUD is an acronym for the *a*mine *p*recursor *u*ptake and
*d*ecarboxylation characteristic of these cells. Uncommonly,
these paragangliomas have been documented as having endocrine activity.[7,23,24] Tumors with endocrine activity occur
more commonly in males than females and tend to present in
younger patients. Both glomus jugulare tumors and carotid
body tumors have been shown on occasion to have active
endocrine function. Most of the reports have indicated a
syndrome of severe hypertension similar to that caused by
pheochromocytoma. Farrior et al. recently reported a tumor
presenting with a carcinoid syndrome with excessive secretion of serotonin.[7] They emphasize that in the management
of a patient with a glomus jugulare tumor or a carotid body
tumor, the possible activity of the lesion should be determined. Although endocrine activity is a rare occurrence, this
step ensures adequate preoperative planning and management. The carcinoid syndrome can be suspected in a patient
who has a history of explosive diarrhea, violent headaches,
facial flushing, and possibly mild hypertension. The more
common pheochromocytoma syndrome should be suspected
in a patient with a history of severe hypertension, headaches, or palpitations. On the other hand, hypertension may
not be present initially but may suddenly be stimulated by
tumor manipulation, so careful preoperative evaluation of
urine levels for vanillylmandelic acid and metanephrines is
recommended. Occasionally, direct blood levels of catecholamines can be obtained during retrograde jugular venous
studies.

These tumors may be multicentric and are not uncommonly bilateral. There is a clear hereditary incidence in
some families.[11,32] Women more commonly have the tumors
than men, and the incidence appears to be greater in persons
living at high altitudes or subject to hypoxia. In the case of
carotid body tumors, 6 percent of patients develop second
primary tumors, mostly other paragangliomas. When familial, carotid body tumors are transmitted by autosomal dominant genetic transmission.

Tumors of the carotid body, glomus jugulare, or glomus
tympanicum characteristically have a slow and unpredictable growth. A small percentage—under 10 percent[4,6,16]—
may be malignant. The malignant features may produce regional and distant metastasis, usually to lymph nodes and
lung.[4] Occasional tumors of the glomus jugulare will grow
down the jugular vein into the superior vena cava. Farr, in a
retrospective study, estimated the growth rate of a typical
carotid body tumor to be 2 centimeters in 5 years.[6]

Pathologically the tumors are also similar, containing polyhedral epithelioid chief cells with centrally located nuclei and fine grandular cytoplasm. The cells are arranged in clusters interspersed in a network of fibrous tissue. The degree of cellularity varies, but all are associated with multiple vascular channels. They generate an extensive blood supply. With carotid body tumors or tumors arising from the vagus nerve, the vasa vasorum and vasa nervorum increase remarkably. In glomus jugulare and glomus tympanicum cases, the tumors are discolored by their rich blood supply and attract numerous collateral vessels not only from the external carotid system but also from intrathecal vessels. The blood supply of the glomus jugulare tumor is predominantly from the ascending pharyngeal artery, with additional supply from the posterior auricular artery via the stylomastoid branch and from branches of the occipital, internal maxillary, and internal carotid arteries.[30] The tumor is thought to arise in the adventitia of the jugular bulb; it may ultimately extend intra- and extravascularly. In the author's experience, the intravascular portion of the tumor, which often blocks the jugular bulb and may grow down or up in the involved vein, seems to be entirely separate from the tumor that extends out into the temporal bone and surrounding tissues.[8-10,26]

Carotid Body Tumors

A carotid body tumor usually presents as a painless, slow-growing, rubbery, compressible mass in the upper neck which is attached to the carotid sheath and easily movable laterally but markedly limited in vertical movement. Such tumors may pulsate and often have a bruit. They almost never produce total occlusion of the carotid arteries. There may be associated symptoms of syncope, dizziness, pulsating tinnitus, visual blurring, hoarseness, local pain, dysphagia, or headache or, occasionally, transient ischemic attacks.[20] Since the tumors are uncommon, the surgeon must make every effort to distinguish a carotid body tumor from other more common lesions presenting as neck masses. The tumors are not uncommonly bilateral. The diagnosis is best confirmed by angiography.

Management of these tumors continues to be controversial because of their slow growth, their biological behavior, the risk of operative morbidity and mortality, and the conflicting reports on the role of radiation therapy.[6,16,20,22] Mortality rates have ranged from 5 to 13 percent, stroke rates from 8 to 20 percent, and the rates of operative injury to the hypoglossal and vagal nerves from 32 to 44 percent. Biologically, the association between histological evidence of malignancy and the incidence of metastasis correlate poorly. The incidence of metastasis is stated to be approximately 2.1 percent in one leading review, whereas the incidence of histologically malignant changes has been reported to be as high as 50 percent.

Surgical excision in the otherwise good risk patient who has a symptomatic or enlarging mass is considered the treatment of choice.[6,16,20,22] Shamblin et al. recommend that the tumors be considered in three groups:[28] group I tumors, small and easily dissected from adjacent vessels; group II tumors, more adherent and partially surrounding the vessel; and group III tumors, large and adhering intimately to the entire circumference of the carotid or involving perivascular structures. Careful preoperative angiographic evaluation allows tumor classification. Carotid body surgery should be approached with detailed preoperative evaluation.

The patient should be operated on under general intratracheal anesthesia, with wide exposure of the carotid bifurcation. This should include sharp dissection, with careful isolation of the proximal common carotid artery, the distal external carotid artery, and the distal internal carotid artery. The hypoglossal nerve should be carefully dissected and mobilized superiorly, and meticulous dissection between the posterior aspect of the internal carotid and carotid bifurcation should free these structures from the vagus nerve and superior laryngeal nerve. Proximal and distal control of the carotid vessels should be achieved by umbilical tapes and a careful subadventitial excision of the tumor effected. The extensive collateral circulation of the vasa vasorum requires careful obliteration as the tumor plane is approached. With small tumors, a relatively avascular cleavage plane between the artery and the tumor can be recognized as a white line. Excessive bleeding can often be minimized by ligation of the major tumor feeder artery on the posterior aspect of the carotid bifurcation. In dealing with the larger tumors, ligation and division of the external carotid artery is often helpful to effect mobilization and reduce the blood supply of the tumor.

Preoperative angiography, particularly in the large group III tumors, should include cross compression to be certain about the collateral circulation through the circle of Willis. In very large tumors, it is not infrequently necessary to excise the involved carotid after placing a bypass shunt and then, after tumor excision, to replace the involved segment of the carotid artery with a saphenous vein graft. Occasional cases may warrant consideration of a superficial temporal to middle cerebral artery bypass immediately prior to attempted excision. During occlusion of the carotid system, the patient should be given heparin to prevent the formation of thrombi and subsequent distal embolization. If regional nodes appear to be involved, they should be excised.

With the application of appropriate newly established vascular surgical techniques, the morbidity and mortality from this procedure has steadily decreased. This is reflected in recent reports from large centers experienced in vascular surgical techniques which have learned to avoid x-ray therapy and operations on asymptomatic elderly patients. External radiation of this tumor is not an effective mode of treatment but may occasionally be indicated with unresectable masses or for poor risk surgical patients.

On occasion, a patient presents with both a glomus jugulare or tympanicum tumor and a carotid body tumor ipsilaterally. It is strongly recommended that the carotid body tumor be resected initially and that the procedure be staged to ensure patency of the carotid system before the glomus jugulare or tympanicum is operated on.[14]

Occasional large tumors extend into the carotid canal, necessitating consideration of carotid artery sacrifice and a cranial bypass procedure or, in the case of a patent circle of Willis, simple carotid sacrifice. These patients may be treated by postoperative radiation therapy or a more extensive procedure in which, through the use of a temporal craniotomy and superior neck exposure, the tumor may be removed from the carotid canal.

Glomus tumors involving the vagus nerve which are extracranial should be excised by wide exposure, with careful preservation of the remaining cranial nerves and vessels, but sacrifice of the vagus nerve will nearly always be required. Tumors that extend into the jugular foramen may require a more extensive combined procedure.

Glomus Jugulare Tumors of the Temporal Bone

Patients with a glomus tumor may present with the complaint of a pulsating tinnitus followed, in tympanicum tumors, by conductive hearing loss.[8-10,26] With careful otoscopic examination, the lesion can be visualized behind an intact eardrum. The lesion can be seen to pulsate, and often the otologic surgeon is able to determine the margins of the tumor. Appropriate diagnostic studies include audiometric and vestibular testing and special x-ray studies of the temporal bones, augmented by computed tomography and arteriographic studies with magnification and subtraction views. Tumors limited to the middle ear are surgically treated.

On the other hand, tumors of the glomus jugulare often present with the same symptom complex, and the tumor is frequently visualized through the intact eardrum. These tumors, however, because of their extension, often are associated with glossopharyngeal, vagal, spinal accessory, and hypoglossal nerve palsies. Not infrequently the facial nerve is involved. On rare occasions these lesions present with increased intracranial pressure, and this may occur with or without significant intracranial extension.[1] Some degree of ear pain is not uncommon. With massive lesions, the patient may have symptoms and signs of ataxia or hydrocephalus.

The patient with a glomus tumor deserves an intense neurological and otologic evaluation, with great emphasis on specific neuroradiological studies. Computed tomography with contrast enhancement and with careful evaluation of soft tissue and bone detail is essential.[2] This may be supplemented by polytomography, and it is essential that four-vessel selective angiography and retrograde jugular venography complement the evaluation. These studies allow an accurate determination of tumor size and the extent of the tumor invasion of surrounding tissues. With tumors of the glomus jugulare, the jugular bulb and vein are nearly always partially or completely occluded by the intravascular portion of the tumor. The combination of the CT scan and the arteriogram clearly delineates the extension of the tumor into the cranial cavity as well as the temporal bone.[2,33]

Spector et al. recently discussed the patterns of invasion of the temporal bone.[31] Since the glomus jugulare tumor arises in the jugular bulb area or along Jacobson's nerve, it has access to the recesses of the temporal bone, including the fissures and foramina of the base of the skull. The tumor slowly extends along the lines of least resistance and frequently follows the major vessels in the temporal bone.

Regarding tumors of the glomus jugulare, the modified classification of Jackson et al. should be applied, after appropriate diagnostic studies, in order to determine the extent of the surgical approach.[14] These authors classify glomus jugulare tumors as follows: type I—a small tumor involving the jugular bulb, middle ear, and mastoid; type II—a tumor extending under the internal auditory canal that may have intracranial extension; type III—a tumor extending into the petrous apex that may have intracranial extension; type IV—a tumor extending beyond the petrous apex into the clivus or infratemporal fossa that may have intracranial extension.

It is the author's belief that tumors of the glomus jugulare should be managed by a neurosurgical, otologic, and head and neck surgical team. The relevant experience has been reported in detail elsewhere.[8-10,26]

Glomus jugulare tumors have a fascinating history of therapeutic approaches over the last forty years. Both otologic surgeons and neurosurgeons have been involved in the development of the surgical therapy, and various approaches have been used. Radiation has been used as a pre- or postoperative adjunct in the care of these tumors. Some recommend that glomus jugulare tumors have primary treatment by radiotherapy and that only tumors that do not respond be considered for secondary radical surgical treatment. Cole reported that following adequate radiotherapy, glomus jugulare tumors may remain unchanged for many years; in his series of 20 glomus jugulare tumors, he did not encounter any case of nonresponse to high-voltage x-ray therapy in the dose range of 4000 to 5000 rad.[3] This should clearly be a consideration of therapy, particularly in the otherwise impaired or aged patient.[3,29]

The author's routine, after considerable experience in the development of an operative approach, has been to pretreat the patient with approximately 4500 rad of x-ray therapy, with subsequent 4- to 6-month delayed neuroradiological evaluations. If the tumor does not respond, enlarges, or becomes more symptomatic, surgery is then employed. If response occurs, even with persistent tumor, the patient is not operated on routinely. If this course of therapy is followed, close long-term follow-up of the patient is mandatory. In patients who are operated on, radiation therapy is a definite adjunct in reducing the vascularity of the tumor, and wound healing has not been found a major problem.[26]

More recent methods of decreasing the blood supply of the tumor prior to surgery or, on occasion, as a form of therapeutic infarction of the tumor have been reported.[13,30] When the blood supply has been decreased as a therapeutic measure, tumor response has unquestionably been demonstrated, but long-term follow-up on this form of therapy is not presently available. However, embolization can be considered a therapeutic approach and may be combined with radiation therapy. Preoperative embolization, delayed or immediate, has been shown to be a great asset in the subsequent surgical excision of these tumors.

Simpson et al. consider combined embolization and immediate surgery the best approach for the treatment of a resectable glomus jugulare tumor.[30] The technique of absorbable gelatin sponge embolization unquestionably reduces bleeding problems at the time of operation. One of the patients reported on by these authors sustained a cerebral vascular accident during the angiographic procedure; this was thought to be due to a reaction to the contrast medium, however, rather than to embolic particles.

Pandya et al. reported a death following external carotid artery embolization for a huge epinephrine-norepinephrine–secreting glomus jugulare tumor.[23] Postmortem examination showed a markedly compressed and distorted cerebellum with tonsillar herniation and a greatly swollen, infarcted tumor. They also discussed other causes of the marked hypotension that occurred after tumor embolization. In the case of very large glomus tumors with marked intracranial extension, they suggest that the surgeon consider a posterior fossa decompressive craniectomy before embolization.

Kempe reported on the extensive collateral circulation in a nonoperated autopsy specimen of a very large tumor of the glomus jugulare.[15]

It is clear that embolization carries the risk not only of tumor infarction with swelling but also of brain stem or cerebellar infarction. Tumor infarction with marked swelling has produced compression of vital structures.

Surgical Technique for Removal of Glomus Jugulare Tumors

A review of the historical development of the surgical approaches to glomus jugulare tumors reveals that successful therapy did not result from a pure intracranial approach to these tumors. The neurosurgical approach by suboccipital craniectomy usually reveals a pulsating red mass around the jugular foramen extending to varying degrees anteriorly and medially. One is struck by the extensive vascularity of the covering dura and the relative rarity of sizable dural penetration. Surgical attempts to remove the tumor by this approach usually result in extensive blood loss and nearly always in inadequate excision of the tumor, because that portion in the temporal bone and beneath the jugular foramen as well as inside the venous system cannot be removed. For this reason, neurosurgeons should think of this tumor as primarily an extradural tumor. Even though collateral supply to the tumor develops from intrathecal sources, if one adopts the philosophy that this is primarily an extradural mass, a more complete surgical excision can be effected, with brain exposure and retraction limited markedly. For this reason, the author's service has developed the technique and team described below for the surgical removal of glomus jugulare tumors. This technique has been well illustrated and reported.[8–10,26]

The surgical team consists of a neurosurgeon, an otologic surgeon, and a head and neck surgeon. The procedure is divided into three phases: (1) exposure of the base of the skull through the neck; (2) exposure of the tumor within the temporal bone and jugular fossa; (3) removal of the tumor and closure of the wound with or without reconstruction of the sound-conducting system.

The skull base is exposed by an oblique skin incision made in the upper neck that extends from the postauricular region almost to the hyoid bone below the level of the tail of the parotid gland. The facial nerve is identified at the stylomastoid foramen, and the sternocleidomastoid muscle is detached from the mastoid bone. The posterior belly of the digastric muscle is detached from the mastoid bone, and

subsequently the mastoid tip is removed with a Gigli saw. The occipital artery is ligated and the styloid process removed to the skull base after the attached muscles are divided. Meticulously, the neurovascular structures of the upper neck are mobilized as a unit to the carotid canal and jugular foramen. The tributaries of the internal jugular vein are dissected and ligated. The jugular vein is preserved in continuity, and small vascular loops are placed around the neural and vascular structures for identification and mobilization. The soft tissues of the base of the skull are divided to permit exposure of the posterior three-fourths of the circumference of the jugular foramen. At times, this requires exposure and dissection of the transverse process of the first cervical vertebra, with careful identification and protection of the vertebral artery. The rectus capitis lateralis muscle and the atlanto-occipital ligament are detached from the jugular process of the occipital bone. The internal jugular vein is separated with an elevator from the posterior margin of the jugular foramen and partially from the neurovascular bundle anteriorly.

The temporal bone exposure is effected by a circumferential skin incision in the external ear canal at the bony cartilaginous junction, and the earlier neck incision is extended superiorly into the postauricular region. The external ear is retracted forward. A simple mastoidectomy is performed, with careful skeletonization of the sigmoid sinus and the mastoid segment of the facial nerve. The upper two-thirds of the sigmoid sinus and the mastoid and tympanicum segments of the facial nerve are then carefully isolated with a diamond burr. If the tumor extends posteriorly into the mastoid air cells, either superficially or deep to the facial nerve, great care may be required to differentiate the nerve from the glomus tissue in order to preserve the nerve. Obviously, microscopic assistance is mandatory. Every effort is made to preserve the facial nerve in continuity, although occasionally, with facial nerve paralysis and extensive invasion of the nerve, a segment of the facial nerve may require resection with subsequent grafting or end-to-end suture. The posterior wall of the external bony canal is removed unless the tumor is extremely small. The facial nerve is elevated with its periosteum from the facial canal and is carefully retracted anteriorly in continuity with the extratemporal segment of the nerve. The bone is then removed from the posterior lateral skull base, including the base of the lateral aspect of the temporal bone and the jugular process of the occipital bone. This is effected by removing the lower half of the occipital-mastoid suture line, the digastric groove, the stylomastoid foramen, the inferior aspect of the anterior wall of the bony canal, the base of the styloid process, the posterior lip of the jugular foramen, and the lateral wall of the jugular fossa. After bone removal, the soft tissue of the lower one-third of the sigmoid sinus, the jugular bulb, and the tumor is exposed. If the tumor extends anteriorly to the internal carotid artery, bone over the lower aspect of the anterior wall of the mesotympanum may be removed in order to expose the tumor. Occasionally the ascending ramus of the mandible is resected to facilitate exposure in the region of the carotid.

At this point the internal jugular vein is ligated and is carefully dissected superiorly in continuity with the jugular bulb to the sigmoid sinus. The carotid artery is exposed up to the carotid canal, and formal tumor removal begins. A suboccipital craniectomy is done, exposing the dura of the posterior fossa as well as the anterior end of the lateral sinus and its junction with the sigmoid sinus. Prior to making an incision in the upper end of the sigmoid sinus above the tumor, a small purse-string suture is placed around the site of incision, using 4-0 or 5-0 suture. A Fogarty catheter of the necessary size is passed superiorly into the lateral sinus and inflated, and another Fogarty catheter is passed inferiorly toward the tumor and inflated. The lateral sinus is opened and carefully sutured to its medial wall above the tumor, and just prior to closure the catheter is deflated and removed. The remaining lateral sinus and sigmoid sinus are packed quite tightly with absorbable hemostatic material, allowing occlusion of the petrous veins and the sinus. At this point the inferior Fogarty catheter is deflated and removed. The tumor is then removed along with the attached lateral wall of the sigmoid sinus, the jugular bulb, and the upper end of the internal jugular vein, carefully dissecting the jugular bulb and upper vein from the neurovascular bundle. An effort is made to remove this portion of the tumor and venous system intact. The inferior petrosal sinus is usually torn as this is removed; the bleeding is easily controlled with the use of hemostatic material. After removal of the immediate intra-vascular and extravascular portion of the tumor, the additional tumor remaining in the temporal bone and middle ear is removed separately, along with the tympanic membrane and the skin of the ear canal. No attempt is made in large tumors to reconstruct the conduction hearing chain. The facial nerve is placed in a bed of soft tissue anteriorly.

Usually the tumor extending into the temporal bone along the posterior fossa dura is mainly an extradural tumor. If it extends intracranially, the dura may require wider opening with tumor removal. This approach minimizes cerebellar retraction. The dura must be sutured or grafted. If the tumor is mainly extradural, it is unusual for a dural tear to occur. However, if it does, meticulous suture or closure with tissue adhesive is essential. Subsequent to tumor removal, a free abdominal fat graft is placed in the cavity and the wound is closed in layers. Drains with suction are placed and wound closure effected.

The patient's postoperative care is that of a standard craniotomy patient, with meticulous attention to pre- and postoperative facial and lower cranial nerve paresis. Using this technique, and with expanded experience, the author's department has steadily reduced operating time and blood loss. This technique has evolved as a planned and successful surgical means of tumor removal. With extensive fingers of tumor growth, particularly into and around the carotid artery and into the bone, complete removal of the tumor can never be certain, but gross tumor removal is usually achieved.

Complications and Results

There has been no death in the author's series of patients, and other surgeons using similar or slightly modified results report a low surgical mortality rate. The complications that have occurred include spinal fluid leakage with or without meningitis. Spinal fluid leakage can be prevented by meticulous dural closure, but if it occurs, it can be treated by tem-porary spinal drainage. On occasion, reoperation may be required. Meningitis, which may occur as a result of the spinal fluid leak or simply as a result of wound infection, should be recognized promptly and treated. It is the author's belief that infection can be minimized by meticulous surgical technique, and preoperative broad spectrum antibiotic therapy continued during the operation and for 2 to 3 days is recommended in cases requiring several hours.

With this technique, some degree of facial nerve paresis may occur. When the facial nerve has been sacrificed because of tumor involvement, paresis may be treated by facial nerve grafting or a simultaneous spinal accessory or hypoglossal to facial nerve anastomosis. A temporary paresis with an intact nerve usually has a satisfactory recovery. In facial nerve palsy, meticulous postoperative care of the eye, with an occasional tarsorrhaphy, is required. Patients who awaken with postoperative tenth, eleventh, and twelfth nerve palsies may require tracheostomy; they should be treated in an intensive care unit for 24 to 48 h with airway and nursing care.

References

1. Beck DW, Kassell NF, Drake CG: Glomus jugulare tumor presenting with increased pressure. J Neurosurg 50:823–825, 1979.
2. Caughran M, White TJ III, Gerald B, Gardner G: Computed tomography of jugulotympanic paragangliomas. J Comput Assist Tomogr, 4:194–198, 1980.
3. Cole JM: Panel discussion: Glomus jugulare tumors of the temporal bone. Radiation of glomus tumors of the temporal bone. Laryngoscope 89:1623–1627, 1979.
4. Davis JM, Davis KR, Hesselink JR, Greene R: Case report: Malignant glomus jugulare tumor. Case with two unusual radiographic features. J Comput Assist Tomogr 4:415–419, 1980.
5. Dickison AM, Traver CA: Carotid body tumors: Review of the literature with report of two cases. Am J Surg 69:9–11, 1945.
6. Farr HW: Carotid body tumors: A 40-year study. CA 30:260–265, 1980.
7. Farrior JB III, Hyams VJ, Benke RH, Farrior JB: Carcinoid apudoma arising in a glomus jugulare tumor: Review of endocrine activity in glomus jugulare tumors. Laryngoscope 90:110–119, 1980.
8. Gardner G, Cocke EW Jr, Robertson JT, Trumbull ML, Palmer RE: Glomus jugulare tumours—combined treatment: Part I. J Laryngol Otol 95:437–454, 1981.
9. Gardner G, Cocke EW Jr, Robertson JT, Trumbull ML, Palmer RE: Glomus jugulare tumours—combined treatment: Part II. J Laryngol Otol 95:567–580, 1981.
10. Gardner G, Robertson JT, Cocke EW Jr: Surgical therapy of tumors of the glomus jugulare, in Schmidek HH, Sweet WH (eds): *Current Techniques in Operative Neurosurgery*. New York, Grune & Stratton, 1977, pp 57–66.
11. Grufferman S, Gillman MW, Pasternak LR, Peterson CL, Young WG: Familial carotid body tumors: Case report and epidemiologic review. Cancer 46:2116–2122, 1980.
12. Guild SR: A hitherto unrecognized structure, the glomas jugularis in man. Anat Rec 79 (Suppl 2):28, 1941 (abstr).
13. Hilal SK, Michelsen JW: Therapeutic percutaneous embolization for extra-axial vascular lesions of the head, neck, and spine. J Neurosurg 43:275–287, 1975.
14. Jackson CG, Glasscock ME III, Nissen AJ, Schwaber MK: Glomus tumor surgery: The approach, results, and problems. Otolaryngol Clin North Am 15:897–916, 1982.

15. Kempe LG: Collateral circulation in a tumor of the glomus jugulare. Neuroradiology 20:193–195, 1980.

16. Krupski WC, Effeney DJ, Ehrenfeld WK, Stoney RJ: Cervical chemodectoma: technical considerations and management options. Am J Surg, 144:215–220, 1982.

17. Lahey FH, Warren KW: A long term appraisal of carotid body tumors with remarks on their removal. Surg Gynecol Obstet 92:481–91, 1951.

18. Lattes R, Waltner JG: Nonchromophin paraganglioma of the middle ear (carotid-body-like tumor; glomus-jugulare tumor). Cancer 2:447, 1949.

19. Lawson W: The neuroendocrine nature of the glomus cells: An experimental, ultrastructural, and histochemical tissue culture study. Laryngoscope 90:120–144, 1980.

20. Lees CD, Levine HL, Beven EG, Tucker HM: Tumors of the carotid body: Experience with 41 operative cases. Am J Surg 142:362–365, 1981.

21. Mulligan RM: Chemodectoma in the dog. Am J Pathol 28:680–681, 1950 (abstr).

22. Padberg FT Jr, Cady B, Persson AV: The carotid body tumor: The Lahey clinic experience. Am J Surg 145:526–528, 1983.

23. Pandya SK, Nagpal RD, Desai AP, Purohit AV: Death following external carotid artery embolization for a functioning glomus jugulare chemodectoma: Case report. J Neurosurg 48:1030–1034, 1978.

24. Parkinson D: Intracranial pheochromocytoma (active glomus jugulare): Case report. J Neurosurg 31:94–100, 1969.

25. Pearse AGE: The APUD cell concept and its implications in pathology. Pathol Annu 9:27–41, 1974.

26. Robertson JT, Gardner G, Cocke EW Jr, Gerald BE, Trumbull ML, Palmer RE: Glomus jugulare tumors, in Schmidek HH, Sweet WH (eds): Operative Neurosurgical Techniques: Indications, Methods, and Results. New York, Grune & Stratton, 1982, pp 649–670.

27. Rosenwasser H: Carotid body tumor of the middle ear and mastoid. Arch Otolaryngol 41:64–67, 1945.

28. Shamblin WR, ReMine WH, Sheps SG, Harrison EG: Carotid body tumor (chemodectoma): Clinicopathologic analysis of ninety cases. Am J Surg 122:732–739, 1971.

29. Simko TG, Griffin TW, Gerdes AJ, Parker RG, Tesh DW, Taylor W, Blasko JC: The role of radiation therapy in the treatment of glomus jugulare tumors. Cancer 42:104–106, 1978.

30. Simpson GT II, Konrad HR, Takahashi M, House J: Immediate postembolization excision of glomus jugulare tumors: Advantages of new combined techniques. Arch Otolaryngol 105:639–643, 1979.

31. Spector GJ, Sobol S, Thawley SE, Maisel RH, Ogura JH: Panel Discussion: Glomus jugulare tumors of the temporal bone. Patterns of invasion in the temporal bone. Laryngoscope 89:1628–1639, 1979.

32. Veldman JE, Mulder PHM, Ruijs SHG, de Haas G, van Waes PFGM, Hoekstra A: Early detection of asymptomatic hereditary chemodectoma with radionuclide scintiangiography. Arch Otolaryngol 106:547–552, 1980.

33. Wright JW Jr, Wright JW III, Hicks GW: Panel discussion: Glomus jugulare tumors of the temporal bone. Radiological appearance of glomus tumors. Laryngoscope 89:1620–1622, 1979.

SECTION I

Sellar and Parasellar Tumors

90

Hypothalamic Control of Anterior Pituitary Function: Surgical Implications

Robert B. Page

Three efferent systems emerge from the brain and spinal cord. Two are neural—the somatic and visceral efferent systems. The third is humoral—the neuroendocrine system. The somatic efferent system employs striated muscle cells to move the organism or its component parts in response to environmental stimuli. The visceral efferent system employs smooth muscle cells and exocrine gland cells to regulate vascular function and to assimilate nutrients. The neuroendocrine system employs the pituitary gland to regulate the function of selected visceral organs (kidney, uterus, and breast), to regulate growth, and to trophically support and regulate the function of specific target organs of internal secretion—the thyroid gland, adrenal gland, and gonads. Through the pituitary gland the brain affects the growth and development of the organism, maintains its internal milieu, regulates its metabolism, and assures its reproduction.

Pituitary Anatomy: Assembly from Components

The pituitary gland is also called the *hypophysis cerebri* (from the Greek *hypo-*, below, and *phuein*, to grow). It is composed of glandular and neural tissue and hence is subdivided into an adeno- and a neurohypophysis. The glandular cells which make up the adenohypophysis may be viewed as the effector cells of the neuroendocrine system.

The adenohypophysis is not generally believed to be a neural diverticulum but to arise from the primitive foregut—the stomodeum. A diverticulum of stomodeum is thought to migrate cranially, pinch off from the foregut, and become applied to a neural diverticulum emerging from the diencephalon—the neurohypophysis.[4] With the establishment of vascular connections between the neurohypophysis and the displaced foregut tissue, differentiation of the stomodeal remnant into the adenohypophysis occurs.

Recently this classic schema has been challenged with the recognition that some adenohypophyseal cells are capable of amine precursor uptake and decarboxylation and thus can be considered part of the APUD system.[32] Cells in this system are believed to be of neural origin (frequently from the neural crest). Takor and Pearse[41] have suggested that the "ventral neural ridge" gives rise to the adenohypophysis and thus that the adenohypophysis is of neuroectodermal, not stomodeal, origin. The finding that some hypothalamic neurons are capable of synthesizing adrenocorticotropic hormone and melanocyte-stimulating hormone, hormones that are also synthesized in adenohypophyseal cells, strengthens the argument that at least some adenohypophyseal cells migrate from the brain to the adenohypophysis. The observation that adenohypophyseal cells appear epithelial (glandular) does not vitiate the argument, as adrenal medullary cells (neural crest derivatives) are also glandular in appearance.

The adenohypophysis is made up of connective tissue, fenestrated capillaries, and epithelial cells. These cells secrete eight known hormones—growth hormone (GH), prolactin (Pro), follicle-stimulating hormone (FSH), luteinizing hormone (LH), thyroid-stimulating hormone (TSH), adrenocorticotropic hormone (ACTH), melanocyte-stimulating hormone (α-MSH), and β-endorphin (End). The epithelial cells which secrete these hormones are organized into a glandular pattern and can be characterized on the basis of their reaction with acid or basic dyes. In the human, most cells (52 percent) contain clear cytoplasm which does not stain with these dyes (chromophobes); 34 percent are characterized by the presence of granules within their cytoplasm which stain with acid dyes (acidophils or eosinophils); 14 percent contain granules within their cytoplasm that stain with basic dyes (basophils).[31] It has long been recognized that acidophils secrete GH or Pro and that basophils secrete TSH, FSH, LH, or ACTH. Elaborate classification schemes based upon tinctorial properties of cells after complex staining procedures have been proposed to further relate epithelial cell structure to secretory function, but all have failed. Transmission electron microscopy has demonstrated that these epithelial cells contain large nuclei with dense chromatin and a single nucleolus. Their cytoplasm is characterized by the presence of a well-developed Golgi apparatus, abundant rough endoplasmic reticulum, and large, dense core vesicles which are sites of hormone storage (Fig. 90-1). Functional classification of adenohypophyseal cells on the basis of their electron microscopic appearance (cell shape, size, and distribution of vesicles) is possible but is a difficult and time-consuming task. With the advent of immunohistochemical procedures which stain hormones within cells, a method was developed to identify functional cell types within the adenohypophysis. At least seven cell types have been identified (somatotropes, lactotropes, gonadotropes, thyrotropes, corticotropes and melanotropes).

The adenohypophysis is, in most species, divided into three regions—the pars tuberalis, pars intermedia, and pars distalis (Fig. 90-2). The pars tuberalis is applied to the surface of the median eminence and the upper infundibular stem—rostral regions of the neurohypophysis. It is made up of epithelial cells, fenestrated capillaries, and stromal cells.

No nerve terminals are present in the pars tuberalis. The epithelial cells have been histochemically identified as thyrotropes and gonadotropes. Other cell types have thus far not been found.

In many species a pars intermedia is present and is applied to the lower portion of the lower infundibular stem and the infundibular process—caudal regions of the neurohypophysis. It is made up of epithelial cells, with only a few capillaries and stromal cells. Dopaminergic nerves are found in the pars intermedia and terminate near glandular cells. Immunohistochemical and physiological studies have demonstrated that its epithelial cells contain α-MSH and β-endorphin. The pars intermedia is present in the fetal human and in the pregnant adult female but is absent in adult human males and nonpregnant females. However, in adults basophilic epithelial cells are frequently found invading the neural lobe and immunohistochemical procedures demonstrate many cells containing α-MSH closely apposed to the neurohypophysis. It appears likely that these cells form a functional unit analogous to the pars intermedia of lower species.

The pars distalis forms the bulk of the adenohypophysis. It too is composed of epithelial cells arranged in a glandular pattern, stromal cells, and fenestrated capillaries. Like the pars tuberalis, the pars distalis contains no axon terminals. Immunohistochemistry has revealed lactotropes, somatotropes, gonadotropes, thyrotropes, corticotropes, and melanotropes within the pars distalis. Several studies have demonstrated that lactotropes and somatotropes lie predominantly in the lateral wings of the pars distalis, whereas thyrotropes and gonadotropes lie in the medial third—the

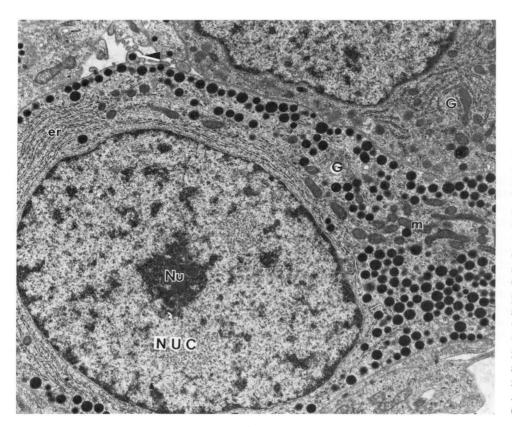

Figure 90-1 Transmission electron micrograph of an adenohypophyseal cell. The large nucleus (NUC) contains a single nucleolus (Nu). The cytoplasm contains abundant rough endoplasmic reticulum (er) and mitochondria (m). The Golgi apparatus (G) is prominent in this and the adjacent cell. Dense core vesicles are abundant in the cytoplasm and range from 200 to 600 nm in diameter. They contain adenohypophyseal hormones. A vesicle is being extruded (*arrowhead*). ($\times$7700.)

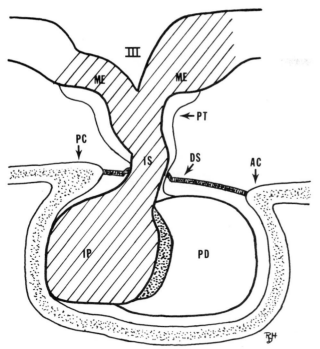

Figure 90-2 Midsagittal section of the human pituitary gland. The neurohypophysis (*hatching*) consists of the median eminence (ME), infundibular stem (IS), and infundibular process (IP), of the neural lobe. The adenohypophysis consists of the pars tuberalis (PT), which is applied to the median eminence and infundibular stem and lies in the subarachnoid space above the diaphragma sellae (DS), and the pars distalis (PD), which is within the sella turcica beneath the DS. The region of aggregated melanotropes corresponding to the pars intermedia of lower forms is indicated by the stippled area between the PD and the IP. Anterior clinoid (AC); posterior clinoid (PC); third ventricle (III).

"mucoid wedge"—so called because the secreted hormones contain glycoproteins (TSH, LH, FSH). As this median zone is continuous with the pars tuberalis and contains similar functional cell populations, it is also termed the *zona tuberalis*. Corticotropes lie anteriorly in the mucoid wedge and over the surface of the lateral wings.[5] Melanotropes lie posteriorly near the neural lobe, with a small number scattered throughout the pars distalis [42] (Fig. 90-3).

Pituitary peptide hormones are synthesized on rough endoplasmic reticulum. The sequence of amino acids making up the hormones is encoded in nuclear DNA. Through the mediation of messenger RNA (mRNA), this information is conveyed to the cytoplasm. Protein assembly occurs in the cytoplasm with the interaction of mRNA with ribosomes, with the mRNA dictating the sequence of amino acids. This process is termed *translation*. The assembled protein is transported to the Golgi complex and packaged in large vesicles, which can be visualized with the electron microscope[14] (Fig. 90-1).

Growth hormone and prolactin are peptide hormones with similar structures. Growth hormone affects the metabolic processes in all body tissues by stimulating protein synthesis. Some of its actions are mediated by somatomedins believed to be synthesized in the liver. Prolactin stimulates protein synthesis (milk production) in the primed breast. TSH, LH, and FSH are glycoproteins made up of two subunits—an α and a β chain. The α chain, which is not biologically active, is common to the three hormones. Rarely, a "nonfunctioning" pituitary adenoma is found to secrete the α chain. The β chain is unique to each hormone and is biologically active. TSH supports thyroid structure and secretion. FSH supports growth of the ovarian follicle and spermatogenesis. LH supports the corpus luteum and estrogen and progesterone secretion in females and the Leydig cells and testosterone production in males. ACTH is a peptide of 39 amino acids secreted by corticotropes. α-MSH is a 13-amino acid peptide secreted by melanotropes. The structure of α-MSH is the same as that of the first 13 amino acids of ACTH. ACTH supports the structure and function of the adrenal cortex to regulate secretion of glucocorticoids. α-MSH acts to disperse melanophores in amphibian skin, but its role in humans is not well established.

The neurohypophysis is a diverticulum of brain which makes its appearance in the human early in fetal life (between 10 and 14 mm crown-to-rump length).[4] The mature neurohypophysis is made up of axon terminals, specialized glial cells, and blood vessels. Several features are common throughout the neurohypophysis and serve to distinguish it from the hypothalamus. The neurohypophysis contains no neuronal cell bodies—only axons and axon terminals. Axons terminate in the perivascular space of fenestrated capillaries, not on neurons or their processes. The neurohypophysis lacks a blood-brain barrier.[18,45] It regulates the function of the adenohypophysis, which is applied to it.

The neurohypophysis is subdivided into three regions on the basis of regional morphological specializations: (1) the median eminence, (2) the infundibular stem, and (3) the neural lobe[35] (Fig. 90-2). The median eminence, with the paired lateral eminences, makes up the tuber cinereum and is a visible structure on the inferior surface of the brain, lying caudal to the optic chiasm and rostral to the paired mamillary bodies.[28] As the median eminence forms the funnel-shaped floor of the third ventricle, it is also called the *infundibulum*. It is the rostral region of the neurohypophysis. The infundibular stem is the neural portion of the pituitary stalk. The neural lobe (infundibular process) is the caudal region of the neurohypophysis. The classification of the neurohypophysis into the infundibulum (median eminence), infundibular stem, and infundibular process (neural lobe) stresses the observation that the neural portion of the pituitary gland is a diverticulum of brain but is distinct from the hypothalamus with which it is contiguous.

The infundibulum, the floor of the third ventricle, is separated into an ependymal layer, an internal zone, and an external (or palisade) zone (Fig. 90-4). Its ependymal layer is made up of specialized epithelial cells. They are united by zonulae occludentes (tight junctions) which inhibit the passive exchange of materials between the third ventricle and the interstitial fluid of the infundibulum. These cells lack cilia at their ventricular surface. In some regions their apical surface is characterized by the presence of large blebs as well as numerous smaller microvilli. Some of these ependymal cells ("tanycytes") are stretched, with their apical surface facing

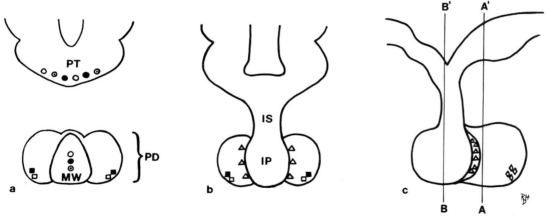

Figure 90-3 Human pituitary (schematic) in coronal and sagittal section, indicating the distribution of cell types. *a.* Far anterior section (plane *A–A'* in *c*). Cells containing TSH (*clear circles*), FSH (*clear circles with central dot*), and LH (*dark circles*) lie in the pars tuberalis (PT) and mucoid wedge (MW) of the pars distalis (PD). Somatotropes (*dark squares*) and lactotropes (*clear squares*) aggregate in the lateral wings. *b.* Posterior section (plane *B–B'* in *c*). Melanotropes (*clear triangles*) aggregate near the junction of the pars distalis and the infundibular process (IP). *c.* Sagittal section. Melanotropes (*clear triangles*) lie posteriorly near the neural lobe. Corticotropes (*clear diamonds*) predominate anteriorly.

ventricular fluid and their basilar processes terminating in the perivascular space of fenestrated capillaries on the median eminence surface. Such cells do not resemble the ependymal cells lining the walls of the third ventricle, which are cuboidal in shape, have cilia at their apical surface, lack apical blebs, and are united by gap junctions and desmasomes. The ependymal cells lining the infundibulum resemble the ependymal cells lining the rudimentary neural tube during embryonic development.[18]

The median eminence internal zone is made up of axons of the supraopticohypophyseal tract, which originate in the hypothalamic supraoptic and paraventricular nuclei and pass through the median eminence to terminate in the neural lobe. This supraopticohypophyseal tract is selectively stained by acid fuchsin techniques for light microscopic studies. Its axons are typically large and are characterized by the presence of dense core vesicles (150 to 300 nm in diameter) on transmission electron microscopic examination.[7] In addition, noradrenergic fibers and terminals have been demonstrated in the internal zone by formaldehyde fluorescence techniques. These fibers are believed to originate outside the hypothalamus in the brain stem and to represent the terminus of the ascending reticuloinfundibular tract.[8]

The median eminence external zone is made up of glial cells, axons, and axon terminals. Light microscopic studies demonstrate that the dopaminergic tuberoinfundibular tract (originating in the hypothalamic tuberal nuclei) terminates in this region. Transmission electron microscopy demonstrates three groups of terminals in this region: (1) terminals containing only small, lucent synaptic vesicles (~50 nm), (2) terminals containing small, lucent synaptic vesicles and large granular vesicles (~100 nm), and (3) terminals containing small synaptic vesicles with dense cores (~50 nm), with or without large granular vesicles after pretreatment

with 5-hydroxydopamine. These latter terminals contain dopamine in their small, dense synaptic vesicles. Few synaptic contacts are found in the median eminence. Axons terminate in the perivascular space of median eminence capillaries.[1]

The infundibular stem lies between the infundibulum and the infundibular process. It is characterized by the presence of axons of the supraopticohypophyseal tract. The dopaminergic tuberohypophyseal tract is also present in this region.

The infundibular process (neural lobe) is the terminus of the supraopticohypophyseal tract. Here axons of the supraopticohypophyseal tract terminate in the perivascular space of neural lobe capillaries. Near the adjacent adenohypophysis, terminals of the dopaminergic tuberohypophyseal tract may also be found.[23]

Pituitary Control: Information Transfer by Vessels

In the somatic efferent system information is carried as a pattern of neural impulses by ventral horn cells which are the final common pathway to striated muscle cells. The pattern of impulses carried along the ventral horn cells is determined by segmental and suprasegmental (descending) input across chemical synapses. The information thus channeled into the final common pathway reaches the target (muscle) cell through a chemical synapse at the myoneural junction. The central nervous system employs the mechanism of neurotransmission to cause the effector organ (striated muscle) to exert a force over a distance—to perform mechanical work—with considerable precision.

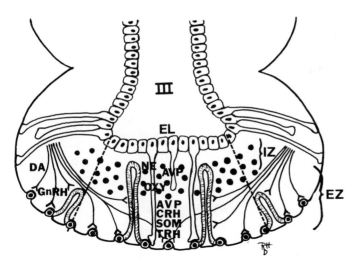

Figure 90-4 Median eminence (schematic) in coronal section. The ependymal layer (EL) is composed of specialized cells. Some stretch to reach capillaries on the median eminence external surface. The internal zone (IZ) is made up of large neurons of the supraopticohypophyseal tract (*large dots*) and smaller axons of the noradrenergic reticular infundibular tract (not shown). The external zone (EZ) is made up of small axons and terminals which lie in the perivascular space of median eminence capillaries. The dopaminergic tuberohypophyseal tract and neurosecretory systems arising in the hypothalamus terminate in this region. The capillary bed of the median eminence is subdivided into an external plexus lying on the median eminence surface and an internal plexus of capillary loops arising from the external plexus. These vessels provide a large surface area for neurohemal contact.

The dashed lines separate the median eminence into medial and lateral thirds. In the lateral third dopamine (DA)- and gonadotropin-releasing hormone (GnRH) fibers predominate. In the medial third norepinephrine (NE)-, arginine vasopressin (AVP)-, and oxytocin (OXY)-containing fibers are found in the internal zone. Arginine vasopressin, corticotropin-releasing hormone (CRH), somatostatin (SOM), and thyrotropin-releasing hormone (TRH) are present in the external zone, predominantly in the medial third.

In the visceral efferent system a similar arrangement is found. Suprasegmental and reflex (segmental) inputs converge upon cell bodies in the intermediolateral cell column (or in visceral efferent cranial nerve nuclei), which serve as the final common pathway to the effector organ. In the case of cardiovascular regulation, the effector organ is again a muscle cell (smooth or cardiac muscle). The visceral efferent system also regulates glandular secretion—for example, gastrointestinal, salivary, lacrimal, pineal, and choroid plexus secretions. In this system, postganglionic neurons make synaptoid contact with secretory epithelial cells. In the case of the adrenal medulla, preganglionic neurons make synaptoid contact with cells originating in the neural crest and modified to become secretory epithelium. Secretory activity of glandular cells is regulated by the central nervous system in a manner analogous to regulation of the motor activity of muscle cells. Descending (suprasegmental) and reflex (segmental) inputs are integrated into the final common pathway to regulate the performance of chemical work by secretory epithelial cells (as opposed to mechanical work by muscle cells).

The third efferent system—the neuroendocrine system—may be viewed in an analogous manner. In this system the effector organ is a secretory epithelial organ which performs the chemical work of synthesizing and releasing hormones. These secretory epithelial cells, like the muscle cells or the exocrine glandular cells, lie at some distance from the central neural elements which control their function. The final common pathway to these endocrine cells, unlike the pathway to the muscle cells or the exocrine cells, is not neural but vascular. The information carried to the pituitary (effector) cell is not carried by neurotransmission in a pattern of neural impulses along an axon; it is carried by neurohormones released in a pulsatile pattern from neurohypophyseal axon terminals by the process of neurosecretion into restricted vascular channels passing to the adenohypophysis. The blood vessels in the pituitary gland bear the same relation to the epithelial cells in the adenohypophysis as the ventral horn cells bear to striated muscle cells. They are the final common pathway.

Information in the form of neurosecretions from axon terminals is carried from the neurohypophysis to the adenohypophysis by vascular routes. The three neurohypophyseal regions share a common capillary bed. It is supplied rostrally at the median eminence by the superior hypophyseal arteries which arise from the intracranial internal carotid artery, the proximal (A_1) segments of the anterior cerebral arteries, and the posterior communicating arteries. It is supplied caudally at the neural lobe by the inferior hypophyseal arteries. In several species there is a third source of arterial supply variously called the trabecular artery, the loral artery, the anterior hypophyseal artery, or the artery to the infundibular stem, depending upon the species studied. As this vessel supplies the infundibular stem and rises along the course of the internal carotid artery between the superior and inferior hypophyseal arteries, the name *middle hypophyseal artery* seems appropriate.

The neurohypophyseal capillary bed is specialized at its rostral pole into a complex median eminence (primary) capillary plexus. This plexus is subdivided into an external (mantle) plexus and an internal plexus of complex capillary loops and coils. The external plexus lies on the median eminence surface, interposed between the median eminence and the pars tuberalis. Its fenestrated capillaries lie in close proximity to axon terminals in the median eminence external zone. The internal plexus arises from the external plexus. Its complex vascular formations penetrate the median eminence neuropil. Some (short) capillary loops penetrate only through the external zone. Other (long) capillary loops penetrate through the external and internal zones to the subependymal region before turning back and retreating to the median eminence surface (Fig. 90-4).

The neurohypophysis is drained rostrally by a series of fenestrated portal vessels which lie interposed between the median eminence primary plexus and the pars distalis secondary plexus. These portal vessels drain both the external and the internal plexus. Capillary connections between the median eminence and pars distalis are also ample. In addition, drainage routes from the median eminence to the hypothalamus and to the veins at the cerebral base have recently been demonstrated in several species. The rostral region of the neurohypophysis has access to limited drainage routes to the general circulation but ample local drainage routes to the pars distalis.

The neurohypophysis is drained caudally (at the level of the neural lobe) by paired posterior hypophyseal veins. These vessels course parallel to the inferior hypophyseal arteries and drain to the posterior cavernous sinus lateral to the midline. In addition, capillary connections unite the neural lobe with the adjacent pars distalis; and in some species (for example, the rat), a series of short portal vessels also unites the neural lobe and the pars distalis. The caudal region of the neurohypophysis has access to ample drainage routes to the general circulation but somewhat limited local routes to the adjacent pars distalis.

The adenohypophysis does not receive a direct arterial supply. Blood entering the adenohypophysis first passes through the neurohypophysis. The venous drainage of the adenohypophysis is from the pars distalis to the adjacent cavernous sinus. The primary drainage routes are through the same posterior hypophyseal veins which drain the neurohypophysis. These veins are Y-shaped, with one limb draining the caudal neurohypophysis and another draining the caudal pars distalis. These limbs unite into a common channel which drains into the posterior cavernous sinus. In addition, small lateral hypophyseal veins course from the lateral wings of the pars distalis into the lateral cavernous sinus.[29]

The direction of blood flow in the pituitary gland has been deduced from histological examination of the gland after stalk section and from direct observation of blood flow from the median eminence down the anterior surface of the pituitary stalk to the pars distalis in living animals. Only recently has the pattern of blood flow on the surface of the entire gland been studied (Fig. 90-5). Blood enters the neurohypophysis at each end (the median eminence and the neural lobe) almost simultaneously. However, as the inferior hypophyseal arteries lie closer to the heart than the superior hypophyseal arteries, blood enters the neural lobe just prior to entering the median eminence. Within the neurohypophysis, blood flow between different regions occurs. It flows retrograde from the neural lobe into the lower infundibular stem and anterograde from the median eminence into the upper infundibular stem. The site within the infundibular stem where the ascending and descending wave fronts meet varies. The infundibular stem is a watershed zone which receives blood from both the median eminence and the neural lobe. Rostrally the median eminence drains rapidly to the pars distalis. Caudally the neural lobe and infundibular stem drain to the cavernous sinus through posterior hypophyseal veins. Some blood does cross from the neural lobe into a small zone of the adjacent pars distalis. The bulk of the pars distalis, however, receives its blood from the median emi-

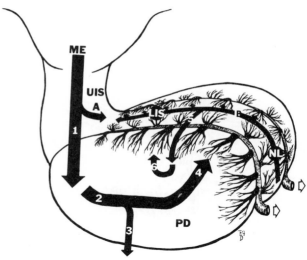

Figure 90-5 Blood flow in the (porcine) pituitary gland (schematic). Blood enters the neurohypophyseal capillary bed at each end. Blood flow within the neurohypophyseal capillary bed is retrograde (B) from the neural lobe (NL) into the lower infundibular stem (LIS) and anterograde (A) from the median eminence (ME) into the upper infundibular stem (UIS). The site within the neurohypophysis where the ascending and descending wave fronts meet varies. The infundibular stem is a watershed zone between the two sources of arterial supply.

Blood flow from ME to pars distalis (PD) is by portal and capillary routes (1). Blood flow from the NL and LIS into the adjacent PD also occurs (5) by capillary routes, but the territory of the PD thus supplied is small. Blood from the ME sweeps into the lateral regions of the PD (2). A small lateral region drains to the adjacent cavernous sinus by lateral hypophyseal veins (3). Most of the blood entering the PD sweeps dorsomedially (4) to drain into Y-shaped pituitary veins draining the pars distalis. Blood which has coursed from the neural lobe and lower infundibular stem (5) by capillary routes into the adjacent PD also drains into these veins (6). Y-shaped pituitary veins drain the LIS and NL as well as the PD. Drainage of these caudal neurohypophyseal regions is more rapid than drainage of the pars distalis and occurs in a caudal-to-rostral pattern. The Y-shaped veins carry blood containing neuro- and adenohypophyseal hormones to the posterior region of the cavernous sinus and join it lateral to the midline. (From Page.[29])

nence. Blood passes down the pituitary stalk into the medial third of the pars distalis and courses into the lateral wings. A small region in the lateral wings of the pars distalis drains to the lateral cavernous sinus through lateral hypophyseal veins. Most of the blood sweeps dorsomedially to the junction of the pars distalis and neural lobe, where it drains into the Y-shaped pituitary veins, which in turn drain to the posterior cavernous sinus. With stalk section the pattern of blood flow is markedly altered. No blood enters the pars distalis through portal routes from the median eminence. The small territory of the pars distalis supplied from the neural lobe is diminished if the blood pressure falls.[29]

The physiology of pituitary blood flow has only recently come under close scrutiny, and a composite picture cannot as yet be presented. Pars distalis blood flow (in the rat and dog) is about 70 cm^3/100 g per minute. Neurohypophyseal blood flow (in the sheep) is much higher—about 450 cm^3/100 g per minute. This flow is about 8 times cortical blood flow and 10 times hypothalamic blood flow in these same animals. Flow in the median eminence does not differ from neural lobe flow. Neurohypophyseal blood flow is autoregulated and is decreased with hypocarbia. In these respects it is similar to cerebral blood flow, a finding that should not be unexpected in a brain diverticulum.[29] As neurosecretory cells terminate upon median eminence capillaries which drain to the pars distalis via portal routes and upon capillaries in the infundibular stem and neural lobe which drain to the adjacent pars distalis, the entire neurohypophyseal capillary bed may be viewed as the final common pathway to the pars distalis. The vascular arrangements in the pituitary gland assure the delivery of neurosecretions from the neurohypophysis to the adenohypophysis over local routes at high rates of flow.

Neurosecretion provides the mechanism by which the brain controls adenohypophyseal function. In 1947 Green and Harris[12] demonstrated that the pars distalis lacked axon terminals, and they suggested that a neurovascular link between the median eminence and pars distalis controlled anterior pituitary function. They postulated the release of chemical messengers from axon terminals in the median eminence about the fenestrated median eminence capillaries, passage of these humors into median eminence capillaries, and transport by restricted portal routes to target cells in the pars distalis. The Scharrers[37] had previously proposed the concept of neurosecretion. They had suggested that some neurons could function as glandular cells—they could synthesize and release hormones. Subsequently hormones (oxytocin and vasopressin) were isolated from the neural lobe and the hypothalamic supraoptic and paraventricular nuclei. With demonstration that oxytocin (OXY) and arginine vasopressin (AVP) were synthesized in these hypothalamic regions, transported by axoplasmic flow through fibers in the supraopticohypophyseal tract to axon terminals in the neural lobe, and released under appropriate physiological conditions, the concept of neurosecretion was established and the means by which the brain controls neural lobe function was clarified.

Hormones were also found in the median eminence and medial basilar hypothalamus which supported adenohypophyseal function. Several of these peptide hypothalamic hypophysiotropic hormones were subsequently isolated, sequenced, and synthesized. Gonadotropin-releasing hormone (GnRH) stimulates both FSH- and LH-secreting adenohypophyseal cells. Thyrotropin-releasing hormone (TRH) stimulates TSH release by thyrotropes. Corticotropin-releasing hormone (CRH) stimulates ACTH release by corticotropes. Somatostatin (SOM) inhibits GH release by somatotropes. In addition, evidence is accumulating that dopamine is a physiological prolactin-inhibiting factor.

With the chemical synthesis of these peptide hypothalamic hormones, it has been possible to identify them by immunohistochemistry in neurosecretory cells whose cell bodies lie in the hypothalamus and whose terminals lie in the median eminence. It has also been possible to demonstrate that these neurohormones are synthesized in the cell soma and are transported to axon terminals by axoplasmic flow and that they are released into portal blood under appropriate physiological conditions.

Neural hormones are synthesized in the cell soma (on rough endoplasmic reticulum) by the same series of steps involved in pituitary peptide synthesis within adenohypophyseal cells. The sequence of amino acids is determined by nuclear DNA, and the information is carried to the cytoplasm by messenger RNA (mRNA). The prescribed sequence is formed by the interaction of mRNA with ribosomes. Amino acids are united through peptide bond formation by the mediation of transfer RNA (tRNA)—an energy-requiring process. The translated protein hormones are transported to the Golgi apparatus and packaged in large, granular vesicles. Vesicles containing the hormones are transported by axoplasmic flow from the cell soma to the axon terminal lying in the perivascular space of a fenestrated capillary in the neurohypophysis. Recent evidence suggests that the hormone translated from mRNA is frequently a prohormone—considerably larger than the final biologically active product. Post-translation modification of the prohormone by cleavage of peptide bonds at selective sites occurs during axoplasmic transport of hormones within vesicles.[9,26]

Several differences may be cited between neurotransmission and neurosecretion. In neurosecretion the active product is released from axon terminals into the perivascular space of a fenestrated capillary and is carried by vascular routes to a target cell at a considerable distance (millimeters to meters) from the axon terminal. In neurotransmission the final product is released into a synaptic cleft and carried by diffusion to a target cell extremely close to the axon terminal (200 nm). In neurosecretion the peptide hormone is synthesized in the cell soma and carried to the axon terminal by axoplasmic flow; post-translation modification of the peptide may occur. In neurotransmission the (amine) transmitter is synthesized in the axon terminal, and post-translation modification does not occur. In neurosecretion, reuptake of the secretory product does not occur; in neurotransmission, reuptake of amine neurotransmitters does occur. The duration of action of the neurosecretory product upon its target cell is far longer (minutes) than the duration of action of the neurotransmitter (msec).

Two peptidergic neurosecretory systems terminate in the neurohypophysis (Fig. 90-6). The first is the magnocellular system with cell bodies in the hypothalamic supraoptic and paraventricular system. This system projects to the infundibular process (neural lobe) through the supraopticohypophyseal tract. Cells in this system contain oxytocin and vasopressin and their associated neurophysins (I and II, respectively). Oxytocin and vasopressin are found in both the supraoptic and paraventricular nuclei but are found in different cells within those nuclei. As noted above, the supraopticohypophyseal tract forms the internal zone of the median eminence. The cells and axons are typically large, stain selectively with acid fuchsin dyes, and are characterized by the presence of large dense core vesicles which contain either oxytocin and neurophysin I or vasopressin and neurophysin II.

The second neurosecretory system is the parvocellular

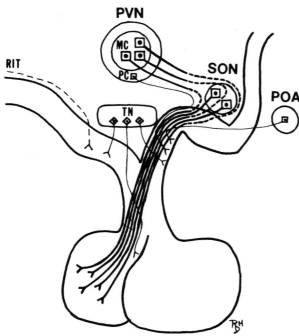

Figure 90-6 Peptidergic and aminergic systems terminating in the neurohypophysis: sagittal view. Magnocellular systems containing arginine vasopressin (AVP), oxytocin (OXY), and neurophysin originate in the supraoptic nucleus (SON) and paraventricular nucleus (PVN) and terminate in the neural lobe. Projections from the magnocellular region (MC) of the paraventricular nucleus are also believed to terminate in the median eminence (not shown). Projections from the parvocellular (PC) region of the PVN and from periventricular sites project to the medial third of the median eminence and contain CRH, TRH, and somatostatin (see text). Parvocellular projections from the preoptic area (POA) contain GnRH and terminate in the lateral thirds of the median eminence. Aminergic systems also terminate in the neurohypophysis. The dopaminergic tuberoinfundibular and tuberohypophyseal tracts originate in the tuberal nuclei (TN) and terminate in the external zone of the median eminence (predominantly in the lateral thirds) and in the superficial regions of the infundibular stem and process adjacent to the adenohypophysis. The noradrenergic reticuloinfundibular tract (RIT) arises in the brain stem and terminates in the medial third of the median eminence. Dashed lines indicate uncertainty as to the exact course of fiber tracts passing from the PVN in the vicinity of the SON.

system. The cells in this system originate in several hypothalamic cell groups and terminate in the median eminence in the perivascular space of fenestrated capillaries. Its terminals are mostly found in the median eminence external zone. The neurons are typically small, and their axon terminals contain small synaptic and large granular vesicles. By immunohistochemical techniques, GnRH, TRH, SOM, and CRH have been localized within cells of the parvocellular peptidergic system.

Two aminergic systems also terminate in the neurohypophysis. One originates in the hypothalamic tuberal (arcuate) nucleus and terminates in the median eminence external zone (tuberoinfundibular tract) or in the infundibular stem and process (tuberohypophyseal tract). These tracts are dopaminergic. The other—the noradrenergic reticular infundibular tract—originates in the brain stem and terminates in the median eminence internal zone.

The secretion of hypothalamic hypophysiotropic releasing factors and catecholamines into median eminence capillaries and their transport via portal vessels to the pars distalis is not the only mechanism by which the brain can control anterior pituitary function. The neural lobe hormone AVP released from peptidergic terminals in the median eminence can be carried by portal routes to the pars distalis to play a role in regulation of ACTH release by corticotropes. AVP and oxytocin can be transported by vascular (capillary) routes from the neural lobe to the pars distalis to participate in the regulation of α-MSH and prolactin release by melanotropes and lactotropes[33] (Fig. 90-5). The entire neurohypophysis appears to participate in controlling adenohypophyseal function.

Mechanisms to Assure Specificity of Adenohypophyseal Response

In the somatic efferent system, specificity of response is assured by the close proximity of the axon terminal to the muscle cell, isolation of the synapse at the myoneural junction, and specificity of receptor sites on the muscle cell membrane. In the pars distalis, epithelial cells are virtually bathed in blood containing a host of hypothalamic-releasing and -inhibiting hormones. These hormones interact with specific receptors on the cell surface of target pituitary epithelial cells to modify the production of intracellular cyclic AMP (cAMP) and alter protein kinase activity. There is accumulating evidence that the releasing hormones (GnRH and TRH) stimulate intracellular cAMP production in gonadotropes and thyrotropes and that the inhibiting hormones (somatostatin and dopamine) inhibit cAMP production in somatotropes and lactotropes. The brain causes a specific pituitary hormone response by the release of specific hypothalamic stimulating and inhibiting hormones which interact with specific receptors on pituitary target cells. These hypothalamic hormones regulate adenohypophyseal hormone secretion through the second messenger system.[20]

This schema rests upon three assumptions: (1) that the specificity of receptors at the adenohypophyseal cell surface is absolute, (2) that only one stimulating and/or releasing hormone governs the secretory activity of each functional pituitary cell type, and (3) that a single releasing hormone releases only one pituitary hormone. Regarding the first assumption, however, specificity of hypothalamic hypophysiotropic hormones is not absolute. TRH administration stimulates not only TSH release but also Pro release, although the role of TRH in the physiological control of Pro secretion has not as yet been established. Somatostatin inhibits the synthesis and release of hormones other than growth hormone. In certain pathological conditions, for example adenoma formation, cellular receptors apparently lose their specificity. In some acromegalic persons, growth hormone secretion is stimulated by TRH infusion and is inhibited by the administration of dopamine agonists.

As for the second assumption, some adenohypophyseal cells respond to two or more hypothalamic peptidergic hormones. ACTH secretion by the pituitary gland is stimulated by CRH, but it is also stimulated by vasopressin (AVP). The response of corticotropes to CRH is much greater than their response to AVP on a molar basis. However, when the two are combined, the effect on ACTH secretion is not simply additive but is synergistic. In addition, ACTH release can be increased by the stimulation of β-adrenergic receptors on corticotropes by levels of catecholamines which can be achieved by adrenal medullary secretion under conditions of stress.

Regarding the third assumption, although receptor specificity on the adenohypophyseal cell surface is a mechanism that would appear to guarantee that a specific pituitary hormone is released in response to a specific brain hormone, CRH apparently stimulates both ACTH and MSH secretion from corticotropes and melanotropes, respectively, in the rat pituitary.[34] The explanation for this discrepancy lies in different post-translational processing of a prohormone common to both functional cell lines (Fig. 90-7). Both corticotropes and melanotropes translate the same prohormone—pro-opiomelanocortin—from mRNA. Both cleave this 31,000-dalton prohormone into a precursor hormone containing 130 amino acids. Corticotropes further cleave this precursor to form ACTH (1–39) and β-lipotropin (1–91). Within melanotropes, ACTH (1–39) is further cleaved into α-MSH (1–13) and corticotropin-like intermediate peptide (CLIP). β-LPH (1–91) is cleaved to form γ-LPH (1–58) and β-endorphin (61–91).[14,25]

Within the median eminence, peptidergic and aminergic nerve terminals segregate in an endocrinotopic manner (Fig. 90-4). Dopaminergic systems (from the arcuate nucleus) terminate in the external zone, principally in the lateral

third. Norepinephrine-containing terminals of neurons arising in the brain stem terminate in the medial third of the median eminence, principally in the internal zone. CRH projections terminate in the medial third (internal and external zone), and AVP systems pass through the median eminence internal zone to the neural lobe but also terminate in the external zone in the medial third. Somatostatin-containing fibers terminate diffusely in the medial third, and TRH-containing fibers terminate in the external zone of the middle third. Hence the lateral thirds of the median eminence contain neurosecretory and catecholamine terminals involved in the regulation of reproduction (GnRH and dopamine) through regulation of FSH, LH, and Pro secretion. The medial third contains releasing hormones involved with the regulation of metabolism (somatostatin and TRH) through GH and TSH secretion and with mediation of the organisms response to stress (CRF and AVP) through regulation of ACTH secretion. It is interesting that dopamine systems terminate in the lateral thirds of the median eminence and lactotropes predominate in the lateral wings of the pars distalis. CRH, TRH, and AVP systems terminate in the medial third of the median eminence, and corticotropes and thyrotropes are found in the medial third of the pituitary.[2]

Vascular elements need not be interposed between the neural terminal and adenohypophyseal secretory cells. The dopaminergic tuberohypophyseal tract terminates along the ventral surface of the infundibular stem and process, near melanotropes in the adjacent pars distalis whose secretory and adenyl cyclase activity are negatively coupled to dopamine concentration. The proximity of these nerve terminals to melanotropes provides another mechanism for specific control of adenohypophyseal function by the brain.

Receptor specificity at the adenohypophyseal cell surface for corresponding peptidergic hypothalamic hormones, genetically determined translational pathways of protein (pro-) hormone synthesis, and differential post-translational processing of protein prohormones are the key mechanisms in assuring a specific adenohypophyseal response to neurohumoral instructions from the brain. The close relation of melanotropes to aminergic terminals obviates the need for vascular transport of humoral signals and is a fourth mechanism which ensures specificity of response. The possibility that specific regions in the median eminence "project" by portal vessels to corresponding pituitary regions adds another potential mechanism of neural control of anterior pituitary function and is presently being investigated (Table 90-1).

Surgical Correlates of Pituitary Anatomy

This anatomical survey has constructed a pituitary gland composed of a neurohypophysis (median eminence, infundibular stem, and neural lobe) and an adenohypophysis (pars tuberalis, pars intermedia, and pars distalis). The concepts proposed are quite different in some respects from the traditional teaching that the pituitary gland lies within the sella turcica bounded superiorly by the diaphragma sellae, that the median eminence is part of the hypothalamus, and

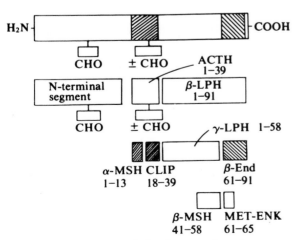

Figure 90-7 Post-translational processing of pro-opiomelanocortin (schematic). (From Gainer H, Brownstein MW: Neuropeptides, in Siegel GJ, Albers RW, Katzman R, Agranoff BW: *Basic Neurochemistry*. Boston, Little, Brown, 3d ed. 1981, chap 14.)

TABLE 90-1 Neurosecretory Systems Which Regulate Pituitary Function

RH/IH*	Pit. Hormone	Hypothalamic Origin†	Neurohypophyseal Terminus‡	Location of Pituitary Target Cell	Hypothalamic Neural Projection
			Reproductive Systems		
GnRH	FSH	POA	ME (lateral third)	PT	Amygdala
	LH			PD (mucoid wedge)	Mesencephalon
Dopamine	Pro	TN	ME (lateral third)	PD (lateral wings)	?
			Metabolic Systems		
TRH	TSH	PVN	ME (medial third)	PT	?
			Neural lobe	PD (mucoid wedge)	
SOM	GH	PVN	ME (diffuse)	PD (lateral wings)	?
CRH	ACTH	PVN	ME (medial third)	Central; anterior	?
AVP	ACTH	PVN	ME (medial third)	Central; anterior	Medulla
AVP	ACTH	SON PVN	NL (central)	Central; anterior	?
OXY	? ACTH	PVN	NL (peripheral, next to pars distalis)	Next to neural lobe	Medulla Spinal cord
Dopamine	MSH	TN	NL (next to pars distalis)	Near neural terminals	?

*RH = releasing hormone, IH = inhibiting hormone.
†POA = preoptic area, TN = tuberal nuclei, PVN = paraventricular nuclei, SON = supraoptic nuclei.
‡ME = median eminence, NL = neural lobe.
§PT = pars tuberalis, PD = pars distalis.

that the pars tuberalis can be dismissed. Such a conceptualization arose from the dividing of the pituitary stalk during removal of the brain from the skull by anatomists and pathologists. In making this division, they conceptually divided the pituitary gland in half, leaving the median eminence and pars tuberalis with the brain and the pars distalis and neural lobe within the sella turcica.

The construction presented here raises two points of surgical interest. First, total hypophysectomy by the transsphenoidal route is a difficult if not dangerous task that would require removal of the median eminence and pars tuberalis. As infarction of the median eminence and pars tuberalis does not occur (in monkeys and rats) following either stalk section or removal of the pars distalis and neural lobe, functioning tissue capable of secreting FSH, LH, and TSH is left behind. Indeed, in the rat, growth of this tissue occurs after hypophysectomy with an increase in the number and size of functioning gonadotropes.[13] Second, the distribution of cell types within the adenohypophysis allows prediction of the sites of development (and hence the localization) of small functioning pituitary tumors.[15] Tumors secreting GH or Pro will be found in the lateral wings of the pars distalis. Tumors secreting TSH or gonadotropins will be found more medially in the mucoid wedge or above the diaphragma sellae in the pars tuberalis. Tumors secreting α-MSH or β-endorphin may be expected to be closely apposed to the neural lobe, whereas ACTH-secreting tumors may be expected to begin anteriorly and inferiorly near the median plane.

Several points of surgical relevance also become apparent when one considers the portal system:

1. In hemorrhagic shock the infusion of vasopressors will raise mean arterial blood pressure (MABP) and restore cerebral blood flow (if MABP is below the limit of autoregulation). Because of the blood-brain barrier, the infused pressor agent has no effect on cerebral vascular resistance. As there is no blood-brain barrier in the pituitary gland, pressor agents can reach the smooth muscle cells of resistance arterioles, causing them to constrict and decrease pituitary blood flow, with resultant pituitary infarction even while cerebral blood flow is being restored. This may be the genesis of Sheehan's syndrome of postpartum pituitary necrosis.

2. Superior hypophyseal arteries lie in the subarachnoid space and vascularize the median eminence and medial basilar hypothalamus. Subarachnoid hemorrhage with spasm of the vessels of the circle of Willis may be expected to reduce pituitary blood flow and alter pituitary function.

3. Venous drainage routes from the pars distalis to the cavernous sinus lie lateral to the midline. Selective bilateral inferior petrosal sinus catheterization with blood sampling for determination of hormone levels may be expected to lateralize small secretory pituitary tumors poorly visualized by radiological studies.

4. Venous drainage routes to the cerebral base from the median eminence are apparently adequate to prevent venous infarction of the median eminence after stalk section or removal of the neural lobe and pars distalis. Hence, following destruction of the pituitary gland within the sella by neoplasm, aneurysm, or traumatic stalk section, pituitary transplantation to sites beneath the median eminence is feasible, as it requires not the re-establishment of neural connections but the re-establishment of portal vascular connections between the graft and the preserved median eminence.

Descending Fiber Systems to the Neurohypophysis

The neurosecretory systems which project to neurohypophyseal capillaries (the final common pathway to adenohypophyseal cells) have been clarified with the application of immunohistochemical, autoradiographic, and horseradish peroxidase tracing techniques (Fig. 90-8). Most of the work has been carried out in experimental animals such as the rat, hence extrapolation to the human condition may be premature. These studies reveal a morphological segregation of functionally discrete neurosecretory cell groups. They also reveal projections from these cell groups to brain regions outside the hypothalamus as well as to capillaries in the neurohypophysis (Table 90-1).

Vasopressin-secreting neurons are found in the supraoptic, paraventricular, and suprachiasmatic nuclei. In the supraoptic and paraventricular nuclei, vasopressin is present in magnocellular neurons which project to the neurohypophysis.[3] Projections from the supraoptic and paraventricular nuclei to the neurohypophysis are segregated. Fibers from the supraoptic nucleus pass through the internal zone of the median eminence and terminate in the central region of the neural lobe. Fibers from the paraventricular nucleus terminate more rostrally and ventrally in the median eminence external zone and the ventral aspect of the infundibular stem and process.[2] Vasopressin is present in small neurons within the suprachiasmatic nucleus which project to neural targets outside the hypothalamus, not to vascular targets in the neurohypophysis.[38]

Oxytocin-secreting neurons are found in the supraoptic and paraventricular nuclei. This oxytocin magnocellular system projects to the neural lobe.[3] A small number of oxytocin-containing fibers are also found in the median eminence and may originate in the parvocellular portion of the paraventricular nucleus.[39]

Neuronal cell bodies containing immunoreactive CRH have been demonstrated in the parvocellular portion of para-

ventricular nucleus.[11] These cells project to the median eminence, entering it from the anterolateral preoptic regions.[30]

Immunoreactive TRH neuronal networks have been demonstrated in hypothalamic and extrahypothalamic brain regions. Extrahypothalamic TRH systems appear to function independently of hypothalamic ones. Within the (rat) brain TRH has been localized by immunohistochemical techniques within perikarya lying in the medullary raphe magnus nucleus and in the hypothalamic suprachiasmatic preoptic nucleus, preoptic periventricular nucleus, dorsomedial nucleus, and (anterobasal) lateral hypothalamus. A few TRH neurons are present in the posterior region of the arcuate nucleus. The largest population of immunoreactive neurons is found in the parvocellular division of the paraventricular nucleus.[21] The origin of TRH fibers projecting to the median eminence has not been completely clarified; but it would appear that they arise in the parvocellular division of the paraventricular nucleus and course with vasopressin-, oxytocin-, and CRH-containing fibers to the median eminence.[21,30]

Somatostatin (SOM)-containing perikarya are also found in extrahypothalamic sites (neocortex, hippocampus, caudate nucleus), as well as in the hypothalamus. Within the hypothalamus, somatostatin-containing neuronal cell bodies are found in the organum vasculosum of the lamina terminalis (OVLT), the anterior preoptic area, the periventricular nucleus, the parvocellular division of the paraventricular nucleus, and the arcuate nucleus.[1,17] The densest accumulation of neuronal cell bodies is found along the third ventricular wall in the preoptic and anterior hypothalamic regions.[6] These periventricular neurons are the origin of axons terminating in the median eminence.[1]

GnRH-containing perikarya are concentrated in the medial preoptic area rostral and dorsal to the chiasma.[1] A few scattered neuronal cell bodies are also present in the arcuate nucleus, but these cells do not contribute substantially to the axons terminating in the median eminence. GnRH-containing cells in the preoptic area project through the preopticoinfundibular tract to terminate in the median eminence.[27] This fiber bundle joins projections from the periventricular cell system (predominantly the parvocellular portion of the paraventricular nucleus) carrying TRH, CRH, AVP, and SOM fibers to the median eminence.[30]

In addition to the parvocellular peptidergic system which secretes hypothalamic releasing and inhibiting hormones, there is a second peptidergic system in the hypothalamus. This system contains the processed products of pro-opiomelanocortin (ACTH, β-LPH, α-MSH and β-endorphin) in its cell bodies, which are located predominantly within the arcuate nucleus.[10] It projects to the median eminence. In addition, ACTH-containing projections from the arcuate nucleus to the parvocellular regions of the paraventricular nucleus have been demonstrated,[36] as have projections containing α-MSH, β-endorphin, ACTH, and LPH to extrahypothalamic brain areas.

Afferent pathways to the median eminence have been studied in the rat by horseradish peroxidase (HRP) tracing techniques. After injection into the median eminence, HRP is found in the arcuate nucleus, preoptic area, periventricular area, and parvocellular regions of the paraventricular nucleus.[22,44] These observations, combined with immunohistochemical studies, demonstrate that:

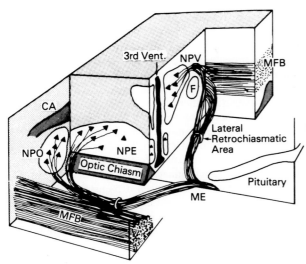

Figure 90-8 Topography of the lateral retrochiasmatic area and cell groups which project axons through it to the median eminence (schematic). Medial preoptic nucleus (NPO); periventricular nucleus (NPE); paraventricular nucleus (NPV); medial forebrain bundle (MFB); median eminence (ME); anterior commissure (CA).
(From Palkovits M: Neuropeptides in the median eminence: Their sources and destinations. Peptides (Fayetteville) 3:299-303, 1982.)

1. The arcuate (tuberal) nucleus is not the origin of neuro-secretory cells which secrete hypothalamic-releasing and -inhibiting hormones in portal blood, although fibers containing these neurohormones pass through it.
2. The dopaminergic tuberoinfundibular tract originates in the arcuate nucleus and projects to the median eminence.
3. CRH, TRH, and SOM systems originate in the periventricular region and parvocellular region of the paraventricular nucleus. It appears that these systems project anterolaterally to the level of the chiasm and then turn medially to enter the median eminence from this region and terminate in its medial third.
4. GnRH fibers originate in the preoptic area and join the fibers coursing from the periventricular zone at the level of the chiasm to distribute to the lateral third of the median eminence. The preoptic area, just ventral to the septum and dorsal to the diagonal band of Broca and the anterior perforated space, contains a "funnel" of hypophysiotropic hypothalamic neuronal systems which control anterior pituitary function.[30]

Surgical Correlates of Hypothalamic Anatomy

Several corollaries to these findings are applicable to surgery of the hypothalamic area if extrapolation to the human patient is justified:

1. Tumors of the medial sphenoid ridge may alter anterior pituitary function without direct pituitary involvement by compressing hypothalamic-hypophysiotropic pathways.
2. As pathways projecting from the paraventricular nucleus to the median eminence lie close to the third ventricle, they will be susceptible to injury by surgical procedures carried out within the third ventricle, as will the periventricular cell bodies.
3. The anterior surgical approach to the third ventricle through the lamina terminalis must be kept strictly midline to avoid damaging fibers passing to the median eminence and neural lobe.
4. Damage to small vessels entering the anterior perforated space during aneurysm dissection will damage pituitary function as well as autonomic function and consciousness.
5. Hydrocephalus with stretching of periventricular fibers will alter pituitary function.
6. The periventricular location of these hypophysiotropic fiber systems and the recovery of hypothalamic hormones from cerebrospinal fluid suggest that transplantation of pituitary tissue into the third ventricle, as well as beneath the median eminence, is feasible.[43]

Integration of Efferent Systems

In this presentation the adenohypophyseal cells are viewed as constituting a motor organ analogous to skeletal muscle cells. The neurohypophyseal capillaries and the portal system are viewed as the final common pathway to these cells, analogous to ventral horn cells. The fiber tracts containing neurosecretory peptides, which originate in the periventricular region of the hypothalamus (particularly in the paraventricular nucleus and the preoptic region) and terminate near neurohypophyseal capillaries, are presented as analogous to fiber tracts descending through the spinal cord from the brain to synapse with ventral horn cells. The tasks remaining are (1) to determine the neural inputs to hypothalamic neurosecretory cell groups, in order to clarify the mechanism by which the humoral responses to changes in the internal and external milieu are integrated; and (2) to determine the neural output of these hypothalamic cell groups in order to clarify the mechanism by which autonomic, motor, and mental activities are correlated with neuroendorine function.

The mechanism by which the brain integrates a humoral response of the pituitary is vaguely understood. On a rudimentary level it is appreciated that in the rabbit, preoptic stimulation in the region containing GnRH cell bodies stimulates GnRH release into portal vessels, with elevation of plasma LH levels and ovulation. It is also appreciated that amygdaloid lesions or division of the stria terminalis (which terminates in the sexually dimorphic nucleus of the stria terminalis in the preoptic area) alters the estrus cycle in the rat. In primates the relation between the medial temporal lobes and reproductive function is not clear. No change in neuroendocrine function was reported in adult female monkeys that had undergone bilateral anterior temporal lobectomy.[24] However, alterations in the control of LH secretion have been reported in humans with temporal lobe epilepsy.[16]

With the exception of feedback mechanisms, it is unusual for the organism to respond to a stimulus from the internal or external milieu with the secretion of only one pituitary hormone. For instance, in hypotensive shock, ACTH, β-End, and AVP are released from the pituitary gland. In addition, compensatory adjustments are made by the visceral efferent (autonomic) system. The response to hypotension provides a model which permits insight into the mechanisms by which neuroendocrine and visceral responses are integrated (Fig. 90-9).

With hypotension there is an increase in neural traffic over the glossopharyngeal nerves, with increased input into the tractus and nucleus solitarius. Radioautographic studies demonstrate connections between the nucleus solitarius and the dorsal motor nucleus of the vagus. Ascending noradrenergic systems originating in this nucleus and in the lateral reticular nucleus have been demonstrated in the rat by the use of formaldehyde fluorescence techniques. These neurons terminate in the paraventricular nucleus, and some terminate directly on small neurons in the parvocellular region and on AVP-containing neurons. There are neural connections between the parvocellular and magnocellular divisions of the paraventricular nucleus and between the paraventricular and supraoptic nucleus. AVP is present in large neurons in the supraoptic nucleus which project to the neural lobe and in paraventricular neurons which project to the median eminence. The ascending noradrenergic tracts may thus regulate AVP secretion into median eminence and neural lobe capillaries, for transport locally to the adenohypophysis and for transport distantly to target organs (kid-

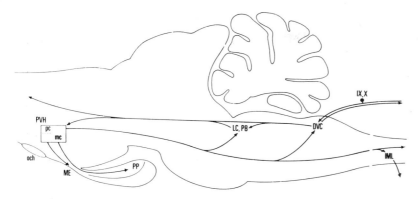

Figure 90-9 Summary of the major longer connections of the paraventricular nucleus (PVH) in the rat, emphasizing the relation between the PVH and cell groups associated with the autonomic nervous system. Dorsal vagal complex (DCV); intermediolateral cell column (IML); locus ceruleus (LC); magnocellular division (MC) of the PVH; median eminence (ME); optic chiasm (OCH); parabrachial nucleus (PB); parvocellular division (PC) of PVH; glossopharyngeal nerve (IX); vagal nerve (X). From Swanson and Sawchenko.[40]

neys, systemic arterioles). CRH is present in axon terminals whose cell bodies lie in the parvocellular divisions of the paraventricular neurons. It is released by axon terminals lying in the median eminence and carried to the pars distalis to stimulate ACTH release. CRH release might thus be regulated by the same ascending noradrenergic pathways that regulate AVP secretion when the organism is faced with a decrease in systemic arterial blood pressure.

In the pars distalis, the effects of the increased AVP and CRH secretion on ACTH release under hypotensive conditions would be synergistic, maximizing ACTH secretion and stimulation of the adrenal cortex to secrete cortisol. AVP released from the neural lobe will be carried by systemic vascular routes to receptors on precapillary arterioles and to renal parenchymal cells to elevate mean arterial blood pressure and to increase renal water conservation, respectively. In addition, AVP secreted by the neural lobe may be carried by capillary routes to the adjacent pars distalis to stimulate ACTH release. In this manner a coordinated neuroendocrine response to a single stimulus, hypotension, may be carried out by the pituitary gland.

Within the paraventricular nucleus, neurons containing AVP project caudally and terminate in the dorsal motor nucleus of the vagus upon noradrenergic cells. A loop is thus formed with noradrenergic cells in the dorsal motor nucleus of the vagus projecting to AVP-containing neurons in the paraventricular nucleus and AVP-containing neurons projecting back to the dorsomotor nucleus of the vagus. In addition, paraventricular neurons containing oxytocin project to brain stem sites and to the intermediolateral cell column of the spinal cord—the site of the final common pathway for the sympathetic (visceral) efferent system. Although the details of this system are far from clear, the paraventricular nucleus would appear to be a "site for the integration of neuroendocrine and autonomic mechanisms."[40]

The sites for regulating the response of specific functional adenohypophyseal cell populations and for integrating the responses of several populations of adenohypophyseal cells are found at several levels but understood well at only a few. At the level of the adenohypophyseal cell, feedback responsive to the level of peripheral target hormones occurs. For example, ACTH secretion is depressed by elevated cortisol levels. TSH secretion is depressed by elevated levels of thyroid hormone. Adenohypophyseal cells also respond to neurosecretions from the median eminence and neural lobe,

as the entire neurohypophyseal capillary bed serves as the final common pathway to the adenohypophysis. Specific releasing and inhibiting hormones regulate the activity of specific adenohypophyseal cell populations.

Within the median eminence there is a morphological integration of separate neurosecretory systems to form functional regions. Reproduction is mediated laterally in the median eminence, whereas neurohormones involved in the regulation of the internal milieu, metabolism, and response to stress are segregated medially. Thus there is a suprahumoral organization of converging input in the median eminence, analogous to the suprasegmental convergence of input within the spinal cord.

The organization of input into the hypothalamus is at this time poorly understood, and no organizing conceptual framework has been constructed. For the time being the surgeon's scope of endeavor is limited to direct approaches to the pituitary to normalize its function. The understanding that releasing hormone systems do not require direct contact with their target cells and that these systems project toward the ventricular system in their transit from their sites of origin will permit investigation of the possibilities of pituitary transplantation into the sella turcica or even into the ventricular system.[43] Even transplantation of hypothalamic neurosecretory cell systems may be possible.[19] Further clarification of the organization of the hypothalamus and of its input may permit the employment of stereotaxic procedures to modify pituitary function. In the future it is to be expected that the pituitary surgeon will employ a broad range of procedures in the brain as well as in the pituitary gland to treat disorders of the neuroendocrine system.

References

1. Ajika K: Relationship between catecholaminergic neurons and hypothalamic hormone-containing neurons in the hypothalamus, in Martini L, Ganong WF (eds): *Frontiers in Neuroendocrinology*, vol 6. New York, Raven Press, 1980, pp 1–32.
2. Alonso G, Assenmacher I: Radioautographic studies on the neurohypophysial projections of the supraoptic and paraventricular nuclei in the rat. Cell Tissue Res 219:525–534, 1981.
3. Antunes JL, Zimmerman EA: The hypothalamic magnocellular system of the rhesus monkey: An immunocytochemical study. J Comp Neurol 181:539–566, 1978.
4. Atwell WJ: The development of the hypophysis cerebri in man,

with special reference to the pars tuberalis. Am J Anat 37:159–193, 1926.

5. Baker BL: Functional cytology of the hypophysial pars distalis and pars intermedia, in Greep RO and Astwood EB (eds) *Handbook of Physiology*, sec 7: Endocrinology, vol 4, *The Pituitary Gland and Its Neuroendocrine Control*, pt 1. Washington, American Physiological Society, 1974, pp 45–80.

6. Bennett-Clarke C, Romagnano MA, Joseph SA: Distribution of somatostatin in the rat brain: Telencephalon and diencephalon. Brain Res 188:473–486, 1980.

7. Bergland RM, Torack RM: An electron microscopic study of the human infundibulum. Z Zellforsch 99:1–12, 1969.

8. Björklund A, Moore RY, Nobin A, Stenevi U: The organization of tubero-hypophyseal and reticulo-infundibular catecholamine neuron systems in the rat brain. Brain Res 51:171–191, 1973.

9. Brownstein MJ, Russell JT, Gainer H: Synthesis, transport, and release of posterior pituitary hormones. Science 207:373–378, 1980.

10. Bugnon C, Bloch B, Lenys D, Fellmann D: Infundibular neurons of the human hypothalamus simultaneously reactive with antisera against endorphins, ACTH, MSH and B-LPH. Cell Tissue Res 199:177–196, 1979.

11. Bugnon C, Fellmann D, Gouget A, Cardot J: Corticoliberin in rat brain: Immunocytochemical identification and localization of a novel neuroglandular system. Neurosci Lett 30:25–30, 1982.

12. Green JD, Harris GW: The neurovascular link between the neurohypophysis and adenohypophysis. J Endocrinol 5:136–146, 1947.

13. Gross DS, Page RB: Luteinizing hormone and follicle-stimulating hormone production in the pars tuberalis of hypophysectomized rats. Am J Anat 156:285–291, 1979.

14. Habener JF: Principles of peptide-hormone biosynthesis, in Martin JB, Reichlin S, Bick KL (eds): *Neurosecretion and Brain Peptides* (Advances in Biochemical Psychopharmacology, vol 28). New York, Raven Press, 1981, pp 21–34.

15. Hardy J, Beauregard H, Robert F: Prolactin-secreting pituitary adenomas: Transsphenoidal microsurgical treatment. Clin Neurosurg 27:38–47, 1980.

16. Herzog AG, Russell V, Vaitukaitis JL, Geschwind N: Neuroendocrine dysfunction in temporal lobe epilepsy. Arch Neurol 39:133–135, 1982.

17. Johansson O, Hökfelt T: Thyrotropin releasing hormone, somatostatin, and enkephalin: distribution studies using immunohistochemical techniques. J Histochem Cytochem 28:364–366, 1980.

18. Knigge KM, Scott DE: Structure and function of the median eminence. Am J Anat 129:223–244, 1970.

19. Krieger DT, Perlow MJ, Gibson MJ, Davies TF, Zimmerman EA, Ferin M, Charlton HM: Brain grafts reverse hypogonadism of gonadotropin releasing hormone deficiency. Nature 298:468–471, 1982.

20. Labrie F, Godbout M, Lagacé L, Massicotte J, Ferland L, Barden N, Drouin J, Lépine J, Lissitzky J-C, Raymond V, Borgeat P, Beaulieu M, Veilleux R: Mechanism of action of hypothalamic hormones and interaction with peripheral hormones at the pituitary level, in Motta M (ed): *The Endocrine Functions of the Brain* (Comprehensive Endocrinology). New York, Raven Press, 1980, pp 207–231.

21. Lechan RM, Jackson IMD: Immunohistochemical localization of thyrotropin-releasing hormone in the rat hypothalamus and pituitary. Endocrinology 111:55–65, 1982.

22. Lechan RM, Nestler JL, Jacobson S, Reichlin S: The hypothalamic "tubero-infundibular" system of the rat as demonstrated by horseradish peroxidase (HRP) microiontophoresis. Brain Res 195:13–27, 1980.

23. Lederis K: Neurosecretion and the functional structure of the neurohypophysis, in Greep RO and Astwood EB (eds): *Handbook of Physiology*, sec 7: Endocrinology, vol 4: *The Pituitary Gland and Its Neuroendocrine Control*, pt 1. Washington, American Physiological Society, 1974, pp 81–102.

24. Louis KM, Cogen P, Manasia A, Ferin M, Antunes JL: Endocrine function in the Klüver-Bucy syndrome: Studies in adult female rhesus monkeys. Neurosurgery 9:287–291, 1981.

25. Mains RE, Eipper BA: Synthesis and secretion of ACTH, B-endorphin, and related peptides, in Martin JB, Reichlin S, Bick KL (eds): *Neurosecretion and Brain Peptides* (Advances in Biochemical Psychopharmacology, vol 28). New York, Raven Press, 1981, pp 35–47.

26. McKelvy JF, Charli J-L, Joseph-Bravo P, Sherman T, Loudes C: Cellular biochemistry of brain peptides: Biosynthesis, degradation, packaging, transport, and release, in Motta M (ed): *The Endocrine Functions of the Brain*. New York, Raven Press, 1980, pp 171–193.

27. Merchenthaler I, Kovács G, Lovász G, Sétáló G: The preoptico-infundibular LH-RH tract of the rat. Brain Res 198:63–74, 1980.

28. Nauta WJH, Haymaker W: Hypothalamic nuclei and fiber connections, in Haymaker W, Anderson E, Nauta WJH (eds): *The Hypothalamus*. Springfield, Ill., Charles C Thomas, 1969, pp 136–209.

29. Page RB: Pituitary blood flow, a review. Am J Physiol 243:E427–442, 1982.

30. Palkovits M, Eskay RL, Brownstein MJ: The course of thyrotropin-releasing hormone fibers to the median eminence in rats. Endocrinology 110:1526–1528, 1982.

31. Pearse AGE: Observations on the localisation, nature and chemical constitution of some components of the anterior hypophysis. J Pathol 64:791–809, 1952.

32. Pearse AGE, Takor TT: Neuroendocrine embryology and the APUD concept. Clin Endocrinol 5:229s–244s, 1976.

33. Peters LL, Hoefer MT, Ben-Jonathan N: The posterior pituitary: Regulation of anterior pituitary prolactin secretion. Science 213:659–661, 1981.

34. Proulx-Ferland L, Labrie F, Dumont D, Cote J, Coy DH, Sveiraf J: Corticotropin-releasing factor stimulates secretion of melanocyte-stimulating hormone from the rat pituitary. Science 217:62–63, 1982.

35. Rioch DM, Wislocki GB, O'Leary JL: A précis of preoptic, hypothalamic and hypophyseal terminology with atlas. Res Publ Assoc Res Nerv Ment Dis 20:3–30, 1939.

36. Sawchenko PE, Swanson LW, Joseph SA: The distribution and cells of origin of ACTH(1–39)-stained varicosities in the paraventricular and supraoptic nuclei. Brain Res 232:365–374, 1982.

37. Scharrer E, Scharrer B: Secretory cells within the hypothalamus. Res Publ Assoc Res Nerv Ment Dis 20:170–194, 1939.

38. Sofroniew MV, Weindl A: Projections from the parvocellular vasopressin- and neurophysin-containing neurons of the suprachiasmatic nucleus. Am J Anat 153:391–430, 1978.

39. Swanson LW, Kuypers HGJM: The paraventricular nucleus of the hypothalamus: Cytoarchitectonic subdivisions and organization of projections to the pituitary, dorsal vagal complex, and spinal cord as demonstrated by retrograde fluorescence double-labeling methods. J Comp Neurol 194:555–570, 1980.

40. Swanson LW, Sawchenko PE: Paraventricular nucleus: A site for the integration of neuroendocrine and autonomic mechanisms. Neuroendocrinology 31:410–417, 1980.

41. Takor TT, Pearse AGE: Neuroectodermal origin of avian hypothalamo-hypophyseal complex: The role of the ventral neural ridge. J Embryol Exp Morphol 34:311–325, 1975.

42. Visser M, Swabb DF: Alpha-MSH in the human pituitary. Front Horm Res 4:42–45, 1977.

43. Weiss S, Bergland R, Page R, Turpen C, Hymer WC: Pituitary cell transplants to the cerebral ventricles promote growth of hypophysectomized rats. Proc Soc Exp Biol Med 159:409–413, 1978.
44. Wiegand SJ, Price JL: Cells of origin of the afferent fibers to the median eminence in the rat. J Comp Neurol 192:1–19, 1980.
45. Wislocki GB, King LS: The permeability of the hypophysis and hypothalamus to vital dyes, with a study of the hypophyseal vascular supply. Am J Anat 58:421–472, 1936.

91

Anatomy and Physiology of the Neurohypophysis

William A. Shucart
Ivor M. D. Jackson

The hypothalamus forms the inferior and lateral walls of the third ventricle, extending from the optic chiasm to the caudal border of the mamillary bodies (a distance of about 10 mm in the adult) and is divided into three regions: (1) the supraoptic area dorsal to the optic chiasm, (2) the central tuberal region, and (3) the caudal mamillary region.[6] The neurohypophysis consists of a portion of the base of the hypothalamus, the neural stalk, and the neural (posterior) lobe of the pituitary gland. The median eminence of the tuber cinereum, while anatomically part of the neurohypophyseal portion of the hypothalamus, is involved primarily in the regulation of anterior pituitary function.

Nerve cells scattered throughout the hypothalamus have been designated as small, or parvocellular (10 to 15 mm), with no distinguishing features, while others are large, or magnocellular (20 to 35 mm) and clustered together to form prominent nuclei. These magnocellular neurons are located in the paired supraoptic nuclei (SON) situated above the optic tract and paraventricular nuclei (PVN) immediately beneath the ependyma of the third ventricle.[4,13] The unmyelinated nerve fibers from these large cells descend through the infundibulum and neural stalk to end in the neural lobe of the pituitary gland, forming the supraopticohypophyseal and paraventriculohypophyseal tracts.[10] The vasopressinergic and oxytocinergic fibers in the external lamina of the median eminence appear to arise primarily from the medial parvocellular group in the PVN. This neuronal system is the probable source of the vasopressin transported in the portal vessel circulation to the anterior pituitary. Magnocellular neuronal perikarya that stain for vasopressin predominate in both the SON and the PVN. However, only scanty oxytocinergic cell bodies are found in the SON, most being located in the PVN.

Recently vasopressin and the opioid peptide dynorphin have been localized to the same magnocellular neuron by immunohistochemical techniques.[15] Glucagon, cholecystokinin, and angiotensin II-like immunoreactivities have also been identified in magnocellular neurosecretory systems, but the functional significance of this coexistence has not yet been established. The neurohypophyseal hormones are synthesized as part of a large precursor glycopeptide (propressophysin and pro-oxyphysin), which also contains carrier proteins (nicotine-sensitive neurophysin for vasopressin and estrogen-sensitive neurophysin for oxytocin). These are then transported in secretory vesicles (packets of hormone and carrier protein) down the axons for storage in the posterior pituitary gland.

Experimental section of the hypophyseal stalk results in the accumulation of colloid substance granules varying from 500 to 2000 nm in diameter above and their disappearance below the transection. The stored vesicles in the nerve endings are situated on delicate membranes which are separated from the basement membranes of adjacent capillaries by a narrow perivascular space. This anatomical juxtaposition allows the posterior lobe neurons to act as endocrine organs, i.e., they become cells of the type referred to as *neuroendocrine transducers*, which convert neural information to hormonal information. Indeed, the impetus for release of these stored posterior lobe hormones is an action potential originating in the neuronal cell body.

The neurons of the neurohypophysis are primarily regulated by β-adrenergic (inhibitory) and cholinergic (stimulatory) neurotransmitters. α-Adrenergic agonists and prostaglandins of the E group also release ADH. However, magnocellular neurons are also stimulated by neuropeptides, particularly angiotensin II and endogenous opiates (endorphins), which may function as physiological modulators of posterior pituitary hormone secretion.

Vasopressin

While it is now clear that vasopressin has a wide distribution throughout the central nervous system, where it may act as a neurotransmitter or neuromodulator quite unrelated to posterior pituitary function,[5] its only established function is its role as the antidiuretic hormone (ADH). Following its release, ADH is transported in the blood to the distal renal tubule and collecting ducts, where, after binding to specific receptors on the cell membrane, it activates adenyl cyclase;

this leads to the generation of cyclic AMP (cAMP), which operates as an intracellular second messenger. The hormonal activity causes a change in the configuration of the luminal membrane of the cells of the distal renal tubules and collecting ducts, altering their permeability to water, urea, and possibly sodium. The net effect of this chain of events is increased reabsorption of water from the nephron back into the circulation.[2]

Endogenous prostaglandins (mainly E_2) appear to antagonize the effect of vasopressin-activated (cAMP), while inhibitors of prostaglandin synthesis such as indomethacin enhance the effect of vasopressin. Other substances or conditions which impair the generation or action of vasopressin include hypercalcemia, hypokalemia, lithium, and the antibiotic demeclocycline. This effect of lithium and demeclocycline accounts for their therapeutic effect in clinical states of vasopressin "excess," as in the syndrome of inappropriate ADH secretion (SIADH).

The interplay between thirst and antidiuretic hormone—the two most important factors in maintaining fluid balance—is controlled by information received from both osmoreceptors and volume receptors. The osmoreceptors are situated in the anterior hypothalamus but appear to be outside the blood-brain barrier. When plasma osmolality rises, these receptors cells shrink, and the formation and release of ADH into the circulation is stimulated. A decrease in osmolality has the opposite effect. As first demonstrated by Verney, the prime factor regulating ADH secretion is plasma osmolality.[14] In the event of severe hypovolemia (a loss of more than 10 to 15 percent of blood volume) the maintenance of volume takes priority over the maintenance of osmotic balance. There is some evidence that volume receptors themselves may have a regulatory effect on osmoreceptor function.

The volume receptors affecting ADH secretion are located peripherally, in the left atrium, in the pulmonary veins, and, as stretch receptors, in the arterial circulation. These receptors respond to changes in volume and arterial pressure and, through neuronal pathways, lead to an increase or decrease in ADH secretion in order to maintain normal volume.

The renin-angiotensin system is also concerned with the preservation of volume. If renal perfusion is decreased (e.g., as a result of decreased blood volume), more of the enzyme renin is released. Renin activates the conversion of angiotensinogen to angiotensin I (decapeptide), which in turn is converted to angiotensin II (octapeptide). Angiotensin II acts on the hypothalamus not only to promote ADH secretion but also to increase thirst, both effects designed to restore volume.

It should be noted that within the hypothalamus there is an independent neuronal renin-angiotensin system, all the components of which arise in situ. It appears likely that both central and peripheral angiotensin II regulate thirst and vasopressin secretion, but the relative physiological importance of each system has not been established.

A wide variety of pharmacological agents affect the release or action of ADH. Thyroid hormone and cortisol appear to modulate the osmotic set point for the release of ADH. Thus hypothyroidism and hypoadrenocorticism enhance ADH release and contribute to the hyponatremia seen

in these disorders. Glucocorticoid excess raises the osmotic threshhold for ADH release and can exacerbate a borderline diabetes insipidus. Some drugs which enhance ADH release the nicotine, chlorpropamide, cholinergic drugs, clofibrate, barbiturates, morphine, anesthetic agents, and carbamazepine. Agents which decrease release of ADH include water, ethanol, phenytoin, and anticholinergic agents.

"Higher" neural centers have an effect on ADH secretion, as evidenced by the increased ADH release seen in pain, nausea, and stress (both emotional and physical) and the ability experimentally to bring about either diuresis or antidiuresis by hypnotic suggestion or psychological conditioning.

It is of interest, and perhaps of some clinical importance, that when the neurohypophyseal system is isolated from the neural input of other parts of the brain, the system is more active electrically and ADH secretion is increased. This isolation or "denervation" hyperfunction of the neurohypophyseal system may explain in part some of the abnormalities of ADH secretion seen in some patients with brain injuries.

Oxytocin

Oxytocin, like vasopressin, is a member of the family of neuropeptides, now numbering over thirty, which are distributed throughout the CNS. In extrapituitary locations oxytocin probably functions as a neurotransmitter or neuromodulator;[5] this role is quite separate from its established physiological role related to reproduction. The hormone has a selective effect on the smooth muscle of the uterus and plays a major role in the expulsion of the fetus and placenta. Labor can begin in a patient with deficient posterior pituitary function but may be prolonged. It is possible that other hormonally induced changes in the uterus make it sensitive to normal concentrations of oxytocin, and uterine contraction becomes enhanced only when the proper hormonal priming has taken place.

Oxytocin also causes contraction of the myoepithelial cells of the breast. These cells cause the glands to express their contents into ducts so that the milk will accumulate in the nipples. Once nursing has started, the release of oxytocin appears to be stimulated via a neural reflex arc which is activated by sensory nerve endings in the nipple.

The secretion of vasopressin and of oxytocin are independent of each other. This has been demonstrated in lactating women in two ways: (1) the normal sucking stimulus will induce milk letdown without accompanying antidiuresis, and (2) intravenous hypertonic saline infusion will increase ADH production without producing milk letdown.

Diabetes Insipidus

The requirements for normal water balance include adequate ADH production, normal osmoreceptors in the hypothalamus, normally functioning nephrons, a relatively normal renal medulla such that the osmolar gradient necessary for water reabsorption can be maintained, a normal thirst center, and the ability to respond to thirst in an appropriate way.[12] It becomes clear that the clinical picture of diabetes insipidus (DI; polyuria secondary to water diuresis and polydipsia) may result from dysfunction in any of these areas.[8]

Central (neurogenic) DI is caused by insufficient ADH production in the hypothalamus.[11] Inability to secrete ADH results in excretion of a dilute urine. Failure to counter this fluid loss results in dehydration, hemoconcentration, and hypovolemia. Destruction of the hypothalamic centers or division of the supraoptic tract above the median eminence causes permanent diabetes insipidus. Transection below the median eminence, including removal of the posterior pituitary lobe, causes only a transient polyuria: It appears that sufficient ADH can be released from fibers at the level of the median eminence. Nephrogenic diabetes insipidus (impaired activity of vasopressin at the level of the kidney) may be the expression of a congenital abnormality or may result from an acquired disorder (e.g., chronic renal disease, electrolyte disorders, administration of certain drugs).

Diabetes insipidus usually becomes clinically apparent because of polyuria. The differential diagnosis of polyuria includes diabetes mellitus, hypercalcinuria, psychogenic polydipsia, chronic renal failure, and the various forms of diabetes insipidus. Abnormalities of glucose metabolism, electrolyte balance and renal function can usually be ruled out with routine laboratory studies. The next step is to determine whether solute or water excretion is causing the diuresis.

When solute excretion is responsible for the diuresis, the urinary specific gravity is usually between 1.010 and 1.035; urine osmolality is usually greater than 300 mosm/kg; and serum sodium is variable—e.g., it may be low in hyperglycemia with glucose diuresis or high in subjects dehydrated by high-protein tube feedings. In mild solute diuresis the urine osmolality may be high, e.g., 800 mosm/L; as the rate of solute excretion increases, however, an increasing amount of water will escape reabsorption in the proximal tubule and the urine will approach isotonicity. In the neurosurgical patient population the major causes of solute diuresis are osmotic diuretics, hyperglycemia, and corticosteroid deficiency leading to an inability to retain sodium.

If polyuria is secondary to water diuresis, as in diabetes insipidus, the urinary specific gravity is usually between 1.001 and 1.005; urine osmolality is usually between 50 and 150 mosm/kg; serum sodium is normal or, if there is a water balance deficit, increased; and thirst is usually a prominent clinical feature. The common causes of water diuresis in the neurosurgical patient include (1) diabetes insipidus (Table 91-1) (2) chronic renal insufficiency—the patient is usually azotemic with abnormal renal function studies; (3) nephropathy secondary to multiple myeloma, amyloidosis, sickle cell disease, radiation nephritis, or systemic lupus erythematosus or following the relief of obstructive uropathy; (4) recovery phase of acute tubular necrosis—may be secondary to ischemic or toxic injury; and (5) fluid overload—this is a particularly important consideration in the perioperative period, when the patient's fluid intake is parenterally administered and not regulated by the thirst mechanism.

Simultaneous measurement of urine and serum osmolality can provide valuable information. In all instances of water diuresis the urine is hypo-osmolar, but the serum

TABLE 91-1 Types and Causes of Diabetes Insipidus

Type	Cause
Neurogenic (central):	
Primary	Familial; idiopathic
Secondary	Head trauma; neurosurgical procedures; hypothalamic disease
Nephrogenic (congenital)	Unresponsive renal tubules in males (sex-linked)
Nephrogenic (acquired)	Electrolyte disorders: hypercalcemia, hypokalemia Chronic renal disease Drugs, e.g., lithium, demeclocycline Excess water intake

osmolality is normal or increased in DI and usually reduced in compulsive water drinking (Table 91-2). When the serum is hyperosmolar, the administration of ADH will differentiate between central diabetes insipidus (there will be a response of water conservation) and nephrogenic diabetes insipidus (no response to ADH). Patients with psychogenic polydipsia may be resistant to exogenous vasopressin because of diminished renal medullary tonicity from chronic water intake. Compulsive polydipsia is most often secondary to a behavioral disorder, but the possibility of habitual water drinking secondary to an organic abnormality of the thirst center should also be considered.

It should be kept in mind that hyperosmolality of the serum seen in association with hyperosmolality of the urine is caused by lack of water intake and not DI. This situation can be seen in patients with defective thirst mechanisms or with impaired levels of consciousness such that they do not recognize their thirst and in those who either have no access to water or are unable to drink water.

The diagnosis becomes difficult in patients with mild or compensated diabetes insipidus, in whom the serum osmolality may be relatively normal despite a hypo-osmolar urine.[7] It is in these less obvious cases that provocative testing is required; a modified dehydration test is usually adequate.

The patient is deprived of all fluids until three consecutive hourly urine specimens have the same specific gravity, usually 6 to 12 from the start of testing in patients with partial DI, less in patients with severe DI. The body weight is measured before and during the test, and no more than a 3 to 4 percent loss of body weight is allowed. The serum and

TABLE 91-2 Abnormalities of Urine and Serum Osmolality and Their Most Common Causes

Osmolality Change from Normal		
Urine	Serum	Most Common Cause
Decreased	Normal	Mild or compensated DI, excess water intake
Decreased	Increased	Any cause of water diuresis, most commonly DI
Decreased	Decreased	Psychogenic polydipsia
Increased	Increased	Dehydration

urine osmolality are measured simultaneously, 1-deamino-8-D-arginine vasopressin (desmopressin, DDAVP) is given (10 μg intranasally), and the serum and urine osmolality are then measured hourly for an additional 2 to 4 h. Patients with diabetes insipidus from any cause will show an abnormally high serum osmolality (more than 295 mosm/kg, and often much higher) prior to DDAVP. In central diabetes insipidus a 10 percent or greater increase in the urine osmolality will occur, whereas in nephrogenic diabetes insipidus the DDAVP will have no effect. In some cases measurement of endogenous plasma vasopressin and its responsiveness to dehydration can help to distinguish cases of compulsive water drinking or nephrogenic DI from central DI.[16]

The clinical expression of diabetes insipidus in postoperative and post-traumatic situations can be variable, and the permanence of the diabetes insipidus cannot always be predicted in the early stages. It is well documented that an occasional patient may require months, or even years, to regain an adequate level of ADH function. It should also be kept in mind that patients who do not have clinically obvious problems may, given the appropriate stimuli, have a transient appearance of diabetes insipidus. This latter phenomenon can be seen with increased ethanol intake or a significant increase in corticosteroid dosage.

The clinical course of diabetes insipidus following head injury or surgery in the hypothalamic area usually follows one or four major patterns:

1. The most common situation is transient polyuria starting 1 to 3 days after surgery and lasting 1 to 7 days. This may follow traction on the pituitary stalk and seems to be an expression of hypothalamic rather than pituitary dysfunction. The onset and duration of this syndrome are compatible with the onset and dissolution of local edema.

2. A triphasic pattern has been described both in humans and in experimental animals. Polyuria beginning 1 to 2 days after surgery lasts 1 to 7 days and is followed by a period of normal urinary output lasting up to several days; abnormally large urinary output then resumes and persists. This triphasic response was produced in experimental animals by transection of the pituitary stalk and destruction of the hypothalamic median eminence if the posterior lobe of the pituitary gland was left in place; if the posterior lobe was removed, there was an immediate and permanent polyuria. The interphase of normal urinary output appears to be secondary to the release of ADH stored previously in the posterior pituitary gland: when the previously stored ADH has been completely utilized, permanent diabetes insipidus ensues.

3. Polyuria may begin within the first 2 to 3 postoperative days and be followed by a small decrease in total urinary volume over the next several days. This is seen in patients with a partial ADH deficiency which is magnified in the initial stages because of superimposed local edema.

4. Permanent polyuria develops within the first 2 to 3 postoperative days and continues thereafter with no interphase and no significant change in urinary output volumes. This is seen in patients with immediate, extensive damage to the hypothalamus. After previously formed ADH has been used up, there is no recovery of borderline viable cells to produce ADH and modify the postoperative course.

Treatment of Acute Diabetes Insipidus

The several patterns of expression of clinical diabetes insipidus mentioned above should be kept in mind when formulating a postoperative treatment plan. Therapeutic regimens need to be flexible, since the degree and duration of the disease process are uncertain.

Patients with significant diabetes insipidus preoperatively seldom have any postoperative improvement. In that group of patients it is reasonable to resume preoperative medical treatment as soon as practical.

Patients likely to develop diabetes insipidus following surgery (i.e., those with surgery in and around the hypothalamic and pituitary area) are treated expectantly. Until polyuria becomes apparent, the patient is treated with standard parenteral fluid replacement. Urinary output should be closely monitored, with volume and specific gravity readings every 1 to 2 h if the patient has an indwelling bladder catheter, otherwise as urine specimens are obtained. The body weight should be recorded prior to surgery and at least once a day in the postoperative period. The patient who is able to take liquids by mouth in the prepolyuria phase is allowed to drink at will, but careful charting of intake and output must continue.

When polyuria appears, treatment is determined primarily by the patient's clinical status and the urine volume. A patient who is alert and taking food by mouth may be able to regulate the fluid intake satisfactorily as dictated by thirst. Body weight and serum electrolytes are measured daily. If the urinary output exceeds an average of 250 ml/h for two consecutive hours or 3 to 4 liters per day, or if the patient is unable to maintain adequate intake orally, medication is given. If the patient is awake and there is no contraindication to intranasal agents, DDAVP is administered. If the surgery has been trans-sphenoidal or if there is some other contraindication to intranasal medication, Pitressin (vasopressin injection, Parke-Davis, Morris Plains, N.J.) is used. The most difficult management problem is the patient unable to maintain adequate oral intake, particularly the lethargic or obtunded patient. In the latter the clinical parameter of thirst is lost and meticulous fluid intake and output records become essential. Twice-daily weight records provide a valuable guide to the state of hydration. If fluid intake and output are approximately equal, the patient may maintain the weight or occasionally lose a small amount of weight but will never gain weight. If the urinary output is very large or there is concern about the patient's status, the serum electrolytes, blood urea nitrogen (BUN), and hematocrit are measured twice a day. If the level of urinary output is relatively low, once-a-day measurement of these various indexes is adequate. The serum osmolality is best measured directly but can be estimated (within 5 percent) if the serum electrolytes, BUN, and blood sugar are known:

$$\text{Serum osmolality} = 2 \times \text{Na (meq/L)} + \frac{\text{blood glucose}}{18} \text{ (mg/dl)} + \frac{\text{BUN}}{3} \text{ (mg/dl)}$$

With normal blood sugar, a fairly reliable rough estimate is 2 times the serum sodium (mEq/L) plus 10. An attempt should be made to equalize fluid intake with fluid output. The equalization can be done at intervals varying from 1 h to 1 day, depending on the degree of polyuria. If the patient has a large urinary output (over 300 ml/h) it is best to maintain balance on an hourly basis; if the urinary output is less than that it is reasonable to maintain fluid balance on a 4 to 6 h basis.

Since fluid replacement should be as free water, intravenous fluids should consist almost solely of dextrose-in-water solutions and oral fluids such as tap water. The only electrolyte replacement required in the postoperative period is what would normally be given to a postoperative patient; this should be administered as 1 liter of a balanced electrolyte solution and should not be divided in several infusions.

If salt solutions are used continuously, they deliver a continuing solute load to the kidneys which will aggravate the renal loss of water. Solute concentration cannot be increased in the absence of ADH. The administration of saline solutions as replacement for the urinary loss in diabetes insipidus is probably the commonest error in the management of this problem.

In the awake patient with an intact thirst mechanism it is possible to replace by oral intake very large urinary outputs, particularly if some intravenous supplementation is also used. In the very young or in older patients with associated medical problems, it is preferable to keep fluid intake at lower levels. Pitressin or one of its analogues can be used at any time in the postoperative period if there is careful monitoring of fluid balance.

A so-called iatrogenic inappropriate ADH syndrome can be created in patients given exogenous Pitressin and excess water by mouth or parenterally. This complication can and should be avoided with careful management. The two most important things to remember in managing acute diabetes insipidus are that the primary problem is water loss and that the process is not static but dynamic.

Treatment of Chronic Diabetes Insipidus

Posterior Pituitary Hormone Preparations

Aqueous vasopressin is a sterile solution of synthetic 8-arginine vasopressin available in 0.5 and 1-ml ampules of 20 IU/ml. The short duration of action (4 to 6 h) makes this preparation unsuitable for prolonged use. In the acute stage a slow, continuous infusion of not more than 3 IU/h or intermittent intramuscular injections of 0.1 to 1.0 ml are usually effective.

Pitressin tannate in oil is a water-insoluble compound of vasopressin obtained from animal sources and supplied in 1-ml ampules with a strength of 5 IU/ml. It is given intramuscularly and is effective in doses of 0.25 to 1 ml. This agent has a variable but long duration of action (24 to 72 h) and is therefore suitable for chronic severe cases. If the vial is not warmed and shaken thoroughly prior to administration, the active moiety may precipitate out. Local or systemic allergic reactions may occur in hypersensitive persons.

Lysine vasopressin (Diapid, Sandoz Pharmaceuticals, East Hanover, N.J.) nasal spray is a synthetic preparation of vasopressin 8-lysine. It is supplied in a plastic bottle (5 ml) containing 50 IU/ml. Administration of one or two sprays up each nostril three or four times a day may produce good control of the diabetes. Each spray delivers approximately 2 IU. This agent is most effective in mild cases.

Arginine vasopressin (desmopressin acetate, DDAVP, Armour Pharmaceutical Co., Tarrytown, N.Y.), a vasopressin analogue, is a synthetic preparation which is administered intranasally once or twice per day in a dose of 5 to 20 μg (0.05 to 0.2 ml).[3] Its altered chemical structure, relative to vasopressin, retards its degradation, and it has high antidiuretic-to-pressor potency (2000:1). This agent is now the drug of choice for vasopressin-sensitive diabetes insipidus. It is usually self-administered intranasally through a calibrated plastic catheter but may be given even to the unconscious patient (the end of the tube is attached to an air-filled syringe). Intranasal preparations are not practical for a time after trans-sphenoidal surgery, and alternate parenteral preparations for ADH must be given. Intravenous DDAVP, not yet available in the United States, has been reported from Europe as being effective.

Nonpituitary Preparations

In recent years it has been appreciated that a number of drugs may be effective in reducing urine volume when given orally.[9] Among these is chlorpropamide, an oral hypoglycemic agent that may effectively reduce the polyuria in hypothalamic but not in nephrogenic diabetes insipidus. The drug appears to act by potentiating the antidiuretic effect of low levels of endogenous ADH. It is most effective in mild cases, in which the usual dosage is 50 to 250 mg per day. Antabuse-like symptoms and hypoglycemia occasionally cause problems as side effects of this drug.

Paradoxically, thiazide diuretics are the only effective drugs for the treatment of congenital nephrogenic diabetes insipidus. The presence of vasopressin is not required for action, and the mechanism is probably contraction of the extracellular fluid volume secondary to loss of sodium. Hydrochlorothiazide should be used in doses of 50 to 100 mg per day. Potassium supplements may be required. The use of chlorpropamide and hydrochlorothiazide together, often in only small doses, may be effective in neurogenic diabetes insipidus because of a synergistic effect. Further, the thiazide diuretic helps to counteract the hypoglycemia which may be a problem in patients with growth hormone or ACTH deficiency when they are treated with chlorpropamide alone.

Other agents include carbamazepine (used as an anticonvulsant and in the treatment of tic douloureux), the antineoplastic agents vincristine and cyclophosphamide, the hypolipidemic agent clofibrate, and the analgesic acetaminophen. All may be effective in mild diabetes insipidus by effecting the release of vasopressin and/or enhancing its effect on the kidney. Carbamazepine, in particular, may potentiate the action of chlorpropamide.

Pharmacological and Physiological Interactions with ADH

1. **Diphenylhydantoin.** This commonly used agent suppresses the release of both ADH and insulin. The enhancement of free water clearance seldom leads to a significant enough water diuresis to be clinically important,

but occasional severe hyperglycemic episodes have been reported. In patients with partial or difficult-to-control diabetes insipidus, this drug should probably not be used.

2. **Glucocorticoids.** Glucocorticoid administration frequently leads to the full clinical expression of an underlying ADH deficiency. The DI does not disappear when the doses of glucocorticoids are decreased, although there may be a lessening of severity. The effect of high steroid dosages on patients with trauma affecting the hypothalamus or with surgery in the hypothalamic-pituitary area may, on the contrary, benefit DI by reduction of local edema.

3. **Thyroid hormone.** It should also be pointed out that not only cortisol but also thyroid hormone affects the secretion of ADH. Patients with severe hypothyroidism frequently have hyponatremia due to an "inappropriate ADH-like" syndrome, and thyroid deficiency as well as adrenocortical deficiency may alleviate the severity of concomitant DI.

Syndrome of Inappropriate Secretion of Antidiuretic Hormone (SIADH)

This syndrome was initially proposed to explain the occurrence of renal salt loss and hyponatremia in patients having neither renal nor adrenal disease. The basis of the syndrome is an overexpansion of extracellular fluid (ECF) resulting from abnormal secretion of ADH. The primary features of SIADH remain those described initially:[1]

1. Hyponatremia with corresponding hypo-osmolality of the serum and extracellular fluid
2. Continued renal excretion of sodium (>20 meq/L)
3. Absence of fluid volume depletion (serum creatinine and BUN are usually low, in contradistinction to hyponatremia from ECF depletion)
4. Greater osmolality of the urine than is appropriate for the osmolality of the plasma
5. Normal renal function and normal adrenal function
6. Absence of peripheral edema

The syndrome is characterized by (1) persistence of the hyponatremia despite the administration of sodium (even if several hundred milliequivalents of sodium per day is infused, nearly all of it is lost in the urine) and (2) an abnormal response to a water load: excess water is retained and not promptly eliminated.

In the broadest classification, SIADH is a form of dilutional hyponatremia, and the sine qua non of SIADH is increased ECF volume. The size of the increase is usually 3 to 4 liters, so peripheral edema is not present. Because of the expanded extracellular volume, the glomerular filtration rate is increased and the renin-angiotensin-aldosterone mechanism suppressed, leading to a decrease in the renal reabsorption of sodium. Another factor, the hypothetical "third factor," is also of importance in explaining the salt loss in SIADH. The third factor effect is suppression of proximal tubular reabsorption of sodium when extracellular fluid volume is expanded; this appears to be brought about by renal

hemodynamic changes. A state is reached in which patients with SIADH excrete essentially all their dietary intake of sodium, and this tends to stabilize the ECF expansion. The determining factor in the degree of hyponatremia as well as fluid volume expansion is water intake.

SIADH can occur in a wide variety of CNS disorders, including encephalitis, stroke, head trauma, and brain tumors. It has also been described in pulmonary disorders such as fungal, viral, and bacterial pneumonia. The ADH is secreted from the neurohypophysis but is no longer under its normal regulatory influences. Whether there is a functional alteration in osmo-receptor function, or inappropriate information is being transmitted centrally from peripheral volume receptors, or some other situation prevails is uncertain. In some instances SIADH may result from the ectopic production of ADH from a tumor such as oat cell carcinoma of the bronchus. Since surgical stress, morphine, barbiturates, and anesthetics may all stimulate ADH secretion, a transient form of SIADH can occur in the immediate postoperative period.

Symptoms in SIADH are related to hyponatremia, which becomes a problem primarily because of hypo-osmolality. Pseudohyponatremia can be seen in association with increased blood glucose, hyperlipidemia, administration of mannitol, etc.; in these cases the effective osmolality of the serum is not reduced.

SIADH usually causes no symptoms until the serum sodium concentration falls below 120 meq/L, but if there is progressive retention of water with rapid reduction in serum sodium, significant symptoms can appear with a serum sodium concentration of more than 120 meq/L. Symptoms are often nonspecific and include anorexia, nausea, irritability, and an accentuation of focal neurological deficits if there is underlying structural brain damage. If the serum sodium concentration drops to less than 110 meq/L, severe neurological dysfunction due to brain edema may occur, with areflexia, diffuse muscle weakness, seizures, and stupor. The appearance of symptoms varies greatly from one patient to another and with the rate of development of the hyponatremia. Rapidly developing hyponatremia (hours) is much more serious than slowly developing hyponatremia (days), since the cell volume regulatory mechanisms may not have time to act before cerebral edema occurs.

The treatment of SIADH is determined by the severity of the symptoms. The basis of all treatment is elimination of excess water and treatment of the underlying disease. In patients with minor symptoms, restriction of fluid intake to about 500 ml per day is adequate. A weight loss of 5 to 10 pounds is generally needed before serum sodium returns to normal. In senile patients or those with behavior disorders, in whom it is difficult to control oral fluid intake, the use of demeclocycline (600 to 1200 mg per day) or lithium carbonate (600 to 900 mg per day), both of which block the renal tubular response to ADH, can be helpful. Furosemide, a loop diuretic which facilitates free water clearance, may also be useful at 40 to 60 mg per day.

If symptoms are acute and severe, the patient's serum osmolality should be raised quickly. Hypertonic saline infusions and the use of diuretics will expedite the water loss; 1000 ml of 3% NaCl or 500 ml of 5% NaCl is infused over 4 to 6 h. Furosemide, 40 to 60 mg, can be given intravenously at the beginning of the infusion and may be repeated in 3 to

4 h. Mannitol infusion can also be used to accelerate the water loss.

The differentiation of SIADH from the hyponatremia seen in salt depletion is straightforward: none of the signs of hypovolemia, such as decreased blood pressure, decreased tissue turgor, and elevated BUN, are present. The clinical picture most often confused with SIADH is that of the patient with an isotonic fluid loss, usually due to the administration of diuretics, who is treated with hypotonic fluid replacement. In that case the body will sacrifice the maintenance of tonicity for the sake of preserving volume—really a form of hypotonic dehydration. Once again it should be stressed that the absence of an increase in extracellular volume precludes a diagnosis of SIADH.

References

1. Bartter FC, Schwartz WB: The syndrome of inappropriate secretion of antidiuretic hormone. Am J Med 42:790–806, 1967.
2. Buckalew VM Jr, Walker BR, Puschett JB, Goldberg M: Effects of increased sodium delivery on distal tubular sodium reabsorption with and without volume expansion in man. J Clin Invest 49:2336–2344, 1970.
3. Cobb WE, Spare S, Reichlin S: Neurogenic diabetes insipidus: Management with dDAVP (1-desamino-8-D arginine vasopressin). Ann Intern Med 88:183–188, 1978.
4. Defendini R, Zimmerman EA: The magnocellular neurosecretory system of the mammalian hypothalamus. Res Publ Assoc Res Nerv Ment Dis 56:137–152, 1978.
5. Eiden LE, Brownstein MJ: Extrahypothalamic distributions and functions of hypothalamic peptide hormones. Fed Proc 40:2553–2559, 1981.
6. Joseph SA, Knigge KM: The endocrine hypothalamus: Recent anatomical studies. Res Publ Assoc Res Nerv Ment Dis 56:15–47, 1978.
7. Miller M, Dalakos T, Moses AM, Fellerman H, Streeten DHP: Recognition of partial defects in antidiuretic hormone secretion. Ann Intern Med 73:721–729, 1970.
8. Moses AM: Diabetes insipidus and ADH regulation. Hosp Prac 12:37–44, 1977.
9. Moses AM, Miller M: Drug-induced dilutional hyponatremia. N Engl J Med 291:1234–1239, 1974.
10. Reichlin S: Anatomical and physiological basis of hypothalamic-pituitary regulation, in Post KD, Jackson IMD, Reichlin S (eds): The Pituitary Adenoma, New York, Plenum, 1980, pp 3–28.
11. Robertson GL, Aycinena P, Zerbe RL: Neurogenic disorders of osmoregulation. Am J Med 72:339–353, 1982.
12. Schrier RW, Bichet DG: Osmotic and nonosmotic control of vasopressin release and the pathogenesis of impaired water excretion in adrenal, thyroid, and edematous disorders. J Lab Clin Med 98:1–15, 1981.
13. Swanson LW, Kuypers HGJM: The paraventricular nucleus of the hypothalamus. J Comp Neurol 194:555–570, 1980.
14. Verney EB: Absorption and secretion of water: The antidiuretic hormone. Lancet 2:739–744, 781–783, 1946.
15. Watson SJ, Akbil H, Fischli W, Goldstein A, Zimmerman E, Nilaver G, Van Wimersma Greidarus TB: Dynorphin and vasopressin: Common localization in magnocellular neurons. Science 216:85–87, 1982.
16. Zerbe RL, Robertson GL: A comparison of plasma vasopressin measurements with a standard indirect test in the differential diagnosis of polyuria. N Engl J Med 305:1539–1546, 1981.

92
Microsurgical Anatomy of the Sellar Region
Albert L. Rhoton, Jr.

The purpose of this chapter, based on previously reported studies by the author,[1–8] is to review the microsurgical anatomy important to performing the various transcranial and subcranial approaches to the sellar region.

Chiasmatic Configuration and Tuberculum Sellae

The relation of the chiasm to the sella (Figs. 92-1, 92-2) is an important determinant of the ease with which the pituitary fossa may be exposed by the transfrontal surgical route. The normal chiasm overlies the diaphragma sellae and the pituitary, the prefixed chiasm overlies the tuberculum sellae, and the postfixed chiasm overlies the dorsum sellae. In approximately 70 percent of cases the chiasm is in the normal position. Of the remaining 30 percent, about half are prefixed and half postfixed.[4]

A prominent tuberculum sellae may restrict access to the sella even in the presence of a normal chiasm. The tuberculum may vary from being almost flat to protruding upward as much as 3 mm toward the anterior margin of a normal chiasm.[4]

Carotid Artery, Optic Nerve, and Anterior Clinoid Process

An understanding of the relations between the carotid artery, optic nerve, and anterior clinoid process is fundamental to all surgical approaches to the sellar and parasellar areas

A

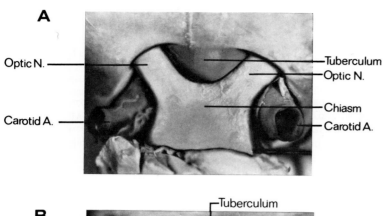

Optic N.

Carotid A.

Tuberculum
Optic N.
Chiasm
Carotid A.

B

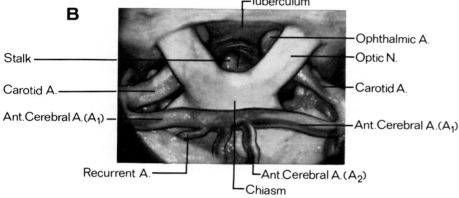

Tuberculum

Stalk

Carotid A.

Ant.Cerebral A.(A₁)

Recurrent A.

Ophthalmic A.
Optic N.
Carotid A.
Ant.Cerebral A.(A₁)
Ant.Cerebral A.(A₂)
Chiasm

C

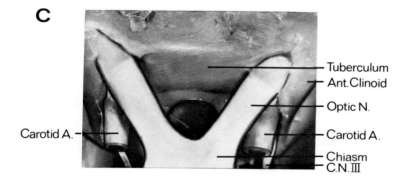

Carotid A.

Tuberculum
Ant.Clinoid
Optic N.
Carotid A.
Chiasm
C.N.III

Figure 92-1 Superior view of the sellar region. *A.* Prefixed chiasm. *B.* Normal chiasm. The ophthalmic artery protrudes medial to the right optic nerve. The anterior cerebral arteries pass dorsal to the chiasm. The left recurrent artery arises from the A_1 segment of the left anterior cerebral artery. The pituitary stalk lies between the optic nerves. *C.* Postfixed chiasm. The diaphragma sellae and pituitary gland have been removed. Cranial nerve III lies ventral to the carotid artery. (From Renn and Rhoton.[4])

(Fig. 92-3). The carotid artery and the optic nerve are medial to the anterior clinoid process. The artery exits the cavernous sinus beneath and slightly lateral to the optic nerve. The optic nerve pursues a posteromedial course toward the chiasm, and the carotid artery a posterolateral course toward its bifurcation into the anterior and middle cerebral arteries.

Optic Canal

The optic nerve proximal to its entrance into the optic canal (Fig. 92-1) is covered by a reflected leaf of dura, the falciform process, which extends medially from the anterior

clinoid process across the top of the optic nerve. The length of nerve covered by dura only at the intracranial end of the optic canal may vary from less than 1 mm to as much as 1 cm. Coagulation of the dura above the optic nerve just proximal to the optic canal on the assumption that bone separates the dura from the nerve could lead to nerve injury. Compression of the optic nerves against the sharp edge of the falciform process may result in a visual field deficit even if the compressing lesion does not damage the nerve enough to cause visual loss. The full length of the optic canal must be unroofed before its narrowest point is passed, because the narrowest part is closer to the orbital than to the intracranial end. The optic canals average 5 mm in length and are of conical configuration, tapering to a narrow waist

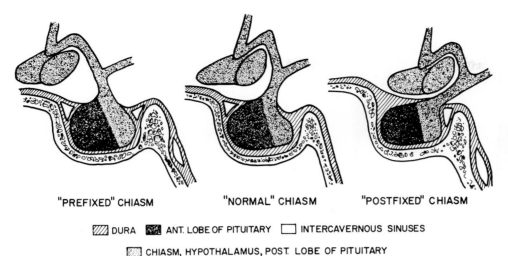

"PREFIXED" CHIASM   "NORMAL" CHIASM   "POSTFIXED" CHIASM

▨ DURA   ▦ ANT. LOBE OF PITUITARY   ☐ INTERCAVERNOUS SINUSES

▨ CHIASM, HYPOTHALAMUS, POST. LOBE OF PITUITARY

Figure 92-2 Three sagittal sections of sellar region. The prefixed chiasm is above the tuberculum, the normal chiasm is above the diaphragma, and the postfixed chiasm is above the dorsum. (From Renn and Rhoton.[4])

near the orbit. The ophthalmic artery is found inferolateral to the optic nerve when the periosteum lining the optic canal is opened.[4]

Suprasellar Arteries

All the arterial components of the circle of Willis and the adjacent carotid artery give origin to multiple perforating branches which may become stretched over suprasellar tumors[7,8] (Fig. 92-3). The supraclinoid portion of the carotid artery, in addition to giving off the posterior communicating and anterior choroid arteries, also gives off perforating branches, which include the superior hypophyseal artery and other branches passing to the optic nerve, chiasm, anterior hypothalamus, and anterior perforated substance. The posterior part of the circle of Willis and the upper centimeter of the basilar artery also send a series of perforating arteries through the suprasellar area into the diencephalon and midbrain which may become stretched around suprasellar tumors. The largest perforating branches arising from the posterior part of the circle of Willis are the thalamoperforate and medial posterior choroid arteries.

The origin and proximal segment of the ophthalmic artery may be visible below the optic nerve without retracting the nerve, although elevation of the optic nerve away from the carotid artery is usually required to see the preforaminal segment (Fig. 92-1). The artery arises above the cavernous sinus in most cases, but it may also arise within the cavernous sinus or be absent in a few cases.[2,4]

The posterior communicating artery arises from the posteromedial wall of the carotid artery (Fig. 92-3). It courses posteromedially above the oculomotor nerve toward the interpeduncular fossa and gives rise to multiple perforating branches which may be stretched over the tip of a suprasellar tumor.

The origin and initial segment of the anterior choroid artery may be visible between the posterior communicating artery and the bifurcation of the internal carotid artery. The initial segment of the anterior choroid artery, which

is directed posterolaterally below the optic tract, may be displaced upward and laterally by sellar tumors (Fig. 92-3).

Each anterior cerebral artery (Fig. 92-3) courses over the superior surface of the optic chiasm or nerve to join the anterior communicating artery.[3] The junction of the anterior communicating artery with the right and left A_1 segments is usually above the chiasm rather than above the optic nerves. The shorter A_1 segments are stretched tightly over the chiasm, and the longer ones pass anteriorly over the nerves. In some cases displacement of the chiasm against these arteries may result in visual loss before that caused by direct compression of the visual pathway by the tumor. The arteries with a more forward course are often tortuous and elongated, and some may course forward and rest on the tuberculum sellae or planum sphenoidale. The anterior cerebral and anterior communicating arteries give rise to multiple branches which terminate in the superior surface of the optic chiasm, the anterior hypothalamus, the anterior perforated substance, and the region of the optic tract.

The recurrent artery of Heubner also arises from the anterior cerebral artery in the region of the anterior communicating artery and runs above the chiasm adjacent to the anterior cerebral artery. The recurrent artery courses anterior to the anterior cerebral artery and is seen when the frontal lobe is elevated prior to visualizing the anterior cerebral artery in about two-thirds of cases.[3]

Diaphragma Sellae

The diaphragma sellae (Fig. 92-4) forms the roof of the sella turcica. It covers the pituitary gland, except for a small central opening which transmits the pituitary stalk. The diaphragma is more rectangular than circular, tends to be convex or concave rather than flat, and is thinner around the infundibulum and somewhat thicker at the periphery. The opening in its center is large compared to the size of the pituitary stalk. The diaphragma is frequently a thin, tenu-

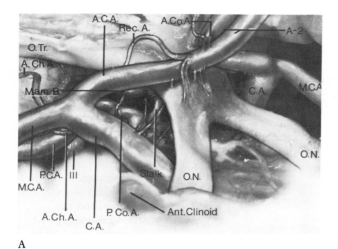

A

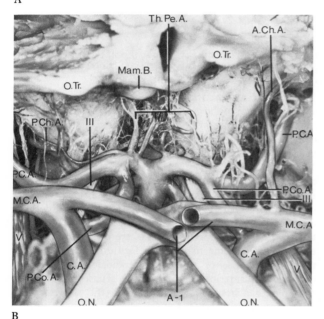

B

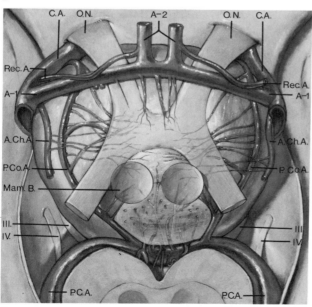

C

Figure 92-3 Arterial relationships of the suprasellar area. *A.* Right anterolateral view. The anterior clinoid process (Ant. Clinoid) is lateral to the carotid artery (C.A.) and the optic nerve (O.N.). Perforating arteries pass from the carotid to terminate in the optic chiasm and tract (O.Tr.) and the hypothalamus anterior to the mamillary body (Mam.B.). The right posterior communicating artery (P.Co.A.) is medial to the carotid artery. The anterior choroid artery (A.Ch.A.) arises from the carotid artery and passes above the posterior cerebral artery (P.C.A.). The third nerve (III) lies below the right posterior cerebral artery. The right recurrent artery (Rec. A.) arises from the anterior cerebral artery (A.C.A.) proximal to the anterior communicating artery (A.Co.A.). Middle cerebral artery (M.C.A); anterior cerebral artery distal to the anterior communicating artery (A-2). *B.* Superior view of the suprasellar area. The posterior part of the optic chiasm has been split at the junction with the optic tracts to give this view. The proximal portion of each anterior cerebral artery (A-1) arises from the carotid artery and passes above the optic nerve and chiasm. The anterior third ventricle lies above the mamillary bodies. The thalamoperforate arteries (Th.Pe.A.) terminate in the retromamillary area and the interpeduncular fossa. The right posterior choroid artery (P.Ch.A.) originates from the posterior cerebral artery. Small branches arise from the posterior cerebral artery and terminate in the peduncle. The left third nerve courses medial to the posterior communicating artery. The right posterior communicating artery joins the posterior cerebral artery medial to the third nerve. The left anterior choroid artery passes lateral to the peduncle and optic tract. The trigeminal nerves (V) are lateral to the carotid arteries. *C.* Superior view of the suprasellar area. Arterial branches of the carotid, basilar, anterior and posterior communicating, anterior and posterior cerebral, recurrent, and anterior choroid arteries are stretched around the superior extension of a pituitary tumor. The anterior cerebral arteries send branches to the superior surface of the optic nerves and chiasm. The posterior communicating, internal carotid, and posterior cerebral arteries send branches into the area below and behind the chiasm. Trochlear nerve (IV). (From Saeki and Rhoton.[7])

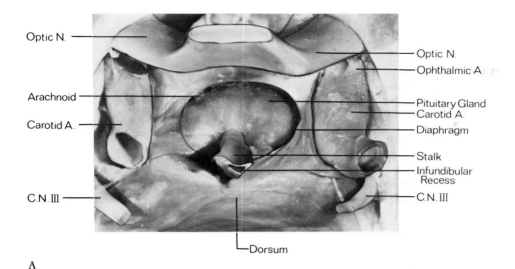

Optic N.

Arachnoid

Carotid A.

C.N. III

Optic N.
Ophthalmic A.
Pituitary Gland
Carotid A.
Diaphragm
Stalk
Infundibular Recess
C.N. III

Dorsum

A

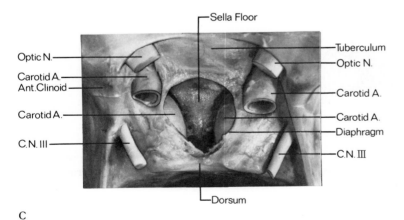

Ophthalmic A.

Carotid A.

Meningo-hypophyseal A.

Tentorial A.
Inferior Hypophyseal A.

Ostium C N III

Carotid A.

Dorsal Meningeal A.

C N VI

Ophthalmic A.

Carotid A.

Anterior Pituitary

C N III

Meningo-hypophyseal A.

Posterior Pituitary

C N VI

B

Sella Floor

Optic N.

Carotid A.
Ant. Clinoid

Carotid A.

C.N. III

Tuberculum
Optic N.

Carotid A.

Carotid A.
Diaphragm

C.N. III

Dorsum

C

Figure 92-4 *A.* Superior view of the sellar region. The optic chiasm is reflected forward. A congenitally absent diaphragma exposes the superior surface of the gland. Cranial nerve III is posterior to the carotid artery. The right ophthalmic artery arises below the optic nerve. (From Renn and Rhoton.[4]) *B.* Superior view of the cavernous sinus, anterior and posterior lobe of the pituitary, intracavernous portion of the carotid artery, and meningohypophyseal trunk with its three branches: the inferior hypophyseal, tentorial, and dorsal meningeal arteries. The ophthalmic artery arises from the anterior surface of the carotid artery above the clinoid and enters the optic canal under the optic nerve. The dorsum has been removed to expose the posterior lobe of the pituitary. Cranial nerve VI receives a branch from the dorsal meningeal artery and courses laterally around the carotid artery. The dural ostium of cranial nerve III (*left*) is in the roof of the cavernous sinus, and cranial nerve III (*right*) enters its dural ostium. The carotid artery is exposed in the medial part of the foramen lacerum (*left*). (From Harris and Rhoton.[2]) *C.* Superior view of the sellar region showing optic nerves, carotid arteries, and cranial nerve III. Carotid arteries bulge into the pituitary fossa. (From Renn and Rhoton.[4])

ous structure which would not be an adequate barrier for the protection of the suprasellar structures during trans-sphenoidal surgery. An outpouching of the arachnoid protrudes through the central opening in the diaphragma into the sella

turcica in about half the specimens. Although this diverticulum can usually be retracted unruptured during trans-sphenoidal surgery, it represents a potential source of postoperative cerebrospinal fluid leakage.

Pituitary Gland

The surface of the posterior lobe of the pituitary gland is lighter in color than the anterior lobe. The upper part of the anterior lobe wraps around the lower part of the pituitary stalk to form the pars tuberalis. When the gland is removed from the sella, the posterior lobe (Fig. 92-4) will be found to be more densely adherent to the sellar wall than the anterior lobe. The gland's width is equal to or greater than either its depth or its length in most specimens. Its inferior surface usually conforms to the shape of the sellar floor, but its lateral and superior margins vary in shape, because these walls are composed of soft tissue rather than bone. If there is a large opening in the diaphragma, the gland tends to be concave superiorly in the area around the stalk. The superior surface may become triangular as a result of being compressed laterally and posteriorly by the carotid arteries. As the anterior lobe is separated from the posterior lobe, there is a tendency for the pars tuberalis to be retained with the posterior lobe. Intermediate lobe cysts are frequently encountered during separation of the anterior and posterior lobes.

The distance separating the medial margin of the carotid artery and the lateral surface of the pituitary gland usually varies from 1 to 3 mm; however, in some specimens the artery protrudes medially and indents the gland (Fig. 92-4). Heavy arterial bleeding during trans-sphenoidal hypophysectomy has been reported to be caused by injury to a branch of the carotid artery (e.g., the inferior hypophyseal artery) or by avulsion of a small capsular branch from the carotid artery.

If the carotid arteries indent the lateral surface of the gland, the gland loses its rounded shape and conforms to the wall of the artery, often developing protrusions above or below the artery. Separation of these protrusions from the main mass of gland or tumor may explain cases in which functioning gland or tumor remains after hypophysectomy and tumor removal.

Intercavernous Venous Connections

Venous sinuses may be found in the margins of the diaphragma and around the gland. The intercavernous connections (Figs. 92-5, 92-6) within the sella are named on the basis of their relation to the pituitary gland: the anterior intercavernous sinuses pass anterior to the hypophysis, and the posterior intercavernous sinuses pass behind the gland. Actually, these intercavernous connections may occur at any site along the anterior, inferior, or posterior surface of the gland. The anterior sinus is usually larger than the posterior sinus, but either or both may be absent. If the anterior and posterior connections coexist, the whole structure constitutes the circular sinus. Entering an anterior intercavernous connection which extends downward in front of the gland during transsphenoidal surgery may produce brisk bleeding. However, this usually stops with temporary compression of the channel or with light monopolar diathermy, which serves to glue the walls of the channel together.

A large intercavernous venous connection called the *basilar sinus* consistently passes posterior to the dorsum sellae and upper clivus. The basilar sinus connects the posterior aspect of both cavernous sinuses and is the largest and most constant intercavernous connection across the midline. The superior and inferior petrosal sinuses join the basilar sinus. The abducens nerve often enters the posterior part of the cavernous sinus by passing through the basilar sinus.

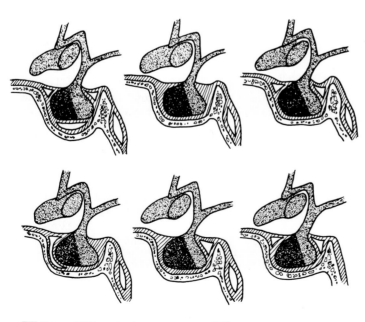

▨ Dura ■ Anterior lobe of pituitary ▢ Intercavernous sinuses

▨ Chiasm, hypothalamus, posterior lobe of pituitary

Figure 92-5 Six sagittal sections of the sellar region showing variations in the intercavernous venous connections within the dura. The variations shown include combinations of anterior, posterior, and inferior intercavernous connections and the frequent presence of a basilar sinus posterior to the dorsum. Either the anterior (*lower center*) or posterior (*lower left*) intercavernous connection or both (*top center*) may be absent. The anterior intercavernous sinus may extend along the whole anterior margin of the gland (*lower left*). The basilar sinus may be absent (*lower right*). (From Renn and Rhoton.[4])

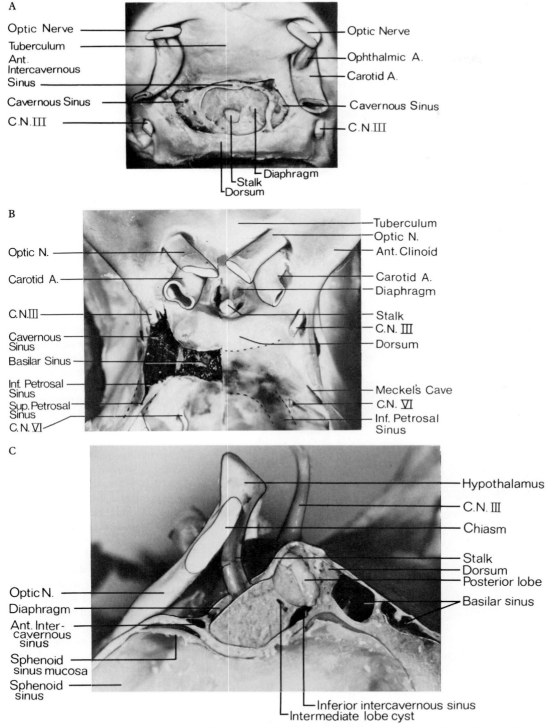

Figure 92-6 Superior views of the sellar region. *A.* The ophthalmic artery arises from the superior aspect of the carotid artery and courses laterally beneath the optic nerve to the optic foramen. The dura over the cavernous and anterior intercavernous sinuses has been removed to show the venous connection across the midline. *B.* Superior view of the sellar region showing optic nerves, carotid arteries, cranial nerves III and VI, and pituitary stalk. The basilar sinus connects the posterior portion of the two cavernous sinuses. The dura over the posterior aspect of the left cavernous sinus and the left half of the basilar sinus has been removed. The course of the basilar, inferior petrosal, and superior petrosal sinuses within the dura is shown by the dotted lines. *C.* Midline sagittal section of the sellar region showing the optic nerve and chiasm, cranial nerve III, inferior part of the hypothalamus, and pituitary stalk and gland. The anterior and inferior intercavernous sinuses are small. The basilar sinus, dorsal to the clivus and joining the posterior aspect of the two cavernous sinuses, is the largest connection across the midline. The anterior sellar wall bulging into the sphenoid sinus is very thin. (From Renn and Rhoton.[4])

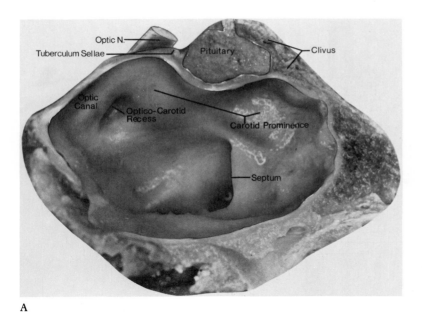

A

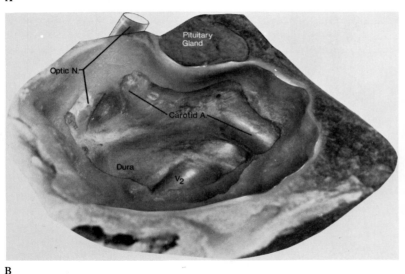

B

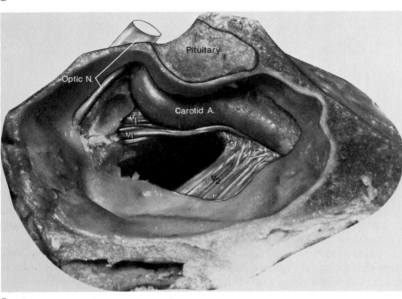

C

Figure 92-7 Stepwise dissection of the lateral wall of the right half of a sellar-type sphenoid sinus and adjacent structures. *A*. The sphenoid sinus and sellar area are divided in the midsagittal plane. The optic nerve (Optic N.) is seen proximal to the optic canal. The opticocarotid recess separates the carotid prominence and the optic canal. The septum in the posterior part of the sinus is incomplete. *B*. The sinus mucosa and thin bone of the lateral sinus wall have been removed to expose the dura covering the carotid artery (Carotid A.), the second trigeminal division (V_2) just distal to the trigeminal ganglion, and the optic nerve. *C*. The dura has been opened to expose the carotid artery, the optic nerve in the optic canal, the second trigeminal division below the carotid artery, and the abducens nerve (VI) between the first trigeminal division (V_1) and the carotid artery. *D*. Lateral view of the specimen showing the area of the cavernous sinus. The oculomotor (III) and trochlear (IV) nerves are seen above. The intracavernous portion of the carotid artery is seen medial to the trigeminal root (V) and the ophthalmic, maxillary, and mandibular (V_3) divisions of the trigeminal nerve. The petrous portion of the carotid artery is seen in cross section below the trigeminal nerve. The opening into the sphenoid sinus is located between the first and second trigeminal divisions. *E*. The trigeminal nerve is reflected forward to expose the carotid artery, trigeminal impression, artery of the inferior cavernous sinus (Art. Inf. Cav. Sinus), and abducens nerve; the last splits into three bundles as it passes around the carotid artery. (From Fujii et al.[1])

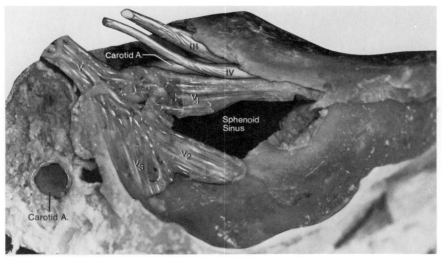

D

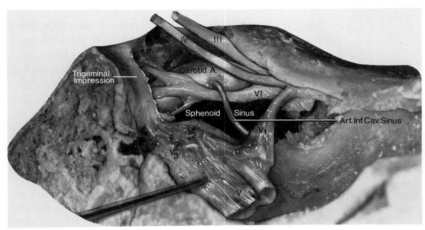

E

Sphenoid Sinus

The sphenoid sinus is subject to considerable variation in size and shape and to variation in the degree of pneumatization[1,4,5] (Figs. 92-7, 92-8). It is present as minute cavities at birth; its main development takes place after puberty. In early life, it extends backward into the presellar area and subsequently expands into the area below and behind the sella turcica, reaching its full size during adolescence. As the sinus enlarges, it may partially encircle the optic canals. As age advances, the sinus frequently undergoes further enlargement associated with absorption of its bony walls. Occasionally there are gaps in its bone, with the mucous membrane lying directly against the dura mater. In a study in adult cadavers, this sinus was found to be of the presellar type in 24 percent and of the sellar type in 75 percent.[1,4] In the infrequent conchal type, the thickness of bone separating the sella turcica from the sphenoid sinus is at least 10 mm.

The carotid artery frequently produces a serpiginous prominence into the sinus wall below the floor and along the anterior margin of the sella (Figs. 92-7, 92-8). The optic canals usually protrude into the superolateral portion of the sinus, and the second and third divisions of the trigeminal nerve into the inferolateral part. A diverticulum of the sinus, called the *opticocarotid recess*, often projects laterally between the optic canal and the carotid prominence.

Removing the mucosa and bone from the lateral wall of the sinus exposes the dura covering the medial surface of the cavernous sinus and optic canals (Figs. 92-7, 92-8). Opening this dura exposes the carotid arteries and optic and trigeminal nerves within the sinus. The sixth cranial nerve is located between the lateral side of the carotid artery and the medial side of the first trigeminal division. The second and third trigeminal divisions are seen in the lower margin of the opening through the lateral wall of the sphenoid sinus. In half the cases the optic and trigeminal nerves and the carotid arteries have areas where bone 0.5 mm or less in thickness separates them from the mucosa of the sphenoid sinus, and

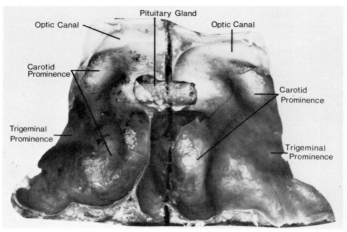

A

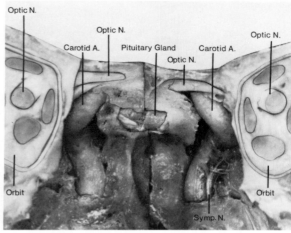

B

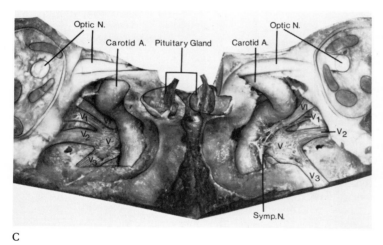

C

Figure 92-8 Anterior views of a sellar-type sphenoid sinus. *A.* The anterior wall of the sella has been removed to expose the pituitary gland. The specimen was split in the midline. The air cavity is wider below than above, as is typical in a well-pneumatized specimen. The optic canals are above. Carotid prominences are lateral to the sella. The trigeminal prominence is below the carotid prominence. *B.* The mucosa, dura, and bone of the lateral walls of the sinus have been removed to expose the parasphenoidal segments of the carotid artery. Sympathetic nerves (Symp. N.) are anterior to the left carotid artery. Orbital contents appear laterally. *C.* The specimen is spread slightly to show the abducens nerve (VI) and the ophthalmic (V_1), maxillary (V_2), and mandibular (V_3) divisions of the trigeminal nerve (V) on each side. (From Fujii et al.[1])

in a few cases the bone separating these structures from the sinus is absent.[1,4,6] The absence of such bony protection within the walls of the sinus may explain some of the cases of cranial nerve deficits and carotid artery injury reported following trans-sphenoidal surgery. The bone is often thinner over the carotid arteries than over the anterior margin of the pituitary gland.

The septa within the sphenoid sinus (Fig. 92-9) vary greatly in size, shape, thickness, location, completeness, and relation to the sellar floor. The cavities within the sinus are seldom symmetrical from side to side and are often subdivided by irregular minor septa. The septa are often located

off the midline as they cross the floor of the sella. In a previous study,[4] a single major septum separated the sinus into two large cavities in only 68 percent of specimens, and even in these cases the septum was often located off the midline or was deflected to one side. The most common type of sphenoid sinus has multiple small cavities in the large paired sinuses. The smaller cavities are separated by septa oriented in all directions.

Computed tomography of the sella is routinely used to define the relation of the septa to the floor of the sella for trans-sphenoidal surgery. Major septa may be found as much as 8 mm off the midline.[4]

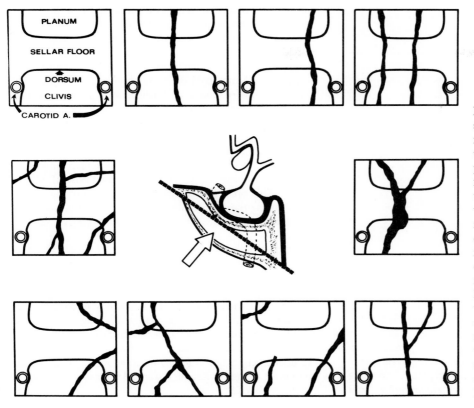

Figure 92-9 Schematic representation of septa in the sphenoid sinus. The broken line in the center diagram depicts the plane of section of each specimen from which drawings were taken, the large arrow the direction of view of the specimens. The planum is above, the dorsum and clivus below, and the sella in an intermediate position on each diagram. Carotid arteries are represented as double circles; the heavy dark line shows the location of septa in the sphenoid sinus. A wide variety of septa separate the sinus into cavities which vary in size and shape, seldom being symmetrical from side to side. (From Renn and Rhoton.[4])

References

1. Fujii K, Chambers SM, Rhoton AL Jr: Neurovascular relationships of the sphenoid sinus: A microsurgical study. J Neurosurg 50:31–39, 1979.
2. Harris FS, Rhoton AL Jr: Anatomy of the cavernous sinus: A microsurgical study. J Neurosurg 45:169–180, 1976.
3. Perlmutter D, Rhoton AL Jr: Microsurgical anatomy of the anterior cerebral-anterior communicating-recurrent artery complex. J Neurosurg 45:259–272, 1976.
4. Renn WH, Rhoton AL Jr: Microsurgical anatomy of the sellar region. J Neurosurg 43:288–298, 1975.
5. Rhoton AL Jr, Hardy DG: Microsurgical anatomy of the sphenoid bone, cavernous sinus, and sellar region, in Tindall GT, Collins WF (eds): *Clinical Management of Pituitary Disorders.* New York, Raven Press, 1979, pp 1–73.
6. Rhoton AL Jr, Hardy DG, Chambers SM: Microsurgical anatomy and dissection of the sphenoid bone, cavernous sinus and sellar region. Surg Neurol 12:63–104, 1979.
7. Saeki N, Rhoton AL Jr: Microsurgical anatomy of the upper basilar artery and the posterior circle of Willis. J Neurosurg 46:563–578, 1977.
8. Zeal AA, Rhoton AL Jr: Microsurgical anatomy of the posterior cerebral artery. J Neurosurg 48:534–559, 1978.

93

Radiology of Sellar and Parasellar Lesions

James C. Hoffman, Jr.

The radiographic investigation of sellar and parasellar lesions has undergone rapid change in the last several years. High-resolution CT scanning has replaced invasive neuroradiological studies such as angiography and pneumoencephalography. For many years polytomography has been used as a screening procedure for pituitary adenomas; however, it has been shown that the findings of subtle erosion, focal ballooning, and asymmetry of the sellar floor may be normal.[1,10] Thus there is a high degree of false-positive and false-negative results with polytomography. The radiation dosage from tomography can be as high as 20 rad, whereas the radiation dosage from CT is about 4 rad. At the present time sellar and parasellar diseases can be evaluated radiographically by high-resolution CT scanning, metrizamide cisternography, and angiography in certain patients to rule out aneurysm or involvement of the carotid arteries or cavernous sinuses by a lesion. Polytomography is no longer necessary or indicated. Routine anterior-posterior and lateral films of the skull are helpful for planning the surgical approach to a lesion and determining the overall size and configuration of the sella.

Technique

In order to adequately study the sellar and parasellar region, a CT scanner capable of producing multiple thin slices (1.5 mm) in both axial and coronal planes is necessary, along with the ability to obtain a lateral skull image to localize the level of the slices and obtain the proper angle for coronal slices. In order to obtain parallel slices through the area of interest, the scans are performed at a zero angle from the canthomeatal line for the axial cuts. Coronal slices are obtained with the patient in a prone position with the head hyperextended. In some patients this position is not obtainable, so the scans are performed with the patient in the supine posi-

tion and the head extended. The lateral skull image is used to determine the proper angle for the coronal slices. It is necessary to obtain the coronal slices in a retromandibular position to keep artifacts from the teeth at a minimum. If the patient is unable to remain in either of these positions for the scan, then 1.5-mm axial slices are obtained and sagittal and coronal reconstruction is performed through the sellar and parasellar region (Fig. 93-1).

Intravenous contrast enhancement is routinely used on all patients unless there is a strong history of allergy. A 50-ml bolus of iothalamate meglumine 52% and iothalamate sodium 26% is given initially, followed by a drip infusion of 100 ml during the study. This gives a total dose of 60 g of iodine. This procedure keeps the blood level of iodine elevated during the entire study and gives good visualization of the cavernous sinus, carotid arteries, and pituitary infundibulum.

Metrizamide cisternography is indicated after the contrast CT if it cannot be determined whether the lesion is intra- or extra-axial in location. Cisternography is also indicated in a patient with clinical findings of optic chiasm disease and a normal contrast CT. This study is done by performing a lumbar puncture with a 22-gauge needle and instilling 4/ml metrizamide in a concentration of 190 mg/ml into the subarachnoid space. The patient is then placed in a Trendelenberg position for 1 min to allow the metrizamide to migrate to the suprasellar cistern. Axial and coronal scans are then obtained.

Anatomy of the Sellar and Parasellar Region

The structures in the sellar and parasellar region that must be visualized in evaluating patients with lesions of this region are the suprasellar cistern, the pituitary gland, the infundibulum of the pituitary gland, the optic chiasm, the carotid arteries, the cavernous sinus, and the anterior recesses of the third ventricle. The bony margins of the sella and sphenoid sinus should also be evaluated by viewing the scans on a wide window width.

The normal suprasellar cistern has the configuration of a five-pointed star. The points of the star are formed by the interhemispheric fissure, the sylvian fissures, and the ambient and crural cisterns (Fig. 93-2). On higher slices through the suprasellar cistern, the cistern has the configuration of a six-pointed star, with the sixth point formed by the interpeduncular fossa.

The anterior border of the suprasellar cistern is formed by the inferior-posterior aspect of the frontal lobes, and the lateral border is formed by the uncus and medial aspect of the temporal lobe. On the lower slices the posterior border of the suprasellar cistern is formed by the pons and on higher sections by the interpeduncular fossa. On contrast scans performed with axial sections, the circle of Willis is well visualized, and the pituitary infundibulum can be seen lying in the center of the cistern. The normal pituitary infundibulum measures 1 mm in diameter. The optic chiasm is a rectangular structure lying in the center of the cistern. The normal transverse diameter is 18 mm. On coronal CT

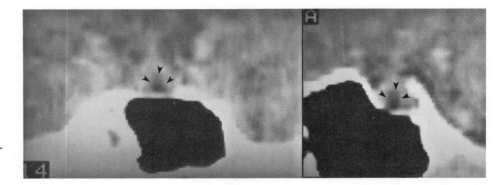

Figure 93-1 Coronal (*left*) and sagittal (*right*) reconstruction in patient with prolactinoma (*arrows*).

the vertical diameter is 4 mm.[2] Any enhancement in the suprasellar cistern other than that of the optic chiasm, pituitary infundibulum, and carotid arteries should be viewed with suspicion. Occasionally the anterior recesses of the third ventricle can be recognized as two low-density areas lying within the cistern.

The pituitary gland is visualized best on coronal CT slices (Fig. 93-3). The normal pituitary gland has a height of 5 mm in males and 7 to 8 mm in females.[11] The superior surface should be concave or flat. Following contrast enhancement, the gland has a homogeneous appearance, with a density the same or slightly greater than that of normal brain tissue. The infundibulum is usually in the midline but occasionally may lie to the left or right of the midline.

The cavernous sinus can be evaluated on axial and coronal contrast CT scans. On coronal scans the oculomotor, trochlear, and abducens nerves plus the ophthalmic and maxillary divisions of the trigeminal nerve can be seen as filling defects in the cavernous sinus.[6]

Metrizamide cisternography gives the best visualization of structures within the suprasellar cistern. The pituitary infundibulum can be visualized as a structure measuring 1 mm in diameter lying adjacent to the optic chiasm (Fig. 93-4). The normal infundibulum is slightly smaller than the basilar artery on the cisternogram. The optic chiasm appears as a boomerang-shaped structure on high sections through the cistern. On lower sections it may appear as a linear area of density lying in front of the pituitary infundibulum.

Diseases of the Sellar and Parasellar Region

Table 93-1 lists the conditions that can be identified in the sellar and parasellar area by neuroradiological studies.

TABLE 93-1 Tumors and Other Conditions Involving Sellar and Parasellar Regions

Common:
   Pituitary adenoma
   Empty sella syndrome
   Glioma, optic chiasm or hypothalamus
   Craniopharyngioma
   Aneurysm
   Meningioma
Uncommon:
   Arachnoid cyst
   Germinoma
   Nasopharyngeal carcinoma
   Sarcoid
   Histiocytosis X
   Metastatic carcinoma
   Chordoma
   Lymphoma
   Choristoma
   Abscess
   Pituitary carcinoma
   Chondroma

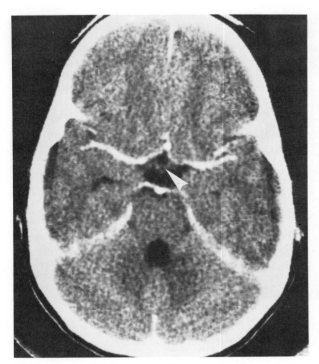

Figure 93-2 Axial contrast CT demonstrating normal configuration of suprasellar cistern. Optic chiasm is in the center of the cistern (*arrow*).

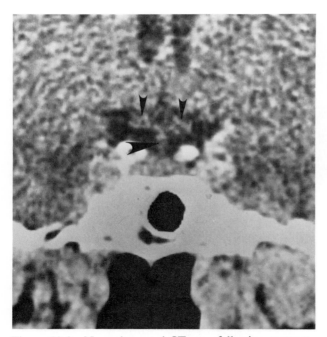

Figure 93-3 Normal coronal CT scan following contrast enhancement. Optic chiasm is well visualized (*small arrowheads*). Pituitary infundibulum can be seen lying in midline (*large arrowhead*).

Pituitary Adenoma

The most common tumors in this region are pituitary adenomas. Clinically, they may be divided into secreting and nonsecreting tumors. The secreting tumors cause the clinical diseases of acromegaly, Cushing's syndrome, and the amenorrhea-galactorrhea syndrome. The nonsecreting tumors have been designated pathologically as *chromophobe adenomas.*

Since patients with secreting tumors tend to seek medical help earlier than those with nonsecreting tumors, they usually have smaller tumors at the time of diagnosis. In our series of patients with tumors less than 1 cm in size (microadenoma), CT scan correctly identified the tumor in 70 percent.

On CT, the usual appearance of a microadenoma shows a gland more than 8 mm in height with a convex superior surface.[11] Most microadenomas appear as discrete low-density areas in the gland if the scan is performed immediately after contrast injection. However, an occasional tumor may enhance or have calcification in it (Fig. 93-5). Erosion of the cortical floor is of little help, since this may be a normal finding. Hyperplasia or a cyst of the pituitary gland may have an appearance similar to that of a microadenoma on CT, so one must also rely on the prolactin level. In the author's experience, a prolactin level of more than 125 ng/ml is almost always associated with a microadenoma.

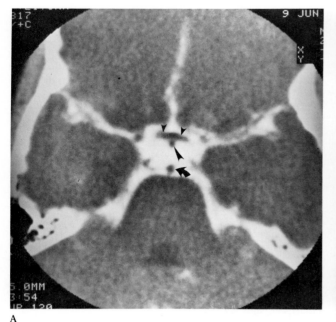

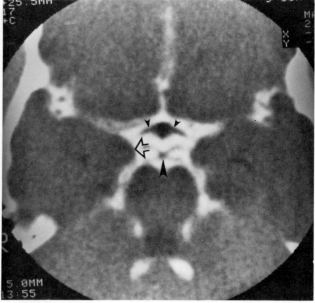

A   B

Figure 93-4 Normal metrizamide cisternogram. *A.* Section through the lower part of the optic chiasm (*small arrowheads*). Shown are the pituitary infundibulum (*large arrowhead*) and basilar artery (*curved arrow*) *B.* Section through the upper part of the optic chiasm (*small arrowheads*). Shown are the basilar artery and its branches (*large arrowhead*). The medial aspect of the uncus forms the lateral border of the cistern (*open arrow*).

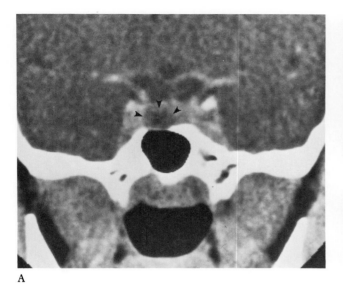

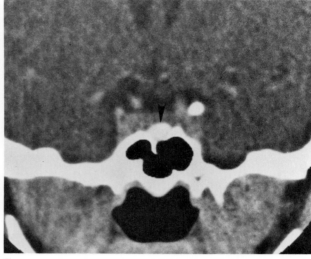

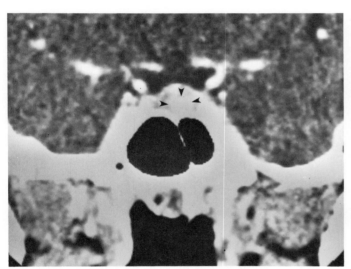

Figure 93-5 Prolactinomas. *A.* Low-density area represents the typical appearance of prolactin-secreting tumor (*small arrowheads*). *B.* Prolactin tumor with calcospherites (*large arrowhead*). *C.* Enhancing prolactinoma (*small arrowheads*).

When the tumor reaches a size of more than 1 cm, CT is very accurate in detecting it. In our series of patients with both secreting and nonsecreting tumors, the CT was 95 percent accurate in detection of the tumor. The CT appearance of secreting and nonsecreting tumors is similar. The contrast CT will usually demonstrate a dense area of enhancement extending from the sella and into the suprasellar cistern.[7] There may also be cystic areas within the tumor from either previous hemorrhage or necrosis (Fig. 93-6). There is usually some erosion of the floor of the sella, and frequently the tumor may extend into the sphenoid sinus. When the tumor erodes into the sphenoid sinus, the patient may develop CSF rhinorrhea or pneumocephalus.

A large invasive tumor may cause considerable erosion of the skull base and may present as a nasopharyngeal mass (Fig. 93-7). Nasopharyngeal carcinoma may also erode and destroy the base of the skull and present as a pituitary mass.

When this occurs it may be difficult to differentiate this tumor from a pituitary adenoma (Fig. 93-8).

In patients with large tumors, angiography is indicated to rule out an aneurysm. Digital venous imaging (DVI) can be used in place of arterial studies to rule out an aneurysm (Fig. 93-9).

Invasion of the cavernous sinus has been difficult to determine with CT, since the medial wall of the sinus cannot be differentiated from the pituitary gland on CT. If there is bowing of the lateral wall of the cavernous sinus, this probably indicates that there has been tumor invasion of the sinus.

Hyperostosis has occasionally been demonstrated with pituitary tumors. Calcification has rarely been reported.[7]

Pituitary apoplexy is a clinical emergency, since it may threaten both vision and the patient's life. Patients with this condition usually present with a clinical history of sudden onset of headache, nausea, and vomiting. They may have

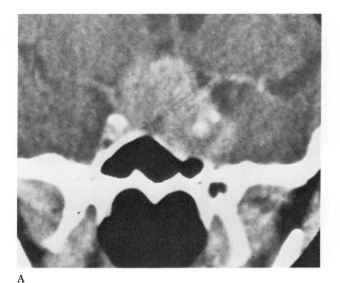

A

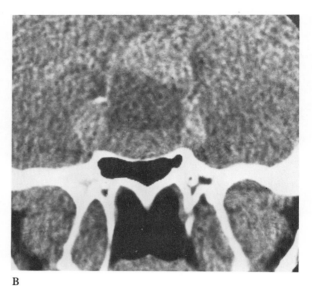

B

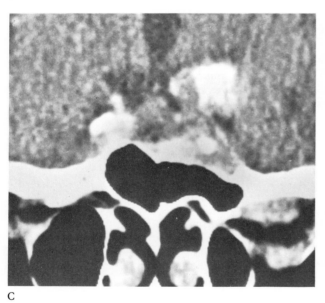

C

Figure 93-6 Chromophobe adenomas. *A*. Coronal CT scan demonstrating large enhancing tumor. *B*. Enhancing cystic tumor. *C*. Chromophobe adenoma with calcification.

fever, decreased mental status, visual loss, and signs of meningeal irritation. If there has been hemorrhage into the gland, then the noncontrast CT scan may be pathognomonic, since acute hemorrhage may be demonstrated lying within either the pituitary gland or the suprasellar cistern.[8] Acute hemorrhage will usually have a density from 40 to 90 Hounsfield units (HU). Contrast CT may demonstrate an enhancing tumor mass. Frequently patients with pituitary apoplexy are extremely sick and uncooperative, and extreme care must be exercised to obtain good quality CT scans in the region of the pituitary gland.

If there has been infarction of the gland, the CT scan may demonstrate low-density areas in the tumor mass. Contrast CT may show a ring enhancement pattern. The CT scan pattern is not pathognomonic of infarction of the pituitary gland, since it may be difficult to differentiate infarction from cystic changes within the gland; however, in a patient with the appropriate clinical findings, low-density areas should arouse suspicion of acute infarction.[8]

The CT scan appearance following trans-sphenoidal surgery will demonstrate the surgical defect in the anterior aspect of the sella. There is usually opacification of the sphenoid sinus, with variable amounts of fat demonstrated in the sella and sphenoid sinus. A scan in the immediate postoperative period will demonstrate the thickened tumor capsule, with some enlargement of the pituitary fossa contents; for this reason it is difficult to estimate whether there is residual tumor. After 4 to 6 weeks there is a decrease in the size of the gland and retraction of the capsule. A baseline CT at this time is recommended so that the patient may be followed for tumor recurrence.

Empty Sella Syndrome

Empty sella syndrome (ESS) is a distinct radiological and clinical entity that results from herniation of the suprasellar cistern into the sella through an incompetent diaphragma

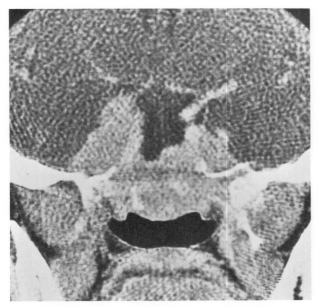

Figure 93-7 Invasive pituitary adenoma. Contrast coronal CT demonstrating large tumor with destruction of the skull base.

sellae. ESS may also result from pituitary tumor that undergoes necrosis following radiation therapy or from previous pituitary surgery. On skull films or tomograms of the sella, ESS may simulate a pituitary tumor. Occasionally the patients may have endocrine abnormalities or symptoms of optic chiasm compression.

Prior to high-resolution CT scanning, pneumoencephalography was necessary to diagnose this entity. The CT appearance is usually characteristic and is, therefore, the definitive study for diagnosing it. On axial CT scans a low-density region will be seen in the sella that has the same density as CSF, and on contrast CT the pituitary infundibulum is displaced posteriorly against the dorsum sellae.[4] On axial CT it is frequently difficult to be sure whether the low-density area in the sella region actually represents empty sella syndrome or a low-lying suprasellar cistern. Coronal CT is more accurate in diagnosis, since it can be determined whether the sella is filled with a low-density area (Fig. 93-10). On posterior coronal cuts the infundibulum is seen to be displaced posteriorly, and there may be a small amount of soft tissue density along the posterior-inferior aspect of the sella. This soft tissue represents the posteriorly displaced and compressed pituitary gland. If the pituitary infundibulum is not identified, then other lesions such as an intrasellar arachnoid cyst or a pituitary adenoma with necrosis should be considered (Fig. 93-11). A metrizamide cisternogram should be performed if the displaced pituitary infundibulum cannot be clearly identified.

Occasionally a secreting adenoma may occur in a patient with ESS. In this situation it can be difficult to diagnose the adenoma on CT.

Optic Chiasm or Hypothalamic Glioma

Since optic chiasm gliomas and hypothalamic gliomas are difficult to differentiate clinically and pathologically, they are discussed together. On a noncontrast CT scan, the only

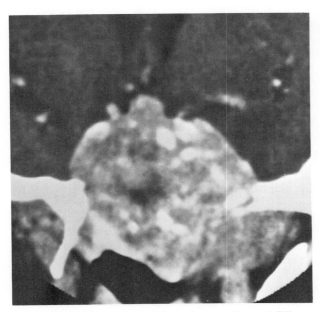

Figure 93-8 Nasopharyngeal carcinoma. Coronal CT demonstrating destruction of the base of the skull with tumor mass extending into the pituitary fossa. Areas of calcification are noted within the tumor.

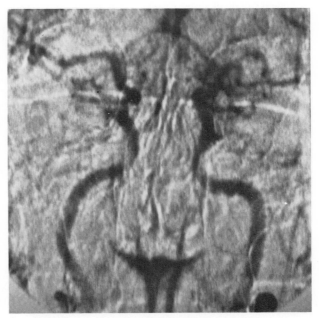

Figure 93-9 Towne's projection of digital venous imaging in a patient with a pituitary adenoma, demonstrating elevation of the anterior cerebral arteries and lateral displacement of the supraclinoid portion of each internal carotid artery.

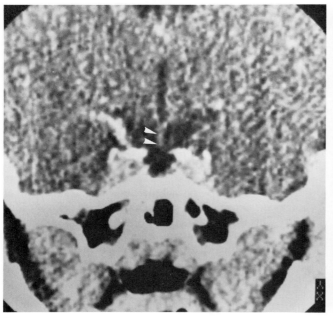

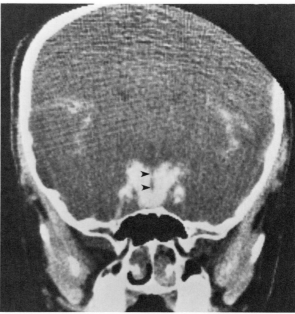

A   B

Figure 93-10 Empty sella syndrome. *A*. Coronal CT scan demonstrating CSF density within pituitary fossa. Pituitary infundibulum is displaced posteriorly (*arrowheads*). *B*. Metrizamide cisternogram demonstrating metrizamide in pituitary fossa. The pituitary infundibulum is shown (*arrowheads*).

indication of tumor may be obliteration or deformity of the suprasellar cistern. If there is gross enlargement of the optic chiasm, this may be detected on the noncontrast CT. Following contrast enhancement there can be a variable amount of enhancement of these lesions. Some tumors show little enhancement, and others develop a homogeneous enhancement.[9] It is frequently difficult to differentiate these lesions from an extra-axial mass such as a meningioma or a

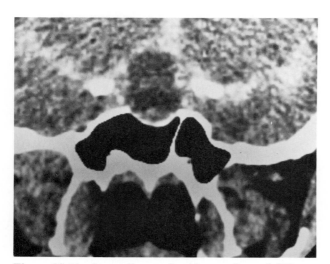

Figure 93-11 Intrasellar arachnoid cyst. Coronal CT scan following introduction of metrizamide demonstrates a cystic mass extending from the sella into the suprasellar cistern. No metrizamide is noted in the mass.

pituitary tumor. The author has found metrizamide cisternography helpful in determining whether the lesion in the suprasellar space is intra- or extra-axial in location. If the lesion arises from the hypothalamus or optic chiasm, enlargement of the chiasm will be seen on the cisternogram (Fig. 93-12). If the tumor is extra-axial, there will be displacement of the chiasm and anterior third ventricle. Since minimal enlargement of the optic chiasm cannot be detected on either a non-contrast or a contrast CT scan, a metrizamide cisternogram is the recommended study in a patient with clinical findings of chiasmatic tumor if the contrast CT is normal. Calcification has been reported in large tumors. Since these tumors spread along the optic tracts and nerves, it is important to obtain good visualization of the optic nerves by obtaining thin axial sections through the optic nerves.

Craniopharyngioma

Craniopharyngioma usually has a typical appearance on CT scanning. There is usually calcification and cyst formation within the tumor.[3] The calcification may appear as a large conglomerate mass or as a ringlike peripheral rim (Fig. 93-13). The cyst usually has the same density as CSF but may occasionally have the density of the brain (12 to 23 HU). Some of the cysts may be of high density because of high protein content. After contrast enhancement there may be only enhancement of the peripheral rim of the tumor, or occasionally a more solid enhancement pattern may be noted, with a cystic area within the tumor. Rarely, the enhancement pattern may be completely solid.

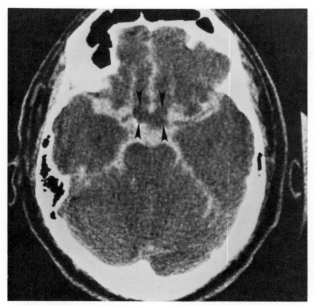

Figure 93-12 Optic chiasm glioma. Axial CT scan performed as part of metrizamide cisternography demonstrates an enlarged, lobulated optic chiasm (*arrowheads*).

Craniopharyngiomas usually begin in the suprasellar cistern and extend inferiorly into the sella turcica or superiorly into the third ventricle. Sagittal reconstruction may be useful in determining the full extent of the tumor (Fig. 93-14). When there is extension into the sella, there is almost always destruction of the bony margins of the sella and dorsum sellae. When there is extension into the third ventricle, there

is frequently an associated hydrocephalus from block at the foramen of Monro. Rarely, craniopharyngiomas have been reported lying totally within the third ventricle.

Aneurysm

Aneurysms that involve the sella and parasellar area may arise from either the cavernous portion or the supraclinoid portion of the carotid artery (Fig. 93-15). Occasionally a large aneurysm arising from the basilar tip presents as a mass in the suprasellar cistern (Fig. 93-16). If the aneurysm is large, a noncontrast CT scan will usually show an area of increased density; however, if the aneurysm is filled with clot, then areas of decreased density may also be seen. Occasionally large aneurysms calcify, and curvilinear areas of calcification on a noncontrast CT may suggest the diagnosis. Following contrast infusion there is usually a dense homogeneous enhancement of the aneurysm; however, if the aneurysm contains a thrombus, the enhancement will be seen only in the nonthrombosed portion of the aneurysm. In patients with giant aneurysms, the CT scan frequently demonstrates the size of the lesion better than angiography.

Angiography is the definitive procedure in the evaluation of a patient with an aneurysm; however, digital venous angiography may be used to follow the size of a large aneurysm.

Suprasellar Meningioma

Meningiomas involving the sella and parasellar region may arise from the planum sphenoidale, anterior clinoid, tuberculum sellae, posterior clinoid, or medial wing of the sphe-

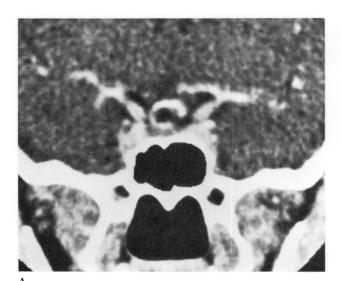
A

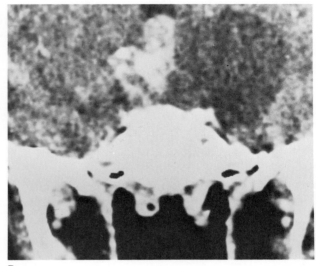
B

Figure 93-13 Craniopharyngiomas. *A.* Coronal CT scan following contrast enhancement demonstrates a small, calcified cystic mass lying in the suprasellar cistern. *B.* Coronal CT scan following contrast enhancement demonstrates enhancing mass extending into third ventricle. Note the large cyst extending laterally.

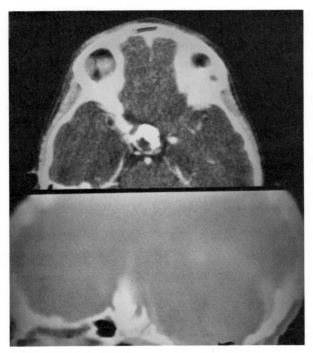

Figure 93-14 Craniopharyngioma. Axial CT scan (*top*) demonstrates calcified mass lying within suprasellar cistern. Sagittal reconstruction (*bottom*) demonstrates expanded sella turcica with a calcified tumor mass extending into the hypothalamus.

noid bone. Rarely, a meningioma may present as a totally intrasellar mass, but the usual presentation is as a mass lying in the suprasellar cistern. On noncontrast CT it usually presents as an isodense lesion or one slightly denser than normal brain tissue. Following contrast enhancement there is a homogeneous enhancement pattern that is well circumscribed (Fig. 93-17). Since these meningiomas are extra-axial in location, they displace and deform the structures lying in the suprasellar cistern. Without the characteristic psammomatous calcification or hyperostosis that occurs with meningiomas, these lesions can be difficult to differentiate from pituitary adenoma or hypothalamic glioma. Angiography may be helpful if the characteristic blush of meningioma is visualized; however, meningiomas located at the base of the skull frequently do not have a vascular blush. The angiogram will help to determine whether there has been involvement of the internal carotid artery or cavernous sinus.

Germinoma

Germinoma is a tumor that occurs primarily in the pineal region, but it may occasionally arise in the suprasellar region or involve the anterior third ventricle and suprasellar area by direct spread. When this tumor involves the suprasellar region, a noncontrast CT scan may show a mass of slightly increased density or a deformity of the suprasellar cistern. Following contrast enhancement there is usually a dense homogeneous blush (Fig. 93-18). Occasionally low-density areas that represent cystic change may occur. Calcification has not been demonstrated in the author's series of germinomas. These tumors may spread into the ventricular system and present as a cast of the ventricle on contrast CT. In a young patient with diabetes insipidus and a suprasellar mass, germinoma should be the strongest consideration.

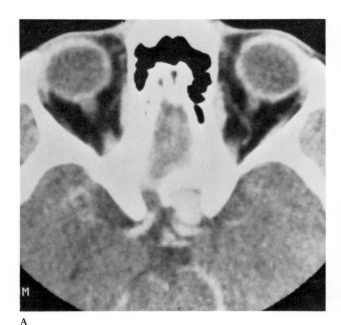

A

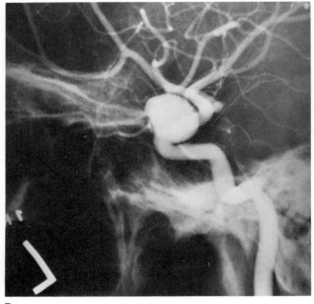

B

Figure 93-15 Suprasellar aneurysm. *A.* Axial CT scan demonstrating enhancing lesion at the origin of the left optic canal, with erosion of the canal. *B.* Lateral view of the internal carotid angiogram demonstrates a supraclinoid aneurysm.

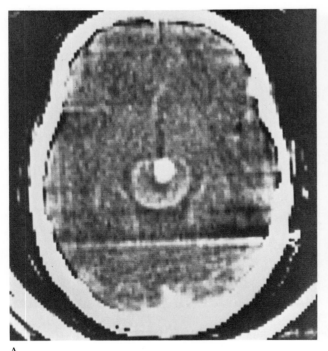

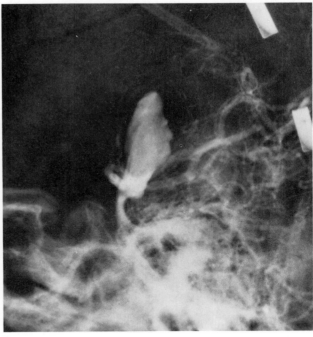

A   B

Figure 93-16 Giant basilar tip aneurysm. *A*. Contrast CT demonstrates enhancing mass lying in suprasellar cistern and indenting the third ventricle. Central area of enhancement represents the nonthrombosed portion of the aneurysm. The peripheral enhancing rim represents wall of the aneurysm. *B*. Lateral view of vertebral angiogram demonstrates a large basilar tip aneurysm.

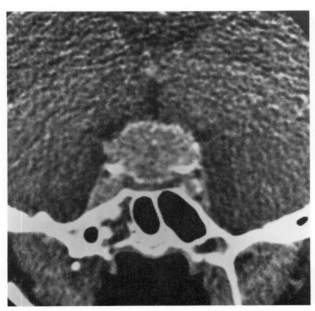

Figure 93-17 Meningioma. Coronal contrast CT scan demonstrates mass lying in the suprasellar cistern above the pituitary gland. No calcification or hyperostosis is noted.

Sarcoidosis

Involvement of the central nervous system by sarcoidosis is unusual. The reported incidence is 4 to 7 percent. When the CNS is involved there are two patterns of involvement. In the first pattern there is a granulomatous leptomeningitis which may be diffuse or more circumscribed to involve the optic chiasma, pituitary gland, anterior third ventricle, and hypothalamus. In the second pattern the granulomas may coalesce in the brain parenchyma to produce a solid mass simulating a primary brain tumor. If there is meningeal involvement, the only CT finding may be a communicating hydrocephalus. When the pituitary gland and hypothalamus are involved, the CT scan may demonstrate enlargement of the pituitary gland and pituitary infundibulum (Fig. 93-19). The CNS may be the only organ system involved.

Chordoma

Chordoma is an uncommon tumor which accounts for less than 1 percent of all intracranial tumors. Forty per cent of the tumors are of the cranial variety, with the remainder occurring in the spinal column.[5] The most common finding is bone destruction, usually involving the clivus and sella turcica. Calcification has been reported in 34 to 70 percent of the tumors. The CT scan demonstrates the bony destruction and calcification. Frequently it is necessary to visualize

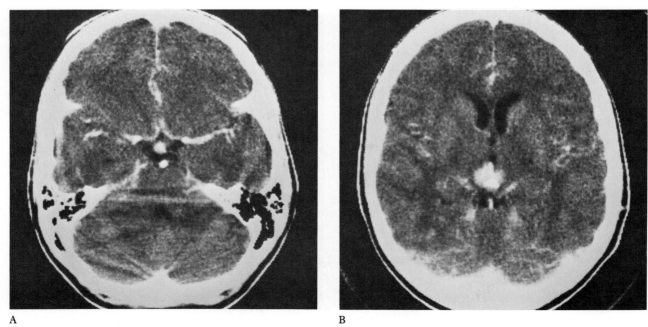

A   B

Figure 93-18 Germinoma. *A.* Axial contrast CT scan at the level of the suprasellar cistern demonstrates an enhancing mass involving the pituitary infundibulum. *B.* Higher section through the posterior third ventricle demonstrates an enhancing mass indenting the posterior third ventricle.

the scan on a wide window setting in order to adequately visualize the bony destruction. Following contrast enhancement, varying amounts of enhancement of the tumor may be seen. Some tumors show little enhancement, while others may be quite vascular (Fig. 93-20). Angiography is indicated in order to demonstrate the location of the vertebral artery and to determine whether there is involvement of the cavernous sinuses. An abnormal vascular pattern is seen in about 25 percent of cases. Rarely, the tumor may present as a completely intrasellar mass.

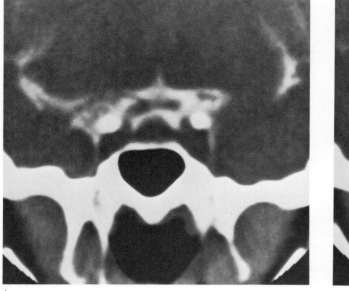
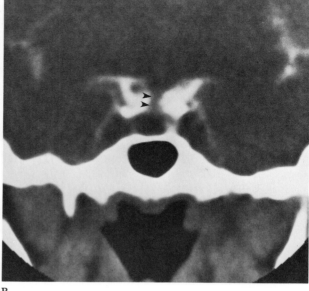

A   B

Figure 93-19 Sarcoidosis. *A.* Coronal CT scan as part of metrizamide cisternography demonstrates an enlarged pituitary gland with a convex upper border. *B.* Posterior coronal CT scan demonstrates an enlarged pituitary infundibulum (*arrowheads*).

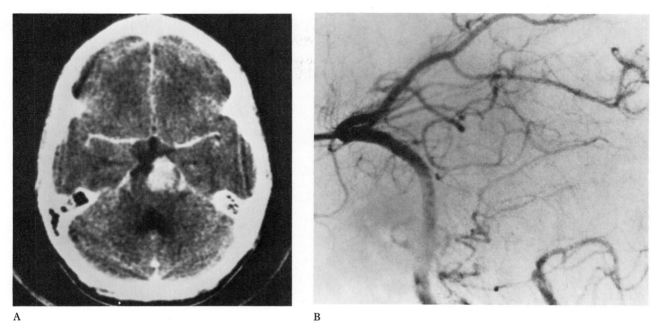

A   B

Figure 93-20 Chordoma. *A*. Axial CT scan following contrast enhancement demonstrates an enhancing mass lying in posterior aspect of suprasellar cistern. *B*. Lateral view of a vertebral angiogram demonstrates posterior displacement of the basilar artery characteristic of an extra-axial mass.

Other Conditions

Many other uncommon lesions involve the pituitary gland and surrounding structures, but most of these do not have specific neuroradiological findings. The CT scan may dem-

onstrate nonspecific enlargement of both the pituitary gland and the pituitary infundibulum (Fig. 93-21).

Deformity of the suprasellar cistern may also be caused by herniation of the uncus and temporal lobe in a patient with a supratentorial intracranial mass.

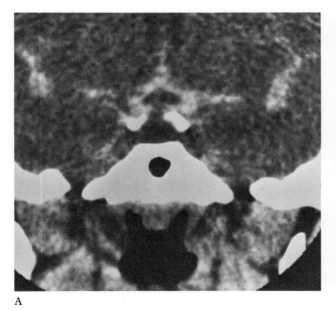
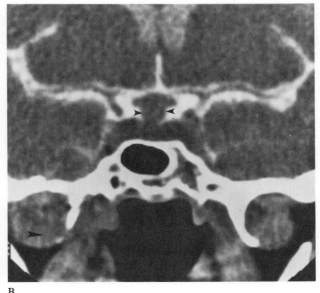

A   B

Figure 93-21 *A*. Coronal CT scan with cisternography demonstrates enlarged pituitary gland and pituitary infundibulum in a patient with histiocytosis X. *B*. Coronal CT scan with cisternography in a patient with metastatic disease. Mass is demonstrated lying between the optic chiasm and the superior surface of the pituitary gland (*arrowheads*).

References

1. Burrow GN, Wortzman G, Rewcastle NB, Holgate RC, Kovacs K: Microadenomas of the pituitary and abnormal sellar tomograms in an unselected autopsy series. N Engl J Med 304:156–158, 1981.
2. Daniels DL, Haughton VM, Williams AL, Gager WE, Berns TF: Computed tomography of the optic chiasm. Radiology 137:123–127, 1980.
3. Fitz CR, Wortzman G, Harwood-Nash DC, Holgate RC, Barry JF, Boldt DW: Computed tomography in craniopharyngiomas. Radiology 127:687–691, 1978.
4. Haughton VM, Rosenbaum AE, Williams AL, Drayer B: Recognizing the empty sella by CT: The infundibulum sign. AJR 136:293–295, 1981.
5. Kendall BE, Lee BCP: Cranial chordomas. Br J Radiol 50:687–698, 1977.
6. Kline LB, Acker JD, Post MJD, Vitek JJ: The cavernous sinus: A computed tomographic study. AJNR 2:299–305, 1981.
7. Leeds NE, Naidich TP: Computerized tomography in the diagnosis of sellar and parasellar lesions. Semin Roentgenol 12:121–135, 1977.
8. Post MJD, David NJ, Glaser JS, Safran A: Pituitary apoplexy: Diagnosis by computed tomography. Radiology 134:665–670, 1980.
9. Savoiardo M, Harwood-Nash DC, Tadmor R, Scotti G, Musgrave MA: Gliomas of the intracranial anterior optic pathways in children. Radiology 138:601–610, 1981.
10. Swanson HA, du Boulay G: Borderline variants of the normal pituitary fossa. Br J Radiol 48:366–369, 1975.
11. Syvertsen A, Haughton VM, Williams AL, Cusick JF: The computed tomographic appearance of the normal pituitary gland and pituitary microadenomas. Radiology 133:385–391, 1979.

94

Classification and Pathology of Pituitary Tumors

Kalman Kovacs
Eva Horvath
Sylvia L. Asa

Pituitary neoplasms represent approximately 15 percent of all intracranial tumors. The majority of these are pituitary adenomas, histologically benign lesions which originate in adenohypophyseal cells. Occasionally, tumors composed of adenohypophyseal cells give rise to distant metastases and are called *pituitary carcinomas*. Nonendocrine tumors also occur in the sella turcica; many tissues, varying in structure and function, are found in the sellar region, and the neoplasms which may derive from them are numerous and often difficult to identify.

The many types of tumors and tumorlike conditions occurring in the sellar region are listed in Table 94-1, and a few representative abnormalities are illustrated in the photomicrographs. While some of these lesions are incidental autopsy findings, others are of considerable clinical significance. Some may cause conspicuous endocrine symptoms with distinct biochemical abnormalities. Visual defects, cranial nerve palsies, and headache may result from increased intracranial pressure or may be due to tissue destruction by compression, invasion, or vascular injury. Some of these tumors are effectively treated with drugs or surgery; others are incurable and may be fatal.

TABLE 94-1 Classification of Pituitary Tumors and Tumorlike Conditions

Tumors derived from adenohypophyseal cells:
Adenoma
Carcinoma
Other primary tumors of the sella turcica:
Angioma and angiosarcoma
Chordoma
Choristoma
Craniopharyngioma
Fibroma and fibrosarcoma
Glioma (optic nerve, infundibulum, posterior lobe, hypothalamus)
Granular cell tumor (posterior lobe, pituitary stalk)
Ganglioglioma
Ganglioneuroma
Germinoma (ectopic pinealoma)
Hamartoma (hypothalamus)
Meningioma
Paraganglioma
Sarcoma
Teratoma
Metastatic tumors:
Carcinoma
Sarcoma, leukemia, lymphoma, histiocytosis X
Tumorlike conditions:
Inflammatory
Infectious
Lymphocytic hypophysitis
Sarcoidosis, giant cell granuloma
Infiltrative
Amyloidosis
Hemochromatosis
Mucopolysaccharidosis

Space does not allow a detailed discussion of all entities. This chapter concentrates on those lesions which are unique to the sella turcica. For additional reading, several recommended recent reviews dealing in detail with the diseases of the sellar region are listed in the References.

Pituitary Adenomas

Pituitary adenomas are frequently occurring epithelial neoplasms composed of and deriving from adenohypophyseal cells. They represent approximately 10 percent of intracranial tumors. Histological studies of pituitary glands obtained from unselected routine adult autopsies show the presence of incidental adenomas in 8 to 23 percent.

Like tumors of other endocrine glands, pituitary adenomas vary considerably in size, growth rate, radiological appearance, clinical presentation, endocrine function, cellular composition, and morphology. In the majority of cases they are histologically benign, slow-growing, small neoplasms confined to the sella turcica. Some tumors, however, exhibit a more rapid growth rate, invade surrounding tissues, and cause local symptoms such as visual disturbances and headache.

Pituitary adenomas are usually well demarcated and are separated from the adjacent compressed nontumorous adenohypophysis by a pseudocapsule which consists of condensed reticulin fibers (Fig. 94-1). Unlike many benign tumors of other locations, these lesions have no fibrous capsule. Some histologically benign tumors may have an indistinct border, and clusters of adenoma cells may be found to spread deeply into the adjacent nontumorous adenohypophysis.

Pituitary adenomas can be classified according to their size, radiographic appearance, endocrine function, morphology, and cytogenesis.

Neurosurgeons frequently classify pituitary adenomas according to their size. Microadenomas measure less, macroadenomas more, than 1 cm in their largest diameter. The pathologist cannot determine the size of the surgically removed adenoma, since the tissue is received in fragments. In autopsy material, pituitary adenomas can be divided into small, medium, and large tumors. Small tumors occupy less than 25 percent, large tumors more than 75 percent, of the gland. This is a rather inaccurate but useful classification. The largest diameter of the tumor can be measured accurately only on serial sections.

Classification of pituitary adenomas by radiographic appearance (Table 94-2) is more useful. With sophisticated radiographic techniques (polytomography, computed tomography, angiography, metrizamide cisternography), the size of the tumor and its spread into neighboring tissue can be conclusively assessed.

Classification of pituitary adenomas on the basis of their endocrine function (Table 94-3) is most valuable to the clinical endocrinologist. With radioimmunoassays, minute quantities of pituitary hormones can be detected in blood and tissues. With the availability of stimulating hormones—insulin for growth hormone (GH) and adrenocorticotropic hormone (ACTH), corticotropin-releasing factor

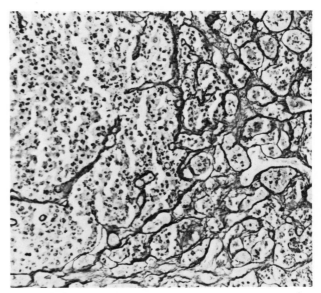

Figure 94-1 The regular reticulin network seen in the nontumorous adenohypophysis (*right*) is absent in the sharply demarcated, small microadenoma (*left*), found incidentally at autopsy. (Gordon-Sweet technique for reticulin, ×100.)

(CRF) for ACTH, thyrotropin-releasing hormone (TRH) for thyroid-stimulating hormone (TSH) and prolactin (PRL), gonadotropin-releasing hormone (GnRH) for follicle-stimulating hormone (FSH) and luteinizing hormone (LH)—responses of adenohypophyseal cells can be evaluated reliably.

Classification of pituitary adenomas according to their morphological features (Tables 94-4 and 94-5) has undergone a substantial change. On the basis of the staining properties of the cell cytoplasm, pituitary adenomas were previously divided into three morphological entities: chromophobic, acidophilic, and basophilic adenomas. Chromophobic adenomas were assumed to be endocrinologically inactive tumors not capable of secreting hormones. Acidophilic adenomas were thought to secrete GH and to be associated with acromegaly or gigantism. Basophilic adenomas were regarded as ACTH-producing tumors accompanied by Cushing's disease. Since the tinctorial characteristics of adenoma cells cannot be correlated with their secretory activity and cytogenesis, classifications based on the staining affinities of the cytoplasm lost their significance.

TABLE 94-2 Classification of Pituitary Adenomas According to Radiographic Appearance

Grade 1	Intrapituitary adenoma: diameter <1 cm, normal sella, minimal configurational changes
Grade 2	Intrasellar adenoma: diameter >1 cm, enlarged sella, no erosion
Grade 3	Diffuse adenoma: enlarged sella, localized sellar erosion
Grade 4	Invasive adenoma: extensive destruction of bony structures, "ghost" sella

TABLE 94-3 Classification of Pituitary Adenomas According to Endocrine Function

Adenomas with growth hormone excess
Adenomas with prolactin excess
Adenomas with ACTH excess
Adenomas with TSH excess
Adenomas with FSH/LH excess
Plurihormonal adenomas
Adenomas with no apparent hormonal function

Progress in methodology, especially the introduction of immunocytology and electron microscopy, has resulted in a new and more meaningful morphological classification which separates pituitary adenomas into distinct entities on the basis of hormone content, cellular composition, fine structural features, and cytogenesis. Immunocytologic procedures have permitted specific and reliable demonstration of the hormones present in the cell cytoplasm. The immunoperoxidase technique has proved to be especially valuable; this method can be used on formalin-fixed and paraffin-embedded material, even on pituitary glands harvested at autopsy and stored for several years. At the electron microscopic level, the immunoperoxidase technique can reveal subcellular sites at which the various hormones are located. Electron microscopy has shed light on the ultrastructural features of the cell; the result has been the distinction of various cell types, the classification of adenomas, and a deeper insight into the details of the secretory process.

From the endocrinologic point of view, pituitary adenomas are either accompanied by or unaccompanied by clinical and biochemical evidence of excessive hormone secretion. They may secrete growth hormone (GH), prolactin (PRL), adrenocorticotropic hormone (ACTH), thyrotropic hor-

TABLE 94-4 Classification of Pituitary Adenomas According to Staining Properties: Correlation with Cytogenesis

Chromophobic adenoma:
  Sparsely granulated GH cell adenoma
  Sparsely granulated PRL cell adenoma
  Mixed GH–PRL cell adenoma
  Acidophil stem cell adenoma
  Corticotropic cell adenoma, functioning
  Corticotropic cell adenoma, silent
  TSH cell adenoma
  FSH/LH cell adenoma
  Null cell adenoma
  Oncocytoma
  Plurihormonal adenoma
Acidophilic adenoma:
  Densely granulated GH cell adenoma
  Densely granulated PRL cell adenoma
  Mixed GH–PRL cell adenoma
  Acidophil stem cell adenoma
  Mammosomatotropic cell adenoma
  Oncocytoma
  Plurihormonal adenoma
Basophilic adenoma:
  Corticotropic cell adenoma
    Functioning
    Silent

TABLE 94-5 Classification of Pituitary Adenomas According to Cytogenesis

	Prevalence, %
Growth hormone cell adenoma:	
Densely granulated	7.0
Sparsely granulated	9.0
Prolactin cell adenoma:	
Densely granulated	0.3
Sparsely granulated	28.6
Corticotropic cell adenoma:	
With ACTH excess	8.4
With no ACTH excess	6.0
Thyrotropic cell adenoma	0.5
Gonadotropic cell adenoma	3.3
Plurihormonal adenoma:	
Mixed growth hormone cell–prolactin cell adenoma	4.6
Acidophil stem cell adenoma	3.1
Mammosomatotropic cell adenoma	1.5
Unclassified	2.8
Null cell adenoma	18.2
Oncocytoma	6.7

mone (TSH), follicle-stimulating hormone (FSH), luteinizing hormone (LH), and α subunits of the glycoprotein hormones. Some pituitary adenomas, called plurihormonal adenomas, produce more than one hormone. More than 20 percent of pituitary adenomas appear to be inactive clinically and biochemically. These silent tumors invariably contain cytoplasmic secretory granules, suggesting the production of substances, whether unidentified hormones, biologically inactive precursors, or hormone fragments. Some of the silent tumors are revealed by immunocytologic techniques to contain hormones but do not discharge them in sufficient amounts to affect endocrine equilibrium.

Morphological Features

GH-Producing Adenomas

These tumors consist of growth hormone cells and are accompanied by acromegaly or gigantism. They can be divided into densely and sparsely granulated growth hormone cell adenomas. Densely granulated growth hormone cell adenomas are slow-growing, well-differentiated tumors which can be removed with a high surgical cure rate. Sparsely granulated growth hormone cell adenomas are more aggressive and are composed of more poorly differentiated cells. They show a faster pace of growth, may invade neighboring tissues, are more prevalent in women, and have a less favorable surgical cure rate. There is no correlation between the granularity, blood GH levels, and clinical activity of GH-producing tumors.

Densely granulated growth hormone cell adenomas are identified as acidophilic adenomas by light microscopy. The cytoplasm of adenoma cells shows positive staining with various acid dyes and exhibits a diffuse positivity for GH by the immunoperoxidase technique. Seen by electron microscopy, densely granulated adenomatous growth hormone cells closely resemble nontumorous growth hormone cells; they contain well-developed, rough-surfaced endoplasmic reticulum membranes, Golgi complexes, and numerous spherical, evenly electron-dense secretory granules measuring 300 to 600 nm (Fig. 94-2).

Sparsely granulated growth hormone cell adenomas are diagnosed as chromophobic adenomas by light microscopy. The cytoplasm of adenoma cells exhibits positive staining for GH by the immunoperoxidase technique. The characteristic fine structural features include irregular nuclei, dispersed rough-surfaced endoplasmic reticulum profiles, aggregates of smooth-surfaced endoplasmic reticulum membranes, conspicuous Golgi complexes, and fibrous bodies composed of type 2 microfilaments and smooth-walled tubules, as well as several centrioles and cilia. The secretory granules are sparse, spherical, and evenly electron-dense and measure 100 to 500 nm (Fig. 94-3).

PRL Cell Adenomas

PRL-producing adenomas consist of prolactin cells and are, in some cases, associated with amenorrhea, galactorrhea, infertility, loss of libido, and impotence. In other cases, mainly in men and postmenopausal women, the endocrine symptoms are inconspicuous or absent, and only an elevation of blood PRL level may indicate PRL production by the tumor. It must be emphasized, however, that hyperprolactinemia itself provides no direct evidence that PRL is synthesized by the adenoma cells; compression or damage of certain hypothalamic structures and the pituitary stalk may interfere with the production or release of hypothalamic PRL-inhibiting factors or their transport to the anterior lobe and thus cause hyperprolactinemia. Morphological investi-

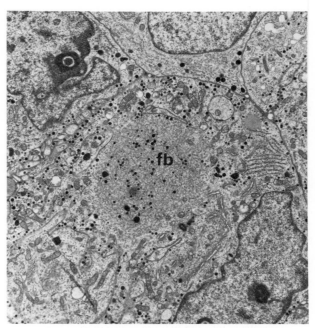

Figure 94-3 This incompletely differentiated, sparsely granulated growth hormone cell adenoma consists of irregular cells with crescent-shaped eccentric nuclei, scattered RER and fibrous body (fb) consisting of smooth-surfaced endoplasmic reticulum and type 2 microfilaments in the Golgi region. (×6600.)

gation can determine whether PRL is produced by the adenoma, underlining the significance of morphological studies in the diagnosis of pituitary adenomas. Blood PRL levels over 200 ng/ml are almost always due to PRL-secreting adenomas. Moderately high blood PRL levels (under 200 ng/ml), however, can be secondary to many other conditions, such as corticotropic cell adenoma, null cell adenoma, oncocytoma, TSH cell hyperplasia, lymphocytic hypophysitis, metastatic carcinoma, and craniopharyngioma. There is a correlation between tumor size and the degree of hyperprolactinemia: larger tumors are accompanied by higher blood PRL levels.

Two types of PRL cell adenomas—densely and sparsely granulated variants—can be distinguished. Densely granulated prolactin cell adenomas are rare. They are acidophilic adenomas by light microscopy, indistinguishable from densely granulated GH cell adenomas. The cytoplasm of adenoma cells exhibits positive staining with Herlant's erythrosin and Brookes' carmoisin. The immunoperoxidase technique reveals the presence of PRL in the cytoplasm of adenoma cells (Figs. 94-4, 94-5). By electron microscopy, densely granulated adenomatous prolactin cells resemble their resting nontumorous counterparts and are characterized by the presence of numerous spherical, oval or irregular, evenly electron-dense secretory granules, measuring 300 to 700 nm. The rough-surfaced endoplasmic reticulum and the Golgi complexes are well developed.

Sparsely granulated prolactin cell adenomas are identified as chromophobic adenomas by light microscopy. Herlant's erythrosin and Brookes' carmoisin stains usually re-

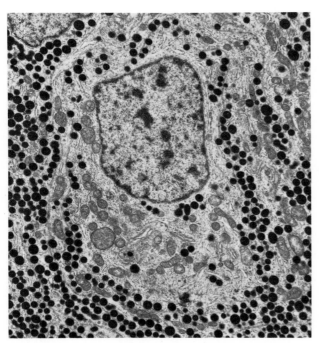

Figure 94-2 This densely granulated growth hormone cell adenoma is composed of well-differentiated uniform cells with prominent RER and Golgi complex and numerous evenly dense secretory granules. (×7900.)

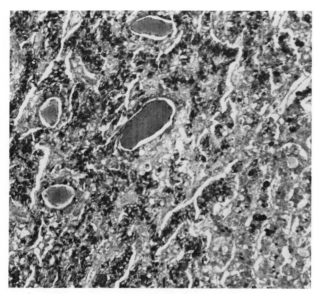

Figure 94-4 This prolactin-producing microadenoma has an indistinct border, and fingerlike projections of tumor tissue penetrate into the nontumorous anterior lobe (*right*). (Immunoperoxidase technique for prolactin, ×100.)

veal a few small secretory granules in the cytoplasm of adenoma cells. The immunoperoxidase technique is of fundamental importance in the diagnosis of this tumor type, since it clearly demonstrates the presence of PRL in the cytoplasm of adenoma cells. The fine structural features of sparsely granulated prolactin cell adenomas are similar to those of stimulated nontumorous prolactin cells and include prominent rough-surfaced endoplasmic reticulum mem-

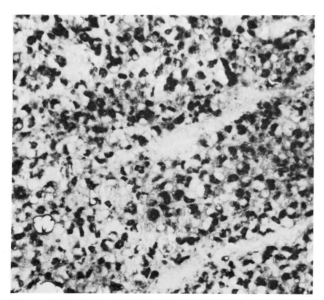

Figure 94-5 Prolactin cell adenoma, showing strong immunostaining for prolactin. (Immunoperoxidase technique, ×250.)

branes often forming whirls, conspicuous Golgi complexes, and misplaced exocytosis, i.e., extrusion of secretory granules on the lateral cell surfaces, distant from capillaries and intercellular extensions of basement membrane. The secretory granules are sparse, spherical, oval or irregular, and evenly electron-dense and measure 150 to 300 nm (Fig. 94-6).

Calcification is not uncommon in PRL-producing adenomas. Amorphous calcium apatite deposits and psammoma bodies are easily noticeable under the light microscope. If extensive, calcification is often accompanied by fibrosis. In some cases the tumor is transformed into a calcified fibrous mass; these lesions are called *pituitary stones*. Marked calcification can also be demonstrated by various x-ray techniques. Calcification as well as amyloid deposition, although characteristic features of PRL-producing adenomas, may be found in other adenoma types; reasons for the more common occurrence of these changes in prolactin-producing adenomas are not known.

Some PRL-producing microadenomas have a very slow growth rate and never turn into macroadenomas. Other PRL-producing adenomas grow relentlessly, often eroding the sella and invading neighboring tissues. Differences in biological behavior are not reflected in the morphological features, which show little variation from case to case. Thus the search continues to find morphological changes which can predict the pace of growth of PRL cell adenomas.

ACTH-Producing Adenomas

ACTH-secreting tumors are composed of corticotropic cells. They produce ACTH, β-LPH, and endorphins and are associated with Cushing's disease or Nelson's syndrome. By light microscopy, the majority of corticotropic cell adenomas are basophilic adenomas and contain secretory granules which stain positively with aniline blue, the periodic acid Schiff method (PAS) and lead hematoxylin. A few corticotropic cell adenomas are chromophobic and have little or no aniline blue, PAS, or lead hematoxylin positivity. The presence of ACTH can be demonstrated in the cytoplasm of adenoma cells by the immunoperoxidase technique. Positive immunostaining is also noted for β-LPH and endorphins. By electron microscopy, adenomatous corticotropic cells resemble those found in the nontumorous pituitary, having well-developed rough-surfaced endoplasmic reticulum membranes and conspicuous Golgi complexes. The secretory granules are spherical or slightly irregular, vary in electron density, often line up along the cell membranes, and measure 250 to 450 nm. In corticotropic cell adenomas associated with Cushing's disease, bundles of type 1 microfilaments are frequently observed in the cytoplasm, principally adjacent to the nucleus (Fig. 94-7). They are identical to Crooke's hyaline material noted in nontumorous corticotropic cells in patients treated with pharmacological doses of cortisol or its derivatives, and in cases of the ectopic ACTH syndrome. Type 1 microfilaments are inconspicuous or absent in corticotropic cell adenomas of patients with Nelson's syndrome, i.e., in those who have undergone bilateral adrenalectomy for pre-existing hypercorticism. Adenomas in association with Cushing's disease are often microadenomas, whereas tumors in patients with Nelson's syndrome are usu-

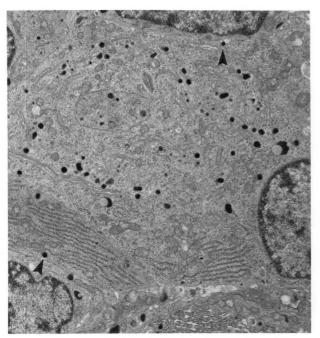

Figure 94-6 The characteristic features of prolactin cell adenoma can be seen—abundant RER, prominent Golgi complex, and misplaced exocytoses (*arrowheads*). (×9700.)

ally large, aggressive, rapidly growing neoplasms which often invade adjacent tissues.

Some corticotropic cell adenomas are unassociated with clinical and biochemical evidence of ACTH excess. These tumors show positive immunostaining for ACTH; however, biologically active ACTH is not released into the circulation in sufficient amounts to cause endocrine abnormalities. The reasons for the lack of ACTH hypersecretion are not understood. In a few cases, crinophagy—i.e., uptake of secretory granules—by accumulated lysosomes is seen by electron microscopy, suggesting an intracellular degradation of the hormone. Underdevelopment of the Golgi complex may also be a conspicuous finding, indicating a defect in hormone synthesis. It may well be that in silent corticotropic cell adenomas an abnormal hormone is produced which has ACTH immunoreactivity but no biological activity. By electron microscopy, some silent corticotropic cell adenomas closely resemble nontumorous corticotropic cells or actively secreting adenomatous corticotropic cells. In other cases, however, silent corticotropic cell adenomas differ considerably in their ultrastructure from corticotropic cells seen in the nontumorous adenohypophysis or in adenomas associated with Cushing's disease or Nelson's syndrome. Although the cytogenesis of these unusual tumors remains to be established, it is obvious that they represent a heterogenous group. It is important to distinguish silent corticotropic cell adenomas from tumors which do not secrete known hormones, such as null cell adenomas and oncocytomas; the differences are not only of theoretical but also of practical significance, since silent corticotropic cell adenomas have a rapid growth rate, tend to recur, and are often complicated by apoplexy, making emergency operation necessary.

TSH-Producing Adenomas

TSH-secreting pituitary adenomas are rare and consist of thyrotropic cells showing various degrees of cellular differentiation. They are usually accompanied by high blood TSH levels and are discovered chiefly in patients with long-standing primary hypothyroidism. This association is consistent with the view that deficiency of thyroid hormones causes stimulation of thyrotropics and may lead to thyrotropic cell hyperplasia and subsequently to the formation of an adenoma. Thyrotropic cell adenomas may occasionally be associated with hyperthyroidism. In these patients, hyperthyroidism is attributed to excessive amounts of TSH discharged from the adenoma cells. By light microscopy, thyrotropic cell adenomas are shown as chromophobic, possessing a few small cytoplasmic secretory granules, and staining positively with PAS, aldehyde fuchsin, and aldehyde thionin; they may contain immunoreactive TSH. By electron microscopy, poorly differentiated thyrotropic cell adenomas are seen to be composed of small elongated or angular cells with long cytoplasmic processes. Abundance of microtubules is a characteristic finding. The rough-surfaced endoplasmic reticulum membranes are scanty, and the Golgi apparatus is moderately developed. Secretory granules are sparse and spherical, frequently line up along the cell membrane, and measure 100 to 250 nm. The limiting membranes of the secretory granules are often separated from the electron-dense core by a wide, conspicuous electron-lucent halo. The well-differentiated adenomatous thyrotropic cells resemble their nontumorous counterparts.

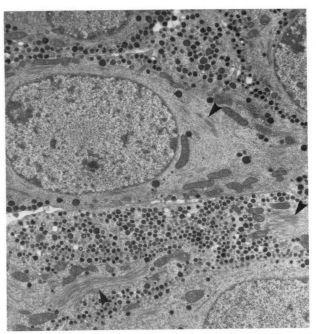

Figure 94-7 Corticotropic cell adenoma, associated with Cushing's disease, contains a large number of slightly irregular secretory granules with varying electron opacity and bundles of type 1 microfilaments (*arrowheads*). (×7900.)

FSH- and/or LH-Secreting Adenomas

These pituitary tumors consist of gonadotropic cells which may vary markedly in differentiation. Clinically, no specific symptoms or signs are evident; biochemically, blood FSH and/or LH levels are elevated. By light microscopy, gonadotropic cell adenomas are identified as chromophobic. The presence of a few PAS-positive granules can usually be noted in the cytoplasm of some of the adenoma cells, and immunohistochemistry may reveal positivity for FSH and/or LH. Immunocytologic techniques are valuable in the diagnosis, since in some cases the adenoma cells may be so immature that their derivation cannot be established even by detailed ultrastructural studies. By electron microscopy, especially in men, gonadotropic cell adenomas may be seen to differ considerably from gonadotropic cells of the nontumorous adenohypophysis. They are characterized by a few rough-surfaced endoplasmic reticulum cisternae, a prominent Golgi apparatus, and numerous microtubules. The secretory granules are spherical, evenly electron-dense, often line up along the cell membranes, and measure 50 to 150 nm. Some adenomas, mainly in women, are well differentiated; the adenoma cells resemble nontumorous gonadotropic cells and contain very small secretory granules.

Plurihormonal Adenomas

Plurihormonal adenomas produce two or more separate adenohypophyseal hormones. Endocrinologically, the most common combination is growth hormone and prolactin. These two hormones can be secreted simultaneously by three pituitary tumor types: mixed growth hormone cell–prolactin cell adenoma, acidophil stem cell adenoma, and mammosomatotropic cell adenoma.

The mixed growth hormone cell–prolactin cell adenoma consists of two distinct cell types: growth hormone cells which produce GH and prolactin cells which produce PRL. The adenoma cells may be densely or sparsely granulated; every combination may occur (Fig. 94-8). The patients have acromegaly or gigantism, with elevated blood GH concentrations and hyperprolactinemia. In some cases blood PRL levels are within the normal range, indicating synthesis of PRL without discharge into the circulation.

Acidophil stem cell adenomas consist of immature cells which are assumed to represent the common committed precursor of growth hormone cells and prolactin cells. They are rapidly growing tumors frequently spreading outside the sella turcica and infiltrating neighboring tissue such as the sphenoid bone, the optic nerve, and even the brain. As seen by light microscopy, they are chromophobic adenomas and consist of one cell type which contains both GH and PRL, as shown by the immunoperoxidase technique. The characteristic fine structural features of the adenoma cells are immature cytoplasm, poorly developed rough-surfaced endoplasmic reticulum, giant mitochondria with alterations in their internal compartment and oncocytic change, sparse secretory granules measuring 150 to 300 nm, fibrous bodies, and misplaced exocytosis. Clinically, the most important finding is hyperprolactinemia and its sequelae. Blood PRL levels, however, even with very large tumors, may be only moderately elevated. The patients may show acromegalic

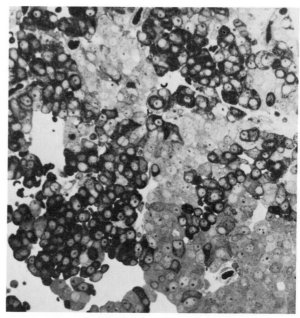

Figure 94-8 Mixed adenoma, composed of densely granulated growth hormone cells and sparsely granulated prolactin cells. (Epon section, toluidine blue stain, ×250.)

features, but blood GH levels are usually within the normal range.

Mammosomatotropic cell adenomas are thought to be the mature counterpart of acidophil stem cell adenomas. Clinically the patients have acromegaly or gigantism. Blood PRL levels are either moderately elevated or within the normal range. These slowly growing benign tumors consist of one cell type, the mammosomatotropic cell, which contains both GH and PRL as seen by the immunoperoxidase technique. Ultrastructurally, the tumor cells are characterized by densely granulated cytoplasm, spherical or oval secretory granules measuring 300 to 2000 nm, exocytosis, and large extracellular deposits of secretory material.

In some patients with pituitary adenomas, more than one adenohypophyseal hormone can be demonstrated in the tumor cells and blood levels of more than one adenohypophyseal hormone may be elevated. Unusual combinations may occur, such as GH and TSH; GH, PRL, and TSH; PRL and α subunit; or GH, PRL, and ACTH. These plurihormonal tumors are either monomorphous or plurimorphous. Monomorphous adenomas are composed of one cell type containing two or more hormones in the same cell; electron microscopy reveals only one cell type. Plurimorphous adenomas consist of more than one cell type; immunocytologic techniques demonstrate different hormones in different cell populations which can also be distinguished ultrastructurally. In some cases the cells are well differentiated and resemble their nontumorous counterparts; in other cases the cellular derivation of the tumor cannot be established. It is difficult to understand the formation of a cell type which produces several distinct hormones, different in chemical composition, immunoreactivity, and biological action. These unusual plurihormonal pituitary adenomas have been insufficiently explored, and more cases must be investigated to elucidate their cytogenesis.

Corticotropic cell adenomas, like nontumorous corticotropic cells, secrete not only ACTH but also the related peptides β-LPH and endorphins, which are part of the pro-opiomelanocortin molecule, the prohormone of ACTH. Gonadotropic cell adenomas often secrete FSH and LH simultaneously. This, however, is not surprising, since nontumorous gonadotropic cells are capable of synthesizing and discharging FSH and LH as well. Hence corticotropic cell adenomas and gonadotropic cell adenomas, although they secrete more than one hormone, are not regarded as plurihormonal tumors and are not classified as such.

Null Cell Adenomas

These adenomas lack immunocytochemical or fine structural markers, and their cellular origin cannot be established. They are diagnosed in older patients; surgery is usually performed on patient's over 40 years of age. They are clinically unassociated with hormone excess, although in some cases mild hyperprolactinemia may be present. This is due to stalk section effect; i.e., excessive PRL is secreted by nontumorous prolactin cells and not by the tumor. Null cell adenomas, when operated on, are usually large tumors showing suprasellar extension and invasion of neighboring tissues. Various degrees of hypopituitarism may be caused by a reduction in the number of hormone-producing nontumorous adenohypophyseal cells due to compression by the tumor or suppression of blood flow to the non-adenomatous anterior lobe. Morphologically, null cell adenomas are chromophobic and exhibit negative staining for all adenohypophyseal hormones by immunocytologic techniques. In some tumors, however, a few cells may contain different adenohypophyseal hormones, suggesting that, during neoplastic transformation or subsequent cellular proliferation, adenohypophyseal cells dedifferentiate and lose their ability to synthesize hormone or, alternatively, that null cells tend to differentiate into a specific hormone-producing cell line. By electron microscopy, null cell adenomas are seen to be composed of polyhedral cells with poorly developed cytoplasm, inconspicuous rough-surfaced endoplasmic reticulum membranes and Golgi apparatus, numerous microtubules, and sparse, small secretory granules measuring 100 to 250 nm (Fig. 94-9). Although secretory granules frequently line up along the cell membranes, no exocytoses are seen.

Pituitary oncocytomas occur mainly in older men and women and clinically are unassociated with hormone excess. In some cases hyperprolactinemia is evident, which is interpreted as a result of stalk section effect. The tumors are slow-growing, benign, chromophobic or acidophilic tumors, characterized by an abundance of mitochondria; they are similar to oncocytomas of other organs, such as Hürthle cell tumors of the thyroid, oxyphil cell adenomas of the parathyroid, and oncocytic tumors of the salivary glands and kidneys. The accumulation of mitochondria may be so great that they almost completely fill the cytoplasm (Fig. 94-10). Oncocytomas usually do not contain immunoreactive adenohypophyseal hormones and can be diagnosed easily by electron microscopy.

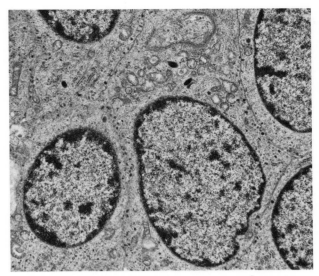

Figure 94-9 Null cell adenoma, showing poorly developed cytoplasm, few membranous organelles, and sparse, small secretory granules. (× 7900.)

Pituitary Carcinomas

Adenohypophyseal cells rarely give rise to carcinoma. The histological criteria of malignancy are not well established, and the morphological diagnosis is often difficult. Cellular pleomorphism and mitotic figures indicate a rapid growth rate but can be apparent also in benign tumors. Invasion of adjacent tissue is not regarded as unequivocal proof of malignancy. The diagnosis of carcinoma can be made only when distant metastases occur. Pituitary carcinomas may secrete hormones such as GH, PRL, and ACTH.

Craniopharyngiomas

Craniopharyngiomas are epithelial neoplasms which occur exclusively in the region of the sella turcica and are thought to derive from squamous cell nests of the pars tuberalis.

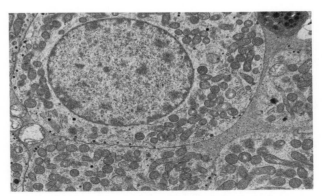

Figure 94-10 The morphological marker of pituitary oncocytoma is the abundance of mitochondria, as documented in this electron micrograph. (× 7900.)

They produce no hormones, account for approximately 3 percent of intracranial neoplasms, and are most frequent in childhood and adolescence. Craniopharyngiomas may be intrasellar or suprasellar and may cause various degrees of hypopituitarism by compression of the adenohypophysis, pituitary stalk, or hypothalamus. They are almost always benign; however, surgical extirpation is difficult and postoperative recurrence is common.

The histological appearance of craniopharyngiomas is distinctive, with cords of squamous and columnar epithelium, keratin pearls, and cystic areas filled with necrotic debris. Calcification is common, and bone formation may occur. Special stains and electron microscopy are usually not required to confirm the diagnosis. Immunohistochemistry reveals keratin in epithelial cells and yields negative results for adenohypophyseal hormones. Electron microscopy shows that the epithelial cells have prominent bundles of tonofibrils, with desmosomes but no secretory granules.

Other Primary Tumors

Primary neoplasms, which occur rarely in the neurohypophysis, include gliomas and granular cell tumors. The latter, the most common tumor in the posterior lobe, is composed of large, acidophilic granular cells whose histogenesis is uncertain. The characteristic large granules in the cytoplasm of the tumor cells are strongly positive with the PAS method and represent lysosomes, as demonstrated by electron microscopy. Granular cell tumors are usually incidental autopsy findings. They are small and, in the majority of cases, can be recognized by histological examination of the posterior lobe and the pituitary stalk. Occasionally they become large and cause local symptoms, increased intracranial pressure, and diabetes insipidus. In these rare cases, surgical intervention may become necessary. Other primary neoplasms in the sella turcica include the rare angiomas, fibromas, meningiomas, chordomas, germinomas and teratomas. These tumors produce no hormones, are often slow-growing, and may be found incidentally post mortem. However, they may cause local symptoms and hypopituitarism.

Occasional rapidly growing, pleomorphic sarcomas have been reported following irradiation for pituitary adenomas, suggesting the etiologic significance of such exposure.

Metastatic Tumors

Metastatic carcinoma involves the pituitary in patients with advanced, widely disseminated malignant disease. Autopsy series have documented adenohypophyseal metastases in 1 to 5 percent of cancer patients; however, clinical diagnosis is rare, since adenohypophyseal insufficiency implies significant destruction of the gland, and patients usually succumb to the disease before this becomes manifest. Neurohypo-

physeal metastases may cause diabetes insipidus.

The most common secondary tumor found in the pituitary is from breast carcinoma; metastases may also originate in bronchogenic, colonic, and prostatic carcinomas.

Lymphomas, leukemias, and various sarcomas may be noted in the pituitary, mainly in the posterior lobe. In cases of widespread tissue destruction, diabetes insipidus may develop.

Tumorlike Conditions

Massive destruction and enlargement of the pituitary may occur with various non-neoplastic conditions, listed in Table 94-1. These can mimic pituitary tumors, particularly when mass lesions cause functional impairment such as varying degrees of hypopituitarism or hyperprolactinemia. In most instances, elevation of blood PRL concentration is due to injury to the stalk or hypothalamus caused by an enlarged gland; when associated with lymphocytic hypophysitis, it may be related to the frequent association of this disorder with pregnancy.

References

1. Ezrin C, Kovacs K, Horvath E: Pathology of the adenohypophysis, in Bloodworth JBM Jr (ed): *Endocrine Pathology: General and Surgical*, 2d ed. Baltimore, Williams & Wilkins, 1982, pp 100–132.
2. Horvath E, Kovacs K: Ultrastructural classification of pituitary adenomas. Can J Neurol Sci 3:9–21, 1976.
3. Horvath E, Kovacs K: Pathology of the pituitary gland, in Ezrin C, Horvath E, Kaufman B, Kovacs K, Weiss MH (eds): *Pituitary Diseases*. Boca Raton, Fla., CRC Press, 1980, pp 1–83.
4. Kovacs K, Horvath E: Pituitary adenomas: Pathologic aspects, in Tolis G, Martin JB, Labrie F, Naftolin F (eds): *Clinical Neuroendocrinology: A Pathophysiological Approach*. New York, Raven Press, 1979, pp 367–384.
5. Kovacs K, Horvath E, Ezrin C: Pituitary adenomas. Pathol Annu 12 (pt 2): 341–382, 1977.
6. Kovacs K, Horvath E, Ryan N: Immunocytology of the human pituitary, in DeLellis RA (ed): *Diagnostic Immunohistochemistry*. New York, Masson, 1981, pp 17–35.
7. Landolt AM: Ultrastructure of human sella tumors: Correlations of clinical findings and morphology. Acta Neurochir (Wien) [Suppl] 22:1–167, 1975.
8. Robert F: Electron microscopy of human pituitary tumors, in Tindall GT, Collins WF (eds): *Clinical Management of Pituitary Disorders*. New York, Raven Press, 1979, pp 113–131.
9. Scheithauer BW: Surgical pathology of the pituitary and sellar region, in Laws ER Jr, Randall RV, Kern EB, Abboud CF (eds): *Management of Pituitary Adenomas and Related Lesions with Emphasis on Transsphenoidal Microsurgery*. New York, Appleton-Century-Crofts, 1982, pp 129–218.
10. Sheehan HL, Kovacs K: Neurohypophysis and hypothalamus, in Bloodworth JMB Jr (ed): *Endocrine Pathology: General and Surgical*, 2d ed. Baltimore, Williams & Wilkins, 1982, pp 45–99.

95

Endocrine Diagnosis in Neurosurgery

Nicholas T. Zervas

The reader is referred to other chapters for the mechanisms and basic biology of the hypothalamic-pituitary endocrine axis. The following sections describe the assessment of hypopituitarism as a result of disease states or pituitary ablation. Later paragraphs deal with the endocrine diagnosis of the major pituitary adenomas.

Assessment of Normal Pituitary Function

Testing for each of the primary hormones secreted by the adenohypophysis can be complicated. Each of the six major hormones requires basal and dynamic testing to portray accurately the reserve potential of the adenohypophysis.[4,16] Patients with hypopituitarism might display no outward evidence of pituitary insufficiency, since a small amount of tissue can sustain adequate function. However, impaired reserve capacity can become apparent during periods of stress. The detection of inadequate reserves requires provocative tests, as basal hormonal levels can be misleading. It is not unusual to find normal reserves of several pituitary hormones, whereas others are marginal or absent. In practice, the determination of thyroid and adrenal function is more important, since failure only of these two glands is life-threatening. The failure or insufficiency of gonadotropic, somatotropic, or lactotropic function might or might not be pertinent to the health of the patient, depending on age, sex, psychological needs, and other determinants. As more information concerning the role of pituitary peptides becomes available, it becomes increasingly possible to prevent systemic changes that can impair health many decades later. For example, hyperprolactinemia, while known to affect fertility, libido, and potency, also can produce osteopenia as a result of estrogen deficiency,[13] and, if not corrected in young women, may ultimately cause osteoporosis later in life. The succeeding paragraphs outline the basal and dynamic testing that should give an accurate portrayal of the adequacy of the adenohypophysis. Table 95-1 gives the major screening tests used to prove total hypophysectomy, and Table 95-2 lists normal endocrine values.

Somatotropic Function

The endocrine evaluation of the somatotropes centers on measuring serum levels of growth hormone both in the fasting state and after the administration of stimulatory or inhibitory agents.[8,18] Growth hormone is released in a pulsatile fashion by the adenohypophysis, and serum levels are variable. In hypopituitary individuals, the mean level of growth hormone can be marginal, and the reserve must be tested. In normal persons, the level of growth hormone rises after insulin-induced hypoglycemia or the administration of arginine or dopamine precursors (L-dopa) or agonists (apomorphine).

Insulin hypoglycemia is the most commonly used provocative test. After the intravenous administration of regular insulin (0.1–0.15 U/kg) plasma glucose levels in normal individuals usually fall to less than 40 mg/dl. This result plus a growth hormone level greater than 5 ng/ml indicates normal somatotropic function. Some normal subjects demonstrate levels as high as 25 ng/ml. Any response indicates surviving somatotropes.

Arginine stimulates the release of growth hormone through the alpha-adrenergic receptor mechanism and is more effective in women than in men. After its infusion in normal individuals, growth hormone levels generally rise to more than 5 ng/ml. Again, any detectable level indicates the presence of surviving somatotropes.

L-Dopa also elicits a rise in human growth hormone. A level greater than 5 ng/ml indicates normal somatotrope reserve, and any detectable level of human growth hormone indicates surviving somatotropes.

The tests described above can cause nausea and hypotension and must be administered under closely monitored conditions. The most commonly used test, insulin hypoglycemia, can be hazardous in hypopituitary patients with inadequate adrenal reserve. It should be avoided in elderly patients and in those with vascular or cerebrovascular disease or a history of convulsive disorders.

From a pragmatic point of view, insulin stimulation is the best single test to verify total ablation or loss of somatotropes. The absence of growth hormone in the serum following adequate stimulation by insulin indicates that all somatotropic cells are dead or absent. Inadequate levels of growth hormone are considered a blunted response. Hepatic, renal, and central nervous system diseases as well as cancer and poor nutrition also can blunt the response to insulin.

Prolactin Function

Prolactin cells make up most of the adenohypophysis. In most laboratories, 15 to 20 ng/ml is the upper limit and 5 ng/ml is the lower limit of normal. Prolactin secretion is pulsatile during the day and rises during sleep. In hypersecretory states associated with amenorrhea or pituitary tumors, prolactin levels are usually above 30 ng/ml, but patients without pituitary tumors can have levels as high as 100 ng/ml.[4,15,16,26,29]

The dynamic test employed most often is the thyrotropin-releasing hormone (TRH) stimulation test. TRH administration (200 μg intravenously) should cause at least a

TABLE 95-1   Screening Tests to Prove Total Hypophysectomy

	ACTH Cortisol	Growth Hormone	Thyroid Stimulating Hormone	Prolactin	Follicle Stimulating Hormone
Insulin stress	None	—	—	—	—
TRH stimulation	—	None	None	None	—
GnRH stimulation	—	—	—	—	None

twofold rise in prolactin levels within an hour; any rise over 100 percent is considered normal. Failure to obtain a rise is almost always abnormal. A blunted response with a low basal level usually indicates inadequate lactotrope reserve. An elevated basal prolactin level with a subnormal response to TRH is consistent with a prolactin-secreting adenoma. However, a blunted rise is not pathognomonic of a tumor. After total hypophysectomy, no prolactin should be detectable after stimulation with TRH.

A low level of prolactin should be present in the hypopituitary state and can also be seen in patients taking dopaminergic drugs such as L-dopa or bromocriptine. High levels can be due to a number of factors, the most common being pregnancy, breast feeding, hypothyroidism, or the ingestion of drugs such as phenothiazines or estrogens.

Thyroid Function

Routine tests of thyroid function generally indicate an adequate pituitary-thyroid axis. Today, many factors can be measured such as T_3, T_4, and free thyroxine. The free T_4 index is a good screening test of thyroid function, because it takes into account both T_3 uptake and total T_4 in the serum. Radioactive iodine uptake should not be used as a screening test of thyroid function. Table 95-2 shows the physiological levels of these factors.

When these factors are low, one must measure serum thyroid-stimulating hormone (TSH) directly to distinguish primary from secondary hypothyroidism. However, a normal level of TSH is not a satisfactory indication of adequate thyrotrope reserve. In order to measure TSH reserve, TRH (200 μg) is administered intravenously. The adenohypophysis generally is considered normal if TSH values rise to 6 to 20 μU/ml. A blunted response indicates diminished reserve and, therefore, diminished activity of the adenohypophysis, presumably with depopulation of thyrotropic cells. After total hypophysectomy, the administration of TRH should result in no measurable level of TSH. A decreased response to TRH stimulation also occurs in a variety of clinical settings, including glucocorticoid therapy, hyperthyroidism, renal failure, and depression.[4,16]

Adrenocorticotropic Hormone (ACTH)

ACTH is secreted in pulsatile fashion and is highest at 8 A.M. and lowest at midnight. ACTH is difficult to measure, and plasma or urinary cortisol levels also must be measured to assess basal conditions. The mean plasma cortisol level of four to six samples collected from normal individuals over a 24-h period should be 5 to 25 μg/dl. The urinary free cortisol level should be less than 100 μg per 24 h and 17-hydroxysteroids should be 3 to 8 mg per 24 h.

The presence of circulating cortisol is evidence that some ACTH is being secreted from the pituitary gland and thus indicates incomplete hypophysectomy. However, levels may be undetectable despite the presence of a very few remaining cells. ACTH reserve can be demonstrated using the metyrapone test or insulin-induced hypoglycemia. Totally hypophysectomized patients produce no cortisol in response to either of these provocative tests.

Metyrapone inhibits 11-β-hydroxylase in the adrenal cortex, thus blocking the conversion of 11-deoxycortisol to cortisol. The attendant drop in serum cortisol stimulates ACTH secretion by surviving corticotropes. The release of ACTH stimulates the synthesis of 11-deoxycortisol, and the metabolites of this compound can be measured in the urine. Hence, over a 1- or 2-day period, measurable amounts of urinary 17-hydroxycorticoids indicate production of ACTH by the pituitary gland. In normal individuals, 24 h urinary 17-hydroxycorticoid levels measured after metyrapone administration are usually two to three times higher than baseline. The level is lower in hypophysectomized patients, and, if hypophysectomy is complete, no 17-hydroxycorticoids are found in the urine.

A quick test involves the administration of metyrapone (2.0 to 3.0 g) at midnight and the measurement of plasma 11-deoxycortisol and plasma cortisol levels at 8 A.M. In normal subjects, the plasma cortisol value is usually less than 5.0 μg/dl, and plasma 11-deoxycortisol is greater than 7.5 μg/dl. In completely hypophysectomized patients, the plasma deoxycortisol level is negligible. Insulin-induced hypoglycemia also can be used to elicit a rise in cortisol or metabolites, but this has limitations in patients with cardiovascular disease or convulsive disorders.[2,4,16]

Gonadotropic Function

The plasma levels of follicle-stimulating hormone (FSH), luteinizing hormone (LH), estradiol, and testosterone depict the status of the gonadotropic elements of the hypophysis. Where plasma levels of these hormones are not measurable or are low, stimulation with gonadotropin-releasing hormone (GnRH) can help to determine the presence of adequate pituitary reserve.[4,16] Administration of GnRH should produce no detectable level of these hormones in patients with total hypophysectomy, and low levels when reserves are low. Any detectable level of FSH or LH indicates some remaining gonadotropic cells.

High levels of the pituitary hormones and low levels of

TABLE 95-2 Normal Endocrine Values

Adrenocorticotropin (ACTH)	< 80 pg/ml	
Growth hormone (GH)	2–5 ng/ml	Resting
Prolactin (PRL)		
Male	0–10 ng/dl	
Female	0–15 ng/dl	
Thyroid stimulating hormone (TSH)	0.5–3.5 μU/ml	
Luteinizing hormone (LH)		
Male	6–30 mIU/ml	
Female	5–30 mIU/ml	Follicular
	40–200 mIU/ml	Midcycle
	5–40 mIU/ml	Luteal
Follicle stimulating hormone (FSH)		
Male	5–25 mIU/ml	
Female	5–30 mIU/ml	Follicular
	28–94 mIU/ml	Midcycle
	5–30 mIU/ml	Luteal
Alpha subunits		
Male and female	0.5–2.5 ng/ml	
Menopausal female	0.5–5.0 ng/ml	
Somatomedin C		
Male	0.34–1.9 U/ml	Ages 18–64
Female	0.45–2.2 U/ml	Ages 18–64
Thyroxine (T$_4$)	4.0–12.0 μg/dl	
T$_3$ resin uptake	25–35%	
Free T$_4$ index	1.0–4.0	
Cortisol		
8 A.M.	5–25 μg/dl	
8 P.M.	≤ 10 μg/dl	
11-Deoxycortisol	≥ 7.5 μg/dl	After metyrapone
Urinary cortisol	20–70 μg/24 h	
17-Hydroxysteroids	3.0–8.0 mg/day	
17-Ketosteroids		
Male	6.0–21.0 mg/24 h	Age 20
	8.0–26.0	Age 30
	5.0–18.0	Age 50
	2.0–10.0	Age 70
Female	4.0–16.0 mg/24 h	Age 20
	4.0–14.0	Age 30
	3.0–9.0	Age 50
	1.0–7.0	Age 70
Testosterone		
Male	300–1100 μg/dl	
Female	25–90 μg/dl	
Unbound testosterone		
Male	3.06–24.0 ng/dl	
Female	0.09–1.28 ng/ml	
Progesterone		
Male	< 1 ng/ml	
Female	0.21–3.1 ng/ml	Follicular
	5.7–33.6 ng/ml	Luteal

the end organ hormones testosterone or estradiol indicate end organ failure. When the levels of both pituitary and end organ hormones are high, rare pituitary adenomas secreting gonadotropins or pituitary hormone resistance states may be present.

Prolactin-Secreting Tumors

Prolactin is under tonic inhibition by the hypothalamus and thus is unique among pituitary hormones. Dopamine is the hypothalamic agent primarily implicated in the inhibition of prolactin. Pituitary stalk section and a variety of substances can over-ride tonic inhibition, thus causing secretion of prolactin by the adenohypophysis. In addition, a number of substances act directly on lactotropes or the hypothalamus to negate the influence of dopaminergic inhibition.[9,16,23,29]

The principal prolactin-stimulating factors are estrogen and TRH. Estrogen acts directly at the level of the pituitary lactotrope to stimulate the synthesis and release of prolactin. In normal subjects, the administration of either estrogen or TRH causes a prompt two- to three-fold rise of the prolactin level. The administration of serotonin or its precursors (e.g., 5-hydroxytryptophan or L-tryptophan) also increases prolactin levels. Agents like γ-aminobutyric acid, the phenothiazines, metoclopramide, opiate agonists, and intravenous cimetidine have a variable effect, whereas serotonin blockers, L-dopa, and other dopaminergic agents can reduce the level of prolactin.

Diagnosis

Men and women with large prolactin-secreting tumors present no major diagnostic problem because a positive CT scan and an elevated level of prolactin together are diagnostic, especially if the prolactin level is greater than 200 to 300 ng/ml. Lower levels may be found with non-neoplastic lesions that functionally sever the pituitary stalk or with other lesions such as mixed prolactin and growth hormone–secreting tumors.[3,9,15,23,26,29]

Hyperprolactinemia is a common finding in infertility clinics, especially in women with amenorrhea and galactorrhea, but can be associated with a number of conditions besides pituitary tumors; 20 to 30 percent of patients with amenorrhea may have such tumors. The diagnosis of a microadenoma generally demands great experience and judgment, since endocrine and radiological tests can be misleading. The diagnosis generally is suspected when women begin to experience menstrual irregularity or amenorrhea and galactorrhea. Amenorrhea can be the sole sign of a prolactin-secreting tumor, whereas galactorrhea alone accompanied by normal menstrual function is seldom the sole expression of such a tumor. Some patients have mild rises of prolactin and growth hormone and report not only amenorrhea and galactorrhea but also fatigue, weakness, and slight swelling of hands and feet. Their tumor may demonstrate both prolactin and growth hormone secreting cells. Removal is followed by a return to well being and resumption of normal menstrual function. These can be termed clinically active dual secretory adenomas.

The single most useful endocrine maneuver is determination of the basal serum prolactin level. In most laboratories the normal level ranges from 5 to 20 ng/ml. Minimal elevations must be confirmed by averaging several samples taken during the day in patients who have taken no medication during the previous week. When an elevated prolactin level is confirmed but radiological verification is absent, great care must be exercised in making decisions regarding therapy.

The higher the prolactin level, the more likely it is that a tumor is present. When the level is much lower than 100 ng/ml, the likelihood of finding an identifiable tumor drops by as much as 50 percent. With levels as high as 350 ng/ml, a tumor is almost always found.

The size of the prolactin-secreting tumor also is related to the level of serum prolactin, but with wide variations.[14] Microadenomas can secrete levels as high as 550 ng/ml, whereas larger tumors (i.e., with a diameter of 2 cm or greater) can secrete levels lower than 100 ng/ml. One must keep in mind that prolactin levels as high as 150 to 200 ng/ml can be caused by partial or total functional pituitary stalk section resulting from some other process or tumor. Thus, a small craniopharyngioma, a null cell tumor, an oncocytoma, or a vascular, granulomatous, or other type of lesion can account for hyperprolactinemia. In such cases, the hyperprolactinemia can revert to normal with bromocriptine therapy while the nonsecretory lesion grows to invasive size. In view of this possibility, it is necessary to ensure after operation that a presumed prolactinoma in fact contains prolactin granules as demonstrated by immunocytochemistry.

Ancillary Tests

Various stimulation and suppression tests provide ancillary aid in arriving at a diagnosis.[3,15,16,23,28,29] In a pragmatic sense, no dynamic endocrine test is totally reliable for the diagnosis of a prolactin-secreting adenoma. TRH is an excellent stimulus of pituitary lactotropes and causes hypersecretion by normal cells. However, in patients with prolactinomas, additional secretion generally does not occur, thus the level of prolactin during the hour following the administration of TRH does not rise significantly, whereas in normal patients it may rise by two- or even three-fold. A flat TRH response is consistent with, but not exclusively diagnostic of, a pituitary tumor, since approximately 10 percent of patients with tumors demonstrate an additional rise in prolactin level after TRH administration.

Several other tests have been evaluated. The administration of 500 mg of L-dopa suppresses prolactin levels by 50 percent in normal subjects; patients with prolactinomas do not always exhibit the same degree of suppression. However, marked suppression with L-dopa can occur, and the existence of considerable overlap of normal and abnormal results negates the value of this test.

Chlorpromazine often increases prolactin levels in normal individuals, but not in patients with tumors. The response, however, is variable, and hence unreliable. Metoclopramide stimulates prolactin secretion and usually doubles the resting prolactin level in normal individuals. Trials in patients with prolactin-secreting tumors usually show a blunted response. Although advocated as an ancillary test, it is not unfailingly accurate.

Nomifensine, a dopaminergic antidepressant, inhibits dopamine reuptake and/or stimulates dopamine release, thus reducing serum prolactin to less than 30 or 40 percent of the baseline level. Most patients with tumors exhibit less suppression, but some show as much as normal individuals, negating the value of the test. In addition, about 30 to 40 percent of normal individuals do not exhibit significant suppression with nomifensine. Although the results may be of interest, L-dopa, chlorpromazine, metoclopramide, or nomifensine testing is not done in the routine evaluation of hyperprolactinemia.

The criteria mentioned above apply to both sexes, as there is no consistent difference between normal serum prolactin levels in men and nonpregnant women. Prolactinomas are common in men (60 percent of all adenomas), but usually are found only when large, since systemic complaints often are ignored for many years. Thus, men may not seek early attention despite loss of libido and potency, headache, or fatigue. Only when visual loss or disturbing endocrine symptoms are present do they seek medical attention, by which time the opportunity for early endocrine diagnosis is lost.

Differential Diagnosis

Hypothyroidism, pregnancy, and depression as well as chronic disease of the liver and renal failure must be excluded, as these entities also can be associated with hyperprolactinemia.[6] In addition, prolactin levels are sometimes elevated in hypoglycemia, during stress, and in the postpartum period. Acromegaly can be associated with modest elevations in prolactin levels, sometimes as high as 150 to 200 ng/ml. Hyperprolactinemia also can accompany Cushing's disease. Since some commonly used drugs enhance prolactin secretion, especially psychotropic drugs, estrogens, and some antihypertensives,[24] a complete drug history is mandatory.

Postoperative Evaluation

Total removal of a prolactin-secreting microadenoma returns prolactin levels to normal within a day or two. If the level is lower than 10 ng/ml, the surgeon can feel confident of prolonged remission, if not outright cure. When the level of prolactin is normal, ovulation and menstruation return in at least 75 percent of women and galactorrhea ceases. These findings are evidence of total remission, although recurrence is still possible. Failure of prolactin to fall to normal levels usually is caused by incomplete tumor removal. However, it also can result from injury to the pituitary stalk. If the surgeon suspects a retained fragment of tumor in the first few weeks after operation in a straightforward case, early re-exploration is warranted.[22]

Clinical evidence of late recurrence is much more sensitive. Thus, if menses and ovulation again begin to fail and if galactorrhea resumes, endocrine verification must be undertaken quickly.

Acromegaly

Patients thought to have acromegaly on clinical grounds must undergo verification by endocrine testing and CT scanning. The differential diagnosis must exclude individuals with a genetically determined physiognomy similar to that of the acromegalic but who do not have the disease. All individuals with true acromegaly harbor a growth hormone–secreting adenoma or, more rarely, an ectopic tumor producing growth hormone–releasing factor (GRF).[9,15,16,23,29]

The level of growth hormone is governed by the interplay of GRF, a 41–amino acid peptide characterized in 1983, and somatostatin, an inhibitory 14–amino acid peptide. The balance between these two peptides is regulated by neighboring hypothalamic neurons. Other substances that can stimulate growth hormone release are: enkephalin, glucagon, α-melanocyte-stimulating hormone, vasopressin, diazepam, and estrogens. Variations during the day are quite striking. High levels of growth hormone are found during the first few hours of sleep, with smaller rises occurring during the day. For many hours no secretion is evident. The ventromedial and infundibular nuclei of the hypothalamus are involved with the pulsatile nature of the secretion.[8,18]

Stimulation of growth hormone release is mediated through alpha-adrenergic and dopaminergic mechanisms. Therefore, in normal individuals, the growth hormone level increases after the administration of norepinephrine, L-dopa, clonidine, and apomorphine. In addition, behavioral conditions that stimulate alpha-adrenergic mechanisms, such as stress, hypoglycemia, and exercise, also enhance the secretion of growth hormone. The limbic system participates in growth hormone release through serotonergic mechanisms. Thus, the administration of serotonin precursors such as L-tryptophan or 5-hydroxytryptophan also causes growth hormone release.

Beta-receptor mechanisms inhibit the secretion of growth hormone. Therefore, isoproterenol blocks secretion, whereas propanolol, its antagonist, enhances secretion to a certain extent in response to glucagon, vasopressin, and L-dopa. Growth hormone release also is inhibited by the administration of glucocorticoids and in patients who are obese or have elevated levels of free fatty acids.

The somatomedins mediate the stimulation of cell growth by growth hormone.[19,20] Two somatomedins have been identified, and their secretion by the liver depends largely on the level of growth hormone. Somatomedin C possesses properties similar to those of insulin, and its level is increased in acromegaly.

Once acromegaly is suspected, endocrine diagnosis depends on the demonstration of elevated levels of human growth hormone that fail to decrease to less than 5 ng/ml during a glucose tolerance test. It must be remembered, however, that normal adolescents sometimes do not demonstrate this suppression. Almost all acromegalics have levels of growth hormone greater than 10 ng/ml, but a few have levels between 4 and 10 ng/ml. Measurement of somatomedin C is helpful in equivocal cases. Levels of somatomedin C are almost never normal in active acromegaly, and they are elevated in acromegalics with low (4 to 10 ng/ml) levels of human growth hormone. The clinical disturbances of acromegaly are related more closely to the level of somatomedin C than to the level of growth hormone.[5]

Acromegalic patients do not display normal regulatory responses to certain agents, and often their growth hormone response is described as "parodoxical."[8,12] For example, in 10 to 20 percent of patients, glucose ingestion does not cause the fall in growth hormone levels seen in normal individuals, but rather causes a paradoxical rise. L-Dopa increases growth hormone values in normal subjects, but in most acromegalics it induces a fall. Similarly, the dopaminergic agonist bromocriptine, while increasing growth hormone levels in normal individuals, causes a decrease in some acromegalics. This finding is the basis of bromocriptine therapy for acromegaly. TRH does not affect the growth hormone level in normal subjects, but increases it in 70 to 80 percent of acromegalics. The serotonergic agonist L-tryptophan, while increasing human growth hormone values in normal subjects, causes no change in patients with acromegaly. Taken together, these factors help to clarify the diagnosis in doubtful cases. They are especially helpful in adolescents and in patients thought to have gigantism.

The endocrine diagnosis of acromegaly has received much attention, and some consensus has been reached. In the normal individual, plasma levels of growth hormone show considerable variation over a 24 h period with a sleep associated rise. Several samples usually have no measurable level of growth hormone, and the mean value is 4 ng/ml or less. In the acromegalic, basal levels vary from 5 ng/ml to levels in the hundreds or, rarely, thousands. In most patients with microadenomas or small tumors, the mean level is greater than 10 ng/ml; levels as high as 40 ng/ml have been recorded. When the serum concentration is greater than 40 ng/ml, a large tumor, perhaps with suprasellar extension or invasion of the sphenoid sinus or surrounding areas, may be present. Since the mean values are sometimes high in normal individuals, the diagnosis requires further verification when the sella turcica appears normal.

Hyperglycemia fails to suppress the hypersecretion of growth hormone in acromegalics. Therefore, endocrinologists rely on the oral glucose tolerance test as the best screening and diagnostic test for acromegaly. If the elevated basal level of growth hormone fails to fall below 5 ng/ml during the test, it is safe to conclude that the patient has acromegaly. In normal patients the level of growth hormone usually drops to 0 to 3 ng/ml. The untreated acromegalic does not exhibit this suppression, and even may show a paradoxical rise in growth hormone values. In many patients with untreated acromegaly, but not in normal individuals, TRH stimulates the release of growth hormone. Surgical cure of acromegaly should eliminate this response.

The somatomedin C level is always elevated in active acromegaly. Normal levels are 0.34 to 1.97 IU/ml in males and 0.45 to 2.2 IU/ml in females. Higher levels suggest acromegaly.

In summary, the endocrine diagnosis of acromegaly rests on the determination of sustained high levels of human growth hormone, the failure of glucose loading to suppress the level of growth hormone to less than 5 ng/ml, and the presence of elevated levels of somatomedin C.

Evaluation of patients after operation, radiotherapy, or pharmacologic treatment demands the same testing. These therapies rarely return human growth hormone dynamics completely to normal. Nevertheless, if the mean value of growth hormone is less than 5 ng/ml, clinical remission is almost certain in all spheres save those in which permanent changes have already taken place. Thus, bone changes and cardiac disease rarely reverse, but should not progress. Absolute cure of acromegaly is accompanied by a full return of normal dynamics, i.e., the mean value of growth hormone on four to six determinations during the day would not be higher than 2 to 4 ng/ml, oral glucose would suppress growth hormone levels to below 5 ng/ml, and somatomedin C levels would return to normal. Use of the term "cure" or "remission" when resting levels of growth hormone are greater than 4 ng/ml and are not suppressed to less than 5 ng/ml with glucose loading is misleading and inaccurate.

Recurrence also can be detected by these examinations. The first indication of recurrence may be the return of a paradoxical response of growth hormone to glucose intake or TRH infusion despite low mean basal levels. It is necessary to remember that any therapy that results in apparent normalization of growth hormone levels may be accompanied by continued or later growth of the tumor. Consequently, even when endocrine testing is normal, if the patient reports a return of symptoms, every effort should be made to detect a possible recurrence so that appropriate therapy can be instituted as soon as possible.

Cushing's Disease

Cushing's disease can be defined as hypersecretion of cortisol caused by an abnormality of the pituitary gland. The lesion most commonly responsible for the disease is an adenoma. More rarely, pituitary hyperplasia is the cause.

Hypercortisolemia also can be caused by a number of different systemic lesions such as ectopic tumors that produce ACTH or adrenal cortical lesions that produce cortisol.[11,17] The general syndrome caused by excess cortisol is, by convention, called *Cushing's syndrome*. The term *Cushing's disease* is used for parasellar etiologies.[25]

The diagnostic problem thus is twofold: (1) the verification of hypercortisolemia, and (2) the identification of the primary cause of the hypercortisolemia.[1,4,7,9,15,16,21,23,29]

Corticotropin-releasing factor is produced in neurons in the anterior median eminence of the hypothalamus and regulates normal ACTH secretion by the pituitary gland.[2,21] ACTH secretion has a diurnal rhythm, which is regulated by the central nervous system. The highest levels are found early in the morning, with spiking later during the day, especially in midafternoon. The diurnal rhythm of cortisol secretion must be taken into account when resting or sporadic sampling of plasma is undertaken. The secretion of ACTH is dependent on serotonergic mechanisms and can be blocked by serotonin-blocking agents. Many forms of stress, including hypoglycemia, also increase the production of ACTH through mechanisms mediated by the hypothalamus. Negative feedback on ACTH secretion is due primarily to the action of plasma cortisol, which exerts its effect directly on the pituitary gland and probably also on the hypothalamus.

The stimulation of the adrenal gland by ACTH causes the secretion of cortisol and some adrenal androgens and estrogens. Because of similarities in structure between ACTH and melanocyte-stimulating hormone, ACTH possesses some melanocytic stimulating activity as well.

The Demonstration of Hypercortisolemia

Basal Levels

Screening tests can be used to determine whether cortisol secretion is within the range of normal. Plasma cortisol levels vary widely and are therefore rarely useful as a screening test. A 24-h urine collection can be tested for free cortisol and 17-hydroxycorticosteroids. Elevation of either raises the suspicion of Cushing's syndrome. An amount of free cortisol above 100 μg per 24 h or of 17-hydroxycorticosteroids above 12 mg per 24 h suggests hypersecretion of cortisol.

Cortisol Dynamics

The demonstration of abnormal cortisol dynamics is also valuable in making the diagnosis of Cushing's syndrome. In normal individuals, serum cortisol is highest at 8 A.M. and, despite pulses of secretion during the day, is lowest between 6 P.M. and midnight. This fluctuation (termed the *diurnal rhythm*) is lost in Cushing's syndrome, where the midnight level might be 8 μg/dl or higher (normal is <8 μg/dl). Conversely, re-establishment of a normal diurnal pattern is a reliable demonstration of remission of the disease.

Suppression of Cortisolemia

In normal individuals, the administration of a small quantity of a glucocorticoid such as dexamethasone lowers the level of cortisol in plasma or 17-hydroxysteroids and free cortisol in the urine. When Cushing's syndrome is caused by a pituitary disorder, the hypothalamic "set point" for dexamethasone inhibition of ACTH secretion is believed to be raised, thus requiring a higher dose of dexamethasone to suppress ACTH and cortisol secretion. When an excess of cortisol is suspected, a quick overnight test is carried out as follows. At 11 P.M., 1 mg of dexamethasone is given by mouth. The following morning (8 A.M.), serum cortisol is determined again. If the cortisol level is less than 5 μg/dl, Cushing's syndrome can be eliminated as a possibility.

An overnight dexamethasone test is the best screening test for Cushing's syndrome. An abnormal test does not establish the diagnosis; however, it indicates the need for additional testing, since stress, estrogen therapy, phenytoin, and failure to do the test properly all can cause abnormal results. If Cushing's syndrome is suspected, a low dose of oral dexamethasone (0.5 mg four times a day for 2 days) is then given. In normal individuals, the urinary free cortisol and 17-hydroxysteroid values fall over a 24 h period to less than half of baseline levels. In patients with Cushing's syndrome, cortisol levels and urinary steroids fail to suppress.

If the low-dose dexamethasone test is abnormal, the patient is given a 2-day high-dose dexamethasone test. This requires the administration of four 2-mg doses daily for 2 days. The plasma and urinary factors should be reduced by more than 50 percent to signify suppressibility. On some occasions, more than 8 mg of dexamethasone are necessary to suppress pituitary-based Cushing's syndrome. Consistent suppression of cortisol production by high-dose dexamethasone is diagnostic of ACTH-dependent Cushing's syndrome. Recently, an overnight test has been used in which 8 mg of dexamethasone is given at midnight, and plasma cortisol is measured at 8 A.M. and compared with the level obtained the previous morning.

The key point is the failure of low doses of dexamethasone to suppress cortisol but the ability of high doses to suppress cortisol to 50 percent of the baseline level. Under these circumstances, a pituitary lesion can be implicated with a confidence level of 90 percent in the face of a normal CT scan or plain sellar tomography.

Many lesions causing Cushing's syndrome are independent of pituitary influence, and these require diagnostic measures to prove that manipulation of endogenous ACTH fails to alter hypercortisolemia. In these cases, the use of higher and higher doses of dexamethasone to suppress the hypothalamic-pituitary axis never suppresses cortisol secretion.

Plasma ACTH Levels

Although Cushing's disease is accompanied by hypersecretion of ACTH, the levels of ACTH in plasma are often normal or only slightly elevated. Therefore, they cannot be used to make the diagnosis. ACTH levels in normal individuals vary from 50 to 100 pg/ml; in Cushing's disease, they can range from 50 to 250 pg/ml. Moreover, the radioimmunoassay for ACTH is difficult, can be unreliable, and is not as valuable as dexamethasone suppression testing.

β-Lipotropin synthesis is accompanied by equimolar ACTH synthesis, as each of these agents is derived from the same molecule, pro-opiocortin. In the future, the assay for β-lipotropin might prove to be a useful test for Cushing's disease.

A patient's response to exogenous ACTH can also help to diagnose Cushing's disease. In patients with Cushing's disease, cortisol shows an exaggerated response to ACTH, whereas in those with ectopic ACTH tumors the response is variable.

In doubtful cases, measurement of ACTH in venous blood taken from the sigmoid sinus on each side might show an ACTH gradient, the level being higher than that in blood taken from an arm vein. This test is not used very often, but it can be helpful.

Differential Diagnosis

As discussed above, Cushing's disease is associated with hypercortisolemia, loss of the diurnal rhythm of cortisol secretion, and normal to slightly raised levels of ACTH in plasma. The definitive diagnosis is based on the failure of low-dose dexamethasone (0.5 mg orally, four times a day for 2 days) to suppress the level of cortisol by 50 percent, whereas high doses (2.0 mg orally, four times a day for 2 days) are successful in suppressing it.

However, a number of lesions cause hypercortisolemia, and detection of them rules out Cushing's disease.[1,7] Diagnosis by exclusion and inclusion is often necessary in doubtful cases. If the laboratory testing for Cushing's disease is inconsistent, one should be careful in making this diagnosis, especially if the neuroradiological picture is not diagnostic of a pituitary tumor.

Some adrenal lesions and ectopic ACTH-producing tumors have pulsatile secretory behavior that can confuse the results of dexamethasone suppression testing. Also, hypersecretion can be sporadic in Cushing's disease, necessitating long-term repeated testing. A false-positive diagnosis of Cushing's disease is observed sometimes in alcoholics (alcoholic pseudo-Cushing's disease). More important, depressed patients can exhibit hypercortisolemia and, to a certain extent, may appear to be "cushingoid" when, in fact, they are simply obese. These individuals may show loss of diurnal variation and increased cortisol levels during the day. They can be distinguished from those with Cushing's disease by their lack of true clinical signs of excessive cortisol and their response to insulin-induced hypoglycemia. Patients with Cushing's disease have no noticeable increases in plasma cortisol during periods of hypoglycemic stress, whereas depressed or normal individuals demonstrate the usual rise in cortisol levels. Some depressed patients fail to suppress after dexamethasone administration.

Ectopic ACTH-Secreting Tumors

A number of malignant tumors can secrete ACTH, including oat cell carcinoma of the lung, some bronchial adenomas, medullary carcinoma of the thyroid, pancreatic carcinoma, and carcinoid tumors.[11] In these cases the production of ACTH is autonomous and fails to respond to increasing doses of dexamethasone. Whereas pituitary adenomas may produce moderately increased amounts of ACTH, ectopic ACTH tumors produce very high levels. Localization of the ectopic ACTH tumor, which is often small, requires CT scanning or other imaging techniques in other organs.

Hypercortisolemia also can be caused by adrenal lesions such as independent adenomas and adrenal carcinoma. These lesions are independent of ACTH, and thus hypercortisolemia is resistant to the administration of dexamethasone (no suppression) or of ACTH (no elevation). Also, resting ACTH levels in these diseases are usually low or undetectable.

ACTH-independent Cushing's syndrome is also resistant to metyrapone, i.e., to induced hypocortisolemia. With ACTH-independent Cushing's syndrome, administration of metyrapone fails to cause a rise in ACTH levels because of chronic suppression of the pituitary ACTH function. Consequently, urinary 17-hydroxysteroids and plasma 11-deoxycortisol values do not increase after the administration of metyrapone. In contrast, the response to metyrapone usually is exaggerated in Cushing's disease.

The early diagnosis of Cushing's disease can be difficult, but is being done with increasing frequency today because of heightened awareness on the part of physicians. Early cases can lack the classic stigmata, and hypercortisolemia may be marginal. Classic features often help to identify true Cushing's disease and differentiate the various causes of the syndrome. Cushing's disease is commonest in young to middle-aged women and has a slow progression. In early cases, abnormal menstrual cycles, abnormal striae, spontaneous bruising, and hypertension may be absent. The progression is slow, and androgen excess or hirsutism may be minimal. The classic ectopic ACTH syndrome, on the other hand, is found typically in older males who smoke to excess. Recent weight loss, anemia, low serum potassium levels, and severe hypertension are prominent. Adrenal adenomas are relatively slowly progressive; cortisol excess is mild, and very often androgen features are minimal. Adrenal carcinoma has a rapid onset with very high levels of adrenocorticoid hormones. Adrenal carcinomas and adenomas that produce cortisol cause atrophy of the contralateral adrenal. Consequently, asymmetry of the adrenals should warn against the diagnosis of a pituitary adenoma.[1,7,11,17]

It is well to remember that the accuracy of endocrine testing for Cushing's disease is not absolute, but is in the range of 90 percent. Consequently, in the absence of confirmation by CT or other imaging modality, errors will be made, and this must be stressed to the patient and family in the context of discussions surrounding operation.

Postoperative Evaluation

Early postoperative evaluation is limited to measuring serum cortisol levels. All patients require replacement therapy of adrenal cortisol hormones because the normal corticotropes are suppressed. Following the removal of the adenoma, it is necessary to use dexamethasone in the early postoperative period to confirm the adequacy of the operative procedure. Dexamethasone does not cross react significantly with the serum cortisol testing procedure. Several days after operation, when the patient is on maintenance doses of dexamethasone, the plasma cortisol level should be determined. If it is 2 to 5 μg/dl, one can have some confidence that the procedure was successful and that satisfactory removal of the tumor has been accomplished. True remission, as measured by endocrine testing as opposed to clinical examination, demands the following: (1) normal or low serum cortisol levels; (2) return of diurnal rhythm; (3) normal 24-h urinary output of free cortisol and 17-hydroxysteroids; (4) normal dexamethasone suppressibility.

When these criteria are met, especially if clinical remission has occurred as well, one's confidence of total removal can be high. As time goes on, the need for replacement therapy lessens as normal endogenous cortisol secretion returns. At this time, formal testing should detect normal cortisol dynamics and basal levels.

TSH-Secreting Pituitary Adenomas

Pituitary adenomas that secrete thyroid-stimulating hormone are unusual and account for less than 1 percent of all adenomas.[15,16,23,29] Diagnosis requires judicious interpreta-

tion of serum TSH levels. These can range from 1.6 to 480 μU/ml in the presence of clinical hyperthyroidism. In approximately 30 percent of these cases, TSH levels are lower than 10 μU/ml.

In addition, TSH-secreting adenomas commonly release excessive quantities of the alpha subunit of this glycoprotein hormone.[27] In terms of molarity, the alpha subunit exceeds the TSH beta subunit, the other half of the molecule. The ratio of the alpha subunit to TSH is greater than 1.

In normal individuals, TRH stimulation causes a rise in TSH. In patients with TSH-secreting pituitary adenomas, the response to TRH is negligible, with few exceptions. This blunting of the response is not seen exclusively in TSH-secreting adenomas, but helps in making the diagnosis. Thyroid hormone generally suppresses TSH secretion in normal persons. However, the administration of thyroid hormone may fail to suppress TSH and the free alpha subunit when the tumor is a TSH-secreting adenoma.

Gonadotropin-Secreting Pituitary Adenomas

The gonadotropin-secreting pituitary adenomas usually produce FSH and/or LH. One recent problem in diagnosis has been the sensitivity of the radioimmunoassay for FSH and LH. Other problems involve the high serum concentration of gonadotropins normally observed in menopause. Since these tumors have few systemic effects, they rarely are diagnosed until headache and loss of vision have been reported. Three types of tumor have been recorded: LH-secreting, FSH-secreting, and FSH- and LH-secreting. Many difficulties arise in making the diagnosis, as other factors such as testicular failure may be the cause of elevated levels of FSH or LH. Thus, serum testosterone concentrations must be obtained to verify the diagnosis. This diagnosis is complex and is beyond the scope of this chapter. The reader is referred to more comprehensive examinations of the subject.[10,23]

Alpha Subunit–Secreting Pituitary Adenomas

The glycoprotein hormones are composed of alpha and beta subunits. The alpha subunit is the same for all of these hormones. The beta subunit is unique to each hormone and confers biological and immunologic specificity. Some rare pituitary adenomas have been associated solely with the production of the alpha subunit. The laboratory tests used to determine the alpha subunit and to restrict the diagnosis convincingly to this entity are complex. Nevertheless, this entity must be considered, especially in patients with large, apparently nonsecreting tumors. The serum alpha-subunit level can be measured directly by radioimmunoassay. For further confirmation, immunocytochemical staining of the tissue should be carried out to demonstrate the presence of the alpha subunit alone in the secretory granules.

Future Trends

As this chapter is written, major advances are being made in the synthesis of factors such as corticotropin-releasing hormone and somatotropin-inhibiting hormone, and the assay of ACTH and other fragments of pro-opiocortin. It is to be expected that as these and other new techniques are developed, the diagnosis and management of pituitary tumors will undergo further improvements.

References

1. Aron DC, Tyrrell JB, Fitzgerald PA, Findling JW, Forsham PH: Cushing's syndrome: Problems in diagnosis. Medicine (Baltimore) 60:25–35, 1981.
2. Baxter JD, Tyrrell JB: The adrenal cortex, in Felig P, Baxter JD, Broadus AE, Frohman LA (eds): *Endocrinology and Metabolism.* New York, McGraw-Hill, 1981.
3. Boyd AE III, Reichlin S, Turksoy RN: Galactorrhea-amenorrhea syndrome: Diagnosis and therapy. Ann Intern Med 87:165–175, 1977.
4. Christy NP, Warren MP: Disease syndromes of the hypothalamus and anterior pituitary, in Degroot LJ, Cahill GF Jr, Odell WD, Martini L, Potts JT Jr, Nelson DH, Steinberger E, Winegrad AI (eds): *Endocrinology.* New York, Grune & Stratton, 1979, pp 215–252.
5. Clemmons DR, Van Wyk JJ, Ridgway EC, Kliman B, Kjellberg RN, Underwood LE: Evaluation of acromegaly by radioimunoassay of somatomedin-C. N Engl J Med 301:1138–1142, 1979.
6. Cowden EA, Ratcliffe WA, Ratcliffe JG, Dobbie JW, Kennedy AC: Hyperprolactinaemia in renal disease. Clin Endocrinol (Oxf) 9:241–248, 1978.
7. Crapo L: Cushing's syndrome: A review of diagnostic tests. Metabolism 28:955–977, 1979.
8. Eddy RL, Gilliland PF, Ibarra JD Jr, McMurry JF Jr, Thompson JQ: Human growth hormone release: Comparison of provocative test procedures. Am J Med 56:179–185, 1974.
9. Faglia G, Giovanelli MA, McLeod RM: *International Symposium on Pituitary Microadenomas.* London, Academic, 1980.
10. Harris RI, Schatz NJ, Gennarelli T, Savino PJ, Cobbs WH, Snyder PJ: Follicle-stimulating hormone-secreting pituitary adenomas: Correlation of reduction of adenoma size with reduction of hormonal hypersecretion after transsphenoidal surgery. J Clin Endocrinol Metab 56:1288–1293, 1983.
11. Imura H, Matsukura S, Yamamoto H, Hirata Y, Nakai Y, Endo J, Tanaka A, Nakamura M: Studies on ectopic ACTH-producing tumors: II. Clinical and biochemical features of 30 cases. Cancer 35:1430–1437, 1975.
12. Irie M, Tsushima T: Increase of serum growth hormone concentration following thyrotropin-releasing hormone injection in patients with acromegaly or gigantism. J Clin Endocrinol Metab 35:97–100, 1972.
13. Klibanski A, Neer RM, Beitins IZ, Ridgway EC, Zervas NT, McArthur JW: Decreased bone density in hyperprolactinemic women. N Engl J Med 303:1511–1514, 1980.
14. Klijn JGM, Lamberts SWJ, DeJong FH, Docter R, Van Dongen KJ, Birkenhäger JC: The importance of pituitary tumour size in patients with hyperprolactinaemia in relation to hormonal variables and extrasellar extension of tumour. Clin Endocrinol (Oxf) 12:341–355, 1980.
15. Linfoot JA (ed): *Recent Advances in the Diagnosis and Treatment of Pituitary Tumors.* New York, Raven Press, 1979.
16. Martin JB, Reichlin S, Brown GM (eds): *Clinical Neuroendocrinology.* Philadelphia, Davis, 1977.
17. Meador CK, Bowdoin B, Owen WC Jr, Farmer TA Jr: Primary adrenocortical nodular dysplasia: A rare cause of Cushing's syndrome. J Clin Endocrinol Metab 27:1255–1263, 1967.
18. Merimee TJ: Growth hormone: Secretion and action, in De Groot LJ, Cahill GF Jr, Odell WD, Martini L, Potts JT Jr, Nelson DH, Steinberger E, Winegrad AI (eds): *Endocrinology.* New York, Grune & Stratton, 1979, pp 123–132.
19. Phillips LS, Vasilopoulou-Sellin R: Somatomedins: First of two parts. N Engl J Med 302:371–380, 1980.
20. Phillips LS, Vasilopoulou-Sellin R: Somatomedins: Second of two parts. N Engl J Med 302:438–446, 1980.
21. Pieters GFFM, Hermus ARMM, Smals AGH, Bartelink AKM, Benraad TJ, Kloppenborg PWC, Kloppenborg PWC: Responsiveness of the hypophyseal-adrenocortical axis to corticotropin-releasing factor in pituitary-dependent Cushing's disease. J Clin Endocrinol Metab 57:513–516, 1983.
22. Post KD, Biller BJ, Adelman LS, Molitch ME, Wolpert SM, Reichlin S: Selective transsphenoidal adenomectomy in women with galactorrhea-amenorrhea. JAMA 242:158–162, 1979.
23. Post KD, Jackson IMD, Reichlin S (eds): *The Pituitary Adenoma.* New York, Plenum, 1980.
24. Reyniak JV, Wenof M, Aubert JM, Stangel JJ: Incidence of hyperprolactinemia during oral contraceptive therapy. Obstet Gynecol 55:8–11, 1980.
25. Salassa RM, Kearns TP, Kernohan JW, Sprague RG, Mac Carty CS: Pituitary tumors in patients with Cushing's syndrome. J Clin Endocrinol Metab 19:1523–1539, 1959.
26. Schlechte J, Sherman B, Halmi N, VanGilder J, Chapler F, Dolan K, Granner D, Duello T, Harris C: Prolactin-secreting pituitary tumors in amenorrheic women: A comprehensive study. Endocr Rev 1:295–308, 1980.
27. Smallridge RC, Smith CE: Hyperthyroidism due to thyrotropin-secreting pituitary tumors: Diagnostic and therapeutic considerations. Arch Intern Med 143:503–507, 1983.
28. Sowers JR, McCallum RW, Hershman JM, Carlson HE, Sturdevant RAL, Meyer N: Comparison of metoclopramide with other dynamic tests of prolactin secretion. J Clin Endocrinol Metab 43:679–681, 1976.
29. Zervas NT, Martin JB, Ridgway EC, Black PMcL (eds): *Tumors of the Pituitary Gland.* New York, Raven Press (in press).

96

Prolactinomas

George T. Tindall
Daniel L. Barrow

The prolactinoma is a pituitary tumor that autonomously secretes prolactin, a polypeptide hormone whose amino acid sequence was recently discovered. It is secreted by the erythrosinophilic subtype of acidophilic cells in the adenohypophysis under the dual control of hypothalamic neurohormones that act as releasing and inhibiting factors.

Hypothalamic modulation of prolactin, unlike that of other anterior pituitary hormones, is predominantly one of inhibition. A prolactin inhibitory factor (PIF), required to prevent an unrestrained release of prolactin by the adenohypophysis, has been demonstrated in hypothalamic extracts but not purified and characterized. Thus pituitary stalk section or certain hypothalamic lesions that interfere with the normal delivery of PIF to the anterior lobe increase serum prolactin levels. The prolactin inhibitory mechanism is mediated by the hypothalamic catecholamines dopamine and norepinephrine and blocked by dopaminergic blocking agents such as phenothiazines, tricyclic antidepressants, methyldopa, and reserpine. There is some evidence that dopamine is the naturally occurring PIF.

A prolactin-releasing factor (PRF), possibly regulated by serotonin, has been identified in hypothalamic extracts but has not been characterized. Thyrotropin-releasing hormone (TRH) is a potent stimulator of prolactin release from the pituitary but is not believed to be the physiological PRF.

A variety of hormones and endocrine disorders affect serum prolactin levels. Prolactin secretion is increased by the administration of estrogens and is diminished following oophorectomy. Patients with primary hypothyroidism may have hyperprolactinemia stemming from an increased responsiveness to the prolactin-releasing activity of TRH. Hyperthyroid patients, on the other hand, do not respond to TRH with elevated serum prolactin levels.

In humans, prolactin is essential for stimulation of breast tissue growth and for initiation and maintenance of lactation, provided that the glandular breast tissue has been appropriately primed by the interaction of several other hormones, including estrogen, progestins, corticosteroids, growth hormone, and insulin. Small amounts of prolactin are also necessary for progesterone production by granulosa cells, but hyperprolactinemia inhibits progesterone production.

Although the function of prolactin in males is unclear, the hormone appears to be necessary for normal sperm production. Hyperprolactinemia has been shown to inhibit 5α-reductase, which converts inactive testosterone to the biologically active dihydrotestosterone, a hormone necessary in high concentrations within the testicular tubules for spermatogenesis to occur.

In the past, hyperprolactinemia was not considered a health hazard. However, in view of a report by Klibanski et al. describing decreased bone density in 14 hyperprolactinemic women,[6] the traditional concept of hyperprolactinemia as a benign condition must be questioned. In their study, the decreased density correlated with the relative or absolute estrogen deficiency that can accompany hyperprolactinemia. As the serum prolactin values were not excessively elevated (they ranged from 22 to 99 ng/ml) in the study by Klibanski et al., it would seem that further studies are necessary to clarify this important issue.

Pathology

Classically, pituitary tumors were identified histologically as chromophobe, acidophil, basophil, or mixed adenomas, depending on their staining characteristics with hematoxylin and eosin. Though attempts were made to correlate secretory characteristics of the tumor with its hematoxylin-eosin pathology, this correlation was not reliable. Over the past several years the introduction of radioimmunoassay techniques, electron microscopy, and immunocytochemistry have permitted closer study of the pathology of pituitary adenomas,[7] as outlined elsewhere in this text.

Pituitary tumors are divided according to their size into microadenomas (less than 10 mm in greatest diameter) and macroadenomas (more than 10 mm in greatest diameter). The authors believe that a third category—the invasive adenoma—should be recognized. This group would include those tumors that invade the cavernous sinus and are thus not totally resectable.

Prolactin may be secreted by several types of pituitary adenoma. Hyperprolactinemia has also been attributed to hyperplasia of the prolactin-producing cells of the anterior pituitary in the absence of an actual adenoma.

Clinical Presentation

Considered rare prior to the availability of radioimmunologic assay of prolactin concentration in blood, prolactinomas have been found to be the most common hyperfunctional pituitary tumor, accounting for approximately 25 percent of all pituitary neoplasms. The exact incidence of prolactinomas is unknown, as is the natural history of the neoplasm. It is not uncommon for small incidental pituitary adenomas to be found during postmortem examination in patients who had no recognizable endocrinopathy.

There has been a definite increase in the number of pituitary adenomas in women of childbearing age, while the incidence in men and older women appears to have remained stable. Whether this increase is due to exposure to etiologic factors is controversial. The administration of estrogen to laboratory animals has been associated with an increased incidence of pituitary adenomas, but the role of oral contraceptives in the production of human prolactinomas is unknown. It seems unlikely that such a low dosage of estrogen as that contained in birth control pills would stimulate the development of an adenoma, and no clear relationship has yet been identified between oral contraceptives and prolactinomas during a time of widespread use of the drugs.

As with other hyperfunctional pituitary tumors, prolactin-secreting tumors may present with symptoms of endocrinopathy or mass effect. The resultant hyperprolactinemia may result in gonadal dysfunction in both sexes. The major clinical features in females are amenorrhea and galactorrhea (AG, Forbes-Albright syndrome), usually resulting from a microadenoma. Prolactinomas tend to be larger in men than in women at the time they come to medical attention. The reason for this difference in size at the time of presentation is unknown, but it may be related to the fact that tumors in females are detected earlier because of the more apparent symptoms resulting from the endocrinopathy. Since the tumors are usually larger in males at the time of presentation, the clinical picture is often dominated by hypopituitarism and symptoms resulting from mass effect, namely, headaches, decreased visual acuity, visual field defects (bitemporal hemianopia), and, more rarely, other cranial nerve palsies (III, IV, V, VI), hypothalamic dysfunction, or hydrocephalus.

The endocrinopathy associated with prolactinomas is due to the hyperprolactinemia and is symptomatically identical to that produced by any other cause of elevated serum prolactin levels. While several different conditions can cause hyperprolactinemia, in practice the three most commonly identifiable are ingestion of certain drugs, particularly phenothiazines; primary hypothyroidism; and pituitary tumors. Thus, in the diagnostic workup of patients with hyperprolactinemia due to a suspected pituitary tumor, it is essential to obtain a detailed history and to perform appropriate tests in order to identify the cause of the elevated serum prolactin value.

Elevated serum prolactin levels (>25 ng/ml) in patients with a pituitary tumor may occur as a result of autonomous secretion of excessive quantities of prolactin or through impingement on the hypothalamus and/or pituitary stalk in such a manner as to diminish the secretion and delivery of PIF, thus resulting in unrestrained overproduction by normal, nontumorous cells in the adenohypophysis.

Elevated levels of serum prolactin in females may suppress or interfere with the menstrual cycle and result in primary or secondary amenorrhea and infertility. Spontaneous galactorrhea occurs in about 30 percent of women and less frequently in men with prolactinomas. It is not known why only some patients develop galactorrhea, but its occurrence does not appear to be related to serum prolactin levels. Men with prolactinomas may present with decreased libido and potency and oligospermia.

Advances in Diagnosis and Treatment

Over the past several years, many significant diagnostic and therapeutic advances have been made in the clinical management of pituitary disorders. These advances have resulted

TABLE 96-1 Endocrine Tests for Evaluation of Suspected Prolactinoma

1. Pituitary-thyroid axis: TSH, T_3, T_4
2. Pituitary-adrenal axis: cortisol
3. Pituitary-gonadal axis: LH, FSH, estrogen, testosterone
4. Serum prolactin ($\times 2$)

from important progress in neuroendocrinology, neuroradiology, neuropharmacology, and neurosurgery and include the availability of a precise and sensitive radioimmunoassay for prolactin, the widespread employment of computed tomography (CT), the introduction of new pharmacological agents such as the ergot alkaloids for the treatment of certain conditions, and the increasing sophistication of microsurgical operative techniques and equipment. As a result of these important advances, the diagnostic and therapeutic approach to the patient with a pituitary disorder is now more aggressive and more effective.

Diagnostic Evaluation

In patients with pituitary tumors, it is frequently difficult to identify the underlying mechanism for elevated prolactin levels when the values are only moderately elevated (i.e., up to 100 ng/ml). Elevations of this magnitude in patients with pituitary tumors can result from compression of the stalk and/or hypothalamus as well as autonomous secretion by the tumor. Thus a lesion such as an intrasellar craniopharyngioma, an aneurysm, or a nonfunctional pituitary adenoma could cause modest elevations of prolactin values. On the other hand, a fasting level of prolactin above 150 ng/ml almost certainly indicates that the mechanism for the elevated prolactin value is autonomous secretion by a pituitary adenoma. Very high serum prolactin levels (> 1000 ng/ml) are believed to indicate invasiveness, and this implies that the tumor has extended into the cavernous sinus.

Diagnostic evaluation for a suspected prolactinoma is divided into endocrine testing and neurodiagnostic studies. Endocrine studies should include baseline pituitary target organ tests and at least one determination (preferably two) of the fasting serum prolactin level. A recommended protocol is shown in Table 96-1. The pituitary target organ tests serve two purposes: (1) they determine whether pituitary endocrine function is disturbed before treatment for the prolactinoma is instituted, (2) they supply a baseline to be compared with post-treatment values to determine whether the treatment caused any loss of pituitary endocrine function.

Provocative tests have been utilized to determine prolactin reserve both in prolactin deficiency states and in cases of autonomous prolactin release. TRH stimulation is the most efficient test for determining prolactin reserve. Baseline fasting TSH and prolactin levels are determined and 500 ng of TRH is given intravenously over 30 sec. The serum prolactin and TSH levels are determined at 15, 30, 45, and 60 min, with the patient in the supine position to prevent orthostatic hypotension. A less than twofold increase in the level of prolactin or TSH is indicative of loss of pituitary reserve. Chlorpromazine, a dopamine antagonist that inhibits PIF, can also be used to assess prolactin reserve. The chlorpromazine test is performed by determining fasting serum prolactin levels before and 60, 120, and 180 min after an intramuscular injection of 50 mg chlorpromazine. A less than twofold increase of prolactin levels from the baseline after injection of chlorpromazine is considered to show loss of reserve if the baseline prolactin value is low and loss of hypothalamic control if the baseline level is high.

While the prolactin response to provocative tests such as chlorpromazine and TRH has been useful in identifying structural lesions in the vicinity of the stalk and gland, these tests have not served to differentiate between the different mechanisms responsible for elevated prolactin levels in patients with pituitary tumors. The response (in serum prolactin levels) to provocative tests is blunted or absent in all such situations. Failure of prolactin to rise to two to three times the baseline value is characteristic of virtually all pituitary tumors or other space-occupying lesions of the sella, whether their mechanism of action is related to autonomous secretion or to disruption of the PIF pathways. These tests are unnecessary when prolactin levels are more than 150 ng/ml or when a tumor is identified on CT, as the diagnosis is already made and the tests would add little to the investigation. When the prolactin levels are mildly elevated and the CT scan is equivocal or nondiagnostic, the provocative tests are more useful; in these instances the tests confirm that elevated prolactin levels are due to abnormal prolactin secretion rather than being a variation of normal.

Neurodiagnostic studies have undergone tremendous evolution in recent years. The test that has had the greatest impact in this area has been the CT scan—an impact seen in diagnosis, in planning and executing surgery, and in postoperative follow-up for early identification of recurrent tumor. A high-resolution coronal scan without and with contrast enhancement is the only neurodiagnostic test required in the majority of cases. The diagnostic accuracy of the scanner, while not perfect, is superior to multidirectional polytomography and pneumoencephalography and thus has replaced these tests. The authors believe that cerebral angiography is usually not indicated in the neurodiagnostic evaluation, particularly when the level of serum prolactin is more than 150 ng/ml. However, when the level is less than 150 ng/ml and there is a nagging possibility of an intracranial aneurysm with intrasellar extension, visualization of the intracranial circulation becomes important. The newer technique of intravenous digital subtraction angiography will confirm or eliminate the presence of an aneurysm and avoid the arterial injections of conventional arteriography.

Medical vs. Surgical Management

There is continuing controversy over the ideal method of therapy for prolactinomas, since medical treatment (e.g., bromocriptine) and surgical treatment (e.g., trans-sphenoidal microsurgery) can each provide either effective control or cure in a majority of cases.

In the past, many different hormonal therapies were utilized in patients with amenorrhea and galactorrhea, most

without affecting the syndrome. More recently, dopamine agonists such as L-dopa and ergot alkaloids have undergone therapeutic trials. The most noteworthy, bromocriptine, is a potent inhibitor of the synthesis and release of prolactin by the pituitary gland and has been demonstrated to effect significant structural change (i.e., shrinkage) in prolactinomas. This reduction in size has been noted to be reversible; the tumors will rapidly return toward their pretreatment size within days of bromocriptine withdrawal.[12] This observation, combined with absence of pathological evidence of cell necrosis, infarction, or vascular injury, indicates that the reduction in the size of prolactinomas treated with bromocriptine is explained by reduction of cell size and not by cell loss secondary to necrosis.

The enthusiasm among some clinicians over the initial results with bromocriptine therapy of prolactinomas has led to the suggestion that the drug be used as primary treatment of these neoplasms, reserving surgery for the therapeutic failures. The authors believe this approach to be unsound, as the data currently available are insufficient to support the notion that prolactinomas can be cured by bromocriptine, despite the sporadic case reports of successful medical treatment of prolactinoma patients with bromocriptine. The many advantages of trans-sphenoidal microsurgery, with its low morbidity and mortality, give it preference over the use of a drug that as yet has not been proved to eradicate the tumor.

A relatively common diagnostic and therapeutic problem is the patient with an elevated serum prolactin level without a radiographically demonstrable tumor. In this situation the results of the chlorpromazine stimulation test make it possible to determine whether a mass exists within the sella. Should this provocative test indicate that a neoplasm is the source of the hyperprolactinemia, some reasonable options are available. One approach is to follow the patient with serial serum prolactin levels, ophthalmologic examinations, and CT scans at 6- to 12-month intervals. A second option is to treat the patient with bromocriptine, again with chemical and radiographic follow-up. Still a third option is to perform exploratory trans-sphenoidal surgery. The decision is made only after extensive discussion with the patient and determination of the patient's wishes. On the authors' service, a very small adenoma has usually been found in this group of patients if the chlorpromazine response was blunted. More rarely, a grossly abnormal area in the gland has been found which microscopically proved to be an area of "hyperplasia."

Another clinical situation that presents difficulty in management is the rare patient with a prolactinoma who becomes pregnant. If the tumor is a microadenoma without any evidence of mass effect, the authors would elect to institute no form of medical or surgical treatment until the end of the pregnancy. These patients should be followed closely to check for evidence of mass effect during the pregnancy, which may occur as a result of physiological pituitary enlargement during pregnancy, tumor expansion, or both. If the pregnant patient presents with a macroadenoma or a tumor producing symptoms from its mass (e.g., visual loss), trans-sphenoidal microsurgical removal of the tumor would be recommended.

Trans-sphenoidal Surgery

Indications

While realizing that a medical option is available for the treatment of certain prolactinomas, the authors believe that trans-sphenoidal microsurgery is a safe and effective means of therapy. Trans-sphenoidal microsurgery is a reasonable choice for a woman with a verified prolactinoma causing the amenorrhea-galactorrhea syndrome who desires pregnancy. Such a patient will usually have a microadenoma, and it is in this group that surgery achieves the best results. The macro-adenoma, particularly with suprasellar extension, should also be treated surgically; the lesion has already demonstrated that it has growth potential, and, while medical therapy can shrink the lesion, it does not eradicate it, and surgery is the only method offering a reasonable chance of cure. Prolactinomas causing mass effect, especially those producing visual loss, should be treated surgically without delay; and the rare prolactinomas that are associated with pituitary apoplexy require emergency operation. These indications for surgery—which are followed at our institution—are summarized in Table 96-2.

Technique

Currently, trans-sphenoidal microsurgery is the most appropriate surgical procedure for the majority of pituitary tumors, including prolactinomas. The technical details of the exposure along the nasal septum, entry into the sphenoid sinus and floor of the sella turcica, and method of tumor removal are well covered elsewhere.[3,4,8,11,13] Intraoperative televised fluoroscopy is not routinely used on the authors' service. A satisfactory surgical approach is one in which the surgeon develops a plane along one side of the nasal septum, thus allowing this structure to be spared.[13] This technique minimizes the risk of creating a postoperative nasal deformity and, more importantly, reduces the technical difficulties of a future trans-sphenoidal operation should one be necessary. Since many tumors associated with abnormalities in prolactin secretion are less than 10 mm in diameter, it is important not to damage the pituitary gland during opening of the dura. Lacerations in the gland with attendant subcapsular bleeding make it extremely difficult, if not impossible, to detect the subtle differences between the normal gland and a small tumor that must be determined if the surgeon is to remove the tumor successfully and spare the gland. Also, the less the gland is manipulated the greater the chance for

TABLE 96-2 Indications for Surgical Treatment of Prolactinoma

1. Verified prolactinoma causing AG syndrome and infertility in woman who desires pregnancy
2. Macroadenoma (particularly with extrasellar extension)
3. Prolactinoma causing mass effect (visual loss, pituitary insufficiency)
4. Prolactinoma associated with pituitary apoplexy

preservation of pituitary function. The dura mater can be opened safely by making a slow, deliberate incision with a no. 11 blade on a bayonet knife holder under relatively high magnification. Once an adequate opening is made, it can be enlarged appropriately with fine angled microscissors.

In the authors' series, the prolactin microadenomas were nearly always situated laterally in the gland. Larger pituitary tumors usually eroded the floor of the sella turcica, and in these cases the tumor commonly extruded into the operative wound upon removal of the floor of the sella and opening of the dura mater. Frequently the pituitary gland was compressed and flattened against the dorsum sellae or diaphragma sellae by the tumor.

After total or subtotal removal of the tumor, absolute alcohol is applied to the tumor bed for approximately 5 min for cytotoxic effect if the tumor capsule is intact and thus provides a barrier between the tumor site and the subarachnoid space.

Adipose tissue taken from the abdominal wall is inserted loosely into the tumor bed to prevent prolapse of the optic chiasm into the sella turcica. After withdrawal of the speculum, the incision in the gingival mucosa is closed with a single catgut suture. Soft airway tubes are inserted into each nostril for 24 h, in order to reapproximate the nasal mucosa.

Low operative mortality rates and the ability to remove the tumor and spare the normal pituitary gland in the majority of patients are the primary advantages of modern trans-sphenoidal microsurgery. It is recommended in all prolactinoma patients in whom an operation is to be done except when there is:

1. Extrasellar extension of the tumor into the anterior and/ or middle fossa as determined by CT scan or other reliable neurodiagnostic tests. Suprasellar extension of tumor directly above the sella turcica, even in cases where the extrasellar extension reaches 2 to 3 cm, can be managed by the trans-sphenoidal technique.
2. A suprasellar tumor with a normal or only slightly abnormal sella turcica. This is likely to be the unusual "collar-button" type extension in which the tumor extends through a relatively small opening in the diaphragma sellae and then expands into a larger suprasellar component.

In both these situations the lesion is best exposed and managed by craniotomy.

Some surgeons believe that a conchal type of sphenoid sinus, i.e., a sphenoid sinus with little or no pneumatization, is a contraindication to the trans-sphenoidal approach. However, by the use of air-driven, high-speed angled drills, the bone can be removed safely and the dura mater over the pituitary gland and/or tumor exposed. Under these circumstances intraoperative skull films or televised fluoroscopy are essential for localization.

Results

The three main factors that influence the results of surgery are tumor size, preoperative levels of prolactin, and the direction of extrasellar tumor extension if the tumor extends outside the confines of the sella turcica. Tumor size, best measured by a high-resolution CT scan, is probably the most important of the three factors. Numerous workers have shown that the best results are obtained in patients with microadenomas.[1-5] Macroadenomas are also amenable to cure by surgery provided that the extrasellar extension does not involve the cavernous sinus or the middle and/or posterior cranial fossa.

Another factor that has a bearing on surgical results is the preoperative level of serum prolactin. For this reason, patients on the authors' service are divided into two groups: group 1 includes those patients whose preoperative prolactin levels are less than 200 ng/ml and group 2, patients with preoperative levels above 200 ng/ml. Patients in group 1 usually have tumors that are less than 10 mm in greatest diameter and those in group 2, over 10 mm. Among a total of 100 women with verified prolactinomas treated at Emory, 81 percent of the 72 patients in group 1 had microadenomas, and 86 percent of the 28 group 2 patients had tumors more than 10 mm in diameter.[4] Thus the level of preoperative serum prolactin is related to the size of the tumor, and both these factors have a distinct bearing on the results of surgery.

The authors' criteria of cure in prolactinomas are summarized as follows:

Normalization of serum prolactin below 25 ng/ml. This indicates that all hypersecreting tumor tissue was removed by the surgery. If the value remains normal for a long period of time, preferably longer than 5 years, one can assume that cure was achieved, with little chance that the tumor will recur. Persistent hyperprolactinemia following trans-sphenoidal resection of a prolactinoma may be due to persistent tumor or to damage to the pituitary stalk either by the tumor or by surgery or both. When the postoperative value is less than 100 ng/ml, the persistent hyperprolactinemia may reflect stalk damage, which results in impairment in delivery of PIF to the adenohypophysis, which in turn allows an unrestrained release of prolactin from the normal gland.

Cessation of galactorrhea and resumption of normal menstrual periods. These clinical indicators of cure nearly always coincide with normalization of serum prolactin values. In exceptional cases menstrual periods return and galactorrhea ceases even with levels of prolactin slightly above normal; in other cases these symptoms may continue despite normalization of serum prolactin levels.

The observations of the surgeon. In the case of a moderate size or small tumor confined to the sella, an experienced neurosurgeon can usually determine whether gross total removal of tumor has been accomplished. Patients who do not have a progressive increase in serum prolactin and, more importantly, who have negative high-resolution coronal CT scans for a period of at least 5 years may appropriately be considered cured by the surgical procedure.

As shown in Table 96-3, a number of workers have reported results of trans-sphenoidal microsurgery for prolactinoma. Hardy et al.[5] showed that trans-sphenoidal surgery for these tumors was followed by normalization of prolactin levels in 59 (74 percent) of 80 cases. Menses returned in 50 (63 percent) of these 80 patients, and 29 patients (36 percent) became pregnant. Similar results were obtained by Chang et al.,[2] who reported return of menses in 16 of 17

women with prolactin-secreting microadenomas and in 2 of 7 with macroadenomas.

The wide range in results obtained in different surgical series of patients with prolactinomas treated by trans-sphenoidal surgery reflects differences in patient selection. In several series, the results were better with patients who had microadenomas than in those with larger tumors. Faria and Tindall[4] reported normalization of prolactin levels following trans-sphenoidal surgery in 55 of 72 patients whose preoperative prolactin level was less than 200 ng/ml and in only 13 of 28 patients in whom the preoperative prolactin level was more than 200 ng/ml. In the series of Hardy et al.,[5] serum prolactin levels were normal following trans-sphenoidal surgery in 90 percent of patients with localized microadenomas, in 53 percent of those with enclosed adenomas, and in 43 percent of those with invasive adenomas. Domingue et al.[3] defined *therapeutic failure* as failure of amenorrhea to resolve within a follow-up period of at least 18 months. Therapeutic failure was encountered in 32 percent (29 of 91) of their patients with prolactinomas. They found that therapeutic failure occurred in patients who had higher preoperative serum prolactin levels (i.e., prolactin levels > 200 ng/ml) and in those in whom total removal was not achieved.

To summarize the above, patients with microadenomas are more likely to have preoperative prolactin levels below 200 ng/ml, and it is in this group that trans-sphenoidal surgery has its best results, with a cure rate on the order of 75 percent. Patients with macroadenomas usually have preoperative prolactin levels above 200 ng/ml, and the cure rate in this group is approximately 50 percent.

Effect on Pituitary Endocrine Function

The potential effect of trans-sphenoidal surgery on pituitary endocrine function is an important consideration. For instance, if one or more pituitary target organ axes were damaged in a significant number of patients during removal of a prolactin microadenoma, particularly if surgery was aimed at restoring fertility, surgery would not be a good therapeutic option to consider. To answer the question

TABLE 96-3 Achievement of Normal Postoperative Prolactin Levels: Summary of Published Surgical Series

Author	Year	Evaluable Patients*	Normal Postoperative Prolactin Level	
			No.	Percent
Chang et al.[2]	1977	23	11	48
Hardy et al.[5]	1978	80	59	74
Post et al.[11]	1979	30	21	70
Aubourg et al.[1]	1980	90	39	43
Domingue et al.[3]	1980	91	62†	68
Faria and Tindall[4]	1982	100	69	69

*Evaluable patients are those for whom preoperative and postoperative data were complete and for whom, in the opinion of the report authors, the follow-up period was adequate for analysis of the results of surgery.

†In this series, resolution of amenorrhea within a follow-up period of 18 months after trans-sphenoidal surgery was considered "therapeutic success." Pre- and postoperative prolactin levels were not reported.

raised, complete endocrine tests were performed before and 10 days after trans-sphenoidal surgery in 97 women with prolactinomas, 70 (72 percent) of which were microadenomas.[9] The results of the study are shown in Table 96-4. Of 65 patients who had normal pituitary endocrine function preoperatively, 50 had normal function postoperatively, 10 had a temporary impairment in one or more axes that fully recovered, and 5 had permanent damage to one or more axes. Of 32 patients who had impairment of at least one axis preoperatively, 11 showed documented improvement in endocrine function, 19 showed no change, and 2 were worse. It can be concluded from these data that approximately 7 percent (i.e., 7 of 97) will experience damage to one or more pituitary target organ axes as a sequel to trans-sphenoidal surgery performed by an experienced surgeon.

Mortality and Morbidity

Patients and endocrinologists often question the safety of trans-sphenoidal microsurgery. In an effort to provide an answer, several neurosurgeons with considerable trans-sphenoidal experience were polled as to the mortality and morbidity rates in their series. Any death within 30 days of surgery was counted as an operative death. Complications included CSF rhinorrhea which required reoperation (i.e., leaks that did not stop spontaneously or after one or more lumbar punctures), meningitis, and nonfatal arterial injury. The data, which were obtained from eight neurosurgeons, included all pituitary tumor surgery and were not restricted to prolactinomas. Some 4876 trans-sphenoidal operations were performed by these eight surgeons, with an operative mortality of only 0.4 percent. Among the 19 deaths occurring as a result of or in association with the operation, there were mitigating circumstances in nearly every case; for instance, some patients had undergone previous treatments such as craniotomy, had extremely large tumors, or were in marginal health. It is significant that none of the eight neurosurgeons had an operative death of a patient with a microadenoma. The complication rate of only 2.3 percent, or 110 of the total of 4876 operations, is acceptably low.

Recurrence Rate

The recurrence rate of prolactinoma following modern trans-sphenoidal microsurgery has been cited in a few articles in the literature, but realistically the true rate is pres-

TABLE 96-4 Effect of Trans-sphenoidal Surgery on Pituitary Endocrine Function in 97 Patients

Postoperative Result	No. of Patients
Patients with Normal Preoperative Values	
Normal postoperative values	50
Temporary deficit in one or more axes	10
Permanent deficit in one or more axes	5
*Patients with Abnormal Preoperative Values**	
Postoperative improvement	11
No postoperative change	19
Postoperative deterioration	2

*I.e., deficit in one or more axes.

ently unknown, as the follow-up period in most patients is simply not long enough to adequately assess this parameter. Also, a distinction needs to be made between cases of incomplete removal because of invasiveness or inaccessibility and cases in which an experienced surgeon effected gross total removal. The recurrence rate in this latter group is approximately 5 percent.[3,4,8,10] In the past the diagnosis of recurrence was made on the basis of a progressive rise in serum prolactin levels and/or radiographic changes such as increased sellar destruction on polytomography or increased mass effect on pneumoencephalography. However, with the availability of high-resolution CT scanners, the diagnosis of recurrence will undoubtedly be made with more precision. Thus with the passage of time and the availability of high-resolution scanners, the incidence of recurrence of prolactinoma following trans-sphenoidal microsurgery may be recognized as higher than present figures suggest.

Postoperative Irradiation

The authors believe that routine irradiation after trans-sphenoidal microsurgical gross total removal of a pituitary tumor is not warranted and that irradiation should be reserved for tumors associated with mass effect in which recurrence becomes evident or for tumors found at the first operation to be invasive. Since clinical data on the irradiation of prolactinomas in patients with the amenorrhea-galactorrhea syndrome are limited, routine irradiation of these tumors is not advised.

Patients with persistent postoperative hyperprolactinemia who continue to have amenorrhea and galactorrhea on the basis of disruption of PIF pathways are good candidates for medical treatment with bromocriptine. Patients with persistent hyperprolactinemia from suspected persistent or recurrent tumors not associated with mass effect may also be considered for bromocriptine therapy, provided close medical supervision is available.[10]

The Role of Bromocriptine as a Surgical Adjuvant

Although bromocriptine is not tumoricidal, its ability to produce dramatic reduction in the size of a prolactinoma makes it a useful preoperative adjunct to make excision of the tumor not only easier but probably more certain. This hypothesis has been tested in a small number of patients with macroadenomas, both prolactin-secreting and non-prolactin-secreting. A 6-week course of bromocriptine effected measurable reduction in the size of all prolactinomas thus treated and failed to reduce the size of the nonfunctional tumors. Furthermore, in two patients who discontinued the therapy due to side effects, the reduction in the size of the prolactinoma documented by CT was reversed and tumors were restored to their original size within days of drug withdrawal. This observation further supports the conclusion that bromocriptine interferes with prolactinoma cell metabolism but does not have tumoricidal properties. Tumors in patients treated with bromocriptine appeared to be softer, wetter, and more easily removed than the usual pituitary adenoma, although this is difficult to document objectively. Because of the variable gross state of prolactinomas, this preliminary observation will require documentation in many more cases before it can be concluded that the changes induced by the drug truly facilitate surgical removal.

The optimal duration of bromocriptine therapy prior to surgery is still under investigation. Ideally, the operation should be performed at the point of maximal shrinkage of the tumor. Preliminary investigations with serial CT examinations indicate that about 3 weeks of treatment is ideal. It is theoretically possible that bromocriptine continued for too long a period may actually interfere with surgery. If, for example, fibrotic changes developed in the tumor, total removal might be hindered. Because of the rapid return of responsive tumors to their original size following cessation of therapy, it is essential to maintain the patient on bromocriptine up to the time of surgery.

References

1. Aubourg PR, Derome PJ, Peillon F, Jedynak CP, Visot A, LeGentil P, Balagura S, Guiot G: Endocrine outcome after transsphenoidal adenomectomy for prolactinoma: Prolactin levels and tumor size as predicting factors. Surg Neurol 14: 141–143, 1980.
2. Chang RJ, Keye WR Jr, Young JR, Wilson CB, Jaffe RB: Detection, evaluation, and treatment of pituitary microadenomas in patients with galactorrhea and amenorrhea. Am J Obstet Gynecol 128: 356–363, 1977.
3. Domingue JN, Richmond IL, Wilson CB: Results of surgery in 114 patients with prolactin-secreting pituitary adenomas. Am J Obstet Gynecol 137: 102–108, 1980.
4. Faria MA, Tindall GT: Transsphenoidal microsurgery for prolactin-secreting pituitary adenomas: Results in 100 women with the amenorrhea-galactorrhea syndrome. J Neurosurg 56: 33–43, 1982.
5. Hardy J, Beauregard H, Robert F: Prolactin-secreting pituitary adenomas: Transsphenoidal microsurgical treatment, in Robyn C, Harter M (eds): *Progress in Prolactin Physiology and Pathology.* Amsterdam, Elsevier/North-Holland Biomedical Press, 1978, pp 361–370.
6. Klibanski A, Neer RM, Beitins IZ, Ridgway EC, Zervas NT, McArthur JW: Decreased bone density in hyperprolactinemic women. N Engl J Med 303: 1511–1514, 1980.
7. Kovacs K, Horvath E: Pathology of pituitary adenomas. Bull Los Angeles Neurol Soc 42: 92–110, 1977.
8. Laws ER Jr, Kern EB: Pituitary tumors treated by transnasal microsurgery: 7 years of clinical experience with 539 patients, in Sano K, Takakura K, Fukushima T (eds): *Functioning Pituitary Adenoma: Proceedings of the First Workshop on Pituitary Adenomas.* Tokyo, 1980, pp 25–34.
9. McLanahan CS, Christy JH, Tindall GT: Anterior pituitary function before and after transsphenoidal microsurgical resection of pituitary tumors. Neurosurgery 3: 142–145, 1978.
10. Pelkonen R, Grahne B, Hirvonen E, Karonen S, Salmi J, Tikkanen M, Valtonen S: Pituitary function in prolactinoma: Effect of surgery and postoperative bromocriptine therapy. Clin Endocrinol 14: 335–348, 1981.
11. Post KD, Biller BJ, Adelman LS, Molitch ME, Wolpert SM, Reichlin S: Selective transsphenoidal adenomectomy in women with galactorrhea-amenorrhea. JAMA 242: 158–162, 1979.
12. Thorner MO, Perryman RL, Rogol AD, Conway BP, Macleod RM, Login IS, Morris JL: Rapid changes of prolactinoma volume after withdrawal and reinstitution of bromocriptine. J Clin Endocrinol Metab 53: 480–483, 1981.
13. Tindall GT, Collins WF Jr, Kirchner JA: Unilateral septal technique for transsphenoidal microsurgical approach to the sella turcica: Technical note. J Neurosurg 49: 138–142, 1978.

97

Cushing's Disease and Nelson's Syndrome

James E. Boggan
Charles B. Wilson

I ventilated myself mildly on the subject before this H. C. Society group, someone of whom I hope and believe will ere long venture in surgically upon a case and suck out the small adenoma which is usually visible on the upper surface of the pars anterior.

Harvey Cushing
Letter to Sir Geoffrey Jefferson,
May 30, 1935

Pituitary-dependent hypersecretion of adrenocorticotropic hormone (ACTH) results in two clinical conditions that are of particular interest to the neurosurgeon—Cushing's disease and Nelson's syndrome. Cushing's disease is the hypersecretion of ACTH by a pituitary source, usually a pituitary adenoma, that causes bilateral adrenal cortical hyperplasia and consequent hypercortisolism. Nelson's syndrome, which some patients develop after undergoing adrenalectomy for the treatment of Cushing's disease, is the hypersecretion of ACTH by a pituitary adenoma that results in cutaneous hyperpigmentation. Nelson's syndrome differs from Cushing's disease in that hypercortisolism cannot occur because of the adrenalectomy and in that, by definition, a pituitary tumor is known to be present.

Historical Perspective

In 1932, Cushing reported his detailed study of 12 patients who manifested signs of hypercortisolism during their lifetime.[3] On the basis of the demonstration of pituitary basophilic adenomas in six of the eight patients studied at autopsy, Cushing suggested that there was a causal relationship between the pituitary tumor and the characteristic bilateral adrenocortical hyperplasia. A year later, Howard

Naffziger performed the first craniotomy for the removal of a pituitary adenoma in a patient with Cushing's disease.[12] The resection produced a dramatic resolution of symptoms—but despite postoperative pituitary irradiation, the patient's disease recurred and she died in 1940, seven years after the operation. The convincing implication of a link between pituitary adenoma and hypercortisolism provided by this case and subsequent case studies did not dispel skepticism that a pituitary adenoma was the primary defect in Cushing's syndrome. The doubts were based on the high incidence (10 to 20 percent) of asymptomatic basophilic pituitary adenomas found at autopsy and on the recognition of—but inability to distinguish biochemically between the different causes of—hypercortisolism. They remained unresolved, primarily because of technological difficulties in the radiological detection of small pituitary tumors.[5,7,17] Many investigators believed that the primary defect lay in the adrenal glands.[10,19] After the introduction of cortisone in 1950, adrenalectomy became the preferred mode of therapy for all cases of Cushing's syndrome.

The efficacy of pituitary irradiation in some cases of hypercortisolism, the lack of consistent pathological findings among patients who underwent adrenalectomy, and the recognition of Nelson's syndrome[10] fostered renewed interest in the concept of a pituitary origin. These observations supported the notion that at least two types of Cushing's syndrome exist, one of adrenal origin and one of pituitary origin. Clayton, in 1958, may have been the first to provide direct evidence of pituitary hyperfunction in Cushing's syndrome by her report of two patients with elevated plasma ACTH levels who were found to have pituitary tumors and adrenal hyperplasia.[2] In the same year, Nelson reported the development of a pituitary tumor, hypersecretion of ACTH, and cutaneous hyperpigmentation in a patient who had undergone bilateral adrenalectomy for the treatment of Cushing's syndrome.[15] In that case, surgical removal of the pituitary adenoma resulted in resolution of the hyperpigmentation and apparently complete resolution of ACTH hypersecretion, as reflected in the finding of no detectable ACTH in the plasma. The subsequent report by Salassa et al. substantiated Nelson's findings, and provided radiological evidence that in some patients, pituitary tumors were present before adrenalectomy.[19] These authors suggested that adrenalectomy had enhanced the growth of the adenoma and the secretion of ACTH. Their study suggested that approximately 10 percent of patients undergoing adrenalectomy for Cushing's syndrome would subsequently develop signs of a pituitary tumor and cutaneous melanosis. Their findings also emphasized the existence of complex feedback loops between pituitary corticotropes and the adrenal gland.

The subsequent clarification of the different biochemical factors involved in the development of Cushing's syndrome has permitted the development of therapies specific to the particular cause of hypercortisolism in most patients.[10,16] These endocrinologic methods and the results obtained with pituitary microsurgery, which can achieve lasting remission of disease while preserving normal pituitary function after the selective removal of a corticotropic adenoma,[1,6,9] have firmly established Cushing's disease as a distinct clinicopathological entity.

Pathogenesis

The pathophysiology of Cushing's disease is as complex as Cushing predicted in summarizing his cases as being "so many and varied as to baffle analysis." Although the hormonal mechanisms that produce the observed clinical features are poorly understood, it is known that chronic exposure of tissues to excessive quantities of cortisol, which influences cytoplasmic and nuclear receptors, results in Cushing's syndrome. At least two-thirds of all cases of Cushing's syndrome can be ascribed to a pituitary cause and are examples of pituitary Cushing's syndrome (Cushing's disease). ACTH-secreting nonpituitary neoplasms that cause secondary hypercortisolism (ectopic Cushing's syndrome) and the adrenal disorder causing primary hypercortisolism (adrenal Cushing's syndrome) are responsible for approximately equal proportions of the remaining cases of spontaneous Cushing's syndrome.

The periodic or continuous oversecretion of ACTH by a pituitary source is now recognized as the hormonal dysfunction underlying Cushing's disease. There is loss of the normal diurnal secretory pattern and reduced sensitivity to glucocorticoid feedback suppression. The increased stimulation of the adrenal cortices causes hyperplasia and secondary hypercortisolism. Plasma ACTH levels usually are normal or modestly elevated in the presence of a high serum cortisol level, although the high levels of serum cortisol cause some continued suppression of ACTH secretion by normal and neoplastic corticotropes; this is the basis for the use of dexamethasone suppression tests in the diagnostic differentiation of this from other causes of Cushing's syndrome. Perhaps in synergy with the overproduction of ACTH, the adrenal glands are also more sensitive to stimulation by ACTH.

In Nelson's syndrome, the loss of partial cortisol inhibition as a consequence of the adrenalectomy allows the pituitary tumor to secrete tremendous amounts of ACTH and may also promote growth of the adenoma. The resulting high levels of plasma ACTH stimulate cutaneous melanocytes to produce the hyperpigmentation characteristic of this condition; β-lipotropin (βLPH) and melanocyte-stimulating hormone have not been shown to contribute to the hyperpigmentation. In contrast to Cushing's disease, the tumors of Nelson's syndrome do not suppress ACTH secretion in response to the administration of high-dose dexamethasone. This difference is presumably a consequence of prolonged "inadequate" cortisol stimulation (suppression) after the adrenalectomy.

Among patients with Cushing's disease, as many as 80 percent have a pituitary adenoma.[7] Other pituitary lesions reported in association with the disease include diffuse or multinodular hyperplasia of corticotropes; multiple, separate pituitary adenomas; and coexisting corticotrope hyperplasia and adenoma.[7,8,13] In some cases, total hypophysectomy has resulted in remission of disease, and serial sections through the excised gland have revealed no abnormality. These variations in the pathology of the pituitary, and clinical data suggesting that certain neurotransmitters may influence the course of the disease, have been considered evidence that hypothalamic dysfunction is a factor in Cushing's disease.[5,7,8,13] However, the failure of a pituitary stalk section to prevent ACTH secretion or to induce remission of Cushing's disease seems to contradict the theory of a hypothalamic cause of Cushing's disease.[10] Furthermore, the return of normal pituitary function after a prolonged period of hypocortisolism following selective removal of a pituitary microadenoma implies that the hypothalamus and normal pituitary corticotropes were chronically suppressed rather than hyperactive. The evidence that hypothalamic corticotropin-releasing factor (CRF) or inhibitory factors have a role in the pathophysiology of Cushing's disease or Nelson's syndrome is not conclusive. Despite the ongoing debate about the role of the hypothalamus in the pathogenesis of Cushing's disease, pituitary tumors are now considered its main cause.

The corticotropic pituitary adenomas responsible for the hypersecretion of ACTH are most often microadenomas averaging 5 mm in diameter. In Nelson's syndrome more often than in Cushing's disease (approximately 50 percent compared to less than 20 percent of cases, respectively), the responsible tumor is a macroadenoma, occasionally one with invasive tendencies. The typical corticotropic adenoma can be recognized intraoperatively as soft, sometimes semiliquid, white-to-reddish tissue that is distinct from the normal yellow anterior lobe. However, the adenoma may be difficult to distinguish from the posterior lobe. Although it has been suggested that corticotropic adenomas have a predilection for the central mucoid core of the anterior lobe,[6,17] they may be located anywhere in the sella. Lamberts et al. have suggested that corticotropic adenomas originate in either the anterior or the intermediate lobe.[8] They postulated that tumors originating within the intermediate lobe contain interspersed axons, are sensitive to a dopamine agonist, have a greater tendency toward recurrence after surgery, and are an expression of hypothalamic dysfunction.

Microscopically, corticotropic tumors are composed of compact sheets of uniform polygonal cells having round to oval nuclei with prominent nucleoli. Often a radial arrangement of tumor cells around capillaries is noted. The surrounding gland and acini are compressed or destroyed, and the tumor may or may not be well circumscribed. There are usually no mitoses or other signs of malignancy, but local invasiveness, subarachnoid dissemination, and distant metastasis occur more frequently with corticotropic tumors than with any other pituitary adenoma.

When examined with routine histological techniques, the tumor cells may exhibit the classic basophilic staining reported by Cushing. These densely granulated cells stain positively with periodic acid Schiff (PAS) stain and lead hematoxylin and usually are indistinguishable from normal corticotropes. A review of Cushing's original report[3] and subsequent experience[18] indicates that the tumors may be chromophobic, mixed, or eosinophilic. Variations in the histological appearance of the cells may be a result of minor differences in staining technique, but they may in some cases relate to the volume of secretory granules within the tumor cells. The long-standing classification of pituitary tumors as chromophobic, basophilic, or eosinophilic is known to be inadequate, however, in that this designation has no correlation with the in vivo secretory product, activity, or cellular origin of the lesion. Tumors are now classified according to the secretory product or the cell of origin (e.g., lactotrope, somatotrope, corticotrope).

Ultrastructural and immunohistochemical studies of corticotropic adenomas reliably reveal distinct identifying features. Characteristically, there are spherical or slightly irregular dense core secretory granules that average 450 nm in diameter and tend to line up along cell membranes. These granules stain selectively when anti-ACTH and anti-β-lipotropin immunohistochemical techniques are used. Also characteristic is the presence of bundles of microfilaments, 7 nm in diameter, arranged in a perinuclear distribution. Robert et al. believe that these perinuclear microfilaments represent the ultrastructural morphology of Crooke's hyaline change.[17] When examined by light microscopy, Crooke's hyaline change is seen only in nonadenoma corticotropes, and only when hypercortisolism is present. The microfilaments are found in minimal numbers in the tumor and normal corticotropes of Nelson's syndrome, presumably because there is no hypercortisolism to induce their deposition. Secretory granules may be slightly smaller (approximately 200 nm) in these cells, but otherwise there is no significant ultrastructural difference between normal corticotropes and the adenoma corticotropes of Nelson's syndrome. Similarly, there is no significant histopathologic difference between the adenomas seen in Cushing's disease and those of Nelson's syndrome.

Even though there are no well-established criteria for the diagnosis of corticotrope hyperplasia, it is claimed that this condition accounts for as many as 25 percent of cases of Cushing's disease in some series.[7,13] These reports contrast markedly with other series in which there has been no incidence of corticotrope hyperplasia.[1,9] Definitive criteria for the recognition of this entity have been proposed by McKeever et al. in their report of a case of Cushing's disease resulting from multinodular corticotrope hyperplasia.[13] In general, one would expect to find an increase in ACTH-laden corticotropes interspersed among fewer than 10 percent noncorticotrope secretory cells, and no evidence of compressed or destroyed acini. Expanded acini may be seen if the process is focal. Light microscopy should show no evidence of Crooke's hyaline change.

Clinical Features

Cushing's disease is a serious endocrinopathy, the natural course of which is unpredictable. Of the hypersecretory pituitary disorders, Cushing's disease has the highest incidence of morbidity and of persistence after therapeutic intervention. Untreated, the disease has been associated with a 5-year survival rate of less than 50 percent. Death most often results from cardiovascular or infectious complications. Women constitute over 75 percent of patients with Cushing's disease; in contrast, there is a predominance of children (65 percent) in cases of adrenal Cushing's syndrome and of men (60 percent) in cases of ectopic Cushing's syndrome. Most patients with Cushing's disease are between 30 and 40 years old at the time of diagnosis.

Nelson's disease appears unpredictably months to years after adrenalectomy; its incidence is highest in patients who underwent adrenalectomy during childhood.[14] Nelson's syndrome seems to occur as frequently in men as in women, but its incidence may be less among patients who received pituitary irradiation after their adrenalectomy.

No one clinical feature is singularly diagnostic of Cushing's disease, and the clinical presentation is diagnostic in less than 50 percent of cases. The classic findings are moon facies, centripetal obesity, buffalo hump, hypertension, thin skin, purple abdominal striae, and ecchymoses. The prominent supraclavicular and mandibular fat pads seen in cases of Cushing's disease are not present in the "pseudocushingoid" patient with exogenous obesity who occasionally presents with complaints and laboratory findings suggestive of Cushing's disease. Frequently the patients have emotional disorders, most often depression and psychosis, menstrual irregularities or impotence, osteoporotic back pain, and symptoms referable to glucose intolerance.

In comparison with the symptoms of endogenous Cushing's disease, only obesity, acne, and mental symptoms (typically hyperactivity and elation) occur as frequently in patients who are given high-dose glucocorticoids (exogenous Cushing's syndrome) as part of a therapeutic regimen for unrelated disease. In this same group, less than 20 percent of patients develop hypertension, and hyperpigmentation does not occur at all. A similarly low incidence of hypertension is noted in patients with ectopic Cushing's syndrome, despite their having the highest levels of ACTH and cortisol observed in any of the groups. However, in 25 percent of cases of ectopic Cushing's syndrome, cutaneous hyperpigmentation occurs.

Other hormones probably contribute primarily or secondary to the clinical syndrome. For example, plasma testosterone, presumably from the adrenals, is significantly elevated in females who have Cushing's disease and may contribute to hirsutism, acne, and mental disorders. In contrast, testosterone is less than one-third the normal value in males and may be the cause of oligospermia and impotence. A hormonal basis for the hypertension is yet to be demonstrated. In many cases, hypertension, mental illness, and obesity persist despite adrenalectomy.[5]

The history of Cushing's disease that has been treated by adrenalectomy in a patient who complains of increased cutaneous pigmentation and has an enlarged sella turcica is diagnostic of Nelson's syndrome. Compared with patients with Cushing's disease, who have a very low incidence of headaches or visual symptoms, those with Nelson's syndrome are more likely to have headaches or visual system impairment as a consequence of mass effect or tumor invasion. A significant proportion of patients with Nelson's syndrome have died from the direct effects of their tumors.[22]

Diagnostic Evaluation

The diagnosis of Cushing's disease is established by endocrinologic criteria. If doubt regarding the cause persists, or if microsurgical exploration of the pituitary is negative, selective venous sampling for ACTH should be performed.[4] Plasma ACTH levels in samples from the inferior petrosal sinus, jugular bulb, thyroidal veins, and superior and inferior vena cava are compared with a peripheral venous sample obtained simultaneously. An inferior petrosal sinus to peripheral ACTH ratio of more than 2:1 is a reliable indicator of Cushing's disease and may support a recommendation of total hypophysectomy for a patient in whom a negative pituitary exploration has been performed.

The radiological evaluation of the sella may be restricted to studies with hypocycloidal polytomography and high-resolution computed tomography (CT) scanning with sagittal and coronal reformations. These studies should delineate the sella and localize any focal abnormalities. A high incidence of incidental bone abnormalities found on polytomography and changes in pituitary parenchymal attenuation seen on CT scans emphasizes the need to rely on endocrinologic criteria for diagnosis.[1] If endocrinologic criteria are met, radiological studies showing no abnormalities should not dissuade the surgeon from performing a trans-sphenoidal exploration.

Medical Management

For the patient with Cushing's disease or Nelson's syndrome who is not considered a candidate for surgical intervention or who has an unresectable or incompletely treated tumor, medical therapy may be an option. Medical therapy is only palliative, however, and should be reserved for use in preparation for surgery, in conjunction with pituitary irradiation, or after both these modalities have failed to achieve a cure. Drug therapy is directed at reducing the secretion of ACTH by the pituitary or at interrupting adrenal steroidogenesis.

Cyproheptadine, a serotonin antagonist, and bromocriptine, a dopaminergic agonist, are thought to alter hypothalamic neurotransmitters that regulate CRF. Cyproheptadine reportedly has achieved remission in more than 50 percent of patients with Cushing's disease.[7] A dosage of 24 mg per day is attained gradually, and if effective, chemical and clinical remission should be evident within 2 to 6 months. A relapse while the patient is under treatment, and the side effects of somnolence and hyperphagia—especially in children, may limit the usefulness of the drug in some cases.

The reported results with the use of bromocriptine to treat Cushing's disease have been contradictory. Lamberts et al.[8] have presented evidence that patients whose corticotropic adenomas originate in the intermediate lobe suppress ACTH secretion in response to 10 mg per day of bromocriptine. After the discontinuation of cyproheptadine or bromocriptine therapy, a relapse can be expected in virtually all cases. The recent finding that naloxone selectively suppresses ACTH hypersecretion in patients with Cushing's disease, Nelson's syndrome, or Addison's disease holds promise for improved medical therapy in the future.[21]

Aminoglutethimide, metyrapone, o,p'-dichlorodiphenyl-dichloroethane (o,p'-DDD), and trilostane have been used to direct pharmacological therapy to the adrenal cortices. These adrenoactive agents do not suppress either the secretion of ACTH or the growth of the pituitary lesion. ACTH levels in plasma may increase during effective antiadrenal therapy in a manner analogous to the increase of ACTH levels in patients with Addison's disease or during the development of Nelson's syndrome. Although o,p'-DDD is toxic to the adrenal cortices, it has been used at a reduced dosage to block steroidogenesis chronically. Its side effects include sedation, depression, gastrointestinal problems, and permanent adrenal damage. Aminoglutethimide, which inhibits the conversion of cholesterol to pregnenolone, blocks the first step in steroidogenesis. It has been used successfully alone as well as in combination with metyrapone. Metyrapone (250 to 750 mg orally every 6 h) blocks the 11-hydroxylase step in cortisol production in response to ACTH stimulation, but aminoglutethimide is often added to prevent "adrenal escape" from the inhibition, as ACTH levels increase in response to decreased serum cortisol. Hirsutism has been a problem with the prolonged use of metyrapone, and 20 to 30 percent of patients develop skin rash, goiter, somnolence, or gonadal toxicity while taking aminoglutethimide. Mineralocorticoid and glucocorticoid replacement is required when o,p'-DDD or aminoglutethimide is used.

Surgical Therapy

The goals of definitive therapy should be (1) to eliminate the inappropriate ACTH secretion and/or hypercortisolism; (2) to eradicate the responsible lesion; and (3) to prevent permanent dependence on hormonal replacement by averting endocrine deficiency.

As primary therapy, irradiation of the pituitary gland, either with heavy particles or from a megavoltage source, produces remission of disease in 50 to 80 percent of patients with Cushing's disease, and in a much smaller percentage of those with Nelson's syndrome.[11,20] Children appear to respond better than adults to this form of therapy. The efficacy of pituitary irradiation, however, is qualified by the delay in response and by the inclusion of normal structures in the treatment fields. In addition, most patients who undergo radiation therapy subsequently have varying degrees of hypopituitarism.

Selective microsurgical removal of corticotropic microadenomas has proved to be the most effective method of achieving the goals of definitive therapy. The refinement of trans-sphenoidal pituitary microsurgery constitutes the single most important advance contributing to the successful treatment of Cushing's disease and Nelson's syndrome. This procedure, when performed by an experienced surgeon, involves an extremely low incidence of morbidity and mortality.

The microadenomas are rarely located on the surface of the anterior lobe and must be exposed by a systematic, thorough dissection through an apparently normal gland.[1,6,9,22] For consenting adults, total hypophysectomy should be considered an option if no abnormality is demonstrated at the time of operation, as an undetectably minute adenoma may be presumed to be the source of disease. Craniotomy should be restricted to those cases in which suprasellar or parasellar extension of tumor, a small sella turcica, or both preclude adequate access to a large tumor by the trans-sphenoidal route. Adrenalectomy should be used only as a last resort, after pharmacological therapy, pituitary surgery, and irradiation have failed to produce a cure.

TABLE 97-1 Results of Trans-sphenoidal Microsurgical Treatment of ACTH-secreting Pituitary Adenomas in Four Series

	No. of Patients	No. Cured (%)	No. with Persistent Tumor (%)	No. with Recurrent Tumor (%)
Hardy:[6]				
Cushing's disease	38			
Nelson's syndrome	12			
Combined	50	32 (64)	16 (32)	2 (4)
Laws et al.:[9]				
Cushing's disease	65	51 (79)	12 (18)	2 (3)
Nelson's syndrome	26	4 (15)	18 (69)	4 (15)
Wilson et al.:[1,22]				
Cushing's disease	96	74 (77)	18 (19)	4 (4)
Nelson's syndrome	19	4 (21)	15 (79)	
Overall	256	165 (64)	79 (31)	12 (5)

The results of trans-sphenoidal microsurgical management of ACTH-secreting pituitary tumors derived from four representative reports in the literature are summarized in Table 97-1. In these series, the rate of cure obtained by the selective removal of microadenomas was more than 90 percent. Extrasellar extension of tumor, macroadenomas, the presence of Nelson's syndrome, or any combination of these, was associated with a comparatively poorer outcome. In each series, long-term remission of disease was associated with a prolonged (more than 3 months) period of hypocortisolism after successful microsurgery; during this period, steroid replacement was required for at least 6 months. Hypopituitarism occurred only in those patients in whom hypophysectomy was performed intentionally. Among the patients initially considered cured, less than 5 percent have had recurrent tumors.

In contrast, less than 30 percent of patients with Nelson's syndrome who undergo surgery can be expected to have remission of disease, regardless of tumor size. The high incidence of cranial nerve dysfunction, the tendency toward invasion of surrounding structures by tumor, and the poor response to all treatment modalities associated with Nelson's syndrome emphasize that adrenalectomy should be used to treat Cushing's disease only after all other therapy has failed.

The specificity of treatment by trans-sphenoidal microsurgical exploration of the pituitary gland and the high likelihood of cure following selective trans-sphenoidal microsurgery make this approach the present treatment of choice. It should be the primary treatment for all patients with Cushing's disease or Nelson's syndrome.

References

1. Boggan JE, Tyrrell JB, Wilson CB: Transsphenoidal microsurgical management of Cushing's disease: Report of 100 cases. J Neurosurg 59:195–200, 1983.
2. Clayton BE: Some observations on adrenocorticotropin in blood. Proc R Soc Med 51:558–560, 1958.
3. Cushing H: The basophil adenomas of the pituitary body and their clinical manifestations (pituitary basophilism). Bull Johns Hopkins Hosp 50:137–195, 1932.
4. Findling JW, Aron DC, Tyrrell JB, Shinsako JH, Fitzgerald PA, Norman D, Wilson CB, Forsham PH: Selective venous sampling for ACTH in Cushing's syndrome: Differentiation between Cushing's disease and ectopic ACTH syndrome. Ann Intern Med 94:647–652, 1981.
5. Gold EM: The Cushing syndromes: Changing views of diagnosis and treatment. Ann Intern Med 90:829–844, 1979.
6. Hardy J: Microsurgery of pituitary disorders, in Sano K, Takakura K, Fukushima T, Teramoto A (eds): *Functioning Pituitary Adenoma and Bromocriptine: Proceedings of the Second Workshop on Pituitary Tumors.* Tokyo, Sandoz Pharmaceuticals, 1981, pp 41–46.
7. Krieger DT: Pharmacological therapy of Cushing's disease and Nelson's syndrome, in Linfoot JA (ed): *Recent Advances in the Diagnosis and Treatment of Pituitary Tumors.* New York, Raven Press, 1979, pp 337–340.
8. Lamberts SWJ, de Lange SA, Stefanko SZ: Adrenocorticotropin-secreting pituitary adenomas originate from the anterior or the intermediate lobe in Cushing's disease: Difference in the regulation of hormone secretion. J Clin Endocrinol Metab 54:286–291, 1982.
9. Laws ER Jr, Ebersold MJ, Piepgras DG, Randall RV, Salassa RM: The results of trans-sphenoidal surgery in specific clinical entities, in Laws ER Jr, Randall RV, Kern EB, Abboud CF (eds): *Management of Pituitary Adenomas and Related Lesions: With Emphasis on Trans-sphenoidal Microsurgery.* New York, Appleton-Century-Crofts, 1982, pp 277–305.
10. Liddle GW: Pathogenesis of glucocorticoid disorders. Am J Med 53:638–648, 1972.
11. Linfoot JA: Heavy ion therapy: Alpha particle therapy of pituitary tumors, in Linfoot JA (ed): *Recent Advances in the Diagnosis and Treatment of Pituitary Tumors.* New York, Raven Press, 1979, pp 245–267.
12. Lisser H: Hypophysectomy in Cushing's disease (Report of a case operated upon by Dr. HC Naffziger, December 1933). J Nerv Ment Dis 99:727–733, 1944.
13. McKeever PE, Koppelman MCS, Metcalf D, Quindlen E, Kornblith PL, Strott CA, Howard R, Smith BH: Refractory Cushing's disease caused by multinodular ACTH-cell hyperplasia. J Neuropathol Exp Neurol 41:490–499, 1982.
14. Moore TJ, Dluhy RG, Williams GH, Cain JP: Nelson's syndrome: Frequency, prognosis, and effect of prior pituitary irradiation. Ann Intern Med 85:731–734, 1976.
15. Nelson DH, Meakin JW, Dealy JB Jr, Matson DD, Emerson K Jr, Thorn GW: ACTH-producing tumor of the pituitary gland. N Engl J Med 259:161–164, 1958.
16. Nelson DH, Sprunt JG, Mims RB: Plasma ACTH determinations in 58 patients before or after adrenalectomy for Cushing's syndrome. J Clin Endocrinol Metab 26:722–728, 1966.
17. Robert F, Pelletier G, Hardy J: Pituitary adenomas in Cushing's disease. Arch Pathol Lab Med 102:448–455, 1978.
18. Rovit RL, Berry RG: Cushing's syndrome and the hypophysis: A re-evaluation of pituitary tumors and hyperadrenalism. J Neurosurg 23:270–295, 1965.
19. Salassa RM, Kearns TP, Kernohan JW, Sprague RG, MacCarty CS: Pituitary tumors in patients with Cushing's syndrome. J Clin Endocrinol Metab 19:1523–1539, 1959.
20. Sheline GE: Conventional radiation therapy in the treatment of pituitary tumors, in Tindall GT, Collins WF (eds): *Clinical Management of Pituitary Disorders.* New York, Raven Press, 1979, pp 287–314.
21. Tolis G, Jukier L, Wiesen M, Krieger DT: Effect of naloxone on pituitary hypersecretory syndromes. J Clin Endocrinol Metab 54:780–784, 1982.
22. Wilson CB, Tyrrell JB, Fitzgerald PA, Pitts LH: Cushing's disease and Nelson's syndrome. Clin Neurosurg 27:19–29, 1980.

98

Acromegaly and Gigantism

Edward R. Laws, Jr.

Acromegaly represents the somatic manifestation of a pathological excess of growth hormone secretion. When this condition is present in childhood, before the closure of the epiphyses of the long bones, it leads to gigantism. Acromegalic persons and giants have been described in literature and art throughout history. The unfortunate people afflicted with this condition have been held in awe, and enormous strength and physical powers have been attributed to them, although these are rarely present, at least for any extended period of time.

Historical Aspects

Pierre Marie described acromegaly as a medical syndrome in 1886. The causative role of the pituitary gland was not recognized at that time, however, and the enlarged pituitaries found at autopsy were thought by many to be just another feature of the hypertrophy which affected many parts of the body. By 1900, pathophysiological correlations by Benda and others had suggested that the hypertrophy or hyperplasia of the pituitary might be the cause of acromegaly, and the adenomatous nature of pituitary enlargement was ultimately documented.

Pathogenesis and Natural History

The vast majority of cases of acromegaly are produced by neoplasms of the somatotrophic cells of the anterior pituitary. These tumors appear to arise independently of known alterations of other hormones and tropic factors. Some tumors (20 to 30 percent) have the ability to produce excessive amounts of both growth hormone (GH) and prolactin. Acromegaly can also occur as a result of hyperplasia of the somatotropes either independently or in response to excessive amounts of growth hormone–releasing factor. This latter syndrome has been seen in association with a hypothalamic hamartoma, a pancreatic adenoma, and a mediastinal carcinoid tumor.

Spontaneous remission of acromegaly may occur but is rare and usually is associated with infarction or hemorrhage within the tumor. Spontaneous hemorrhage may also present as pituitary apoplexy, threatening vision and life; fortunately, apoplexy also occurs rarely. Persistent active acromegaly is the usual course associated with a growth hormone–secreting pituitary tumor. The cumulative effects of excess growth hormone shorten life and interfere with its quality. Structural changes occur in the cardiovascular system and are frequently associated with hypertension and severe atherosclerosis. Diabetes mellitus and its many complications are common in these patients. In addition to morphological changes in soft tissues with enlargement of the digits and loss of dexterity, joints are commonly affected, resulting in severe and progressive osteoarthritis. Early therapy is recommended to forestall these pathophysiological changes.

Therapy

Trans-sphenoidal Surgery[2–5,7,9,10]

The first operation on the pituitary for acromegaly was performed in Vienna in 1908 by Hochenegg using Schloffer's trans-sphenoidal approach. In the United States, the first such operation was performed by Harvey Cushing in 1909 (Fig. 98-1).[4] The patient, a farmer from South Dakota, was referred to Cushing in Baltimore by C. H. Mayo of Rochester, Minnesota. This was Cushing's first trans-sphenoidal operation for a pituitary tumor, and he used a superior transnasal approach, resecting the upper septum and the turbinates. He soon perfected the sublabial rhinoseptal submucosal approach and operated on some 60 acromegalic patients using this method.

Radiation

Radiation therapy for acromegaly also began in 1909 and has been applied with considerable success. The majority of patients have been treated with conventional photon therapy, currently best delivered by a linear accelerator using multiple ports and appropriate shielding of the eyes. Interstitial radiation by implantation of ^{198}Au or ^{90}Y sources has been used in the past, and heavy particle external therapy using neutrons and alpha particles has also been effective.

Craniotomy

Craniotomy in the acromegalic patient is made difficult by the thick cranial bone and exuberant frontal sinuses characteristic of this condition. Large lesions with significant suprasellar or parasellar extension may still require craniotomy if adequate removal of the tumor is to be accomplished. Bronson Ray became extraordinarily skilled in the transfrontal approach and reported his excellent results in a large series of patients.[11] Currently, when craniotomy is indicated, it is usually accomplished by either the transfrontal or pterional approach, depending on the anatomy of the lesion.

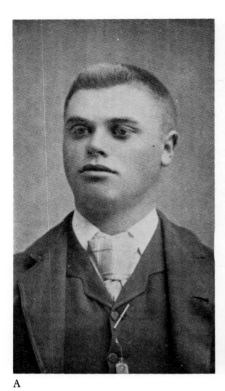

A

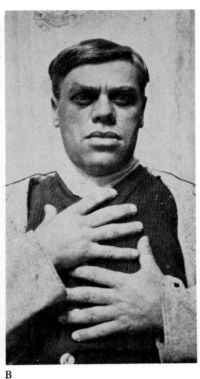

B

Figure 98-1 An acromegalic from South Dakota upon whom Harvey Cushing performed his first trans-sphenoidal operation. *A*. The patient some years before onset of symptoms. *B*. The patient upon admission to the hospital.

Medical Treatment

The discovery and isolation of somatostatin (growth hormone release-inhibiting factor) gave great promise for medical control of acromegaly. Unfortunately, the effects of this peptide are so transient as to make it ineffective for control of excessive GH secretion. Subsequent discovery of the fact that GH release is under significant dopaminergic control has led to the use of the dopamine agonist bromoergocriptine, or bromocriptine, in the management of acromegaly. Approximately 75 percent of patients with active acromegaly, when treated with bromocriptine, will respond with a decrease in GH production. Unfortunately, high doses (20 to 60 mg/day) are usually required, and reduction of GH levels to normal is rare. The response to bromocriptine appears to be most dramatic in acromegalic patients who also have hyperprolactinemia. These patients commonly will show shrinkage of the bulk of the tumor after bromocriptine therapy. Although manifestations of the tumor return after bromocriptine therapy is discontinued, continued bromocriptine therapy is thought by many to protect against further growth of the tumor.

Clinical Manifestations

Patients with active acromegaly present with a wide spectrum of symptoms and signs. Those who have elevated growth hormone in childhood develop gigantism, with long arms and legs and nearly proportional increases in size of other body parts. The tallest accurately measured acromegalic giant was 7 ft 6 in (2.3 m) tall, but others undoubtedly have been taller. Once the epiphyses close, excessive growth hormone produces acromegaly with focal enlargement of bones and soft tissues in various parts of the body. There is thickening of the heel and palm pads and soft tissues of the fingers and toes. The facial features become characteristically coarse, and enlargement of the nose and lips occurs. The jaw enlarges, and the teeth become maloccluded. The tongue and heart both enlarge, leading to partial airway obstruction on the one hand and decreased cardiac output on the other. The scalp may become hypertrophic enough to appear corrugated. There is exuberant enlargement of the air sinuses in the thickened skull, leading to a "beetle brow" appearance. Bone density is generally increased, and joints and costochondral junctions undergo hypertrophy. Later in life, severe degenerative osteoarthritis and spinal stenosis may occur. The ligaments thicken, and median thenar neuropathy from the carpal tunnel syndrome is a common presenting complaint. The generalized effect on the cardiovascular system leads to hypertension.

Abnormalities in glucose metabolism are common, and diabetes mellitus is a frequent finding. Associated hypothyroidism may occur, and a small but significant number of patients (about 5 percent) will have a multiple endocrine neoplasia (MEN) syndrome, most commonly with parathyroid and pancreatic adenomas. These patients with MEN may suffer from hypercalcemia and urolithiasis, hyperinsulinemia, and gastric ulcer. Because about 20 percent of acromegalic patients also have hyperprolactinemia, premenopausal women may develop oligomenorrhea, amenorrhea, and galactorrhea. Other symptoms related to prolactin include loss of libido in both sexes and impotence in men.

Large tumors may produce hypopituitarism with fatigue, anemia, pallor, poor response to stress, and hypogonadotropism.

Compression of the optic apparatus from suprasellar extension of the tumor may lead to photophobia, progressive visual loss (usually a bitemporal hemianopsia), and optic atrophy. Sudden loss of vision secondary to apoplexy within the pituitary adenoma (hemorrhage and/or necrosis) may occur. Compression of the cavernous sinus from lateral expansion of the tumor may lead to complaints of trigeminal pain and diplopia. Invasive tumors may produce cerebrospinal rhinorrhea.

Acromegaly undoubtedly has direct effects on the nervous system, perhaps related to abnormalities of peptide neurotransmitters. Acromegalic patients may have a greater than normal incidence of neuropathies and myopathies, epilepsy, dementia, and psychopathy.

The relative incidence of these symptoms and signs in a surgically treated series is presented in Table 98-1. Men represented 59 percent of the series of women 41 percent. The mean age at the time of the operation was 42 years.

The endocrinologic evaluation of patients with acromegaly has been discussed elsewhere.[1]

Results

Surgical Management

Since 1972, all acromegalic patients treated surgically at the Mayo Clinic have been operated on initially with the trans-sphenoidal microsurgical approach.[6] Criteria for satisfactory results are clinical improvement in the symptoms and signs of acromegaly and normalization of GH secretion. The latter is measured by fall in serum GH values to less than 3 ng/ml during a glucose tolerance test. The results are discussed within the limits of these rigid criteria.

Clinical improvement has occurred in 97 percent of the patients. Endocrinologic success has been more difficult to achieve and is related to the biological and morphological classification of the tumor and to the preoperative level of human growth hormone (hGH). Those patients with basal hGH values less than 50 ng/ml have the best chance for nor-

malization after surgery. Tumors are classified as microadenomas ($\leq$ 10 mm in diameter), diffuse adenomas, and invasive adenomas according to their size and the findings at operation. Those patients with microadenomas have the best prospects for "cure" following surgery. The worst results are in patients with invasive tumors and markedly elevated hGH values.

The author's surgical philosophy has been to perform a radical removal of all tumor and a rim of adjacent normal gland. Planned total hypophysectomy has been performed only once, in an acromegalic giant with diabetic retinopathy. Alcohol or Zenker's solution has not routinely been used to treat the tumor bed.

The results of trans-sphenoidal microsurgery in this series are given in Table 98-2. When more liberal criteria are used for "cure" (hGH $\leq$ 10 ng/ml), satisfactory results are obtained in more than 90 percent of patients with microadenoma, and this has been the experience of others as well.[2,3,5]

Other Forms of Primary Management

Critical summaries of other forms of primary management are not readily available, but reports have been published of "success" rates of 64 percent for craniotomy, 27 to 41 percent for radioactive implants, 76 to 86 percent for cryotherapy, 88 percent for thermocoagulation, 23 to 81 percent for conventional radiation therapy, and 53 to 91 percent for proton and heavy particle therapy. These reports were summarized by Laws et al. in 1982.[9]

Adjunctive Management of Acromegaly

It has been the general policy at the Mayo Clinic to recommend postoperative radiation in all patients with tumors having suprasellar extension and those with invasive characteristics. When elevation of postoperative growth hormone levels increases over time, radiation therapy is also usually recommended. Bromocriptine therapy is considered in cases in which active acromegaly persists despite surgery and radiation therapy and in cases of invasive tumors that appear to remain active or enlarge over time. Relatively large doses (20 to 60 mg per day) of bromocriptine are usually necessary for hormonal control.

Complications of Trans-sphenoidal Surgery for Acromegaly[8]

There have been no operative (30-day) deaths in the Mayo Clinic series. Two arterial injuries occurred, one of the carotid artery, which was directly repaired, and one of the anterior cerebral artery, which was clipped. One patient with compromised vision from a large tumor developed further loss of vision which was later recovered. Another patient developed optic nerve type visual loss, which resolved after craniotomy and radiation therapy. One patient devel-

TABLE 98-1 Symptoms and Signs in 170 Surgically Treated Acromegalic Patients

Clinical Feature	Percent Incidence
Acromegaly	100
Gigantism	4
Headache	50
Arthralgias, osteoarthritis	66
Diabetes mellitus	50
Hypertension	46
Hyperprolactinemia	20
Carpal tunnel syndrome	19
Thyroidopathy	4
Visual loss	8
Multiple endocrine neoplasia	4

TABLE 98-2 Results of Trans-sphenoidal Surgery in the Management of Acromegaly

Tumor Category	Mean Preoperative hGH Level (ng/ml)	Percent "Cure" (hGH≤3 ng/ml)
Microadenoma	29.1	65
Diffuse adenoma	56.2	55
Invasive adenoma	65.2	52

oped cerebrospinal rhinorrhea, which was successfully repaired with a second trans-sphenoidal procedure. Significant intraoperative bleeding occurred in three patients; in two the procedure was abandoned, with later successful surgery in one, and in the third, multiple transfusions allowed completion of the original procedure. Loss of preoperative normal anterior pituitary function occurred in six patients, and permanent diabetes insipidus in four. One patient developed severe sinusitis in the postoperative period, and another developed a nasoseptal perforation. Fortunately, major postoperative complications have been rare.

References

1. Abboud CF, Laws ER Jr: Clinical endocrinological approach to hypothalamic-pituitary disease. J Neurosurg 51:271–291, 1979.

2. Balagura S, Derome P, Guiot G: Acromegaly: Analysis of 132 cases treated surgically. Neurosurgery 8:413–416, 1981.

3. Baskin DS, Boggan JE, Wilson CB: Transsphenoidal microsurgical removal of growth hormone–secreting pituitary tumors: A review of 137 cases. J Neurosurg 56:634–641, 1982.

4. Cushing H: Partial hypophysectomy for acromegaly. Ann Surg 50: 1002–1017, 1909.

5. Hardy J, Somma M, Vezina JL: Treatment of acromegaly: Radiation or surgery? in Morley T (ed): *Current Controversies in Neurosurgery*. Philadelphia, Saunders, 1976, pp 377–391.

6. Laws ER Jr: Transsphenoidal approach to lesions in and about the sella turcica, in Schmidek HH, Sweet WH (eds): *Current Techniques in Operative Neurosurgery*. New York, Grune & Stratton, 1977, pp 161–172.

7. Laws ER Jr: Transsphenoidal microsurgery in the management of acromegaly, in Smith JL (ed): *Neuro-Ophthalmology Focus, 1980*. New York, Masson Publishing, USA, 1979, pp 289–293.

8. Laws ER Jr: Complications of transsphenoidal microsurgery for pituitary adenomas, in Brock M (ed): *Modern Neurosurgery*. New York, Springer-Verlag, 1982, pp 181–186.

9. Laws ER Jr, Piepgras DG, Randall RV, Abboud CF: Neurosurgical management of acromegaly: Results in 82 patients treated between 1972 and 1977. J Neurosurg 50:454–461, 1979.

10. Laws ER Jr, Randall RV, Abboud CF: Surgical treatment of acromegaly: Results in 140 patients, in Givens J (ed): *Hormone-Secreting Pituitary Tumors*. Chicago, Year Book, 1982, pp 225–228.

11. Ray BS, Horwith M, Mautalen C: Surgical hypophysectomy as a treatment for acromegaly, in Astwood EB, Cassidy CE (ed): *Clinical Endocrinology*. New York, Grune & Stratton, 1968, pp 93–102.

99

Perioperative Endocrine Management of Patients with Pituitary Tumors

Kalmon D. Post
William Cobb

Pituitary hormone deficiencies are of significant concern in the management of patients with pituitary tumors. Fortunately, most patients undergoing trans-sphenoidal surgery have microadenomas and do not have significant pre- or postoperative endocrine deficiencies. However, those patients with larger tumors and some of those with hypersecreting states have abnormalities that need endocrine attention before surgery, immediately after surgery, and on a continuing basis. This is always true in patients undergoing hypophysectomy for endocrine-dependent cancer. The routine use of corticosteroids and the long plasma half-life (7 days) of thyroxine mean that the appearance of adrenocorticotropic hormone (ACTH) and/or thyroid-stimulating hormone (TSH) deficiency in the immediate postoperative period may be of little importance, whereas acute deficiency of the posterior pituitary octapeptide, vasopressin, may result in a life-threatening disturbance of water balance. Beyond the immediate postoperative period, the management of ACTH, TSH, gonadotropin, and growth hormone (GH) deficiencies assumes a greater significance in the long-term follow-up of patients.

Preoperative Hormone Therapy

Preoperative assessment includes attention to specific problems associated with pituitary tumors, including diabetes mellitus, hypertension, diabetes insipidus (DI), hypothyroidism (rarely hyperthyroidism), and adrenal insufficiency. Many tests are available for the evaluation of pituitary function, and these are discussed elsewhere in this textbook. In the preoperative period, the most informative studies are those for ACTH reserve, thyroid function, and electrolyte balance.

Because the surgical procedure may involve either manipulation or removal of the anterior lobe of the pituitary gland, all patients, regardless of preoperative hypothalamic-pituitary-adrenal (HPA) axis testing, receive steroid replacement to provide adequate glucocorticoid concentrations during the perioperative period. The benefit of supplementing steroids in patients with normal preoperative function has not been established, particularly when high doses are given to patients undergoing adenomectomy. However, supplemental steroids are routinely administered preoperatively (50 to 100 mg cortisone acetate p.o. or hydrocortisone parenterally or p.o. the evening prior to surgery) to all patients, including those with microadenomas.[9,11] Although this approach is probably not necessary in most instances, it provides steroid coverage for patients who show partial or complete ACTH deficiency on preoperative testing, as well as those who become deficient during surgery.

If diabetes mellitus is present, appropriate insulin coverage will be necessary. The hypothyroid patient receives thyroid replacement beginning 4 to 6 weeks before elective surgery to achieve an euthyroid state. Thyroid replacement is never given without complete adrenal reserve function testing, since thyroid therapy increases the need for adrenal function and may precipitate an adrenal crisis. Diabetes insipidus can be controlled with aqueous pitressin or with 1-deamino-8-D-arginine vasopressin (DDAVP).

Intraoperative Hormone Therapy

Steroids such as hydrocortisone sodium succinate in a dose of 100 mg/1000 ml crystalloid solution are given early in the operative procedure and are repeated in 4 h if the operation lasts that long.

Administration of fluids during trans-sphenoidal procedures is calculated to include maintenance requirements and replacement of blood loss and fluid deficit. Some patients may have taken nothing by mouth for as long as 12 to 15 h before surgery. It is therefore important that they receive additional fluid during induction of anesthesia to replace the deficit and in anticipation of blood loss. Although operative blood loss is usually 200 to 300 ml, it can be extensive and acute, so blood should be available. If diabetes insipidus is present, the urinary losses must be replaced as well.

Diabetes insipidus is not an uncommon sequela of trans-sphenoidal procedures, particulariy hypophysectomy. Although its onset is usually on the first or second postoperative day, DI occasionally occurs during anesthesia or in the recovery room. Measurement of urine output is important, but insertion of a urinary catheter is usually unnecessary.

Immediate Postoperative Replacement Therapy

Pituitary-Adrenal Dysfunction

Glucocorticoids are routinely administered to all patients following surgery for a pituitary tumor, regardless of preoperative HPA axis testing.

If the pituitary-adrenal function is normal prior to microadenoma surgery (i.e., for treatment of prolactinomas and acromegaly), it is normal afterward in most cases.[9,11] Moderate-dose dexamethasone (4 to 8 mg per day) is commonly used in these patients during and immediately after surgery. This is rapidly tapered to maintenance levels (0.75 mg) by the third and fourth postoperative days. This rapid tapering usually averts adrenal suppression and decreases the incidence of glucose intolerance. In the past, patients on the authors' service have been routinely maintained on replacement steroids (prednisone 7.5 mg per day) until postoperative evaluation was carried out 4 to 6 weeks later. Currently, however, following microadenoma surgery where the normal gland is well seen and not overly manipulated, the patient is discharged without replacement medication. The possible need for steroids and the symptoms of insufficiency are discussed with the patient and family upon discharge; the patient is given prednisone tablets and the physician's telephone number in case of an emergency.

Patients with an ACTH-secreting microadenoma (Cushing's disease) are not totally withdrawn from steroids. Rather, if a total adenomectomy has been achieved, normal or slightly greater than normal replacement therapy is required for several months.[5]

Patients with preoperative pituitary-adrenal insufficiency usually require replacement steroids following surgery. In these patients and in those subjected to total hypophysectomy, the high-dose steroids (dexamethasone 16 mg per day) are tapered to replacement levels, which are adjusted prior to discharge. Patients receiving adrenal replacement are always informed of the probable need for additional hormones in times of stress.

In patients with significant suprasellar tumor extension, the dosage is tapered more slowly, since high-dose steroids may offer the additional benefit of reducing local brain swelling caused by the tumor and the manipulation of surgery. (See below for steroid usage during radiation therapy.)

Pituitary-Thyroid Dysfunction

Following surgery for a pituitary tumor, the patient who is preoperatively euthyroid may become deficient in thyroid-stimulating hormone; this is not important in the immediate postoperative period, however, because thyroxine has a plasma half-life of 7 days. In contrast, a patient whose chronic preoperative secondary hypothyroidism has been untreated or treated inadequately with replacement thyroid medication may develop complications in the immediate postoperative period due to or aggravated by thyroid deficiency.

The hypothyroid patient may exhibit impaired consciousness postoperatively, ranging from mild lethargy to coma, because of the various effects of thyroid deficiency on drug metabolism, respiratory function, fluid and electrolyte balance, and cardiac output. Hypothyroidism may reduce drug metabolism, potentiating the effects of sedative, analgesic, and anesthetic medications; may reduce the ventilatory drive to a hypoxic and, in the severely hypothyroid state, a hypercapneic stimulus;[2] and may impair urinary dilution and sodium excretion, an effect that may produce hyponatremia and cause a reduced myocardial contractility, decreasing cardiac output and cerebral perfusion. The author prefers to treat hypothyroid patients for a minimum of 4 to 8 weeks preoperatively with sodium L-thyroxine to avoid postoperative complications associated with hypothyroidism. When this is not possible, a daily dose of thyroxine (0.025 to 0.1 mg p.o.) is started in the immediate postoperative period. The age of the patient, duration of hypothyroidism, and evidence of coexisting coronary artery disease determine the precise initial dosage. Sodium L-thyroxine may be administered intravenously when the patient is unable to take medication orally. This dose is one-half to three-fourths the oral dose, since only 60 to 80 percent of the oral sodium L-thyroxine is absorbed from the gastrointestinal tract. The management of myxedema coma has been most successful when up to 0.5 mg of intravenous sodium L-thyroxine is given first to replete the total body thyroxine pool.

Patients requiring preoperative thyroid medication or those who have had a total hypophysectomy are usually started on replacement thyroid as soon as they can take oral medications. Thyroid hormone therapy is rarely needed after microadenoma surgery. A slight fall of T_3 and T_4 values can be seen 1 week after operation, probably secondary to a transient disturbance in pituitary TSH function. A falsely low T_4 can also be due to phenytoin administration. Adrenal reserve function should always be tested prior to initiation of thyroid replacement, because institution of thyroid therapy increases the need for adrenal hormone and may precipitate an adrenal crisis. When thyroid replacement is needed, adrenal replacement is usually required as well.

Hypogonadism

Gonadotropin deficiency does not require treatment in the immediate postoperative period.

Diabetes Insipidus

The incidence of DI in the immediate postoperative period varies with the nature of the procedure. In total hypophysectomy patients, it may be as high as 37 percent.[7] In 250 microsurgical procedures for adenoma, the incidence of DI reported by Wilson and Dempsey was 9.2 percent; of these, 3.6 percent had partial and 2.0 percent had total persistent DI.[11] After most trans-sphenoidal procedures, DI is self-limited and resolves within a week to 10 days. This may simply reflect the extreme sensitivity of the hypothalamic-neurohypophyseal unit to local alterations in blood flow, edema, and traction on the pituitary stalk. Permanent disturbance of ADH secretion is due to direct damage to the neurohypophyseal unit and depends much more on the original size and location of the tumor and the extent of surgical resection. High-dose glucocorticoids and phenytoin may interfere with the secretion of vasopressin as well.

Prompt, accurate diagnosis and aggressive treatment are essential to prevent the extreme alterations in electrolyte and water balance that may accompany these syndromes. Usually DI is easily recognized by the polyuria in the early postoperative period. It commonly occurs 12 to 24 h after pituitary surgery. Urine volume is frequently more than 150 ml/h, with an abnormally high serum osmolality (>295 mosm/kg) and an inappropriately dilute urine (<300 mosm per liter).

In a patient undergoing water diuresis due to overhydration during surgery and the early postoperative period, an erroneous diagnosis of DI is avoided by allowing the diuresis to continue until a state of mild serum hyperosmolality is achieved. A normal or high serum osmolality and high urine osmolality suggest an osmotic diuresis, most often due to osmotic agents such as mannitol or to glycosuria in a diabetic patient. Basic requirements of successful management include meticulous intake and output records, once- or twice-daily measurements of weight and of serum electrolytes and serum and urine osmolalities, and replacement of fluid loss as free water (5% dextrose in water if given intravenously).[10] Patients who are not very sick and who can take oral fluids should be allowed to regulate their own intake and water balance. As soon as possible, their intravenous fluids should be removed and their glucocorticoid dosages tapered. By the second or third postoperative day, the polyuria and polydipsia have usually attenuated to several liters a day and do not require treatment. If the patient can self-regulate fluid intake, it is best not to overuse vasopressin; in this situation the diabetes insipidus is more of an annoyance. Only when adequate fluid intake cannot be maintained because of lethargy or an impaired thirst mechanism is specific drug therapy instituted in the early postoperative period. The rationale for this approach is that DI may be transient or may progress rapidly to the interphase of endogeneous ADH secretion. However, since the consumption of large quantities of fluid may be poorly tolerated and may interfere significantly with sleep, hormonal substitution therapy may be indicated, regardless of the urinary volume.

The preferred agent for treating acute postoperative DI in the patient who has had a trans-sphenoidal procedure is aqueous vasopressin (20 U/ml), because its action is of brief duration. The usual dose is 0.1 to 0.3 ml every 4 to 6 h. The longer-acting vasopressin tannate in oil (5 U/ml) is also used in the treatment of acute postoperative DI, and the author has achieved good results with a starting dose of 0.25 to 0.5 ml I.M. (1.25 to 2.5 U). The lower dose may produce a more diluted urine, and its effect is dissipated more rapidly, minimizing the potentially dangerous complication of water intoxication and the less dangerous, albeit disturbing, problem of rapid shifts in serum sodium concentration. As the effect wears off, water diuresis is allowed to persist up to several hours in anticipation of a return of endogenous ADH secretion.

In the long-term management of DI, 1-deamino-8-D-arginine vasopressin (desmopressin; DDAVP), has replaced other hormonal preparations.[3] Administered intranasally through a calibrated plastic catheter, its usefulness is limited in acute DI following trans-sphenoidal surgery by the potential risk of irritating acutely injured nasal mucosa. Its efficacy is further limited by the packing of nasal passages soon after surgery. Following transfrontal craniotomy for large pituitary tumors with eccentric suprasellar extension, however, DDAVP may be readily administered, even in an unconscious patient. An initial dose of 2.5 to 5 μg is recommended. Repeat doses in the acute setting are determined in

a manner similar to that discussed earlier for vasopressin tannate in oil.

Triphasic DI is unusual with microadenoma surgery but may occur with larger tumors. After several days, DI may disappear and be followed by the syndrome of inappropriate secretion of ADH (SIADH). If this is unanticipated, the patient may rapidly become water-intoxicated and severely hyponatremic on parenteral fluids.[6] Several days of inappropriate vasopressin secretion are usually followed by reappearance of transient or permanent diabetes insipidus.[10]

Syndrome of Inappropriate ADH (SIADH) Secretion

Preoperative medications (narcotics and barbiturates), anesthetic agents, and surgical stress stimulate ADH secretion and may cause hyponatremia and low urinary volume in the early postoperative period. SIADH resulting from surgical irritation of the hypothalamic neurohypophyseal unit must be considered in the absence of an identifiable explanation for hyponatremia. The diagnosis is supported by the demonstration of low serum osmolality, inappropriate high urine osmolality, and a urinary sodium concentration above 20 meq per liter.

SIADH is usually transient, occurring independently of or during the interphase of DI, and may persist for months or years following surgery. Appropriate management, similar to that for DI, requires frequent measurements of body weight, urine and serum osmolality, and serum sodium concentration and accurate intake and output records. Fluid intake should be restricted to maintain serum sodium in the normal range (usually 0.5 to 1.5 liters per day). Fluid restriction alone is inadequate therapy if severe water intoxication occurs with severe hyponatremia (115 to 120 meq per liter or less) and mental changes or seizures; furosemide diuresis with electrolyte replacement (3% NaCl) should be instituted. The concurrent use of hypertonic saline (three times normal) and furosemide has been proposed as a way to raise serum osmolality without the risk of a large fluid accumulation.[1,6] Furosemide, because it acts by blocking active sodium transport in the ascending limb of Henle's loop (concentrating segment) and early distal tubule (diluting segment), results in a urine of high volume with an osmolality that approximates that of plasma. The combined effect of hypertonic solute load and high-volume isosthenuric urine leads to a rapid rise in serum osmolality.

Chronic Pituitary Hormone Therapy

Pituitary-Adrenal Dysfunction

Patients are usually retested for HPA function 4 to 6 weeks after surgery. Significant drug-related HPA axis suppression has not occurred in the author's patients receiving prednisone for this period of time. If replacement steroids were used, they are discontinued 48 h prior to testing.

If adrenal gland unresponsiveness is suspected, the serum cortisol response to ACTH 1-24 (Cortrosyn, Organon

Pharmaceuticals, West Orange, N.J.) should first be assessed. Patients who respond poorly to Cortrosyn are excluded from further testing of the HPA axis and are maintained on replacement steroids. A normal or impaired cortisol response to insulin or metyrapone may be exhibited by patients not tested with Cortrosyn or those who show a normal cortisol response to Cortrosyn. Under stress, patients with an impaired response but normal basal cortisol levels are at risk of developing acute ACTH deficiency. They are instructed in the use of supplemental steroids and are routinely retested at 12- to 24-month intervals. Patients with low basal levels and impaired HPA responsiveness are placed on daily physiological steroid replacement.

Exceptions to this plan of steroid management and postoperative testing include patients severely deficient in HPA function preoperatively and those who have had such extensive tumor resection that the probability of permanent hypopituitarism is high. These patients are maintained on replacement steroids for life. Patients undergoing radiotherapy after incomplete removal of a large pituitary adenoma are maintained on twice the usual physiological replacement dose of corticosteroid (e.g., prednisone 10 to 15 mg daily in divided doses) throughout the course and for 1 week after completion of radiotherapy. The stress of radiotherapy justifies the use of supplemental steroids in patients who may have underlying ACTH deficiency. Dosage is then tapered to physiological levels over 1 to 2 weeks. Although minor physical changes resulting from glucocorticoid excess may occur during the period of radiotherapy, the transient side effects of steroid excess appear to be outweighed by the improved energy level and sense of well-being seen with this regimen. The prolonged use of supraphysiological doses of prednisone increases the likelihood of drug-induced HPA axis suppression. Therefore, postoperative HPA axis testing is delayed for 6 months or more in this group of patients.

Prednisone 5 mg daily in single or divided doses is adequate maintenance therapy for most patients with secondary adrenocortical insufficiency. An increase in steroid dosage under stress is required by all ACTH-deficient patients, including those with normal basal cortisol levels but impaired ACTH reserve (and not receiving daily replacement steroids). Patients are advised to increase prednisone to 10 to 15 mg daily for minor stress (e.g., an upper respiratory infection) and 15 to 25 mg daily for intermediate stress (e.g., an infectious illness with fever or a dental or minor surgical procedure). Major stress (e.g., major trauma or surgery) usually requires parenteral steroids: 100 mg hydrocortisone three or four times daily or its intravenous equivalent. All patients should be provided with Medicalert identification (necklace or bracelet) indicating deficiency in adrenocortical function, and they should be instructed in the use of an injectable corticosteroid (e.g., 4 mg dexamethasone phosphate) in the event that vomiting precludes ingestion of an oral preparation. If the patient is unconscious, a relative or friend may administer the intramuscular dose of dexamethasone prior to seeking medical care. Patients are also advised not to travel great distances from convenient access to health care facilities unless accompanied by someone knowledgeable in the parenteral administration of glucocorticoids. Mineralocorticoid replacement is not needed in ACTH deficiency.[12]

Pituitary-Thyroid Dysfunction

The optimum replacement dose of sodium L-thyroxine for management of chronic central hypothyroidism is 0.1 to 0.2 mg daily, the variability partly due to the dependence of dose on body size. The use of a synthetic thyroxine preparation is preferred, because thyroxine, administered once daily, results in constant levels of T_4 and T_3 in blood. Serum levels of T_4 and T_3 obtained with thyroxine can be used to adequately assess thyroid hormone dosage, but those obtained with preparations containing triiodothyronine cannot be used because of the shorter (24-h) half-life of T_3.

Hypogonadism

Gonadotropin assay, prolactin level, and testosterone assay in males are useful guides to treatment. The most sensitive tests of fertility are the sperm count in the male and menstrual cycles with evidence of ovulation (temperature rise at midcycle or progesterone elevation at late cycle) in the female. Gonadotropin (luteinizing hormone, follicle-stimulating hormone) concentrations are frequently in the normal range in pituitary hypogonadism.[12] Androgen concentration partly determines libido in both sexes. Women with pituitary insufficiency usually do not achieve normal libido after estrogen replacement alone, because ACTH deficiency results in a loss of adrenal androgens; approximately one-fourth (or less) of the testosterone dose given to men is usually required to compensate for this loss. It may be necessary to inquire specifically about sex drive, because many patients hesitate to complain about decreased libido, believing that this is an effect of their illness for which there is no treatment.

Chronic replacement therapy consists of 200 to 300 mg testosterone propionate intramuscularly every 2 to 4 weeks in men and ethinyl estradiol 20 to 50 μg or conjugated estrogens (Premarin, Ayerst Laboratories, New York, N.Y.) 0.625 to 2.5 mg daily in women. Estrogen treatment is administered to women for 25 days each month, with oral medroxyprogesterone, 5 to 10 mg daily, added for the last 5 days. This induces menstrual flow and reverses the endometrial hyperplasia which may occur when estrogens are administered alone. Alternative treatments are buccal testosterone propionate (Oreton propionate, Schering Corp., Kenilworth, N.J.), 5 to 20 mg sublingual daily in men, or one of the combination oral contraceptives in women.[8]

Successful treatment of infertility using sequential combinations of human menopausal gonadotropin (hMG) and human chorionic gonadotropin (hCG) in patients who have undergone hypophysectomy is now well established,[4] so that hypophyseal deficiency need not preclude the possibility of parenthood. Because of its great expense and the occurrence, in some women, of ovarian hyperstimulation, this form of therapy should be administered only by physicians who are familiar with its application. After treatment, males may successfully impregnate their partners even when sperm concentration does not exceed 10×10^6 ml. Although clomiphene citrate enhances gonadotropin secretion by blocking estrogen receptors and therefore the negative feedback of estrogen, it is of no value in many patients who are infertile after hypophysectomy, since gonadotropin reserve is often reduced or absent.

Growth Hormone Deficiency

In the United States, hGH replacement therapy is offered at many major medical centers under protocols sponsored by the National Pituitary Agency. Eligibility generally requires that patients be less than 60 in. tall and have a growth rate of less than 1.5 in. (4 cm) per year, a bone age 2 years or more below chronological age, and a diagnosis of GH deficiency confirmed by results of at least two standard tests of GH stimulation. In most protocols treatment is continued until the child is 5 ft 6 in. (168 cm) tall or until full growth potential has been realized. The maximum effect is generally seen in the first 3 months, the so-called catch-up growth period. After the first and each subsequent year of treatment, growth velocity usually decreases.[2]

Chronic Diabetes Insipidus

Persistence of DI beyond the immediate postoperative period presages a poor long-term outlook for recovery, particularly after transfrontal surgery. It is unusual to see permanent DI in a patient following trans-sphenoidal pituitary surgery. We have seen several cases of partial ADH reserve deficiency which may become more symptomatic during alcohol ingestion or after an increase in corticosteroid dosage. Both alcohol and corticosteroids cause a central inhibition of ADH release.

If a postoperative patient complains of mild polyuria and polydipsia and if there is a possibility of partial DI, a modified dehydration test is performed. All fluids are withheld until the specific gravity of three consecutive hourly urine collections remains constant, usually 6 to 15 hours after the start of the test in patients with partial DI. (In more severe DI, this end point may be attained very quickly; it is important to monitor body weight before and during the test, and dehydration should be terminated when 3 to 5 percent of body weight has been lost). Serum and urine osmolality are measured simultaneously, and DDAVP, 10 μg intranasally, is given. Serum and urine osmolality are then measured for an additional 2 to 4 hours. Prior to DDAVP administration, patients with central or nephrogenic DI show an abnormally high serum osmolality (>295 mosmol/kg) and inappropriately low urine osmolality (<600 mosmol/kg and often much lower). Following DDAVP, there is a 10 percent or greater increment in urine osmolality in patients with central, but not with nephrogenic, DI. The treatment of choice for chronic DI is DDAVP,[3] which is virtually free of side effects except for the headache that may occur in some patients. Moreover, in the doses usually prescribed, DDAVP does not raise blood pressure and pulse rate or cause abdominal pain. Good control is usually achieved with 2.5 to 20 μg twice a day, although once daily may suffice and occasionally three doses per day may be needed. Therapy is best initiated at night. When an evening dose that controls nocturia has been established, a second daily dose is added, usually in the morning.

Chlorpropamide (an oral sulfonylurea used to treat diabetes mellitus), clofibrate (an agent used to treat hyperlipidemia), and carbamazepine (an anticonvulsant drug useful in the management of tic douloureux), have demonstrated an antidiuretic effect that is useful in the treatment of patients with chronic DI.[3] Chlorpropamide (50 to 500 mg. daily) alone is effective in mild degrees of DI, but its use has been limited by life-threatening hypoglycemic reactions, particularly in patients with panhypopituitarism, and over-hydration resulting in symptomatic hyponatremia. The usual daily dose of clofibrate is 500 mg 2 to 4 times and of carbamazepine 400 to 600 mg.

The older hormonal preparation, vasopressin tannate in oil, at a dose of 2.5 to 5 U (0.5 to 1.0 ml) every 24 to 48 h provides good control of DI. Its major disadvantage is the requirement that it be administered intramuscularly. Common problems, particularly in children, are sterile abscess formation and painful injection sites. Side effects due to the action of vasopressin on smooth muscle (such as abdominal pain in children or aggravation of coronary artery disease in adults) and allergic reactions due to animal-protein contamination of vasopressin preparations are common problems associated with the chronic use of vasopressin tannate in oil. A short-acting (2 to 4 h) nasal spray of synthetic lysine vasopressin (Diapid, Sandoz Pharmaceuticals, East Hanover, N. J.), 50 U/ml, may be used to treat mild DI or as an adjunct to vasopressin tannate in oil or nonhormonal preparations.

Chronic SIADH

Fluid restriction is an effective means of maintaining serum sodium levels in the normal range. Lithium carbonate and demeclocyline have also been used in SIADH because of their action on the renal tubule leading to nephrogenic DI. The therapeutic dose for demeclocyline is 600 to 1200 mg daily (in divided doses) and for lithium carbonate, 600 to 900 mg per day. Patients receiving lithium should have frequent determinations of serum levels, and the dose should be adjusted to maintain a therapeutic range.

References

1. Bartter FC: The syndrome of inappropriate secretion of antidiuretic hormone (SIADH). DM pp 1–47, Nov 1973.
2. Cobb WE: Endocrine management after pituitary surgery, in Post KD, Jackson IM, Reichlin S (eds): *The Pituitary Adenoma.* New York, Plenum, 1980, pp 417–435.
3. Cobb WE: Spare S, Reichlin S: Neurogenic diabetes insipidus: Management with dDAVP (1-desamino-8-D-arginine vasopressin). Ann Intern Med 88:183–188, 1978.
4. Glass RH: Infertility, in Yen SSC, Jaffe RB (eds): *Reproductive Endocrinology: Physiology, Pathophysiology and Clinical Management.* Philadelphia, Saunders, 1978, pp 413–417.
5. Fitzgerald PA, Aron DC, Findling JW, Brooks RM, Wilson CB, Forsham PH, Tyrrell JB: Cushing's Disease: Transient secondary adrenal insufficiency after selective removal of pituitary microadenomas: Evidence for a pituitary origin. J Clin Endocrinol Metab 54:413–422, 1982.
6. Hantman D, Rossier B, Zohlman R, Schrier R: Rapid correction of hyponatremia in the syndrome of inappropriate secretion of antidiuretic hormone: An alternative treatment

to hypertonic saline. Ann Intern Med 78:870–875, 1973.

7. Hardy J: Transsphenoidal hypophysectomy: Pathophysiology and results, in Tindall GT, Collins WF (eds): *Clinical Management of Pituitary Disorders*. New York, Raven Press, 1979, pp 409–412.

8. Martin JB, Reichlin S, Brown GM: *Clinical Neuroendocrinology*. Philadelphia, Davis, 1977, pp 370–372.

9. Post KD, Biller BJ, Adelman LS, Molitch ME, Wolpert SM, Reichlin S: Selective transsphenoidal adenomectomy in women with galactorrhea-amenorrhea. JAMA 242:158–162, 1979.

10. Shucart WA, Jackson I: Management of diabetes insipidus in neurosurgical patients. J Neurosurg 44:65–71, 1976.

11. Wilson CB, Dempsey LC: Transsphenoidal microsurgical removal of 250 pituitary adenomas. J Neurosurg 48:13–22, 1978.

12. Zimmerman EA, Postoperative management following pituitary surgery, in Tindal GT, Collins WF (eds): *Clinical Management of Pituitary Disorders*. New York, Raven Press, 1979, pp 425–434.

100

Bromocriptine

William S. Evans
Michael O. Thorner

It is perhaps surprising that a textbook of neurosurgery should contain a chapter on the medical approach to the treatment of certain pituitary tumors. The inclusion of such a review has, however, been prompted by the extraordinary success which has accompanied the management of prolactin-secreting pituitary tumors with the dopamine agonist drugs. The question of primary therapy for such tumors (i.e., surgical versus medical) is currently a subject of some controversy. The authors welcome the opportunity to present their personal views on the topic but recognize that only time will tell whether these opinions or those of others regarding optimal management of prolactin- and growth hormone–secreting tumors will prove to be correct.

Since the observation was made over ten years ago that prolactin exists in humans separate from growth hormone, much attention has focused on the etiology, pathophysiology, and clinical ramifications of nonphysiological hyperprolactinemia. An understanding of the pathological mechanisms involved in states of prolactin hypersecretion and approaches to treatment are of more than simple academic interest, in that 40 percent of all pituitary tumors are associated with hyperprolactinemia.[5] Although symptoms such as headache and visual field defects may result from local expansion of a prolactin-secreting pituitary macroadenoma, the presenting complaints in the majority of patients stem from the effects of overproduction of the hormone itself. For example, although many women with hyperprolactinemia have diminished libido, dyspareunia, and galactorrhea, most present with amenorrhea, oligomenorrhea, and/or infertility.[18] In men, symptoms related to compressive effects of the tumor are more common, but a history of decreased libido and impotence is often obtained, although frequently only in retrospect following successful treatment.[2] Of premier importance is the fact that, provided the normal anterior pituitary is not damaged in the process, successful lowering of circulating prolactin levels often results in reversal of the hypogonadal state with restoration of normal sexual and reproductive function. Therefore the clinician must be aware of the clinical manifestations of hyperprolactinemia, methods of proper diagnostic evaluation, and available treatment modalities with their advantages and disadvantages. The purpose of this review is to outline one method of treatment—the use of the dopamine agonists—with emphasis on patient selection, expected results, and specific concerns. It should be noted that although several dopamine agonists are currently being tested in clinical trials, the first agonist, bromocriptine, has been used most extensively. The majority of studies cited have involved treatment with bromocriptine, but it is reasonable to assume that the mechanisms of action and results of other dopamine agonists may be similar.

Bromocriptine: Clinical Pharmacology and Applications

Control of Prolactin Secretion

Compared to the other anterior pituitary hormones, the secretion of prolactin by the lactotrope is unique in that it is primarily under tonic inhibitory control by the hypothalamus. A significant body of evidence implicates the catecholamine dopamine as the most important physiological prolactin inhibitory factor.[14] Secreted by the tuberoinfundibular neurons with cell bodies in the arcuate nucleus, dopamine is released into the hypothalamic hypophyseal portal circulation, by which it is transported to the anterior pituitary. Dopamine receptors on the lactotrope, when stimulated appropriately, set into motion a series of intracellular events which ultimately result in the inhibition of prolactin secretion. Thus any abnormality in the dopaminergic pathway, such as diminished secretion by the hypothalamus, interruption of the transport system, or decreased lactotrope receptor number or sensitivity to dopamine, could account for lessened or absent tonic inhibition and thus enhanced prolactin secretion. It is indeed the inhibitory nature of dopaminergic control of prolactin release which has provided the foundation for the medical therapy of hyperprolactinemia using dopamine agonists.

Effects on Elevated Circulating Prolactin Concentrations

The prototype dopamine agonist, bromocriptine (2 bromo-ergocryptine, CB-154), was developed as a specific inhibitor of prolactin secretion. However, it was some years later before it was recognized that bromocriptine exerted its effect directly at the pituitary level by stimulating dopamine receptors on the lactotrope.[7] Thus, while chemically an ergot alkaloid, bromocriptine may be considered a potent analogue of dopamine.

Following its introduction into clinical trials in 1971, bromocriptine was found capable of lowering serum prolactin levels in patients both with and without obvious pituitary tumors.[19] Concomitant with the reduction of circulating prolactin, galactorrhea was found to be abolished in 90 percent of women and normal ovulatory cycles restored in over 80 percent. In men, the majority of whom have macroadenomas, as with women harboring large tumors, the results are similarly encouraging. Among patients who have not undergone either surgery or irradiation, the hypogonadal state is reversed in more than 80 percent.

Effects on Tumor Size

Recently, an unexpected clinical result of dopamine agonist therapy has been demonstrated: between 60 and 80 percent of large prolactin-secreting adenomas undergo size reduc-tion during medical treatment with the agonists.[15] In a recent study at our institution, 18 patients with large prolactinomas were treated with bromocriptine (2.5 mg tid). Using radiological techniques, reduction in tumor size was demonstrated in 15 (83 percent), with such changes beginning as early as 5 days after the initiation of treatment (Fig. 100-1). In the same patients, clinical improvement began as early as 48 h after initiation of treatment and was maintained as long as therapy was continued. Patients so treated reported fewer or no headaches, less visual disturbance (Fig. 100-2), and, with time, improved libido and return of sexual function. Neuro-opthalmologic evaluation revealed partial or complete resolution of the visual field defects, and serial computed tomography scanning confirmed the clinically apparent sustained reduction in tumor size.

Although the mechanism involved in tumor reduction is far from clear, recent evidence[23] shows that such changes may not be due to diminished tumor cell mitotic activity, as has been proposed. For several weeks prior to trans-sphenoidal surgery, patients with prolactin-secreting macroadenomas were treated with bromocriptine. Following tumor removal, detailed light and electron microscopic examination of the tissue revealed a marked reduction in both nuclear and cytoplasmic volumes, accounting for the observation of overall decreased cell volume. Moreover, the amount of rough endoplasmic reticulum and the size of the Golgi apparatus were reduced. Thus, compared to the hypersecretory prolactinoma cells observed in untreated patients, the morphology of the bromocriptine-treated cells was compatible with that of biologically quiescent cells and was reminiscent of the histological picture of normal lactotropes. Such findings are more consistent with the concept of deranged control mechanisms than with a primary abnormality in the cell itself resulting in pathological growth and division.

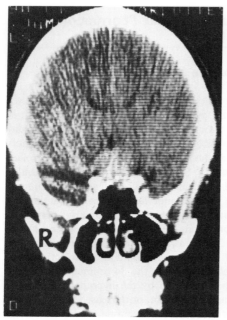

A

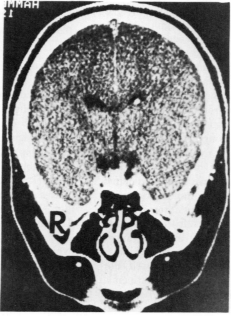

B

Figure 100-1 Coronal CT head scans after enhancement. *A.* Before therapy (on Delta 25 scanner). A large enhancing mass in the pituitary fossa extends inferiorly into the sphenoid sinus and superiorly into the chiasmatic cistern and abuts on the third ventricle. *B.* Two weeks after starting bromocriptine therapy. Scan (GE8800 scanner) shows marked reduction in tumor size, with regression of the suprasellar extension. The chiasmatic cistern is now largely free of tumor, apart from a fingerlike process to the left of midline. The intrasellar high density was present in the pre-enhancement scan and represents calcification within the tumor. (From Thorner et al.[21])

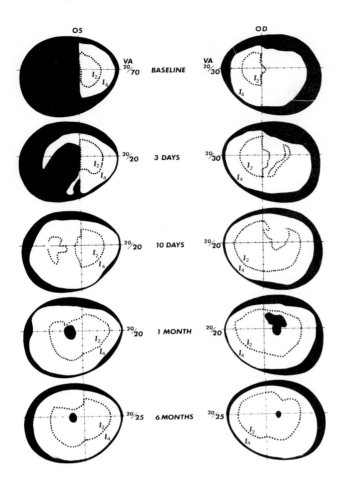

Figure 100-2 Visual acuity and diagrammatic representation of visual field plots before and during 6 months of bromocriptine therapy. The visual fields were plotted by one observer using the Goldmann apparatus under identical conditions with a 0.25-mm² object at two different light intensities, 1000 apostilb (I₄) and 100 apostilb (I₂). The black periphery indicates a normal visual field for comparison. Before therapy, a complete temporal hemianopsia in the left eye and an incomplete hemianopsia in the right eye were present, with reduced visual acuity in both. After 3 days, the left visual field had improved and visual acuity was restored to 20/20. Thereafter, progressive improvement in the visual fields was noted; the only abnormality at 6 months was an equivocal superior bitemporal quadrantic defect to the low-intensity object. (From Thorner et al.[21])

Clinical Manifestations of Withdrawal

It must be stressed that treatment with bromocriptine or the other dopamine agonists does not result in sustained normoprolactinemia or reduction in tumor size following discontinuation of therapy.[21] Indeed, withdrawal of agonist therapy is associated with re-expansion of the tumor, which can best be seen in macroadenomas (Fig. 100-3), and the return of hyperprolactinemia. Dopamine agonist administration must therefore be considered similar to other forms of replacement therapy: when used as the primary mode of treatment, it must be continued indefinitely in order for appropriate suppression of hyperprolactinemia to be maintained.

Treatment of Prolactinomas: Surgery Versus the Medical Approach

As with all treatment of pituitary tumors, the goals of therapy for prolactinomas are (1) decompression or removal of the tumor mass, (2) preservation or restoration of anterior pituitary function; (3) reduction of circulating levels of tumor hormonal product to normal; and (4) prevention of tumor recurrence. Surgery offers the theoretical possibility

of complete cure if selective removal of the tumor can be achieved. Representative surgical results for both micro- and macroadenomas are shown in Table 100-1. Although there is a significant amount of variability, it can be appreciated that the cure rate (defined as postoperative normalization of serum prolactin levels) is related to tumor size. While cure rates for small tumors are in the range of 50 to 100 percent, the rates for large tumors are much less impressive, averaging about 37 percent. The largest series, which has been provided by Hardy,[10] perhaps deserves particular comment. His results reflect the position that the degree of success is inversely related to the preoperative level of serum prolactin, which is, in turn, a function of tumor size. Of those patients with serum prolactin values of less than 250 ng/ml, 78 percent were cured. When this value was greater than 250 ng/ml, however, the cure rate fell significantly and was related to the invasive qualities of the tumor; postoperative normalization of serum prolactin level was 29 percent when the tumor was noninvasive and less than 20 percent when it was invasive. Moreover, no male patient with an invasive tumor experienced a cure.

Another finding described by Hardy requires attention. When followed for up to 5 years, the group considered cured postoperatively demonstrated a 14 percent recurrence rate. These results, when considered in the context of the histological assessment described above, emphasize the concern that a significant number of prolactinomas may well not

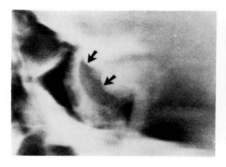
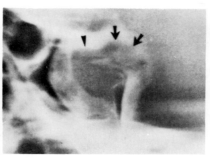
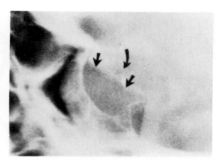

12 months on   **12 days After Withdrawal**   **36 days After Restarting**

Figure 100-3 *Left:* Midline tomogram during metrizamide cisternography 12 months after commencement of treatment. There is extension of the chiasmatic cistern downward into the pituitary fossa (*arrows*), demonstrating a partially empty pituitary fossa. *Middle:* Midline tomogram during metrizamide cisternography 12 days after withdrawal of bromocriptine. There is almost complete obliteration of the chiasmatic cistern, with only a trace of contrast between the inferior surface of the chiasm and the pituitary fossa. The superior margin of the chiasm is identified (*arrowhead*). The summit of the suprasellar extension of the tumor is outlined by contrast (*arrows*). *Right:* Midline tomogram during metrizamide cisternography 36 days after recommencement of bromocriptine therapy. There is again extension of the chiasmatic cistern into the pituitary fossa (*arrows*). This intrasellar extension is not as marked as seen before bromocriptine withdrawal. A small defect is seen in the chiasmatic cistern posteriorly (*curved arrow*), indicating a persistent small suprasellar mass. (From Thorner et al.[22]).

behave in an autonomous manner. If the pathological process indeed relates to an absolute or functional dopamine deficiency, then recurrence, with time, may be the rule rather than the exception.

With the above factors in mind, it is understandable why no well-accepted recommendation has been made concerning the role of surgery in the treatment of prolactinomas. It seems clear that, since the chance of a successful outcome from surgical treatment of a prolactin-secreting macroadenoma is poor, dopamine agonist therapy should be primary. In most instances such treatment should lead to reduction of both circulating prolactin levels and tumor size. Whether surgery will have a role following such reduction in

the size of the tumor remains to be seen. When dealing with prolactin-secreting microadenomas, the choice is less clear. Ideally, selective removal of an adenoma, which is often technically feasible, would be expected to result in permanent cure. If, however, the recurrence rate turns out to be as high as that reported by Hardy or higher, then attention needs to be focused on identification and surgical removal of only those tumors not expected to recur. Currently, no data are available on this. The authors, therefore, take the position that until such guidelines have been established, patients with microadenomas should be offered medical treatment, provided they understand that such therapy must be considered to be lifelong.

TABLE 100-1 Representative Surgical Series: Treatment of Hyperprolactinemia

Series (First Author and Year)	Sex	Microadenomas		Macroadenomas	
		Number of Subjects	Subjects with Normal Postoperative PRL Levels (%)	Number of Subjects	Subjects with Normal Postoperative PRL Levels (%)
Chang[3] (1977)	F	17	10 (59)	7	0 (0)
Franks[6] (1977)	F	5	4 (80)	4	2 (50)
Gomez[9] (1977)	F	7	6 (86)	—	—
Tindall[24] (1978)	F	20	11 (55)	10	5 (50)
	M	2	1 (50)	5	4 (80)
Post[17] (1979)	F	17	13 (76)	13	7 (54)
Tucker[25] (1981)	F	27	20 (74)	18	8 (44)
Hardy[10] (1981)	F	196	151 (77)	97	37 (38)
	M	8	8 (100)	47	12 (26)
Woosley[29] (1982)	F	22	14 (64)	13	4 (23)
	M	—	—	1	0 (0)

Potential Concerns Regarding Bromocriptine Therapy: Pregnancy

Infertility is the primary complaint of many women presenting with hyperprolactinemia. Since the success rate of bromocriptine in restoring normal ovulatory function is high and pregnancy is often achieved, questions about the potential teratogenic effects of bromocriptine and about tumor expansion during pregnancy must be addressed.

In order to minimize exposure of the fetus to bromocriptine, the authors recommend that women use mechanical contraceptive precautions for several months after the initiation of treatment. Once a regular menstrual cycle has developed, contraceptive measures are withdrawn and the patient is instructed to discontinue bromocriptine when an expected menstrual period is 48 h overdue. As a result, fetal exposure to the drug is kept to a minimum. It must be pointed out, however, that no teratogenic sequelae have been associated with bromocriptine in any studies to date in animals. Furthermore, in over 1400 pregnancies in women being treated with bromocriptine at the time of conception, no increase in fetal abnormalities has been found.[26] Thus the outcomes of the pregnancies to date are reassuring concerning bromocriptine and fetal development.

Although few data are available concerning the risk of tumor expansion during pregnancy, it has been estimated that tumor enlargement occurs in less than 1 percent of patients with microadenomas and in 5 to 20 percent with macroadenomas.[8] Such enlargement appears to be associated with the pregnancy itself rather than with the mode of induction; i.e., expansion may occur in women who conceive spontaneously as well as in those who have been treated with clomiphene, the gonadotropins, or bromocriptine. Treatment of tumor enlargement during pregnancy may take one of several forms. Therapeutic abortion and premature delivery have been uniformly successful in reducing tumor expansion but may be neither applicable nor acceptable in a given situation. Trans-sphenoidal surgery has been utilized but carries the associated concerns of any surgical procedure performed during pregnancy. High-dose steroids have been successfully employed and may, in addition to their primary effects on the pituitary tumor, reduce the problems encountered with the fetal respiratory distress syndrome. Bromocriptine has been administered to a limited number of women during pregnancy with favorable results: further tumor expansion is prevented and tumor size reduced. Although the number of offspring born to women treated during pregnancy with bromocriptine is small, no fetal abnormalities have been detected thus far. Thus when considering alternatives, treatment with bromocriptine during pregnancy when tumor expansion has occurred may be the most rational approach.

Bromocriptine and Acromegaly

Under normal circumstances the pituitary growth hormone (GH)–secreting somatotrope is under both stimulatory and inhibitory hypothalamic control by growth hormone releasing hormone (GRH) and by growth hormone release inhibiting hormone (somatostatin), respectively. When excessive GH is secreted by a pituitary adenoma or, much more rarely, by hyperplastic somatotropes, the syndrome of acromegaly occurs. Although symptoms such as thickening of soft tissues, coarsening of the features, excessive sweating, paresthesias, and arthralgias are important, the major concern is that acromegaly is associated with reduced life expectancy: premature death results from cardiovascular and cerebrovascular disease and respiratory dysfunction. Thus it is imperative that every effort be made to bring about normalization of circulating GH levels.

Acromegaly has classically been treated by ablative surgery or radiotherapy. If cure is defined as the reduction of basal GH to values to less than 10 ng/ml, conventional[4] and heavy particle[11] radiotherapy are successful in 60 to 81 percent and 50 to 82 percent of the cases, respectively. Such therapy, however, may take years to reach its maximum effectiveness and is sometimes associated with hypopituitarism. Trans-sphenoidal surgical excision of a well-defined somatotrope adenoma is safe, is not associated with significant postoperative complications, and is effective: 44 to 92 percent of patients are cured by such surgery.[12,27] The authors' position, therefore, is that surgery should be the primary mode of therapy for acromegaly resulting from a somatotrope adenoma.

Defining "cure" as above may, however, not be entirely justifiable. It has been argued that normalization of circulating somatomedin C levels and suppression by glucose of GH to less than 2 ng/ml may reflect the normal situation and thus be more accurate criteria for defining cure. A number of acromegalic patients do not achieve these goals postoperatively and thus are candidates for further treatment. In this situation, bromocriptine may be quite useful.

The role of dopamine in the regulation of GH secretion is not well understood. Clearly, dopamine receptors are present on both normal and adenomatous somatotropes. In the normal subject, dopamine and its agonists stimulate GH release; the mechanism accounting for this stimulation remains unclear, however, and it may well occur at the hypothalamic level. In acromegaly, GH secretion is inhibited by dopaminergic agents. This paradoxical observation has promoted clinical investigation, which in turn has led to the development of medical therapy for acromegaly. Bromocriptine, like dopamine, stimulates GH secretion in normal subjects but inhibits release of the hormone in acromegalic patients. Unlike its effects in hyperprolactinemia, bromocriptine rarely normalizes serum GH when used as primary treatment for acromegaly.[28] Thus, except in the unusual patient in whom surgery and irradiation are not viable forms of treatment, medical therapy should be considered adjunctive. There is, in fact, some debate as to whether bromocriptine is actually useful in the treatment of acromegaly even as a secondary mode of therapy.[13] It has, however, been the authors' experience and that of several other groups that patients who fail to be cured by surgery or who are awaiting the full effects of irradiation often benefit from bromocriptine administration.[20] Of interest is the fact that, even in those patients in whom bromocriptine does not normalize serum GH levels, significant clinical and metabolic improvement occurs.[1]

Size reduction of GH-secreting tumors following dopamine agonist therapy is much less impressive than is seen with prolactinomas, having been said to occur in only 10 percent of patients.[16] Further clinical trials are needed to address this question.

Future Prospects

At the present time, although other dopamine agonists are undergoing clinical trials, bromocriptine is the only agonist widely available in the United States. It must be noted that bromocriptine is currently recommended by the Food and Drug Administration for use only in cases of hyperprolactinemia not associated with a pituitary tumor. Until FDA approval is issued for its use in treating pituitary tumors, it is recommended that the situation be discussed with each patient on an individual basis prior to treatment; it is to be hoped that such approval will be forthcoming shortly.

Several groups have expressed concern that some patients do not tolerate the drug and hence there is a need for other agonists with fewer side effects. In the experience at our institution, acceptable suppression of prolactin and GH can be achieved with bromocriptine (2.5 mg tid for the former and qid for the latter). Although side effects, including nausea, dizziness, headaches, and postural hypotension, may occur, when the medication is begun in a gradual manner (e.g., 2.5 mg upon retiring, slowly increased over the next several days) and in a supervised setting, significant problems are unusual. Tolerance of these side effects develops quickly, and thereafter problems associated with continuation of the drug are rare.

References

1. Besser GM, Wass JAH, Thorner MO: Bromocriptine in the medical management of acromegaly, in Goldstein M, Calne DB, Lieberman A, Thorner MO (eds): *Ergot Compounds and Brain Function: Neuroendocrine and Neuropsychiatric Aspects.* New York, Raven Press, 1980, pp 191–198.
2. Carter JN, Tyson JE, Tolis G, Van Vliet S, Faiman C, Friesen HG: Prolactin-secreting tumors and hypogonadism in 22 men. N Engl J Med 299:847–852, 1978.
3. Chang RJ, Keye WR, Young JR, Wilson CB, Jaffe R: Detection, evaluation, and treatment of pituitary microadenomas in patients with galactorrhea and amenorrhea. Am J Obstet Gynecol 128:356–363, 1977.
4. Eastman RC, Gorden P, Roth J: Conventional supervoltage irradiation is an effective treatment for acromegaly. J Clin Endocrinol Metab 48:931–940, 1979.
5. Faglia G, Moriondo P, Beck-Peccoz P, Travaglini P, Ambrosi B, Spada A, Nissim M: Use of neuroactive drugs and hypothalamic regulatory hormones in the diagnosis of hyperprolactinemic states, in Müller EE: *Neuroactive Drugs in Endocrinology.* Amsterdam, Elsevier, 1980, pp 263–278.
6. Franks S, Jacobs HS, Hull MGR, Steele SJ, Nabarro JDN: Management of hyperprolactinemic amenorrhea. Br J Obstet Gynecol 84:241–253, 1977.
7. Flückiger E, Wagner HR: 2-Br-α-ergokryptin: Beeinflussung von Fertilität und Laktation bei der Ratte. Experientia 24:1130–1131, 1968.
8. Gemzell C, Wang CF: Outcome of pregnancy in women with pituitary adenoma. Fertil Steril 31:363–372, 1979.
9. Gomez F, Reyes FI, Faiman C: Nonpuerperal galactorrhea and hyperprolactinemia: Clinical findings, endocrine features and therapeutic responses in 56 cases. Am J Med 62:648–660, 1977.
10. Hardy J: Le prolactinome prolactinoma. Neurochirugie 27 (Suppl 1):1–110, 1981.
11. Lawrence JH, Tobias CA, Linfoot JA, Born JL, Chong CY: Heavy-particle therapy in acromegaly and Cushing disease. JAMA 235:2307–2310, 1976.
12. Laws ER Jr, Piepgras DG, Randall RV, Abboud CF: Neurosurgical management of acromegaly: Results in 82 patients treated between 1972 and 1977. J Neurosurg 50:454–461, 1977.
13. Lindholm J, Riishede J, Vestergaard S, Hummer L, Faber O, Hagen C: No effect of bromocriptine in acromegaly: A controlled trial. N Engl J Med 304:1450–1454, 1981.
14. MacLeod RM, Lehmeyer JE: Studies on the mechanism of the dopamine-mediated inhibition of prolactin secretion. Endocrinology 94:1077–1085, 1974.
15. McGregor AM, Scanlon MF, Hall K, Cook DB, Hall R: Reduction in size of a pituitary tumor by bromocriptine therapy. N Engl J Med 300:291–293, 1979.
16. Oppizzi G, Liuzzi A, Chiodini PG, Dallabonzana D, Spelta B, Rainer E, Horowski R: Dopaminergic treatment of large GH secreting pituitary adenomas. Presented at the 64th Annual Meeting of the Endocrine Society, 1982.
17. Post KD, Biller BJ, Adelman LS, Motlitch ME, Wolpert SM, Reichlin S: Results of selective transsphenoidal adenomectomy in women with galactorrhea-amenorrhea. JAMA 242:158–162, 1979.
18. Thorner MO: Prolactin: Clinical physiology and the significance and management of hyperprolactinemia, in Martini L, Besser GM (eds): *Clinical Neuroendocrinology.* New York, Academic, 1977, pp 319–361.
19. Thorner MO, Besser GM: Bromocriptine treatment of hyperprolactinaemic hypogonadism. Acta Endocrinol [Suppl.] (Kbh) 216:131–146, 1978.
20. Thorner MO, Besser GM, Wass JAH, Liuzzi A, Hall R, Muller EE, Chiodini PG: Bromocriptine in acromegaly. N Engl J Med 305:1092, 1981.
21. Thorner MO, Martin WH, Rogol AD, Morris JL, Perryman RL, Conway BP, Howard SS, Wolfman MG, MacLeod RM: Rapid regression of pituitary prolactinomas during bromocriptine treatment. J Clin Endocrinol Metab 51:438–445, 1980.
22. Thorner MO, Perryman RL, Rogol AD, Conway BP, MacLeod RM, Login IS, Morris JL: Rapid changes of prolactinoma volume after withdrawal and reinstitution of bromocriptine. J Clin Endocrinol Metab 53:480–483, 1981.
23. Tindall GT, Kovacs K, Horvath E, Thorner MO: Human prolactin-producing adenomas and bromocriptine: A histological, immunocytochemical, ultrastructural, and morphometric study. J Clin Endocrinol Metab 55:1178–1183, 1982.
24. Tindall GT, McLanahan CS, Christy JH: Transsphenoidal microsurgery for pituitary tumors associated with hyperprolactinemia. J Neurosurg 48:849–860, 1978.
25. Tucker H St G, Grubb SR, Wigand JP, Taylon A, Lankford HV, Blackard WB, Becker DP: Galactorrhea-amenorrhea syndrome: Follow-up of forty-five patients after pituitary tumor removal. Ann Intern Med 94:302–307, 1981.
26. Turkalj I, Braun P, Krupp P: Surveillance of bromocriptine in pregnancy. JAMA 247:1589–1591, 1982.
27. U HS, Wilson CB, Tyrrell JB: Transsphenoidal microhypophysectomy in acromegaly. J Neurosurg 47:840–852, 1977.
28. Wass JAH, Thorner MO, Morris DV, Rees LH, Mason AS, Jones AE, Besser GM: Long-term treatment of acromegaly with bromocriptine. Br Med J 1:875–878, 1977.
29. Woosley RE, King JS, Talbert L: Prolactin-secreting pituitary adenomas: Neurosurgical management of 39 patients. Fertil Steril 37:54–60, 1982.

101
Pituitary Apoplexy
Richard L. Rovit

Acute hemorrhagic necrosis of a pituitary adenoma in a young patient with acromegaly was first documented as a pathological entity by Bleibtreu in 1905.[2] The clinical syndrome associated with massive infarction, necrosis, and hemorrhage of a pituitary tumor received little attention until the report of Brougham et al. in 1950,[3] which described five postmortem cases of acute degenerative changes in pituitary adenomas, together with the pertinent clinical data, and called the clinical-pathological entity *pituitary apoplexy*. The authors suggested that the apoplectiform event was the culmination of the outstripping of its blood supply by a rapidly growing adenoma.

There are now hundreds of case reports of pituitary apoplexy in the literature, and these have provided useful data on the incidence, predisposing factors, pathological findings, putative pathophysiological mechanisms, clinical features, radiological concomitants, and treatment of this fascinating condition.

The term *pituitary apoplexy* represents a form of medical shorthand describing a complex series of clinical events occurring as a consequence of the fulminant expansion of a pituitary tumor by infarction, hemorrhage, or hemorrhagic infarction of the tumor and the adjacent pituitary tissue. It should be recognized that the pathological process may be relatively circumscribed, producing a sudden, albeit restricted, increase in the volume of the tumor. Under these circumstances the accompanying clinical symptoms may be minimal (e.g., a transient episode of headache or diplopia) or may even be absent. On the other hand, a massive hemorrhagic infarction of a large pituitary tumor may present as an acute medical catastrophe.

Incidence

Cysts, many containing old or recent hemorrhages, within pituitary tumors examined pathologically are relatively common. In Henderson's review of Cushing's series of 338 pituitary tumors,[10] 17 percent of 260 chromophobe adenomas and 6 percent of 67 eosinophilic adenomas were largely cystic. Lopez, in 1970, collected cases of pituitary tumor from the literature and estimated that there were 135 instances of

pituitary apoplexy, an incidence of about 6 percent.[12] Wakai et al., in 1981, reviewing their own series of 560 verified pituitary tumors, found the incidence of pituitary apoplexy to be unexpectedly high, 93 cases (16.6 percent);[25] a major attack was documented in 6.8 percent of cases, a minor attack in 2.3 percent and asymptomatic hemorrhages in 7.5 percent of proven cases. Müller-Jensen and Lüdecke reported an incidence of extended cystic necrotic areas, frequently containing a hemorrhagic component, in 72 cases (12.3 percent) of 586 pituitary tumors operated on by the transnasal route.[16] In only 10 instances (1.7 percent of the entire series) had the hemorrhagic area ruptured through the tumor capsule into the chiasmatic cistern, producing meningeal irritation. These authors postulated that the incidence of pituitary apoplexy was highest in hormonally inactive adenomas, although they included prolactinomas within this category. Other authors have suggested that patients harboring endocrinologically active adenomas (e.g., those associated with acromegaly and Cushing's disease) are at increased risk for the development of pituitary apoplexy.[19]

Predisposing Factors

In most instances the syndrome of pituitary apoplexy occurs *de novo* without the occurrence of an identifiable precipitating factor. In many patients the apoplectiform attack may represent the first definitive indication that either a pituitary tumor or an endocrinopathy is present. Mohanty et al. have suggested that the incidence of intratumoral hemorrhage is directly related to the size and vascularity of the pituitary tumor.[14] This correlation has not been corroborated in other series.

On the other hand, a variety of potential insults have been associated with documented instances of pituitary apoplexy. The common denominator is the pre-existence of naturally occurring conditions, artificial agents, or manipulations that can result in rapid tumor expansion, usually accompanied by ischemia or hemorrhage. Instances of pituitary apoplexy have been associated with pregnancy, endocrinologic manipulations such as estrogen administration,[5] bromocriptine medication,[13,25] head injury,[12] chronic coughing and sneezing,[6] anticoagulant drugs,[20] cerebral angiography,[22] and radiation therapy of a pituitary tumor.[23,27]

Symptoms and Signs

There are many reports of surgically verified but clinically asymptomatic cases of pituitary apoplexy.[15,25] In these instances obvious hemorrhage, relatively acute or chronic, or the residua of old hemorrhage and/or infarction (cysts containing xanthrochromic fluid, empty sella, etc.) are found at operation, yet the patient cannot recall any clinical event to match up with the pathological data.

The symptoms and corresponding signs are consistent with precipitous enlargement of and/or hemorrhage within the pituitary tumor. Sudden headache, nausea, vomiting, diplopia, and visual impairment are all concomitants of rapid expansion of a tumor, first laterally, with compression of the cranial nerves within one or both cavernous sinuses, then by superior extension of the tumor, with compression of the visual apparatus. Paresis of the oculomotor nerve followed by abducens weakness and in some instances trigeminal impairment and proptosis are the signs of cavernous sinus compression. These may occur unilaterally or bilaterally. Compression of the visual apparatus by suprasellar tumor expansion results in diminished visual acuity on one or both sides, progressing occasionally to blindness. Scotomas and/or field defects are dependent on direct pressure on or ischemia of the optic nerves, chiasm, or rarely, the optic tracts. In some series,[20] ophthalmoplegias were the major sign of visual system impairment, while in others loss of vision predominated.[25]

Other symptoms of an abrupt and potentially catastrophic intracranial ictus, possibly secondary to acutely increased intracranial pressure and/or hypothalamic involvement, are lethargy, stupor, and coma. Meningeal irritation with neck stiffness and photophobia, accompanied by bloody CSF, occurs when an acute hemorrhage within a pituitary tumor breaks through the tumor capsule into the neighboring chiasmatic cistern.

Signs and symptoms of a pre-existing endocrinopathy may be present: acromegaly, Cushing's syndrome, or the amenorrhea-galactorrhea syndrome of a prolactinoma. On the other hand the particular tumor presenting as a neurological catastrophe may be a non-functioning adenoma which has produced pressure on normal pituitary tissue and resulted in hypopituitarism. Occasionally, acute but restricted necrosis of a functioning adenoma may have a salutary effect on a pre-existing endocrinopathy, resulting in improvement of pituitary hormone hypersecretion with or without the development of hypopituitarism.[4,8,11] In many instances the apoplectiform insult constitutes the first conclusive evidence that a pituitary tumor is present.[20]

Possible Pathophysiological Mechanisms in Pituitary Apoplexy

It is possible for any tumor, especially at times of rapid growth, to outstrip its blood supply with resultant ischemia, necrosis, and hemorrhage—the more so if the tumor is confined within an enclosed bony or membranous space such as the sella turcica, where tumor expansion is limited by relatively unyielding structures. An additional factor which may render a pituitary tumor peculiarly vulnerable to ischemic necrosis may be its somewhat tenuous blood supply.

The anterior lobe of the pituitary gland (pars distalis) is supplied exclusively by a hypophyseal–portal system of vessels consisting of a capillary network originating from branches of the internal carotid which terminate in the neural lobe of the pituitary gland and infundibular stem.[29,30] It has been hypothesized that an expanding pituitary tumor may squeeze its way through the diaphragmatic notch, distorting and impacting the infundibular stem between the tumor and the firm, fibrous walls of the diaphragma sellae.[20] If this occurs, the afferent blood supply to the tumor and surrounding pituitary tissue may be severely compromised at the infundibulum, resulting in acute necrosis and infarction of the anterior lobe of the pituitary.

Clinical and Laboratory Diagnosis

Sudden excruciating headache, nausea, vomiting, or meningismus, accompanied by a decreased state of consciousness with visual impairment and ophthalmoplegia, suggests an acute process localized primarily at the base of the brain around the chiasmal–hypophyseal region. The differential diagnosis includes ruptured cerebral aneurysm, meningitis, mesencephalic infarction and/or hemorrhage, chiasmal apoplexy, and transtentorial uncal herniation secondary to a cerebral mass lesion. The possibility of pituitary apoplexy is not usually entertained unless the patient's previous history or general physical examination suggests the presence of a pituitary tumor.

In those patients in whom apoplexy constitutes the initial definitive indication of a pituitary disorder—a not unappreciable number—plain roentgenograms of the skull invariably provide the key diagnostic clue.[9,16] A large eroded sella turcica, thinning or erosion of the dorsum sellae, undercutting of the clinoid processes, a double floor of the sella, and occasionally a soft tissue mass projecting into the sphenoid sinus are all highly suggestive of a pituitary tumor. These radiographic changes, seen more clearly with tomographic techniques, are not specific for the apoplectiform event but are characteristic of a pituitary mass, usually an adenoma.

The next diagnostic step should be computed tomography without and with contrast enhancement, supplemented if possible with thin slices centered around the sella turcica and utilizing coronal cuts when feasible. In instances of acute hemorrhage, provided the examination is performed within a short time after the insult, a high-density, nonenhancing area should be seen, comprising a portion of a soft tissue mass within an expanded sella which often extends into the suprasellar cistern (Fig. 101-1). On occasion the hemorrhage may occupy virtually the entire tumor mass (Fig. 101-2). In instances of infarction or necrosis of a pituitary tumor, rather than acute hemorrhage, or in those cases in which the apoplectiform insult has occurred days to weeks prior to computed tomography, the mass within and above the sella may be of normal to low density surrounded by a complete or fragmented ring of contrast enhancement (Fig. 101-3). The latter is consistent with a necrotic or cystic area within a pituitary tumor, the enhancing ring being the result of increased vascularity or increased permeability. With large suprasellar masses or extreme hemorrhagic insults, hydrocephalus may be present.

Since the advent of computed tomography, the role of angiography in the diagnostic workup of patients with pituitary tumors, including those with apoplexy, has undergone substantial modification. The angiographic features of pituitary apoplexy are not dissimilar to those of pituitary tumors: displacement of vessels consistent with an expanding intrasellar tumor having a variable degree of suprasellar extension and occasionally associated with hydrocephalus. Extreme narrowing of the supraclinoid portion of the internal

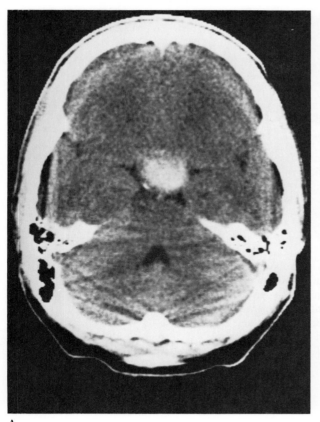
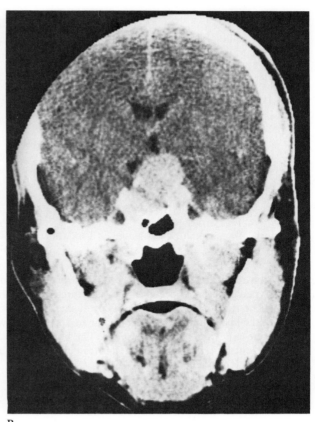

A   B

Figure 101-1   On a plain axial CT scan (*A*) and on a coronal projection with contrast enhancement (*B*), a hyperdense area occupies the sella turcica. The mass contains a large suprasellar extension effacing and displacing the chiasmatic cistern and projects inferiorly into the sphenoid sinus on the right. There is no hydrocephalus. (Courtesy of Dr. Michael Ebersold, Mayo Clinic.)

carotid artery and anterior cerebral vessels has been reported with this syndrome, a consequence both of rapid tumor expansion and sudden pressure on contiguous vessels.[20] Vasospasm secondary to blood breaking through into the basal cisterns may also contribute to the narrowed cerebral vasculature.

In general, the diagnosis of pituitary apoplexy can be established by computed tomography, with cerebral angiography utilized to rule out a ruptured or associated aneurysm, especially a giant intrasellar aneurysm.[24] Angiography may also be helpful in delineating the course and configuration of the intracavernous carotid vessels prior to trans-sphenoidal surgery. For these purposes, the use of intravenous digital computerized angiographic techniques will probably assume a dominant role in the future. Pneumoencephalography in the diagnosis of most pituitary tumors has been almost entirely superseded by computed tomography.

The correct diagnosis should be established on clinical and radiographic grounds; routine lumbar puncture is neither necessary nor advisable. Lumbar puncture may be performed when the patient presents with a sudden devastating headache, rapid deterioration of consciousness, fever, and severe meningismus. In these circumstances the possibility of meningitis must be entertained, especially in those rare

instances in which the sella turcica is normal or only slightly enlarged.[20] With pituitary apoplexy the CSF may be grossly bloody, xanthrochromic, or occasionally clear. Elevated CSF pressure and protein levels have been encountered.

Management and Treatment

The treatment of pituitary apoplexy is no different from the management of any patient with a rapidly enlarging pituitary tumor. Bleeding or infarction within a pituitary tumor invariably compromises the secretion of endogenous pituitary hormones, as well as those hypothalamic factors regulating the appropriate release of pituitary hormones. Prompt administration of corticosteroids is necessary, concomitant with rapid laboratory investigation of the patient's endocrinologic status. The latter survey requires determination of serum prolactin, growth hormone, and cortisol levels; assessment of thyroid status; and occasionally provocative tests to evaluate the functional integrity of the hypothalamic–hypophyseal axis.

Whether a patient with pituitary apoplexy should be managed solely with corticosteroids or should undergo

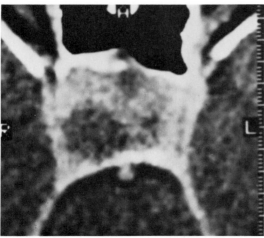
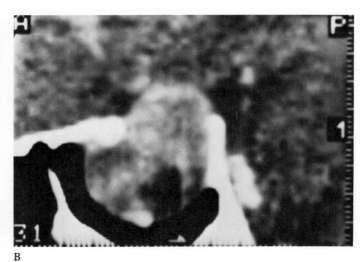

A   B

Figure 101-2 Enlarged CT scan of the region of the sella turcica in both axial (A) and sagittal reconstructed (B) views with contrast enhancement. A moderately large, mostly hyperdense, mass occupies the sella turcica and has significant suprasellar extension. The mass has displaced the floor of the sella turcica inferiorly, partially obliterating the sphenoid sinus. Several hypodense areas are within this mass and represent necrosis or resolving hemorrhage. The basilar artery and prepontine cistern are seen in their normal positions. (Courtesy of Dr. Nicholas T. Zervas, Massachusetts General Hospital.)

prompt surgical decompression depends almost exclusively on the status of and impending threat to the visual apparatus. Those patients with severe and/or rapid deterioration in visual acuity or with constricted visual fields require prompt decompression of a swollen, necrotic, or hemorrhagic pituitary tumor, usually utilizing a trans-sphenoidal approach. Corticosteroids must be given before and during surgery and in the postoperative period. The goal of the operation is to decompress the optic nerves and chiasm primarily, as well as

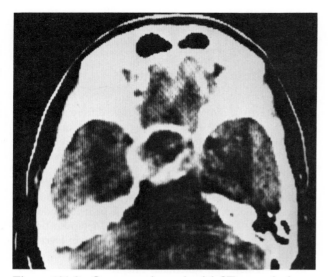

Figure 101-3 Contrast-enhanced axial CT scan. A ring of contrast enhancement surrounds a hypodense mass which occupies the sella turcica.

those lateral expansions of pituitary tumor compressing the cavernous sinuses. It may be neither necessary nor desirable to remove all the pituitary tumor, but sufficient pathological tissue must be evacuated to provide a thorough decompression of the visual apparatus. Adequate trans-sphenoidal decompression of an acutely swollen pituitary tumor will usually relieve acute hydrocephalus, the result of large or sudden suprasellar tumor extension. On occasion, supplemental ventricular drainage or shunting procedures may be required.

Prompt and adequate trans-sphenoidal decompression is usually followed by resolution of pre-existing ophthalmoplegia. Generally there is also an improvement or at least a stabilization of visual deficits, but this is dependent largely on the degree of irreversible neuropathy which existed prior to surgery. It should be emphasized that the trans-sphenoidal route for evacuation of an acutely swollen pituitary tumor is usually the surgical procedure of choice; but on occasion (e.g., where pituitary apoplexy occurs in a patient with a normal sella turcica), technical considerations might favor the transfrontal approach to the pituitary.[25]

Those patients in whom the apoplectiform attack does not pose an immediate threat either to vision or to consciousness may be followed closely and treated expectantly. Sudden, albeit restricted, pituitary hemorrhage or infarction may occur in patients with pituitary tumors more often than is generally believed.[25] In many of these cases the apoplectic event is recalled only retrospectively, e.g., when the surgeon who has removed a cystic or necrotic pituitary tumor reviews the history in detail with the patient. Sudden headache, with or without meningismus, with minimal impairment of visual acuity and fields in an alert patient who has a pituitary tumor verified by computed tomography may be treated medically with corticosteroids, at least over the short term, unless it is apparent that vision is threatened. After the apoplectiform event has been successfully managed medically, with resolution of headache and ophthalmoplegia, the long-term management of these patients is the same as that of the usual patient with a pituitary tumor. The primary treatment options, utilized singly or in combination, are medical management of any endocrinopathy, surgery with tumor removal, radiation therapy, and pharmacological manipulation (e.g., bromocriptine administration).[3,26] Since documented cases of pituitary apoplexy have developed during or after radiation treatment of a pituitary tumor, it has been suggested that this modality not be used for patients known to have had an attack of pituitary apoplexy with recovery.[23,27] No data supporting this conclusion are available, and radiation therapy of pituitary tumors has been successfully used in patients who have previously recovered from apoplexy.[20]

References

1. Berti G, Heisey WG, Dohn DF: Pituitary apoplexy treated by stereotactic transsphenoidal aspiration. Cleve Clin Q 41:163–175, 1974.
2. Bleibtreu L: Ein Fall von Akromeglia (Zerstörung der Hypophysis durch Blutung). Munch Med Wochenschr 52:2079–2080, 1905.
3. Brougham M, Heusner AP, Adams RD: Acute degenerative changes in adenomas of the pituitary body—with special reference to pituitary apoplexy. J Neurosurg 7:421–439, 1950.
4. Corkill G, Hanson FW, Sobel RA, Keller TM: Apoplexy in a prolactin microadenoma leading to remission of galactorrhea and amenorrhea. Surg Neurol 15:114–115, 1981.
5. David M, Philippon J, Bernard-Weil E: Les formes hémorragiques des adénomes hypophysaires: Aspects cliniques et étiologiques. Nouv Presse Med 77:1887–1889, 1969.
6. Dawson BH, Kothandaram P: Acute massive infarction of pituitary adenomas: A study of five patients. J Neurosurg 37:275–279, 1972.
7. Epstein S, Pimstone BL, de Villiers JC, Jackson WPU: Pituitary apoplexy in five patients with pituitary tumours. Br Med J 2:267–270, 1971.
8. Findling JW Jr, Tyrrell JB, Aron DC, Fitzgerald PA, Wilson CB, Forsham PH: Silent pituitary apoplexy: Subclinical infarction of an adrenocorticotropin-producing pituitary adenoma. J Clin Endocrinol Metab 52:95–97, 1981.
9. Fitz-Patrick D, Tolis G, McGarry EE, Taylor S: Pituitary apoplexy: The importance of skull roentgenograms and computerized tomography in diagnosis. JAMA 244:59–61, 1980.
10. Henderson WR: The pituitary adenomata: A follow-up study of the surgical results in 338 cases (Dr. Harvey Cushing's series). Br J Surg 26:811–921, 1939.
11. Jacobi JD, Fishman LM, Daroff RB: Pituitary apoplexy in acromegaly followed by partial pituitary insufficiency. Arch Intern Med 134:559–561, 1974.
12. Lopez IA: Pituitary apoplexy, J Oslo City Hosp 20:17–27, 1970.
13. McGregor AM, Scanlon MF, Hall K, Cook DB, Hall R: Reduction in size of a pituitary tumor by bromocriptine therapy. N Engl J Med 300:291–293, 1979.
14. Mohanty S, Tandon PN, Banerji AK, Prakash B: Haemorrhage into pituitary adenomas. J Neurol Neurosurg Psychiatry 40:987–991, 1977.
15. Mohr G, Hardy J: Hemorrhage, necrosis and apoplexy in pituitary adenomas. Surg Neurol 18:181–189, 1982.
16. Müller-Jensen A, Lüdecke D: Clinical aspects of spontaneous necrosis of pituitary tumors (pituitary apoplexy). J Neurol 224:267–271, 1981.
17. Post MJD, David NJ, Glaser JS, Safran A: Pituitary apoplexy: Diagnosis by computed tomography. Radiology 134:665–670, 1980.
18. Ramamurthi B, Anguli VC, Narasimhan ST: Pituitary apoplexy. Neurol India 1:60–64, 1954.
19. Rovit RL, Duane TD: Cushing's syndrome and pituitary tumors: Pathophysiology and ocular manifestations of ACTH-secreting pituitary adenomas. Am J Med 46:416–427, 1969.
20. Rovit RL, Fein JM: Pituitary apoplexy: A review and reappraisal. J Neurosurg 37:280–288, 1972.
21. Rushworth RG: Pituitary apoplexy. Med J Aust. 1:251–254, 1971.
22. Steimle R, Royer J, Oppermann A, Patard G, Jacquet G, Gehin P: Hématome post-angiographique dans un adénome de l'hypophyse: Cécité et troubles oculomoteurs régressant apres intervention d'urgence. Neurochirurgie 20:599–608, 1974.
23. Uihlein A, Balfour WM, Donovan PF: Acute hemorrhage into pituitary adenomas. J Neurosurg 14:140–151, 1957.
24. Wakai S, Fukushima T, Furihata T, Sano K: Association of cerebral aneurysm with pituitary adenoma. Surg Neurol 12:503–507, 1979.
25. Wakai S, Fukushima T, Teramoto A, Sano K: Pituitary apoplexy: Its incidence and clinical significance. J Neurosurg 55:187–193, 1981.
26. Wass JAH, Moult PJA, Thorner MO, Dacie JE, Charlesworth M, Jones AE, Besser GM: Reduction of pituitary-tumour size in patients with prolactinomas and acromegaly treated with bromocriptine with or without radiotherapy. Lancet 2:66–69, 1979.
27. Weisberg LA: Pituitary apoplexy: Association of degenerative change in pituitary adenoma with radiotherapy and detection by cerebral computed tomography. Am J Med 63:109–115, 1977.
28. Wright, RL, Ojemann RG, Drew JH: Hemorrhage into pituitary adenomata: Report of two cases with spontaneous recovery. Arch Neurol 12:326–331, 1965.
29. Xuereb GP, Prichard MML, Daniel PM: The arterial supply and venous drainage of the human hypophysis cerebri. Q J Exp Physiol 39:199–217, 1954.
30. Xuereb GP, Prichard MML, Daniel PM: The hypophysial portal system of vessels in man. Q J Exp Physiol 39:219–230, 1954.

102

Empty Sella Syndrome

Peter W. Carmel

The term *empty sella* was first applied to an anatomical finding at autopsy by Busch in 1951.[4] He found that in 40 cases of patients with no known pituitary disease, the pituitary gland was severely flattened against the floor of the sella (5.6 percent of the series); the diaphragma sellae was restricted to a thin rim of tissue around a huge infundibular foramen (Fig. 102-1). He also noted that an incomplete diaphragma might leave the pituitary gland intact but with its superior surface fully exposed and covered by arachnoid or might leave the pituitary indented and eccentrically placed within the sella. This latter condition resulted in a partially empty appearance. Busch pointed out that an empty sella was far more frequent in females than in males (34:6).

Little clinical attention was initially paid to Busch's interesting findings. Both radiologists and neurosurgeons usually regarded nontumoral sellar enlargement as reflecting pressure due to intrasellar arachnoidal cysts. However, Kaufman, in 1968, demonstrated that the "empty" sella was a manifestation of an enlarged intrasellar subarachnoid space.[14] He noted that when the diaphragma sellae was incomplete or incompetent the subarachnoid space could expand, thus enlarging, deepening, and reshaping the sella.

The term *empty sella syndrome* appeared in two articles published in 1968. One of these papers applied the term to a patient with an enlarged sella that filled with air on pneumoencephalography, who had no known or demonstrable pituitary lesion.[12] The other used the term for patients who had undergone prior surgery or radiation for proven pituitary tumors and who were later investigated for possible tumor recurrence when visual symptoms returned.[15] An air study showed no tumor and an empty sella in each case. Current usage is to call cases of sellar enlargement which are not related to a previously treated pituitary tumor *primary empty sella syndrome*, whereas those found following treatment of a pituitary tumor are denoted by *secondary empty sella syndrome*.

Clinical Presentation

Clinical studies of patients with primary empty sella syndrome have revealed a variety of associated problems, and it seems likely that several etiologic factors are involved in producing an empty sella. Despite this diversity, patients with primary empty sella syndrome are a surprisingly homogeneous group. Over 80 percent of these patients are women, more than 75 percent are obese, and the majority become symptomatic in the decade from age 40 to 49, with over 80 percent presenting between 30 and 59 years of age.[22] An intrasellar problem is seldom suspected when the diagnostic studies are started.

Initial complaints fall into three categories; neurological, endocrinologic and systemic. Headache is the most common presenting symptom, occurring in 50 to 80 percent of these patients. Other neurological complaints include memory loss, balance impairment, dizziness, seizures, rhinorrhea, papilledema, and, rarely, decreased visual acuity or visual field loss. Endocrine complaints leading to investigation include amenorrhea, galactorrhea, loss of libido, and diabetes. Systemic complaints such as obesity or hypertension lead to radiological studies, initially by skull films in almost all cases, and sellar abnormalities are revealed.

Radiological Diagnosis

Plain skull film or polytome measurements of the sella turcica should normally not exceed a length of 17 mm and a depth of 13 mm.[21] Di Chiro and Nelson have stated that the normal volume of the sella should not exceed 1092 mm^3.[5] In most patients with empty sellas, these measurements are greatly exceeded, and in a recent series of 20 patients the mean sellar volume was 2770 mm^3.[7] However, volume measurements within normal limits do not rule out an empty sella, and sellar depth measurements greater than the anteroposterior diameter call for further investigation.

Plain roentgenographic changes typically include symmetrical ballooning of the sella, which still maintains a "closed" configuration (Fig. 102-2). Although the floor may be considerably thinned, the clinoids are usually not attenuated. In the anteroposterior view, the sellar floor is symmetrical, in both position and bone thickness.

The definitive radiological procedure for diagnosis of the empty sella has been the demonstration of air within the sella during pneumoencephalography. Air rarely fills the entire sella, and the proportion of intrasellar herniation is often expressed as a percentage of the lateral sellar area or as the extension below the diaphragmatic line (Fig. 102-3). It may be technically difficult to fill the sella with air, even when the sella is empty. Considerable maneuvering of the patient, with frequent injections of aliquots of air, is often necessary to demonstrate the empty sella. This procedure is associated with a high degree of discomfort in most patients. Suprasellar structures, including the optic chiasm, may be forced downward into the empty sella, preventing the entrance of air.

Computed tomographic scanning may be helpful in diagnosing an empty sella (Fig. 102-4). Advanced generation machines and coronal sections are often useful. To demonstrate that fluid density within the sella is an extension of the subarachnoid space, many neuroradiologists currently employ metrizamide cisternography.[23] Metrizamide is a nonionic water-soluble compound. Its increased specific gravity

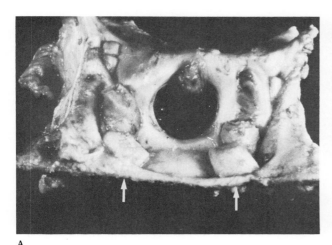

A   B

Figure 102-1 *A.* Sella turcica of a patient with an empty sella, viewed from above. In this autopsy specimen the sella has been removed en bloc. The diaphragma sellae is seen as a thin rim of tissue around a large infundibular foramen. The pituitary stalk may be identified at the posterior portion of the sella. The optic nerves are seen anteriorly (*arrows*). *B.* Coronal view of the sella turcica, sectioned in a midsellar plane. The stalk and posterior pituitary are compressed posteriorly against the wall of the sella. The anterior pituitary is severely compressed downward and is reduced to a thin rim of tissue at the base of the sella (*arrow*). Lines indicate the level of the diaphragma sellae, and the large foramen is apparent.

compared with that of CSF allows gravitational manipulation within the subarachnoid space. This manipulative capacity is limited by the fairly rapid dilution of metrizamide by CSF. The intrathecal dose of metrizamide for cisternography is usually much less than that required for myelography. Patients tolerate this dosage level well, and the complications and discomfort are less than with pneumoencephalography. Contrast enhancement with metrizamide is used to delineate the subarachnoid cisterns on plain films, on planar tomograms, or in conjunction with CT scanning.

Endocrine Studies

Clinical endocrine dysfunction is rare in patients with empty sella syndrome;[7,17] however, significantly altered pituitary function tests are noted in up to 30 percent of these patients.[17] The most commonly observed abnormality has been deficient growth hormone (GH) secretion during stimulation tests. In some of these patients an impaired GH response to glucagon may be attributed to associated obesity. Abnormalities of secretion of ACTH, LH, and TSH have also been reported in association with an empty sella.[7]

Hyperprolactinemia or intermittent increases in prolactin (PRL) levels have both been associated with the primary empty sella.[3] The degree of hyperprolactinemia found in empty sella syndrome is usually moderate; PRL values are more elevated with prolactinomas. In some series, as many as 25 percent of women with an empty sella have elevated serum prolactin levels. Patients with empty sellas have a normal PRL rise when stimulated with thyroid-releasing hormone (TRH), while patients with prolactinomas do not.

Finally, the normal nocturnal peak PRL release is preserved with primary empty sella syndrome but is blunted with prolactinoma.[16]

Radiological demonstration of an empty sella does not preclude the presence of a pituitary tumor. Functional pituitary tumors in "empty" sellas have been reported in acromegaly, Cushing's disease, and prolactinemia. In fact, intrasellar arachnoid herniation appears to be more common with coexistent pituitary tumors than in the normal population. Intrasellar CSF extension has been observed in 14 percent of patients with acromegaly and in 17 percent of patients with prolactin-secreting tumors.[6] This finding sug-

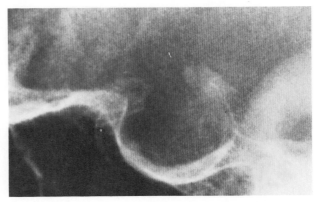

Figure 102-2 Lateral skull film of a woman with an empty sella. The sella is ballooned and its volume greatly increased, while the "closed" configuration of the sella is maintained. The floor is eroded and thinned, but the clinoids are not undercut or attenuated.

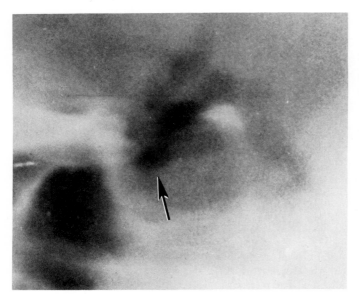

Figure 102-3 Pneumoencephalogram (lateral view) of a patient with a partially empty sella. Air fills only the most rostral portion of the sella (*arrow*). This 30-year-old obese woman was studied because of headaches and visual field loss. The optic chiasm is in a slightly more inferior position than usual and seems to be pushed toward the empty sella. However, the patient was not operated on, and her headaches spontaneously improved and field deficits cleared.

gests that infarction of a pre-existing pituitary tumor may be important in the pathogenesis of the empty sella in these patients.

Normal pituitary function may persist despite extensive

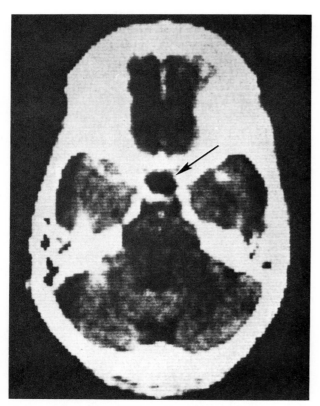

Figure 102-4 Axial unenhanced CT scan of patient with empty sella. The large volume of the sella may be appreciated (*arrow*). This is the same patient as in Figure 102-3; the scan was obtained when her headaches returned 5 years after the initial investigation.

arachnoidal herniation with severe compression and flattening of the pituitary gland. However, cases of nontumoral hyperprolactinemia and of diabetes insipidus seen with primary empty sella syndrome suggest disruption of normal hypothalamic-pituitary pathways. It is possible that the arachnoidal herniation compresses the pituitary stalk at the rim of the diaphragma or upper portion of the bony sella.[7] A similar mechanism has been proposed for certain visual problems associated with the empty sella.

Pathogenesis

The primary empty sella is evidently a heterogeneous and multicausal syndrome, arising from several different pathogenetic processes. Three of the factors to be considered in the formation of the primary empty sella are pituitary cysts, arachnoidal cysts, and increased intracranial pressure.

Busch, in his early description of the empty sella, noted an unusually high incidence of cysts of the pars intermedia of the pituitary gland, usually microscopic in size, in females.[4] He postulated that these small cysts might become confluent and rupture superiorly into the subarachnoid space. A deficient diaphragma sellae was needed to permit this rupture and thus create an "empty sella." This mechanism must be distinguished from the rare intrasellar epithelial cysts described by Fager and Carter.[8] These epithelial cysts apparently arise from Rathke's pouch and are true mass lessions that may cause sellar destruction and optic nerve compression. They are not in free communication with the subarachnoid space.

Arachnoid cysts, either congenital or acquired, may extend from the suprasellar region downward into the sella if there is an incompetent diaphragma sellae. Friedmann and Marguth described eight arachnoid cysts that had been operated on[11] and suggested that with basal arachnoiditis a collateral pathway for the cerebrospinal fluid may result in sellar enlargement.

A primary empty sella has been encountered with several conditions that cause increased intracranial pressure, and this is an important pathogenetic factor in some patients.[10] Benign increased intracranial pressure (pseudotumor cerebri) also disproportionately affects obese females, and the similarity of this group of patients to those with empty sella probably reflects the causality of increased pressure. In addition, intracranial pressure rises with systemic hypertension, and it has been suggested that severe hypertension may give rise to intermittent increases of intracranial pressure and thus to the empty sella.[14]

Various other intracranial conditions that elevate cerebrospinal fluid pressure have been associated with the empty sella syndrome, including hydrocephalus, brain tumors, and the Arnold-Chiari malformation.[1] Recent studies by Brismar and Bergstrand,[2] using CT scanning, pneumoencephalography, and cisternography with isotope or metrizamide, have demonstrated impaired CSF circulation in the majority (>80 percent) of patients with a primary empty sella. They pointed out the "obvious similarity" between the symptoms presented by these patients and those with normal pressure hydrocephalus, including headache, moderate dementia, balance disturbances, and psychiatric symptoms. One of their patients benefited from a shunting procedure, and four others had temporary help from lumbar punctures.

CSF Rhinorrhea

In 1968, Ommaya et al. reported two cases of CSF rhinorrhea associated with the empty sella syndrome,[18] pointing out the relation between elevation of CSF pressure and eventual rhinorrhea. They suggested that increased intracranial pressure might force open an anatomical defect not previously apparent, and thought that CSF leaks from the sella might result from persistence of the craniopharyngeal canal. Elevation of CSF pressure, combined with pulsations of the intrasellar arachnoid diverticulum, are likely causes of progressive sellar erosion and leakage.[14]

Accurate figures on the incidence of CSF leakage in patients with primary empty sella syndrome are not readily available. Relatively few cases of trans-sellar leakage have been reported, in view of the high incidence of empty sellas in autopsy material. Weisberg et al. had two patients with rhinorrhea in their group of 25 empty sellas.[22] In cases of nontraumatic CSF rhinorrhea, the sella is a far less frequent site of leakage than the cribriform plate.[19]

Establishing the correct site of CSF rhinorrhea is of prime importance, and identification of an arachnoidal intrasellar herniation alone is not diagnostic; rather, it is necessary to demonstrate the actual site of leakage. Many elaborate schemes employing isotopic localization have been described, but it is likely that the use of a water-soluble contrast medium (metrizamide) injected intrathecally will replace these earlier methods. Metrizamide may be used in conjunction with polytomography or with high-resolution computed tomography.

Several of the above points are illustrated by the following case report.

The 62-year-old patient was a hypertensive, obese woman who was admitted to the hospital because of CSF rhinorrhea of 4 weeks' duration. She had had vague vertex headaches for several years but specifically denied significant head trauma. Neurological examination showed a diminished sense of smell, greater on the right side.

Skull films revealed an enlarged sella, with thinning of the bone of the sellar floor but not of the clinoids (Fig. 102-2). Hypocycloidal polytomograms of both the sella and cribriform plate regions failed to reveal a fracture or other discontinuity of bone. Study with intrathecal metrizamide enhancement showed an empty sella (Fig. 102-5). However, there was no evidence of penetration of metrizamide through the sellar floor, nor was there any collection in the sphenoid sinus. Polytomograms of the cribriform plate were repeated, and metrizamide was seen draining through a hole in the cribriform plate and collecting in the right ethmoid sinus (Fig. 102-6).

At operation a funnel-shaped hole in the dura and bone at the medial border of the right olfactory bulb was readily identified. It was closed with muscle and acrylic, and a pericranial graft was sutured above the repair. The patient has had no further leakage for 5 years.

Surgical Treatment

Surgery is not indicated for the great majority of patients with empty sella syndrome. The initial complaints of some of these patients are related to hypertension or obesity and require only medical treatment. The endocrinopathy associ-

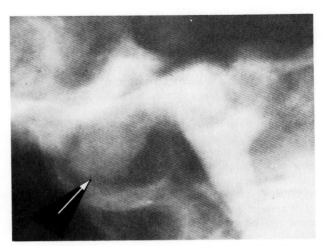

Figure 102-5 Lateral x-ray view of the sella after cisternal injection of metrizamide (same patient as in Fig. 102-2). The contrast fills the greater part of the sella (*arrow*), while the pituitary gland is shown to be compressed posteriorly. Contrast material does not leak through the sellar floor, and none is seen in the sphenoid sinus beneath the sella.

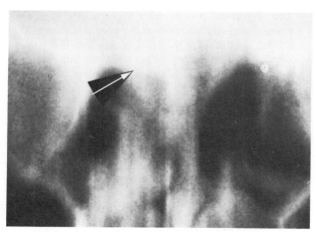

Figure 102-6 Coronal polytomographic view of the cribriform region (same patient as in Figs. 102-2 and 102-5). Contrast material leaks through the right cribriform plate (*arrow*) and fills much of the right ethmoid sinus. At operation, a funnel-shaped defect of dura and bone was found at this location.

ated with primary empty sella syndrome is usually slight and rarely requires replacement therapy.

Benign intracranial hypertension (pseudotumor cerebri) is usually a self-limited process and is treated by nonsurgical methods. An occasional patient may require a shunting procedure employing lumboperitoneal diversion to control papilledema or debilitating headache; subtemporal decompression has also been advocated in the past for relief of optic nerve pressure. Patients who have communicating hydrocephalus with elevated CSF pressures and an empty sella should be treated by shunting without undue delay. When hydrocephalus is caused by a tumor or an Arnold-Chiari malformation, surgical correction of the underlying pathological lesion is indicated.

CSF rhinorrhea via an empty sella requires surgical intervention. Like other nontraumatic CSF leakage, this type of rhinorrhea seldom stops spontaneously. The first step in diagnosis is to determine whether a high pressure or normal pressure mechanism underlies the rhinorrhea. When the pressure is elevated by a tumor, diagnosis and surgical therapy is primarily directed at tumor diagnosis and removal. However, it is not enough to correct the cause; usually the leak must be repaired as well. When the leakage is due to hydrocephalus, shunting procedures may lead to development of tension pneumocephalus.[13] Trans-sphenoidal repair, followed shortly by a shunting procedure, may serve to avoid this problem.

When the intracranial pressure is normal, several treatment methods are available. Continuous external lumbar subarachnoid drainage of CSF has been successfully employed to treat both postoperative and post-traumatic CSF fistulas.[9] However, in both the postoperative and post-traumatic situations some repair of the fistula might be expected during the healing process. There is little information on the use of external drainage for spontaneous fistulae, but one would expect it to be less effective than in other types of leakage. Continuous drainage is not without risk

and may result in pneumocephalus. Several methods have been proposed to minimize this problem, including flow-regulated drainage.[20]

References

1. Brismar K, Bajraktari X, Goulatia R, Efendić S: The empty sella syndrome—intrasellar cisternal herniation—in "normal" patients and in patients with communicating hydrocephalus and intracranial tumors. Neuroradiology 17:35–43, 1978.
2. Brismar K, Bergstrand G: CSF circulation in subjects with empty sella syndrome. Neuroradiology 21:167–175, 1981.
3. Brismar K, Efendić S: Pituitary function in the empty sella syndrome. Neuroendocrinology 32:70–77, 1981.
4. Busch W: Die Morphologie des Sella turcica und ihre Beziehungen zur Hypophyse. Virchows Arch [Pathol Anat] 320:437–458, 1951.
5. Di Chiro G, Nelson KB: The volume of the sella turcica. AJR 87:989–1008, 1962.
6. Dominque JN, Wing SD, Wilson CB: Coexisting pituitary adenomas and partially empty sellas. J Neurosurg 48:23–28, 1978.
7. Ekblom M, Ketonen L, Kuuliala I, Pelkonen R: Pituitary function in patients with enlarged sella turcica and primary empty sella syndrome. Acta Med Scand 209:31–35, 1981.
8. Fager CA, Carter H: Intrasellar epithelial cysts. J Neurosurg 24:77–81, 1966.
9. Findler G, Sahar A, Beller AJ: Continuous lumbar drainage of cerebrospinal fluid in neurosurgical patients. Surg Neurol 8:455–457, 1977.
10. Foley KM, Posner JB: Does pseudotumor cerebri cause the empty sella syndrome? Neurology 25:565–569, 1975.
11. Friedmann G, Marguth F: Intraselläre Liquorzysten. Zentralbl Neurochir 21:33–41, 1961.
12. Gabriele OF: The empty sella syndrome. AJR 104:168–170, 1968.
13. Ikeda K, Nakano M, Tani E: Tension pneumocephalus complicating ventriculoperitoneal shunt for cerebrospinal fluid rhinorrhea: Case report. J Neurol Neurosurg Psychiatry 41:319–322, 1978.
14. Kaufman B: The "empty" sella turcica—a manifestation of the intrasellar subarachnoid space. Radiology 90:931–941, 1968.
15. Lee WM, Adams JE: The empty sella syndrome. J Neurosurg 28:351–356, 1968.
16. Malarkey WB, Goodenow TJ, Lanese RR: Diurnal variation of prolactin secretion differentiates pituitary tumors from the primary empty sella syndrome. Am J Med 69:886–890, 1980.
17. Neelon FA, Goree JA, Lebovitz HE: The primary empty sella: Clinical and radiographic characteristics and endocrine function. Medicine (Baltimore) 52:73–92, 1973.
18. Ommaya AK, Di Chiro G, Baldwin M, Pennybacker JB: Nontraumatic cerebrospinal fluid rhinorrhea. J Neurol Neurosurg Psychiatry 31:214–225, 1968.
19. Shugar JMA, Som PM, Eisman W, Biller HF: Non-traumatic cerebrospinal fluid rhinorrhea. Laryngoscope 91:114–120, 1981.
20. Swanson SE, Kocan MJ, Chandler WF: Flow-regulated continuous spinal drainage: Technical note with case report. Neurosurgery 9:163–165, 1981.
21. Taveras JM, Wood EH: *Diagnostic Neuroradiology*. Baltimore, Williams & Wilkins, 1964.
22. Weisberg LA, Zimmerman EA, Frantz AG: Diagnosis and evaluation of patients with an enlarged sella turcica. Am J Med 61:590–596, 1976.
23. Zull DN, Falko JM: Metrizamide cisternography in the investigation of the empty sella syndrome. Arch Intern Med 141:487–489, 1981.

103

Trans-sphenoidal Approach to the Pituitary Gland

J. Hardy

Historical Review

Historically, the first successful removal of a pituitary tumor was performed by Schloffer in 1907, using an extracranial trans-sphenoidal approach through a superolateral nasoethmoidal route. Although Hirsch from Vienna pioneered in 1909 an inferolateral endonasal approach, Harvey Cushing ingeniously introduced a new method in 1910 combining the advantages of previous technical modalities and deserves the credit for having standardized an oronasal midline rhinoseptal trans-sphenoidal approach.[14,16] He routinely used this method during a 20-year period in over 247 cases of pituitary tumor, remaining faithful to an early statement that "the important factor seems to me a direct extracranial midline approach by the shortest possible route."[1]

Nevertheless, by 1929, Cushing began using the intracranial transfrontal operation which was initially described by Frazier, who performed the first such operation in 1912. The reason for changing from the trans-sphenoidal to the intracranial operation was not the operative results but rather a consideration of the indications. The occasional discovery of other kinds of lesions about the sella turcica, such as a meningioma or a craniopharyngioma, was so much emphasized that, noted Henderson: "The intracranial approach was eventually used . . . for nearly all pituitary tumors irrespective of whether the growth of the tumor was chiefly upwards or downwards as well (with a large sella)."[12] Another reason was the higher incidence of recurrence with the trans-sphenoidal operation because of incomplete tumor removal; with this method "in the average favorable case probably one third or even two thirds of the tumor was removed," wrote Cushing.

Norman Dott from Edinburgh remained faithful to Cushing's approach and used the trans-sphenoidal operation throughout his career in over 120 cases. Guiot of Paris learned the procedure from Dott and deserves the credit for reviving and popularizing the method in Europe by the early 1960's.[2] Until then, the indications for surgical treatment remained the classic criteria which had been used over the previous forty years, chiefly the presence of visual disturbance secondary to a large pituitary adenoma with suprasellar

expansion. The procedure was a massive debulking of the tumor in order to relieve pressure on the optic nerves, which indeed was successful in the majority of cases; the alternatives were subtotal removal of the tumor followed by radiation therapy, or total sellar cleanout, or nonselective tumor removal. The attempt to perform a complete radical excision of the tumor did not permit distinction between normal and pathological tissues; both were excised, resulting in panhypopituitarism, which required total pituitary hormonal substitution therapy.

In 1962, Hardy of Montreal, returning from Paris where he had learned the trans-sphenoidal approach from Guiot, reintroduced the procedure in North America.[3] He provided further advancement in technique by introducing the combined use of televised radiofluoroscopic control, optical magnification with the surgical microscope, and microsurgical techniques of dissection.[4] He demonstrated the possibility of achieving complete tumor removal (including the suprasellar extension) by direct television monitoring of the fluoroscopic control during surgery and by observing the refilling of the chiasmatic cistern with air after tumor removal. A direct magnified view with excellent illumination of the operative field overcame the major criticism in the past that the trans-sphenoidal approach was a blind procedure. The main advantage was to assure complete tumor removal in the majority of the cases, thus avoiding postoperative radiotherapy.[5] Striking progress in microsurgery made it possible to clearly distinguish between normal and pathological tissues, thus opening the field of histological functional microsurgery. Selective microsurgical adenomectomy with preservation of the normal gland became possible, so that the pituitary function could be preserved or even restored without hormonal substitution therapy.[6] Hardy first reported the possibility of recognizing intrapituitary lesions measuring a few millimeters in diameter, which he called *microadenomas*. The concept of selective microadenomectomy has contributed to better understanding of the pathophysiology of hypersecretory pituitary disorders and of the causes of tumor formation and has cast new light on the therapeutic approach to pituitary endocrine disorders.[7-11] Current refinements in technique have clarified the indications for the intracranial versus the trans-sphenoidal approach to sellar lesions.[13,15,17]

Indications

Basically, there are two major clinical endocrinologic pituitary syndromes. The first involves hyposecretion secondary to a pituitary tumor: Progressive loss of pituitary hormone secretions secondary to compression of the gland by a nonfunctional tumor may result in panhypopituitarism, requiring lifelong multihormonal substitution therapy. Surgical decompression of the gland interrupts this process and may even favor restoration of function. Most often, this hyposecretion syndrome is found in association with a large intrasellar mass—a nonsecreting cystic or oncocytic pituitary adenoma, a Rathke's pouch cyst, or a craniopharyngioma; occasional meningiomas, germinomas, and epidermoid tumors are also found in the sella. Further tumor growth may even encroach upon the adjacent optic pathways and cranial nerves. The accurate final diagnosis can only be reached by exploratory biopsy, for which the trans-sphenoidal approach is the least traumatic and most convenient method. The incidental radiological finding of a nonfunctional tumor in the sella without endocrinologic or visual disturbance does not require immediate surgical treatment. Progressive impairment of function, however, may render surgery mandatory.

The second major pituitary syndrome is the hypersecreting pituitary adenoma, which has now emerged as the most frequent tumor of the pituitary.[8] It gives rise to well-known clinical pictures such as galactorrhea-amenorrhea and infertility in the female and sexual impotence and loss of libido in the male secondary to a prolactin-secreting adenoma; gigantism or acromegaly; and Cushing's disease. These hypersecretory syndromes are usually isolated but occasionally are combined. They can be detected early with radioimmunoassay methods for the measurement of pituitary hormones, methods which have clearly defined the association of the clinical syndromes with specific hormones. Refinement in neuroradiological diagnostic procedures, using hypocycloidal tomography of the sella turcica and high-resolution CT scanning, now permits the detection of lesions smaller than the pituitary gland itself—those originally called *microadenomas*. In the present state of medical knowledge, a preoperative predicted pathological diagnosis is accurate in over 90 percent of cases.

According to the author's radiological classification,[11] pituitary adenomas are divided into two major groups: enclosed tumors and invasive lesions. These may be associated with suprasellar or parasellar extensions. The trans-sphenoidal approach is the recommended approach for the majority of enclosed tumors even with large suprasellar extension, provided the tumor extends symmetrically in the midline above the sella turcica. Downward extension into the sphenoid sinus and lateral extension toward the cavernous sinus from a locally or diffusely invasive tumor are also suitable for trans-sphenoidal surgery, since the procedure allows a massive debulking of the tumor prior to radiation therapy. Irregular multinodular, fungating tumors or eccentric extensions into the frontal, temporal, or posterior fossa dictate an intracranial transfrontal approach.[15]

Technique

Among the various approaches to the sphenoid sinus and sella turcica, such as the lateral orbital, lateral endonasal, and transmaxillary, the sublabial midline rhinoseptal transsphenoidal approach stands out as the most convenient and practical for neurosurgeons, as it is the safest and simplest procedure (devised and adopted by Harvey Cushing beginning in 1909). However, as Cushing wrote:

> The mere technical triumph of exposing the contents of the sella turcica by one or another method is far from the most important consideration. The "crux" of the situation lies in the manner of dealing with the pathologically modified gland when it has been brought into view.[1]

The procedure described below can be learned and performed by a single neurosurgeon unless other considerations require the assistance of a "nose" surgeon.

After induction with intravenous thiopental sodium, an endotracheal tube placed in the angle of the mouth is used to produce light general anesthesia. To prevent bronchial aspiration, the oropharyngeal cavity is packed with moist sponges. The patient is placed in a semisitting position, with the head firmly affixed to a horseshoe headrest and the neck slightly flexed at an angle of 20 degrees from the horizontal and then tilted 40 degrees onto the left shoulder. In this manner, the patient's body on the operating table is out of the way and the surgeon is in front of the face, working in a strictly median sagittal plane (Fig. 103-1).

A portable image intensifier is then positioned on the side of the patient's head in such a way that the horizontal beam is centered on the sella turcica. The television monitor is placed behind and just above the patient's head. This enables the surgeon to look at the screen in line with the binocular of the microscope, so that only a slight head movement is required for observing either the operative field or the screen. Radiofluoroscopic control is used only as needed during the operation; its proper placement limits radiation to only a few seconds at each stage of the procedure. The image intensifier is switched on and off with a foot pedal controlled by the surgeon or an assistant. Lead shielding and aprons are used to protect operating room personnel from radiation. Television input from the microscope and radiofluoroscopy from the image intensifier can be monitored on two separate channels of a video tape recorder.

The patient's face, mouth, and nasal cavities are prepared with an aqueous antiseptic solution. Infiltration of the nasal mucosa and upper gum with 0.5% procaine containing epinephrine (1:200,000) facilitates the subsequent elevation of the mucosa and diminishes oozing of blood. An adhesive plastic drape is used to cover the face, and additional draping of the entire operative field ensures complete isolation and sterility. A hole is made in the drape at the level of the upper lip, and sterile sponges are introduced into the mouth so that only the upper gingival margin is exposed.

The surgical procedure begins with a horizontal sublabial incision above the gingival margin, extending from one canine fossa to the other (Fig. 103-2). After the incised upper lip and submucosal tissues are elevated to expose the nasal bony cavity, the mucosa of the floor of the nose is elevated on both sides. The anterior spinous process is resected and the sharp edge of the maxilla sheared off. The mucosa of the nasal septum is elevated on one side until the entire nasal septum is exposed. At this point there is a unilateral rhinoseptal submucosal cavity which can be used whenever possible in the absence of septal deviation. The plane of cleavage is on the left side for a right-handed surgeon, and the mucosa is further detached from the posterior wall and the lateral edge of the vomer. The base of the septal cartilage is separated from the palatine crest, and the posterior vertical attachment to the vomer is separated with sharp dissection or a swivel knife moving in an upward direction. Then the entire nasal septum is tilted laterally toward the right side, although it remains attached to the upper part of the perpendicular plate of the ethmoid bone, which serves as a hinge. When there is marked septal deviation or when the

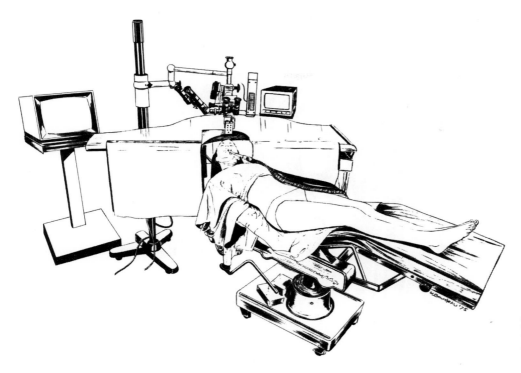

Figure 103-1 Position of the patient. (From Hardy.[7])

cartilaginous septum breaks in pieces at the lower portion, it is preferable to remove the loose parts or the inferior third (resected with a swivel knife) and preserve the pieces for further use in closure of the sella floor.

The sphenoid rostrum or the vomer comes into view, having the appearance of the keel of a boat. A special double-bladed nasal speculum is introduced into the newly formed submucosal cavity, and the blades are widely opened to hold the retracted mucosa out of the field (Fig. 103-3). Ordinarily, only minimal pressure is required to open the blades of the speculum; additional pressure with a dilator is not required. When the blades cannot be opened widely enough because of a narrow bony nasal orifice, the latter should be enlarged by shearing off the ascending branches of the maxilla. Occasional hypertrophy of the turbinates in acromegalic patients may require the use of a dilator. The

vomer is then detached, and further resection of the sphenoid floor gives wide exposure of the entire sinus cavity. After the mucosa is pierced and deflected and the bony septa are removed, the entire posterior aspect of the sinus and the floor of the sella turcica are brought into view (Fig. 103-4). The boundaries of the sella are carefully determined under direct vision and on lateral views with fluoroscopic control. At this stage, the binocular surgical microscope is moved into place.

After the main portion of the procedure within the sella is accomplished, the rhinoseptal closure is simple. Nasopharyngeal tubes are placed in the patient's nostrils to ensure free nasal airways. Then the septal mucosa is reapproximated with endonasal packs, using petrolatum (Vaseline) gauze impregnated with steroids and antibiotic ointment. A few loose catgut sutures are placed along the sublabial gingival incision; these are well tolerated and painless because of the temporary numbness due to the section of small nerve endings. With this approach there is no visible postoperative scar. The procedure described here can be carried out by a single surgeon, although other considerations may make the assistance of a nasal surgeon desirable.

Removal of Microadenoma

In patients suffering from a hypersecretory pituitary syndrome with a normal-size sella turcica (Cushing's disease, gigantism-acromegaly, galactorrhea-amenorrhea), trans-sphenoidal microsurgical exploration makes it possible to identify an intrapituitary lesion smaller than 10 mm in diameter (microadenoma).[4-6] These lesions are located in specific areas of the gland: growth hormone microadenomas are usually located in the anterior portion of the lateral wing, pro-

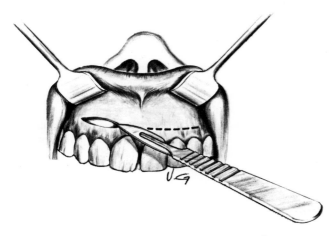

Figure 103-2 Gingival incision. (From Hardy.[7])

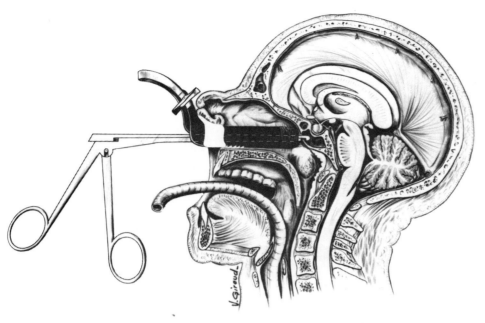

Figure 103-3 Side view: The bivalve speculum with the lip retractor in place. The sphenoid floor is opened with a rongeur. (From Hardy.[7])

lactin-secreting microadenomas in the posterior inferior portion of the lateral wing, and ACTH-secreting microadenomas in the central portion of the mucoid zone of the

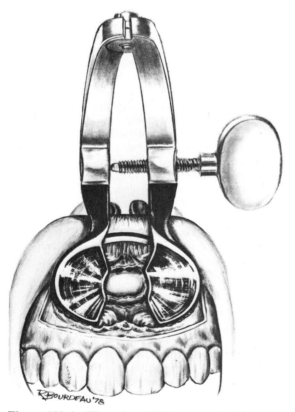

Figure 103-4 The sphenoid floor opening is enlarged to give wide exposure of the sphenoid sinus. After deflection of the mucosa, the sellar floor comes into view. (From Hardy.[7])

gland, deep in the parenchyma, just in front of the posterior lobe (Fig. 103-5).

When the floor of the sella is exposed, it is usually opened only on the side of the lesion which is suspected from tomographic or CT scan studies. Usually the floor appears slightly lower and thinner on the side of the lesion. After a cruciform incision is made in the dura, a growth hormone microadenoma is readily exposed, since it usually is bulging at the surface of the lateral wing of the gland. Gentle pressure on the gland will squeeze out the microadenoma. Residual tumor tissue is further removed with a small pituitary spoon and microcurettes especially designed with 45- and 90-degree angles to allow scraping of the lateral walls of the sella and particularly of the anterior corner, where some abnormal tissue can be hidden and easily overlooked.

A prolactinoma which is smaller than 5 mm in diameter is not readily visible at the surface, because it is usually located deep in the posterior inferior portion of the lateral wing of the gland. A vertical incision is therefore made lateral to the midline, and the pituitary parenchyma is opened and dissected gently until the tumor tissue is found posteriorly. The microcurette is introduced under televised control, and upon withdrawal the grayish purple tissue of the tumor is identified and resected (Fig. 103-6). This maneuver often results in separation of the anterior portion of the lateral wing, which is also removed and serves as a control biopsy of the normal gland. This allows better exposure and facilitates removal of the remaining tumor tissue.

An ACTH microadenoma is more difficult to find and to remove completely. When the tumor is not visible at the surface, it is located most often, in the author's experience, in the central core of the midportion of the gland in front of the posterior lobe; only occasionally is it eccentric.[9] The exploration of the pituitary in such cases is more tedious. A stepwise procedure is recommended. First, a horizontal incision is made in the midportion of the anterior lobe deep into the parenchyma. Second, a vertical incision is made on the midline from the superior to the inferior surface of the

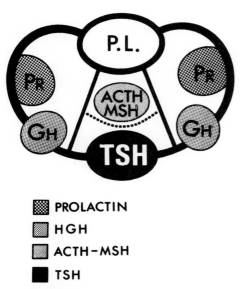

- ⊞ PROLACTIN
- ▨ HGH
- ▨ ACTH−MSH
- ■ TSH

Figure 103-5 Specific locations of hypersecretory pituitary microadenomas. P.L., posterior lobe. (From Hardy.[7])

gland, and a fragment of anterior lobe is taken for frozen histological study. As the parenchyma is further dissected deeply, the microadenoma will be encountered and identified as a grayish purple tissue. After it is removed with a microcurette, the cavity is further examined at 25-power magnification and any doubtful residual tumor tissue further excised; the margin of the tumor cavity is then biopsied. As the posterior lobe is difficult to distinguish clearly from the tumor tissue, the last fragment biopsied should be normal neural lobe tissue. The normal adenohypophyseal tissue is yellowish orange and is usually firmer than the tumor tissue, so it is not readily removed by low-pressure suction. Occasionally the margin of the tumor cavity is composed of a thin layer resembling a pseudocapsule between the tumor and the normal tissue. This membrane is also peeled off in one or several pieces (Fig. 103-7).

If the surgeon is in doubt about having achieved total tumor removal, it is recommended that intraoperative frozen biopsies be performed with histological verification. It must be stressed that for complete and selective functional histological microsurgical removal of pituitary hypersecretory lesions, help of a qualified neuropathologist is indispensable in the operating room during surgery. The risk of leaving pathological tissue or removing too much of the normal gland requires immediate histological tissue examination during surgery. Additional sterilization of the tumor bed may be accomplished by the temporary application of a cotton pad soaked in sterile 90% alcohol.

After removal of the microadenoma, the tumor cavity can be measured by placing in it a piece of Gelfoam (absorbable gelatin sponge, the Upjohn Co., Kalamazoo, Mich.) soaked in barium sulfate solution and x-raying it. Incidentally, this contrast substance has been found useful also in achieving hemostasis. After removal of the barium-impregnated Gelfoam, the cavity is packed with plain Gelfoam. If a CSF leak is present, a watertight closure can be achieved with a piece

of fascia and muscle or lyophilized dura. The sellar window should be closed with a small piece of cartilage from the nasal septum.

Removal of Macroadenoma with Suprasellar Extension

Before the patient is positioned, a catheter is inserted into the lumbar subarachnoid space so that air may be injected as desired to outline the suprasellar contour of the tumor during the operation.

Once the floor of the sphenoid sinus has been opened, the sinus is frequently noted to be partially or completely filled by the bulging sellar floor. The floor is usually thinned and can be opened easily, producing a large window into the sella. The dural sheet also has been thinned by pressure from the growing tumor. At this step, a transdural puncture, using a 22-gauge needle mounted on a syringe, may be carried out to aspirate a possible cystic or semiliquid necrotic adenoma. Intratumoral metrizamide injection is also useful at this point to outline the tumor contour (Fig. 103-8). Rupture of the superior dural capsule may also be detected by the extension of the contrast medium outside the tumor into the subarachnoid space. When the dura is incised in cruciform fashion, the gelatinous grey-purple tissue of the tumor will burst forth into the sphenoid sinus to be removed by further aspiration.

It should be emphasized that no capsule other than the previously opened dura is found around the pituitary adenoma. The dura is in fact the "capsule" of the tumor. It is contiguous with the lateral wall of the sella, it forms the inner layer of the cavernous sinus, and it is continuous with the diaphragma sellae. No attempt should be made to remove the "capsule," since any tear in the cavernous sinus wall will result in profuse bleeding. Further removal of the tumor is by curettage in all directions, using a malleable spoon and various types of curettes and suction tubes (Fig. 103-9).

In large tumors some pathological tissue may be hidden in the lateral corners of the sella. Using a 45-degree angle fiberoptic mirror, this tissue may be identified and removed with a 90-degree angle curette and suction tube.

Once the enlarged sella has been partially emptied of tumor, the suprasellar extension usually collapses into the sella as a result of normal intracranial pulsations. If this does not occur, curettes should be introduced under televised radiofluoroscopic control and the suprasellar bulge detached piecemeal until the diaphragm or superior capsule is seen to collapse downward, pulsating and hanging freely in the sella. The gradual passage of air into the suprasellar cistern is seen on the television screen, while the anterior third ventricle returns to its normal position above the sella. Thus immediate pneumographic control is obtained during surgery, proving the completeness of tumor removal.

In the unusual circumstance of a fibrous adenoma (accounting for about 5 percent of cases), it is necessary to use the electrical loop to remove the lesion because of its firm consistency. Oozing may occur during tumor removal and may persist until the last fragment has been detached. It

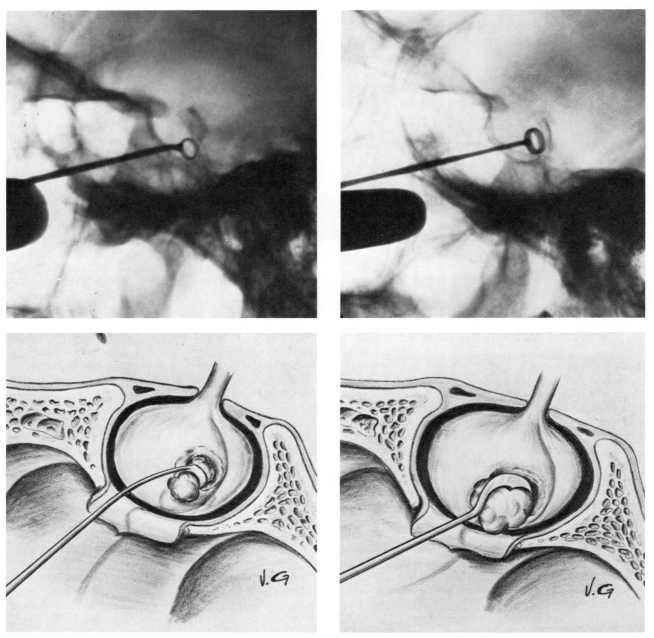

Figure 103-6 Prolactin-secreting microadenomas located in the posterior inferior region of the lateral wing. *Left:* A 3-mm microadenoma. *Right:* A 5-mm microadenoma. Ring curettes appropriate to the size of the microadenomas are used. (From Hardy and Mohr.[10])

stops after the temporary packing of Gelfoam into the cavity. This oozing is of no real consequence, since it drains into the sphenoid sinus and the submucosal nasal opening.

Cerebrospinal fluid leakage rarely occurs during tumor removal, since the distention produced by the tumor generally causes the diaphragm to adhere to the arachnoid. The diaphragm is itself a natural protection against fistula formation, which will not occur if surgical maneuvers are performed gently under televised radiofluoroscopic control.

After exploration of the cavity to make certain that all pathological material has been removed, a Gelfoam pledget soaked in radiopaque barium sulfate solution is applied underneath the diaphragma sellae to serve as an opaque marker for periodic postoperative radiological assessment. (Silver clips are no longer used because of the artifacts they produce on CT scans). Tumor recurrence will eventually be signaled by the slight elevation of the opaque contour as well as by CT scan.

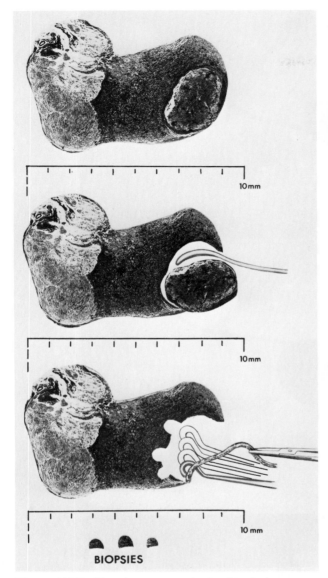

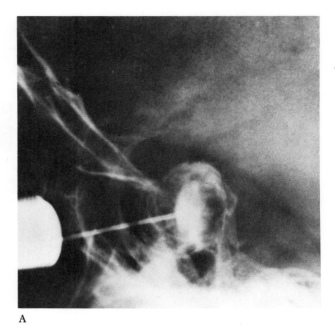

A

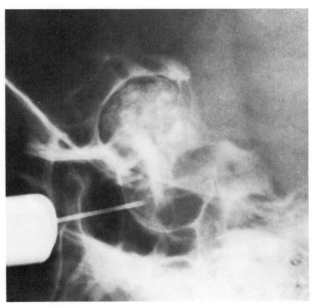

B

Figure 103-7 *Top:* Autopsy specimen of a pituitary containing a 4-mm microadenoma. (From Hardy.[7]) *Middle:* Enucleation of the microadenoma. (From Hardy and Mohr.[10]) *Bottom:* Peeling off the pseudocapsule and biopsies of the surrounding normal pituitary tissue. (From Hardy and Mohr.[10])

Figure 103-8 Intraoperative delineation of pituitary adenoma with metrizamide injection. *A.* Intrasellar adenoma. *B.* Large suprasellar extension.

If blood oozing persists after complete removal of the tumor, a catheter is left in the sphenoid cavity, fixed in place with a silk ligature at the gum margin. The catheter is connected to a low-pressure suction apparatus and is removed on completion of drainage.

Ordinarily, the larger the pituitary tumor extending downward into the sphenoid sinus the easier it is to remove. For this reason, neurosurgeons with little or no experience in trans-sphenoidal pituitary surgery would do well to try to remove this type of lesion as their first attempt—even before attempting ablation of a normal gland (or a microadenoma,

which is a much more difficult procedure). With tumors extending above the sella, considerable experience is needed to properly assess the amount of curettage needed to accomplish the required manipulation of the superior "capsule" without producing a tear. It must be emphasized that no attempt should be made to pull down the "capsule." It will come down of its own accord, as a result of intracranial pulsation, once the tumor has been totally removed. In accomplishing this, assistance may be obtained from the anesthesiologist, who can produce a temporary increase in the thoracic pressure (Valsalva maneuver) or can inject fluid

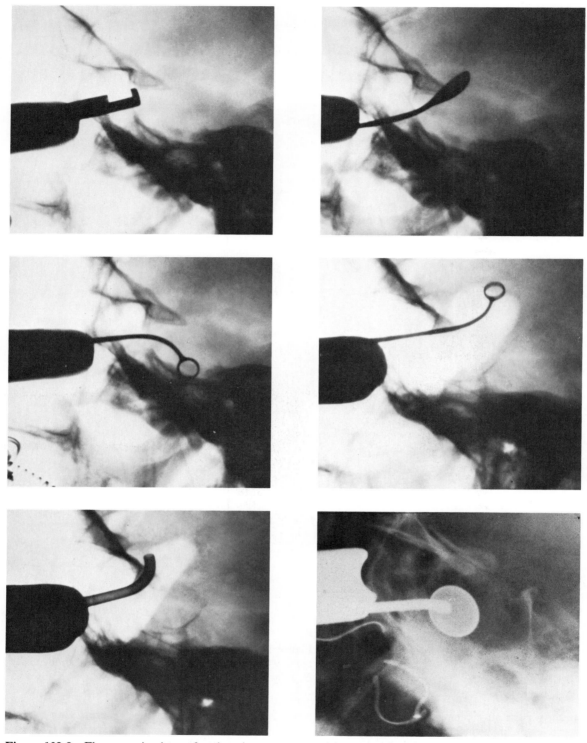

Figure 103-9 Fluoroscopic views of various instruments used in trans-sphenoidal removal of large pituitary tumors with suprasellar extension: malleable spoon, downward and upward ring curettes, 90-degree angle suction, and fiberoptic angled mirror. (From Hardy.[7])

through the lumbar catheter; either will increase the pressure in the cranial cavity and will help to push the capsule down into the sella.

In the case of large tumors with considerable suprasellar extension, collapse of the "capsule" far down in the sella may give rise to the empty sella syndrome. This can be prevented by placing a piece of muscle in the cavity in order to prevent downward herniation of the relaxed diaphragm, a procedure called *preventive chiasmapexy*.

Removal of Craniopharyngiomas and Other Sellar Tumors

The surgical management of craniopharyngioma will remain a challenging problem. Although usually a benign embryological tumor, it is deceptive in that subtotal removal is often followed by recurrence. The only curative approach is total excision of the tumor at the time of the first operation. With the present medical knowledge of the clinical picture and radiographic features of this tumor, the surgical anatomy of the growing lesion has been clarified so that the indications for trans-sphenoidal versus intracranial approach are now better defined.

There are three anatomical varieties of craniopharyngioma. A pure intrasellar lesion, as evidenced by intrasellar calcification and a long history of hypopituitarism, suggests that the neoplasm is located beneath the diaphragma sellae and has extended into the sphenoid sinus, with enlargement of the floor of the sella turcica. This is the major indication for the trans-sphenoidal approach in an attempt to achieve total excision of the tumor. The striking difference between a pituitary adenoma and a craniopharyngioma is evident as soon as the dural sheet of the floor of the sella has been opened. With a craniopharyngioma, a second membrane abuts on the inner surface of the dura. This is the capsule of the craniopharyngioma. Once the capsule has been punctured and the brownish fluid containing cholesterol crystals drained, the capsule collapses. The tumor content is further removed with various curettes (Fig. 103-10*A, B*). Then the capsule is grasped with a forceps, and a blunt enucleator is used to gently separate it from its attachment to the dura. Slight traction and dissection with cotton pledgets are used to detach the superior reflection of the capsule, particularly in instances when it is attached to the inferior aspect of the diaphragma sellae (Fig. 103-10*C*). When dealing with craniopharyngiomas, it is important to be aware of the fact that

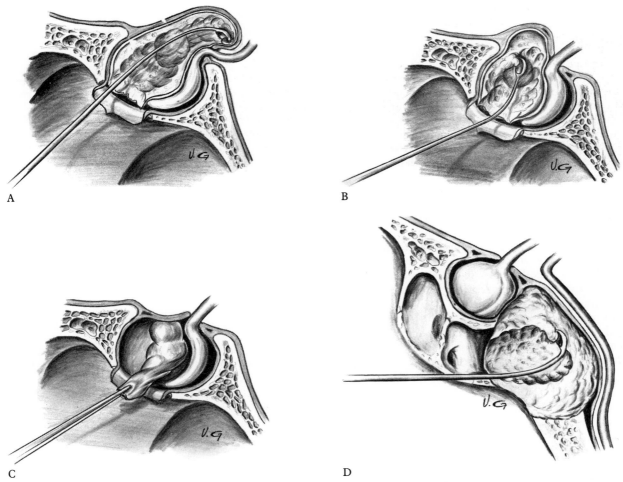

A
B
C
D

Figure 103-10   *A*. Intracapsular removal of a craniopharyngioma using a downward-curved curette. *B*. Intracapsular removal of a craniopharyngioma using an upward-curved curette. *C*. Excision of a craniopharyngioma capsule. *D*. Excision of a clivus chordoma. (From Hardy.[7])

the normal pituitary gland is outside of the capsule and can be identified with the microscope. It can therefore be left in the sella to prevent further hypopituitarism and even favor restoration of hormonal secretion. Because of its firm adherence to the diaphragma sellae and arachnoidal sheet of the chiasmatic cistern, the detachment of tumor at this point may occasionally produce a tear in the arachnoid, resulting in a cerebrospinal fluid leak. The tear is closed with a piece of fascia lata and the sellar cavity packed with muscle; further closure can be achieved with a cartilaginous septal graft applied with biological glue.

The second variety of craniopharyngioma is the one that is located only intracranially, above the diaphragma sellae, extending upward along the pituitary stalk either posterior or anterior to the chiasm and optic nerves. In this case, the transcranial subfrontal approach is absolutely mandatory.

The third variety of craniopharyngioma is the one that has its origin within the sellar cavity, as evidenced by a long history of hypopituitarism, but extends upward to result in a recent visual disturbance. This lesion is associated with a large sella turcica; its suprasellar extension is most often covered by the diaphragma sellae. This case presents a controversial indication. In the author's experience, it has been possible to approach the lesion by a trans-sphenoidal route and achieve total excision. However, if the suprasellar extension does not collapse down into the sella during the first procedure, a second must be tried approximately 1 month later, after repeated radiographic studies. If the capsule has collapsed down into the sella, it is still possible to achieve total excision by a trans-sphenoidal route. If the capsule remains attached to the hypothalamus and the surrounding neurovascular structures, however, the second operation should use an intracranial transfrontal approach.

Finally, occasionally an emergency procedure is required because of development of an acute intracranial pressure effect before an endocrine workup has been completed. Using intravenous cortisone replacement, a trans-sphenoidal approach can be carried out rapidly and a large cystic craniopharyngioma punctured and evacuated. Residual fluid will eventually drain into the sphenoid sinus, preventing recurrence of cystic dilatation and pressure upon neurovascular structures. A decision concerning the ideal surgical treatment and further radical excision of the lesion can be postponed until after this temporary relief has been obtained and the endocrine workup completed.

Other nonpituitary lesions of the sella turcica can also be approached trans-sphenoidally: meningiomas, germinomas, granulomas, and intrasellar cystic lesions can best be so approached. Tumors destroying the posterior wall of the sella turcica and the clivus, such as chordomas, are located just below the sella turcica in the posterior wall of the sphenoid sinus (Fig. 103-10D). After the usual trans-sphenoidal approach is carried out, the maneuvers along the posterior clivus are performed under televised radiofluoroscopic control, making possible extensive removal of the tumor, although most often this is incomplete. Nevertheless, radiation therapy may prevent or delay recurrence of this unusual lesion.

References

1. Cushing H: *Pituitary Body, Hypothalamus and Parasympathetic Nervous System.* Springfield, Ill, Charles C Thomas, 1932.
2. Guiot G (ed): *Adénomes Hypophysaires.* Paris, Masson, 1958.
3. Hardy J: L'exérèse des adénomes hypophysaires par voie transsphénoïdale. Union Med Can 91:933–945, 1962.
4. Hardy J: Transsphenoidal microsurgery of the normal and pathological pituitary. Clin Neurosurg 16:185–217, 1969.
5. Hardy J: Transsphenoidal hypophysectomy: Neurosurgical techniques. J Neurosurg 34:582–594, 1971.
6. Hardy J: Transsphenoidal surgery of hypersecreting pituitary tumors, in Kohler PO, Ross GT (eds): *Diagnosis and Treatment of Pituitary Tumors.* New York, American Elsevier, 1973, pp 179–194.
7. Hardy J: *Transsphenoidal Operations on the Pituitary.* Randolph, Mass., Codman & Shurtleff, 1975.
8. Hardy J: Microsurgery of pituitary disorders. Ann R Coll Physicians Surg Con 13:294–298, 1980.
9. Hardy J: Cushing's disease: 50 years later. Presidential address XVII Canadian Congress of Neurological Sciences. Can J Neurol Sci. 9:375–380, 1982.
10. Hardy J, Mohr G: Le prolactinome aspects chirurgicaux. Neurochirurgie 27 (supp. 1): 41–60, 1981.
11. Hardy J, Vezina JL: Transsphenoidal neurosurgery of intracranial neoplasm. Adv Neurol. 15:261–274, 1976.
12. Henderson WR: The pituitary adenomata: A follow-up study of the surgical results in 338 cases (Dr Harvey Cushing's series). Br J Surg 26:811–921, 1939.
13. Laws ER Jr, Randall RV, Kern EB, Abboud CE (eds): *Management of Pituitary Adenomas and Related Lesions with Emphasis on Transsphenoidal Microsurgery.* New York, Appleton-Century-Crofts, 1982.
14. Rosegay H: Cushing's legacy to transsphenoidal surgery. J Neurosurg 54:448–454, 1981.
15. Symon L, Jakubowski J, Kendall B: Surgical treatment of giant pituitary adenomas. J Neurol Neurosurg Psychiatry 42:973–982, 1979.
16. Walker EA: *A History of Neurological Surgery.* Baltimore, Williams & Wilkins, 1982.
17. Wilson CB, Dempsey LC: Transsphenoidal microsurgical removal of 250 pituitary adenomas. J Neurosurg 48:13–22, 1978.

104

Stereotactic Treatment of Pituitary Tumors

Robert W. Rand

Few surgeons disagree with the recommendation of prompt and aggressive intervention in a case of acromegaly or Cushing's disease, in view of the morbidity associated with the clinical and metabolic manifestations of these diseases. However, the efficacy of various surgical and radiotherapeutic techniques in the treatment of these diseases has been debated for many years. According to Evans and his associates, acromegaly is progressive, disfiguring, and potentially fatal, with a 50 percent death rate before middle age and 90 percent before the sixth decade.[3] The cause of death ranges from intracerebral tumor extension to diabetic coma; Wright et al. considered cardiovascular disease the most frequent cause.[9] In the choice of treatment, the preferred modalities at present include microsurgical trans-sphenoidal tumor resection, conventional radiotherapy, heavy particle irradiation, and stereotactic cryohypophysectomy. The author favors cryohypophysectomy for its simplicity, safety, and effectiveness in both these diseases.

Stereotactic Cryohypophysectomy

Between 1963 and 1974, a total of 54 patients with a diagnosis of acromegaly were studied at the UCLA Medical Center. The diagnosis was based on metabolic and clinical criteria. The average age of the patients was 43 years for the 28 men and 46 years for the 26 women.

Comprehensive evaluation to confirm the initial clinical impression was performed. Physical examination revealed several acromegalic features in each patient, the most common being enlargement of the facial features. Next in order of frequency were headache, hypertension, diminished libido, fatigue, and arthralgia. Radiological studies showed heel pad enlargement from 23 mm to 34 mm in more than 95 percent of the patients, as well as prominent distal tufts with hypertrophy of osseous and soft tissue structures in the hands. In 70 percent of the patients, skull x-ray films demonstrated an abnormal sella turcica, and chest examination showed cardiomegaly in 28 percent. Pneumoencephalography in every case ruled out excessive suprasellar adenoma extension, a specific contraindication to cryohypophysectomy.

Radioimmunoassay of serum human growth hormone (hGH) level was used for a definitive endocrinologic diagnosis regardless of the clinical aspects. A major criterion of acromegaly was considered to be an elevated fasting level of hGH which was not suppressed during glucose tolerance testing. At our hospital, normal hGH levels are considered to be those values below 10 ng/ml in the fasting basal state or below 5 ng/ml nonfasting which are suppressed by the glucose tolerance test. To determine the degree of associated diabetic involvement, blood sugar levels were measured simultaneously.

For those patients with evidence of pituitary apoplexy, sudden or marked loss of either visual acuity or peripheral fields, or significant suprasellar tumor extension associated with cranial nerve palsies or obstructive hydrocephalus, transfrontal craniotomy was the treatment of choice at that time. (Currently a transnasal trans-sphenoidal operation is preferred in these cases.) All other acromegalic patients were treated by trans-sphenoidal cryohypophysectomy during that period. To evaluate the efficacy of this therapy, hGH levels were obtained pre- and postoperatively in every patient. To determine the adequacy of other pituitary functions, the pituitary adrenal axis was studied by measurement of urinary hydroxy- and ketosteroids and thyroid output by measurement of protein-bound iodine (PBI), T_3, and ^{131}I thyroid uptake. Serological tests are also used currently.

The stereotactic cryohypophysectomy procedure uses cryoprobes 2.7 to 4.3 mm in diameter, cooled by liquid nitrogen and guided into the sella turcica under stereotactic manipulation with fluoroscopic and teleroentgenographic control. At the cryoprobe tip, temperatures ranging from -170 to $-180°C$ are reached, producing several overlapping cryogenic lesions on either side of the midline over a period of 10 to 15 min. An average of five lesions are made unless (as is rarely the case) the tumor is very large.

The temperature gradient rises sharply to a range of -5 to $+10°C$ at 8 to 10 mm from the freezing site. The patient is under local anesthesia and sedation but is awake while the lesions are being created. The extraocular movements, visual acuity, and visual fields are monitored carefully. As the cranial nerves adjacent to the tumor become cooled to below $15°C$, about 15 percent of patients are apt to develop incipient palsies, which disappear as the probe warms. In this series of 54 patients there was no postoperative evidence of residual deficit, although a number of the patients had transient decrease in vision or function of the extraocular nerves.

The efficacy of cryohypophysectomy was judged on the basis of substantial overall clinical improvement and regression of acromegalic features, improvement of the glucose tolerance curve, and a reduction of hGH to below 10 ng/ml in a 10- to 20-year follow-up study.

Significant subjective and objective improvement was observed in many of the patients during the first 24 h and continued for several months. Facial feature enlargement diminished substantially in 61 percent and acral enlargement in 63 percent. hGH levels were lowered, but radiographic studies demonstrated little if any change in osseous deformities. It was therefore concluded that the regression of acromegalic features was due to loss of excess fluid from hypertrophic collagenous structures and gradual reduction of excessive soft tissue. Heel pad thickness following cryohypophysectomy decreased to a range of 20 to 30 mm, and hand volume decreased by almost 15 percent as measured by water displacement.

Blood pressure after therapy averaged 128/86, whereas before the procedure 63 percent of the patients demonstrated hypertension, with an average blood pressure of 164/101. In 56 percent of those with skin signs such as oiliness, coarseness, and increased pigmentation, these characteristics either disappeared altogether or were markedly improved. Headache vanished in more than a third, and body weight returned to the premorbid status in 50 percent. In at least 40 percent there was no further need for medication for relieved or lessened arthralgias and acroparesthesias. Two complaints, however, hyperhidrosis and diminished libido, were not alleviated by the operative procedure to any significant degree.

All patients were evaluated for fasting blood sugar (FBS) and glucose tolerance. Glucose tolerance was tested, after oral intake of 100 g of glucose, at 30, 60, 120, and 180 min and averaged for determination of the mean. It soon became evident that at least 34 percent of the acromegalic patients demonstrated severe chemical diabetes, with an average FBS of 198 mg/100 ml and a mean glucose tolerance of 250 mg/100 ml before surgery. These figures rapidly improved to 137 m/100 ml and 158 mg/100 ml, respectively, after surgery. Those patients who before surgery had had a normal glucose tolerance continued to have a normal glucose tolerance curve after cryohypophysectomy. There appeared to be little difference between presurgery diabetic and nondiabetic patients in regard to the intensity and duration of the initial clinical symptoms, but the diabetic patients showed greater morbidity, for example, hypertension with an average blood pressure of 153/99 and an almost doubled incidence of cardiomegaly. After surgery the blood pressure approached a more normal range of 128/82. Visual impairment (36 percent in diabetic patients and only 11 percent in the nondiabetic) was associated with definite though not excessive suprasellar tumor extension in both groups.

Lowering the fasting basal hGH level to below 10 ng/ml is the metabolic criterion of successful endocrinologic therapy. The 10- to 20-year follow-up has showed that 56 percent of the patients had hGH levels below 5 ng/ml and 21 percent had levels between 5 and 10 ng/ml. In those who had been successfully treated, preoperative hGH values had ranged from 13 to 185, with a mean of 50 ng/ml, and postoperative values averaged 4.05 ng/ml. Patients who had not benefited from cryohypophysectomy had had preoperative hGH levels between 30 and 140, with a mean value of 66 ng/ml; the postoperative mean of 39 ng/ml was far greater than the acceptable therapeutic range, even though the preoperative values were similar to those of the patients in the successful group.

The majority of the patients in this series had undergone previous unsuccessful courses of radiation at other institutions, which made it difficult to evaluate the function of the remaining pituitary tropic hormones postoperatively. Maintenance thyroid therapy had been administered to 24 percent of the patients before they came to UCLA, and 28 percent had had some form of exogenous steroid. Half the patients in the series ultimately employed supplemental therapy after surgery. Of the 27 patients who postoperatively demonstrated pituitary dysfunction, 24 had required some type of endocrine replacement even before cryohypophysectomy. Of the 26 patients treated solely by cryosurgery and with no previous history of radiation treatment, only 7, or 27 percent, required postoperative exogenous hormones. These results seem to indicate the degree of residual pituitary function to be expected when cryohypophysectomy is the initial procedure in acromegalic patients of otherwise normal endocrine status.

The only complications were transient and infrequent. Diabetes insipidus developed in 13 percent of the patients and rhinorrhea in 7 percent, neither lasting more than 4 days. Inflammatory noninfectious meningitis, usually clearing within a week, occurred in 3 patients.

The technique of stereotactic cryohypophysectomy has been used in several patients who had Nelson's syndrome as a result of development of a pituitary adenoma following adrenalectomy. Although the results in these patients have not been as striking as those in the acromegalic patients, two of four patients have had lasting improvement, with depigmentation and resolution of other symptoms.

Although the technique of stereotactic cryohypophysectomy would seem to be ideally suited to the treatment of primary Cushing's disease, in which the basophilic adenoma can now be identified by high-resolution computer tomography, most neurosurgeons prefer to use a surgical transnasal trans-sphenoidal approach to this condition rather than cryohypophysectomy.

The operation has been applied to microadenomas that cause galactorrhea and amenorrhea where the prolactinoma is identifiable by neuroradiological tests. The results in one typical patient show striking and lasting 7-year improvement of the syndrome and preservation of pituitary function. The tumor was located in the right lobe of the pituitary gland, and it was possible, using a small (2.7-mm) probe, to discretely destroy the right side of the gland only. The patient quickly recovered from the operation and was discharged from the hospital within a few days, with her problem resolved.

Stereotactic cryohypophysectomy thus has a role to play in the treatment of carefully-selected secretory or nonsecretory pituitary tumors. There have been no operative deaths and no permanent extraocular or optic nerve palsies. The procedure is well tolerated by patients but is tedious for the surgeon to perform and requires an anesthesiologist who can exercise the fine control necessary to keep the patient pain-free during the intervals between the production of the lesions and yet alert enough at the time of freezing for the functioning of the extraocular and optic nerves to be tested.

Interstitial Irradiation

An alternative to external beam irradiation is the stereotactic implantation of interstitial radioactive substances, as performed by Molinatti et al. in 16 patients using radioactive yttrium (^{90}Y).[5] While maintaining normal residual pituitary function, half their patients had clinical improvement with respect to acromegalic features, headaches, and fatigue. However, the possibility of recurrence was not reported, and the follow-up period was too short for any judgment to be made. Hartog et al., using both radioactive gold (^{198}Au) and ^{90}Y, noted a beneficial hGH response in only five of nine patients.[4] However, in another study of 22 cases, within 19 months of implantation 32 percent of the patients had a satisfactory response, i.e., loss of symptoms, recognizable regression of acromegalic facies, and return to a normal glucose tolerance curve. A second implantation was performed on nine patients, raising the number achieving a successful result to 60 percent. Some form of endocrine replacement therapy was ultimately required by 41 percent of the patients.

Eighty patients who had received implants between 1958 and 1967 were evaluated by Wright et al., who observed that 53 percent showed clinical improvement of headaches, paresthesias, and acromegalic appearance.[8,9] In 45 percent of the cases with previous evidence of diabetes, glucose tolerance tests returned to normal. A majority of the patients (59 percent) continued to show hGH levels above 10 ng/ml, although the hGH level fell an average of 54 percent. Bloom noted that hGH levels did not regularly return to normal values even when they were greatly reduced.[2]

Among the hazards of this technique are cranial nerve palsies, reported by Molinatti et al. in 13 percent, and diabetes insipidus, found in 38 percent of their cases.[5] The most frequent complications reported by Hartog and his associates were pituitary abscess, rhinorrhea, meningitis, diabetes insipidus, and visual impairment.[4] Wright et al. reported three operation-related deaths, although the above noted complications occurred in only 13 percent of their cases.[8]

The author's results with radioactive yttrium were disappointing, primarily because of a 12 to 15 percent complication rate similar to that of Molinatti et al. However, more recently Mundinger and Busam reported excellent results using different isotopes stereotactically implanted into pituitary tumors.[6] Stereotactic radiosurgery has also been employed successfully by Backlund et al. in treating nonsecre-

tory pituitary adenomas and prolactinomas.[1] With the same technique, Rahn et al. have reported excellent results in Cushing's disease.[7]

References

1. Backlund EO, Bergstrand G, Hierton-Laurell U, Rosenborg M, Wajngot A, Werner, S: Tumor changes after single dose irradiation by stereotactic radiosurgery in 'non-active' pituitary adenomas and prolactinomas in Szikla G (ed): *Stereotactic Cerebral Irradiation* (INSERM Symposium No 12). Amsterdam, Elsevier/North Holland, 1979, pp 199–212.

2. Bloom HJG: Radiotherapy of pituitary tumors, in Jenkins JS (ed): *Pituitary Tumors*. London, Butterworth, 1973, pp 165–197.

3. Evans HM, Griggs JH, Dixon JS: The physiology and chemistry of growth hormone, in Harris GW, Donovan BT (eds): *The Pituitary Gland*, vol 1. Berkeley/Los Angeles, University of California Press, 1966, pp 439–491.

4. Hartog M, Doyle F, Fraser R, Joplin GF: Partial pituitary ablation with implants of gold-198 and yttrium-90 for acromegaly. Br Med J 2:396–398, 1965.

5. Molinatti GM, Camanni F, Massara F, Olivetti M, Pizzini A, Giuliani G: Implantation of yttrium 90 in the sella turcica in sixteen cases of acromegaly. J Clin Endocrinol Metab 22:599–611, 1962.

6. Mundinger F, Busam B: Stereotactic interstitial iridium-192 permanent implantation of pituitary adenomas, in Szikla G (ed): *Stereotactic Cerebral Irradiation* (INSERM Symposium No 12). Amsterdam, Elsevier/North Holland, 1979, pp 187–197.

7. Rahn T, Thorén M, Hall K, Backlund EO: Stereotactic radiosurgery in the treatment of MB Cushing, in Szikla G (ed): *Stereotactic Cerebral Irradiation* (INSERM Symposium No 12). Amsterdam, Elsevier/North Holland, 1979, pp 207–212.

8. Wright AD, Hartog M, Palter H, Tevaarwerk G, Doyle FH, Arnot R, Joplin GF, Fraser TR: The use of yttrium 90 implantation in the treatment of acromegaly. Proc R Soc Med 63:221–223, 1970.

9. Wright AD, Hill DM, Lowy C, Fraser TR: Mortality in acromegaly. Q J Med 39:1–16, 1970.

105

Subfrontal Approach to the Pituitary Gland

Russel H. Patterson, Jr.

The shortest distance from the frontal or temporal region of the head to the sella turcica is along the sphenoid ridge rather than over the roof of the orbit. This fact, the reluctance of some surgeons to open the frontal sinuses, and the fear of finding short optic nerves account for the popularity of the temporal approach for surgery of tumors in the region of the pituitary. However, the transtemporal approach has deficiencies that can be hard to overcome. For example, the approach along the sphenoid ridge places the optic nerves and carotid artery in the line of the tumor, leaving only a small space in which to operate. The opposite optic nerve and carotid artery are poorly visualized, and the required rotation of the head puts the nerves and arteries at an odd angle that can confuse the surgeon (Fig. 105-1).

The straight frontal approach was popularized by Ray in the 1950s for the performance of hypophysectomy.[3] The principal advantage of the approach along the falx is that the surgeon can work readily between the optic nerves and easily identify the pituitary stalk and carotid arteries (Fig. 105-1). As outlined later in this chapter, the frontal sinuses are easy to manage, and short optic nerves are not a major roadblock; the answer is to remove the tuberculum and to work behind the chiasm between the optic tracts. Neither of these maneuvers is difficult, as will be shown later.

The main disadvantage of the approach is that the frontal lobe of the brain falls into the olfactory groove, adding to the bulk of brain that needs to be retracted. The possible consequences of heavy retraction led Ray to advocate an oblique approach over the roof of the orbit for the simple pituitary adenoma. In this approach the retraction is less but the access to the pituitary fossa between the optic nerves is angled rather than straight.

Indications

Transphenoidal surgery has distinct advantages over a transcranial operation for hypophysectomy and in the management of most pituitary adenomas. It is unsuitable if the pituitary adenoma is markedly eccentric and spills over either

into the temporal or frontal fossa. In such cases the transcranial operation allows better access to the tumor as it does in most cases of craniopharyngioma and parasellar meningioma. A transcranial operation is also suitable for treating chordoma and meningioma of the clivus as well as carotid and basilar aneurysms.

Surgical Technique

Midline Subfrontal Approach

In positioning the head, the trick is to mentally visualize the roof of the orbit, which is the path to the pituitary. If the surgeon is using a microscope with angled eyepieces, then the head must be positioned so that the roof of the orbit is not far from the vertical. Straight eyepieces have the advantage that their use allows the orbital roof to be tilted 30 degrees from vertical toward the surgeon. This allows the brain to fall back from the orbital roof, which lessens the need for retraction. The head should be positioned straight up, because most surgeons find orientation easier if the head is straight rather than turned. The optic nerves are more elusive and the carotid and anterior cerebral arteries assume unexpected locations when the head is rotated.

In most cases the approach will be from the right side, the most convenient for a right-handed surgeon. The incision is made in the hairline and can be quite low for a patient with a low hairline but needs to be quite far back for a patient who is bald. It extends from the right temple at about the level of the lateral canthus of the eye to perhaps 5 to 8 cm to the left of the midline. The opening in the skull need not be more than 5 cm on a side, but it must reach the midline and must be flush with the roof of the orbit. The most important bone cut starts from a burr hole placed at

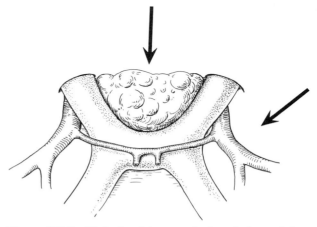

Figure 105-1 If the head is rotated, the relations of the optic nerves and major arteries are complex. In addition, the surgeon must operate over or between the nerves and arteries on the near side and is blind to the nerves and arteries on the far side. A straight frontal approach puts the optic nerves and arteries in a familiar orientation, but the frontal sinus must be opened.

the point of attachment of the zygoma to the orbital ridge and parallels the orbital ridge flush with the roof of the orbit to another opening made with a trephine over the sagittal sinus just above the nose. In the process, the frontal sinuses usually are opened. Another saw cut follows the sagittal sinus posteriorly for about 4 cm and curves laterally, eventually terminating at the first burr hole.

Opening the dura and retracting the frontal lobe is facilitated by draining spinal fluid through a previously placed lumbar needle. This relaxes the brain, reduces the need for retraction, and prevents spinal fluid from welling up into the operative field. If the head is thrown back sufficiently, the brain tends to fall away from the roof of the orbit. Additional room can be achieved by using osmotic diuretics and hyperventilation. An effort should be made to preserve draining veins from the frontal lobe to the sagittal sinus, even if they are on the stretch.

The approach is either along the falx or over the roof of the orbit. If along the falx, the olfactory nerve is coagulated and divided. If the brain is particularly full or the operation is anticipated to be long or extensive exposure is required, it may be prudent to resect a few grams of the undersurface of the frontal lobe in order to gain early exposure of the sellar region. The biggest danger of the surgery is edema or swelling in the frontal lobe. The degree of swelling is directly related to the force and duration of retraction.

The olfactory tract leads to the optic nerves as the brain is gradually retracted. Once the optic nerve is located, the arachnoid that binds the frontal lobe to the nerves is divided with microscissors or a sharp dissecting instrument, thereby exposing both optic nerves and the chiasm. In dealing with pituitary adenomas and tuberculum sellae meningiomas, it is best to completely expose both optic nerves and the chiasm early in the operation to avoid inadvertently injuring an unseen nerve. Often exposure of the chiasm can be facilitated by dividing the arachnoid over the carotid artery and out the sylvian fissure. This separates the frontal and temporal lobes, which allows the frontal lobe to fall back farther.

Access to the sella turcica may be blocked by short optic nerves and a large tuberculum, particularly in cases of craniopharyngioma. Ray reported that in about 8 percent of patients undergoing transfrontal hypophysectomy the tuberculum had to be removed to gain adequate working space. To do this, a flap of dura is peeled off the tuberculum and a chisel is used to knock a hole through the thin bone into the sphenoid sinus. The sphenoid mucosa is fairly thick and often can be pushed away without being perforated. Long, delicate bone instruments or a diamond drill are used to remove the tuberculum and anterior wall of the sella. Care must be taken in separating the dura from the bone to avoid entering the venous sinuses. After the bone is removed, it is possible to coagulate the circular sinus and divide the dura, which provides a good view of the contents of the sella. The pituitary stalk is identifiable by its shape and orientation and also by the portal veins, which impart a longitudinally striped appearance to the stalk.

Entrance into the sella is achieved in the rarely performed operation of transfrontal hypophysectomy by dilating the hole in the diaphragma sellae after dividing the stalk flush with the diaphragm. The contents of the sella then are

removed with a variety of ring curettes, paying particular attention to the region under the right optic nerve, where fragments of gland are most likely to be left behind. The cavity of the sella can be treated with alcohol or some other fixative after the gland is removed.

In large subfrontal meningiomas, it may be necessary to remove a small portion of frontal lobe to "uncap" the tumor. On the author's service it has never been found necessary to perform a bifrontal exposure of these tumors, even those as large as 200 g. There always seems to be adequate space to remove all the tumor from a unilateral approach. If the surgeon feels more comfortable with a bifrontal exposure, then the falx is cut above the crista galli. The frontal lobes can both be retracted or can even be retracted separately as Lougheed has recommended for anterior communicating artery aneurysms. The tumor is evacuated by means of a cutting loop, a laser, or the ultrasonic aspirator. An effort is made early to interrupt the tumor's blood supply, which springs from the floor of the frontal fossa.

In the surgery of subfrontal meningiomas, the greatest risk to the patient comes from injury to the anterior and middle cerebral arteries. Sometimes the mass greatly stretches these arteries, which leads to their mistaken identification as inconsequential feeders of the tumor. The surgeon should not cut or divide any arteries attached to the tumor capsule unless it is absolutely certain that they do not supply an important area of the brain.

It is sometimes possible to remove craniopharyngiomas between the optic nerves without any further exposure. However, in many cases the optic nerves will be short. If they are, the tuberculum sellae should be removed so that fragments of tumor can be pushed down into the sphenoid sinus rather than being pulled between short optic nerves with resultant trauma to the nerves (Fig. 105-2). A second trick that facilitates removal is to expose the tumor between the optic tracts behind the optic chiasm and through the lamina terminalis. The tumor then can be pushed down away from the chiasm and hypothalamus and out through

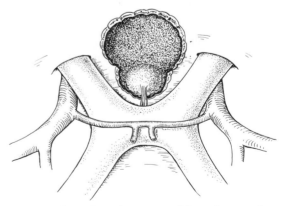

Figure 105-2 Exposing a retrochiasmal tumor in the presence of short optic nerves by opening the sphenoid sinus and removing the tuberculum sellae. Operating between the optic tracts can provide additional exposure. The pituitary stalk sometimes can be recognized by its portal system, which lends a striated appearance.

the sphenoid sinus. The main problem comes with cystic tumors, because tugging on a thin cyst wall is likely to result in a tear that leaves a fragment behind in the hypothalamus.[1]

In closing the wound, the principal challenge is the open sinuses. Fat can be packed into the sphenoid sinus and a few stitches taken in the dural flap to hold the fat in place. The frontal sinus can be closed with a plug of fat or gelatin foam and then a flap of periosteum turned down from the underside of the scalp flap and sutured to the dura. It is not necessary to remove the mucosa from the sinus; it need only be pushed down into the sinus and the packing then placed on top of the mucosa. Spinal fluid which has been kept in sterile syringes is reinjected through the spinal needle at the end of the procedure to flush out air and any blood that may have run down into the basilar cisterns.

Oblique Subfrontal Approach

The incision and flap are exactly the same as described above, except that the approach is over the roof of the orbit instead of along the midline. This requires less retraction of the frontal lobe and possibly carries less risk of stretching the opposite olfactory tract with consequent anosmia. The disadvantage is that the cavity of the sella is less accessible, so the surgeon must work over the right optic nerve. In most pituitary adenomas this is not an important compromise, and the approach can be recommended.

In dealing with a pituitary adenoma, it is important to make a large opening in the stretched diaphragma sellae that comprises the capsule of the tumor, in order to prevent any postoperative bleeding in the tumor cavity from reinflating the tumor and causing sudden loss of vision. With a large opening, any blood or exudate is free to leak into the subarachnoid spaces rather than becoming loculated within the tumor capsule. The tumor itself is evacuated by the use of suction, laser, and ring curettes.

In many cases the capsule of the tumor will fall away from the optic nerves, but if it does not, it is wise to leave the capsule adherent to the nerves. Sometimes stripping the capsule from the nerves will strip away their blood supply, thereby damaging vision. Normal optic nerves can stand a fair amount of manipulation, but this is not true of nerves stretched by tumor. The slightest trauma may result in visual loss.

Pterional Approach

This approach, which has been widely used for the surgery of aneurysms, is described elsewhere in this textbook. It consists of drilling off the sphenoid ridge to the landmark of the orbitomeningeal artery. The sylvian fissure then is split either from the medial to the lateral aspect or from the lateral to the medial. Splitting the fissure allows retraction of the frontal lobe with less distortion of the brain. In the surgery of lesions around the sella, this approach is most useful for lesions behind the clivus. The difficulties with the alter-

native approach under the temporal lobe, which is another possibility, are that it requires heavy retraction of the temporal lobe and provides poor visualization of the structures in the prepontine cistern. The surgeon can see the ipsilateral posterior cerebral and superior cerebellar arteries well enough, but their counterparts on the opposite side and the opposite third nerve are difficult or impossible to see. Also, the ipsilateral third and fourth nerves are in the way and are therefore prone to injury. In the pterional approach, the medial side of the temporal lobe is dissected free of the third nerve and the edge of the tentorium, and the carotid artery is retracted medially, using a narrow self-retaining retractor. For adequate exposure, the sylvian fissure must be split much more widely than is necessary for aneurysms of the anterior circulation. Unless the fissure is widely split, the posterior clinoid process may appear to block the exposure. Most of the clivus can be seen, and chordomas and meningiomas, which occur in this location, can be removed totally or in part. At New York Hospital, this has been found the safest approach to aneurysms of the upper basilar artery.

Operative Complications

The principal operative complication of the subfrontal approach is excessive brain retraction. This must be avoided at all costs. If mannitol and spinal drainage do not provide sufficient exposure, then it is safer to resect a few grams of frontal lobe than to apply heavy retractor pressure for an hour or two.

Other preventable complications include injury to the optic nerve, the third nerve, and the cerebral arteries. As emphasized above, a stretched or impaired optic nerve should never be manipulated; to do so is to risk further visual loss. The damage to the arteries occurs because the surgeon fails to recognize them for what they are. The anterior cerebral and other arteries may be imbedded in a meningioma or may be so stretched and distorted that they are taken for a tumor vessel. Any artery on or in the tumor must be preserved until it is confirmed as an artery feeding only the tumor.

Anosmia is a distinct risk in subfrontal surgery. The olfactory tract on the right often is divided, and if osmotic diuretics, spinal drainage, and old age cause the left frontal lobe to fall back, the other olfactory nerve may suffer avulsion.

References

1. Patterson RH Jr, Danylevich A: Surgical removal of craniopharyngiomas by a transcranial approach through the lamina terminalis and sphenoid sinus. Neurosurgery 7:111–117, 1980.
2. Rand RW: Transfrontal transsphenoidal craniotomy in pituitary and related tumors, in Rand RW (ed): *Microneurosurgery*. St. Louis, Mosby, 1978, pp 93–104.
3. Ray BS: Intracranial hypophysectomy. J Neurosurg 28:180–186, 1968.

106

Cranio-
pharyngiomas

Peter W. Carmel

Controversy has surrounded the craniopharyngioma as it has almost no other tumor affecting the brain. Debate has arisen concerning its origin, natural history, operative removability, response to radiation, and optimal therapy. Many of these questions remain unresolved, and the conclusions reported in this chapter must be regarded as only tentative answers in the ongoing history of treatment of this tumor.

Origin

At the end of the 19th century pathologists were intrigued by a strange group of epithelial tumors encountered above and within the sella turcica. Mott and Barrett, in 1899, postulated that these tumors might arise from the hypophyseal duct or Rathke's pouch.[32] This amazingly prescient theory, based on three cases of third ventricular tumor, continues to be widely held. Histological characteristics of these tumors were well described in 1904 by Erdheim, who pointed out similarities between craniopharyngiomas and adamantinomas, tumors known to be primitive neoplasms of buccal origin.[13] He thought this close resemblance proved that craniopharyngiomas arose from ectoblastic remnants of Rathke's duct. In addition, the anterior wall of Rathke's pouch forms both the pars tuberalis and the anterior lobe of the pituitary, the most common sites for craniopharyngiomas. Since that time craniopharyngiomas have been found along the path of development of Rathke's pouch from the pharynx to the floor of the sella,[36] as well as above and within the sella.

However, while craniopharyngiomas and adamantinomas have a similar appearance,[12] the histological picture differs greatly between a Rathke's cleft cyst and a craniopharyngioma, although they are postulated to have a common origin.[39] The Rathke's cleft cyst may be a simple cystic enlargement and may lack the changes induced by neoplastic transformation found in craniopharyngiomas.

Some investigators have demonstrated histological differences between adult and childhood craniopharyngiomas which might indicate separate origins.[18] They stress that almost half the adult tumors are made up of squamous epithelium without the palisading or other adamantinomatous characteristics of the childhood tumor. Squamous epithelial

rests in the hypophysis were described in autopsy material by Carmichael more than fifty years ago.[10] However, these cell rests are found in only 3 percent of neonates[14] and are found with increasing frequency in each succeeding decade.[27] This finding suggests that an embryonic origin need not be postulated for such cells, which may appear later in life because of cellular alteration or metaplasia of pituitary cells, which are also of ectodermal origin.

Pathology

Craniopharyngiomas may vary greatly in size. Small intrasellar tumors only 6 or 7 mm in diameter may be detected in amenorrheic young women and may be mistaken for prolactin-secreting adenomas (Fig. 106-1), whereas large tumors may occupy a significant portion of the intracranial volume (Fig. 106-2). Almost all these tumors have both solid and cystic portions, and even portions that appear densely calcified on diagnostic studies usually contain small cysts. Fluid within these cysts may appear yellow, light tan, greenish, dark black (like machinery oil), or even milky white and may range in viscosity from watery to sludgelike. Cystic craniopharyngioma fluid contains suspended cholesterol crystals, recognized by their characteristic birefringency.

The microscopic appearance typically shows an external layer of high columnar epithelium, a variable portion of polygonal cells, and a central network of epithelial cells. These epithelial bands are supported by a mesodermal connective tissue stroma. Papillary structures are common, recognized

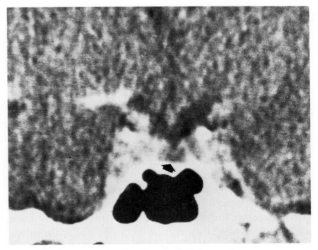

Figure 106-1 Coronal enhanced CT scan in a young woman with the complaint of amenorrhea and with mild serum prolactin elevation. The scan shows a lucent lesion in the midsellar region (*arrow*), without erosion of the sellar floor or elevation of the diaphragma sellae. The preoperative diagnosis was a prolactin-secreting tumor, but at surgery a 10-mm-diameter tumor filled with dark black cyst fluid and walls with typical craniopharyngioma tissue was found and removed.

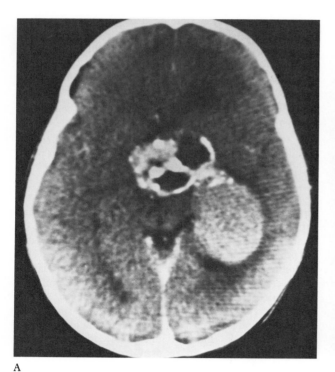

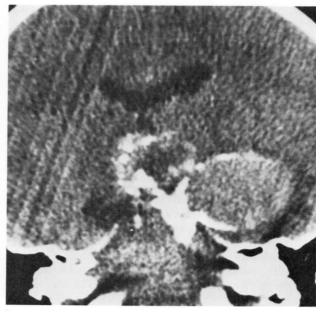

A   B

Figure 106-2 *A.* Axial enhanced CT scan in 4-year-old boy with visual loss and headaches. A large calcified mass with several large cysts is seen. The suprasellar mass is continuous with a large mass in the right temporal lobe. *B.* Coronal enhanced CT scan. A large calcification in the interpeduncular fossa extends into both the suprasellar and intratemporal portions of the tumor. The tumor has pushed through the choroid fissure to enter the right temporal horn. Distortion of the right thalamus was caused by another cystic component rostral to this section. (Compare with postoperative scans in Fig. 106-12.)

as islands of squamous cells showing stellate forms in their interior. Regressive changes in the epithelial cells may vary from cellular liquefaction to cellular swelling with deposition of keratin-like material. The central stroma may degenerate and lead to cyst formation. Cysts may coalesce to produce large cystic components. Cyst walls may vary from thin, diaphanous membranes to thick, tough structures which may be hard and rigid because of calcium salt deposition. Calcification is found on microscopic examination in approximately half of adult craniopharyngiomas and in almost all those in children.[40]

Craniopharyngiomas often cause an intense glial reaction in subjacent brain. This is particularly dense around small papillary tumor projections toward the hypothalamus. Some authors have stated that traction on this glial attachment will always lead to hypothalamic infarction and thus preclude safe total removal of the tumor.[19] However, the attachment to the nervous system has proved to be very limited in some cases. Hoffman et al. reported autopsy findings in two children with large tumors in which the only attachment of the tumor was at the tuber cinereum.[17] Others have reported similar experiences, especially in cystic tumors of the papillary type.[35] Moreover, others have found that this "glial envelope" often provides a plane in which to dissect without damaging neural tissue.[41]

Craniopharyngiomas may be adherent to major arteries at the base of the brain. The internal carotid artery was the only site of attachment preventing total removal in 6 of a series of 23 children.[17] In the author's experience, tumor remaining after attempted total removal was more likely to be adherent to a major artery than to the hypothalamus or chiasm.[8] It may be that the mesenchymal reaction of the vessel wall to tumor produces a tougher and more tenacious attachment than glial proliferation does.

Craniopharyngiomas in the suprasellar region derive their blood supply from small arterial feeders arising from the anterior cerebral and anterior communicating arteries or from the internal carotid and posterior communicating arteries. Pertuiset makes the important point that craniopharyngiomas do not receive blood supply from the posterior cerebral arteries or from the basilar artery bifurcation unless the blood supply of the floor of the third ventricle is parasitized,[35] a fact basic to removal of retrosellar portions of tumors. Within the sella, the tumor may be supplied via small arteries penetrating the dura of the cavernous sinuses.

Occasional cases of extremely aggressive craniopharyngiomas with rapid growth and recurrence are reported, but it is generally held that these tumors do not undergo malignant degeneration. Matson and Crigler specifically denied that craniopharyngiomas invade the brain.[29]

Incidence

Craniopharyngiomas are variously reported to constitute between 2.5 and 4 percent of all brain tumors.[11,20] Since almost half these tumors occur in childhood, their incidence in children is higher; they constituted 9 percent of Matson's series of childhood tumors, in which craniopharyngioma was the most common nonglial tumor.[28] When the differential diagnosis is limited to tumors of the sellar-chiasmatic region, craniopharyngiomas constitute a majority in children (54 percent) but only 20 percent in adults.[23]

The age distribution in a series of 109 patients[8] is shown in Figure 106-3. This graph shows the preponderance in childhood years, with peak incidence from age 5 to 10 years. However, craniopharyngiomas may become symptomatic at any age, with the oldest in this series being 71 at time of operation.[40] The tumor occurs with equal frequency in both sexes throughout life. Although a male preponderance in children has been reported,[23] this is not supported by two recent reports of large series of children with equal sex distribution.[8,17]

Symptoms and Signs

Although the suprasellar region has a high potential for production of neurological deficits with expanding lesions, there may be some variation in presenting complaints, and adults and children have dissimilar clinical syndromes. These differences are summarized in Tables 106-1 and 106-2. Since craniopharyngiomas are slow-growing, extra-axial tumors, they may reach quite large size before causing symptoms, especially in children. Many of these tumors in children obstruct CSF pathways and present with increased intracranial pressure. In addition, children will tolerate surprising degrees of visual loss without complaint and may continue school and watch television without arousing the suspicions of parents or teachers despite severe deficits (in one case complete visual loss in one eye and a major field cut in the other).

Adults are much more sensitive to visual impairment, and it is almost a uniform complaint of adult patients. A

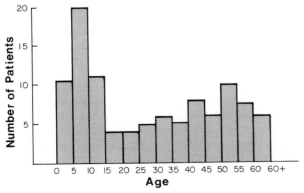

Figure 106-3 Age distribution in a series of 109 patients operated on for craniopharyngioma.

TABLE 106-1 Initial Complaints in Craniopharyngioma *

	Children,%	Adults,%
Headache	80	30
Nausea/vomiting	60	20
Visual loss	40	80
Short stature	30	15
Mentation disturbance	5	15
Diplopia	10	20

*Based on data from Banna,[4] Banna et al.,[5] Cobb and Youmans,[11] and Carmel.[8]

notable exception are patients with purely intrasellar lesions. In institutions treating large numbers of women with complaints of amenorrhea or infertility, a higher proportion of intrasellar tumors is now found than was reported in series of even a decade ago.

Psychiatric symptoms are difficult to diagnose in children, and most examples are found in adults, usually in association with hydrocephalus. Decreases in mentation (especially memory), apathy, incontinence, depression, and hypersomnia may be noted. Long-standing mentation deficits or depression are associated with a poor prognosis.[6] Kahn and coworkers found the marked mental changes of Korsakoff's syndrome in 3 of 12 adult patients.[18]

Diagnosis

Contemporary x-ray technology allows accurate preoperative diagnosis in almost all cases of craniopharyngioma. Two-thirds of the adults and almost all the children will have pathological changes on plain skull films.[4,30,35] The most common plain film changes are enlargement or erosion of the sella and tumor calcification either within or above the sella (Fig. 106-4A). Half of all patients will have sellar enlargement, and those with major suprasellar components show erosion of the dorsum sellae and anterior clinoids. Radiographically identifiable plain film tumor calcification is found in approximately 85 percent of childhood craniopharyngiomas, while only 40 percent of adults had similar calcification.[30,40]

The CT scan has dramatically changed the diagnostic workup for these tumors and in some cases, especially in younger children, has been the sole diagnostic study other than plain films. Computed tomographic scanning distinguishes areas of dense calcification, often identifies cysts, and allows delineation of soft tissue portions of a tumor following intravenous injection of a contrast agent (Fig. 106-4).

TABLE 106-2 Initial Findings in Craniopharyngioma *

	Children,%	Adults,%
Papilledema	40	10
Visual defects	70	85
Endocrine dysfunction	90	70
Cranial nerve palsy	25	25
Psychiatric abnormality	<10	20

*Based on data from Banna,[4] Banna et al.,[5] Cobb and Youmans,[11] and Carmel.[8]

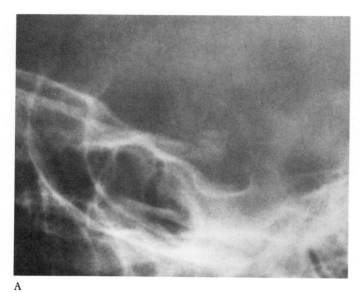

A

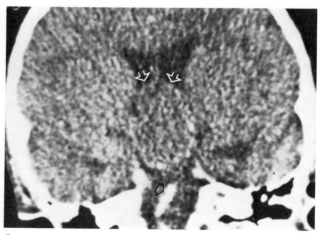

Figure 106-4 A 6-year-old boy with visual loss, hydrocephalus, and growth arrest. *A.* Lateral skull film shows posterior clinoids and dorsum sellae eroded and sellar floor distorted. Large calcification is seen at tip of a sharpened anterior clinoid. *B.* Coronal enhanced CT scan. Hydrocephalus had been controlled by a shunting procedure 10 days earlier. A large piece of calcium is seen at the inferior border of the tumor, and there is calcification throughout the tumor wall. The calcification and distorted vessels of the circle of Willis serve to outline the tumor (*arrows*). Despite its rounded appearance, this tumor was only partially cystic. *C.* Coronal enhanced CT scan, in a plane caudal to that of *B.* The tumor has completely filled the third ventricle from below, obstructing both foramina of Monro (*white arrows*). The basilar artery is seen in the interpeduncular fossa below the tumor (*black arrow*), but it did not supply the tumor. (See also Figs. 106-8 and 106-10.)

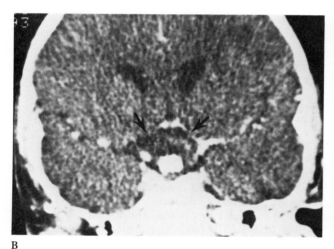

B   C

Cyst fluid may be of low density, indistinguishable from CSF, or may appear densely solid if it contains sufficient suspended calcium salts.[33] Coronal scanning should be employed to identify intrasellar extension, relation to the third ventricle, degree of obstruction of CSF pathways, and, perhaps most important, impingement of tumor on the basal subarachnoid spaces. Almost all craniopharyngiomas may be reached via a subfrontal approach, but coronal scanning will reveal those rare wholly intraventricular tumors that may require a transcallosal route.

Angiography may be useful in helping to plan the operative approach to these tumors but is rarely diagnostic. Some authors have found it helpful in determining the arterial supply to the tumor. However, the vessels that directly supply this lesion are usually quite small, and the author has not been able to identify them.

Radioisotope scanning is usually positive in these patients[30] but cannot distinguish craniopharyngiomas from many other suprasellar tumors and does not delineate the relation of the tumor to neural structures. Electroencephalography is abnormal in most patients with craniopharyn-

giomas,[35] but this abnormality is diffuse, not diagnostic, and of limited usefulness. A possible exception is in those patients who present with seizure disorders and who may have structural lesions within the medial temporal lobe.

Until the advent of CT scanning, the diagnostic procedure of choice was air encephalography, using either lumbar or ventricular injection. Positive contrast injection was also employed via ventriculography. These methods are quite sensitive, and several excellent descriptions of them are available.[29,35] The risks of tonsilar herniation with lumbar puncture in patients who have increased pressure, and the need for a surgical procedure with ventriculography, have made both less desirable methods than CT scanning. In those adult patients who do not have increased intracranial pressure, computed tomography after injection of water-soluble contrast material into the CSF may be employed. This method is useful in outlining isodense cysts or those which have poor enhancement with intravenous contrast injection (Fig. 106-5).

Endocrine assessment is usually employed preoperatively. These tests are not diagnostic but indicate those pa-

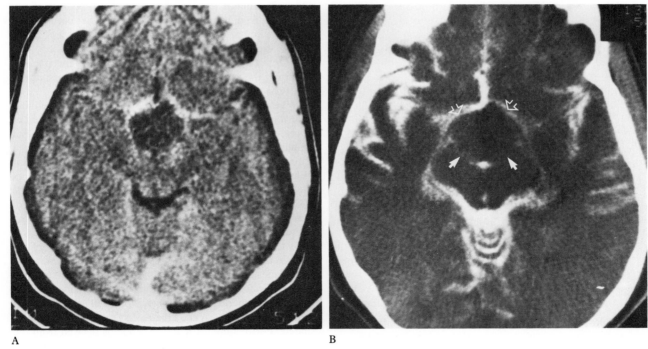

A   B

Figure 106-5   *A.* Axial enhanced scan of 24-year-old man with visual loss. The large mass enhances poorly, and the only real definition is provided by the enhanced vessels of the circle of Willis. No calcification was seen on the unenhanced scan. *B.* Axial scan following intrathecal metrizamide injection. The tumor is delineated anterior to the mesencephalon. The cerebral peduncles are pushed apart by the posterior aspect of the tumor (*closed arrows*), while the basal vessels are stretched over its anterior surface (*open arrows*).

tients at higher risk endocrinologically. Both hypoadrenalism and hypothyroidism may contribute to poor intra- or postoperative results.[8] Hypoadrenalism is correctable and is adequately treated by the high dosages of steroid used in contemporary cranial surgery. Hypothyroidism takes longer to correct, and correction should be attempted preoperatively if the patient shows clinical manifestations of decreased thyroid function or has mentation deficits and if the need for surgical intervention is not pressing. If endocrine results are not available and if the need to decrease intracranial pressure is urgent, shunting or external drainage may be employed and the major operation deferred.

Surgical Treatment

Operative Procedure

Hydrocephalus is present in many craniopharyngioma patients, and this complicating factor must be considered before definitive therapy is attempted. Ventricular drainage can decompress preoperative hydrocephalus, aid in obtaining necessary retraction intraoperatively, and control postoperative pressure if CSF pathways are not re-established. An alternative method is to perform a ventricular shunt, delaying a definitive procedure until the ventricles have decompressed and the patient has stabilized. Bilateral shunting

may be required if the tumor has obstructed both foramina of Monro.

Craniopharyngiomas are usually approached through a large right frontotemporal flap. This restricts retraction to the nondominant hemisphere and allows greater freedom for the right-handed surgeon. However, a left frontal or (rarely) a bifrontal approach may be indicated if there is major tumor extension into the left frontal or middle fossa. The bone flap should be as low as possible along the base of the frontal fossa, but the medial burr hole may be placed higher to avoid the frontal sinus. The lateral portion of the sphenoid wing is extensively removed with rongeurs or an air drill before the dura is opened. The approach to the tumor is extra-axial, through either a subfrontal or a frontotemporal route. The subfrontal approach allows better exposure of both optic nerves but does not give good access to the area beneath the ipsilateral optic nerve and tract. The frontotemporal route, opening the rostral sylvian fissure, is the most direct route to the parasellar region and allows visualization of the retrosellar area.[2] Once the suprasellar region is exposed, the operating microscope is brought into position, and dissection may employ several of the available pathways (Fig. 106-6). These include:

1. **The subchiasmatic pathway**   This is the traditional approach between the optic nerves.
2. **The opticocarotid pathway**   This is an excellent route, between the right internal carotid artery and the right

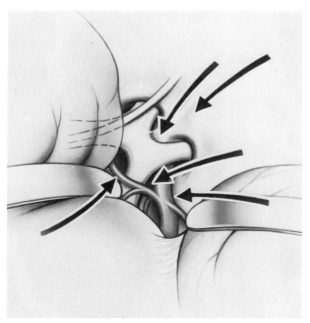

Figure 106-6 Subfrontal approach to the suprasellar region indicating the modifications available to expose the tumor. The top two arrows indicate (1) the subchiasmatic route and (2) the approach by drilling away a portion of the tuberculum sellae. Approaches lateral to the optic nerve and tract, shown by lower arrows on right, include routes (1) between the nerve and the carotid artery and (2) lateral to the carotid. The arrow on the left indicates the approach by opening the lamina terminalis. (From Antunes et al.[2])

optic nerve and tract, when the chiasm has been pushed forward by tumor and appears to be prefixed with shortened optic nerves.

3. **The lamina terminalis** The lamina terminalis may be exposed above the chiasm and divided between the optic tracts. Opening the lamina does not often expose the tumor, as it is covered by the thinned floor of the third ventricle. However, it is then possible to displace the mass downward and remove it subchiasmatically or laterally as described by Matson.[28]

4. **Lateral to the carotid artery** Opening the arachnoid at the rostral end of the sylvian fissure and retracting the temporal pole may give access to the lateral tumor surface.

5. **The transfrontal-trans-sphenoidal pathway** This route has recently been described by Patterson and Danylevich.[34] It requires drilling or chiseling away the tuberculum sellae, opening the sphenoid sinus, and removing the anterior sellar wall. This is useful when the chiasm is prefixed and may be employed with opening of the lamina terminalis. The author finds a more restricted drilling of the tuberculum to be adequate and tries not to enter the sphenoid sinus, leaving its mucosa intact.

As the tumor is approached, each of the possible routes is evaluated and the greatest possible exposure of the tumor surface is sought. When the tumor is retrochiasmatic in po-

sition, the chiasm will appear to be prefixed because of displacement from behind (Fig. 106-7). Much has been written of "short" optic nerves, but some of the "prefixity" is lost during the course of operation (Fig. 106-8). Lateral displacement of the optic tract is due to a similar mechanism, distorting the tract and decreasing the space between its lateral surface and the carotid artery.

When a portion of the tumor is exposed, the arachnoid covering the tumor is carefully opened. Care is taken not to coalesce the arachnoid with the tumor capsule by the use of cautery, as preservation of the subarachnoid CSF plane is a requisite for safe and total tumor removal. A needle is inserted into the tumor and the cyst is aspirated. All tumors should be aspirated, even those which appear solid on the CT scan, since these may be partially cystic, and removal of only 1 or 2 ml may provide room for dissection. Entering the tumor with a small microsuction tip will further decompress the tumor. As the tumor mass decreases, more of the capsule may be exposed by dissecting in the subarachnoid CSF plane around the tumor. Small arterial feeders from the anterior circulation to the tumor may be coagulated and divided, remembering that the plexus of small arterial feeders to the undersurface of the chiasm and optic tracts must be spared. Fortunately, little blood supply is derived from the posterior portion of the circle of Willis, and the caudal surface of these tumors is usually, but not always, less adherent. The interior of the tumor is entered and the solid portion removed piecemeal. As these fragments are removed, care must be taken to protect the optic nerve and tract, especially from the calcified fragments. Larger calcifications should be crushed to appropriate size for removal. As the tumor is progressively gutted, portions of the capsule may be resected. It is important however, not to "lose the handle," for the capsule will retract upward out of sight and may prove impossible to retrieve. After tumor attachments

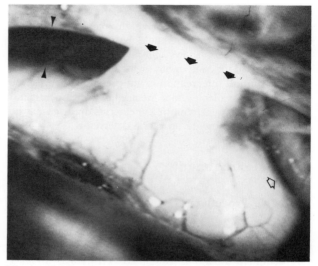

Figure 106-7 Exposure of chiasm, right optic nerve, and tract (same case as in Fig. 106-4). The right optic nerve (*closed arrows*) appears short, and the prechiasmatic opening between the arrowheads measured approximately 1.5 mm. The optic tract is distorted laterally (*open arrow*). (Compare with Fig. 106-8.)

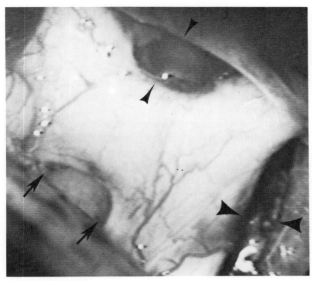

Figure 106-8 Operative exposure of the anterior visual system and floor of the third ventricle (same case as in Fig. 106-7). An angled micromirror had revealed residual tumor beneath the ventricle. The lamina terminalis was opened (*black arrows*), and the tumor fragment was manipulated through the floor and prechiasmatic space. The fragment was then removed via the space between the nerve and the carotid artery (*large arrowheads*). Note that the chiasm has moved away from the tuberculum sellae (*small arrowheads*) and the nerves are no longer "short." (See also Fig. 106-10.)

to the optic apparatus, hypothalamus, and basal arterial vessels are dissected with higher microscopic magnification, the tumor remnant usually delivers easily. Small angled dental mirrors are then used to inspect the undersurface of the chiasm and the median eminence region for tumor remnants.

Preserving the Pituitary Stalk

The pituitary stalk is necessary for the resumption of normal pituitary responses, and its preservation is now technically possible with microscopic visualization.[16,35] Even if damaged, a remnant of stalk reaching from the median eminence to the pituitary will serve as a matrix upon which the important portal system may re-form.[9] Recognition of the stalk is basic to its preservation. Under higher powers of magnification the stalk has a striate pattern that is distinctive among neural structures (Fig. 106-9). This striation is caused by the parallel arrangement of the long portal veins and is maintained despite severe distortion of the stalk. Once the stalk is visualized, it is often possible to dissect the tumor away without sacrificing the stalk (Fig. 106-10). While the stalk has been described as lying on the posterior surface of the tumor,[35] it may be found displaced laterally or anterolaterally as well. Patients with an intact stalk appear to regain endocrine function more quickly and completely than other patients, and a case has been described of total removal without postoperative diabetes insipidus.[16]

Staged Procedures

It may occasionally be desirable or necessary to perform a two-stage procedure in order to achieve total tumor removal. Koos and Miller have described a procedure in which intracranial removal of the suprasellar portion of the tumor was followed by trans-sphenoidal removal of intrasellar tumor at a later operation.[23] The author has used this method in order to preserve the stalk and pituitary displaced by a tumor with both intrasellar and suprasellar components, as shown in Figure 106-11.

Portions of the tumor may extend in a manner that may make access to the entire tumor by any single route hazardous or unfeasible. The tumor illustrated in Figure 106-2 had large suprasellar, retrosellar, and third ventricular components. A portion of the tumor had pushed laterally through the choroid fissure, and a large component was located within the temporal horn. Midline portions of the tumor were removed via a subfrontal approach at the first operation, and the temporal cyst was aspirated through its medial surface (Fig. 106-12A). The calcified portion within the temporal horn and a large calcified interpeduncular fragment were excised in a subsequent transtemporal procedure (Fig. 106-12B).

False Cure

Virtually every large series of craniopharyngiomas has reported recurrences of tumor after "total" removal. Amacher has reviewed several series and has documented 17 recurrences after 92 total removals.[1] Other reports show that even use of the operating microscope and careful examination with micromirrors may not prevent the operator from thinking that total removal has been achieved when it has not.[7] Routine use of CT scanning postoperatively will reveal many, if not all, of these residual tumor fragments. When CT scanning in the postoperative period is required as an additional criterion of total removal, the false cure rate may be expected to fall.

Postoperative Management

Most patients who undergo total or radical subtotal removal of tumor will have either temporary or permanent disruption of neurohypophyseal axis function. Damage to the stalk or pituitary may result in various endocrine deficiencies, of which loss of ACTH and antidiuretic hormone (ADH) will be notable in the immediate postoperative period. Loss of other endocrine functions is important in the long-term management of these patients.

Lack of corticosteroid production secondary to loss of ACTH production is rarely a problem in patients who are receiving large doses of high-potency synthetic corticosteroids, used in most centers to control cerebral swelling. Because these synthetic steroids have little mineralocorticoid effect, some have advocated use of cortisone acetate in physiological doses in addition to the high-potency agents. As the risk of edema lessens, the synthetic steroids are progressively tapered off, and cortisone replacement in physiological dosage is given. These patients must be regarded as

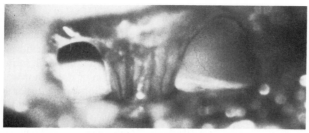

Figure 106-9 Striate pattern of long portal vessels on the pituitary stalk, seen in an operative exposure in the rhesus monkey. The appearance in humans is quite similar, and this striation is unique among suprasellar neural structures.

being hypoadrenal at all times, and death of a patient during a metyrapone test has been reported.[17]

Diabetes insipidus is noted shortly after operation but may begin during the surgical procedure; it is initially best managed by fluid replacement. If excessive thirst or fluid replacement problems become difficult for the patient, vasopressin may be given, preferably in a short-acting form. Patients who have diabetes insipidus due to stalk section may have subsequent involution of neurohypophyseal axons or infarction of a portion of the pituitary, caused by interruption of the blood supply from the portal vessels. ADH may then be released from the degenerating axon terminals in supraphysiological amounts. These events, when they occur, usually take place from 48 to 96 h after stalk damage. Patients who have been given long-acting vasopressin may be at risk for renal shutdown under these circumstances.

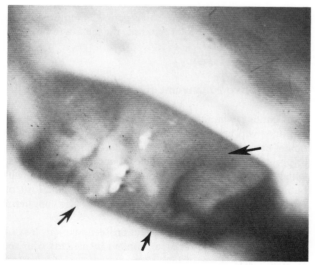

Figure 106-10 Pituitary stalk preserved after removal of tumor (same case as in Figs. 106-4, 106-7, and 106-8). The stalk is seen beneath the optic chiasm (*double arrows*) and runs down to penetrate the diaphragma sellae (*single arrow*). Instruments gently retract the medial surfaces of both optic nerves.

Experience at many centers, including the author's, with synthetic DDAVP (desmopressin acetate) spray has been satisfactory. Determinations of intake and output of fluid, urine specific gravity, and rate of urinary excretion at 2-h or 3-h intervals are helpful in the immediate postoperative period. Daily or twice daily blood counts, serum electrolyte determinations, and accurate patient weight measurements are also needed.

Operative deaths are usually attributed to hypothalamic injury, which causes a clinical syndrome characterized by hyperpyrexia and somnolence. Damage to osmoreceptors in the anterior hypothalamus may lead to loss of the sensation of thirst.[7] Patients are then difficult to manage, as thirst is a major factor in the treatment of the concomitant diabetes insipidus. Other postsurgical hypothalamic deficits may include disturbance of caloric balance, changes in wakefulness, changes in affective behavior, and disturbances of memory.[7]

Results

Mortality rates following attempts at surgical removal of craniopharyngiomas vary widely but range from 5 to 10 percent in most series.[38] There is little doubt that total excision is the treatment of choice, if it can be achieved without injury to the patient. Excellent results with attempted radical removal are reported, including some series with zero mortality[8,29] or very low risk.[15,17,41] Other workers regard craniopharyngiomas as malignant tumors because of their location and manner of growth and think that no forceful attempt at total extirpation should be made.[31] They regard operation as merely palliative and believe that partial resection followed by radiation therapy should be the rule.

Subtotal or partial resection alone is rarely satisfactory treatment for these tumors, which are likely to recur over a period of time. Recurrence has a strong adverse affect on survival, as shown in Table 106-3. These data indicate that less than 10 percent of both adults and children are still recurrence-free 10 years after subtotal removal. Craniopharyngiomas have been reported to be quiescent for years after partial resection,[35] but most that are subtotally removed recur within a few years (Fig. 106-13). Those tumors which are radically removed but recur do so after a much longer time interval.[8,41] Patients with subtotal removal of the tumor will probably require further therapy by either radiation or reoperation.

TABLE 106-3 Course after Partial Tumor Removal*

Follow-up Interval, Years	Percent Surviving	Percent Relapse-free
Children (n=15)		
5	71.4	14.3
10	52.1	7.1
Adults (n=25)		
5	36.9	16.4
10	30.7	9.8

*Data from Sung et al.,[40] expressed on an actuarial basis.

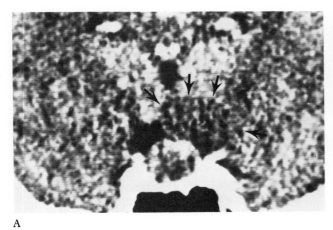

A

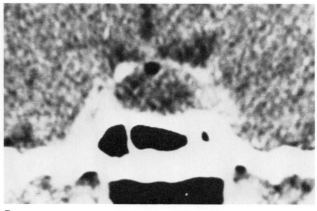

B

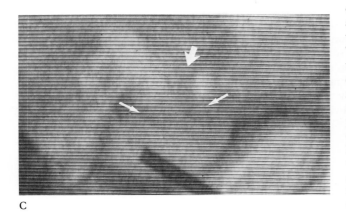

C

Figure 106-11 *A.* Coronal enhanced scan in young man with supra- and intrasellar tumor. The thalamic region is distorted by the suprasellar portion, which extends upward and to the right (*arrows*). After this portion of the tumor was removed, the intrasellar cyst was entered from above. The solid intrasellar tumor could not be totally removed while sparing the stalk, and a two-stage procedure was elected. The diaphragma sellae was closed with a pericranial graft. *B.* Coronal scan 1 month after the first operation. The intrasellar cyst has refilled, pushing the diaphragm upward. The stalk is intact above the sella. The dark lucency at the diaphragm is a small piece of fat adherent to the pericranial graft. *C.* Lateral image-intensified view taken during subsequent trans-sphenoidal operation. Air has been injected intrathecally and outlines the pituitary stalk (*upper arrow*). The sella has been emptied, and the diaphragm curves downward (*lower arrows*).

Radiation

It was long doubtful whether radiation therapy could destroy craniopharyngioma epithelium[17] and whether it had a role in treatment of these tumors. In 1961, Kramer and his colleagues reported a group of six children and four adults who had been treated with radiation therapy prior to 1954. All six of the children survived at follow-up periods approaching 20 years. Results in adults were much poorer. Since this initial report, many have indicated that radiation therapy both increases survival and prolongs the interval before tumor recurrence.[15,24,25,37,40] The survival rates for patients treated with surgery and radiotherapy are better than for those treated with surgery alone; the recurrence-free survival rates are improved to an even greater extent.[40] Comparison of surgery alone and surgery with radiotherapy in the series of Sung et al. is shown in Figure 106-14.

The effectiveness of radiotherapy has led some groups to advocate a conservative operative approach for craniopharyngioma.[37] However, Shapiro and coworkers have described better recurrence-free rates for patients under-

going "radical subtotal removal" before radiotherapy than for those with biopsy and cyst drainage prior to radiation.[38]

Radiotherapy is not without hazard. Radiation necrosis, endocrine deficiency, optic neuritis, and dementia have all been reported as complications of radiation therapy.[8] Many neurosurgeons have expressed concern for intellectual performance after irradiation in children.[1] Conservative operation followed by radiation therapy probably sacrifices the potential for cure. An attempt at radical surgical resection may result in greater damage to the hypothalamus and neuroendocrine axis, and recent reviews have stressed that radical removal of these tumors is strongly dependent on the experience of the surgeon.[11,35] Final agreement on the optimum initial therapy for craniopharyngioma certainly has not been reached.

There has not been any greater unanimity of opinion for radiotherapy in the treatment of recurrent tumors than for radiotherapy as the initial treatment. Some surgeons who advocate radical tumor resection at initial operation advise against reoperation for recurrence as being unduly hazardous,[41] and radiation therapy following CT scan evidence of recurrence has been recommended.[17] In recent years there

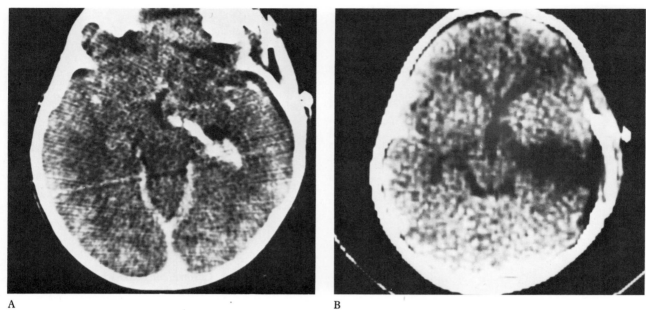

A   B

Figure 106-12 *A*. Postoperative axial enhanced scan of the same patient as in Figure 106-2. The suprasellar portion of the tumor has been removed, as well as much of the temporal mass. A large solid piece of calcification is adherent to the right cerebral peduncle and extends into the temporal horn. *B*. Axial scan after a second operation. The tumor has been approached through the temporal horn of the right lateral ventricle. After the intraventricular portion of the tumor was removed, the choroid fissure was opened and the interpeduncular portion was also removed.

has been an increasing tendency at the author's institution to reoperate on children with recurrence. The experience there indicates that reoperation can be undertaken successfully, either electively or in the presence of renewed tumor symptoms, with only slightly higher risk than for the primary operation.[8] This treatment protocol must be regarded as experimental until greater numbers of patients have been treated in this fashion.

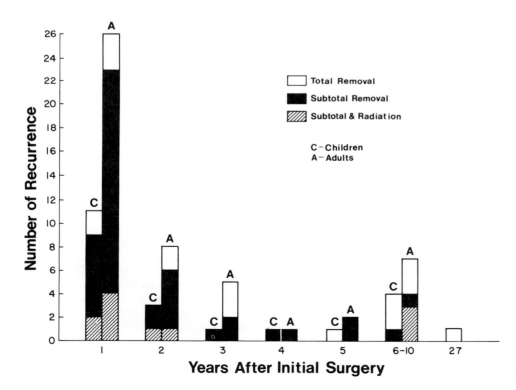

Figure 106-13 Time of recurrence of craniopharyngioma in 22 children and 49 adults. The majority of recurrences occurred in the first postoperative year, and relatively few occurred more than 3 years after operation. Exceptions were those tumors that recurred after "total" removal, a situation in which late recurrences are more common.

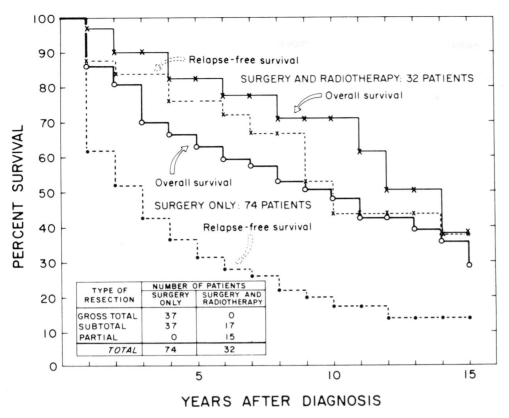

Figure 106-14 Actuarial survival and relapse-free survival rates. Lines with *x* indicate surgery and radiotherapy as initial therapy; lines with *o* indicate surgery only as initial therapy. Overall survival (*solid lines*); relapse-free survival (*dashed lines*).

Cystic tumors may be treated by the introduction of radioisotopes into the cavity. This technique was pioneered by Leksell more than thirty years ago and was coupled with stereotactic placement in the treatment of a wide variety of tumor types.[26] The initial agent used was phosphorus (^{32}P), and dosage was determined by an ingenious volume dilution method. ^{32}P is a beta-emitting isotope and was aspirated with the cyst fluid. ^{32}P was later replaced with ^{90}Y, which has somewhat greater tissue penetration. ^{198}Au was also used in earlier therapy, but because of its emission of gamma as well as beta rays, radiation occasionally penetrated beyond the tumor capsule. Recent advances in dosimetry and administration have refocused attention on this isotope.[21,22] Intracystic isotope treatment is limited to those craniopharyngiomas which have a large volume cystic component and is not applicable to solid tumors or tumors with very thick or calcified walls. Reports on this therapy indicate the advantages of little operative trauma and less long-term endocrine and intellectual deficit than with external radiation therapy.[22] Further experience with a greater number of patients at many centers will be required to compare this method with other forms of therapy.

References

1. Amacher AL: Craniopharyngioma: The controversy regarding radiotherapy. Childs Brain 6:57–64, 1980.
2. Antunes JL, Muraszko K, Quest DO, Carmel PW: Surgical strategies in the management of tumours of the anterior third ventricle, in Brock M (ed): *Modern Neurosurgery*. Berlin, Springer-Verlag, 1982.
3. Backlund EO: Studies on craniopharyngiomas: III. Stereotaxic treatment with intracystic yttrium-90. Acta Chir Scand 139:237–247, 1973.
4. Banna M: Craniopharyngioma in adults. Surg Neurol 1:202–204, 1973.
5. Banna M, Hoare RD, Stanley P, Till K: Craniopharyngioma in children. J Pediatr 83:781–785, 1973.
6. Bartlett JR: Craniopharyngiomas: An analysis of some aspects of symptomatology, radiology and histology. Brain 94:725–732, 1971.
7. Carmel PW: Surgical syndromes of the hypothalamus. Clin Neurosurg 27:133–159, 1979.
8. Carmel PW, Antunes JL, Chang CH: Craniopharyngiomas in children. Neurosurgery 11:382–389, 1982.
9. Carmel PW, Antunes JL, Ferin M: Collection of blood from the pituitary stalk and portal veins in monkeys, and from the pituitary sinusoidal system of monkey and man. J Neurosurg 50:75–80, 1979.
10. Carmichael HT: Squamous epithelial rests in the hypophysis cerebri. Arch Neurol Psychiatry 26:966–975, 1931.
11. Cobb CA, Youmans JR: Brain tumors of disordered embryogenesis in adults, in Youmans JR (ed): *Neurological Surgery*, 2d ed. Philadelphia, Saunders, 1982, pp 2899–2935.
12. Critchley M, Ironside RN: The pituitary adamantinomata. Brain 49:437–481, 1926.
13. Erdheim J: Ueber Hypophysengangsgeshwülste und Hirncholesteatome. Sitzungsber Akad Wiss (Wien) 113:537–726, 1904.
14. Goldberg GM, Eshbaugh DE: Squamous cell nests of the pituitary gland as related to the origin of craniopharyngiomas: A

study of their presence in the newborn and infants up to age four. Arch Pathol Lab Med 70:293–299, 1960.

15. Hoff JT, Patterson RH Jr: Craniopharyngiomas in children and adults. J Neurosurg 36:299–302, 1972.

16. Hoffman HJ: Comment on paper by Patterson RH Jr, Danylevich A. Neurosurgery 7:116–117, 1980.

17. Hoffman HJ, Hendrick EB, Humphreys RP, Buncic JR, Armstrong DL, Jenkin RDT: Management of craniopharyngioma in children. J Neurosurg 47:218–227, 1977.

18. Kahn EA, Gosch HH, Seeger JF, Hicks SP: Forty-five years experience with the craniopharyngiomas. Surg Neurol 1:5–12, 1973.

19. Kempe LG: Operative Neurosurgery: vol. I. Cranial, Cerebral and Intracranial Vascular Disease. New York, Springer-Verlag, 1968, pp 90–93.

20. Kernohan JW: Tumors of congenital origin, in Minckler J (ed): Pathology of the Nervous System. New York, McGraw Hill, 1971, pp 1927–1937.

21. Kobayashi T, Kageyama N, Ohara K: Internal irradiation for cystic craniopharyngioma. J Neurosurg 55:896–903, 1981.

22. Kodama T, Matsukado Y, Uemura S: Intracapsular irradiation therapy of craniopharyngiomas with radioactive gold: Indication and follow-up results. Neurol Med Chir (Tokyo) 21:49–58, 1981.

23. Koos WT, Miller MH: Intracranial Tumors of Infants and Children. Stuttgart, Thieme, 1971.

24. Kramer S: Craniopharyngioma: The best treatment is conservative surgery and postoperative radiation therapy, in Morley TP (ed): Current Controversies in Neurosurgery. Philadelphia, Saunders, 1976, pp 336–343.

25. Kramer S, Southard M, Mansfield CM: Radiotherapy in the management of craniopharyngiomas: Further experiences and late results. AJR 103:44–52, 1968.

26. Leksell L: Stereotaxis and Radiosurgery: An Operative System. Springfield, Ill., Charles C Thomas, 1971.

27. Luse SA, Kernohan JW: Squamous-cell rests of the pituitary gland. Cancer 8:623–628, 1955.

28. Matson DD: Neurosurgery of Infancy and Childhood, 2d ed. Springfield, Ill., Charles C Thomas, 1969, pp 544–574.

29. Matson DD, Crigler JF Jr: Management of craniopharyngioma in childhood. J Neurosurg 30:377–390, 1969.

30. Michelsen WJ, Mount LA, Renaudin J: Craniopharyngioma: A thirty-nine year survey. Acta Neurol Latinoam 18:100–106, 1972.

31. Mori K, Handa H, Murata T, Takeuchi J, Miwa S, Osaka K: Results of treatment for craniopharyngioma. Childs Brain 6:303–312, 1980.

32. Mott FW, Barrett JOW: Three cases of tumor of the third ventricle. Arch Neurol (Lond) 1:417–440, 1899.

33. Naidich TP, Pinto RS, Kushner MJ, Lin JP, Kricheff II, Leeds NE, Chase NE: Evaluation of sellar and parasellar masses by computed tomography. Radiology 120:91–99, 1976.

34. Patterson RH Jr, Danylevich A: Surgical removal of craniopharyngiomas by a transcranial approach through the lamina terminalis and sphenoid sinus. Neurosurgery 7:111–117, 1980.

35. Pertuiset B: Craniopharyngiomas, in Vinken PJ, Bruyn GW (eds): Handbook of Clinical Neurology: vol 18. Tumours of the Brain and Skull, Part III. Amsterdam, North-Holland, 1975, pp 531–572.

36. Podoshin L, Rolan L, Altman MM, Peyser E: "Pharyngeal" craniopharyngioma. J Laryngol Otol 84:93–99, 1970.

37. Richmond IL, Wara WM, Wilson CB: Role of radiation therapy in management of craniopharyngiomas in children. Neurosurgery 6:513–517, 1980.

38. Shapiro K, Till K, Grant DN: Craniopharyngiomas in childhood: A rational approach to treatment. J Neurosurg 50:617–623, 1979.

39. Shuangshoti S, Netsky MG, Nashold BS: Epithelial cysts related to sella turcica: Proposed origin from neuroepithelium. Arch Pathol Lab Med 90:444–450, 1970.

40. Sung DI, Chang CH, Harisiadis L, Carmel PW: Treatment results of craniopharyngiomas. Cancer 47:847–852, 1981.

41. Sweet WH: Recurrent craniopharyngiomas: Therapeutic alternatives. Clin Neurosurg 27:206–229, 1980.

107

Optic Gliomas

Edgar M. Housepian
Merlin D. Marquardt
Myles Behrens

Astrocytomas of the visual pathways are being recognized with increasing frequency; the clinical diagnosis is not difficult, particularly in children, and the advent of computed tomography has made the precise diagnosis of optic nerve tumors relatively commonplace. As the natural course of the disease and the results of various forms of therapy have become better known, there has come to be less controversy regarding treatment of optic nerve and chiasmal gliomas.

Histopathology

The optic nerve is a myelinated extension of the central nervous system, invested with dura, arachnoid, and pia. The myelinated axons of the optic nerve, extensions of the retinal ganglion cells, are supported by oligodendroglia and astroglia. The optic nerve with its meninges has a slightly sinuous course in the orbit, the length allowing for unrestricted movement of the eye. Throughout most of its course the approximately one million fibers of each optic nerve are incompletely separated into about a thousand fascicles by fibrovascular pial septa that are internal extensions of the relatively thick fibrous pia that intimately invests the nerve.

Fine fibrous trabeculae traverse the subarachnoid space between the pia and arachnoid. There is a continuous subarachnoid space from the cranial cavity through the optic canal to the sclera. This subarachnoid space is partially obliterated at the annulus of Zinn, where the meninges are partially fused with the origins of the extraocular muscles. The arachnoid is closely but loosely apposed to the thick, fibrous dura. Clusters of meningothelial cells, so called arachnoidal cap cells, are found in the arachnoid of the normal optic nerve. These cells are believed to give rise to primary meningiomas of the optic nerve.

Optic gliomas apparently arise from the astroglia of the optic nerve.[12,15,18] Oligodendroglial elements are occasionally present, but neoplastic astrocytic cells are usually the predominant component. Astrocytomas of the optic nerve share certain histological features with astrocytomas of the cerebellum and brain stem. Most optic gliomas are histologically benign neoplasms; this, in association with their frequently indolent course, gave rise to consideration of a hamartomatous process. Occasional malignant optic gliomas have been reported in both adults and children.[9,19] The clinical aggressiveness of optic gliomas seems to be partly or perhaps largely related to the primary location of the glioma, which may in turn be associated with the presence or absence of neurofibromatosis.[6,14] The more aggressive chiasmal gliomas tend to invade the hypothalamus and produce hydrocephalus by foraminal obstruction.

Most astrocytomas of the optic nerve are composed of highly elongated astrocytic cells with long, fine fibrillary processes. Because of the latter feature they are often called *pilocytic astrocytomas, juvenile pilocytic astrocytomas,* or *piloid astrocytomas.* In addition to the elongated bipolar cells with long hairlike processes, multipolar or stellate forms may be present. Especially in regions of transition from neoplasm to nerve, neoplastic astrocytes may be nearly indistinguishable from reactive astrocytes. Nuclei of neoplastic astrocytes are slightly hyperchromatic and mildly to moderately pleomorphic. Cells in mitosis are extremely rare. The fibrillar astrocytic processes stain blue with phosphotungstic acid hemotoxylin stain. Rosenthal fibers—intensely staining irregular hyaline structures composed of electron-dense material and associated glial filaments—are frequently present in the astroglial processes of the neoplastic astrocytes in pilocytic astrocytomas of the optic nerve. The neoplastic astrocytes proliferate within the fascicles of the optic nerve, tending to be aligned with their long processes nearly parallel to the long axis of the nerve. The processes may also form a mesh with small cystic spaces containing mucoid material demonstrable with an alcian blue stain;[1] this extracellular material may be elaborated by the neoplastic astrocytes.

Neoplastic astrocytes may invade and thicken the pial septa of the nerve. Proliferation and expansion of both the fascicles and pial septa may occur, with enlargement and preservation of the general structure of the optic nerve. In some instances there may be remarkable sparing of nerve fibers within fascicles that are extensively and diffusely infiltrated by neoplastic astrocytes. The sparing of these neural elements may be demonstrated with appropriate special stains for axons and myelin sheaths.

The neoplasm in the nerve may extend through the pia surrounding the nerve and into the subarachnoid space, where it characteristically provokes an exuberant proliferation of reactive fibroblasts and hyperplasia of meningothelial cells. In the leptomeninges the histological appearance of the astrocytoma is usually somewhat different from its appearance in the optic nerve. The fascicular pattern is less evident. Neoplastic astrocytes become intermixed with reactive fibroblasts, collagenous fibers, reticulin fibers, and meningothelial cells. Neoplastic astrocytes may be so intimately intermingled with fibroblasts as to be difficult to recognize and identify. There may be quite marked and extensive fibrosis in the subarachnoid space. Although invasion of the leptomeninges by an astrocytoma of the optic nerve is common, infiltration of the dura and extradural extension of an astrocytoma is extremely rare. However, recurrence with invasion of orbital tissues after incomplete resection of an optic glioma has been seen.

Hyperplasia of the arachnoidal meningothelial cells, with accompanying leptomeningial fibrosis, has been reported[13] in cases of astrocytoma but has not been proved in the absence of tumor.

Optic nerve gliomas have two different patterns of growth (Fig. 107-1). In one, growth is largely confined to the optic nerve, with minimal involvement of the leptomeninges and little or no reactive alteration in the leptomeninges. In the other there is extensive invasion and growth in the subarachnoid space, often with a marked proliferative fibroblastic response and hyperplasia of meningothelial cells. It has been suggested that the pattern of extraneural growth of the glioma in the subarachnoid space is especially characteristic of optic gliomas in patients with neurofibromatosis, and that the glioma tends to remain confined to the optic nerve in patients without neurofibromatosis.[15]

Clinical Diagnosis

Astrocytoma of the optic nerves and chiasm accounts for 2 percent of central nervous system tumors in adults and 7 percent of tumors in children. Optic gliomas occur with equal frequency in males and females, most commonly in childhood but also in adults; 75 percent of cases occur in the first decade and 90 percent in the first two decades. Neurofibromatosis has been associated in 20 to 30 percent. It is now recognized that there is a relatively high incidence of neurofibromatosis in patients harboring single (71 percent) or multicentric (100 percent) optic nerve astrocytomas and a low incidence of neurofibromatosis (8 percent) in patients with chiasmal glioma (Table 107-1).[6]

The diagnosis of optic nerve glioma is suggested in a child with neurofibromatosis who has painless proptosis (Fig. 107-2). There usually is a variable degree of visual loss, which may be accompanied by disc swelling or optic atrophy on ophthalmoscopy. An enlarged optic foramen or a J-shaped sella in an otherwise normal skull x-ray add confirmation.

In the majority of children with chiasmal glioma but without neurofibromatosis, the diagnosis is more difficult. Monocular or binocular visual impairment with or without optic disc pallor, often with hemianopsia, or a homonymous field defect if there is primarily optic tract involvement, may occur. An afferent pupillary defect is frequently present. However, even large chiasmal gliomas are often not associated with visual impairment. When visual loss presents in

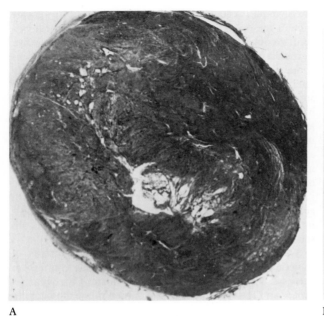

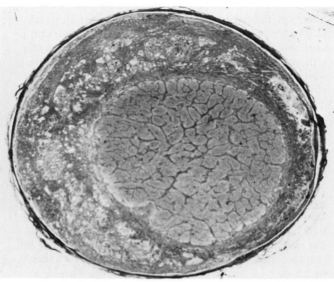

A   B

Figure 107-1 Low-power cross-sectional photomicrographs of optic nerve astrocytomas. (Hematoxylin and eosin.) *A.* Astrocytoma, with areas of microcyst formation,
disrupting fascicular configuration of the nerve; typical pattern of optic nerve tumor
in patient without neurofibromatosis. *B.* Extensive tumor infiltration of the subarachnoid space seen classically in patients with neurofibromatosis.

very young children, it may be manifested by pendular nystagmus.

Chiasmal glioma in a child[3,11] may be difficult to differentiate from hypothalamic glioma, and in some cases an
early presentation may be that of an anterior third ventricular mass with foraminal obstruction causing hydrocephalus.
Endocrinopathies in children, such as precocious puberty
and the diencephalic syndrome,[4] have also been associated
with large chiasmal gliomas. A partially calcified or cystic
chiasmal glioma may be confused with a craniopharyngioma. A chiasmal glioma in an adult can also present a diagnostic problem. The differential diagnosis in primary optic
nerve tumor is essentially between meningioma and optic
glioma, whereas chiasmal glioma must be distinguished
from other lesions, chiefly pituitary adenoma, hypothalamic
glioma, craniopharyngioma, diaphragma sellae meningioma, aneurysm, or ectopic pinealoma.

The CT scan (Fig. 107-3) has been of great help in the
diagnosis of orbital tumors because of the low-density fat

within the orbital cavity, which provides a high contrast to
the optic nerve, ocular adnexa, and extraocular muscles.[17]
Primary optic nerve tumors, gliomas, and meningiomas can
best be identified by a good quality, high-resolution CT
scan. Pneumoencephalography, however, may still provide
critical definition in cases of small chiasmal lesions. Positive
contrast studies, angiography, and venography are of little
help in the diagnosis of optic glioma. Multidirectional polytomography of the sella and optic canals may still be helpful
to define deformity, hyperostosis, dissolution, or destruction.

Treatment

In the past there was considerable disagreement as to the
efficacy of radiotherapy in the treatment of optic glioma.[2,8,16] Although reduction of proptosis and improve-

TABLE 107-1 Neurofibromatosis and the Locus of Optic Glioma

Locus of Glioma	With Neurofibromatosis		Without Neurofibromatosis		Combined Total	
	No.	%	No.	%	No.	%
Chiasm	7	8	81	92	88	69
Single optic nerve	24	71	10	29	34	26
Multicentric (both optic nerves)	6	100	0	0	6	5
	—		—		—	—
Total	37		91		128	100

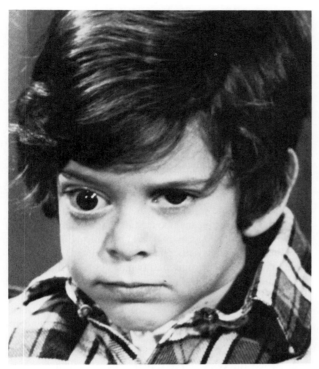

Figure 107-2 Five-year-old child with right optic nerve glioma producing proptosis and diminished visual acuity.

ment of vision was reported prior to CT scanning, objective evidence of response to radiation was difficult to document, probably because the young age of many patients made accurate visual field and acuity testing difficult. Now reduction in tumor size documented by CT scanning before and after radiation therapy has been reported.[5] The recent recognition that the natural history may differ between patients with single or multiple optic nerve tumor and non-neurofibromatosis patients with chiasmal glioma (the majority of optic glioma patients) may have some bearing on response or lack of response to radiation therapy. There is no longer any controversy regarding the treatment of chiasmal glioma with

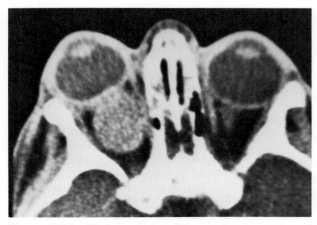

Figure 107-3 High-resolution CT scan showing tumor of the right optic nerve. Same patient as in Figure 107-2.

progressive visual symptoms: the recommended course is 4500 rad in 4 weeks by opposing ports restricted to the region of the tumor.

Nor is there much controversy regarding the appropriate treatment of solitary optic nerve tumors when they present with disfiguring proptosis and severe visual loss. Ophthalmologists and neurosurgeons concede that transcranial orbital exploration for resection of the tumor from behind the globe to the chiasm is the primary procedure of choice.[7,10] Intraoperative biopsy of a primary optic nerve tumor in an adult may be necessary to differentiate glioma from other lesions, most commonly meningiomas, inasmuch as surgical objectives and technique for the two differ. Limited direct orbital exploration and resection are not acceptable because of the potential extension of residual tumor through the optic canal to involve the chiasm. Enucleation of the globe is not usually warranted.

The place of surgery in the treatment of chiasmal lesions is simply one of definition when there is serious question as to the primary diagnosis. Although limited resection of an optic nerve tumor extending to the chiasm may be reasonable, major resection of the chiasm with attendant blindness is not acceptable. When tumor is found at the proximal stump of an optic nerve resected for appropriate indications, radiotherapy to the residual tumor at the chiasmal margin has been recommended.

The advantage of transcranial orbital exploration is obvious. It allows resection of tumor-bearing nerve from the globe to the chiasm while retaining the globe for an excellent cosmetic result (Fig. 107-4). To accomplish this, a unilateral frontal craniotomy is required. The most medial trephinations must be at the midline to allow access to the medial part of the orbit. Prior to orbital exploration, an intradural inspection of the optic nerve and chiasm is mandatory. If tumor is grossly evident, the nerve may be sectioned at this time close to the chiasm.

In many cases of optic nerve glioma, arteriolar hypervascularity surrounding the proximal optic nerve near the chiasm is seen upon intracranial inspection. Tumors extending to the prechiasmal nerve frequently appear grayish and discolored as opposed to the normal whitish nerve. If the nerve appears normal, an epidural approach to the orbit must then be made prior to nerve section. The epidural approach helps protect the underlying brain and the olfactory nerve. Orbital unroofing is started with a chisel or high-speed diamond burr and extended with small double-action bone instruments through the optic canal. Care should be taken to avoid the medially located posterior ethmoid air cells.

In the presence of an intraorbital lesion, the normal structures are flattened and blanched and difficult to see through the periorbita. A landmark structure therefore is the frontalis nerve, whose whitish appearance signals the location of the underlying levator and superior rectus muscles. The trochlear nerve is frequently seen coursing over the levator and superior rectus muscles but cannot be saved when the annulus of Zinn is to be opened for resection of tumor-bearing nerve in one piece. When vision is lost, however, there is no evident functional deficit or visible cosmetic deformity from fourth nerve paralysis.

The fine nerves to the extraocular muscles enter the mus-

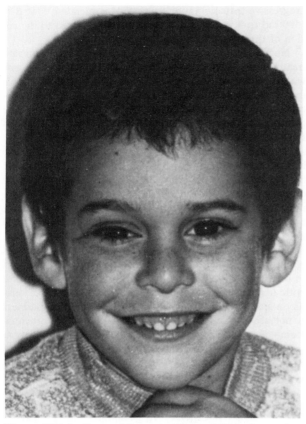

Figure 107-4 Same child as in Figure 107-2, 3 months after transcranial orbital exploration and resection of the tumor from the globe to the chiasm, showing a good cosmetic result.

cle cone through the superior orbital fissure and the oculomotor foramen and then course in a lateral to medial direction to the levator and superior rectus muscles over the optic nerve and to the inferior and medial rectus muscles below it; thus the preferred approach to the optic nerve is through the medial orbit. This allows direct access to the optic nerve without intrusion on the nerves to the extraocular muscles.

Using bayonet forceps, narrow cottonoids, and fine, malleable retractors, a plane must be developed directly on the tumor capsule and strictly adhered to (Fig. 107-5A). It is important that orbital fat not be dissected, as the fine structures within will be injured. When an orbital tumor is large and difficult to remove through a small roof defect, it must be incised and internally decompressed to allow collapse and delivery. Once the junction of the globe and tumor is palpated or visualized, it may be clamped with a fine mosquito clamp and sectioned proximal to the clamp (Fig. 107-5B).

When the diagnosis of optic glioma is proved, it is permissible to remove the specimen in two pieces from the globe to the annulus and from the intracranial optic canal to the chiasm. Residual astrocytoma in the region of the annulus may be simply electrocoagulated. In infants this technique is far simpler than that required to open the annulus and remove the tumor as a single specimen from the globe to the chiasm. This procedure is not acceptable technique, however, when the optic nerve tumor proves to be a meningioma. In this case it is mandatory to section the levator origin at the annulus of Zinn, incise the annulus and the optic canal dura, and remove the entire tumor-bearing nerve from within. Failure to observe this step will result in recurrence of meningioma at the apex or in the canal. Once the tumor is removed, the levator origin is resutured to the annulus with a figure-of-eight 6.0 silk suture (Fig. 107-5C). Bleeding from the ophthalmic artery at the time of resection may be simply controlled by bipolar electrocautery.

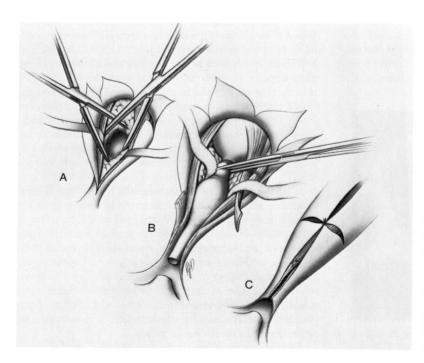

Figure 107-5 Steps in operative removal of optic nerve tumor. *A.* Finding a plane between the orbital areolar tissue and the optic nerve dura using malleable retractors and cottonoids. *B.* Junction of the optic nerve tumor and sclera is crushed with fine mosquito forceps prior to sectioning. To remove an optic nerve tumor in one piece from globe to chiasm, the annulus must be opened and levator origin sectioned. However, an optic nerve glioma may be removed in two pieces (globe to annulus and chiasm to canal). The residual intracanalicular tissue is simply electrocoagulated. *C.* Following removal of the tumor, including the intracanalicular portion of the nerve, the levator origin is sutured with a 6.0 figure-of-eight suture and the periorbita reapproximated.

An attempt should be made to reapproximate the periorbita. Gelfoam (absorbable gelatin sponge, The Upjohn Company, Kalamazoo, Mich.) is then placed over the exposed periorbita and a wire mesh screen fashioned to bridge the orbital root defect to avoid postoperative pulsation of the globe. It should be curved in such a way as to reapproximate the arched roof, to avoid reduction of orbital volume and accompanying downward proptosis. This screen may simply be placed in the epidural space and covered with Gelfoam; the dural stay sutures then suffice to hold it in place.

A temporary tarsorrhaphy is recommended whenever there is extensive orbital exploration, in order to allow safe application of a pressure dressing. Osmotic diuretics and steroids are used to facilitate the procedure and reduce the swelling in the postoperative period.

Complications are rare but, in a series of 52 cases, have included seizure disorder in one patient, denervation of the globe necessitating enucleation in two, mild residual ptosis in two, and orbital recurrence of glioma in one.

References

1. Anderson DR, Spencer WH: Ultrastructural and histochemical observations of optic nerve gliomas. Arch Ophthalmol 83:324–335, 1970.
2. Chang C, Wood EH: The value of radiation therapy for gliomas of the anterior visual pathway, in Brockhurst RJ, Boruchoff SA, Hutchinson BT, Lessel S (eds): *Controversy in Ophthalmology*. Philadelphia, Saunders, 1977, pp 878–886.
3. Chutorian AM, Schwartz JF, Evans RA, Carter S: Optic gliomas in children. Neurology 14:83–95, 1964.
4. DeSousa AL, Kalsbeck JE, Mealey J Jr, Fitzgerald J: Diencephalic syndrome and its relation to opticochiasmatic glioma: Review of twelve cases. Neurosurgery 4:207–209, 1979.
5. Gould RJ, Hilal SK, Chutorian AM: Efficacy of radiotherapy in optic gliomas. Ann Neurol 10:285, 1981 (abstr).
6. Housepian EM: Management and results in 114 cases of optic glioma. Neurosurgery 1:67–68, 1977 (abstr).
7. Housepian EM: Intraorbital tumors, in Schmidek HH, Sweet WH (eds): *Current Techniques in Operative Neurosurgery*. New York, Grune & Stratton, 1977, pp 143–160.
8. Hoyt WF, Baghdassarian SA: Optic glioma of childhood: Natural history and rationale for conservative management. Br J Ophthalmol 53:793–798, 1969.
9. Hoyt WF, Meshel LG, Lessell S, Schatz NJ, Suckling RD: Malignant optic glioma of adulthood. Brain 96:121–132, 1973.
10. Iraci G, Gerosa M, Tomazzoli L, Pardatscher K, Fiore DL, Javicoli R, Secchi AG: Gliomas of the optic nerve and chiasm. Childs Brain 8:326–349, 1981.
11. Lloyd LA: Gliomas of the optic nerve and chiasm in childhood. Trans Am Ophthalmol Soc 71:488–535, 1973.
12. Marquardt MD, Zimmerman LE: Histopathology of meningiomas and gliomas of the optic nerve. Human Pathol 13:226–235, 1982.
13. Spencer WH, Borit A: Diffuse hyperplasia of the optic nerve in von Recklinghausen's disease. Am J Ophthalmol 64:638–642, 1967.
14. Stern J, DiGiacinto GV, Housepian EM: Neurofibromatosis and optic glioma: Clinical and morphological correlations. Neurosurgery 4:524–528, 1979.
15. Stern J, Jakobiec FA, Housepian EM: The architecture of optic nerve gliomas with and without neurofibromatosis. Arch Ophthalmol 98:505–511, 1980.
16. Taveras JM, Mount LA, Wood EH: The value of radiation therapy in the management of glioma of the optic nerve and chiasm. Radiology 66:518–528, 1956.
17. Trokel SL, Hilal SK: Computerized tomography in ophthalmology: Sect. 5. Neuroanatomy and neuro-ophthalmology, in *Ophthalmology Basic and Clinical Science Course*. Rochester, Minn, American Academy of Ophthalmology, 1977.
18. Verhoeff FH: Primary intraneural tumors (gliomas) of the optic nerve. Arch Ophthalmol 51:120–140, 239–254, 1922.
19. Wilson WB, Feinsod M, Hoyt WF, Nielsen SL: Malignant evolution of childhood chiasmal pilocytic astrocytoma. Neurology 26:322–325, 1976.

108
Suprasellar Germinomas

John W. Walsh

Germinomas are tumors of germ cell derivation. They occur primarily in adolescents and young adults and most commonly develop in the ovary and testis. However, occasionally they develop intracranially. There they may occur in the region of the pineal gland; in the suprasellar-retrochiasmal area; within the pituitary fossa; in the posterior third ventricular, interpeduncular, and quadrigeminal plate regions; in the cerebellar vermis; or in the thalamus and walls of the lateral and third ventricles. This chapter covers suprasellar[11] and infrasellar germinomas.

It has been estimated that in the United States and Europe germ cell tumors account for 0.5 to 2.0 percent of all primary intracranial tumors.[7] They are more prevalent in Japan, constituting 2.1 to 4.5 percent of brain tumors detected there.[13] Approximately 20 percent of these germ cell tumors are suprasellar or infrasellar in location,[7] and the large majority are germinomas or mixed germ cell tumors with a predominant germinoma component.

Pathology

Germinomas arising in the region of the anterior third ventricle and sella turcica have been termed *suprasellar* and *infrasellar*, also *ectopic pinealomas*. The last designation is rarely used today, because it is not accurately descriptive: the tumors do not arise from pineal parenchyma, and only a few form as secondary or metastatic deposits of a separate pineal region tumor.[9]

Since suprasellar germinomas are usually quite large and therefore in proximity to a number of structures by the time they are first recognized, it has not been possible to establish with certainty their exact sites of origin. However, they have been classified into three types according to their anatomical and clinical presentation.[9] Type I develops as a metastasis to the floor of the third ventricle from a primary germinoma in the pineal region and infiltrates widely into the hypothalamus, pituitary stalk, neurohypophysis and optic nerves, tracts, and chiasm. Type II is indistinguishable in appearance, site of development, and clinical presentation from Type I, but this suprasellar tumor is primary; a separate germinoma at another site is not found. Type III is also primary but develops more inferiorly and principally infiltrates into the optic chiasm and tracts, the pituitary stalk and gland, and the floor of the third ventricle. A large portion of it may even be intrasellar and severely displace the adjacent normal pituitary gland. Suprasellar germinomas are not encapsulated. They infiltrate so extensively that complete surgical excision is not possible without producing unacceptable neurological deficits. For example, they sometimes infiltrate into the optic chiasm and tracts so completely that it is not possible to distinguish them from primary optic system tumors. Or they can disseminate throughout the craniospinal subarachnoid space and form deposits of tumor on the walls of the lateral and third ventricles.[8] In rare instances they can give rise to metastatic deposits in the retroperitoneum and adjacent soft tissue.[2]

When examined histologically, pure germinomas are composed of two types of cells in a dense, fibrous, and sometimes granulomatous connective tissue stroma. The cells are not arranged in a characteristic architectural pattern but are scattered irregularly throughout a connective tissue stroma with the lymphocytes occurring in clumps (Fig. 108-1). The resulting overall microscopic appearance is thus identical to that of ovarian dysgerminomas and testicular seminomas.[4] The larger, more numerous cells are epithelioid in appearance, polygonal or spheroidal in shape, and do not stain with the silver methods that usually impregnate cells of neural derivation such as the parenchymal cells in true pinealomas. Their nucleus is large, round, and hyperchromatic and contains coarsely granular chromatin and sometimes also a prominent nucleolus. The cytoplasm is pale and eosinophilic and is sometimes filled with PAS-staining vacuoles. Mitotic figures are common, and Langerhans-type multinucleated giant cells are also sometimes seen. The smaller cells are darkly stained and have been shown to be lymphocytes by the demonstration of lymphocyte membrane surface markers on the cell surface.[10]

Other germ cell tumors, such as yolk sac (endodermal sinus) tumors, choriocarcinomas, embryonal carcinomas, and immature teratomas can also arise in the suprasellar and infrasellar regions. They can occur either as homogeneous entities or as parts of mixed germ cell tumors. In the mixed tumors, most of the cells have the appearance of a typical germinoma, but areas having the histological features of one

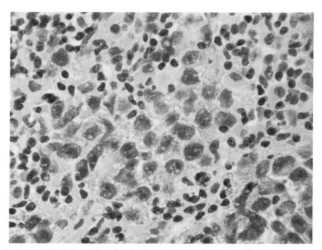

Figure 108-1 Histological pattern of suprasellar germinoma. The tumor is composed of large polygonal or spheroidal germinal cells and clusters of lymphocytes scattered throughout a dense connective tissue stroma. (Hematoxylin and eosin, × 1050.)

or more of these other germ cell tumors can usually be seen. Thus areas having the "festoon pattern" with glomerulus-like structures (Schüller-Duval bodies) and papilloma typical of yolk sac tumors, the cytotrophoblasts and syncytiotrophoblasts typical of choriocarcinoma, or the embryoid bodies seen in embryonal carcinomas may be seen.[3] The presence of these other germ cell tumor cells in a homogeneous or mixed tumor can also be demonstrated by measuring the amount of alpha fetoprotein (AFP) and human chorionic gonadotropin (hCG) that they secrete. Yolk sac tumor cells secrete AFP, choriocarcinoma cells secrete hCG, and embryonal carcinoma cells secrete both AFP and hCG. The extent of such tumor marker secretion can be detected in the patient's CSF or serum or by staining tissue sections of the tumor for the presence of these markers using specific immunofluorescent- or immunoperoxidase-labeled antiserum. Pure germinomas and mature teratomas do not produce these markers.[1]

The extent of the lymphocytes appears to be significant. The clusters of lymphocytes are much more numerous in pure germinomas than in mixed tumors or tumors forming from these other germ cell derivatives and are thought to indicate host immune resistance and, therefore, a better long-term prognosis.[7]

The embryological derivation of intracranial germinomas has not been fully elucidated, but some information is available. In a variety of animals, primitive germ cells have been shown to arise from endoderm situated in an arc just rostral to the head region of the embryo. They have been observed between yolk sac endoderm and the area pellucida of the embryo as early as the fifth segment stage of development. A short time later they migrate centripetally into the adjacent developing mesoderm, stimulate primitive blood vessel formation, and disseminate within these vessels throughout the embryo. Shortly thereafter they become concentrated in greatest number in the splanchnic region, where, because of their ameboid nature, they pass by diapedesis across the vessel walls and migrate to the region of the primordial ovary and testis.[4] In one study such primitive germ cells were also seen in a blood vessel of the forebrain,[12] and this observation suggests that germinomas and other germ cell tumors become intracranial in location because the cells which give rise to them are dispersed throughout the entire circulatory system during embryogenesis. Why these tumors occur in the midline and in pineal, suprasellar, and other perithird ventricular sites is not known, but the particular distribution of the cranial blood vessels during embryogenesis may be important in this regard.

Another hypothesis is that this family of intracranial tumors arises from misplaced multipotential fragments of the embryonic primitive streak.[4] The hypothesis is attractive because the most rostral portion of the primitive streak is in close proximity to the pineal anlage, but it does not explain the formation of tumors in the hypothalamic and retrochiasmal regions. Furthermore, since choriocarcinoma cells of trophoblast derivation form part of this group and since they are of maternal origin, it would seem unlikely that these tumors are derived from misplaced fragments of the primitive streak, even if such fragments have trigerminal potential.

Radiological Features

Probably the most useful radiological procedure for preoperatively confirming the diagnosis of suprasellar germinoma is the computed tomography (CT) scan. With this test, a large, slightly dense or isodense noncalcified suprasellar mass is seen. The tumor is usually of such size that it obliterates the suprasellar cistern and anterior third ventricle and thus is difficult to differentiate from a craniopharyngioma or optic chiasm–hypothalamic glioma. With intravenous contrast infusion, the tumor image is markedly enhanced. Occasionally, a second and entirely separate contrast-enhancing mass can be seen in the pineal region; the location suggests that in such cases the suprasellar mass may be an ectopic pineal germinoma, the result of tumor dissemination. At present most neurosurgeons use the CT scan as the principal, and sometimes only, radiological aid before proceeding with craniotomy and biopsy.[13]

X-ray films of the skull are usually normal. Occasionally, a mild to moderate degree of erosion of the sella turcica is seen. Actual enlargement of the sella is rarer and is only seen with intrasellar germinomas. Cerebral angiography usually gives confirmatory evidence of a suprasellar mass and sometimes also shows the presence of small pathological vessels within the tumor or a tumor stain during the arterial phase. Air and positive contrast ventriculography and pneumoencephalography show irregular filling defects on the floor of the third ventricle or an obliteration of the optic and infundibular recesses. Tumor deposits on the ventricular walls or in the cranial or spinal subarachnoid space can also sometimes be seen. These radiographic procedures were widely used before the CT scan became commonplace but are now used only rarely.

Clinical Features

Most patients with suprasellar germinomas date the onset of their symptoms to the end of the first decade or sometime in the second decade of life. In almost all patients the onset occurs before the age of 25. The diagnosis is usually made a few months to years later, with most cases coming to medical attention between ages 5 and 25. Unlike germinomas in the pineal region, which have a male to female ratio of 4:1 or 5:1, no sex preference has been found for patients with suprasellar lesions, except that patients under 10 years of age are slightly more often females and young adults over age 20 are more often males.[13]

In most patients, the earliest and most prominent symptom is diabetes insipidus. The polydipsia and polyuria that occur are usually striking: 3 to 6 liters of urine may be excreted per day. The development of this symptom usually indicates that the neoplasm has invaded the floor and walls of the third ventricle and infundibulum, has almost totally replaced the neurohypophysis, and in many instances has infiltrated and compressed the adenohypophysis. Diabetes insipidus may be the only symptom to develop for many months or even years. The patient may experience repeated episodes of dehydration and hypernatremia which, if the thirst mechanism and mental capacities of the patient are intact, can be managed with control of fluid intake and antidiuretic hormone replacement. But if the thirst mechanism and mental capacity are impaired—usually the result of an infiltration of tumor into the hypothalamus—the patient can develop seizures and alterations in blood pressure, heart rate, temperature, respiratory patterns, and gastric motility and can even become comatose.

Almost as common as diabetes insipidus are visual field defects and optic atrophy. These have been reported to develop in 85 to 90 percent of patients and usually are the result of infiltration and compression by the neoplasm of the optic tracts, nerves, and chiasm. Most often the tumor produces a bitemporal hemianopsia, but sometimes concentric or other field cuts are seen. Papilledema is rare. Diplopia and impaired accommodation, the result of tumor infiltration of the parasellar regions, may also be seen.

Another clinical feature characteristic of this tumor is hypophyseal dysfunction. Usually this is manifested by an insufficiency of pituitary function. If the patient is prepubertal, growth failure and dwarfism are seen; in older patients, hypogonadism is frequent. Pituitary, thyroid, and adrenocorticoid function may also be abnormal. In rare cases, symptoms associated with hyperfunction of the pituitary such as precocious puberty or galactorrhea are seen, but these are probably secondary to a hypothalamic injury or, in patients with precocious puberty, to the presence of hCG-secreting choriocarcinoma cells within the tumor.

Other less common symptoms associated with suprasellar germinoma are those associated with hydrocephalus (headache, nausea, and vomiting) or a second tumor in the pineal region (Parinaud's syndrome, pupillary inequality, and Argyll Robertson pupils). Ataxia may occur as a result of hydrocephalus, neoplastic involvement of the brain stem, or tumor growth into the cerebellar cortex.

Therapy

Surgery

The principal objectives of surgery are to decompress the optic nerves, tracts, and chiasm and to confirm the histological diagnosis. An extensive surgical procedure for complete or partial tumor resection has been associated with much greater morbidity and mortality. The tumor infiltrates so widely that excision almost always produces hypothalamic injury, leading to seizures, hypernatremic coma, or blindness. It is often difficult to distinguish suprasellar germinomas from craniopharyngiomas and optic chiasm–hypothalamic gliomas, especially if the tumor has infiltrated extensively into the optic nerves or chiasm,[9] which is more often the case for type I and type II suprasellar germinomas. A biopsy of the tumor makes this distinction and allows recognition of the presence within the tumor of other types of germ cells, a fact that strongly influences treatment and long-term prognosis. Type III tumors additionally compress the visual system inferiorly and the adenohypophysis, and therefore a more extensive resection for decompression is sometimes warranted. A partial removal of tumor lying below the chiasm has been reported to be effective in restoring vision and does not have as high a rate of morbidity and mortality as removal of a hypothalamic tumor.[5]

Occasionally patients with suprasellar germinomas present with acute hydrocephalus, and a CSF shunt must be placed before any other therapy can safely be carried out. The ventricular CSF obtained during such a procedure should be examined cytologically because it may contain tumor cells and thus serve as a diagnostic aid. Tumor cells may be identified by staining or may be established in cell culture for later study. The spinal fluid almost always shows a pleocytosis and elevated protein content. The CSF should also be assayed for levels of AFP and hCG even though higher levels are usually obtained with lumbar CSF. High levels of either of these markers might obviate the need for surgery.[1]

Radiation

Pure germinomas, including those occurring primarily or secondarily in the suprasellar region, have been shown to be exquisitely sensitive to radiation. In fact, they are so radiosensitive that they simply melt away over a 1- to 3-month period, thus any indication for surgery, other than biopsy for histological diagnosis, has been strongly questioned.[13] Some authors have gone so far as to suggest that adolescents or young adults with diabetes insipidus, visual field deficits, hypothalamic-pituitary dysfunction, and a noncalcified, contrast-enhancing mass on CT scan should be given radiation therapy initially and only be submitted to craniotomy and biopsy if the tumor is not dramatically reduced in size after administration of the first 1000 to 1500 rad.[13] However, if mixed germ cell tumors are to be controlled with the combined use of radiation and chemotherapy, an early histological diagnosis is essential, and the risks associated with the neurosurgical procedure for biopsy are very small.

Since intracranial germ cell tumors have been shown to disseminate through the ventricular system and metastasize throughout the cranial and spinal subarachnoid space, high-dose radiation must be given to the entire craniospinal axis. For example, Takeuchi et al. have recommended giving 2500 to 3000 R to the suprasellar region, 3000 R to the whole brain, and 2000 to 3000 R to the spinal cord;[13] and Jenkin et al. have contended that a total of 5000 rad is necessary.[8] The total dose should be given over 5 to 6 weeks at 150 to 200 rad per day, 5 to 6 days a week.[8]

The efficacy of radiation therapy for mixed germ cell tumors or pure germ cell tumors other than germinoma has not been established. Only a few cases have thus far been reported. For yolk sac tumors, radiation therapy appears to be much less effective than for pure germinomas, and a more aggressive tumor resection followed by administration of chemotherapeutic agents such as vincristine, actinomycin D, and cyclophosphamide has been necessary.

Long-Term Results

Very little has been reported on the long-term survival of patients with suprasellar germinoma. Only a few studies include assessments of the 5- or 10-year survival of more than a few irradiated versus nonirradiated patients, the incidence of dissemination of tumor cells to the ventricles and subarachnoid space, or the incidence of tumor recurrence. Furthermore, the incidence of complications after full craniospinal irradiation (such as diminished IQ and attention span, behavioral disturbances, and short stature observed after irradiation for medulloblastoma[6]) has not been addressed at all in these few reports.

From the data that are presently available, it appears that radiation is effective and probably increases the chances of long-term survival in the majority of patients, with periods of survival ranging from 1 to 16 years.[13] However, it must be emphasized that very high doses and full craniospinal radiation are essential, and the long-term effects of this therapy have not been reported.

Patients who receive radiation therapy and are generally not among the long-term survivors are those who have a preexisting hypothalamic injury or who subsequently develop widespread dissemination of tumor. Most patients who do not receive radiation therapy do not survive.

References

1. Allen JC, Nisselbaum J, Epstein F, Rosen G, Schwartz MK: Alphafetoprotein and human chorionic gonadotropin determination in cerebrospinal fluid: An aid to the diagnosis and management of intracranial germ-cell tumors. J Neurosurg 51:368–374, 1979.
2. Delahunt B: Suprasellar germinoma with probable extracranial metastases. Pathology 14:215–218, 1982.
3. Eberts TJ, Ransburg RC: Primary intracranial endodermal sinus tumor: Case report. J Neurosurg 50:246–252, 1979.
4. Friedman NB: Germinoma of the pineal: Its identity with germinoma ("seminoma") of the testis. Cancer Res 7:363–368, 1947.

5. Ghatak NR, Hirano A, Zimmerman HM: Intrasellar germinomas: A form of ectopic pinealoma. J Neurosurg 31:670–675, 1969.
6. Hirsch JF, Renier D, Czernichow P, Benveniste L, Pierre-Kahn A: Medulloblastoma in childhood: Survival and functional results. Acta Neurochir (Wien) 48:1–15, 1979.
7. Jellinger K: Primary intracranial germ cell tumours. Acta Neuropathol (Berl) 25:291–306, 1973.
8. Jenkin RDT, Simpson WJK, Keen CW: Pineal and suprasellar germinomas: Results of radiation treatment. J Neurosurg 48:99–107, 1978.
9. Kageyama N, Belsky R: Ectopic pinealoma in the chiasma region. Neurology 11:318–327, 1961.
10. Neuwelt EA, Smith RG: Presence of lymphocyte membrane surface markers on "small cells" in a pineal germinoma. Ann Neurol 6:133–136, 1979.
11. Simson LR, Lampe I, Abell MR: Suprasellar germinomas. Cancer 22:533–544, 1968.
12. Swift CH: Origin and early history of the primordial germ-cells in the chick. Am J Anat 15:483–516, 1914.
13. Takeuchi J, Handa H, Nagata I: Suprasellar germinoma. J Neurosurg 49:41–48, 1978.

109
Diencephalic Syndrome
John E. Kalsbeck

"A diencephalic syndrome of emaciation in infancy and childhood" was described by A. Russell in 1951.[6] Over 90 cases have been reported since 1951, and the literature has been reviewed extensively by Choux et al.,[3] Slooff and Krugsman,[7] Pelc,[5] and Burr et al.[2]

The constant and most striking feature of this condition is the appearance of emaciation with a uniform loss of body fat (Fig. 109-1). Children with this syndrome often appear muscular because of loss of fat over relatively normal muscles. Linear growth at the time of diagnosis is usually normal or above normal. Rotary nystagmoid eye movements are also striking but are present in only 50 to 60 percent of the reported cases. The nystagmoid eye movements, however, may be the first sign of the central nervous system origin of the "failure to thrive." These children may appear inappropriately happy or even euphoric.

Less consistent clinical features of the diencephalic syndrome are pallor, hyperkinesis, hypertension, hypoglycemia, and hyperhidrosis. Disproportionately large hands and feet have been described in three cases. Although optic atrophy is frequently present at the time of diagnosis, visual loss occurs late in the course of the disease. Vomiting, irritability, and an enlarging head due to hydrocephalus are late symptoms. The emaciated appearance, however, is always disproportionate to the anorexia and vomiting.

Russell, in his initial description, stated that all cases had as a common pathological basis a neoplasm predominantly involving the anterior thalamus. With few if any exceptions, the lesion causing diencephalic syndrome is a tumor involving the anterior hypothalamus and optic chiasm. Seven cases of diencephalic syndrome have been reported with lesions in the posterior fossa. However, these lesions have been questioned because of the frequency of anorexia, vomiting, and weight loss associated with posterior fossa tumors. All other reported patients have had tumors in the area of the anterior third ventricle. Pelc reviewed 40 cases plus two of his own and found evidence of optic pathway involvement in 70 percent, with lesions in 20 percent limited to the optic chiasm area.

Of the cases reported, 80 percent have been astrocytic tumors. These tumors are usually grossly soft, transparent, and gelatinous in appearance. The most frequent histological pattern seen is one of moderate cellularity with an open honeycomb background with microcysts. The tumor cells are multipolar, and vascular proliferation is usually minimal. Four reported tumors have had the histological features of an ependymoma. One craniopharyngioma and one suprasellar germinoma have been reported to produce diencephalic emaciation. There was no histological confirmation in 11 percent of the reported cases.

In 95 percent of cases, the onset of symptoms occurs before the age of 2 years. This early onset appears to be significant. The pathophysiology of the lipolysis occurring in this syndrome has not been established. Bauer, in reviewing 60 cases of hypothalamic disease, listed emaciation as occurring in only 2. Of these 60 patients, 8 were below the age of 2 years; 7 of these had precocious puberty.

Growth hormone levels have been elevated in all cases where it has been measured. The response of this elevated growth hormone level to hyperglycemia and hypoglycemia is inappropriate, and the normal diurnal rhythm is lost.[4] Although the elevated growth hormone level has been implicated in the lipolysis found in the diencephalic syndrome, lipolysis has not been reported in acromegaly or gigantism. Elevated growth hormone levels are also seen in anorexia nervosa and starvation, but the levels correlate closely with the degree of malnutrition and return to normal rapidly when the deficient caloric intake is corrected. The elevated growth hormone level in patients with diencephalic syndrome, on the other hand, does not drop with increased caloric intake and may persist for months after the subcutaneous fat returns.

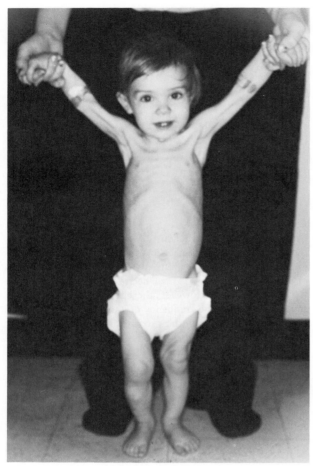

Figure 109-1 Fourteen-month-old female infant with 3-month history of "failure to thrive" and nystagmoid eye movements. There is loss of subcutaneous fat and a muscular appearance of the calves.

The diagnostic evaluation of the patient presenting with diencephalic emaciation may include skull films with views of the optic foramina. The optic foramina are enlarged in somewhat less than half the cases. The absence of subcutaneous fat is seen on soft tissue x-ray films. The CT scan shows a midline suprasellar mass that may be limited to the optic chiasm or optic pathways or may be large, extending subfrontally and temporally. CT bone windows may also show enlarged optic canals. The nuclear magnetic resonance (NMR) scan is of value when approved for use in infants and in children.

Additional studies provide little further information. An isotope brain scan shows increased uptake in over half the cases. Angiography confirms the presence of an avascular suprasellar tumor. Electroencephalography may show diffuse slowing, particularly when the tumor encroaches on the area of the foramen of Monro. The CSF protein content is usually elevated, and tumor cells may occasionally be identified in the CSF. Endocrine evaluation shows elevated growth hormone levels not influenced by hyperglycemia or hypoglycemia. Somatomedin values are low or low normal. ACTH stimulation and metyrapone tests indicate an abnor-

mality in the hypothalamic-hypophyseal-adrenocortical axis. Thyroid function studies are usually normal.

In the differential diagnosis of the patient with "failure to thrive," inadequate caloric intake and malabsorption problems must be excluded. Inflammatory lesions of the hypothalamic area as a cause of this syndrome are rare. Other suprasellar tumors such as craniopharyngioma, germinoma, and epidermoid or other types of suprasellar cyst rarely produce diencephalic emaciation but do enter into the differential diagnosis of a suprasellar mass.

Histological confirmation of this lesion is recommended, although improved imaging techniques make this unnecessary in selected cases. Radiation therapy is recommended, with the ports determined from computed tomography. Chemotherapy using nitrosourea compounds may delay the progression of symptoms.

Regression of the diencephalic syndrome has occurred rarely without irradiation therapy. With radiation therapy, return of subcutaneous fat can be noted in 8 to 12 weeks after completion of treatment. Growth hormone levels may drop below normal following treatment, and linear growth may be delayed. Hypothyroidism is frequently found in survivors. Precocious puberty has occurred following treatment. Radiation therapy in the age group of patients who

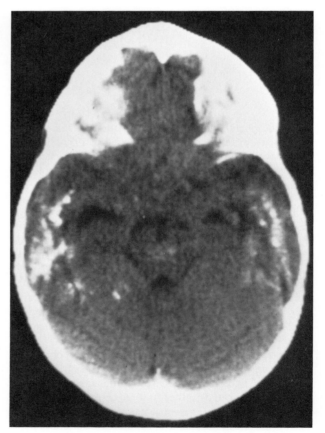

Figure 109-2 CT scan without contrast enhancement in a 7-year-old 6 years after biopsy and irradiation. He has moderate psychomotor retardation and seizures. Dystrophic calcifications are present, and the suprasellar cistern is obliterated.

present with diencephalic syndrome may result in psycho-motor delay, seizures, or progressive visual loss (Fig. 109-2).

Without treatment, the average survival is between 6 months and 2 years; however, Russell reported survivals of 8, 11, and 12 years without treatment. With surgery and radiation, 50 percent survive more than 2 years, and 10- to 12-year survivors are not uncommon; however, even after this length of time, tumor regrowth occurs.

References

1. Bauer HG: Endocrine and other clinical manifestations of hypothalamic disease: A survey of 60 cases, with autopsies. J Clin Endocrinol Metab 14:13–31, 1954.

2. Burr IM, Slonim AE, Danish RK, Gadoth N, Butler IJ: Diencephalic syndrome revisited. J. Pediatr 88:439–444, 1976.

3. Choux M, Baurand C, Pierron H, Vigouroux RP: Lipo-atrophie cachectisante par tumeur de la partie antérieure du plancher du IIIe ventricle ("Syndrome de Russell"). Neurochirurgie 15:59–74, 1969.

4. Drop SLS, Guyda HJ, Colle E: Inappropriate growth hormone release in the diencephalic syndrome of childhood: Case report and 4 year endocrinologic follow-up. Clin Endocrinol 13:181–187, 1980.

5. Pelc S: The diencephalic syndrome in infants: A review in relation to optic nerve glioma. Eur Neurol 7:321–334, 1972.

6. Russell A: A diencephalic syndrome of emaciation in infancy and childhood. Arch Dis Child 26:274, 1951 (abstr).

7. Slooff JP Sr, Krugsman H: Over een Patient met het hypothalamisch-hypophysaire Syndroom van Vermagering. Maandschr Kindergeneeskd 40:14–36, 1972.

110

Cranial Chordomas

Edward R. Laws, Jr.

Cranial chordomas are uncommon lesions, representing 0.15 to 0.2 percent of primary brain tumors. They are more frequent in men than in women (2:1) and may present at any age, with the mean age at diagnosis being 38 years.[2,5,7]

Nearly all the chordomas arising in the skull are related to the clivus, though an occasional apparently isolated tumor in the sella or the petrous bone has been reported. Virchow, in 1846, described the incidental finding at postmortem examination of excrescences of cartilaginous tissue related to the clivus which he termed *ecchondrosis spheno-occipitalis physaliphora*. Similar findings were noted by Luschka, Hasse, and Zenker in 1856 and 1857. Müller suggested in

1858 that these areas of heterotopic tissue might be related to the notochord, and this concept was well established by Ribbert in 1894. The histogenesis and evolution of chordomas was described in detail by Alezais and Peyron in 1914.[8]

The notochord is thought to be epithelial in origin, beginning as a hollow tube, then condensing to a solid cord of undifferentiated epithelioid cells. These cells then undergo vacuolation and fibrillation, become capable of mucin formation, and allow the notochord to become a supporting structure around which the sacrum, vertebrae, and base of the skull may form. The nucleus pulposus of the intervertebral discs is believed to be derived from the notochord. Within the clivus, the notochord runs a characteristically sinuous course, projecting superiorly, ventrally, or dorsally, usually (but not always) in the midline.

Undoubtedly, the sinuous nature of the notochord remnants at the base of the skull explains the various sites of predilection of cranial chordomas. Those tumors related to the most rostral extension of the notochord in the dorsum sellae will present as sellar or parasellar chordomas. Tumors related to the ventral aspect of the clivus will present as nasopharyngeal chordomas; those related to the body and dorsal aspect of the clivus, as spheno-occipital or petrosal chordomas; and those related to the basion or inferior aspect of the clivus, as inferior clival chordomas at the ventral aspect of the foramen magnum.

The clinical presentation of cranial chordomas depends on the location of the tumor (Table 110-1). Traditionally,

TABLE 110-1   Symptoms of Chordoma Related to Origin of Lesion

Location of Notochordal Remnants	Type of Chordoma	Clinical Presentation
Dorsum sellae	Sellar	Pituitary endocrinopathy, chiasmal syndrome
	Parasellar	Visual loss, cavernous sinus syndrome
Body of the clivus	Spheno-occipital:	
	Ventral	Nasopharyngeal mass
	Dorsal	Abducens nerve palsy, multiple cranial nerve palsies, brain stem syndrome, hydrocephalus
	Lateral (petrosal)	Cerebellopontine angle syndrome
Basion	Inferior clival	Hypoglossal nerve palsy, foramen magnum syndrome

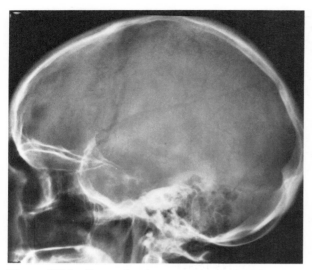

Figure 110-1 Large chordoma, spheno-occipital area, with sellar, suprasellar, and petrosal extension.

the most common presenting symptom is lateral rectus palsy, either unilateral or bilateral, related to stretching of the sixth cranial nerve as it follows a relatively long course in the dura of the clivus. Larger midclival (spheno-occipital) chordomas may present with multiple cranial nerve palsies, brain stem compression syndromes (ataxia, dysarthria, vertigo, pyramidal signs), syndromes of the cerebellopontine angle, and obstructive hydrocephalus. Sellar and parasellar chordomas may present with visual loss, pituitary endocrinopathy, a chiasmal syndrome, or a cavernous sinus syndrome. Inferior clival tumors may present with twelfth nerve palsy, dysphagia, and a foramen magnum syndrome.

The diagnosis of cranial chordoma, once suspected, is confirmed by radiological studies (Figs. 110-1 to 110-3). Plain skull films, polytomography of the clivus and adjacent structures, angiography, high-resolution CT scans, and nuclear magnetic resonance (NMR) scans may all be helpful both in establishing the diagnosis and in planning the therapeutic approach.

The most prominent radiological feature of a chordoma is destruction of bone, along with expansion of the area of destroyed bone. The lesion may have a ground-glass appear-

ance speckled with calcium from residual fragments of sequestrated bone. Rarely it may produce sclerosis of the clivus. Ventrally projecting chordomas may produce a soft tissue mass in the nasopharynx. The destruction and expansion of bone and the soft tissue masses in the nasopharynx and air sinuses may be seen on plain roentgenograms (Fig. 110-1), polytomograms (Fig. 110-2), or CT scans. Angiography will show displacement of the basilar artery in large spheno-occipital lesions and can be used to guide the surgical approach (Fig. 110-3). Pneumoencephalography, which was helpful in outlining the posterior wall of the clivus, has been replaced by CT scanning. Metrizamide CT cisternography has also proved quite useful (Fig. 110-3). Very few cranial chordomas have yet been examined by NMR scanning, but this technique should provide excellent anatomical information.

It is likely that Harvey Cushing performed the first successful operation on a cranial chordoma in 1909. This was reported initially as an interpeduncular teratoma (Case XVII) in his monograph, *The Pituitary Body and Its Disorders*. Dr. W. Welch diagnosed the lesion, removed by the trans-sphenoidal approach (Eiselsberg's superior transethmoidal-trans-sphenoidal approach), as a "mixed tumor from a congenital anlage." Bailey and Bogdasar later reviewed the tissue and were able to confirm the histology as typical of chordoma.[1]

The surgical approaches to chordoma are varied, again depending on the location of the lesion. They also depend, at least in part, on the philosophy of the surgeon. It is probable that the majority of chordomas are not surgically curable. Long-term follow-up of successfully treated cases reveals excellent survival in a number of patients treated by partial removal, both with and without adjunctive radiation therapy. Autopsy study of some patients who have died after radical "total" surgical removal of a clival chordoma has revealed residual tumor infiltrating the remaining bone of the base of the skull.

Chordomas of the ventral aspect of the clivus can be biopsied by transnasal surgery. Tumors of the body of the clivus may be approached by the trans-septal trans-sphenoidal route described by Guiot et al.[4] Some sellar and parasellar tumors may also be approached trans-sphenoidally, but others require a subfrontal or pterional craniotomy, especially if they project posterolaterally. Craniotomy ap-

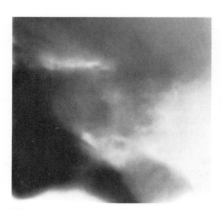
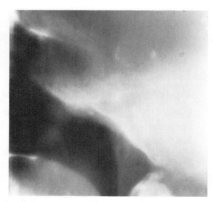
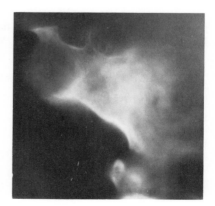

Figure 110-2 Lateral polytomograms of three spheno-occipital chordomas.

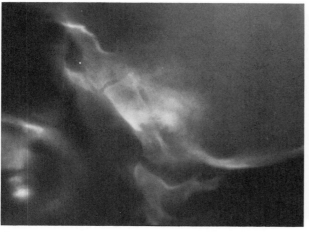

A

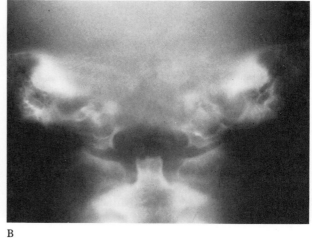

B

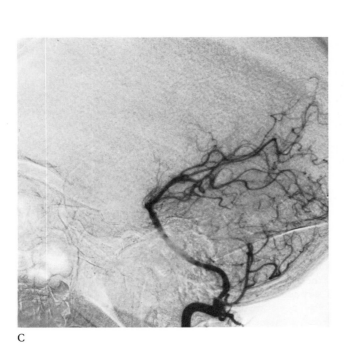

C

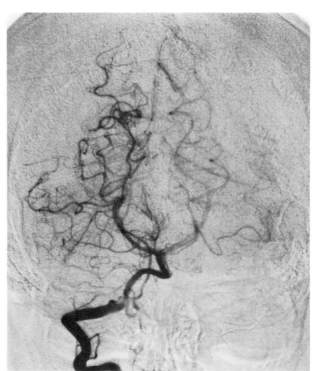

D

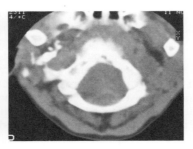

E

Figure 110-3 Six-year-old boy with bilateral twelfth nerve palsies, dysphagia, and ataxia due to chordoma of the inferior clivus. Lateral (*A*) and posteroanterior (*B*) polytomograms showing lesion of the clivus eroding the tip of the odontoid. Lateral (*C*) and anteroposterior (*D*) right vertebral angiogram views, showing displacement of the basilar artery. CT scan (*E*) following lumbar intrathecal metrizamide injection, showing mass lesion ventral to the medulla, more prominent on the right.

proaches to spheno-occipital chordomas include the subtemporal route of Petit-Dutaillis et al.,[6] the parieto-occipital approach with division of the tentorium (Olivecrona, Van Wangenen), and bilateral suboccipital craniectomy. Transcervical (Stevenson), transoral, and transpalatal (Scoville) approaches have been described.[7]

More recently, aggressive approaches for radical removal of chordomas have become possible utilizing the techniques of microsurgery, craniofacial surgery, and otoneurosurgery. Derome has described a bifrontal interorbital approach which allows exposure of the entire base of the skull for removal of a clivus chordoma, followed by iliac bone graft reconstruction.[3] Lateral approaches to the clivus through the infratemporal fossa (Fisch) and through the petrous bone (transcochlear, House and Hitselberger) have been described.

For practical purposes, the preferred current approaches are the trans-septal trans-sphenoidal for ventral lesions of the midclivus, pterional craniotomy for parasellar lesions, subtemporal transtentorial craniotomy for high dorsal lesions of the clivus, and suboccipital craniectomy for low dorsal lesions of the clivus. Other approaches may be useful from time to time, depending on the location and extent of the tumor to be treated.

The histopathology of the tumor is important with respect to prognosis, with the chondroid variant chordoma having a significantly more favorable outlook than the typical physaliferous chordoma.[5] Although chordomas are generally considered resistant to radiation, long-term survival has occurred in patients treated with biopsy and subsequent radiation. It has been the author's policy to recommend postoperative radiation therapy in virtually every case. Chemotherapy has not been utilized in any significant number of patients. Metastatic disease rarely occurs with chordoma, but metastases have been documented in liver, lungs, and heart.

References

1. Bailey P, Bagdasar D: Intracranial chordoblastoma. Am J Pathol 5:439–449, 1929.
2. Dahlin DC, MacCarty CS: Chordoma: A study of fifty-nine cases. Cancer 5:1170–1178, 1952.
3. Derome PJ: The transbasal approach to tumors invading the base of the skull, in Schmidek HH, Sweet WH (eds): *Operative Neurosurgical Techniques: Indications, Methods and Results*, vol 1. New York, Grune & Stratton, 1982, pp 357–380.
4. Guiot G, Rougerie J, Bouche J: The rhinoseptal route for the removal of clivus chordomas. Johns Hopkins Med J 122:329–335, 1968.
5. Heffelfinger MJ, Dahlin DC, MacCarty CS, Beabout JW: Chordomas and cartilaginous tumors at the skull base. Cancer 32:410–420, 1973.
6. Petit-Dutaillis D, Messimy R, Berdet H, Bennaim J: Contribution au diagnostic des chordomes sphéno-occipitaux. Sem Hop Paris 27:2663–2676, 1951.
7. Schisano G, Tovi D: Clivus chordomas. Neurochirurgia (Stuttg) 5:99–120, 1962.
8. Stewart MJ, Morin JE: Chordoma: A review, with report of a new sacrococcygeal case. J Pathol Bacteriol 29:41–60, 1926.

111

Parasellar Granular Cell Tumors

Dennis H. Becker

Although small, asymptomatic, intrasellar granular cell tumors (pituicytomas, myoblastomas, infundibulomas, choristomas, tumorettes) are frequently found at autopsy after the second decade (up to a 17 percent incidence), there have been only about 30 clinically symptomatic cases reported. All have presented with either visual loss from compression of the pregeniculate visual pathways, dementia, adenohypophyseal insufficiency, or diabetes insipidus.[6]

Neuroradiological investigations have revealed either a normal or a ballooned sella turcica on skull films. Lack of calcification has been uniform and helps to distinguish these tumors from craniopharyngiomas. Cerebral angiography most commonly reveals a suprasellar blush, in contrast to the avascular mass of most optic chiasmal gliomas or pituitary adenomas. An avascular suprasellar granular cell tumor has, however, been reported.[1] Computed tomography often demonstrates a surprisingly large suprasellar mass which is denser than normal brain, is sharply demarcated, produces no edema in adjacent brain and may extend down into and enlarge the sella turcica. Post-contrast-infusion CT has revealed dense, often homogenous, enhancement which may suggest an aneurysm or meningioma. A central area may fail to enhance in large lesions (Fig. 111-1).

Histologically, granular cell tumors are rather uniform in appearance. They consist of large cells 30 to 40 nm in diameter containing a distinctive granular cytoplasm. The granules stain positively with both phosphotungstic acid-hemotoxylin (PTAH) and periodic acid Schiff (PAS) stains. Mitotic figures and calcification are uniformly absent. Nuclei are usually small and strongly stained by hematoxylin. In 1981 a series of six clinically symptomatic granular cell tumors was reported.[1] All but Case 2 were typical in presen-

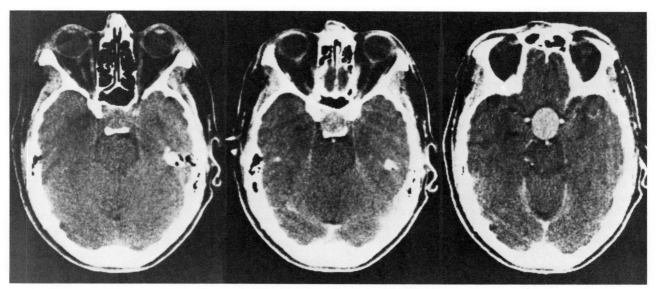

Figure 111-1 A 42-year-old man with visual disturbance for 1 year. *Left:* An unenhanced CT scan demonstrates a slightly hyperdense round lesion enlarging the sella. *Middle:* After contrast infusion, enhancement is seen within the sella. *Right:* The lesion extends into the suprasellar cistern, where it is sharply demarcated and rather homogeneous in appearance.

tation, location, surgical appearance, histology, and clinical course. The tumor in the second case was composed of cells which contained PAS-positive granules, but the location (third ventricle) and general histological appearance were unusual. Subsequent to that report, cells from all six tumors were stained with glial fibrillary acidic protein (GFAP) immunoperoxidase. The five typical granular cell tumors were completely negative, while the atypical second case was positive. From these data it would seem that the lesion in Case 2 should be rejected as a granular cell tumor and should be considered an astrocytoma. Granular cell tumors are GFAP-negative, and this helps differentiate them from tumors of fibrillary astrocytic origin in the parasellar region.

There are many theories concerning the cell of origin of these tumors. They are referred to by some as choristomas, implying an origin from the groups of large, oval, faintly granulated eosinophilic cells often found in the pars nervosa or pituitary stalk. Burston et al. noted similarities to granular myoblastomas found extracranially, noting that the cytoplasmic granules are both PTAH- and PAS-positive.[2] Others believe the lesions arise from the pituicytes of the pars nervosa and therefore are of glial lineage.[5] An altered Schwann cell has been implicated, leading to the hypothesis that the granular material represents altered myelin and axoplasm.[4] The hope is, by designating these tumors simply *parasellar granular cell tumors*, to remove prejudice concerning their cell of origin.

Recently all 20 patients in previously reported cases of symptomatic parasellar granular cell tumor were contacted or the cases reviewed. It was discovered that the natural history of these tumors is unknown. Seven of the twenty patients died either without operation or soon after initial craniotomy. Only three reported patients had had subtotal

resection, were given no postoperative radiation therapy, and survived the postoperative convalescent period. The details of these cases are presented elsewhere and represent early knowledge of the extended natural history of this lesion.[1] Two of these three patients failed to demonstrate new symptoms 16 and 9 years after operation, while the third required four subtotal resections over a 15-year period to maintain normal neurological function. The implication of these three cases is, at worst, slow progression after subtotal resection without radiation therapy.

The larger granular cell tumors that have not ballooned the sella are best approached subfrontally. Since they are usually symmetrical and straddle the midline, the right side is most commonly chosen for the surgical approach. However, if the tumor is skewed off the midline or if the patient presents with an asymmetric acuity loss, a bicoronal incision behind the hairline with elevation of a unilateral low frontal free bone plate on the side of the more marked tumor bulk is advised. This approach can easily be converted into a bifrontal approach if the initial exposure proves wanting. At surgery these tumors appear dull white, gray, light orange, or gray-red and are firm and rubbery. They are often highly vascular and bleed rather more than a glioma, craniopharyngioma, or pituitary adenoma normally would on biopsy. Lack of dural attachment distinguishes them from tuberculum meningiomas.

If a frozen section demonstrates a granular cell tumor, the surgeon should make decompression of the visual apparatus the immediate surgical goal. If it appears safe to remove the entire lesion, this should of course be done. If, however, the dissection in any way jeopardizes the hypothalamus or other vital centers, subtotal resection should be accepted. As in the case of Poppen, these lesions may be debulked many times over decades, with preservation of normal life.[1]

Lesions that balloon the sella may first be encountered by the surgeon trans-sphenoidally. Through the normal gland below, the firm, vascular, red-gray granular cell tumor will be discovered. If frozen section reveals a granular cell tumor, the tumor may be removed and the visual apparatus decompressed from below.[3] It is not wise to attempt total removal if bleeding obscures the surgeon's vision or if excessive traction must be applied to fragment the lesion. Some surgeons have abandoned the trans-sphenoidal resection of large tumors after a simple biopsy.[1]

The role of radiation therapy in these lesions remains controversial. Only four reported patients have had subtotal resection, postoperative x-ray therapy, and extended follow-up (5 to 22 years). The details of these cases are given elsewhere.[1] Since few data suggest that x-ray therapy provides any significant benefit, and since the risks of radiation therapy to the brain are well known and not inconsequen-

tial, it has been suggested that x-ray therapy not be used in these patients; but this advice has not been uniformly accepted.[3]

References

1. Becker DH, Wilson CB: Symptomatic parasellar granular cell tumors. Neurosurgery 8:173–180, 1981.
2. Burston J, John R, Spencer H: "Myoblastoma" of the neurohypophysis. J Pathol Bacteriol 83:455–461, 1962.
3. Cusick JF, Ho KC, Hagen TC, Kun LE: Granular-cell pituicytoma associated with multiple endocrine neoplasia type 2: Case report. J Neurosurg 56:594–596, 1982.
4. Kobrine AI, Ross E: Granular cell myoblastoma of the pituitary region. Surg Neurol 1:275–279, 1973.
5. Liss L, Kahn EA: Pituicytoma: Tumor of the sella turcica: A clinicopathological study. J Neurosurg 15:481–488, 1958.
6. Schlachter LB, Tindall GT, Pearl GS: Granular cell tumor of the pituitary gland associated with diabetes insipidus. Neurosurgery 6:418–421, 1980.

112
Benign Pituitary Cysts

Howard M. Eisenberg
Richard L. Weiner

Although cysts of the sellar and suprasellar region constitute a diverse group of pathological entities, these differences are often indistinguishable on the basis of clinical and radiological findings, and the diagnosis can often be determined only by gross and histological examination. A cystic lesion commonly encountered is the cystic pituitary adenoma; other solid tumors undergo degeneration and also become cystic. Epithelial cysts, including craniopharyngioma, Rathke's cleft cyst, and epidermoid cyst, represent another group of tumors that differ from the first in that they can be considered primarily cystic. Mucocele, abscess, and parasitic and arachnoid cysts are included in a miscellaneous group clearly not neoplastic. This chapter focuses on the various epithelial cysts and specifically the Rathke's cleft cyst. Although these cysts have traditionally been thought of by neurosurgeons as separate entities, there are convincing reasons for considering them as a group.[4,8,10,13,15] It is likely, although not

proved, that these lesions have a common ancestry; histologically, they appear to make up a spectrum ranging from craniopharyngioma, the most complex, to the single-cell-layered Rathke's cleft cyst, the simplest. The craniopharyngioma, the most common and no doubt the most often studied, is reviewed in detail in another chapter and is considered here only as it relates to the group as a whole. Epidermoid cysts, uncommon in this location, are also reviewed in other chapters.

Pathogenesis and Histology

Although the pathogenesis of these lesions is by no means certain, it is generally believed that the cells of origin are derived from or are remnants of Rathke's pouch. Rathke's pouch appears during the third or fourth week of embryonic life as an outgrowth of the stomodeum and elongates dorsally to form the craniopharyngeal duct. By the eleventh week, the proximal end of this duct is obliterated, while the cranial portion comes into contact with the infundibulum, a protrusion of the third ventricle. The anterior wall of the pouch proliferates to form the anterior lobe of the pituitary gland and the pars tuberalis; the posterior wall becomes the pars intermedia. Retention of the lumen as a cleft has been observed in humans and in several other species. Shanklin found clefts in 13 of 100 human autopsy specimens;[11] most were small, the largest measuring 2 × 3 mm. Surprisingly, formation or retention of the cleft was found relatively more often in adults than in children. Small nests of squamous epithelium, particularly at the junction of the pars tuberalis and the stalk, often seen as incidental findings in human autopsies, have been widely accepted as remnants of Rathke's pouch and are thought to be the cells of origin of the craniopharyngioma and the suprasellar epidermoid cyst. Rathke's cleft cysts are believed to originate from within the sella as expansions of the cleft. Lined by a single layer of epithelium (frequently ciliated and often containing goblet cells), the cleft wall is histologically similar to the single-cell-layered Rathke's cleft cyst. Noting, however, that the single-cell-layered Rathke's cleft cysts are also histologically similar to colloid cysts of the third ventricle, Shuangshoti and his colleagues postulated that the Rathke's cleft cyst may also arise from neuroepithelium derived from the precursor of the posterior lobe of the pituitary gland.[12] Reverse metaplasia from pituitary acinar cells has also been suggested as the mechanism for the pathogenesis of these epithelial tumors.

In their most typical forms, Rathke's cleft cysts and craniopharyngiomas are histologically distinct. The craniopharyngioma is composed of stratified squamous epithelium; keratinization, calcification, and the presence of cholesterol crystals are also characteristic. The simple single-cell-layered Rathke's cleft cyst is characterized by a layer of cuboidal or columnar epithelium on a basement membrane. These cells are frequently ciliated, and often many goblet cells are seen. However, a number of pituitary cysts have been described that appear to contain a mixture of both histological types.[8,10,13,15] Stratified squamous epithelium and columnar or cuboidal epithelium may exist at separate locations within the cyst wall, or a layer of cuboidal and columnar cells may be seen overlying stratified squamous epithelium. These complex multilayered cystic tumors are also classified as Rathke's cleft cysts. They appear, however, to represent a transitional form between the simple single-cell-layered cyst and the craniopharyngioma. Further, these tumors raise the possibility that all these cystic epithelial tumors arise from a multipotential stem cell that matures in two different directions. Two observations are interesting in this regard. Russell and Rubinstein reported two cases in which the cyst was dumbbell-shaped, consisting of an intrasellar portion lined by a single layer of cuboidal and columnar cells and a suprasellar portion lined by stratified squamous epithelium.[10] An abrupt transition occurred at the level of the diaphragma sellae. Yoshida et al. described a complex Rathke's cleft cyst containing columnar as well as stratified squamous epithelium.[15] In tissue culture, this tumor and a craniopharyngioma both grew prickle cells with microvilli and desmosomes; the authors suggested that both tumors had a common cell origin. Other overlapping features of craniopharyngioma and Rathke's cleft cysts have also been found. Rathke's cleft cyst generally contains mucoid or opalescent material, while a craniopharyngioma generally contains yellow, brown, or green fluid with cholesterol crystals. However, fluid similar to that contained in a craniopharyngioma has been found in Rathke's cleft cysts. In addition, calcification has been reported in a case of Rathke's cleft cyst.[1]

Clinical Presentation

The incidence of Rathke's cleft cyst is not known, but it is certainly less common than craniopharyngioma. In the approximately 60 cases reviewed in the literature, there is a slight female predominance. The lesion may become symp-tomatic in childhood, but most reported cases have been in adults. Like other tumors arising in this region, the clinical presentation is related to the extent of compression of the pituitary gland and surrounding structures; suprasellar extension is thought to occur in approximately one-third of cases. Hypopituitarism, when it occurs, cannot be distinguished from that caused by other lesions. Gonadatropin failure generally produces early symptoms; failure of growth hormone secretion, thyroid and adrenal dysfunction, and diabetes insipidus generally occur later. Mild to moderate elevations of serum prolactin levels, also seen with other nonsecreting tumors arising in this location, are presumably due to interference with prolactin-inhibiting factor at the stalk level or above.[14] When the tumor expands beyond the confines of the sella, visual field abnormalities and increased intracranial pressure, secondary to hydrocephalus due to deformation of the foramen of Monro, may occur. Aseptic meningitis, presumably due to leakage of cyst contents into the subarachnoid space, has been reported in Rathke's cleft cyst,[13] as well as craniopharyngioma. The irritants have not been defined but may include cholesterol crystals, keratin, and desquamated epithelial debris.

Radiological Features

Plain x-ray films of the skull have shown the usual abnormalities associated with sellar and suprasellar lesions: ballooning of the sella and destruction of the anterior and posterior clinoids. Pluridirectional tomography using 1-mm interval cuts allows elucidation of subtle changes not easily seen on plain films. Calcification, although usually associated with craniopharyngioma, has been seen in a Rathke's cleft cyst.[1] Computed tomography (CT) typically shows an enlarged sella containing a low-density nonenhancing lesion that may extend into the suprasellar spaces. Neither the images nor the density coefficients are adequate to accurately differentiate small collections of CSF from cyst contents, lipid, keratin, or mucoid material. Furthermore, contrast enhancement has been reported in Rathke's cleft cyst,[6] so CT examination alone is not sufficient to differentiate Rathke's cleft cysts from craniopharyngiomas, cystic adenomas, or other intrasellar or suprasellar cystic lesions. Occasionally more detailed information about the anterior third ventricle and suprasellar cisterns is necessary. Metrizamide cisternography with high-resolution CT scanning has recently supplanted pneumoencephalography for visualization of these spaces. This is particularly helpful in differentiating a cyst from an empty sella. Carotid angiography is generally used to determine the location of the intracavernous portions of the carotid arteries and for the diagnosis of aneurysms.

Differential Diagnosis

The differentiation of these epithelial cysts may be difficult or impossible on the basis of clinical and radiological findings alone. Frequently the preoperative diagnosis is either cystic pituitary adenoma or craniopharyngioma, depending on the clinical and radiological features in the individual case. Other conditions to be differentiated include empty sella syndrome, arachnoid cyst, cysticercosis, pituitary abscess, and aneurysm. Generally, the diagnosis of Rathke's cleft cyst cannot be made until the tumor is visualized at operation or, in some cases, after histological examination.

Surgical Therapy

Since Rathke's cleft cyst is an uncommon condition and is usually not diagnosed before operation, the operative approach chosen will depend on the presumptive diagnosis and the preference of the surgeon. Both transfrontal and transsphenoidal approaches have been successfully used in treating the lesion. These lesions, unlike craniopharyngioma, have been successfully treated by drainage and partial excision of the cyst wall; total removal is not recommended if it requires extensive retraction and dissection around the hypothalamus, visual system, or carotid arteries or their branches. A simple single-cell-layered uncalcified Rathke's cleft cyst can frequently be diagnosed by gross inspection, but in those cases in which the contents of the cyst, its calcification, or the thickness of its wall suggest that the lesion may be a craniopharyngioma, a frozen section should be made.[3] A potential drawback to the trans-sphenoidal approach is the difficulty of fenestrating the cyst into the subarachnoid space. This was the reason postulated for two recurrences that occurred within 2 years of trans-sphenoidal partial excision and drainage.[7]

Among 61 cases in the literature, seven have had reported recurrences.[2,5,7-9,15] In five of these patients, the lesion had at least one feature that was typical of craniopharyngioma. In some, the fluid was green to dark brown in color; others had multilayered cyst walls; and in one patient, cholesterol crystals were identified within the cyst. If Rathke's cleft cyst and craniopharyngioma present a continuum, it seems likely that those cysts which appear more like craniopharyngiomas would have, at least to a degree, the craniopharyngioma's potential for regrowth. If, at operation, a complex cyst is found, the patient should receive careful follow-up with serial CT scans. In case of recurrence, a second operation with excision and drainage is recom-

mended. The role of radiation therapy has not been determined, but after repeated recurrences (an unlikely situation), this alternative may be worth considering.

References

1. Adelman LS, Post KD: Calcification in Rathke's cleft cysts. J Neurosurg 47:641, 1977.
2. Berry RG, Schlezinger NS: Rathke-cleft cysts. Arch Neurol 1:48–58, 1959.
3. Eisenberg HM, Sarwar M, Schochet S Jr: Symptomatic Rathke's cleft cyst: Case report. J Neurosurg 45:585–588, 1976.
4. Fager CA, Carter H: Intrasellar epithelial cysts. J Neurosurg 24:77–81, 1966.
5. Iraci G, Giordano R, Gerosa M, Rigabello L, DiStefano E: Ocular involvement in recurrent cyst of Rathke's cleft: Case report. Ann Ophthalmol 11:94–98, 1979.
6. Kapcala LP, Molitch ME, Post KD, Biller BJ, Prager RJ, Jackson IMD, Richlin S: Galactorrhea, oligo-amenorrhea and hyperprolactinemia in patients with craniopharyngiomas. J Clin Endocrinol Metab. 51:798–800, 1980.
7. Marcincin RP, Gennarelli TA: Recurrence of symptomatic pituitary cysts following transsphenoidal drainage. Surg Neurol 18:448–451, 1982.
8. Matsushima T, Fukui M, Ohta M, Yamakawa Y, Takaki T, Okano H: Ciliated and goblet cells in craniopharyngioma: Light and electron microscopic studies at surgery and autopsy. Acta Neuropathol (Berl) 50:199–205, 1980.
9. Raskind R, Brown HA, Mathis J: Recurrent cyst of the pituitary: 26-year follow-up from first decompression: Case report. J Neurosurg 28:595–599, 1968.
10. Russell DS, Rubinstein LJ: *Pathology of Tumours of the Nervous System*, 4th ed. Baltimore, Williams & Wilkins, 1977.
11. Shanklin WM: On the presence of cysts in the human pituitary. Anat Rec 104:379–407, 1949.
12. Shuangshoti S, Netsky MG, Nashold BS Jr: Epithelial cysts related to sella turcica: Proposed origin from neuroepithelium. Arch Pathol Lab Med 90:444–450, 1970.
13. Steinberg GK, Koenig GH, Golden JB: Symptomatic Rathke's cleft cysts: Report of two cases. J Neurosurg 56:290–295, 1982.
14. Trokoudes KM, Walfish PG, Holgate RC, Pritzker KPH, Schwarz ML, Kovacs K: Sellar enlargement with hyperprolactinemia and a Rathke's pouch cyst. JAMA 240:471–473, 1978.
15. Yoshida J, Kobayashi T, Kageyama N, Kanzaki M: Symptomatic Rahtke's cleft cyst: Morphological study with light and electron microscopy and tissue culture. J Neurosurg 47:451–458, 1977.

SECTION J

Third Ventricular Tumors

<h1 style="font-size:3em">113</h1>

Masses of the Third Ventricle

J. Lobo Antunes

No other area of the central nervous system harbors a wider variety of lesions than the third ventricle.[4,5,8,10] This chapter covers the pathological entities affecting the anterior segment of this region; lesions of the posterior part or pineal area will be dealt with separately.

Types of Third Ventricular Tumors

Tumors of the third ventricle always present difficult surgical challenges because of their intimate relations to the hypothalamopituitary axis as well as to the neurovascular elements of the base. It is of practical importance to distinguish two major groups of lesions according to their site of origin.

Primary third ventricular tumors arise from structures that form the ventricular walls, or from embryonic rests that are contained in them. These tumors are attached to the walls by pedicles of variable width through which they receive their blood supplies. Colloid cysts, which are discussed in detail below, are probably the most frequent type. Astrocytomas are relatively common in childhood. Usually of a low-grade type, they arise from the hypothalamus or optic chiasm, grow into the lumen of the ventricle, and cause obstructive hydrocephalus, as well as hypothalamic dysfunction and visual symptoms. Rarely, they are pedunculated, connected with the ventricular wall by a narrow attachment and not extending much beyond the subependymal layer; these are, obviously, more amenable to surgical excision. Glial hamartomas are not uncommon in patients with tuberous sclerosis, they grow from the head of the caudate nu-

cleus, and compromise the CSF flow through the foramen of Monro. Certain gliomas originating in the thalamus or adjacent areas and secondarily extending to the ventricular wall should not be considered among the third ventricle tumors. Ependymomas are less common here than in other segments of the neuroaxis. They are often invasive and occasionally show malignant changes. Papillomas of the choroid plexus represent only 10 to 15 percent of third ventricular tumors. They occur mostly in the first two decades. They are usually quite vascular, but are accessible to surgical excision. Meningiomas of the tela choroidea are quite rare. Truly intraventricular craniopharyngiomas may originate from remnants of Rathke's pouch, attached to the tuberal region, that grow into the subependymal area; they are, however, exceptional. Teratomas with embryonic features or of a more mature type and epidermoid or dermoid tumors have also been found in this area.

Non-neoplastic processes that may involve the third ventricle include ependymal cysts, mycotic or parasitic granulomas (such as cysticercosis or hydatid cysts), and vascular malformations.

Secondary third ventricle tumors arise from the sellar or parasellar region and impinge upon, or invade, the wall of the third ventricle. It is sometimes hard at operation or even by pathological examination to determine the site of origin of some lesions, such as certain gliomas and craniopharyngiomas. These and pituitary adenomas are the most common in this group. Epidermoid and dermoid tumors, meningiomas, metastases, and deposits from medulloblastomas or tumors of the pineal region can all be found in this area. Atypical teratomas and ectopic pinealomas have been described in the suprasellar region in the absence of a primary pineal tumor.

Non-neoplastic lesions include sarcoidosis, histiocytosis X, arachnoid cysts, and large intracranial aneurysms.

Presentation and Management

From the clinical standpoint, third ventricular tumors often cause only a syndrome of obstructive hydrocephalus by blocking the foramina of Monro or the posterior third ventricle and aqueduct. Mental changes are not uncommon, in association with increased intracranial pressure or compromise of septohypothalamic structures. Tumors arising from the hypothalamus may cause changes in the state of consciousness, sleep-wake cycle, appetite, thirst regulation, or endocrine function by disrupting the hypothalamopituitary axis. Impairment of vision is also frequent as these lesions are intimately related to the optic pathways. Motor or sensory symptoms are more frequent when the tumor originates from the thalamic area.

When dealing with tumors of the third ventricle, it is important to try to determine preoperatively the type of lesion, the site of attachment, the blood supply, and the pattern of growth.[3] In general, primary intraventricular tumors are better approached dorsally through a transcortical or transcallosal route, whereas secondary tumors should be exposed by a subfrontal or frontotemporal procedure. The appropriate choice depends most on a thorough clinical and neuroradiological evaluation, including computed tomography, with axial and coronal cuts, and angiography.

Colloid Cysts

The colloid cyst, also called a paraphysial or neuroepithelial cyst, represents the paradigm of the primary third ventricle tumor. Its incidence has been variably estimated as between 0.6 and 15 percent of all brain tumors. With the introduction of computed tomography, more cases are being recognized, and these lesions are probably more frequent than was commonly thought.[2]

Colloid cysts usually present between the ages of 30 and 50 years, but they have been found in children as young as 2 months of age, and are not uncommon in the older population. They seem to affect both sexes equally, although in some series there seems to be a slight male predominance.

These tumors are usually spherical or ovoid, measuring from 1 to 3 cm in diameter, but they may fill the whole third ventricle. They are located in the roof of the third ventricle, usually attached to the tela choroidea, or more rarely to the choroid plexus, by a narrow pedicle (Fig. 113-1). They present between the foramina of Monro, just behind the fornices. Some are found more posteriorly and block the posterior segment of the third ventricle and aqueduct.

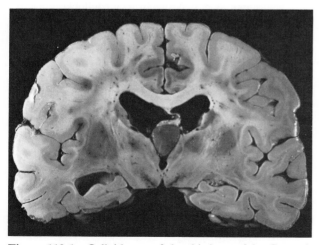

Figure 113-1 Colloid cyst of the third ventricle. Coronal section through the level of the foramina of Monro, which are clearly enlarged by the lesion.

The capsule of these lesions is usually smooth, grayish or greenish in color, and of variable thickness. The content is typically gelatinous, although at times it may be quite fibrous and vascular.

Microscopically, the capsule is made of an outer layer of connective tissue often rich in blood vessels. Signs of an inflammatory reaction, with deposits of hemosiderin and calcium, are observed at times. Inside is an epithelial layer composed of cuboidal or columnar cell epithelium, frequently ciliated, arranged in a single layer or in a pseudostratified fashion. The colloid material is homogeneous, although some cell remnants can be identified as well.

The pathogenesis of these lesions has been a matter of some controversy. On the basis of extensive histological analysis and data from comparative anatomy, Shuangshoti et al. concluded that colloid cysts of the third ventricle originate from abnormal folding of the neuroepithelium that makes up the roof of the diencephalon.[9] The paraphysis, which in man has a very ephemeral existence, is also a neuroepithelial structure, like an extraventricular choroid plexus, so it is possible that indeed some colloid cysts originate from that structure. This pathogenic mechanism also explains why some of these tumors grow dorsally between the leaves of the septum pellucidum.

Xanthogranulomas of the third ventricle may start as typical colloid cysts, in which proliferation and desquamation of the epithelial cells, with subsequent disintegration and release of the cellular lipids, gives rise to an inflammatory reaction with macrophages and multinucleated giant cells.[1]

The clinical presentation of colloid cysts of the third ventricle usually follows one of three forms:[7] (1) a syndrome of increased intracranial pressure without specific features or localizing signs. Headaches are usually present, often in the frontal region, and the sudden onset and intensity of a headache may closely simulate the picture of a subarachnoid hemorrhage; (2) a progressive or fluctuating dementia, with or without signs of increased intracranial pressure (it is of interest to mention that a number of patients have presented with the picture of the so-called normal-pressure hydrocephalus); (3) paroxysmal attacks with short periods of obtundation or loss of consciousness, or a loss of tone of the lower extremities. It has been strongly emphasized in the past that symptoms such as headaches are frequently precipitated by certain positions of the head, but this phenomenon is only observed in a minority of the cases. This has been attributed to a "ball valve" effect of the tumor, which would intermittently occlude the foramina of Monro. This mechanism implies a mobility of the lesion that is hardly ever confirmed at operation. Other, more rare symptoms include seizures, extrapyramidal phenomena, vegetative crises, and cerebrospinal fluid rhinorrhea.

Clinical examination usually reveals only the ocular signs of increased intracranial pressure, often associated with increased deep tendon reflexes and pyramidal signs. Ataxia and an organic mental syndrome are also present in many instances.

The course is rather variable: some patients experience symptoms for more than twenty years whereas others may have coma of sudden onset. Although it is generally believed that the hydrocephalus that is invariably present in these patients is due to an obstruction of the foramina of Monro, this is not always so, and a secondary stenosis of the aqueduct may be the cause of the ventricular dilatation in a number of cases.

The diagnosis of colloid cyst depends on accurate radiological evaluation. Plain radiographs of the skull are not usually helpful, but they may show the marks of increased intracranial pressure. Calcification of the lesion is exceptional. Computed tomography is now the diagnostic technique of choice.[6] These lesions present as rounded masses located at the level of the foramina of Monro (Fig. 113-2). Most often they are homogeneous and hyperdense, showing mild enhancement with contrast medium, although the xanthogranuloma type may be heterogeneous in appearance. Other associated features include widening of the septum pellucidum, slight separation of the posterior inferior segments of the frontal horns, and collapse of the posterior part of the third ventricle.

Ventriculography with the use of air is now rarely justifiable. It may help, however, when the lesion is quite small, or when it is necessary to determine the site of obstruction of the spinal fluid pathways.

The classic angiographic features of these lesions consist of an elevation of the anterior third of the internal cerebral vein, with a curve concave downward, and of a flattening

and depression of the posterior two-thirds, associated with signs of ventricular dilatation. Angiography should always be obtained when a direct surgical attack is entertained, since it is important to exclude a vascular lesion such as an aneurysm of the tip of the basilar artery. Angiography will also provide information about the anatomy of the venous system, which is particularly relevant when a transcallosal approach is adopted.

It is important to emphasize that none of the radiographic signs described above is pathognomonic for a colloid cyst; therefore, surgical verification of the lesion is recommended. The other goal of the treatment is to open the cerebrospinal fluid pathways and resolve the associated hydrocephalus. Since some of these patients have an associated aqueductal stenosis, this cannot always be achieved even when the patency of the foramina of Monro is clearly ascertained at operation. In such cases, a shunting procedure is necessary. Some have advocated a shunt operation as the sole procedure; however, such a decision requires the support of radiographic data, and such data are not always reliable.

The surgical excision of these tumors requires the exposure of one or both foramina of Monro.[2,3] This can be done through a transcallosal or transcortical approach. Both are effective and safe ways to deal with these tumors, although whenever the ventricles are small, the transcallosal route is safer. It requires a frontal craniotomy and a 2- to 3-cm incision in the corpus callosum; the transcortical approach follows an opening through the midfrontal gyrus. A colloid cyst usually widens the foramen of Monro; after the capsule has been opened, the contents can be aspirated, and the tumor capsule slowly delivered through the foramen. At times, this opening has to be enlarged further: either anteriorly by dividing one fornix, or posteriorly by coagulating the thalamostriate vein and then dissecting posteriorly between the thalamus laterally and the choroid plexus and the internal cerebral vein medially. An alternative route is between the fornices, following the midline and then incising the tela choroidea. This is ideal for the tumors that are located more posteriorly and do not show through the foramina. In general, the removal of these lesions is relatively easy, but occasionally the vascularity of the capsule, its adherence to the adjacent structures, or the viscosity of its contents make the operation quite difficult; it is often preferable to leave behind a small fragment of the capsule rather than to pursue it through a wide opening made in the roof of the third ventricle.

Complications of these procedures include collapse of the ventricular system, accumulation of subdural hygromas, and damage to the fornices, which even when apparently unilateral may lead to severe amnestic deficits. Section of a small part of the anterior segment of the corpus callosum does not cause any obvious neuropsychological deficit. Seizures occur in about 5 percent of the patients that have undergone a transcortical approach.

In the past the surgical mortality of these procedures was relatively high, due on the one hand to the inability to control increased intracranial pressure in the postoperative period, and on the other hand to the fact that not infrequently the tumor was not found at operation, or the diagnosis was

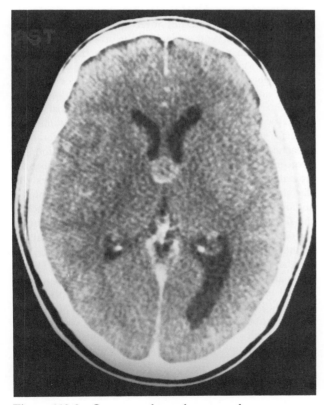

Figure 113-2 Contrast-enhanced computed tomogram showing a typical colloid cyst of the third ventricle. Note the widening of the septum pellucidum and collapse of the posterior segment of the third ventricle.

missed. With better shunting devices and the advent of microsurgical techniques, the results of surgical removal of colloid cysts are excellent.

References

1. Antunes JL, Kvam D, Ganti SR, Louis KM, Goodman J: Mixed colloid cysts: Xanthogranulomas of the third ventricle. Surg Neurol 16:256–261, 1981.
2. Antunes JL, Louis KM, Ganti SR: Colloid cysts of the third ventricle. Neurosurgery 7:450–455, 1980.
3. Antunes JL, Muraszko K, Quest DO, Carmel PW: Surgical strategies in the management of tumours of the anterior third ventricle, in Brock M (ed): *Modern Neurosurgery*. Berlin, Springer-Verlag 1982, pp 215–224.
4. Cassinari V, Bernasconi V: Tumori della parte anteriore del terzo vetricolo. Acta Neurochir (Wien) 11:236–271, 1964.
5. Dandy WE: *Benign Tumors in the Third Ventricle of the Brain: Diagnosis and Treatment*. Springfield, Ill., Charles C Thomas, 1933.
6. Ganti SR, Antunes JL, Louis KM, Hilal SK: Computed tomography in the diagnosis of colloid cysts of the third ventricle. Radiology 138:385–391, 1981.
7. Kelly R: Colloid cysts of the third ventricle: Analysis of twenty-nine cases. Brain 74:23–65, 1951.
8. Pecker J, Ferrand B, Javalet A: Tumeurs du troisième ventricule. Neurochirurgie 12:7–136, 1966.
9. Shuangshoti S, Roberts MP, Netsky MG: Neuroepithelial (colloid) cysts: Pathogenesis and relation to choroid plexus and ependyma. Arch Pathol Lab Med 80:214–224, 1965.
10. Stein BM: Third ventricular tumors. Clin Neurosurg 27:315–331, 1980.

114
Operative Approaches to the Third Ventricle

Albert L. Rhoton, Jr.
Isao Yamamoto

Numerous operative approaches to the third ventricle have been described since the pioneering work of Walter Dandy[2] (Fig. 114-1). The selection of the best operative approach is determined by the location of the lesion in relation to the lateral and third ventricles and other structures, including the foramen of Monro, aqueduct of Sylvius, optic nerves and chiasm, pineal gland, sella turcica, pituitary gland, fornix, midbrain, and thalamus.[8,9,13] The operative approaches are divided on the basis of whether they are suitable for reaching the anterior or posterior half of the third ventricle. Before considering the specific operative approaches, we will review some general principles.

Principles Underlying Operative Approaches

The craniotomy flap should be placed so as to minimize the need for brain retraction. The sites of retraction used to reach the walls of the third ventricle include the orbital surface of the frontal lobe to reach the chiasmatic area; the frontal and parietal parasagittal cortex for the transcallosal approaches; the anterior and inferior part of the temporal lobe and the inferior surface of the frontal lobe for the frontotemporal and subtemporal approaches; the inferior and medial surface of the occipital lobe for the occipital approaches; and the superior surface of the cerebellum for the infratentorial approaches. To minimize the need for brain retraction, the surgeon should place the craniotomy as follows: for the subfrontal, frontotemporal, and subtemporal approaches, the flap should have its lower margin on the floor of the anterior and/or middle cranial fossae; for the parasagittal approaches, the flap should have its medial margin on the midline; for the occipital approaches, the flap should reach the margins of the sagittal and transverse sinuses and the torcular; and for the suboccipital approaches, the opening should reach the margins of the transverse sinus and the torcular.

Self-retaining, rather than hand-held, retractors should be used. The extracerebral space is increased and the need for retraction is further reduced by draining cerebrospinal fluid through a ventriculostomy if hydrocephalus is present, or through a lumbar puncture needle if there is no ventricular obstruction and if the operation is not done with the patient in the sitting position.

Incisions in neural tissue and sacrifice of neural structures should be minimized. It is impossible to reach the cavity of the third ventricle without incising some neural structures. The brain may be retracted to expose an external wall of the third ventricle, but then the wall must be incised to reach its cavity. The fornix and lamina terminalis are common sites of

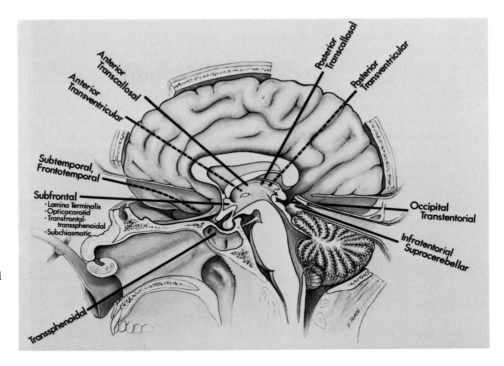

Figure 114-1 Midsagittal view of the head showing the operative approaches to the third ventricle. The approaches that are directed along or near the midline are shown as solid lines, and those that approach the third ventricle away from the midline are shown as dotted lines. (From Rhoton et al.[9])

incision in the wall of the third ventricle. In other cases, the cerebral cortex or corpus callosum is incised to reach the lateral ventricle, and then another neural incision is frequently needed to adequately expose the third ventricle from the lateral ventricle. The consequences of injury to the neural structures incised in reaching the third ventricle have been reviewed in a prior report.[13]

Tissue should be removed from within the capsule of a third ventricular tumor before trying to separate the capsule from adjacent structures. If the tumor could be cystic or the mass could possibly be an aneurysm, the initial step is aspiration with a needle. If the tumor is encapsulated, the capsule is opened, the tumor is biopsied, and an intracapsular removal is completed. The capsule is separated from the neural and vascular structures after its contents have been removed. The most common reason that a tumor appears to be tightly adherent is not that adhesions are present between the capsule and surrounding structures; rather, it is that residual tumor within the capsule wedges the tumor into position. As the intracapsular contents are removed, the tumor collapses, making it possible to remove more tumor through the small exposure. Only rarely is a tumor so densely adherent that it defies easy removal after its contents are removed. If the tumor does not separate easily from the neural tissue after the intracapsular contents have been removed, a brief wait often allows the pulsation of the brain to dislodge the tumor into the exposure, and then more tumor can frequently be removed from within the capsule. Under magnification, individual adhesions between vital structures and the tumor can be divided with microinstruments. This technique has been especially helpful in removing craniopharyngiomas because they are more densely adherent to surrounding structures than are chromophobe adenomas. It is frequently possible to remove the capsules of craniopharyngiomas and

epidermoid tumors, but not those of chromophobe adenomas. The capsule of the chromophobe adenoma is the dura mater of the cranial base, which has been stretched upward over the tumor. The stretched dura over the dome of the chromophobe adenoma may be excised, but an attempt to pull this pseudocapsule of dura mater from its attachment to the cranial base may cause severe vascular and neural injury. A remnant of the tumor capsule may be left if it is attached firmly to vital structures such as the optic nerves or chiasm, colliculi, thalamus, or hypothalamus. The response of craniopharyngiomas, chromophobe adenomas, pinealomas, and some gliomas to radiation therapy is sufficiently good that this may be relied upon to deal with residual neoplasm. Removal is frequently limited to biopsy only or to an internal decompression if the tumor is malignant or infiltrative.

The arteries that pass over the tumor capsule to neural tissues should be preserved. Any vessel that stands above the surface of the capsule should be dealt with initially as if it were a vessel supplying the brain. An attempt should be made to displace the vessel off the tumor capsule using a small dissector after tumor tissue has been removed from within the capsule. Numerous arteries are exposed in removing tumors of the third ventricle: the posterior part of the circle of Willis and the apex of the basilar artery are below the floor; the anterior part of the circle of Willis and the anterior cerebral and anterior communicating arteries are related intimately to the anterior wall; the posterior cerebral, pericallosal, superior cerebellar, and choroidal arteries pass adjacent to the posterior wall; both the anterior and the posterior cerebral arteries send branches into the roof; and the internal carotid, anterior choroidal, anterior and posterior cerebral, and anterior and posterior communicating arteries give rise to perforating branches that reach the walls of the third ventricle. Only infrequently should any of these be sacrificed during the removal of a tumor. Occlusion of these major trunks or their perforating branches at the anterior part of the circle of Willis is likely to result in disturbances in memory and personality, and occlusion of those at the posterior part of the circle of Willis is more likely to result in disorders of the level of consciousness and extraocular motion.

The number of veins sacrificed should be kept to a minimum because of the undesirable consequences of their loss. Obliteration of certain of the deep veins, including the vein of Galen, basal veins, and internal cerebral veins and their tributaries, and the bridging veins from the cerebrum and cerebellum to the dural sinuses, is inescapable in reaching and removing some tumors. Before sacrificing the bridging veins, the surgeon should try placing them under moderate or even severe stretch (accepting the fact that they may be torn) if this will allow satisfactory exposure and yield some possibility of the veins being saved. Before sacrificing the basal, internal cerebral, or great veins, the surgeon should try working around them or displacing them out of the operative route, or try dividing only a few of their small branches, which may allow the displacement of the main trunk out of the operative field.

A shunt may be needed, if obstruction to the flow of cerebrospinal fluid at the foramen of Monro, aqueduct of Sylvius, third ventricle, or tentorial incisura persists at the end of the operation. If the initial operation causes an opening from the third ventricle through the lamina terminalis, floor of the third ventricle, or pineal region into the subarachnoid space, this may suffice. In other cases, one end of a Silastic (Dow Chemical Co., Midland, Mich.) tube may be inserted through the opening into the third ventricle while the other end is led into the subarachnoid space. If a suboccipital exposure has been used to approach a tumor of the pineal region, a tube may be led from the lateral ventricle or from an opening in the posterior part of the third ventricle to the cisterna magna, creating a Torkildsen shunt.

Anterior Operative Approaches

The approaches suitable for lesions within or compressing the anterior portion of the third ventricle are the (1) transsphenoidal, (2) subfrontal, (3) frontotemporal (4) subtemporal, (5) anterior transcallosal, and (6) anterior transventricular (Fig. 114-1).

Trans-sphenoidal Approach

This approach is used for all tumors involving the anteroinferior part of the third ventricle that are located above a pneumatized sphenoid sinus and extend upward out of an enlarged sella turcica (Fig. 114-2).[3,7,8] The trans-sphenoidal approach is reviewed only briefly because the neural and vascular structures surrounding the third ventricle are infrequently exposed and visualized by this approach, even when the tumor extends into the third ventricle. Removal of the tumor by this approach is commonly confined to the removal of tissue within the tumor capsule, thus allowing the capsule to collapse away from the neural structures without

permitting the surgeon to visualize them. If the capsule is opened, the area directly above the sella turcica can be visualized. In relation to the tumor, the optic nerves, chiasm, and tracts, the circle of Willis, and the floor of the third ventricle are above; the oculomotor, trochlear, trigeminal, and abducens nerves, the cavernous sinuses, and the intracavernous portion of each carotid artery are lateral; and the basilar artery and midbrain are posterior (Fig. 114-2).

Potential sources of neural and vascular complications during trans-sphenoidal operations are stretch injury to the infraorbital nerves during the sublabial incision and the insertion of the nasal speculum; injury to the olfactory mucosa and olfactory nerve at the cribriform plate if the intranasal portion of the procedure is directed too far superiorly; optic nerve injury due to a fracture through the optic foramen caused by a forcefully opened speculum; injury to the optic, trigeminal, and abducens nerves and the carotid artery in the lateral wall of the sphenoid sinus caused by forcefully opening the trans-sphenoidal speculum with the tips in the sinus, or caused during dissection in the wall of the sphenoid sinus if absence of bone in the sinus wall exposes the nerves and arteries beneath the sinus mucosa; and injury to the walls and floor of the third ventricle, the first through sixth cranial nerves, the circle of Willis, and the internal carotid and basilar arteries in the subarachnoid space above the tumor.

Subfrontal Approach

This approach is used for those tumors involving the anteroinferior part of the third ventricle that are not accessible by the trans-sphenoidal approach because they do not extend into the sella turcica, are separated from the sella turcica by a layer of neural tissue, are located entirely within the third ventricle, extend upward out of a normal or small sella, or are located above a nonpneumatized (conchal) type of sphenoid bone. The subfrontal route provides the space for four different approaches to tumors involving the third ventricle (Fig. 114-3).[8,9] These are (1) the subchiasmatic approach between the optic nerves and the optic chiasm; (2) the opticocarotid approach directed through the triangular interval between the optic nerve medially, the carotid artery laterally, and the anterior cerebral artery posteriorly; (3) the lamina terminalis approach directed above the optic chiasm through the thin anterior lamina of the third ventricle; and (4) the transfrontal–trans-sphenoidal exposure obtained by removing the tuberculum sellae, planum sphenoidale, and anterior wall of the sella turcica through a frontal craniotomy.

For these subfrontal approaches the patient is placed in the supine position. The head is turned slightly to the opposite side and is extended slightly so that the frontal lobe will fall away from the floor of the anterior cranial fossa. A coronal scalp incision is used. A small, four-hole frontal bone flap, usually on the right side or on the side of the greater optic nerve or chiasmal compression, is placed to reach up to the midline just above the eyebrow and is cut so that its anterior margin is flush with the floor of the anterior fossa. The frontal sinus is not avoided if entering it allows a lower placement of the flap. If the frontal sinus is entered, the

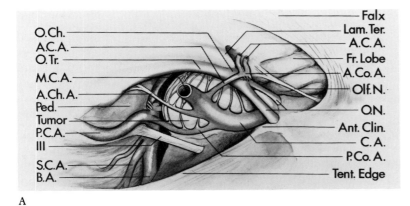

A

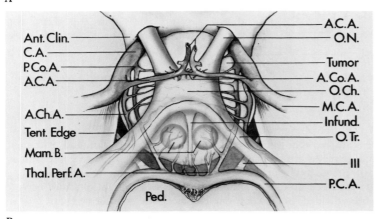

B

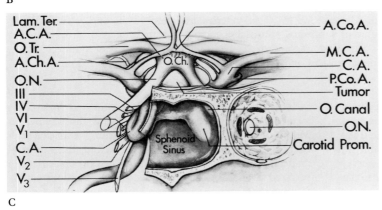

C

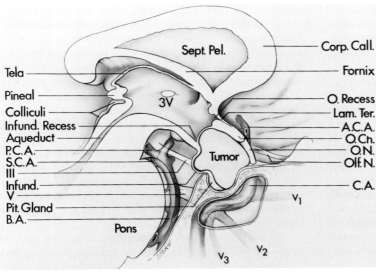

D

Figure 114-2 Relationships of a sellar tumor with suprasellar extension. *A.* Right lateral view. The tumor extends upward out of the sella turcica and stretches the optic nerves (O.N.), optic tracts (O.Tr.), and optic chiasm (O.Ch.) upward. The olfactory nerve (Olf.N.) is above and the oculomotor nerve (III) is posterior to the tumor. The carotid (C.A.), posterior communicating (P.Co.A.), anterior choroidal (A.Ch.A.), and middle cerebral (M.C.A.) arteries are lateral; the anterior cerebral (A.C.A.) and anterior communicating (A.Co.A.) arteries are above; and the basilar (B.A.), superior cerebellar (S.C.A.), and posterior cerebral (P.C.A.) arteries are posterior to the tumor. The cerebral peduncles (Ped.) are posterior to the tumor and the lamina terminalis (Lam.Ter.) and frontal lobe (Fr.Lobe) are above. The tentorial edge (Tent.Edge) is attached to the anterior clinoid process (Ant.Clin.). *B.* Superior view. The tumor stretches the optic nerves, chiasm, and tracts upward. The anterior cerebral and anterior communicating arteries are stretched upward and the carotid, anterior choroidal, and posterior communicating arteries are stretched laterally. The infundibulum of the hypophysis (Infund.) is stretched posteriorly, and the mammillary bodies (Mam.B.) are elevated. The thalamoperforating (Thal.Perf.A.) and posterior cerebral arteries and the oculomotor nerves are on the posterior margin of the tumor. *C.* Anterior view showing structures along the trans-sphenoidal operative approach to a sellar tumor. The suprasellar structures are stretched above the tumor. The carotid arteries form prominences (Carotid Prom.) in the lateral walls of the sphenoid sinus. The optic canals (O.Canal) form prominences in the superolateral margins of the sphenoid sinus. The oculomotor, abducens (VI), and trochlear (IV) nerves and the ophthalmic (V₁), maxillary (V₂), and mandibular (V₃) divisions of the trigeminal nerves are lateral to the sphenoid sinus. The structures near the lateral wall of the sphenoid sinus may be injured in the trans-sphenoidal approach to sellar tumors if the bone in the lateral wall of the sphenoid sinus is very thin or absent. *D.* Midsagittal section. The tumor extends upward into the anteroinferior part of the third ventricle (3V). The infundibulum and pituitary gland (Pit.Gland) are stretched around the posterior margin of the tumor. The optic (O.Recess) and infundibular (Infund.Recess) recesses are partially obliterated. The structures above the third ventricle are the tela choroidea (Tela), fornix, septum pellucidum (Sept.Pel.), and corpus callosum (Corp.Call.). The pineal gland (Pineal) and colliculi are near the posterior wall of the third ventricle. The trigeminal nerve (V) divides lateral to the carotid artery and sphenoid sinus. (From Rhoton et al.[9])

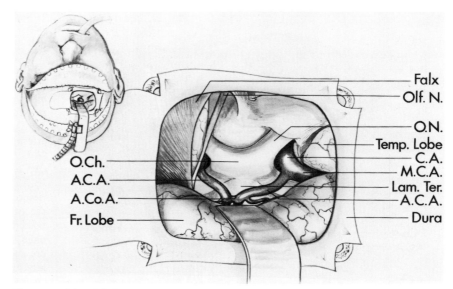

Figure 114-3 Subfrontal approach to the anteroinferior part of the third ventricle. *Left:* The scalp incision, right frontal bone flap, dural incision, and placement of self-retaining retractor are shown. *Center:* Intracranial exposure with the frontal lobe (Fr.Lobe) retracted. The optic nerves (O.N.), optic chiasm (O.Ch.), and optic tracts are stretched upward if a tumor is present. The right olfactory nerve (Olf.N.) has been divided, but the left one is intact. The anterior cerebral (A.C.A.) and anterior communicating (A.Co.A.) arteries cross the optic tracts and the lamina terminalis (Lam.Ter.). The temporal lobe (Temp.Lobe) and carotid (C.A.) and middle cerebral (M.C.A.) arteries are lateral to the optic chiasm. *Facing page:* Different subfrontal approaches to the anteroinferior part of the third ventricle. *A.* Subchiasmatic approach. The tumor is exposed between the optic nerves, the optic chiasm, and the tuberculum sellae (Tub.Sellae). A knife

mucosa is pushed inferiorly, a thin layer of soft acrylic is applied over the opening, and a flap of pericranium or dura is reflected over the sinus and sutured into place. The frontal lobe is retracted to expose the olfactory nerve and the arachnoid over the chiasmatic cistern. The olfactory nerve, if stretched to the point of tearing, is divided posterior to the olfactory bulb.

For the subchiasmatic approach, the arachnoid of the anterior wall of the chiasmatic cistern is incised so that it falls backward over the nerves and chiasm and provides a protective layer during the operation. The optic nerves and chiasm are not retracted. Retraction of stretched nerves, even though gentle, may increase visual loss. The tumor is aspirated with a small lumbar puncture needle before incision of the capsule. Tissue is removed from within the capsule of the tumor until the capsule collapses away from the nerves and chiasm according to the principles outlined previously.

The opticocarotid approach is used if asymmetrical superolateral extension of the tumor widens the interval between the carotid artery and optic nerve and if the tumor cannot be reached by the subchiasmatic approach. Tumor tissue is removed from within the capsule until it collapses away from the optic nerves and carotid artery. An attempt is made to preserve the perforating branches of the internal carotid artery that cross the interval between the artery and the optic nerve.

The lamina terminalis approach is favored for tumors located above the sella turcica and below the foramen of Monro in the anteroinferior part of the third ventricle, especially if there is a prefixed chiasm blocking the subchiasmatic approach or if the tumor has pushed the chiasm into a prefixed position and has distended and stretched the lamina terminalis so that the tumor is visible through it. Craniopharyngioma is the tumor removed most frequently by this approach. By stretching the walls of the third ventricle, the tumor makes more room available for its manipulation. When retracting the anterior cerebral arteries to expose the lamina terminalis, the surgeon should preserve the branches from the anterior communicating and anterior cerebral arteries penetrating the anterior walls of the third ventricle. The tumor will usually bulge forward through the lamina terminalis. An opening is made through the thinned lamina. Meticulous attention is given to preventing damage to the anterior commissure and the rostrum of the corpus callosum above, the optic chiasm below, and the optic tracts, columns of the fornix, and hypothalamic walls laterally. With the descent of the tumor from the foramina of Monro, a gush of cerebrospinal fluid will be seen. The basilar artery and part of the circle of Willis may be seen through the floor of the third ventricle.

Use of the transfrontal–trans-sphenoidal approach is considered if the transfrontal exposure is limited by a prefixed position of the optic chiasm, the sphenoid sinus is aer-

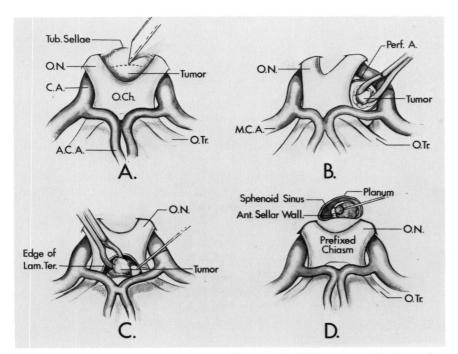

incises the tumor capsule. *B.* Opticocarotid approach. This approach is directed through the interval between the optic nerve and the anterior cerebral and carotid arteries. A cup forceps reaches through a hole in the tumor capsule. Perforating arteries (Perf.A.) cross the interval between the carotid artery and the optic nerve. *C.* Lamina terminalis approach. The lamina terminalis is above the optic chiasm and between the optic tracts. The lamina terminalis has been opened, and a cup forceps reaches between its edges (Edge of Lam.Ter.) to remove tumor in the anteroinferior part of the third ventricle. *D.* Transfrontal–trans-sphenoidal approach. A prefixed optic chiasm blocks the subchiasmatic approach to a tumor. The tumor is exposed by removing the posterior part of the planum sphenoidale and the tuberculum sellae to expose the sphenoid sinus. The sinus mucosa is depressed inferiorly and the anterior sellar wall (Ant. Sellar Wall) is removed to expose the tumor. (From Rhoton et al.[9])

ated, and the tumor does not stretch the lamina terminalis or widen the opticocarotid space. In such cases, the tumor is exposed by removing the planum sphenoidale, tuberculum sellae, and anterior wall of the sella. The mucosa in the sphenoid sinus is depressed inferiorly. This exposure allows free access to the sellar portion of the tumor without trauma to the optic chiasm. Removal of the tumor is completed according to the principles outlined previously. After the tumor removal is complete, the opening into the sphenoid sinus is closed by packing the holes with muscle and covering the area with dural or pericranial grafts.

Frontotemporal and Subtemporal Approaches

These approaches are considered together because the subtemporal craniotomy, as advocated by Symon[11] and Kempe[5] for the removal of third ventricular tumors, is similar to the conventional frontotemporal craniotomy, except that it extends further posteriorly in the temporal region (Figs. 114-4, 115-5). We would use these approaches only if a tumor involving the third ventricle is centered lateral to the sella or

extends into the middle cranial fossa. Symon advocated the use of the subtemporal approach for the removal of craniopharyngioma, stating that it provides "the least difficulty in a highly complex and dangerous field."[11] For either the frontotemporal or the subtemporal approach, the patient is placed in the supine position and the head is tilted a bit backward and turned away from the side of operation: 30 degrees away for the frontotemporal approach and 60 degrees away for the subtemporal approach. For the frontotemporal approach, small scalp and bone flaps are elevated, and for the subtemporal approach the flaps are extended further posteriorly above the ear. The scalp, temporalis muscle and fascia, and pericranium are reflected as a single layer. The lateral aspect of the sphenoid ridge is removed with a rongeur or a drill. The dura is opened, with the main flap pulled down anteroinferiorly along the region of the pterion. The frontal and temporal lobes are retracted to expose the area along the sphenoid ridge. In the subtemporal approach, the tip of the temporal lobe may be elevated to expose the edge of the tentorium. The bridging veins from the sylvian fissure and temporal tip are coagulated and divided only if necessary. It may be possible to preserve

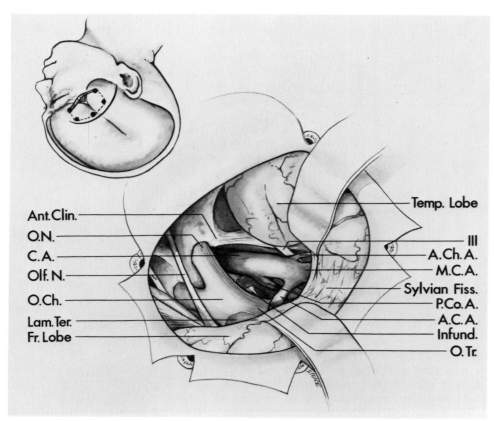

Figure 114-4 Frontotemporal approach to the anteroinferior part of the third ventricle. *Top left:* The scalp incision (*solid line*), bone flap (*dashed line*), and craniectomy (*oblique lines*) have their lower margin centered at the pterion and the lateral part of the sphenoid ridge. *Center:* The frontal (Fr.Lobe) and temporal (Temp.Lobe) lobes are retracted to expose the area along the sylvian fissure (Sylvian Fiss.). The olfactory nerves (Olf.N.) are above the optic nerves (O.N.). The carotid artery (C.A.) is medial to the anterior clinoid process (Ant.Clin.). The anterior choroidal (A.Ch.A.), posterior communicating (P.Co.A.), anterior cerebral (A.C.A.), and middle cerebral (M.C.A.) arteries arise from the carotid artery. The lamina terminalis (Lam.Ter.) is above the optic chiasm (O.Ch.) and medial to the optic tracts (O.Tr.). The infundibulum of the pituitary gland (Infund.) is below the optic chiasm. The oculomotor nerve (III) is posterior to the carotid artery. (From Rhoton et al.[9])

these bridging veins if the frontotemporal approach is entirely above the sphenoid ridge or if the subtemporal approach is entirely below the sphenoid ridge. The arachnoid membrane is opened to expose the carotid artery, the optic nerve, and the origin of the posterior communicating and anterior choroidal arteries. The tumor is exposed through the triangle between the optic nerve and the internal carotid and anterior cerebral arteries in the frontotemporal approach, or below the floor of the third ventricle through the interval between the carotid artery and the oculomotor nerve in the subtemporal approach. The third ventricle may be entered through the floor if the nuclear masses are pushed laterally by the tumor and the floor consists of only a glial membrane. The temporal lobe may be elevated in the subtemporal approach to expose an area as far posteriorly as the anterior and lateral aspect of the midbrain and the upper part of the basilar artery. Special attention is given to preserving the perforating arteries arising from the circle of Willis. Symon noted that in the subtemporal approach it is often difficult to avoid sacrificing some of the perforating arteries arising from the posterior communicating artery, especially in removing a craniopharyngioma.[11] The tumor, once exposed, is removed according to the principles outlined previously.

Anterior Transcallosal Approach

This approach is suitable for lesions located in the anterosuperior part of the third ventricle or extending out of the superior part of the third ventricle into one or both lateral ventricles near the foramen of Monro (Fig. 114-6).[10] It is easier to expose the opening of the foramen of Monro into each lateral ventricle through this approach than through the anterior transventricular approach if the ventricles are of a normal size or are minimally enlarged.

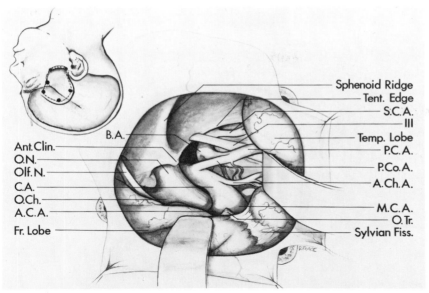

Figure 114-5 Subtemporal approach to the floor of the third ventricle. *Top left:* The head is turned 50 degrees to the opposite side. The scalp incision (*solid line*), bone flap (*dashed line*), and craniectomy (*oblique lines*) are located at the lateral margin of the sphenoid ridge over the tip of the temporal lobe. *Center:* Operative exposure. The dura has been opened, and the frontal (Fr.Lobe) and temporal (Temp.Lobe) lobes are retracted to expose the area along the sphenoid ridge and sylvian fissure (Sylvian Fiss.). The optic nerve (O.N.) and carotid artery (C.A.) are exposed medial to the anterior clinoid process (Ant.Clin.). The olfactory nerve (Olf.N.) is stretched as the frontal lobe is retracted. The posterior communicating (P.Co.A.), anterior choroidal (A.Ch.A.), and middle cerebral (M.C.A.) arteries arise from the carotid artery. The oculomotor nerve (III) passes forward between the superior cerebellar (S.C.A.) and the posterior cerebral (P.C.A.) arteries. The anterior cerebral artery (A.C.A.) passes medially over the optic chiasm (O.Ch.). The optic tract (O.Tr.) extends posteriorly from the optic chiasm. Perforating branches of the various arteries pass upward from the circle of Willis to enter the floor of the third ventricle. The basilar artery (B.A.) is medial to the edge of the tentorium (Tent. Edge). (From Rhoton et al.[9])

The patient is positioned supine with the head elevated 20 to 30 degrees. An alternative is the lateral position with the right side down, so that gravity will assist the retraction of the medial surface of the right cerebral hemisphere away from the right side of the falx. A coronal, horseshoe, or S-shaped skin incision is used. A bone flap extending to the midline is centered on the coronal suture. The dura is opened with the base on the sagittal sinus. The cortical veins entering the superior sagittal sinus are protected; some, usually no more than one, may have to be divided in order to retract the medial surface of the right frontal lobe away from the falx. The arachnoid membrane, encountered deep to the free edge of the falx, is opened to expose the corpus callosum and the anterior cerebral arteries. The corpus callosum is usually approached between the two pericallosal arteries. Short and occasionally long callosal arteries, and even the trunks of the anterior cerebral artery, may cross the midline above the corpus callosum. It may infrequently be necessary to divide some of these branches in order to reach the surface of the corpus callosum. If both pericallosal arteries are retracted to one side, frequently some of the branches that run laterally from the pericallosal arteries to the corpus callosum and the cingulate gyrus must be sectioned in order to reach the corpus callosum.

The anterior part of the corpus callosum is split along the midline. An incision 3 cm in length extending forward to the genu provides satisfactory access to both lateral ventricles. A line from the coronal suture in the midline to the external auditory meatus will roughly bisect the corpus callosum. The foramen of Monro is found by following the choroid plexus and thalamostriate vein to the point where they converge at the foramen of Monro anteriorly. The choroid plexus is attached along the choroidal fissure between the lateral margin of the fornix and the thalamus. The thalamostriate vein passes forward in a more lateral position in the groove between the thalamus and caudate nucleus near the stria terminalis.

Entry into a cavum between the leaves of the septum pellucidum may be confusing until one realizes that no intraventricular structures are present. If the septum pellucidum is complete, it may be opened to provide access to the left lateral ventricle and to the openings of the foramina

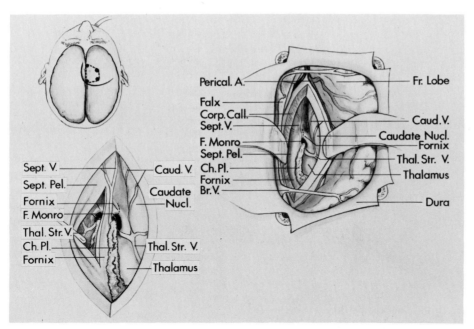

Figure 114-6 Anterior transcallosal approach to the anterosuperior part of the third ventricle. *Top left:* The scalp incision (*solid line*) and the bone flap (*dashed line*) extend up to the midline in the frontal region. *Right:* The dura has been opened, and one bridging vein (Br.V.) has been sacrificed and several others are placed on a stretch to complete the transcallosal exposure. The frontal lobe (Fr.Lobe) is retracted away from the falx. The corpus callosum (Corp.Call.) has been opened below the pericallosal arteries (Perical.A.). The septal vein (Sept.V.) crosses the septum pellucidum (Sept. Pel.) and passes through the foramen of Monro (F.Monro). The caudate veins (Caud.V.) cross the caudate nucleus (Caudate Nucl.). The thalamostriate vein (Thal.Str.V.) passes posteriorly between the caudate nucleus and thalamus. The choroid plexus (Ch.Pl.) is attached along the choroidal fissure, which is located between the fornix and the thalamus. *Bottom left:* The septum pellucidum has been opened to expose the openings of the foramina of Monro into both lateral ventricles. Only one-half of the fornix (*dashed line*) should be divided to enlarge the opening into the anterosuperior part of the third ventricle. (From Rhoton et al.[9])

of Monro into each lateral ventricle. The left rather than the right lateral ventricle may be entered, but the anatomy makes this obvious. An incision is made anteriorly through one column of the fornix at the anterosuperior edge of the foramen of Monro only if needed to explore a deeper portion of the anterior part of the third ventricle. The tumor is removed according to the principles outlined previously. The callosal opening provides an outlet for the escape of fluid from the lateral ventricles into the subarachnoid space.

A modification of the transcallosal approach, called the *interfornicial approach*, has the advantage of giving access to the central portion of the third ventricle by dividing between the paired bodies of the fornix (Fig. 114-7).[1] This approach is uniquely suited to lesions below the roof of the third ventricle and posterior to the foramen of Monro. The interfornicial incision extends posteriorly from the foramen of Monro. The right and left halves of the fornix are each displaced to the ipsilateral side, and the ependyma and tela choroidea below the fornix are opened until the internal cerebral vein comes into view. The remaining strands of tela choroidea are divided, and the roof of the third ventricle is entered through the resulting longitudinal opening.

Anterior Transventricular Approach

This approach is suitable for tumors in the anterosuperior part of the third ventricle, especially if the tumor has a major extension into the anterior part of the lateral ventricle on the side of the approach (Fig. 114-8). It is more difficult to expose the anterior part of the lateral ventricle on the contralateral side when using the transventricular approach than when using the transcallosal approach. The transventricular approach is facilitated if the lateral ventricles are enlarged.

With the patient in the supine position, the head is rotated slightly to the left. The bone and scalp flaps are positioned over the midfrontal area, anterior to the precentral motor cortex of the nondominant hemisphere. The dominant hemisphere is selected only if the tumor has a major extension into the lateral ventricle of the dominant hemisphere. If the approach is through the dominant hemisphere, care is taken to place the cortical incision above and anterior to the expressive speech centers on the inferior frontal gyrus and anterior to the precentral motor strip. The dilated frontal horn is reached through a 4-cm linear cortical incision located in the long axis of the middle frontal gyrus.

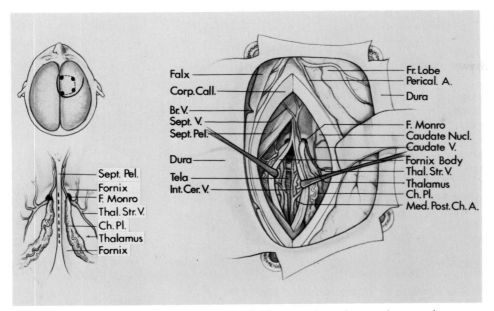

Figure 114-7 Anterior transcallosal interfornicial approach to the anterior superior part of the third ventricle. *Top left:* The approach is along the medial surface of the nondominant right hemisphere. The scalp incision (*solid line*) and the bone flap (*dashed line*) extend up to the midline in the frontal region. *Bottom left:* The interfornicial incision (*dashed line*) is directed through the roof of the third ventricle in the midline between the fornices. *Right:* The frontal lobe (Fr.Lobe) is retracted away from the falx. The corpus callosum (Corp.Call.) has been opened below the pericallosal arteries (Perical.A.), and the septum pellucidum (Sept.Pel.) has been opened to expose both lateral ventricles. The choroid plexus (Ch.Pl.) is attached along the choroidal fissure situated between the thalamus and the fornix. The roof of the third ventricle is opened by an incision between the paired bodies of the fornix beginning at the level of the foramina of Monro and extending posteriorly. The layers of tela choroidea (Tela) in the roof of the third ventricle form the outer walls of the velum interpositum in which the medial posterior choroidal arteries (Med.Post.Ch.A.) and the internal cerebral veins (Int.Cer.V.) course in the roof of the third ventricle. The internal cerebral veins receive the septal (Sept.V.) and thalamostriate veins (Thal.Str.V.). The caudate nucleus (Caudate Nucl.) is lateral to the thalamus. The interfornicial exposure has the advantage of displacing, rather than dividing, the fornix to allow entry into the roof of the third ventricle. After completion of the interfornicial incision, the tela choroidea is opened until the internal cerebral vein comes into view. The right and left fornices are displaced to the right and left sides, respectively, the remaining strands of the tela choroidea are divided, and the roof of the third ventricle is entered.

Upon opening the anterior horn of the lateral ventricle, the thalamostriate, septal, and caudate veins and the choroid plexus are seen to converge at the foramen of Monro; the fornix and septum pellucidum are above and anterior, the thalamus is posterior and inferior, and the caudate nucleus is lateral. The close relationship of the genu of the internal capsule to the foramen of Monro should be kept in mind when operating in this area. The genu of the internal capsule approaches the wall of the ventricle in the area lateral to the foramen of Monro near the anterior pole of the thalamus. It is difficult to expose the anterior part of the third ventricle through the foramen of Monro, and thus it may be necessary to incise the ipsilateral column of the fornix at the anterosuperior margin of the foramen of Monro to gain adequate exposure; but this should be done only on the ipsilateral side because sectioning both sides may cause memory disturbances.[13] To prevent the complications associated with sectioning of the fornix, Hirsch et al. sectioned the thalamostriate vein at the posterior margin of the foramen of Monro, rather than damaging the fornix, to enlarge the opening into the roof of the third ventricle.[4] They stressed that the interruption of this vein was harmless; however, some of their patients developed drowsiness, hemiplegia, and mutism. Furthermore, occlusion of the veins at the foramen of Monro has caused hemorrhagic infarction of the basal ganglia.[13] The tumor, once exposed, is removed according to the principles outlined previously.

A modification of the frontal transventricular approach, called the *subchoroidal approach*, has the advantage of giving access to the central portion of the third ventricle by displac-

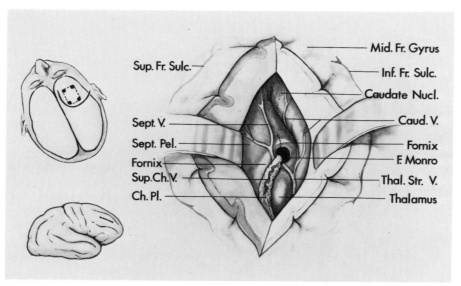

Figure 114-8   Anterior transventricular approach to the anterosuperior part of the third ventricle. *Top left:* The approach is through the nondominant hemisphere if possible. The scalp incision (*solid line*) and bone flap (*dashed line*) are centered over the middle frontal gyrus. *Bottom left:* The cortical incision (*dotted line*) used to reach the ventricle is through the middle frontal gyrus anterior to the motor strip and above the speech areas. *Right:* Intraventricular exposure. The cortical incision is in the middle frontal gyrus (Mid.Fr.Gyrus) between the superior frontal (Sup.Fr.Sulc.) and inferior frontal (Inf.Fr.Sulc.) sulci. The cortical opening exposes the anterior part of the lateral ventricle and the foramen of Monro (F.Monro). The choroid plexus (Ch.Pl.) is attached between the thalamus and the fornix. A superior choroidal vein (Sup.Ch.V.) courses on the surface of the choroid plexus. The thalamostriate vein (Thal.Str.V.) courses posteriorly between the thalamus and the caudate nucleus. A septal vein (Sept.V.) crosses the septum pellucidum (Sept.Pel.). Several caudate veins (Caud.V.) cross the caudate nucleus (Caud.Nucl.). (From Rhoton et al.[9])

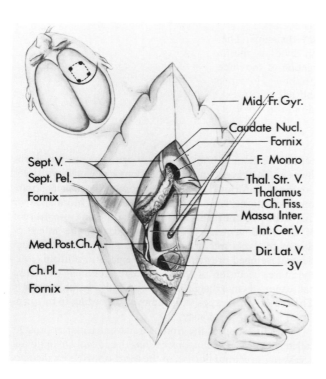

Figure 114-9   Anterior transventricular subchoroidal approach to the anterior superior part of the third ventricle. *Top left:* The approach is through the nondominant right hemisphere if possible. The scalp incision (*solid line*) and the bone flap (*dashed line*) are centered over the middle frontal gyrus. *Bottom right:* The cortical incision (*dotted line*) is directed through the middle frontal gyrus anterior to the motor strip. *Center:* The cortical incision is through the middle frontal gyrus (Mid.Fr.Gyr.) The subchoroidal approach is directed through the choroidal fissure (Ch.Fiss.). The choroid plexus (Ch.Pl.) is attached along the choroidal fissure in the interval between the thalamus and the fornix. The choroidal fissure is opened between the choroid plexus and the thalamus to expose the third ventricle (3V) posterior to the foramen of Monro (F.Monro). The massa intermedia (Massa Inter.) projects into the third ventricle. The medial posterior choroidal arteries (Med.Post.Ch.A.) and the internal cerebral veins (In.Cer.V.) course in the roof of the third ventricle. The internal cerebral veins receive the direct lateral (Dir.Lat.V.), septal (Sept.V.), and thalamostriate (Thal.Str.V.) veins. The caudate nucleus (Caudate Nucl.) is lateral to the thalamus. The subchoroidal exposure has the advantage of displacing, rather than dividing, the fornix to allow entry into the third ventricle. (From Rhoton et al.[9])

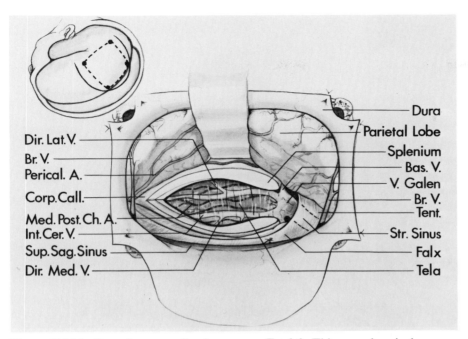

Figure 114-10 Posterior transcallosal exposure. *Top left:* This procedure is done with the patient in the left lateral decubitus position with the right parietal region uppermost. The scalp flap (*solid line*) and bone flap (*dashed line*) extend up to the midline. An alternative position is to place the right side down so that gravity will assist in retracting the medial surface of the right cerebral hemisphere away from the falx. *Center:* The dura is opened with the pedicle along the midline. The exposure extends up to the medial surface of the superior sagittal sinus (Sup.Sag.Sinus). Several bridging veins (Br.V.) are placed on a stretch, and one has been sacrificed in retracting the medial surface of the parietal lobe away from the falx. The branches of the pericallosal artery (Perical.A.) are exposed above the splenium of the corpus callosum (Corp.Call.). The internal cerebral veins (Int.Cer.V.) and their tributaries, the direct lateral (Dir.Lat.V.), direct medial (Dir.Med.V.), and basal (Bas.V.) veins, and the medial posterior choroidal arteries (Med.Post.Ch.A.) are exposed within the leaves of the tela choroidea (Tela). The vein of Galen (V.Galen) enters the straight sinus (Str.Sinus) at the anterior margin of the tentorium (Tent.). (From Rhoton et al.[9])

ing, rather than dividing, the fornix and choroid plexus, and also provides a more favorable angle for visualization of the third ventricle than does the transcallosal approach (Fig. 114-9).[12] This approach is uniquely suited to lesions in the superior half of the third ventricle below the roof and posterior to the foramen of Monro. The incision through the right middle frontal gyrus is directed to the area above the body of the fornix. The ependyma and tela choroidea between the fornix and choroid plexus above and the thalamus below are opened until the internal cerebral vein comes into view. The right half of the fornix and the choroid plexus are displaced to the left side, the remaining strands of tela choroidea are divided, and the lateral border of the roof of the third ventricle is entered through the resulting longitudinal opening. A wider opening of the third ventricle may be provided by dividing the thalamostriate vein and extending the opening into the foramen of Monro. However, occlusion of the veins at the foramen of Monro may result in hemorrhagic infarction of the basal ganglia, as noted previously. A continuous arch formed by the thalamostriate and internal cerebral veins outlines the access route into the third ventricle. The

maximal limits of the opening into the third ventricle are determined by the limits of displacement of these vessels and their branches. After the lesion is exposed, it is removed according to the principles outlined previously.

Posterior Operative Approaches

The approaches suitable for lesions in the posterior part of the third ventricle are the (1) posterior transventricular, (2) posterior transcallosal, (3) occipital transtentorial, and (4) infratentorial supracerebellar (Fig. 114-1). These approaches are reviewed in greater detail in other chapters in this text.

The posterior transcallosal approach, although used by Dandy for pineal tumors, has been replaced in most cases by the occipital transtentorial or the infratentorial supracerebellar approach (Fig. 114-10).[2] The approach is best suited for a third ventricular tumor that has a major upward extension into the posterior part of the corpus callosum, or that

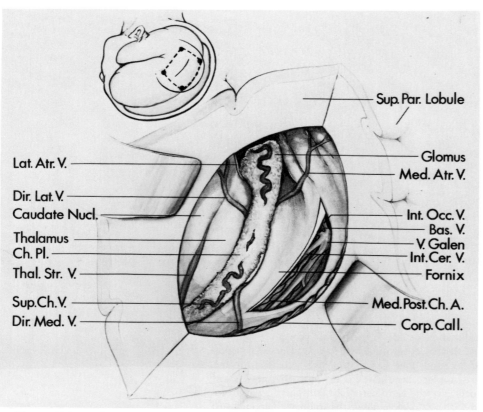

Figure 114-11 *Posterior parietal transventricular approach. Top:* The procedure is done with the patient in the lateral decubitus position with the hemisphere and ventricle through which the approach is to be directed uppermost. The scalp incision (*solid line*) and bone flap (*dashed line*) are centered over the superior parietal lobule posterior to the postcentral somatosensory cortex. *Center:* The cortical incision is through the superior parietal lobule (Sup.Par.Lobule). The ventricle is opened to expose the choroid plexus (Ch.Pl.) and its attachment along the choroidal fissure between the thalamus and the fornix. The thalamostriate vein (Thal.Str.V.) courses in the groove between the caudate nucleus (Caudate Nucl.) and the thalamus. A superior choroidal vein (Sup.Ch.V.) courses on the surface of the choroid plexus. The lateral atrial (Lat.Atr.V.) and the medial atrial (Med.Atr.V.) veins drain the atrium of the ventricle. The direct lateral vein (Dir.Lat.V.) crosses the caudate nucleus and thalamus and passes through the choroidal fissure. The direct medial vein (Dir. Med.V.) crosses the fornix. The incision through the medial wall of the ventricle is through the crus of the fornix below the corpus callosum (Corp.Call.). The opening in the fornix exposes the vein of Galen (V.Galen) and the internal cerebral (Int.Cer.V.), basal (Bas.V.), and internal occipital (Int.Occ.V.) veins and the medial posterior choroidal arteries (Med.Post.Ch.A.) (From Rhoton et al.[9])

appears to arise in the corpus callosum above the great vein and extends into the posterior part of the third ventricle.

The posterior transventricular approach provides adequate exposure of the atrium and posterior portions of the body of the lateral ventricle; this may be the preferred approach to a lesion involving the third ventricle if the tumor extends into the posterior part of the lateral ventricle or if the lesion predominantly involves the atrium or the glomus of the choroid plexus (Fig. 114-11). The transventricular exposures are more difficult to perform if the ventricle is not dilated. They do not provide satisfactory exposure of the

typical midline pineal tumor and are unsuited to the pineal tumor that extends posteroinferiorly through the tentorial opening toward the quadrigeminal plate and the cerebellum.

The occipital transtentorial approach is suitable for tumors in the pineal region, especially if they are centered at the tentorial edge or above and if there is no major extension to the opposite side or into the posterior fossa.

The infratentorial supracerebellar approach is suitable for midline pineal tumors that grow into both the posterior part of the third ventricle and the posterior fossa, displacing the quadrigeminal plate and the anterior lobe and the cerebellum. An advantage of this approach is that the deep venous system that caps the dorsal and lateral aspects of most pineal tumors does not obstruct access to the tumor.

References

1. Apuzzo MLJ, Chikovani OK, Gott PS, Teng EL, Zee CS, Giannotta SL, Weiss MH: Transcallosal, interfornicial approaches for lesions affecting the third ventricle: Surgical considerations and consequences. Neurosurgery 10:547–554, 1982.

2. Dandy WE: *Benign Tumors in the Third Ventricle of the Brain: Diagnosis and Treatment*. Springfield, Illinois, Charles C Thomas, 1933.

3. Hardy J, Vezina JL: Transsphenoidal neurosurgery of intracranial neoplasm. Adv Neurol 15:261–274, 1976.

4. Hirsch JF, Zouaoui A, Renier D, Pierre-Kahn A: A new surgical approach to the third ventricle with interruption of the striothalamic vein. Acta Neurochir (Wien) 47:135–147, 1979.

5. Kempe LG: *Operative Neurosurgery*. New York, Springer-Verlag, 1968, vol 1.

6. King TT: Removal of intraventricular craniopharyngiomas through the lamina terminalis. Acta Neurochir (Wien) 45:277–286, 1979.

7. Laws ER Jr: Transsphenoidal microsurgery in the management of craniopharyngioma. J Neurosurg 52:661–666, 1980.

8. Rhoton AL Jr, Hardy DG, Chambers SM: Microsurgical anatomy and dissection of the sphenoid bone, cavernous sinus and sellar region. Surg Neurol 12:63–104, 1979.

9. Rhoton AL Jr, Yamamoto I, Peace DA: Microsurgery of the third ventricle: Part 2. Operative approaches. Neurosurgery 8:357–373, 1981.

10. Shucart WA, Stein BM: Transcallosal approach to the anterior ventricular system. Neurosurgery 3:339–343, 1978.

11. Symon L: The temporal approach for resection of craniopharyngioma, in Symon L (ed): *Operative Surgery: Neurosurgery*. London, Butterworth, 1979, pp 185–186.

12. Viale GL, Turtas S: The subchoroid approach to the third ventricle. Surg Neurol 14:71–76, 1980.

13. Yamamoto I, Rhoton AL Jr, Peace DA: Microsurgery of the third ventricle: Part 1. Microsurgical anatomy. Neurosurgery 8:334–356, 1981.

Tumors of the Orbit

115

Radiology of the Orbit and Its Contents

Richard E. Latchaw
William E. Rothfus

Diagnostic x-ray procedures have a threefold function: to define the location and extent of pathological changes, to determine the most likely pathological possibilities, and to guide surgical tools and biopsy needles for tissue characterization and/or treatment. Accordingly, this chapter has three goals.

First, we wish to discuss the types of radiographic techniques that are most useful for evaluating diseases of the orbit. Many types of radiography have been utilized to evaluate the orbit and its contents, ranging from plain films to highly technical methods such as computed tomography (CT), ultrasonography, and angiography. For the radiologist, computed tomography has proven to be the best and most useful technique for evaluating the majority of orbital abnormalities, with angiography and ultrasonography being of lesser value. Our discussion includes all of the various radiographic techniques that have been utilized, indicating their advantages and disadvantages for specific disease processes.

The second goal, a listing of the radiographic findings of specific disease processes and points of differential diagnosis, is oriented toward surgeons. Therefore, there is an emphasis upon the typical radiographic features of intraorbital neoplastic lesions. However, there are a number of inflammatory conditions, such as pseudotumor and Graves' disease, that clinically mimic an intraorbital neoplasm. In most cases the radiographic findings distinguish such non-neoplastic processes from neoplastic disease.

Third, both ultrasonography and computed tomography allow rapid visualization of the intraorbital contents. These radiographic modalities facilitate localization for the biopsy of intraorbital lesions. Such biopsy techniques obviate the need in many cases for direct surgical intervention.

Techniques of Radiographic Evaluation

Plain Films

Plain films of the orbit are at best nonspecific in the diagnosis of particular pathological processes. However, they do demonstrate the general features of many disease states, including diffuse orbital enlargement, calcification, and change in the bony walls. Orbital enlargement is usually indicative of long-standing increased intraorbital pressure, such as from a slowly growing benign tumor like a hemangioma, from a non-neoplastic expansion such as an intraorbital varix, or from enlargement of the globe itself (buphthalmos). Obviously, the finding of orbital enlargement is most marked when a chronic process during childhood has produced changes in the developing orbit.

Intraorbital calcification is another nonspecific finding. Retinal calcifications are common with retinoblastoma, and some lacrimal gland tumors tend to calcify. Phleboliths may be present with an intraorbital varix or hemangioma. Focal bony erosion may indicate the site of pathological change, such as may be seen in the superolateral aspect of the orbit when there is a lacrimal gland neoplasm. Sclerosis of the orbital walls may accompany an intraorbital meningioma, but can also be seen with malignant lacrimal gland tumors, metastases, and Paget's disease. Fibrous dysplasia produces a densely sclerotic and expanded bony contour when the orbit is involved; depending upon the degree of involvement, it may be difficult to distinguish a focal area of fibrous dysplasia from the reactive bone of a meningioma. Osteomas of the paranasal sinuses are extremely dense and are obvious on plain films.

By and large, plain film evaluation of the orbit is an outmoded examination method except in cases of trauma. Evaluation of an intraorbital expansion, whether neoplastic or non-neoplastic, or an intraorbital inflammatory process is much more complete and specific with computed tomography.

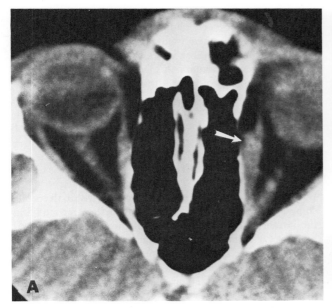

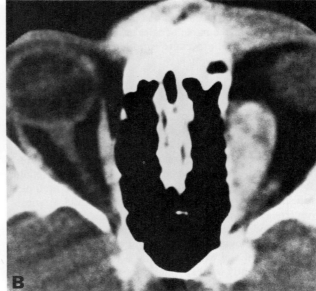

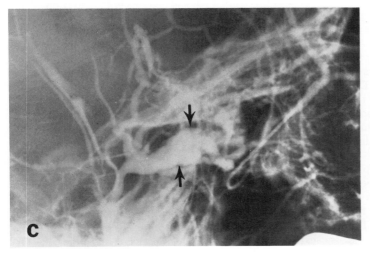

Figure 115-1 Intraorbital venous varix. *A*. The axial scan of the orbits with the patient supine and resting comfortably demonstrates an elongated soft tissue mass (*white arrow*) medial to the medial rectus muscle. *B*. The patient has been scanned in a supine position, but during a Valsalva maneuver following 5 minutes of head down positioning and following the infusion of contrast material. The scan demonstrates the "swelling" of the extraconal mass with these maneuvers, characteristic of a venous varix. *C*. The lateral view of an orbital venogram demonstrates the venous varix (*black arrows*).

Orbital Venography

Orbital venography became very popular in the pre-CT era of the late 1960s and early 1970s for the evaluation of an intraorbital expansion. The technique is usually performed by first placing a scalp vein needle in a vein of the forehead. Contrast material is then injected while the veins draining the scalp are compressed by a tourniquet and the angular veins near the medial aspects of the orbits are compressed manually. Contrast material subsequently fills the superior and inferior ophthalmic veins, with posterior flow into the cavernous sinuses. Displacement of various portions of the superior ophthalmic vein gives only indirect evidence for the location of a mass lesion. Abnormalities of a cavernous sinus can also be evaluated with this technique. An alternative method consists of a transfemoral venous approach to selective catheterization of the petrosal veins draining into the sigmoid sinus. Contrast material flows anteriorly to fill the cavernous sinuses and subsequently the superior ophthalmic veins.

The technique has largely been replaced by computed tomography because of the specificity of CT in determining the location and type of an intraorbital lesion. Orbital venography may still prove helpful in evaluating venous abnormalities such as an intraorbital varix (Fig. 115-1). The presence of a varix, however, can be validated on CT by comparing scans performed before and after either the Valsalva maneuver or exercise. Compression of the superior ophthalmic vein at the orbital apex by an inflammatory condition such as the Tolosa-Hunt syndrome may be proven with orbital venography, and occasionally abnormalities of a cavernous sinus are still evaluated by this technique.

Positive Contrast Orbitography

The injection of a water-soluble contrast material into the retro-ocular soft tissues with subsequent plain film radiography was utilized before orbital venography became popular. Such a technique allowed the direct visualization of an intraorbital mass lesion. Unfortunately, the technique was associated with a high complication rate, specifically secondary infection, and a number of cases of subsequent blindness were reported. The procedure is no longer performed.

Angiography

Orbital angiography became particularly useful with the advent of selective catheterization of the internal and external carotid vasculature, the introduction of magnification techniques to geometrically enlarge the small vessels within the orbit, and the development of high-quality subtraction film. The blood supply to the orbit consists of multiple branches of the ophthalmic and external carotid arteries. Numerous anastomotic channels are available between the internal and external carotid transorbital circulations. Therefore, angiographic evaluation of the orbit requires selective internal and external carotid artery injections. The orbit is frequently overexposed during routine filming; the blood vessels within the orbit are extremely small; and vascular displacement may be quite subtle. All of these factors make mandatory the use of direct magnification angiography and high-quality subtraction in addition to selective arterial catheterization.

Orbital angiography has proved of value primarily for the evaluation of vascular intraorbital mass lesions, such as an intraorbital meningioma or hemangioma (Fig. 115-2). Diseases of blood vessels can obviously be studied with this technique; they include an aneurysm of either the intracranial or intraorbital vasculature, a retro-orbital pial or dural arteriovenous malformation, and a carotid–cavernous sinus fistula.

A less invasive technique for performing angiographic studies is digital subtraction angiography. This technique consists of the acquisition of radiographic information on either a fluoroscopic screen or a solid-state diode array, following the intravascular injection of contrast material. The image is digitized and processed in a computer, similar to the way CT scan data are used, with subsequent edge enhancement, signal amplification, and subtraction of background densities. Contrast material may be injected into an arm vein, with subsequent dissemination to the orbit. While this may represent a potentially easy way to evaluate the orbit, the simultaneous filling of the vessels of the orbit, face, and brain, with an overlap of densities rather than the selective visualization of the orbit itself, may prove far too detrimental to be useful for study of the orbit. Spatial resolution is less than that of typical film-screen combinations, further decreasing the potential for this technique. Intra-arterial injections with digital subtraction techniques may prove to be of far greater value. The ability of computer algorithms to enhance the tiny intraorbital vessels may prove valuable.

Ultrasonography

Ultrasonic evaluation of the orbit has become very popular in recent years, particularly among ophthalmologists. The technique is noninvasive and is excellent for the evaluation of intraocular lesions and diseases involving the anterior portions of the retrobulbar space. Abnormal tissues may be characterized as cystic, solid, or vascular. The technique is not as good as computed tomography for the more posterior portion of the retrobulbar region. However, the two techniques are complementary in many disease processes. For example, a tumor beginning within the globe may be identified and characterized by ultrasonography, whereas computed tomography is used to evaluate the retrobulbar extension of the mass.

Computed Tomography

Because of the inherent contrast differences within the orbit, computed tomography is an excellent method for studying the intraorbital soft tissues. One of the fundamental attributes of CT is its ability to distinguish the densities of various soft tissues. The orbit contains an orderly arrangement of muscle, fat, nervous tissue, and the dense fibrous tissues of the sclera and lens. The inherent contrast differences between these soft tissues allows them to be distinctly separated by CT. Most disease processes can be readily identified without the infusion of contrast material. However, contrast enhancement may aid in the identification and characterization of certain masses, and in the identification of vascular abnormalities. In addition, because the intracranial CT evaluation of a tumor or infection is highly dependent upon an abnormality of the blood-brain barrier, as visualized following the infusion of contrast material, the evaluation of the intracranial extension of a primary intraorbital tumor or inflammation is aided with contrast enhancement.

Multiple CT projections are useful in studying intraorbital disease. The axial scan is the easiest to obtain, and is performed with the patient in a supine position and the scan angle parallel to the longitudinal axis of the orbit. Coronal views may be obtained with hyperextension of the head and neck with the patient either prone or supine. These coronal views are particularly helpful for evaluating diseases of the extraocular muscles or when localizing an intraorbital foreign body. In addition, coronal views are extremely helpful in evaluating complex fractures involving the orbit and in defining the relationships of an intraorbital mass to various anatomical structures.

Contiguous 5-mm cuts are usually obtained in either the axial or direct coronal projections. Thinner slices, of less than 2 mm, may be obtained for better spatial resolution. Reformatted sagittal and off-axis oblique views may also be generated with computer processing of direct axial or coronal data.

Radiographic Characteristics of Intraorbital Lesions

Neoplasms

Optic Nerve

Optic Sheath Meningioma Primary optic sheath meningioma originates in the arachnoid layer attached to the dura. Spread is along the arachnoid sheath of the nerve,

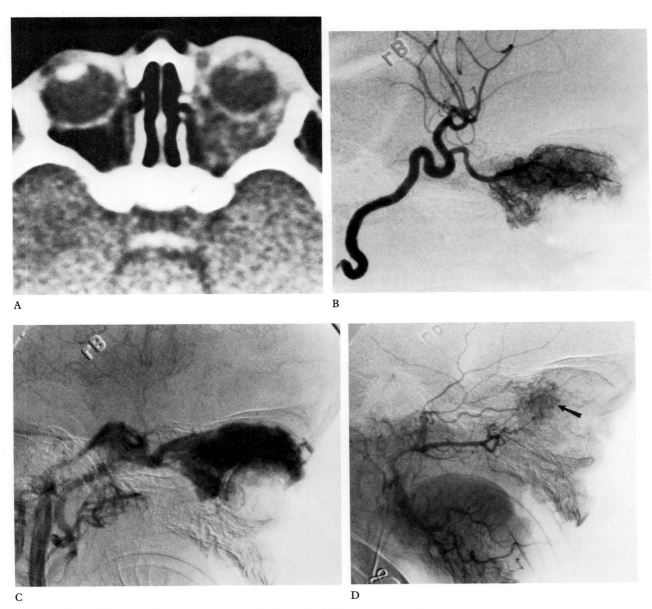

A

B

C

D

Figure 115-2 Orbital capillary hemangioma. *A*. An orbital CT scan demonstrates a diffuse mass in the retro-ocular space, surrounding the lateral and medial portions of the globe and producing soft tissue swelling anteriorly. There is a mild degree of proptosis. The mass is of mixed high and low density. A selective internal carotid artery injection (*B,C*) demonstrates the vascular intraorbital mass with hypertrophic and densely compacted arteries, arterioles, and capillaries (*B*). The capillary and early venous phase (*C*) demonstrates an intense and homogeneous enhancement of this capillary hemangioma. *D*. A selective external carotid artery injection demonstrates numerous branches of the internal maxillary artery supplying the vascular network of the tumor (*arrow*).

encircling the nerve and compressing it without actual invasion in most instances. However, the tumor may invade the neural tissue or break through the dura.[1]

The characteristic of encirclement and compression of the optic nerve means that optic nerve meningioma commonly presents with visual loss and optic atrophy. Other symptoms, such as proptosis and pain, occur late, after the

tumor has grown to a considerable size.[1,14] The linear mode of spread may allow microsurgical stripping of the tumor from the optic nerve, preserving vision.[1]

CT scanning usually demonstrates a fusiform widening of the optic nerve–sheath complex (Figs. 115-3, 115-4).[4] Because the tumor is external to the optic nerve itself, the lucency of the normal underlying nerve is seen with an ap-

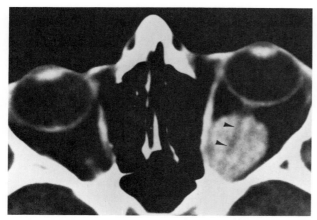

Figure 115-3 Optic sheath meningioma. There is a fusiform mass surrounding the optic nerve. The optic nerve (*arrowheads*) is seen through the mass on this scan, which has been "windowed" for this purpose. This indicates that the mass has arisen outside the nerve itself. The mass is well-marginated and stains intensely and homogeneously, as is typical of an intraorbital meningioma.

propriate CT window (Figs. 115-3, 115-4).[12] This appearance is in contradistinction to that of an optic nerve glioma, which has a homogeneous density throughout. This appearance of dense tumor surrounding a more lucent optic nerve is nonspecific for optic sheath meningioma, since the same appearance may be produced by any type of lesion that grows around the nerve, such as a metastatic tumor or an inflammatory condition like sarcoidosis.

The meningioma is usually dense on the preinfusion scan, and there is marked contrast enhancement (Fig. 115-3), analogous to the changes seen with an intracranial meningioma. It may extend into the optic canal, producing bony hyperostosis (Fig. 115-4). Further extension posteriorly along the optic nerve produces a suprasellar-parasellar intracranial mass lesion.[4,12]

Optic Nerve Glioma Most optic nerve gliomas occur during childhood, with the most common sites of origin being the intracranial portion of the optic nerve and the optic chiasm. The least common site of origin is the intraorbital portion of the optic nerve. The rare optic nerve glioma occurring during the adult years generally presents posterior to the orbit. The optic nerve glioma is a common tumor in

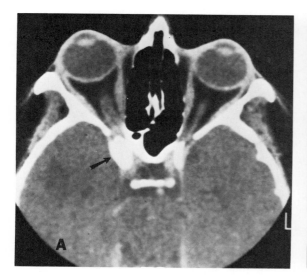

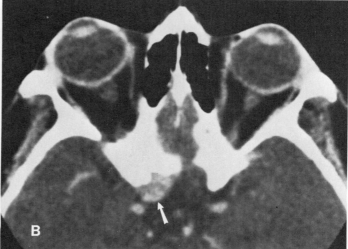

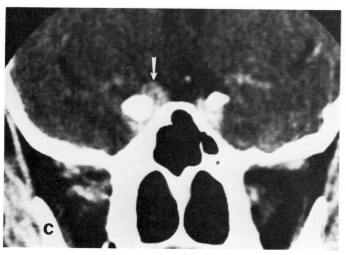

Figure 115-4 Optic sheath meningioma with intracranial extension, producing hyperostosis. *A.* Enhanced axial scan demonstrates tubular enlargement of the optic nerve–sheath complex. That the mass originated outside the optic nerve is indicated by the visualization of the nerve as a lucency coursing through the tubular mass. The neoplasm has produced hyperostosis of the ipsilateral anterior clinoid process (*arrow*). *B.* Slightly higher cut than (*A*) again demonstrates the hyperostotic anterior clinoid process and sharply marginated, densely enhancing tumor (*white arrow*) extending into the anterolateral suprasellar space. *C.* Coronal projection also demonstrates the enlarged anterior clinoid process and intracranial extension of the tumor (*white arrow*).

patients with neurofibromatosis, although it may also occur spontaneously. The usual presenting symptom is that of decreased visual acuity.

The typical CT scan appearance of an intraorbital optic nerve glioma is that of fusiform (Fig. 115-5) or tubular (Fig. 115-6) widening of the optic nerve. The least common CT appearance is that of an eccentric bulge from the nerve. The CT appearance results from growth of the tumor along the axis of the optic nerve without penetration of the overlying dura. The tumor may extend posteriorly through the optic foramen into the optic chiasm; it may further extend into the optic tract or contralateral optic nerve. Subtle chiasmal involvement may be evaluated with CT scanning in both the axial and coronal projections following the intrathecal deposition of a small volume of metrizamide.

The differential diagnosis of a fusiform optic nerve glioma includes optic sheath meningioma and neurofibroma of the nerve sheath. Optic sheath meningioma generally occurs during adulthood, whereas optic nerve glioma is primarily a tumor of childhood. Utilizing CT criteria only, an optic sheath meningioma generally enhances dramatically following the intravenous infusion of contrast material; an optic nerve glioma enhances to a lesser degree. An optic sheath meningioma frequently has a central lucency along the axis of the optic nerve, as previously discussed, but there is no lucency within the homogeneous density of an optic glioma. Both the optic glioma and the nerve sheath neurofibroma are common tumors in children who have neurofibromatosis. The neurofibroma is usually a large, eccentric mass relative to the more fusiform-appearing optic nerve glioma.[3]

Retro-ocular Tumors Outside the Optic Nerve

Meningioma of the Orbital Wall   A meningioma originating from the orbital wall is probably more common than a primary optic sheath meningioma. It is seen as a well-circumscribed, rounded mass projecting into the orbital contents. Characteristically, it is dense on the preinfusion CT scan and shows marked contrast enhancement of a homogeneous character, similar to the pattern of an intracranial meningioma. The bony wall may be sclerotic or have a mixed pattern of sclerosis and osteolysis.

Neurofibroma and Schwannoma   Neurofibromas and schwannomas may arise from either the optic nerve sheath, as previously discussed, or from other nerves within the orbit. Neurofibromas may be of two types, solid or plexiform. Solid neurofibromas usually occur in adults and may not be associated with neurofibromatosis. They are usually well-encapsulated and are therefore easily removed at the time of surgery. The lesion may be calcified on the preinfusion CT scan. Uniform enhancement usually occurs on the enhanced scan, but the degree of enhancement is usually less than that of the typical intraorbital meningioma (Fig. 115-7).

The plexiform type of neurofibroma is always associated with neurofibromatosis. This lesion is not encapsulated, but grows in a diffuse manner by surrounding other intraorbital structures. This presents an extremely difficult surgical problem, and recurrence is common. The CT scan generally shows a diffuse, multinodular lesion insinuating itself among intraorbital anatomical structures. A contiguous facial plexiform component is common.

A patient with neurofibromatosis may present with proptosis that is not caused by an intraorbital tumor. Because neurofibromatosis is a diffuse dysplasia involving bony structures, the posterolateral wall of the orbit (greater wing of the sphenoid) may be dysplastic, allowing the temporal lobe to herniate into the orbit, thereby causing proptosis and mimicking an intraorbital tumor.

Hemangioma   Hemangiomas are the most common primary tumors of the orbit, and may be of either the capillary or cavernous type.[8] The two types of hemangiomas differ in their age of presentation and in their degree of encapsulation.

The capillary hemangioma, which is found primarily in childhood, is made up of a myriad of vessels of capillary size,

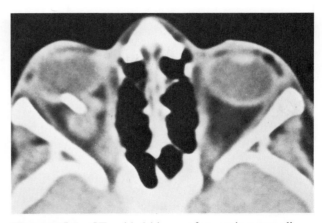

Figure 115-6   CT-guided biopsy of an optic nerve glioma. There is a sharply marginated but somewhat irregular tubular mass involving the optic nerve. The high-density elongated structure in the mass is a portion of the biopsy probe. CT scanning provides an easy method for visualizing deep orbital structures undergoing biopsy.

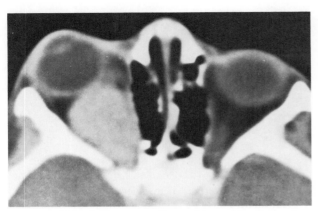

Figure 115-5   Optic nerve glioma. The axial enhanced CT scan demonstrates a sharply marginated fusiform mass involving the optic nerve–sheath complex and extending to the posterior margin of the globe. Appropriate windows did not allow the optic nerve to be seen through the mass.

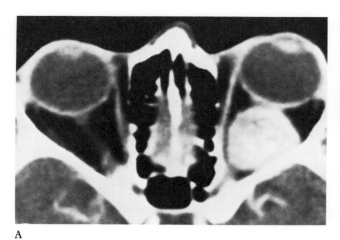
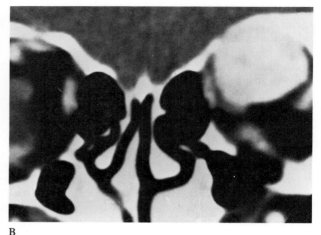

A   B

Figure 115-7   Solid intraorbital neurofibroma. The enhanced axial (*A*) and coronal (*B*) scans demonstrate a deeply enhancing, sharply marginated mass lesion in the superior portion of the orbit. While the degree of enhancement in this case is equal to that of a meningioma, many intraorbital neurofibromas enhance to a lesser degree.

and stains intensely at angiography (Fig. 115-2). It is a soft, nonencapsulated lesion that infiltrates around or through normal intraorbital structures, and growth outside the orbit may occur. CT scanning demonstrates a poorly marginated lesion that is dense on the preinfusion scan due to the presence of a large "blood pool." There is generally an intense and homogeneous degree of enhancement. The extreme degree of vascularity and the infiltrative nature of the lesion make surgery extremely difficult. Fortunately, many of these lesions will involute over time in a fashion similar to facial hemangiomas.

A cavernous hemangioma, which is more commonly found in adulthood, is made up primarily of large sinusoidal vascular channels. Because of the stasis of blood within these sinusoids, contrast material injected at the time of angiography may be diluted so that the lesion appears to be relatively avascular. There may be pooling of contrast material on the venous phase. The lesion is well encapsulated and is therefore seen as a sharply marginated mass on CT scan (Fig. 115-8). Multiple calcifications (phleboliths) may be seen, along with increased density on the preinfusion scan secondary to the increased blood pool within the lesion.[8] Enhancement may be either homogeneous or heterogeneous. Heterogeneity of tissues, including vascular channels of differing sizes, calcification, and variable amounts of supporting stroma, in part leads to this heterogeneous CT appearance. There is dilution of injected contrast material within the larger sinusoids, adding to the heterogeneity.

Hemangiopericytoma   The hemangiopericytoma originates from the supporting pericyte of a capillary.[5] It is usually a well-encapsulated lesion containing many fine tumor vessels. There is usually an intense degree of enhancement on the postinfusion CT scan. Although the enhancement is frequently homogeneous in character, a heterogeneous appearance may be seen with immediate scanning after a bolus injection.

It may be impossible to radiographically distinguish a

hemangiopericytoma from either an intraorbital meningioma or a cavernous hemangioma, but there are a number of findings that may be of value. First, the lesion is relatively aggressive and may invade surrounding structures. Second, there may be metastases to extraorbital sites; there may be a relatively long latent period before these metastases are manifest. Orbital hemangiopericytoma may therefore be suspected on a preoperative radiographic evaluation when there is a lesion that simulates hemangioma, but appears to be more aggressive and/or has metastasized.

Dermoid Cyst   The intraorbital dermoid cyst most commonly involves the lacrimal gland; its slow growth produces remodeling of the bony walls, particularly the superolateral portion of the orbit. The dermoid cyst produces a

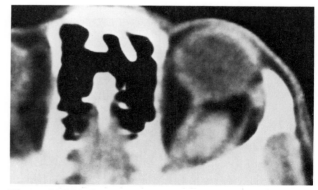

Figure 115-8   Cavernous hemangioma. The well-circumscribed, moderately enhancing mass within the orbit was proven histologically to be a cavernous hemangioma. Although the mass is near the optic nerve and enhances in a homogeneous fashion, it does not spread in a circumferential perineural manner as would a meningioma. Many cavernous hemangiomas do not stain as homogeneously as in this case, and many contain phleboliths.

distinctive CT scan appearance. The lesion has a marked degree of low density in the region of −50 to −100 Hounsfield units on the CT scan, typical of any fatty lesion.

Metastases Metastatic tumor may involve any portion of the orbit. Metastasis to the orbital walls is the most common form of involvement (Fig. 115-9). Metastasis to the vascular choroid of the globe is the next most common, with involvement of retrobulbar structures such as muscle the least common. The most common metastatic solid tumors in adults are adenocarcinomas of the breast, lung, GI tract, and GU tract.[6] In children, neuroblastoma and Ewing's sarcoma are the most common lesions.

A rapidly expanding soft tissue mass and bone destruction are the radiographic hallmarks of metastatic disease in the orbit, as in other parts of the body. Proptosis is common, although scirrhous carcinoma of either the breast or lung may produce a retraction of the globe. Metastasis to the choroid leads to enhancement of the wall of the globe on the enhanced scan, with or without visualization of a retro-ocular mass. Metastatic involvement of an optic nerve leads to enlargement of that nerve. Muscle enlargement may be secondary to compression of venous structures by metastatic tumor at the orbital apex, or to direct infiltration.

Lymphoma Lymphoma is a common type of intraorbital tumor, third in incidence after hemangioma and optic nerve tumors in one series.[3] There is a spectrum of CT scan appearances of lymphoma. The tumor may appear as a localized mass; it may be primarily infiltrative, producing a poorly marginated mass; or there may be involvement of only the extraocular muscles. Generally, there is a marked degree of homogeneous enhancement on the postinfusion CT scan. There may be extension around, and infiltration of, the globe, producing enhancement of the margins of that structure (Fig. 115-10).

Both on the CT scan and at pathological examination, it may be extremely difficult, if not impossible, to distinguish lymphoma from orbital pseudotumor. Both lesions contain lymphocytes and both may have the similar spectrum of CT scan appearances described above. Pseudotumor is discussed in greater detail later in this chapter.

The Globe

The common primary tumors of the globe are melanoma in the adult, originating in the pigmented cells of the retina, and retinoblastoma in the child. Metastases to the globe are primarily the carcinomas, as previously discussed.

Retinoblastoma usually begins within the first 2 years of life and is bilateral in one-third of cases. The lesion is malignant and invasive, and it may spread back along the optic nerve toward the apex of the orbit. Occasionally, the lesion may extend into the optic chiasm and other intracranial structures. However, retinoblastoma grows very slowly, allowing treatment of the lesion. Enucleation of the affected eye, with radiation therapy if optic nerve extension is present, produces a cure in a very high percentage of cases. Therefore, orbital and intracranial CT scanning is essential before undertaking therapy.

The CT scan demonstrates nodular calcification within the globe (Fig. 115-11). There may be a dense intraocular

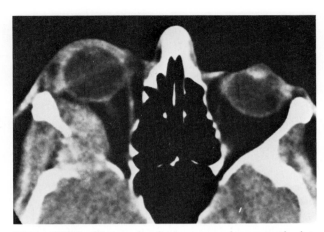

Figure 115-9 Metastasis of a breast carcinoma to the lateral orbital wall. A metastatic deposit produces extensive destruction of the greater wing of the sphenoid and the anterior wall of the middle cranial fossa. A large tumor extends into the orbit, producing proptosis. Tumor extends into the subtemporal fossa; there is also a small amount of intracranial tumor.

mass that enhances slightly. Scanning of the intracranial structures must be performed with contrast enhancement in order to exclude intracranial extension.

Non-neoplastic Lesions

Bony Walls

The most common non-neoplastic lesion of the bony walls is fibrous dysplasia. This is a congenital dysplasia of bone characterized by thickening and sclerosis of the involved bone to produce a homogeneous, "ground glass" texture (Fig. 115-12). Such an appearance simulates the hyperostotic bone of a meningioma, but no soft-tissue mass is

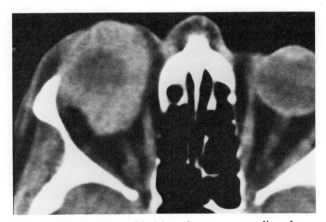

Figure 115-10 Intraorbital lymphoma surrounding the globe. The enhanced axial scan demonstrates an extensive, well-marginated, homogeneously enhancing neoplasm surrounding the globe. This appearance is typical of lymphoma.

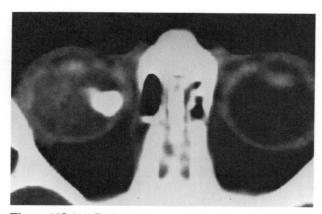

Figure 115-11 Retinoblastoma of the globe. The axial scan in this child demonstrates a large nodule of calcification along the medial aspect of the retina, with diffuse soft tissue density throughout the vitreous. The findings are pathognomonic of retinoblastoma. (Courtesy of K. Shaffer, M.D., Medical College of Wisconsin, Milwaukee, Wis.).

detected on CT scanning as with meningioma. The bony abnormality may be seen as an incidental finding on a skull film or CT scan performed for other reasons. Pronounced thickening of the bony wall may produce proptosis and/or narrowing of the foramina.

Inflammatory Conditions of the Soft Tissues

Graves' Disease Involvement of the orbit by Graves' disease may be a difficult clinical diagnosis because of the presence of normal thyroid function tests in some patients. The CT scan, however, may be extremely helpful in the diagnosis of Graves' disease, since there are a number of characteristic CT scan findings. In addition, the CT scan is extremely important in the evaluation of the extent of intraorbital structural involvement, both to determine management and to evaluate responsiveness to therapy.

The most prominent CT scan finding in Graves' disease is extraocular muscle enlargement. The process is most frequently bilateral and symmetrical, with bilaterality but asymmetry within an orbit the next most common presentation. The least common appearance is that of unilateral involvement, with asymmetry within the orbit and/or single

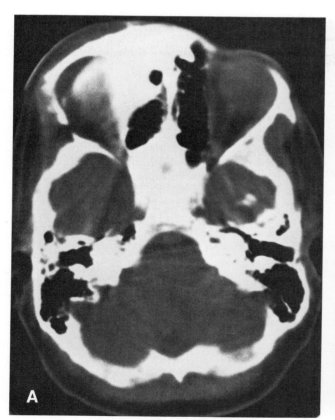
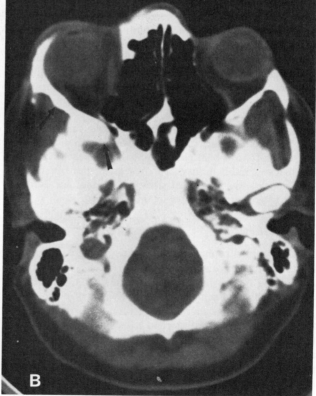

Figure 115-12 Fibrous dysplasia of the orbital walls; CT scan sections. *A.* Diffuse sclerosis and thickening of the body of the sphenoid bone, the ethmoid at its junction with the roof of the orbit, and the inferior and medial portion of the frontal bone. *B.* A lower cut demonstrates bony thickening of the greater wing of the sphenoid (*arrows*). No mass was demonstrable on enhanced views (not shown) to implicate meningioma. The findings are typical of fibrous dysplasia.

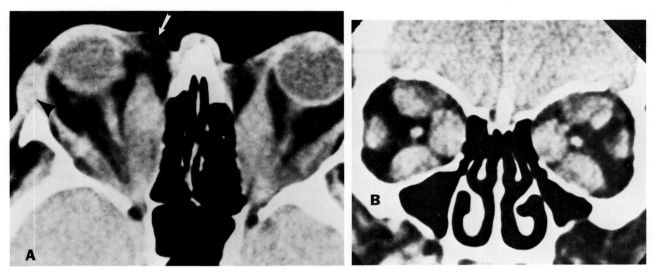

Figure 115-13 Extraocular muscle enlargement in Graves' disease. A moderate degree of bilateral proptosis is present secondary to diffuse extraocular muscle enlargement, as seen on the axial (*A*) and coronal (*B*) CT scans. The medial and inferior rectus muscles show the greatest enlargement. There is anterior displacement of the orbital septum (*A, white arrow*) by the prolapsing orbital fat. The axial scan (*A*) passes through the inferior portion of the lacrimal gland (*black arrowhead*), which is displaced anteriorly by the increase in orbital soft tissues. Involvement of the lacrimal gland by Graves' disease has produced enlargement and enhancement.

muscle involvement. The medial and inferior rectus muscles are the most frequently and most severely involved.[2] Both coronal and axial CT scanning are essential in the evaluation of muscle enlargement (Fig. 115-13). Usually there is diffuse and homogeneous enhancement of those muscles involved.

Edema and cellular infiltration of the retro-ocular fat may produce a change in its appearance on the CT scan. There may be an increased volume of fat, leading to prolapse of fatty tissue behind the orbital septum (Fig. 115-13). Increased density of the fat may also occasionally be seen. Another but less common finding in Graves' disease is mild swelling of the optic nerve secondary to its compression at the orbital apex by the enlarged muscles.[13] Enlargement and enhancement of the lacrimal gland may also occur (Fig. 115-13).

Pseudotumor The term *pseudotumor* refers to a group of noninfectious inflammatory conditions originating within different tissues of the orbit. The condition may begin in and be localized to the lacrimal gland, the extraocular muscles (myositic pseudotumor), or the retro-ocular fat. The condition may also be diffuse and involve multiple intraorbital structures. Histologically, pseudotumor is characterized by a diffuse collection of lymphocytes and therefore has the nonspecific appearance of many chronic inflammatory conditions.[11] Pseudotumor either may be idiopathic or may be associated with systemic disease processes such as sarcoidosis, polyarteritis nodosa, Wegener's granulomatosis, retroperitoneal fibrosis, and a number of other similar inflammatory conditions.

It may be extremely difficult, if not impossible, to distinguish myositic pseudotumor from Graves' disease either clinically or radiographically. Generally, however, pseudotumor has a more abrupt onset, more pain, and more erythema, and is more steroid-responsive than is Graves' disease. Radiographically, myositic pseudotumor is generally unilateral and asymmetrical, in contrast to the bilateral and symmetrical appearance of Graves' disease. Muscle enlargement and enhancement is present (Fig. 115-14), as in Graves' disease; however, the degree of muscle enlargement

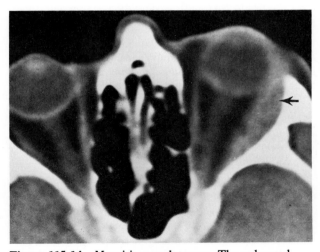

Figure 115-14 Myositic pseudotumor. The enhanced axial scan demonstrates diffuse enhancement and enlargement of the lateral rectus muscle and contiguous soft tissues (*arrow*). Myositic pseudotumor is generally unilateral and asymmetrical, in contrast to the bilateral and symmetrical appearance of Graves' disease.

is usually not as pronounced, nor is prolapse of intraorbital fat as dramatic in myositic pseudotumor as in Graves' disease. Finally, involvement of the tendinous insertions of the extraocular muscles onto the globe is said to be characteristic of pseudotumor and uncommon in Graves' disease.[13] In our experience, this has not been a reliable differentiating characteristic. No single radiographic finding allows a definite differentiation of the various myositic inflammatory conditions, and clinical history must often be correlated with the radiographic appearance.

Nonmyositic pseudotumor may present as a homogeneous mass on the CT scan. While the mass may be relatively well circumscribed along the majority of its contours, irregularity of some margins is common (Fig. 115-15). If such an appearance is present, it may be impossible to distinguish pseudotumor from other types of infiltrative primary or secondary expansions, such as lymphoma. Biopsy is therefore essential.

Tolosa-Hunt Syndrome The Tolosa-Hunt syndrome is a pachymeningitis leading to painful ophthalmoplegia that rapidly clears with steroids. The original description of this syndrome included narrowing of the carotid artery, as noted on cerebral angiography, secondary to the diffuse pachymeningitis. Orbital venography has demonstrated obstruction of the ophthalmic veins at the orbital apex and decreased opacification of the cavernous sinus.[10] As far as we are aware, no definitive findings in this syndrome have been described using computed tomography.

Vascular Lesions of the Orbit

Venous Varix The venous varix is a congenital venous "pouch" that is suggested clinically by the presence of positional or exertional exophthalmos. The Valsalva maneuver, dependency of the head, or exertion produces increased venous pressure leading to dilatation of the varix. The characteristic oval or round enhancing mass within the orbit can be shown to change size and shape on the CT scan with these provocative maneuvers (Fig. 115-1).

Aneurysm Aneurysms of the intraorbital ophthalmic artery are rare. More commonly, aneurysms originate from the cavernous and supraclinoid portions of the internal carotid artery and affect cranial nerves leading to the orbit.

Carotid–Cavernous Sinus Fistula CT scanning may be the initial technique that suggests the presence of a carotid-cavernous sinus fistula. Scanning of the orbits demonstrates a triad of findings. Because of the increased venous outflow from the cavernous sinus through the ophthalmic veins, particularly the superior ophthalmic vein, dilatation of this vein is seen on both the pre- and postcontrast CT scans. The increased orbital volume due to venous distention leads to proptosis. Muscle thickening is the least common of the three findings, but also results from venous distention.[9]

Arteriovenous Malformation If an arteriovenous malformation (AVM) is located within the orbit or in the immediate retro-orbital region, the clinical findings of chemosis, proptosis, and a bruit will be present in a similar fashion to those of a carotid–cavernous sinus fistula. CT scanning will demonstrate tortuous densities representing enlarged arteries and veins within the orbit. A true intraorbital AVM appears as a markedly enhancing mass within the orbit. Angiography is necessary for further evaluation.

Lesions of the Paranasal Sinuses Involving the Orbit

Neoplasms

Primary tumors of the sinuses that secondarily affect the orbit range from the benign osteoma to the malignant carcinoma and sarcoma. The most common location for the paranasal osteoma is the frontal sinus, with the ethmoid sinus second in incidence. Both plain films and the CT scan demonstrate a very dense lesion within the sinus that may become large enough to project into the orbit. The osteoma may also produce blockage of the outflow ostium of a sinus, resulting in a mucocele of the sinus with expansion into the orbit, as described below.

A primary malignant tumor of the paranasal sinus produces bone destruction and an infiltrating soft tissue mass typical of any malignant tumor. It is essential to evaluate orbital involvement with both axial and coronal CT scans. Bone involvement may not be appreciated unless the plane of the scan is perpendicular to the bony structures. In addition, anatomical relationships may only be appreciated with scanning in multiple projections. For example, extension of

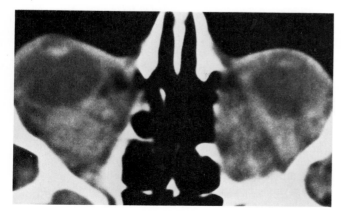

Figure 115-15 Retro-ocular pseudotumor. Soft tissue masses of mixed density are seen bilaterally in the retro-ocular spaces. The margins are irregular and there is infiltration of contiguous anatomical structures. The differential diagnosis includes lymphoma, which frequently demonstrates homogeneous and relatively intense enhancement.

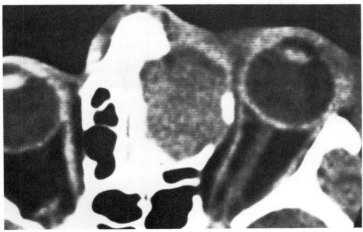 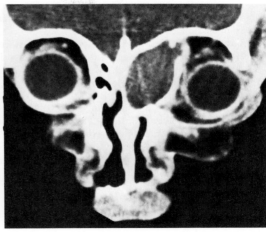

A   B

Figure 115-16 Mucocele of the ethmoid sinus. A long-standing expansion has produced "ballooning" of the ethmoid sinus. There is marked thinning of the medial orbital wall and pronounced lateral, inferior, and anterior displacement of the globe as demonstrated on the axial (A) and coronal (B) CT scans. The contents of the expansion are of a density equal to that of the brain, as is typical in a mucocele. The density is usually greater in a mucopyocele.

a tumor of the maxillary antrum into the superior portion of that antrum may appear to extend into the orbit on axial CT scans. Coronal views will allow a visual separation of the superior antrum from the inferior orbit.

Mucocele and Mucopyocele

A mucocele is a diffuse expansion of a paranasal sinus secondary to blockage of its ostium. Blockage may be secondary to chronic inflammatory disease, scarring from trauma, or a mass such as a polyp or osteoma. The sinus expands slowly over time because of the continuing production of secretions by the mucosa of the sinus. The slow expansion produces a "ballooning" of the sinus walls, which may project into the orbit (Fig. 115-16). While this ballooning has been said to produce a characteristic thin "eggshell" rim of remaining sinus wall, the bone may be so thin that it is difficult to perceive on the CT scan. Generally, CT scanning will demonstrate the contents of the sinus to be of a density equal to that of brain. Infection of the fluid leads to a mucopyocele. The pus and inflammatory tissue produce attenuation coefficients on the CT scan that are greater than those of the fluid of a noninfected mucocele. There may also be a rim of marginal enhancement, analogous to enhancement of the margins of a cerebral abscess.

Fine Needle Aspiration Biopsy

Besides simply imaging an abnormality in the orbit, CT and ultrasound can be used to establish a diagnosis more definitively. Specifically, they can be used to guide a small (22- or 23-gauge) needle into the abnormality.[7] When negative pressure is then applied to the needle while it is being gently agitated, a small aspiration biopsy is obtained. In many cases

this small sample of tissue is adequate to establish or confirm a diagnosis, thus saving the patient a more complicated open biopsy.[7]

Fine needle aspiration biopsy is useful in a wide variety of orbital disease processes. It is particularly useful for inoperable masses, deep orbital masses, and metastatic and inflammatory diseases. With a minimum of trauma, enough tissue can often be obtained to allow appropriate therapy to be begun quickly. Lesions of the optic nerve are amenable to CT-guided biopsy in selected patients (Fig. 115-6). Meningiomas, gliomas, and/or inflammation can be suggested on the basis of the tissue sample. Lesions that are well defined, like hemangiopericytoma, and lesions of the lacrimal gland are usually not biopsied for fear of spreading the tumor. Suspected lymphomatous lesions are not often biopsied by this method because histological differentiation between benign and malignant is very difficult with such a small tissue sample. Complications of fine needle aspiration include hemorrhage, nerve damage, and orbital empyema.

References

1. Alper MG: Management of primary optic nerve meningiomas: Current status—therapy in controversy. J Clin Neuro Ophthalmol 1:101–117, 1981.
2. Enzmann DR, Donaldson SS, Kriss JP: Appearance of Graves' disease on orbital computed tomography. J Comput Assist Tomogr 3:815–819, 1979.
3. Forbes GS, Earnest F IV, Waller RR: Computed tomography of orbital tumors, including late-generation scanning techniques. Radiology 142:387–394, 1982.
4. Forbes GS, Sheedy PF II, Waller RR: Orbital tumors evaluated by computed tomography. Radiology 136:101–111, 1980.
5. Henderson JW, Farrow GM: Primary orbital hemangiopericytoma: An aggressive and potentially malignant neoplasm. Arch Ophthalmol 96:666–673, 1978.

6. Hesselink JR, Davis KR, Weber AL, Davis JM, Taveras JM: Radiological evaluation of orbital metastases, with emphasis on computed tomography. Radiology 137: 363–366, 1980.

7. Kennerdell JS, Dekker A, Johnson BL: Orbital fine needle aspiration biopsy: The result of its use in 50 patients, in Lessell S, van Dalen JTW (eds): *Neuro-Ophthalmology*. Amsterdam, Excerpta Medica, 1980, vol. 1, pp 117–121.

8. Lloyd GAS: Vascular anomalies in the orbit: CT and angiographic diagnosis. Orbit 1:45–54, 1982.

9. Merrick R, Latchaw RE, Gold LHA: Computerized tomography of the orbit in carotid-cavernous sinus fistulae. Comput Tomogr 4:127–132, 1980.

10. Muhletaler CA, Gerlock AJ Jr: Orbital venography in painful ophthalmoplegia (Tolosa-Hunt syndrome). AJR 133:31–34, 1979.

11. Nugent RA, Rootman J, Robertson WD, Lapointe JS, Harrison PB: Acute orbital pseudotumors: Classification and CT features. AJNR 2:431–436, 1981.

12. Swenson SA, Forbes GS, Younge BR, Campbell RJ: Radiologic evaluation of tumors of the optic nerve. AJNR 3:319–326, 1982.

13. Trokel SL, Jakobiec FA: Correlation of CT scanning and pathologic features of ophthalmic Graves' disease. Ophthalmology (Rochester) 88:553–564, 1981.

14. Wright JE, Call NB, Liaricos S: Primary optic nerve meningioma. Br J Ophthalmol 64:553–558, 1980.

116
Tumors of the Orbit

Joseph C. Maroon
John S. Kennerdell

Since 1975 we have used a combined neurosurgical and neuro-ophthalmologic approach in the diagnosis and treatment of patients with tumors in and about the orbit.[11] During that period, 300 patients (Table 116-1) with orbital tumors and pseudotumors have been evaluated. Our indications for surgery, surgical approaches, and surgical technique continue to be modified because of the remarkable technical innovations in submillimeter resolution CT scanning, and diagnostic ultrasound, and the development of lasers, ultrasonic aspirators, and microsurgical instrumentation and techniques.

In this chapter we will briefly outline the surgical anatomy of the orbit and illustrate our surgical approaches to the most commonly encountered orbital tumors.

Surgical Anatomy

The Orbit

The orbits are pear-shaped, bony cavities which taper posteriorly to the apex and optic canal. The optic canal is 5 to 10 mm long and approximately 4.5 mm wide. The average height of the canal is 5 mm. The roof of the canal is approximately 2 mm thick. The proximal opening of the optic canal is formed dorsally by the falciform process, a thin fold of dura overlying the optic nerve. This process is 3 to 5 mm long.

The total intraorbital length of the optic nerve is approximately 30 mm. This is 5 mm longer than the distance from the orbital apex to the posterior margin of the globe. This additional length allows for proptosis or for slight intraorbital manipulation of the nerve during surgery.

The canal itself lies between the two struts or roots of the lesser sphenoid wing. Laterally is the anterior clinoid process which may be aerated and communicate with the sphenoid sinus. Medially is the thinner portion of the sphenoid strut, which also abuts the sphenoid sinus (Fig. 116-1).

The roof of the orbit is composed of the frontal bone, which is of variable thickness. The lateral wall is composed of the zygomatic and frontal bones anteriorly and the greater wing of the sphenoid posteriorly. The medial wall is formed by the thin ethmoid, frontal, lacrimal, maxillary, and sphenoid bones, and borders the ethmoid and sphenoid sinuses and the nasal cavity. The floor of the orbit is formed by the roof of the maxillary sinus.

The orbital walls are perforated by the superior orbital fissure, the inferior orbital fissure, the ethmoid foramina, the zygomaticotemporal and zygomaticofacial canals, the nasolacrimal canal, and the optic canal.

TABLE 116-1 Orbital Tumors Evaluated from 1975 to 1982

Adenoid cystic carcinoma	5
Dermoid cyst	30
Hemangioma	17
Hemangiopericytoma	3
Lymphangioma	18
Meningioma	34
Neurofibroma	3
Optic nerve glioma	6
Rhabdomyosarcoma	2
Metastatic tumor	75
Pseudotumor	72
Dysthyroidal exophthalmos	35
Total	300

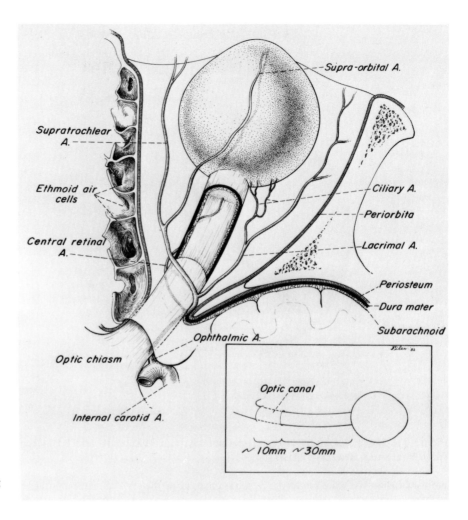

Figure 116-1 Intraorbital relations of the optic nerve, blood vessels, and bony elements. (From Maroon JC and Kennerdell JS, J Neurosurg 60:1226–1235, 1984.)

The superior orbital fissure divides the greater and lesser wings of the sphenoid bone and transmits the third, fourth, and sixth cranial nerves and the ophthalmic division of the fifth cranial nerve (V_1) together with sympathetic fibers. Most of the venous drainage from the orbit passes through this fissure within the superior ophthalmic vein and then into the cavernous sinus (Fig. 116-2).

The inferior orbital fissure transmits the maxillary division (V_2) of the fifth cranial nerve, the zygomatic nerve, and branches of the inferior ophthalmic vein. A branch of the maxillary nerve, the infraorbital nerve, enters the inferior orbital notch and infraorbital canal to provide sensation to the lower lid, cheek, and upper lid. The ethmoid foramina in the medial orbital wall transmit the anterior and posterior ethmoidal arteries. The zygomaticofacial and zygomaticotemporal canals transmit vessels and branches of the maxillary nerve through the lateral orbital wall to the cheek and temporal fossa. The nasolacrimal canal transmits the nasolacrimal duct between the lacrimal sac and inferior nasal meatus.

Figure 116-3 illustrates several important surgical observations, as emphasized by Maniscalco and Habal.[9] The optic canal is narrowed distally as it approaches the orbit, and the medial distal wall of the canal is quite dense relative to the

more proximal segment. This thick distal portion of the optic canal is called the *optic ring*. Complete surgical decompression of the canal must include this narrow distal segment and this can only be done safely using microdissecting techniques. Also, removal of this bone may result in entering the ethmoid or sphenoid air sinuses; such defects must be dealt with appropriately at the conclusion of any operation.

Optic Nerve Layers and Vascularization

The optic nerve continues anteriorly from the chiasm, travels 10 to 15 mm through the intracranial subarachnoid space, and enters the optic canal. Within the optic canal the nerve is invested by its pial layer. The intracranial dura mater also continues through the canal as a dural-periosteal layer and then splits into a dural layer, which forms the dura of the optic nerve, and a periosteal layer, which becomes the periorbita (Fig. 116-1). The intracranial arachnoid and the subarachnoid space are maintained along the entire length of the nerve. At the orbital apex, the pia and arachnoid fuse with the dura and the fibrous annulus of Zinn. The patency of the subarachnoid space is maintained throughout to its

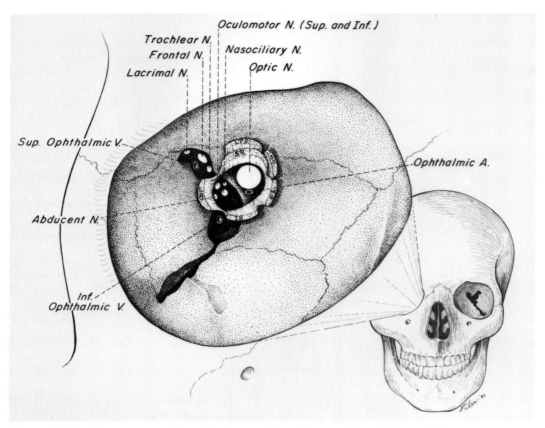

Figure 116-2 The anatomy of the orbital apex. (From Maroon JC and Kennerdell JS, J Neurosurg 60:1226–1235, 1984.)

point of fusion with the pia at the posterior margin of the globe.

The major blood supply of the optic nerve is derived from the ophthalmic artery. Branches include pial vessels and intraneural branches of the central retinal artery. The ophthalmic artery is approximately 1.25 mm wide, and in over 90 percent of the cases arises from the internal carotid artery above the cavernous sinus. In the majority, it arises

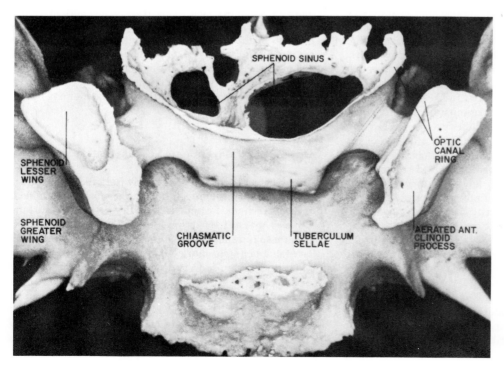

Figure 116-3 The sphenoid bone, horizontal section, demonstrating the anatomy of the optic canals and the dense bone that surround the distal segment of the optic canal. (From Maniscalco and Habal.[9])

anteromedial to the optic nerve, then passes into the optic canal and the orbit lateral and inferior to the nerve (Fig. 116-1).

As it enters the orbit, the ophthalmic artery curves laterally around the optic nerve to take up a more medial position. Eight to fifteen millimeters behind the globe, the ophthalmic artery gives off the central retinal artery. This artery traverses the dural sheath obliquely for a few millimeters and then penetrates into the midportion of the optic nerve. It may send a few small blood vessels to anastomose with the vascular pial network, but this contribution to optic nerve circulation is minimal. This artery primarily contributes to the laminal or retinal vascularization and not to the intraorbital nerve itself.

The intraorbital portion of the optic nerve derives much, if not all, of its blood supply from the tight vascular plexus in the pia mater. This pial network arises primarily from the arterial perforating branches from the posterior ciliary arteries, which are posterior to the entry of the central retinal artery into the optic nerve. A second contribution to this pial network is from the recurrent branches of the long and short posterior ciliary arteries. A third contribution, as mentioned, is from the central retinal artery. There is, therefore, an axial arterial supply in the pia to the optic nerve and a laminar supply derived from multiple sources.[2]

More distally, the ophthalmic artery gives off six or more short posterior ciliary arteries which anastomose with the long posterior ciliary arteries to form the circle of Zinn-Haller. The vessels of this anastomotic ring provide most of the capillaries to the lamina cribrosa and to the adjacent pial vasculature, and supply much of the adjacent optic nerve.

In addition to the laminar and retrolaminar arterial branches, the ophthalmic artery gives off the following vessels in its intraorbital course: the supratrochlear, supraorbital, dorsal nasal, lacrimal, and anterior and posterior ethmoidal arteries. All of the vessels are capable of anastomosis with branches from the external carotid artery.

In summary, the intraorbital portion of the optic nerve derives much, if not all, of its arterial blood supply from a plexus in the pia mater. The intraocular portion of the optic nerve, or the optic nerve head itself, derives its blood supply primarily from the posterior ciliary arteries that enter the sclera adjacent to the optic nerve head and the central retinal artery. The primary venous drainage of the orbit is through the superior and inferior ophthalmic veins. The superior ophthalmic vein passes on the dorsal aspect of the lateral rectus muscle and exits through the superior orbital fissure into the cavernous sinus. The inferior ophthalmic vein drains the medial aspect of the orbit and divides with one branch passing through the inferior orbital fissure and a second anastomosing with the superior ophthalmic vein prior to its entry into the superior orbital fissure.

Annulus of Zinn

At the orbital apex, a fibrous, double-pierced, tendinous funnel gives rise to five of the six extraocular muscles. As seen in Figure 116-2, the annulus is firmly fused to the optic nerve dorsally and then extends laterally and is divided by a dural plane into two compartments. The more medial compartment contains the optic nerve and the ophthalmic ar-

tery. The lateral compartment, or oculomotor foramen, is bounded laterally by the two heads of the lateral rectus muscle. This foramen transmits the superior oculomotor nerve, the abducens nerve, the inferior oculomotor nerve, and the nasociliary nerve. The trochlear nerve, the frontal and lacrimal branches of the fifth nerve, and the ophthalmic vein pass through the superior orbital fissure but not through the oculomotor foramen.

From Figure 116-2, one can see that the most direct approach to the optic nerve is medially between the superior rectus and levator muscles and the medial rectus. This approach obviates potential trauma to the nerves passing through the oculomotor foramen.

When the optic nerve is approached transcranially, it is of significance that the trochlear nerve crosses from lateral to medial above the optic nerve and immediately under the periorbita. This nerve is almost impossible to spare when the annulus is opened for tumor removal.

Types and Incidence of Orbital Tumors

Table 116-1 summarizes the types of tumors we have encountered over the last 8 years. The following discussion will deal with those tumors confined to the intraorbital compartment.

Optic Glioma

Optic nerve gliomas arise from the optic nerve, chiasm, or tract—the anterior visual pathways. The majority become manifest in the first decade of life with progressive visual loss and proptosis. There also is an increased incidence in patients with neurofibromatosis. Histologically, most of these tumors are of a low-grade malignancy with a histological picture varying from a predominantly fibrillar pattern to one that is microcystic. Rosenthal fibers are a frequent finding. As the tumor enlarges, reactive proliferation of the meninges occurs, contributing to the increased size.[14]

There are two distinct clinical courses. The majority of the patients have an indolent course with little change in the size or extent of the tumor. It is in this group that the incidence of neurofibromatosis is higher. In the second group, there is progressive enlargement of the tumor, with blindness, proptosis, and extension intracranially. A lower incidence of neurofibromatosis is found in this progressive group.[4]

The recognition of two different clinical courses is important in patient management. Approximately half of the patients with optic nerve gliomas will undergo a progressive course; this emphasizes the need for close monitoring of function and tumor size with visual field testing and CT scanning, respectively. The decision to operate is determined by the progression of the tumor. In the child with stable or normal vision and CT scans that do not demonstrate progressive enlargement, watchful waiting is indicated. In the child with progressive deterioration of vision or tumor enlargement demonstrated on the CT scan, a transcranial operation for a complete excision of the nerve from the chiasm to the globe is performed. We do not believe that a lateral orbitotomy approach should be used for this tumor.

We have, on occasion, used a fine needle aspiration biopsy technique to confirm the histology of a suspected optic nerve glioma in a patient with markedly impaired or absent vision.[7] Particularly when chiasmatic involvement is present, we use this biopsy technique to confirm the diagnosis and then recommend radiation therapy.

Malignant gliomas usually develop in adults and present a most difficult problem. When possible, they are confirmed histologically by fine needle aspiration biopsy of the optic nerve or by craniotomy. Treatment consists of shunting if the CSF pathways are obstructed, followed by radiation therapy. In our experience, this is a uniformly lethal tumor.

Optic Nerve Meningioma

Optic nerve meningiomas arise from the meningothelial cells, which line the undersurface of the dura and are also found in the arachnoid and pia. The first symptom is usually visual loss. Additional findings include proptosis, impaired movement of the globe, papilledema, or optic atrophy with shunt vessels and an afferent pupillary defect.[1] For unexplained reasons, the majority of these tumors occur in women. The clinical course of progressive visual loss and/or proptosis becomes understandable when one considers the three ways in which these tumors grow (Figure 116-4). If the tumor arises from the cells in the dura mater and grows in a centrifugal manner, an exophytic mass effect may develop with proptosis before vision is severely impaired. If, however, the tumor arises from the arachnoid or the undersurface of the dura and remains confined to the subdural space, progressive visual loss may be the only symptom. Early papilledema occurs with the secondary development of optic atrophy later in the course. "Chronic optic neuritis" is a frequent misdiagnosis. The third clinical presentation is the combined intradural and extradural type. These tumors

originate from the arachnoid and subsequently burst through the limiting outer dural membrane and become exophytic into the orbit. Coincidentally, they may compress the optic nerve, causing progressive visual loss.

With high-resolution CT scanners, it is possible to detect these tumors early in their clinical course and to determine radiographically if they are (1) subdural with axial extension, (2) primarily extradural, or (3) combined extradural and subdural (Fig. 116-5).

The management of optic nerve meningiomas is dependent upon the tumor's location and the visual findings (Table 116-2). Those patients whose tumors are located in the mid- to anterior segment of the optic nerve and whose visual acuity is stable are observed with serial visual function studies and CT scans. If progressive visual loss develops, we prefer the lateral microsurgical approach for decompressive purposes and tumor removal. If the tumor is located in the apex of the orbit and there is nearly normal or normal vision, we will observe the patient. If the tumor is confined to the apex and there is demonstrated progressive visual loss, radiation therapy may be considered, as suggested by Smith et al.[12] An alternative is a craniotomy. If the vision is subtotally or totally lost, a needle biopsy is done to confirm the diagnosis and the patient is allowed the choice of either craniotomy with attempt at total removal or observation.

There remains considerable controversy regarding the management of these lesions.[1,13] We think that, because of the unpredictable and relatively slow growth rate of a meningioma, subtotal removal and decompression to preserve vision is reasonable.[6,8,10] This subtotal type of surgery has been practiced routinely in the past for intracranial meningiomas attached to the sagittal sinus or invading the skull base. Only the lack of detection and the failure to use microsurgical techniques in the orbit have prevented similar decompression of optic nerve meningiomas. Preliminary results suggest that these tumors may be controlled by radiation therapy in some instances, thus obviating the need

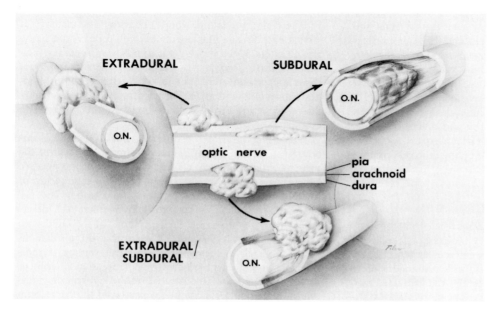

Figure 116-4 Different sites of origin and growth characteristics of optic nerve meningiomas. (From Maroon JC and Kennerdell JS, J Neurosurg 60:1226–1235, 1984.)

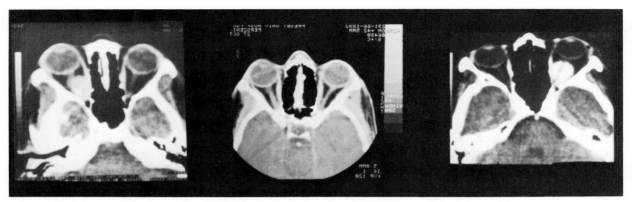

Figure 116-5 CT appearance of meningiomas of the optic nerve. *Left:* Exophytic. *Middle:* Subdural. *Right:* Exophytic and subdural.

to radically resect the optic nerve and, at times, other orbital structures.[12]

If the tumor is located in the apex with intracranial extension and progressive visual loss, a transcranial approach is used to remove the intracranial portion of the tumor as well as the optic nerve and the intraorbital tumor component.

Our failures have occurred in those patients with posterior axial extension and in those with medial and posterior tumors. In two patients in whom we have attempted to remove tumors from the posterior medial portion of the optic nerve, we have compromised the central retinal artery, thus producing blindness in both. We therefore avoid dissection in this area whenever possible.

Cavernous Hemangioma

This is the most common primary benign tumor occurring in the orbit of adults. Its clinical course is one of painless proptosis; remarkably, the eye is able to maintain normal function and motility despite a large and unyielding mass. It occurs most commonly in the second and fourth decades of life and may enlarge during pregnancy.[3]

It is an encapsulated tumor with an excellent cleavage plane from surrounding structures. It is readily palpated

when the orbital structures are exposed and is easily dissected from surrounding tissue. Microscopically, there are large cavernous spaces within which blood is relatively stagnant because of the isolation of the lesion from the systemic circulation. Carotid angiography is not helpful in diagnosis despite the nature of the tumor. Ultrasonograms and CT scans show characteristic abnormalities.

The treatment is complete removal whenever possible, through a lateral orbital approach if the tumor is superior, inferior, or lateral to the optic nerve, as it usually is. A cryoprobe is very helpful for retraction once the dome of the tumor is identified. Bleeding is rarely a problem, and with microdissecting techniques the tumor can be safely removed from surrounding neural and muscular tissue.

Neurofibroma

Neurofibromas of the orbit are divided into solitary orbital forms and diffuse or multicentric types. The solitary orbital neurofibroma occurs in the older age group and is characterized by a slowly progressive, painless proptosis. A several-year history of proptosis may be obtained, depending on the patient's concern about the condition. Visual loss is frequently minimal. Usually the tumor is in the superior and posterior part of the orbit, thus producing weakness in upward gaze. They are usually well-encapsulated, firm tumors that are relatively easy to dissect from adjacent orbital tissue.

The diffuse or multicentric type represents a congenital problem affecting many systems and organs and is most commonly detected in children and infants. Progressive disfiguring proptosis is the usual initial symptom. Aside from total orbital exenteration, it is usually impossible to remove these tumors completely. Recurrence is the rule. For cosmetic appearances, most surgeons remove whatever is considered safe and easily accessible.

Dermoid and Epidermoid Cysts

These are the most frequent of developmental cysts which involve the orbit. Of dermal origin, they are usually found in children and constitute 4 to 6 percent of orbital tumors.

TABLE 116-2 The Management of Optic Nerve Meningiomas According to Location and Visual Acuity

Location	Visual Acuity	Treatment
Mid to anterior	Stable	Observation
Mid to anterior	Progressive loss	Lateral microsurgical operation
Apical	Nearly normal or normal	Observation
Apical	Progressive loss	Radiation and/or craniotomy
Apical	No light perception (or large tumor or intracranial extension)	Craniotomy

They are the most common orbital tumors of childhood, but they may be encountered up to the age of 50.

Epidermoid cysts or cholesteatomas affect an older age group, are usually located deeper in the orbit, and grow in the diploe of bone. They tend to occur in the upper portion of the orbit, and may protrude forward beneath the upper orbital rim and be readily palpable. The lesion is usually painless, not attached to the skin, and causes little or no displacement of the globe. On occasion it may transgress bone and extend into the intracranial cavity or adjacent sinus. The defects in bone are radiolucent with a sclerotic or well-corticated margin.

The surgical approach to these lesions is dependent on their location. Those tumors in the apex near the optic foramen or superior orbital fissure or extending transcranially require a transcranial approach. The majority, however, can be removed through a lateral orbital approach because of their propensity to be located in the lateral aspect of the orbit. Whatever the surgical approach, it is usually impossible to remove the cyst intact. The dermoid cyst is composed of sebaceous glands, hair follicles, fat globules, and collagen. The epidermoid cyst contains an oily liquid with cheesy yellow or white material. A meticulous removal should be carried out, but even this does not guarantee that there will be no recurrence.

Osteoma

These are the most common tumors of bone or cartilage which affect the bony orbit. They comprise approximately 1 percent of all orbital tumors. They are most commonly found in the frontal and ethmoid sinuses, protruding into the orbit. A hard, nontender, space-occupying lesion that displaces the eye is the most common presentation. The diagnosis may be made solely on the basis of plain radiographs of the skull. CT scans are confirmatory.

When symptomatic, osteomas should be removed through the appropriate exposure. If the tumor arises from the intracranial compartment and extends into the orbit, a transcranial approach is used. If it arises from the lateral wall, a lateral approach may be used, and similarly, if it arises from the ethmoid or sphenoid sinuses, a rhinologic approach is best. A high-speed drill greatly simplifies the technical removal from any of these positions. Recurrences are most prevalent in those young patients in whom the initial surgery was incomplete.

Hemangiopericytoma

Although relatively uncommon in the orbit (3 of our 300 cases), this is a slow-growing, painless, circumscribed neoplasm that usually presents with painless proptosis. Symptoms may persist for years to decades and the tumors attain very large size before symptoms become prominent.

These may be quite vascular tumors. Histologically, they may be classified as benign, of borderline malignancy, or malignant, depending on the cellular anaplasia, vascular pattern, shape of pericytes, and mitotic figures present. Grossly, they are red to reddish blue and appear to be encap-

sulated. When incomplete removal is performed, recurrences can be expected. They may metastasize and every effort should be made to remove the tumor completely.

Fibrous Dysplasia

Fibrous dysplasia is a non-neoplastic bony lesion of childhood and adolescence. When involving the orbit, the dysplasia usually affects the maxillary, zygomatic, ethmoid, frontal, or sphenoid bones. Depending on which bone is involved, there may be progressive visual loss from sphenoid bone dysplasia or unsightly proptosis and orbital distortion from involvement of the orbital maxilla. The growth of the lesion is usually painless.

Radiographic changes may demonstrate small translucent zones in the cranial bones or large diffuse areas of sclerosis. The latter may closely resemble a meningioma. Histological changes are found which are consistent with an arrest in the development of immature woven bone into more mature lamellar bone.

The treatment is determined by the severity of the condition. If there is optic nerve compression, a transcranial approach with microscopic techniques should be used to decompress thoroughly the optic nerve in its canal, using extreme care in removing the roof and bony struts of the optic canal. Radiation is not recommended for fear of inducing a malignant transformation.

Mucocele

A mucocele is a cystic tumor, covered by mucous membrane, arising either from an obstructed sinus or from small cysts within the mucous membrane of the air sinuses. Although primarily a rhinologic condition, it may produce orbital symptoms, including proptosis, ophthalmoplegia, visual disturbance, headache, and, at times, a palpable mass. Proptosis is the most common feature. Plain radiographs, a CT scan, and the clinical findings allow a presumptive presurgical diagnosis in most cases. Complete removal of the cyst lining and restoration of drainage from the occluded sinus are the goals of treatment. Recurrence does occur; thus, long-term follow-up is essential.

Mucoceles of the posterior ethmoid and sphenoid sinuses may have protean clinical manifestations, which include headache and ocular motor palsies. Visual loss of a remitting and relapsing course similar to ophthalmoplegic migraine may occur and be of a unilateral, bilateral, or chiasmatic type. Facial pain, loss of sensation in the first or second trigeminal nerve distributions, and vague paresthesias all may be found.

Metastatic Tumors

Neuroblastoma and Ewing's sarcoma are the most common childhood tumors which metastasize to the orbit. More than half of all neuroblastomas originate in the retroperitoneal area and most occur before the age of 7 years. They typically present with abrupt exophthalmos and ecchymosis, which may be bilateral. There may also be bone destruction, particularly in the lateral orbit.

Ewing's sarcoma is a rare tumor, which metastasizes more often to a single orbit than to both. Again, ecchymosis can occur in association with sudden exophthalmos. Testicular tumors, leukemia, and Ewing's sarcoma all may present as orbital masses in children.

In adults, although nearly any malignancy of the internal organs and some skin tumors can metastasize to the orbit, the majority of orbital metastases are from breast and lung cancers. Development of exophthalmos with bone destruction and early ophthalmoplegia should always bring this diagnosis to mind in a woman. Bronchogenic carcinoma is the most frequent source of orbital metastasis in men.

The diagnosis of these tumors is now relatively easily confirmed by fine needle aspiration biopsy.[6] We have done over 125 of these procedures with 92 percent diagnostic results.

Pseudotumor

Pseudotumor or idiopathic orbital inflammation is a confusing term that has been applied to many different orbital inflammatory processes. The condition is characterized by orbital pain of sudden onset and associated edema of the lids and conjunctiva. Ultrasonic evaluation shows diffuse hyperplasia with molding of abnormal tissue to the posterior margins of the globe and possibly to the orbital walls. High-resolution CT scanning demonstrates that this condition may involve specific structures such as the lacrimal gland, muscles, and optic nerve. In such cases, it is best to define the inflammatory process according to the specific focus most involved—for example, acute or chronic orbital myositis, dacryoadenitis, perineural inflammation, or periscleritis.

This disease usually responds to steroids, and, at times, to x-ray therapy. Although we have, on two occasions, operated upon patients we suspected of having neoplasms, we have not made this error in several years due to greater use of fine needle aspiration biopsy, more experience with diagnostic ultrasound, and also better delineation with computed tomography.

Tolosa-Hunt Syndrome

This syndrome usually presents in a middle-aged patient as a painful ophthalmoplegia involving the third, fourth, or sixth nerves, or the first division of the trigeminal nerve. Other cranial nerves, such as the first and seventh, may be involved, which suggests that the syndrome may better be characterized as a cranial polyneuropathy with tendencies for spontaneous resolution and for recurrence. Orbital venography shows occlusion of the superior ophthalmic vein and partial obliteration of the cavernous sinus. CT scans may also show some increased radiodensity in the cavernous sinus area. Mildly elevated sedimentation rates are common and there is frequently a positive clinical response to corticosteroids. Tumors involving the superior orbital fissure and skull base must be considered in the differential diagnosis. A CT scan usually eliminates these possibilities.

Choice of Surgical Approach

We determine the size and location of an orbital tumor and its relationship to the optic nerve by the history, the clinical findings, and, to a major extent, the CT scan. If there is evidence of intracranial extension or involvement of the posterior walls of the orbit, or if the tumor is located medial to the optic nerve in the apex, we use a transcranial approach. If the tumor is clearly circumscribed and located superior, lateral, or inferior to the optic nerve and if it does not involve the sphenoid bone posteriorly, a lateral orbitotomy approach is chosen. If the tumor is located medial to the optic nerve but in the anterior half of the orbit, we will perform a medial micro-orbitotomy.

Anterior Medial Orbitotomy

The anterior medial orbitotomy is indicated for biopsy, decompression, or removal of tumors of the medial intraconal space, the area between the optic nerve and the medial rectus muscle. It is also useful for creating an opening in the optic nerve sheath in patients with chronic papilledema secondary to benign intracranial hypertension, or for performing a distal optic nerve biopsy of a tumor of the optic nerve in the immediate retrobulbar space.

We prefer to place the patient under general anesthesia with the usual ophthalmic preparation of the orbital and periorbital region. A small lid speculum is inserted to begin the operation. A 360 degree peritomy is done around the cornea, and conjunctival relaxing incisions angled away from the muscle are made superior and inferior to the medial rectus. A muscle hook is placed under the medial rectus muscle and it is freed from its inner muscular septa and check ligaments distally. A 6.0 double-arm Vicryl (polyglactin, Ethicon Inc, Somerville, N.J.) suture which is doubly locked at both borders is placed into the medial rectus muscle near its insertion and the muscle is severed from the insertion site in the usual manner of an extraocular muscle recession. A clamp is placed on the suture and the muscle is retracted medially. At this point, the standard lid retractor is removed and a Druck-Mueller retractor, which we have modified, with an attached enucleation spoon is placed into the medial orbital compartment by placing the teeth superiorly and inferiorly under the conjunctiva to spread the conjunctiva and Tenon's capsule superiorly and inferiorly medial to the globe. The handle of the retractor is then angled so that it rests firmly on the temporalis muscle lateral to the eye. The enucleation spoon is angled over the globe and placed in a medial position on the globe, which is then retracted gently laterally. The enucleation spoon handle is then tightened to maintain the lateral retractions of the globe (Fig. 116-6).

At this point, the universal joints are attached to the inferior peg on the retractor, with the surgeon operating from the superior position, as is usual in eye surgery. A malleable retractor is then placed medially to retract the medial rectus and is fitted into place with adjustment of the bars and universal joints, which are attached to the retractor base. The medial orbital compartment is, therefore, exposed, and one

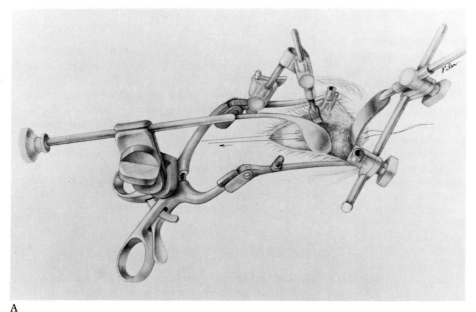

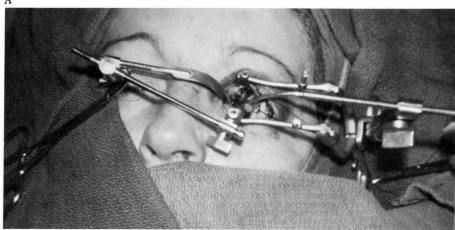

A

B

Figure 116-6 *A.* Specially designed retractor. *B.* Exposure for medial orbitotomy.

can see the orbital fat between the globe and the medial rectus.

The operating microscope is used with a 300 mm objective. Dissection is begun down through the orbital fat using bipolar cauterization and sharp and blunt dissection until the surgeon exposes the tumor or the optic nerve. As the dissection proceeds deeper, the fat is retracted superiorly and inferiorly with cottonoids and additional malleable retractors attached to the base of the Druck-Mueller retractor as needed. It is surprising how much space can be obtained without removing the lateral wall of the orbit. The latter can be done, however, if more space is required for removal of a large mass from the medial orbital compartment.

Following biopsy, subtotal or total removal of a tumor, or decompression of the optic nerve, the area is carefully inspected and complete hemostasis is obtained. The retractors are then gently removed from the deep orbit and again the area is inspected for bleeding. When hemostasis is complete, the retractor is removed and the globe is allowed to resume its position. The medial rectus muscle is then reat-

tached to the globe with the double-arm 6.0 Vicryl sutures at the original insertion site. The conjunctiva is closed with purse-string sutures through the conjunctiva near the limbus at the area of the superior and inferior conjunctival relaxing incisions. An antibiotic ointment is then applied to the eye and the eye is firmly patched as it would be following ocular surgery.

Morbidity following this procedure is minimal and can be compared with extraocular muscle surgery if the surgical manipulation is not excessive.

Lateral Micro-orbitotomy

The patient is placed in the supine position with the head turned to the side contralateral to the lesion. A transverse skin incision 35 to 40 mm long is made, beginning just posterior to the lateral canthal margin and extending posteriorly toward the pinna of the ear. Additional exposure may be obtained by curving the anterior limb of the incision superi-

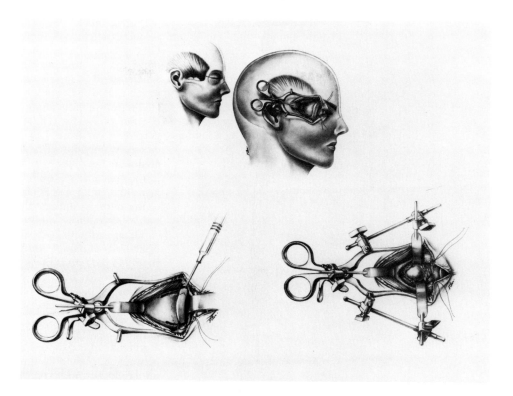

Figure 116-7 The steps in the performance of a lateral orbitotomy. (From Maroon JC and Kennerdell JS, J Neurosurg 60:1226–1235, 1984.)

orly into the eyebrow along the frontal portion of the zygomatic arch (Fig. 116-7). An incision is then made through the temporalis fascia beginning at the midportion of the frontozygomatic rim and extending posteriorly the length of the skin incision. The muscle itself is not incised. A curved incision is made along the frontal zygomatic bone down to the periosteum. Using a periosteal elevator, the periosteum is removed from the anterior and posterior surfaces of the zygomatic bone. The muscle in the temporal fossa is dissected subperiosteally, elevated but not cut, and then retracted posteriorly. The periorbital fascia is then dissected over the anterior portion of the rim of the zygomatic bone.

A reciprocating saw is used to incise the lateral rim of the orbit superiorly and inferiorly. This rim is broken posteriorly with a heavy rongeur. At this point, the self-retaining orbital retractor is inserted and the temporalis fascia and muscle are retracted posteriorly to expose the deep portion of the lateral wall of the orbit. Additional bone is rongeured away with the surgeon taking care to protect the periorbital fascia with cottonoids and a hand-held malleable retractor.

If it is necessary to obtain proximal exposure of the optic nerve or the deep portion of the muscle cone, additional bone is removed from the greater wing of the sphenoid with an air drill and small-angled rongeurs. One may expose the temporal as well as the frontal dura through this approach to obtain visualization deep in the orbital apex.

The periorbital fascia is next incised parallel to the lateral rectus muscle, which is put on stretch by traction on a previously placed 4.0 Vicryl suture at its point of insertion onto the globe anteriorly. After the muscle is retracted, the operating microscope is brought into use and the other two blades of the self-retaining orbital retractor are positioned.

The most expeditious way of proceeding through the ubiquitous orbital fat is to use the self-retaining orbital retractor blades over cottonoids. With an assistant aspirating any blood and holding one of the retractor blades and the primary surgeon retracting with the other blade and using microdissecting techniques, it is possible to rapidly identify the optic nerve or tumors without injuring fine neural or vascular structures in the lateral compartment of the orbit.

If the operation is to remove a tumor in the superior lateral or inferior compartment of the orbit, standard microdissecting techniques are used to dissect the tumor from its surrounding structures. With encapsulated tumors, blunt dissection with the self-retaining retractor blades over cottonoids will expose the dome of the tumor. An ophthalmic cryoprobe is very effective in retracting the tumor while dissection continues. This instrument provides gentle bloodless traction which frequently results in deliverance of the tumor (Fig. 116-8). Fine neural and vascular structures are dissected from the capsule of the tumor and preserved whenever possible. If it is impossible to remove the tumor completely, then the laser or an ultrasonic aspirator is used to reduce its bulk as much as is safely possible.

If the purpose of the operation is to remove a tumor attached to the optic nerve, proximal and distal exposure of the nerve is obtained using the same dissecting techniques with the retractor blades and cottonoids (Fig. 116-9). Exophytic or extradural meningiomas are readily found by palpation and subsequent dissection. The mass is usually easily dissected from the surrounding tissue and exposed. If it is large and fibrotic, an ultrasonic aspirator or laser is used to debulk the mass and obtain proximal and distal exposure. The use of electrocautery is contraindicated in these tumors.

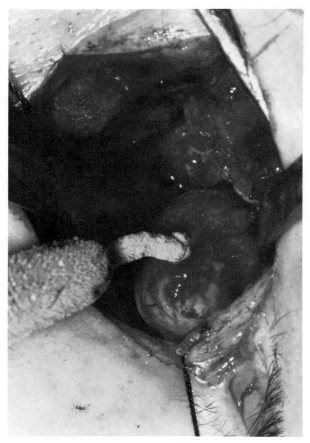

Figure 116-8 Use of the cryoprobe to remove an intraorbital tumor through a lateral micro-orbitotomy.

In our recent experience, the laser provides the most delicate and controlled method for reducing the bulk of the tumor down to its origin from the optic nerve sheaths.

Once the mass is reduced in size, a plane may be seen between the normal dura and tumor. This plane is exploited and the tumor is removed from its dural attachment with microdissecting techniques. If no plane is seen, it then becomes necessary to incise the surrounding dura of the optic nerve and attempt removal of the intradural component. It is also necessary to remove, circumferentially, the involved dura and exophytic tumor using various right- and left-angle scissors, bipolar coagulation, and the laser. Considerable judgment and extreme care are used at this point to avoid traumatizing the optic nerve or its precarious blood supply.

If the tumor is primarily intradural, upon exposing the optic nerve from the lateral approach one may see only a slight elevation of a few millimeters or so above the more proximal or distal normal nerve (Fig. 116-10). If the tumor has spread axially along a larger portion of the intraorbital subdural space, the entire nerve may appear uniformly "fattened." Initially, we had considerable trepidation about incising the dura for fear not only of a negative exploration but also of the potential for injuring the optic nerve. We have found, however, that a careful longitudinal incision in the lateral portion of the dura covering the optic nerve is well tolerated even if small vessels in the dura are transected.

Furthermore, tumor usually immediately exudes through the incision (Fig. 116-11). In two patients with tumors located in the middle and distal portion of the optic nerve, upon incising the dura we found a capacious proximal subarachnoid space and the associated tumor obstruction which caused the papilledema.

To remove these tumors, one must circumferentially incise the dura. This can be done safely in the anteriormost portion of the orbit. The essential retinal artery, however, enters the dura 8 to 15 mm behind the globe on the nerve's medial surface (Fig. 116-1). This artery must be protected. If the tumor arises from the medial portion of the optic nerve and an attempt is made to remove it from the surface of the dura, this artery will be jeopardized. We have had blindness result in two such cases.

Other perforating arteries which arise from the posterior ciliary arteries may be sacrificed if necessary, since the blood supply to the retrolaminar portion of the optic nerve is primarily through the rich anastomotic vascular network located in the pia.

After the dura is incised, the laser, microbipolar forceps, or ultrasonic aspirator may be used effectively to remove the tumor from the surface of the optic nerve and the underlying arachnoid. In our experience there has always been a plane between the pia and the tumor, much as one finds in removing a convexity meningioma of the brain. With careful, tedious dissection these tumors can be traced proximally and distally and removed, in some cases entirely.

In some cases, the dura may be extensively involved with adherent tumor, and technically it may be impossible to remove it completely. In these, bipolar coagulation or the laser is used to cauterize any visible remnants of tumor. In others, there may be small finger-like extensions extending posteriorly toward the intracanalicular portion of the optic nerve. If these cannot be reached through a lateral approach and the tumor is minimal, as visualized through the microscope, we have elected to follow these patients with CT scans rather than perform a craniotomy. We also consider the administration of x-ray therapy.[12]

After any tumor is removed through the lateral approach, the periorbital fascia is reapproximated and the lateral orbital rim is reinserted. The periorbital fascia and the fascia over the temporalis muscle are then reapproximated over the lateral rim of the orbit to maintain it in position. Fixation wires or sutures are not used. The skin is closed in the usual fashion. A firm compressive dressing is applied for 48 h and then removed. Corticosteroids are used for 24 h preoperatively and for 2 to 3 days postoperatively.

Transcranial Approach

Our transcranial approach is closely patterned after that well described by Housepian et al.[4] With the patient in the supine position, enough hair is shaved frontally to allow a bicoronal skin incision to be made with approximately 2 cm of shaved scalp posteriorly. A free bone flap is elevated after a subperiosteal dissection down to the orbital rim. If considerable apical exposure may be necessary for any reason, we use the technique described by Jane for removing the frontal bone at this stage.[5] Otherwise, a four-hole frontal bone flap

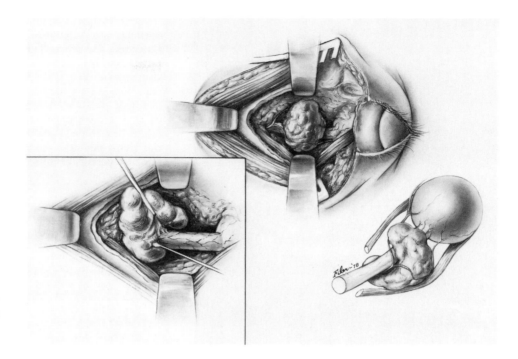

Figure 116-9 The micro-technique for removing an exophytic meningioma attached to the optic nerve.

is elevated with the medial holes on the midline. If the frontal sinus is exposed, which frequently occurs, the mucosa is removed or impacted into the frontal ostia. Temporalis muscle is then used to fill the sinus, and a flap of pericranium is elevated and sutured to the dura to maintain the muscle in place. If the tumor is confined to the orbit, an epidural approach is used. The dura is stripped from the floor of the frontal fossa to expose the orbital roof. Orbital unroofing is

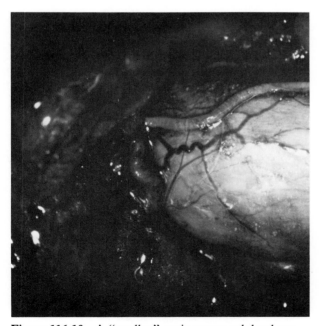

Figure 116-10 A "swollen" optic nerve; subdural meningioma is distal and normal nerve is proximal. (From Maroon JC and Kennerdell JS, J Neurosurg 60:1226–1235, 1984.)

performed initially with a high-speed drill, and then rongeurs of various types and angles are used. The optic canal, however, is unroofed not with rongeurs, but only with a high-speed diamond air drill. The orbitotomy extends medially to within approximately 1.5 cm of the midline and laterally to within 0.5 cm of the orbital margin.

When the orbital unroofing is complete, the transparent periorbita displays the frontal branch of the fifth nerve overlying the superior rectus and levator muscles. The trochlear nerve may be visualized through the operating microscope, but is usually not seen in its position deep in the apex.

To avoid injury to the nerves to the extraocular muscles, it is best to use a medial approach to the intraorbital part of the nerve. Therefore, meningiomas or optic gliomas are best approached by retracting the superior rectus and levator muscles laterally. Dissection through the fat is performed with small retractors and cottonoids. We prefer not to cut, remove, or coagulate the fat to decrease its bulk. With gentle palpation, the tumor will frequently be located, and then it is dissected with the above technique.

If the optic nerve is to be excised completely for a meningioma or optic glioma, it is sharply transected anteriorly between forceps or hemostats and followed posteriorly to the annulus of Zinn. At this point, the attachment of the levator muscle is transected; after sutures have been placed for later closure, the annulus itself is transected. The optic nerve is transected within a few millimeters of the chiasm and the entire optic nerve may be removed. An alternate technique for optic glioma removal in children is not to open the annulus, but rather to transect the nerve intraorbitally as far posteriorly as possible and then pull the proximal section of the optic nerve into the cranial cavity through the annulus of Zinn.

In removing optic nerve sheath meningiomas, it is preferable to do a one-stage operation, opening the annulus

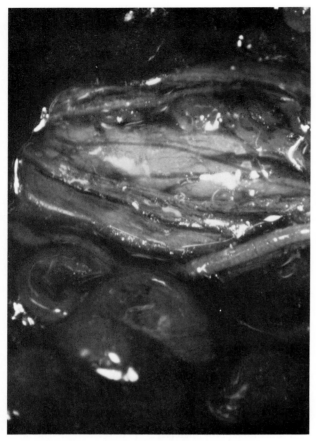

Figure 116-11 A subdural perioptic nerve meningioma exposed by incising the dura. Note the normal glistening arachnoid.

of Zinn and removing the nerve in its entirety. There is frequently tumor in the intracanalicular portion, which must be thoroughly coagulated.

Repair of the annulus of Zinn may be quite difficult, particularly in children or when the cranial exposure has not been adequate medially and inferiorly. For this reason, when it is anticipated that the annulus will be opened, removal of the superior orbital rim in one piece at the time of craniotomy allows excellent exposure with virtually no cerebral retraction.

In the closure, it is imperative to obliterate any iatrogenic openings into the ethmoid or sphenoid sinuses to obviate a CSF leak. The dura is closed in a water-tight fashion. The orbital roof may be reconstituted with a piece of stainless steel mesh or bone taken from the inner surface of the bone flap. We have not used a prosthesis routinely and have not had, to date, any noticeable pulsating proptosis in over 70 cases. A tarsorrhaphy is not usually done, but a compressive orbital dressing is used. Weakness of the levator and superior rectus muscle is routine when the annulus is opened; this may persist for up to three months.

References

1. Alper MG: Management of primary optic nerve meningiomas: Current status—therapy in controversy. J Clin Neuro Ophthalmol 1:101–117, 1981.
2. Hayreh SS: Blood supply of the optic nerve head and its role in optic atrophy, glaucoma, and oedema of the optic disc. Br J Ophthalmol 53:721–748, 1969.
3. Henderson JW: *Orbital Tumors*, 2d ed. New York: Brian C Decker, 1980.
4. Housepian EM, Trokel SL, Jakobiec FO, Hilal SK: Tumors of the orbit, in Youmans JR (ed): *Neurological Surgery*, 2d ed. Philadelphia, Saunders, 1982, pp 3024–3064.
5. Jane JA, Park TS, Poberskin LH, Winn HR, Butler AB: The supraorbital approach: A technical note. Neurosurgery 11:537–542, 1982.
6. Kennerdell JS: Tumors of the optic nerve, in Lessell S, Van Dalen JTW (eds): *Neuro-Ophthalmology* 1980. Amsterdam, Excerpta Medica, 1980, vol 1, pp 31–39.
7. Kennerdell JS, Dubois PJ, Dekker A, Johnson BL: CT-guided fine needle aspiration biopsy of orbital optic nerve tumors. Ophthalmology 87:491–496, 1980.
8. Kennerdell JS, Maroon JC: Microsurgical approach to intraorbital tumors. Arch Ophthalmol 94:1333–1336, 1976.
9. Maniscalco JE, Habal MB: Microanatomy of the optic canal. J Neurosurg 48:402–406, 1978.
10. Maroon JC: Orbital involvement by tumors: Types, recognition, and treatment. Contemp Neurosurg 7:1–6, 1979.
11. Maroon JC, Kennerdell JS: Lateral microsurgical approach to intraorbital tumors. J Neurosurg 44:556–561, 1976.
12. Smith JL, Vuksanovic MM, Yates BM, Bienfang DC: Radiation therapy for primary optic nerve meningiomas. J Clin Neuro Ophthalmol 1:85–99, 1981.
13. Wright JE, Call NB, Liaricos S: Primary optic nerve meningioma. Br J Ophthalmol 64:553–558, 1980.
14. Wright JE, McDonald WI, Call NB: Management of optic nerve gliomas. Br J Ophthalmol 64:545–552, 1980.

SECTION L

Tumors of the Scalp and Skull

117

Noninvasive Tumors of the Scalp

B. Thomas Harter, Jr.
Kathleen C. Harter
Donald Serafin

Noninvasive tumors of the scalp are derived from structures commonly found in this region (Fig. 117-1). In addition to the epidermis and dermis, the most common structure found in this region is the hair follicle. Closely associated with the hair follicle are three different glandular structures: the sebaceous gland, the apocrine gland, and the eccrine sweat gland. All of these are of dermal origin.

The sebaceous gland continuously forms a complex lipoidal mixture, the sebum, which is excreted to the skin surface from the opening of the hair follicle. A common congenital tumor arising from rests of sebaceous cells is the nevus sebaceous of Jadassohn. Another benign neoplasm is the adenoma sebaceum.

The apocrine gland is a vestigial skin appendage of no known physiological significance. It may be responsible for certain body odors when its milky secretion is acted upon by skin bacteria. Its greatest concentration is found in the axilla. Its secretion is also discharged from the orifice of the hair follicle. Although ectopic apocrine glands can be found in the scalp, this is unusual.

The eccrine sweat glands have a more uniform and generalized distribution pattern than do either sebaceous or apocrine glands. These glands are essential to thermal regulation, and discharge their secretion from a separate and distinct pore. The dermal eccrine cylindroma can be traced to rests of eccrine sweat glands.

Hair growth takes place as a holocrine process by the continuous formation of new cells, which move upward and gradually cornify. As indicated above, hair-bearing follicles are closely associated with sebaceous glands and are often referred to collectively as the pilosebaceous apparatus. A pilomatrixoma is thought to arise from a primitive cell which normally would differentiate into a hair matrix cell. Trichillemal cysts are thought to be derived from the trichillema, or external root sheath of the hair follicle.

Most noninvasive scalp tumors can be treated by simple excision. Because the scalp is an unyielding structure lacking distensibility, wound coverage can be a problem following excision of larger tumors. Primary wound closure can be accomplished by undermining and mobilizing a large area of scalp tissue with primary closure. Additional distensibility can be created artificially by making multiple parallel incisions through the galea on the undersurface of the elevated scalp. Larger defects can be closed using a variety of rotation advancement flaps. Excessively large defects usually require closure with split-thickness skin grafts.

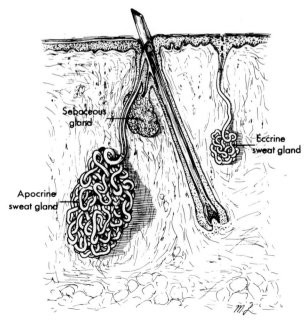

Figure 117-1 Illustration depicting a cross section of hair-bearing skin.

Nevus Sebaceous

The nevus sebaceous was first described by Jadassohn in 1895 to characterize a lesion consisting of an excess of sebaceous glands. Its clinical course can be divided into three stages: childhood, puberty, and tumor development.

The nevus sebaceous is usually present at birth or in early childhood on the scalp or face. In childhood, the nevus usually appears as a yellow or yellow-brown, slightly raised, waxy, hairless plaque with a velvety texture. Histologically, it consists of underdeveloped sebaceous glands and hair roots.

Puberty ushers in the second phase of development, with the lesion becoming verrucose, and in some cases nodular. The surface is firm or rubbery, with either few or no hairs present. At this time there is enlargement of the lesion, which often achieves a linear rather than a circular form. Microscopically, this second phase is characterized by the proliferation of mature sebaceous glands in the dermis. Hair roots either completely disappear or remain small. In many cases apocrine glands become hyperplastic and cystic. The epidermis becomes more verrucose (Fig. 117-2).

The third phase is characterized by the development of neoplasms within the original nevus. In one series of 150 cases of nevus sebaceous where 52 tumors were found, 21

patients developed basal cell carcinomas and 8 developed pipilliferous syringadenomas.[7]

Because of the natural course of this tumor, with proliferation during puberty and the possibility of later malignant change, it is advisable to perform excision during childhood.

Adenoma Sebaceum

Adenoma sebaceum was first described by Balzer and Ménétrier in 1885. It is an uncommon benign tumor which occurs most often in middle age on the nose, cheek and scalp. Sebaceous adenomas appear clinically as discrete, small, flesh-colored or yellow nodules which may be several millimeters to several centimeters in size. The lesions are usually slow-growing and may have been present for a long period of time before the patient seeks treatment.

Microscopically, the tumors are arranged in lobules. Masses of small cells resembling basal cells line the periphery of the lobule. Larger cells containing fat vacuoles and cysts containing sebaceous material are found centrally. The adenoma is usually surrounded by a connective tissue layer.

Sebaceous adenomas should be excised (Fig. 117-3).

Pilomatrixoma (Calcifying Epithelioma of Malberle)

Pilomatrixoma usually occurs on the scalp, face, neck, and upper arms. It usually presents as an asymptomatic, solitary, firm nodule located in the dermis, although at times it may occur in the subcutaneous tissue. Varying in diameter from 0.5 to 5 cm, this lesion may develop at any age.

Microscopically, the tumor is encased by compressed collagen, and consists of folding sheets and bands of basophilic and shadow cells. The basal cells are small, with large, round, deeply basophilic nuclei and scanty cytoplasm. The cytoplasm of the shadow cells stains slightly, but the nucleus does not stain. The cells thus appear with an unstained "shadow" at the site of the nucleus, and hence their name, *shadow cells*. Basophilic cells develop into shadow cells, and older tumors usually show decreasing numbers of basophilic cells.[3]

It is postulated that this tumor arises from a primitive cell which is differentiating toward a hair matrix cell. Calcification is frequently seen in these tumors (84 percent in the study by Forbit and Helwig) and occurs in the areas of the shadow cells.[3]

Malignant change has not been shown to occur, and the pilomatrixoma is best removed by excision.

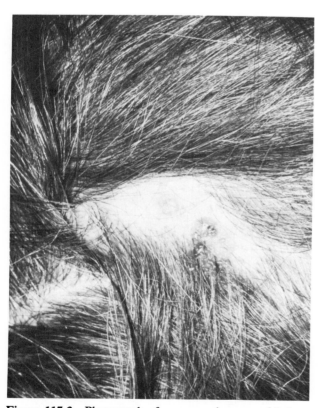

Figure 117-2 Photograph of a nevus sebaceous of Jadassohn. The lesion consists of a yellow or yellow-brown, slightly raised, waxy, hairless plaque. With advancing age, this tumor may undergo malignant change to a basal cell epithelioma.

Figure 117-3 A sebaceous adenoma. *A*. Note that the large size of the lesion precludes simple excision and primary closure. *B*. Outline of rotation advancement flaps following tumor excision. *C*. Flaps elevated, exposing the periosteum of the cranium. *D*. Early postoperative result following successful wound closure.

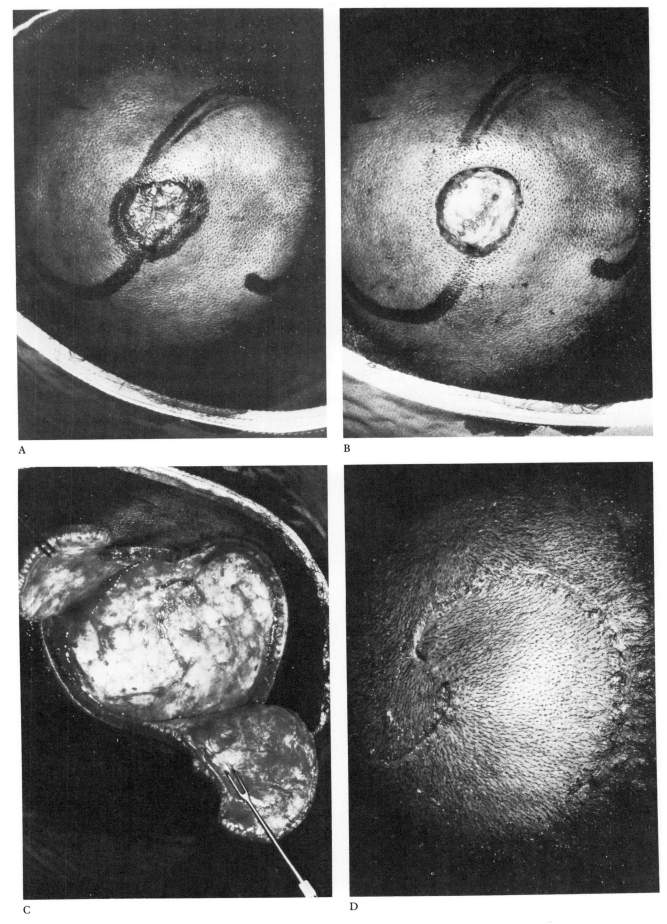

A

B

C

D

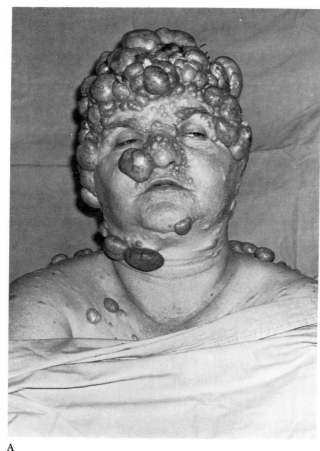

A

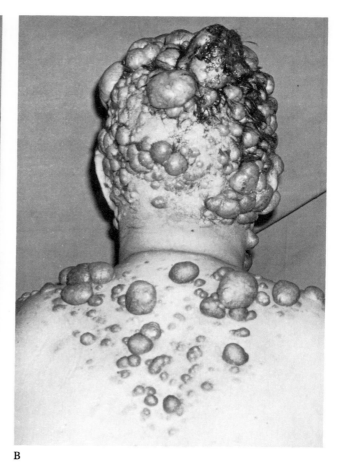

B

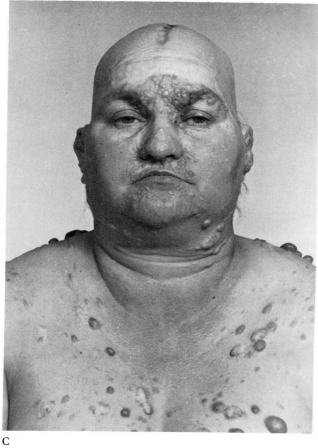

C

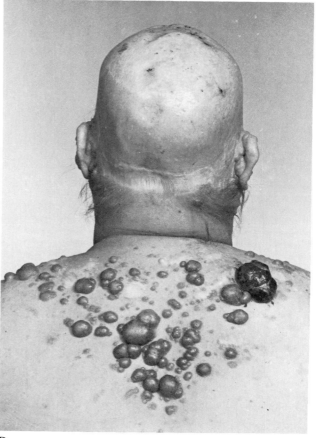

D

980

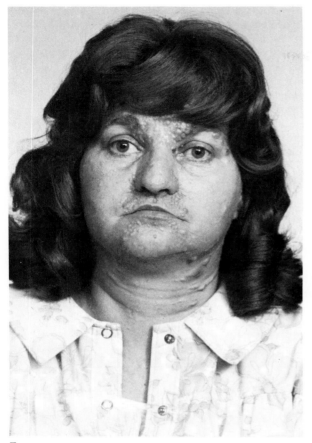

E

Figure 117-4 *A, B*. Preoperative photographs of a patient with a dermal eccrine cylindroma. This tumor is commonly called a turban tumor. *C, D*. Postoperative photographs after excision of entire scalp with application of a split-thickness skin graft. *E*. Late postoperative result following completion of reconstruction, with that patient wearing an artificial hairpiece. (Photographs kindly supplied by Dr. Kenneth L. Pickrell.)

upper dermis. Microscopically, closely packed cords of basophilic round or oval cells are separated into lobules by strands of hyaline material. Cystic and ductlike spaces are also seen within the tumor.[2]

Biopsy is indicated to establish the diagnosis when a single lesion is present, and is often needed to differentiate multiple cylindromas from epidermal cysts.

These tumors usually require excision and skin grafting is often needed if the area involved is large. It is not uncommon for these tumors to recur after excision in adjacent areas of uninvolved skin.

Keratoses

The keratoses represent localized hyperplastic changes in the epidermis. Both seborrheic and solar keratoses are commonly found on the scalp.

Seborrheic Keratoses

These lesions commonly develop during middle age and are most frequently found on the scalp, face, and trunk. They may occur singly or in large numbers, and appear as slightly raised, soft, greasy, brownish, circumscribed papules. Usually they measure only several millimeters, but may attain sizes up to several centimeters.

The epidermis is thickened in seborrheic keratoses. Cells resembling basal cells penetrate into the epidermis, forming a flat or irregular epithelial mass, or develop a reticular pattern with horn cysts or pseudocysts.[11]

The seborrheic keratosis may at times be difficult to distinguish from a solar keratosis or basal cell carcinoma. If the lesion is darkly pigmented, it may resemble a melanoma. In these cases, biopsy is needed to establish the diagnosis.

These lesions do not undergo malignant change and may be removed for cosmetic reasons by currettage, dermabrasion, or freezing with liquid nitrogen.

Solar Keratoses

Solar keratoses (also referred to as actinic keratoses) develop commonly on the sun-exposed areas of skin, most often in fair-complexioned individuals. These lesions usually occur in middle to old age as a function of the cumulative effect of solar radiation.

Dermal Eccrine Cylindroma

The dermal eccrine cylindroma has also been called Spiegler's tumor, cylindroma, and turban tumor since it was first described by Ancell in 1842. These tumors usually begin as small nodules in adolescence or early adulthood, and continue to grow slowly into mushroom-shaped rubbery masses measuring up to several centimeters. They are nonpainful, freely movable, and usually a red-blue or pink color.

The tumors most commonly appear on the scalp and face, and are usually multiple. They have been given the name *turban tumor* because they sometimes cover the entire scalp like a turban (Fig. 117-4).

The dermal eccrine cylindroma occurs more often in women than in men, and there is a positive family history in about 30 percent of the cases. These tumors usually do not bother the patient except as a cosmetic problem, and usually run a benign course.

Cylindromas of the scalp and facial trichoepitheliomas have been reported to occur as a single genetic entity with inheritance determined by an autosomal dominant gene with variable expression.[12] Another syndrome of trichoepitheliomas, milia, and cylindromas has also been reported.[10]

A dermal eccrine cylindroma originates from an eccrine sweat gland. It is usually unencapsulated and lies in the

The lesions begin as dry, hard patches, usually less than 1 cm in diameter, which develop scales on an erythematous base. When the scales are removed, bleeding usually occurs, followed by further scale development.

Microscopically, the epidermis is parakeratotic and has lost its granular layer. The prickle cells have lost their orderly stratified arrangement and have become edematous. The basal layer no longer consists of small, darkly staining cells, but is now composed of cells resembling prickle cells. The dermoepidermal junctions may be flat and the epidermis thin, or the epidermis may be hyperplastic and acanthotic. The regular pattern of rete ridges and papillae is lost. The border of the keratosis is sharp and slants upward and away from the adjoining normal skin.[8]

Skin keratoses are considered premalignant lesions because they may undergo malignant degeneration. If induration or ulceration exists in a lesion, the diagnosis of squamous cell carcinoma must be entertained, and biopsy done to establish the diagnosis.

Removal of these lesions may be accomplished by curettage or liquid nitrogen. If many keratoses are present, 5-fluorouracil cream may be applied topically to the involved area.

Hemangiomas

Hemangiomas are benign vascular tumors and are the commonest tumors of childhood. They are subdivided by their histology into capillary hemangiomas and cavernous hemangiomas. Capillary hemangiomas are formed by aggregations of abnormal capillaries. Two types of capillary hemangiomas are found on the scalp—the port-wine stain and the strawberry mark.

Port-Wine Stain (Nevus Flammeus)

The port-wine stain is a flat, bright pinkish-red to bluish-purple lesion present at birth. It blanches with pressure, and refills when the pressure is released. The tumor is composed of masses of intradermal capillaries lined by mature endothelium. These vessels may follow a dermatome distribution. When trigeminal ophthalmic distributions involve an associated intracranial collection of capillary blood vessels, the Sturge-Weber syndrome must be considered.

These lesions do not undergo spontaneous involution, nor do they grow; but their surface area increases with the growth of the area involved.

Although some port-wine stains may fade slightly with time, most small lesions are treated by excision or by the use of cosmetic covering agents. Recently the argon laser has proved efficacious in treatment.

Strawberry Mark

The strawberry mark is a bright red or purplish red, slightly raised lesion consisting of capillaries lined by embryonic endothelium. On palpation the strawberry mark feels firm and rubbery, and it blanches incompletely with pressure.

The hemangioma is usually not present at birth, but appears within a few weeks as a pink or red spot. It then begins a period of very active growth usually lasting about 6 months. Following a dormant period, the tumor begins to undergo a spontaneous involution during the next 6 to 12 months. With this involutional phase, small grey islets develop within the lesion. During the next 2 to 3 years, these islets increase and become confluent, and the hemangioma decreases in size. Eventually normal or atrophic skin remains in the area.[6]

The diagnosis of strawberry mark can usually be made by careful history and observation.

In dealing with these hemangiomas, it is important to remember that 85 percent will undergo spontaneous resolution by the age of 5 years. Therefore, in most cases no treatment is necessary, and parents are best advised to wait until the involutional phase begins.

Surgical resection may be indicated in cases involving obstruction or loss of function of an organ, bleeding, or ulceration. The use of systemic steroids may also prove helpful in certain cases.

Scalp Cysts

Four types of cysts are found in the scalp: epidermoid inclusion cysts, trichilemmal cysts, dermoid cysts, and branchiogenic cysts. In the past the term *sebaceous cyst* was used to describe the common wen. However, studies have shown that these cysts are either epidermoid or trichilemmal cysts, and do not contain elements of the sebaceous gland. Hence, the term *sebaceous cyst* is not used in this discussion of scalp cysts.

Epidermoid Inclusion Cysts

Epidermoid cysts are slow-growing, rounded, subcutaneous masses. They lie in the dermis but are attached to the epidermis, and a central punctum may be seen on the overlying skin. The cysts vary in size from several millimeters to several centimeters. On palpation, the cyst may feel soft or firm, depending on its contents. Epidermoid cysts may undergo calcification or become inflamed and infected, leading to the development of an abcess.

These cysts commonly develop during adolescence and adulthood. Multiple epidermal cysts of the scalp and face are a component of Gardner's syndrome, which is also characterized by polyposis of the colon, fibromas, and lipomas of the skin.

Histologically, the wall of the cyst is composed of stratified squamous epithelium. It contains laminated keratin or an amorphous material with a high lipid content.[5] Pressure from these contents may cause flattening of the cyst wall.

These cysts are best handled by surgical excision, and the entire cyst must be removed to avoid recurrence. When the cyst is infected, incision and drainage may initially be undertaken, with excision planned at a later date after the inflammation has subsided.

Trichilemmal Cysts

Trichilemmal cysts occur most commonly on the scalp during the adult years and occur more frequently in females than in males. Cysts are often found within families, and inheritance is determined by an autosomal dominant gene.

These smooth, rounded cysts are located within the dermis. They may occur as a single lesion, but usually are multiple and increase very slowly in size. About 50 percent of the affected individuals will develop increasing numbers of cysts with time, but it is unusual to find a large number of cysts on one person. In one study, only 10 percent of the patients had more than 10 cysts.[4] Multiple cysts usually appear all over the scalp and originate independently, but they may derive from one cyst or appear as recurrences following the removal of a cyst.

These cysts are derived from the trichilemma, or external root sheath of the hair follicle. The cyst wall consists of stratified epithelium and shows a characteristic lining of pale cells. These cells increase in vertical diameter as they lose their nuclei, and mature into keratin without the formation of a granular layer. The cyst is filled with keratin.[9]

Trichilemmal cysts show fewer inflammatory changes than do epidermoid cysts. These cysts are usually excised for cosmetic reasons.

Congenital Inclusion Dermoid Cysts

Displaced dermal cells along the lines of embryonic fusion may develop into dermoid cysts. In the scalp, they originate as the developing cranial bones grow toward each other. Dermal cells may become isolated from the overlying epithelium, creating the dermoid cyst.

Although these lesions are congenital, they usually enlarge later in life and may reach a diameter of several centimeters. The overlying skin is freely movable and the lesion feels cystic upon palpation. Stratified squamous epithelium lines the cyst wall and the cyst may contain a greasy keratinized material and hair.

Dermoid cysts occur frequently on the head and neck; only a small percentage appear on the scalp. In one study, the three dermoid cysts found on the scalp from among a total of 36 head and neck cases were located at the right parieto-occipital suture line, at the anterior fontanel, and at the bregma.[1]

These cysts are excised with careful attention to the possibility of a connection of the cyst wall to the underlying meninges, or of intracranial extension of the cyst.

Branchiogenic Cysts

Branchiogenic cysts and sinuses result from the failure of the branchial arches to close completely during embryonic development. The only branchiogenic cysts found in the scalp area involve lesions of the first branchial cleft, which appear anterior to the upper part of the external ear.

Although present at birth, these cysts may not become apparent until later in life, often in the third decade. They usually appear as smooth, painless lumps, slowly increasing in size.

The cyst is lined by stratified squamous or columnar epithelium, and contains caseous fluid. These cysts should be completely excised.

References

1. Colcock BP, Sass RE, Staudinger L: Dermoid cysts. N Engl J Med 252:373–379, 1955.
2. Crain RC, Helwig EB: Dermal cylindroma (dermal eccrine cylindroma). Am J Clin Pathol 35:504–515, 1961.
3. Forbis R Jr, Helwig EB: Pilomatrixoma (calcifying epithelioma). Arch Dermatol 83:606–618, 1961.
4. Leppard BJ, Sanderson KV: The natural history of trichilemmal cysts. Br J Dermatol 94:379–390, 1976.
5. Lund HZ: *Tumors of the Skin*. Armed Forces Institute of Pathology, Washington, D.C. 1957.
6. Margileth AM: Developmental vascular abnormalities. Pediatr Clin North Amer 18:773–800, 1971.
7. Mehregan AH, Pinkus H: Life history of organoid nevi. Arch Dermatol 91:574–588, 1965.
8. Pinkus H: Keratosis senilis. Amer J Clin Pathol 29:193–207, 1958.
9. Pinkus H: "Sebaceous cysts" are trichilemmal cysts. Arch Dermatol 99:544–555, 1969.
10. Rasmussen JE: A syndrome of trichoepitheliomas, milia, and cylindromas. Arch Dermatol 111:610–614, 1975.
11. Rook A, Dawber R: *Diseases of the Hair and Scalp*. Oxford, Blackwell, 1982.
12. Welch JP, Wells RS, Kerr CB: Ancell-Spiegler cylindromas (turban tumours) and Brooke-Fordyce trichoepitheliomas: Evidence for a single genetic entity. J Med Genet 5:29–35, 1968.

118

Tumors of the Skull

Rand M. Voorhies
Narayan Sundaresan

Malignant bone and soft tissue tumors account for less than 1 percent of cancers diagnosed annually in the United States; approximately 1,900 primary malignant tumors of bone and 5,000 soft tissue sarcomas are diagnosed each year.[7] The skull as a primary site accounts for less than 2 percent of these malignancies.[49] Precise figures do not exist for the incidence of benign skull tumors. Many benign skull tumors are asymptomatic lesions that never come to medical attention; others present with radiological features that are so typical that continued observation is all that is necessary. Two relatively old comprehensive reviews of calvarial tumors indicate that the most common benign tumors are osteoma and hemangioma, while the most common malignant lesion is osteogenic sarcoma.[20,49] In the pediatric age group, dermoid and epidermoid cysts are the most common benign lesions.[11] Primary sarcomas of the vault are rare in childhood, and are usually fibrosarcomas.[27]

Any type of tumor which occurs in the skeletal system may originate in the skull. Because of the rarity of these tumors, the literature consists of single case reports or small series restricted to a single histological entity. Various classifications of skull tumors have been proposed: benign vs. malignant, osteoblastic vs. osteolytic, site of origin in the diploe vs. origin in the tables of the skull, and location at the skull base vs. in the vault. This last classification is based on the embryological development of the skull: the bones of the base are formed by endochondral ossification, whereas the bones of the vault are formed by membranous ossification. This accounts for the propensity of certain tumors to arise at particular sites, e.g., chondromas at the skull base.

In this chapter we have catalogued the multitude of skull tumors along the lines of the pathological classification suggested by Huvos[17] (Table 118-1). There are many areas of controversy among bone tumor pathologists concerning the characteristics and clinical behavior of some of the rarer or more recently described tumors. The discussion of each tumor type is concise, although in some instances an oversimplified view is presented. Several common tumors and tumor-like conditions (i.e., dermoid and epidermoid cysts, eosinophilic granuloma, chordoma, fibrous dysplasia, and Paget's disease) are discussed elsewhere in this volume.

From a clinical standpoint, primary calvarial tumors present special problems by virtue of their location. Neurological symptoms and signs are related to the degree of intracranial extension. Careful preoperative radiographic examination of the lesion is helpful in establishing the diagnosis, but often the radiographic features are misleading. The CT scan appearance of osteogenic sarcoma, for example, may be extremely variable, and may mimic benign and otherwise more common tumors. In a recent series of four patients, the CT scan appearance suggested osteoma in one, giant cell tumor in another, and meningioma in the third; only in the fourth, where Paget's disease coexisted, was the correct diagnosis of osteogenic sarcoma made preoperatively.[42]

TABLE 118-1 Classification of Skull Tumors

I. Bone-forming tumors
  A. Benign
    1. Osteoma
    2. Ossifying fibroma
    3. Osteoid osteoma
    4. Osteoblastoma
  B. Malignant
    1. Osteogenic sarcoma
II. Cartilage-forming tumors
  A. Benign
    1. Chondroma
    2. Chondroblastoma
    3. Chondromyxoid fibroma
  B. Malignant
    1. Chondrosarcoma
    2. Mesenchymal chondrosarcoma
III. Tumors of fibrous connective tissue
  A. Benign
    1. Intradiploic meningioma*
  B. Malignant
    1. Fibrosarcoma
IV. Tumors of histiocytic or fibrohistiocytic origin
  A. Benign
    1. Nonossifying fibroma
    2. Giant cell tumor†
  B. Malignant
    1. Malignant fibrous histiocytoma
V. Tumors and tumor-like lesions of blood vessels or the hemopoietic system
  A. Benign
    1. Hemangioma
    2. Aneurysmal bone cyst
  B. Malignant
    1. Angiosarcoma
    2. Solitary osseous myeloma (plasmacytoma)
    3. Ewing's sarcoma
    4. Non-Hodgkin's lymphoma
VI. Fat-forming tumors
  A. Benign
    1. Lipoma
VII. Miscellaneous tumors and tumor-like lesions
    Dermoid cyst
    Epidermoid cyst
    Eosinophilic granuloma
    Chordoma
    Fibrous dysplasia
    Paget's disease

*The cell of origin is believed to be an arachnoid cell.
†The distinction between benign and malignant varieties is especially vague.

Although the CT scan has in many instances supplanted tomograms and special views, the plain skull roentgenogram remains an important tool in patient evaluation (Fig. 118-1). Thomas and Baker found that about 7 percent of the patients undergoing radiographic examination of the skull at the Mayo Clinic had clinically suspicious lytic lesions.[45] A few general conclusions of their study were that lytic lesions with smooth edges, even if irregular in contour, were usually benign; the presence of circumferential sclerosis and expansion of the diploic space were also favorable. The size of the lesion by itself was not a reliable indicator of malignancy, whereas a large number, especially more than half a dozen, and location off the midline, often pointed to malignancy. Osteoblastic lesions are much less common, with osteoma and metastatic prostate carcinoma being two examples. A variety of metabolic, endocrine, and infectious conditions can produce diffuse changes, but are beyond the scope of this discussion.

Angiography is useful in the assessment of tumor vascularity, and in some cases may lead to a consideration of preoperative tumor embolization to reduce blood loss at surgery.[37] Technetium pertechnetate radionuclide scans may have a role in selected cases in following the response to therapy or local recurrence; this is particularly true in osteoid osteoma[52] and osteogenic sarcoma. Occasionally a bone scan may be useful in providing preoperative localization of lesions which are poorly visualized on either skull films or CT scans (Fig. 118-2). Usually, however, it is possible to precisely localize a small, nonpalpable skull tumor with the aid of a scalp marker placed under CT scan guidance.

The treatment of primary calvarial tumors is generally surgical. Although distant metastases can occur with sarcomas, the major problem is local recurrence with intracranial extension. For this reason, adequate preoperative planning is necessary to prepare for radical en bloc resection that will not disseminate tumor and will obtain adequate margins. When the scalp is involved, rotational flaps and skin grafting may be required. Therefore, consideration should be given to obtaining preoperative pathological diagnosis, if the location of the tumor makes this feasible, by either needle biopsy or small-incision biopsy. On the other hand, if the lesion proves to be a highly radio-sensitive tumor such as a primary lymphoma of bone, radiation therapy or chemotherapy would be the initial treatment. If biopsy reveals a metastasis, then an extent-of-disease workup is indicated (Fig. 118-3). If widespread metastatic disease is found, indicating a short life expectancy, then mutilating surgical excision of the skull lesion might be deferred.

Preoperative chemotherapy has shown some promise in the treatment of osteogenic sarcoma and other sarcomas.[36] If a lesion is extremely bulky, a possible approach would be to establish the diagnosis with incisional biopsy and then give preoperative chemotherapy to shrink the tumor. This technique has produced impressive results with paraspinal sarcomas, where reduction in size occurred, and at operation largely necrotic non-viable tumor was found.[43] Further experience with this treatment modality is necessary.

Radiation therapy is often recommended in the management of patients with malignant bone tumors. Sarcomas, however, are generally radiation-resistant and require doses

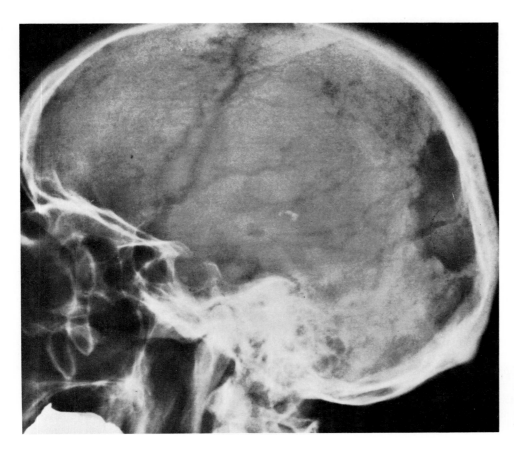

Figure 118-1 A lytic skull lesion with irregular, undermined edges. This appearance is suggestive of a malignant tumor.

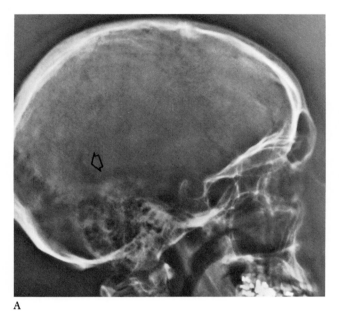

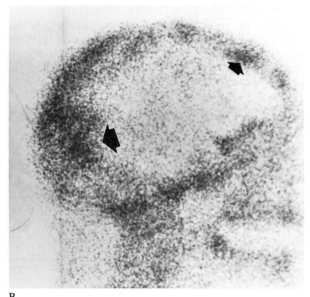

A   B

Figure 118-2 *A.* A plain lateral roentgenogram showing minimal irregularity (*arrow*) which could not be demonstrated with bone windows on computed tomography. *B.* A radionuclide bone scan shows several areas of increased uptake (*arrows*). The biopsy site was selected by placing a scalp marker over the larger abnormal area. (Courtesy of Richard Benua, M.D.).

greater than 5,000 rad. Since this dose carries a potential risk to the underlying brain, newer techniques have been advocated, including the use of implanted radioactive seeds and electron beam therapy, which permits the delivery of high-intensity energy precisely to a preselected depth. More recently, proton beam treatment with computerized dosimetry has allowed dosages in excess of 7,000 rad to be delivered to the base of the skull for chondrosarcoma, with sparing of adjacent normal tissues.[41]

Osteoma

Sporadic Osteomas

Osteomas are benign, slowly growing lesions composed of mature dense cortical bone, arising from either table in bone that is formed by intramembranous ossification. They are fairly common, with as many as 1 percent of the patients seen in large otolaryngology clinics having osteomas of the paranasal sinuses. The true incidence is unknown, since most are asymptomatic, but osteomas were the most common primary bone tumor found in the cranial vault in two large series.[20,49] Osteomas occur in the vault, the paranasal and mastoid sinuses, and the mandible (Figs. 118-4 to 118-6).

Those located in the vault present as a painless swelling. Osteomas in the paranasal sinuses can present with headache and recurrent sinusitis. Extension into the orbit can cause exophthalmos. Intracranial extension can occur, and a reported case arising from the mastoid sinus caused brain stem compression.[48]

Radiographically, osteomas are dense, well-demarcated lesions arising from either the inner or outer table. They may be sessile or pedunculated. Several conditions must be considered in the differential diagnosis. A solitary osteoblastic metastasis is rare but can occur with prostate carcinoma. The solitary or monostatic form of fibrous dysplasia can be purely sclerotic, but this is more common at the skull base. Hyperostosis frontalis interna stops at the midline and does not form over large cortical veins. Meningiomas are usually associated with increased vascular markings and will be visualized on arteriography.

An osteoma is composed of mature lamellar bone and is arranged either in compact, trabecular, or mixed patterns. An osteoma can be distinguished from fibrous dysplasia since the latter has no osteoblasts lining the spicules of bone, and initially involves the diploe rather than the cortices. Meningioma hyperostosis is identified by the infiltrating meningothelial cells, or by the presence of an underlying dural meningioma.

Asymptomatic osteomas do not require treatment. Lesions of the vault may be resected locally. If only the outer table is involved, the inner table may be spared. Use of a CO_2 laser has been recommended,[22] although conventional techniques are adequate. For large tumors involving the orbit, a combined craniofacial approach may be necessary.[34]

Gardner's Syndrome

This condition is inherited as a mendelian dominant disorder and consists of polyps of both the small and large intestine; multiple osteomas, especially of the frontal bone and mandible; soft tissue fibromas; and sebaceous cysts of the

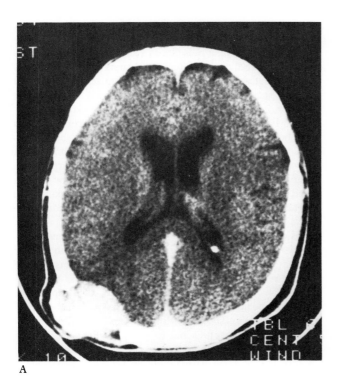

A

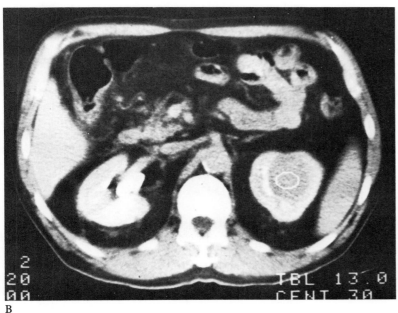

B

Figure 118-3 *A*. A CT scan of the lesion shown in Figure 118-1 reveals both extradural and soft tissue extension of the tumor. Needle biopsy revealed a clear cell carcinoma. *B*. A CT scan of the abdomen revealed a hypernephroma in the right kidney.

skin. There is an abnormal proliferative connective tissue disorder in this syndrome, which frequently results in keloids, fibromas, or desmoid tumors arising after surgical intervention. Postoperative dural fibromatosis has been reported in this setting.[44] Less than 10 percent of the patients have the complete tetrad. The bony abnormalities occur at a young age and precede the other manifestations. The clinical significance of this syndrome rests in the virtual certainty that these patients will develop colonic carcinoma later in life. Patients with multiple osteomas should undergo complete gastrointestinal tract evaluation. Recently, tissue cul-

ture of skin fibroblasts has shown abnormalities in karyotyping that allow preclinical detection of this syndrome. Siblings of these patients should also be examined.

Ossifying Fibroma

Ossifying fibroma is a slow-growing benign tumor composed of a fibrous stroma with varying amounts of immature woven and mature lamellar bone. Its synonyms are os-

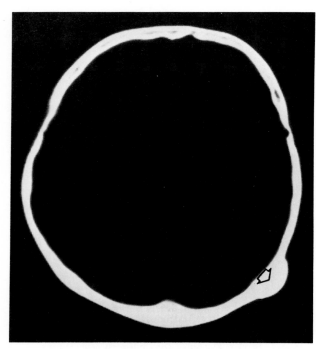

Figure 118-4 A CT scan with a skeletal window setting shows an osteoma arising from the outer table (*arrow*). The homogeneous dense appearance is characteristic.

teofibroma, fibro-osteoma, and benign nonodontogenic tumor of the jaw.

This tumor most commonly occurs in the mandible and maxilla. It is very rare, possibly more common in females, with a peak incidence in the third or fourth decades. The

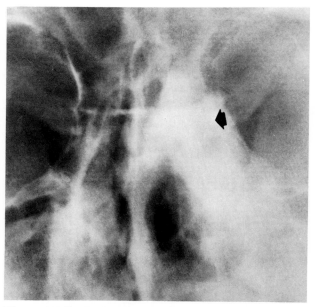

Figure 118-5 A skull film showing an osteoma of the paranasal sinuses (*arrow*). The radiographic differential diagnosis includes fibrous dysplasia and meningioma.

most common site in the skull is the frontal bone, near the orbital roof.[38]

Ossifying fibroma presents as a slowly growing, painless mass that produces symptoms and signs dependent on its location, such as nasal obstruction, anosmia, or proptosis. It is radiolucent initially, and later presents with varying amounts of calcification. It often appears to expand the involved bone, usually with preservation of the cortex, which may be very thin. Sometimes a densely sclerotic bony reaction is produced, giving an appearance similar to that of fibrous dysplasia. However, the margins are sharper with ossifying fibroma. Dilated vascular channels may be seen on skull films when the lesion is located in the convexity. The ^{99m}Tc scan may be positive, and scalp and dural feeding vessels may be shown with angiography.[40]

Microscopically, an ossifying fibroma shows a uniformly cellular, fibrous spindle cell growth arranged in a whorled or matted pattern. There are spicules of bone composed of immature woven bone but with mature lamellar bone peripherally. The bony fragments can be small spherules which can be mistaken for meningioma psammoma bodies.[39] Ossifying fibroma should be differentiated from fibrous dysplasia: fibrous dysplasia occurs at an earlier age, usually within the first two decades; it is composed entirely of immature woven bone with randomly arranged birefringent lines when viewed under polarized light; twisted, tangled, and disoriented fibers are seen with a silver reticulin stain; no osteoblasts or osteoclasts are present; and there are areas of hemorrhage with associated inflammation and giant cell reaction.

Juvenile ossifying fibroma occurs in the maxilla of children under the age of 15, and is histologically identical to the adult tumor. However, it grows very rapidly, and may cause death by aggressive local invasion (Fig. 118-7).[47]

The usual ossifying fibroma is a slowly growing, painless mass. The preferred surgical treatment is complete excision, which is easily accomplished in tumors of the vault. When the tumor is located at the skull base, subtotal removal provides excellent results for 10 years or more.[39]

Osteoid Osteoma

This is a benign lesion consisting of a small nidus, usually less than 1 cm in diameter, surrounded by dense reactive sclerosis. Osteoid osteoma accounts for about 10 percent of benign bone tumors. It is most commonly located in the long bones of the lower extremeties, but has been reported in almost every bone, and rarely in the skull; 75 percent of the cases occur before 25 years of age, and it is twice as common in males.

Osteoid osteoma may cause localized pain and tenderness, particularly at night, which is characteristically relieved by aspirin. However, some cases are asymptomatic or produce only vague discomfort, such as mild headache.[13,33]

The nidus is most often radiolucent, with a surrounding area of dense sclerosis. Occasionally, a lesion located in the cortical bone will have a radiopaque center with a ringlike outer band of radiolucency, which in turn is surrounded by a sclerotic reaction. The sclerosis is less marked in flat bones

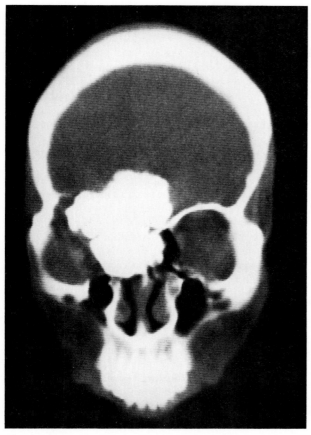

Figure 118-6 A CT scan in the coronal plane showing a large osteoma which originated in the frontal sinus but grew to involve the orbit and the maxillary and ethmoid sinuses. Note the marked extension into the anterior cranial fossa. Complete surgical resection requires a craniofacial approach.

than in tubular bones. These tumors are readily detected by radionuclide bone scans.[52]

The development of this lesion can be subdivided into three stages which differ histologically, but are not correlated with a particular clinical presentation. The initial stage is characterized by actively proliferating, densely packed, prominent osteoblasts in a background of highly vascularized stroma. The intermediate phase, which is the most characteristic appearance, is one in which osteoid is deposited between the osteoblasts. The patches of intercellular osteoid and osteoid trabeculae show various degrees of calcification. In the mature, or osteoma, stage, the osteoid is composed of well-calcified, compact trabeculae of atypical bone, which is typically neither woven nor lamellar. Surrounding the nidus in all stages is a region of thickened cortical bone.

Osteoid osteoma is a benign tumor; treatment is indicated to relieve pain. Surgical excision, either en bloc or by curettage of the nidus and surrounding sclerotic bone, is curative. Amelioration of symptoms has been reported even if the nidus is left but the overlying bony cortex is unroofed. Rare cases of recurrence following en bloc resection have been reported; recurrence is more likely, but still rare, after thorough curettage. Poorly documented cases of spontaneous regression of this tumor have been reported.

Osteoblastoma

Osteoblastoma is a benign tumor histologically similar to osteoid osteoma, but larger, with less peripheral reactive sclerosis. It is often very vascular. Its synonyms include giant cell osteoma and spindle cell variant of giant cell tumor.

Osteoblastomas comprise about 1 percent of all primary bone tumors; 75 percent occur in the second and third decades, with a 2:1 male preponderance. They are most commonly located in the posterior vertebral elements, and 8 percent are located in the calvaria or maxilla.[17]

Osteoblastoma typically produces a dull, aching, poorly localized pain, which is neither characteristically worse at night, nor relieved by aspirin. When the tumor occurs in the vertebral column it can cause spinal cord compression. In

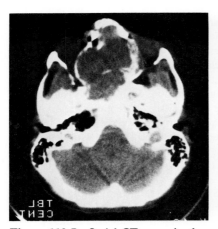
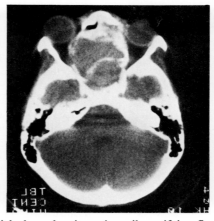
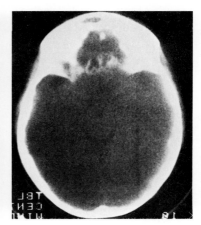

Figure 118-7 Serial CT scans in the axial plane showing a juvenile ossifying fibroma of the paranasal sinuses with early extension through the cribriform plate. (From Tomita et al.[47])

the skull, it presents as a slowly growing, moderately tender mass.[51]

Osteoblastoma is a predominantly osteolytic, expanding lesion with varying degrees of calcification. It is larger (greater than 2 cm), and has a less marked peripheral sclerosis than osteoid osteoma. Bone scans are positive and arteriography may show a vascular supply from both dural and scalp arteries.[51]

Pathologically, osteoblastoma may be confused with osteogenic sarcoma. However, examination reveals stromal cells that are small and slender and do not resemble sarcomatous spindle cells; mitoses are rare, anaplastic tumor cells are not present, tumor cartilage is not formed, and the tumor cells present in the osteoid matrix are small and inconspicuous. Osteoblastoma may be differentiated from osteoid osteoma by its abundant fibrous stroma and by the presence of many multinucleated giant cells which congregate around vascular channels, extravasated blood, and osteoid or newly formed bone. The vascularity may be so pronounced as to give the appearance of an aneurysmal bone cyst in places (Fig. 118-8).

Osteoblastoma is a benign tumor, but local recurrences have been reported following subtotal resection. When the tumor is located in the vault, en bloc resection is recommended. The scalp, pericranium, bone, and dura may be highly vascular.[51] Tumors at the skull base involving the sinuses and orbit may be approached in a combined procedure, with surgeons from the disciplines of neurosurgery, otolaryngology, and ophthalmology taking part. Postoperative radiation therapy for subtotally excised tumors has been effective in some cases. Malignant transformation in osteblastoma has been reported to occur both spontaneously and following radiation treatment.

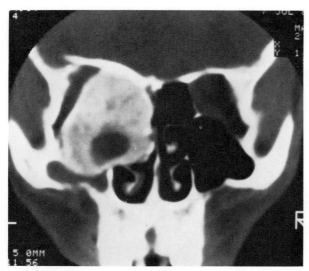

Figure 118-8   A CT scan in the coronal plane shows a partially cystic lesion involving the paranasal sinuses. Pathologically this proved to be an osteoblastoma with areas of aneurysmal bone cyst.

Osteogenic Sarcoma

This is the most common primary malignant tumor of bone, in which the malignant proliferating spindle cell stroma directly produces osteoid or immature bone. This tumor occurs approximately twice as frequently as chondrosarcoma and is three times more common than Ewing's sarcoma. An annual incidence rate of 1 per 100,000 population in the United States is reported. Although it can occur at any age, 50 percent of the patients are adolescents in the second decade of life. The average age of patients with calvarial tumors is about 39 years, and is slightly higher than that noted for extremity lesions. Osteogenic sarcoma may arise de novo, or in association with other pre-existing bone lesions, such as Paget's disease, fibrous dysplasia, or other benign bone tumors, or may be induced by radiation therapy.[28] A slight predominance of males is noted in most series.

The majority of patients with calvarial tumors usually present with a mass on the skull, with or without associated pain. The history is relatively brief and often of less than 3 months' duration. On occasion, when the tumor arises predominantly from the inner table, it may simulate an intracranial neoplasm. There is one report of a tumor originating predominantly within the brain substance without apparent attachment to the dura or skull.

Unlike extremity tumors, most skull lesions usually present with irregular destruction of both the outer and inner tables, which are usually nonspecific findings of malignancy. The characteristic "sun-ray" appearance suggesting extension of ossification into soft tissues is rarely present (Fig. 118-9). For this reason, the diagnosis of osteogenic sarcoma is rarely entertained unless a pre-existing condition such as Paget's disease is present (Fig. 118-10). The computed tomographic appearances of this tumor are highly variable, and in our experience may mimic the appearances of other benign bony tumors.[42]

Huvos has divided osteogenic sarcoma into four main histological types: fibroblastic, chondroblastic, osteoblastic, and telangiectatic.[17] This subclassification is based on the predominant cell forming the lesion, or the microscopic pattern of growth in the case of the telangiectatic variety. In most instances, a spindle cell malignant stroma is seen that may imitate fibrosarcoma, but focal production of osteoid by tumor cells is pathognomonic. Many chondrosarcomas that show secondary ossification or metaplastic bone formation may be wrongly classified as osteogenic sarcoma; this has important prognostic significance since patients with chondrosarcomas have a much more favorable survival rate. Although no definite or consistent differences in survival are noticed between the various types, there is some tendency suggesting a poorer prognosis in patients with osteoblastic osteogenic sarcoma. The histological differential diagnosis includes chondrosarcoma, fibrosarcoma, malignant fibrous histiocytoma, and a rapidly growing osteoblastoma.

Osteogenic sarcomas of the skull are noted to have a poor prognosis compared to extremity lesions.[9] Occasional long-term survivors have been reported following radical surgery alone.[46] Nevertheless, this tumor has a marked tendency toward local recurrence and distant metastases. For this reason, aggressive chemotherapy along the lines used for osteo-

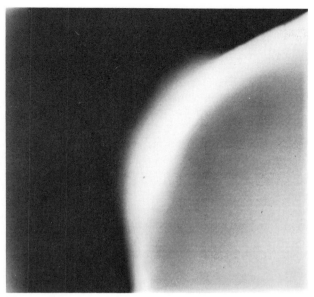

Figure 118-9 A tangential view of the skull showing an osteogenic sarcoma involving both tables with irregular new bone formation.

sarcoma of the extremity is advocated. If a rapidly growing mass in the skull is suspected of being an osteogenic sarcoma by its clinical and radiographic features, incisional biopsy is suggested to establish a diagnosis. Following this, several cycles of chemotherapy using high-dose methotrexate may allow both marked regression in size of the original tumor

and treatment of systemic micrometastases while definitive surgery is being contemplated.[36] Wide resection of the scalp, underlying muscles, and periosteum and resection of the cranium wide of the primary tumor is necessary. Such extensive procedures may require close collaboration with a plastic surgeon. Aggressive combined-modality therapy has resulted in several long-term survivors in our experience. Although radiation therapy has been advocated for the treatment of incompletely resected lesions, there is little evidence in the literature to suggest that this tumor is responsive to radiation in the dosages currently employed.

Chondroma

This is a benign tumor composed of mature hyaline cartilage. When a cartilaginous tumor arises in the peripheral skeleton, it is classified according to its relationship to the cortex of a long bone. If it is located within the medullary cavity it is termed an enchondroma. It is most commonly found in the small bones of the hands and feet and may be present in an asymptomatic form in about 1 percent of the general population. Ollier's disease is multiple enchondromatosis. A rare form of cartilage-forming tumor is the juxtacortical periosteal chondroma, which is located between the periosteum and cortex, causing erosion of the latter. When the tumor grows outward from the cortex and presents as a cartilage-capped bony protrusion on the external surface of the bone, the term osteochondroma is applied. This variety accounts for 10 to 15 percent of all primary

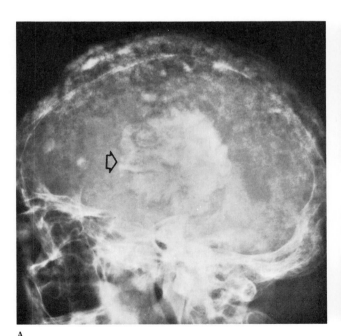

A

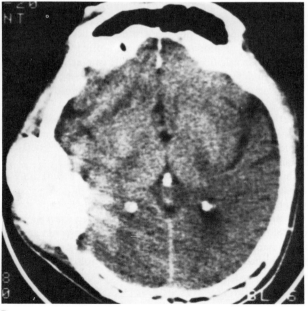

B

Figure 118-10 *A.* The sudden appearance of a rapidly growing skull mass in a patient with Paget's disease is classic for osteogenic sarcoma (*arrow*). *B.* A contrast-enhanced CT scan of an osteogenic sarcoma shows both intracranial extension and invasion of the soft tissues of the scalp. For complete surgical excision, wide resection of the scalp, skull, and dura with adequate margins is necessary.

bone tumors. The relevance of this classification for cartilage-forming tumors which occur in the bones of the skull is not clear. Consequently, these tumors will be considered here simply as chondromas.

Chondromas are rare, comprising roughly 0.1 to 0.2 percent of the intracranial tumors in several large series, and are most common in the second through fifth decades, with a female predominance.[23] They arise in bones formed by enchondral ossification. Since the bones of the vault are formed by membranous ossification, these tumors are rarely found there, although chondromas have been reported in a number of diverse locations including the vault, choroid plexus, dura, arachnoid, and brain. More common sites for these tumors are the skull base and the paranasal sinuses.

Chondromas are painless, slow-growing tumors that produce symptoms and signs dependent on their location. Those arising in the sinuses can produce nasal obstruction, exophthalmos, and pituitary or chiasmal symptoms. Chondromas that arise at the basilar synchondroses are extradural and the majority lie in the parasellar area or in the middle cranial fossa. More rarely they occur below the tentorium in the cerebellopontine angle in the region of the petro-occipital synchondrosis. Primary sellar chondromas have also been reported.[14]

These tumors are primarily lucent, with bone destruction at the base as well as avascularity on angiography. More than half of these tumors will have some degree of intralesional calcification ranging from granular to massive, which is helpful in distinguishing them from metastases or nasopharyngeal carcinoma. Chondromas which occur in the cerebellopontine angle apparently have much less tendency to calcify, whereas those arising in the parasellar area are more likely to be calcified.[30] Radiological differentiation between clivus chordoma and clivus chondroma may be impossible. When the tumor is in the suprasellar region, confusion with a craniopharyngioma is possible. Although the radiological appearances of craniopharyngioma more often include peripheral linear calcification outlining the tumor, it can present with nodular calcification very similar to that of a chondroma. Associated bone destruction, if widespread, would favor the diagnosis of chondroma.

Histologically, there are lobules of hyaline cartilage, which usually contain only one cell per lacuna. Areas of myxoid degeneration may be present. Calcification and ossification take place near blood vessels.

Chondromas are slow-growing, benign tumors with only a small risk of malignant transformation in the absence of multiple enchondromatosis. Krayenbühl and Yasargil surveyed the literature in 1975 and recommended surgical removal of the tumors since even subtotal excision could ameliorate symptoms for several years. They thought that radiation therapy had no place in the treatment of these tumors.[23]

Ollier's Disease (Multiple Enchondromatosis)

Multiple enchondromas occur most commonly in the phalanges and metacarpals. Intracranial involvement has also been reported.[4,18] This syndrome occurs sporadically with no inheritance pattern, but in contrast to the solitary form, is often reported as more common in males. The histology of these tumors is similar to that of the solitary enchondroma, but it is more cellular, the nuclei of the chondrocytes are slightly larger, more binucleate forms are seen, and the cartilage matrix appears less calcified. The significance of this entity is that the risk of malignant transformation is believed to be higher, and is estimated at 50 percent by Jaffe, although Huvos believes this figure is too high.[17]

Maffucci's Syndrome

This is similar to Ollier's disease with the additional findings of multiple hemangiomas. These may be 5 cm or more in diameter; are soft, lobulated or nodular; are located in the deeper layers of the skin or subcutaneous tissue; and may give a bluish discoloration to the skin. These lesions are painless. Intracranial involvement has been reported.[18] Huvos believes that the risk of malignant transformation is higher than with Ollier's disease, and rates it at approximately 15 percent.[17]

Chondroblastoma

Chondroblastoma is a primary benign bone tumor of immature cartilage cell derivation with preferential localization in the epiphyses of long bones. Its synonyms are calcifying giant cell tumor and Codman's tumor. These tumors are rare, comprising less than 1 percent of all bone tumors. They are most common in males in the second decade. Location in the skull is very rare.[8]

Symptoms and signs are usually nonspecific. These tumors may be painful; they may produce neurological signs depending on location.

Chondroblastomas are characterized by well-demarcated osteolytic areas, often with foci of mottled calcification. These tumors may expand the cortex of the bone, causing a periosteal "eggshell" bone production. Periosteal reaction is usually a feature only of malignant tumors. The presence of intralesional calcification rules out a diagnosis of giant cell tumor. However, if the calcification is pronounced, then the lesion is more likely to be a chondroma or chondrosarcoma. The bone scan may be positive. In those chondroblastomas with an associated component of aneurysmal bone cyst, the angiogram may also be positive.

Chondroblastomas are composed of uniform, polyhedral, closely packed cells which may sometimes be difficult to distinguish from plasma cells. Pericellular lattice-like calcification is characteristic. As calcification builds up, necrosis results. Multinuclear giant cells are found either singly or in small collections, especially around areas of hemorrhage and necrosis, but are not as numerous or evenly dispersed, and are not located in viable portions of the lesion as they are in giant cell tumors. Large patches of collagenous hyaline or chondroid tissue may replace the necrotic tissue. In about one-quarter of cases, there are associated areas which display the microscopic features of aneurysmal bone cyst engrafted onto the basic pattern of chondroblastoma.

In a series from our institution, the recurrence rate for

chondroblastomas was 20 percent, whereas it was 100 percent for those tumors with an aneurysmal bone cyst component.[17] The tumor is best treated by en bloc resection when possible, and in the peripheral skeleton curettage followed by liquid nitrogen cryotherapy has reduced the recurrence rate. These tumors are thought to be radiosensitive, but there is a risk of malignant transformation following radiation therapy.[17]

Chondromyxoid Fibroma

This is a benign tumor of bone characterized by chondroid and myxoid differentiation and growth in a lobular pattern. Its synonyms include myxoma, fibromyxoma, myxofibroma, chondromyxoma, and fibromyxochondroma.

Chondromyxoid fibroma is rare, and is most commonly found in the second decade, usually in a long bone of the lower extremities. It is often painful. Occurrence in the skull has been reported.[19,35]

This is a radiolucent lesion with sharp margins and a sclerotic rim. Intralesional calcifications are rarely seen on x-ray studies.

The histological appearance of a chondromyxoid fibroma is characterized by great variability, with a predominance of myxomatous fields in some areas and chondroid zones of differentiation in others. There is sometimes sharp demarcation into a lobular arrangement. Giant cells may be seen. Unlike chondroblastomas, calcification is rare.

Myxoma of the facial skeleton is considered a separate entity by Huvos.[17] It is found in the mandible and maxilla of young adults and is locally aggressive, with a 25 percent recurrence rate.

Chondromyxoid fibroma is generally benign and nonaggressive, although malignant transformation has been reported. Subtotal excision results in a 10 to 15 percent recurrence rate. The efficacy of radiation therapy is not certain.

Chondrosarcoma

Chondrosarcoma is a malignant tumor in which the neoplastic tissue is fully developed cartilage. Secondary myxoid changes, calcification, and ossification may be present.

Chondrosarcomas comprise 17 to 22 percent of primary bone tumors, of which approximately 9.4 percent arise from the craniofacial bones.[17] Chondrosarcoma may arise de novo in normal bone, or result from sarcomatous changes in a pre-existing cartilaginous tumor. Secondary malignant changes have been described in Ollier's disease (multiple enchondromatosis), multiple hereditary exostoses, chondromyxoid fibroma, and chondroblastoma. Chondrosarcoma has also been reported in Maffucci's syndrome, which is characterized by subcutaneous cavernous hemangiomas, phlebectasia, and a dyschondroplasia identical with Ollier's disease.[12] This syndrome is characterized by disturbance in the formation of bone and cartilage, particularly at the growing ends of the bone. Most lesions reported in the skull arise in the base, because these bones are preformed in carti-

lage.[3] Preferential sites include the parasellar and retrosellar areas, cerebellopontine angle, and paranasal sinuses. The average age at presentation is 32 years, with two-thirds of patients being male.

A combination of lytic and sclerotic changes may be present on plain radiography. Stippled calcification is commonly seen. Distinguishing between benign chondromas and chondrosarcomas may be difficult, even using computed tomography. Especially when the tumor is large, it is important to remember that, in the craniofacial bones, malignant cartilaginous lesions outnumber benign lesions by two to one.[17]

Chondrosarcomas are bluish-white, pearly, translucent lesions that are frequently lobulated. Areas of calcification and ossification are represented by yellow or white areas of speckling. A mucoid, slimy character is seen when secondary myxomatous changes supervene. Slowly growing lesions elicit more reactive new bone formation. The histological appearance has to be correlated with both the clinical and radiographic features in arriving at a diagnosis of a benign versus a malignant tumor. Age is a major consideration since chondrosarcomas are very uncommon in patients less than 20 years old. Furthermore, large lesions more than 6 to 10 cm in diameter are almost invariably malignant despite an innocent-looking histology. In addition, two tumors with identical features may behave entirely differently. The criteria for malignancy include the presence of an increased number of cartilage cells having plump nuclei, more than occasional binucleated cells, and mononuclear or multinucleated giant cartilage cells. Two or more cells within a cartilage lacuna in more than an occasional microscopic field characterizes a low-grade chondrosarcoma. The presence of myxomatous changes and cystic degeneration correlates well with lower-grade lesions, whereas the microscopic absence of cartilage lobules and the presence of spindle-cell sarcomatous areas are characteristic of high-grade variants. Occasional ossification of the cartilage matrix may cause confusion with osteogenic sarcoma. The histological grading into grades 1 to 3 has some prognostic importance because low-grade lesions rarely metastasize, whereas more than 70 percent of the high-grade lesions are reported to have metastases.[17] In the skull, chondrosarcoma must be distinguished from chondroblastic osteogenic sarcoma. This malignant cartilage tumor should not show direct osteoid or bone production by the sarcomatous stroma; careful examination of the entire specimen may be necessary. As a practical guide, it is important to remember that primary chondrosarcomas in children and adolescents are extremely rare. On occasion, an aggressive chondromyxofibroma may be mistaken for a chondrosarcoma. In addition, large, locally aggressive, benign mixed tumors of the salivary glands with prominent cartilaginous components may cause diagnostic difficulty if only a small biopsy is examined. The cartilage component in a benign mixed salivary gland tumor closely resembles well-differentiated hyaline cartilage with foci of myxochondroid growth streaks.

Since the majority of chondrosarcomas arise from the base of the skull, complete surgical resection presents a formidable challenge. Many of these lesions may involve the sinuses and may require a combined craniofacial approach for tumors involving the anterior cranial fossa or the temporal bone. Curative resections may not always be possible, but debulking operations may be useful in palliation. There is very little evidence to suggest that radiotherapy or chemotherapy is useful in these tumors.

Mesenchymal Chondrosarcoma

A recently described variant of chondrosarcoma is the mesenchymal chondrosarcoma. This tumor is a distinct clinicopathological entity which differs from the usual chondrosarcoma by its generally unfavorable outcome, its predilection for unusual sites, and its frequent origin in soft tissues. More than 100 cases have been reported in the world literature, and the central nervous system represents the second most common site of origin. These lesions have been reported to arise from the calvarial bone, dura, orbit, and the base of the skull (Figs. 118-11, 118-12). The majority of patients are in the second and third decades of life, with an age range from 5 to 70 years. A slight female predilection is noted. Histologically, the tumor is characterized by a biphasic population, with sheets of undifferentiated small round cells, similar to those of Ewing's sarcoma, and lobules of cartilage showing the general characteristic features of chondrosarcoma. In some areas, the pattern of the tumor may indicate a hemangiopericytoma. Areas of calcification or ossification may be present.

On angiography, the presence of numerous arteriovenous shunts may simulate an arteriovenous malformation. The treatment of this tumor is primarily surgical. The tumor does not respond to radiation therapy; both local re-

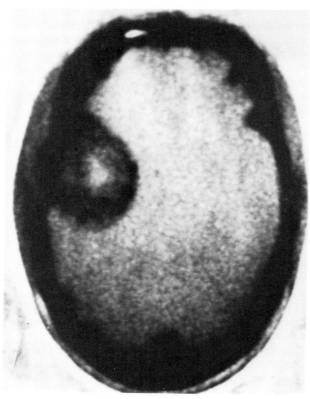

Figure 118-12 A CT scan of a mesenchymal chondrosarcoma arising from the temporal bone, with intracranial extension. Following subtotal excision, the tumor responded to combination chemotherapy.

currences and distant metastases have been reported following incomplete excision. More recently, an encouraging response to combination chemotherapy was observed in two patients treated at this institution.

Intradiploic Meningioma

Intradiploic meningiomas are tumors of arachnoid origin, and present as either an osteolytic or osteoblastic skull defect. They are very rare and occur at all ages; a case was reported in a 7-month-old infant.[11] No particular site within the vault is favored. These lesions may cause nonspecific headache or local tenderness.

Intradiploic meningioma is usually associated with an osteoblastic reaction, and can be mistaken for an osteoma or a solitary osteoblastic metastasis. More rarely, a purely osteolytic defect can be seen on skull films, usually without a sclerotic rim.[11,29,31] Brain scans may be negative, but bone scanning using ^{99m}Tc diphosphonate is often positive.[29] The radiological differential diagnosis of a lytic skull defect is discussed in the introduction.

Although their histology is typical for meningioma, it is suggested in the literature that purely lytic meningiomas are

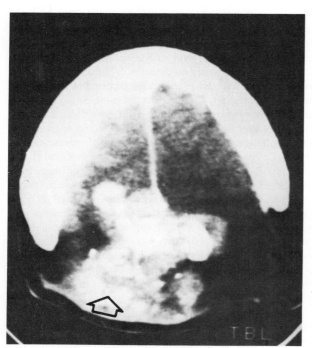

Figure 118-11 A CT scan of a mesenchymal chondrosarcoma involving the occipital bone, dura, and falx. Note the irregular, stippled calcifications (*arrow*).

more aggressive than other meningiomas. Treatment is by en bloc resection with cranioplasty if indicated.

Fibrosarcoma

This is a malignant tumor characterized by a varying amount of collagen production and lacking any tendency to produce tumor bone, osteoid, or cartilage, either in its primary site or in its metastases. Fibrosarcomas account for less than 5 percent of malignant bone tumors. In a series of 130 cases reviewed by Huvos, only two lesions were located in the skull.[17] These lesions arise de novo, or may be secondary to fibrous dysplasia, Paget's disease, bone infarcts, or osteomyelitis. Radiation-induced tumors may be predominantly fibroblastic. A wide range of age groups between 4 and 83 years may be affected, with an average age of 38 years. The sex distribution is approximately equal. Depending on the precise site of origin, these tumors are classified as parosteal or medullary types, with the former having the better prognosis.

Most patients present with a mass, and pain may be noticed if the cortex and medullary cavity are involved. Often, the precise site of origin from scalp or bone may be impossible to determine. Intracranial extension is unusual.

These tumors usually present as a lytic lesion in the skull with little periosteal reaction. A computed tomographic scan in the coronal plane is helpful in delineating the actual extent of tumor (Fig. 118-13).

Grossly, fibrosarcomas are grayish white and rubbery, with areas of hemorrhagic necrosis in larger lesions. On histological examination, the low-grade well-differentiated tumor exhibits ample intercellular collagen with a distinctive herringbone pattern. Mitoses are rare. Increased mitoses and pleomorphism usually suggest a higher-grade malignancy. Silver impregnation stains usually demonstrate a close relationship between individual tumor cells and the fine reticulum. In the presence of numerous giant cells, malignant fibrous histiocytoma is an important consideration. Other entities which may mimic fibrosarcoma are fibroblastic osteogenic sarcoma, in which histochemical examination for alkaline phosphatase may be helpful in the differential diagnosis, and, occasionally, the spindle cell variant of renal cell carcinoma, which may present as a solitary skeletal lesion.

Wide excision of the scalp, skull, and dura is advocated; radiation therapy is not very effective in this tumor. Some chemotherapeutic agents used in the treatment of other soft tissue sarcomas may have a role in this neoplasm. Only a few cases have been reported in the skull, and the major cause of treatment failure in these patients was local recurrence.[26]

Nonossifying Fibroma

Nonossifying fibroma appears as a well-demarcated lytic lesion composed of benign fibrous tissue. Its synonyms are metaphyseal fibrous cortical defect, healing variant of giant

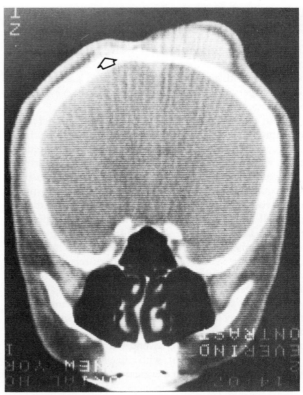

Figure 118-13 A coronal CT scan showing a fibrosarcoma involving the scalp and skull, with a satellite nodule (*arrow*).

cell tumor, and solitary xanthoma or xanthogranuloma of bone.

Fibrous cortical defects are seen in 30 to 40 percent of normal children between 4 and 8 years of age as lucencies in the cortex of the metaphysis of long bones, and are asymptomatic. Most of these heal spontaneously. When the lesion is larger, is actively growing, and involves the medullary cavity of a long bone, the term *nonossifying fibroma* is used. Only rarely has it been reported in the cranial vault.[1]

The great majority are asymptomatic, although pathological fracture through the lesion can occur. In the skull it is likely to present as a painless swelling.

In long bones the lesion is radiolucent, with sclerotic margins and interior bony trabeculae giving the appearance of soap bubbles or a bunch of grapes. In the skull the surrounding sclerosis suggests an epidermoid or dermoid cyst.

Spindly fibroblastic cells are arranged in matted whorls in a storiform pattern (*storea* means rope mat or straw mat in Latin). Scattered giant cells and lipid-laden cells of the xanthoma variety are present. Some of these lesions are probably synonymous with "benign" fibrous histiocytoma, although the latter lesions occur in atypical locations in older age groups, and may be more aggressive. The histological appearance is similar to that of the stromal tissue of both ossifying fibroma and fibrous dysplasia, but there is no bone formation in nonossifying fibroma.

These are benign tumors and can be cured by curettage or block excision.

Giant Cell Tumor

Giant cell tumor of bone is an aggressive lesion characterized by well-vascularized tissue composed of plump, spindly, or ovoid cells with numerous multinucleated giant cells uniformly dispersed throughout the tumor tissue. A synonym is osteoclastoma.

Giant cell tumor accounts for approximately 5 percent of all primary bone tumors and occurs most commonly in the third and fourth decades. There is a slight female predominance with benign forms, whereas the malignant variety is more common in males. More than 75 percent are situated at or near the articular end of a long tubular bone. The spine is a relatively common site of involvement, with 8 percent of giant cell tumors involving either the anterior or posterior elements. Location in the skull is infrequent, with the temporal and sphenoid bones being the preferred sites.[2,5,15,16,32] Location in the sellar region has also been reported.[50] Most cases of giant cell tumor of the calvaria present as complications of Paget's disease.

Giant cell tumor presents as an enlarging mass which may or may not be tender. Specific neurological signs depend upon its location. The duration of symptoms may range from a few weeks to several years.

The lesion is radiolucent, with expansion of the overlying cortex. There is usually no marginal sclerosis. There may be a multilocular or cystic component, especially if there is a coexisting region of aneurysmal bone cyst. In those cases the angiogram will be positive. Bone scanning is routinely positive. CT scans show an enhancing mass with erosion and expansion of bone (Fig. 118-14).

Histologically, there are large numbers of giant cells

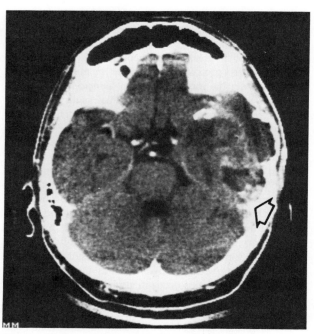

Figure 118-14 A CT scan with contrast enhancement, showing a giant cell tumor of the temporal bone with significant extension into the middle cranial fossa (*arrow*). (From Epstein et al.[15])

evenly dispersed among inconspicuous mononuclear stromal cells with indistinct cellular outlines. An attempt can be made to grade these tumors as follows: grade I lesions are dominated by multinucleated giant cells; grade II lesions are characterized by a diminished number of giant cells, by stromal cells that are spindly and elongated, and by a moderate number of mitotic figures; grade III tumors have only sparse giant cells with large fields of dense collagenous scarring and a stroma characteristic of a sarcoma. There are many bone tumors which feature giant cells (Table 118-2), but in giant cell tumor the giant cells are evenly distributed throughout the viable portions of the lesion.

The biological behavior of giant cell tumors is unpredictable despite histological grading.[17] About 20 percent of the histologically benign lesions invade through the bony cortex and extend into adjacent soft tissues. Overall, about 30 percent recur locally within 2 years following curettage, and close to half recur within 5 years. In the peripheral skeleton, the use of liquid nitrogen cryotherapy has decreased the recurrence rate to about 12 percent.[17] Radiation therapy is palliative in some cases, but there is a substantial risk of malignant transformation.

Giant Cell "Reparative" Granuloma

This lesion can be histologically indistinguishable from giant cell tumor. The clinical significance is that the prognosis of these lesions is favorable. It occurs in a younger age group, with three-fourths of the patients under 30. Often there is history of trauma. This lesion is more frequent in females, and involves the mandible more often than the maxilla. Treatment is by enucleation or curettage, with an approximate 15 percent recurrence rate.

Brown Tumor of Hyperparathyroidism

Osteitis fibrosa can be due to primary, ectopic, or secondary hyperparathyroidism. Severe bone disease is usually found either with parathyroid carcinoma, or secondary to chronic renal failure. Cysts of osteitis fibrosa are of two kinds: true cysts, which consist of unusually large resorptive cavities filled with fluid; and pseudocysts, which consist of masses of osteoclasts and fibrous tissue, called the brown tumor because of its gross appearance. Histological examination reveals that the giant cells are smaller than those found in giant cell tumor, and tend to be clumped together, especially about regions of hemorrhage, rather than evenly spread out. There is also evidence of osseous metaplasia. The diagnosis can be confirmed by documenting an elevated serum calcium level. Treatment is directed toward the underlying cause of hyperparathyroidism, with resolution of the brown tumor expected to follow within months (Fig. 118-15).

Malignant Fibrous Histiocytoma

This is a malignant pleomorphic mesenchymal tumor which consists of a bicellular population of fibroblasts and histiocytes in varying proportions. Most of these tumors arise from soft tissues, but occasionally the primary site may be

TABLE 118-2 Differential Diagnosis of Giant Cell Lesions of the Skull

Lesion	Most Common Age Group	Radiological Appearance	Sex (M:F) Distribution	Microscopic Features	
				Giant Cells	**Stromal Cells**
Giant cell tumor	3rd and 4th decades	Irregular expanded radiolucency	M<F	Abundant number uniformly distributed	Plump and polyhedral with abundant cytoplasm
Nonossifying fibroma	1st decade	Oval defects	2:1	Focal in distribution; small with few nuclei	Slender and spindly with little cytoplasm
Aneurysmal bone cyst	1st and 2nd decades	Irregular "soap bubble" appearance	M=F	Focal around vascular channels	Large vascular channels; slender to plump cells with hemosiderin granules
Brown tumor of hyperparathyroidism	Any age	Absent lamina dura of teeth	M=F	Focal around hemosiderin pigment	Fibrous stroma with slender cells
Chondroblastoma	2nd decade	Radiolucency with spotty opacities	M>F	Few and focal	Large, plump, and round with pericellular calcifications
Fibrous dysplasia	1st and 2nd decades	"Ground glass" appearance	M>F	Few and focal	Woven bone and fibrous tissue
Ossifying fibroma	2nd and 3rd decades	Radiopaque	M<F	Few and focal	Lamellar bony trabeculae in fibrous tissue
Osteogenic sarcoma	2nd and 3rd decades	Radiolucent	M>F	Focal distribution	Malignant spindle cells with direct osteoid formation
Chondromyxoid fibroma	2nd and 3rd decades	Eccentric with expanded cortex	M<F	Focal distribution	Chondroid and myxoid components
Osteoblastoma	2nd and 3rd decades	Radiolucent or dense	2:1	Focal distribution	Abundant osteoblasts between osteoid trabeculae

SOURCE: Modified from Huvos.[17]

bone. Dahlin noted that only 4 of 35 cases from bone arose in the calvaria.[13] This tumor may also be induced by radiation therapy. The average age of patients is approximately 45 years with an age range from 7 to 57 years. A slight male predominance is noted.

Most patients present with a mass which may or may not be painful. Intracranial extension of a temporal bone tumor was recently reported.[10]

Radiographically, these tumors usually present as poorly circumscribed lytic lesions, with occasional areas of calcification. The presence of a periosteal reaction may cause confusion with osteogenic sarcoma or fibrosarcoma of bone (Fig. 118-16, and 118-17).

Malignant fibrous histiocytomas are extremely pleomorphic and exhibit a definite storiform pattern of growth, with spindle cells appearing in a pinwheel configuration. They are predominantly fibrous, with occasional tumor giant cells scattered throughout. Often the histiocytic components incorporate lipid, hemosiderin, or erythrocytes, thereby manifesting phagocytic activity. On occasion, numerous mitotic figures may be seen, and the overall appearance may resemble a highly anaplastic sarcoma. The level of mitotic activity in these tumors may not correlate well with the biological behavior of this tumor.[6] Both local recurrences and systemic metastases have been noted. The histological differential diagnoses includes malignant giant cell tumor, osteogenic sarcoma, histiocytic lymphoma, and metastatic carcinoma.

Wide surgical excision is the treatment of choice. This tumor has a variable response to radiation therapy, and may respond to systemic chemotherapy.

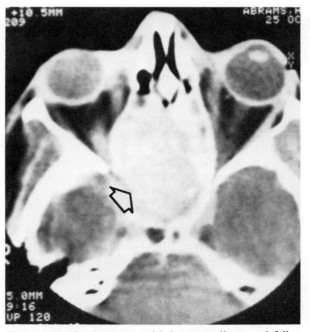

Figure 118-15 A patient with long-standing renal failure and known severe secondary hyperparathyroidism who had refused parathyroidectomy. A previous transnasal biopsy provided the diagnosis of brown tumor. The CT scan shows an expansile tumor of the ethmoid and sphenoid sinuses with destruction of the anteromedial border of the right middle cranial fossa (*arrow*).

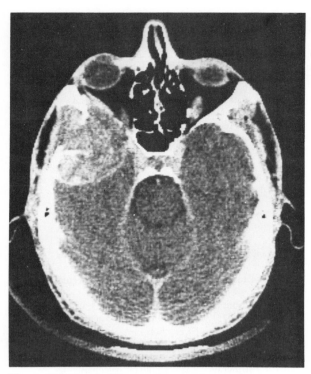

Figure 118-16 A CT scan shows a destructive tumor of the temporal bone with extradural extension along the floor of the middle cranial fossa. The pathological diagnosis was malignant fibrous histiocytoma.

sional bone remnants are visualized in 80 percent of hemangiomas, but in only 20 percent of epidermoids and 10 percent of histiocytomas. About half of the hemangiomas show the well-known honeycomb or trabecular pattern, but only 10 to 15 percent reveal classic striations of the sunburst variety with tangential soft tissue technique roentgenograms.[45] When present, the sunburst pattern of hemangiomas appears to radiate from a central point, while that observed with some meningiomas has spicules which are arranged parallel to each other. Futhermore, meningiomas often have associated enlarged vascular markings in the skull, a finding which is not usually present with hemangiomas. Angiography will show a tumor blush in about one-half of the cases, whereas direct puncture of the lesion for injection of contrast will give visualization of the tumor in all cases.[21]

Hemangiomas are classified according to the size of the vascular channels, with capillary hemangiomas being rare in the skull. The blood vessels are usually similar to those of a cavernous angioma, thin-walled, without muscle or elastic tissue. This tumor is distinguished from the aneurysmal bone cyst since the latter does not have radiating bone spicules and has more soft tissue osteoid, granulation tissue, and giant cells.

Hemangiomas are benign lesions totally cured by en bloc resection. Occasionally external carotid ligation will be necessary to minimize blood loss, especially for the rare globular hemangioma found at the base of the skull.[37] In those tumors which cannot be completely resected, radiation therapy has been recommended. However, this mode of treatment has been found ineffective by some.[21]

Hemangioma

This is a benign lesion of bone composed of either capillary or cavernous vascular channels. Hemangiomas comprise 0.7 percent of neoplasms of bone. The most common site is the vertebral column, with the cranial vault the second most favored location.[53] Hemangiomas were the second most frequent primary calvarial neoplasm (after osteoma) in two large series.[20,49] One large series of calvarial hemangiomas showed a peak incidence in the second to fourth decades, with most located in the parietal bone and with a female predominance.[53] Another series showed a peak incidence in the first and second decades, the most common location being the frontal bone and a male predominance.[21]

Usually these neoplasms present as a swelling which is tender to palpation. Headache, often nonspecific, is present in perhaps one-quarter of patients. Occasionally, these lesions are completely asymptomatic and are discovered incidentally on skull films.

Calvarial hemangiomas occur in two forms: (1) the very rare globular variety, which arises from the skull base on a broad stalk, and acts like a space-occupying lesion,[37] and, (2) the more common sessile type, which causes expansion of the diploe of the vault. The sessile type is characterized by a well-defined lytic lesion on plain skull films (Figs. 118-18, 118-19). Peripheral sclerosis occurs in one-third, in contrast to epidermoid cysts where it is almost always seen. Intrale-

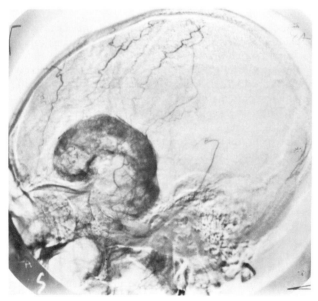

Figure 118-17 A subtraction angiogram that reveals a highly vascular malignant fibrous histiocytoma involving the temporal bone with extradural extension. (From Chitale et al.[10])

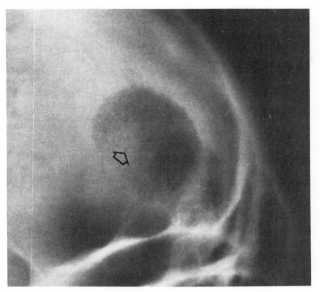

Figure 118-18 A skull film showing a well-demarcated, partially honeycombed (*arrow*) lytic lesion without significant marginal sclerosis. This appearance is classic for hemangioma.

Aneurysmal Bone Cyst

Aneurysmal bone cyst is a benign lesion composed of large vascular spaces separated by trabeculae of connective tissue and bone. Aneurysmal bone cyst may occur by itself, or in association with other tumors, or after trauma.

This rare tumor tends to occur in the second and third decades with equal sex distribution. In approximately 50 percent of the cases, aneurysmal bone cysts are found near one end of the shaft of a long bone, and in 25 percent of the cases they are associated with vertebrae. Location in the skull accounts for about 5 percent of the cases; a recent review of the literature described 22 cases of aneurysmal bone cyst of the skull.[25] The occipital bone was the most common site in this series, although all bones of the vault are susceptible.

Usually these tumors present as a painful swelling which is tender to palpation. Focal neurological signs were present in 5 of 13 cases, and signs of increased intracranial pressure were found in 4 of 13 cases. The duration of symptoms is usually about 6 months.[25]

An aneurysmal bone cyst is classically a lytic lesion that arises in the diploe and usually expands both the inner and outer table, which are quite thinned but usually intact. CT scans may show a multilocular lesion with regions of high and low density, with the regions of high density showing enhancement with contrast. In four of seven cases studied with angiography, the lesion was completely avascular.[25]

After opening through the thin wall of bone, the surgeon is confronted by a hole containing fluid blood. The interior is honeycombed with meager amounts of stringy tissue. Microscopically, this tissue contains delicate thin-walled capillaries or distorted vascular spaces that are lined by en-dothelial-like cells, but do not have muscular coats. Between and around some of the larger vascular spaces are trabeculae of connective tissue and bone. Giant cells may be seen, especially around areas of hemorrhage. Aneurysmal bone cyst may coexist with other bone tumors, so it is important that the pathologist be given as much specimen as possible to examine. In a review of 57 cases, the most commonly associated lesions were unicameral bone cyst in 18, giant cell tumor in 14, and osteosarcoma in 12. Other associated lesions were nonossifying fibroma, osteoblastoma, hemangioendothelioma, and hemangioma. Five cases of aneurysmal bone cyst were reported to be the direct result of bone trauma which had occurred from 3 weeks to 5 months previously. Other underlying lesions reported in the literature include chondroblastoma, fibrous dysplasia, and fibromyxoma.[24]

The recurrence rate in a series of 35 extracranial aneurysmal bone cysts was 50 percent following subtotal resection.[17] Complete removal can usually be achieved by en bloc resection when the lesion is located in the cranial vault, and recurrence is rare if the dura is not involved. If the lesion is highly vascular on angiography, preoperative embolization or ligation of the external carotid can be considered.

Miscellaneous Tumors

On occasion, the skull may be a primary site for a number of extremely rare malignancies. These include angiosarcoma, hemangiopericytoma, Ewing's tumor, non-Hodgkin's lymphoma, and many others.

Angiosarcoma, also known as malignant hemangioendothelioma, is characterized by the formation of irregular anastomosing vascular channels, which are lined by atypical anaplastic endothelial cells. In a review of malignant vascular tumors at our institution, 1 of 39 cases involved the calvaria.[17] These tumors are purely osteolytic, and angiography will reveal abnormal tumor vessels, although the degree of

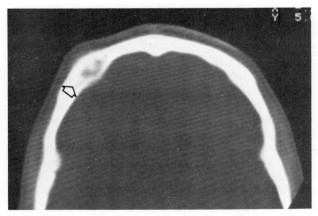

Figure 118-19 A CT scan with a skeletal window setting reveals the smooth expansion of both the inner and outer tables. This suggests a primary benign intradiploic lesion. At operation a hemangioma was found. (Courtesy of Dr. Michael Lavyne.)

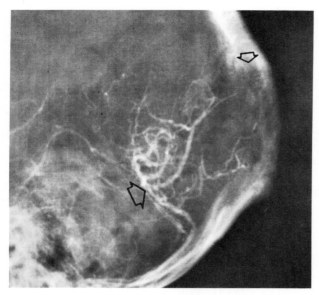

Figure 118-20 Angiogram of a malignant occipital bone tumor (*small arrow*) showing intracranial extension and neovascularity (*large arrow*). At operation a primary angiosarcoma of the occipital bone was resected.

vascularity is variable (Fig. 118-20). The histological differential diagnoses include aneurysmal bone cyst, telangiectatic osteogenic sarcoma, and metastatic renal carcinoma. This condition may on occasion present with multifocal bone involvement, which, oddly enough, seems to carry a better prognosis. Complete resection is the treatment goal, but radiation therapy may be beneficial when surgical excision is impossible.

Ewing's sarcoma is characterized by uniform, densely packed small cells, with round nuclei, but without distinct cytoplasmic borders or prominent nucleoli. It comprises 10 to 15 percent of primary malignant bone tumors, and is extremely rare in blacks, or in patients over 30 years of age. Due to extremely rapid growth, many such tumors present with local pain and fever and an increased sedimentation rate, suggesting an infectious process. The histological finding of a small, round cell malignancy always poses diagnostic problems because the differential diagnosis includes Ewing's sarcoma, non-Hodgkin's lymphoma, metastatic neuroblastoma, and embryonal rhabdomyosarcoma. Special stains, including those for glycogen, electron microscopy, and tissue markers, may be helpful in providing a definitive diagnosis. Although the majority of these neoplasms are considered radiosensitive, there is currently a great deal of interest in the use of aggressive chemotherapy prior to radiation. Although radiation therapy is still considered important in local control, surgery may be needed for persistent residual or recurrent disease. Many of these new concepts in treatment are somewhat controversial, and still have to stand the test of time. Nevertheless, whenever confronted with an aggressively growing skull lesion, diagnosis by incisional biopsy is suggested to rule out tumors that might respond primarily to other treatment modalities such as chemotherapy or radiation therapy.

References

1. Ando S, Tsuchida T, Hayakawa I: Diploic fibroma of the skull. Surg Neurol 10:108–109, 1978.
2. Arseni S, Horvath L, Maretsis M, Carp N: Giant cell tumors of the calvaria. J Neurosurg 42:535–540, 1975.
3. Bahr AL, Gayler BW: Cranial chondrosarcomas: Report on four cases and review of the literature. Radiology 124:151–156, 1977.
4. Bakdash H, Alksne JF, Rand RW: Osteochondroma of the base of the skull causing an isolated oculomotor nerve paralysis. J Neurosurg 31:230–233, 1969.
5. Bitoh S, Takimoto N, Nakagawa H, Namba J, Sakaki S, Gohma T: Giant cell tumor of the skull. Surg Neurol 9:185–188, 1978.
6. Blitzer A, Lawson W, Zak FG, Biller HF, Som ML: Clinical-pathological determinants in prognosis of fibrous histiocytomas of the head and neck. Laryngoscope 91:2053–2070, 1981.
7. Cancer Statistics, 1982. CA32:15–31, 1982.
8. Cares HL, Terplan KL: Chondroblastoma of the skull: Case report. J Neurosurg 35:614–618, 1971.
9. Caron AS, Hajdu SI, Strong EW: Osteogenic sarcoma of the facial and cranial bones: A review of forty-three cases. Am J Surg 122:719–725, 1971.
10. Chitale VS, Sundaresan N, Helson L, Huvos AG: Malignant fibrous histiocytoma of the temporal bone with intracranial extension. Acta Neurochir (Wien) 59:239–246, 1981.
11. Choux M, Gomez A, Choux R, Vigouroux RP: Diagnostic and therapeutic problems concerning tumors of the vault. Childs Brain 1:207–216, 1975.
12. Cook PL, Evans PG: Chondrosarcoma of the skull in Maffucci's syndrome. Br J Radiol 50:833–836, 1977.
13. Dahlin DC: *Bone Tumors: General Aspects and Data on 6221 Cases.* Springfield, Ill., Charles C Thomas, 1978.
14. de Divitiis E, Spaziante R, Cirillo S, Stella L, Donzelli R: Primary sellar chondromas. Surg Neurol 11:229–232, 1979.
15. Epstein N, Whelan M, Reed D, Aleksic S: Giant cell tumor of the skull: A report of two cases. Neurosurgery 11:263–267, 1982.
16. Geissinger JD, Siqueira EB, Ross ER: Giant cell tumors of the sphenoid bone. J Neurosurg 32:665–670, 1970.
17. Huvos AG: *Bone Tumors: Diagnosis, Treatment and Prognosis.* Philadelphia, Saunders, 1979.
18. Imagawa K, Hayashi M, Toda I, Asai A, Nomura T: Intracranial chondroma. Surg Neurol 8:268–272, 1977.
19. Inoue K, Sugiyama Y, Ishii R: Intrasellar fibromyxochondroma. Surg Neurol 10:167–170, 1978.
20. Jelsma F: *Primary Tumors of the Calvaria with Specific Consideration of the Clinical Problems.* Springfield, Illinois, Charles C Thomas, 1959.
21. Kirchhoff D, Eggert HR, Agnoli AL: Cavernous angiomas of the skull. Neurochirurgia 21:53–62, 1978.
22. Kosary IZ, Shacked I, Farine I: Use of surgical laser in the removal of an osteoma of the skull. Surg Neurol 8:151–153, 1977.
23. Krayenbühl H, Yasargil MG: Chondromas. Prog Neurol Surg 6:435–463, 1975.
24. Levy WM, Miller AS, Bonakdarpour A, Aegerter E: Aneurysmal bone cyst secondary to other osseous lesions: Report of 57 cases. Am J Clin Pathol 63:1–8, 1975.
25. Luccarelli G, Fornari M, Savoiardo M: Angiography and computerized tomography in the diagnosis of aneurysmal bone cyst of the skull. J Neurosurg 53:113–116, 1980.
26. Mansfield JB: Primary fibrosarcoma of the skull: Case report. J Neurosurg 47:785–787, 1977.
27. Matson DD: *Neurosurgery of Infancy and Childhood.* Springfield, Ill., Charles C Thomas, 1969.

28. McKenna RJ, Schwinn CP, Soong KY, Higinbotham NL: Sarcoma of the osteogenic series (osteosarcoma, fibrosarcoma, chondrosarcoma, parosteal osteogenic sarcoma, and sarcomata arising in abnormal bone): Analysis of 552 cases. J Bone Joint Surg [Am] 48A:1–26, 1966.

29. McWhorter JM, Ghatak NR, Kelly DL: Extracranial meningioma presenting as lytic skull lesion. Surg Neurol 5:223–224, 1976.

30. Minagi H, Newton TH: Cartilaginous tumors of the base of skull. AJR 105:308–313, 1969.

31. Pearl GS, Takei Y, Parent A, Boehm WM Jr: Primary intraosseous meningioma presenting as a solitary osteolytic skull lesion: Case report. Neurosurgery 4:269–270, 1979.

32. Pitkethly DT, Kempe LG: Giant cell tumors of the sphenoid: Report of 2 cases. J Neurosurg 30:301–304, 1969.

33. Prabhakar B, Reddy DR, Dayananda B, Rao GR: Osteoid osteoma of the skull. J Bone Joint Surg [Br] 54B:146–148, 1972.

34. Rawe SE, VanGilder JC: Surgical removal of orbital osteoma: Case report. J Neurosurg 44:233–236, 1976.

35. Richardson RR, Deshpande VS, Thelmo WL, Rothballer A: Chondromyxoma of the middle cranial fossa: Case report. Neurosurgery 8:707–711, 1981.

36. Rosen G, Caparros B, Huvos AG, Kosloff C, Nirenberg A, Cacavio A, Marcove RC, Lane JM, Mehta B, Urban C: Preoperative chemotherapy for osteogenic sarcoma: Selection of postoperative adjuvant chemotherapy based on the response of the primary tumor to preoperative chemotherapy. Cancer 49:1221–1230, 1982.

37. Schneider RC, Gabrielsen TO, Hicks SP: Calvarial hemangioma: The value of selective external carotid angiography in surgical excision of the lesion. Neurology 23:352–356, 1973.

38. Schwarz E: Ossifying fibromas of the face and skull. AJR 91:1012–1016, 1964.

39. Scott M, Peale AR, Croissant PD: Intracranial midline anterior fossae ossifying fibroma invading orbits, paranasal sinuses, and right maxillary antrum: Case report. J Neurosurg 34:827–831, 1971.

40. Seitz W, Olarte M, Antunes JL: Ossifying fibroma of the parietal bone. Neurosurgery 7:513–515, 1980.

41. Suit HO, Goitein M, Munzenrider J, Verhey L, Davis KR, Koehler A, Linggood R, Ojemann RG: Definitive radiation therapy for chordoma and chondrosarcoma of the base of the skull and cervical spine. J Neurosurg 56:377–385, 1982.

42. Sundaresan N, Huvos A, Rosen G: Computerized tomography in osteogenic sarcoma of the skull. In press.

43. Sundaresan N, Rosen G, Fortner J, Lane JH, Hilaris B: Preoperative chemotherapy for paraspinal sarcomas. J Neurosurg 58:446–450, 1983.

44. Terao H, Sato S, Kim S: Gardner's syndrome involving the skull, dura, and brain: Case report. J Neurosurg 44:638–641, 1976.

45. Thomas JE, Baker HL Jr: Assessment of roentgenographic lucencies of the skull: A systematic approach. Neurology 25:99–106, 1975.

46. Thompson JB, Patterson RH Jr, Parsons H: Sarcomas of the calvaria: Surgical experience with 14 patients. J Neurosurg 32:534–538, 1970.

47. Tomita T, Huvos AG, Shah J, Sundaresan N: Giant ossifying fibroma of the nasal cavity with intracranial extension. Acta Neurochir (Wien) 56:65–71, 1981.

48. Van Dellen JR: A mastoid osteoma causing intracranial complications: A case report. S Afr Med J 51:597–598, 1977.

49. Vandenberg HJ, Coley BL: Primary tumors of the cranial bones. Surg Gynecol Obstet 90:602–612, 1950.

50. Viale GL: Giant cell tumours of the sellar region. Acta Neurochir (Wien) 38:259–268, 1977.

51. Williams RN, Boop WC Jr: Benign osteoblastoma of the skull: Case report. J Neurosurg 41:769–772, 1974.

52. Winter PF, Johnson PM, Hilal SK, Feldman F: Scintigraphic detection of osteoid osteoma. Radiology 122:177–178, 1977.

53. Wyke BD: Primary hemangioma of the skull: A rare cranial tumor. AJR 61:302–316, 1949.

119

Craniofacial Resection for Advanced Head and Neck Cancers

James P. Neifeld
Harold F. Young

Cancers of the skin, soft tissues, and paranasal sinuses with involvement of the cranium are difficult to treat with local surgery and/or radiation therapy. Local recurrences are common, and bony erosion will eventually result in meningeal involvement. Massive hemorrhage or meningitis may then result in the patient's demise. In order to prevent these complications and to effect local disease control, a combined intracranial-extracranial (craniofacial) approach to these neoplasms is often appropriate.

The purpose of a combined craniofacial approach to these tumors is to allow tumor resection with a clear margin in all directions, while at the same time protecting the intracranial contents and minimizing the risks of hemorrhage or subsequent infection. Therefore, the optimal approach to these tumors requires the participation of a neurosurgeon, an oncologic surgeon, and, for reconstruction, a plastic surgeon. Postoperative rehabilitation is greatly facilitated by a prosthodontist.

Indications for Operation

Carcinomas

Paranasal Sinus

Cancers arising in the maxillary, ethmoid, sphenoid, or frontal sinuses are rarely diagnosed early due to their lack of early symptoms. Accordingly, they tend to grow to a large size with invasion of surrounding tissues before diagnosis. Symptoms include those of chronic sinusitis, with nasal "stuffiness," obstruction, and discharge being prominent. Epistaxis is frequent, especially in those cancers that arise in ethmoid air cells or those arising in the maxillary sinus with medial wall involvement. Pain is not usually a prominent symptom but, when present, may seem obscure in origin; its origin may be difficult to diagnose, even radiologically. Anosmia is a common symptom of cancers arising in the ethmoid air cells, but its onset is so gradual that it may only be noticed very late. Other symptoms also relate to the insidious growth of these tumors; proptosis and decreased vision or even blindness are frequent findings in patients with large maxillary sinus cancers which grow through the floor of the orbit to involve the orbital contents. When the tumor grows laterally to involve the pterygoid plate and pterygoid muscles, trismus may result. Lymph node metastases are rare, usually occurring only when the tumor has eroded through the skin or the palate; thus, prophylactic treatment of the cervical lymph nodes (by radiation or radical neck dissection) is not indicated.

Physical examination of patients with cancers arising in the paranasal sinuses is most often unrewarding. For advanced cancers of the maxillary sinus, however, in addition to the findings mentioned above, tumor may be seen eroding through skin (Fig. 119-1) or palate (Fig. 119-2), into the nasopharynx, or even into the nasal cavity. Anesthesia of the cheek and adjacent portion of the nose may be present and is due to involvement of the infraorbital nerve. Cancers arising in the ethmoid air cells may involve the medial orbit, with resulting loss of extraocular movements. Thus, knowledge of the anatomy of this region will allow proper evaluation of the patient's symptoms and signs when they present, thereby aiding in determination of the primary tumor site.

Traditional management of paranasal sinus cancers has been operative resection and/or radiation. Although radiation and surgery have both been effective treatment modalities for small cancers, especially of the maxillary sinus, more advanced cancers have high rates of local treatment failure.[2,3,6,7] The addition of radiation therapy, either before or after radical surgery, has not resulted in a significant improvement in survival. A problem with analyzing the results of many series, however, is in the definition of "radical" surgery; most authors treat even advanced cancers with an extracranial approach, thus providing inadequate resection margins. Furthermore, few authors report their treatment results according to tumor stage. Long-term disease-free survivals have been reported in the range of 20 to 30 percent for T_3 and T_4 cancers of the maxillary sinus, and a high rate of recurrence has been noted in the infratemporal (pterygomaxillary) space, an area not encompassed by the

Figure 119-1 A 60-year-old farmer presented with a facial squamous cell carcinoma present for 10 years. *A.* The tumor involved the entire left maxillary sinus but preoperative workup suggested no intracranial extension. *B.* Resection included the left maxilla, the floors of the anterior and middle cranial fossae, the entire bony orbit, the medial canthus of the right eye, the medial wall of the right maxilla, the entire parotid gland, the nose, and half of the upper lip. *C.* Reconstruction included a large scalp flap to cover the dura and split-thickness skin grafts for the soft tissue and remaining walls of the right maxilla. *D.* The prosthesis in place 3 months following resection. The local tumor was controlled but the patient eventually died of pulmonary metastases.

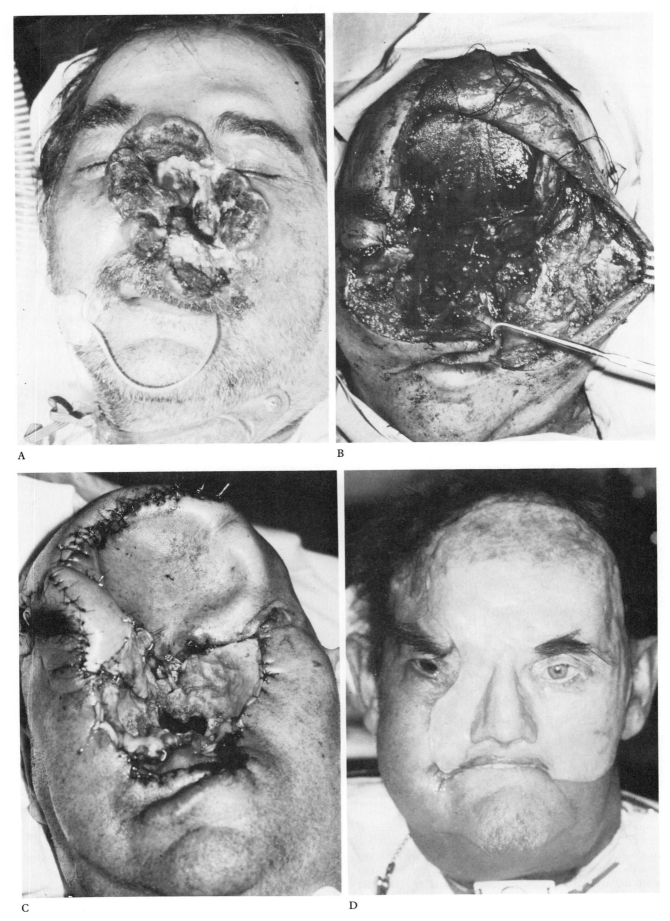

A

B

C

D

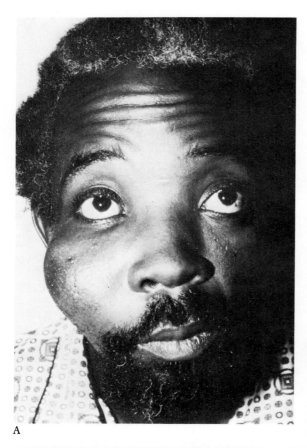

A

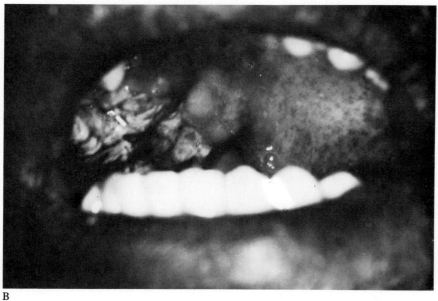

B

Figure 119-2 A 38-year-old male presented with trismus, a large right facial mass (*A*), and tumor extension to the mandible along the lateral pharyngeal wall (*B*). The tumor originated in the maxillary sinus and was locally controlled by resection of the floors of the anterior and middle cranial fossae, maxillectomy, hemimandibulectomy, and radical neck dissection. The patient died later of pulmonary metastases.

usual maxillectomy or when resecting the floor of the anterior cranial fossa.[4] Resection of the floor of the middle cranial fossa to remove the pterygoid fossa en bloc with the maxilla (see below) for selected cancers of the maxillary sinus has markedly diminished the local recurrence rate and improved survival in our patients.[10]

Skin Cancer

An unusual indication for combined intracranial-extracranial resection is advanced squamous cell or basal cell carcinoma of the skin or, even more infrequently, melanoma. Tumors requiring this approach are usually recurrent cancers which have been operated upon several times previously and have often been irradiated.[8,9] They are adherent to and invade bone; many tumors are close to the orbit and, in an effort to save the eye, have had previous inadequate excisions. Severe pain is frequent, and adequate resection may obviate the need for postoperative analgesics. Cosmesis may also be an important consideration in these patients; previous inadequate resections may have been performed in an effort to minimize cosmetic deformity. At the time of presentation with the recurrent tumor, however, a large, ulcerated, foul-smelling mass may be present. Resection may be necessary just to palliate the patient's symptoms, even though the resulting deformity will be severe.

Other Carcinomas

Even less frequent indications for combined intracranial-extracranial resection include cancers of the middle ear, orbit, and lacrimal gland. Middle ear carcinomas are squamous cell cancers histologically and invade adjacent bone; temporal bone resection is required to obtain an adequate margin. Cancers of the external auditory canal may be squamous cell carcinomas or adenoid cystic carcinomas.[5] Presenting symptoms include ear pain, the presence of a mass, hearing loss, sanguinous discharge, tinnitus, and facial paralysis. Wide resection performed through an extracranial approach will often cut through tumor; if the margin has tumor within it, the tumor will recur. Radiation therapy may be effective for squamous cell carcinoma, but adenoid cystic carcinomas are relatively radioresistant. Advanced cancers of the external auditory canal that cannot be adequately resected locally should be treated by a temporal bone resection (see below), which will minimize the risk of local recurrence.

Lacrimal gland cancers are often adenoid cystic carcinomas histologically; these cancers spread along nerve sheaths and vessels and through haversian canals, thus requiring wide resection including bone (Fig. 119-3). Even with this approach, late local recurrence or hematogenous metastases may occur.

Sarcomas

A small group of tumors arising from the primitive mesoderm, sarcomas, may be situated so that their removal will require a combined intracranial-extracranial approach. Although the orbit is one of the most common primary sites of rhabdomyosarcoma in children, recent advances pioneered through the Intergroup Rhabdomyosarcoma Study have shown that the major role of surgery for this primary site is biopsy to establish the histological diagnosis. Therefore, since these patients are usually cured by the combination of radiation and chemotherapy, radical surgery is no longer necessary. Bone and cartilage sarcomas, as well as most other soft tissue sarcomas, are relatively resistant to radiation and chemotherapy, and adequate resection with wide margins remains the treatment of choice; most patients with tumors adjacent to the skull will require a combined intracranial-extracranial approach.

Benign Disease

Few indications exist for a combined intracranial-extracranial approach to benign lesions. Occasional recurrent benign tumors, such as benign mixed tumors of the parotid, may recur in an area requiring bone resection to remove the tumor entirely. Inverted papillomas of the paranasal sinuses, when recurrent or, rarely, when primary and advanced, may require craniotomy in order to remove the tumor in toto. Resections performed in such circumstances should be as conservative as possible, with orbital preservation and retention of the palate and vigorous curettage of the bone close to resection margins.

Necrotizing infection is a very rare indication for combined intracranial-extracranial resection. Mucormycosis, a fungal infection often resistant to antifungal medications, is a rapidly progressive infection almost uniformly fatal in its craniofacial form. Adequate surgical debridement is a prerequisite for cure, but is often difficult to attain because of ethmoid air cell and sphenoid sinus involvement and progression through the cribriform plate to involve the dura. In the one patient we have treated with a combined approach, the mucormycosis had progressed after initial debridement and was resistant to all antifungal agents. It involved the ethmoid, maxillary, and sphenoid sinuses, caused blindness due to orbital invasion, and eroded through the cribriform plate to the anterior cranial fossa. Surgery, including total maxillectomy, resection of the ethmoid complex, orbital exenteration, debridement of frontal lobe, resection of dura, and curettage of the posterior wall of the sphenoid sinus until bleeding was observed, cured this patient.

Patient Management

Preoperative Management

Evaluation of patients with tumors involving the cranium must begin by obtaining a tissue diagnosis. Skin cancers are easily biopsied using local anesthesia, but deep-seated tumors, such as those in the pterygoid space or paranasal sinuses, may require general anesthesia for biopsy. It is generally advisable not to use aspiration cytology but to obtain a tissue biopsy to establish the histology. In order to avoid contaminating the planes for a future definitive resection, a limited-incisional biopsy should be performed. During the same anesthetic, patients with maxillary sinus cancers should undergo careful nasopharyngoscopy with biopsies of the posterior nasopharynx and the area around the eustachian tube; when tumor has extended to this area it cannot be encompassed surgically.

Prior to tumor resection, evaluation of tumor extent is of paramount importance. Plain roentgenograms may be useful in demonstrating bony erosion; they are especially useful in evaluating paranasal sinus cancers, and may show involvement of the pterygoid plate, the wall of the maxillary sinus, or the floor of the orbit.

Even more useful than the plain films are polytomograms, especially for paranasal sinus cancers or carcinomas arising

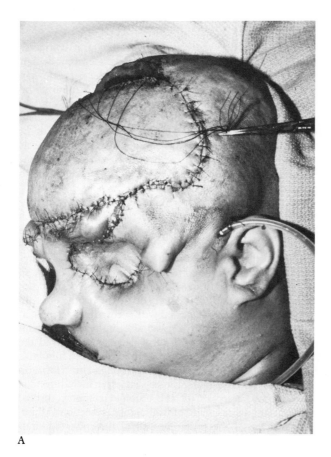

A

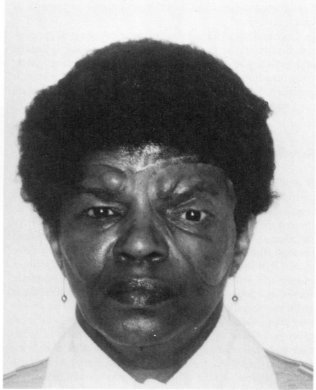

Figure 119-3 This 51-year-old woman presented with an adenoid cystic carcinoma of the lacrimal gland. Resection included the entire bony orbit and both eyelids. *A*. Reconstruction included a forehead flap sutured to the lateral nose, buccal skin, and eyebrow. A large scalp flap was rotated to cover the frontal craniotomy site and the posterior scalp was skin grafted. *B*. Five months following resection. *C*. Orbital prosthesis in place.

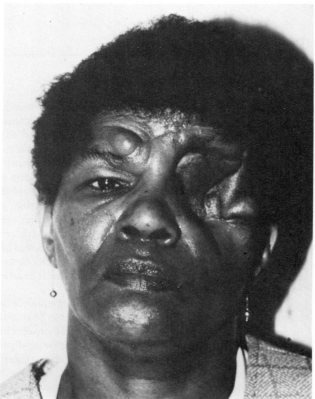

B

C

in the middle ear. Detail not evident on plain x-rays may be evident on tomography; tomograms will demonstrate masses within the sinuses and delineate tumor size as well as show early bony changes.

Computed tomographic (CT) scans are usually the most helpful preoperative tests. It is important to obtain the proper CT examination; the usual head CT scan will not provide the proper views of the paranasal sinuses and will not accurately assess the bones at the base of the skull. The CT examination should be specifically directed to these areas and should include coronal views. When the appropriate CT examination has been performed, accurate delineation of tumor location and extent are possible and bone involvement is easy to assess. In addition, intracranial involvement by tumor not readily apparent on plain x-rays or polytomograms can be detected by CT scans. The CT scan is relatively easy to interpret, especially when compared to polytomography. A potential problem with CT scans, however, is the occasional overestimation of tumor size; sinusitis due to tumor obstruction of mucus drainage may be interpreted as proximal tumor involvement. Thus, histological confirmation of tumor extent is usually required even when radiological evaluation suggests tumor extension to the sphenoid sinus.

Prior to operation for tumors of the paranasal sinuses, cultures of the nasal cavity should be obtained. Because a craniotomy is part of the procedure, appropriate antibiotics (i.e., those that cross the blood-brain barrier) should be used. Unless the culture results suggest other antibiotics or the patient is allergic, we routinely administer aqueous penicillin and chloramphenicol preoperatively, intraoperatively, and for up to 7 days postoperatively.

Intraoperative Management

After induction of anesthesia, a Foley catheter should be inserted into the bladder, an arterial catheter should be placed into a radial artery, and two large-bore venous catheters, including a central venous catheter, should be inserted. If a palatectomy is anticipated, as for cancers of the maxillary sinus, a tracheostomy should be performed prior to craniotomy. Mannitol, 1.5 to 2 g per kilogram of body weight, is then rapidly infused to provide for cerebral decompression and to allow an easier dissection of the dura from the appropriate area of the skull.

Postoperative Management

The course of most patients following surgery is relatively smooth. Antibiotics are continued for 7 days or until drainage catheters below the flaps are removed. Platelet counts should be obtained every other day, but chloramphenicol-induced thrombocytopenia has not been observed in our patients.

Most patients not requiring tracheostomy can be extubated early in the recovery room; some patients do, however, require overnight ventilator assistance. For those not undergoing palate resection, a diet is begun on the first postoperative day; when the palate has been resected, a nasogas-

tric tube is inserted in the operating room and the patient begun on tube feedings on the first postoperative day. Ambulation is begun on the first postoperative day, and for those patients with tracheostomies, the tracheostomy tube is usually removed about the fifth postoperative day. Patients undergoing resection of the palate with the craniofacial resection are usually hospitalized 3 to 4 weeks following surgery; when the resection is performed entirely superior to the palate, most patients are discharged in 10 to 12 days.

Types of Resection

Anterior Cranial Fossa Resection

Tumors originating in the maxillary sinus, ethmoid air cells, or orbit, or other tumors with involvement of the orbit or in apposition to the anterior bone of the skull may be candidates to have some or all of the floor of the anterior cranial fossa resected with the tumor. A frontal craniotomy is performed; the bone flap removed is saved for replacement at the end of the procedure. The dura mater is stripped from the bone to the crista galli; the cribriform plate is exposed, and the dura is taken back as far as the optic chiasm, if necessary. At this point entrance is made into the sphenoid sinus, either with a small burr or a small osteotome; the sphenoid sinus mucosa is sent for frozen section, and if tumor is present the operation is terminated. If there is no tumor in the sphenoid sinus, the necessary resection of the floor of the anterior cranial fossa can proceed. This may include the area between the orbits, which would encompass the anterior wall of the sphenoid sinus as well as the ethmoid air cells; the entire roof of the orbit can be resected with this area, if necessary.

Pitfalls with this resection may include proceeding too far posteriorly with damage to the internal carotid artery; major bleeding is otherwise not a problem. When it is necessary to remove the eye, the optic nerve should be divided sharply in the optic canal and the ophthalmic artery should be carefully clipped.

Middle Cranial Fossa Resection

Tumors in the infratemporal fossa or extensions of maxillary sinus cancer to the infratemporal fossa have a high incidence of local recurrence with the standard operative approach. Thus, the concept of combined intracranial-extracranial resection of these tumors was extended to include the floor of the middle cranial fossa.

A subtemporal craniectomy is performed and the dura is dissected posteriorly and medially to expose the foramina spinosum, ovale, and rotundum. This approach can also give exposure of the superior orbital fissure when resection of the entire bony orbit is required. The middle meningeal artery is clipped, and the floor of the fossa is resected through the three foramina. This transects the second and third branches of the trigeminal nerve; therefore, postoperative pain is usually minimal. Transection of the zygomatic bone and the coronoid process of the mandible allows the pterygoid muscles and infratemporal contents to be removed en bloc with the appropriate facial resection.

The major potential complication of this resection is hemorrhage; clipping the middle meningeal artery prior to bone resection prevents significant bleeding. Resection posterior and medial to the foramina is inadvisable due to the presence of the internal carotid artery and the cavernous sinus.

Temporal Bone Resection

This type of resection is indicated for middle ear tumors, mastoid cancer, some cancers of the external auditory canal, advanced skin cancers of the ear or adjacent skin, and some advanced parotid tumors. A temporal craniectomy is performed and the bone rongeured posteriorly to expose the posterior fossa. The sigmoid sinus is mobilized with the dura from the bone, and the condyle of the mandible resected for anterior exposure. The resection is concluded by fracturing the base of the petrous bone with an osteotome.

Massive blood loss is not uncommon during this procedure. It may be due to entrance into the sigmoid sinus, laceration of the bony portion of the internal carotid artery, or bone bleeding. Following removal of the specimen, hemostasis is fairly easy to obtain.

Reconstruction

Closure of the dura mater is one of the most important, as well as one of the most difficult, steps in the procedure. Every attempt should be made to perform the entire operation without penetration of the dura. Yet, in at least two situations, this is impossible: (1) where the tumor invades or penetrates the dura, requiring dura removal or resection of intradural tumor, and (2) in the course of exposure of the anterior cranial fossa in planned removal of the orbit, or in exposure of the sphenoid sinus. In this latter instance, the cribriform plate area must be exposed and the dura will need to be slightly opened at the exit of the olfactory nerves. It is impossible to expose the midline anterior cranial fossa extradurally without opening the dura at the cribriform plate area. Awareness of this fact will permit preoperative planning and preparation for closure.

The dura may be inadvertently opened or torn in the exposure or the performance of the craniotomy, such as during the burr hole placement, or when using the Gigli saw or a craniotome. The dura may also be penetrated when it is being dissected from the inner table of the skull if the patient is elderly or has had previous irradiation to the cranium. The dural dissections may be extremely difficult and multiple holes may be made. Failure to recognize each hole in the dura may lead to postoperative CSF leakage, meningitis, and death of the patient.

Closure of the dura is generally done by one of three methods: primary closure, the use of a muscle or fascial plug for a small rent, or the use of a fascia lata graft for a large defect. Primary closure of the dura is the preferred technique and is applicable to the closure of the dural openings

at the cribriform plate area as well as for closure of small holes. Careful sharp dissection of the dura at the cribriform plate will produce two small 1-to-2-cm-long narrow slits in the dura, one on either side of the falx. Upon completion of tumor resection, with the brain retracted and relaxed by mannitol, re-approximation of the dura by running suture is easily performed to provide a watertight clearance. In the past, we have used the standard dural 4-0 silk suture (Ethicon, Somerville, N.J.) but, more recently, have used Vicryl (polyglactin, Ethicon) because of less adhesion formation with the surface of the brain.[11]

When the dura is opened near its attachment to the anterior clinoid processes or tuberculum sellae or in the area of the optic nerves, primary closure is impossible. The dura is usually very thin and there will be no attachments for suture. In this case, one or two sutures will draw the dural ends together and a fascial graft or muscle plug can be sutured in place, though usually not in a perfectly watertight fashion. In such instances, careful attention is placed to any evidence of a postoperative CSF leak, and a lumbar subarachnoid drain is used immediately if a CSF leak is observed. The drain is usually removed on the fifth postoperative day. This has been uniformly successful in stopping CSF leakage, and no reoperations have been necessary in our experience for closure of the dura.

When a large area of dura is removed or sacrificed in the course of the operation, a fascia lata graft is necessary. This is usually necessary only when the tumor invades or penetrates the dura and wide resection of the dura is required. A large section of fascia lata from the thigh is obtained and sutured in place in a watertight fashion. The use of fascia lata is preferred over any artificial substitute for dura because of the higher risk of infection with the latter.

Appropriate extradural reconstruction following the combined intracranial-extracranial resection depends upon the location of the defect, the amount of soft tissue and skin removed, and the location of the bony defect. The major goal of the immediate reconstruction is to obtain good coverage of the dura. Secondary goals are to provide a palatal replacement (if resected) and to provide external cosmesis; these can be readily accomplished with prostheses.

We have employed many different flaps for reconstruction, depending upon the location of the defect. Temporal bone resections done for recurrent parotid tumors or skin cancers have a large soft tissue defect which must be closed for good dural coverage. Large superiorly based scalp flaps with or without a pectoralis major musculocutaneous flap (Fig. 119-4) have proven very useful in closing these defects.[1]

Patients undergoing resection of the floor of the anterior cranial fossa with orbital preservation can be reconstructed using a flap of pericranium; this is based anteriorly and the blood supply is through branches of the supraorbital and supratrochlear vessels which have been preserved by development of a bicoronal flap. The pericranial flap will line the floor of the resected anterior cranial fossa and provide excellent support for the brain.

The temporalis muscle is particularly useful in supplying coverage to the floor of the middle cranial fossa. While raising the skin flap, care should be taken to preserve the branch of the superficial temporal artery which supplies the muscle. The muscle is raised from the temporal bone and taken down from its attachments on the zygomatic arch and coronoid process, thus providing a wide, fan-shaped muscle which can be skin grafted and can easily cover the floor of the middle cranial fossa (and the undersurface of the orbital contents if necessary).

When tumor involves the orbit and orbital exenteration is required along with a large skin resection, reconstruction is more difficult and not as cosmetically satisfying. Elevation of a forehead flap (to the midline) will provide excellent exposure for the frontal craniotomy; the flap can then be rotated to cover the base of the brain, a scalp flap can be rotated to cover the craniotomy defect, and the posterior scalp can be covered with a split-thickness skin graft. Occasionally, the nasal septum can be rotated to provide a replacement for the hard palate. Although this is a cosmetically disfiguring operation, very acceptable results can be obtained prosthetically.

Complications

Intraoperative

The major complication occurring during the performance of a combined intracranial-extracranial resection is hemorrhage. The risk of hemorrhage is diminished when the operation is performed by a skillful surgeon who has good knowledge of anatomy. However, sufficient quantities of cross-matched blood should be available for use in the event of major bleeding. Careful monitoring and fluid replacement by the anesthesiologist can reduce the chances of development of hypotension. Careful preoperative assessment should demonstrate if the tumor has extended posteriorly to involve the carotid artery or cavernous sinus; if it has, resection usually should not be attempted. Internal carotid artery ligation can be performed if a combined extracranial-intracranial bypass to the middle cerebral artery is performed, which would require additional preoperative evaluation and is rarely indicated.

Another problem which can occur intraoperatively is that of inadequate wound closure. Avoidance of this potentially disastrous complication begins in the preoperative period; knowledge of operations previously performed and blood vessels which may have been divided, as well as the blood vessels to be divided during the planned procedure with their skin supply, is an absolute requirement. Evaluation by the entire operative team will ensure the proper incisions for the tumor resection and wound closure.

Postoperative

A major complication occurring in the postoperative period is that of wound infection. With careful surgical technique ensuring a good blood supply to all flaps, prophylactic antibiotics, and closed suction drainage to prevent fluid accumulations, infections are rare. When they do occur, they are usually extradural and can be treated by drainage.

More serious, however, is infection developing below the skin flaps due to inadequate blood supply. Recognizing that the skin is not viable may be difficult in the early postoperative period, and such delay will contribute to slough of the

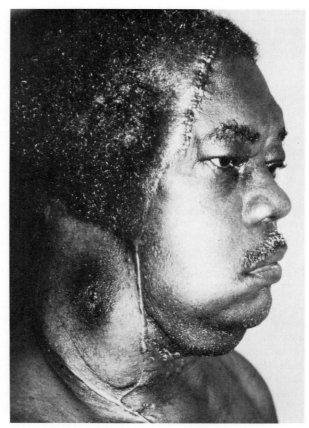

Figure 119-4 A 69-year-old man who had previously undergone total parotidectomy and 6600 rad for an undifferentiated parotid malignancy. He presented with a massive local recurrence and cervical nodal metastases. Temporal bone resection was performed in conjunction with radical neck dissection; reconstruction included both a large scalp flap and a pectoralis major musculocutaneous flap.

dura and subsequent meningitis. Sloughing is best treated by prompt debridement; the area can be covered by using a free omental graft with anastomosis of the right gastroepiploic vessels to the superficial temporal vessels or to branches of the external carotid artery and jugular vein in the neck. The omentum will seal the wound quickly, dura does not have to be replaced, and a skin graft will always be successful. The omentum is so successful in closing the wound, however, that meningitis may result; prophylactic intrathecal aminoglycosides should be considered. Two deaths in our series occurred when the patients developed meningitis after successful omental grafts; antibiotics begun after the onset of meningitis, although effecting a cure, were too late to reverse severe brain damage.

A less serious complication occurring in the postoperative period is that of a cerebrospinal fluid leakage. This is due to incomplete closure of small holes made in the dura. These leaks are usually small, and may present as CSF appearing in the suction catheters or through the nose; they can be treated with lumbar punctures twice daily or with an

TABLE 119-1 Indications for Craniofacial Resection

Primary Lesion	Histology	No. of Cases
Skin tumor	Basal cell carcinoma	7
	Squamous cell carcinoma	17
	Melanoma	3
Paranasal sinus tumor	Squamous cell carcinoma	28
	Adenoid cystic carcinoma	4
	Other	5
Sarcoma		5
Other		18

indwelling lumbar drain. The leak usually closes after 2 to 3 days of drainage.

Results of Craniofacial Resection

Our updated series of craniofacial resections includes 87 patients with a variety of diagnoses (Table 119-1).[9,10] The age range was 7 to 85 years, with a median age of about 65; most nonmelanoma skin cancer patients were male (23 male to 1 female). Eight patients underwent temporal bone resection and the remainder underwent resection of the anterior and/or middle cranial fossae.

Nonfatal complications occurred in 16 (18 percent) of the patients. Eleven patients had a CSF leak, but none required reoperation. Two had meningitis and three had miscellaneous minor complications.

There have been 13 deaths (15 percent); most were early in our experience. Two deaths were from hemorrhage of oropharyngeal carcinomas that extended into the pterygoid space, which we no longer consider an indication for craniofacial resection. Two patients had flap necrosis with resultant meningitis, two had incomplete tumor resection, three died from pulmonary emboli, one died of a myocardial infarction, and three died of miscellaneous causes.

Long-term results have been very encouraging. Patients with maxillary sinus cancers treated by this approach have not had any local recurrences; this shows the benefit of resecting the floor of the middle cranial fossa and therefore removing the contents of the pterygoid space en bloc with the specimen. Overall survival has also been improved when compared to other series.[10]

The relatively small number of patients with other diagnoses who underwent craniofacial resection precludes meaningful analysis of their survival rates, but only five patients have had local recurrences and two could be retreated for cure.

References

1. Ariyan S, Sasaki CT, Spencer D: Radical en bloc resection of the temporal bone. Am J Surg 142:443–447, 1981.
2. Bush SE, Bagshaw MA: Carcinoma of the paranasal sinuses. Cancer 50:154–158, 1982.
3. Cheng VST, Wang CC: Carcinomas of the paranasal sinuses: A study of sixty-six cases. Cancer 40:3038–3041, 1977.
4. Ketcham AS, Wilkins RH, Van Buren JM, Smith RR: A combined intracranial facial approach to the paranasal sinuses. Am J Surg 106:698–703, 1963.
5. Perzin KH, Gullane P, Conley J: Adenoid cystic carcinoma involving the external auditory canal: A clinicopathologic study of 16 cases. Cancer 50:2873–2883, 1982.
6. Robin PE, Powell DJ: Treatment of carcinoma of the nasal cavity and paranasal sinuses. Clin Otolaryngol 6:401–414, 1981.
7. Sako K: Management of cancer of the maxillary sinus. J Surg Oncol 6: 325–333, 1974.
8. Sypert GW, Habal MB: Combined cranio-orbital surgery for extensive malignant neoplasms of the orbit. Neurosurgery 2:8–14, 1978.
9. Terz JJ, Young HF, Lawrence W Jr: Combined craniofacial resection for locally advanced carcinoma of the head and neck: I. Tumors of the skin and soft tissues. Am J Surg 140:613–617, 1980.
10. Terz JJ, Young HF, Lawrence W Jr: Combined craniofacial resection for locally advanced carcinoma of the head and neck: II. Carcinoma of the paranasal sinuses. Am J Surg 140:618–624, 1980.
11. Vällfors B, Hansson HA, Svensson J: Absorbable or nonabsorbable suture materials for closure of the dura mater? Neurosurgery 9:407–413, 1981.

120

Surgical Resection of Tumors of the Skull Base

Leonard I. Malis

Various techniques have been used for the removal of the tumors of the skull base, and these differ for the anterior, middle, and posterior cranial fossas. I have used a bifrontal intradural approach for most of the suprasellar tumors, a pterional approach for most of the parasellar tumors, and a transnasal approach mainly for the chordomas of the clivus. The petrosal (combined subtemporal and posterior fossa) approach has been used for most clivus and clivotentorial tumors. The posterior fossa approach has been used for various tumors of the cerebellopontine angle, and is essentially like that used for acoustic neuromas, which will not be further discussed here. The unilateral frontal flaps and the temporal flaps are reserved for the relatively easier lesions. Derome's transbasal approach has produced excellent results in his hands[2] and should be understood by surgeons dealing with basal lesions.

General Principles

All patients are under general anesthesia, and all are fully monitored, including via arterial and central venous lines. The head is always fixed in a pin headrest. The intraoperative antibiotic regimen previously described is used in every case and has essentially eliminated the incidence of infection.[4] All procedures are carried out under controlled hypotension, usually at a mean of 70 to 80 mmHg. Urea is given after the induction of anesthesia in every case, and spinal drainage is never used. Wide arachnoid dissection permits sufficient additional room and yet permits cerebrospinal fluid below the level of the surgical procedure to remain available to lyse any blood leakage from the operative field in order to avoid postoperative adhesive processes due to clotted subarachnoid blood. All procedures are begun with headlamp and loupes for more precise openings, and all intradural operative technique is carried out through the operating microscope at magnifications of 10 to 25 $\times$. The supine position with the table flexed and the head somewhat elevated is used for the subfrontal approach. The patient is placed in the supine oblique position for the pterional procedures. We have preferred to use the semisitting position for the petrosal combined approach and for the posterior fossa approaches. In the sitting positions, the pressure suit and the Doppler monitor are routinely used.

Bifrontal Approach

The bifrontal approach is carried out with the larger part of the exposure either on the nondominant side or the side where the lesion is significantly larger. The curved incision following the hairline begins at the zygoma, very close to the tragus, curves forward near the midline, and then backward again and down on the opposite side, about halfway to the zygoma. After separating the muscle along the zygomatic process of the frontal bone, a burr hole is made near the pterion. The dura is separated and the bone flap is cut from this single burr hole, right along the orbital roof and through the frontal sinus to within a centimeter of the midline, then turning backward parallel to the midline and then laterally again anterior to the coronal suture and into the temporal squama. This unilateral flap is then broken on the hinge of temporal muscle. Now, from the area of the flap under direct vision, the dura may be freed with a dissector across the midline over the top of the sagittal sinus to a point about 3 or 4 cm to the opposite side of the midline. A rectangular free flap is now cut with the craniotome across the midline. This technique avoids additional burr holes and prevents the possibility of injury to the sagittal sinus. Before the dura is opened, the frontal sinus mucosa is completely exenterated bilaterally; the interior of the sinus, including the area of the nasofrontal duct, is stroked with the unipolar coagulating current; and then the sinuses are packed with strips of temporalis muscle. At the time of closure, the muscle-packed sinus will be oversewn with a split layer of the galea, with periosteum, or with the lower limb of the dura.

The dura is opened parallel to the frontal base to reach the sagittal sinus bilaterally. The frontal polar veins are visualized, sealed with the bipolar coagulator, and cut. The sagittal sinus is doubly ligated with sutures passed through the falx just above the crista and is cut between the ligatures. The rest of the falx is cut backward along the crista through the free margin.

Self-retaining retractors are now fastened to the posterior calvarial margins bilaterally, and a pair of broad-bladed retractors, one on each side, is brought in for more even support. It has been well demonstrated that retractor pressure must not exceed 10 torr in the hypotensive patient, and preferably the retractors are used more for support than retraction. Since the microscope is able to provide stereoscopic visualization and good light through a small opening, retraction should be just sufficient to permit the insertion of a finger (Fig. 120-1). The minimal displacement of brain has allowed the development of a far less traumatic approach to structures at the base as compared with unmagnified surgery. Self-retaining retractors are essential, since they can support the brain and provide the minimal separation

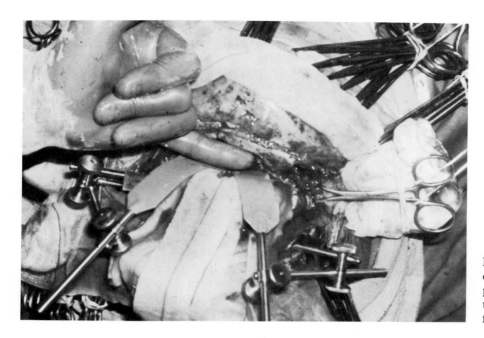

Figure 120-1 Bifrontal craniotomy showing retractor placement and minimal elevation of frontal lobes required for the microprocedure.

required without the risk of movement or extra pull of the hand-held retractors. Microsurgical instrumentation scarcely needs rediscussion, but it is essential for working in these fields. Long, bayonetted instruments, properly balanced and suitably fine at the working ends, must interface with the hands of the surgeon, which are rendered no smaller just because the tip of the instrument is tiny. Despite the small field of approach vertically, the field is wide horizontally along the plane of the base, allowing an entry from many directions, and the microscope must be able to move freely across this arc. The retractors should lie flat against the head and should never be permitted to build up an obstruction to the field. One must be able to smoothly and rapidly move instruments in from any angle of the arc without the interference of obstructive levels of instrumentation. Tactile sense plays almost no part in the microdissection, which is virtually entirely a visual technique. Accordingly, a bloodless field must be maintained, both by the prevention of vascular injury and by the proper use of gentle bipolar coagulation under saline. An essential instrument is the regulated soft suction, a true pressure regulator in the suction line, not just a constriction or a calibrated leak; this permits the suction to be maintained at a fixed level of 80 mmHg. With a size 7 or smaller sucker, the suction tip may now be used to retract, dissect, or support structures without the danger of aspirating delicate neural and vascular tissue but will still allow adequate visualization.

The patients are informed that they will lose their senses of smell and of taste. Occasionally, one olfactory nerve may be spared if the lesion is modest, but where this is possible most lesions do not require bifrontal exposure and can be handled easily unilaterally. Accordingly, for the more difficult lesions that are now being discussed, both olfactory nerves are sectioned, usually with the bipolar coagulator, leaving the bulbs intact to avoid bleeding deep in the cribriform plate. By this point, the tumors that extend anteriorly have come into view and those in the suprasellar area arising behind the tuberculum will be seen behind the optic nerves. Wide arachnoid opening is now carried out into the sylvian fissures bilaterally, as this will permit the frontal lobes to separate backward without retraction as well as release the excess of spinal fluid at the level of the surgery.

Removal of the tumor may now be started. Unlike tumors of the rest of the body, tumors of the central nervous system, with rare exceptions, are cored in the initial stage of their removal. The object, of course, is to have a perfectly normal looking nervous system and a miserable, cut-up, fragmented tumor as the end specimen rather than vice versa. Nowhere is this more important than in tumors of the base. Coring is done with the idea of slowly bringing the deepest part of the tumor outward to the surface so that the visualization of the final dissection can be carried out without enlarging the space of the retraction additionally. Coring should be carried out in an area to devascularize as much of the tumor as possible as the coring continues. In the basal meningiomas, most of the blood supply will come up through the dural attachment. In the tumors of the planum, olfactory groove, and orbital roof, most of the supply is likely to be from perforating branches of the ophthalmic artery. Proceeding further backward, meningohypophyseal branches, posterior branches of the ophthalmic, and medial branches of the middle meningeal arteries are the most likely sources of supply to the suprasellar tumors. Accordingly, coring along the base of the tumor will tend to devascularize the deeper portions that lie above the base. Coring is carried out, using the bipolar coagulator under saline solution, to make millimeter-by-millimeter necrotization within the tumor, allowing bits of the tumor to be removed without bleeding. The Cavitron ultrasonic surgical aspirator (Cooper Medical Devices, Mountain View, Calif.) can speed up this process if the lesion is relatively avascular or has already been partly devascularized. Always carried out under direct vision, this process brings the deeper part of the tumor closer and closer down to the base into the field until finally the extracapsular dissection can be carried out.

Many of these basal meningiomas are out of the capsule or have no distinct capsule and fungate out into the subarachnoid space. Here, they regularly engulf blood vessels and neural structures in this area (e.g., the carotid arteries, optic nerves, chiasm, and anterior cerebral arteries). It is generally feasible to shrink the tumor away from these structures. In most cases, the adventitia of the carotid system is well separated, and often the arachnoid of the posterior surface of the chiasmatic cistern protects the pituitary stalk. Engulfed anterior cerebral arteries can be followed through the tumor by shrinking the tumor away, millimeter by millimeter, with the microbipolar coagulator and achieving complete separation with preservation of the vessels and their fine striatal branches. Most of the suprasellar tumors splay the optic nerves widely apart so that the carotid and ophthalmic arteries at their origins now appear medial to the optic nerves in the prechiasmal region and then cross beneath the optic nerves to come up in their usual lateral position. They can be freed of tumor at this point, and tumor may be taken from the optic foramen along the ophthalmic artery beneath the optic nerve to complete the resection of the intracranial part of the tumor (Fig. 120-2).

In most of these tumors, there is still the hyperostotic base, which may involve the cribriform plate, planum sphenoidale, anterior clinoids, or dorsum sellae. Sometimes the tumor invades through to the sphenoid or ethmoid sinuses or into the nose itself, along the cribriform plate. In any case, the classical procedure of coagulating the base has resulted in what appears to be too high a percentage of recurrences. Accordingly, the high-speed diamond drill is used to carve away all of the hyperostotic bone and then to permit exposure and resection of the invaded mucosa and the portion of the tumor that enters the sinuses or nasal cavity. At times, this requires resection of turbinates and septum, and occasionally tumor can be followed down even into the antra and resected. If the tumor surrounds the optic nerve and the optic foramen, resection of the medial orbital wall and ethmoid allows the exposure of this portion of the tumor under direct vision so that it may be resected without damage to the optic nerve or to the ophthalmic artery, thereby preserving vision (Fig. 120-3).

Of course, this leaves a large cranial defect that requires repair. My policy has been to pack the nasal cavity transcranially with Vaseline gauze, pushing the gauze down far enough so that it may be removed later through the nostrils and bringing the pack up to fill the nasal and sinus cavities as a support for the graft that is now to be placed. The patient has been previously informed that a graft will be taken from the thigh, and the thigh has been prepared and draped for the taking of the graft. However, the graft is not taken until it is ready to be used. While it would be more convenient to take it at the beginning of the procedure before even opening the head, this would result in a piece of graft sitting and deteriorating as a culture medium at room temperature throughout a long operative procedure. The graft itself consists of a sandwich of a layer of fascia lata, a layer of muscle, and a final layer of fascia lata. The first layer of fascia is tacked in place with a few sutures. A thin layer of

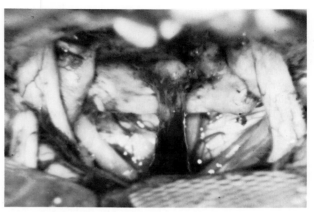

Figure 120-2 The patient is supine with the brow up. A suprasellar meningioma has been totally removed through a bifrontal craniotomy. The retractors support the frontal lobes at the lower part of the picture. The proximal carotid arteries may be seen medial to the two optic nerves. The pituitary stalk is preserved, running backward over the posterior clinoid and concealing all but a small part of the basilar artery, which is just to the right of the stalk. The third nerve on the left is seen medial to the posterior part of the optic nerve, while on the right the superior cerebellar artery, third nerve, and posterior cerebral artery are seen medial to the posterior portion of the right optic nerve. The tuberculum has not yet been resected.

crushed muscle is placed over the fascial layer, and a final sheet of fascia is placed to cover the muscle and overlap the entire repair intradurally. Fascia lata is a surprising structure when seen under the microscope. It looks like a cross-

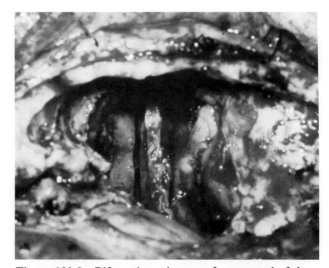

Figure 120-3 Bifrontal craniotomy after removal of the intranasal portion of the tumor. The brow is up. The cribriform plate and tuberculum have been removed. The medial orbital walls have been removed. The crista galli and the upper portion of the nasal septum, the ethmoids, and the superior and middle turbinates, as well as the medial walls of the antra, have been resected.

woven canvas, has almost no stretch, and is remarkably adhesive when placed on other structures (Fig. 120-4). The success rate in waterproof sealing with this type of closure has been virtually 100 percent in the nonmalignant tumors. Foreign bodies, nonautogenous tissue, wax, acrylics, or glues are not used, and it is not necessary to reinforce the opening with rib segments or segments of other bone. The nasal packing is removed on about the fifth postoperative day, by which time the sealing and support are fairly complete.

In the repair of the bifrontal craniotomy, the free flap is sewn to the osteoplastic portion of the flap with sutures through multiple drill holes, and the combined flap is replaced after the dural repair. One principle, long adhered to in neurosurgery, states that the dura should always be closed watertight except in the posterior fossa, where it is usually left open. My technique is exactly the reverse of this time-honored custom. We rarely close the dura under the bone flap, merely covering the defect with a sheet of Gelfoam (absorbable gelatin sponge, The Upjohn Company, Kalamazoo, Mich.) On the other hand, in the posterior fossa where the bone is often not replaced, the dura is always closed watertight, the difference being entirely a matter of whether the bone is replaced.

Again, on general principles, it is expected that blood loss will be minimal and rarely reach 200 ml and that transfusion will virtually never be used. It is expected that there will be a negative fluid balance of 600 to 800 ml and that the immediate postoperative osmolarity will be about 310 to 315 mosm per liter.

Pterional Approach

Tumors arising from the medial sphenoid ridge, the superior orbital fissure, the anteromedial temporal surface, or the cavernous sinus region are approached through a pterional exposure.[3,6] The scalp incision begins at the zygoma, close

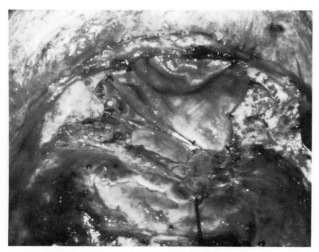

Figure 120-4 The frontal floor has been repaired with a layer of fascia lata, which will now be covered with a layer of muscle and another layer of fascia lata.

to the tragus, and then curves upward and forward within the hairline, usually looping backward for a centimeter or two on the opposite side of the midline. This somewhat S-shaped curve allows sufficient length to keep the incision off the forehead and yet allow an adequate subgaleal dissection of the flap forward. A triangular segment of temporalis muscle with its base against the zygoma and its apex at the top of the zygomatic process of the frontal bone is incised, separated subperiosteally, and pulled downward by traction sutures. This permits a good exposure of the pterion itself, and the placement of a single burr opening in the lesser wing of the sphenoid at the pterion. Through this burr hole, the middle meningeal artery can be sealed with the bipolar coagulator. The bone flap is cut forward along the orbit, then upward, backward, and around, then down beneath the temporal muscle to the zygoma, and then forward so that the flap can be hinged on the posterior portion of the temporalis muscle. Resection of the lesser wing of the sphenoid is now carried inward to reach the superior orbital fissure using either Leksell rongeurs or high-speed nitrogen-driven burrs. Coagulation of the dural fold at the superior orbital fissure is avoided for fear of producing a sixth nerve palsy.

The usually described method of opening the dura suggests a rather straight line parallel to the base of the incision and a centimeter or so away from it. I have generally preferred to open the dura in the opposite direction, cutting along the superior margin of the flap and turning the dura on a downward hinge, which completely covers the cut surface of the lesser wing and the deep portion of the temporal muscle, thereby providing a cleaner field.

Now, with microtechnique, the sylvian fissure arachnoid is opened, and as cerebrospinal fluid flows out, the self-retaining retractor is clamped to the bony margin antero-superiorly and a broad-bladed retractor is used to support the frontal lobe. The wider the arachnoidal dissection, the better the exposure of deep structures. Again, it must be emphasized that microtechnique is a subarachnoid technique, not a subdural operative system. Of course, the size and position of the lesion determines what will be achieved in the arachnoidal opening early on. If the tumor is quite large and extends far laterally as well as deeply medially, the opening of the arachnoid of the sylvian fissure may be only superficial and may not even progress medially past the trifurcation of the middle cerebral artery until after the tumor has been adequately cored.

The sylvian veins drain into the dura at the temporal pole close to the orbital fissure. While they may be spared if the tumor is mainly anterior, a tumor that extends posteriorly will be much better exposed if the bridging veins are sealed with the bipolar coagulator and cut. Any bridging vein to the dura that is to be divided should be coagulated over a segment of length beginning almost directly at the brain surface and should be cut as far away from the dural end of the bridging vein as possible as a matter of safety, since the point of entrance into a dural channel is much more difficult to seal than the other end of the vein. This particular group of sylvian veins has at no time caused any problem after sealing and always seems to have an adequate collateral flow, regardless of the angiographic difficulty in demonstrating this flow. A second retractor may be necessary to support the temporal lobe and draw it backward.

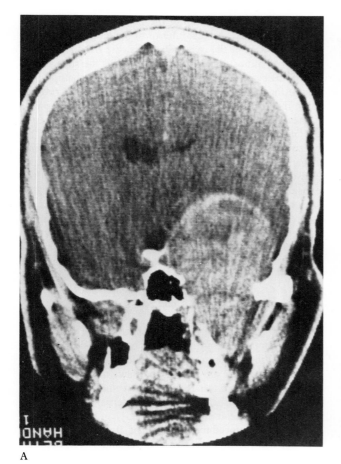

A

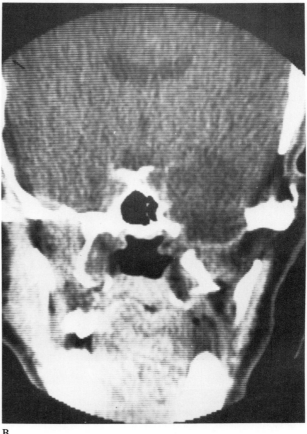

B

Figure 120-5 *A.* A coronal CT scan shows a large left gasserian neuroma eroding through the base, the sella, and the sphenoid sinus. *B.* The tumor has been completely resected through a pterional approach. The sphenoid wall and the floor of the skull have been replaced with a sheet of fascia lata.

While I will be describing here the use of this technique mainly for the meningiomas, it can also be used for craniopharyngiomas, particularly those associated with a prefixed chiasm, for lateral extensions of invasive pituitary tumors, and for most aneurysms of the circle. It has been indispensable for the removal of gasserian ganglion neuromas. An example of a huge gasserian neuroma on CT, pre- and postoperatively, is shown in Fig. 120-5. In this case, the exposure permitted me to follow the tumor down through the massively eroded temporal floor where the foramen lacerum, foramen ovale, and foramen rotundum had become one single opening. I was able to complete the removal down along the carotid sheath in the neck. The wall of the cavernous sinus, the sphenoid sinus, and the base of the skull were patched with a single sheet of fascia lata after the completion of the removal of the tumor, preventing cerebrospinal fluid leakage. For this area, the three-layer sandwich described for the frontal region was not necessary because of the adequate support of the underlying tissues.

With the bipolar coring technique, it is possible to progressively necrotize medial-third meningiomas and shrink them away from the carotid artery and its branches where these structures are completely engulfed. By this technique, using low coagulator power settings under continuous saline irrigation, tumors that have been routinely thought to permit only partial removal can be resected completely with preservation of the vessels, including the striate, choroidal, and posterior communicating branches. Such a patient is shown in Fig. 120-6 where an inner-third sphenoid ridge meningioma completely engulfed the carotid artery up past its bifurcation, including the A_1 and M_1 segments as well as the choroidal and striatal branches. The microbipolar technique permitted freeing of the entire vascular tree without damage and with the retention of completely normal neurological function.

When the tumor has extended into the cavernous sinus, the problems are by no means comparable in difficulty to those of carotid cavernous fistulas. Venous channels within the cavernous sinus are under only normal venous pressure and so offer very little problem, as contrasted to the arterial pressure encountered in the patients with fistulas. Additionally, in many of these patients, the interior of the cavernous dura is filled with tumor, which collapses the venous channels. It is essential to know the anatomical course of the carotid artery through the skull base and then through the cavernous sinus to its point of emergence. The carotid artery

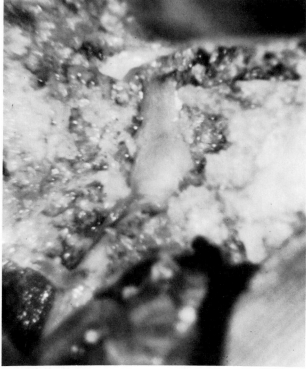

A

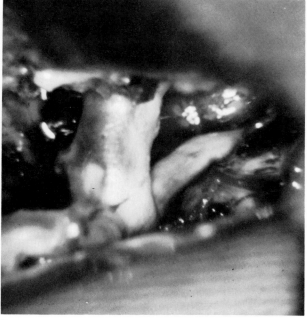

B

Figure 120-6 *A.* A right pterional craniectomy has been done. The patient is supine. The vertex is down, the base up. Posterior is on the left of the picture, and anterior on the right. An inner-third sphenoid ridge meningioma totally engulfing the carotid artery is being removed from around the carotid and middle cerebral arteries and their branches. *B.* The meningioma has been removed from around the engulfed carotid, middle, and anterior cerebral arteries.

lies against the medial wall of the cavernous dura. Just lateral to the carotid and just inferior to the tentorial margin at the upper edge of the cavernous dura, the third and fourth nerves run almost directly forward toward the superior orbital fissure, where they are joined by the ophthalmic division of the fifth nerve. The sixth nerve has a course running along the lower part of the cavernous sinus, angling upward to eventually reach the superior orbital fissure, just deep to the ophthalmic division. In the meantime, it crosses between the carotid wall and the outermost layer of the cavernous sinus inferiorly and is overlaid by the gasserian sheath. The space above the gasserian sheath and the ophthalmic division of the fifth nerve forms the inferior margin of Parkinson's triangle, while the line of the fourth nerve parallel to the tentorial edge is the upper margin. This anatomical triangle is critically important for a direct approach to carotid-cavernous fistulas.[5] When tumors invade this area, the anatomy can be markedly distorted, but again because of the low venous pressure it is possible to work readily, and as the tumor is dissected, venous bleeding is controlled by simply sliding strips of Surgicel (oxidized regenerated cellulose, Johnson & Johnson Products Inc., New Brunswick, N.J.) ahead of the operative plane. Indeed, the major difficulty is neither venous bleeding nor injury to the carotid artery but is preservation of the much more delicate neural structures. Nevertheless, there are tumors that have not only engulfed the carotid artery in this region but have invaded its wall so that there is no structural wall to preserve, thus requiring the sacrifice of the artery. At times, this can be a contraindication to the procedure if sufficient flow is still coming through the partially occluded vessel and is required for brain function, particularly if this cannot be made up by carrying out an external to internal anastomosis. An example would be a situation where striatal branches were being fed through such a partly occluded carotid artery but the tumor had occluded the middle cerebral bifurcation.

From this pterional approach, the anterior clinoid may be resected quite as readily as it can from the subfrontal direction, and the preparation can be carried across with opening of the arachnoid along the anterior cerebral arteries, even to expose the carotid of the opposite side from above the chiasm. Much more frequently the carotid of the opposite side has been visualized from beneath a markedly elevated chiasm in the course of the resection of the opposite end of an inner-third tumor.

Transnasal Approach

The clival chordomas begin as epidural lesions and expand anteriorly and posteriorly, often causing large bulges into the nasal and oral pharynx and displacing the dura backward. Locally invasive, they may erode through the dura and go into the subdural space or go through the arachnoid and be truly intracranial tumors. A series of chordomas too large and extensive to remove by the trans-septal trans-sphenoidal route that is normally used for pituitary tumors has now been operated upon by a transnasal approach.[1] For me the transcranial approaches of various types for chordomas have allowed only palliative partial tumor removals. On the other hand, by the transnasal approach a significant percentage of patients have had radical tumor removal without recurrence over the long term, particularly in those tumors that were epidural as well as in some of the tumors that had extended subdurally but had not penetrated the arachnoid.

The contents of the chordoma, frequently covered by destroyed remnants of clival bone, are mucinous, glairy, usually quite soft, and relatively avascular, though there may be a great deal of vascularity in contiguous tissues. Clival meningiomas, on the other hand, are generally highly vascular, frequently fibrous, very rarely soft, virtually always subarachnoid in their extension, and covered with a thickened or at least a normal bone, and they do not lend themselves to a transnasal approach well.

The patient is placed in the same position generally used for trans-septal trans-sphenoidal pituitary surgery with the head supported in the pin headrest and the storage image intensifier in position. The incision is begun at the inner edge of the eyebrow of either eye and carried down around the base of the nose, surrounding both alae and crossing the columella. The incision is carried upward on the opposite side, not quite to the top of the alar fold in order to preserve the alar artery. The incisions are carried into the nasal cavity, and the nose is hinged upward with suture retraction toward the side of the lesser incision. In short, a standard lateral rhinotomy approach has been extended across the midline and up the other side a bit (Fig. 120-7A). The base of the nasal septum is then cut free from the palate all the way back through its free margin. The nasal choanae are widened by opening laterally into the antra. The medial wall of the antrum is removed, usually with the inferior turbinate, although sometimes, if the room is sufficient, these structures may be hinged laterally. The septum is now tilted into the antrum on the same side to which the nose has been reflected. This provides a wide exposure from the sphenoid sinus superiorly all the way down to the second cervical vertebra. No speculum or retractor is used in this exposure. The mucosa of the posterior wall of the nasal and oral pharynx is now opened, usually in the midline, but occasionally as a curvilinear flap, depending upon the extension of the tumor (Fig. 120-7B).

After the surface of the tumor has been exposed, it is dissected up and down and generally cored in order to provide more dissection room so that the carotid artery and jugular sheath on each side may be freed of tumor up to the skull base or to the point where the tumor invades the bone. Removal of the bone with its invaded tumor can now be carried out with cup forceps and punches or, if it is really soft and gelatinous, with hard suction alone. If the tumor is indeed epidural, the resection may reach normal tissue in all directions. The surface of the dura then may be coagulated for further security. If the dura is involved but the arachnoid remains intact, resection of the involved dura, attempting to spare the arachnoid insofar as possible, is carried out. Intra-arachnoid extension that may engulf the basilar artery and its branches and the sixth nerves intracranially has not been successfully handled with adequate removal, although on several occasions the structures have been exposed and tumor removed from their undersurface when they have not been engulfed.

Repair again is carried out with the fascia-muscle-fascia

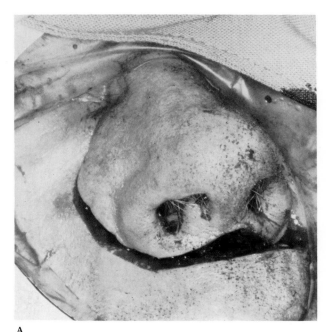

A

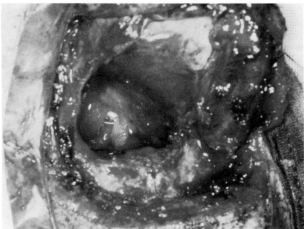

B

Figure 120-7 *A.* Incision for the transnasal approach to a clivus chordoma. A right lateral rhinotomy has been carried across the midline and up the other alar fold. *B.* The nose has been lifted up to the left, the septum cut, the antra opened, the posterior pharyngeal mucosa incised, and the chordoma visualized.

sandwich taken at this time from a previously prepared area of the thigh. Here, the three layers of the repair sandwich are not sutured or otherwise fastened into place but are merely tucked into position, with the innermost layer intradural and the outermost layer on the surface of the remaining clival bone. The pharyngeal mucosa is now closed with sutures of an absorbable material, providing some support and coverage for the fascial grafts. Since the graft is large in area and the mucosa is thin, this would rarely be adequate on its own, and thus it is supported by nasal packing. The septum is replaced in the midline, and the nasal packing is then placed bilaterally. The septal position is supported with just a few sutures at the junction of the septum and the anterior palatal spine. Closure of the skin incision is carried out with fine absorbable subcuticular sutures and a minimum number of nonabsorbable skin sutures in order to assure the best cosmetic result.

Combined Suboccipital-Subtemporal or Petrosal Approach

The vein of Labbé has been a major factor in the determination of posterior subtemporal and transtentorial operations. While the vein of Labbé has been called the great anastomotic vein by anatomists, I know of no vein within the head that so regularly produces hemorrhagic venous infarction when it is occluded. We have learned that the vein of Labbé must be preserved regardless of how good the collateral flow may appear angiographically. Accordingly, I designed a procedure to preserve the vein of Labbé and allow a wide petrosal approach. I first carried out this technique in 1970 and have since used it more than 50 times for clival, clivotentorial, and basilar tumors, mostly for meningiomas but also for epidermoids, dermoids, trigeminal neuromas, hemangiopericytomas, sarcomas, and intra-arachnoid chordomas, and occasionally for midbrain astrocytomas with

exophytic extension. A preoperative CT scan of a clivotentorial meningioma is shown in Fig. 120-8A and a corresponding postoperative scan in Fig. 120-8B.

The scalp incision begins medial and inferior to the mastoid process, goes up behind and above the ear, and turns forward to the anterior hairline above the brow and then backward and downward to curve back to the zygoma in front of the tragus. This large scalp flap is turned downward almost to the external auditory canal, and the posterior fossa portion is exposed very much as it would be for an angle tumor. The mastoid process is removed, and the bone resection is carried completely across the sigmoid sinus and up across the lateral sinus. Now, the dura is separated and a high-speed craniotome is used to turn the temporal portion of the flap and hinge it forward on the temporal muscle. This exposes the lateral and sigmoid sinus at their junction. Then the dura is opened in a curved flap with its base medially in the posterior fossa, coming just beneath the line of the lateral sinus, and the temporal dura is opened parallel to the base, extending backward over the first anterior centimeter of the lateral sinus. The entrance of the vein of Labbé from the temporal lobe is posterior to this point on the lateral sinus.

Now the tentorium can be visualized from below and from above, and suture-ligatures are used to doubly ligate the lateral sinus between the entrance of the vein of Labbé posteriorly and the sigmoid sinus and petrosal sinus anteri-

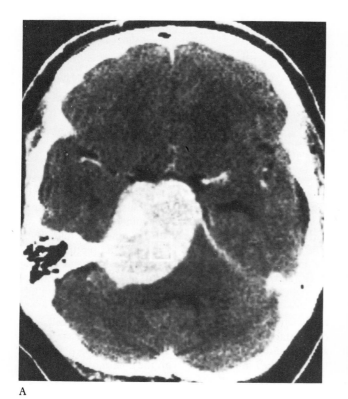

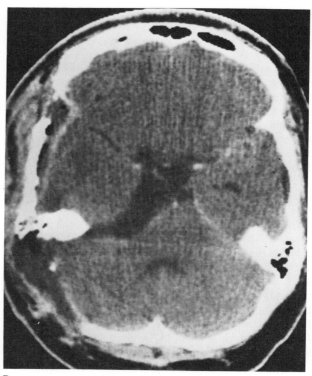

A   B

Figure 120-8 *A.* Preoperative CT scan of a clivotentorial meningioma. *B.* CT scan several days after surgery, verifying tumor removal and providing a baseline for follow-up scans. The scan shows the extent of the craniotomy and craniectomy. There is a fluid lake where the tumor had been. A few air bubbles are unabsorbed under the flap.

Figure 120-9 Right-sided approach, vertex up. Combined suboccipital, subtemporal petrosal approach. The lateral sinus has been ligated at its junction with the sigmoid sinus and divided, with the division carried forward along the petrous pyramid through the free edge of the tentorium. The self-retaining retractor elevates the tentorium with the temporal lobe and the vein of Labbé. The vein of Labbé continues to drain through the lateral sinus across through the torcular and out through the opposite lateral sinus. The anterior and superior surface of the cerebellum and the clivus can now be visualized.

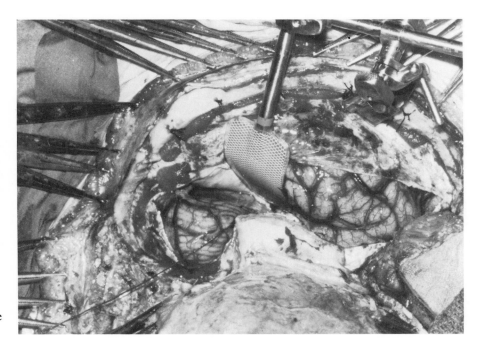

orly. The sinus is now divided, and the tentorium can be divided along the petrosal apex a few millimeters from the bone so as to avoid the petrosal sinus. This part of the division is carried out under the microscope with a retractor placed above the cerebellum on the undersurface of the tentorium, which lifts the tentorium, the lateral sinus, the temporal lobe, and the vein of Labbé together. After the incision goes through the free margin of the tentorium, the exposure is now quite wide from well forward subtemporally, extending all the way down the clivus toward the foramen magnum (Fig. 120-9). The vein of Labbé is able now to drain through the medial part of the lateral sinus, across the torcular, and then through the opposite lateral and sigmoid sinus down through the opposite jugular vein.

It is, of course, essential to know that the two lateral sinuses join through the torcular and that the jugular vein of the opposite side is indeed open. There have been several patients in whom all of the venous drainage from the sagittal sinus was to a single lateral sinus with no communication across to the other lateral sinus. Of course, with this anomaly this procedure is contraindicated. Additionally, patients have been referred for this approach after previous posterior fossa operation had failed to achieve complete removal of the tumor, only to find that the previous approach had led to a lateral sinus occlusion, making this technique impossible. Good bilateral venous phases of angiography are therefore required prior to planning this operative procedure.

For the clivotentorial meningiomas, the incision along the petrosal sinus may run into tumor at the petrous apex and then will be curved up toward the tentorial apex to whatever extent is necessary to cut through free tentorium. Again, coring of the tumor is essential since many of these tumors rise high up under the brain stem, deforming it, and having the seventh and eighth nerves curved backward and downward behind the tumor while the fifth nerve is frequently pressed down to the posterior fossa floor, perhaps

even overlapping or touching the sixth nerve. Depending on the point of origin, the fifth nerve might be pushed upward and backward. In any case, the bringing down of the superior medial capsule is carried out by coring the tumor rather than attempting to retract or dissect around the tumor until the room has been achieved by dropping the superior surface of the tumor with its coring internally. Again, this is done with the bipolar coagulator as the major tool to shrink down and necrotize bits of the tumor. Blood supply to these tumors arising from the petrous apex and clivus and the medial tentorial margin often comes from multiple sources, although usually it is from the anteroinferior aspect of the tumor. These vessels are the tentorial meningeal artery, the meningohypophyseal branches of the carotid artery, the middle meningeal artery, and, surprisingly, branches of the ophthalmic artery that turn backward and run along the cavernous dura, very much like a tentorial meningeal artery. Devascularization of these tumors is achieved by coring close to the dura, as deeply as feasible, and then taking down the more medial portions. Again, after partial devascularization, the use of the Cavitron ultrasonic surgical aspirator may speed up the resection.

Frequently these tumors have respected the membrane of Liliequist and have lifted the apex of the basilar artery backward, stretching the superior cerebellar and posterior cerebral arteries of the larger side, which is the side of approach, much higher than the arteries of the other side, and permitting a view of the pituitary stalk from behind through the stretched membrane of Liliequist above the posterior clinoids (Fig. 120-10). For most of these tumors it has regularly been possible to take the tumor down after adequate coring, from the membrane of Liliequist, from the opposite third nerve, from the opposite superior cerebellar and posterior cerebral arteries, and from the basilar artery, as well as from the structures of the more involved side. Occasionally, the membrane of Liliequist is involved, and the dissection

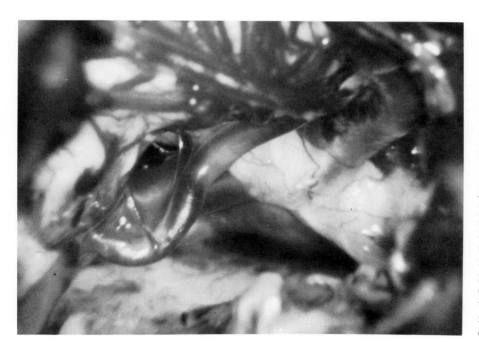

Figure 120-10 The patient, sitting in the same position as in the previous figure, is shown after clivotentorial tumor removal. At the left edge of the photograph, the basilar artery can be seen coming up into the field along the pons, branching into the posterior cerebral and superior cerebellar arteries. The third nerve is flattened and thinned out over the posterior cerebral artery where the tumor had compressed it. The fourth nerve can be seen at the upper right corner of the photograph, running along the line of the posterior cerebral artery. Inferiorly, the posterior clinoids are visible, separated from the third nerve by the membrane of Liliequist.

may follow along the posterior communicating arteries, the optic tracts, and the carotid arteries bilaterally.

Unfortunately, unlike the tumors of the anterior or middle fossa, a clival tumor that engulfs blood vessels is rarely truly separable. When the basilar artery is engulfed within such a meningioma, the perforating vessels are essentially not able to be spared and multiple neural structures will be engulfed as well. Accordingly, when in the course of the dissection one finds that major vessels and nerves are totally within the tumor in the posterior fossa, it nearly always means that the operation will have to be terminated without further attempt at completion of the resection lest unacceptable damage or fatality occur. There are occasional exceptions, and if it is clear that tumor separates readily from engulfed vessels, the procedure may be continued. Rather strikingly, those tumors in which this has been feasible have separated readily even from the very first engulfed vessel, so that they were demonstrably operable all along.

For the fifth nerve neuromas, which may be of very large size in the posterior fossa and in the subtemporal region, the procedure is significantly easier. Their vascularity is regularly less, the Cavitron aspirator can be used more readily to debulk the tumor, and the capsule can be brought down with the posterior fossa portion separated from the brain stem and the posteriorly displaced seventh and eighth nerves and from the basilar artery. Within the temporal fossa, such tumors tend to vastly expand Meckel's cave. The ones that are larger in the posterior fossa tend to end in the foramen ovale and rarely go forward through the cavernous sinus into the superior orbital fissure involving the first division of the fifth nerve, although when this does occur, it is possible to carry out this entire dissection through the same approach. The fourth nerve will frequently be sacrificed in such patients, but the other neural and vascular structures can generally be preserved.

A special word need be said for the clival cholesteatomas,

where the tumors go deeper into the cerebellar fissures and must be approached in many directions since there will be hidden masses of tumor surprisingly well concealed. In these tumors, displacements of vessels and nerves are far less than the size of the tumor, which engulfs all structures in its path. Totally avascular, they may be emptied piecemeal, and then the membrane from which the desquamated flakes are produced may be peeled progressively from all of the involved structures. The membrane looks like slightly thickened arachnoid but is separable from the arachnoid, and, indeed, both arachnoid and membrane may be taken together. Use of small platinum stainless razorblade bits working against the counterpressure of microsuction or fine forceps often permits this dissection to follow out along engulfed vascular branches or neural structures without stretching or tearing. In other areas, allowing the gentle spring tension of the opening force of microforceps separates the membrane gently enough to permit its resection. This is probably the only tumor where I do not core with the bipolar coagulator, nor do I use the Cavitron ultrasonic aspirator through fear of taking a nerve or blood vessel within the mass.

Secondary Operations

A final word about secondary operations. Many of these more difficult tumors, particularly if they are reasonably well encapsulated and do not engulf major vessels, can be successfully removed even at secondary procedures. On the other hand, meningiomas, after partial removal, may fungate outward and both engulf and scar, making their separation from vital structures impossible. In the cholesteatomas, for example, what would have been a painstaking, lengthy, meticulous but utterly reasonable operative procedure may become impossible because of scarring in an area where partial membrane removal has been previously carried out. Secondary procedures are less likely to be successful in terms of achieving cure, and they will, indeed, carry a higher morbidity and mortality and will require a great deal more time for their consummation even if they can be carried out. It is therefore incumbent to be as diagnostically accurate as possible in advance; and it is necessary to know (as much as can be ascertained with reasonable cost effectiveness) the full extent of the tumor, its nature, and its blood supply. The operative decision should include the full knowledge both of the features of the tumor and of the special capabilities and experience in microtechnique required for a successful approach. This is particularly important since secondary procedures are so much more difficult.

References

1. Decker RE, Malis LI: Surgical approaches to midline lesions at the base of the skull. J Mt Sinai Hosp 37:84–102, 1970.
2. Derome PJ: The transbasal approach to tumors invading the base of the skull, in Schmidek HH, Sweet WH (eds): *Current Techniques in Operative Neurosurgery.* New York, Grune & Stratton, 1977, pp 223–245.
3. Malis LI: Tumors of the parasellar region. Adv Neurol 15:281–299, 1976.
4. Malis LI: Prevention of neurosurgical infection by intraoperative antibiotics. Neurosurgery 5:339–343, 1979.
5. Parkinson D: A surgical approach to the cavernous portion of the carotid artery. J Neurosurg 23:474–483, 1965.
6. Stern WE: Meningiomas in the cranio-orbital junction. J Neurosurg 38:428–437, 1973.

SECTION M

Miscellaneous Intracranial Tumors

121

Primary Lymphoma of the Central Nervous System

Milam E. Leavens
John T. Manning
Sidney Wallace
Moshe H. Maor
William S. Velasquez

Primary lymphomas of the central nervous system (CNS) are malignant neoplasms of lymphocytic derivation which are localized to the CNS, at least on initial presentation. The possibility of systemic lymphoma must be excluded by clinical staging or by autopsy. The synonyms that have been used to denote primary lymphoma of the nervous system include malignant lymphoma, non-Hodgkin's lymphoma, reticulum cell sarcoma, microgliomatosis, microglioma, reticulum cell sarcoma–microgliomatosis, perithelial sarcoma, perivascular sarcoma, reticuloendothelial cell sarcoma, malignant reticulosis, malignant reticuloendotheliosis, histiocytic lymphoma, immunoblastic sarcoma, and granulomatous encephalitis.

Incidence

Primary and secondary lymphomas in the CNS are rare entities. In a review of the pathological material obtained from 8,070 patients with brain tumors, Kernohan and Uihlein found that only 40 (0.5 percent) of the patients had reticu-

lum cell sarcoma or lymphoma of the brain.[32] Freeman et al. reported that 23 (0.18 percent) of 12,447 lymphoma patients had primary lymphoma in the CNS, and Henry et al. reported 83 (0.7) similar patients among 11,712 lymphoma patients in the Armed Forces Institute of Pathology files.[13,24] CNS lymphoma was primary in 8 (7.6 percent) of 105 patients with non-Hodgkin's CNS lymphoma reported by Mackintosh et al.[40] The incidence of secondary lymphoma in the CNS in 592 patients with non-Hodgkin's lymphoma was found to be 9 percent according to Levitt et al.[37] The lymphoma involvement of the CNS in those patients was in the meninges in 4 percent, in the epidural space in 3.3 percent, and in the parenchyma of the brain in 1.3 percent.

Location and Gross Pathology

Primary CNS lymphomas occur in all areas of the brain;[8,36,53] however, primary lymphomas of the spinal cord are extremely rare.[7,30,44,53,62] The cerebral hemispheres are the most commonly involved sites, but the basal ganglia, thalamus, brain stem, and cerebellum are all sites of occurrence. A solitary mass was the most common lesion in some series,[8,36] whereas a high incidence of multifocal or diffuse involvement has been emphasized by others.[4,39,62] A predilection toward involvement of the corpus callosum has been found by some.[4,27,53] "Butterfly tumors," involving the corpus callosum and extending symmetrically and bilaterally into the perivascular and deep white matter of the cerebral hemispheres, have been frequent in some series.[9,27]

A common gross appearance is a gray-pink, homogeneous, circumscribed mass that is firmer than the surrounding brain parenchyma. The appearance and texture will be more heterogeneous if necrosis, hemorrhage, or cavitation is present. The tumor mass is usually surrounded by marked edema in the region of the brain involved. This pattern of brain involvement produces a mass lesion effect with increased intracranial pressure, midline displacement, and herniation of brain structures.[8,33] A less common gross appearance is an ill-defined area that looks swollen but lacks a distinct tumor mass.[1,4,62]

Microscopic Pathology

The central part of the tumor mass is characterized by high cellularity. Necrosis may be present. Diffuse infiltration of the parenchyma for some distance beyond the grossly evident tumor has often been emphasized.[4,12,24,49] The infiltrating tumor cells at the advancing edge often have a strikingly perivascular orientation. Infiltration and distention of perivascular (Virchow-Robin) spaces is a highly characteristic feature which is usually most easily seen near the tumor border (Fig. 121-1). Perivascular cuffing of lymphoma cells is associated with an increase of reticulin, which appears as concentric rings in reticulin stained sections.[24,49] Some investigators interpret this as evidence of the perivascular origin of the tumors and refer to these neoplasms as perithelial or perivascular sarcomas.[2,24] While it is a helpful diagnostic feature, vascular and perivascular infiltration is not specific for lymphoma; granulocytic sarcoma (myeloblastoma) can infiltrate in exactly the same manner.

Besides perivascular extension, diffuse parenchymal, leptomeningeal, and subpial spread are characteristic, and the choroid plexus may be involved.[24,49,53] Reactive gliosis may be prominent either at the periphery or in the center of the tumor.

The majority of primary CNS lymphomas are classifiable as diffuse, large cell lymphomas and are essentially indistinguishable from lymphomas of the same type arising in lymph nodes or extranodal sites outside the CNS (Fig. 121-2). There are, however, several notable differences between the relative occurrence rates of lymphomas of histological types originating within and types originating outside the CNS. A larger percentage of lymphomas arising in the CNS, particularly those arising in association with primary or acquired immunodeficiency, appear to be B-cell immunoblastic sarcomas.[14,41,58] Another difference is the absence in the CNS of nodular (follicular) lymphoma, a type of non-Hodgkin's lymphoma that is common outside the CNS.[22,30,36,58] And third, examples of Hodgkin's disease restricted to the CNS are rare or nonexistent.[30,36,58] Although such cases were reported in earlier series with some

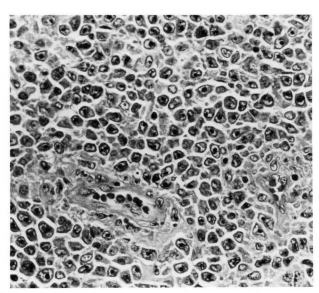

Figure 121-2　Same case as Figure 121-1. Diffuse, large cell lymphoma (B-immunoblastic sarcoma) of the brain, with high cellularity in the central area of the left posterior frontal lobe mass. The plasmacytoid features of the tumor cells are apparent (H & E, ×380).

frequency, most if not all were probably B-cell immunoblastic sarcomas.[36,56,58]

Lymphomas having the histological features of undifferentiated Burkitt's lymphoma or lymphoblastic (convoluted cell) lymphoma have been reported.[17,22,30,58]

Terminology and Origin

A semantic disagreement over terminology existed for a number of years, and even today there is considerable lack of uniformity in reporting cases. Bailey provided perhaps the earliest description of these tumors and regarded them as perivascular sarcomas and perithelial sarcomas, for reasons mentioned above.[2] Yuile considered them to be indistinguishable from reticulum cell sarcomas originating outside the CNS, and preferred that term.[61] Kinney and Adams also preferred that term and thought that such tumors originated from primitive reticulum cells.[33] Russell and other British pathologists were impressed by the affinity of tumor cells for the silver carbonate stain, which they regarded as being specific for microglia. They argued that *reticulum cell sarcoma* was not appropriate, since the primitive reticulum cell should not show affinity for the silver carbonate stain, and thought *microgliomatosis* to be a more accurate name.[50] Burstein et al. concluded that the dispute was basically one of semantics caused by different interpretations given to the term *reticulum cell*, since both sides agreed that the tumors were derived from brain histiocytes. They therefore proposed *reticuloendothelial cell sarcoma* as a name denoting the basic histiocytic nature of the tumors.[8] Rubinstein preferred the term *reticulum cell sarcoma–microglioma* as a better compromise.[49]

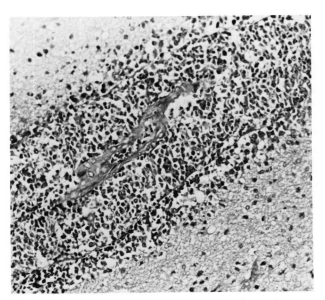

Figure 121-1　Tumor cells infiltrate the perivascular (Virchow-Robin) space at the periphery of the lesion (H & E, ×150).

An assumption made by workers on both sides of the dispute was that these tumors derived from the reticular component of the reticuloendothelial (lymphoreticular) system and not from lymphocytes, since only the former were intrinsic to the CNS. In the light of modern knowledge it is now apparent that this assumption was incorrect. Virtually all lymphomas, including those restricted to the CNS, derive from lymphocytes. Intracytoplasmic immunoglobulin has been demonstrated in a high percentage of primary CNS lymphomas by immunoperoxidase staining of tissue sections for light and heavy chains, and primary lymphoma cell suspensions and cell cultures have shown B-lymphocyte membrane markers.[2,27,45] Electron microscopy has shown them to have the ultrastructural features of immunoblasts.[59]

The terms *reticulum cell sarcoma*, *microglioma*, and *microgliomatosis* are therefore all inappropriate in view of current knowledge. *Histiocytic lymphoma*, a term still in wide usage among experienced hemopathologists, is also misleading since very few of these lymphomas are of histiocytic derivation.[60] To this date, lymphocyte marker studies of primary intracranial lymphomas have not shown any to be T-cell lymphomas.[45]

The high reported incidence of CNS lymphomas in renal transplant recipients and in patients with primary immunodeficiency diseases has recently generated considerable interest about the cause of these tumors.[3,14,23,46,47,54] It has been proposed that the various lymphoproliferative disorders occurring in individuals with primary and acquired immunodeficiency are caused by proliferation of B lymphocytes infected by Epstein-Barr virus (EBV).[48,51] EBV, the B-lymphocytotrophic herpes virus, is the cause of infectious mononucleosis (IM). During acute EBV infection the B-lymphocytic proliferation is controlled by, and EBV forced into latency in large part by, the cell-mediated (T-lymphocyte) immune system, as well as by specific antibodies to viral-related antigens and possibly by natural killer cell activity.[50,51] Viral genomes remain present in the B-lymphocytes of asymptomatic seropositive individuals, and immortal lymphoblastoid cell lines can be readily established from the blood of such individuals.[16,51] There is now substantial evidence that the lymphoproliferative disorders (fatal IM and malignant lymphoma) occurring after renal transplantation in patients with X-linked lymphoproliferative syndrome and in other diverse types of immunodeficiency are caused by EBV infection (either primary or reactivation).[21,48,51] Following renal transplantation, patients develop high antibody titers to EBV and shed large numbers of virus particles in their oropharyngeal secretions. Tumor biopsy specimens from renal transplant recipients contain lymphoma cells with Epstein-Barr nuclear antigen and EBV genomes.[21] Similarly, the tissues of patients with X-linked lymphoproliferative syndrome, an affliction of young males who are unable to mount an immune response to EBV and who usually die at an early age from a lymphoproliferative process such as IM or immunoblastic sarcoma, as well as the tissues of patients with various other primary immunodeficiency states, contain significant numbers of EBV genomes in their cells.[51] Lymphomas arising in X-linked lymphoproliferative syndrome, in Wiskott-Aldrich syndrome, and in renal transplant recipients all have similar features with regard to histology and type of presentation. Most are

B-cell immunoblastic sarcomas, and they frequently have localized extranodal presentations. There is a high rate of CNS involvement, and the occurrence of primary CNS lymphoma in association with these immunodeficiency states has been reported in a number of instances.[3,14,21,23,41,46-48,51,54] Its occurrence has also been reported in association with other abnormal immune states, such as Waldenström's macroglobulinemia and immunoglobulin A (IgA) deficiency, and in immunosuppressed patients with immunoinflammatory diseases such as necrotizing vasculitis.[18,19,29]

The high rate of CNS occurrence of lymphomas associated with immunodeficiency could be related to the fact that the brain is an immunologically privileged site where the cell-mediated immune response is weak compared to that in other tissues. Such lymphomas could well arise in the systemic tissues but favor growth in the CNS.[10,16] This could also help explain how lymphomas arise in an organ which does not contain lymphatics or lymphoid tissue.

Clinical Characteristics

The clinical presentations of 193 patients have been reported in the literature.[8,12,20,24,27,38,52,53] The presentations of an additional 4 patients treated at our institution have been included for review.

Age and Sex Incidence

The patients studied included 121 males and 76 females. Their ages at the time of diagnosis ranged from 2 months to 90 years. The greatest incidence was in the fourth through sixth decades of life, with a mean age of about 55 years; there was a separate early peak incidence in the first decade.[4,8,12,24,36,53]

Considerable variation in the duration of symptoms prior to diagnosis was detected in these patients. The symptom duration in the majority was 2 to 7 months. Four had symptoms for only 1 to 2 weeks prior to diagnosis. Seven had symptoms ranging from 1 to 20 years. One patient had intermittent depression and diplopia for 20 years before exhibiting progressive neurological symptoms and signs. Still another patient had intermittent neurological complaints over an 8-year period before a definitive diagnosis was made.

Clinical Presentation

The clinical presentations of patients with primary lymphoma in the brain differ due to variations in tumor involvement of the brain and meninges and to variations in the biological behavior of these tumors. The various clinical presentations seen in such patients may be catalogued as follows: (1) symptoms and signs of a rapidly expanding intracranial mass lesion, (2) a clinical course suggestive of encephalitis, (3) a course suggestive of a demyelinating disease, (4) symptoms suggestive of cerebrovascular disease, and (5) symptoms and signs indicative of meningeal involvement by tumor.

An estimated 60 percent of the patients with primary lymphoma of the brain present clinically with a rapidly growing mass lesion in the brain similar to that seen in patients with glioblastoma multiforme or metastatic carcinoma.[52] Such patients usually have a circumscribed lymphoma in the brain surrounded by marked edema; the disease is fatal and its course is relatively rapid.[12] Symptoms and signs indicate raised intracranial pressure, and focal symptoms and signs are indicative of specific site involvement in the brain. Usually, the symptoms and signs are such that a diagnosis of an expanding lesion above or below the tentorium can be made and lateralized correctly.[20]

Approximately 25 percent of the patients with primary lymphoma in the brain have a clinical course that suggests an erroneous diagnosis of either a viral encephalitis or a demyelinating disease. Seven reported patients had a clinical course suggestive of influenza or encephalitis.[8,52] Each patient had several of the following symptoms and signs: fever, chills, vertigo, insomnia, fatigue, malaise, anorexia, sore throat, dizziness, somnolence, lethargy, headache, vomiting, diarrhea, and neck stiffness. Early in the course of the disease, some patients underwent carotid arteriography and pneumoencephalography. Neither of these procedures revealed evidence of an intracranial mass lesion. Spinal fluid pressures were normal; CSF total protein content was elevated; the glucose level was low; there was CSF lymphocytosis; and cultures were negative. Late in the disease, some patients developed specific neurological deficits or symptoms and signs of increased intracranial pressure which led to a diagnosis of a space-occupying intracranial lesion. The duration of symptoms prior to diagnosis varied from 2 weeks to 9 months (mean, 3.4 months). The tumor location varied (temporal lobe, thalamus, frontal and parietal lobes, bilateral frontal lobes and corpus callosum, and cerebellum). In some patients the tumor was diffuse. Two patients had multiple brain lesions.

A few patients, including one of our patients who had primary lymphoma of the brain, had exacerbations and remissions of neurological symptoms for 8 to 20 years, resulting in the erroneous initial diagnosis of a demyelinating disease.[52,53] These patients, 1 to 2 years prior to being diagnosed as having lymphoma in the brain, developed progressive neurological symptoms and signs. One patient had diffuse lymphoma in the brain stem, thalamus, and cerebellar vermis and peduncle. Another patient had a frontal lobe lymphoma.

The clinical course of lymphoma of the brain may simulate cerebrovascular disease in approximately 7 percent of patients.[52] One such patient was 70 years old when she developed aphasia and a right homonymous hemianopsia.[52] Angiography was negative for a mass or abnormal vascularity. Postmortem examination revealed diffuse lymphoma in both frontal lobes, the corpus callosum, the basal ganglia, and the frontal horn of the lateral ventricle.

Primary lymphoma may occur in the meninges and may be manifested by a clinical course similar to that seen in patients with meningeal carcinomatosis or gliomatosis.[53] Patients with such a condition have a clinical course of 4 to 7 months during which they may develop headache, nausea, neck stiffness, multiple cranial nerve palsies, and spinal root and/or spinal cord involvement.

There are a few reports in the literature of the duration of life after appearance of the first symptom in patients with primary lymphoma of the brain who had only supportive care or no treatment at all. Twenty-four patients who did not undergo definitive treatment had symptoms 3 weeks to 21 months (means, 5.6 months) prior to death.[8,52,53] Fifteen similar patients had symptoms an average of 3.3 months prior to death.[24]

Clinical Diagnosis

All patients who have the clinical diagnosis of localized lymphoma in any area should undergo complete staging including basic radiological studies, such as chest radiography and lymphangiography, as well as bone marrow biopsy. Abdominal and pelvic computed tomography (CT) may also add valuable information about the status of mesenteric and retrocrural nodes not visualized by lymphangiography. Any suspicious peripheral nodes should be biopsied to confirm and complement the histological diagnosis. Systemic chemotherapy treatment will be needed if other sites of involvement are present.[26,31]

The cerebrospinal fluid is usually abnormal in patients with central nervous system lymphoma. Increased pressure and protein content (58 to 900 mg/100 ml) are common. The white blood cell count may be normal but is usually higher in cases of encephalitic or meningeal symptomatology. In this latter group, CSF sugar levels may be found to be below the normal range (0 to 36 mg/100 ml).

Cytological examination of the spinal fluid is essential and may reveal the presence of malignant lymphoma, with a sensitivity level of 50 to 70 percent.[26,40] Repeat CSF examinations are required in many patients before a positive diagnosis is made.[6,40] The determination of beta-2-microglobulin has proved to be of value in evaluating lymphoma patients. A level of beta-2-microglobulin which is higher in CSF than in serum has correlated well with the presence of lymphoma in the CNS.[42] Lumbar puncture is contraindicated in patients suspected of having a brain tumor until an intracranial mass can be ruled out by means of a CT examination.

Radiological Features

A characteristic radiological picture of primary lymphoma of the brain has not as yet evolved. The radiological features naturally reflect the gross and microscopic changes created by the disease.

Conventional radiography of the skull seldom helps to establish a diagnosis. Pneumoencephalography, although rarely employed, might demonstrate a mass effect when the tumor is obvious, as well as distortion of the contour of the ventricular system by subependymal invasion. Cerebral angiography presents a gamut of possible results, which include a negative study; local irregularity, narrowing, or even occlusion of vessels; or an avascular or hypervascular mass. The hypervascularity, described as "shaggy" arteries and veins, is considered characteristic but not pathognomonic.

Computed tomography, although nonspecific, is now the procedure of choice in defining the presence and extent of primary lymphoma of the brain.[55,57] Early in the course of the disease a normal study is not uncommon. An area of decreased attenuation which fails to enhance after the infusion of contrast material may simulate a vascular accident. The area of decreased attenuation may enhance in the center of the lesion with little mass effect. At times a focus of increased attentuation, not necessarily due to hemorrhage, may be present. This area of increased attenuation is usually enhanced after contrast infusion and is usually surrounded by an area of decreased density. Primary lymphoma of the brain may be manifested by a single lesion or by multiple lesions, may invade the corpus callosum and the contralateral hemisphere, and may eventually involve the meninges (Figs. 121-3 and 121-4).

The differential diagnoses include vascular disease, infection, inflammation, parasitic infestation, histiocytosis X, multiple sclerosis, and primary and secondary neoplasms.[34] A primary lymphoma may simulate an infiltrating glioma.

Surgical Treatment

Tumor biopsy, subtotal or total removal, and Ommaya reservoir placement are indicated, depending on the size and location of the lymphoma in the brain and meninges.

Biopsy is indicated in many patients with unresectable tumors in the brain and meninges, or in patients with brain masses or lesions of unknown pathology. Small, deep lesions beneath the motor cortex or speech areas or in the basal

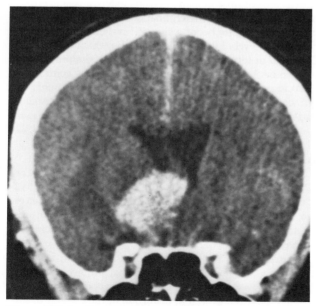

Figure 121-3 Contrast-enhanced CT scan demonstrates an enhancing solitary lymphoma located in the region of the third ventricle, floor of the lateral ventricles, hypothalamus, and base of the frontal lobe. (Courtesy of R.N. Bryan, M.D.)

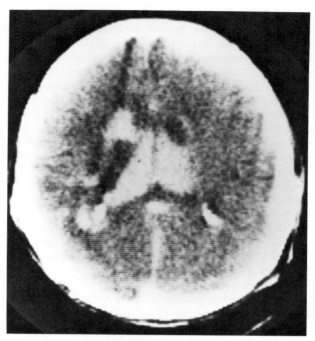

Figure 121-4 Contrast-enhanced CT scan of an enhancing lymphoma located bilaterally in the corpus callosum and periventricular region. (Courtesy of Francis K. Lee, M.D.)

ganglia, thalamus, or brain stem should be biopsied using a sterotactic technique. Patients with tumor believed to involve the meninges, but not so proved with certainty by CSF examination, can be further studied by biopsy of the meninges and cortex, as well as examination of the ventricular fluid at the time of Ommaya reservoir placement.[35] The Ommaya reservoir can be used in such patients for intraventricular chemotherapy and for control of ventricular pressure. Patients whose ventricular pressure cannot be controlled by radiotherapy and chemotherapy may require a shunt procedure.

In some patients, part of the tumor is located in functionally nonsensitive regions of the brain and may cause significant mass effect because of size and surrounding edema. Tumors may also invade regions such as the corpus callosum, speech areas, and posterior frontal regions. These patients may be treated surgically by removing only that part of the tumor which is accessible and causing the mass effect. This should ameliorate increased intracranial pressure and establish a tissue diagnosis.

Either removal of an accessible tumor or tumor biopsy is indicated in order to ascertain a tissue diagnosis in patients with multiple brain tumors. Total removal of a solitary, accessible, and seemingly noninvasive primary lymphoma is advisable.

The results of treating patients who have primary lymphoma in the brain by surgery alone are available in a few reports in the literature.[8,12,24,53] The postoperative survival of 12 patients was between 1 day and 9 months (mean, 1.4 months).[8,12,53] In another report, the mean postoperative survival of 28 patients was 4.6 months.[24] The results are poor and substantiate the opinion that patients with primary lymphoma in the brain require additional postoperative treatment for improved tumor control.

The operative morbidity and mortality can be expected to be high when attempts are made to remove lymphoma which has invaded sensitive and functional areas of the brain. Extensive surgery alone has been responsible for the demise and severe morbidity of many patients.[38] If reasonable criteria for patient selection are utilized, then the operative mortality rate for biopsy and subtotal and total tumor removal should be no greater than 3 to 5 percent.

Radiotherapy

Previous treatment with limited fields and moderate doses of radiation has led to recurrences both in and out of the treatment fields.[38] The multicentricity and the wide invasiveness of this disease dictate the need for whole brain irradiation, including the base of the skull and all cranial meninges. A dose of 4500 rad in 5 weeks (180 rad per day, 5 fractions per week) is delivered to this volume. (An additional dose of 1000 rad in 5 fractions is added to a reduced volume of the known area of the gross tumor.) If the tumor is very infiltrating or there are multiple foci, the whole cranial contents should be treated to 5400 rad in 30 fractions over a 6-week period. Localization of the portal for the boost can be aided by CT scanning.

Elective irradiation of the spinal canal is unjustified at the present as very few patients have evidence of seeding on presentation, and all reported failures are confined to the brain. In the case of spinal metastases as evidenced by clinical symptoms or myelography, the entire canal is treated to the level of S2. The recommended dose for the spinal axis is 3500 rad with a boost of 1000 rad to known areas of gross tumor. If the only evidence of spinal spread is a positive cytology, the surgeon should consider combining cranial irradiation with intrathecal instillation of a chemotherapeutic agent(s).

There are a number of reports in the literature that indicate the value of postoperative radiotherapy in patients with lymphoma in the brain.[8,20,24,38,52,53] Burstein et al. reported the average survival of such patients as 3 years and 9 months.[8] Three were still living 2, 10, and 17 years following treatment.

Ten patients reported by Hanbery and Dugger had postoperative radiotherapy restricted to the region of the neoplasm.[20] They survived 3 to 48 months (mean, 11.7 months). Three patients were still living 3, 13, and 48 months after treatment. Twenty patients reported by Henry et al. survived an average of 15.2 months; one survived 6 years.[24] Schaumburg et al. reported 12 patients who had surgery followed by the delivery of 4,000 rad to the region of the tumor.[53] Ten survived 12 to 67 months (mean, 33 months).

Littman and Wang reported the results of the treatment of 19 patients.[38] Eight patients lived 3 years or more following surgery and radiotherapy. All deaths except one were preceded by deterioration of the patient's neurological status. Necropsy of two patients revealed tumor in the brain but not in the original site. One patient had two recurrences in nonirradiated parts of the brain. Another had received whole brain radiotherapy, plus a boost to the tumor site. At the time of their report, Littman and Wang found in the literature reports of 131 patients with lymphoma in the brain. Of those, only five patients were disease-free survivors for 5 years or longer. All had undergone surgery and had postoperative radiotherapy. Three survived 5 to 10 years. Two were still alive 10 and 17 years following treatment.

Chemotherapy

Advances in chemotherapy have recently led to the development of effective drug therapy for the treatment of relapsing metastatic CNS lymphoma.[5,6,28,40] In patients with solid lymphoma in the brain, chemotherapy is begun 1 month after completion of radiotherapy; in patients with meningeal lymphoma, chemotherapy is given first, and radiotherapy is started 1 month after the initiation of chemotherapy. Methotrexate (MTX) and cytosine arabinoside (Ara-C) are given intrathecally or intraventricularly. The dose of MTX in adults and children is 12 mg/m^2. The maximum dose is 12 mg when the patient's surface area is over 1 m^2.[40] The dose of Ara-C in adults and children is 100 mg/m^2 with the maximum dose being 100 mg.

MTX and Ara-C should be given alternately to diminish the possibility of CNS complications from the treatment. In meningeal or solitary CNS lymphoma, intrathecal or intraventricular MTX or Ara-C is given biweekly until the CSF cell count and protein content are normal, then weekly for 1 month, and then once a month for 2 years. This treatment has been very effective in bringing about complete remissions in most patients with relapsing CNS lymphoma. Only a few patients with primary CNS lymphoma have been treated in this manner. However, its effectiveness in primary CNS lymphoma should be similar to its effectiveness in relapsing CNS lymphoma. High-dose intravenously administered MTX, which reaches therapeutic levels in the CSF, has also been given with good results.[11,25,43]

CNS toxic reactions to therapy with MTX and Ara-C can be serious and include seizures, dementia, and paraplegia.[15] Mackintosh et al. reported that 4 of 11 patients who survived for 1 year had severe functional impairment secondary to therapy.[40]

The relapse rate is high following the treatment of CNS lymphoma. However, survival of patients with CNS lymphoma is expected to improve, as it has in patients with lymphoma localized in other sites, with the use of combined-modality programs which alternate radiotherapy and chemotherapy.

Neuwelt et al. have reported the first successful chemotherapy treatment of CNS lymphoma in which a reversible blood-brain barrier (BBB) opening was used to enhance drug delivery to the tumor.[46a] They treated three patients with primary central nervous system lymphoma with multiple courses of chemotherapy. The patients received intra-arterial (carotid or vertebral artery) 25% mannitol (250 ml) for BBB disruption followed by 500 to 1000 mg of intra-arterial MTX. The chemotherapy courses also included cyclophosphamide (15 mg/kg I.V.) and procarbazine (150 mg/day orally). Leucovorin rescue and dexamethasone were initiated on the day following intra-arterial MTX. These investigators showed that drug (contrast) delivery to the tumor as well as to the surrounding brain is enhanced after BBB modification. They also found that discontinuing steroids prior to BBB disruption increased delivery of the contrast agent to the tumor.

An objective tumor response was obtained in all three patients. One patient was neurologically intact and without evidence of disease 16 months after the onset of symptoms. Another patient had a 50% tumor regression following chemotherapy and a complete tumor regression after radiation treatment but later refused further chemotherapy and died 12 months after diagnosis. The third patient, after two courses of chemotherapy, improved neurologically. A CT scan showed resolution of the tumor in the left basal ganglia, where the tumor had been noted prior to radiotherapy. Morbidity with this technique was low in these three patients. One patient had focal motor seizures due to the iodinated contrast material used to enhance the CT scan during the period the BBB was open. Another patient developed sepsis during a period of leukopenia.

This combination of chemotherapy and BBB opening appears to be an advancement in the treatment of primary lymphoma of the central nervous system. More experience is needed with BBB openings along with better chemotherapy agents for improved survival rates and, hopefully, an eventual cure for patients with such tumors.

References

1. Adams JH: The classification of microgliomatosis with particular reference to diffuse microgliomatosis. Acta Neuropathol [Suppl] (Berl) 6:119–123, 1975.
2. Bailey P: Intracranial sarcomatous tumors of leptomeningeal origin. Arch Surg 18:1359–1402, 1929.
3. Bale JF Jr, Wilson JF, Hill HR: Fatal histiocytic lymphoma of the brain associated with hyperimmunoglobulinemia-E and recurrent infections. Cancer 39:2386–2390, 1977.
4. Barnard RO, Scott T: Patterns of proliferation in cerebral lymphoreticular tumours. Acta Neuropathol [Suppl] (Berl) 6:125–130, 1975.
5. Bleyer WA, Dedrick RL: Clinical pharmacology of intrathecal methotrexate: I. Pharmacokinetics in nontoxic patients after lumbar injection. Cancer Treat Rep 61:703–708, 1977.
6. Borowitz M, Bigner SH, Johnston WW: Diagnostic problems in the cytologic evaluation of cerebrospinal fluid for lymphoma and leukemia. Acta Cytol (Baltimore) 25:665–674, 1981.
7. Bruni J, Bilbao JM, Gray T: Primary intramedullary malignant lymphoma of the spinal cord. Neurology (Minneap) 27:896–898, 1977.
8. Burstein SD, Kernohan JW, Uihlein A: Neoplasms of the reticuloendothelial system of the brain. Cancer 16:289–305, 1963.
9. Ebels EJ: Reticulosarcomas of the brain presenting as butterfly tumors: Possible implications for treatment. Eur Neurol 8:333–338, 1972.
10. Epstein AL, Herman MM, Kim H, Dorfman RF, Kaplan HS: Biology of the human malignant lymphomas: III. Intracranial heterotransplantation in the nude, athymic mouse. Cancer 37:2158–2176, 1976.
11. Ervin T, Canellos GP: Successful treatment of recurrent primary central nervous system lymphoma with high-dose methotrexate. Cancer 45:1556–1557, 1980.
12. Foncin J F, Faucher J N: Primary and borderline brain lymphosarcoma: A neuropathological review of nine cases. Acta Neuropathol [Suppl] (Berl) 6:107–113, 1975.
13. Freeman C, Berg JW, Cutler SJ: Occurrence and prognosis of extranodal lymphomas. Cancer 29:252–260, 1972.
14. Frizzera G, Rosai J, Dehner LP, Spector BD, Kersey JH: Lymphoreticular disorders in primary immunodeficiencies: New findings based on an up-to-date histologic classification of 35 cases. Cancer 46:692–699, 1980.
15. Gagliano RG, Costanzi JJ: Paraplegia following intrathecal methotrexate: Report of a case and review of the literature. Cancer 37:1663–1668, 1976.
16. Giovanella B, Nilsson K, Zech L, Yim O, Klein G, Stehlin JS: Growth of diploid, Epstein-Barr virus–carrying human lymphoblastoid cell lines heterotransplanted into nude mice under immunologically privileged conditions. Int J Cancer 24:103–113, 1979.
17. Giromini D, Peiffer J, Tzonos T: Occurrence of a primary Burkitt-type lymphoma of the central nervous system in an astrocytoma patient. Acta Neuropathol (Berl) 54:165–167, 1981.
18. Gregory MC, Hughes JT: Intracranial reticulum cell sarcoma associated with immunoglobulin A deficiency. J Neurol Neurosurg Psychiatry 36:769–776, 1973.
19. Gunderson CH, Henry J, Malamud N: Plasma globulin determinations in patients with microglioma: Report of five cases. J Neurosurg 35:406–415, 1971.
20. Hanbery JW, Dugger GS: Perithelial sarcoma of the brain: A clinicopathological study of thirteen cases. Arch Neurol Psychiatry 71:732–761, 1954.
21. Hanto DW, Frizzera G, Purtilo DT, Sakamoto K, Sullivan JL, Saemundsen AK, Klein G, Simmons RL, Najarian JS: Clinical spectrum of lymphoproliferative disorders in renal transplant recipients and evidence for the role of Epstein-Barr virus. Cancer Res 41:4253–4261, 1981.
22. Hassoun J, Andrac L, Gambarelli D, Toga M: Lymphomes malins primitifs du systeme nerveux central: Etude anatomoclinique, ultrastructurale et immunocytochimique. A propos de 23 cas. Ann Pathol 1: 193–203, 1981.
23. Heidelberger KP, LeGolvan DP: Wiskott-Aldrich syndrome and cerebral neoplasia: Report of a case with localized reticulum cell sarcoma. Cancer 33:280–284, 1974.
24. Henry JM, Heffner RR Jr, Dillard SH, Earle KM, Davis RL: Primary malignant lymphomas of the central nervous system. Cancer 34:1293–1302, 1974.
25. Herbst KD, Corder MP, Justice GR: Successful therapy with methotrexate of a multicentric mixed lymphoma of the central nervous system. Cancer 38:1476–1478, 1976.
26. Herman TS, Hammond N, Jones SE, Butler JJ, Byrne GE Jr, McKelvey EM: Involvement of the central nervous system by non-Hodgkin's lymphoma: The Southwest Oncology Group experience. Cancer 43:390–397, 1979.
27. Houthoff HJ, Poppema S, Ebels EJ, Elema JD: Intracranial malignant lymphomas: A morphologic and immunocytologic study of twenty cases. Acta Neuropathol (Berl) 44:203–210, 1978.
28. Jacobs A, Clifford P, Kay HEM: The Ommaya reservoir in chemotherapy for malignant disease in the CNS. Clin Oncol 7:123–129, 1981.
29. Jellinger K, Kothbauer P, Weiss R, Sunder-Plassmann E: Primary malignant lymphoma of the CNS and polyneuropathy in a patient with necrotizing vasculitis treated with immunosuppression. J Neurol 220:259–268, 1979.
30. Jellinger K, Radaskiewicz TH, Slowik F: Primary malignant lymphomas of the central nervous system in man. Acta Neuropathol [Suppl] (Berl) 6:95–102, 1975.

31. Jones SE, Grozea PN, Metz EN, Haut A, Stephens RL, Morrison FS, Butler JJ, Byrne GE Jr, Moon TE, Fisher R, Haskins CL, Coltman CA Jr: Superiority of adriamycin-containing combination chemotherapy in the treatment of diffuse lymphoma: A Southwest Oncology Group study. Cancer 43:417–425, 1979.

32. Kernohan JW, Uihlein A: *Sarcomas of the Brain.* Springfield, Ill., Charles C Thomas, 1962.

33. Kinney TD, Adams RD: Reticulum cell sarcoma of the brain. Arch Neurol Psychiatry 50:552–564, 1943.

34. Kolar OJ: Differential diagnostic aspects in malignant lymphomas involving the central nervous system. Acta Neuropathol [Suppl] (Berl) 6:181–186, 1975.

35. Leavens ME, Aldama-Luebert A: Ommaya reservoir placement: Technical note. Neurosurgery 5:264–266, 1979.

36. Letendre L, Banks PM, Reese DF, Miller RH, Scanlon PW, Kiely JM: Primary lymphoma of the central nervous system. Cancer 49:939–943, 1982.

37. Levitt LJ, Dawson DM, Rosenthal DS, Moloney WC: CNS involvement in the non-Hodgkin's lymphomas. Cancer 45:545–552, 1980.

38. Littman P, Wang CC: Reticulum cell sarcoma of the brain. Cancer 35:1412–1420, 1975.

39. Lukin R, Tomsick TA, Chambers AA: Lymphoma and leukemia of the central nervous system. Semin Roentgenol 15:246–250, 1980.

40. Mackintosh FR, Colby TV, Podolsky WJ, Burke JS, Hoppe RT, Rosenfelt FP, Rosenberg SA, Kaplan HS: Central nervous system involvement in non-Hodgkin's lymphoma: An analysis of 105 cases. Cancer 49:586–595, 1982.

41. Matas AJ, Hertel BF, Rosai J, Simmons RL, Najarian JS: Post-transplant malignant lymphoma. Am J Med 61:716–720, 1976.

42. Mavligit GM, Stuckey SE, Cabanillas FF, Keating MJ, Tourtellotte WW, Schold SC, Freireich EJ: Diagnosis of leukemia or lymphoma in the central nervous system by beta$_2$-microglobulin determination. N Engl J Med 303:718–722, 1980.

43. Meadows AT, Evans AE: Effects of chemotherapy on the central nervous system: A study of parenteral methotrexate in long-term survivors of leukemia and lymphoma in childhood. Cancer 37 (Suppl 2):1079–1085, 1976.

44. Mitsumoto H, Breuer AC, Lederman RJ: Malignant lymphoma of the central nervous system: A case of primary spinal intramedullary involvement. Cancer 46:1258–1262, 1980.

45. Miyoshi I, Kubonishi I, Yoshimoto S, Hikita T, Dabasaki H, Tanaka T, Kimura I, Tabuchi K, Nishimoto A: Characteristics of a brain lymphoma cell line derived from primary intracranial lymphoma. Cancer 49:456–459, 1982.

46. Model LM: Primary reticulum cell sarcoma of the brain in Wiskott-Aldrich syndrome: Report of a case. Arch Neurol 34:633–635, 1977.

46a. Neuwelt EA, Balaban E, Diehl J, Hill S, Frenkel E: Successful treatment of primary central nervous system lymphomas with chemotherapy after osmotic blood-brain barrier opening. Neurosurgery 12:662–671, 1983.

47. Pattengale PK, Taylor CR, Panke T, Tatter D, McCormick RA, Rawlinson DG, Davis RL: Selective immunodeficiency and malignant lymphoma of the central nervous system. Acta Neuropathol (Berl) 48:165–169, 1979.

48. Purtilo DT: Epstein-Barr-virus–induced oncogenesis in immune-deficient individuals. Lancet 1:300–303, 1980.

49. Rubinstein LJ: *Tumors of the Central Nervous System.* Washington, D.C. Armed Forces Institute of Pathology, 1972, pp 215–234.

50. Russell DS, Marshall AHE, Smith FB: Microgliomatosis: A form of reticulosis affecting the brain. Brain 71:1–15, 1948.

51. Saemundsen AK, Purtilo DT, Sakamoto K, Sullivan JL, Synnerholm A C, Hanto D, Simmons R, Anvret M, Collins R, Klein G: Documentation of Epstein-Barr virus infection in immunodeficient patients with life-threatening lymphoproliferative diseases by Epstein-Barr virus complementary RNA/DNA and viral DNA/DNA hybridization. Cancer Res 41:4237–4242, 1981.

52. Samuelsson SM, Werner I, Ponten J, Nathorst-Windahl G, Thorell J: Reticuloendothelial (perivascular) sarcoma of the brain. Acta Neurol Scand 42:567–580, 1966.

53. Schaumburg HH, Plank CR, Adams RD: The reticulum cell sarcoma–microglioma group of brain tumours: A consideration of their clinical features and therapy. Brain 95:199–212, 1972.

54. Schneck SA, Penn I: De-novo brain tumours in renal-transplant recipients. Lancet 1:983–986, 1971.

55. Scully RE, Mark EJ, McNeely BU: Case records of the Massachusetts General Hospital. N Engl J Med 307:359–368, 1982.

56. Sparling HJ Jr, Adams RD: Primary Hodgkin's sarcoma of the brain. Arch Pathol 42:338–344, 1946.

57. Tadmor R, Davis KR, Roberson GH, Kleinman GM: Computed tomography in primary malignant lymphoma of the brain. J Comput Assist Tomogr 2:135–140, 1978.

58. Taylor CR, Russell R, Lukes RJ, Davis RL: An immunohistological study of immunoglobulin content of primary central nervous system lymphomas. Cancer 41:2197–2205, 1978.

59. Varadachari C, Palutke M, Climie ARW, Weise RW, Chason JL: Immunoblastic sarcoma (histiocytic lymphoma) of the brain with B cell markers: Case report. J Neurosurg 49:887–892, 1978.

60. Warnke R, Miller R, Grogan T, Pederson M, Dilley J, Levy R: Immunologic phenotype in 30 patients with diffuse large-cell lymphoma. N Engl J Med 303:293–300, 1980.

61. Yuile CL: Case of primary reticulum cell sarcoma of the brain. Relationship of microglia cells to histiocytes. Arch Pathol 26:1036–1044, 1938.

62. Zimmerman HM: Malignant lymphomas of the nervous system. Acta Neuropathol [Suppl] (Berl) 6:69–74, 1975.

122

Intracranial Sarcomas

J. F. Ross Fleming
John H. N. Deck
Mark Bernstein

Primary intracranial sarcomas are uncommon, representing only 1 to 2 percent of all intracranial neoplasms. Because this group of tumors is so rare, and because there are several subgroups of sarcomas, their nature has not been well understood. Early classifications were somewhat confusing and included several tumors that are no longer considered to be sarcomas.

The commonest intracranial sarcoma that a neurosurgeon is likely to encounter is gliosarcoma, which is a sarcoma arising in continuity with a malignant glioma and occurring in up to 8 percent of malignant gliomas. The next most common intracranial sarcoma is primary sarcoma arising de novo in the brain and meninges; this sarcoma is exceedingly rare, and occurs most commonly in infants and children. In this chapter we present a simple working classification of intracranial sarcomas and review their pathological features. The clinical features and management will be reviewed briefly, although most of the clinical features of intracranial sarcomas are shared by other more common malignant neoplasms and are not particularly distinctive.

Classification

Intracranial sarcomas may be classified according to their origin as (1) sarcomas arising in the brain and meninges, (2) primary sarcomas of the skull, or (3) metastatic sarcomas of the brain, secondary to primary sarcomas elsewhere in the body. Only sarcomas arising in the brain and meninges will be covered in this chapter.

Sarcomas of the brain and meninges are those malignant tumors which arise from the mesenchymal tissues present within the cranial cavity, that is, from dura mater, from pia-arachnoid, from blood vessels of the subarachnoid space and brain, and from the tela choroidea. These sarcomas can be classified into four groups.

A. Primary sarcoma of the brain and meninges arising de novo
   1. Fibrosarcoma
   2. Spindle cell sarcoma
   3. Polymorphic cell sarcoma
   4. Variants (better differentiated cell types)
B. Sarcoma arising in continuity with a malignant glioma (gliosarcoma)
C. Sarcoma arising in a meningioma
D. Sarcoma arising after cranial irradiation

Sarcomas arising from the skull and presenting as intracranial tumors are excluded from this chapter; they are discussed separately in another chapter. Also excluded from this chapter are the rare sarcomas which are metastatic to the brain; these tumors have few clinical features to distinguish them from other metastatic tumors and they are discussed elsewhere. Lymphomas of the brain, formerly referred to as reticulum cell sarcomas, are highly distinctive tumors which share few features with the non lymphoreticular sarcomas; they are therefore excluded from this chapter and are discussed in another chapter. Also excluded are the rare examples of malignant tumors arising from cranial nerves, such as malignant schwannomas and neurofibrosarcomas.

There are, in addition, some highly undifferentiated tumors that in the past were classified as sarcomas by some pathologists, but for which alternative designations are now widely preferred. These tumors include the "circumscribed sarcoma of the cerebellum" and "monstrocellular sarcoma". The circumscribed sarcoma of the cerebellum was classified as a sarcoma because of its prominent reticulin formation; however, it is now generally accepted as a subtype of medulloblastoma that has stimulated leptomeningeal proliferation or desmoplasia. The monstrocellular sarcoma was so called because of the prominence of reticulin and of vascular structures. The nature of its giant cells was quite uncertain until their glial nature was demonstrated by stains for glial fibrillary acidic protein (GFAP); this tumor is now widely accepted as a giant cell variant of glioblastoma multiforme. The use of GFAP as a glial cell marker has resulted in the reclassification of yet another tumor, "meningeal fibrous xanthosarcoma," which has proven to be a pleomorphic xanthoastrocytoma and not a sarcoma.

Primary Sarcoma of the Brain and Meninges

Primary sarcomas arising de novo in the meninges or brain constitute fewer than 1 percent of all intracranial tumors. These tumors tend to occur in children and are extremely rare in adults. The more histologically malignant tumors tend to occur in younger patients. They affect males and females with equal frequency.

These sarcomas form a spectrum of tumors in which the degree of malignancy varies widely. Christensen and Lara have divided them into three histological subgroups of increasing malignancy: fibrosarcoma, spindle cell sarcoma, and polymorphic cell sarcoma.[1] Fibrosarcoma represents a low-grade malignancy, and survival of patients with fibrosarcoma in Christensen and Lara's series averaged 74 months, with occasional very long term survival. Survival of patients with spindle cell sarcoma averaged 27 months, and with polymorphic cell sarcoma it was less than 1 year.

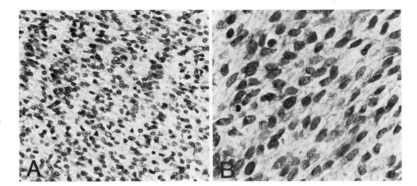

Figure 122-1 Spindle cell sarcoma. Tumor cells are elongated with oval nuclei. Note the streaming pattern and the tendency to palisading of nuclei. Mitotic figures are numerous and stroma is scant. (H & E; original magnifications: *A*, ×10; *B*, ×25.)

Gross and Microscopic Features

A sarcoma usually appears as a discrete mass involving the meninges and compressing and invading the underlying brain. Occasionally, a sarcoma may lie entirely within the brain parenchyma, presumably arising from perivascular pia-arachnoid sheaths. A rare form of sarcoma that occurs exclusively in infants is meningeal sarcomatosis, in which an extensive sheet of highly anaplastic tumor extends widely over the intracranial and spinal dura.

Sarcomas tend to be large, clearly demarcated masses. The fibrosarcomas, especially, may be sufficiently clearly delineated to make gross total surgical removal possible. The production of collagen may give fibrosarcomas a relatively firm texture, whereas the more cellular sarcomas tend to be soft and friable. They are usually homogeneous and pale, and foci of necrosis occur, since vascular stroma is sparse.

The presence of reticulin and a characteristic pattern of infiltration into adjacent brain tissue typify these sarcomas. Fibrosarcomas are firm, with abundant reticulin and collagen, and are moderately cellular with mostly spindle-shaped tumor cells. Spindle cell sarcomas (Fig. 122-1) are more densely cellular, and reticulin is easily demonstrated, but there is less collagen; the cells tend to be arranged in parallel bundles, and microscopic areas of necrosis and pseudopalisades may be seen. Polymorphic cell sarcomas (Fig. 122-2) are the least differentiated and most malignant variant, with highly variable, large, irregularly shaped cells and little stroma; reticulin stroma may be fine or absent, and the tumor is usually very soft and extensively necrotic.

Sarcomas infiltrate the brain in a characteristic way.

Tongues of tumor penetrate irregularly into adjacent parenchyma, and collars of sarcoma cells surround blood vessels; the advancing tumor encompasses distinct islands of neuroglia. Adjacent astrogliosis may be quite marked.

Histological Variants

Rare examples of primary sarcoma of the brain and meninges showing different histological patterns of differentiation have been reported. Such tumors include myxosarcoma (Fig. 122-3), leiomyosarcoma, rhabdomyosarcoma, osteosarcoma, chondrosarcoma, mesenchymal chondrosarcoma, and liposarcoma. Rarely, mixed patterns of differentiation suggest an origin from incompletely differentiated mesenchymal cells, giving rise to the mixed malignant mesenchymoma.

Sarcomas of the brain and meninges often give rise to conspicuous reactive gliosis in adjacent brain tissue. A number of cases have been reported in which the view has been taken that the reactive gliosis has progressed to glial neoplasia. The development of such a "sarcoglioma" must be an extremely rare event. Such a development is very difficult to distinguish from the relatively common and widely accepted development of sarcoma secondary to glioma, termed *gliosarcoma*, a tumor which is discussed below.

Management

The principles for treatment of patients with intracranial sarcomas are the same as those for patients with any malignant intracranial tumor. The goal is surgical removal of all,

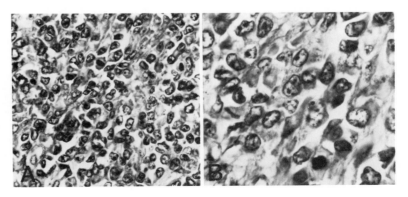

Figure 122-2 Polymorphic cell sarcoma. Tumor cells with scant cytoplasm have highly variable nuclei with a coarse pattern of nuclear chromatin. Mitotic figures are numerous; stroma is scant. Extensive necrosis was present but is not shown in these views. (H & E; original magnifications: *A*, ×25; *B*, ×40.)

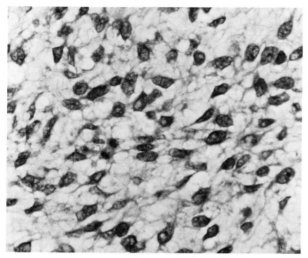

Figure 122-3 Fibrosarcoma with extensive areas of myxoid stroma. This stroma separates tumor cells and the cellularity is thus reduced. The frequent mitotic figures are the principal histological indication of malignancy. (H & E, original ×25.)

or as much as possible, of the tumor, and gross total removal may be achieved in some of the fibrosarcomas. Little but temporary palliation can be achieved in patients with the highly malignant polymorphic cell sarcoma, and meningeal sarcomatosis will run its rapid course in spite of all endeavors to arrest it. There is no definite evidence that radiation therapy or chemotherapy, either alone or in combination, will affect the survival time of patients with intracranial sarcomas, although these treatment measures may be appropriate in the management of some patients.

Sarcoma Arising in Continuity with Malignant Glioma (Gliosarcoma)

One of the cardinal features of glioblastoma multiforme is the presence of hyperplasia of tumor blood vessels with proliferation of both endothelial and adventitial cells. Such vascular hyperplasia is believed to reflect the production of an angiogenic factor by the tumor, and although it is not unique to glioblastoma multiforme, vascular hyperplasia is more prominent in this than in any other brain tumor. The stimulation of vascular proliferation is such that hyperplasia may progress to neoplasia, and the mesenchymal proliferation acquires both the cellular atypia and the aggressive growth characteristic of sarcomatous malignancy. The result is a mixed tumor often known as gliosarcoma. This entity is now generally accepted, and although earlier reports suggested that sarcoma was an uncommon development in glioblastoma, with increased awareness of the process, it is now reported in as many as 8 percent of glioblastomas.[2] Since glioblastoma multiforme is the commonest primary brain tumor and the incidence of sarcoma secondary to it is substantial, sarcomas of the brain occurring in this way represent the great majority of intracranial sarcomas.

Histology

The sarcomatous areas of gliosarcoma usually exhibit a pattern of spindle-shaped cells with reticulin formation, and glial cells are lacking. Two distinct but intermingled tumor patterns are thus produced (Fig. 122-4), a gliomatous pattern and a sarcomatous pattern. The gliomatous component consists of astrocytes which are readily identified by GFAP stains and by the absence of reticulin and collagen. The sarcomatous component is rich in reticulin and collagen but is

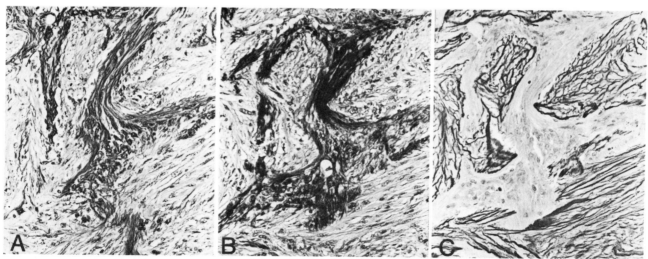

Figure 122-4 Gliosarcoma. Identical fields from three serial sections of the tumor are stained as follows: *A*, PTAH; *B*, GFAP; *C*, reticulin. Dark-staining areas are composed of astrocytes rich in glial fibrils which are PTAH positive (*A*) and GFAP positive (*B*). *C.* The astrocytic areas are pale, since they are devoid of reticulin. (Original ×10.)

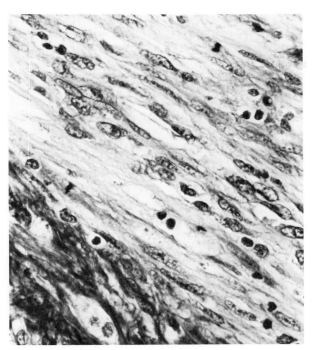

Figure 122-5 Gliosarcoma. High-power view of sarcoma showing streaming pattern of somewhat pleomorphic spindle-shaped cells and numerous mitotic figures. (H & E, original ×25.)

devoid of GFAP–positive cells. Cellular atypia and mitotic figures are prominent in both areas, since both are malignant tumor patterns (Fig. 122-5). Occasionally, the intimate admixture of glioma and sarcoma produces such a confusing histological picture that the sarcomatous tumor may be completely overlooked. The amount of collagen in the sarcoma is variable but is usually sufficient to produce a tumor of quite firm consistency. The sarcoma may become the dominant tumor and overgrow the glioma, so that the pre-existing glioma may become obscured. Gliosarcoma is much more prone to metastasize to extracranial sites (such as the liver and lung) than the original glioblastoma. The metastases may contain either the gliomatous or the sarcomatous elements or both.

Variants

The majority of sarcomas arising in continuity with gliomas exhibit no specialized differentiation and can be described as spindle cell sarcomas or fibrosarcomas. However, smooth muscle differentiation may occur, and myofibrils in the cytoplasm that stain positively with phosphotungstic acid hematoxylin (PTAH) may easily be mistaken for glial fibrils, which also stain positively with PTAH; this error in interpretation was almost unavoidable prior to the advent of GFAP stains. The development of leiomyosarcoma may well reflect the participation of smooth muscle cells from the vascular media in the neoplastic process.

The development of chondroid or osteoid differentiation within the sarcoma is much less common. Here, the cartilage and bone exhibit the malignant features of chondrosarcoma and osteosarcoma and are thought to represent a type of metaplasia of the sarcomatous cells (Fig. 122-6).

Clinical Features

The clinical features of gliosarcoma are similar to those of anaplastic astrocytoma or glioblastoma multiforme. As with glioblastoma there is a slight male predominance; in 24 patients with gliosarcoma reviewed by Morantz et al. there were 14 men and 10 women ranging in age from 37 to 68 years.[2] Gliosarcomas occur more often in the temporal lobe

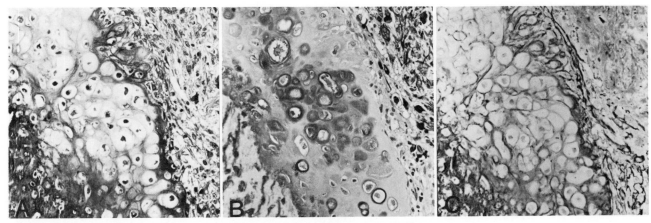

Figure 122-6 Gliosarcoma showing chondroid and osteoid differentiation. The astrocytic component of the tumor is on the right in each picture. Identical fields from three serial sections of the tumor are stained as follows: *A*, Masson's trichrome; *B*, GFAP; *C*, reticulin. *B*. Astrocytes in the upper right stain darkly for GFAP. The dark staining of bone and cartilage is due to the hematoxylin counterstain. *C*. The absence of reticulin in the astrocytic tumor is noted at the upper right (Original ×10).

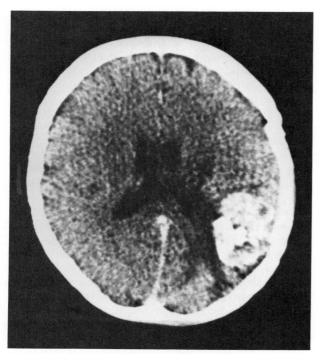

Figure 122-7 An enhanced CT scan of a 35-year-old female. The first symptom was a seizure 4 years before her first operation. A partial removal of an anaplastic astrocytoma was performed, followed by radiation therapy. The tumor recurrence (2 years later), as shown here, was a gliosarcoma.

than in any other part of the brain; in 10 of the 24 patients, the tumor was confined to the temporal lobe, and in another 4 a substantial portion was in the temporal lobe; 6 tumors were parietal and 4 were frontal. This temporal predominance is confirmed in other published series, and is not seen in glioblastoma. CT scans of typical gliosarcomas are shown in Figures 122-7 and 122-8.

The diagnosis of gliosarcoma was first made at the time of a repeat craniotomy done for the removal of a tumor recurrence in several of our own cases; in these cases, the diagnosis at the initial operation had been glioblastoma multiforme; upon review of some cases, however, sarcomatous features could be found in the tissue that had been removed at the initial operation. In other cases, it is possible that the sarcomatous change had not yet occurred at the time of the first operation, or that the tissue biopsied was remote from the sarcomatous area of the tumor. With increasing awareness of its features, the diagnosis of gliosarcoma is now being made more frequently.

Gliosarcomas are usually firm or even hard, and are often well-circumscribed. They commonly present at the surface of the brain, and may be firmly attached to the dura. The outer surface may be lobulated, and the tumor may be dissected fairly readily from the surrounding brain substance. Because of these features, a gliosarcoma may be mistaken for a meningioma at the time of operation. A superficially located gliosarcoma may have a rich external carotid blood supply, so that its angiographic appearance also resembles that of a meningioma. The tumor center is often necrotic, and of course, the gross features may be quite variable and

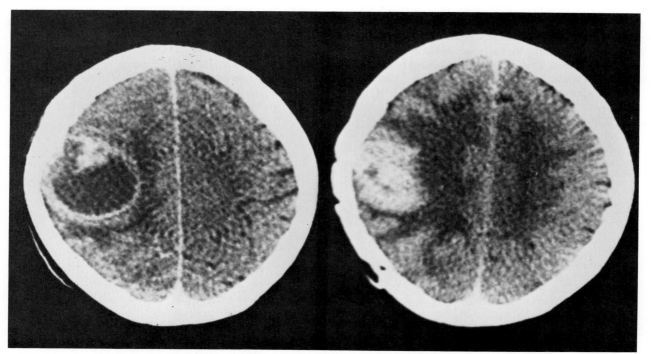

Figure 122-8 Evolution of a gliosarcoma in a 68-year-old woman. An enhanced CT scan at the time of the first symptom (*left*) showed a tumor cyst with a mural nodule which was found to be a highly anaplastic astrocytoma. Radiotherapy was given 4 months later. The tumor recurred 1 year after the initial symptom, as shown on the right (enhanced CT scan). It contained some anaplastic astrocytoma but was mostly a mixed fibrochondro-osteosarcoma.

include those commonly seen in glioblastoma multiforme.

Survival time is similar to that of patients with glioblastoma multiforme. The average survival time in the 24 patients reported by Morantz et al. was 26 weeks after the onset of symptoms, and 21 weeks after surgery. The survival rate at 6 months was 75 percent and at 1 year 19 percent.[2] These figures are quite similar to those reported in other series.

Half of the patients reported by Morantz et al. lived long enough to complete a radiation therapy dose of 6000 rad; in this selected group, the survival rate was somewhat longer, being 37 weeks from the onset of symptoms and 33 weeks after surgery. Chemotherapy in addition to radiation made no significant difference in survival rate. However, these treatment groups were biased by the selection of only patients who had survived at least 5 weeks postoperatively. There is, as yet, no statistical evidence to show that either radiation therapy or chemotherapy confers any benefit or prolongs the survival time in patients with gliosarcoma.

With our present knowledge, the principles of management of patients with gliosarcoma are exactly the same as for those with glioblastoma multiforme. In addition, it must be remembered that gliosarcomas not uncommonly metastasize to extracranial sites.

Sarcoma Arising in Meningioma

Malignancy in meningiomas is uncommon, but on rare occasions a benign meningioma may change into a tumor which has features of malignancy or even of frank sarcoma.[3,4] Meningiomas are subclassified on the basis of histological appearance, but these categories do not reflect differences in behavior except in the case of angioblastic meningiomas. Almost all angioblastic meningiomas are now recognized to be histologically identical to hemangiopericytomas; they have the rather unpredictable tendency to aggressive growth characteristic of the hemangiopericytoma, but are not generally regarded as sarcomas.

There are, however, meningiomas which deserve the designation of malignant meningioma. These tumors are not

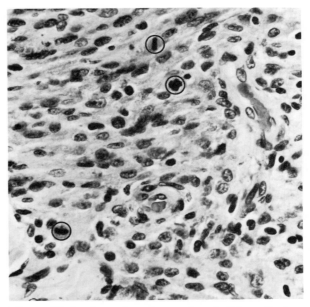

Figure 122-9 A portion of a meningothelial meningioma undergoing malignant change. As many as six mitotic figures were seen per high power field. The three mitotic figures in this field are indicated by circles (H & E, original ×25.)

sharply distinguished from their benign counterparts; in fact, there may over time be a gradual evolution from a picture which appears entirely benign to one which, while retaining the general histological picture of meningioma, has additional features of malignancy. This malignant change is characterized by pattern of infiltration into brain tissue, frequent mitoses (Fig. 122-9), and the development of a distinctive papillary epithelioid pattern rarely if ever seen in benign meningiomas (Fig. 122-10). The malignant meningioma provokes a marked hyperplastic astroglial reaction in the invaded brain tissue, unlike the very limited astroglial reaction in the compressed brain adjacent to a benign meningioma.

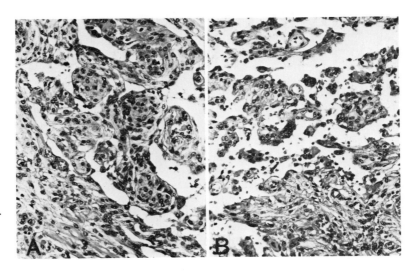

Figure 122-10 Malignant meningioma. *A* and *B* are from the same case. Note the typical whorling pattern (*A*), interrupted by cleftlike spaces to produce a papillary pattern, more developed in *B*. (H & E, ×10.)

The process of malignant evolution of a meningioma progresses on rare occasions to a frankly sarcomatous appearance in which all histological evidence of the pre-existing meningioma is lost. The tumor is then difficult to distinguish from a primary meningeal sarcoma.

Treatment of the sarcomatous meningioma consists of radical surgical removal of the initial tumor and of any and all recurrences, as long as it is feasible to do so. While there is some evidence that radiation therapy may retard the growth rate of benign meningiomas, no information is available as to the benefit of radiation therapy in patients with malignant meningiomas.

Sarcoma Arising After Cranial Irradiation

The development of sarcoma many years after radiation therapy is uncommon but well-recognized, and has been reported in a number of different tissues of the body. Intracranial sarcomas have occurred following radiation of a variety of intracranial tumors, but most commonly following radiation of pituitary tumors. Postradiation sarcomas are usually fibrosarcomas, although other types, including osteogenic sarcoma and malignant meningioma, have occurred.

Sarcomas that develop following radiation therapy of pituitary tumors arise in the field of radiation in or near the sella, where the dose was maximal, but are not necessarily contiguous with the radiated tumor. Waltz and Brownell reviewed 10 such cases from the literature, and described three more cases of their own.[5] The time interval between radiation and the diagnosis of sarcoma ranged from 2 to 20 years, with an average of 10.1 years; this latent interval is similar to that encountered in the development of sarcomas at the site of radiation elsewhere in the body. The minimum radiation dose which was followed by subsequent sarcoma development was 3000 rad (cGy), and multiple courses of radiation greatly increased the risk of developing sarcoma.

The clinical features of postradiation sarcomas are similar to those of other intracranial sarcomas and will not be detailed here. The clinician must be alert to the possible diagnosis of sarcoma in a patient with symptoms that suggest recurrence of a pituitary adenoma some years following radiation; further radiation to such a lesion might well be unwise. Surgical removal of the sarcoma, if possible, is the treatment of choice.

References

1. Christensen E, Lara DE: Intracranial sarcomas. J Neuropathol Exp Neurol 12:41–56, 1953.
2. Morantz RA, Feigin I, Ransohoff J: Clinical and pathological study of 24 cases of gliosarcoma. J Neurosurg 45:398–408, 1976.
3. Rubinstein LJ: Sarcomas of the nervous system, in Minckler J (ed): *Pathology of the Nervous System*. New York, McGraw-Hill, 1971, vol 2, pp 2144–2164.
4. Rubinstein LJ: *Tumors of the Central Nervous System (Atlas of Tumor Pathology, Series 2, Fasc 6)*. Washington, D.C., Armed Forces Institute of Pathology, 1972, pp 74–78, 186–188, 190–204.
5. Waltz TA, Brownell B: Sarcoma: A possible late result of effective radiation therapy for pituitary adenoma: Report of two cases. J Neurosurg 24:901–907, 1966.

123
Lipoma of the Corpus Callosum
Doyle G. Graham

slightly more frequently in males, over half are located within and around the corpus callosum; others have been seen beneath the third ventricle, associated with the choroid plexus, on the cerebellum or quadrigeminal plate, and, rarely, in other sites, such as the cerebellopontine angle.[1–6]

Lipoma of the corpus callosum was first described by Rokitansky in 1856; these tumors were observed only as incidental findings at autopsy until 1939, when Sosman described their appearance using plain skull x-ray films.[5] Slightly more than 100 cases have been reported to date, but it is expected that these lesions will be recognized more frequently with computed tomography. Indeed, in one series of 13,000 consecutive computed tomography studies, four lipomas of the corpus callosum were detected.[2,4,6]

Incidence

While lipomas are common in the rest of the body, lipomas within the central nervous system are rare and constitute fewer than 0.1 percent of intracranial tumors. Found

Pathological Findings and Histogenesis

The deeply yellow lipomas vary from less than a millimeter to several centimeters in greatest dimensions. They are composed of adult fat cells with peripheral, sometimes indented, nuclei. Large vessels, such as the anterior cerebral artery, commonly course through the lesion. The mass of fat cells is surrounded by a fibrocollagenous capsule, which may be intimately bound to surrounding structures. The capsule and surrounding parenchyma frequently contain calcifications, which are sometimes associated with bone formation (Fig. 123-1).

Lipomas of the corpus callosum and elsewhere in the central nervous system are most accurately described as lipomatous hamartomas.[1] The term *lipoma* implies that the biology of this lesion is that of an enlarging neoplasm. The term *hamartoma,* on the other hand, connotes a congenital origin and suggests that the lesion is best viewed as a malformation composed of an abnormal mixture of tissues indigenous to the CNS. One can argue that there is never adult fat within the developing or mature CNS. However, both the meninx primitiva and early pericapillary parenchyma have been proposed as cells from which fat cells could differentiate. The facts that lipomas are sometimes multiple and do occur in other than midline locations favor this mode of origin. The opposing argument, that dermal anlage are included in the CNS during embryogenesis, derives its greatest support from the occasional association with dysraphic disturbances (more often seen with spinal than cranial lesions) and from the preferred midline location. The latter genesis results in lesions called *choristomas,* i.e., masses of tissue not indigenous to that organ.[1] Thus, the simplest term to use is *lipoma* while acknowledging that this lesion is not a true neoplasm.

While one would expect intracranial lipomas to grow during early life, it is important to note that the biology of such lipomas is not that of an expanding lesion. Furthermore, there have been no reports of malignant transformation.[1,5]

Clinical Manifestations

More than half of the patients reported to date with lipomas of the corpus callosum have had seizures or a history suggestive of a seizure disorder.[2] Twenty percent have a mild to severe mental deficit, and 13 percent show hemiparesis. Signs of increased intracranial pressure are rare. Associated subcutaneous lipomas over the vertex or frontal area are seen in 10 percent of the patients. Other presenting features have been headache, vomiting, fainting spells, episodic leg weakness, blurred vision, sleepwalking, and diencephalic disturbances such as adiposogenital dystrophy and hypothermia. Nonetheless, a significant number of people with lipomas of the corpus callosum are asymptomatic.[2-5]

Neuroradiological Findings

The larger lipomas of the corpus callosum are often recognized on plain skull films as radiolucent zones in the frontal region in the midline, best demonstrated in the lateral view. The lesion is surrounded by curvilinear calcification (Fig. 123-2); the calcification may be punctate in the capsular region and rarely may resemble tumor calcification. Small areas of bone formation may be seen. Associated findings may be asymmetry of the skull or midline skull defects.

Carotid angiography may reveal enlarged and tortuous anterior cerebral arteries, which may lack a pericallosal curve. There may be only a single pericallosal artery. Rarely, pathological neovascularity has been seen.

Pneumoencephalography may reveal separation and deformity of the bodies and anterior horns of the lateral ventri-

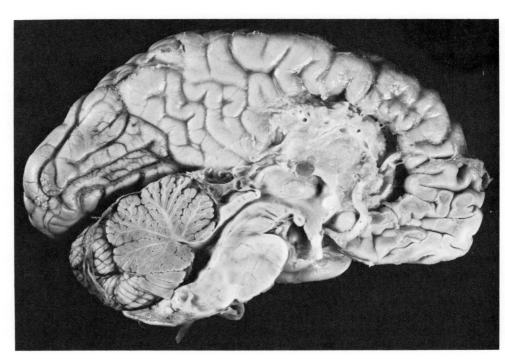

Figure 123-1 The brain of a 56-year-old man who died of renal cell carcinoma contained this asymptomatic lipoma in the region of a congenitally absent corpus callosum. The lesion was canary yellow except for the unusual nodule of cartilage seen just superior to the massa intermedia. (From Burger PC, Vogel FS: *Surgical Pathology of the Nervous System and Its Coverings,* 2d ed. New York, Wiley, 1982, p 109.)

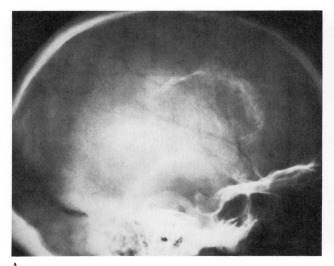
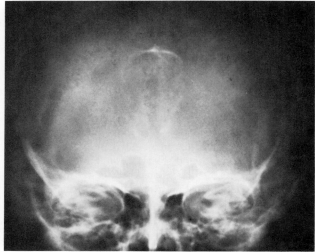

A   B

Figure 123-2   Lateral (*A*) and anteroposterior (*B*) skull films showing a rim of calcification in the periphery of a lipoma of the corpus callosum.

cles or agenesis of the corpus callosum with or without hydrocephalus. In agenesis of the corpus callosum the third ventricle is elevated and enlarged. Associated porencephalic cysts may be seen.

Radionuclide scans may or may not show nonspecific uptake.

Computed tomography is the most accurate method for the diagnosis of a collosal lipoma because of the low attenuation valves of fat (except with very small lesions, with which an average of the lipoma and surrounding tissue may be obtained) and because of the ability of this technique to delineate calcification. Lipomas do not demonstrate contrast enhancement. CT scans not only define the location and extent of the lesion but also detect associated abnormalities, such as agenesis of the corpus callosum, meningocele, hydrocephalus, porencephalic cysts, and additional lipomas. Thus, in the view of most radiologists, CT is the only study required to establish the diagnosis.[3,4]

Treatment

Among symptomatic patients the most significant problem is seizures, which are often serious, frequent, and resistant to medical therapy.[2] Surgical removal of the lipoma has been attempted but with generally poor results. The incorpora-

tion of the anterior cerebral arteries in the mass and the dense adherence to surrounding brain make the procedure technically difficult, and removal is considered unlikely to improve a seizure disorder or dementia when these are present. Shunting for hydrocephalus has likewise been of questionable benefit.[2–5]

References

1. Budka H: Intracranial lipomatous hamartomas (intracranial "lipomas"): A study of 13 cases including combinations with medulloblastoma, colloid and epidermoid cysts, angiomatosis and other malformations. Acta Neuropathol (Berl) 28:205–222, 1974.
2. Gastaut H, Regis H, Gastaut JL, Yermenos E, Low MD: Lipomas of the corpus callosum and epilepsy. Neurology (NY) 30:132–138, 1980.
3. Kazner E, Stochdorph O, Wende S, Grumme T: Intracranial lipoma: Diagnostic and therapeutic considerations. J Neurosurg 52:234–245, 1980.
4. Nabawi P, Dobben GD, Mafee M, Espinosa GA: Diagnosis of lipoma of the corpus callosum by CT in five cases. Neuroradiology 21:159–162, 1981.
5. Tahmouresie A, Kroll G, Shucart W: Lipoma of the corpus callosum. Surg Neurol 11:31–34, 1979.
6. Zettner A, Netsky MG: Lipoma of the corpus callosum. J Neuropathol Exp Neurol 19:305–319, 1960.

SECTION N

Spinal Tumors

124

Radiology of Spinal Canal Neoplasia

Andrew L. Tievsky
David O. Davis

The mode of evaluation of spinal cord tumors is in transition at this time. Previously in the United States and Britain there was heavy reliance on myelography with use of iophendylate (Pantopaque, Lafayette, Alcon Laboratories, Humacao, Puerto Rico). The recent availability of safe water-soluble myelographic agents and high-resolution computed tomography (CT) adds preoperative anatomical information previously unobtainable. This is causing a significant change in the way patients with symptoms secondary to spinal cord tumors are being evaluated.

Plain Film Findings

The plain film remains an important first step for the detection of spinal cord tumors. Malignant bony changes may be distinguished from benign conditions and the lesion localized to a specific vertebral segment. The cervical and lumbar regions should be evaluated with multiple views, including oblique projections, and laminography may be useful. High-resolution CT is probably going to decrease the need for routine laminograms, however.

Lytic bone changes are commonly due to metastatic disease and myeloma, whereas the most common focal blastic metastases include carcinoma of the prostate and lymphoma. Lung, renal, and breast tumors are more commonly lytic but may be blastic in appearance. Often presenting a

permeative appearance, myeloma tends to spare the vertebral pedicle, a factor often used as a differential point. In the presence of a compression fracture it may be difficult to demonstrate the bony pathology even with tomography. As a useful general rule, disc spaces are preserved in neoplasia, while infectious disease is often centered at a narrowed disc space, with destruction of adjacent vertebral end plates.

Specific findings associated with intraspinal tumors include changes in the appearance of the pedicles and of the dorsal surface of the vertebral body. The distance between the pedicles on the frontal projection is a guide to the transverse dimension of the thecal sac. Interpediculate widening involving several segments with flattening or erosion of the medial surface of the pedicles suggests an intramedullary mass effect of long standing. In particular this finding is common with cervical cord glioma. Ependymoma of the conus medullaris may cause a similar appearance in the thoracolumbar region. Thinning of pedicles at T12-L2 is a normal variant in 7 percent of the population, especially in young women.[12] Differentiation from an expanding intraspinal mass may require tomography to demonstrate a normal interpediculate distance and convex, intact cortical margins of the pedicles. A slightly oblique plain film may also mimic thinning of pedicles, and may be corrected by obtaining optimal views.

The size of the neural foramen distal to C2-3 increases caudally and is well-evaluated by oblique radiography, tomography, or CT. Foraminal widening is often an indication of an intradural nerve root sheath tumor or less frequently a dumbbell meningioma. However, enlargement of foramina in neurofibromatosis may be secondary to dural ectasia as well as to tumor; these cannot be differentiated by plain film examination. Other causes of vertebral foramen enlargement include dilatation of vertebral or, rarely, radicular arteries, the latter related to intrathecal tumor or arteriovenous malformation. The C2-3 neural foramen is normally larger than the others in the cervical area. Apparent enlargement of the foramen caused by congenital hypoplasia of a pedicle should not be confused with widening secondary to tumor, a distinction possible on plain films.

Although scalloping of the posterior surface of vertebral bodies may be due to connective tissue disorders such as neurofibromatosis, or to increased intracranial pressure, a focal occurrence of this finding should lead to the suspicion of intradural neoplasia.

Primary bone tumors of the axial skeleton are generally first diagnosed on plain films. If there is no nerve root or cord impingement, pain may be the only presenting complaint. Hemangioma of the vertebral body is a common disorder with a pathognomonic appearance characterized by coarse vertical trabeculations and is usually asymptomatic. Rarely there may be posterior extradural extension. This characteristic extradural mass is well demonstrated on CT, but may be difficult to appreciate on routine myelography. Other primary bone tumors of the vertebrae are unusual. Osteoblastoma or osteoid osteoma presents as a well-defined sclerotic lesion with a lytic nidus, often confined to the posterior elements. Aneurysmal bone cyst, giant cell tumor, chondrosarcoma, and osteogenic sarcoma occur less commonly and all may cause extradural indentation on myelography. Radiographic evaluation with conventional tomography may help to assess the extent of disease; but in order to fully appreciate the relationship to the spinal canal, high-resolution computed tomography is the procedure of choice. In addition to routine examination of the soft tissues, CT images also must be studied with window widths of 500 to 2,000 Hounsfield units (bone windows) in order to fully evaluate the bony architecture.

Myelography

Historically, myelography has been the definitive radiological procedure for the diagnosis of spinal cord tumors. Ease of examination and the ability to investigate long lengths of the thecal sac provide a straightforward method for tumor localization with respect to specific vertebral segment and superficial landmarks. In addition to its proven safety, utilization of readily available standard radiographic apparatus suggests that this technique will remain a definitive procedure in the foreseeable future for the diagnosis of spinal cord tumors.

Traditionally in the United States and Great Britain, myelography has been performed with iophendylate. This viscous iodized oil possesses virtually no acute toxicity but may cause chronic arachnoiditis, an effect that may be enhanced by blood in the spinal fluid. As its absorption from the subarachnoid space is extremely slow, removal of this material is required at the end of myelography. Residual intrathecal iophendylate droplets may interfere significantly with subsequent CT examinations of the skull or spine.

For these reasons and others, a long-standing search for a satisfactory replacement has resulted in a new, relatively nontoxic water-soluble myelographic agent, metrizamide (Amipaque, Winthrop Laboratories, New York, N.Y.), which has been available in this country only since 1978.[11] Previously available water-soluble materials, including sodium methiodal (Abrodil), iothalamate (Conray), and iocarmate (Dimeray), exhibited differing toxicities and are not in current use for myelography. Metrizamide does possess some neurotoxicity, manifested by the rare occurrence of seizures (0.02 percent) and cranial or peripheral nerve palsies. In order to minimize these side effects, concentration and total dose should be limited and care should be taken to maintain patient hydration before and after the procedure. In all cases, maximum dosage of this drug is one 6.75 g vial (3.1 g iodine) which may be dissolved to varying concentrations and volumes to be tailored to the specific examination. Patients with a pre-existing seizure disorder or those receiving epileptogenic drugs present a relative contraindication to metrizamide; iophendylate is preferred in this patient population. Less toxic and possibly less costly water-soluble intrathecal contrast agents (iopamidol, Squibb; iohexal, Winthrop; iogulamide, Mallinckrodt) are undergoing clinical tests at this time and promise to reduce the patient intolerance now occasionally seen with metrizamide.

The nonionic water-soluble agents possess significant advantages compared with iophendylate.[11] To date we know of no reports of clinically detectable chronic arachnoiditis, even if metrizamide is instilled in the presence of bloody cerebrospinal fluid. As the contrast material is considerably less radiopaque than iophendylate, visualization of the spinal cord and nerve roots is facilitated. Lower viscosity often permits flow beyond a region of high-grade obstruction and distally in the nerve root sheaths. Since it is miscible with cerebrospinal fluid, the entire diameter of the subarachnoid space may be opacified. This enables the diagnosis of small tumors and decreases the potential misdiagnosis of spinal cord widening perceived because of inadequate filling of the thecal sac. Water-soluble myelography may be followed with immediate or delayed CT examination for further delineation of lesions in the axial projection, optimal evaluation of the craniocervical region, or the differentiation of intramedullary tumor from hydrosyringomyelia.

When a limited area of the spine, especially the thoracolumbar region, is to be evaluated and there are no specific contraindications, metrizamide is considered to be the agent of choice. Cervical metrizamide myelography may be performed by way of lumbar puncture, but a lateral cervical approach is preferred for those patients with less flexibility of the neck, in order to minimize unnecessary intracranial spillage with the resultant increased risk of complication or failed examination. Unfortunately, the water-soluble nature of metrizamide provides its most significant disadvantage: time limitation for optimal examination without the option to use additional contrast material. For this reason, many neuroradiologists prefer iophendylate for all cervical studies. While complete water-soluble myelographic examination of the cooperative patient is generally successful for the evaluation or exclusion of compressive cord lesions, the temporally last portion of the examination may be suitable only for screening purposes. Regular tomography may help salvage these examinations and accompanying computed tomography may eliminate the need for re-examination. On the other hand, a search for multiple spinal lesions may require a prolonged examination, for which iophendylate often is preferred. In patients with advanced metastatic disease it is advantageous to leave a small quantity of iophendylate in the thecal sac in order to facilitate noninvasive follow-up of compressive lesions.

Myelographic characterization of spinal cord tumors has been traditionally divided into intramedullary, extramedullary-intradural, and extradural components.[12] The importance of true frontal, lateral, and oblique projections and utilization of optimal radiographic technique cannot be overly stressed. Sufficient contrast material must be present to outline a lesion in its entirety. The more irregular the shape of a tumor, the more difficult it may be to determine its exact relationship to the cord and meninges.

Evaluation of a clinically suspected total block requires

specific precautions.[11,12] All efforts should be made to avoid inadvertent puncture of the tumor during myelography. As disturbance to the CSF hydrodynamics may cause worsening of clinical findings after the procedure, only a few drops of cerebrospinal fluid should be removed in order to verify subarachnoid needle position. Most physicians in the United States prefer to use iophendylate, as 1 to 3 ml will establish the level of blockage as well as compartmentalize the lesion. If total obstruction is found, then introduction of a small amount of water-soluble contrast or air with the patient in the Trendelenburg position can force the iophendylate past the lesion so it will outline the upper margin of the mass. Otherwise, a lateral C1-2 puncture with additional contrast injection is required for this purpose. At the termination of the procedure, the skin should be marked under fluoroscopic guidance with indelible material or a scratch (just off the midline and slightly away from the location of a possible later surgical incision) at the upper and lower limits of the block. The iophendylate is not removed under these circumstances; it remains in the subarachnoid space for followup evaluation with fluoroscopy.

Other physicians prefer to use metrizamide for evaluation of total blockage.[11] Complete obstruction seems to be less frequently encountered with water-soluble agents, which may be due to their lower viscosity. Hence, cervical puncture may not be required. Furthermore, concomitant computed tomography may facilitate precise delineation of the mass as well as the bony canal and paraspinal soft tissues. Spinal seizures in response to metrizamide present an extremely rare complication and are generally self-limited, responding to intravenous diazepam.

Fusiform cord enlargement is the hallmark of an intramedullary mass (Fig. 124-1). Cord widening must be observed on both frontal and lateral projections. Generally, the involved region is several segments long, with thinning of the adjacent subarachnoid contrast column and often with partial blockage. The most common intramedullary tumor is ependymoma, which occurs twice as often as astrocytoma. Together these tumors account for the vast majority in this compartment. Less common tumors include other gliomas, hemangioblastoma, and rarely metastatic melanoma and lung and breast carcinomas. A small number of cases of primary intramedullary melanoma have also been described. Other causes of swollen cord, such as intramedullary hematoma, transverse myelitis, abscess or granuloma, and sarcoidosis cannot be radiologically distinguished from tumor. Clinical and laboratory findings usually help elucidate these causes of cord widening.

While there is no reliable radiological differentiation of intramedullary tumors, all must be distinguished from hydrosyringomyelia. In the past, air myelography was employed in order to demonstrate positional changes in cord diameter. Presently, metrizamide computed tomography of the spine is the procedure of choice. The central cavity in hydrosyringomyelia usually fills with metrizamide either immediately or on 6-h delayed scans. Accordingly, this procedure is recommended for postmyelographic evaluation of all cervicothoracic intramedullary lesions. Although the most common cause of central cord filling with metrizamide is hydrosyringomyelia, cystic cavities within intramedullary tumors may also be seen on the CT performed after myelog-

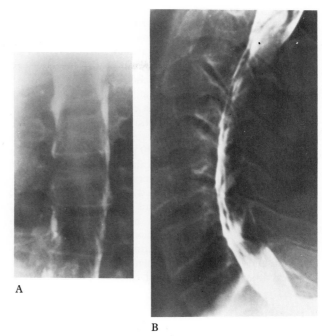

A

B

Figure 124-1 An intramedullary tumor shown by anteroposterior (A) and lateral (B) myelogram views. Diffuse cervical cord widening is due to an intramedullary metastasis from a bronchogenic carcinoma which cannot be distinguished by radiographic criteria from other more common tumors that widen the spinal cord, such as ependymoma or astrocytoma.

raphy with water-soluble agents. Some of these cysts may extend for most of the length of the cord. Additionally, intramedullary cord tumors may cause dilatation of the central canal and mimic hydromyelia similar to that seen occasionally with the Arnold-Chiari malformation. In some instances, when the distinction is difficult, it may be advantageous to percutaneously puncture the cord with a thin (22 to 25-gauge) needle and inject metrizamide (170 mg I per ml) into the cord in an attempt to demonstrate the tumor mass itself as well as to localize the cyst, which may not be possible with metrizamide CT or myelography.

The largest number of intrinsic spinal tumors, predominantly benign, occur in the extramedullary-intradural compartment. Since these masses are within or contiguous to the subarachnoid space they present a well-defined interface with the contrast column. Hence, they produce a sharply defined, rounded defect associated with contralateral displacement of the spinal cord. This displacement causes ipsilateral widening of the contrast column. Determination of the site of dural attachment of these tumors, an important preoperative consideration, is facilitated by multiple views; it will generally be opposite the point of maximal cord displacement. In cases of complete block there is a "cap" at the tumor margin at this location. Very bulky intradural tumors may not be readily compartmentalized by myelography.

The most common tumors in this category are those that originate from Schwann cells in the nerve sheath: neurilemmoma and neurofibroma; the latter is associated with von Recklinghausen's disease and is the most common cause of multiple intradural tumors.[7,10] Inasmuch as they arise from the nerve root, approximately 16 percent penetrate the extradural space to produce a "dumbbell" tumor, which may present a significant paravertebral component (Fig. 124-2). An extreme example is a posterior mediastinal mass due to a thoracic neurilemmoma. Occasionally, a nerve root sheath tumor may be entirely extradural.[7]

Meningioma, the second most common tumor in the intradural compartment, is indistinguishable from schwannoma by conventional myelographic means (Fig. 124-3). Generally smaller in size, over 80 percent occur in the thoracic spinal canal. Microscopic calcification is detectable in less than one-third of these tumors by conventional tomography, but is often demonstrated by CT. These are more frequent in women than men and the finding of a calcified extramedullary-intradural lesion in an elderly female is virtually pathognomonic of meningioma. Uncommonly, spinal meningiomas may be entirely extradural or possess both intradural and extradural components.[10]

Less frequently encountered extramedullary-intradural

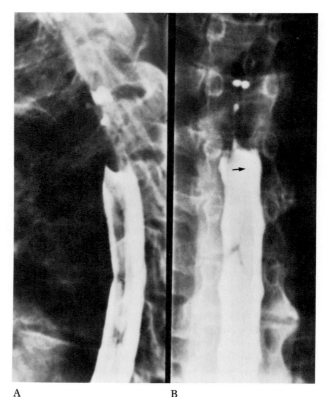

A   B

Figure 124-3   An extramedullary-intradural spinal tumor. Lateral (*A*) and frontal (*B*) views demonstrate a thoracic meningioma causing incomplete obstruction to the flow of iophendylate. The characteristic features of this extramedullary-intradural mass include spinal cord displacement and ipsilateral broadening of the contrast column (*arrow*) with a "cap" or meniscus around the caudal pole of the tumor.

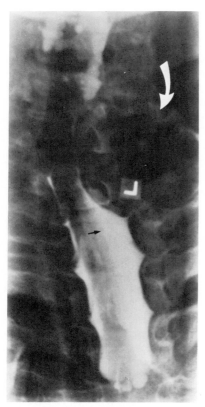

Figure 124-2   An extramedullary-intradural spinal tumor. This oblique view demonstrates an "hourglass" or "dumbbell" schwannoma at C7. The tumor is both intradural and extradural. The ipsilateral contrast column is widened (*black arrow*) due to obvious cord displacement and the neural foramen is markedly enlarged (*white arrow*).

neoplasms include "drop" metastases from brain tumors. In the adult, such metastases occur most frequently from glioblastoma, ependymoma, and melanoma. In the child, medulloblastoma, pineoblastoma, and ependymoma may cause this; ectopic pinealoma is a rare cause. Rarely, in the adult, metastatic melanoma, or breast or bronchogenic carcinoma presumably spread by the hematogenous route, will present intradural metastases located on the dorsal surface of the cord and best detected at myelography on supine views.

Extradural masses displace both the thecal sac and the spinal cord. As the contrast column does not directly encounter the tumor, its margin appears unsharp. There is ipsilateral thinning of the adjacent subarachnoid contrast with tapering. Complete blockage below the conus medullaris may result in an asymmetrical feathered appearance to the thecal sac ("paintbrush" sign), related to compression of the underlying nerve roots.

In contemporary medical practice, extradural tumors are the most commonly encountered, usually due to metastatic disease to the adjacent bone. The most common epidural tumors include metastatic breast, lung, and prostate carcinomas, myeloma, and lymphoma. In view of the high frequency of associated bone changes, inspection of plain films of the entire spine is mandatory prior to myelography in the patient with known malignancy. Epidural hematoma simulating metastasis should be considered in the differential diagnosis of a thrombocytopenic patient receiving chemotherapy. CT of the spine and retroperitoneal space may be useful in this circumstance.

The previously described classification of myelographic compartments is functional but simplistic. Combined intradural-extradural lesions may present a mixed picture or, if a mass is bulky and causes a complete block, it may be impossible to categorize. Occasionally, an extradural lesion such as a herniated disc may cause midsagittal cord enlargement on the frontal projection and mimic an intramedullary mass. Narrowing of the cord on the lateral view may be difficult to appreciate. Even oblique views may not clarify the diagnosis. It is extremely important to evaluate the course of the contrast medium at the site of a block categorized as intramedullary, especially in the cervical or thoracic region. If the contrast is elevated away from the vertebral body, the lesion is extradural and may represent a herniated disc if appropriately situated. Metrizamide CT provides an axial view to confirm the presence of extradural compression in these cases. Thoracic disc herniation with cord compression remains a difficult diagnosis and relative pitfall of myelography (Fig. 124-4).[12]

Subdural iophendylate injection may mimic the appearance of intrathecal carcinomatosis, epidural tumor, or complete block.[1] In the lumbar region there may be a very thin layer of contrast anteriorly, forming a featureless mold of the arachnoidal sac. The major portion of contrast remains in the dorsal subdural space, stripped away from the bone and contained ventrally by ligamentous attachments which produce a serrated appearance in the cervical and thoracic regions. Characteristically, the subdural space is displaced far posteriorly by the dorsal root of the second cervical nerve and its ganglion. In a combined subarachnoid-subdural con-trast injection a large "filling defect" is produced posteriorly between the first and second cervical vertebrae. This must not be mistaken for a tumor.

On occasion, adhesive arachnoiditis, whether related to previous surgery, trauma, intrathecal injection, or myelography, may present with an appearance which simulates spinal neoplasia.[9] Deformity of the thecal sac may mimic epidural tumor. Intradural or extradural arachnoidal CSF cysts may prove to be indistinguishable clinically and radiographically from tumor. Intradural fibrosis producing nerve root thickening and encasement may simulate carcinomatosis. Distinguishing arachnoiditis from tumor is facilitated by the presence of other signs of scarring, e.g., generalized nerve root sleeve blunting, pseudomeningocele formation, or retained loculated iophendylate.

Conus Medullaris and Cauda Equina

Ependymoma (Fig. 124-5) is the most frequent primary tumor of the conus medullaris and upper cauda equina.[3,12] Of 169 cases examined at the Mayo Clinic, 99 (56.5 percent) were located in the cauda equina, presenting as a loculated, intradural mass. The remaining 70 (43.5 percent) were intramedullary, located in the conus medullaris. Of these, 15 percent presented with bony alterations, most commonly widening of the distance between pedicles. Frequently, these tumors may become large, bulky lesions, extending over several segments and at times simulating extramedullary masses. Of the benign intradural tumors, schwannomas are more commonly found in the cauda equina than are meningiomas, which account for only 1 to 2 percent in large series. Other cauda equina tumors include metastatic implants from primary brain tumors and rare hematogenous spread of non-CNS malignancy to the intradural compart-

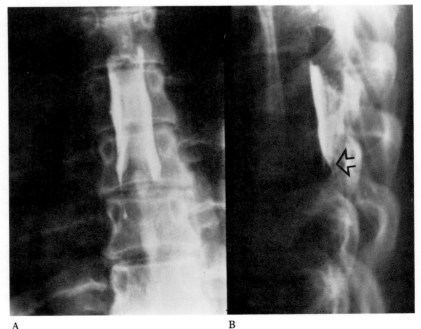

Figure 124-4 An extradural thoracic disc herniation. Frontal (*A*) and lateral (*B*) views depict a complete block to the flow of the contrast medium, which was introduced via C1–2 puncture. On the frontal projection, the cord is widened and there is tapering of the contrast column on either side. On the lateral view, the contrast column is stripped away from the dorsal surface of the vertebral bodies, especially on one side (*arrow*). This extradural sign must be searched for on all patients with the suggestion of cord widening. The cord is displaced posteriorly as well. As the blockage appears to be centered about the disc, herniation is the most likely etiology. Obviously, an extradural tumor or inflammation may present a similar picture, but the bone is usually abnormal in these situations.

A   B

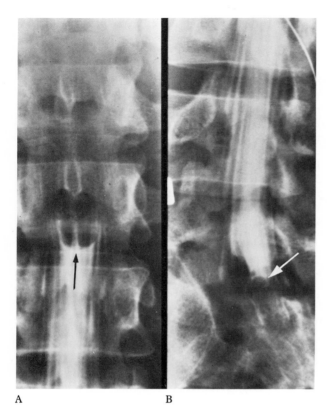

A   B

Figure 124-5 *A*. Lumbar myelography reveals an intradural high lumbar filum ependymoma (*black arrow*).
Compressed and displaced nerve roots surround the lower
edge of the primary tumor. *B*. In the same patient an
intradural "drop metastasis" (*white arrow*) compresses the
sacral roots.

ment.[8] Tumor and lymphomatous (leukemic) implants may
present as discrete or diffuse thickening of the nerve roots
and meninges (Fig. 124-6).

The Foramen Magnum

Mass lesions of the foramen magnum region often present an
elusive clinical and diagnostic picture which may mimic
demyelinating disease. Frequently, routine cranial computed tomographic examination and cervical myelography
fail to examine this region, contributing to the high frequency of false-negative diagnostic evaluations during the
initial presentation of the patient. Accordingly, in patients
with other than clear-cut radicular symptoms and signs, the
standard cervical myelogram should include frontal and lateral views of the contrast column at the level of the clivus.
Oblique or supine views of the foramen magnum with contrast pooled in this region will demonstrate posteriorly located masses and the position of the cerebellar tonsils. Occasionally, if iophendylate is used, some will remain in the
basal cisterns, although a long-term clinical effect is rare or
nonexistent. A significant advantage to the use of metrizamide for cervical myelography is that it may be supple-

mented by CT of the craniocervical junction and cisterns.
Metrizamide CT examination of this region is considered by
many to be the definitive radiological procedure. Axial images may be supplemented by coronal and sagittal reformatting in order to demonstrate the precise characteristics of
masses in this region.[5] Computed tomography of the foramen magnum with intravenous contrast is also of value;
however, spectral changes in the x-ray beam due to the effect of extreme bone density of the skull base do not permit
optimal demonstration of subarachnoid soft tissues.

Approximately one-third of tumors occurring in the foramen magnum region are benign, hence, potentially curable.[6]
Meningioma is the most common intradural mass in this
location (Fig. 124-7). Most often this tumor arises from the
anterior dura of the upper cervical spine and extends superiorly into the foramen magnum, displacing the spinal cord
posteriorly. Tumors arising from the posterior aspect of the
foramen magnum may be differentiated from low-lying cerebellar tissue of the Arnold-Chiari malformation by the cleft
usually seen in the latter. Schwannomas account for most
other intradural foramen magnum masses. Extramedullary-
intradural tumors of the craniocervical junction may occasionally be simulated by posterior fossa tumors such as
hemangioblastoma, metastases, or rarely, acoustic neuromas

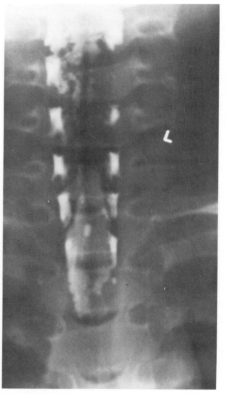

Figure 124-6 Diffuse leukemic infiltration of the leptomeninges produces
marked thickening of the cervical nerve
root sleeves. Multiple intradural defects
can also be due to neurofibromatosis,
sarcoidosis, or hypertrophic interstitial
neuritis.

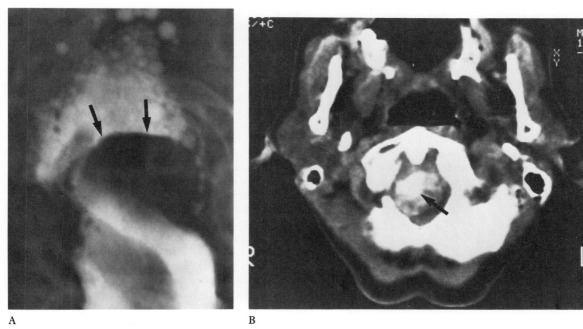

A   B

Figure 124-7   This 66-year-old woman with severe quadriparesis progressive for 5 years was thought to have a demyelinating disorder. *A*. Myelography demonstrates a large mass (*arrows*) at the foramen magnum with posterolateral displacement and thinning of the spinal cord. *B*. CT after the intravenous injection of a contrast agent reveals a large calcified enhancing tumor (*arrow*) probably arising from the dura. A meningioma was completely removed at operation, with a subsequent fair recovery.

which protrude through the foramen magnum and compress the cord. Accordingly, intravenous contrast CT examination of the entire head with thin sections of the infratentorial region should be performed when a foramen magnum tumor is suspected. If an extramedullary mass is discovered by myelography or CT, vertebral angiography should be considered in order to exclude aneurysm. Intramedullary masses occurring at the foramen magnum include brain stem glioma with caudal extension. Metastases arising in adjacent bone are the most common extradural tumors in this location. Chordoma of the upper cervical spine or lower clivus is a rare anterior extradural tumor. Plain films and tomograms will characteristically (but not invariably) reveal midline osseous destruction with adjacent prolific nodular soft tissue calcification. CT reveals the extent of the tumor quite graphically and should be performed prior to surgery or radiation therapy.

Hemangioblastoma of the Spinal Cord

Hemangioblastoma of the spinal cord is radiographically and histologically similar to its cerebellar counterpart, and when seen with a retinal lesion is part of the Hippel-Lindau complex. Accordingly, spinal hemangioblastomas should be sought in patients with cord symptoms associated with the presence of cerebellar or retinal lesions. Not infrequently, multiple spinal tumors, varying in size from a few millimeters to up to 10 cm, are detected. These tumors are often

first detected by myelography, but at times it is difficult to accurately characterize these lesions or their locations with this technique.

In a compilation of 80 well-documented cases, Djindjian et al. noted that nearly all had abnormal myelograms.[2] The most characteristic findings occurred in 20 percent, with diffuse cord swelling and associated vascular filling defects, but this could not be differentiated from arteriovenous malformation (AVM) with hematomyelia. Another 70 percent presented with partial or complete blockage as well as vascular filling defects. Hemangioblastomas may have an exophytic component; often the characteristic tortuous draining veins may cause a block and/or suggest the appearance of a benign intradural tumor. As these retromedullary vessels may extend the entire length of the spinal cord, their location does not facilitate tumor localization. Approximately 10 percent of the cases demonstrated vascular shadows without a mass; these cases are indistinguishable from arteriovenous malformation.

Selective spinal arteriography is the definitive procedure for the diagnosis of spinal hemangioblastoma. As multiple tumors are not infrequently encountered, evaluation of the entire length of the thecal sac may be required. The angiographic appearance of hemangioblastoma is pathognomonic and readily differentiated from AVM. Characteristically, a sharply defined, hypervascular mass with an intense blush appears early and persists into the late venous phase. Heterogeneous enhancement suggests cystic cavitation within the tumor. While anterior or posterior spinal arteries are usually slightly hypertrophied, the numerous tortuous dilated veins may reach gargantuan proportions. There is no arteriovenous shunting in hemangioblastoma; rather, venous filling is extremely slow, requiring prolonged filming sequences in order to demonstrate these characteristic structures.

Two newer techniques hold promise for the evaluation of this disorder. Dynamic computed tomographic angiography accurately depicts the axial configuration of the tumor and its precise relationship to the cord, and distinguishes draining veins over limited lengths of the spine. Also, digital subtraction radiographic techniques, such as intravenous angiography and mini-dose arterial aortography, show great potential for screening purposes, antecedent to total spinal arteriography (Fig. 124-8). Furthermore, these minimally invasive techniques may facilitate postoperative follow-up.

Computed Tomography

Although already useful, the full diagnostic potential of this technique has not yet been realized. The primary attributes of CT, cross sectional imagery and exquisitely sensitive detection of minimal differences in x-ray attenuation, are optimally suited for evaluation of tumor effect upon the axial skeleton, thecal sac, and paraspinal soft tissues. The segmental level of a lesion in question can be determined elec-

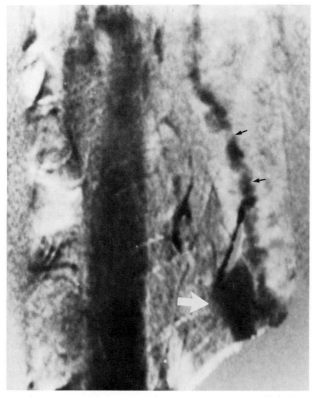

Figure 124-8 Lateral view from an intravenous digital angiogram of the cervical region demonstrates the sharply defined "stain" of an intramedullary hemangioblastoma (*white arrow*) with a tortuous enlarged posterior draining vein (*black arrows*) flowing cephalad.

tronically by utilizing a scan projection (digital) radiograph generated while the patient is moved through the gantry. Computerized image manipulation allows coronal or sagittal reformatting for evaluation of longitudinal extent. For example, these features are useful in the demonstration of the extraspinal portions of dumbbell tumors. Extradural neoplasms frequently cause profound bone destruction underestimated by conventional radiography. Usually the more discrete, "moth-eaten" pattern of vertebral tumor involvement can be distinguished from the pattern of irregular, multifocal destruction of cancellous and cortical bone typical of osteomyelitis. Tumor infiltration of paraspinal fat and muscle planes as well as adjacent viscera may be optimally demonstrated with CT (Fig. 124-9). Often the exact anatomical relationship of an epidural tumor to the thecal sac can be determined.[4]

Evaluation of the patterns of tumor density and enhancement for the purpose of differentiation of histology has not yet been fully investigated. However, of the intradural tumors, meningioma often demonstrates increased attenuation on noncontrast scans related to microscopic calcification, and exhibits moderate enhancement after intravenous infusion of contrast material. On the other hand, spinal hemangioblastoma enhances intensely, often with the demonstration of associated prominent tortuous draining veins (Fig. 124-10). Intradural lipoma presents as a lobulated, nonenhancing radiolucent lesion which is particularly well suited for CT evaluation. As well as assessment of the degree of cord compression, tethering and bony dysraphism are readily demonstrated, as well as the relationship to extraspinal lipomas. Although unpredictable, intramedullary gliomas rarely enhance after intravenous contrast administration.[4]

A significant limitation is the inability of CT to distinguish soft tissue detail within the spinal canal below the upper cervical region. Without the intrathecal introduction of a contrast agent, the cord cannot be distinguished below this level, nor can the conus medullaris be differentiated from emerging roots of the cauda equina. Since many tumors prove isodense relative to the cord, some intradural and small extradural masses will be missed completely on routine spinal CT examination. For the most part, intramedullary gliomas are not distinguishable from normal tissue and do not enhance with intravenous contrast. Unless intrathecal contrast agents are introduced for the demonstration of the spinal cord widening, such lesions may be missed by computed tomography. The distinction of intramedullary tumors from syrinx with metrizamide CT has been previously noted.

Metrizamide CT of the entire spine proves to be a lengthy and generally impractical procedure. The location of a lesion should be suspected from specific symptoms and signs and by assessment with plain films and myelography so that a directed examination can be performed.

An additional problem is encountered in the patient with spinal curvature. Images not parallel to the vertebral end plates prove difficult to interpret and, if scoliosis is severe, there may be difficulty in determination of precise vertebral levels.

Obviously, metrizamide CT is not a preferred primary diagnostic modality for evaluation of spinal cord tumors. For the most part, myelography continues to play that key

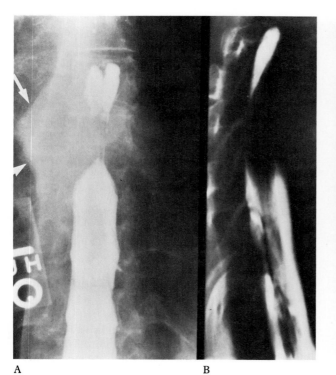
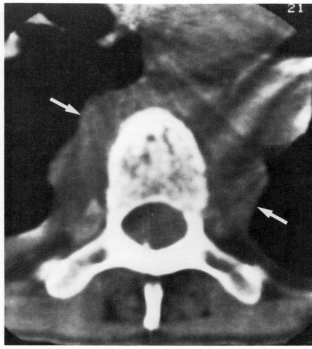

A   B   C

Figure 124-9 Frontal (*A*) and lateral (*B*) views from a myelogram demonstrate an extradural mass causing a partial block in the midthoracic region. The diffusely narrowed contrast column is associated with a paraspinal mass on the frontal projection (*A, arrows*). The spinal cord and thecal sac are displaced posteriorly (*B*). *C.* CT readily demonstrates vertebral body destruction with associated paraspinal adenopathy (*arrows*) due to lymphoma.

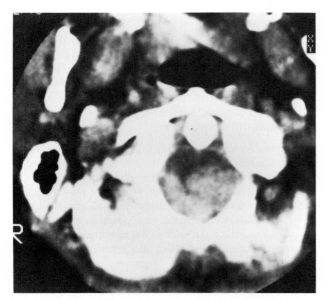

Figure 124-10 CT of the craniocervical region after the intravenous injection of contrast material demonstrates a huge, posteriorly located, enhancing hemangioblastoma in a patient with the Hippel-Lindau complex. This massive tumor extended from the posterior fossa to the upper cervical cord.

role. Nevertheless, CT adds hitherto unobtainable anatomical information; the importance of this technique may well eclipse the traditional myelogram in the future.

Nuclear Magnetic Resonance

Finally, nuclear magnetic resonance (NMR) imaging, in which the patient's body is placed in a strong, graded magnetic field so that its protons align with the field and are perturbed by a radio-frequency (RF) beam, allows reconstruction of body images utilizing the RF signals returning from the body after the perturbation ceases. Various techniques for this procedure (spin-echo, inversion-recovery) are presently undergoing evaluation in order to determine which is optimal for use. Early work shows great promise for the detection of brain and spinal cord lesions. Specifically, intramedullary tumors and Arnold-Chiari malformations have been optimally analyzed by this method. In addition to significant improvement in the methodology in the next few years, development of paramagnetic contrast media may also aid the detection and analysis of spinal cord neoplasms. It is distinctly possible that in the next few years all spinal symptoms and signs will be evaluated primarily by NMR imaging.

References

1. Azar-Kia B, Batnitzky S, Liebeskind A, Schechter MM: Subdural Pantopaque: A radiologist's dilemma. Radiology 112:623–627, 1974.
2. Djindjian R, Merland JJ, Djindjian M, Stoeter P: Neuroradiological study of intraspinal hemangioblastomas, in Djindjian R, Merland JJ (eds): *Angiography of Spinal Column and Spinal Cord Tumors.* Stuttgart, Thieme-Stratton, 1981.
3. Fischer G, Tommasi I: Spinal ependymomas, in Vinken PJ, Bruyn GW (eds): *Handbook of Clinical Neurology.* Amsterdam, North-Holland, 1976, vol 20, pp 353–387.
4. Haughton VM, Williams AL: *Computed Tomography of the Spine.* St. Louis, Mosby, 1982.
5. LaMasters DL, Watanabe TJ, Chambers EF, Norman D, Newton TH: Multiplanar metrizamide-enhanced CT imaging of the foramen magnum. AJNR 3:485–494, 1982.
6. Marc JA, Schechter MM: Radiological diagnosis of mass lesions within and adjacent to the foramen magnum. Radiology 114:351–365, 1976.
7. Nittner K: Spinal meningiomas, neurinomas and neurofibromas and hourglass tumours, in Vinken PJ, Bruyn GW (eds): *Handbook of Clinical Neurology.* Amsterdam, North-Holland, 1976, vol 20, pp 177–322.
8. Prentice WB, Kieffer SA, Gold LHA, Bjornson RGB: Myelographic characteristics of metastasis to the spinal cord and cauda equina. AJR 118:682–689, 1973.
9. Quencer RM, Tenner M, Rothman L: The postoperative myelogram. Radiology 123:667–679, 1977.
10. Rasmussen TB, Kernohan JW, Adson AW: Pathologic classification, with surgical consideration, of intraspinal tumors. Ann Surg 111:513–530, 1940.
11. Sackett JF, Strother CM: *New Techniques in Myelography.* Hagerstown, Md, Harper & Row, 1979.
12. Shapiro R: *Myelography.* Chicago, Year Book, ed 3, 1975.

125

Spinal Intradural Tumors

Bennett M. Stein

Credit is given to Victor Horsley for the first successful removal of a spinal cord tumor.[9] The tumor was extramedullary-intradural and typed as a fibromyxoma. The condition had been diagnosed by William Gowers; Horsley proceeded with the surgery with a great deal of trepidation, since even the successful performance of laminectomy at that time (1887) was rare. The patient was a captain in the British army who suffered relentless progression of the disease to a paraplegia. The operation was performed under ether anesthesia with the patient in a semiprone position. The performance of the laminectomy was a topic of detailed discussion.

> The spinous processes of the vertebrae whose laminae are to be removed are cut through close to their base by a very powerful bone forceps. This is readily done in a few seconds and we then have the laminae forming a continuous if irregular plate, and this can be perforated with a trephine with the usual precautions. The trephine should be almost as large as the diameter of the neural canal, this, of course, varying with the region operated on, the age of the patient, &c.

The localization being solely on a clinical basis, the laminectomy had to be modified to include additional laminae after the dura had been opened in order to fully expose the tumor.

> Another lamina was removed at each end of the wound, the dura mater as before slit up, and the cord still further exposed, but still nothing pathological was discovered. At this juncture it appeared as if sufficient had been done, but I was very unwilling to leave the matter undecided, and my friend Mr. Ballance being strongly of the opinion that further exposure of the cord was indicated, I determined to go further—I removed another lamina at the upper part of the incision. On opening the dura mater, I saw on the left side of the subdural cavity a round, dark, bluish mass about three millimeters in diameter, resting upon the left lateral column and posterior root-zone of the spinal cord. I recognized it at once to be the lower end of a new growth, and therefore quickly cut away the major part of the lamina next above. This enabled me to see almost the whole extent of the tumour when the dura mater was divided.

Subsequently the entire tumor was removed, which alleviated the pressure on the spinal cord. Interestingly, one of the patient's major postoperative problems was incessant pain keeping him without sleep, a problem that is not uncommon in contemporary neurosurgery of spinal cord tumors. The patient subsequently made excellent progress and became ambulatory. Horsley's conclusion regarding spinal cord tumors was, "there is but one treatment, viz. removal of the source of pressure by operation."

Although Cushing[4] is given credit for the first successful removal of an intramedullary ependymoma, the technique of intramedullary spinal cord tumor surgery as well as the diagnosis and treatment of all spinal tumors is epitomized by Elsberg's masterpiece on this subject in 1925.[6] He pointed out, "Not so many years ago 'chronic myelitis' and 'transverse myelitis' were considered diseases of frequent occurrence; we now know that, excluding the secondary and traumatic forms, they are rare." Symptoms and findings leading to these erroneous diagnoses were in fact due to tumors of the spinal cord. Elsberg underscored the tremendous advance from the first diagnosis and successful removal of a spinal cord tumor by Gowers and Horsley in 1887 to his review in 1924.

> Then and now! In the thirty-seven years that have passed, our knowledge of the symptomatology of the spinal-cord tumors and their surgical treatment has made rapid strides. Then, spinal-cord tumors were considered rare; now, the diagnosis is frequently made in every neurological clinic! Then, the neurologist was victorious if he successfully determined the level of a spinal new growth. Now, we are able to diagnosticate from the progress of the symptoms and from the signs of interference with function, not only the level of the cord lesion, but also the location of the growth in relation to the cord, ventral and dorsal roots, and dentate ligament!

> Then the operation of laminectomy was a hazardous procedure; now, the exposure and removal of a spinal neoplasm is an operation without great danger!

> It is, perhaps, not too daring to prophesize that the day is not too far distant when the early symptoms and signs of a spinal tumor will be so well understood that the diagnosis and localization of the growth and its removal will be possible at a stage when little paralysis and few sensory disturbances have occurred.

Elsberg's prophecy has become a reality with our current ability to clinically and radiographically diagnose spinal cord tumors with precision during the early stages of their growth. With advances in imaging techniques, it is not unrealistic to assume that spinal cord tumors may be uncovered at the stage of minimal symptoms or as a serendipitous finding while the spine is being evaluated for an unrelated pain syndrome, much as we now experience with the use of intracranial computed tomography (CT).

Remarkable as was the progress made in spinal tumor surgery during the 37 years cited by Elsberg, it is notable and ironic that little progress[13] in the treatment of intramedullary tumors was made during a hiatus of 43 years from Elsberg's pioneering work until Greenwood reported a large series of patients in which successful removal of intramedullary tumors was performed.[10,11]

Incidence

Tumors of the spinal canal are generally divided into the following categories: (1) extradural, (2) extramedullary-intradural, and (3) intramedullary. Depending on situational factors, the incidences of these three major types vary somewhat. In a setting dealing with cancer patients, extradural tumors will be most common. Some surgeons have taken a particular interest in intramedullary tumors, and in their series these tumors will have a disproportionately higher incidence.[7,8,11,20,27] As a group, intradural tumors are uncommon (approximately 20 percent as common as cerebral

tumors), with an incidence of from 3 to 10 per 100,000 population.[2,3,17,36] The ratio of intradural to extradural tumors is approximately 3 to 2. This discussion is primarily related to tumors located intradurally, including the extramedullary-intradural tumors and the intramedullary tumors. The ratio of intramedullary to extramedullary tumors is somewhat higher in children than in adults, approximately 30 percent in children and 15 percent in adults.[5,22,25]

These tumors occur predominately in the middle decades and except for the unusually high incidence of meningiomas in females, the sex ratio is about equal. Because of the relative proportions of cord substance, the most common location is the thoracic region, with the cervical region next and the lumbosacral region the least likely location for tumors. The ependymoma, besides being intramedullary, has a predilection for occurrence at the conus medullaris, where it may be both intra- and extramedullary, with an ectophytic component extending into the cauda equina. Dermoids, epidermoids, and teratomas are found in intra- and extramedullary locations.

The most common extramedullary-intradural tumors are the neurilemmomas, which comprise approximately 30 percent of spinal tumors, and the meningiomas, which comprise approximately 25 percent of tumors. The most common intramedullary tumors, with about equal incidence, are the astrocytomas and ependymomas. A variety of other intramedullary tumors, including hemangioblastomas, dermoids, epidermoids, and mixed tumors, are uncommon.

As a group, a high percentage, approaching 90 percent, of all intradural spinal cord tumors are benign and potentially resectable. Therefore, the outlook after surgical therapy is excellent. Similarly, severe defects due to spinal cord compression in relatively young individuals can be reversed by the removal of these tumors, with the expectation of return of neurological function.

Clinical Symptoms and Signs

In interpreting symptoms, the surgeon must take into account certain factors including (1) anatomical discrepancies between segmental levels of the spinal cord and of the vertebral bodies; (2) variations produced by a blood supply predominantly to specific regions of the spinal cord, producing a watershed effect that may result in relative ischemia in other areas of the spinal cord distant from the primary lesion; (3) an anchoring of the spinal cord to its adjacent structures, which may produce unpredictable stresses within the cord structure, perhaps at some distance from the tumor; and (4) known anatomical features such as the two- to three-level crossing of the anterolateral spinothalamic tract.

The fact that the spinal cord is shorter than the vertebral canal results in a discrepancy between spinal cord segments and their analogous vertebral bodies. This discrepancy increases caudally. For example, the C8 spinal cord level lies between vertebral bodies C6 and C7. The fourth thoracic segment of the spinal cord is opposite the third thoracic vertebra. The twelfth thoracic cord segment is opposite the T10-T11 interspace, and the L5-S1 spinal cord segment lies opposite the L1 vertebral body. In searching for appropriate changes in the bone structure the surgeon must take into account these discrepancies.

The arterial blood supply to the spinal cord derives from different sources at different levels.[18,32,35] The anterior spinal artery is supplied predominantly by branches of the intracranial portions of the vertebral arteries and it nourishes the upper cervical spinal cord, assisted by a major radicular artery at C6; in the thoracic region the major arterial supply is at T7; and in the lower spinal cord segments, the predominant supply is via the artery of Adamkiewicz, which may enter the cord from T9 to L2. Therefore, the intermediate areas of the spinal cord have a watershed blood supply and if the predominant arterial supply related to this watershed is compromised by tumor, the watershed area at some distance from the primary lesion will be the first to suffer. These vascular relationships may explain the necrosis of central areas of the spinal cord in the lower cervical region at some distance from tumors of the high cervical area.

The spinal cord is anchored to some extent by the dentate ligaments and the dorsal and ventral roots. Masses displacing the spinal cord will produce stresses within the interior of the spinal cord that may be lessened by these tethering structures.[14]

The anatomical particularity that fibers of the pain pathway mediated by the anterolateral spinothalamic tract take from two to three segments to cross before they enter the ascending tract has significance in terms of neurological localization.

Irrespective of the location of tumors, symptoms precede the discovery of the tumor by an average of 2 years. Pain is an early signature whether the tumor is extra- or intramedullary.[3,6,24,36] The clinical syndrome depends primarily on the longitudinal rather than the coronal location of the tumor, i.e. on whether the tumor is intra- or extramedullary, although there are a few classic discrepancies. In general, extramedullary tumors tend to be eccentric, lying to the side of the spinal cord either dorsally or ventrally. Therefore, the compressive effect is asymmetrical. This results in a higher incidence of Brown-Séquard's syndrome, whereby the corticospinal tract and the dorsal columns are affected ipsilateral to the lesion while the involvement of the spinothalamic tract, which receives crossed fibers, produces contralateral sensory abnormalities. Conversely, intramedullary tumors because they involve the interior of the spinal cord are not commonly associated with Brown-Séquard's syndrome. Rather, there results a dissociated sensory loss due to the interruption of the crossing pain fibers. The result is an impairment of pain and temperature appreciation at certain segmental levels, with relative sparing of the position, light touch, and vibratory sensations. Because of the topographic arrangement of the spinothalamic tract, intramedullary tumors are associated with a relative sparing of the lumbosacral pain- and temperature-conducting fibers, which are located more externally. This is a theoretical consideration, and although sacral sparing would be expected with intramedullary tumors, this is not always found to be the case.

Most spinal cord tumors produce symptoms and signs with a combination of local or segmental and distant features. Segmental involvement of the dorsal root entry zone or the anterior motor cells and roots results in specific sensory and lower motor neuron defects. Distant features are related to involvement of the longitudinally oriented ascending and descending tracts, which interrupts function below the level of the tumor. In the case of the corticospinal tract, this results in upper motor neuron defects; in the spinothalamic tract, a decrease in pain and temperature sensation; and in the dorsal columns, a decrease in position and vibratory sensation. Involvement of the descending autonomic pathways, which are located between the corticospinal and spinothalamic tracts, results in both sympathetic and parasympathetic disturbances below the level of the lesion. This is most important when the lesion affects function bilaterally and thereby impairs respiratory, bowel, bladder, and sexual function. The volume of the tumor in terms of longitudinal and transverse orientation dictates to some extent the degree of involvement of these systems. However, the clinical presentation can be variable and seemingly inconsistent. Theoretically, other factors such as age, vascular distributions, relative size of the spinal column, and tethering structures may modify the clinical course. The surgeon is always amazed to find large tumors, either intrinsic or extrinsic, with severe spinal cord compression that produce very few abnormalities.

Specific syndromes related to the rostrocaudal site of the tumor can be identified. Lesions of the upper cervical spine or foramen magnum region produce a unique syndrome characterized by (1) a disproportionate loss of position and vibration sense in the upper as compared to the lower extremities, and (2) atrophy of the intrinsic muscles of the hands.[30] This finding has been the topic of speculation. It has been suggested that compromise of the arterial blood supply to the spinal cord results in central necrosis of the anterior gray matter at C8-T1. However, this is inconsistent with the pattern of blood supply to the cervical spinal cord. Similarly, pressure on the central canal at the high cervical level has been incriminated in this syndrome, and the hypothesis has been forwarded that a central hydromyelia or cystic degeneration is created at lower levels. Perhaps the most attractive hypothesis surmises interruption of the venous channels by the high cervical lesion, with venous infarction and central necrosis at lower levels.[33] Involvement of the dorsal roots of C2 results in both pain and sensory loss over the occipital region. Nystagmus has been attributed to pressure on the sulcomarginal fibers, which are an extension of the medial longitudinal fasciculus. Involvement of the other pathways of the spinal cord eventually leads to a host of neurological abnormalities below the level of the lesion.

Involvement of the middle and lower cervical regions by intramedullary tumors produces a suspended, capelike sensory loss, with pain which involves the upper extremities, most often the shoulders or fingers. Horner's syndrome may be seen unilaterally or bilaterally, depending on the degree of involvement of the sympathetic system.

Involvement of the upper thoracic region evokes pain in a girdle-type distribution, sometimes mistaken for angina pectoris, coronary thrombosis, or pleurisy. Similarly, in the middle and lower thoracic regions pain may in error suggest an abdominal lesion.

Tumors at the lumbosacral or conus medullaris regions of the spinal cord affect the parasympathetic innervation of the bladder, bowel, and sexual organs. The ensuing symptoms and signs, including enuresis and disturbances in sexual capacity, may precede other overt neurological abnormalities by many months or years. These are often misdiagnosed as psychological problems, as cystocele in women of child-bearing age, and as prostatic disease in men. Involvement of the lumbosacral interface may lead to the fascinating neurological picture of upper motor neuron neurological deficits in the sacral myotomes and lower motor neuron deficits in the affected lumbar myotomes.

Tumors of the cauda equina may selectively impair the function of a single dorsal root for many months. This leads to persistent, discrete dermatomal appreciation of pain, which may be mistaken for disc prolapse or psychological symptoms.

Although it may seem reasonable to assume that intramedullary tumors produce a syndrome different from that produced by extramedullary tumors, in practical experience it is often difficult to differentiate these two conditions on clinical grounds alone.

In the adolescent child the clinical syndromes are often similar to those of the adult. In the younger child, tumors frequently present as extremity weakness or as growth deformities and are recognized first by the orthopedic surgeon who sees the child for kyphoscoliosis. This is especially

common with extensive intramedullary astrocytomas. Beside deformities of the spine, gait abnormalities or deformities of the feet, such as talipes equinovarus or pes cavus, may be witnessed in the young child. Enuresis in the previously toilet-trained child is another symptom of a caudal tumor.[5,22,25] Although rare, congenital tumors such as the teratomas, dermoids, and epidermoids have a higher incidence in children than in adults; there may be associated abnormalities such as a sinus tract or hairy or pigmented cutaneous lesions.

Pathology

Neurilemmomas or neurofibromas arise from the dorsal roots at the various segmental levels of the spinal cord. These tumors are relatively avascular, globoid in configuration, and relatively soft, without calcification. The dorsal root is intimately involved in the matrix of the tumor and can rarely be spared in the surgical removal of these tumors (Fig. 125-1). When associated with von Recklinghausen's

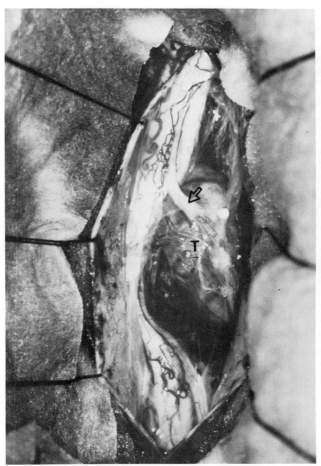
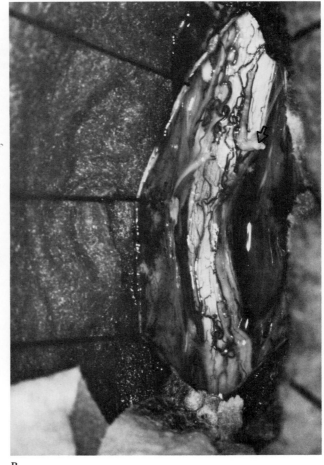

A   B

Figure 125-1 *A*. Operative photograph showing a discrete neurofibroma (T) lateral to the thoracic cord. The parent nerve root is indicated by an arrow. *B*. Operative photograph after removal of the neurofibroma showing the cut end of the sacrificed nerve root (*arrow*).

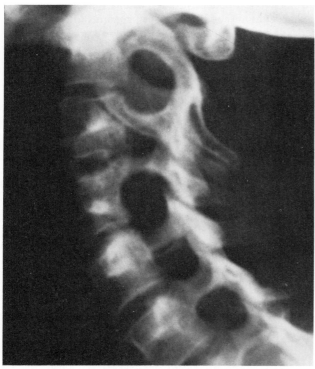
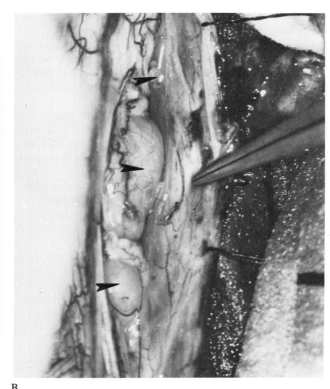

A   B

Figure 125-2 *A.* Lateral x-ray film of the cervical spine showing multiple enlargements of the neural foramina. *B.* Operative photograph showing multiple neurofibromas (*arrowheads*) in a case of von Recklinghausen's disease.

disease, the tumors are multiple, occurring at numerous levels of the spinal canal in various stages of growth (Fig. 125-
2). The protein content of the spinal fluid is often elevated
beyond a range ascribable to CSF block. When occurring in
the region of the cauda equina, these tumors may have some
degree of mobility because of the elasticity of the parent
nerve root. Only when these tumors have a dumbbell configuration, following the nerve root through the dural sleeve
into the extradural space, do they have an attachment to and
blood supply from the dura. In the case of the dumbbell
neurofibroma, the size of the extradural mass may exceed
that of the intradural mass. This may result in a large soft
tissue mass visible on chest or abdominal x-ray films or a
mass palpable in the cervical region.

Rare instances have been described of wholly intramedullary neurilemmomas presumably arising from aberrant
nerve roots, with growth predominately into the spinal
cord.[21] These tend to be museum cases; however, it is important to recognize this possibility because these are eminently resectable tumors, unlike some of the other intramedullary tumors.

Meningiomas occur most commonly in the thoracic region in women, may be calcified, and have an intimate attachment to, if not permeation of, the dura, frequently over
more than one segment. They presumably arise from arachnoid cluster cells and therefore are located at the exit zones
of nerve roots or the entry zones of arteries into the spinal
canal. They are often located lateral or ventrolateral, (uncommonly dorsal) to the spinal cord (Fig. 125-3). The
growth of a foramen magnum meningioma is intimate to the

entry of the vertebral artery into the subarachnoid space.
Meningiomas caudal to the level of the conus medullaris are
uncommon. In spite of their relationship to root entry and
exit zones, they can often be separated from the nerve roots
and do not bear the same intimate relationship to these roots
that is apparent with the neurilemmomas.

The ependymoma is primarily an intramedullary tumor,
occurring most frequently in the thoracic region but not excluded from other regions of the spinal cord. An alternative
site is the conus region, where the tumor may be partially
intramedullary and partially exophytic, in the latter instance
involving the nerve roots of the cauda equina. These tumors
are rarely malignant and are often associated with intramedullary cysts containing fluid of high protein content. Rarely,
when the tumor is malignant, it may seed throughout the
spinal as well as the cranial axis. In cases of exophytic components of this tumor, the protein content of the CSF is
disproportionately elevated and has been associated with the
occurrence of papilledema.[1] These tumors are encapsulated
and relatively avascular. When involving the filum terminale—presumably arising from the ependyma of the central
canal—they may be mobile and change position during
myelography (Fig. 125-4). This accentuated mobility may
make differentiation from a neurofibroma difficult. Grossly
at operation it may also be hard to distinguish a neurofibroma attached to a nerve root of the cauda equina from a
globoid ependymoma attached to a thin filum.

The astrocytoma is invariably intramedullary, relatively
avascular, usually distinguishable from neural tissue in color
and contour, and soft, without calcification. In adults, ap-

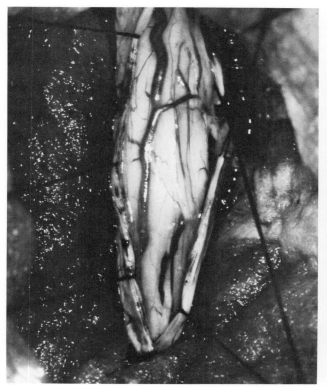

A

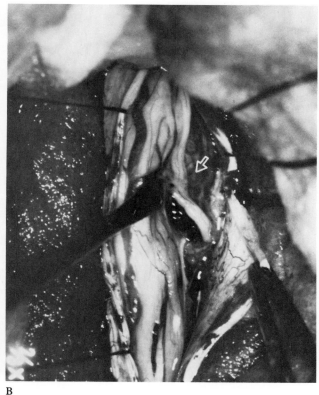

B

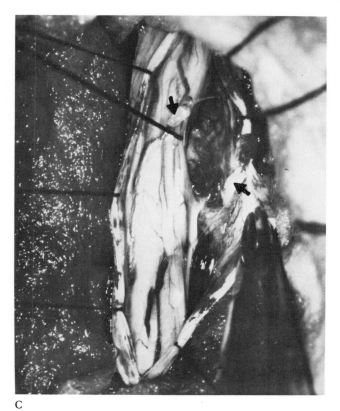

C

Figure 125-3 *A.* Operative photograph showing a widened spinal cord but no obvious tumor. *B.* Operative photograph showing retraction of the cord and visualization of the tumor (*arrow*) underlying a dorsal nerve root. *C.* Operative photograph following removal of the tumor showing the cut ends (*arrows*) of a thoracic dorsal root, sacrificed to expedite the removal of this tumor.

instances, the plane between the tumor and the spinal cord may be indistinguishable around most of the tumor; however, the characteristic features of the tumor may allow it to be gutted without injuring the surrounding spinal cord. This is frequently feasible in the case of the holointramedullary astrocytoma of childhood. Epstein and Epstein have debulked these low-grade astrocytomas, either grade I or grade II with associated cysts, in a majority of cases, leading to improved neurological function and possibly to long-term cure.[7] Rarely, the intramedullary astrocytoma is malignant—grade III or grade IV. In such cases the growth of the tumor is rapid, the color and contour differences between neural tissue and tumor are absent, and the tumor has a propensity for seeding the spinal and in some cases the intracranial subarachnoid spaces. Interestingly, the low-grade astrocytomas, although extensive, do not often violate the junction between the spinal cord and the brain stem. The sister tumor occuring within the cerebellar hemisphere is similar in terms of growth, histological features, and anatomical division between tumor and neural tissue.

Uncommon intradural tumors include the dermoids, epi-

proximately 50 percent of astrocytomas have a well-defined plane between tumor and neural tissue and are often associated with cysts, and accordingly can be resected. In other

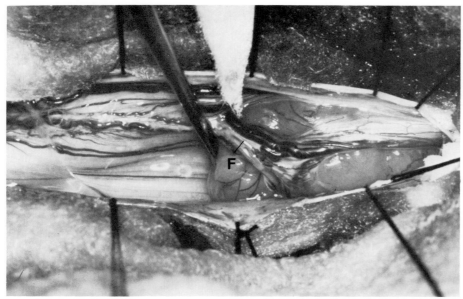

A

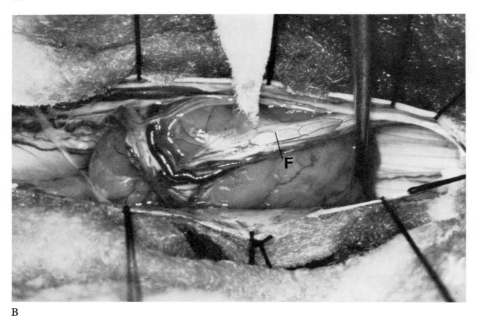

B

Figure 125-4 Operative photograph showing an ependymoma of the filum (F). The white cottonoid marker remains static in position, demonstrating the mobility of this tumor.
A. Tumor displaced caudally.
B. Tumor displaced rostrally.

dermoids, and teratomas. The rare teratomas are intramedullary. The dermoid and epidermoid tumors occur both in an intramedullary location and in the region of the cauda equina. In the latter instance, the occurrence of an epidermoid tumor has been attributed to one or more preceding lumbar punctures presumably carrying cutaneous tissue into the spinal canal. The capsule of these tumors creates a reaction in the surrounding neural tissue that may thwart total removal of the capsule and contents. Nevertheless, these tumors are slow-growing, avascular, and encapsulated, and for the most part should be resectable. Experience indicates that residual diaphanous portions of the capsule apparently remain static or grow at such a slow rate that cures for a decade or more have been recorded.

Hemangioblastomas as solitary tumors or as part of the broader syndrome of the von Hippel-Lindau complex do involve the spinal cord but are rare.[12,23,38] They most commonly involve the cervical or thoracic regions. Their vascularity varies; however, they are the most vascular variety of intradural tumor. They may be wholly intramedullary, but frequently gain the dorsal surface of the spinal cord and are visible upon initial exposure of the involved area (Fig. 125-5). They are discrete and encapsulated, and rarely involve more than one or two segments of the spinal cord. They are often associated with cysts that may extend some distance from the body of the tumor. These tumors are benign and are amenable to surgical resection. In two cases, we have witnessed an unexplained widening of the spinal cord below the

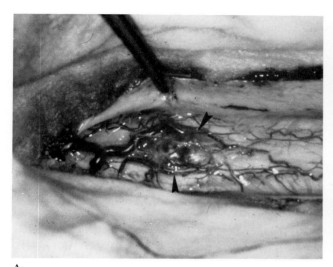
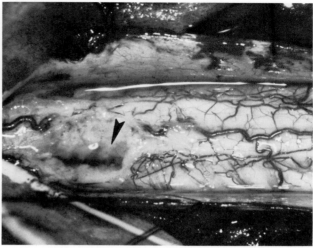

A   B

Figure 125-5 *A.* Operative photograph showing a cervical hemangioblastoma (*ar-rowheads*), intramedullary but with a portion reaching the surface. *B.* Operative photograph following tumor removal. A small cyst is marked by an arrowhead. The widening of the cervical cord below the level of the tumor remains unexplained.

level of the lesion without an associated cyst or another hemangioblastoma. Following the total removal of the tumor, this widening regressed, as shown on follow-up myelography.

Rare types of spinal tumors include intramedullary carcinomatous metastases, mixed tumors that include malignant elements of a variety of tumors, and neurenteric cysts, which often compress the cord from a symmetrical ventral location and mimic an intramedullary tumor upon initial exploration of the spinal cord.[16,31] These latter tumors are very rare and are discussed elsewhere in this textbook.

Lipomas have been excluded from this discussion since purely intramedullary lipomas are rare.[34] The more common variety of lipoma, associated with lipomeningocele, is a different entity, congenital in nature and associated with extradural components; these often manifest neurological abnormalities due to tethering of the spinal cord and local mass effect.

Differential Diagnosis

A mass within the spinal canal presenting with insidious development and progression of clinical symptoms and signs is invariably a tumor and has little rival in a differential diagnosis. The most confusing differential diagnosis is between intramedullary tumor and syringomyelia. Both produce gradual, progressive symptoms over many years and are associated with spinal cord widening. Syringomyelia, however, is often associated with other abnormalities such as an Arnold-Chiari malformation, hydrocephalus, and congenital deformities of the cervical spine. A diagnosis should be made by myelography in combination with CT scanning. Inflammatory conditions involving the spinal cord may mimic a spinal tumor; however, the course is more rapid and

is often associated with severe pain, fever, tenderness of the spine, and other evidence of a rapidly progressive inflammatory process or primary focus. Certain parasitic conditions, especially schistosomiasis, involve the spinal cord, producing a widening, vascular occlusion, and a progressive clinical picture. Fortunately, because of their rarity in the western hemisphere these present little problem in differential diagnosis.

Surgical Considerations

Although the clinical picture is important in suggesting a spinal tumor and assisting in the localization of the process, the radiographic diagnosis is the key to preparing for and performing surgery. Plain spine radiography often reveals abnormalities at the site of the tumor (Fig. 125-2A) and additional information acquired by myelography (Fig. 125-6), combined with routine radiographs and CT scanning, makes the diagnosis secure in virtually all cases. Armed with the clinical and radiographic information, the surgeon is able to design exposures that minimize the removal of bone and maximize the potential for removal of the benign tumors afflicting the spinal cord.[6,19] Generally, the earlier the recognition of the problem at a time of minor neurological deficit, the better the prognosis and surgical result. Patients who are neurologically devastated, especially older people, are unlikely to gain satisfactory resolution of neurological defects.

The patient is prepared for surgery by steroid medication and a medical evaluation that is aimed at turning up any coagulation deficiencies or any pulmonary problems, especially in association with cervical tumors, where the surgeon may be confronted by additional respiratory problems postoperatively. It is pertinent that many of these patients have

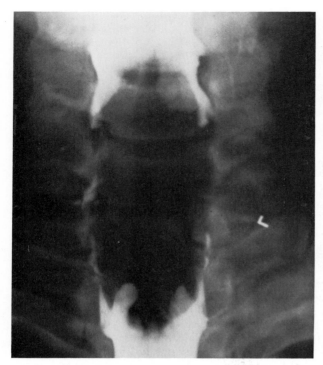

Figure 125-6 A cervical myelogram showing typical widening of the spinal cord by a large intramedullary tumor encompassing most of the cervical region. This requires a broad laminectomy of all cervical and upper thoracic segments for exposure.

taken aspirin or other platelet-inhibiting medications to relieve their pain and do not make the physician aware of these circumstances prior to operation. Such medications may create problems with hemostasis. The operation is discussed in detail with the patient and family, emphasizing that these tumors often occupy a high percentage of the spinal space, severely compressing spinal cord tissue, and that their symptoms and signs may not truly reflect the huge extent of the tumor. The implication of this is that any additional injury or compression to the spinal cord may lead to a neurological disaster during or immediately after the operation. In the case of cervical tumors, the patient should be warned that it may be necessary to maintain intubation for 24 to 48 h postoperatively to insure an adequate airway. Furthermore, because flexion of the head on the cervical spine is necessary for operations involving the cervical region, a preoperative test in flexion should be carried out for 15 to 20 min with the patient awake in order to see if the flexion is tolerated. The area to be operated on is kept relatively high above the heart in order to maximize venous drainage and prevent any congestion around the area of the surgery. A free abdomen or chest, as well as excellent ventilation, is absolutely essential. A midline incision is utilized and a relatively wide laminectomy sparing the intervertebral articulations is carried out.

Because of the confined nature of the spinal canal and the size of tumors relative to the diameter of the spinal cord, the use of the operating microscope is advisable. I prefer the

prone position in most cases, since this maximizes the use of the surgical assistant working via the binocular sidearm of the microscope, face-to-face with the operating surgeon. Some surgeons prefer the sitting position for tumors located in the cervical or upper thoracic region; however with this position it is almost impossible to use the assistant effectively. The spinal exposure should encompass the area of the pathological process, leaving a modest amount of space at the rostral and caudal margins in order to prepare for mobilization of the tumor. In children, there is controversy regarding the use of laminotomy versus laminectomy.[24] Theoretically, replacement of the spinous processes and laminae minimizes progressive spinal deformities in the postoperative period. Spinal stability is always an important consideration in operations on these tumors, especially those that are more extensive in rostrocaudal dimension. In adults, laminotomy is not a practical consideration and in all cases laminectomy is performed. If the tumor is intradural but extramedullary, the laminectomy must be wide on the ipsilateral side and may include the joint facets and the intervertebral foramen, especially in the case of a dumbbell neurofibroma. A similar situation exists in the case of a meningioma, where the attachment to the dura may demand removal of a segment of dura in order to ensure total removal of the tumor. While preserving bone and ligamentous structures wherever possible, nerve roots and radicular arteries must also be preserved when feasible in the removal of even the largest tumors. The dorsal roots, which are often impediments to tumor removal, may be sacrificed over a number of segments in the thoracic region; however, the surgeon should attempt to preserve the dorsal roots in the midcervical region wherever possible (Fig. 125-7). Nevertheless, it has been shown in physiological experiments that all but one or two of the dorsal roots to an upper extremity may be sacrificed without significant impairment in the neurological function of that extremity, including fine movements of the fingers.[29] This apparent paradox exists because of the substitution of eye-motor coordination. However, the loss of anterior roots in the cervical or lumbosacral enlargements is associated with severe consequences which are not compensated. All of these roots must be spared wherever possible. In the thoracic region, anterior roots may be sectioned without severe neurological consequences.

In the case of extramedullary-intradural tumors, surgical principles employed elsewhere for benign tumors also apply to the spinal region. It is important to create traction only on the lesion and not on the neural tissue. This may be accomplished in larger tumors by an intracapsular decompression prior to removal of the tumor, sparing nerve roots and other vital structures. The use of a CUSA unit (Cavitron ultrasonic surgical aspirator; Cooper Medical, Stamford, Conn.) in such tumors is most beneficial as this creates a rapid debulking without displacement of neural or tumor tissue. The surgeon is advised to seek out the vascular supply, no matter how minimal this may be, prior to the debulking or final removal of the tumor in order to create a relatively avascular situation. Keeping the operative field free of blood assists in the removal of the tumor because the anatomical and color planes between the tumor and neural tissue are maintained in a virgin state, without staining of the tissues by blood. In those extramedullary tumors located predominantly ventral

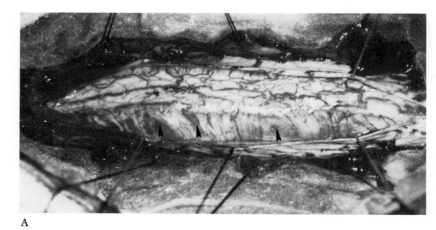

A

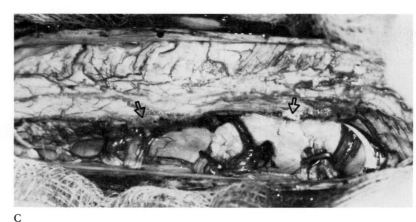

B

Figure 125-7 *A*. Operative photograph showing a large, ventrolaterally located meningioma barely visible (*arrowheads*) between the dorsal roots of the midcervical region. *B*. Operative photograph showing two cut dorsal roots (*arrows*). This allows better visualization of the tumor (T) and facilitates removal. *C*. Operative photograph showing the cavity left by tumor removal. The two cut dorsal roots are marked by arrows and the ventral roots are intact.

C

or ventrolateral to the spinal cord, a wide laminectomy with transverse cutting of the dura facilitates an undercutting and debulking of the tumor and permits the surgeon to maneuver it out from under the critical ventral area of the spinal cord. In most instances, meningiomas and neurilemmomas receive little blood supply and are attached by few adhesions to the spinal cord. In the case of the foramen magnum meningioma, the tumor often encases or envelopes the vertebral artery. Here great care must be taken not to injure this structure. When the tumor extends above the foramen magnum, it often incorporates the twelfth cranial nerve and it

may be impossible to remove the tumor without sacrificing this nerve.

In surgery for conus medullaris and cauda equina tumors, especially ependymomas, which occur both in and out of the spinal cord, first the exophytic portion of the tumor is removed, and then the intramedullary portion may be separable from the conus medullaris region. The tumor often is situated like a cork in a bottle, coming away from a cystic extension within the conus medullaris region of the spinal cord with relative ease. In removing an ependymoma of the filum terminale, it is often necessary to remove the latter as

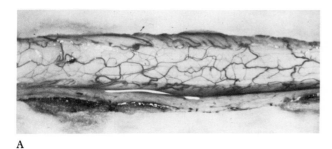

A

Figure 125-8 *A.* Operative photograph of a widened cervical cord caused by an intramedullary ependymoma. *B.* A drawing showing the steps in the removal of an intramedullary tumor, including bipolar cautery under irrigation. *C.* Intact specimen of an ependymoma removed from the intramedullary position. *D.* Cavity left by removal of the intramedullary ependymoma (*diamonds*). Arrowheads indicate fine traction sutures in the pia that maintain the opening in the spinal cord. *E.* Drawing showing the cavity left by the removal of an intramedullary tumor. Note that the tumor tends to grow in a dorsal position.

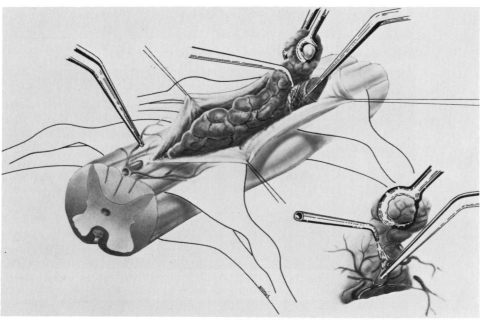

B

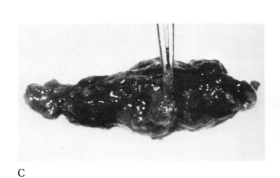

C

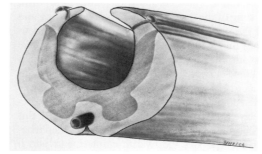

D

E

well (without consequent neurologic deficit). A neurofibroma of the cauda equina is easily removed, usually with sacrifice of a single dorsal root (with no consequence). Dermoid and epidermoid tumors occurring in the cauda equina region present a unique problem. The surgeon must be careful not to spill the noxious contents of these tumors into the subarachnoid space because this will result in an arachnoiditis and adhesions around the conus, leading to distressing pain and neurological deficits in the postoperative period. Therefore, these tumors must be carefully debulked and a persistent, careful attempt made to remove the capsule from the surrounding nerve roots. This may present difficulties, and in some cases it may be necessary to leave diaphanous portions of the capsule adherent to the roots so as not to sacrifice them. The result should be good.

The removal of intramedullary tumors has undergone evolution over many decades, as previously mentioned (Fig. 125-8).[4,6–8,10–13,20,27,28,38] These tumors tend to be avascular and in the majority of instances can be totally removed, resulting in a cure. It is essential that the exposure encompass the entire extent of the intramedullary process whether it be cystic or solid. In most instances the tumor spans a number of segments. The dura will be tense due to the underlying compression by the tumor and should be opened at either extreme of the tumor. At the caudal end of the tumor, the surgeon is more apt to encounter dilated veins and therefore it may be safer to open the dura from the rostral end. Once the entire area of spinal cord widening has been exposed, the surgeon must select a site for myelotomy. In a minority of instances, the tumor will be visible through the translucent dorsal or dorsolateral portion of the spinal cord. However, in most instances, the tumor lies beneath the surface so that it is not readily visible. A myelotomy should be carried out as close to the midline as possible. The incision must be straight and parallel to the longitudinal plane of the spinal cord. With the ladder-like arrangement of arteries and veins that occurs over the dorsal surface of the spinal cord, in performing a myelotomy it will be necessary to interrupt a number of small vascular channels. This is accomplished with a bipolar cautery set at low level under irrigation, and the myelotomy is then made by a sharp dissection. The myelotomy should be carried over the entire extent of widening of the spinal cord so that any planes between the tumor and the spinal cord will not be missed. Once this has been performed, the pial margins are held back with fine sutures under tension, opening the cord as one would open a book. If the myelotomy has been extensive, a plane between the tumor and the spinal cord will be readily visible. This is then further developed by gentle use of dissectors, bipolar cautery, and cottonoids. If the surgeon is fortunate enough to encounter a cyst at either one or both ends of the tumor, this significantly facilitates the removal of the tumor. In many instances, it may not be necessary to debulk the interior of the tumor in order to effect a total removal. In terms of debulking the interior of the tumor, care must be taken not to allow any bleeding, which spills over and obscures the plane between the external surface of the tumor and the spinal cord. It is absolutely essential that this area be kept dry so that the surgeon can carefully follow the contour and coloration provided by the margin of a resectable tumor. Combining these maneuvers allows the surgeon to remove the tumor expeditiously. In the case of the astrocytoma there may be a plane which encompasses most of the tumor but in some places tends to fade into the surrounding spinal cord. In this instance, judgment must be used in defining where this plane is or should be, and removal is carried out radically. Epstein and Epstein have recently reported the use of the CUSA in the removal of intramedullary astrocytomas in children.[7] They state that these tumors are probably different from those in adults; the childhood astrocytoma is more indolent in growth and can usually be debulked to give an excellent postoperative result.

In the case of intramedullary dermoid tumors, it may be impossible to remove every filament of the fine tumor capsule; the surgeon should attempt the most radical removal possible without injury to the surrounding spinal cord tissue. Recently we have utilized sensory evoked potential monitoring during radical tumor removal. The potentials are recorded from the spinal cord above the site of operation and from the cortex. The usefulness of this procedure is yet to be determined. It appears to warn when cord function is affected during the removal of tumor. However, if the surgeon is carefully dissecting with the microscope it may not be necessary to give up at this point, since the loss of potentials appears to be reversible on occasion.

I have found no need to appose the pial margins of the opened spinal cord. These are released and tend to collapse together. I have not had the development of cysts under tension within the spinal cord following these resections.

In dealing with an intramedullary hemangioblastoma, the area of the tumor is exposed by appropriate laminectomy and dural opening, care being taken not to injure any of the vasculature in the performance of this initial exposure. The arterial supply to the tumor, which is easily recognized, is interrupted first; this is similar to the technique used in the removal of an arteriovenous malformation from either the spinal cord or the brain. After a myelotomy directed rostrally and caudally in the midline a short distance from the tumor, a bipolar cautery is utilized to caress the margin of the tumor, around which a circumscribing incision is then made. Gradually the vascular adhesions to the tumor are interrupted, preserving a large, easily visible draining vein until the final removal of the tumor, which is swung out on this venous pedicle that is then cauterized and divided between clips. Any associated cysts are drained in the process.

Following the removal of a spinal tumor, the dura is closed or a dural substitute (preferably fascia or freeze-dried dura) is used to close the opening. I prefer not to cover the exposed spinal cord with Gelfoam (absorbable gelatin sponge; The Upjohn Co, Kalamazoo, Mich.) alone, although this has been recommended by others as a satisfactory means of closure. In those patients that have been previously operated on and given radiation, the surgeon is doubly concerned about the integrity and watertightness of the closure. Any leakage from the area of operation may lead to a disastrous infection, or at the very least to a nagging inflammatory reaction in the surrounding tissues and agony for both the surgeon and the patient in the postoperative period. If a laminotomy has been done, then these fragments are wired or sewn back into position and the muscles and fascia are then closed in meticulous fashion. I generally use drains in the epidural space if the integrity of the dura has been reconstituted. These drains are left for a period of 12 h. The muscle layers are carefully approximated, with the surgeon taking care that these heavy sutures are not placed too close to the dorsal surface of the cord, which might lead to a guillotine-like compression of the spinal cord with motion of the spine. In the instance of thoracic lesions, a brace of heavy tape is applied to the shoulders and the back to prevent postoperative stretching of the incision by movements of the patient or by the nursing staff in moving the patient.

In the instance of high cervical lesions, whether they be

intra- or extramedullary, it is often advisable to leave the endotracheal tube in position until the surgeon is assured of normal respiratory function. This may require a 24- to 48-h interval of careful monitoring of respiratory function before the endotracheal tube can be removed. Special care in the postoperative period must be given to bladder function if these areas are involved. The surgeon must also remember that extensive tumors (whether intra- or extramedullary) above the lumbosacral region, especially cervical and high thoracic tumors, may lead to sympathetic denervation and therefore to postural hypotension as the patient is mobilized postoperatively.

The use of a two-stage operation, as originally proposed by Elsberg[6] and carried out in a minority of his intramedullary tumor cases, is not now widely accepted.[20,28] The theory is that performance of a myelotomy over an intramedullary tumor followed by closure of the wound with the dura open will allow the tumor to extrude from the spinal cord and therefore permit it to be removed at a second-stage operation. It is my opinion that with the use of the operating microscope, the best opportunity to remove such tumors is at the primary operation, and if they cannot be removed at that time then a secondary operation performed on the heels of the first will not lead to additional removal of a significant amount of tumor. Experience with malignant astrocytomas has been discouraging. These tumors are not completely resectable and in my experience the effect of radiation has been nil, with the tumors continuing to grow and with frequent seeding throughout the subarachnoid space in spite of extensive radiotherapy.

The use of radiotherapy in the treatment of intramedullary tumors is controversial. Optimistic reports of the effect of radiation on intramedullary tumors, such as ependymomas and low-grade astrocytomas, appear to be without foundation.[26,37] In analyzing these reports, it is noted that the follow-up period is purely clinical and is too short relative to the normal evolution of these tumors. It is quite feasible that the beneficial results attributed to this treatment are related more to the decompressive laminectomy. Unfortunately, follow-up myelograms have not been performed in the vast majority of these cases to indicate resolution or involution of the tumor following radiation therapy. Orthopedists have also reported that radiotherapy has a deleterious effect on growth of the spine.[15] Additionally, in many instances I have observed deleterious effects from radiation to central areas of the spinal cord adjacent to the tumor when these patients have been operated upon some time after a course of radiotherapy.[27,28] Lacking definitive evidence for a beneficial effect of radiation upon benign intramedullary tumors, I have not recommended such treatment. Rather, I prefer to observe these patients and consider a second operation should the clinical and radiographic situation so dictate.

Prognosis and Results

The immediate results and future prognoses in the common extramedullary-intradural tumors, including meningiomas and neurilemmomas, have been well established. These tumors are benign and if such a tumor is carefully and thoroughly removed, the patient should be cured, with an excellent prognosis.[11,20,28] Even in patients that have been devastated neurologically by the growth of these tumors prior to surgical intervention, there is some hope, especially in young individuals, that many of the neurological abnormalities may resolve slowly in the postoperative period. It may take 18 months to 2 years to maximize the resolution of these neurological deficits, and in some instances there has been progressive improvement beyond this time frame.

The majority of intramedullary tumors are benign and resectable. Paradoxically, in the rare intramedullary lipomas, total removal is rarely possible; however, because of their extremely slow growth the long-term prognosis is encouraging.[34]

In my series of 31 intramedullary tumors (32 operations), there has been no mortality. Postoperative deterioration has occurred in seven patients. The result of the surgery is predicated on the preoperative neurological condition of the patient. Those individuals who have maximum neurological deficits prior to the operation have made no significant functional recovery following successful tumor removal. In those individuals with mild to modest neurological deficits, when the tumor has been totally removed excellent functional recovery may be expected. In those instances where only a portion of the tumor has been removed, the subsequent course depends upon the growth pattern of the tumor. If the tumor is static or indolent, the neurological deficits may improve or may remain chronic. In the case of malignant tumors the postoperative course tends to be disastrous, with rapid growth and seeding of the tumor. I have not as yet used a second-look operation to remove more of these incompletely removed tumors. This, however, is a viable option and in my estimation is preferable to radiotherapy. If cysts in association with an incompletely removed tumor recur, these may be tapped percutaneously to alleviate symptoms and reduce pressure within the spinal cord.

I have had no instance of recurrence in those cases of totally removed tumors that comprise the majority of this series over a follow-up period which varies from 6 months to ten years. Few conclusions can be drawn from this statement since this disease process, as previously mentioned, may span not only years but decades.

One problem unique to intramedullary tumor surgery has been the increase in pain syndromes following successful surgery. The physiological mechanism for this phenomenon is poorly understood and the treatment defies the grasp of most physicians dealing with these problems. The pain is often comprehensive and involves many portions of the body. It is almost impossible to control except by psychological preparation and treatment of the patient pre- and postoperatively. I have seen no ameliorative effect from the use of various drugs or stimulators that are useful in other pain problems of spinal origin.

References

1. Arseni C, Maretsis M: Tumors of the lower spinal cord associated with increased intracranial pressure and papilledema. J Neurosurg 27:105–110, 1967.
2. Austin G: *The Spinal Cord: Basic Aspects and Surgical Consider-*

ations, 2d ed. Springfield, Ill., Charles C Thomas, 1972, pp 281–283.

3. Connolly ES: Spinal cord tumors in adults, in Youmans JR (ed): *Neurological Surgery*, 2d ed. Philadelphia, Saunders, 1982, pp 3196–3214.

4. Cushing H: The special field of neurological surgery. Bull Hopkins Hosp 16:77–87, 1905.

5. DeSousa AL, Kalsbeck JE, Mealey J Jr, Campbell RL, Hockey A: Intraspinal tumors in children: A review of 81 cases. J Neurosurg 51:437–445, 1979.

6. Elsberg CA: *Tumors of the Spinal Cord and the Symptoms of Irritation and Compression of the Spinal Cord and Nerve Roots: Pathology, Symptomatology, Diagnosis, and Treatment*. New York, Paul B Hoeber, 1925.

7. Epstein F, Epstein N: Surgical management of holocord intramedullary spinal cord astrocytomas in children: Report of three cases. J Neurosurg 54:829–832, 1981.

8. Garrido E, Stein BM: Microsurgical removal of intramedullary spinal cord tumors. Surg Neurol 7:215–219, 1977.

9. Gowers WR, Horsley V: A case of tumour of the spinal cord: Removal; recovery. (Wilkins RH (ed): Neurosurgical classics XI). J Neurosurg 20:815–824, 1963.

10. Greenwood J Jr: Intramedullary tumors of spinal cord: A follow-up study after total surgical removal. J Neurosurg 20:665–668, 1963.

11. Greenwood J Jr: Surgical removal of intramedullary tumors. J Neurosurg 26:276–282, 1967.

12. Guidetti B, Fortuna A: Surgical treatment of intramedullary hemangioblastoma of the spinal cord. Report of 6 cases. J Neurosurg 27:530–540, 1967.

13. Horrax G, Henderson DG: Encapsulated intramedullary tumor involving the whole spinal cord from medulla to conus: Complete enucleation with recovery. Surg Gynecol Obstet 68:814–819, 1939.

14. Kahn EA: The role of the dentate ligaments in spinal cord compression and the syndrome of lateral sclerosis. J Neurosurg 4:191–199, 1947.

15. Katzman H, Waugh T, Berdon W: Skeletal changes following irradiation of childhood tumors. Bone Joint Surg [Am] 51A:825–842, 1969.

16. Klump TE: Neurenteric cyst in the cervical spinal canal of a 10-week-old boy: Case report. J Neurosurg 35:472–476, 1971.

17. Kurland LT: Frequency of intracranial and intraspinal neoplasms in the resident population of Rochester, Minnesota. J Neurosurg 15:627–641, 1958.

18. Lazorthes G, Gouaze A, Zadeh JO, Santini JJ, Lazorthes Y, Burdin P: Arterial vascularization of the spinal cord: Recent studies of the anastomotic substitution pathways. J Neurosurg 35:253–262, 1971.

19. Love JG: Laminectomy for the removal of spinal cord tumors. J Neurosurg 25:116–121, 1966.

20. Malis LI: Intramedullary spinal cord tumors. Clin Neurosurg 25:512–540, 1978.

21. Mason TH, Keigher HA: Intramedullary spinal neurilemmoma: Case report. J Neurosurg 29:414–416, 1968.

22. Matson DD: *Neurosurgery of Infancy and Childhood*, 2d ed. Springfield, Ill., Charles C Thomas, 1969, pp 647–693.

23. Otenasek FJ, Silver ML: Spinal hemangioma (hemangioblastoma) in Lindau's disease. Report of six cases in a single family. J Neurosurg 18:295–300, 1961.

24. Raimondi AJ, Gutierrez FA, di Rocco C: Laminotomy and total reconstruction of the posterior spinal arch for spinal canal surgery in childhood. J Neurosurg 45:555–560, 1976.

25. Rand RW, Rand CW: *Intraspinal Tumors of Childhood*. Springfield, Ill., Charles C Thomas, 1960.

26. Schwade JG, Wara WM, Sheline GE, Sorgen S, Wilson CB: Management of primary spinal cord tumors. Int J Radiat Oncol Biol Phys 4:389–393, 1978.

27. Stein BM: Surgery of intramedullary spinal cord tumors. Clin Neurosurg 26:529–542, 1979.

28. Stein BM: Management of intramedullary spinal cord lesions. Neurol Neurosurg Update Ser 4(13):1–12, 1983.

29. Stein BM, Carpenter MB: Effects of dorsal rhizotomy upon subthalamic dyskinesia in the monkey. Arch Neurol 13:567–583, 1965.

30. Stein BM, Leeds NE, Taveras JM, Pool JL: Meningiomas of the foramen magnum. J Neurosurg 20:740–751, 1963.

31. Stein BM, Richardson EP Jr: Spinal-cord disorder in a 19-year-old man. N Engl J Med 293:33–38, 1975.

32. Suh TH, Alexander L: Vascular system of the human spinal cord. Arch Neurol Psychiatry 41:659–677, 1939.

33. Taylor AR, Byrnes DP: Foramen magnum and high cervical cord compression. Brain 97:473–480, 1974.

34. Thomas JE, Miller RH: Lipomatous tumors of the spinal canal: A study of their clinical range. Mayo Clin Proc 48:393–400, 1973.

35. Turnbull IM, Brieg A, Hassler, O: Blood supply of cervical spinal cord in man: A microangiographic cadaver study. J Neurosurg 24:951–965, 1966.

36. Webb JH, Craig WM, Kernohan JW: Intraspinal neoplasms in the cervical region. J Neurosurg 10:360–366, 1953.

37. Wood EH, Berne AS, Taveras JM: The value of radiation therapy in the management of intrinsic tumors of the spinal cord. Radiology 63:11–24, 1954.

38. Yasargil MG, Antic J, Laciga R, de Preux J, Fideler RW, Boone SC: The microsurgical removal of intramedullary spinal hemangioblastomas: Report of twelve cases and a review of the literature. Surg Neurol 6:141–148, 1976.

126

Spinal Epidural Tumors

Perry Black

Incidence

Metastatic lesions of the spine make up a large majority of spinal epidural tumors. Approximately 5 percent of cancer patients develop spinal epidural tumor deposits, although not all of these become clinically evident.[1] Spinal metastasis as a clinical problem is likely to increase in the future as the life expectancy of cancer patients is prolonged with advances in therapy. Benign tumors such as neurilemmomas, neurofibromas, and meningiomas are generally intradural but occasionally have an extradural component or may be limited to the extradural space (Fig. 126-1).

Pathology

Origin of Metastatic Lesion

The three most common primary lesions are carcinoma of the lung, carcinoma of the breast, and lymphoma. In almost one-tenth of cases, the patient is not known to have cancer, and the spinal cord compression is the initial symptom of malignancy; in an additional one-tenth of cases, the primary lesion cannot be identified, even after diagnostic study.[8]

Latent Interval

The time interval between the original diagnosis of cancer and the occurrence of spinal metastasis varies widely. In one series the range was 0 to 19 years, with the longest interval occurring in patients with breast carcinoma.[8]

Sex and Age Distributions of Metastatic and Benign Tumors

For metastatic tumors, there is a slight preponderance of males (60 percent) over females.[8,14] All ages may be affected, but the period of highest incidence coincides with the relatively high cancer risk period of 40 to 65 years of age. Males and females are equally affected by neurilemmomas;

these tumors occur predominantly from 30 to 50 years of age. Eighty percent of spinal meningiomas occur in females in the age range of 40 to 70 years.[13]

Route of Metastatic Spread to the Spinal Canal

Extraspinal malignant tumors are believed to metastasize to the spine and extradural space by hematogenous spread via the paravertebral and extradural venous plexus, as described by Batson.[2] Tumors may also gain entry to the spinal extradural space by bony erosion and direct extension from adjacent vertebrae.

Distribution of Spinal Metastases and Benign Tumors

Metastatic deposits may occur in any portion of the spinal canal. For each portion of the canal, the rate of involvement corresponds roughly to the proportion of that part to the total length of the spine; thus the thoracic spine is involved in about 60 percent of the cases. A large majority of the tumors are localized to one or two vertebral segments; 17 percent of the patients in one large series, however, showed evidence of compression of the spinal cord or cauda equina at two or more sites at some time during the course of their disease.[8] The possibility of multiple sites of involvement points to the desirability of radiological examination of the entire spinal canal in patients suspected of having spinal metastatic lesions. Metastasis to the vertebral column may involve any portion of one or more vertebral elements, including the vertebral body, pedicle, lamina, or spinous process. Although the vertebral body may be destroyed, the intervertebral disc is maintained because it is resistant to invasion by tumor; this feature is a useful radiographic diagnostic aid in distinguishing neoplastic destruction of a vertebral body from infection (vertebral osteomyelitis), in which the disc is often destroyed along with the vertebral body.

When metastasis invades the spinal canal, it is usually restricted to the extradural space. The dura mater is a barrier to penetration of tumor cells into the subdural or subarachnoid space; for this reason surgeons are generally reluctant to open the dura when resecting an epidural metastasis. Within the epidural space there is variable tumor involvement of the anterior (ventral) compartment, the lateral gutters, and the posterior compartment (or any combination of these sites). The location of the extradural metastatic lesion has important surgical implications, in that a metastatic tumor mass in the posterior extradural compartment is easily accessible to the surgeon by a posterior laminectomy approach, whereas a ventral mass is technically more difficult to remove by this approach.

Intradural extramedullary metastasis is uncommon, with a reported incidence of 1 to 4 percent.[6,10,15] Invasion of the spinal cord parenchyma is even less common; in one series, intramedullary metastasis formed only 2 percent of the spinal metastases.[6]

With respect to benign epidural tumors, neurilemmomas and neurofibromas are intradural and extramedullary in

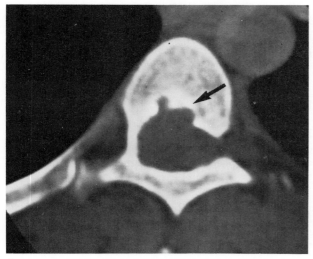

A

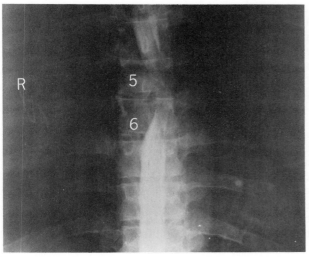

B

Figure 126-1 Epidural neurilemmoma at T5–6 in 34-year-old man with 1-year history of pain in midthoracic and upper lumbar regions and progressive weakness and sensory impairment in the lower extremities. He also had difficulty with gait and micturition. *A.* CT scan (without contrast enhancement) at T5 shows involvement (*arrow*) of the posterior portion of the vertebral body. *B.* Myelogram shows a subtotal block at T5–6 suggestive of extradural mass lesion. Microsurgical total excision of an extradural neurilemmoma was carried out, with rapid postoperative recovery of neurological function.

approximately 70 percent of cases, and the remaining 30 percent are equally divided between a strictly extradural location and a dumbbell or hourglass configuration (involving the intradural and/or extradural compartment with extension into the paraspinal space); 1 percent are intramedullary.[11] Half of all neurilemmomas and neurofibromas are located in the thoracic spine; the next most frequent site is the cervical region, and the least frequent site the lumbar area.

Meningiomas are generally intradural and extramedullary, but 15 percent are extradural. They are often attached to the insertion of the dentate ligaments and may be seen as multiple lesions in von Recklinghausen's disease. Meningiomas may be located in any portion of the spinal canal, but two-thirds are found in the thoracic region.

Symptoms and Signs

Metastatic Tumors

The onset of symptoms of spinal cord or nerve root compression may be acute or insidious. The duration of symptoms before diagnosis by myelography varies from 5 days to 2 years (with a median of 2 months).[8] Pain is usually the initial symptom (96 percent of cases), preceding other symptoms by 5 days to 2 years (with a median of 7 weeks).[8] Local pain in the vertebral column is generally located close to the site of the lesion. Radicular pain, less common than local spinal pain, is also of localizing value, as it radiates in the dermatomal distribution of the compressed or tumor-infiltrated nerve roots.

Weakness, usually in the lower extremities, rarely occurs as a first symptom but is common (76 percent of cases) by the time the diagnosis is made.[8] Despite an antecedent history of spinal or radicular pain, some 15 percent of patients present with paraplegia;[8] this points to the importance of placing a high index of suspicion on spinal or radicular pain in following patients with known cancer.

More than half the patients with spinal cord compression secondary to metastatic disease have bladder and bowel dysfunction at the time of diagnosis. Sphincter dysfunction is usually associated with motor and sensory loss, although a few patients with compression limited to the conus medullaris do not have weakness or sensory impairment of the lower limbs.

Sensory symptoms such as numbness or paresthesias in the extremities or trunk do not generally occur as initial symptoms but are present in about half the patients at the time of diagnosis.[8]

In the presence of paraplegia, the neurological deficit is clear-cut and a presumptive diagnosis of spinal cord compression is readily made. There is flaccid paralysis of the lower limbs and a distended bladder; the level of motor or sensory loss approximates the site of spinal cord compression. The deficit may be more subtle, however, in cases of early spinal cord compression. Anterior (ventral) cord compression is suspected when there is weakness in the extremities and loss of spinothalamic tract function (pain and temperature sense) below the level of the lesion, with preservation of dorsal column sensation (touch, position, vibration).[3] The loss of dorsal column sensation with preservation of other sensory or motor functions suggests pressure on the posterior spinal cord.

The level of motor loss, except in thoracic cord involvement, is a somewhat more reliable indicator of the spinal cord segment involved than is the sensory loss level. The level of sensory loss on the chest or abdomen is the most useful localizing sign in thoracic spinal cord compression.

The abdominal reflexes may also help in localization, because their innervation originates from segments T_8 to T_{12}. The motor and sensory deficits are generally symmetrical, but occasionally asymmetrical compression of the spinal cord or interference with its blood supply produces Brown-Séquard's syndrome.

The lumbar and sacral nerve roots of the cauda equina are loosely arranged in the spinal canal. Compression of the cauda equina is, therefore, often irregular, giving rise to patchy and asymmetrical motor and sensory loss in the lower limbs. By comparison, compression of the lower spinal cord (conus medullaris) may be identified by a more complete and symmetrical distribution of neurological signs. Compression of the conus or cauda equina characteristically produces saddle anesthesia and loss of sphincter control.

In a spinal examination, the patient's characteristic pain is commonly reproduced by spinal movement or by gentle fist percussion over the vertebral spinous processes at the affected level.

When there is some question regarding bladder dysfunction, the situation can be clarified by having the patient void, then introducing a urinary catheter to measure the volume of residual urine. Neurogenic bladder may be assumed to be present if the residual urine volume is more than 150 ml.

Benign Tumors

When it is located in the epidural space, a benign tumor (neurilemmoma, neurofibroma, or meningioma) is likely to cause nerve root irritation with associated radicular pain or dysesthesias. As the tumor enlarges and produces spinal cord compression, segmental sensory or motor disturbances develop. Brown-Séquard's syndrome is more apt to occur in benign tumors than in epidural metastatic tumors, because benign tumors are more commonly confined to one side. Besides the absence of a history of malignant disease, patients with benign epidural tumors are likely to have symptoms of longer duration—months to years—than those of patients with metastatic tumors.

Diagnostic Studies

The radiological appearance of spinal tumors is discussed in another chapter of this textbook. However, some general principles concerning selection of diagnostic studies, of particular relevance to epidural tumors, are discussed here.

Spine Films

Plain x-ray films of the suspected portion of the vertebral column show evidence of metastatic involvement in about 60 percent of the patients who are subsequently shown to have spinal cord or nerve root compression.[14] The radiographic lesion corresponds approximately to the level of spinal cord or nerve root compression, although tumor may be present without radiographic evidence of vertebral involvement. Because there may be multiple sites of tumor deposit in almost one-fifth of cases,[8] it is worthwhile to obtain plain x-ray films of the entire spine, not just the region of primary suspicion.

Radioisotope Bone Scan

Abnormal uptake of isotope may "light up" a metastatic deposit in the spine before it becomes radiographically evident. An additional advantage of a skeletal isotope survey is the early identification of extraspinal bony metastasis.[7]

Myelography

Myelography is the single most valuable diagnostic tool for the evaluation of spinal cord and nerve root compression. Osteolytic or osteoblastic changes in the spine adjacent to an intraspinal mass lesion make the diagnosis of metastatic tumor highly likely. Myelography should be carried out as a preliminary step to aid in accurate localization for either surgery or radiotherapy. "Blind" radiotherapy or "blind" surgical decompression, relying on clinical examination and plain spine films alone, risks missing multiple tumor deposits that might be readily revealed by myelography (Fig. 126-2).

In the presence of a complete myelographic block, it is important to visualize the upper limit of the block. Although an extradural tumor deposit is usually limited to one or two adjacent vertebral segments, there are exceptions in which clinically unsuspected multiple separate tumor deposits occur in different portions of the spinal canal (Fig. 126-2). It is useful to have as much myelographic information as possible regarding the entire spinal axis before instituting treatment; this would include identification of the upper end of a complete myelographic block. This can sometimes be achieved by placing the patient on the fluoroscopy table with the head inclined downward and injecting a few milliliters of air, which slightly increases the pressure in the subarachnoid space and thereby forces a small quantity of the contrast medium past the obstruction (Fig. 126-3). Another possible maneuver is the intravenous administration of a diuretic agent such as mannitol to shrink the tumor and spinal cord and permit the contrast medium to bypass the obstruction. If such measures fail to identify the upper end of the block, then contrast medium can be injected into the spinal subarachnoid space laterally between C1 and C2 or posteriorly in the midline into the cisterna magna.

With respect to the choice of a contrast medium, water-soluble agents such as metrizamide have become popular. However, in cancer patients suspected of having a metastatic spinal tumor, there is good reason to use the oily contrast medium iophendylate (Pantopaque). First, in the interest of visualizing the entire spinal axis, the dense contrast iophendylate offers a better chance of visualizing the lesion with less chance of absorption or dilution on moving the medium to different parts of the spinal canal. A second advantage is that in cancer patients it is desirable to leave all the contrast material permanently in the subarachnoid space as a marker

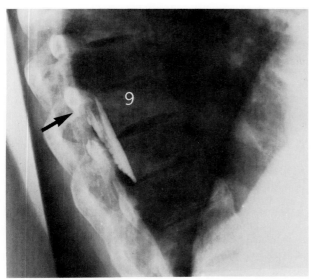

Figure 126-2 A case illustrating the desirability of *complete* myelographic visualization of the spinal canal prior to radiation therapy or surgery. This patient was a 65-year-old man with a history of prostatic carcinoma who presented with low back pain and mild weakness in the legs. Plain x-ray films showed multiple osteolytic lesions in the midlumbar region for which he received a course of radiation therapy, but without a prior myelogram. Lumbar pain was relieved, but 3 weeks after completion of radiotherapy he was referred to the neurosurgical service with a 1-week history of rapid development of paraparesis. This myelogram showed a complete block at T8–9 (*arrow*), several segments above the uppermost limit of the radiotherapy exposure. If the patient had had the myelogram prior to radiotherapy, the T8–9 metastatic lesion would probably have been identified and the radiation port would have been extended to include the thoracic metastatic deposit. Radiotherapy to the thoracic region was now out of the question, since the radiotherapy port would be adjacent to an area of the cord that had already been maximally exposed to radiation. Consequently, surgical decompression was carried out with only slight improvement in the paraparesis. Myelography to visualize the entire spinal canal, and not restricted to the area of obvious clinical concern, is recommended, in order to identify multiple tumor deposits which may have a bearing on management by radiotherapy or surgical decompression.

to provide a subsequent fluoroscopic or plain film check on the postsurgical or postradiotherapeutic status of the intraspinal tumor. Leaving the oily contrast medium as a permanent radiographic marker is also helpful in the follow-up of cancer patients in whom the original myelogram revealed no evidence of metastatic tumor.

On rare occasions, an acute increase in neurological deficit may occur after myelography, which is generally thought to be the result of downward herniation of the spinal cord induced by a reduction of CSF pressure below the lesion. Administration of an intravenous diuretic (such as mannitol) and steroids may help to reverse the deficit, but urgent surgical decompression may be necessary. Apart from the advantage of leaving iophendylate in the subarachnoid space as a marker for follow-up purposes, removal of the medium should be avoided in cases of myelographic block, because aspiration of the agent may alter CSF dynamics, with resultant risk of additional compression of the spinal cord.

The Queckenstedt test has been used as part of myelography or simple lumbar puncture to detect a spinal fluid block, which, when present, would suggest spinal cord compression. In recent years, however, the value of the test has been questioned, because significant spinal cord or root compression may be present even though spinal fluid dynamics as measured by the Queckenstedt test may be recorded as normal. The routine use of this test is therefore not recommended, particularly in view of the clear superiority of myelography in defining cord compression.

CSF Examination

A specimen of CSF obtained at myelography is submitted for cytopathological examination; this may reveal the nature of a tumor if it lies within the subarachnoid space. Cytological examination may also reveal leptominingeal carcinomatosis (carcinomatous meningitis), which is being recognized in cancer patients with increasing regularity. In the presence of a myelographic block, it is best to avoid removing more than a few drops of CSF because of the hazard of spinal cord herniation.

Lumbar Puncture

Because myelography is the definitive diagnostic study in most cases of suspected tumor compression of the spinal cord or nerve roots, lumbar puncture for examination of the CSF is best carried out as part of the myelographic study.

Spinal CT Scan

When spinal metastasis is suspected, CT scan is of limited value, particularly since myelography provides the best diagnostic overview of the spinal axis and precisely localizes the lesion. In situations in which screening myelography fails to reveal the diagnosis, however, CT scanning following intrathecal administration of metrizamide is sometimes invaluable. Similarly, in cases of benign epidural tumors, CT scanning may be helpful in supplementing the information obtained from routine myelography (Fig. 126-1).

Management

Metastatic Epidural Cancer

Complexity of the Problem

Because cure is usually beyond expectation, palliation is a reasonable goal in the management of patients with spinal metastasis. Preservation or restoration of neurological func-

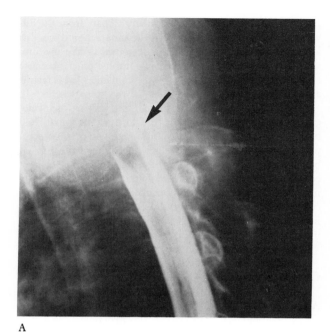

A

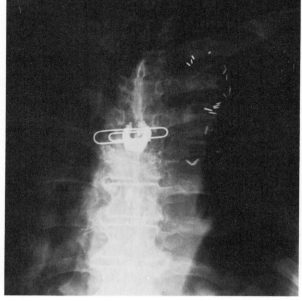

B

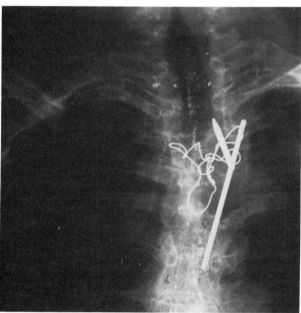

C

Figure 126-3 Spinal epidural metastasis from multiple myeloma. The patient was 65-year-old woman with known multiple myeloma, presenting with a 1-month history of progressive paraparesis. *A.* Myelogram showed a complete block in the upper thoracic region (*arrow*). *B.* In order to visualize the upper end of the block, several milliliters of air were injected via the lumbar puncture needle, resulting in displacement of contrast medium, which was seen fluoroscopically to bypass the block and thereby permit visualization of the top end of the lesion (indicated by a paperclip taped on the patient's skin). *C.* In view of the radiosensitivity of multiple myeloma, the patient was started on course of radiotherapy. Several days later the paraparesis increased, so that surgical intervention was undertaken. A myelogram suggested a ventral component of the epidural tumor, and this was supported by evidence from plain thoracic spine films showing marked destruction of the adjacent vertebral body. A costotransversectomy approach was therefore undertaken, and the bulk of the tumor lying ventral to the dural sac was removed, along with destroyed portions of the vertebral body. In order to provide stability, a fusion was performed by introducing a Steinmann pin into vertebral bodies above and below the site of the tumor resection and filling the cavity with methyl methacrylate. In addition, spinous processes were wired and further secured with methyl methacrylate. Surgery was followed by a course of radiotherapy, and the patient eventually was able to ambulate with a walker. However, she died several months later from further extension of the disease.

tion—ambulation and bladder control—are the criteria of successful therapy. Pain relief is also an important, but secondary, goal which may often be achieved by treatment of the metastatic tumor. In situations in which the decision is not to treat the metastatic tumor, control of pain becomes a primary concern.

Radiotherapy and surgical decompression are the keystones of management. Despite long experience with both therapeutic modalities, individually and in combination, the relative merits of each for spinal metastases have not yet been clarified. Much of the difficulty in analysis relates to sorting out the influence of factors such as the biological

activity, radiosensitivity, and systemic spread of the primary tumor; the rate of progression and degree of neurological deficit; and the associated involvement of the vertebral column. This multiplicity of factors is compounded by the fact that to date there have not been any large, prospective, controlled series comparing radiotherapy and surgery.

Radiotherapy

Radiotherapy to the area of the spine involved by a metastatic tumor may be expected to produce significant neurological improvement in about 45 percent of patients.[4] The results are a little better for radiosensitive tumors, such as Hodgkin's disease, non-Hodgkin's lymphoma, multiple myeloma, seminoma, and neuroblastoma, with an improvement rate of about 50 percent.[4] The outlook is not as favorable for those tumors less sensitive to radiotherapy, including the carcinomas, melanomas, and soft tissue sarcomas.[8]

There has been concern that radiation therapy may result in neurological deterioration, presumably by inducing radiation edema in the tumor and/or spinal cord. This concern has been an important factor prompting the use of decompressive laminectomy before starting the patient on a course of radiotherapy. Experimental studies, however, do not support the concept of radiation edema. Rubin has postulated that the increase in tumor volume following small daily radiation doses is caused by the inadequacy of such doses to slow tumor growth rather than by radiation edema.[12]

Surgical Decompression

Neurosurgical attitudes regarding surgery for metastatic tumor compression of the spinal cord or cauda equina have varied widely over the years. The proportion of patients significantly benefited by surgical decompression alone ranges from 14 to 42 percent, with a pooled improvement rate of 30 percent.[4] It is important to note that surgical decompression in the past has almost always implied wide laminectomy in the region of the tumor mass; in some cases the decompression has been limited to a laminectomy or hemilaminectomy, without any tumor resection. These factors may account, to an unknown degree, for the wide variability in surgical results and for the overall relatively low rate of improvement (30 percent) after surgical decompression. The fact that decompression has almost always been carried out by the posterior approach (laminectomy) limits the neurosurgeon's ability to remove tumors other than those located in the posterior portion of the epidural space. Removal of tumors in the lateral and particularly in the ventral compartment is technically difficult by the posterior approach. In a series of 118 patients with spinal metastasis, Hall and Mackay reported that posterior decompression (laminectomy) improved 39 percent of the patients when the tumor was posterior, 35 percent when the lesion was lateral, 25 percent when the tumor was circumferential, and only 9 percent when the lesion was in ventral anterior epidural space.[9] This suggests that, because laminectomy is effective primarily for posteriorly and laterally placed tumors, neurosurgeons should consider an anterior or lateral surgical approach to the spine when the tumor mass is located ventrally (Fig. 126-3).

The location of a tumor may often be determined preoperatively by a combination of neurological findings and myelography; the appearance of vertebral body involvement on plain x-ray films also suggests tumor or bone extension into the anterior spinal compartment. In this regard, the majority of epidural tumors are believed to arise in a vertebral body.[1,14]

Operative mortality—death within the first month after surgical decompression—has ranged from 3 to 14 percent in various series, with an average mortality rate of 9 percent.[4] Included in varying proportions in these series were patients in generally poor condition with disseminated cancer, so the expected mortality rate might be less if surgery were limited to patients whose general medical status was satisfactory. In addition to mortality, surgical morbidity must be evaluated when considering operative risk. Worsening of neurological status has been reported in 7 to 22 percent of patients in different studies, with an overall mean of 12 percent. Besides neurological worsening, surgical morbidity includes postoperative complications such as wound infection, CSF leak, and instability with subluxation of the spine. The frequency of these complications has ranged from 8 to 42 percent, with a mean of 11 percent.[4] In summary, the hazards of operation consist of an estimated 9 percent risk of death, 12 percent risk of neurological worsening, and 11 percent risk of developing other complications. These risks must be weighed against the potential benefit in the individual patient and must be taken into account when comparing surgical decompression with other forms of therapy.

Combined Therapy: Surgical Decompression Plus Radiotherapy

Combined therapy consisting of surgical decompression followed by local irradiation of the involved area is another management option. A laminectomy is carried out initially to effect prompt relief of cord compression. Postoperative radiation therapy is intended to eradicate or suppress the regrowth of residual tumor tissue. In various reported series of combined therapy, significant improvement was observed in 43 to 61 percent of patients, with a mean improvement rate of 51 percent.[4] In studies restricted to tumors of the lymphoma group, the results after combined therapy were still better, with benefit in 60 to 83 percent of patients and a pooled improvement rate of 68 percent.[4]

Comparison of Radiotherapy and Surgery

Although there are obvious limitations to retrospective comparison of nonrandomized treatment groups, a statistical comparison among the various modalities—radiation vs. surgical decompression (by laminectomy) vs. combined radiation and surgery—revealed that radiotherapy alone seems to be superior to surgery alone. Furthermore, it appears that radiotherapy alone is as effective as the combination of radiotherapy and surgical decompression.[4,8] Analysis by various authors also suggests that the radiosensitivity of the tumor is more important in determining outcome than the modality of treatment.[5,8] Although the available evidence suggests that radiotherapy is superior to surgical decompression, it should be noted that the surgical experience to date, as mentioned earlier, has been based upon the standard laminectomy approach, without taking into account the ventral, lateral, or posterior location of the tumor in the epidural space. It may be that surgical decompression, individualized for each patient on the basis of the specific location of the tumor, may improve surgical results in the future.

Recommended Guidelines for Management

The following guidelines are proposed as tentative criteria for management, to be modified in the future in response to new clinical experience and research.

Radiotherapy may be viewed as the primary or basic mode of treatment for most patients presenting with metastasis to the spine. It is most clearly indicated for radiosensitive tumors, such as the lymphomas and myeloma; its advantages are less clear-cut for radioresistant neoplasms.

There are six indications for surgical intervention:

1. **Spinal instability or compression by bone** When spinal instability endangers spinal cord or nerve root function or when a pathological fracture produces direct compression of the neural structures, surgical decompression and possible fusion may be essential.
2. **Failure to respond to radiotherapy** In the case of relatively radiosensitive tumors, further decline in neurological function or failure to improve during the course of radiotherapy should prompt early consideration of surgical decompression.
3. **Known radioresistance of the tumor** When the tumor is known to be radioresistant, decompressive surgery might be considered as the primary mode of therapy, supplemented by postoperative radiation, in the hope that it might retard tumor regrowth.
4. **Previous radiation exposure of the spinal cord** Surgical decompression may have to be considered when the patient has had a previous course of radiotherapy to the spine such that further radiotherapy might exceed the spinal cord tolerance for radiation (Fig. 126-2). This applies even in the case of highly radiosensitive tumors.
5. **Diagnosis in doubt** Surgical decompression is advisable to establish a tissue diagnosis when the nature of the intraspinal lesion is in doubt. Surgery in these cases should generally be followed by radiotherapy.
6. **Repeat surgical decompression for recurrent tumor** When radiotherapy cannot be used, reoperation for removal of recurrent tumor is warranted for relapse occurring months or years after previous spinal decompression for metastatic tumor.

Surgical Technique

Decompressive laminectomy, with or without tumor removal, has been the standard surgical approach for spinal metastatic lesions, but it is important to individualize the approach on the basis of the location of the tumor mass or bony compression in the spinal canal. Lesions situated in the posterior compartment of the spinal canal are approached through a standard wide laminectomy. Ventral lesions, however, call for a modification in technique. In the cervical or thoracic region, an anterior (ventral) lesion should be approached by an anterior or lateral route to assure decompression of the site of direct pressure (Fig. 126-3). In the lumbar area, in view of the greater mobility of the cauda equina, it is generally possible to achieve satisfactory decompression by a posterior (laminectomy) approach even when the mass is located ventral to the dural sac. When there is associated instability in the cervical, thoracic, or lumbar area, a fusion is carried out during the same operation (Fig. 126-3).

There seems to be a greater than average risk of wound infection in patients who have had previous radiotherapy to the same area of the spine. The use of short-term prophylactic intraoperative antibiotics may help reduce this risk.

Vertebral Metastasis Without Neurological Deficit

When there is metastatic involvement of the vertebral column but no associated compression of the spinal cord or nerve roots, radiotherapy is usually the preferred treatment. If spinal stability is preserved, some additional support may be provided by an external brace. However, when there is a question regarding stability, internal fixation by fusion, followed by postoperative irradiation, should be considered.

Steroids

Corticosteroids are recommended for their protective effect on the spinal cord and nerve roots and serve as a supplement to radiotherapy or surgical decompression.

No Active Treatment Warranted

When a patient is terminally ill with widely disseminated cancer, there seems to be little value in aggressive management with radiotherapy or surgery. Despite the probability, however, that life expectancy in such patients is limited to a matter of weeks or possibly a few months, radiotherapy may be of value if spinal pain is a problem. An alternative for pain managment in such patients is the use of the spinal morphine pump or similar device, which is usually effective in the control of cancer pain.

Benign Epidural Tumors

The treatment of neurilemmomas, neurofibromas, and meningiomas is surgical excision, and this can generally be achieved completely. Microsurgical technique contributes considerably to the safety of their removal. Occasionally, meningiomas with a broad attachment cannot be completely removed. Radiation therapy is not indicated for these benign tumors.

Prognosis

For both benign and malignant epidural tumors, the rapid onset and progression of neurological symptoms are associated with a worse prognosis than are gradual onset and slow progression. There is a positive correlation between the pretreatment motor status and the functional outcome; 60 percent of patients who can walk at the time of diagnosis retain that ability after treatment, whereas only 35 percent of those who are initially paraparetic (mild to moderate weakness) become ambulatory.[5] Only 0 to 25 percent (in different series) who present with paraplegia regain the ability to walk.[8–10,15] These observations emphasize the value of early diagnosis and treatment.

References

1. Barron KD, Hirano A, Araki S, Terry RD: Experiences with metastatic neoplasms involving the spinal cord. Neurology (Minneap) 9:91–106, 1959.
2. Batson OV: The function of the vertebral veins and their role in the spread of metastases. Ann Surg 112:138–149, 1940.
3. Black P: Injuries of the vertebral column and spinal cord: Mechanisms and management in the acute phase, in Zuidema GD, Rutherford RB, Ballinger WF II (eds): *The Management of Trauma*, 3d ed. Philadelphia, Saunders, 1979, pp 226–253.
4. Black P: Spinal metastasis: Current status and recommended guidelines for management. Neurosurgery 5:726–746, 1979.
5. Bruckman JE, Bloomer WD: Management of spinal cord compression. Semin Oncol 5:135–140, 1978.
6. Chade HO: Metastatic tumours of the spine and spinal cord, in Vinken PJ, Bruyn GW (eds): *Handbook of Clinical Neurology*, vol 20. Amsterdam, North-Holland Publishing Company, 1976, pp 415–433.
7. Charkes ND, Sklaroff DM, Young I: A critical analysis of strontium bone scanning for detection of metastatic cancer. AJR 96:647–656, 1966.
8. Gilbert RW, Kim JH, Posner JB: Epidural spinal cord compression from metastatic tumor: Diagnosis and treatment. Ann Neurol 3:40–51, 1978.
9. Hall AJ, Mackay NNS: The results of laminectomy for compression of the cord or cauda equina by extradural malignant tumour. J Bone Joint Surg [Br] 55:497–505, 1973.
10. Livingston KE, Perrin RG: The neurosurgical management of spinal metastases causing cord and cauda equina compression. J Neurosurg 49:839–843, 1978.
11. Nittner K: Spinal meningiomas, neurinomas and neurofibromas and hourglass tumours, in Vinken PJ, Bruyn BW (eds): *Handbook of Clinical Neurology*, vol 20. Amsterdam, North-Holland Publishing Company, 1976, pp 177–322.
12. Rubin P: Extradural spinal cord compression by tumor: Part I. Experimental production and treatment trials. Radiology 93:1243–1248, 1969.
13. Slooff JL, Kernahan JW, McCarty CS: *Primary Intramedullary Tumors of the Spinal Cord and Filum Terminale*. Philadelphia, Saunders, 1964.
14. Törmä T: Malignant tumours of the spine and the spinal extradural space: A study based on 250 histologically verified cases. Acta Chir Scand [Suppl] 225:1–176, 1957.
15. Wright RL: Malignant tumors in the spinal extradural space: Results of surgical treatment. Ann Surg 157:227–231, 1963.

127

Spinal Chordomas

Narayan Sundaresan
Ralph C. Marcove

Chordomas are rare primary osseous tumors that arise from the axial skeleton. They are traditionally considered relatively slowly growing neoplasms that tend to be locally invasive and have little disposition to metastasize; more recent reviews suggest considerable metastatic potential, and sometimes very aggressive clinical behavior despite an innocuous histology.[2,5,8,13,15,23,24,28]

Luschka in 1856 is credited with the earliest descriptions of jelly-like excrescences of tissue around the clivus. Virchow subsequently rendered a more complete histological description of these lesions, and coined the term *physaliphorous* to describe the large vacuolated cells that are characteristic of the tumor. He believed that these tumors were of cartilaginous origin. In 1858, Muller noted their resemblance to notochord, and suggested that they be called chordoid tumors. His view did not gain support until 1894, when Ribbert produced an experimental tumor resembling chordoma by puncturing the intervertebral disc of rabbits. Willis noted that these embryonic rests around the clivus are found in 0.5 to 2.0 percent of autopsies; it is uncertain whether the tumors encountered clinically actually arise from such ectopic rests.[14,31,32]

Although the presumed origin of chordomas from the primitive notochord is generally accepted, it is curious that this is the only embryonic neoplasm that manifests itself clinically in the latter decades of life. The notochord, which is associated with the development of the axial skeleton, appears in the fourth week of embryonic life and regresses by the seventh. The spinal column is derived by condensation of mesoderm around the notochord; in the adult axial skeleton, only the centrum of the nucleus pulposus remains as the derivative of the notochord. As the surrounding mesoderm begins to lay down cartilage, the notochord evolves into a sigmoid curve in the midsagittal plane. It lies in close apposition to the developing cartilage at various points: near the dorsal surface in the hypophyseal fossa, and on the clivus just caudal to it. It may actually come into close contact with the developing pharynx, where ectopic rests of tissue may be incorporated. It is at these sites that clival chordomas may be found. Further evidence supporting the notochordal origin of chordomas was provided in 1952 by Congdon,[4] who duplicated Ribbert's experiments, and by recent electron microscopic observations that suggest a similarity between nucleus pulposus and chordoma.[18,22] In the clinical situation, however, it is extremely rare for tumors to arise from the actual disc tissue itself; the majority appear to originate from the vertebral body. More recently, Ulich and Mirra have reported finding a microscopic ectopic remnant of notochord and hyaline cartilage within a vertebral body, and postulate that these remnants may be related to the development of chordomas in the spine.[30]

Anatomical Distribution and Clinical Features

Chordomas occur in almost all age groups, although they are predominantly tumors of the fifth through seventh decades of life. The mean age in two of the largest single-institution series reported was 47 years (range 8 to 76 years) in the series of Utne and Pugh from the Mayo Clinic,[31] and 51 years (range 2.5 to 74 years) in the series reported from the Memorial Sloan-Kettering Cancer Center.[28] They have occasionally been reported in infants.[19] Approximately 50 percent of all chordomas originate in the sacrococcygeal region, 35 percent from the base of skull region of the clivus, and 15 percent from vertebrae above the sacrum (Fig. 127-1). Lesions originating in the vertebrae seem to have a predilection for the cervical region, according to Utne and Pugh; this was not noted in our series, and may represent sampling variation. In comparison to sacral lesions, vertebral chordomas tend to occur in a younger age group and behave somewhat more aggressively. The male:female ratio shows a preponderance of tumors in males, often exceeding the 2:1 ratio noted in the Memorial Sloan-Kettering series.

Although chordomas represented approximately 3 to 4 percent of all primary osseous tumors in Dahlin and MacCarty's series from the Mayo Clinic,[7] Huvos believes that this figure is too high and that a more realistic estimate would be closer to 1 percent.[14] Chordoma is an important diagnostic consideration whenever a primary neoplasm of the axial skeleton is encountered. Cody et al. noted that chordoma was the most common primary neoplasm of the sacrum (close to 40 percent) in a retrospective review of sacral tumors spanning a 28-year period.[3] Unfortunately, the age group in which they occur is the same in which metastatic disease to the spine is often seen; accurate diagnosis has therefore seldom been made preoperatively. Current radiographic techniques should enable this tumor to be diagnosed with reasonable certainty.

Symptoms and Signs

The symptoms and signs of the tumor are related to its location and are often nonspecific. Surprisingly, a history of trauma to the involved region may be present in 40 percent of the patients. In our review of sacral lesions, we found that symptoms were present for about a year before the diagnosis of tumor was entertained.[28] Pain in the low back or coccyg-

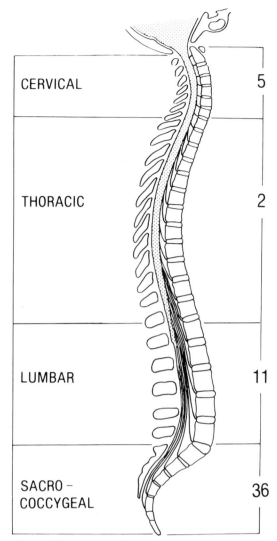

Figure 127-1 Distribution of 54 spinal chordomas treated at Memorial Sloan-Kettering Cancer Center between 1949 and 1976. (From Sundaresan et al.[28])

eal region was the most frequent symptom, occurring in 72 percent of the patients. Rectal dysfunction, consisting of alteration of bowel habits, tenesmus, or bleeding, occurred in 42 percent; 6 of 36 patients (17 percent) presented with a mass over the sacrum. Early radicular symptoms and signs were unusual, appearing in 11 percent. Many patients, therefore, are misdiagnosed as having degenerative disc disease, coccygodynia, or hemorrhoids for several months before the true diagnosis is suspected. Rectal examination in these patients was the most important diagnostic test on physical examination, since a palpable presacral mass that did not involve the mucosa was evident in all sacral lesions.

Vertebral chordomas are diagnosed relatively sooner, because they produce cord compression early. Symptoms in such lesions are often present for a few months and consist of radicular pain and sensory symptoms. Unfortunately, the majority of these patients still present with subacute cord compression; diagnostic investigations and treatment have to be undertaken on an emergency basis. Atypical findings include dysphagia for retropharyngeal cervical lesions, or the presence of a neck mass. On occasion, a lumbar tumor may grow to an extremely large size and present as an intra-abdominal tumor.

Radiology

The conventional radiographic findings in chordoma have been described in several recent reviews.[10,28,31] Sacral lesions are characterized by an expansile, destructive tumor occupying several segments (Figs. 127-2 and 127-3). The presence of a presacral mass and calcification, which are helpful diagnostic features, may be difficult to appreciate on plain x-ray films because of overlying gas shadows. Lesions involving the true vertebrae are characterized by destructive changes primarily involving the vertebral body, often with a peripheral rim of osteosclerosis. Involvement of adjacent bodies was noted in seven of eight patients in the series of Firooznia et al.; this finding, together with involvement of the disc space, is typical of chordoma.[10] Later in the course of the disease, complete collapse of the vertebral body may occur. By far the most important finding is the presence of a prevertebral soft tissue mass (Fig. 127-4). This finding is readily noticeable in cervical lesions, but may not be appreciated in lesions lower down unless it is looked for specifically. Until recently, indirect evidence of anterior extension had to be obtained by barium swallow, intravenous pyelogram, or barium enema. This prevertebral extension is often much larger than the area of destruction noted on spine films, suggesting that in most cases the predominant tumor mass is ventral to the spinal cord. Angiography may be useful in selected cases to demonstrate encasement or displacement of important vascular structures, such as the vertebral artery in the neck. Chordomas are characteristically avascular lesions, although hypertrophied tumor vessels with a

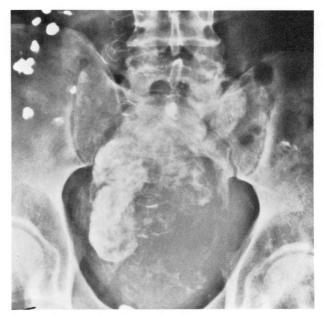

Figure 127-2 Plain x-ray film showing destruction of the sacrum over several segments.

tumor blush may be seen on subtraction films. Myelography is important to rule out epidural extension; virtually every patient with a lesion above the sacrum will have some degree of epidural extension of the tumor (Fig. 127-5).

Computed tomography is currently the radiographic examination of choice for chordoma.[16] This technique can elegantly demonstrate the presence of a soft tissue tumor, or a variable degree of calcification, that is associated with osseous destruction and epidural extension (Fig. 127-6). The reported incidence of calcification varies from 40 to 80 percent. Krol et al. noted that amorphous calcification was most often a feature of sacral lesions, and that this was usually located peripherally.[16] The degree of involvement of the epidural space could often be suspected when obliteration of epidural fat was noted, or if there was soft tissue tumor den-

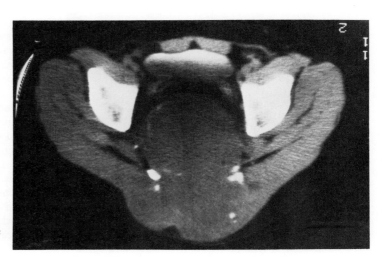

Figure 127-3 CT scan demonstrating a presacral mass displacing the rectum, with destruction of the sacrum and amorphous peripheral calcification.

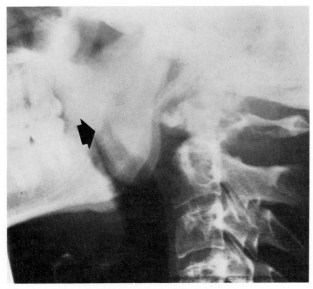

Figure 127-4 A high cervical chordoma presenting as a retropharyngeal mass (*arrowhead*). Note the early destruction of the anterior tubercle of the atlas.

sity posterior to the vertebral body. Soft tissue extensions had the same tissue density as adjacent muscle and did not enhance with contrast media. Krol et al. therefore recommended routine use of contrast media–enhanced scans only to detect intracranial extensions of tumors located at the clivus. Despite the fact that these soft tissue extensions had the same density as muscle, they were often clearly distinguishable from adjacent structures, suggesting the presence of a well-preserved pseudocapsule. Exceptionally, the tumor may present predominantly as a soft tissue mass without apparent osseous involvement.

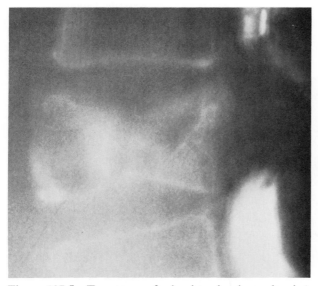

Figure 127-5 Tomogram of a lumbar chordoma showing the combination of lytic destruction, collapse, and epidural extension of tumor.

Pathology

Grossly, chordomas are well-demarcated, lobulated tumors varying considerably in size. They have a well-formed pseudocapsule in soft tissue, but this apparent capsule is not present in bone. Within the bone itself, the boundary between tumor and destroyed bone is indistinct, although tumors may be covered by intact periosteum. The consistency varies considerably from soft or jellylike in most areas to firm or even cartilaginous in other areas of the tumor. Recurrent lesions, especially those modified by radiation, tend to infiltrate muscle and soft tissues with satellite nodules. Areas of hemorrhage and necrosis may predominate, giving a firm, almost sarcomatous appearance to the tumor.[14]

Microscopically, chordomas are characterized by tumor cells arranged in sheets, cords, or lobules. The characteristic cell is the so-called physaliphorous cell, with its ample, vacuolated cytoplasm (Fig. 127-7). Signet-ring cells, in which the nuclei are displaced to the periphery by intracytoplasmic vacuoles, may sometimes simulate a mucin-producing adenocarcinoma. A dense, often incomplete layer of fibrous septa may be seen; these septa are occasionally infiltrated by tumor cells or lymphocytes. Intracytoplasmic droplets may stain positively for both mucin and glycogen. Occasional giant cells may be observed, but mitotic figures are rarely seen.

Sometimes the distinction between chordomas and chondrosarcomas poses a problem. According to Crawford, chondrosarcomas stain positively with phosphotungstic acid hematoxylin and are readily impregnated with silver reticulin.[6] These classic features notwithstanding, the histological diagnosis may be confused with mucinous adenocarcinoma, myxosarcoma, reticulum cell sarcoma, or chondrosarcoma. Recurrent lesions, especially those modified by radiotherapy, may show spindle cell anaplasia with occasional transformation into spindle cell sarcoma; such sarcomatous transformation was seen in three patients in our series.[28] Heffelfinger et al. have also reported this malignant transformation in two patients, in one of whom the pulmonary metastases from a chordoma showed foci of chondrosarcoma, osteosarcoma, fibrosarcoma, and chordoma.[12] To add to the diagnostic confusion, areas of cartilage may sometimes be seen in chordomas, resulting in a histological variant called chondroid chordoma.[14] Occasionally, tumors resembling chordoma may be noted at ectopic sites, especially adjacent to tendons and bone. These tumors, called chordoid sarcomas or parachordomas, resemble chordomas at the light microscopic level but seem morphologically closer to chondrosarcoma at the electron microscopic level.[20]

Electron microscopy has shown that the tumor is predominantly of two cell types, the more compact stellate cell and the physaliphorous cell, with many transitional forms.[9,18,22] The physaliphorous cell is believed to represent extreme vacuolization of the stellate cell. Erlandson et al. noted that the most striking feature was the association of mitochondria with endoplasmic reticulum in a structurally ordered fashion: single mitochondria alternated with single rough endoplasmic reticulum cisternae at intervals of 50 nm. These complexes may serve as convenient morphological markers.[9] Murad and Murthy noted the presence of virus-like particles in the cytoplasm, the significance of which is unclear.[18]

Metastatic Potential

While the propensity of chordomas to recur locally is well established, the tendency of these tumors to metastasize is less well appreciated. Early reports indicated that less than 10 percent of patients with chordoma developed metastases. In Utne and Pugh's review of 72 cases from the Mayo Clinic, only three patients were discovered to have metastatic lesions.[31] More recently, in the Memorial Sloan-Kettering series, 40 percent of the patients were found to have metastases, which occurred uniformly throughout the clinical course of the disease.[28] Eleven of 18 vertebral lesions and 10 of 36 sacrococcygeal lesions were found to have metastases. Metastatic foci occurred predominantly in lungs, bones, soft tissues, and liver. Chambers and Schwinn found an incidence of 30 percent in 27 cases, but curiously the metastasis in their study was predominantly to skin and bone.[2] In two of three patients with dermal metastases, the lesions in the skin were diagnosed prior to diagnosis of the primary tumor. While the presence of locally aggressive diseases and a history of radiotherapy were positively correlated with the presence of metastases, the histological appearance of the primary tumor was not. Although foci of fibrosarcoma, noted in four patients in their series, were seen in patients who developed metastatic disease, our own observations indicate that anaplasia and spindle cell features suggesting malignant transformation are often the result of prior treatment (especially radiation). Metastatic lesions in chordoma occur throughout the course of the disease, but may have little impact on overall survival.

Treatment

The two major treatment modalities in the management of chordomas are surgical resection of the tumor and radiation therapy. Unfortunately, curative surgical resection is precluded in most patients because of the extent of tumor at the initial diagnosis; furthermore, many of these tumors occur in the older age groups and concomitant medical problems may not allow definitive resection. At the present time, the overall cure rate is less than 10 percent, although it is possible that neuroradiological diagnostic tools now available may help bring about better results.

A variety of surgical approaches have been described for sacrococcygeal tumors.[3,8,15,17] For extremely small lesions located in the coccyx and lower sacral segments, the transperineal or transcoccygeal approach may suffice. The proportion of patients who presented with such small tumors was less than 10 percent in our series, but these patients have the best prospects for cure. For lesions extending up to the second sacral segment, Dahlin and MacCarty described a strictly posterior approach for radical sacrectomy. However, involvement of the second sacral segment remained the

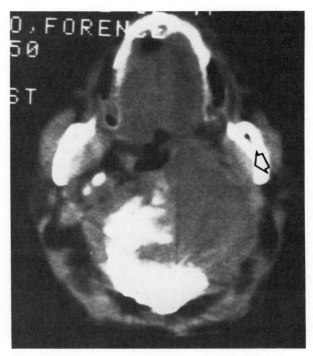

Figure 127-6 A recurrent high cervical chordoma located predominantly anterolateral to the spine (*arrow*). The operative approach was through a median mandibuloglossotomy (see text).

major contraindication for this operation, since bilateral sacrifice of the second sacral nerve roots would result in both bladder and bowel incontinence.[8] Cody et al. suggested a combined anterior-posterior approach, since uncontrollable hemorrhage was a major problem with the strictly posterior

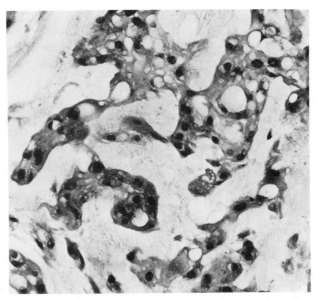

Figure 127-7 Tumor cells arranged in sheets and cords, with individual cells showing marked vacuolation (physaliphorous cells). (Hematoxylin-eosin, ×280; courtesy of Andrew G. Huvos, M.D.).

approach.[3] Preliminary laparotomy offers the opportunity to assess operability; mobilize the rectum, ureters, and iliac vessels; and permit bilateral internal iliac artery ligation (helpful in control of blood loss during the operation). Localio et al. suggested a simultaneous one-stage abdominosacral approach, with the patient positioned in the lateral position.[17] The abdomen is entered through an oblique incision between the iliac crest and costal margin. The colon and rectum are mobilized, the left ureter is identified, and tapes are placed around the iliac vessels. The dissection is continued down to the levator ani, and both middle sacral vessels and the lateral sacral veins are ligated. Attention is then directed posteriorly, where a transverse incision is made and skin flaps developed. The sacral resection is completed by severing muscular and ligamentous attachment of the sacrum. Operative mortality for this operation in this series was low (5 percent), with four of five patients living more than 5 years; there was one local recurrence. Stener and Gunterberg have more recently described surgical techniques for high radical sacrectomies in a series of patients with malignant tumors of the sacrum, five of whom had chordomas.[26] They stated that no disturbance of bowel or bladder function was noted with unilateral sacrifice of the sacral nerve roots. Furthermore, amputation of the sacrum above the second sacral segment did not impair the pelvic girdle's ability to resist a vertical load without breaking. All of these radical surgical resections have yielded long-term disease-free intervals without the use of postoperative radiation, which was only used to treat recurrent disease.[3,8,17,25,26]

Surgical treatment of vertebral chordomas is less satisfactory because virtually all patients present with epidural tumor extension at the time of diagnosis. Most surgical procedures described have been limited to debulking through a posterior laminectomy approach. In view of the radiological findings that suggest an anterior or anterolateral tumor

mass in most cases, consideration should be given to an anterior operative approach whenever feasible. For cervical lesions, which are often located in the upper cervical segments, the surgical approach described by Arbit and Patterson may provide a more extensive exposure than does the traditional submental approach.[1] In this approach, termed the median labiomandibular glossotomy, the lower lip and chin are incised in the midline inferior to the hyoid bone. The mandible is split with a power saw. The tongue is then split in the medial raphe to the glossoepiglottic fold, and the floor of the mouth is split between the submaxillary ducts as far as the hyoid bone. The uvula may be retracted laterally or split. The upper cervical vertebrae are then exposed by an incision in the posterior pharynx. Additional exposure to the clivus may be provided by removal of a portion of the hard palate. This operation is well tolerated, with surprisingly little cosmetic deformity or functional loss.

Lesions in the thoracic vertebrae may require formal thoracotomy for exposure, and for lesions in the lumbar region a retroperitoneal approach may be necessary to gain full access to the vertebral bodies.[11] Following resection, stability should be ensured with either bone grafts or methyl methacrylate. In selected patients, an additional posterior fusion may be indicated either before or after a major anterior resection.

Despite surgery and radiation, recurrences within the first few years are common; this is especially so in vertebral lesions for which the operative procedure was decompressive laminectomy. Useful palliation and pain relief may be obtained by repeated decompressions, whenever feasible. Sacral lesions may recur, producing tumor masses in the gluteal region and severe radicular pain. If resection is not feasible, cordotomy may be required for pain relief.

Although chordoma is considered a relatively radioresistant tumor, external radiation therapy has been advocated both for palliation of recurrent tumors and for otherwise

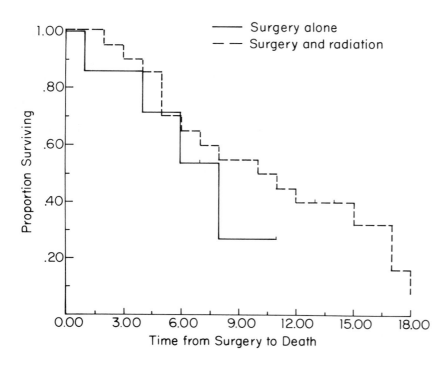

Figure 127-8 Survival of 36 patients with sacral chordoma treated at Memorial Sloan-Kettering Hospital; no difference in survival was seen following postoperative radiation therapy (x axis indicates years).

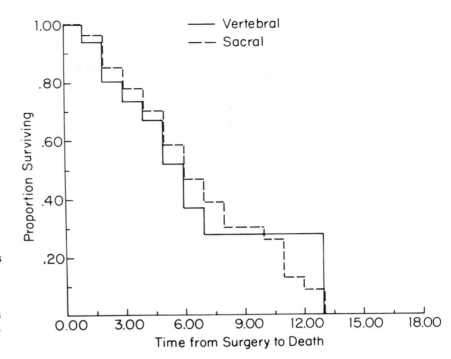

Figure 127-9 Survival of 36 patients with sacral chordomas compared to 18 patients with vertebral lesions. Overall median in both groups was 5 years, with 40 percent of the patients with sacral tumors surviving 10 years (x axis indicates years).

inoperable lesions.[8,13,15,21,23,24,29] Doses ranging from 6,000 to 7,000 rad given over 6 to 10 weeks are used for curative treatment, and lesser doses of 4,000 to 5,000 rad are given for palliation.[28,29] A number of recently developed techniques deliver precise treatment to the tumor while sparing normal structures; these include the use of wedge filter techniques and of rotational beam therapy using gravity-oriented blocks. More recently, the local dose of radiation has been increased by the use of iridium 192 seeds, which are implanted in the tumor and subsequently removed. Suit et al. have used proton beam therapy, in which doses up to 76 Cobalt Gray Equivalents (7600 rad) can be delivered next to the spinal cord for high cervical lesions. These treatments have proved safe, but their long-term effectiveness remains to be established.[27]

Other treatment modalities include systemic chemotherapy, which to date has been largely unsuccessful. Both radioactive sulfur and cryosurgery have been used in the palliative treatment of recurrent lesions, but these techniques have not gained widespread acceptance. It has been suggested that cryosurgery could be used to treat sacral involvement in situations where further resections might produce bony instability.[3] The actual impact of any form of treatment on chordoma is difficult to gauge, primarily because of the slow-growing nature of the tumor in most cases. Analysis of the survival of patients in the Memorial Sloan-Kettering series showed an overall median survival of 5 years for both sacral and vertebral lesions; at 10 years the survival rate for sacral lesions was approximately 40 percent, although less than 10 percent were actually free of disease.[28] Figures 127-8 and 127-9 show that there is no significant difference between the survival rates of patients with sacral chordomas who received surgical treatment alone and those who received surgery followed by radiation therapy. Patients with vertebral lesions tended to have a shorter sur-

vival, with the tumor having a more aggressive course, but again a statistically significant difference in survival rates could not be demonstrated. These results are consistent with those reported in several recent reviews, and it is possible that with the use of combined-modality therapy and more aggressive surgery, a higher proportion of patients with disease-free survival might be obtained.[15,23,24,27,28] Unfortunately, the rarity of the tumor precludes the design of clinical trials to evaluate the relative merits of different treatment modalities.

References

1. Arbit E, Patterson RH Jr: Combined transoral and median labiomandibular glossotomy approach to the upper cervical spine. Neurosurgery 8:672–674, 1981.
2. Chambers PW, Schwinn CP: Chordoma: A clinicopathologic study of metastasis. Am J Clin Pathol 72:765–776, 1979.
3. Cody HS, Marcove RC, Quan SH: Malignant retrorectal tumors: 28 years' experience at Memorial Sloan-Kettering Cancer Center. Dis Colon Rectum 24:501–506, 1981.
4. Congdon CC: Proliferative lesions resembling chordoma following puncture of the nucleus pulposus in rabbits. J Nat Cancer Inst 12:893–907, 1952.
5. Congdon CC: Benign and malignant chordomas: A clinico-anatomical study of twenty-two cases. Am J Pathol 28:793–821, 1952.
6. Crawford T: The staining reactions of chordoma. J Clin Pathol 11:110–113, 1958.
7. Dahlin DC: *Bone Tumors: General Aspects and Data on 6,221 Cases*, 3d ed., Springfield, Ill., Charles C Thomas, 1978.
8. Dahlin DC, MacCarty CS: Chordoma: A study of fifty-nine cases. Cancer 5:1170–1178, 1952.
9. Erlandson RA, Tandler B, Lieberman PH, Higinbotham NL: Ultrastructure of human chordoma. Cancer Res 28:2115–2125, 1968.

10. Firooznia H, Pinto RS, Lin JP, Baruch HH, Zauser J: Chordoma: Radiologic evaluation of 20 cases. AJR 127:797–805, 1976.
11. Gregorius FK, Batzdorf U: Removal of thoracic chordoma by staged laminectomy and thoracotomy: Case report. Am Surg 45:535–537, 1979.
12. Heffelfinger MJ, Dahlin DC, MacCarty CS, BeaBout JW: Chordomas and cartilaginous tumors at the skull base. Cancer 32:410–420, 1973.
13. Higinbotham NL, Phillips RF, Farr HW, Hustu HO: Chordoma: Thirty-five year study at Memorial Hospital. Cancer 20: 1841–1850, 1967.
14. Huvos AG: *Bone Tumors: Diagnosis, Treatment and Prognosis.* Philadelphia, Saunders, 1979, pp 373–391.
15. Karakousis CP, Park JJ, Fleminger R, Friedman M: Chordomas: Diagnosis and management. Am Surg 47:497–501, 1981.
16. Krol G, Sundaresan N, Deck M: Computerized tomography in axial chordomas. J Comp Asst Tomogr 7:286–289, 1983.
17. Localio SA, Eng K, Ranson JHC: Abdominosacral approach for retrorectal tumors. Ann Surg 191:555–560, 1980.
18. Murad TM, Murthy MSN: Ultrastructure of a chordoma. Cancer 25:1204–1215, 1970.
19. Occhipinti E, Mastrostefano R, Pompili A, Carapella CM, Caroli F, Riccio A: Spinal chordomas in infancy: Report of a case and analysis of the literature. Childs Brain 8: 198–206. 1981.
20. Pardo-Mindan FJ, Guillen FJ, Villas C, Vazquez JJ: A comparative ultrastructural study of chondrosarcoma, chordoid sarcoma and chordoma. Cancer 47:2611–2619, 1981.
21. Pearlman AW, Friedman M: Radical radiation therapy of chordoma. AJR 108:333–341, 1970.
22. Pena CE, Horvat BL, Fisher ER: The ultrastructure of chordoma. Am J Clin Pathol 53:544–551, 1970.
23. Reddy EK, Mansfield CM, Hartman GV: Chordoma. Int J Radiat Oncol Biol Phys 7:1709–1711, 1981.
24. Saxton JP: Chordoma. Int J Radiat Oncol Biol Phys 7:913–915, 1981.
25. Steckler RM, Martin RG: Sacrococcygeal chordoma. Am Surg 40:579–581, 1974.
26. Stener B, Gunterberg B: High amputation of the sacrum for extirpation of tumors: Principles and technique. Spine 3: 351–366, 1978.
27. Suit HD, Goitein M, Munzenrider J, Verhey L, Davis KR, Koehler A, Linggood R, Ojemann RG: Definitive radiation therapy for chordoma and chondrosarcoma of the base of skull and cervical spine. J Neurosurg 56:377–385, 1982.
28. Sundaresan N, Galicich JH, Chu FCH, Huvos AG: Spinal chordomas. J Neurosurg 50:312–319, 1979.
29. Tewfik HH, McGinnis WL, Nordstrom DG, Latourette HB: Chordoma: Evaluation of clinical behavior and treatment modalities. Int J Radiat Oncol Biol Phys 2:959–962, 1977.
30. Ulich TR, Mirra JM: Ecchordosis physaliphora vertebralis. Clin Orthop 163:282–289, 1982.
31. Utne JR, Pugh DG: The roentgenologic aspects of chordoma. AJR 74:593–608, 1955.
32. Willis RA: *Pathology of Tumours,* 4th ed., London, Butterworth, 1967, p 937.

128
Vertebral Hemangiomas
David C. Hemmy

Incidence

Vertebral hemangioma is the most commonly encountered tumor of the vertebral column. Its incidence has been noted variously from 2 to 12 percent in routine autopsy material. It occurs slightly more commonly in females than males. It is also a disease of advancing age, encountered only infrequently in children and most commonly beyond the fourth decade of life in adults. The hemangioma may involve any portion of the spine, including the sacrum, but occurs most often in the thoracic spine and next most often in the lumbar spine. It rarely occurs in the cervical spine, but cases have been described in which the tumor has caused cord compression or radicular symptoms.

In slightly less than two-thirds of the cases, a single vertebral body is involved. Two to five lesions are encountered in approximately one-third of the cases. Involvement of more than five vertebral bodies is extremely rare.

Pathology

Vertebral hemangiomas can be either cavernous or capillary. Most common is the cavernous form, which consists of large, irregular spaces filled with blood and lined by a single layer of endothelial cells. The capillary hemangioma consists of small blood vessels lined by a single layer of cuboidal cells.

The blood supply to the lesion consists of small branches of the intercostal or lumbar arteries which arise proximal to the radicular branches. The lesion is functionally an arteriovenous shunt.

Radiological and Clinical Features

Frequently, but not always, changes on plain x-ray films are pathognomonic of the lesion. Vertical trabeculae buttressed by new bone produce axial sclerotic strands between areas of rarefaction (Fig. 128-1). Such areas represent the tumor tissue, which is sometimes mingled with fat. The tumor most often involves a vertebral body but may extend into the pedicles, laminae, and transverse and spinous processes. Vertebral end plates are usually preserved, but extension into disc spaces and neighboring ribs has been described. Simulation of destruction by metastasis may appear radiographically if the pedicles are involved and ill-defined.

Extraspinal contiguous extension of the tumor may produce a paravertebral soft tissue shadow that suggests tuberculosis. In hemangioma, however, the disc space usually remains intact. The presence of a paravertebral mass without bone changes usually suggests an inflammatory or neoplastic process. However, hemangioma may present in a similar fashion. Similarities to Paget's disease will be observed when a hemangioma presents with coarse trabeculation that is accentuated at the periphery of a vertebral body. Furthermore, expansion of the vertebral body may occur, as in Paget's disease. The presence of a high alkaline phosphatase value and involvement of other bones will serve to differentiate Paget's disease.

Angiography is most valuable in defining the nature and the blood supply of the tumor. Enlarged intercostal arteries will be noted. Furthermore, contrast medium tends to opacify the vertebral body because of the large blood sinuses within the bone (Fig. 128-2).

The clinical presentation is often insidious. The patient

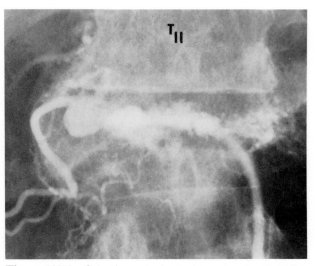

Figure 128-2 Selective spinal arteriography showing rich perfusion. The lesion is supplied by the intercostal vessels. (From Hemmy et al.[2])

may note local pain, radicular symptoms, or a slowly progressive paraparesis. Frequently, trivial trauma will cause the onset of a paraparesis.

Plain film examination of the spine will usually show, in addition to the characteristic features of vertebral hemangioma, loss of vertebral height suggesting recent collapse of the vertebra (Fig. 128-1). To determine the extent of tumor involvement of the spinal canal, and its relationship to the spinal cord, I prefer to use either gas myelography with sagittal polytomography (Fig. 128-3) or CT myelography with

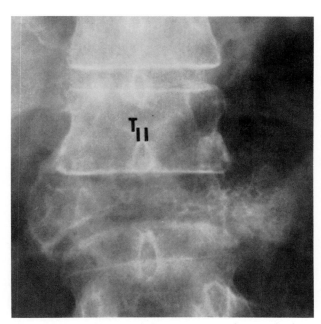

Figure 128-1 Characteristic appearance of a vertebral hemangioma. There is coarse vertical trabeculation and loss of vertebral height with preservation of the interspaces. (From Hemmy et al.[2])

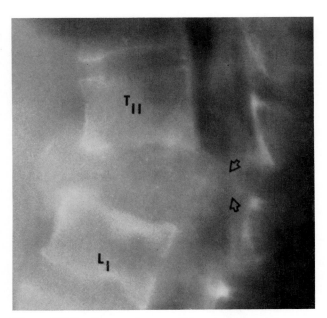

Figure 128-3 Gas myelogram with a sagittal polytomographic section. There is a complete spinal subarachnoid block with cord compression by the tumor (*arrows*). Kyphosis has developed at the site of the lesion. (From Hemmy et al.[2])

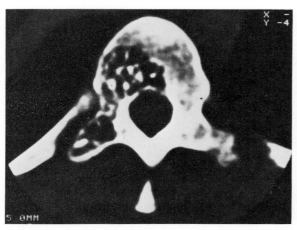

Figure 128-4 A CT section through a vertebral hemangioma, showing involvement of the vertebral body and transverse process.

sagittal reconstruction. The occasional annular constriction of the spinal canal because of involvement of the pedicles, laminae, and vertebral body is best shown by CT studies (Fig. 128-4).

Therapy

Several methods of treatment have been employed when hemangioma causes neurological dysfunction. Surgical therapy alone is quite hazardous and is not to be recommended because of the threat of exsanguination. Furthermore, laminectomy is not recommended except in those cases of annular constriction with hypertrophy of the laminae alone. Most frequently the lesion lies anterior to the spinal cord and proper anatomical reconstruction of the spinal canal cannot be performed through a posterior approach. Because of the hazards of surgery, alternative modes of therapy have been proposed, including radiation therapy and embolization of the mass. Radiation therapy is said to offer arrest of the progression of myelopathy, but generally it has not resulted in significant improvement. Furthermore, radiation treatment offers the added risk of radiation myelopathy.

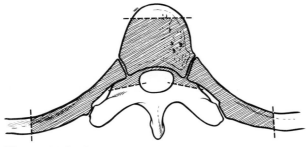

Figure 128-5 Bone to be resected through the lateral extracavitary approach. (From Hemmy et al.[2])

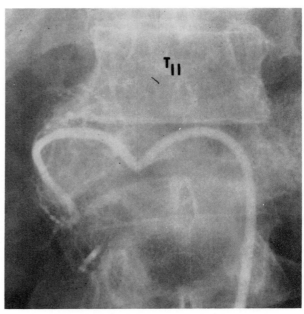

Figure 128-6 Preoperative angiography showing complete obliteration of the blood supply to a hemangioma following embolization. (From Hemmy et al.[2])

Embolization of the tumor through selective arterial catheterization has been employed as a method of treatment.[1] Although improvement has been demonstrated with use of this method, I believe that this improvement is due to the collapse of angiomatous vessels which lie within the epidural space rather than to any effect on the involved vertebral body.

Since most symptomatic patients have collapsed vertebral bodies, significant kyphosis, and encroachment upon the vertebral canal, surgical therapy should be directed toward relief of spinal angulation and restoration of the anatomical continuity of the spinal canal. Since the vertebral body is usually the major offending structure, the surgical approach will be anterior or anterolateral to the spinal canal. I find the lateral extrapleural or lateral extraperitoneal approach preferable because of the paravertebral mass frequently associated with the tumor, which may have an intimate relationship to major thoracic or lumbar vessels. This approach permits subtotal resection of the vertebral body, allowing the surgeon to visualize the dura prior to resecting the tumor, and it permits the anterior portions of the vertebral body, which, as indicated, may be intimately related to great vessels, to remain behind (Fig. 128-5). This approach must, however, be preceded by preoperative embolization of the tumor mass. Embolization should be performed on the day prior to surgery. It is best performed via a transfemoral approach utilizing a nontapered French catheter. The largest catheter which can be completely wedged into the lumen of the proper arterial branch should be selected. This will prevent retrograde reflux of emboli. Complete wedging of the catheter prior to embolization should be confirmed by fluoroscopy.

Since surgery is to follow, embolization with Gelfoam (absorbable gelatin sponge; The Upjohn Company, Kalamazoo, Mich.) emboli can be used. The chief disadvantage of Gelfoam embolization is that later recanalization of the lesion may occur. This usually occurs months after the initial embolization; nonetheless, I think that a rapid angiographic assessment of the site of the lesion should be made on the day of surgery to confirm the continued obliteration of the lesion by the emboli (Fig. 128-6). The 24-hour delay between embolization and surgery is to confirm that the lesion has remained obliterated over this period.

I suggest that the artery of Adamkiewicz be identified at the time of angiography. However, it is unlikely that the artery of Adamkiewicz will arise from the intercostal branches serving the angioma because of its fistulous nature. Following successful embolization, excision of the tumor is quite easy due to the friability of the tumor, and minimal blood loss should be encountered.[2]

Since many of these patients have angular deformities of the spine, application of spinal instrumentation such as Harrington or Luque rods or Weiss springs (Zimmer, Inc, Warsaw, Ind.) will serve to correct the angulation and stabilize the spine. Finally, spinal fusion should be performed between vertebral bodies adjacent to the tumor, utilizing iliac crest donor bone (Fig. 128-7). This technique will permit significant improvement in myelopathy and, in most cases, early ambulation.

In those few cases which are due to angiomatous hypertrophy of the posterior elements, laminectomy following embolization is the procedure of choice.

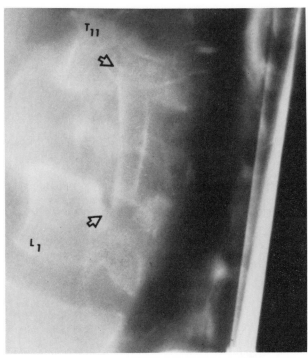

Figure 128-7 Polytomogram showing the extent of the tumor resection, correction of angulation, and placement of the bone graft (*arrows*). (From Hemmy et al.[2])

References

1. Benati A, DaPian R, Mazza C, Maschio A, Perini SG, Bricolo A, Dalleore G: Preoperative embolization of a vertebral hemangioma compressing the spinal cord. Neuroradiology 7:181–183, 1974.

2. Hemmy DC, McGee DM, Armbrust FH, Larson SJ: Resection of a vertebral hemangioma after preoperative embolization: Case report. J Neurosurg 47:282–285, 1977.

129

Masses of the Sacrum

Setti S. Rengachary

Masses occurring in the sacrococcygeal region often present problems that overlap many medical fields, including pediatrics, teratology, neurosurgery, colorectal surgery, ortho-

pedics, gynecology, and genitourinary surgery. The neurosurgeon's role is twofold—first, to diagnose and treat developmental or neoplastic neurogenic lesions occurring in this area; and second, to assist surgeons in other fields in the resection of non-neurogenic lesions, with special emphasis on preserving neural elements within the sacrum.

Clinical Features

The symptoms and signs due to a sacral mass are generally disproportionately mild with respect to the size of the mass. This results from insidious growth of the tumor into the capacious sacral canal, with chronic pressure erosion of the sacral vertebral bodies and further extension into the potentially large retrorectal space. The sacral nerves tend to withstand chronic pressure well, with minimal manifestation of neurological deficit.

The symptoms frequently start with vague, nondescript

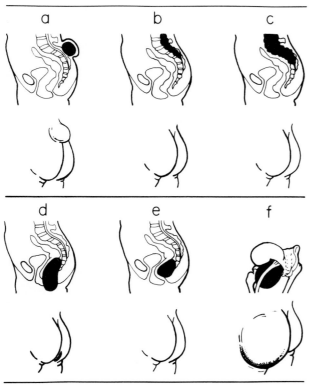

Figure 129-1 Principal anatomical spaces in the sacro-coccygeal region where mass lesions occur. *a.* Subcutaneous space behind the sacrum (lipoma, meningocele, ectopic ependymoma, hemangioma). *b.* Neural canal of the sacrum (ependymoma, neurilemmoma). *c.* Osseous elements of the sacrum (chordoma, giant cell tumor, osteogenic sarcoma, chondrosarcoma, aneurysmal bone cyst). *d, e.* Presacral space, with and without presentation of a mass in the perineum (teratoma, dermoid, ganglioneuroma, neurilemmoma). *f.* Buttock. Unilateral buttock enlargement can be caused by a presacral teratoma, with extension of the mass into the buttock through the greater sciatic notch.

low back pain or pelvic pressure. The pain may radiate to the buttock and the back of the thigh but radiation below the knee is somewhat uncommon. A persistent sensation of fullness in the perineum or pelvis may occur. In malignant infiltrative lesions, the low back pain may be relentlessly persistent. Rectal symptoms may be due either to direct pressure by the mass on the rectum or to neural impairment. Chronic constipation results from the former and incontinence from the latter.

There may be no visible or palpable external mass, but if one is noted it may be in the subcutaneous area behind the sacrum, in the intergluteal cleft, in the buttock, or in the perineum (Fig. 129-1). Proctoscopy and digital examination of the rectum may reveal a retrorectal mass, as evidenced by the ability to glide the rectal mucosa over the mass. The rectal sphincter may be patulous if the S2 and S3 roots are involved. Rarely, a presacral mass may grow large enough to be palpable through the anterior abdominal wall.

Motor weakness and atrophy may be manifest in the gluteal, hamstring, or gastrocnemius-soleus groups. Sensory impairment may be detected in the perianal or saddle area. The ankle reflex(es) may be impaired or absent.

Investigation

Changes in the plain radiographs of the sacrum may be missed unless special attention is paid. Fecal material and bowel gas frequently overlie and obscure the sacrum, particularly when the sacral nerves are compromised. The curvilinear shape of the sacrum makes it difficult to evaluate on standard anteroposterior projections. A modified sacral projection with the x-ray beam angled 15 to 30 degrees cephalad and with the patient's hips flexed can greatly faciliate detection of a bony abnormality. A lateral projection will often yield more useful information than the frontal projection (Fig. 129-2). Pluridirectional tomography will help to define the bony margins of the lesion. Smooth, sclerotic margins tend to denote a long-standing and benign process, whereas irregular, destructive margins suggest a malignant lesion. Bone scanning with bone-seeking radionuclides gives nonspecific positive information when there is bone destruction, bone repair, or increased blood flow in the sacral area, but the principal advantage of bone scanning is to determine whether the pathological process is confined to the sacral area or is disseminated or multifocal. Lumbar myelography

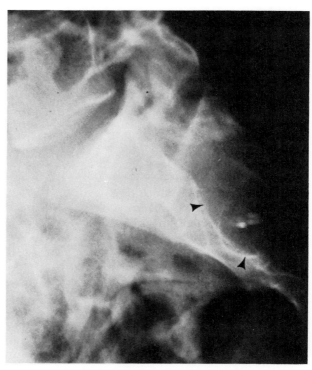

Figure 129-2 Roentgenogram of the sacrum in the lateral projection, showing bony erosion with sclerotic margins (*arrowheads*) caused by an intrasacral cyst.

with a water-soluble contrast agent is especially helpful when the lesion communicates with the subarachnoid space (e.g., a meningocele) (Fig. 129-3). In other lesions, the distal thecal sac may show nonspecific displacement (Fig. 129-4). High-resolution computed tomography (CT) is perhaps the most useful noninvasive diagnostic test; it may be advantageously performed in conjunction with metrizamide myelography. The principal advantage of computed tomography is its ability to distinguish between a far wider spectrum of radiological densities than can conventional radiographs. Thus, soft tissue masses and their relationships to neighboring structures are delineated better by CT than by any other radiological modality (Figs. 129-5 and 129-6). Calcifications not visible on plain radiographs are often clearly visible on CT. Image manipulation with various window width settings optimally demonstrates either the soft tissue component or the bony margin of a tumor. Arteriography seldom adds any useful information in diagnosing sacrococcygeal lesions.

Differential Diagnosis of Sacral Masses

A vast array of mass lesions of different etiologies occur in the sacrococcygeal area (Table 129-1). When confronted with a patient with a sacrococcygeal mass, critical and methodical analysis of certain factors is likely to lead to a logical diagnosis.[1,7]

Precise Anatomical Location

There are five principal anatomical spaces in the sacrococcygeal region where masses may occur (Fig. 129-1). They are (1) the subcutaneous space behind the sacrum, (2) the buttocks, (3) the osseous elements of the sacrum, (4) the sacral canal, and (5) the presacral or retrorectal space.

A mass occurring in the subcutaneous area behind the sacrum may represent a lipoma, meningocele, ectopic ependymoma, pilonidal cyst, or hemangioma. Unilateral buttock enlargement is commonly seen in infants with a presacral teratoma that extends into the buttock through the greater sciatic notch. In adults, a sarcoma arising from the ilium may produce unilateral buttock enlargement. A primary tumor arising from the osseous elements of the sacrum, such as a giant cell tumor, osteogenic sarcoma, chondrosarcoma, osteoma, or aneurysmal bone cyst, may produce a palpable bony mass. Chordoma, thought to arise from notochordal remnants in the osseous element of the sacrum, is discussed in detail elsewhere in this textbook. Metastatic tumors to the sacrum, such as those from the prostate, seldom produce a mass lesion or offer any diagnostic difficulty. Neurogenic tumors (ependymoma, neurilemmoma) most commonly occur in the sacral canal. The presacral space or retrorectal area is a potential space bounded anteriorly by the posterior wall of the rectum, posteriorly by the sacrum and coccyx, superiorly by the peritoneal reflection, and inferiorly by the levator ani and coccygeus muscles of the pelvic floor; the iliac vessels and ureters define the lateral margins. Lesions

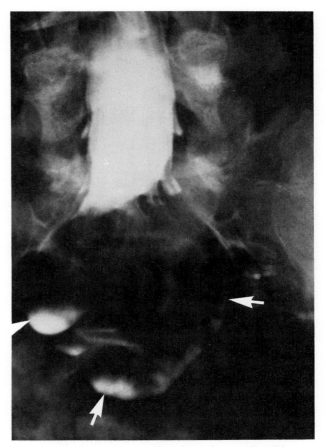

Figure 129-3 Anteroposterior view of a metrizamide lumbar myelogram showing a large multiloculated cyst within the sacrum (*arrows*).

such as dermoid cyst, teratoma, ectopic kidney, ectopic ependymoma, neurilemmoma, ganglioneuroma, or anterior sacral meningocele occur in this area.

Cystic or Solid Form

A purely cystic lesion in this area generally implies a developmental lesion, such as a meningocele, or an inclusion cyst, such as an epidermoid or dermoid cyst. Solid or nodular lesions are usually neoplastic in nature.

Communication of Cystic Mass with Subarachnoid Space

This can be determined in an infant by palpating the mass both when the infant is quiet, especially immediately after a feeding or during sleep, and when it is crying. An increase in tension in the cyst during straining suggests communication with the subarachnoid space. A CT scan will show the cyst to have attenuation values for water, and myelography will demonstrate the communication (Figs. 129-3 and 129-6).

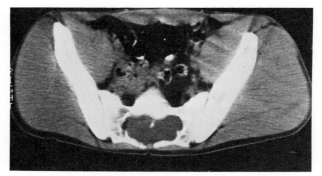

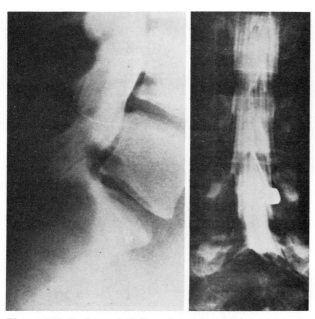

Figure 129-4 Lateral (*left*) and anteroposterior (*right*) views from a metrizamide lumbar myelogram showing a complete block at the lower border of L5, with displacement of the dural sac to the patient's right by a large intrasacral schwannoma. Erosion of the posterior surface of the sacral vertebral bodies is evident in the lateral view.

Age of Patient

Teratoma, meningocele, and lipoma are the most common sacrococcygeal lesions in the neonate. Anterior sacral meningoceles may not be detected until late in adulthood. It is noteworthy that teratomas manifest in the newborn tend to be benign, whereas those occurring after 3 months of age tend to be malignant. Chordomas, although thought to arise from notochordal remnants, are rarely seen in childhood. Ependymomas and neurilemmomas occur in young to middle-aged adults.

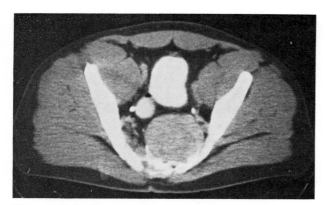

Figure 129-5 Computed tomogram of the lower sacral area shows extension into the presacral space by a large neurilemmoma arising from the neural canal of the sacrum. The mass has a smooth, globular outline.

Figure 129-6 Computed tomogram of the sacrum, showing an intrasacral cyst.

Presence of Neurological Impairment

Neurological impairment is most commonly observed with ependymomas and neurilemmomas. Benign sacrococcygeal teratomas, even when they assume enormous size, seldom produce neurological impairment. Chordomas and osseous neoplasms may produce neurological impairment late in the course of the disease. Meningoceles, because of their low location, produce minimal or no neurological deficit.

Presence of Bone Destruction or Pressure Erosion

Typically, destructive or invasive lesions are malignant neoplasms, whereas a lesion with smooth sclerotic margins is a developmental process or a benign tumor.

Dissemination of Lesion

A disseminated or multifocal lesion generally implies a metastatic or multifocal neoplastic process such as plasmacytoma.

Certain Sacral Lesions of Neurosurgical Interest

Intrasacral Extradural Arachnoid Cyst

Synonyms include intrasacral cyst, occult intrasacral meningocele, expansion of subarachnoid space in the lumbosacral region, and intraspinal meningocele.[6] This is discussed in detail elsewhere in this textbook.

Neurogenic Tumors

The two most common tumors occurring in the cauda equina are neurilemmoma and ependymoma. Most commonly these tumors occur in the lumbar region, but rarely they may occur in the sacral area. An intradural ependy-

TABLE 129-1 Sacral and Presacral Masses

Congenital Masses

Anterior sacral meningocele
Chordoma
Dermoid cyst
Ectopic kidney
Epidermoid cyst
Intrasacral meningocele
Teratoma

Neurogenic Masses

Ependymoma (intraspinal and ectopic)
Ganglioneuroma
Metastatic neuroblastoma
Neurofibroma
Neurilemmoma

Osseous Masses

Aneurysmal bone cyst
Chondroma
Chondrosarcoma
Ewing's sarcoma
Giant cell tumor
Osteogenic sarcoma
Osteoma

Miscellaneous Tumors

Fibrosarcoma
Hemangioendothelioma
Leiomyosarcoma
Liposarcoma
Metastatic carcinoma
Myeloma
Rhabdomyosarcoma

Inflammatory Conditions

Abscess
Granuloma

moma occurring low in the lumbar thecal sac, if highly invasive, may extend into the sacral canal and may present in part as an intrasacral tumor.[8]

Less than 5 percent of all spinal ependymomas occur extradurally in the sacrococcygeal region.[4] The age at onset may range from 3 months to 65 years, with a mean of 26 years. Extradural ependymomas occur in three characteristic locations in the sacrococcygeal area: (1) in the subcutaneous soft tissue posterior to the sacrum. When occurring in this location, the tumor presents as a slow-growing mass in the intergluteal fold; (2) within the sacral canal but lying extradurally. In late stages the tumor may infiltrate and erode the sacrum either anteriorly or posteriorly, with extension into the presacral space or retrosacral tissue, respectively; (3) in the retrorectal (presacral) space. In this location the tumor is usually quite large on initial discovery, since it may attain enormous size without impingement upon any structure that will produce symptoms.

The origin of extradural ependymomas in the sacrococcygeal region has been the subject of debate. No unitary hypothesis would explain all cases. Heterotopic ependymal cell rests may be the source of tumor in some cases, especially those occurring in the subcutaneous tissue. Some have suggested an origin from the coccygeal medullary vestige, which is an ependymal-lined cavity remaining in the caudal portion of the neural tube beneath the skin of the postanal pit. A few have theorized that persistent remnants of the notochordal canal give rise to ependymomas.

Neurilemmomas occasionally occur in the sacral canal; they attain enormous size before symptoms occur (Fig. 129-5). Unlike ependymomas, these are benign tumors and thus cause smooth pressure erosion rather than invasion or destruction of bone.[5]

Surgical Approach to Sacrococcygeal Masses

The surgical approach to the sacrococcygeal lesion will depend greatly upon the exact anatomical site and the nature of the lesion.[2] Subcutaneous masses behind the sacrum are amenable to wide local excision. Neurilemmomas and ependymomas in the sacral canal may be excised after the posterior wall of the sacrum is removed. Chordomas require an attempt at radical resection.[3] In regard to preservation of sacral roots, it is useful to remember that the critical roots are S2 and S3, which subserve sphincter function; saving these roots only on one side will maintain sufficient visceral function. The S1 root subserves significant motor function in the lower extremity and should be preserved. Purely presacral lesions are best approached through the abdomen.

References

1. Luken MG III, Michelsen WJ, Whelan MA, Andrews DL: The diagnosis of sacral lesions. Surg Neurol 15: 377–383, 1981.
2. MacCarty CS, Waugh JM, Coventry MB, Cope WF Jr: Surgical treatment of sacral and presacral tumors other than sacrococcygeal chordoma. J Neurosurg 22:458–464, 1965.
3. Mindell ER: Current concepts review: Chordoma. J Bone Joint Surg 63A:501–505, 1981.
4. Morantz RA, Kepes JJ, Batnitzky S, Masterson BJ: Extraspinal ependymomas: Report of three cases. J Neurosurg 51:383–391, 1979.
5. Rengachary SS, O'Boynick P, Batnitzky S, Kepes JJ: Giant intrasacral schwannoma: Case report. Neurosurgery 9:573–577, 1981.
6. Rengachary SS, O'Boynick P, Karlin CA, Batnitzky S, Price H: Intrasacral extradural communicating arachnoid cyst: Case report. Neurosurgery 8:236–240, 1981.
7. Turner ML, Mulhern CB, Dalinka MK: Lesions of the sacrum: Differential diagnosis and radiological evaluation. JAMA 245:275–277, 1981.
8. Vara-Thorbeck R, Sanz-Esponera J: Intrasacral ependymoma: Case report. J Neurosurg 32:589–592, 1970.

SECTION O

Adjunctive Therapy of CNS Tumors

130

Principles of Radiotherapy of CNS Tumors

K. Thomas Noell
Arnold M. Herskovic

Put simply, all modes of therapeutic irradiation inject energy into biochemical systems such as cellular nuclei. The addition of energy into a previously stable biochemical unit, like heating a strip of bacon, causes rapid and permanent alteration.

The mutual intent of radiotherapy and chemotherapy is to eradicate by nonextirpative means the aberrant cells which form a tumor. If effective, both treatment methods cause a fatal derangement of cellular functions. All chemotherapeutic agents are subject to common pharmacologic considerations, such as binding to plasma proteins, diffusibility, membrane transport, biochemical activation, and excretion, as is any medication. Once within the nuclei of neoplastic cells, these drugs, or their derivatives, may have the intended deranging and lethal effect. Ionizing radiation, which is composed of packets of energy, reaches the cellular targets without pharmacologic processing. The deposited energy causes the creation of new biochemical moieties within the cell. At the level of the therapeutic target, then, radiotherapy and chemotherapy may be roughly comparable. Methods of application and intermediate (processing) steps are very different, however, as are results.

The Nature of Ionizing Radiation

Ionizing radiation deposits energy in absorbing materials such as tissue. Energized electrons are freed from their irradiated atoms; ions are thus formed. Electromagnetic radiation has the physical properties of both waves and subatomic particles (photons). Such radiation may be x-rays or gamma rays. The former are produced by extranuclear events; the sudden deceleration of a stream of electrons in the metallic target of an x-ray tube produces x-rays and heat as the result of the law of conservation of energy. Gamma rays are identical to x-rays except for their source; they are the result of intranuclear rearrangements to a lower, more stable energy state, with the residual energy discharged as gamma rays.[14,17]

In an irradiated medium, energy absorption occurs by processes known as photoelectric absorption, Compton absorption, and pair production, or by combinations thereof, depending on the energy spectrum of the incident photons.[14,16]

Photoelectric absorption predominates at low incident photon energies (40 to 125 keV). A tightly bound electron is escalated to an energized orbit more distant from the atomic nucleus; when this energized electron then falls back to a closer, less energized orbit, its excess energy is released as a stream of photons, which may be in the form of detectable light. Photoelectric absorption varies directly with the cube of the absorbing materials' electron content (atomic number, or Z). Thus, tissues composed of atoms with high atomic numbers distinctly attenuate the radiation beam. This yields the visible contrast, on film, between iodinated contrast agent, bone, and soft tissue in diagnostic roentgenograms (high, medium, and lower Z, respectively).

In Compton interactions, the collision of photons is with outer orbital, or less strongly bound, electrons of the atom, so that the x-rays are mainly scattered rather than absorbed. In contrast to photoelectric absorption, the probability of Compton absorption depends not on the atomic number, but rather upon the electron density. Soft tissue, composed mostly of elements of lower atomic number, has a high electron density.

Pair production requires higher energies than do the other processes described. At photon energies of more than 1.02 MeV, absorption of a photon yields simultaneous production of an electron and its oppositely charged equivalent, the positron; energy has thus been converted into matter. The resultant species then dissipate their remaining energy within the absorbing medium.

X-ray sources, including linear accelerators, produce a continuous spectrum of x-ray energies up to a maximum, or peak, energy. A 250 kilovoltage peak (250,000 volts peak) x-ray unit, for example, produces a spectrum of x-rays with energies ranging from just above 0 to 250,000 electron volts. Six million electron volts (6 MeV) in the accelerator produces a spectrum also, up to a maximum x-ray energy of 6 MeV. The average energy of emitted x-rays is about one-third of the maximum, as a rough generalization. At 50 keV and below, photoelectric absorption predominates in the target material; from 50 to 200 keV, both photoelectric and Compton absorption occur; from 200 keV to 1 MeV, Compton absorption predominates; and with yet higher x-ray, or gamma ray, energy, pair production increasingly occurs.

As their energy increases, photon beams can be thought of as more penetrating: a greater proportion of their incident energy reaches a specific tissue depth. X-ray units yielding up to 125 keV are considered to give superficial irradiation. Orthovoltage radiations were used for the "deep x-ray therapy" of the 1930 to 1950 era. Megavoltage, or supervoltage, radiations (greater than 1 MeV) have become increasingly common since the early 1950s. Megavoltage irradiation has several important advantages over orthovoltage, including greater penetrability and skin sparing in addition to deposit of a relatively lower dose in denser materials, especially bone.

Skin sparing results when the energized electrons are scattered away from the atmosphere-tissue interface and deeper, with reference to the path of the x-rays from their origin. Hence less energy is deposited in the epidermis, and the epidermal reaction is less.

Equilibrium dose is the point in the absorbing medium at which the number of energized electrons arriving is matched by the number of scattered electrons leaving. This is the point of maximum energy dose. In isodose distributions the maximum dose (D_{max}) is normalized at 100 percent, and dosages at greater depth are described as percentages of D_{max}. For cobalt 60 machines, D_{max} is 0.5 cm below the skin surface; for 4 MeV linear accelerators, 1 cm; and for higher beam energies, yet deeper. The reviled radiation burns caused by orthovoltage x-rays essentially disappeared as megavoltage therapy became increasingly available in the 1970s.

The International Commission on Radiation Units and Measurements defined the roentgen (R) as the unit of radiation. One roentgen will produce one electrostatic unit of charge in one cubic centimeter of air. The unit of absorbed dose, the rad, is the energy absorbed per unit mass; 1 rad equals 100 ergs per gram. Lately, another unit, the gray, has been designated; 1 gray equals one joule per kilogram, or 100 rad. As air, water, and muscle have essentially the same effective atomic number and the same number of electrons per gram, the conversion between roentgens and rads remains fairly constant from 0.01 to 10 MeV.

As radiation beams become more energetic, secondary interactions occur, with forward scattering. This allows a buildup to a maximum dose at electronic equilibrium at a depth proportional to energy, accounting for the skin spar-

ing. This is clinically important as it allows the physician to treat the deeper structures to a significant dose. Orthovoltage beams, which were the primary treatment modality prior to the end of the 1950s, gave their maximum dose at the skin surface. More recently, machines using cobalt 60 give their maximum dose at a depth of 0.5 cm. A more energetic linear accelerator may give its maximum dose at a depth of over 3 cm. This physical phenomenon translates into an ability to deliver clinically important doses to significant tumor volumes.

Particle irradiation uses a beam of accelerated particles such as neutrons, nuclei of helium or other atoms, protons, or pions. Usually produced in cyclotrons, these are considered in another chapter. Brachytherapy, in which a radiation source is placed within or next to the tumor by interstitial or intracavitary means, is also discussed in another chapter.

Teletherapy Machines

Teletherapy is treatment with the radiation source at a distance from the patient. Brachytherapy refers to the replacement of radiation sources within the patient, and generally within the tumor itself. Only megavoltage teletherapy units will be discussed in this chapter. Prior to the 1950s, some machines utilizing radium were used for teletherapy, but in fact, it was only in the 1950s that megavoltage therapy became a practical reality. In 1952, Johns and coworkers reported the use of the first cobalt teletherapy machine, which was made possible by the activation of cobalt 59 to cobalt 60 by neutron bombardment in a nuclear reactor.[16] The radioactive cobalt is encapsulated in stainless steel, and is surrounded by a high Z material except for a window in the treatment direction. During treatment, the cobalt 60 source is positioned over this window in the shield, exposing the patient to the gamma rays, which reach the patient after passing a series of beam-shaping collimators. The relatively large size of the source (2 to 3 cm) results in an indistinct beam edge, or penumbra, which becomes more pronounced as the distance from the source increases. As the source-to-target distance increases, the dose per unit time decreases because of the inverse-square law, which states that dose decreases with the square of the distance from the source. Another disadvantage of cobalt units is the relatively large amount of shielding required in the head of the machine, since the radiation source can never be turned off, but just shielded (Fig. 130-1). This may produce mechanical problems as the weight of the shielding must be counterbalanced, and thus these machines have a tendency to be minutely out of line. Because cobalt 60 has a half-life of 5.25 years, the source must be replaced at approximately 5-year intervals. However, cobalt 60 machines still have the advantages of electrical simplicity, operational dependability, and beam uniformity (1.25 MeV).

Cesium 137 teletherapy units are occasionally still used to treat relatively shallow lesions, since the dose distribution in tissue approximates that from 400 kV x-ray machines. Because of the relatively low intensity of the cesium source, treatment usually has to be done at a short distance. However, the half-life is rather long (30 years).

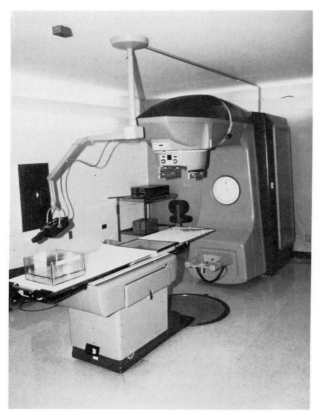

Figure 130-1 A typical isocentric cobalt 60 machine.

By now, most Van de Graaff generators have been phased out of practice. These devices utilized a mechanical transport of electrons to produce a large electrical potential. The accumulated electrons were released to impact on a transmission target which then emitted x-rays at a dose rate of about 80 to 250 rad per min. The Van de Graaff generator had the desirable feature of a relatively small target diameter of 3 mm. However, this was a large, noisy, and cumbersome apparatus which was difficult to use because of its bulk and weight.

In the betatron, electrons from a tungsten filament are injected into an evacuated "doughnut" (a circular chamber) mounted between the poles of an electromagnet which is energized as its alternating voltage oscillates with a frequency of between 50 and 180 Hz. The changing magnetic fields induce increasing acceleration of the electrons. An electron "peeler" made of laminated soft iron shields the accelerated electrons from the residual magnetic field and permits their escape from the doughnut. X-rays are produced as they are stopped by the target. The effective focal spot of the betatron is very small, producing a well-defined, sharp beam. In general, betatrons have relatively small outputs (rad per min) and limited field sizes, but can produce very high energy electron or photon beams. Like the Van de Graaff generator, the betatron is large, cumbersome, and noisy, making it difficult to use clinically.

Since the 1970s, the linear accelerator (Fig. 130-2) has become the principal external beam irradiation machine in

most radiotherapy facilities in the United States, by virtue of its high dose rates and relatively long target-to-patient distances. These are compact and relatively stable machines that can be rotated around the patient. Available at multiple x-ray and electron beam energies, the machine consists of an electron gun, which injects electrons into a wave guide. The electrons accelerated through the wave guide hit a metallic foil target and produce x-rays by a process known as *Bremsstrahlung* (as happens in betatrons and Van de Graaff generators). If the metallic foil is moved out of the path of the electron beam, the electrons themselves emerge from the unit. Linear accelerators provide irradiation pulses of 1 to 5 μsec repeated some 5 to 500 times per second.

The linear accelerator has made use of electron beams practical in most major facilities. The critical property that makes use of electrons appealing is their rapid falloff, or decrease in dose beyond D_{max}. For most electron energies the dose to the surface is approximately 85 percent of D_{max}. The deposited energy may have an effective range of from about 2 cm for a 6 MeV beam to 5 cm for 20 MeV. As the electron beam energy increases, the falloff becomes more gradual and clinically less useful.

The dose distribution of the radiation beam can be described by diagramming a vertical cross section at the central axis (Fig. 130-3). The dose of a representative orthovoltage beam decreases rather rapidly from the maximum at the sur-

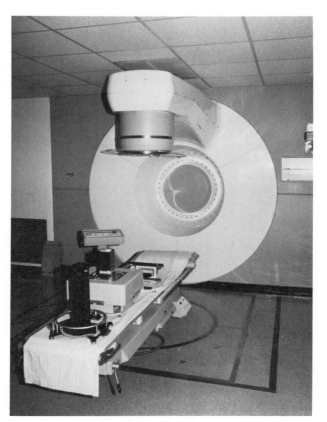

Figure 130-2 A high-energy linear accelerator; several electron beam modifying devices are on the treatment table.

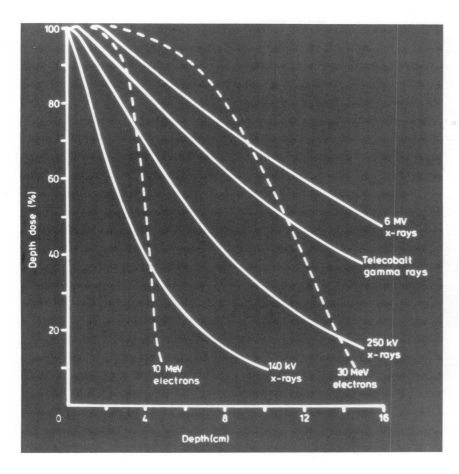

Figure 130-3 Comparison of dose profiles along the central axis. The beam is positioned on the left with the skin at depth = 0. Typical orthovoltage curves are shown for 140 kV and 250 kV x-ray machines; note the relatively high dose at the surface and low dose at depth. Two megavoltage beams, cobalt 60 and 6 MV, are represented. They give a lower dose at the surface (with skin sparing) and a higher dose at depth. Electrons have a rapid falloff. Note that the 10 MeV electrons are almost perfect for treating at a depth of 4 cm and limiting the dose to deeper structures. The higher-energy electrons (e.g., the 30 MeV) fall off more gradually.

face to 50 percent at a depth of about 6 cm; it is the maximum dose at the skin surface which limits the patient's tolerance to treatment. For the cobalt 60 beam there is a buildup zone of 5 mm, and a 50 percent dose at about 10 cm. Isodose distributions will show comparable off-axis doses. The beam edges or penumbras are relatively wide in cobalt and orthovoltage irradiation, whereas the penumbra is narrow for the linear accelerator photon beam, which also offers a significant buildup zone and greater penetration. In comparison, electron beam isodose distributions show a rapid falloff of dose beyond the maximal, and a wider curve, or sideward bulge, near the surface (Fig. 130-4A).

Radiation beams have to be carefully measured; this is usually done in water-filled phantoms with ionization chambers. Other means of measurement are thermoluminescent dosimetry and photographic film densitometry. The beams themselves can be altered by placing various field-shaping blocks, wedges, or compensators in their paths.

After determining the appropriate volume to be irradiated, the physician frequently uses the simulator, a device which mimics the treatment machine's geometry, generates images with conventional x-rays, and frequently has an image intensifier for fluoroscopy. Because the simulator yields x-ray energies in the photoelectric range, it produces a diagnostic-quality radiological image. Using this image, a physician can better define the volumes to be irradiated or spared; the films are also frequently used in making custom-

ized blocks. Recent attempts to marry computed tomography with the simulator, either directly or indirectly, have already proved useful. If a complicated treatment plan will be needed, a contour is frequently taken at several levels through the treatment volume in order to explore possible field variations on a treatment planning computer. When the optimal treatment plan is selected, the patient can be marked with small skin tattoos to identify each field; this is very useful for future reference. Portal verification films are often taken during treatment, but these are of poor imaging quality since there are no differences in Compton absorption between tissues of differing densities. Patients increasingly have computed tomographic scans done in the treatment position at specified levels. This is extremely important because neoplasms are not cooperative geometric shapes like cylinders or spheres; tissue densities and dimensions can be measured. The lung, for example, has a density of approximately one-quarter to one-third that of soft tissue. A beam passing through the lung goes three or four times farther before being absorbed, or, as a corollary, a greater proportion of energy is deposited in tissue beyond the lung as less absorption has taken place by lung than other tissue.

The axis about which a rotational therapy unit moves is called an *isocenter*. In multifield techniques, placement of the isocenter in the volume of interest means that any beam from that machine will pass through the treatment volume. This is thought to decrease the chance and significance of error in the clinical setup of patients. Optimal treatment requires reproducible execution of the treatment plan with respect to field size, beam-modifying devices, beam direction, and patient position. Variations in any parameter may adversely affect the outcome of the treatments. Laser optical pointers mounted on the walls of the treatment room, or on the treatment machine, are aligned with marks on the center and both sides of the patient. This fixes the patient in the same position for each treatment at the same isocenter. Wedge filters and tissue compensators improve dose distribution in the treatment volume by partial attenuation of the radiation beam.

Radiation Fields

Single Field

This is the simplest form of radiotherapy, in which the beam is directly aimed at the tumor. The radiation oncologist accepts a dose gradient as the beam traverses the treatment volume (Fig. 130-4). The gradient would be used in treating tumor volume that is closer to a beam's entry point than to its exit, for example, the spinal cord. The clinician accepts a dosage gradient, from the D_{max} point just under the skin

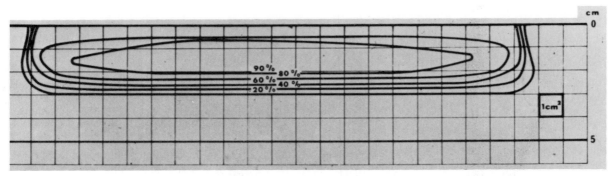

A

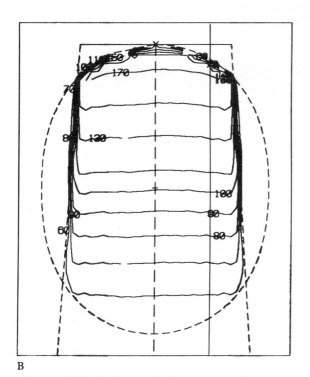

B

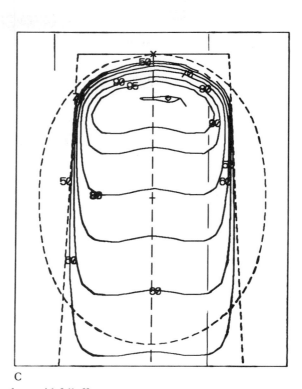

C

Figure 130-4 *A*. A typical electron beam isodose curve; note the rapid falloff at depth. *B*. A typical cobalt 60 beam isodose profile; note the relatively wide beam edge or penumbra and 50 percent isodose at 10 cm depth. *C*. A typical high-energy linear accelerator 15 MeV x-ray beam isodose profile; note the sharper beam edge and greater penetration.

through the defined tumor depth, and actually irradiates tissues on the far side of the treatment volume with a lower dose. The gradient depends on the energy intensity of the treatment beam; for example, a 6 MeV photon beam has less of a dose gradient than does a cobalt beam. The most frequent application of single fields in the central nervous system is in treatment of the spinal cord or spine. However, it should be noted that the lumbosacral vertebrae are an almost midline structure, and parallel opposed fields may be used as an alternative treatment.

Parallel Opposed Fields

This is the most frequently used field arrangement because it produces a relatively homogeneous dose distribution throughout the treatment volume (Fig. 130-5). Such homogeneity is dependent on the distance of separation of the fields and upon beam parameters such as energy and source-to-skin or source-to-axis distances. In comparison to single fields treated with cobalt 60 or lower energy linear accelerators, which irradiate superficial tissues to higher doses, parallel opposed fields yield relatively uniform doses if field separation is less than twice the depth of the 50 percent dose. There is a dose variation at the edges of the field, the amount depending chiefly on the "flatness" characteristic of the beam. A flattening filter can be used for compensation. An anomaly of the flattening filter is that the beam for the

linear accelerator tends to be compensated for 10 cm depth, and that there is an increased dose nearer the surface at the edges of the treatment field. Occasionally one side is treated more heavily than the other, for lateralized lesions. As this "differential loading" produces a higher surface dose on the more heavily irradiated side, it is not frequently used.

The best biological effects are achieved if both fields in a parallel opposing arrangement are treated every day, instead of alternately treating one field per day, with low energy accelerators and cobalt 60.[34] The parallel opposed technique is used for most patients who have whole brain treatment for metastatic foci.

Wedges are frequently used to form a slanted treatment volume. In a like manner a pair of wedge fields, for example, an anterior brain field and a lateral brain field, can be combined to treat one frontal lobe. The two wedge fields added together deposit energy homogeneously within a limited volume and subject the contralateral frontal lobe and ipsilateral posterior parts of the brain to lower exit doses. These lower doses to normal tissue should translate into lower morbidity and therefore a greater therapeutic ratio (Fig. 130-6).

Adjacent Fields

Spinal cord injury is probably the number one cause of radiotherapy malpractice suits, as the morbidity is severe and permanent and may occur in patients who have a long life

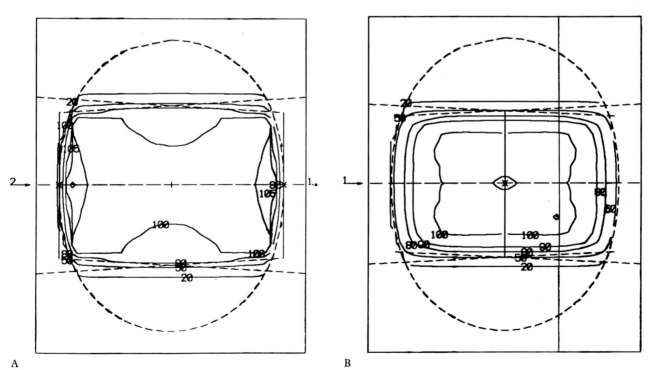

A   B

Figure 130-5 Comparison of the isodose curves of parallel opposing lateral (partial brain) fields: *A.* Cobalt 60; note the higher dose (105 percent) at entrance and exit and narrowed isodose area at mid-depth compared to *B. B.* The curves produced by a 15 MeV x-ray beam.

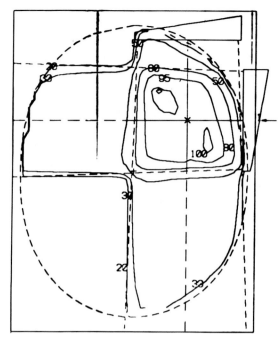

Figure 130-6 A plan that uses lateral and anterior wedged fields. A fairly homogeneous distribution results, with limited irradiation of other brain areas.

expectancy. Most frequently it is related to the use of adjacent, abutting fields without accurate determination of the appropriate gap on the skin between adjacent fields, which is needed because radiation beams diverge. Since this is extremely critical, it may be advisable to move the junctions between fields during treatment so that no single small area receives an unacceptably high dose because of beam overlap.

Arc Rotational Therapy

An isocentric treatment machine lends itself well to arc rotational therapy, in which the arc (or the entire 360 degree rotation) of the machine is used to concentrate the dose in the required treatment volume; the lowered dose to interposed normal tissue reduces treatment morbidity. Such techniques can be modified to become fairly sophisticated, with the placement of wedges, blocks, or compensators in the beam. The arc rotational technique is frequently employed for tumors that have a well-defined, central location, for example, pituitary lesions (Fig. 130-7).

Multifield Technique

Numerous fields can be used to summate the radiation dose at a specified volume: generally pituitary treatment (using wedges) or a three-field technique can be used with essentially the same result as the arc rotational technique. Computer-aided treatment planning is the most efficient method for combining isodose curves; these computers add the

doses to multiple points and can take into consideration variations in tumor volume and beam attenuation (Fig. 130-8).

Tissue compensating systems are presently being developed at several institutions, but the various devices still need further refinement before they can be used clinically. The intention is to produce beam attenuation proportional to differences in the thickness of tissues interposed between the radiation source and the tumor which would otherwise cause undesirable variation in doses. If the compensator is placed near the radiation source (not near the patient), skin sparing effects can be preserved.

Radiobiological Considerations

The exact mechanism of radiation kill remains unknown but is obviously extremely efficient, as the energy equivalent to raise the temperature of the body only 0.0012°C, or 500 rad of total body irradiation, is lethal. All ionizing radiation produces products such as reactive free radicals and ions, with the hydroxyl ion being the most important. This ion has a very short effective range, which suggests that the lesion occurs within or near DNA.

Cells that do not have the ability to reproduce themselves can be considered dead even though they may be morphologically viable. The dose required to reduce the surviving fraction to 37 percent of the original number of cells is the D_0, which is related to the slope of the cell survival curve. The smaller the dose required to reduce the cell population, the greater the cells' sensitivity. The survival curve will show an area of reduced efficiency, or shoulder. Extrapolation of the survival curve to a dose of 0 yields an N, or

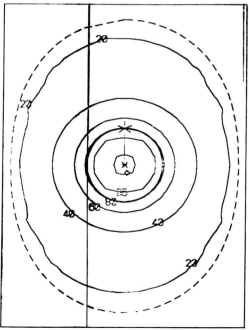

Figure 130-7 Rotational field as for a pituitary tumor. The plan uses a 5 × 5 cm field and 15 MeV x-rays.

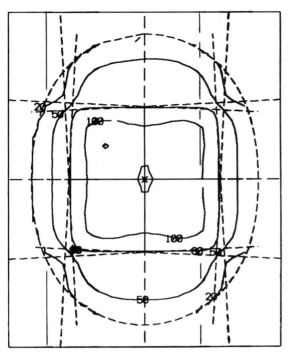

Figure 130-8 A four-field 15 MeV x-ray plan to limit the dose to the areas outside the target volume.

extrapolation number. The shoulder of the survival curve is thought to represent sublethal damage (Fig. 130-9). Elkind and Sutton divided the dose of irradiation and determined that when the radiation doses are given a few hours apart, the shoulder is reproduced.[6] The difference between these two doses represents the effect of repair, which is probably complete in 3 h in most tissue. With multiple treatments there is interference by many factors, such as partial cell cycle synchronization, changes in cellular oxygenation, tumor repopulation and revascularization, and probably selection of clones of different responsiveness to irradiation. As the dose rate of irradiation decreases, the efficiency of cell kill per rad also decreases. This is thought to be due to the repair of sublethal injury, which is believed to be maximal at a dose rate of about 100 rad per hour or less (common in brachytherapy) and minimal above 100 rad per minute (as in external beam teletherapy). The most important modifier of irradiation effect is thought to be oxygen. In 1952, Read demonstrated the need for a greater radiation dose in a hypoxic environment than in an oxic one.[25] The oxygen enhancement ratio (OER) describes the ratio of cell kill in oxic versus hypoxic environments. The exact mechanism is uncertain but the clinical influence is undeniable. Thomlinson and Grey predicted that the diffusion range of oxygen tension was limited to 150 μm from a capillary.[28] It appears that reoxygenation occurs mostly in cells at 100 to 150 μm from capillaries, as cells beyond that distance are essentially anoxic or necrotic. Several clinical studies have defined a benefit from use of hyperbaric oxygen with small numbers of radiation treatments, but the technique was found to be cumbersome and difficult for the patient and treatment staff, prohibiting careful beam definition and beam modifi-

cation and occasionally being hazardous.[32] The use of sensitizers for hypoxic cells is conceptually more attractive and has recently been explored. These compounds may actually reach more areas of the tumor than does hyperbaric oxygen.[24]

Of the phases of the cell cycle, G1, S, G2, and M are extremely sensitive, but late G1 and S phases are relatively radiation resistant. At times mitotic delay induced by radiation synchronizes the cells so that the next dose fraction may come when cells are in their most resistant phase. However, tumor cells usually tend to desynchronize and redistribute themselves within the cell cycle. Chemotherapeutic agents of different toxicities may be combined with irradiation. The combination of multiple-drug chemotherapy and irradiation may produce a clinical response that is additive, synergistic, or even antagonistic. Obviously, the therapeutic ratio is the critical criterion in determining the clinical usefulness of such combinations. Relative biological effectiveness (RBE) is the ratio of tissue doses of two different radiation treatments that produce the same biological effect; this is important in comparing radiation beams with high linear energy transfer (LET) to conventional radiation beams. Clinically, the therapeutic index remains the most important indicator.

Unfortunately, cell survival curve characteristics do not allow the differentiation of normal from malignant cells or sensitive from resistant cells.[33] Dose-response curves can be generated experimentally by implanting tumor cells, allowing the tumor to become palpable, and then testing the ef-

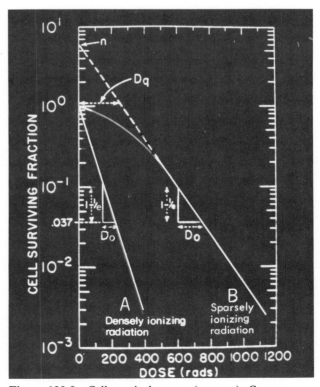

Figure 130-9 Cell survival curves (see text). Conventional irradiation is represented by Line B. High-LET irradiation (e.g., neutrons) is better described by Line A.

fects of different doses of a therapeutic agent. Thus the classic sigmoid curve can be produced, with a relatively constant slope in the middle of the curve; control increases dramatically with dose. Hellman states that the dose necessary to increase the likelihood of tumor control from 10 percent to 90 percent is 3 times the D_0 dose.[13] If tumor cells are relatively radioresistant, the radiation survival curve will become shallow. Then the dose–tumor control curve will be shallow also.

As a generalization, larger tumors have a smaller portion of their cell population proceeding through the cell cycle to division (the *growth fraction*) than smaller tumors, presumably due to chronic metabolic deficiencies which result from an inadequate microvasculature. Interference with a tumor's ability to produce tumor angiogenesis factor may limit tumor growth, as described by Folkman.[8]

Those tissues made of cells that do not divide, particularly neural and muscular tissue, have long been regarded as relatively resistant to irradiation; however, they are supported by vascular and connective tissue cells which do divide, and which may ultimately determine the response to radiation.[26] Filler et al. describe a D_q (shoulder) of 340 rad and D_0 of 170 rad, with $N = 7$ for these endothelial cells, which are similar to epithelial cells.[7]

Total body irradiation in the range of 10,000 rad produces rapid death; this occurs within hours and is characterized by vomiting, diarrhea, nausea, sweating, fever, headache rapidly evolving to obtundation, seizures, and coma. In the range of 500 to 1000 rad, death occurs within several days from gastrointestinal mucosal damage that results in profuse diarrhea, hemorrhage, sepsis, and dehydration. At doses of 100 to 500 rad, hematopoietic failure occurs, with death 2 to 4 weeks later because of the differential survival of end product cells in the marrow and peripheral blood. The number of lymphocytes falls first, the number of platelets and granulocytes in about 5 to 6 days, and the number of red blood cells last.[13]

Radiation has definite effects on the immune response; for example, following whole body irradiation, most of the lymphocytes die immediately. Anderson and Warner reached the following conclusions: B lymphocytes and T-lymphocyte precursor cells are sensitive to irradiation; the homing potential of immunocompetent cells may be altered; resting cells just having been stimulated are less sensitive; and effects of whole body irradiation are different from those of localized irradiation.[1]

Localized radiotherapy will produce a lymphopenia of both T and B cells in humans. However, established immunity recovers quickly. Claims that patients treated after mastectomy have an increased mortality due to immunosuppression have been repudiated.[20]

Normal Tissue Consequences of Therapeutic Irradiation

Radiation carcinogenesis is a subject of considerable concern. After the exposure of a population to irradiation, there is a gradual increase in tumor incidence with time until a plateau is reached, as evidenced by studies of atomic bomb survivors in Japan and of patients irradiated for benign diseases.[4,9,11,27] The tumor induction period can range from 3 to 5 years for leukemia to 10 to 15 years or longer for solid tumors. Patients treated for benign diseases with modest radiation doses (1000 rad or less) to the pelvis have a higher incidence of secondary malignancies than do patients treated with tumoricidal higher doses to the same volume.[2] Radiation is both teratogenic and carcinogenic for in utero exposure.

The basic principle of fractionation of radiation therapy was described by Coutard, who observed a relationship between acute reaction and late effects and established the importance of fractionation.[5] The rationale of fractionation is that normal cells recover better from sublethal radiation damage than do neoplastic cells, and that this recovery takes place between successive treatment sessions. In addition, partial reoxygenation of hypoxic tumor cells probably takes place gradually as multiple radiation doses are administered.

Predictions of late complications on the basis of the severity of acute reactions break down when a few high-dose treatments are given, possibly because delayed reactions are the responses of nonproliferating tissue or slowly proliferating vascular and connective tissue. In comparison, the acute reactions are the result of injury to rapidly renewing epithelial tissues. Also, the ability to recover from an acute reaction is greater if high total doses are given in many, rather than fewer, treatments. Orton and Ellis have developed a method of comparing different time-dose fractionation (TDF) schemes which is useful in clinical practice.[23] Tolerance to irradiation is also related to the anatomical location of the treatment volume, which must be considered in the patient's overall treatment plan.

In certain situations irradiation and surgery are most useful when combined, because irradiation is usually very effective in the (oxygenated) periphery of the tumors, whereas surgery can fail in those areas, particularly when vital structures are involved. The disadvantages of using preoperative radiotherapy are (1) the surgical definition of tumor extent is not known, (2) it is difficult to evaluate the histological specimen obtained at operation for the viability of any remaining tumor cells, and (3) there may be some delay in healing after surgery. If 4000 to 5000 rad are given to a potential operative site, a 4- to 6-week delay prior to surgery is necessary while capillary dilatation subsides. If higher doses are given, even greater healing problems may be evident. A major problem is the combined toxicity of irradiation and surgery; particularly evident is increased fibrosis in the area of scars, which may lead to damage to underlying vessels, muscles, or nerves.

It is probably best that radiation-related cerebral edema be clinically anticipated, since it may be prevented by surgical decompression, medical means, or a combination of both. The clinician does occasionally see patients whose symptoms and signs, such as headache, obtundation, nausea, and vomiting are increased when brain irradiation begins. In the past it has been common to begin with low individual radiation doses and gradually increase the daily dose, but that approach has largely been abandoned with the advent of steroid medication. If patients are irradiated postoperatively, this should be delayed until the wound is healed (usually 7 to 14 days).

It is difficult to determine if necrosis in irradiated brain is related to tumor, treatment, or a combination of the two. Brain tolerance is probably in the range of 6000 rad of conventional irradiation. Frequently brain necrosis is seen in patients who are treated for recurrent disease, an anticipated complication that may be justified because of a desperate situation. The physician is occasionally able to effect a reasonable remission in these patients. There also appears to be a greater incidence of brain necrosis in patients treated with a higher dose per fraction. A third parameter, treatment volume, is seldom mentioned when considering the incidence of brain necrosis but obviously has a major effect (Fig. 130-10).

A common delayed reaction of irradiation to the whole brain is a somnolence syndrome, first described in 1929 in patients irradiated for ringworm of the scalp. Its onset is about 6 to 8 weeks following radiotherapy, and it persists for about 2 weeks. More recently, symptoms have been reported recurring in children several months after completion of treatment for acute leukemia.[10] The symptoms were nonfocal and transient; all of the children had spontaneous complete recovery. Late delayed effects can occur within a range of 4 months to 12 years. They tend to peak in 1 to 3 years and are characterized by insidiously progressive deterioration, focal neurological signs, dementia, and seizures. Differentiation from recurrence of the brain tumor is difficult at times since both may produce increased spinal fluid protein levels, increased uptake in a radioisotope scan, focal EEG dysfunction, and CT scan changes. This is usually due to progressive changes in white matter caused by vasculopathy involving small and large blood vessels (Fig. 130-11).

Investigators involved with pediatric patients in recent years have been concerned about the long-term effects of brain irradiation and chemotherapy. In combined group studies of 108 patients there was no evident decrease in verbal performance IQs found in irradiated children, but several intellectual limitations have been recognized. Other pediatric studies involving patients with brain tumors showed that irradiation resulted in a disproportionate number of patients who were severely disabled mentally. For example, Hirsch et al. compared the IQs of children with medulloblastoma with those of children with cerebellar astrocytoma; the latter were presumed to have a lower chance of having a significant increase in intracranial pressure.

There was a striking difference between these two populations, with a higher IQ in those patients who had cerebellar astrocytoma.[15] A study done at Roswell Park Memorial Institute noted deterioration of full-scale IQ of at least 25 points in each of four children who had intelligence testing before and after treatment. CT scans after brain irradiation may show leukoencephalopathy as evidenced by large ventricles, widened sulci, hypodense areas, and calcifications. The implication of these studies is that brain irradiation in childhood has definite adverse effects which are probably worse in children treated with higher doses.

Endocrine dysfunction (a decrease in growth hormone release) was noted in children treated prophylactically to prevent central nervous system leukemia, but normal FSH, LH, cortisol, and testosterone levels were noted.[29] Thyroid dysfunction resulting from irradiation of the thyroid gland has been well documented.

Irradiation of the spinal axis in children can produce a decrease in sitting height in adulthood. The exact interrelationships of irradiation and intrathecal chemotherapy still need to be defined and are under study by the Pediatric Oncology Group. Patients receiving combined treatment do not have neurological signs, but Lhermitte's sign usually develops 1 to 3 months following completion of radiation therapy and resolves in several weeks. Its precise pathogenesis is unclear because tissue for pathological study has not been available.

Transverse myelitis caused by irradiation is usually irreversible. It develops 6 months to 5 years after treatment, and no effective treatment is known. The likelihood of myelitis tends to increase with the length of spinal cord irradiated, and if doses over 5000 rad are given at 180 to 200 rads per treatment, 5 days per week; if higher doses per treatment are used, spinal cord injury may follow total doses less than 5000 rad. Spinal cord irradiation is particularly a problem at field junctions, where there is a risk of overlapping beams; the upper thoracic spinal cord is most susceptible.

Other potential adverse effects of radiotherapy range from otitis media (if a middle ear is irradiated) to seizures (presumably due to focal gliosis) and cataracts (if a lens is irradiated). These adverse effects can be minimized by careful treatment planning, daily treatment precision, and due consideration of tolerance doses, but not completely eliminated, unless tumor treatment is seriously compromised.

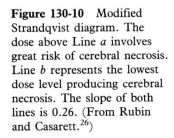

Figure 130-10 Modified Strandqvist diagram. The dose above Line *a* involves great risk of cerebral necrosis. Line *b* represents the lowest dose level producing cerebral necrosis. The slope of both lines is 0.26. (From Rubin and Casarett.[26])

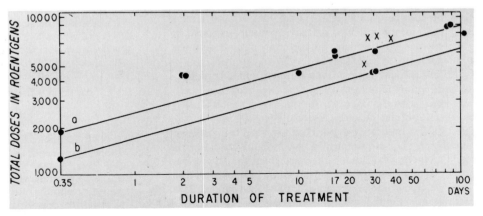

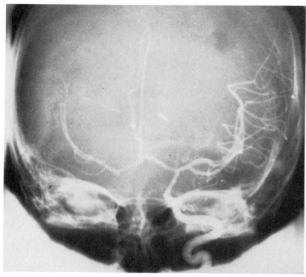

Figure 130-11 Left carotid arteriogram of a child with medulloblastoma treated with external irradiation and intrathecal radioactive gold colloid. Note the narrowing of the intracranial segment of the left internal carotid artery and of the left anterior cerebral artery.

Radiation Sensitizers

The direct effect of irradiation involves the deposition of energy in DNA, whereas the indirect effect involves the creation of short-lived species such as hydroxyl radicals which subsequently interact with DNA, leading to cell death.[23] After the initial radiochemical interaction, the target site contains a free radical (unpaired electron). This can be reduced by a sulfhydryl group or fixed by oxidation by oxygen itself or electronic affinic compounds, etc.

The characteristics of successful hypoxic cell radiosensitizing compounds include high electron affinity, the ability to sensitize hypoxic cells while being nontoxic to oxygenated cells, and a lack of cell cycle specificity.[24] Clinical usefulness is based on a lack of toxicity and the ability to achieve pharmacological concentrations and sensitization with small daily doses.

Two hypoxic cell radiosensitizing compounds have been developed: 5-nitroimidazole (metronidazole) and 2-nitroimidazole (misonidazole). Unfortunately central nervous system toxicity has limited the clinical use of these drugs. These drugs are presently undergoing evaluation in patients suffering from tumors of the lung, cervix, head and neck, and brain (malignant gliomas).

Hyperthermia

Exposure of neoplastic cells to elevated temperatures produces survival curves similar to those with ionizing radiation. A hypoxic, acidic environment enhances hyperthermia cell kill.[12] Hyperthermia would seem a logical supplement to radiation therapy, as confirmed by considerable laboratory and clinical experience, with clinical complete tumor response rates of 27–78 percent to combined thermo- and radiotherapy.[18,21,29] Complete responses to heat alone are infrequent.

Tumor temperatures of at least 42°C are usually required. With each degree above 42°C, heating time for the same fraction of tumor kill is approximately halved. Body core temperature with total body hyperthermia is usually 41.5–42°C. This formidable effort, with an anesthetized patient inspiring heated gases, and heated by immersion, inhalation, or perfusion with extracorporeally warmed blood, must be maintained "at temperature" for several hours. Bull[3] and Larkin[19] obtained partial response rates above 50 percent with such treatment, but they were of short duration and several patients died.

Localized hyperthermia is more attractive. Optimal heating and thermometry methods have not yet been developed. Localized heating is not uniform, since energy is dissipated by several complex variables, especially blood flow. Predictable uniform heating at depth does not yet exist. Invasive thermometry is a requirement of good clinical studies. Primary methods of heating are electromagnetic (radio-frequency and microwave) and ultrasound; in selected situations, electrodes can be implanted for localized current field heating, thus combining hyperthermia and brachytherapy.[30]

Radioprotectors

At the cellular level, repair by reduction competes with fixation of damage by oxidation. Promising radioprotective compounds tend to have a sulfhydryl and an aminopropyl group.[24] Interestingly, the protection is greater in the oxygenated than in the hypoxic cell population. WR 2721, which is one example of a radioprotector, has a differential absorption rather greater in normal than in tumor tissue. Unfortunately, the drug is not lipophilic and therefore is poorly concentrated in central nervous tissue. It affords greater protection for bone marrow, mucous membranes, and gastrointestinal and cutaneous tissue.

References

1. Anderson RE, Warner NL: Ionizing radiation and the immune response. Adv Immunol 24:215–335, 1976.
2. Boice JD, Hutchinson GB: Leukemia in women following radiotherapy for cervical cancer: Ten year follow-up of an international study. JNCI 65:115–129, 1980.
3. Brown WM, Doll R: Mortality from cancer and other causes after radiotherapy for ankylosing spondylitis. Br Med J 2:1327–1332, 1965.
4. Bull J: Summary of the informal discussion of animal models and clinical studies. Cancer Res 39:2262–2263, 1979.
5. Coutard H: Roentgen therapy of epitheliomas of the tonsillar region, hypopharynx and larynx from 1920–1926. AJR 28:313–331, 1932.
6. Elkind MM, Sutton H: Radiation response of mammalian cells grown in culture. 1: Repair of x-ray damage in surviving Chinese hamster cells. Radiat Res 13:556–593, 1960.

7. Filler RM, Tefft M, Vawter GF: Hepatic lobectomy in child-hood: Effects of x-ray and chemotherapy. J Pediatr Surg 4:31–41, 1969.

8. Folkman J: Tumor angiogenesis: A possible control point in tumor growth. Ann Intern Med 82:96–100, 1975.

9. Folley JH, Borges W, Yamawaki T: Incidence of leukemia in survivors of atomic bomb in Hiroshima and Nagasaki, Japan. Am J Med 13:311–321, 1952.

10. Freeman JE, Johnston PGB, Voke JM: Somnolence after pro-phylactic cranial irradiation in children with acute lymphoblas-tic leukaemia. Br Med J 4:523–525, 1973.

11. Gray LH: Radiation biology and cancer, in Cellular Radiation Biology. M.D. Anderson Hospital and Tumor Institute, 18th Sym-posium on Fundamental Cancer Research. Baltimore, Williams & Wilkins, 1965, pp 7–25.

12. Hahn GM: Hyperthermia, in DeVita VT Jr, Hellman S, Ro-senberg SA (eds): Cancer—Principles and Practice of Oncology. Philadelphia, Lippincott, 1982, pp 1811–1821.

13. Hellman S: Principles of radiation therapy, in DeVita VT Jr, Hellman S, Rosenberg SA (eds): Cancer—Principles and Prac-tice of Oncology. Philadelphia, Lippincott, 1982, pp 103–131.

14. Hendee WR: Radiation Therapy Physics. Chicago, Year Book, 1981, pp 1–19, 56–78, 83–114.

15. Hirsch JF, Renier D, Czernichow P, Benveniste L, Pierre-Khan A: Medulloblastoma in childhood: Survival and func-tional results. Acta Neurochir (Wien) 48:1–15, 1979.

16. Johns HE, Bates LM, Watson TA: 1000 Curie cobalt units for radiation therapy: I. Saskatchewan cobalt 60 unit. Br J Radiol 25:296–302, 1952.

17. Johns HE, Cunningham JR: The Physics of Radiology, 3d ed., Springfield, Ill., Charles C Thomas, 1969.

18. Kim JH, Hahn EW: Clinical and biological studies of localized hyperthermia. Cancer Res 39:2258–2261, 1979.

19. Larkin JM: A clinical investigation of total-body hyperthermia as cancer therapy. Cancer Res 39:2252–2254, 1979.

20. Levitt SH, McHugh RB: Early breast cancer and postoperative irradiation. Lancet 2:1258–1259, 1975.

21. Manning MR, Cetas TC, Miller RC, Oleson JR, Connor WG, Gerner EW: Clinical hyperthermia: Results of a phase I trial employing hyperthermia alone or with external beam or inter-stitial radiotherapy. Cancer 49:205–216, 1982.

22. Marmor JB, Kozak D, Hahn GM: Effects of systemically ad-ministered bleomycin or adriamycin with local hyperthermia on primary tumor and lung metastases. Cancer Treat Rep 63:1279–1290, 1979.

23. Orton CG, Ellis F: A simplification in the use of the NSD concept in practical radiotherapy. Br J Radiol 46:529–537, 1973.

24. Phillips TL: Radiation sensitizers and protectors, in DeVita VT Jr, Hellman S, Rosenberg SA (eds): Cancer—Principles and Practice of Oncology. Philadelphia, Lippincott, 1982, pp 1822–1836.

25. Read J: The effect of ionizing radiations on the broad beam group: Part X. The dependence of the x-ray sensitivity on dis-solved oxygen. Br J Radiol 25:89–99, 1952.

26. Rubin P, Casarett GW: Clinical Radiation Pathology. Philadel-phia, Saunders, 1968, p 651.

27. Smith PG, Doll R: Late effects of x irradiation in patients treated for metropathia haemorrhagica. Br J Radiol 49:224–232, 1976.

28. Thomlinson RH, Grey LH: The histological structure of some human lung cancers and the possible implications for radiother-apy. Br J Cancer 9:539–549, 1955.

29. U R, Noell KT, Woodward KT, Worde BT, Fishburn RI, Miller LS: Microwave-induced local hyperthermia in combina-tion with radiotherapy of human malignant tumors. Cancer 45:638–646, 1980.

30. Vora N, Forell B, Joseph C, Lipsett J, Archambeau JO: Inter-stitial implant with interstitial hyperthermia. Cancer 90:2518–2523, 1982.

31. Voorhees M, Brecher ML, MacGillivray M, Hologgitas J, Har-ris M, Dasgupta I, Vasquez M, Glidewell O, Forman E: Effect of different forms of central nervous system (CNS) prophylaxis on pituitary function of children with acute lymphocytic leuke-mia (ALL). Proc Am Soc Clin Oncol 22:396, 1981 (abstr).

32. Watson ER, Halnan KE, Dische S, Saunders MI, Cade IS, McEwen JB, Wiernik G, Perrins DJO, Sutherland I: Hyper-baric oxygen and radiotherapy: A Medical Research Council trial in carcinoma of the cervix. Br J Radiol 51:879–887, 1978.

33. Weichselbaum RR, Nove J, Little JB: X-ray sensitivity of human tumor cells in vitro. Int J Radiat Oncol Biol Phys 6:437–440, 1980.

34. Wilson CS, Hall EJ: On the advisability of treating all fields at each radiotherapy session. Radiology 98:419–424, 1971.

131

Conventional Radiotherapy of Specific CNS Tumors

Steven R. Plunkett

Malignant Gliomas

Until recently there has been some controversy as to the specific role of radiotherapy in the management of patients with malignant gliomas. Although external beam irradiation has been used in the treatment of these high-grade gliomas for a number of years, there have been uncertainties as to the optimum dose, field size, and fractionation scheme which should be used. Fortunately, the use of radiotherapy in the treatment of these malignant gliomas (grades III and IV) has become more clearly defined.

The most comprehensive study relating to the role of radiotherapy in the treatment of these tumors was conducted by the Brain Tumor Study Group (BTSG).[35] In this study, a group of 222 patients with histologically confirmed anaplastic gliomas were studied in a prospective, randomized fashion. The patient population was divided into four groups. The first group received no postoperative radiotherapy or chemotherapy but received the best conventional care; the second group received 1,3-bis(2-chloroethyl)-1-nitrosourea (BCNU) postoperatively; the third group received radiotherapy following surgical resection; and the fourth group received a combination of BCNU and radiotherapy postoperatively. The patient groups were broken down into those who received any amount of therapy (the Valid Study Group, VSG) and those who were deemed to have been adequately treated (the Adequately Treated Group, ATG). The ATG included patients in all four of the treatment arms. Patients who received radiotherapy and/or BCNU were included in the ATG if they received at least 5000 rad of radiotherapy, received at least 2 courses of chemotherapy, and survived a minimum of 8 weeks after treatment.

There were no differences between the four groups in patient age or sex, diagnosis, characteristics and location of tumor, or the amount of corticosteroids used. The results were broken down into median survival times for patients in the VSG and for those in the ATG. Median survival times of patients in the VSG were as follows: best conventional care,

14 weeks; BCNU, 18 weeks; radiotherapy, 35 weeks; and radiotherapy plus BCNU, 34.5 weeks. Median survival times of patients in the ATG were: best conventional care, 17 weeks; BCNU, 25 weeks; radiotherapy, 37.5 weeks; and radiotherapy plus BCNU, 40.5 weeks. Clearly, radiotherapy was found to have a favorable prognostic effect in this study. The median survival time in those patients who received radiotherapy was increased by approximately 150 percent. Although BCNU did not alter the median survival times in either of the patient groups in which it was used, a significantly greater fraction of surviving patients was noted at 18 months in the group that received a combination of BCNU and radiotherapy.

The technique of radiotherapy was delineated rather specifically in the BTSG studies, and this needs to be emphasized. Patients were treated with a dose of 6000 rad over 6 to 7 weeks, using 5 fractions per week. Large parallel opposing lateral fields were used, and the entire cranial contents were encompassed within the irradiated area. The daily fraction size was 170 to 200 rad and the dose was calculated at the midplane of the patient's brain.

The importance of radiotherapy dose in regard to patient survival was emphasized in another study involving a much larger patient population within the Brain Tumor Study Group.[36] This study demonstrated that patient survival increases as the dose of radiotherapy is increased. Six hundred twenty-one patients were analyzed for the median survival times relative to the doses of radiotherapy which were given (Table 131-1). Those patients who received 4500 rad or less had a median survival of 13.5 weeks; 5000 rad, 28 weeks; 5500 rad, 36 weeks; and 6000 rad, 42 weeks. Those patients who received 4500 rad or less comprised a heterogeneous group of patients, and this group as a whole is difficult to analyze. However, the use of radiotherapy at a dose of 6000 rad increased the patients' median life span by 2.3 times as compared to those patients who received no radiotherapy. A 5000-rad dose resulted in an increased life expectancy of 1.6 times, and life expectancy was doubled with a 5500-rad dose. In this study, the difference in toxicity between a dose of 5000 rad and one of 6000 rad was not thought to be clinically significant.

The need for large radiation fields in treating the malignant gliomas was emphasized over twenty years ago.[7] The extent of supratentorial gliomas was analyzed by autopsy studies in 30 patients who expired shortly after admission to the hospital for radiotherapy. The investigators consistently found that the tumor was larger and more extensive than had been anticipated on the basis of clinical and radiographic examinations. Those patients who were treated with large fields had a much greater chance of having the entire tumor volume encompassed within the treated field. This study demonstrated that there is no place for small- or medium-sized treatment volumes in the radiotherapeutic management of malignant gliomas. Indeed, the number of patients in whom, had they survived, tumors would have been missed was greatest in those patients who were being treated with small- or medium-sized fields.

The use of radiotherapy in doses greater than those conventionally used has recently been studied.[29] All patients underwent surgical resection and were then treated with megavoltage equipment. This retrospective analysis in-

TABLE 131-1 Median Survival of Patients in Each Therapeutic Subgroup*

Nominal Dose (rad)	Number Entered	Percentage Failed	Median Survival (weeks)	Wilcoxon Test†			
0	194	98	18.0	+			
≤4500	61	97	13.5	0.346	+		
5000	56	91	28.0	0.001	0.003	+	
5500	33	97	36.0	0.001	0.001	0.174	+
6000	270	89	42.0	0.001	0.001	0.004	0.110

*Results of the Brain Tumor Study Group analysis of median survival relative to the total dose of whole brain irradiation for malignant glioma.
†The Wilcoxon test was applied between the survival time indicated on each line by a dagger and each succeeding survival time below the dagger.
SOURCE: Walker et al.[35] Reprinted with permission.

cluded a group of patients considered to have received very high dose treatment. These patients received 5000 to 6000 rad of whole brain irradiation followed by an additional dose to a smaller volume encompassing the primary lesion. The total dose to the primary region was between 7000 and 8000 rad. Patients in the medium high dose group received 6000 rad of whole brain irradiation. Patients in the conventional dose group received between 5000 and 5500 rad. The patients were analyzed in separate groups, according to the histological grade of their tumors. In those patients who had grade IV lesions, there was statistically significant improvement in median survival in those patients who received the very high doses compared to those who received conventional doses. However, the difference was not maintained after 2 years from the beginning of treatment. Patients with grade III lesions were found to have statistically significant differences in their median survival between each group. These differences were maintained for 4 years after the initiation of treatment. The patients who received the higher doses of irradiation tolerated their treatments fairly well. There were no documented cases of brain tissue necrosis. It is important to realize that the higher doses did not alter the long-term survival of patients. In addition, the patients who received very high (7500 to 8000 rad) doses to the primary region still did not have tumor sterilization.

The technique used in delivering radiotherapy can make a great difference in terms of patient tolerance, patient compliance, and side effects. The use of high-energy x-rays, sometimes in combination with lower-energy sources, is often of benefit. It is often advisable to use CT scans and computerized dose distributions in order to concentrate the dose of irradiation to a specific region of the tumor and reduce the dose to the surrounding soft tissues and normal brain substance. The use of compensating filters and specially cut blocks for each patient can enhance hair growth, even out the dose distribution, and result in improved tumor control, as well as reduce undesirable side effects (Fig. 131-1). In general, since the treatment of malignant gliomas requires whole brain irradiation, the use of high-energy sources with equal loading on each portal results in an adequate dose distribution while minimizing the risk of complications. Certainly as the dose of irradiation is increased, the number of complications to both the cerebral tissue and the overlying soft tissue is increased as well. It is for this reason that some prefer treating the whole brain with a dose of approximately 4500 to 5000 rad, followed by higher doses to a reduced volume encompassing the area of the primary lesion. The efficacy of this technique as compared to whole brain irradiation has not been determined. In making a decision about the dose to be used in treating these patients, the

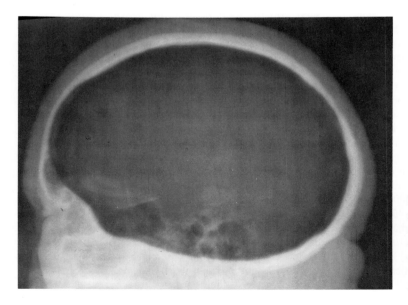

Figure 131-1 Port film of a patient with a malignant glioma who is receiving whole brain irradiation. Specially cut blocks of Cerrobend (Cerro Sales Corp, New York, N.Y.) made for each patient can reduce the dose of irradiation to surrounding soft tissues and decrease the incidence of undesirable side effects.

physician must weigh the benefits of improved tumor control against the greater risk of complications at the higher dose levels.

Low-Grade Astrocytomas

The role of postoperative radiotherapy in the low-grade astrocytomas is not as clear-cut as in the case of the malignant gliomas. It has often been said that the low-grade astrocytomas (grades I and II) are radioresistant and that radiotherapy is not useful in their treatment. However, there are several convincing retrospective studies which indicate that radiotherapy can be effective against these tumors. These studies suggest that postoperative irradiation of incompletely resected low-grade astrocytomas results in prolonged survival. Many of the studies lack a control arm and the radiation doses are often inconsistent. A 5-year survival of 49 percent was reported for a patient population which was studied by Bouchard and Peirce.[5] These patients were described as having received adequate irradiation for their astrocytomas. However, it is unclear exactly how the patients who received postoperative irradiation were selected.

A convincing retrospective analysis which involved 147 patients seen over a 25-year period was reported by Leibel et al.[20] In this study, the patient population consisted of 80 males and 67 females over a wide age range. All patients had histological confirmation of a grade I or grade II astrocytoma, and all patients underwent surgical removal of the primary lesion. Only 14 of these 147 patients were thought by the surgeon to have had complete resection of the tumor. These 14 patients were treated by surgery alone and all survived 5 years or longer. Some of the patients in whom the lesion was considered to be incompletely resected were referred for postoperative irradiation. In reviewing the patient population, the authors did not think that there was any bias regarding which patients were referred for irradiation. However, during the latter portion of the study, a larger percentage of patients were referred for postoperative irradiation. Of the 147 patients, 25 were eliminated because of early postoperative death. These patients did not have the opportunity to receive radiotherapy and were excluded from the analysis. Of the remaining 122 patients, 108 had incompletely resected tumors. Thirty-seven of these patients were treated with surgery alone and the remainder received postoperative radiotherapy. Treatment was administered to fields which included the area of known disease and a margin of several centimeters around the tumor to allow for the possibility of additional tumor extent. No patients received whole brain irradiation. The tumor dose varied from less than 3500 rad to 5500 rad. Only four patients received radiotherapy in doses of less than 3500 rad, and none of these patients survived 5 years. However, there was no difference in survival between those patients who received 3500 to 4500 rad and those who received doses greater than 4500 rad. Overall, patients who received postoperative irradiation for incompletely excised tumors had a longer survival time than those who did not receive treatment (Table 131-2). This was true for both grade I and grade II lesions, but patients with grade I astrocytomas experienced a greater survival rate. In the group as a whole, the 5-year survival rate for those patients who did not receive postoperative irradiation after incomplete resection was 19 percent. When irradiation was given, the 5-year survival rate increased to 46 percent. The authors found no evidence of complications induced by the radiotherapy. The 10- and 20-year survival rates without irradiation were 11 percent and 0 percent, compared to rates of 25 percent and 23 percent, respectively, in the irradiated group.

It would thus appear that postoperative radiotherapy does have a role to play in the incompletely resected low-grade astrocytoma. The optimum dose has not been fully determined, but most radiation oncologists would recommend treating these patients with a dose of 5000 to 5500 rad. There also is some controversy as to the optimum field size to be used in this patient group. Although many radiation oncologists would recommend whole brain irradiation, others think that treatment can be directed to the area of the primary lesion, with an adequate margin. In general, patients with astrocytomas which are completely resected surgically appear not to require postoperative irradiation. In the case of low-grade tumors which are incompletely resected, an advantage of postoperative irradiation may not be identified in short-term survival rates. A survival advantage is more likely to appear in survival rates after several years. In particular, patients who receive postoperative irradiation do seem to have an improved survival rate at the 5-, 10-, and 20-year marks.

Oligodendrogliomas

These tumors of glial cell origin are similar in many ways to the gliomas which have already been discussed. In particular, complete surgical resection is often difficult, and there are good data in the literature documenting the effectiveness of postoperative irradiation in prolonging survival and improving the quality of the patient's life.

The various treatment modalities utilized in a group of 54 patients were recently reported.[6] Follow-up data on 35 of these patients were available for 5-year survival analysis. Eleven patients received surgery only and twenty-four received postoperative irradiation. The 5-year survival rate for the surgery group was 82 percent, and for the radiotherapy group, 100 percent. Tumor doses varied from 5300 to 7000 rad given over a total elapsed time of 49 to 66 days. The surgical procedure included complete tumor excision combined with electroencephalography to indicate if any abnormal areas of tissue remained. If an abnormal corticogram was noted, an additional attempt was made to remove the remaining neoplastic tissue. Thus, the patients had fairly radical surgical excision, but in spite of this the group receiving postoperative irradiation responded more favorably.

Similar data are available in a retrospective view of 37 patients with a histologically confirmed diagnosis of oligodendroglioma.[33] The neurosurgeon made an attempt in each case to remove as much of the tumor as possible. However, complete tumor excision was not thought to have been achieved in any of these patients. Since five patients died within 2 weeks of their operation, they were excluded from

TABLE 131-2   Survival Rates According to Therapy*

| Interval (years) | All Cases† | Surgery Alone | | Surgery + Irradiation |
		Total Resection	Incomplete Resection	Incomplete Resection
1	65% (33/51)	100% (14/14)	51% (19/37)	80% (57/71)
3	47% (24/51)	100% (14/14)	27% (10/37)	59% (42/71)
5	41% (21/51)	100% (14/14)	19% (7/37)	46% (33/71)
10	33% (16/49)	100% (12/12)	11% (4/37)	35% (19/54)
15	24% (9/37)	89% (8/9)	4% (1/28)	25% (8/32)
20	26% (7/27)	88% (7/8)	0% (0/19)	23% (6/26)

*Survival rates in patients with low-grade astrocytoma, according to the therapy received.
†Includes two patients lost to follow-up and considered DOD.
SOURCE: Leibel et al.[20] Reprinted with permission.

the analysis. The 32 remaining patients were divided equally among those who received postoperative irradiation and those who did not. One patient in each group was lost to follow-up. The 5- and 10-year survival rates for the patients who underwent surgical resection only were 31 percent and 25 percent, respectively. Those patients who received postoperative irradiation had a 5-year survival rate of 85 percent and a 10-year survival rate of 55 percent. Analysis revealed that the difference between the 5-year survival rates was statistically significant.

Since complete tumor excision is very difficult in the patient with an oligodendroglioma, postoperative irradiation is indicated. The recommended tumor dose is in the range of 5000 to 6000 rad. Some radiation oncologists recommend whole brain irradiation, while others feel that irradiation to the tumor-bearing volume, with adequate margins, is sufficient. The actual technique of irradiation may vary depending upon the location and size of the tumor. Although there are no data relating to the optimum time over which irradiation should be given, it is recommended that treatments be initiated when the patient has recovered from surgery sufficiently and the surgical incision site is healing satisfactorily.

Metastatic Disease

The value of radiotherapy in the treatment of tumors metastatic to the brain has been known for approximately thirty years. There have been numerous studies documenting the effectiveness of radiotherapy in providing symptomatic improvement in these patients, and a number of different fractionation schemes have been used. Some authors report that a prolonged course of treatment with high doses is the most effective both in symptomatic control of the disease and in prolongation of survival. Others think that a more rapid fractionation scheme is just as effective.

The most extensive clinical trials of irradiation in the treatment of brain metastases were conducted by the Radiation Therapy Oncology Group (RTOG).[19] In the first trial, different doses of whole brain irradiation were delivered with different fractionation schedules. There was also a treatment arm which utilized a single high dose of irradiation to the whole brain. Patient assessment was done on the basis of improvement in the patient's neurological status and

overall condition. Only 12 percent of the total patient population in this study had undergone a prior surgical procedure. This group included those patients who had gross removal of the tumor as well as those who underwent biopsy only.

The dose of whole brain irradiation varied from 1000 rad in a single treatment (optional in this study) to 4000 rad in 4 weeks given at 200 rad per day; patients could be treated with 4000 rad in 3 weeks, 3000 rad in 3 weeks, or 3000 rad in 2 weeks. At the completion of the study, the most favorable treatment arms were found to be those in which 4000 rad were given in 3 weeks and 3000 rad were given in 2 weeks. There was no significant difference between these two arms in terms of patients' general performance or neurological function. Thus, 3000 rad given to the whole brain in 2 weeks (300 rad per fraction) appears to be an optimum dosage schedule. This is not only as effective as the higher-dose treatment, but it also allows the patient to be treated over a shorter time interval and thus could be a factor in improving the quality of the patient's life.

Although the use of corticosteroids was not a controlled factor in the RTOG study, it was considered in the analysis of the results. As a general rule, the patients who had more significant symptoms were given corticosteroids. These patients had a more rapid improvement in their neurological function than did patients who did not receive corticosteroids. However, this improvement was not noted after the fourth week. The patients who received steroids did not have an improved median survival time. Thus, it seems that steroids are effective in alleviating the initial symptoms, but it appears that they have no antitumor effect. However, they are useful agents when used in combination with radiotherapy. It is interesting to note that in 40 percent of the patients analyzed, their ultimate deaths did not appear to be related to the brain metastases.

In an additional prospective randomized trial, a dose of 3000 rad given in 2 weeks was compared to a dose of 1000 rad in a single fraction.[12] All patients received whole brain irradiation with two parallel opposed fields. The dose was calculated at the midline. Of the 101 patients eligible for analysis, there was no significant difference in median survival time between the two groups. A slightly higher percentage of patients in the single-dose group had acute complications of nausea, vomiting, headache, or increased neurological deficit (40 percent, versus 27 percent in the fractionated group). Overall, there was no significant difference in survival rate, frequency or degree of response, or complication rate. Although overall survival rates did not differ significantly between the two groups, the curve delineating probability of survival did appear to slightly favor the group receiving 3000 rad in 10 fractions.

The patient with a solitary metastatic deposit poses an additional therapeutic problem. Certain tumors with a potentially long course do have a propensity for solitary metastatic lesions, and patients with these tumors are sometimes treated with a surgical approach. In particular, malignant melanoma and carcinomas of the colon and uterus sometimes present with solitary metastases and can be managed surgically. In other situations, surgery is the initial treatment because the metastasis may be the only known manifestation of disease before the primary lesion has been found. In cases where a solitary metastatic deposit has been removed surgically, many radiation oncologists would recommend a course of whole brain irradiation following the surgical procedure in order to decrease the incidence of clinical manifestations from micrometastases which may already have been present in other areas of the brain. An effective dose is 3000 rad in 10 fractions.

It is sometimes of benefit to retreat the patient who has previously undergone a course of external beam irradiation for cerebral metastases. In general, the results of reirradiation are not as favorable as those of the initial course of treatment. However, if the patient has had a relatively long interval of symptomatic improvement after the initial course of treatments, it may be of benefit to attempt another trial of whole brain irradiation. The patients are sometimes treated with slightly lower doses and over a slightly longer period of time in order to decrease the chance of radiation complications in the reirradiated brain.

Meningeal Carcinomatosis

Malignant disease involving the meninges is a perplexing and difficult problem. Numerous treatment techniques for meningeal carcinomatosis have been utilized, and the results of treatment have generally been less than encouraging. Despite appropriate treatment, meningeal carcinomatosis often progresses rapidly and results in death of the patient within a fairly short period.

CNS irradiation has been utilized in the treatment of this disorder with varying success. It was probably first used in the treatment of meningeal leukemia. (The meninges were frequently found to be a site of relapse in patients who otherwise had no evidence of disease.) The most encouraging results in the treatment of meningeal carcinomatosis in patients with solid tumors appeared in a group with carcinoma of the breast.[40] In this study, 40 patients with meningeal carcinomatosis underwent treatment with whole brain irradiation combined with intrathecal and intraventricular methotrexate with citrovorum factor rescue. The patients were diagnosed as having meningeal involvement on the basis of the presence of malignant cells in the cerebrospinal fluid and the absence of mass lesions on either radionuclide brain scans or computed tomography. Patients received whole brain irradiation consisting of 3000 rad given over a 2-week period. They also received 16 mg of dexamethasone per day and continued with dexamethasone for 1 week after the completion of treatment. Patients also received intrathecal methotrexate, 20 mg, with citrovorum factor rescue. At the completion of whole brain irradiation, an Ommaya reservoir was inserted for the instillation of intraventricular methotrexate. This was done in 36 of the 40 patients who were in systemic remission or who were thought likely to have a survival time of greater than 8 weeks. In patients who had a complete response, malignant cells disappeared from the cerebrospinal fluid. In addition, the CSF protein, glucose, and carcinoembryonic antigen (CEA) levels returned to normal. Patients also had clinical improvement of their neurological function. Patients defined as having a partial response had complete disappearance of tumor cells from the CSF, but there was not complete normalization of CSF or significant improvement in the patients' functional status. Twenty-six of the forty patients had complete responses and 1 had a partial response. Thus, the overall response rate was an encouraging 67 percent. In patients who responded, the survival time was 23 weeks. This compared favorably to a median survival time of 4 weeks in the patients who did not respond. There did not appear to be a relationship between a patient's response and the initial degree of neurological dysfunction. However, patients who had neurological symptoms for more than 4 weeks were found to have a shorter median survival time (7 weeks) and a lower response rate (47 percent) than those patients who had neurological symptoms for less than 4 weeks; the latter group had response rates greater than 75 percent and survival times longer than 18 weeks.

Comparable results have been obtained in patients with carcinomatous meningitis from primary malignancies other than breast carcinoma.[31] In this study, an Ommaya reservoir was used to treat 67 patients. Thirty of these patients had solid tumors, seven had lymphoma, and thirty had leukemia. Fifty-eight percent of the patients with solid tumors improved, while one hundred percent of the leukemic patients improved from a clinical standpoint, and ninety percent of the leukemic patients improved from the standpoint of normalization of cerebrospinal fluid. It is interesting that in the solid tumor group, patients with breast carcinoma and patients with lymphoma showed the greatest amounts of improvement. All but four of the patients with solid tumors received CNS irradiation, and half of the patients with leukemia received this treatment. Thus, comparable response rates can be obtained in patients who have neoplasms other than carcinoma of the breast.

The actual benefit of whole brain irradiation in patients with meningeal carcinomatosis is difficult to assess, since the vast majority of patients were treated with a combination of radiotherapy and chemotherapy. Because the approach to management of meningeal carcinomatosis has not been consistent in most centers and early diagnosis has been difficult, it has been difficult to assess the actual role of the specific modalities used in treating this disorder. However, there are now reports in the literature that show some encouraging results, and whole brain irradiation with a dose of approximately 3000 rad in 10 fractions combined with intrathecal and/or intraventricular chemotherapy can lead to improved control of this condition.

Meningiomas

The meningiomas are typically considered to be rather slow-growing, benign lesions which are well circumscribed and can often be completely resected. Recurrence after complete tumor removal has been reported and is found to occur in 10 to 15 percent of cases. The recurrence rate after incomplete resection has been reported to be as high as 28.9 percent.[39]

The role of radiotherapy in the treatment of meningiomas, primarily to prevent recurrence, is quite controversial. In 1946, McWhirter indicated that roughly 43 percent of meningiomas are radiosensitive.[23] Since these tumors tend to be slow-growing, patients generally have a long survival time and therefore survival time per se may not be an accurate indication of the value of postoperative irradiation. This problem was circumvented in a report from King et al., who studied the interval between initial treatment and subsequent recurrence (the recurrence interval).[16] Forty-eight of the seventy-nine patients studied were treated with surgery and radiotherapy. Twenty-five patients had surgery alone and six received radiotherapy alone. The tumors were histologically divided into meningiomas, angioblastic meningiomas, and malignant or sarcomatous meningiomas. The mean interval to recurrence for all meningiomas was analyzed; those treated with surgery alone had a recurrence interval of 44.5 months and those treated with a combination of surgery and radiotherapy had a recurrence interval of 54.5 months. The difference is not statistically different. However, when the angioblastic meningiomas were analyzed separately, the average recurrence interval after surgery alone was 39 months as compared to 72 months after treatment with the combined approach. Patients with sarcomatous meningiomas had a 10-month average recurrence interval following surgery alone and an 83-month recurrence interval following surgery and radiotherapy. Thus, the authors suggest that these two subtypes of meningioma do respond to radiotherapy and that radiotherapy is indicated in treating these lesions. However, there were fairly small numbers of patients in both of the histological subtypes. These authors did not find radiotherapy alone to be of benefit as the primary mode of treatment.

Another study involving a fairly large number of patients indicated that histological subtypes did not have a bearing on the response of meningiomas to irradiation.[38] In this study, 188 patients were treated by surgery with or without irradiation. If the patients were thought to have had complete removal of their tumors, no further treatment was given. Forty-four percent of the patients were thought to have had total surgical removal. There was no recurrence in this group of patients. Fifty-eight of the remaining 104 patients who had subtotal removal of tumor did not receive postoperative irradiation. In this patient group the recurrence rate was 74 percent. Ninety-four patients had subtotal resection and had immediate postoperative irradiation. The recurrence rate in this group was 29 percent. There was an additional group of 12 patients who had tumors which were initially not thought to be totally resectable. These patients underwent either limited partial resection or biopsy only, followed by radiotherapy. Patients in this group were scheduled for reoperation about 6 months after completion of the radiation therapy. In this group, eight patients underwent total resection following the course of radiotherapy. Seven of these patients were alive and well with no recurrence at an interval of between 4 and 13 years after surgery.

It would thus appear that complete surgical removal is the treatment of choice in the patient with a meningioma. However, in those cases where the neoplasm cannot be completely resected, radiotherapy may well be effective in either totally preventing or delaying the onset of recurrence. There is some controversy as to whether the histological subtype of the meningioma is related to its sensitivity to irradiation. There has been some indication that the meningiomas which are very vascular may respond favorably to irradiation, and that the resectability of these tumors may be improved with a course of preoperative radiotherapy. The patient with a meningioma should be treated through fields which encompass the known area of disease, with adequate margins around the primary lesion. High-energy equipment should be utilized in the vast majority of cases. The dose should be 5000 to 5500 rad at a rate of 170 to 200 rad per day. If a recurrent meningioma which has not been previously irradiated is not amenable to further surgical resection, radiotherapy may play a very effective role in controlling this tumor for a prolonged period.

Pineal Tumors

Neoplasms in this region are rather uncommon. Because of their anatomical location, surgical excision is often not possible and radiotherapy plays a primary role in their management. There continue to be questions regarding the optimum field size and dose to use in these neoplasms, and the question of neuraxis irradiation for the germinomas occurring in this region remains to be clearly answered.

For those patients in whom neuraxis irradiation is not deemed necessary, the question still remains as to what are the optimum field size and dose for tumor control. In a recent study, 22 patients with a clinical diagnosis of tumor in the pineal region were treated with radio therapy.[28] The patients were thought to have pineal-region tumors when they presented with a combination of increased intracranial pressure and altered pupillary function and upward-gaze paralysis. Air studies and CT scans were obtained and demonstrated a defect in the posterior third ventricle, with associated hydrocephalus. Patients with ectopic tumors generally had diabetes insipidus, visual disturbances, and some amount of hypopituitarism. General radiographic studies showed a defect in the anterior third ventricle, with or without hydrocephalus. These twenty-two patients received irradiation with megavoltage equipment. Patients received a daily dose of 150 to 180 rad given 5 times per week. Twelve patients received whole brain irradiation and ten received less than whole brain treatment. Five of these patients were treated with fields which included the entire ventricular system, and the other five patients had smaller portals which were limited to the primary tumor and an adequate margin.

A review of the results of treatment indicated that the patients who received whole brain irradiation or who received maximum doses greater than 5000 rad had a longer survival time than did those patients who received lower doses or less extensive treatment portals. Three of five patients who were treated with whole brain irradiation had no evidence of disease 10 years after diagnosis, whereas only one of eight patients who were treated with partial brain fields was alive at 10 years.

The authors included a review of the literature in an attempt to further document the effectiveness of irradiation. Adequate radiotherapy data were available for 67 patients. The favorable prognosis in this tumor is reflected by the fact that the median survival time in this patient population was 10 years. Sixty-two percent of the patients had no evidence of disease at 5 years, and 60 percent of all failures had occurred by 4 years after diagnosis. Patients who were treated with fields that included the whole brain had better survival rates than did those patients who received less than whole brain treatment. The difference between those patients receiving whole brain irradiation and those receiving partial brain treatment was maintained for up to 10 years from the date of diagnosis. In the patient group that received treatment with fields that included the entire ventricular system, the survival rate was better for 3 years as compared to that in patients who received treatment to smaller portals. The failure rates were comparable for patients with ectopic tumors and those with pineal-area tumors. There was no difference in failure rates between the patients who were under 12 years old and those who were over 12 years old at diagnosis.

Since the surgical procedure in the vast majority of these patients is limited to a shunting procedure to relieve intracranial pressure, radio-therapy remains the primary treatment modality. It appears that doses in excess of 5000 rad given at conventional fractionation are indicated, and large treatment fields seem to improve the survival. As a minimum, patients should receive treatment to the entire ventricular system, and many radiation oncologists would advocate whole brain irradiation. This can be adequately achieved with opposing bilateral fields. In some institutions, the whole brain is treated with a moderate dose, and then the fields are reduced to bring the dose to the area of tumor volume up to the 5000- to 5500-rad level. Some authorities have suggested that a reduction in total dose by approximately 20 percent should be considered in children who are under 3 years of age. There has been some indication that the cerebral tissue of young children is more sensitive to the damaging effects of irradiation than that of older patients.

The question of neuraxis irradiation is a controversial one. Certainly there are documented instances of spinal cord seeding from primary tumors of this type, and after seeding has occurred, the disease is difficult to control with irradiation. If malignant cells are found in the neuraxis irradiation is indicated. The recommended dose to the spinal cord is approximately 3500 rad. There have been some instances where a patient has been found to have an elevated alpha-fetoprotein level or an elevated human chorionic gonadotropin level in the CSF studies. The question of whether or not to treat the neuraxis in the face of positive markers and in the absence of malignant cells is also controversial. The benefit of neuraxis irradiation in patients with positive markers in the CSF has yet to be proven. In the young child, radiotherapy to the neuraxis can result in significant long-term sequelae. These include the arrest of bone growth, as well as the possibility of long-term growth abnormalities in

the soft tissues and vasculature within the irradiated field. If the physician thinks that inclusion of the entire subarachnoid space is necessary, the treatment field must be extended to the level of S2. Treatment to this inferior border could result in radiation damage to the gonads as well.

In a study by the Childrens Cancer Study Group, the incidence of spinal cord metastases was 8 percent (9 of 118 patients).[37] Two of these nine patients had primary recurrences as well. None of the patients received spinal irradiation. It was not thought that the 8 percent incidence of metastasis warranted prophylactic neuraxis irradiation. However, it is interesting to note that of the patients who had biopsy-proven germinomas, 14 percent developed spinal metastases, in contrast to a 1.7 percent incidence of metastases in the group that did not receive biopsies.

Cerebellar Astrocytomas

Cerebellar astrocytomas are found in the pediatric age group in the vast majority of cases. These lesions generally have a good prognosis, possibly because of the fact that symptoms occur early in neoplasms in this location. In addition, these tumors are commonly cystic and they tend to be relatively noninvasive. These characteristics permit complete surgical removal of the lesion in the majority of patients. These tumors, like the low-grade astrocytomas of the optic nerve, carry a favorable prognosis.

Because of the characteristics of these tumors, there is some controversy as to the specific role of radiotherapy in their management. If the tumor is completely removed, 5-year survival rates as high as 80 percent or better are reported. A fairly recent study included 14 patients who received postoperative irradiation for cerebellar astrocytoma.[4] In this series, 12 patients survived from 5 to 22 years. Only one patient was physically impaired and this was because of an unsteady gait.

There seems to be no role for radiotherapy in cases where the lesion has been completely excised. However, radiotherapy is indicated if the tumor has been incompletely excised. Treatment can be delivered either through bilateral opposed fields or through three fields consisting of a posterior field in conjunction with two lateral fields. The dose should be in the range of 5000 rad, with some consideration for reduction of the total dosage if the patient is under 2 years of age. The solid astrocytoma that is subtotally removed is more likely to recur than a solid tumor that is totally removed or a cystic tumor that is subtotally removed. Although long-term radiation-induced complications in these patients have been difficult to document, utilization of small fields which adequately encompass the tumor volume, along with appropriate fractionation schemes, should reduce any treatment-related morbidity (Fig. 131-2).

Medulloblastomas

This relatively uncommon neoplasm, which primarily affects children, is routinely treated with a combination of surgical resection and postoperative irradiation. It has long

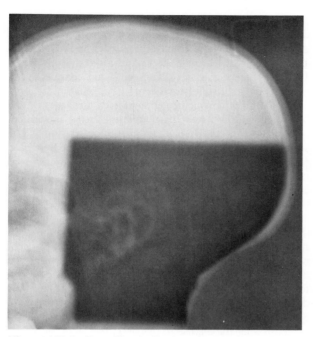

Figure 131-2 Port film indicating the treatment field in a patient with a cerebellar astrocytoma. An individually made Cerrobend block was used to treat the specific area of risk.

been known that surgery alone is ineffective in the management of these patients, resulting in a survival time which averages from 6 to 12 months.

Appropriate irradiation includes treatment to the entire craniospinal axis. It has been known for approximately thirty years that radiotherapy to this volume is necessary, and recent data indicate that survival can be improved in this patient population if postoperative irradiation is administered to the appropriate fields and in appropriate doses. A recent large study looked retrospectively at 122 patients with histological confirmation of medulloblastoma who received radiotherapy postoperatively.[2] Since the review covered 21 years, various doses and treatment techniques were utilized, but some interesting conclusions can be drawn. In this patient population, 36 percent were thought to have had macroscopically complete tumor resection, while 54 percent had subtotal removal, and 10 percent had biopsy only. Most of the patients were treated with cobalt 60, but early in the study, some patients received treatment with kilovoltage irradiation only. In the entire patient group, the median dose to the whole brain was 3500 rad. The posterior fossa received a boost, and median dose to this region was 5000 rad. Patients received a median spinal cord dose of 3500 rad. Survival rates from the date of surgery were 56 percent of the entire group at 5 years and 43 percent at 10 years. The relapse-free rates were 49 percent and 38 percent, respectively. The amount of tumor resection had a bearing on survival rates in that 64 percent of the patients who had what were thought to be total resections survived 5 years, while 33 percent of those patients who received biopsy only survived 5 years. The survival rate for subtotal resection was 56 percent at 5 years. When the dose of irradiation to the posterior fossa was analyzed, no statistical difference was found in

survival rates relative to the dose received. Yet there did seem to be a trend of increasing survival when higher doses were given to the posterior fossa (Figure 131-3). However, the posterior fossa was the site of first relapse in 46 percent of the patients, and there was a relationship between the dose to the posterior fossa and recurrence in this area. The relapse-free rate was 79 percent in patients who received more than 5350 rad, 82 percent in those who received between 5200 and 5350 rad, 74 percent in those who received 5000 to 5100 rad, and only 42 percent in those who received less than 5000 rad. There did not appear to be any difference in survival between the patients for whom radiotherapy was initiated within 10 days of surgical treatment and those patients for whom the initiation of treatment was delayed because of postoperative complications.

Further data indicating a relationship between the dose to the posterior fossa and control of the tumor come from a retrospective study involving 33 children under the age of 20.[8] During the later portion of this study, patients received a dose of 4500 rad to the whole brain, with an additional 1000-rad boost to the posterior fossa. The spinal cord received 4500 rad. Treatments were given at 180 rad per fraction to the brain and 160 rad per fraction to the spinal cord. In those children who were under 3 years of age, the total dose to each area was decreased by 1000 rad. In those patients who received posterior fossa doses of 5500 rad, the local control rate was 86 percent (six of seven patients) while

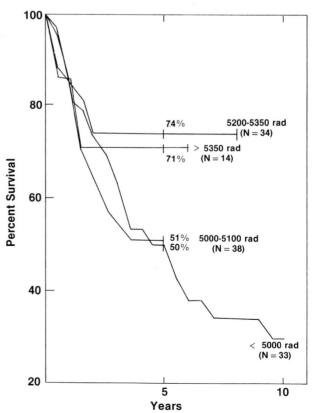

Figure 131-3 Survival rates in medulloblastoma patients relative to the dose of irradiation which was given to the posterior fossa. (From Berry et al.[2] Reprinted with permission.)

local control was achieved in only 17 percent (two of twelve patients) when the posterior fossa doses were less than 5000 rad. Although the incidence of recurrence might be highest in the first 2 to 3 years after treatment, two patients in this series had recurrences at 47 and 62 months. A similar correlation of dose and response was noted in the spinal cord. In those patients who received cord doses of 4000 rad the 5-year control rate was 62 percent (eight of thirteen patients), whereas in those who received less than 3500 rad the 5-year local control rate was 33 percent (two of six patients).

Various techniques have been developed for irradiating the whole brain and spinal cord. In an acceptable technique, the patient is placed in a prone position, with treatment of the brain and upper cervical cord via lateral opposed portals. The spine is treated through a direct posterior field, which can be done in either one or two segments, depending on the length of the patient's spine. In order to avoid a dose overlap between abutting fields, the field junctions are moved at regular intervals during the course of treatment (Figure 131-4). The posterior fossa can be boosted with an additional dose with lateral fields after the completion of the whole brain irradiation.

Since this patient population tends to be fairly young and the radiotherapy is rather extensive, complications can be significant. These patients receive treatment to at least 20 percent of the functioning marrow, and neutropenia and/or

thrombocytopenia can sometimes be a problem. In all patients treated, a moderate depression of the blood counts is expected. If the white blood cell count drops to less than 1000 or the platelet count decreases to significantly below 100,000, some radiation oncologists would consider interrupting treatment until the counts have recovered. Long-range complications include endocrine disturbances caused by irradiation of the hypothalamopituitary axis, impairment of bone growth, and hypoplasia of some of the soft tissue structures which may have been included in the irradiated field. Many radiation oncologists think that a lower dose is justified in patients under 3 years of age because of the decreased myelinization present within the CNS of patients in this age range.

It thus appears that patients with medulloblastoma should be treated first with surgical resection of as much tumor as is reasonably possible without causing significant morbidity. This should be followed by external beam megavoltage irradiation to the entire neuraxis. The posterior fossa should receive a boost to a higher dose. This higher dose appears to be effective in decreasing local recurrences. Since the posterior fossa is a common site of initial relapse, by controlling the disease in this area, the physician might decrease the incidence of disease in other areas. Patient tolerance is generally good, but the patient should be monitored closely during the course of treatment with frequent blood tests. The technique used to deliver treatment is extremely important; it is essential to avoid overlapping fields that increase the risk of spinal cord myelitis due to overdosage to a segment of the cord.

Some physicians perform myelography routinely in these patients, and in some cases defects are noted. In those situations, additional radiotherapy to the area of the abnormality should be considered. It is difficult to determine at this time if the additional treatments to the areas of abnormality result in improved control.

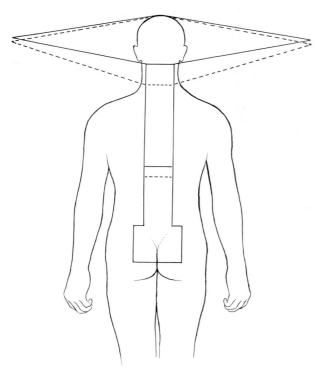

Figure 131-4 Field arrangement utilized in treating the craniospinal axis in patients with medulloblastoma. The brain and upper cervical cord are treated via lateral portals, and the spine is treated posteriorly. Field junctions are moved at regular intervals to avoid overdosing the cord. Solid and dashed lines indicate field arrangements on alternating days.

Brain Stem Gliomas

Brain stem gliomas are often diagnosed on radiographic and clinical grounds, since these tumors are not often surgically accessible. Because of their critical location, the vast majority of these neoplasms have been treated primarily with radiotherapy. Analysis of treatment results relating to brain stem tumors is sometimes difficult because tumors of various anatomical locations are included within this group. Some series include tumors of the thalamus, midbrain, and fourth ventricle, while others are limited to the area of the medulla oblongata and pons. In addition, since biopsy is often not possible, the specific histological subtype is often not known. These tumors occur in patients of a wide age range, and the results of treatment will vary depending on the ages of the patients in the study group. Certainly those studies which include a large proportion of pediatric patients may report a more favorable prognosis than do studies dealing only with adults.

A recent retrospective review reported the results of radiotherapy in treating patients with primary brain stem tumors.[15] Approximately one-half of these patients were under 20 years of age. In 45 patients the primary lesion was located in the pons, in 11 in the medulla oblongata, and in 18 the exact location was not known. Histologically, 54 percent of the patients had low-grade astrocytomas and 38 percent had higher-grade gliomas.

The patients were treated with megavoltage equipment, using fields to the posterior fossa and upper cervical cord. Of the 63 patients who received full courses of radiotherapy, 44 received doses of over 5000 rad. It is interesting to note that the survival rate for those patients who received over 5000 rad was better, and all of the survivors of 5 years or more received doses of at least 5000 rad. There was a correlation between survival rate and response to treatment. Those patients who were poor responders had a poor survival rate, while the long-term survivors all exhibited a good initial response to the radiotherapy.

External beam irradiation remains the mainstay of treatment in patients with brain stem gliomas. Localized fields that include the posterior fossa and upper cervical cord are generally recommended. The dose should be in the range of 5000 to 6000 rad, at a daily dose rate of between 160 and 200 rad per fraction. Various field arrangements have been used in treating these patients, including bilateral opposed fields as well as rotational and three-field techniques. A clear-cut advantage of one treatment plan over another has not been demonstrated. In the younger patient, the physician should consider decreasing the total dose because some think that the developing nervous system in children under the age of 3 is more sensitive to the damaging effects of irradiation.

Reirradiation of a recurrent brain stem glioma carries an increased risk of radiation necrosis. However, in a patient who is deteriorating due to recurrent tumor, reirradiation is sometimes justified, and there have been cases in which retreatment of the primary area has resulted in improved symptoms and probable prolongation of the patient's life.

Ependymomas

Neoplasms of ependymal cell origin are relatively rare. Because of this, it has not been possible to look at the role of radiotherapy in a prospective fashion. However, there are a number of retrospective reports which indicate a clear role for radiotherapy in treating these neoplasms.

In one study, the role of radiotherapy was analyzed in 31 patients who survived 2 months after subtotal surgical removal of ependymomas.[25] Twenty-eight of these patients received radiotherapy. Twenty-five received postoperative irradiation, and three were treated preoperatively. Ten patients either received radiation doses of less than 3500 rad or did not receive any irradiation at all. Only one of these ten patients was a 5-year survivor. In the patient group receiving 4500 rad or more, 13 of 15 were 5-year survivors. The difference between the 5-year survival rates of patients receiving less than 3500 rad and those receiving more than 4500 rad was statistically significant. The overall 5-year survival rate in the entire patient population was 40 percent. The 5-year survival rate was 56 percent for those patients who survived

surgery and 87 percent for the patients who were thought to have adequate radiotherapy, consisting of a dose of at least 4500 rad.

The same study addressed the question of spinal seeding within the subarachnoid space. This is a controversial subject, and there have been conflicting data regarding the need for prophylactic irradiation to the entire neuraxis. The authors of this study found that the incidence of clinically significant subarachnoid seeding was very low, and it was thought that irradiation of the cerebrospinal axis was not indicated. Although some autopsy studies have indicated that the incidence of microscopic subarachnoid seeding is somewhat higher, the low incidence of clinically significant subarachnoid seeding would seem to justify this treatment approach. In some instances, however, neuraxis irradiation may be indicated. In those patients who have very poorly differentiated ependymoma involving the posterior fossa, the incidence of spinal cord seeding might be significantly higher, and neuraxis irradiation should be seriously considered in these situations.

The site of origin of the ependymoma within the central nervous system may have a direct influence on the clinical characteristics of the tumor.[22] In a series of 61 patients with ependymomas located in various areas within the central nervous system, the subgroup of patients with infratentorial lesions was noted to have improved local control with increasing biologically effective doses of irradiation.[22] No such correlation could be demonstrated in patients with tumors in other locations. The incidence of spinal cord seeding was found to be 11 percent in pathological specimens, but it was clinically evident in only 4 percent of these patients. Of the five patients who had pathologically documented spinal metastases, four had infratentorial primary tumors and in one the lesion was located supratentorially. Eight patients in this study had also received intrathecal gold 198 as a part of their therapy. Three of these eight patients developed a radiation myelopathy and/or cauda equina syndrome, from 3.5 to 17 years after treatment.

On the basis of a number of retrospective analyses, it appears that postoperative irradiation has a clear-cut role to play in the treatment of ependymomas. The actual treatment approach will vary depending upon the location and histology of the tumor. In general, the more distally located lesions have more favorable prognoses. That is, lesions of the cauda equina have the most favorable prognosis, whereas supratentorial lesions have the least favorable prognosis. Tumors of the infratentorium and spinal cord have an intermediate prognosis.

The optimum treatment for most ependymomas is surgical removal of as much tumor as is possible without inducing significant morbidity, followed by radiotherapy. The radiotherapy should be given with a generous margin around the primary tumor. Doses in the range of 5000 to 5500 rad at conventional fractionation are appropriate. In some cases, the whole brain can be treated with 4500 to 5000 rad, followed by an additional 500 rad to a reduced volume encompassing the primary lesion. Parallel opposed portals are sufficient for most patients. Whole neuraxis irradiation should be considered in those patients who have histological evidence of spinal cord seeding. The dose to the spinal cord should be in the range of 3000 to 3500 rad at conventional fractionation. This dose is well tolerated and carries a minimal risk of myelopathy.

Pituitary Tumors

Most tumors of the pituitary are histologically benign. However, they are often malignant in their behavior due to their critical anatomical location. It has been reported that normal pituitary tissue is relatively resistant to the effects of ionizing irradiation, and that doses in the usual therapeutic range do not produce significant signs of hypopituitarism.[5] However, it may take many years for the pituitary gland to display any evidence of damage induced by irradiation, and long-term endocrinological follow-up of these patients is often lacking.

External beam irradiation has long been recognized as an effective therapeutic modality in the treatment of pituitary adenomas. A number of different techniques have been utilized in treating these lesions, including use of two parallel opposed fields, three-field techniques, and arc rotational therapy (Fig. 131-5). These lesions require moderate doses for control, generally in the range of 4500 to 5000 rad at conventional fractionation (160 to 200 rad per day). It has been clearly shown that the combination of surgery followed by postoperative irradiation is effective in controlling the chromophobe adenomas. In a study involving 107 patients, Sheline analyzed the determinant control rate in patients treated with surgery alone compared with those who received both surgery and radiotherapy.[32] At 5 years, the control rate with surgery only was 38 percent (9 of 24 patients) versus a control rate of 96 percent (65 of 68 patients) in the group which received surgery plus postoperative irradiation. At 10 years, the control rates were 14 percent and 83 percent, respectively.

External beam irradiation has also been shown to be a very effective technique for treating acromegaly.[11] A group of 47 patients with documented acromegaly made up the study group. The patients received between 4000 and 5000 rad of external beam irradiation and were followed for a period of up to 10 years. This treatment approach was found to be quite effective, but it should be emphasized that the decline in growth hormone levels took place quite gradually, over 5 to 10 years after completion of treatment. In 81 percent of the patients, plasma growth hormone valves were less than 10 ng/ml. As the growth hormone level declined, the objective changes induced by growth hormone (GH) excess improved as well. Although the decline was gradual, conventional irradiation was found to produce the same fall in the GH level as do other forms of treatment for acromegaly. (It is interesting to note that the incidence of hypopituitarism was also noted to increase throughout the follow-up period.) The authors therefore thought that conventional external beam irradiation had fewer serious side effects than do the surgical techniques which are normally employed for the treatment of acromegaly.

Surgical removal of prolactinomas has been found to be an effective method of reducing an elevated prolactin level to the normal range. In those patients who have persistently elevated prolactin levels postoperatively, radiotherapy can be effective in further reducing the serum level.[17] In addition, it has been shown that radiotherapy alone can result in normalization of the serum prolactin level.[10] A group of six women with evidence of prolactin-secreting pituitary adenomas were treated with a course of external beam irradiation consisting of 5000 rad given over 5.5 weeks. Half of these patients had normalization of their serum prolactin levels and two of the patients had normal pregnancies. In the third patient, a normal menstrual cycle was re-established. The fall in the prolactin level was fairly rapid, with five of the six patients having a substantial reduction in the serum prolactin level after a brief period. It is important to realize that after radiotherapy these patients were given maintenance bromocriptine treatments. In the remaining three patients, radiotherapy did not appear to have beneficial effects. All six of the patients in this study had been previously treated with various medications, and the drugs had not been effective in controlling their prolactin-secreting tumors.

In 1932, Dr. Harvey Cushing introduced the use of x-irradiation for a syndrome which he attributed to a basophilic adenoma. Since that time, a number of investigators have documented the beneficial effects of radiotherapy in treating Cushing's disease. As diagnosis of this disease became more specific and advances were made in radiotherapy, there were a number of treatment plans used in the management of this disease. An attempt to establish some correlation between time-dose factors and control of the primary lesion was made in a study of 45 patients with Cushing's disease.[1] This study was limited to patients with hypercortisolism which was caused by excessive pituitary ACTH secretion. These patients were treated with megavoltage equipment, using either a three-field technique (one anterior and two lateral portals), parallel opposed portals, or rotational therapy. Three patients were treated with five to seven isocentric stationary fields. Patients were considered to have been cured of their disease if urinary hydrocortisone excretion was less than 7 mg/g creatinine and the plasma hydrocortisone level was either normal or subnormal. In 39 patients, follow-up observations of from 2 to 15 years were available. Twenty-five percent of the patients were considered cured. An additional 28 percent were found to have improved to the point that they either required aminoglutethimide or no further therapy. Nineteen patients failed and subsequently underwent adrenalectomy or hypophysectomy. Complications developed in three patients (necrosis of the brain stem in one, progressive blindness in another, and blindness of one eye in the third patient).

When the time-dose factors were reviewed, it was found that treatment with less than 4000 rad was not satisfactory. At doses between 4500 and 5000 rad the maximum benefits of radiotherapy were noted. It appears that the complication rate increased as the dose exceeded 4500 rad. It is interesting to note that there were no clear relationships between the field size or the technique used in and the development of complications. In particular, patients who received treatment via opposed lateral fields were not found to have a higher incidence of complications.

Thus, using conventional fractionation and megavoltage equipment and a dose of approximately 4500 rad in 5 weeks (treating 5 times per week), Cushing's disease can be controlled in approximately 50 percent of the patients. Since the tumor tends to occupy a fairly small volume, small treat-

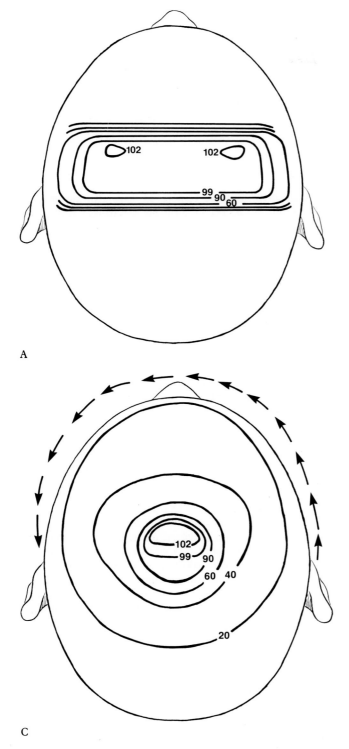

A

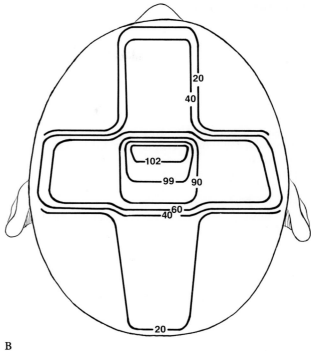

B

Figure 131-5 Isodose distributions for various techniques used in the treatment of pituitary tumors. *A*. Bilateral opposed portals. *B*. Three-field technique utilizing two lateral ports and a single anterior port. *C*. Arc rotational therapy.

C

ment fields can be utilized. It is difficult to assess the advantage of one particular treatment technique over another. Certainly bilateral opposed fields are technically simpler to reproduce, but some radiation oncologists think that the dose distribution is somewhat better when three fields are used. Others prefer the arc rotational technique. Each technique is effective, and no advantage of one treatment method

over another has been demonstrated. An additional technique uses proton beams, and this treatment modality is discussed elsewhere in this text.

Although Cushing's disease is uncommon in childhood, the use of conventional radiotherapy in this patient population has also been studied.[14] Fifteen patients were diagnosed as having Cushing's disease, and all underwent radiotherapy with an 8 MeV linear accelerator, using doses from 3500 to 5000 rad at a daily fractionation of 150 to 200 rad. Most of the patients were treated with opposed lateral fields. Within 11 to 18 months after the initiation of irradiation, 12 of the 15 patients were thought to be cured of their disease. The three patients who failed subsequently underwent bilateral adrenalectomies. Sexual development was normal in all 15 patients, and growth resumed in 12 of the 15 patients treated. Pituitary irradiation was thought to be a safe and effective therapy for Cushing's disease in the pediatric patient population.

Craniopharyngiomas

These histologically benign tumors are malignant by virtue of their location and their locally invasive characteristics. They can produce considerable morbidity and a significant proportion of patients will eventually succumb to their disease process.

The clinical course of the patient with a craniopharyngioma can vary considerably, depending on the size and characteristics of the tumor. This fact has led to some controversy regarding the optimum management of these neoplasms. Some have advocated a radical surgical approach only, while others think that limited surgical excision followed by postoperative irradiation is the treatment of choice. Most of the reports involving limited surgical procedures followed by irradiation indicate that control rates are quite good and treatment complications are less.

A recent report analyzed 35 patients with craniopharyngioma who fell into three separate treatment groups.[21] Nineteen patients had surgery alone and eleven were treated with limited surgery followed by irradiation. Eleven were treated for recurrent disease; four of these were from the group which had originally received surgery only. The minimum follow-up was 3 years in the 35 patients suitable for analysis. Twelve of these patients were older than 18 years and 23 were 18 or younger.

In the group receiving surgery only, three of eight patients who were thought to have had total resection had recurrences. Five of the nine who had partial removal of their tumor had recurrences. Therefore, a 47 percent recurrence rate was noted in these groups. The group receiving both surgery and radiotherapy had a rate of local recurrence of 20 percent (2 of 10 patients). It is interesting to note that one of these recurrences occurred in a patient who had received an inadequate dose of irradiation (3450 rad). There were no recurrences in eight patients who had fairly small tumors and to whom adequate doses of postoperative irradiation were given.

In the group of 11 patients who had recurrent disease, 7 received irradiation with or without limited resection and 4 received surgery only. Five patients from the irradiated group were alive and four showed no evidence of disease within the minimum follow-up period of 3 years. In contrast, only one patient from the group that received surgery alone remained alive without evidence of recurrence. Only three patients from the reirradiated group were thought to have a good initial result following their retreatment. Overall, the complications of treatment were fewer in the group of patients who received both limited surgical resection and postoperative irradiation.

This study confirms several previous reports which indicated that irradiation after surgical excision of as much tumor as possible without inducing significant morbidity seems to be the treatment of choice for patients with craniopharyngioma. The radiotherapy should be given with megavoltage equipment and using field sizes which correspond to the area of tumor volume, with an adequate margin. Communication between the surgeon and the radiation oncologist is extremely important in localizing the tumor, and radiological imaging techniques are very helpful as well.

The dose to the tumor volume should be between 5000 and 6000 rad, delivered in 5 treatments per week in fractions of from 160 to 200 rad. Some have advocated using lateral opposed portals, while others think that a three-field technique using lateral wedged portals and an anterior field is optimum. There have not been any studies which show a significant advantage of one type of field arrangement over another.

Optic Nerve Gliomas

The majority of these tumors are slow-growing astrocytomas, and a number of different therapeutic approaches have been successful in their management. Suggestions for appropriate treatment have included complete excision, inspection and biopsy only, and partial removal followed by radiotherapy. Indeed, there have been cases of long-term control after only incomplete excision. Thus, the optimum management of the optic nerve glioma remains somewhat controversial. Most treatment reports have been retrospective analyses, and have included patients whose gliomas were confined to the optic nerve as well as those whose tumors extended to involve the chiasm or hypothalamus. Certainly those patients with chiasmal and/or hypothalamic involvement have a less favorable prognosis than do those patients with involvement of the optic nerve.

A recent retrospective analysis involved 18 children with optic nerve gliomas who underwent treatment with external beam irradiation.[9] All of these patients had rather extensive disease in that none of them had neoplasms limited to a single optic nerve. Eight patients were noted to have chiasmal lesions; ten had neoplasms which involved the hypothalamus and chiasm, and of these 10, 6 had hydrocephalus as well. Of the entire group of 18 patients, 7 had partial resection, 7 had biopsy, 2 had surgical inspection without biopsy, and 2 patients had the diagnosis made on neuroradiological findings. All the patients received treatment with megavoltage equipment, and received doses of 5000 to 6000 rad. Sixteen of the eighteen patients underwent their radiotherapy when the initial diagnosis was made. The other two patients underwent treatment after they developed signs of disease progression. This occurred 1.5 years after the initial diagnosis had been made.

Five-year survival statistics were available for 12 of the 18 patients. In this group, the 5-year survival rate was 83 percent (10 of 12 patients). The 10-year survival rate was 73 percent (eight of eleven patients). Of the five patients with chiasmal lesions, all survived 5 years, and four of the five survived 10 years. The seven patients who had involvement of the hypothalamus or third ventricle had a 5-year survival rate of 71 percent and a 10-year survival rate of 66 percent. Of the total group, 14 of the 18 patients were thought to have improvement or maintenance of their visual status. The remaining four patients had decreased vision after completion of treatment.

The primary goal in treating the optic nerve glioma is to achieve long-range survival. Above this, it is hoped to either preserve or improve the patient's vision. there are certain clinical situations where total surgical removal of the tumor is not possible, i.e., for those tumors that extend to the chiasm or involve the hypothalamus and/or third ventricle. Thus, there is clearly a patient population that would benefit from postoperative irradiation. In addition, when there is a question of preserving the patient's vision, a biopsy followed by irradiation may be the most appropriate treatment approach.

A number of different techniques have been utilized in the treatment of optic nerve gliomas, including bilateral opposed fields, arc rotational therapy, and a three-field technique. The optimum tumor dose should be in the range of 5000 to 6000 rad at conventional fractionation. It has been recommended by some radiation oncologists that children under the age of 2 years should be treated with lower doses, in the range of 4500 rad, at slightly lower daily dose fractions. For the low-grade gliomas, treatment fields should include the extent of known tumor, with adequate margins. Precise localization of the tumor, using both radiographic and surgical findings, can be extremely important in limiting the total volume of the irradiated field. In those unusual instances where the patient may have a higher-grade glioma, more generous fields should be utilized. In cases where an adult presents with an optic nerve glioma, some radiation oncologists have recommended increasing the tumor dose to the range of 6500 rad. The efficacy of this higher-dose range has not been shown conclusively.

Chordomas

These rare tumors have traditionally been considered to be radioresistant. However, there is recent evidence to indicate that they do respond to irradiation. Because of the difficulty of completely resecting these tumors, radiotherapy is often utilized in their management. The malignancy of these tumors is caused primarily by their locally aggressive nature, high recurrence rate, and critical anatomical location. Although these neoplasms do metastasize, it is the local tissue damage and high recurrence rate that generally lead to the death of the patient.

Although it has been reported that these tumors vary in their sensitivity to irradiation, the consensus is that the chordomas require radical doses for control. The primary limiting factor in treating these tumors is the tolerance of the normal surrounding structures. Recent advances both in image localization of these tumors and in use of high-energy photon and proton beams have resulted in some encouraging results.

The clinical histories of 46 patients with chordoma who

were evaluated over a 35-year period were reviewed by Higinbotham et al.[13] Thirty of the patients in this series had chordomas that were of sacral origin. This incidence is somewhat higher than that reported by others, in which approximately 50 percent of the chordomas are located in the sacrococcygeal area. It is interesting as well that in this series 43 percent of the patients had documented metastases. This is significantly higher than the usually described metastatic rate of approximately 15 percent. Eighteen of the thirty cases with sacrococcygeal chordoma underwent radiotherapy. The authors noted that both the symptomatic relief and the objective tumor response increased as the dose of irradiation was increased. In the eight cases where an objective response was noted, the minimum tumor dose which produced this response was 3900 rad. In addition, five other patients were found to have had significant relief of symptoms. The authors thought that a tumor dose of up to 7000 rad can result in significant benefit for those patients in whom the tumor is incompletely resected.

In an attempt to more clearly define the optimal dosage of irradiation required to control these tumors, a scatter diagram of control rates was constructed.[24] The patients were divided into a group whose tumors were destroyed or who were free of regrowth for a period of 5 years or longer and a group whose tumors persisted after treatment or in whom regrowth occurred, usually within a 2-year period. Tumor doses of less than 4000 rad were of little benefit in controlling the tumors. Doses of 8000 rad or more were found to be most likely to be successful. Eight of eleven patients were thought to have successful treatment with doses in this range. An increasing local control rate is seen with increasing doses (Table 131-3). This particular analysis did not consider the size or location of the tumor. Certainly with doses of 7000 rad and higher, there is a significant risk of damaging normal tissues, and doses in this range make considerations of reirradiation very difficult. The risk of serious radiation sequelae limits the use of these doses to those anatomical regions which are not surrounded by vital structures, in particular the sacrococcygeal area.

Some promising results have been obtained with the use of proton beam irradiation in these tumors.[34] This series of ten patients included six with chordoma, three with chondrosarcoma, and one with a neurofibrosarcoma. The patients were treated with a combination of photons and 160 MeV proton beams. All tumors were located in the base of the skull and/or upper cervical spine region. The proton beam used in treating these patients allowed a higher dose to be given to a very specific area of the tumor volume. Therefore, the patient's tumor was localized very carefully in each case. Overall doses ranged from a dose equivalent to 6500

TABLE 131-3 Radical Radiotherapy of Chordoma*

Tumor Dose (rad)	Failure		Significant Palliation		Success	
	Number	Percentage	Number	Percentage	Number	Percentage
To 4,000	47	85	5	9	3	6
4,001–6,000	18	60	6	20	6	20
6,001–8,000	8	43	5	31	4	26
Over 8,000	2		1		8	80

*Dose-response rates in patients receiving radiotherapy for chordoma.
SOURCE: Pearlman and Friedman.[24] Reprinted with permission.

rad to as high as 7620 rad. In all ten patients, local control was achieved for follow-up periods of up to 6 years. One patient was thought to have a marginal failure because of an error in calculating the actual extent of disease. An additional advantage of the proton beam is that it allows for a fairly rapid falloff of the dose outside of the designated treatment volume, thus sparing much of the surrounding normal tissue.

The relative radioresistance of the chordoma, the increasing risk of complications at higher doses, and frequent presence of critical anatomical structures within the area of the tumor mass make therapeutic considerations in these patients quite difficult. Because of the slow-growing nature of the tumor, the response of the tumor to irradiation is often slow. Patients who present with pain or discomfort caused by their tumors may not have achieved much relief of their symptoms at the completion of treatments. However, over the next few weeks or months the patients may notice decreased pain, and an objective response in terms of tumor regression may be noted as well. This regression may continue for several months after the completion of treatment. Although irradiation in and of itself has not been shown to be a curative modality in these tumors, it often presents the possibility of substantial palliation and either regression or stabilization of the tumor. Most studies indicate that the most effective treatment approach in these tumors is surgical resection of as much tumor as is reasonably possible, with postoperative irradiation in doses which approach normal tissue tolerance.

Primary Lymphomas of the Brain

A malignant lymphoma originating in the central nervous system and without systemic manifestations is an uncommon condition which comprises only 1 to 2 percent of all of the extranodal lymphomas. However, with the recent increase in the use of immunosuppressive drugs for organ transplantation, the incidence of primary CNS lymphoma appears to be increasing.

Primary CNS lymphoma has traditionally had a poor response to treatment. The median survival in these patients has generally been from 4 to 6 months. These lesions have been called by a number of different names, including reticulum cell sarcoma, microglioma, and reticuloendothelial sarcoma. Pathological studies have documented that the histological findings of primary CNS lymphoma are similar to those of malignant lymphomas that originate in the reticuloendothelial system of other organs. More recently, CNS lymphomas have been designated according to the more common terminology utilized for the non-Hodgkin's lymphomas which arise outside the central nervous system.

A report documenting 24 histologically confirmed cases of intracranial lymphoma indicates that there may be a time-dose factor involved in controlling this disease.[27] Twenty-one of these twenty-four patients primarily had involvement of intra-axial structures, and three were found to have extradural and meningeal involvement. Every patient in the study had surgical exploration. Some patients underwent subtotal tumor removal, while others had only biopsy. Four patients died postoperatively and did not receive radiother-

apy. The other 20 patients received postoperative irradiation and 18 of these patients were available for evaluation. In this patient group, there were six who received a tumor dose of less than 3000 rad. The tumor was not controlled locally in any of these patients. The 12 remaining patients received tumor doses in excess of 3000 rad, and local control was achieved in 50 percent. The authors thought that failure to control the disease could have been caused by inadequate tumor dose or by failure to recognize the actual extent of disease. In addition, the presence of multiple involved sites within the central nervous system sometimes led to use of an inadequate field size. Thus, it was concluded that whole brain irradiation would be the most appropriate treatment and that a minimum dose of 3500 rad delivered with conventional fractionation was indicated.

Six patients who were treated for intracranial disease subsequently developed lymphoma involving the spinal canal. Although this suggests that primary irradiation to the entire neuraxis might be indicated, other studies have shown that spinal cord involvement from primary intracranial lymphoma is not a common occurrence, and most radiation oncologists would not recommend neuraxis irradiation. However, in situations where symptoms or abnormal radiographic results indicate that disease involves the spinal canal, the indications for larger fields, possibly including the entire neuraxis, are more clear-cut.

Irradiation to the entire neuraxis has been performed for treatment of primary cerebral lymphomas.[26] Twelve patients with primary CNS lymphoma were studied. Four patients received neuraxis irradiation consisting of 4000 to 4500 rad to the whole brain and 3000 to 3300 rad to the spinal cord. All four patients who received neuraxis irradiation survived for more than 1 year. One patient had no evidence of disease at 3 years, one patient was alive with possible disease at 35 months, and two patients survived for 13 and 16 months. The patients who received whole neuraxis irradiation were thought to have primary lymphoma in an "unfavorable" condition, meaning that the disease was diffuse or multifocal, was located in the vital structures around the brain stem, or had positive CSF cytology.

Even in those patients who do not have a significant prolongation of survival after treatment with irradiation, the symptomatic response to treatment is often good and there is very little morbidity associated with treatment. In most of the reported cases, patients noted an improvement in both neurological symptoms and general physical status. It would thus appear that radiotherapy for primary CNS lymphoma is important not only as a possible modality for prolonging survival, but also for improving the quality of the patient's life.

Spinal Cord Tumors

Primary neoplasms of the spinal cord are relatively rare and there are few published reports involving large series of patients. Thus, the specific role of radiotherapy for the various intramedullary neoplasms is difficult to assess.

A retrospective review of 34 patients who received radiotherapy for primary spinal cord neoplasms indicates that postoperative irradiation is of benefit in many of these patients.[30] The initial diagnoses included 12 patients with ependymoma, 7 with astrocytoma, and 2 with chordoma. Of the 12 patients with ependymoma, 4 received only biopsies, 7 had incomplete resection, and 1 was thought by the surgeon to have had total resection of the tumor. With a minimum follow-up of 2.5 years, all patients with ependymoma were alive. One patient who was alive 16 years after treatment developed a severe neurological deficit and became paraplegic. Three of the seven patients with astrocytoma had subtotal resections and the other four had biopsy only. Four of these seven patients were alive and without evidence of disease at a follow-up time of 4 to 11 years.

It is difficult to delineate a dose-response curve for primary astrocytoma of the spinal cord.[18] In contrast, a dose-response relationship has been noted in patients with primary ependymoma of the spinal cord. This retrospective analysis converted the dose of irradiation and the time over which it was given into a factor termed the time, dose, and fractionation factor (TDF). By doing so, the investigators hoped to determine an optimum dosage for response of these tumors. In this patient population, local control was achieved in five of the seven patients who were treated with irradiation alone. In addition, local control was maintained in one patient who underwent subtotal resection plus irradiation. None of the patients in this study had complete removal of their astrocytoma at operation. Since the intramedullary astrocytomas did not exhibit any significant correlation of control and TDF, it must be assumed that they vary in their sensitivity to irradiation. It is important to remember that this study dealt with a fairly small series of patients. In the ependymoma group, a dose-response relationship was established. In seven of eight ependymoma patients who received irradiation after subtotal resection, tumor control was achieved. The actuarial 5-year survival rates were 100 percent for ependymoma and 58 percent for astrocytoma. At 10 years, actuarial survival figures for ependymoma and astrocytoma were 73 percent and 23 percent, respectively (Fig. 131-6). On the basis of the findings of this study, a dose of 4000 to 4500 rad given in fractions of 180 to 200 rad per treatment was recommended. The authors of this study also analyzed the functional results in the patient population. Most of the deficits that were present prior to surgery either increased or did not change postoperatively. In the 19 irradiated patients, there were 45 deficits present prior to the initiation of treatments. Thirty-four of these forty-five deficits resolved completely and eight of the deficits improved. The implication is that a minimal surgical procedure is indicated for histological confirmation of tumor type, followed by definitive irradiation. Others would argue that surgical removal of as much tumor as is functionally possible should be done and then postoperative irradiation should be given.

The use of neuraxis irradiation for primary ependymomas of the spinal cord is controversial. The question is difficult to answer because CSF cytological studies are generally not obtained in these patients. It appears that the incidence of intracranial recurrence is fairly low. Many radiation oncologists prefer to irradiate only the area of known disease, with a 2 to 3 cm margin around the tumor. Others recommend neuraxis irradiation with a dose of 3500 rad, followed by additional treatment to the area of known tumor. This seems a reasonable approach in patients in whom positive

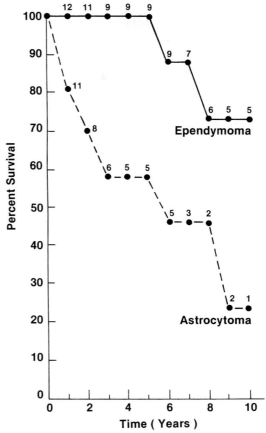

Figure 131-6 Actuarial survival rates for spinal cord ependymoma and astrocytoma. (From Kopelson et al.[18] Reprinted with permission.)

CSF cytology has been demonstrated. Of course, the presence of other abnormal neuroradiological findings during the initial evaluation of the patient with a primary spinal cord tumor would have an additional bearing on the decision to give neuraxis irradiation.

Primary tumors of the spinal cord are treated mainly through direct posterior portals, with the dose generally calculated at the spinal cord. The depth of different segments of the cord varies from 3 to 5 cm in most patients, and the particular segment being irradiated needs to be considered when calculating the depth at which the dose of irradiation is to be given. For the astrocytomas, most radiation oncologists would recommend tumor doses in the range of 4500 to 5000 rad. Many would recommend a similar dose for the ependymomas, but others think that ependymomas might be slightly more sensitive to irradiation, and would prefer a dose in the range of 4000 to 4500 rad. Both of these doses should be fairly well tolerated, and the risk of radiation myelitis at these doses should be minimal. However, if a large segment of the spinal cord is being treated or high daily doses are being utilized, the incidence of myelitis might be considerably higher. Reirradiation of these lesions after documented recurrence has been attempted on several occasions, but the number of patients is too small for meaningful analysis.

Metastatic Epidural Tumors

Metastatic disease involving the epidural space and causing neurological compromise is a fairly common problem. There has been some controversy regarding the optimum management of these patients, and certainly no single treatment approach is optimum for all patients. As the life expectancy of cancer patients increases and their clinical course becomes longer, the incidence of epidural metastases may increase as well. Indeed, metastatic disease is the most common neoplasm which occurs in the spinal canal.

Radiotherapy has been used in the management of metastatic epidural lesions for some time. It has been shown to be effective, resulting in improvement of significant neurological symptoms in one-third to one-half of the patients.[3] In addition, patients who are treated with external beam therapy usually receive significant relief of painful symptoms. There are some data to support the concept that patients with tumors which are more radioresponsive (e.g., lymphomas) have a higher rate of neurological improvement than those patients with tumors which are generally considered relatively radioresistant.

There are no firmly established data regarding the optimum radiation schedule to be used in this patient population. Comparable results have been obtained using various dose and fractionation schedules. Some radiation oncologists advocate using higher doses for the first three treatments, followed by continuation of therapy at more conventional fractionation for the remaining course of treatment. In general, most think that multiple fractions, resulting in a tumor dose of approximately 3000 rad, are more effective than a single high-dose treatment. A common schedule is to deliver 300 to 500 rad daily for 3 days, followed by continuation of treatment at reduced fractionation. The field should include the area of known extradural defect, with an adequate margin. Often, the field is extended to include other areas of bony involvement or other potential extradural defects.

Patients are often treated with dexamethasone concomitantly, and the question of radiotherapy causing edema has often been raised. In experimental models, radiation induced edema has not been shown to be a problem, and, in fact, higher doses of radiation cause more tumor regression without the induction of significant edema.

The diagnosis of spinal cord compression in its early stages requires a high index of suspicion. Once the diagnosis has been made, treatment should be initiated immediately using a combination of steroids and external beam irradiation. In selected cases, laminectomy is done prior to the initiation of treatment, and most radiation oncologists would recommend giving postoperative irradiation when the patient has recovered sufficiently from the surgical procedure.

References

1. Aristizabal S, Caldwell WL, Avila J, Mayer EG: Relationship of time dose factors to tumor control and complications in the treatment of Cushing's disease by irradiation. Int J Radiat Oncol Biol Phys 2:47–54, 1977.

2. Berry MP, Jenkin RDT, Keen CW, Nair BD, Simpson WJ: Radiation treatment for medulloblastoma: A 21-year review. J Neurosurg 55:43–51, 1981.

3. Black P: Spinal metastasis: Current status and recommended guidelines for management. Neurosurgery 5:726–746, 1979.

4. Bouchard J: Radiation Therapy of Tumors and Diseases of the Nervous System. Philadelphia, Lea & Febiger, 1966.

5. Bouchard J, Peirce CB: Radiation therapy in the management of neoplasms of the central nervous system, with a special note in regard to children: Twenty years' experience, 1939–1958. AJR 84:610–628, 1960.

6. Chin HW, Hazel JJ, Kim TH, Webster JH: Oligodendrogliomas: I. A clinical study of cerebral oligodendrogliomas. Cancer 45:1458–1466, 1980.

7. Concannon JP, Kramer S, Berry R: The extent of intracranial gliomata at autopsy and its relationship to techniques used in radiation therapy of brain tumors. AJR 84:99–107, 1960.

8. Cumberlin RL, Luk KH, Wara WM, Sheline GE, Wilson CB: Medulloblastoma: Treatment results and effect on normal tissues. Cancer 43:1014–1020, 1979.

9. Danoff BF, Kramer S, Thompson N: The radiotherapeutic management of optic nerve gliomas in children. Int J Radiat Oncol Biol Phys 6:45–50, 1980.

10. De Schryver A, VandeKerckhove D, Debruyne G: Prolactinsecreting pituitary adenoma: Observations in irradiated patients. Acta Radiol Oncol Radiat Phys Biol 19:169–175, 1980.

11. Eastman RC, Gorden P, Roth J: Conventional supervoltage irradiation is an effective treatment for acromegaly. J Clin Endocrinol Metab 48:931–940, 1979.

12. Harwood AR, Simpson WJ: Radiation therapy of cerebral metastases: A randomized prospective clinical trial. Int J Radiat Oncol Biol Phys 2:1091–1094, 1977.

13. Higinbotham NL, Phillips RF, Farr HW, Hustu HO: Chordoma: Thirty-five-year study at Memorial Hospital. Cancer 20:1841–1850, 1967.

14. Jennings AS, Liddle GW, Orth DN: Results of treating childhood Cushing's disease with pituitary irradiation. N Engl J Med 297:958–962, 1977.

15. Kim TH, Chin HW, Pollan S, Hazel JH, Webster JH: Radiotherapy of primary brain stem tumors. Int J Radiat Oncol Biol Phys 6:51–57, 1980.

16. King DL, Chang CH, Pool JL: Radiotherapy in the management of meningiomas. Acta Radiol Oncol Radiat Phys Biol 5:26–33, 1966.

17. Kleinberg DL, Noel GL, Frantz AG: Galactorrhea: A study of 235 cases, including 48 with pituitary tumors. N Engl J Med 296:589–600, 1977.

18. Kopelson G, Linggood RM, Kleinman GM, Doucette J, Wang CC: Management of intramedullary spinal cord tumors. Radiology 135:473–479, 1980.

19. Kramer S, Hendrickson F, Zelen M. Schotz W: Therapeutic trials in the management of metastatic brain tumors by different time/dose fraction schemes of radiation therapy. Natl Cancer Inst Monogr 46:213–221, 1977.

20. Leibel SA, Sheline GE, Wara WM, Boldrey EB, Nielsen SL: The role of radiation therapy in the treatment of astrocytomas. Cancer 35:1551–1557, 1975.

21. Lichter AS, Wara WM, Sheline GE, Townsend JJ, Wilson CB: The treatment of craniopharyngiomas. Int J Radiat Oncol Biol Phys 2:675–683, 1977.

22. Marks JE, Adler SJ: A comparative study of ependymomas by site of origin. Int J Radiat Oncol Biol Phys 8:37–43, 1982.

23. McWhirter R: Radiation treatment of cerebral tumors. Proc R Soc Med 39:673–679, 1946.

24. Pearlman AW, Friedman M: Radical radiation therapy of chordoma. AJR 108:333–341, 1970.

25. Phillips TL, Sheline GE, Boldrey E: Therapeutic considera-

tions in tumors affecting the central nervous system: Ependymomas. Radiology 83:98–105, 1964.

26. Rampen FHJ, van Andel JG, Sizoo W, van Unnik JAM: Radiation therapy in primary non-Hodgkin's lymphomas of the CNS. Eur J Cancer 16:177–184, 1980.

27. Sagerman RH, Cassady JR, Chang CH: Radiation therapy for intracranial lymphoma. Radiology 88:552–554, 1967.

28. Salazar OM, Castro-Vita H, Bakos RS, Feldstein ML, Keller B, Rubin P: Radiation therapy for tumors of the pineal region. Int J Radiat Oncol Biol Phys 5:491–499, 1979.

29. Salazar OM, Rubin P, Feldstein ML, Pizzutiello R: High dose radiation therapy in the treatment of malignant gliomas: Final report. Int J Radiat Oncol Biol Phys 5:1733–1740, 1979.

30. Schwade JG, Wara WM, Sheline GE, Sorgen S, Wilson CB: Management of primary spinal cord tumors. Int J Radiat Oncol Biol Phys 4:389–393, 1978.

31. Shapiro WR, Posner JB, Ushio Y, Chernik NL, Young DF: Treatment of meningeal neoplasms. Cancer Treat Rep 61:733–743, 1977.

32. Sheline GE: Treatment of nonfunctioning chromophobe adenomas of the pituitary. AJR 120:553–561, 1974.

33. Sheline GE, Boldrey E, Karlsberg P, Phillips TL: Therapeutic considerations in tumors affecting the central nervous system: Oligodendrogliomas. Radiology 82:84–89, 1964.

34. Suit HD, Goitein M, Munzenrider J, Verhey L, Davis KR, Koehler A, Linggood R, Ojemann RG: Definitive radiation therapy for chordoma and chondrosarcoma of base of skull and cervical spine. J Neurosurg 56:377–385, 1982.

35. Walker MD, Alexander E Jr, Hunt WE, MacCarty CS, Mahaley MS Jr, Mealey J Jr, Norrell HA, Owens G, Ransohoff J, Wilson CB, Gehan EA, Strike TA: Evaluation of BCNU and/or radiotherapy in the treatment of anaplastic gliomas: A cooperative clinical trial. J Neurosurg 49:333–343, 1978.

36. Walker MD, Strike TA, Sheline GE: An analysis of dose-effect relationship in the radiotherapy of malignant gliomas. Int J Radiat Oncol Biol Phys 5:1725–1731, 1979.

37. Wara WM, Jenkin RDT, Evans A, Ertel I, Hittle R, Ortega J, Wilson CB, Hammond D: Tumors of the pineal and suprasellar region: Childrens Cancer Study Group treatment results 1960–1975. A report from Childrens Cancer Study Group. Cancer 43:698–701, 1979.

38. Wara WM, Sheline GE, Newman H, Townsend JJ, Boldrey EB: Radiation therapy of meningiomas. AJR 123:453–458, 1975.

39. Yamashita J, Handa H, Iwaki K, Abe M: Recurrence of intracranial meningiomas, with special reference to radiotherapy. Surg Neurol 14:33–40, 1980.

40. Yap HY, Yap BS, Rasmussen S, Levens ME, Hortobagyi GN, Blumenschein GR: Treatment for meningeal carcinomatosis in breast cancer. Cancer 50:219–222, 1982.

132

Heavy Particle Irradiation of Intracranial Lesions

Introduction

John H. Lawrence

Since 1935 there has been continuing interest in this laboratory in the investigation of the radiobiology, the health hazards, and the clinicotherapeutic applications of the dense tissue ionization produced by penetrating neutrons, high-energy penetrating charged particles such as protons and helium nuclei, and heavier particles such as carbon and neon.[1-3] Our early studies led to the use of neutrons in cancer therapy, based on the apparent greater effect of neutrons upon neoplastic tissue than upon normal tissue in mice (later explained by the so-called oxygen effect); neutron therapy is now being carried out at several other centers in the world. The present discussion will concern only positively charged particles.

Our first experience, beginning in the 1950s, involved the use of protons and alpha particles to suppress the function of or ablate the pituitary gland in patients with breast cancer. There are long-term results of particle irradiation in the treatment of hypophyseal tumors, particularly hormone-secreting tumors, where we have had experience extending over a period of more than 25 years.

References

1. Lawrence JH, Aebersold PC, Lawrence EO: Comparative effects of x-rays and neutrons on normal and tumor tissue. Proc Natl Acad Sci USA 22:543–557, 1936.

2. Lawrence JH, Aebersold PC, Lawrence EO: The comparative effects of neutrons and x-rays on normal and neoplastic tissue. Amer Assoc Adv Sci Occas Publ 4:215–219, 1937.

3. Lawrence JH, Lawrence EO: The biological action of neutron rays. Proc Natl Acad Sci USA 22:124–133, 1936.

Radiosurgery with Charged Particles: Physical Principles and Techniques

Cornelius A. Tobias

William Bragg discovered in 1912 that alpha particles emitted from natural radioactive substances and passed through condensed matter deposit more energy near the end of their ionization tracks than at their points of entry. The complete explanation of this property paved the way for important developments in nuclear physics. Thirty-four years later the Bragg ionization property became the basis of a suggestion by Robert Wilson that charged particles such as protons might be used in cancer therapy, where it is important to achieve good depth localization of the ionizing particles.[25]

In 1947, Ernest Lawrence completed construction of the first large synchrocyclotron at Berkeley, making available for the first time beams of nuclear particles with sufficient range to penetrate deep-seated structures in the human body. In the same year, biomedical investigations were started with high-energy protons, deuterons, and helium ions. In 1951, Tobias et al. demonstrated experimentally some of the physical properties of these particles and conducted initial biological experiments.[23] It became clear that the energetic light nuclei have excellent properties for producing clearly delineated lesions in mammalian tissues. Unlike electrons or electromagnetic radiations, which diffuse in tissues because of strong scattering collisions, the nuclei propagated essentially along straight trajectories. It was this property that allowed careful aiming and, eventually, stereotactic localization of the irradiated regions.

Proton beams were first used in clinical patients in 1955; the goal was treatment of metastatic breast carcinoma by particle hypophysectomy. Since that time there has been continuous progress in the methodology of applying particles in basic biomedical research, clinical diagnosis, and therapy (reviewed for example by Tobias[22]). Beginning in 1971, atomic nuclei of carbon, neon, silicon, and argon became available for research studies at the Berkeley Bevalac,[9]

and in 1982 the methods were extended to the acceleration of even the heaviest of the natural nuclei in the periodic table, uranium.[1] Proton irradiation is now being routinely administered at various centers: Harvard University,[12,16,21] the University of Uppsala,[13] and Moscow, Dubna, and Leningrad in the Soviet Union.[10] The applications of heavy particles are too numerous to describe here, but most of them have been reviewed recently.[7,17,18] Plans are in progress in Canada, West Germany, and Japan to build heavy ion accelerators similar to the one in Berkeley, with the chief aim of using heavy charged particles in basic biophysical research and in the diagnosis and therapy of cancer and other diseases.

Basic Physical Properties of Particle Beams

Accelerators usually produce highly monoenergetic and nearly parallel beams of particles. These beams produce a nearly straight path in tissue, and essentially all particles stop at the same depth, creating the so-called Bragg peak. However, the particles do deviate slightly from straight-line paths because of multiple elastic scattering, and their stopping points vary slightly because of straggling, a statistical variation in energy transfer.

The rate of energy transfer from particles to tissue is a function of the atomic number and the energy of the particles. Typical Bragg curves from beams now in use at Berkeley are shown in Fig. 132-1. The left side of this figure is the ionization curve of 225 MeV/u helium particles in water, which is nearly equivalent to that in soft tissue (u = atomic mass unit). This is the beam that has been used in our most

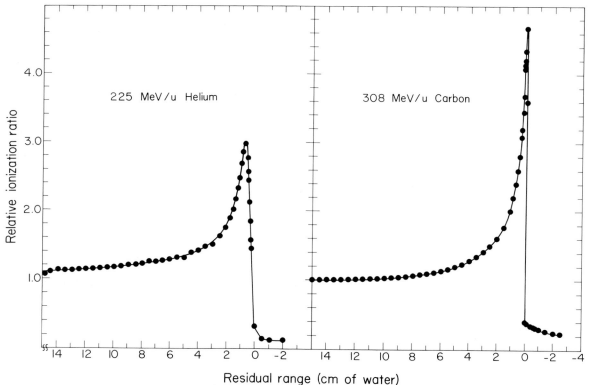

Figure 132-1 Typical Bragg ionization curves. (u = atomic mass unit.)

extensive clinical study, pituitary irradiation, which has gone on for more than twenty years. The right side of Fig. 132-1 shows the Bragg peak of a 308 MeV/u carbon beam from the Bevalac. This carbon beam has properties that make it suitable for heavy ion radiography and it is a candidate for future medical use in the production of highly localized lesions in brain and other body tissues.[2] The heavy particle beams also produce secondary particles of lower atomic and mass numbers through a process of nuclear fragmentation. The dose from fragmentation products acts as a background and extends beyond the peak. For carbon, the relative magnitude of the fragmentation dose is small, but it increases significantly for heavier particles.[3,14,19]

Classification of Particle Lesions

There are several simple methods of applying collimated particle beams to mammalian tissues.

Plateau Lesions

A collimated beam, usually not more than a few millimeters in width, is allowed to pass through the head; the particles stop beyond the head and so only ions produced in the flat part of the Bragg curve, called *plateau ions*, are of use. This method, sometimes called the "atomic knife," can produce sharply limited radiation fields. With the aid of diagnostic x-ray films the beam can be focused in any well-defined region; metal clips left in strategic locations by surgeons can also serve to guide the localization of the beam. A relatively small dose of a few hundred rad causes a transient increase in the permeability of the blood-brain barrier within the irradiated volume; there is no bleeding. At higher doses of possibly several thousand rad, local delayed radionecrosis occurs; the nerve tissue liquifies, glial reactions take place, and scar tissue develops. The scar tissue at the edge of the lesion usually occupies a narrower region than that which forms after surgically produced lesions. Perhaps the most interesting use of this technique so far has been in the cutting of the corpus callosum in cats using a knife-edged beam of helium ions.[8] This was accomplished with no bleeding, and the thalamus, hypothalamus, pituitary, and brain stem were completely protected. When the lesion was wider than 0.4 cm, all neural communication between the two sides of the cerebrum ceased after an appropriate time interval.

Laminar Lesions

Laminar lesions are radiolesions parallel to the surface of the brain. A strictly monoenergetic beam is passed into a specific area of the brain, sometimes after a bone flap is removed. Because radiation effects in brain appear to have a threshold, it is possible to obtain lesions only at the Bragg peak. The sharpness of the Bragg peak and its relative height compared to the plateau region are obviously related to the minimal size of the lesions that can be achieved. The first such lesions were obtained by Malis et al.;[15] Haymaker et al. described many of the properties of such lesions.[11] High-energy carbon beams are probably best suited to de-liver laminar lesions of a minimal size; the width of the lesion can be as little as one-sixtieth of the depth at which the lesion is made.

Focal Lesions

Using a multiport irradiation technique, a number of shaped beams may be passed through the same small region of the body. In this manner small focal neurological lesions can be produced at any location in the head that has well-defined coordinates. This is the technique that has been used in the Berkeley series of pituitary irradiations for the treatment of Cushing's disease and acromegaly, described in detail in this chapter. The pituitary gland, located at the geometrical center of the head, is a quite suitable target for such an approach.

The nominal dose given to the patient is the maximum dose (expressed in rad) at the geometric center of the pituitary. The reason for quoting the nominal dose is that it is convenient to measure: it is the sum total of beam doses passing through the external ion chamber integrator. Biologically, however, a more meaningful measure of dose is the rad dose at the periphery of the pituitary. Numerically, the rad dose is about 50 percent of the nominal dose. The effectiveness of the rad dose given is further modified because of cellular repair between dose installments or fractions. The manner in which a variety of beams impinge on the pituitary over the course of therapy and a three-dimensional dose distribution are shown in Fig. 132-2.

The isodose curves obtained with heavy charged particles are much better than the isodose curves obtained with conventional radiation, which usually cannot avoid sensitive structures adjacent to the pituitary. A typical dose distribution used for an acromegalic patient treated at Berkeley is shown in Fig. 132-3.

Histopathological observations from early pituitary patients who received helium therapy for metastatic mammary carcinoma confirmed that more than 95 percent of the pituitary cells can be eradicated with nominal doses of 18,000 to 22,000 rad delivered over a 2 or 3 week period. Connective tissue replaces the pituitary cells after several months. At lesser doses, it appeared that the magnitude of the histological effects depended on the dose at the periphery of the pituitary gland, where viable, hormone-secreting cells were found. Surviving pituitary cells tended to migrate to the periphery, where the blood supply was best.

The fractionation techniques used often complicate the evaluation of appropriate dose levels. Strandqvist suggested that in a fractionated irradiation scheme, the effective dose D can be expressed as: $D = d\,(T/t)^s$, where d is the dose in each fraction, T is the total number of treatments, and t is the number of days it takes to deliver the entire therapeutic sequence.[20] The exponent s is determined empirically; it is a measure of the repair occurring between dose installments and it is always smaller than unity. For skin, Strandqvist found s to be equal to 0.22, whereas Du Sault later determined s to be equal to 0.27.[6] For humans, where large volumes of the brain were exposed to x-rays in a total of 17 patients, and for rabbits, Linfoot[13a] used a value of 0.27 for s.

Figure 132-4 is a Strandqvist plot of some of the actual

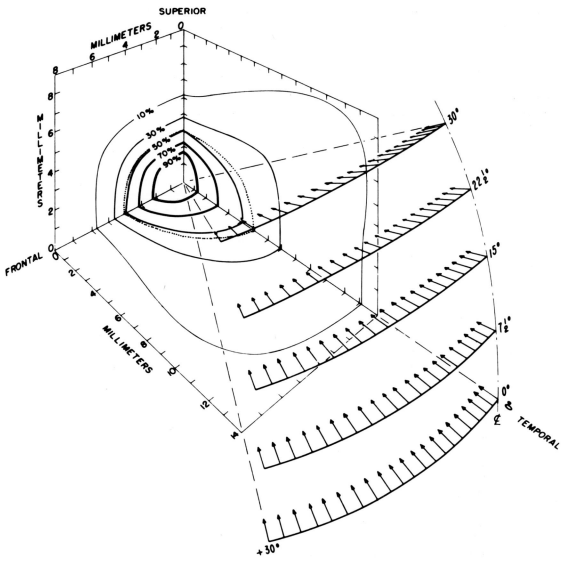

Figure 132-2 An isodose curve for one octant of a radiation field for pituitary radiotherapy.

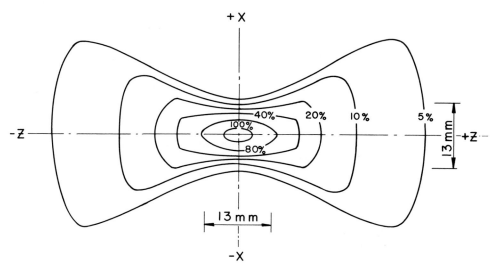

Figure 132-3 A typical isodose curve (lateral plane) for the treatment of an acromegalic patient.

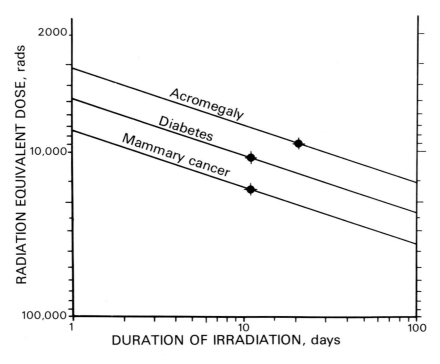

Figure 132-4 A Strandqvist plot of some of the dose schemes used to treat acromegaly, diabetes, and mammary cancer.

dose schemes we used to treat diabetic patients and patients with mammary cancer. The center of the pituitary gland received fractionated doses that were equivalent in effect to a single dose of 4500 to 6500 rad (diabetes) or 8000 to 18,000 rad (mammary cancer). The local doses considered to be without demonstrable effects to the temporal lobe are 1500 rad in 12 days, corresponding to an 800-rad single dose, for patients with diabetes and vascular disease, and 2000 rad in 12 days, or about a 1100-rad single dose, for other patients who have normal vascular structures. These local temporal lobe doses can be calculated for a distance of 2.1 cm from the center of the pituitary. This is the point at which the temporal lobe dose is at its highest; the dose falls very rapidly with distance from the pituitary.

Focal Bragg Peak Lesions

Further depth-dose improvements are reached in focal irradiation if the Bragg peak of the beams is brought into or near the focal region (Fig. 132-5). This focal Bragg peak technique has been used for irradiation of some of the acromegaly patients at Harvard and at Berkeley; however, the proper use of this technique requires an exact knowledge of the stopping power of intervening tissues. For proton and helium beams, this is calculated on the basis of x-ray tomography and measurements of the stopping power of the beam passed through the head. These techniques need further improvement. The quantitative information on electron densities that can be obtained from x-ray tomography may contain errors because of x-ray hardness artifacts and because the x-ray techniques usually measure attenuation coefficients instead of electron-stopping power. There are also limitations to ordinary focal pituitary irradiation; the doses delivered to the cranial nerves and to the temporal lobes are

limiting. Furthermore, because of beam scattering, sometimes the ocular nerves and optic chiasm, lying only a few millimeters from the sella turcica, may get more irradiation than is desired.

The heavier ion beams, particularly carbon and neon, promise to be much more suitable for the delivery of focal Bragg peak irradiations, not only because of reduced scatter and the sharpness of their Bragg peaks, but also because it is possible to obtain beams of some of their radioactive isotopes.[4] When a carbon beam is passed through an absorber of modest thickness, some of the carbon 12 particles change into radioactive carbon 11. The carbon 11 particles can be collected in a beam separate from the parent carbon 12 beam. If irradiation is performed using carbon 11, then the particles first come to a stop in tissue and later decay, with a half-life of 21.5 minutes. Using a special gamma-ray camera, the stopping point of the beam can be located with an accuracy of about 0.1 cm while the irradiation is still in progress. For neon, the [19]Ne isotope is used, which has a half-life of a few seconds. The data obtained from the gamma-ray camera allow a continuous check on the correctness of the depth of the beam's stopping point and should lead to greatly increased accuracy in the delivery of stereotactic microfocal irradiation. Figure 132-6 is an artist's view of the way in which focal Bragg peak radiation might be administered in the future. A special gamma-ray camera has already been built for the purpose of imaging the location of radioactive beam particles in the body. We expect that within a few years the use of radioactive beams will become the treatment of choice in microfocal particle irradiation. It will be then possible to deliver greater doses to smaller structures in the brain than is feasible with protons or with helium, and the adjacent tissues will be better protected from radiation effects than at present.

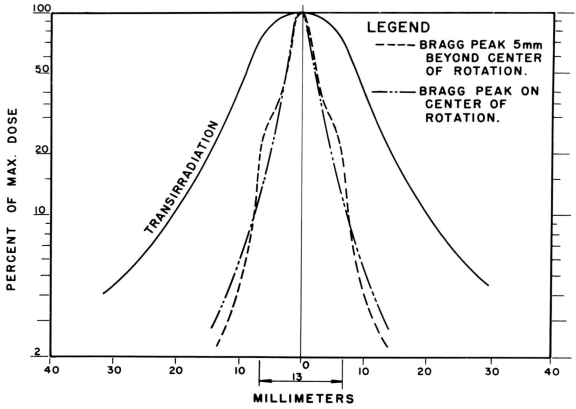

Figure 132-5   Dose distributions that may be reached using the focal Bragg peak technique with bilateral rotation.

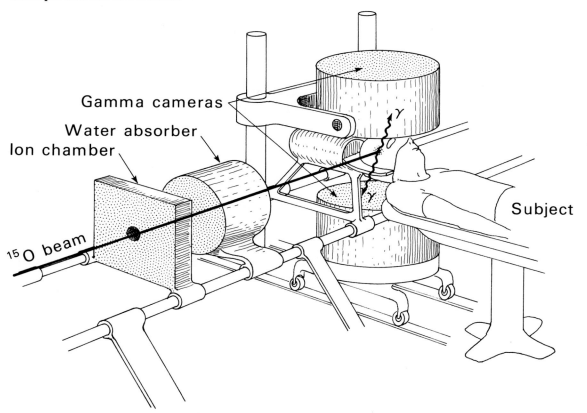

Figure 132-6   Artist's concept of a future method of administering focal Bragg peak radiation.

Localized Tumor Therapy

There is a substantial effort under way at Berkeley to use accelerated heavy ions for localized therapy of tumors. A complex rationale has been developed on the basis of the biological effectiveness of the particles, their ability to reduce the radiobiological oxygen effect, and the extent of intracellular repair and sensitivity changes during the cell division cycle.[24] A special computerized approach that has been created for therapy planning takes into account a variety of diagnostic information, including computed tomography.[5] The depth penetration properties of the particles are also considered in the therapy plan. A detailed study of heavy ion radiobiology indicates that silicon or argon ions might be more effective than lighter ions for localized cancer therapy.

References

1. Alonso JR, Avery RT, Elioff T, Force RJ, Grunder HA, Lancaster HD, Lofgren EF, Meneghetti JR, Selph FB, Stevenson RR, Yourd RB: Acceleration of uranium at the Bevalac. Science 217:1135–1137, 1982.
2. Benton EV, Henke RP, Tobias CA: Heavy-particle radiography. Science 182:474–476, l973.
3. Benton EV, Tobias CA, Blakely EA: Heavy ion fragmentation studies with plastic nuclear detectors. In press.
4. Chatterjee A, Alpen EL, Tobias CA, Llacer J, Alonso J: High energy beams of radioactive nuclei and their biomedical applications. Int J Radiat Oncol Biol Phys 7:503–507, 1981.
5. Chen GTY, Pitluck S: Treatment planning for heavy charged particle radiotherapy in Skarsgard LD (ed): *Pion and Heavy Ion Radiotherapy: Pre-Clinical and Clinical Studies.* Amsterdam, Elsevier Biomedical, 1983, pp 149–158.
6. Du Sault LA: The influence of the time factor on the dose-response curve. AJR 87:567–573, 1962.
7. Fowler JF: *Nuclear Particles in Cancer Treatment.* Bristol, England, Adam Hilger Ltd, 1981.
8. Gaffey CT, Montoya VJ: Split-brain cats prepared by radiosurgery. Int J Radiat Biol 24:229–242, 1973.
9. Ghiorso A, Grunder HA, Hartsough W, Lambertson G, Lofgren E, Lou K, Main R, Mobley R, Morgado R, Salsig W, Selph F: The Bevalac: An economical facility for very high energetic heavy particle research. IEEE Trans Nucl Sci NS-20:155, 1973 (Abstr).
10. Gol'din LL, Chuvilo IV, Ruderman AI: *Application of Charged Heavy Particles in Medicine.* Dubna, USSR, Joint Institute for Nuclear Research, Report JINR P 18-82-117, 1982.
11. Haymaker T: in Haley TJ, Snider RS (eds): *Response of the Nervous System to Ionizing Radiation: Second International Symposium Held at the University of California, Los Angeles.* Boston, Little, Brown, 1964.
12. Kjellberg RN, Kliman B: Lifetime effectiveness—A system of therapy for pituitary adenomas, emphasizing Bragg peak proton hypophysectomy, in Linfoot JA (ed): *Recent Advances in the Diagnosis and Treatment of Pituitary Tumors.* New York, Raven, 1979, pp 269–288.
13. Larsson B, Graffman S: Proton beams in biomedical research: Experience and plans in Uppsala, in *Maria Design Symposium. Vol II: Radiation Oncology Workshop.* Edmonton, Alberta, Medical Accelerator Research Institute in Alberta, 1980.
13a. Linfoot, JA (ed): *Recent Advances in the Diagnoses and Treatment of Pituitary Tumors.* New York, Raven, 1979.
14. Llacer J: Characterization of fragments in heavy ion beams with a simple semi-conduction telescope. In press.
15. Malis I, Loevinger R, Kruger L, Rose JE: Production of laminar lesions in the cerebral cortex by heavy ionizing particles. Science 126:302–303, 1957.
16. Munzenrider JE: Proton therapy at Harvard, in Skarsgard LD (ed): *Pion and Heavy Ion Radiotherapy: Pre-Clinical and Clinical Studies.* Amsterdam, Elsevier Biomedical, 1983, pp 363–372.
17. Pirruccello MC, Tobias CA (eds): *Biological and Medical Research with Accelerated Heavy Ions at the Bevalac, 1977–1980.* Berkeley, Ca., Lawrence Berkeley Laboratory Report LBL-11220, 1980.
18. Raju MR: *Heavy Particle Radiotherapy.* New York, Academic Press, 1980.
19. Schimmerling W, Benton EV, Hildebrand DJ, Henke RP, Heinrich W, Tobias CA: Experimental heavy particle physics: A. Nuclear interactions and radiation dosimetry, in Pirruccello MC, Tobias CA (eds): *Biological and Medical Research with Accelerated Heavy Ions at the Bevalac, 1977–1980.* Berkeley, Ca. Lawrence Berkeley Laboratory Report LBL-11220, 1980, pp 35–41.
20. Strandqvist M: Studien über die kumulative Wirkung der Röntgenstrahlen bei Fraktionierung: Erfahrungen aus dem Radiumhemmet an 280 haut-und Lippenkarzinomen. Acta Radiol [Suppl] (Stockh) 55, 1944.
21. Suit HD, Goitein M: Rationale for use of charged-particle and fast-neutron beams in radiation therapy, in Meyn R, Withers R (eds): *Radiation Biology and Cancer Research.* New York, Raven, 1980, pp 547–565.
22. Tobias CA: Pituitary radiation: Radiation physics and biology, in Linfoot JA (ed): *Recent Advances in the Diagnosis and Treatment of Pituitary Tumors.* New York, Raven, 1979, pp 221–243.
23. Tobias CA, Anger HO, Lawrence JH: Radiological use of high energy deuterons and alpha particles. AJR 67:1–27, 1952.
24. Tobias CA, Blakely EA, Alpen EL, Castro JR, Ainsworth EJ, Curtis SB, Ngo FQH, Rodriguez A, Roots RJ, Tenforde T, Yang TCH: Molecular and cellular radiobiology of heavy ions. Int J Radiat Oncol Biol Phys 8:2109–2120, 1982.
25. Wilson RR: Radiological use of fast protons. Radiology 47:487–491, 1946.

Treatment of Functioning Pituitary Tumors

John A. Linfoot
John H. Lawrence

Our first experience, beginning in 1957, involved the use of protons and alpha particles to suppress the function of or ablate the pituitary gland in the therapy of hypophyseal tumors, particularly hormone-secreting tumors. This work has been reported over the years in considerable metabolic and clinical detail on a large series of patients with acromegaly.

In a recent compendium, a wide spectrum of experts discussed the many advances in the diagnosis and treatment of various hypophyseal tumors.[11] Treatment modalities discussed included surgery (trans-sphenoidal and transfrontal), heavy particle irradiation,[9] conventional irradiation (x-rays or gamma rays), the implantation of radioactive seeds, cryosurgery, and thermocautery.

Since 1957, alpha particles (helium ions) have been used to suppress pituitary function in 807 patients with a variety of neoplastic and metabolic disorders, including mammary carcinoma,[19] diabetes complicated by retinopathy, and functioning and nonfunctioning pituitary tumors.[10,13,15,16] This review presents our experience in the treatment of 314 acromegalic patients with macro- or microadenomas, using alpha particle pituitary irradiation (APPI). The duration of follow-up in these patients ranges from 4 to more than 20 years, with the majority of patients having been followed for 10 years or more.

Radiotherapeutic Technique

A system was developed for pituitary irradiation using a projected physical dose system with a geometric delivery that limits the volume of extrasellar tissue irradiated by the particle beam.[19] A beam is shaped to fit the contour of the sella turcica, and, with multiport exposure with a sequential pendulum motion, a dose distribution is achieved that maximizes the particle beam dose at the center of the pituitary while protecting the basal structures, e.g., the optic chiasm, brain stem, and hypothalamus. In most of the patients the beam is passed through the head; this is referred to as the plateau or "through-and-through" technique. The use of the Bragg peak for selected patients with large tumors was limited, although this method has been used extensively by other investigators.[8] Therapy is administered in four treatments over a 4- to 5-day period. The patients are individually fitted with bivalved head holders which ensure that the head is rigidly fixed to the adjustable treatment table; no more than 1 mm of movement is permitted within the head holder. A brass collimating aperture is selected and fitted according to the size and configuration of the tumor. With the aid of diagnostic x-rays, desired alignment is achieved and the treatment plan is programmed on a computer. The specially designed treatment table allows the head and trunk to be independently rotated during therapy. The high-energy particles have sufficient energy to penetrate the entire thickness of the skull. The skin dose and the dose to the peripheral portions of the brain are minimal, and no epilation occurs. The optic chiasm, hypothalamus, temporal lobes, and outer portions of the sphenoid sinus receive less than 10 percent of the dose received by the central pituitary.

Patient Selection Criteria

Criteria for the selection of patients for alpha particle pituitary irradiation included

1. Presence of a pituitary tumor confirmed by neuroradiological or histological examination
2. Demonstrated pituitary hypersecretion with detectable endocrine or metabolic effect
3. Absent history of prior therapeutic irradiation to the pituitary or parasellar structures
4. Absence of major suprasellar extension
5. CSF growth hormone level under 1.5 ng/ml in patients with pituitary gigantism or acromegaly[14]
6. Pituitary size under 2.5 cm
7. Clearly defined radiological tumor landmarks in the presence of extensive sphenoid extension

8. Adequate localization of the optic chiasm and residual tumor mass in postsurgical patients

Using these criteria, pituitary tumor therapy has been achieved with a high degree of success and a low amount of morbidity.

The invasive grade III and IV tumors were common in the series and were usually associated with marked extension into the sphenoid as well as indeterminate lateral extension into the cavernous sinus.

Goals of Treatment

Four primary goals of APPI are

1. Control of tumor growth
2. Control of hormonal hypersecretion
3. Acceptable hormonal side effects
4. No CNS side effects

APPI has been suitable as a primary treatment in the majority of referred patients. In recent years many patients have been referred following transfrontal or trans-sphenoidal surgery because of recurrence or partial or incomplete tumor removal, thus permitting a comparison of the more recent combined therapy and the prior experience with de novo treatment. Combined therapy is desirable in many patients with invasive tumors. Inability to appreciate early invasion of the dura, and existence of multiple microadenomas and adenomatous hyperplasia are causes of treatment failure with trans-sphenoidal hypophysectomy.[4,17] In the case of large tumors, the inability to visualize and excise pockets of invasive tumor, with resulting inadequate control of hormonal hypersecretion and successful control of tumor regrowth, is a therapeutic limitation for all surgical approaches. Mass control is achieved with conventional radiotherapy, but control of hormonal hypersecretion is often limited.[18]

Acromegaly

A total of 314 patients with acromegaly were treated with APPI. The analyses are based upon those patients having pre- and post-treatment growth hormone studies (299 patients). Figure 132-7 shows the fall in the average fasting growth hormone level, determined on two or three consecutive mornings, of patients treated with APPI. The decrease in plasma growth hormone level has been associated with striking clinical and metabolic improvement (e.g., improved glucose tolerance, loss of insulin resistance, and fall in elevated serum phosphorus levels), and is frequently seen within the first year even before the growth hormone levels fall to under 10 ng/ml. More striking improvement is observed when the growth hormone level falls to 5 to 10 ng/ml. The rate of this fall in patients treated surgically prior to APPI was slower but parallelled that of the de novo group. Growth hormone levels fell to 5 ng/ml in 30 percent of the patients within 2 years, in 68 percent within 6 years, and in 95 percent within 8 years.

In order to evaluate the influence of tumor size, the acro-

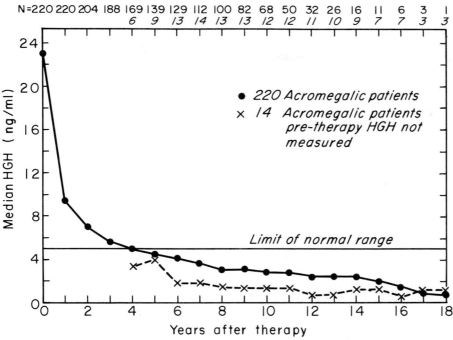

Figure 132-7 Changes in plasma growth hormone level in 234 patients with acromegaly who have been re-evaluated one or more years after completion of heavy particle pituitary irradiation (HPPI). At the top of the graph are the numbers of individuals used in calculating the median for each time interval. Fourteen patients did not have pretreatment growth hormone determinations by radioimmunoassay, but their growth hormone levels determined 4 to 18 years after treatment are consistent with those of the other 220 patients. These data are for patients who had HPPI only. Excluded were 63 patients (20.1 percent of the entire group) who had undergone prior surgical procedures on the pituitary, and 5 patients (1.6 percent) whose pretreatment growth hormone levels were less than 5 ng/ml. The 20 patients who subsequently underwent a second pituitary procedure (surgical operation or irradiation) were included until the time of the second procedure.

megalic patients were categorized into four groups according to sellar volume. Patients in group I had microadenomas; group II included patients with grades II through IV tumors. In spite of progressively increasing mean growth hormone levels with increasing sellar size, there was a great deal of overlap of basal hormone levels in patients with grades II–IV size tumors.

Patients with microadenoma responded extremely well. Invasive tumors (grades III and IV) present difficult therapeutic geometry for heavy particle therapy and have a less favorable prognosis. Similar findings have been seen in patients who had trans-sphenoidal surgery. Combined use of surgery and APPI is probably the optimal therapy in these difficult cases.

Relapse

Relapses or failures are defined as those patients who have failed to show clinical improvement or a fall of growth hormone levels to 10 ng/ml or less. Less than 10 percent of the patients treated with helium nuclei as the primary treatment have required subsequent surgery (Figs. 132-8, 132-9).

Recently, trans-sphenoidal microsurgery has been em-

ployed by a large number of neurosurgeons, with impressive success.[2,6,20,21] In Boston, Kjellberg and Kliman[7] and in Russia, Goldin et al.[5] have been using protons in the therapy of pituitary tumors. Centers in France, Canada, Great Britain, Germany, Japan, Sweden, and the United States are planning to use or are currently using pions or well-collimated photons for intracranial tumors. However, it will be several years before the investigations of any of these surgical or radiotherapeutic methods will have a large enough series with long enough follow-up to be compared or analyzed with the series reported here.

Relapse after alpha particle therapy was usually the result of failure to appreciate the presence of extrasellar extension. Through retrospective analysis, four major reasons for what are referred to as "geometric misses" have been identified.

1. Prior to hypocycloidal polytomography during pneumoencephalography (PEG) and the use of CSF growth hormone measurements to confirm the presence of suprasellar extension, failure to appreciate these extensions accounted for some of the relapses occurring early in our series.
2. Intrasphenoidal extension accounted for 50 percent of the relapses.
3. Mild posteroinferior extension was not considered signif-

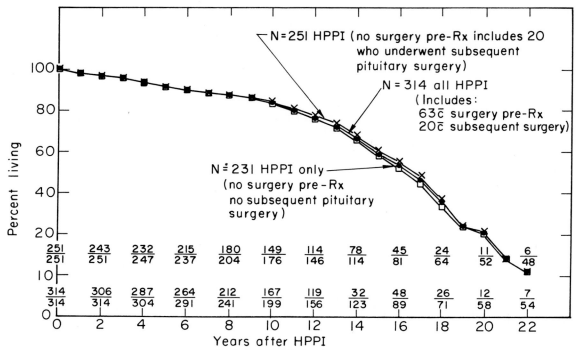

Figure 132-8 Survival of 314 acromegalic patients treated with heavy particle pituitary irradiation (HPPI), with 93 percent follow-up (1958–1978).

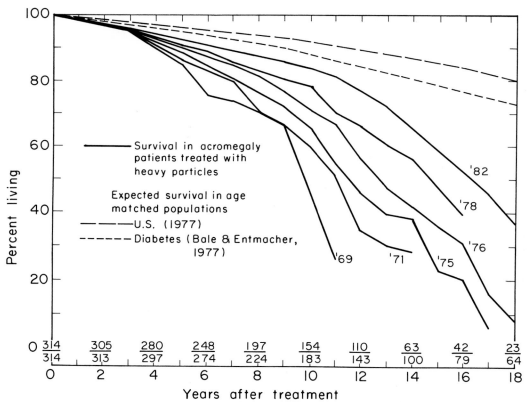

Figure 132-9 Survival of 314 acromegalic patients treated with heavy particle pituitary irradiation (HPPI). Since the majority of the patients are alive, the survival curves will continue to approach the curves of the age- and sex-matched diabetic population and general population.

icant in the treatment of the tumor but in retrospect accounted for some of the relapses in our series of patients.

4. Prior to the advent of newer generation CT scanners, lateral extension into the cavernous sinus was difficult to detect in the majority of cases.

Endocrine Effects

Of the patients who were analyzed, 233 had received APPI as sole or de novo treatment and 65 patients had received APPI following surgical treatment. Adrenal replacement data are shown in Table 132-1. One hundred fifty (65 percent) of the de novo patients, treated only with APPI, are currently on no adrenal replacement; three patients (1 percent) were on adrenal steroids prior to treatment; and eighty patients (34 percent) were placed on adrenal steroids after irradiation. Of the patients who had surgery prior to APPI, 29 percent are on no adrenal replacement; 39 percent were on replacement prior to APPI; and 34 percent required replacement after APPI.

Similar data were observed for thyroid replacement (Table 132-2). Of the de novo patients 61 percent are on no thyroid replacement; 6 percent were on thyroid replacement prior to APPI; and 33 percent are on thyroid replacement after APPI. In the surgical group, 20 patients (31 percent) are on no replacement; 27 patients (41 percent) were on thyroid replacement after surgery; and 18 patients (28 percent) were given thyroid replacement after the combined treatments.

Gonadal steroid replacement (Table 132-3) with estrogen or testosterone is perhaps somewhat less reliable as an estimate of gonadotropin deficiency, since many of the older patients may not be given gonadal steroids in spite of some degree of hypogonadism. Of the de novo patients, 73 percent are on no gonadal steroid replacement; 2 percent were on gonadal steroids before treatment; and 25 percent are on replacement after APPI. Of the patients who had prior surgery, 49 percent are on no replacement; 22 percent were on gonadal steroids prior to APPI; and 29 percent are on replacement after combined treatment.

Location of the extrasellar extension in patients who had geometric misses has assisted trans-sphenoidal microsur-

gery. Patients with persistent tumor activity have been successfully managed by either a trans-sphenoidal or a transcranial subfrontal operation. In a limited number of patients with invasive tumors who were treated prospectively with combined therapy, i.e., trans-sphenoidal surgery followed by APPI, complete normalization of growth hormone levels was achieved.

Complications of Alpha Particle Therapy in Acromegaly

Complications other than endocrine complications have been largely limited to those patients who received previous unsuccessful photon therapy; two of seven patients had partial field cuts which fortunately did not impair visual acuity and were asymptomatic. Three patients developed unilateral extraocular motor nerve (usually third nerve) lesions, which usually cleared and were relatively asymptomatic. Three of these patients developed temporal lobe epilepsy due to focal radiation necrosis of the temporal lobes; this was easily controlled with anticonvulsant therapy. As a result of these early complications, patients who had received prior photon therapy have not been accepted for treatment since 1961.

TABLE 132-1 Replacement Therapy in Acromegaly: Adrenal Replacement

Adrenal Replacement	Percentage of Patients
APPI* primary treatment	
No replacement	65
"F" prior to APPI	1
"F" after APPI†	34
Total	100
Surgery prior to APPI	
No replacement	29
"F" prior to APPI	37
"F" after APPI‡	34
Total	100

*APPI = Alpha particle pituitary irradiation.
†Replacement time average 4.3 years (range 0.2 to 12 years).
‡Replacement time average 3.0 years (range 0.2 to 14.7 years).

TABLE 132-2 Replacement Therapy in Acromegaly: Thyroid Replacement

Thyroid Replacement	Percentage of Patients
APPI* primary treatment	
No replacement	61
T_4 prior to APPI	6
T_4 after APPI†	33
Total	100
Surgery prior to APPI	
No replacement	31
T_4 prior to APPI	41
T_4 after APPI‡	28
Total	100

*APPI = Alpha particle pituitary irradiation.
†Replacement time average 3.9 years (range 0.2 to 11.3 years).
‡Replacement time average 3.5 years (range 0.7 to 15.4 years).

TABLE 132-3 Replacement Therapy in Acromegaly: Gonadal Replacement

Gonadal Replacement	Percentage of Patients
APPI* primary treatment	
No replacement	73
E/T prior to APPI	2
E/T after APPI†	25
Total	100
Surgery prior to APPI	
No replacement	49
E/T prior to APPI	22
E/T after APPI‡	29
Total	100

*APPI = Alpha particle pituitary irradiation; E = estrogen; T = testosterone.
†Replacement time average 4.1 years (range 0.2 to 12.0 years).
‡Replacement time average 2.5 years (range 0.9 to 10.9 years).

A second group of patients with complications are those who were initially treated with Bragg peak therapy. One of eight patients developed small field cuts immediately following treatment which subsequently cleared. Two patients had transient unilateral third nerve lesions which cleared, and one patient developed temporal lobe epilepsy that is controlled by anticonvulsant medication.

Of the 308 patients who were treated by the through-and-through technique, only two patients, who were treated prior to 1961, received higher doses of radiation than are currently used, and both developed temporal lobe symptoms. The overall incidence of CNS complications in 298 acromegalic patients is 4 percent. This complication rate is less than that described for photon therapy; however, lower total doses and lower doses per fraction are now employed.[1,12]

Survival of acromegalic patients treated with alpha particle irradiation was compared with that of an age- and sex-matched set from a diabetic and general population. Figures 132-8 and 132-9 show the increasing survival with the passage of time. Most of the patients are still alive, hence percent survival will increase with the passage of time. There have been 48 deaths in our acromegalic series, the major cause being cardiovascular disease (Table 132-4). The life expectancy of the acromegalic patients has been improved with APPI, which is free of operative morbidity and has caused minimal CNS morbidity and a significant but acceptable incidence of hypopituitarism (Tables 132-2 to 132-4).

In the primary treatment of acromegaly, patients with grade I and grade II tumors appear to do as well as patients who have had trans-sphenoidal operations. The response following APPI is delayed, although more rapid than that seen following photon therapy. The incidence of hypopituitarism is greater than after trans-sphenoidal surgery and probably less than after photon therapy because of the lack of any hypothalamic irradiation with APPI. The response to treatment in grade III and IV lesions is further delayed, but ultimate normalization of growth hormone level as well as tumor control can be achieved if the extent of tumor invasion is fully appreciated. Although the incidence of partial or total hypopituitarism is additive, the combined use of trans-sphenoidal surgery with clear definition of the tumor mass and confirmation of the presence of tumor invasion, followed by APPI, appears to be the optimal approach for grade III and IV lesions.

TABLE 132-4 Cause of Death in Acromegalic Patients Treated with Alpha Particle Pituitary Irradiation

Cause of Death	Number of Patients	Survival Time After Therapy
Cardiovascular or cerebrovascular disease	27	0.5–21.8
Systemic histoplasmosis	1	3.8
Acute myelogenous leukemia	1	4.1
Drug overdose	2	1.6, 4.0
Suicide	1	0.6
Meningioma	1	10.8
Bleeding duodenal ulcer	1	0.2
After surgery	4	2.8–5.8
During surgery	1	3.2
Acute renal failure	1	11.1
Metastatic cancer (breast, lung)	4	0.4–22.9
CNS (exact cause unknown)	1	16.3
Organic brain syndrome★	1	6.6
Accidental (choking, vehicular accident)	2	2.9, 11.0
Total	48	

★As previously reported, this patient was lost to follow-up; at another clinic, he was inadvertently given a second series of pituitary photon irradiation.

The availability of new generation CT scanners should substantially improve treatment planning and further improve precise localization of radiation to the desired tumor volume. Such treatment plans should considerably improve the results of treatment while substantially reducing the incidence of hypopituitarism.

With the improved definition of tumor masses and the ability to collimate charged particle beams accurately, localized tumor destruction using a highly focused, stereotactically delivered microbeam of protons or helium ions, or of heavier ions such as carbon, may eventually be the optimal method for many cases in which selective microadenoma destruction is desired.[3]

Table 132-5 shows the age and sex distributions of patients with acromegaly treated with heavy particle pituitary irradiation; and Table 132-6 summarizes the survival times of all patients with pituitary tumors treated by us.

TABLE 132-5 Age and Sex Distribution of Patients with Acromegaly Treated with Heavy Particle Pituitary Irradiation★

Patients		Age (years)				Duration (years)	
		At Time of Heavy Particle Therapy		At Time of Onset of Symptoms and Signs		At Time of Heavy Particle Therapy	
Sex	Number	Median	(Range)	Median	(Range)	Median	(Range)
Male	191	40.2	(15–69)	31.1	(13–64)	7.6	(1–40)
Female	121	48.3	(15–68)	36.8	(13–63)	9.0	(1–29)
Total	312	42.6	(15–69)	34.5	(13–64)	8.1	(1–40)

★This table illustrates the fact that acromegaly occurs more commonly in males, and that there is usually a long delay before acromegalic patients are referred for treatment.

TABLE 132-6 Survival of Patients with Pituitary Tumors Treated with Heavy Particle Pituitary Irradiation, Feb. 1958–Oct. 1979

Condition	Treated Patients			Survival After Treatment (years)											
	Total	Living	Dead	1 year		3 years		5 years		10 years		15 years		20 years	
				Live	At Risk	Live	At Risk	Live	At Risk	Live	At Risk	Live	At Risk	Live	At Risk
Acromegaly	314	275	39	309	314	297	307	268	290	152	179	50	83	11	49
Cushing's disease	80	76	4	79	80	74	76	51	53	20	23	9	13	1	5
Nelson's syndrome	17	16	1	17	17	17	17	12	13	6	7	3	4	1	2
Chromophobe adenoma	34	27	7	34	34	31	34	27	32	14	20	7	14	2	9
Prolactinoma	22	22	0	22	22	22	22	15	15	2	2	1	1	—	—
Total	467	416	51	461	467	441	456	373	403	194	231	70	115	15	65

References

1. Aristizabal S, Caldwell WL, Avila J: The relationship of time-dose fractionation factors to complications in the treatment of pituitary tumors by irradiation. Int J Radiat Oncol Biol Phys 2:667–673, 1977.

2. Baskin DS, Boggan JE, Wilson CB: Transsphenoidal microsurgical removal of growth hormone–secreting pituitary adenomas: A review of 137 cases. Neurosurg 56:634–641, 1982.

3. Chatterjee A, Alpen EL, Tobias CA, Llacer J, Alonso J: High energy beams of radioactive nuclei and their biomedical applications. Int J Radiat Oncol Biol Phys 7:503–507, 1981.

4. Ganguly A, Stanchfield JB, Roberts TS, West CD, Tyler FH: Cushing's syndrome in a patient with an empty sella turcica and a microadenoma of the adenohypophysis. Am J Med 60:306–309, 1976.

5. Goldin LL, Chuvilo IV, Ruderman AI: *Application of Charged Heavy Particles in Medicine.* Dubna, USSR, Joint Institute for Nuclear Research, Report JINR P 18-82-117, 1982.

6. Hardy J, Somma M, Vezina JL: Treatment of acromegaly: Radiation or surgery? in Morely TP (ed): *Current Controversies in Neurosurgery.* Philadelphia, WB Saunders, 1976, pp 377–391.

7. Kjellberg RN, Kliman B: Radiosurgery therapy for pituitary adenoma, Post KD, Jackson IMD, Reichlin S (eds): in *The Pituitary Adenoma.* New York, Plenum, 1980, pp 459–478.

8. Kjellberg RN, Sweet WH, Preston WM, Koehler AM: The Bragg peak of a proton beam in intracranial therapy of tumors. Trans Am Neurol Assoc 87:216–218, 1962.

9. Lawrence JH: History of pituitary therapy at Donner laboratory, in Linfoot JA (ed): *Recent Advances in the Diagnosis and Treatment of Pituitary Tumors.* New York, Raven, 1979, pp 1–3.

10. Lawrence JH, Tobias CA, Linfoot JA, Born JL, Lyman JT, Chong CY, Manougian E, Wei WC: Successful treatment of acromegaly: Metabolic and clinical studies in 145 patients. J Clin Endocrinol Metab 31:180–198, 1970.

11. Linfoot JA (ed): *Recent Advances in the Diagnosis and Treatment of Pituitary Tumors.* New York, Raven, 1979.

12. Linfoot JA: Alpha particles *versus* conventional radiotherapy to the pituitary region: A comparison of risk-benefit. Clin Neurosurg 27:83–98, 1980.

13. Linfoot JA, Chong CY, Lawrence JH, Born JL, Tobias CA, Lyman J: Acromegaly, in Li CH (ed.): *Hormonal Proteins and Peptides,* New York, Academic Press, 1975 vol 3, pp 191–246.

14. Linfoot JA, Garcia JF, Wei W, Fink R, Sarin R, Born JL, Lawrence JH: Human growth hormone levels in cerebrospinal fluid. J Clin Endocrinol Metab 31:230–232, 1970.

15. Linfoot JA, Lawrence JH, Born JL, Tobias CA: The alpha particle or proton beam in radiosurgery of the pituitary gland for Cushing's disease. N Engl J Med 269:597–601, 1963.

16. Linfoot JA, Nakagawa JS, Wiedemann E, Lyman J, Chong C, Garcia J, Lawrence JH: Heavy particle therapy: Pituitary tumors. Bull Los Angeles Neurol Soc 42:175–189, 1977.

17. Lüdecke D, Kautzky R, Saeger W, Schrader D: Selective removal of hypersecreting pituitary adenomas. Acta Neurochir (Wien) 35:27–42, 1976.

18. Sheline GE: Role of conventional radiation therapy in the treatment of functional pituitary tumors, in Linfoot JA (ed): *Recent Advances in the Diagnosis and Treatment of Pituitary Tumors.* New York, Raven, 1979, pp 289–314.

19. Tobias CA, Lawrence JH, Born JL, McCombs RK, Roberts JE, Anger HO, Low-Beer BVA, Huggins CB: Pituitary irradiation with high energy proton beams: A preliminary report. Cancer Res 18:121, 1958.

20. Wilson CB, Tyrrell JB, Fitzgerald PA, Forsham PH: *Cushing's Disease: Surgical Management.* Chicago, Year Book, 1982.

21. Wilson CB, Tyrrell JB, Fitzgerald PA, Pitts LH: Cushing's disease and Nelson's syndrome. Clin Neurosurg 27:19–30, 1980.

Malignant Glioma and Other Tumors

Joseph R. Castro
William M. Saunders
George T. Chen
J. Michael Collier
Devron Char
Grant Gauger
Kay Woodruff
Sandra Zink

Malignant Glioma

Heavy charged particles offer significant potential advantages for treatment of malignant gliomas of the brain. Physical parameters of heavy charged particle beams offer the opportunity to conform the extended Bragg peak to the tumor target volume, with less delivery of dose to adjacent portions of the brain.[4] This physical advantage is increased by the higher level of biological effectiveness in the stopping region, where most of the heavy charged particles' high linear energy transfer (LET) occurs. Thus, the increased relative biological effectiveness (RBE) in this region represents the ratio of biologically effective dose delivered to the tumor relative to surrounding normal tissues. Use of lighter charged particles such as protons and helium ions offers physical advantages because of the sharp lateral and distal edges of the beam. However, the LET characteristic of these beams is not sufficient to distinguish them from low-LET megavoltage photon beams, at least so far as present radiobiological and clinical studies demonstrate. Heavier charged particles such as nuclei of atomic numbers 10 to 15 offer biological advantages over light particles—specifically, depressed oxygen effect in the region of the extended Bragg peak, diminished variations in sensitivity during different phases of the cell division cycle, depressed enzymatic repair mechanisms, greater-than-expected delays in cell division, and decreased protective effects of neighboring cells in organized systems.[6,9,10,12,13] Because of the greater amount of fragmentation and range straggling in the heavier beams, a significant (although reduced) dose distal to the stopping point of the heavy charged particle beam will be encountered. Nevertheless, compared to exponentially decaying ionizing radiation such as photons or neutrons, the dose-localization advantage lies with heavy charged particles, particularly when the beam is appropriately modified to maximize the biologically effective dose in the target volume relative to areas of normal brain. For tumors such as glioblastoma and anaplastic astrocytoma, the precise dose localization that is available with protons or helium is not required, since present methods of tumor localization are not accurate enough to avoid utilizing a significant volume of clinically uninvolved tissue (ordinarily 2 cm wide) as a margin so that the target volume includes possible microscopic extensions. Thus, use of heavy charged particles with atomic numbers between 10 and 15 is an attractive approach; these beams should retain significant biological potential and still have sufficient physical attributes to be of advantage in tumors likely to be encountered within the brain.[4]

The optimum method of using such heavy charged particle beams has not yet been developed. At present, preliminary studies have been done with lighter ions ranging from helium through neon, utilizing fixed-ridge filters to spread the beam and significant amounts of absorber to spread the beam to a clinically useful diameter. In the future, fragmentation effects may be diminished by alternative methods of beam spreading. Optimization of beam delivery will probably require development of three-dimensional beam scanning in order to best minimize dosage to adjacent normal tissues. While completion of such optimization is several years in the future, we have begun preliminary studies at the Lawrence Berkeley Laboratory, utilizing heavy particle beams in the treatment of anaplastic astrocytoma and glioblastoma of the brain.[1] We are mindful of the experience with neutron irradiation of such tumors and of the effects of neutrons upon normal brain.[3,7,8,14] While the neutron studies focus at present on searching for the optimal dose-time parameters, we intend to study the utilization of heavy charged particles for reduction of dose to normal brain. We will continue to search for improved fractionation schedules as well as optimized beam delivery. We are also interested in possible potentiation that might take place between split-dose delivery separated by less than 30 minutes in time; such split doses might effectively combine high-LET and low-LET irradiation in order to maximize their effect on a tumor while perhaps protecting normal tissues.[9]

Since 1975, 14 patients with primary malignant glioma of the brain have received part or all of their irradiation with neon ions. Six of these patients received boost therapy following photon irradiation, with a small group of eight patients receiving treatment entirely with neon ions. The RBE and dose selected in these early patients were conservative, and consequently the findings to date have not been different from previous results with low-LET megavoltage photon irradiation. The longest survival has been 18 months following therapy, with a mean survival of 8.3 months and a median of 6 months. Of the eight patients treated entirely with neon ions, six had tumor recurrence within 14 months after treatment. All of the patients who received partial treatment with neon ions to a reduced volume after photon irradiation have also failed. In the group treated fully with heavy particle irradiation, only two of eight patients remain alive with follow-up of less than 24 months. Of the six patients dead, five are known to have had persistent tumor. One patient died without evidence of persistent tumor but without clear data to indicate that brain damage by heavy charged particle irradiation was the cause of death. As this was a phase I study beginning with a conservative RBE value and gradually escalating dosage, failure because of tumor persistence is understandable.

As this study proceeds, further dose escalation will take place, with careful clinical and computed tomographic (CT) follow-up of these patients. We are particularly interested in the use of serial quantitative CT analysis to look for evidence of altered function in normal brain as well as to evaluate tumor status.[5] These studies will be augmented by positron emission tomography, to be accomplished at the Lawrence Berkeley Laboratory. The efficacy of neutron irradiation in destroying glioblastoma leads to the hope that heavy charged particles, which have biological potential similar to that of neutrons, can destroy the tumor equally well. The dose-localization advantage of heavy charged particles permits the possibility that optimization of beam delivery will allow the level of damage to normal brain structures to be lower than with neutrons, thus granting improved survival. As the tumor itself has a propensity to tumor-induced necrosis, destruction of the tumor may leave these patients with areas of persistant coagulative necrosis. Improved surgical techniques may be needed to deal with this problem if longer survival and an improved quality of life is to be found.

Other Tumors

One of the critical areas of radiation oncologic research is that of improving local and regional control of resistant tumors through delivery of more effective radiotherapy. Protons[11] and helium ions[2] possess attractive physical characteristics that allow for the maximum delivery of dose to the target volume, with sparing of adjacent normal tissues. There is little increase in relative biological effectiveness and the oxygen enhancement ratio for these beams is virtually the same as for low-LET x-ray therapy. Such beams are of value in the treatment of difficult tumors that lie close to the spinal cord and/or the base of the brain and cannot be completely resected surgically. Tumors such as chordoma, chondrosarcoma, malignant schwannoma, and melanoma of the uveal tract of the eye are among these. At the Lawrence Berkeley Laboratory, helium ions have been tried in a variety of such sites, where improved dose localization might constitute a possible advantage. From 1975 through 1981, 88 patients completed therapy for (1) selected tumors around the base of the skull and spinal cord and in the paranasal sinuses (26 patients), and (2) uveal melanomas (62 patients).

The preliminary data for the first patient group are given in Table 132-7. Since many had fairly low-grade malignancies, long-term follow-up is still needed in order to fully evaluate tumor control and complications. Our goal has been to deliver a minimum dose of 60 to 75 gray equivalents*, at 2.0 GyE per fraction in four fractions per week, while keeping the dose to the spinal cord, brain stem, or small volumes of the brain to below 50 GyE wherever possible. Because the precision of these techniques is gauged in millimeters rather than centimeters, this approach should generate new information concerning the morbidity of small volumes of the spinal cord or brain stem that receive doses higher than the levels usually accepted as safe.

---

*The gray equivalent is the product of the physical dose Gy (which equals 100 rad) and a relative biological effectiveness factor.

TABLE 132-7 Precision High-Dose Therapy with Heavy Charged Particles for Juxtaspinal or Base-of-Skull Tumors

Site of Tumor	Number of Patients		Tumor Dose, GyE	Survival (mos)	
	Treated	Local Control Achieved		Median	Range
Sacrum	6	4	70–75	20	(10–67)
Clivus	9	8	36–74	19	(3–60)
Base of skull, paranasal sinus	7	5	42–70	12	(5–66)
Juxtaspinal	4	4	36–70	7	(4–17)
Total	26	21 (81%)			

SOURCE: Lawrence Berkeley Laboratory.

References

1. Castro JR, Quivey JM, Lyman JT, Chen GTY, Phillips TL, Tobias CA, Alpen EL: Current status of clinical particle radiotherapy at Lawrence Berkeley Laboratory. Cancer 46:633–641, 1980.

2. Castro JR, Saunders WM, Tobias CA, Chen GTY, Curtis S, Lyman JT, Collier JM, Pitluck S, Woodruff KA, Blakely EA, Tenforde T, Char D, Phillips TL, Alpen EL: Treatment of cancer with heavy charged particles. Int J Radiat Oncol Biol Phys 8:2191–2198, 1982.

3. Catterall M, Bloom JG, Ash DV, Walsh L, Richardson A, Uttley D, Gowing NFC, Lewis P, Chaucer B: Fast neutrons compared with megavoltage x-rays in the treatment of patients with supratentorial glioblastoma: A controlled pilot study. Int J Radiat Oncol Biol Phys 6:261–266, 1980.

4. Chen GTY, Castro JR, Quivey JM: Heavy charged particle radiotherapy. Annu Rev Biophys Bioeng 10:499–529, 1981.

5. Fike JR, Cann CE, Davis RL, Phillips TL: Radiation effects in the canine brain evaluated by quantitative computed tomography. Radiology 144: 603–608, 1983.

6. Fu KK, Phillips TL: The relative biological effectiveness (RBE) and oxygen enhancement ratio (OER) of neon ions for the EMTG tumor system. Radiology 120:439–441, 1976.

7. Griffin TW, Laramore GE, Hussey DH, Hendrickson FR, Rodriguez-Antunez A: Fast neutron beam radiation therapy in the United States. Int J Radiat Oncol Biol Phys 8:2165–2168, 1982.

8. Laramore GE, Griffin TW, Gerdes AJ, Parker RG: Fast neutron and mixed (neutron/photon) beam teletherapy for grades III and IV astrocytomas. Cancer 42: 96–103, 1978.

9. Ngo FQH, Blakely EA, Tobias CA: Sequential exposure of mammalian cells to low- and high-LET radiations: 1. Lethal effects following x-ray and neon-ion irradiation. Radiat Res 87:59–78, 1981.

10. Roots R, Yang TC, Craise L, Blakely EA, Tobias CA: Rejoining capacity of DNA breaks induced by accelerated carbon and neon ions in the spread Bragg peak. Int J Radiat Biol 38:203–210, 1980.

11. Suit H, Goitein M, Munzenrider J, Verhey L, Blitzer P, Gragoudas E, Koehler AM, Urie M, Gentry R, Shipley W, Urano M, Duttenhaver J, Wagner M: Evaluation of the clinical applicability of proton beams in definitive fractionated radiation therapy. Int J Radiat Oncol Biol Phys 8:2199–2205, 1982.

12. Tenforde TS, Afzal SMJ, Parr SS, Howard J, Lyman JT, Curtis SB: Cell survival in rat rhabdomyosarcoma tumors irradiated *in vivo* with extended peak silicon ions. Radiat Res 92:208–216, 1982.

13. Tobias CA, Blakely EA, Alpen EL, Castro JR, Ainsworth EJ, Curtis SB, Ngo FQH, Rodriquez A, Roots RJ, Tenforde T,

Yang TCH: Molecular and cellular radiobiology of heavy ions. Int J Radiat Oncol Biol Phys 8:2109–2120, 1982.

14. Tsunemoto H, Arai T, Morita S, Ishikawa T, Aoki Y, Takada N, Kamata S: Japanese experience with clinical trials of fast neutrons. Int J Radiat Oncol Biol Phys 8:2169–2172, 1982.

Stereotactic Heavy Ion Bragg Peak Radiosurgery for Intracranial Vascular Disorders

Jacob I. Fabrikant
John T. Lyman
Yoshio Hosobuchi

Recent advances in diagnostic and microsurgical techniques have made direct neurosurgical treatment of certain intracranial vascular disorders safer and more successful. Surgical treatment of poorly accessible deep arteriovenous malformations (AVMs), including carotid–cavernous sinus fistulas, involves total excision, where possible, or can be combined with ligation or intravascular occlusion. If deep AVMs are inoperable or where other factors preclude neurosurgery, certain stereotactic radiosurgical techniques to induce vascular thrombosis and obliteration have been tried. It appears that if the small shunting vessels of a deep AVM possess hemodynamic flow conditions which differ from flow in normal vessels, then focal beam irradiation of these shunting vessels can lead to thrombosis and hemostasis in the AVM, with eventual complete obliteration.

Leksell[3] and his colleagues in Stockholm introduced stereotactic radiosurgery for inoperable intracranial vascular lesions and other disorders; they use focal gamma radiation from a specially designed unit with 179 cobalt 60 sources, giving rise to narrow radiation beams that are stereotactically directed to a small volume within the brain.[6] Patients with deep AVMs receive single or multiple treatments; presently, doses of approximately 50 Gy are delivered. In their series of AVM patients thus far treated, of the group in which the entire deep AVM was included in the irradiated field, 81 patients have now gone through 1 year and 63 patients have gone through 2 years of follow-up. Total obliteration of the AVM has occurred in about 85 percent of the patients by 2 years. When the deep AVMs were completely covered by the radiation field, partial or complete obliteration led to cure in over 90 percent of the patients, (Steiner L: Personal communication). Partial recovery, presumably with progress to total obliteration in the future, occurred in 10 percent.

However, focal gamma irradiation is limited in its physical characteristics, primarily due to poor isodose distribution, poor beam quality, limited size of treatment volume, and lack of precision and accuracy of dose delivered. Initial studies on the feasibility of proton beam–induced narrow focal lesions in the brain were carried out by Larsson and his colleagues with a 185 MeV cyclotron. Kjellberg and his colleagues introduced stereotactic proton beam Bragg peak radiosurgical treatment of intracranial deep AVMs with a 165 MeV cyclotron.[2] Patients receive a single treatment to larger tissue volumes where necessary; presently, doses are usually well below 30 GyE and are delivered in a single treatment, depending on the location and volume irradiated. The Harvard group has now reported on the follow-up of 205 patients (Kjellberg RN: Personal communication). In 75 patients with 2- to 17-year follow-up, 63 percent have thus far demonstrated reduction in the size of the deep AVM and 20 percent have demonstrated complete obliteration.[3]

Barcia-Saloria has begun to use a cobalt 60 teletherapy beam to induce focal lesions in deep AVMs.

Stereotactic Heavy Ion Bragg Peak Radiosurgery

At the Lawrence Berkeley Laboratory, patients with inoperable intracranial deep AVMs are treated with stereotactic heavy ion Bragg peak radiosurgery, using focal beams of accelerated 230 MeV/u helium ions at the 184-inch Synchrocyclotron.[1] The procedure begins with the fabrication of a vacuum-formed polystyrene head holder adapted to a modified Leksell-type stereotactic frame; this is used for immobilization of the patient during all stereotactic procedures, including cerebral angiography, CT, and heavy ion Bragg peak radiosurgery (Figs. 132-10 to 132-12). Information from stereotactic cerebral angiography and brain CT scans, together with the raw CT data, is transferred to the computer system in our laboratory for use in interactive charged particle treatment planning and provides the basis for delivery of stereotactically directed heavy ion beams to the AVM target contour within the brain. The stereotactic CT data are

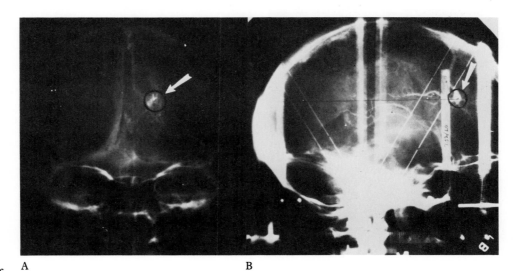

A   B

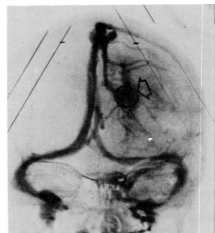

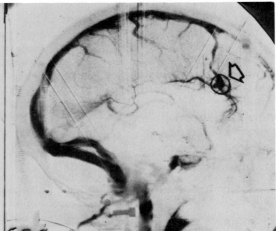

Figure 132-10 Stereotactic cerebral angiogram for stereotactic helium ion Bragg peak radiosurgery of an arteriovenous malformation (AVM) in the left frontal cerebral cortex of a 45-year-old woman. Anteroposterior (*A*) and lateral (*B*) views demonstrate the left frontal AVM (*arrows*) filling primarily from the left anterior cerebral artery; the patient is immobilized in the stereotactic head mask and frame. Subtraction x-ray images (*C, D*) of the stereotactic cerebral angiograms demonstrate the size, shape, and location of the AVM in the frontal pole (*arrows*).

C   D

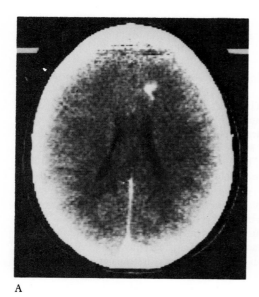

A

Figure 132-11   Stereotactic helium ion Bragg peak radiosurgery of the AVM illustrated in Figure 132-10. *A.* Stereotactic CT scan demonstrating the contrast accumulation in the left frontal region. *B.* Anteroposterior localization roentgenogram of the skull, illustrating isodensity curves of the stereotactic radiosurgical treatment plan. *C.* Lateral localization film and isodensity curves of the treatment plan. Multiple-port stereotactic radiosurgery was delivered over 2 days; the dose was 45 GyE, and the volume of tissue receiving greater than 40 GyE was 1440 mm³.

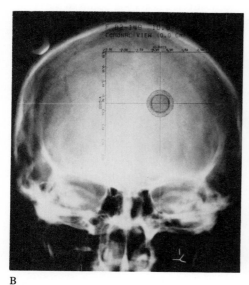

B

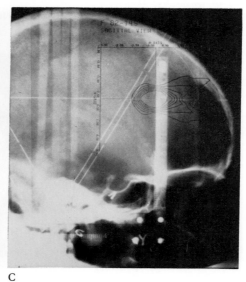

C

used on a pixel-by-pixel basis to design and/or select a collimator aperture for each entry portal, to select the appropriate spread Bragg peak so as to contour the stopping region of the heavy ion beams, and to generate isoeffect and physical dose distributions that match the CT image and can be used to guide stereotactic radiosurgical treatment with accelerated heavy ions. Entry angles and heavy ion beam ports are chosen to confine the Bragg peak region to the defined target volume while carefully protecting adjacent normal brain structures.

Method

A finely focused beamline configuration has been developed at the 184-inch Synchrocyclotron for stereotactic radiosurgery in the brain with the Bragg ionization peak of the 230 MeV/u helium ion beams.[5] The helium ion beam provides improved dose localization and dose distribution for

stereotactic radiosurgery in all patients with intracranial deep AVMs, including carotid–cavernous sinus fistulas, thus far treated. Stereotactic x-ray CT scans and cerebral angiograms are used to calculate the dose distributions of stereotactically directed helium ion beams; these data are used in computer-guided treatment for individual patients. The patient's head is secured in the cyclotron unit by the head immobilizer, which is part of the irradiation stereotactic apparatus for humans (ISAH) system.[4] Computer-controlled head and beam positioning can direct the collimated beam as desired, to within 0.1 mm in the brain.

The greatest density of heavy ions stop in the deep AVM; the spread of the Bragg peak is adjusted so that the amount of radiation to critical adjacent brain structures is less than 10 percent of the nominal radiation dose. The central AVM dose, the aperture size, the number of ports, the angle of delivery of the heavy ion beams, and the Bragg peak spread all determine the isodose contour (Figs. 132-11, 132-12). A

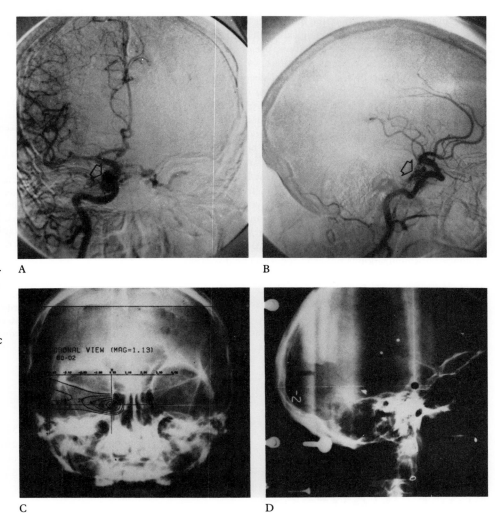

Figure 132-12 Stereotactic helium ion Bragg peak radiosurgery of a right carotid–cavernous sinus fistula (CCF) in a 67-year-old woman. Subtraction images in AP (*A*) and lateral (*B*) views of the stereotactic cerebral angiogram demonstrate the location and size of the CCF (*arrows*); the patient is immobilized in the stereotactic head mask and frame. *C.* An anteroposterior localization roentgenogram of the skull illustrates the isodensity curves of the stereotactic Bragg peak radiosurgical treatment plan. *D.* A lateral localization film demonstrates the helium ion beam port, which is 6 mm in diameter. Multiple-port radiosurgery was delivered in 1 day; the dose was 40 GyE, and the volume of tissue receiving greater than 90 percent of the dose was 280 mm^3.

radiation dose of 45 GyE is delivered to intracranial volumes of from 200 mm^3 to 25 cm^3; treatment usually occurs through one to three entry portals, delivered daily for 1 or 2 days, depending on the treatment volume and the volume of normal brain tissue traversed by the beam. The dose to the critical and sensitive normal brain structures immediately surrounding the AVM is considerably less than 45 GyE; falloff to 10 percent of the central dose occurs within 4 to 6 mm and is much greater (within 2 to 3 mm) along the lateral margins of the helium ion beam (Figs. 132-11, 132-12).[5]

Clinical Results

Cerebral angiography and CT brain scanning are carried out prior to radiosurgery and at 12-month intervals following radiosurgery; extended follow-up to 24, 36, and 60 months is planned for each patient, as necessary. Clinical objectives are to achieve changes in the intracerebral hemodynamic condition, through complete or partial obliteration of the deep AVM, that result in a decrease in neurological deficiencies, subjective complaints, or frequency of seizures. Initial observations in all 55 patients thus far treated indicate that these objectives are being achieved. Radiothera-

peutic objectives are to achieve quantifiable hemodynamic changes; that is, decrease in blood flow through the AVM, with decrease in the size of the AVM until total disappearance. It has been observed by the Stockholm group[6] and the Harvard group[2] that hemodynamic changes occur progressively and are usually observed before morphological vascular alterations. However, in the majority of our patients, a significant decrease in the size of the treated deep AVM has occurred.

Certain conclusions can be drawn from our experience with stereotactic heavy ion Bragg peak radiosurgery in patients with intracranial deep AVMs at the 184-inch Synchrocyclotron at the Lawrence Berkeley Laboratory: (1) Whenever possible, surgical excision remains the treatment of choice for intracranial deep AVMs; when deep AVMs are inaccessible and conditions preclude surgery, stereotactic heavy ion radiosurgery is a safe, reliable, and potentially efficient therapeutic alternative. (2) Stereotactically directed heavy ion Bragg peak irradiation is more advantageous than use of gamma-ray beams, x-ray beams, or proton beams because of the much improved spatial definition and dose distribution of the focal lesion that it induces in the target volume in the brain. (3) Therapeutic failure results from irradiating some, but not all, of the multiple arterial feeders, or where only a part of the pathological cluster of vessels is irradiated; this has not occurred with our use of helium ion Bragg peak beams and dose distributions. (4) Heavy ion focal beam irradiation of the intracranial deep AVMs can induce hemodynamic changes and reduction in the size of the vascular lesion, leading to complete obliteration of the AVM. Neurological changes and improvement have been observed within 3 months, cerebral angiographic changes with decrease in AVM size and flow have been observed within 6 months following radiosurgery. (5) Heavy ion radiosurgery has proved to be a highly selective method for treatment of deep vascular structures within the brain. The advantages of the method are that it is a safe, noninvasive procedure that causes no blood loss; patients under threat of hemorrhage from inoperable or inaccessible AVMs can be treated in cases where neurosurgery is unable to help; and prolonged hospitalization is not required. (6) The disadvantages of the method are that obliteration of irradiated deep AVMs does not begin for some 6 months, and sometimes changes require 18 months or more—thus, patients are under threat of hemorrhage for a long time; and relationships between time, dose, volume, and fractionation for heavy ion focal beam irradiation of brain and other CNS tissues are not fully understood.

References

1. Fabrikant JI, Hosobuchi Y, Lyman JT: Stereotactic heavy-ion Bragg peak radiosurgery for intracranial vascular disorders: Method for treatment of deep arteriovenous malformations. Br J Radiol, in press, 1984.
2. Kjellberg RN, Hanamuva T, Davis KR, Lyons SL, Adams RD: Bragg peak proton beam therapy for arteriovenous malformations of the brain. N Engl J Med 309:269–274, 1983.
3. Leksell LGF: *Stereotaxis and Radiosurgery: An Operative System.* Springfield, Ill., Charles C Thomas, 1971.
4. Lyman JT, Chong CY: ISAH: A versatile treatment positioner for external radiation therapy. Cancer 34:12–16, 1974.
5. Lyman JT, Kanstein L, Yeater F, Fabrikant JI, Frankel KA, Hosobuchi Y: A helium ion beam for stereotaxic radiosurgery. Med Phys, in press, 1984.
6. Steiner L, Backlund EO, Greitz T, Leksell L, Norlen G, Rähn T: Radiosurgery and intracranial arteriovenous malformations, in Carrea R, Le Vay D (eds): *Neurological Surgery: With Emphasis on Non-Invasive Methods of Diagnosis and Treatment.* Amsterdam, Excerpta Medica, 1978, pp 168–180.

133

Fast Neutron Irradiation of Malignant Gliomas

Alexander M. Spence

The standard treatment of malignant supratentorial astrocytic gliomas in adults now consists of surgical excision, which is usually subtotal, followed by a course of high-dose (5500 to 6000 rad) fractionated whole brain photon irradiation. Following this therapy, median survival is close to 35 weeks. The addition of chemotherapy, in particular 1,3-bis(2-chloroethyl)-1-nitrosourea (BCNU), appears to extend median survival to about 52 weeks.[11] In parallel with the development of this treatment there has been an effort at several centers to evaluate cyclotron-generated fast neutron irradiation as an alternative treatment approach.

Rationale for Fast Neutron Therapy

Whereas x-rays and gamma rays are sparsely ionizing and interact with the orbital electrons of atoms, fast neutrons are more densely ionizing and interact with atomic nuclei. In soft tissues, this latter interaction yields chiefly recoil protons since hydrogen is the most abundant atom in tissue and has a large collision cross section. The positively charged recoil protons, in turn, produce further excitation and ionization reactions. There are additional events that contribute to the radiation dose in tissue treated with fast neutrons, such as the production of alpha particles, gamma rays, or heavy nuclear fragments, but only a small fraction of the energy of the neutron beam is involved.

These differences between x-ray and gamma-ray photon irradiation, on the one hand, and fast neutrons on the other correlate with radiobiological investigations which have established that neutrons destroy hypoxic cells more effectively than do photons. Since an area of spontaneous necrosis in malignant brain tumors may well indicate the presence of a hypoxic cell population, fast neutron therapy has a theoretical advantage over the use of photons against such cells. That these cells are potentially clonogenic is suggested by the frequent occurrence of perinecrotic palisading of nuclei.

Besides this theoretical advantage, exposure to fast neutrons instead of photons leads to less repair of sublethal radiation injury in cells and less variation of the radiosensitivity of cells in different phases of the mitotic cycle.

Results of Therapy Trials

Several series have been recorded (Table 133-1).[1,2,5,6,9] Among these there are differences in the proportions of cases in grades III and IV and in how these two groups are combined or separated.[8] There are also differences in the total neutron dosage and in the inclusion of cases with mixed-beam (neutron/photon) whole brain treatment. The later reports show a shift away from large-volume neutron therapy to protocols which combine whole brain photon treatment with neutron boost treatment to a restricted volume containing the neoplasm.[1,5,6]

In these therapy trials it was assumed that the relative biological effect (RBE) of fractionated neutron irradiation compared to photon irradiation for brain tissue was approximately 3, i.e., that one-third as many neutron rad as photon rad produced an equivalent biological effect. It is now thought that this value is low and current estimates of RBE range up to 5.2.[7] Thus, the effectiveness of irradiation with neutrons per rad was greater than originally estimated in these studies. Some unusual clinical and pathological features of the neutron-beam-treated cases may be explained by this RBE discrepancy (see below).

Despite these considerations and the theoretical advantages of fast neutrons, none of these clinical trials has shown that neutron therapy produces better-quality or longer-duration survival than does treatment with whole brain fractionated photons in the dose range of 5000 to 6000 rad.

Currently at our institution, patients with malignant astrocytic gliomas are being treated with fractionated whole brain photon irradiation at a total dose of 4500 rad. In conjunction with this, they receive fractionated neutron irradiation to the tumor volume by means of a "field-within-a-field" method. Initially, the neutron dosages selected totaled 360, 420, or 480 rad, but more recently cases have been randomized into 520-, 560-, or 600-rad groups. This represents an attempt to define a therapeutic window within which there is tumor destruction without unacceptable radiation-induced injury to normal brain. Preliminarily it appears that 360-, 420-, and 480-rad doses do not define such a window. Tumor recurrences with progression have been identified in these cases by clinical, computed tomographic, and postmortem examinations. The results in groups treated with 520, 560, or 600 rad are still accumulating.

Clinical and Pathological Correlations

Many of the patients studied by Laramore et al. became steroid-dependent and showed progressive neurological deterioration with obtundation and unresponsiveness in the weeks and months prior to death.[9] Autopsy studies in 15 of these cases revealed, contrary to expectations, that in most cases the cause of death was not mass effect from regrowth of the neoplasm.[9,12] Rather, the principal neuropathological findings consisted of:

1. Extensive coagulative necrosis in the tumor bed and surrounding white matter.
2. Scarcely any residual tumor tissue that retained the malignant features of the preirradiation biopsy specimens, except for persistent tumor giant cells.
3. Astrocytic cells that appeared to be preserved but frequently showed atypical nuclear and cytoplasmic features. (These cells were interpreted to be non-neoplastic astrocytes showing radiation-induced changes, but the possibility that they represented residual neoplastic astrocytes could not be ruled out.)
4. Diffuse demyelination and gliosis in cerebral, cerebellar, and brain stem white matter.
5. Fibrosis and vascular changes, with only a mild phagocytic response to the necrotic debris.

These observations contrast with the changes which characterize photon-treated malignant astrocytic gliomas, namely, gross and microscopic tumor recurrence associated with significant mass effect and transtentorial herniation.

It was concluded from these autopsy findings that diffuse radiation injury of normal tissue, manifest as gliosis and demyelination, best explains the progressively deteriorating clinical course to death in the neutron-treated cases. The absence of mass effect and the scarcity of viable tumor demonstrated by microscopic analysis suggested good local control of tumor growth with the neutron dosage level supplied. The postmortem results in the cases of Catterall et al.[2] are similar to these, but in the series that examined neutron boost protocols[1,5,6] the autopsy results differed. Battermann[1] and Herskovic et al.[6] reported recurrent tumor and absence of damage to normal brain tissue, whereas Griffin et al.[5] reported the converse, namely, lack of recurrence and presence of changes consistent with neutron injury to normal brain tissue in 9 of 12 cases.

Animal Experiments

In the 36B-10, F-344 rat transplanted-glioma model, we have compared fast neutron and photon radiotherapy and recently have included BCNU in the radiotherapy protocols.[4,13] With or without BCNU chemotherapy, under the conditions of these experiments it has not been possible to demonstrate that neutrons produce better survival results than do photons. Analysis of the gross and microscopic changes in irradiated tumors showed that both neutron and photon treatment produced an essentially identical pattern of extensive areas of confluent necrosis and cytological and vascular changes in a dose-dependent fashion. It must be emphasized that these experiments tested mainly single-dose radiotherapy and that more studies with multiple fractions need to be undertaken in order to define better the efficacy of adding BCNU to neutron radiotherapy.

TABLE 133-1 Survival Data in Neutron-Treated Malignant Astrocytic Gliomas

Authors	Glioma Grade	Number of Patients	Treatment Volume and Dose (rad)*			Mean Survival (mo.)	Control	
			Whole Brain (No.)	3-Field Wedge (No.)	Boost to Tumor		Type	Mean Survival (mo.)
Laramore et al.[9]	III	15	N 1550–1850 (11) MB Varied (4)			18	Historical, photon	26.0
	IV	22	N 1550–1850 (15) MB Varied (6)			7.5		9.9
Catterall et al.[2]	III } IV }	30		N 1560 (18) N 1300 (11) N 1400 (1)		10	Whole brain photon, 5000–5500 rad	11.4
Herskovic et al.[6]	III	9	N 725–1120		N 468–624	11.1		
	IV	8	N 725–1120		N 468–624	6.8		
	III	4	P 5000			11		
	IV	8	P 5000			9.1		
Battermann[1]	III } IV }	22	P 3000		N 1160	7–9		
Griffin et al.[5]	III	9	P 5000		N 450–480	15.8†	P 5000 rad whole brain plus 1500 rad boost	26.3†
	IV	58	P 5000		N 450–480	9.6†		8.5†

*N = neutrons; P = photons; MB = mixed beam (N/P).
†Median survival.

Future Prospects

It is not yet possible to claim that the theoretical advantage of fast neutrons over conventional photon radiotherapy in glioblastoma multiforme has been realized in terms of improved quality or duration of survival.[3,5] With the doses used, local tumor control has been demonstrated in some cases, but the neutron dose necessary to achieve this produces unacceptable injury to normal brain.

If there is a neutron dose low enough to preserve normal brain and high enough to destroy glioblastoma, this so-called therapeutic window should be defined by the present therapy trials. If not, several other approaches may define a place for fast neutrons in brain tumor therapy. Radiosensitizing and radioprotecting agents may open the therapeutic window for fast neutrons by further reducing the tumor-sparing effect of hypoxia or improving the tolerance of normal brain tissue to the destructive effects of neutrons. The near future will see the use of improved cyclotrons that will reduce dose inhomogeneities in the treatment volume. Advances in the sophistication of imaging methods, such as computed tomography, positron emission tomography, and nuclear magnetic resonance scanning, promise to facilitate more accurate tumor localization and provide a means to direct radiation beams into the critical tumor tissue volume. Chemotherapy in combination with fast neutrons remains to be explored systematically in humans. Lastly, californium 252, a fast neutron–emitting radioisotope used for interstitial tumor therapy, is now being studied in therapy of malignant brain tumors.[10] Preliminary results suggest that this novel approach is feasible and perhaps effective.

References

1. Battermann JJ: Fast neutron therapy for advanced brain tumors. Int J Radiat Oncol Biol Phys 6:333–335, 1980.
2. Catterall M, Bloom HJG, Ash DV, Walsh L, Richardson A, Uttley D, Gowing NFC, Lewis P, Chaucer B: Fast neutrons compared with megavoltage x-rays in the treatment of patients with supratentorial glioblastoma: A controlled pilot study. Int J Radiat Oncol Biol Phys 6:261–266, 1980.
3. Geraci JP: Efficacy of neutrons in radiotherapy. Health Phys 40:41–53, 1981.
4. Geraci JP, Spence AM: RBE of cyclotron fast neutrons for a rat brain tumor. Radiat Res 79:579–590, 1979.
5. Griffin TW, Davis R, Laramore G, Hendrickson F, Rodriguez-Antunez A, Hussey D, Nelson J: Fast neutron radiation therapy for glioblastoma multiforme: Results of an RTOG study. Am J Clin Oncol (CCT) 6:661–667, 1983.
6. Herskovic A, Ornitz RD, Shell M, Rogers CC: Glioblastoma multiforme treated with 15 MeV fast neutrons. Cancer 49:2463–2465, 1982.
7. Hornsey S, Morris CC, Myers R, White A: Relative biological effectiveness for damage to the central nervous system by neutrons. Int J Radiat Oncol Biol Phys 7:185–189, 1981.
8. Kernohan JW, Sayre GP: *Tumors of the Central Nervous System* (*Atlas of Tumor Pathology*, Sect. 10, Fasc 35 and 37). Washington D.C., Armed Forces Institute of Pathology, 1952, pp 17-42.
9. Laramore GE, Griffin TW, Gerdes AJ, Parker RG: Fast neutron and mixed (neutron/photon) beam teletherapy for grades III and IV astrocytomas. Cancer 42:96–103, 1978.
10. Maruyama Y, Chin HW, Young AB, Beach JL, Bean J, Tibbs P: Work in progress: ^{252}Cf neutron brachytherapy for hemispheric malignant glioma. Radiology 145:171–174, 1982.
11. Shapiro WR: Treatment of neuroectodermal brain tumors. Ann Neurol 12:231–237, 1982.
12. Shaw CM, Sumi SM, Alvord EC Jr, Gerdes AJ, Spence A, Parker RG: Fast-neutron irradiation of glioblastoma multiforme: Neuropathological analysis. J Neurosurg 49:1–12, 1978.
13. Spence AM, Geraci JP: Combined cyclotron fast-neutron and BCNU therapy in a rat brain-tumor model. J Neurosurg 54:461–467, 1981.

134

Interstitial Brachytherapy of Primary Brain Tumors

Philip H. Gutin

Most malignant gliomas are localized to a single area of the brain, although multifocal disease and metastases can occur.[4] Many systemic tumors that are localized at the time of detection can be cured by surgery and radiotherapy; while this combination is the best known treatment for malignant gliomas, radiation toxicity to normal brain surrounding the lesion makes it impossible to deliver doses of radiation that would sterilize the tumor.

The interstitial implantation of radioactive isotopes (brachytherapy) allows high doses of radiation to be delivered to localized tumor volumes without significant irradiation of surrounding normal brain. The relatively high therapeutic ratio of interstitial irradiation allows aggressive reirradiation of tumors that recur after they have been irradiated by external sources and might allow the delivery of boosts to brain tumors adjuvant to external irradiation.

Increased Therapeutic Ratio of Interstitial Radiation

Radiation from an interstitial source is delivered at low dose rates of approximately 1 to 2 rad/min, compared to dose rates of approximately 200 rad/min from a linear accelerator or cobalt 60 source. A therapeutic dose of low-dose-rate interstitially delivered radiation that can be delivered continuously over several days spares normal tissue; to avoid necrosis of normal tissue, the same total dose delivered at high dose rates from an external source must be divided into multiple fractions that are given over several weeks. The increased therapeutic ratio of interstitial radiation is a result of the relatively superior capacity of normal as opposed to neoplastic cells to repair sublethal radiation damage, a process that occurs during low-dose-rate exposures.[1] Moreover, the rapid decrease in radiation exposure at increasing distance from an implanted radioactive source, because of the in-verse-square law, relatively protects surrounding normal tissues and thereby also improves the therapeutic ratio.

Isotopes

A number of isotopes, particularly [198]Au and ^{192}Ir, have been used for brain tumor brachytherapy,[1] but ^{125}I, an isotope that has only recently been used, seems best suited for this application; purportedly, ^{125}I radiation kills tumor cells more effectively than does radiation from isotopes such as [192]Ir. [125]I emits characteristic x-rays with energies of 27 to 35 keV, which are lower than the energy ranges from other isotopes used for brachytherapy. Low-energy radiation from implanted sources can be attenuated effectively by interposed tissue and less surrounding normal brain is irradiated. In addition, less radiation penetrates through the skull during the time that sources are implanted, and x-rays that do penetrate the skull can be effectively shielded; hence it is easier to protect surgeons, nurses, and other personnel who would be exposed to radiation from implanted sources.

[125]I is provided as a standard low-activity (approximately 0.5 mCi) source that, if implanted in reasonable numbers into fast-growing, malignant brain tumors, delivers radiation at dose rates that are insufficient to delay the growth of tumor. Higher-activity ^{125}I sources (activities of approximately 40 mCi) are available only by special order and at considerable expense. Calibration and dosimetry are problems with ^{125}I sources because of the low energy of the emitted x-rays.

Case Selection

Only solitary primary or metastatic tumors can be effectively treated by brachytherapy. If the CT scan image shows that the lesion is localized, with distinct margins, tumors as large as 6 cm in greatest dimension can be treated. Diffusely infiltrative tumors (e.g., across the corpus callosum), tumors with subependymal spread, or multifocal tumors should not be treated by brachytherapy. Because of the poor biological reserve of structures in the posterior fossa that might be damaged by intense local radiation, in general only supratentorial tumors should be treated by brachytherapy. Cerebral metastases are treated only if they are solitary and have recurred after external irradiation, and if the patient has no documented systemic metastases.

Technique of Implantation

Removable Sources

For successful brachytherapy of rapidly growing (malignant) brain tumors, the radiation dose rate must be sufficiently high that tumor cells receive a critical threshold dose during a complete cell cycle. This condition can be met by using high-activity radioisotopes; however, if such a source remains implanted, normal brain surrounding the source will be exposed to potentially toxic doses of radiation. Radioactive sources that are held in catheters can be removed after the desired dose is delivered, and catheters can hold the source with precision at the target site in the often semisolid or liquid centers of more grossly necrotic malignant brain tumors. We have described a coaxial catheter system for afterloading sources into brain tumors.[2]

Treatment Planning

A preoperative CT scan with contrast enhancement is obtained and the size of the tumor is measured. A target is selected at the center of roughly spherical tumors; to ensure uniform dosimetry, sources held in catheters are implanted along the axis of elongated (prolately ellipsoidal) tumors. [125]I sources sufficient to deliver approximately 1000 rad per day (30 to 50 rad per h) of a minimum (peripheral) tumor dose are implanted.

Stereotactic Techniques

An integrated CT-directed sterotactic system is absolutely essential for effective implantation of isotopes into brain tumors. A number of these integrated systems have been described, all of which appear to be satisfactory. We have adapted the Leksell system because of its simplicity and the great freedom it allows in selecting an approach to the tumor target.[5]

We prefer to implant catheters and load sources in the controlled environment of the operating room rather than in the CT scanner room. After the frame is fixed to the skull, localizing CT scans are taken, and calculation of stereotactic coordinates is completed, the patient is taken to the operating room; there, under local anesthesia, catheters are placed through burr holes, loaded with dummy sources, and localized on intraoperative radiographs. If the catheter(s) appears to be in an acceptable position when compared to reformatted sagittal and coronal CT images of the tumor, it is loaded with the coaxial inner catheter that holds the ^{125}I source. Surgeons and nurses wear lead aprons and radiation exposure badges for this part of the procedure. Surgeons should wear protective leaded glasses.

Dosimetry

On the day after the implantation procedure, source position is localized on orthogonal roentgenograms of the skull. A computer program for ^{125}I generates isodose curves using known source strengths and target sites (Fig. 134-1). A postoperative CT scan is obtained to verify accurate positioning of sources (Fig. 134-2). However, because dosimetry is calculated from source positions determined from plain films, the exact relationship between the isodose curves and tumor margins is unclear. Isodose curves that have been reduced to the magnification of the CT scan can be superimposed on the image of the tumor, but this is at best an approximation. We are adapting a computer program that will generate do-

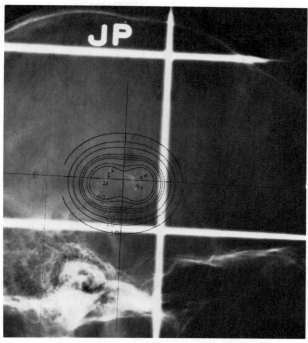

Figure 134-1 Roentgenogram showing two catheters, each containing two high-activity ^{125}I sources, implanted in a recurrent left thalamic glioma. The isodose curves for these sources are superimposed.

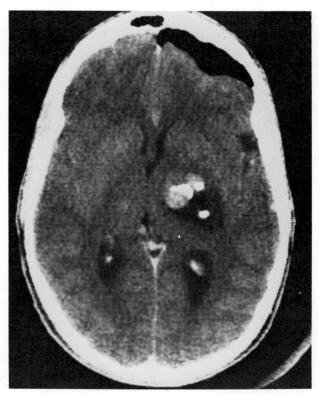

Figure 134-2 CT scan localizing the position of the ^{125}I sources in two catheters placed along the axis of a partially calcified, cystic left thalamic tumor.

simetry from source positions localized on CT scans; isodose curves computed by the program can be directly superimposed onto scan images. Preoperative determination of optimum source placement and final dosimetry, based on source visualization on a postoperative scan, will be obtained with this program.

We delivered minimum (peripheral) tumor doses of 3,000 to 12,000 rad during the early phase of our clinical studies; recently, we have delivered doses of approximately 10,000 rad.

Response to Treatment

Serial CT scans and neurological examinations have been used to evaluate the response of patients treated by chemotherapy for brain tumors. For the evaluation of patients treated by brachytherapy, however, these criteria have been difficult to apply. There can be clear-cut deterioration in the CT scan findings (increased contrast enhancement and brain edema) and neurological status of patients treated with high doses of focal radiation, especially patients who have been treated previously with teletherapy. These changes, which appear to be caused by radiation, begin to appear within 2 to 6 months after brachytherapy. It is not possible to predict which patients will be affected.

We have found that more than half of patients treated for recurrent malignant gliomas will show a clear-cut improvement—for up to 4 months to 1 year—in CT scan appearance and neurological function (Fig. 134-3), and 20 percent of patients who are deteriorating when treated will stabilize for up to 1 year. The remainder will show progression of disease; some will develop disease in distant areas of the brain, and some will develop focal radiation necrosis, which is the apparent cause of the changes in the CT scan and the deterioration in neurological condition described above. Several patients whose condition deteriorated have been reoperated upon 6 to 12 months after implantation, and histological changes consistent with radiation necrosis have been identified, sometimes mixed with apparently viable tumor. Two of these patients, young men treated for recurrent glioblastoma, survive free of disease at 1 year after reoperation, 2 years after the implantation procedure, and 3 years after the initial diagnosis. Two others, who were reoperated upon for necrosis, are free of disease approximately 1 year after the implantation procedure.

Future of Brachytherapy for Malignant Gliomas

The value of interstitial brachytherapy for recurrent (previously irradiated) malignant brain tumors is now evident.[3] To use interstitial irradiation to boost external beam treatment of malignant glioma would seem the next logical step. Walker et al. documented increased survival with each 500-rad incremental step in doses between 5,000 and 6,000 rad;[6] a pilot study is being conducted at our institution for the

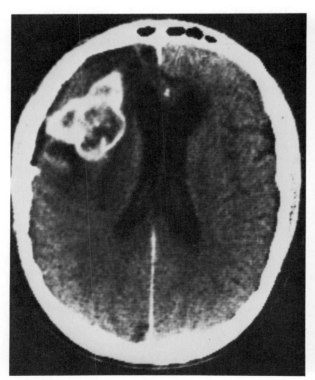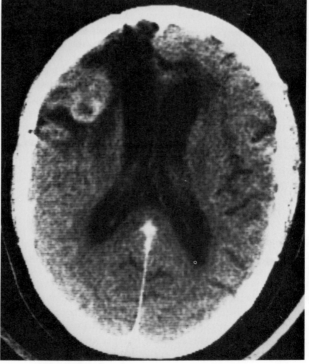

Figure 134-3 CT scan showing a left frontal glioblastoma before (*left*) and 2 months after (*right*) brachytherapy with removable high-activity ^{125}I sources. Tumor volume and midline shift are reduced.

Northern California Oncology Group in order to assess any possible increase in survival that might be caused by a local interstitial boost given adjuvant to standard teletherapy. Doses of both the external beam and the interstitial boost are 6000 rad; while it is too early in the series to evaluate the effects of the protocol, the 12,000-rad tumor dose seems to be well tolerated in the short run. The extent of tumor necrosis and perifocal brain injury caused by this adjuvant treatment will not be known until patients undergo repeat resections or autopsy data are available.

It is clear from our experience with recurrent tumors that a reduction in radiation dose that would decrease the chance of radiation damage of normal brain would be desirable. It may be possible to maintain equal or enhanced capability for local tumor control if the interstitial radiation is delivered concomitantly with tumor hyperthermia or in the presence of radiation sensitizers. Both of these modalities are being studied at our institution.

References

1. Bernstein M, Gutin PH: Interstitial irradiation of brain tumors: A review. Neurosurgery 9:741–750, 1981.
2. Gutin PH, Dormandy RH Jr: A coaxial catheter system for afterloading radioactive sources for the interstitial irradiation of brain tumors: Technical note. J Neurosurg 56:734–735, 1982.
3. Gutin PH, Philips TL, Wara WM, Leibel SA, Hosobuchi Y, Levin VA, Weaver KA, Lamb S: Brachytherapy of recurrent malignant brain tumors with removable high-activity iodine-125 sources. J Neurosurg 60:61–68, 1984.
4. Hochberg FH, Pruitt A: Assumptions in the radiotherapy of glioblastoma. Neurology (NY) 30:907–911, 1980.
5. MacKay AR, Gutin PH, Hosobuchi Y, Norman D: Computed tomography–directed stereotaxy for biopsy and interstitial irradiation of brain tumors: Technical note. Neurosurgery 11:38–42, 1982.
6. Walker MD, Strike TA, Sheline GE: An analysis of dose-effect relationship in the radiotherapy of malignant gliomas. Int J Radiat Oncol Biol Phys 5:1725–1731, 1979.

135

Immunotherapy of Human Gliomas

Michael L. J. Apuzzo

Since the early part of this century, with the observation of rejection of transplanted tumors in animals and the postulation of tumor antigens and immune responses, there has been periodic enthusiasm for immunotherapy as a mode of cancer treatment. During the past two decades, as greater focus on basic mechanisms has emerged, animal tumor systems have been employed to demonstrate that this approach is feasible. In general terms, animal studies have taken two major forms: (1) immunoprophylactic experiments in which immunotherapy is applied before neoplastic cell challenge or oncogenic virus inoculation, with subsequent lower incidence of tumors, and (2) tumor implantation or induction, with subsequent immunotherapy at various schedules in relation to concomitant application of the more common conventional forms of cytoreductive therapy. Within these systems it has become apparent that tumor masses of less than

10^6 cells are more responsive to immunotherapy than are those of more than that number. Therefore, cytoreductive therapy by more conventional means should be a primary undertaking in any immunotherapeutic project.

In view of our current comprehension of immune mechanisms,[1] the primary objectives of immunotherapy should include (1) activation of cell-mediated cytotoxic responses, (2) activation of humorally mediated cytoxic responses, and (3) mitigation of the emergence of blocking factors and suppressor mechanisms.

In a variety of animal models, various immunotherapeutic modalities have shown promise. A number of these have been applied to glioma-bearing human patients. Such endeavors have been prompted by discovery of the following properties of malignant glial tumors: (1) moderate tumor-associated antigenicity, (2) humoral responses which are tumor-associated and capable of initiating complement-mediated cytotoxic responses, (3) depression of cell-mediated immune responses, and (4) the presence of blocking factors in serum components.

Many of the immunotherapeutic studies in glioma patients have used no controls, no assays of specific immune impact, and no external pathological review, and have been undertaken on individuals with excessive tumor burdens; therefore, they provide data which are difficult to evaluate. To date, immunotherapy of gliomas has remained largely within classic categories which relate to techniques of immunization;[9] in addition, restorative immunotherapy has recently been employed.

Active Immunotherapy

This technique attempts to stimulate the intrinsic immune response to the neoplasm. The method may be employed through specific, nonspecific, or combination modes.

Active Specific Immunotherapy

This method utilizes specific immunization of the host with neoplastic cells or cell products. Alteration of tumor cells by the addition of haptenic groups or by treatment with neuraminidase to remove the sialic acid coating (thus revealing membrane antigens) has been undertaken to enhance the generally weak immunogenicity of naturally occurring tumors. Butanol extracts have likewise been employed for this purpose.

Active specific immunotherapy, like active immunization for infectious disease, has promise of emerging as a reliable form of immunotherapy since it elicits memory T cells that permit long-term recognition of offending antigens. However, this form of therapy may also initiate the emergence of tumor-specific suppressor elements and enhancement of tumor progression. This adjunct in glioma-bearing patients creates the risk of concomitant induction of experimental allergic encephalomyelitis (EAE) due to cross-reacting antigenic components shared with brain and brain-derived neoplastic tissues.

Bloom et al. reported tumor growth at 10 of 12 sites of autologous injection in a single patient, with no evidence of immune response peripherally or in the brain.[4] In a comparable study, Grace et al. observed evidence of immune rejection at the peripheral graft site in two of six cases without apparent evidence of alteration in the patient's course.[6]

A randomized prospective trial was reported by Bloom et al. in 1973.[5] All patients had surgery and radiotherapy. Approximately half of the cases had concomitant specific immunotherapy. The immunotherapy group (27 cases) received varying numbers of injections of irradiated autologous tumor cells. No positive therapeutic response was observed. One case of EAE was detected on external pathological review.

Active Nonspecific Immunotherapy

This modality, which represents the category most exploited thus far, employs compounds or materials that do not have an antigenic similarity to the tumor, but which enhance the immune capacity of the host. These include a variety of substances such as microorganisms like Bacillus Calmette-Guérin (BCG) and *Corynebacterium parvum* (*C. parvum*) as well as newer chemical agents such as glucan, pyran, fluorenone derivative, and certain interferon inducers. These materials fundamentally act on macrophages, activating them into the cytotoxic phase and initiating their activity as T-cell stimulators.

In addition to their inherent toxicity, these substances likewise enhance mechanisms of suppression. Whenever a nonspecific modulator is administered, its apparent effects represent the net effect of its sometimes conflicting activities on both the effector and suppressor arms of the immunoregulatory systems. Suppressor macrophages acting via prostaglandins are particularly problematical, as they impede the emergence of cytotoxic T cells.[11]

Utilization of *C. parvum* therapy was reported in six patients with intrinsic glial tumors; intracranial pressure was increased with administration, and no alteration in survival time was apparent.[12] Intradermal BCG was employed in 45 patients who were P.P.D.-negative.[8] Increased survival time was reported in those who converted to P.P.D.-positive, but no external pathological review was presented.

Combination Immunotherapy

Combined specific extracts and potentiating nonspecific adjuvants may be employed concurrently. The use of adjuvants significantly increases the risk of EAE. To date, the most elaborate study in this regard was reported by Trouillas.[16] Immunotherapy consisted of weekly injections of autologous tumor extracts emulsified with complete Freund's adjuvant. Sixty-five patients were randomized after surgery into four groups whose treatment consisted of immunotherapy (10 cases), immunotherapy and radiotherapy (18 cases), radiotherapy (20 cases), or no postoperative treatment (7 cases). A moderate but significant increase in survival time was observed in the immunotherapy groups. Phenomena indicating strong antiglioma immunization were observed. Four of six tumors evaluated showed increased round cell responses. One case of EAE was observed. Bigner et al. think that the threat of EAE induction and the potential difficulty of its detection in a disabled glioma patient receiving active specific or nonspecific immunotherapy warrant the biological screening of immunizing CNS material in experimental animals prior to its administration to patients.[2]

Adoptive Immunotherapy

Sensitized cellular components or fractions thereof may be transferred from one host to another or from the peripheral blood to a tumor site. Takakura et al. have transferred histocompatible adult bone marrow into children with a variety of tumors, with no controls.[13] In addition, the same group infused white cells into tumor beds postoperatively.[14] Once again, the tumor population was mixed and no control data were presented.

Seventeen patients who had failed conventional therapy for glioblastoma were treated by Young et al. with intratumoral infusions of autologous lymphocytes.[17] Eight patients demonstrated unequivocal clinical improvement and were alive as long as 17 months later. No indication of EAE was apparent on clinical or pathological assays.

Subsequent to these efforts, improved in vitro technology has been realized.[8] The ability to clone T cells and preserve their properties of helper or cytotoxic function is due to the identification of T-cell growth factor (interleukin 2). The use of autologous sensitized cells circumvents the ethical issue of donor sensitization and the serious problem of graft-versus-host responses which may be inititated by recognition of minor histocompatibility antigens. Autologous lymphocytes from tumor-bearing patients may be assayed for their in vitro reactivity and then restimulated in vitro by incubation with killer tumor cells. Clonal selection and/or expansion is a potential strategy.

Other currently promising modes of adoptive therapy include: lymphokines, monokines (macrophage source), and various other well-characterized lymphocytic factors. Interleukin 1 (monokine) and interleukin 2 (lymphokine) are discrete biological entities that can be isolated and administered. These substances afford the ability to transfer homogeneous defined materials and to activate lymphocytes and macrophages in vivo.

Restorative Therapy

Efforts in this regard involve direct and indirect restoration of deficient immunological function by any means but direct adoptive transfer of cells. Restoration of depressed cell-mediated immunity may be selectively attempted by the administration of agents such as levamisole. This agent can convert T-cell precursors, including some null cells, into functional T cells.

In a rigidly designed and well-controlled study, Mahaley et al. evaluated levamisole therapy in patients with anaplastic glioma who had undergone surgical resection and who were also treated with radiotherapy and chemotherapy.[7] No significant differences in survival time were observed between the treated and nontreated groups within a group of 85 adequately treated patients. Those who received levamisole did not demonstrate significantly different assays of cellular or humoral immunity from those who did not receive levamisole. The same group reported that the utilization of BCG in combination with levamisole was effective in an animal model and proposed future pilot studies.

Thymic hormones are currently under investigation as agents which, in various fractions, impact selectively upon depressed T-cell function to restore T-cell populations to normal levels and restore physiological mechanisms related to this group of cells. Thymosin in particular has been fractionated and found to cause differentiation of precursors into specific T-cell subfractions in mice. It may soon be possible to selectively augment various components of the T-cell compartment.

Passive Immunotherapy

Transfer of antibodies from immunized individuals to tumor-bearing recipients is passive immunotherapy. Not only is the theoretical danger of tumor enhancement present, but antibodies are short-lived and in general are less important in tumor rejection than is cell-mediated immunity. In addition, technical problems in screening sera of donors and ethical restraints against immunization of individuals has made this form of therapy one of the most restrictive and least desirable approaches. No significant report relating to this form of therapy for malignant gliomas has been advanced. However, the development of hybridoma techniques and the production of monoclonal antibodies have given new impetus toward consideration of this method.[10]

Biological Response Modification

What has been previously termed immunotherapy might more aptly be called biological response modification or biomodulation.[3] All therapeutic approaches to neoplastic disorders which attempt to modify the antigenic structure or growth characteristics of the tumor and thus influence host-neoplasm interplay may be considered within this province. An agent may be considered a biomodulator if it accomplishes one or more of the following actions:

1. Alteration of the characteristics of the cell membrane or the tumor sufficient to increase antigenicity or to increase susceptibility to cytotoxic drugs or immune mechanisms.
2. Enhancement of the host's ability to tolerate injury by cytotoxic modalities, such as by increasing the number of leukocyte precursors in bone marrow.
3. Enhancement of the host's defenses by being an effector or mediator.
4. Decrease in suppressor mechanisms.
5. Direct enhancement of the host's response by stimulating an increase in the amount of effector cells or soluble mediators, such as T-cell lymphokines or macrophage monokines.
6. Prevention or reversal of transformation or increased maturation of the primitive tumor cells.

Biomodulation based on precise comprehension of immune neoplastic mechanisms emerges as a logical province for investigative enterprise in relation to the enigmatic issue of malignant glioma therapy.

Future Perspectives

In order to embark on a rational course for effective mobilization of immune mechanisms, the most sophisticated comprehension of the immune concert is required. This issue is one of the major factors responsible for the paucity of effective efforts in the utilization of adjunctive immunotherapy. As our appreciation of elements of the immune system develops, more precise modes of intervention and manipulation will emerge. Some of the newer emerging concepts of immunotherapy have been detailed previously. In addition, specific removal of blocking antibodies and circulating immune complexes appears to be a logical approach for restoring effective immunity and ultimately improving control of malignant disease. Therefore, the current focus has initiated interest in the therapeutic use of immunoabsorption.[15] Blocking antibodies may compete with cytotoxic antibodies for antigenic loci on tumor cells. Immune complexes ultimately stimulate the emergence of suppressor predominance in T-cell and macrophage populations. The end result of these events is a globally reduced effector immune response in tumor-bearing patients.

Immunoabsorption can be performed through the use of an absorptive column. In this method, antigen and antibody are bound to a column of immobilized charcoal, and the column is then perfused with the patient's plasma. The immune substance complementary to the bound reagent is removed by the column and the filtered plasma is returned to the patient in an immunomodulated state. The concept has been effective in the laboratory and, as employed in a small number of patients with carcinoma of the breast, has shown promising results.

Disclosures of recent investigations related to serum factors, immune complexes, and suppressor mechanisms in glioma-bearing patients would make such therapy logical in these patients. A pilot study is currently underway at our institution in order to evaluate these possibilities.

Antagonism of suppressor influence is a form of immunorestorative therapy.[9] Cyclophosphamide in low doses can specifically inhibit precursors of suppressor T cells, thereby augmenting cytotoxic effector function. In addition, antagonists of prostaglandin synthetase such as indomethacin inhibit the effects of suppressor macrophages, which are mediated through prostaglandin E. Employment of these agents with the immunoabsorption technique logically offers a potential therapy for the reversal of suppressor impact.

The hybridoma technique has proved to be a potent tool in the identification of antigenic determinants and in the production of antibodies specific to those determinants. By employing the capacities of sensitized B cells and a myeloma tumor cell line, large quantities of monoclonally derived antibodies which are specific for cellular determinants can be obtained. In view of this development, it is logical to believe that more specific knowledge and comprehension of the antigenic components of the individual neoplasms will emerge, and also that antibodies more specific to individual neoplasms will be generated and will become available for passive immunotherapy. Specific immunization is conceivable.

The retinoid derivatives of vitamin A have been effective in redirecting the maturation of cells that are metaplastic toward normalcy. When administered with carcinogens, retinoids may prevent and occasionally reverse progression of malignant transformation. Extensive epidemiological evidence supports the protective role of these agents in high-risk cancer populations. These agents can augment the immune response by increasing antibody production and cell-mediated cytotoxicity. In brief, these agents have both direct and indirect effects on transformed cells.

The interferons, a family of inducible secretory glycoproteins, need evaluation in glioma management. These agents exert a number of potential therapeutic effects on neoplastic processes. These include (1) antiviral impact, (2) inhibition of cellular proliferation, (3) alteration of membrane antigenicity and structure, (4) enhancement of lymphocytic cytotoxic responses, (5) augmentation of natural killer cell and macrophage cytotoxicity, and (6) augmentation of antibody-dependent cell-mediated responses. Because of issues related to blood-brain barrier permeability, alternative administration modes and delivery systems are being evaluated in

glioma cases. In addition, a number of interferon inducers such as poly I:C, poly A:U, and pyran require further study.

References

1. Apuzzo MLJ, Mitchell MS: Immunological aspects of intrinsic glial tumors. J Neurosurg 55:1–18, 1981.
2. Bigner DD, Pitts OM, Wikstrand CJ: Induction of lethal experimental allergic encephalomyelitis in nonhuman primates and guinea pigs with human glioblastoma multiforme tissue. J Neurosurg 55:32–42, 1981.
3. Biological Response Modifier Subcommittee Report. JNCI: In press.
4. Bloom WH, Carstairs KC, Crompton MR, McKissock W: Autologous glioma transplantation. Lancet 2:77–78, 1960.
5. Bloom HJG, Peckham MJ, Richardson AE, Alexander PA, Payne PM: Glioblastoma multiforme: A controlled trial to assess the value of specific active immunotherapy in patients treated by radical surgery and radiotherapy. Br J Cancer 27:253–267, 1973.
6. Grace JT Jr, Perese DM, Metzgar RS, Sasabe T, Holdridge B: Tumor autograft responses in patients with glioblastoma multiforme. J Neurosurg 18:159–167, 1961.
7. Mahaley MS Jr, Steinbok P, Aronin P, Dudka L, Zinn D: Immunobiology of primary intracranial tumors. J Neurosurg 54:220–227, 1981.
8. Miki Y, Sano K, Takakura K, Mizutani H: (Adjuvant immunotherapy with BCG for malignant brain tumors.) Neurol Med Chir (Tokyo) 16:357–364, 1976.
9. Mitchell MS, Bertrum JH: Tumor immunology: Current concepts and therapeutic applications in human cancer, in Calabresi P, Schein PS, Rosenger SA (eds): *Medical Oncology.* New York, McMillan, In press.
10. Mitchell MS, Oettgen HF (eds): *Hybridomas in Cancer Diagnosis and Treatment* (Progress in Cancer Research and Therapy, Vol 21). New York, Raven, 1982.
11. Powles TJ, Bockman RS, Honn KV, Ramwell P (eds): *Prostaglandins and Cancer: First International Conference.* New York, Alan R Liss, 1982, vol 2.
12. Selker RG, Wolmark N, Fisher B, Moore P: Preliminary observations on the use of *Corynebacterium parvum* in patients with primary intracranial tumors: Effect on intracranial pressure. J Surg Oncol 10:299–303, 1978.
13. Takakura K, Miki Y, Kubo O: Adjuvant immunotherapy for malignant brain tumors in infants and children. Childs Brain 1:141–147, 1975.
14. Takakura K, Miki Y, Kubo O, Ogawa N, Matsutani M, Sano K: Adjuvant immunotherapy for malignant brain tumors. Jpn J Clin Oncol 2:109–120, 1972.
15. Terman DS, Young JB, Shearer WT, et al.: Preliminary observations of the effects on breast adenocarcinoma of plasma perfused over immobilized protein A. N Engl J Med 305:1195–1200, 1981.
16. Trouillas P: Immunologie et immunothérapie des tumeurs cérébrales: État actuel. Rev Neurol (Paris) 128:23, 1973.
17. Young H, Kaplan A, Regelson W: Immunotherapy with autologous white cell infusions ("lymphocytes") in the treatment of recurrent glioblastoma multiforme. Cancer 40:1037–1044, 1977.

136

Chemotherapy of Primary Brain Tumors

S. Clifford Schold, Jr.
J. Gregory Cairncross
Dennis E. Bullard

Standard forms of treatment for patients afflicted with primary malignant brain tumors have had only limited success. Surgery and radiotherapy prolong survival, but cures are rare. These limitations and the success of chemotherapy against other types of cancer have led to an assessment over the last 15 to 20 years of the value of antineoplastic drug therapy in patients with brain tumors. Although major advances in treatment have not been forthcoming, there has been progress in several areas of clinical importance. Prognostic factors that influence outcome have been identified; the science of prospective controlled clinical trials has been refined; unequivocal antineoplastic activity has been documented in some patients using some forms of chemotherapy; and these initial steps have stimulated detailed investigations of basic aspects of brain tumor chemotherapy. Studies of the blood-brain barrier and its manipulation, of blood flow and metabolic activity in normal and neoplastic brain, and of the molecular basis of drug resistance, as well as the development of chemosensitivity testing of human brain tumors, represent active areas of research with potential for clinical impact.

History and Basic Principles

History

The history of brain tumor chemotherapy begins shortly after the introduction of the first antineoplastic chemicals in the late 1940s and early 1950s. Pioneer neurosurgeons such as B. Woodhall, G. Odom, G. Owens, C. Wilson, J. French, and M. S. Mahaley, among others, used agents such as nitrogen mustard, vincristine, and mithramycin to treat patients with anaplastic gliomas. This early work, which was necessarily based on limited experimental data, demon-

strated the technical feasibility of intracarotid drug administration, the potential brain and eye toxicity of some of these agents, and the limited efficacy of even highly aggressive approaches.[19] However, there were a few apparent responses, and these investigators can be credited with laying the foundation for the modern era of brain tumor chemotherapy.

In 1962 the nitrosoureas were introduced. These drugs were of special importance to those interested in nervous system tumors because of their impressive efficacy in experimental intracranial tumors. 1,3-bis(2-chloroethyl)-1-nitrosourea (BCNU), the most active nitrosourea experimentally, also showed activity in patients with recurrent gliomas, and it was introduced into large-scale clinical trials. The use of the nitrosoureas and the introduction of the randomized clinical trial permanently changed the management of patients with anaplastic brain tumors. A new chemotherapeutic agent is now usually compared to a nitrosourea in carefully controlled trials.

Basic Principles of Cancer Chemotherapy

In the design and interpretation of chemotherapeutic trials, a number of basic principles must be considered (Table 136-1). First, the greater the tumor burden, the less effective are therapeutic maneuvers and the worse is the prognosis. This principle, which is intuitively obvious and which has now been demonstrated repeatedly in experimental systems, is especially important to the neurosurgeon dealing with primary brain tumors. Surgical decompression of a tumor is important not only in order to relieve symptoms and to establish a diagnosis, but also because it allows other forms of therapy to begin under more favorable circumstances. This will become increasingly important as more active drugs are introduced.

Second, there is often a steep dose-response curve with any chemotherapeutic agent.[9] The practical consequence of this principle is that antineoplastic agents should be given in the highest tolerated dose. Bone marrow toxicity is often the dose-limiting factor with anticancer drugs, and a certain degree of hematologic toxicity and risk should be accepted to be certain that as much of the drug as possible is being given. Circumventing the primary site of toxicity, such as by reinfusion of autologous bone marrow, might allow use of higher doses and could further improve therapeutic effects.

Third, it is now clear that, with few exceptions, curative cancer chemotherapy requires drug combinations.[4] There are many explanations for this, including tumor cell heterogeneity and acquired drug resistance, but if two or more drugs are available for the treatment of a particular tumor,

TABLE 136-1 Important Basic Principles of Cancer Chemotherapy

Therapeutic success is inversely related to tumor volume.
Dose-response curves are steep.
Drug combinations improve responses.
Therapeutic scheduling affects outcome.
Drugs must be adequately delivered.
Response must be carefully defined.

their use in combination is likely to be more effective than using one drug alone. When used in combination, drugs again should be given at the maximum tolerated dose. While doses must be modified because of overlapping toxicity, often almost a full dose of each agent can be given without a significant increase in toxicity. Again, the importance of drug combinations in brain tumor chemotherapy will increase as more effective agents are introduced.

Fourth, scheduling of combined-modality therapy can influence results. When surgery, radiotherapy, and multiple-agent (or multiple-route) chemotherapy are considered, the permutations of treatment order are staggering, and it would be impractical to test all of them. Even when drugs alone are considered, certain agents, such as methotrexate, are much more effective in multiple lower doses than in a single high dose; others, such as the alkylating agents, appear to be more effective in a single large dose. The order and timing of single doses of different agents can be important both because of "priming" of the tumor (by altering its kinetics) by one drug and because overlapping toxicity can be avoided.

Fifth, in order to be effective an antineoplastic agent must be delivered appropriately to the tumor cells. The problem of adequate drug delivery is especially complex in tumors of the nervous system because of the variable preservation of the blood-brain barrier in these tumors. To the extent that the barrier is preserved in anaplastic brain tumors, efforts to either disrupt or circumvent it are important in delivering certain chemotherapeutic agents.

Finally, the problem of the evaluation of response to a drug must be addressed very carefully. "Response," "treatment failure," and similar terms must be defined precisely in any study or useful information may be lost. This again is especially difficult in brain tumor therapy because clinical deficits may persist even though the tumor mass is reduced and because computed tomography may not always give an accurate representation of tumor burden.

Even though the introduction of active agents in brain tumor chemotherapy has been painfully slow, many basic principles of combined-modality cancer therapy are now understood. As new agents are introduced and alternate delivery routes refined, an appreciation of these basic principles will permit their optimal implementation in the brain tumor patient.

Development of New Drugs

Preclinical Evaluation of Potential Agents

The National Cancer Institute screens over 10,000 compounds annually for anticancer activity. Substances come from various sources, ranging from folk remedies to research laboratories.[10] The mouse P388 leukemia is the primary experimental tumor used in drug screening because it is the most sensitive of the standard tumor lines. Agents that show activity in this system are then used to treat other experimental tumor lines, including mouse leukemia L1210, the Lewis lung tumor, and B16 melanoma. If the drug

shows activity in any of these systems, it is then used against a battery of more specialized tumor lines, including human tumors growing in congenitally athymic mice.

The standard tumor cell lines used for screening potential brain tumor drugs are the intracranial L1210 leukemia and the mouse ependymoblastoma. Both tumor lines were initiated in the 1940s by the application of a carcinogen, and both are sensitive to nitrosoureas. They have the advantages of highly reproducible growth and an established experimental track record. However, both lines have limitations as models for human brain tumors. The L1210 line is a leukemia or lymphoma and biologically has little resemblance to tumors of the nervous system. Treatment of the intracranial L1210 addresses the drug delivery problem, but it does not necessarily reflect what is likely to be the cellular sensitivity of human brain neoplasms. The mouse ependymoblastoma is a primary brain neoplasm, but it is histologically dissimilar to the most common human brain tumors, and its relation to the human tumor is uncertain. Other experimental brain tumor lines, such as the 9L gliosarcoma and the avian sarcoma virus–induced astrocytoma, have also been used in order to evaluate therapeutic approaches. The use of human brain tumors growing in athymic mice offers significant theoretical advantages over animal tumor lines, but this is a much more expensive model and its value in comparison to the standard screens remains to be demonstrated.

Clinical Evaluation of New Agents

Once drugs show activity in standard experimental tumors and their toxicity in large animals, including primates, has been assessed, they may be introduced into clinical trials. Clinical protocols for new agents are commonly divided into phase I, II, and III studies. Phase I studies are designed to assess toxicity. Standard practice is to begin phase I studies of new drugs in specialized cancer centers, treating patients with extensive disease who have failed on conventional agents. Drug dosages are increased until significant toxicity develops, and the highest tolerated doses are then used in phase II studies. Information about therapeutic efficacy is collected, but it is recognized that drug activity will be underestimated in patients with advanced disease. Phase II protocols are designed to test efficacy. Drugs are given to patients with measurable disease, using a schedule and dose based on phase I results. Criteria for response are carefully defined, and both the percentage of patients responding and the duration of the responses are compared to those achieved with currently available therapy. Phase II studies may of course involve drug combinations as well as single agents. If the new agent compares favorably with conventional drugs, phase III trials may be initiated. In phase III trials the new therapeutic regimen is compared in carefully controlled fashion to the best available conventional treatment. Patient selection and therapeutic schedule are controlled, and usually alternative therapies are chosen by randomization. Relative efficacy is then compared, using a standard measure such as time to tumor recurrence or survival time. Occasionally phase III studies are conducted using historical controls, but this approach is risky.

Human Brain Tumor Chemotherapy

Drug Delivery in Brain Tumor Chemotherapy

Successful cancer chemotherapy requires that tumor cells be properly exposed to cytotoxic agents to which they are sensitive. Intrinsic cellular susceptibility is poorly understood and currently impossible to predict. Consequently, in the last decade attempts to improve therapeutic results using standard agents have emphasized improving drug delivery.

Drug delivery in its broadest sense encompasses basic pharmacologic properties such as absorption, protein binding, metabolism, and excretion. These properties are important in the treatment of any neoplasm in any location, but the blood-brain barrier (BBB) adds unique complexity to the chemotherapy of central nervous system tumors. Molecules that are small, lipid-soluble, and un-ionized are best suited to cross the intact barrier, and these characteristics have been considered essential in the design of agents for the treatment of CNS neoplasms.[21] Yet several lines of evidence show that the BBB is disrupted in anaplastic brain tumors. Both radiographic evidence of abnormal vascular permeability and elevation of CSF protein concentration are crude but definite measures of loss of barrier integrity in patients with brain tumors. More detailed observations using quantitative autoradiographic methods in a rat brain tumor model indicate marked variability of barrier function both within individual tumors and among different tumors.[12] Similar methods applied in patients with brain tumors could, in theory, permit individualization of therapy on the basis of the degree of preservation of the barrier.

The other critical variable in drug delivery to central nervous system tumors is blood flow. Quantitative autoradiographic measurements of blood flow in tumor-bearing rat brain demonstrate marked regional variability in large tumors.[12] Flow is markedly diminished in the necrotic center of a tumor and increases toward normal levels at the periphery. In very small cerebral tumors, blood flow is normal or minimally reduced. These findings support the clinicopathological impression that central necrosis in rapidly expanding cerebral neoplasms reflects relative ischemia. Direct measurement of blood flow in human cerebral neoplasms awaits the application of newer technologies, but findings of regional variability and the tendency to diminished blood flow would have major implications for chemotherapeutic approaches to these diseases. As a result of blood flow alterations, tumor cells may escape cytotoxic drugs or be exposed to sublethal concentrations, the latter a factor that may be important in the emergence of drug resistance. At the same time, tumor cells may survive and proliferate under these relatively ischemic conditions.

Direct intra-arterial administration of chemotherapeutic agents could theoretically improve the therapeutic index of these treatments by exposing the tumor to higher concentrations of drug and by reducing systemic toxicity. It has been demonstrated in animals that higher intracerebral levels of BCNU can be achieved by intracarotid than by intravenous administration of the drug. However, it is not yet clear that systemic toxicity has been reduced or that therapeutic efficacy has been enhanced by this route of administration.

Furthermore, significant ocular and brain toxicity have been produced by intracarotid BCNU administration, and higher tissue levels of BCNU by any route of delivery have been associated with a hemorrhagic encephalomyelitis.[18] The theoretical advantages of improving drug delivery by intra-arterial administration have yet to be convincingly demonstrated in experimental systems.

Improved drug delivery by direct infusion into the ventricles, tumor, or tumor cavities or by transient BBB disruption has also been considered. Again, there is as yet no strong experimental basis for these approaches.

Pharmacology of Specific Chemotherapeutic Agents

Antineoplastic agents may be classified according to their presumed mechanism of action. Traditionally, cytotoxic agents fall into one of two major groups: drugs that act during specific phases of the cell cycle (cell cycle specific, CCS), including the folate antagonists, pyrimidine analogs, purine analogs, and vinca alkaloids; and those whose activity does not depend on the cell cycle phase (cell cycle nonspecific, CCNS), including the alkylating agents, many antitumor antibiotics, and a variety of miscellaneous compounds. CCS drugs arrest proliferating cells by interfering with crucial functions such as DNA replication, protein synthesis, or mitotic spindle formation. CCNS agents are equally toxic to both resting and proliferating cells. Theoretically, cell cycle specific agents are ideally suited to the treatment of CNS neoplasms since tumor cells represent the only actively proliferating cells in the target tissue. However, single-agent chemotherapy using CCS drugs has been disappointing. The most effective drugs to date have been the CCNS drugs, including the nitrosoureas (especially BCNU), procarbazine, dianhydrogalactitol, cisplatin, and diaziquone. The failure of CCS chemotherapeutic agents has been attributed to the low proportion of tumor cells that are actively dividing (i.e., low growth fraction) in many CNS neoplasms. Nevertheless, selected CCS drugs (e.g., hydroxyurea, VM-26, vincristine) may prove useful when administered in combination with the alkylating agents. Table 136-2 lists typical dosage schedules and common toxic effects of some drugs used in brain tumor chemotherapy.

Nitrosoureas

The chloroethylnitrosoureas are small, highly lipid-soluble CCNS alkylating agents with clinical activity against a variety of neoplasms. Many derivatives incorporating this basic structure have been synthesized (including BCNU, CCNU, methyl-CCNU, PCNU, ACNU, streptozotocin, and chlorozotocin). Decomposition of these agents in aqueous solution yields two reactive intermediates, a chloroethyl-diazohydroxide and an isocyanate group. The former alkylates DNA, producing strand breaks and cross-links. The latter has been related to the drugs' toxicity rather than to their antitumor effect. Parent compounds disappear rapidly from plasma after absorption or intravenous infusion. These agents readily cross the intact blood-brain barrier, which

TABLE 136-2 Characteristics of Drugs Commonly Used in Human Brain Tumor Chemotherapy

Drug	Usual Dosage and Route of Administration	Common Toxic Effects
Nitrosoureas		Bone marrow toxicity is delayed and cumulative. BCNU is associated with pulmonary fibrosis in total doses exceeding 1400 mg/m².
BCNU	200 mg/m² IV q 6–8 weeks	
CCNU	130 mg/m² PO q 6 weeks	
meCCNU	125–200 mg/m² PO q 6 weeks	
Procarbazine	100 mg/m² PO daily for 14 days	Bone marrow suppression. Allergic rash occurs in 10 percent of patients.
Dianhydrogalactitol	25–35 mg/m² daily x5 q 4–6 weeks	Myelosuppression
Cisplatin	50–100 mg/m² IV q 4 weeks	Nausea may be severe. Kidney damage can be prevented with hydration. Peripheral neuropathy is uncommon.
Diaziquone	Optimal schedule not yet determined. Maximum tolerated dose is approximately 40–60 mg/m² IV q 4 weeks.	Bone marrow suppression. Nausea is mild.
VM-26	100 mg/m² weekly	Leukopenia. A mild peripheral neuropathy is uncommon.
Vincristine	0.5–1.5 mg/m² IV weekly	Polyneuropathy is the dose-limiting toxic effect. Bone marrow suppression is mild.

may partially explain their efficacy against CNS neoplasms. Myelosuppression, which is both delayed and comulative, is their most notable and consistent toxic effect. Prolonged administration has also been associated with pulmonary fibrosis.

Procarbazine

Procarbazine (PCB) is a water-soluble agent with a molecular weight of 258. It has monoamine oxidase–inhibiting activity, but the mechanism of its antineoplastic action is incompletely understood. The drug requires metabolic activation yielding an end product with alkylating activity. Procarbazine is readily absorbed from the gastrointestinal tract, disappears rapidly from plasma, and readily crosses the intact blood-brain barrier. Cerebrospinal fluid levels are in equilibrium with plasma within minutes of intravenous administration. Nausea and anorexia may be dose-limiting, myelosuppression is mild to moderate in degree, and clinically significant neurotoxicity is very uncommon. A rash appears in approximately 10 percent of the patients taking the drug.

Dianhydrogalactitol

Dianhydrogalactitol (DAG) is a water-soluble, CCNS alkylating agent with a molecular weight of 146. It freely crosses the blood-brain barrier and has been demonstrated in CNS tumor tissue. Its major limiting toxic effect is bone marrow suppression.

Cis-diamminedichloroplatinum (II)

Cis-platinum (cisplatin, CDP) is a water-soluble CCNS agent with a molecular weight of 300. It is the first heavy metal to be used as an anticancer agent. It appears to act through interstrand and intrastrand cross-linking of DNA in a manner similar to that of the bifunctional alkylating agents. After intravenous administration, most of the drug is protein-bound and inactive, and drug not bound to tissues or plasma proteins is excreted in the urine. Cis-platinum pen-

etrates poorly into the central nervous system; the ratio of drug concentration in plasma to CSF is 25:1 or greater. The major dose-limiting effect is renal toxicity. This is minimized by vigorous hydration in conjunction with a mannitol-induced diuresis, but dosage should be reduced in the presence of impaired renal function. Severe nausea and vomiting occur frequently. Ototoxicity and peripheral neuropathy may also complicate cis-platin therapy. Myelosuppression is usually mild, which can be an advantage in patients who are receiving or who have received myelotoxic drugs.

Diaziquone

Diaziquone (AZQ) is a lipid-soluble CCNS drug with a molecular weight of 364. It probably acts as an alkylating agent, although its exact mechanism of action is unclear. It freely crosses the blood-brain barrier and has been shown to have significant antitumor activity against a variety of intracerebral tumors in animals. Preliminary studies indicate that myelosuppression is its major dose-limiting toxic effect.

Hydroxyurea

Hydroxyurea (HU) is a water-soluble CCS drug with a molecular weight of 76. It interferes with DNA synthesis by inhibiting the enzyme ribonucleoside diphosphate reductase. This enzyme catalyzes the conversion of ribonucleotides to deoxyribonucleotides, a process which is necessary for DNA synthesis. In experimental systems, hydroxyurea has been shown to potentiate radiation damage. It readily crosses the blood-brain barrier and is excreted in the urine. Myelosuppression is its major dose-limiting toxic effect.

VM-26

VM-26 is a lipid-soluble CCS agent with a molecular weight of 656. Its parent compound, podophyllotoxin, binds to tubulin and inhibits microtubule assembly, but the exact mechanism of action of VM-26 remains uncertain. It has no discernable effect on microtubule assembly and arrests cells in G2 rather than in mitosis. Despite its high lipid solubility, VM-26 penetrates poorly into the CNS, probably because of extensive protein binding. The primary route of eliminiation of the drug is metabolic. Leukopenia is its dose-limiting toxic effect. Nausea and vomiting, thrombocytopenia, and peripheral neuropathy may occur but are usually mild in degree.

Vincristine

Vincristine (VCR) is a water-soluble CCS agent with a molecular weight of 923. It acts as a mitotic spindle poison, resulting in metaphase arrest. Vincristine is administered intravenously, metabolized in the liver, and excreted via the biliary and gastrointestinal tracts. Under normal circumstances the drug does not cross the blood-brain barrier to any significant extent. Sensory-motor and autonomic neuropathies are usually the dose-limiting toxic effects of vincristine, and the bone marrow is relatively spared.

Chemotherapy of Anaplastic Gliomas

Anaplastic gliomas are a heterogeneous group of primary malignant brain neoplasms, variously referred to as anaplastic astrocytomas, malignant astrocytomas, astrocytomas grades 3 and 4, and glioblastoma multiforme.[3] Also included under this designation are the less common anaplastic oligodendrogliomas, mixed anaplastic gliomas, and gliosarcomas. These are predominantly supratentorial tumors of adults, with a peak incidence in the fifth or sixth decade of life and a slight preponderance in males.

The natural history of the malignant gliomas is remarkably uniform, yet variables independent of treatment significantly influence prognosis. One of the major contributions of the Brain Tumor Study Group (BTSG) of the National Cancer Institute has been the identification of these prognostic variables. Age, duration of symptoms prior to diagnosis, histopathological type, and pretreatment performance status are the most important clinical characteristics influencing outcome. Considering these variables, Walker et al. have identified a favorable-prognosis group in which the expected median survival exceeds 40 months.[30] The design of clinical trials must account for the impact of these factors on results and conclusions.

A partial list of studies of the chemotherapeutic response rates of recurrent malignant gliomas is found in Tables 136-3 and 136-4. Recent studies and studies involving large numbers of patients have been emphasized. In certain instances the results have been edited to permit concentration on anaplastic gliomas, and individual reports should be consulted for details. A number of drugs and drug combinations have produced objective response rates exceeding 20 percent.[6,24,27] These include BCNU, intra-arterial BCNU, high-dose BCNU with autologous bone marrow rescue, CCNU, PCB, CDP, VM-26, AZQ, BCNU plus VCR, BCNU plus PCB, BCNU plus 5-fluorouracil, BCNU plus DAG, CCNU plus VM-26, DAG plus VP-16, CCNU plus PCB plus VCR, and others. In general, response durations rarely exceed 9 months; response rates have been lower in patients previously exposed to chemotherapeutic agents;

and studies in which strict response criteria, especially guidelines with respect to corticosteroid use, have been defined report lower rates of response. Surprisingly, many commonly available chemotherapeutic agents have not been carefully examined for activity against anaplastic glial tumors.

Encouraging results from response studies have led to an analysis of the role of adjuvant chemotherapy in the treatment of patients with anaplastic gliomas. The results of several major studies of adjuvant chemotherapy are summarized in Table 136-5. In most, survival was the therapeutic end point, concurrent randomized controls were used, and at least 5,000 rad were administered to the tumor bed. However, details vary, and the individual reports should be reviewed.

A landmark study was reported by the BTSG in 1978, in which patients were randomized after surgery into one of four arms: no further therapy, BCNU alone, radiotherapy (RT) alone, or RT plus BCNU.[29] These data established unequivocally the benefit of RT in this disease. They also suggested the additional value of BCNU chemotherapy, since the percentage of survivors at 18 months was significantly greater in the group treated with combination therapy than in the group treated with RT alone. Since then, surgery plus RT and BCNU has been considered the standard form of treatment against which new forms of therapy must be compared. Other important observations made in these adjuvant chemotherapy studies include the activity of PCB,[11] the apparent radiosensitizing effect of HU in patients with glioblastoma,[17] and the curious observation that patients in whom CCNU chemotherapy was delayed until the time of clinical recurrence did at least as well as those in whom drug treatment was instituted immediately after diagnosis.[8]

These adjuvant studies are difficult to compare because of different eligibility criteria and because of differences in other forms of therapy, notably radiotherapy. The variable results in the control arms of different studies emphasize this point. Furthermore, many of the earlier studies are difficult to interpret because of the small numbers of patients in each treatment arm and because the importance of non-treatment-related prognostic variables was not appreciated. Clinical trials are now becoming more tightly controlled and their outcomes more rigorously analyzed. Nevertheless, results of these prospective controlled clinical trials support the use of BCNU, CCNU, PCB, or DAG in the management of patients with anaplastic glioma.

A number of additional adjuvant chemotherapy trials are under way in order to examine, among other things, the value of combination chemotherapy using cytotoxic agents that were judged to be effective as single agents in previous adjuvant or response studies. It is likely that currently available drugs will show greater efficacy when used in appropriate combinations or when given by the most effective routes. Although many of these active agents are now commercially available, it is still desirable to refer patients for participation in controlled studies when appropriate so that useful information can be accumulated.

Among the anaplastic gliomas are the malignant brain stem gliomas and the anaplastic ependymomas. An evaluation of chemotherapy in the treatment of these predominantly pediatric tumors is hampered by the small number of

TABLE 136-3 Studies of the Response of Recurrent Anaplastic Gliomas to Single-Agent Chemotherapy

Drug	No. of Patients	% Responding	Response Criteria	Comment	Reference
BCNU	19	37	Clinical improvement	Includes only patients with glial tumors who received at least two courses of chemotherapy	Wilson, 1970*
BCNU	19	47	Clinical improvement	Includes only patients with glial tumors	Walker, 1970*
BCNU, high-dose	11	36	Clinical and CT improvement		Hochberg, 1981*
BCNU, intracarotid	12	58	Clinical improvement with stable or decreasing corticosteroids and no CT deterioration		(20)
CCNU	23	22	Clinical improvement unrelated to corticosteroids	No responders among eight patients previously exposed to BCNU	Fewer, 1972*
CCNU	27	29	Clinical improvement for at least 6 weeks off corticosteroids		EORTC, 1978*
CCNU	12	25	As in EORTC, 1978	Includes only patients receiving at least two courses of treatment; three additional patients stabilized	(7)
CCNU or BCNU	55	7	Clinical improvement off corticosteroids		(2)
PCB	25	32	Clinical and brain scan improvement with stable or decreasing corticosteroids		Kumar, 1974*
cis-DDP	7	29	Clinical and CT improvement	Children	(14)
cis-DDP, intracarotid	11	55	Clinical or CT improvement	CNS and retinal toxicity	(28)
VM-26	10	20	Clinical and radiographic improvement		Spremulli, 1980*
VM-26	20	35	Clinical or CT improvement		Gerosa, 1981*
AZQ	15	20	Clinical and improvement on stable or decreasing corticosteroids		(26)
DDMP	29	3	Neurological improvement lasting 6 weeks off corticosteroids		(7)
Methotrexate, high-dose	6	0	Not stated	Severe toxicity	Shapiro, 1977*
Thio-TEPA	12	0	Improvement in two of: neurological examination, brain scan, or CT	Three patients with stable disease	Edwards, 1979*

*References may be found in Reference 24.

TABLE 136-4 Studies of the Response of Recurrent Anaplastic Gliomas to Multiple-Agent Chemotherapy

Drugs	No. of Patients	% Responding	Response Criteria	Comment	Reference
BCNU, VCR	19	37	Clinical improvement unrelated to corticosteroids		Fewer, 1972*
BCNU, PCB	45	29	Clinical and brain scan improvement with stable or decreasing corticosteroids		Levin, 1976*
BCNU, 5-FU	29	31	Improvement in two of: neurological examination, brain scan or CT on stable or decreasing corticosteroids	Includes only patients completing two courses of therapy. An additional 15 patients had stable disease	Levin, 1978*
BCNU, DAG	17	53	Clinical and CT improvement with stable or decreasing corticosteroids		(5)
CCNU, PCB, VCR	46	26	As in Levin, 1978		Levin, 1980*
CCNU, PCB, VCR	30	40	As in Levin, 1976		Gutin, 1975*
CCNU, VM-26	20	55	Clinical improvement and stable CT with decreasing corticosteroids		Seiler, 1979*
CCNU, VM-26	15	20	Clinical improvement for at least 6 weeks off corticosteroids	Includes only patients receiving at least two courses. In five other patients progressive disease stabilized.	(8)
meCCNU, PCB, VCR	28	32	Clinical and either CT or brain scan improvement off corticosteroids	No prior radiation	Avellanosa, 1979*
DAG, VP-16	15	40	As in (5)	Median age = 35 years	Eagan, 1981*
DAG, VP-16, Triazinate	15	33	As in (5)	Median age = 35 years	Eagan, 1981

*References may be found in Reference 24.

TABLE 136-5 Studies of the Adjuvant Chemotherapy of Anaplastic Gliomas

Treatment	No. of Patients	Median Survival	Comment	Reference
RT, BCNU	124	50 weeks	Survival figures are for valid study group. BCNU, PCB arms both significantly better than methyl-prednisolone alone. RT = 6000 rad.	(11)
RT, methylprednisolone	141	40 weeks		
RT, PCB	128	47 weeks		
RT, BCNU, methylprednisolone	134	41 weeks		
No further treatment	38	5.2 months	RT = 4500 rad; Bleomycin ineffective.	(16)
RT	35	10.8 months		
RT, bleomycin	45	10.8 months		
RT	55	30.7 weeks	Figures indicate time to tumor progression. No significant difference. RT = 5500–6000 rad.	(8)
RT, VM-26, CCNU	61	39.0 weeks		
RT	94	36 weeks	Survival figures are for "valid study group." RT, BCNU not significantly better than RT alone. meCCNU alone significantly worse than other arms. RT = 6000 rad.	(30)
meCCNU	81	24 weeks		
RT, BCNU	92	51 weeks		
RT	50	~ 9 months	No significant differences RT = 5000 rad.	Cianfriglia, 1980*
CCNU	27	~ 9 months		
RT, CCNU	26	~12 months		
RT, BCNU } Glioblastoma	26	31 weeks	Figures indicate time to tumor progression. Differences significant for glioblastoma, but not for malignant glioma. RT = 6000 rad.	(17)
RT, HU, BCNU } Glioblastoma	36	42 weeks		
RT, BCNU } Malignant	20	73 weeks		
RT, HU, BCNU } glioma	17	50 weeks		
RT	20	35 weeks	$p = 0.002$; RT = 5000 rad.	Eagan, 1979*
RT, DAG	22	67 weeks		
RT	32	10.5 months	RT, CCNU significantly better than RT alone ($p = 0.03$). RT = 5000 rad.	Solero, 1979*
RT, BCNU	34	12.0 months		
RT, CCNU	36	16.0 months		
No further treatment	31	14.0 weeks	Survival figures for valid study group. RT vs. no further treatment, $p = 0.001$.	Walker 1978*
RT	68	36.0 weeks		
BCNU	51	18.5 weeks		
RT, BCNU	72	34.5 weeks	RT vs. RT, BCNU—no difference in median survival, but more long-term survivors in RT, BCNU arm ($p < 0.01$). RT = 5000–6000 rad.	
RT	13	21.5 weeks	"Poor risk" patients. $p = 0.01$. RT = 5500–6000 rad.	EORTC, 1978*
RT, CCNU	10	31.0 weeks		
RT, CCNU	42	43 weeks	Favorable prognosis patients. $p = 0.07$. RT = 5500–6000 rad.	EORTC, 1978*
RT, delayed CCNU	39	62 weeks		
RT	15	27 weeks	RT = 4000–4500 rad.	Weir 1976*
CCNU	13	37 weeks	No significant differences.	
RT, CCNU	13	36 weeks		
RT	22	11.5 months	CCNU alone significantly worse ($p = 0.02$). RT vs. RT, CCNU—no significant difference. RT = 5000 rad.	Reagan, 1976*
CCNU	22	6.6 months		
RT, CCNU	19	12.0 months		

*References may be found in Reference 24.

RT = radiation therapy.

patients in any one center and by the absence of a tissue diagnosis in many patients with intrinsic brain stem neoplasms. A variety of single agents and combinations of agents have been used in conjunction with radiotherapy or at the time of tumor progression, and although occasional responses have been described, the role of chemotherapy remains uncertain. Radiotherapy is unquestionably of benefit in the treatment of patients with anaplastic ependymomas, and the tendency for this tumor to seed the subarachnoid space has led to whole neuraxis irradiation following surgical removal. At the present time there is no defined role for

chemotherapy in the management of patients with anaplastic ependymomas.

Chemotherapy of Other Primary Brain Tumors

Perhaps one-third of all primary glial tumors of adults and children are histologically benign. Treatment of these lesions varies among centers but usually includes surgical removal followed by cranial irradiation. The role of chemotherapy in the treatment of these diseases has not been addressed. Since patients with low-grade gliomas may live for many years following conventional treatment, the toxicity and potential long-range complications of cytotoxic agents weigh heavily against their use.

Medulloblastoma is the most common primary malignant CNS tumor of childhood. Conventional treatment includes surgical resection followed by whole neuraxis irradiation. The latter is recommended because of the propensity for this tumor to spread throughout the subarachnoid space. Using this approach, prolonged control of the disease is accomplished in approximately 25 percent of the patients. Relapse usually occurs at the primary site, although occasionally leptomeningeal or systemic metastases are the first indication of tumor recurrence. Until recently, chemotherapy has been reserved for patients with evidence of recurrent or progressive disease. In this setting, response rates of over 50 percent have been achieved for varying periods of time in small series of patients (median duration of response: 6 to 18 months). A number of cytotoxic agents have been used, alone or in combination, including procarbazine, CCNU, vincristine, and methotrexate. Methotrexate has been administered intravenously or into the subarachnoid space via either the lumbar or intraventricular routes. Adjuvant chemotherapy of medulloblastoma is currently being evaluated. A European study, conducted by the International Society of Pediatric Oncology (SIOP), compares conventional radiotherapy with conventional radiotherapy plus CCNU and vincristine. Significantly longer disease-free survival has been observed in the chemotherapy group, although results are still preliminary. In contrast, the Children's Cancer Study Group has compared conventional radiotherapy with radiotherapy plus adjuvant vincristine, CCNU, and prednisone, and no significant differences in disease-free survival have been found. These conflicting results require clarification before adjuvant chemotherapy can be routinely recommended for patients with medulloblastoma. A problem with chemotherapy for this tumor is the limited bone marrow reserve following whole neuraxis irradiation, so that irradiation of the tumor bed alone followed by vigorous chemotherapy might be an alternative if active drugs become available. Attention to prognostic factors, including patient age and the extent of disease following surgery, should play an important role in treatment planning and in design of future studies.

The pineal region tumors are a heterogeneous group of neoplasms that are often indistinguishable from one another on clinical grounds and that may be difficult to biopsy or remove. Astrocytomas, germinomas, and teratomas are the most common pineal region neoplasms, and true neoplasms of pineal cells are rare. At times, these tumors can be distinguished on the basis of CSF tumor markers or CSF cytology. Although pineal region tumors may seed the subarachnoid space, the necessity for whole neuraxis radiation is debated. At the present time, adjuvant chemotherapy in patients with pineal region tumors of unknown histological type cannot be recommended. Rational chemotherapeutic approaches to the treatment of recurrent tumors of known histology are possible, however. CNS germinomas should respond to agents, such as cis-platinum, that are active against gonadal cell tumors, and this has been demonstrated in individual cases.

Other primary malignant CNS neoplasms such as meningeal sarcomas and malignant meningiomas are sufficiently rare that guidelines with respect to the chemotherapy of recurrent disease are wanting.

Therapeutic Sensitivity Testing

One of the major problems in the chemotherapy of human cancer is our limited ability to design treatments for individual patients. Sensitivity testing of individual tumors is in its infancy, so for the most part therapeutic decisions are based on results in large-scale clinical trials. However, neoplasms of similar origin and histological type are often heterogeneous in their therapeutic sensitivity, and it would be very desirable to choose agents based on a tumor's measured drug sensitivity profile. Since currently available antineoplastic agents appear to inhibit the growth of only a minority of anaplastic brain tumors, a rational method of choosing a particular drug for a particular patient and tumor would be a major advance.

In Vitro Chemosensitivity

There has been considerable interest recently in the development of an in vitro assay of therapeutic sensitivity of individual tumors.[13] These assays are based on the presumption that the clonogenic or stem cells that grow in soft agar represent the proliferative cells of a neoplasm and that their sensitivity to agents in vitro will parallel the clinical response of the parent tumor. The assays have largely been used for drug screening, but some promising studies of their direct clinical application have been reported.[23] The studies are limited by the extremely low clonogenicity of most human tumors and by the difficulty of transferring in vitro pharmacologic data into an in vivo setting.

Little information in this regard is available for human brain tumors. Both Rosenblum et al.[22] and Kornblith et al.[15] have developed in vitro chemosensitivity assays using glioma cells, and they have found a correlation between the in vitro response (or lack of response) to BCNU and the response of the tumor in situ to the same agent. Although this observation is important, clonogenicity is less than 1 percent even with the most anaplastic tumors, and the assays are subject to a number of technical factors. Their general applicability is therefore uncertain. Although this work may be important for an appreciation of the biological basis of drug sensitivity and resistance in these tumors, neither group of investigators has used the assays to design therapy for individual patients.

Human Tumor Xenografts

A number of laboratories have now reported successful transplantation of human neoplasms into congenitally or artificially immunosuppressed animals. Anaplastic brain tumors take especially well after heterotransplantation into congenitally athymic mice, and a number of these transplanted tumor lines have been used for therapeutic studies.[25] In general, drugs that show some clinical activity against human brain tumors show efficacy against the transplanted tumors, and such tumor lines are now being used to evaluate new agents in the preclinical stage of development. Used in this manner, an athymic mouse system has considerable potential as a secondary screen for possible new agents.[1] However, xenografted brain tumors usually require many months before therapy can be evaluated, and so far this prolonged latency has limited any attempts to use these animals in order to design therapy for individual patients.

Drug Toxicity and Patient Acceptance

Most chemotherapeutic agents are potent cell poisons that produce toxic effects on normal tissues. In general, toxicity is most prominent in rapidly proliferating tissues, such as gut and bone marrow, but some agents produce distinctive organ toxicity. The neuropathy of the vinca alkaloids, the nephropathy from cisplatin, and pulmonary fibrosis from BCNU are notable examples among the agents used in brain tumor chemotherapy. These complications are usually preventable and may be reversible, and given the overall circumstances, the potential benefits outweigh the risks. However, in patients treated for longer periods, unexpected side effects may appear and must be monitored. Finally, other considerations being equal, patient acceptance is improved by oral rather than parenteral medications and by infrequent treatments. Acceptance of any treatment program will also be enhanced by an open explanation of therapeutic options and expectations, as well as of possible adverse effects.

References

1. Bellett RE, Danna V, Mastrangelo MJ, Berd D: Evaluation of a "nude" mouse-human tumor panel as a predictive secondary screen for cancer chemotherapeutic agents. JNCI 63:1185–1188, 1979.
2. Bloom HJG: Intracranial tumors: Response and resistance to therapeutic endeavors, 1970–1980. Int J Radiat Oncol Biol Phys 8:1083–1113, 1982.
3. Burger PC: Gliomas: Pathology. Chapter 63, this textbook.
4. DeVita VT, Schein PS: The use of drugs in combination for the treatment of cancer: Rationale and results. N Engl J Med 288:998–1006, 1973.
5. Eagan RT, Dinapoli RP, Hermann RC Jr, Groover RV, Layton DD Jr, Scott M: Combination carmustine (BCNU) and dianhydrogalactitol in the treatment of primary brain tumors recurring after irradiation. Cancer Treat Rep 66:1647–1649, 1982.
6. Edwards MS, Levin VA, Wilson CB: Brain tumor chemotherapy: An evaluation of agents in current use for phase II and III trials. Cancer Treat Rep 64:1179–1205, 1980.
7. European Organization for Research on Treatment of Cancer (EORTC) Brain Tumor Group: Effect of DDMP (2,4-Diamino-5-3',4'-dichlorophenyl-6-methylpyrimidine) on brain gliomas—a phase II study. Eur J Cancer Clin Oncol 16:1639–1640, 1980.
8. European Organization for Research on Treatment of Cancer (EORTC) Brain Tumor Group: Evaluation of CCNU, VM-26 plus CCNU, and procarbazine in supratentorial brain gliomas: Final evaluation of a randomized study. J Neurosurg 55:27–31, 1981.
9. Frei E III, Canellos GP: Dose: A critical factor in cancer chemotherapy. Am J Med 69:585–594, 1980.
10. Goldin A, Venditti JM: The new NCI screen and its implications for clinical evaluation. Recent Results Cancer Res 70:5–20, 1980.
11. Green SB, Byar DP, Walker MD, Pistenma DA, Alexander E Jr, Batzdorf U: Comparison of carmustine, procarbazine, and high-dose methylprednisolone as additions to surgery and radiotherapy for the treatment of malignant glioma. Cancer Treat Rep 67:121–132, 1983.
12. Groothuis DR, Molnar P, Blasberg RG: Regional blood flow and blood-to-tissue transport in five brain tumor models: Implications for chemotherapy, in Rosenblum M, Wilson CB (eds): Progress in Experimental Brain Tumor Research. New York, S Karger, In press.
13. Hamburger AW, Salmon SE: Primary bioassay of human tumor stem cells. Science 197:461–463, 1977.
14. Khan AB, D'Souza BJ, Wharam MD, Champion LAA, Sinks LF, Woo SY, McCullough DC, Leventhal BG: Cisplatin therapy in recurrent childhood brain tumors. Cancer Treat Rep 66:2013–2020, 1982.
15. Kornblith PL, Smith BH, Leonard LA: Response of cultured human brain tumors to nitrosoureas: Correlation with clinical data. Cancer 47:255–265, 1981.
16. Kristiansen K, Hagen S, Kollevold T, Torvik A, Holme I, Nesbakken R, Hatlevall R, Lindgren M, Brun A, Lindgren S, Notter G, Andersen AP, Elgen K: Combined modality therapy of operated astrocytomas grade III and IV: Confirmation of the value of postoperative irradiation and lack of potentiation of bleomycin on survival time: A prospective multicenter trial of the Scandanavian Glioblastoma Study Group. Cancer 47:649–652, 1981.
17. Levin VA, Wilson CB, Davis R, Wara WM, Pischer TL, Irwin L: A phase III comparison of BCNU, hydroxyurea, and radiation therapy to BCNU and radiation therapy for the treatment of primary malignant gliomas. J Neurosurg 51:526–532, 1979.
18. Omojola MF, Fox AJ, Auer RN, Viñuela FV: Hemorrhagic encephalitis produced by selective non-occlusive intracarotid BCNU injection in dogs. J Neurosurg 57:791–796, 1982.
19. Owens G: Intraarterial chemotherapy of primary brain tumors. Ann N Y Acad Sci 159:603–607, 1969.
20. Pruitt A, Hochberg FH, Grossman R, Davis K: Intracarotid BCNU therapy for recurrent glioblastomas: A phase II dose escalation study in 12 patients. In press.
21. Rall DP, Zubrod CG: Mechanisms of drug absorption and excretion: Passage of drugs in and out of the central nervous system. Annu Rev Pharmacol Toxicol 2:109–128, 1962.
22. Rosenblum ML, Gerosa MA, Wilson CB, Barger GR, Pertuiset BF, de Tribolet N, Dougherty DV: Stem cell studies of human malignant brain tumors. Part 1: Development of the stem cell assay and its potential. J Neurosurg 58:170–176, 1983.
23. Salmon SE, Hamburger AW, Soehnlen B, Durie BGM, Alberts DS, Moon TE: Quantitation of differential sensitivity of human-tumor stem cells to anticancer drugs. N Engl J Med 298:1321–1327, 1978.
24. Schold SC Jr: Chemotherapy of primary central nervous system neoplasms. Semin Neurol 1:189–201, 1981.
25. Schold SC Jr, Bullard DE, Bigner SH, Jones TR, Bigner DD: Growth, morphology, and serial transplantation of anaplastic human gliomas in athymic mice. J Neuro-Oncol 1:5–14, 1983.
26. Schold SC, Friedman HS, Bjornssen TD, Falletta JM: Treatment of recurrent anaplastic brain tumors with diaziquone (AZQ, NSC-182986). Neurology 33 (Suppl 2): 108–109, 1983 (abstr).
27. Shapiro WR: Treatment of neuroectodermal brain tumors. Ann Neurol 12:231–237, 1982.
28. Stewart DJ, Wallace S, Feun L, Leavens M, Young SE, Handel S, Mavligit G, Benjamin RS: A phase I study of intracarotid

artery infusion of *cis*-diaminedichloroplatinum(II) in patients with recurrent malignant intracerebral tumors. Cancer Res 42:2059–2062, 1982.

29. Walker MD, Alexander E Jr, Hunt WE, MacCarty CS, Mahaley MS Jr, Mealey J Jr, Norrell HA, Owens G, Ransohoff J, Wilson CB, Gehan EA: Evaluation of BCNU and/or radiother-

apy in the treatment of anaplastic gliomas: A cooperative clinical trial. J Neurosurg 49:333–343, 1978.

30. Walker MD, Green SB, Byar DP, et al: Randomized comparisons of radiotherapy and nitrosoureas for the treatment of malignant glioma after surgery. N Engl J Med 303:1323–1329, 1980.

137

Blood-Brain Barrier Modification in Delivery of Antitumor Agents

Edward A. Neuwelt

Several types of disseminated systemic malignancies have demonstrated significant and complete responses to chemotherapy.[2,31] It is noteworthy that when these same (responsive) neoplasms are identified as having metastatic foci in the CNS, the efficacy of systemic chemotherapy on the CNS tumors has been minimal.[31] Compared with treatment of extraneural cancers, the treatment of primary CNS tumors with systemic or intrathecal chemotherapy has resulted in only modest efficacy.

The presence of the blood-brain barrier (BBB) probably partially accounts for the therapeutic ineffectiveness of systemically administered drugs used in the treatment of CNS tumors. This hypothesis proposes that an intact or partially intact BBB is often present in both primary and metastatic CNS tumors, thus inhibiting adequate drug penetration. In this discussion, I shall consider the characteristics of the BBB and examine how it can be modified by osmotic treatment, as originally described by Scandinavian radiologists who were evaluating hypertonic contrast agents used in cerebral angiography.[5] The efficacy of multiagent chemother-

apy when combined with osmotic BBB opening will also be discussed.

Limitation of Drug Delivery by the Blood-Brain Barrier

The BBB is created by tight junctions (*zonulae occludentes*) between endothelial cells in brain capillaries. Diffusion between endothelial cells is restricted at the tight junction. Tight junctions are found where there is physiological evidence of a blood-brain barrier and are absent in the few brain areas that lack a BBB, such as the circumventricular organs.[32]

Vick et al.[41] suggested that "the blood-brain barrier is not a factor in the chemotherapy of brain tumors," because of observations that blood vessels within primary and metastatic cerebral tumors have a fenestrated, discontinuous endothelium.[13] Contrary to this suggestion, brain tumors often have regions in which the BBB is partially or wholly intact. Methotrexate (MTX) uptake by intracerebral ependymoblastomas in mice is much greater at the tumor center than at its edge or in the adjacent brain, indicating a gradient in BBB permeability from the tumor center to the edge.[12,40] In experimental tumors, variable BBB disruption (and in some small tumors, no disruption at all) was demonstrated in studies using intravascular horseradish peroxidase or [^{14}C]α-aminoisobutyric acid as markers.[9,39] Walker and Weiss proposed that a "sink effect" might also contribute to the low drug concentration at the tumor periphery; extra drug that enters the periphery could rapidly diffuse into drug-free surrounding brain because of "mild disruption" or absent BBB disruption.[42]

Previously, two approaches have been utilized to enhance drug delivery to CNS neoplasms. Because most chemotherapeutic agents, like MTX, normally penetrate into the brain, although poorly, very high systemic doses followed by citrovorum factor rescue have been administered in an attempt to achieve therapeutic levels, but with only limited success.[38,39] In another approach, drugs are instilled into the ventricular and subarachnoid spaces. However, when the brain penetration of MTX was examined in monkeys following intraventricular injection, therapeutic levels were not found in the white matter deep to the cortex or ependyma.[11] Uncertain drug dispersal is another problem encountered with intrathecal or intraventricular chemotherapy, especially when there is blockage of the spinal fluid circulation by spinal or supratentorial lesions.

Regulation of Drug Entry into the Brain

A drug's lipid solubility is the most important factor that determines its transfer between the blood and the brain. As demonstrated by Rapoport et al., brain uptake of different drugs is proportional to their octanol/water partition coefficient.[8,37] This is a measure of lipid solubility and thus of the ability of a drug to cross the lipid-containing membranes of the cerebrovascular endothelium. MTX has a pH of 4.7 and is 99.8 percent ionized at a blood pH of 7.4; it is lipid-insoluble and the normal CSF/plasma ratio is only 0.02.[32]

Reversible Modification of the Blood-Brain Barrier

Many different types of insults to the brain can alter BBB permeability.[32] Most cause irreversible BBB disruption or brain damage. Dimethyl sulfoxide and 5-fluorouracil have recently been reported to increase BBB permeability sufficiently to allow their use as adjuncts to increase chemotherapy delivery to the CNS.[4,14] However, we have been unable to open the BBB with either of these agents.[15]

Reversible osmotic BBB modification has been employed successfully in animals and humans to produce therapeutic drug concentrations throughout large brain regions without resulting in long-term brain damage.[10,15-21,23-28,32-37] In this method, a hypertonic solution of a sugar such as arabinose or mannitol is infused for up to 30 s through a major artery of the cerebral circulation. Tracer studies and drug assays indicate that BBB permeability is then increased to poorly permeable agents, such as adriamycin,[27] sucrose,[36] or MTX,[26,28] by 10- to 15-fold. By using electron microscopic examination with intravascular electron-dense tracers, the ultrastructural basis of osmotic barrier modification has been shown to be an increase in permeability at the tight junctions between cerebrovascular endothelial cells.[3,6]

Production of osmotic BBB modification through intracarotid infusion of a hypertonic solution appears to be an all-or-nothing phenomenon. The threshold in the rat for effective BBB modification using arabinose is 1.6 osmolal and the minimum infusion time is 20 to 30 s.[33] A similar threshold has been observed in other species. The BBB remains open to intravascular Evans blue or to ^{14}C-labeled sucrose for about 30 min to 2 h[25,26,33] and then resumes its normal impermeability, indicating the reversibility of osmotic BBB modification.[25,26,33] In addition, barrier closure is more rapid to large than to small molecules following hypertonic infusion.[17,27,43]

Osmotic BBB disruption appears to be a threshold phenomenon dependent on the rate and duration of infusion. Dilution of the infusate by blood from collateral flow at the circle of Willis will result in a subthreshold osmotic exposure at the cerebral capillary bed.[33] Infusion rates sufficient to wash the blood from the capillary bed of the brain should be approximated by inspecting the exposed cortical surface of the ipsilateral hemisphere during infusion.

Although osmotic BBB opening is reversible and is not followed by any long-term brain injury or measurable functional defects, transient changes have been demonstrated in animals. Glucose consumption is frequently elevated in af-

fected brain regions, as measured by the ^{14}C]2-deoxy-D-glucose technique; despite this, regional cerebral blood flow declines.[30,34] The uncoupling of the normal proportionality between brain metabolism and blood flow probably is associated with a concurrent increase in brain water by 1.0 to 1.5 percent of wet weight. This alteration in brain water, which occurs at the expense of the intravascular volume, may prevent vasodilation and lasts less than 24 h. Hypertonic carotid infusion reduces intraocular pressure and severely damages the ciliary epithelium of the eye in monkeys but not in rats (Rapoport SI: Unpublished observations).[29] There has been no evidence of such ocular damage in humans.[18]

Effects of Adrenocortical Steroids and Osmotic BBB Opening upon Methotrexate Delivery

The effects of adrenocortical steroids and osmotic blood-brain barrier modification upon methotrexate delivery were studied in normal and glioma-bearing rats.[16] In animals with avian sarcoma virus-induced glioma, osmotic blood-brain barrier modification resulted in significantly increased delivery of methotrexate to the tumor-bearing hemisphere (including the tumor, the brain around the tumor, and the brain distant from the tumor) compared to delivery to the nonmodified hemisphere or to either hemisphere in control animals. The administration of adrenal steroids, followed by intracarotid methotrexate, resulted in slightly decreased methotrexate delivery to the tumor, to the brain around the tumor, and to the brain distant from the tumor. When adrenal steroids were given prior to barrier modification and methotrexate therapy, the amount of methotrexate delivered to the tumor was significantly less. These studies provide evidence that the blood-brain barrier exists in tumors and is a factor in drug delivery to tumors. Steroid administration greatly interferes with the enhancement of drug delivery that can be achieved with osmotic blood-brain barrier modification.

Modification of the Blood-Brain Barrier in Dogs

As a model for examining osmotic BBB modification, the dog has several advantages over small rodents.[25,26,32,33] The brain is large enough to be scanned by computed tomography (CT) following intravenous administration of iodinated contrast material, and serial CSF samples can be obtained following BBB opening.

In the initial canine studies, hypertonic (25 percent) mannitol was infused through the common carotid artery, but this resulted in variable BBB opening as determined by transudation of Evans blue given intravenously and by variable blanching of the ipsilateral cerebral cortex.[21] A major technical advance was made by altering the site of infusion. The dog has a small internal carotid artery (2 mm in diameter) located distally just under the mandible and has a large distal external-to-internal carotid circulation. When the distally located internal carotid artery was cannulated, 42 ml of hypertonic fluid infused over 30 s completely and consistently blanched the ipsilateral cerebral cortex in 25-kg mongrel dogs. Following osmotic BBB modification and administration of MTX at 100 mg/kg through the internal carotid artery, MTX levels rose as high as 90,000 ng/g of brain tissue as compared to 1000 ng/g in dogs that were infused with saline rather than hypertonic mannitol. Brain staining with intravascular Evans blue was more pronounced and consistent than that following common carotid artery infusion. MTX levels in CSF more accurately reflected brain levels with the internal carotid infusion method than with the common carotid technique. However, this correlation is not a measurement adequate for use as a parameter in pharmacological planning, since osmotic BBB disruption is a very unreliable method of enhancing drug delivery to the CSF.

Osmotic Blood-Brain Barrier Opening in the Posterior Fossa

Transient, reversible osmotic BBB disruption was produced in the posterior fossa of 33 dogs.[23] A new percutaneous catheter technique, rather than the previous open surgical technique, was used for the infusion of the hypertonic mannitol into the vertebral artery. This method permits repeated regional barrier modification in the same dog. Brain stem function was not altered in most of the experimental animals. The extent of BBB modification approximated that seen in the supratentorial parenchyma after osmotic carotid BBB opening via the internal artery. When 100 mg of MTX was infused into the vertebral circulation of a 25-kg dog, MTX uptake was elevated from about 100 to 300 ng/g to 2000 to 3000 ng/g of brain tissue.

Computed Tomography as a Means of Monitoring Blood-Brain Barrier Opening

The enhanced CT scan has proven useful in dogs and humans in monitoring the location and extent of BBB changes seen with brain tumors and following osmotic treatment. Water-soluble iodinated radiocontrast agents penetrate the BBB very slowly.[25] However, significant quantities can be identified within the brain following BBB modification caused by brain tumor growth or by the osmotic method. Numerical densities (CT numbers) can be calculated and used to quantitate the extent of altered BBB permeability. The CT number is linearly related to tissue iodine content.[7]

CT images in dogs reveal contrast enhancement in brain regions where the barrier was disrupted using hypertonic mannitol.[25] At autopsy, these regions were shown to be stained with Evans blue which had been previously injected intravenously. These are attenuation differences of about 20 CT units between normal and osmotically opened areas on the enhanced CT scan; this corresponds to a 2 percent difference in attenuation relative to water.[25,26]

Effects of Blood-Brain Barrier Modification on Pharmacology and Toxicity of Chemotherapeutic Drugs

The effect of osmotic BBB modification on delivery of adriamycin to the brain was studied in rodents and dogs.[27] Pharmacokinetic and toxicological studies were done in these animals after different doses of adriamycin (0.1 to 1.0 mg/kg) were administered into the internal carotid artery following hypertonic mannitol infusion. Immunoreactive adriamycin was not detected in the cerebrums of the control animals. However, in those animals upon which blood-brain barrier modification was performed, up to 4.5 μg of drug and/or metabolites per gram of brain tissue were detected by radioimmunoassay. Optimum tissue levels of adriamycin and its metabolites were achieved following barrier modification when the drug was administered either by a rapid bolus over 30 s or by slow, continuous infusion (for 15 min).

Up to 6 h after administration, immunoreactive drug could still be identified in the brain. Functional neurotoxicity was evident at all dose levels, even at 0.1 mg/kg, a level at which adriamycin in the brain could not be detected by radioimmunoassay but at which neuropathological examination still revealed necrosis and hemorrhagic infarcts. In animals in which the BBB was opened but no adriamycin was given, and in control animals infused with isotonic NaCl rather than hypertonic mannitol (leaving the BBB intact) followed by the administration of adriamycin, no CNS toxicity or pathological change was observed. These studies indicate that adriamycin and/or its metabolites are very neurotoxic in the brain. More recent studies similar to those with adriamycin indicate that cis-platinum and 5-fluorouracil are also very neurotoxic when allowed into the brain following osmotic treatment. Bleomycin and mitomycin C also have significant toxicity, but cyclophosphamide and methotrexate are fairly well tolerated in the brain.[22]

Delivery of Enzymes and Monoclonal Antibodies Across the Blood-Brain Barrier

Studies have been undertaken to see if hexosaminidase A, the enzyme deficient in Tay-Sachs disease, could be effectively delivered to the brain for replacement therapy.[17] By using the rat model, in which blood-brain barrier modification was followed by radiolabeled enzyme administration, increased hexosaminidase A delivery to the brain was clearly demonstrated. It was found that the time of injection of hexosaminidase A after BBB modification is a critical factor for maximum delivery. Rapid (a 30-s bolus) intra-arterial administration of hexosaminidase A immediately after BBB modification markedly increased enzyme delivery to the brain as compared to delivery in controls without prior BBB opening. Fifty percent less hexosaminidase A was delivered when the enzyme was administered 15 to 20 min after opening, and when given 60 to 120 min after blood-brain barrier modification the amount delivered was the same as in the control animals. This critical time factor is very much different from that seen in trials with low molecular weight chemotherapeutic agents such as methotrexate and adriamycin.

Recent studies have focused on hexosaminidase A delivery into the brain cells after BBB modification and upon the drug's intracellular disposition.[19] An antibody to human hexosaminidase A was developed which did not cross react with the rodent enzyme. With this antibody it was shown that human hexosaminidase A administered via the internal carotid artery after BBB modification was taken up by brain

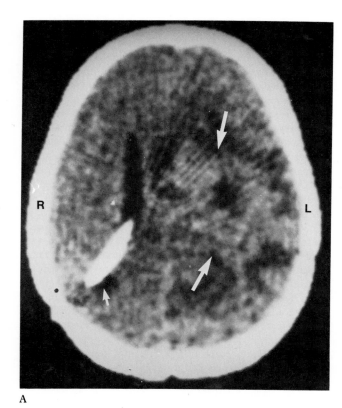

A

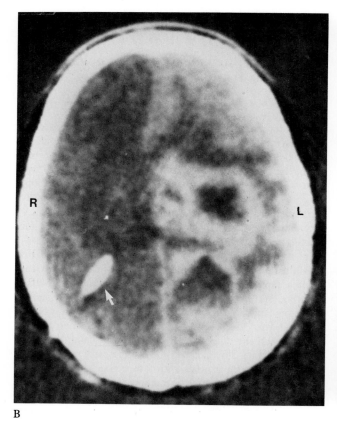

B

C

Figure 137-1 *A.* Enhanced CT scan done 1¼ h after a standard dose of intravenous contrast agent. This is a transverse scan done at the level of the lateral ventricles, and a ventricular catheter can be seen entering the right lateral ventricle (*small arrow*). The large arrows indicate the enhancement due to tumor. There is a surrounding low density due to presence of edema. *B.* Enhanced CT scan after osmotic BBB disruption. It should be noted that there is increased enhancement not only in the region of the tumor, but also in the surrounding brain. There is a low-density region in the center of the tumor which does not enhance, and this probably represents a known cyst. *C.* Enhanced CT scan, after osmotic blood-brain barrier disruption, at the level of the superior cerebellum (*open arrows*) which demonstrates that barrier disruption was also present in the posterior fossa. (From Neuwelt et al.[18])

cells. Latency studies indicated that up to 75 percent of the enzyme that entered the brain (0.2 to 0.5 percent of the total administered dose) was released simultaneously with the ly-

sosomal marker, β-galactosidase. This indicates that human hexosaminidase A is deposited in and remains active within subcellular organelles, possibly lysosomes, after delivery across the BBB. Therefore, enzyme replacement therapy may be a feasible possibility for treating Tay-Sachs disease.[1,17] With regard to brain tumors, these enzyme studies may be applicable in designing a system to deliver tumor-specific monoclonal antibodies across the BBB.

Osmotic Blood-Brain Barrier Opening in Patients with Malignant Brain Tumors

Methotrexate was administered after BBB modification a total of 33 times to 6 patients with different types of brain tumors. No permanent complications were seen.[18] Serial enhanced CT scans and quantification by CT numbers have indicated that the BBB modification increased drug delivery to the tumor and the surrounding brain (Fig. 137-1). Neuroradiological evaluation with radiocontrast agents has demonstrated that the enhancement material persisted in the tumor longer after BBB modification than without modification. MTX levels in cerebrospinal fluid did not correlate with the degree of barrier modification measured by CT and radionuclide scans. In one patient in the series, an anatomical variation in the circle of Willis resulted in barrier modification extending into the posterior fossa without ill effect. Thus, osmotic BBB modification appears to be a nontoxic, reproducible procedure for increasing drug delivery to both malignant brain tumors and surrounding brain parenchyma in humans.

In more recent clinical trials, there has been documented tumor regression in patients with microglioma, medulloblastoma, and glioblastoma.[24] However, there was a significant incidence (about 20 percent) of focal motor and grand mal seizures in these patients following BBB opening with hypertonic mannitol. The seizures could be attributed to the use of meglumine iothalamate, an iodinated contrast agent known to be epileptogenic. An adequate and safer though less sensitive means to monitor barrier modification was employed, using radionuclide brain scanning. Since going to this method of monitoring, we find seizures are much less frequent and indeed rarely seen.

Two patients with primary CNS lymphoma have had complete tumor regression with multiple-agent chemotherapy in association with reversible BBB opening.[20] It is of interest that the extent of the tumor was evident only following BBB modification, thus again clearly demonstrating that some portions of CNS tumors have an effective BBB. These studies also indicate that drug delivery to tumor as well as to the surrounding brain can be augmented by osmotic BBB modification, and that such therapy can result in an objective clinical response. In addition, barrier modification has been carried out in the posterior fossa in one of these patients by mannitol infusion into the vertebral artery, without untoward effects.

References

1. Barranger JA, Rapoport SI, Fredericks WR, Pentcher PG, MacDermot KD, Steusing JK, Brady RO: Modification of the blood-brain barrier: Increased concentration and fate of en-zymes entering the brain. Proc Natl Acad Sci USA 76:481–485, 1978.

2. Benjamin RS, Wiernik PH, Bachur NR: Adriamycin chemotherapy: Efficacy, safety, and pharmacologic basis of an intermittent single high-dosage schedule. Cancer 33:19–27, 1974.

3. Brightman MW, Hori M, Rapoport SI, Reese TS, Westergaard E: Osmotic opening of tight junctions in cerebral endothelium. J Comp Neurol 152:317–325, 1973.

4. Broadwell RD, Salcman M: Expanding the definition of the blood-brain barrier to protein. Proc Natl Acad Sci USA 78:7820–7824, 1981.

5. Broman T, Olsson O: The tolerance of cerebral blood-vessels to a contrast agent of the Diodrast group. Acta Radiol 30:326–342, 1948.

6. Dorovini-Zis K, Sato M, Goping G, Rapoport SI, Brightman M: Ionic lanthanum passage across cerebral endothelium exposed to hyperosmotic arabinose. In press.

7. Drayer BP, Schmeckel DE, Hedlund LW, Lischko MM, Sage MR, Heinz ER, Dubois PT, Goulding PL: Radiographic quantitation of reversible blood-brain barrier disruption in vivo. Radiology 143:85–89, 1982.

8. Fenstermacher JD, Johnson JA: Filtration and reflection coefficients of the rabbit blood-brain barrier. Am J Physiol 211:341–346, 1966.

9. Groothuis DR, Fischer JM, Lapin G, Bigner DD, Vick NA: Permeability of different experimental brain tumor models to horseradish peroxidase. J Neuropathol Exp Neurol 41:164–185, 1982.

10. Hasegawa H, Allen JC, Mehta BM, Shapiro WR, Posner JB: Enhancement of CNS penetration of methotrexate by hyperosmolar intracarotid mannitol or carcinomatous meningitis. Neurology (NY) 29:1280–1286, 1979.

11. Kimelberg HK, King D, Watson RE, Reiss FL, Biddlecome SM, Bourke RS: Direct administration of methotrexate into the central nervous system of primates. Part 1: Distribution and degradation of methotrexate in nervous and systemic tissue after intraventricular injection. J Neurosurg 48:883–894, 1978.

12. Levin VA, Clancy TP, Ausman JI, Rall DP: Uptake and distribution of ^{3}H-methotrexate by the murine ependymoblastoma. JNCI 48:875–883, 1972.

13. Long DM: Capillary ultrastructure in human metastatic brain tumors. J Neurosurg 51:53–58, 1979.

14. MacDonell LA, Potter PE, Leslie RA: Localized changes in blood-brain barrier permeability following the administration of antineoplastic drugs. Cancer Res 38:2930–2934, 1978.

15. Neuwelt EA, Barnett P, Barranger J, McCormick C, Pagel M, Frenkel E: The inability of dimethyl sulfoxide (DMSO) and 5-fluorouracil (5-FU) to open the blood-brain barrier. Neurosurgery 12:29–34, 1983.

16. Neuwelt EA, Barnett PA, Bigner DD, Frenkel EP: Effects of adrenal cortical steroids and osmotic blood-brain barrier opening on methotrexate delivery to gliomas in the rodent: The factor of the blood-brain barrier. Proc Natl Acad Sci USA 79:4420–4423, 1982.

17. Neuwelt EA, Barranger JA, Brady RO, Pagel M, Furbish FS, Quirk JM, Moot GE, Frenkel E: Delivery of hexosaminidase A to the cerebrum after osmotic modification of the blood-brain barrier. Proc Natl Acad Sci USA 78:5838–5841, 1981.

18. Neuwelt EA, Diehl JT, Vu LH, Hill SA, Michael AJ, Frenkel EP: Monitoring of methotrexate delivery in patients with malignant brain tumors after osmotic blood-brain barrier disruption. Ann Intern Med 94:449–454, 1981.

19. Neuwelt EA, Frenkel E, Barranger J, Brady R, Pagel M: Use of antibody to trace hexosaminidase-A activity after blood-brain barrier opening. In press.

20. Neuwelt EA, Frenkel E, Diehl J, Hill S, Balaban E: Successful treatment of primary central nervous system lymphomas (mi-

crogliomas) with chemotherapy after osmotic blood-brain barrier opening. Neurosurgery 12:662–671, 1983.

21. Neuwelt EA, Frenkel EP, Diehl JT, Maravilla KR, Vu LH, Clark WK, Rapoport SI, Barnett PA, Hill SA, Lewis SE, Ehle AL, Beyer CW Jr, Moore RJ: Osmotic blood-brain barrier disruption: A new means of increasing chemotherapeutic agent delivery. Trans Am Neurol Assoc 104:256–260, 1979.

22. Neuwelt EA, Glasberg M, Barnett P: The neuropathologic effects of chemotherapy administered after osmotic brain barrier modification. Ann Neurol 14:316–324, 1983.

23. Neuwelt EA, Glasberg M, Diehl J, Frenkel EP, Barnett P: Osmotic blood-brain barrier disruption in the posterior fossa of the dog. J Neurosurg 55:742–748, 1981.

24. Neuwelt EA, Howieson J, Specht D, Haynes J, Bennett M, Hill S: Comparison of enhanced computerized tomography and radionuclide brain scan to monitor osmotic blood-brain barrier disruption. AJR 147:829–836, 1983.

25. Neuwelt EA, Maravilla KR, Frenkel EP, Barnett P, Hill S, Moore RJ: The use of enhanced computerized tomography to evaluate osmotic blood-brain barrier disruption. Neurosurgery 6:49–56, 1980.

26. Neuwelt EA, Maravilla KR, Frenkel EP, Rapoport SI, Hill SA, Barnett P: Osmotic blood-brain barrier disruption: Computerized tomographic monitoring of chemotherapeutic agent delivery. J Clin Invest 64:684–688, 1979.

27. Neuwelt EA, Pagel M, Barnett P, Glasberg M, Frenkel EP: Pharmacology and toxicity of intracarotid adriamycin administration following osmotic blood-brain barrier modification. Cancer Res 41:4466–4470, 1981.

28. Ohno K, Fredericks WR, Rapoport SI: Osmotic opening of the blood-brain barrier to methotrexate in the rat. Surg Neurol 12:323–328, 1979.

29. Okisaka S, Kuwabara T, Rapoport SI: Selective destruction of the pigmented epithelium in the ciliary body of the eye. Science 184:1298–1299, 1974.

30. Pappius HM, Savaki HE, Fieschi C, Rapoport SI, Sokoloff L: Osmotic opening of the blood-brain barrier and local cerebral glucose utilization. Ann Neurol 5:211–219, 1979.

31. Posner JB: Management of central nervous system metastases. Semin Oncol 4:81–91, 1977.

32. Rapoport SI: *Blood-Brain Barrier in Physiology and Medicine.* New York, Raven Press, 1976.

33. Rapoport SI, Fredericks WR, Ohno K, Pettigrew KD: Quantitative aspects of reversible osmotic opening of the blood-brain barrier. Am J Physiol 238:R421–R431, 1980.

34. Rapoport SI, London ED, Fredericks WR, Dow-Edwards DL, Mahone PR: Altered cerebral glucose utilization following blood-brain barrier opening by hypertonicity or hypertension. Exp Neurol 74:519–529, 1981.

35. Rapoport SI, Matthews K, Thompson HK, Pettigrew KD: Osmotic opening of the blood-brain barrier in the rhesus monkey without measurable brain edema. Brain Res 136:23–29, 1977.

36. Rapoport SI, Ohno K, Fredericks WR, Pettigrew KD: Regional cerebrovascular permeability to ^{14}sucrose after osmotic opening of the blood-brain barrier. Brain Res 150:653–657, 1978.

37. Rapoport SI, Ohno K, Pettigrew KD: Drug entry into the brain. Brain Res 172:354–359, 1979.

38. Rosen G, Ghavimi F, Nirenberg A, Mosende C, Mehta BM: High-dose methotrexate with citrovorum factor rescue for the treatment of central nervous system tumors in children. Cancer Treat Rep 61:681–690, 1977.

39. Shapiro WR, Mehta B, Blasberg RG, Patlak CS, Kobayashi T, Allen JC: Pharmaco-dynamics of entry of methotrexate into brain of humans, monkeys and a rat brain tumor model, in Paoletti P, Walker MD, Butti G, Knerich R (eds): *Multidisciplinary Aspects of Brain Tumor Therapy.* Amsterdam, Elsevier North-Holland, 1979, pp 135–142.

40. Tator CH: Chemotherapy of brain tumors: Uptake of tritiated methotrexate by a transplantable intracerebral ependymoblastoma in mice. J Neurosurg 37:1–8, 1972.

41. Vick NA, Khand-ekar JD, Bigner DD: Chemotherapy of brain tumors: The "blood-brain barrier" is not a factor. Arch Neurol 34:523–526, 1977.

42. Walker MD, Weiss HD: Chemotherapy in the treatment of malignant brain tumors. Adv Neurol 13:149–191, 1975.

43. Ziylan YZ, Robinson PJ, Rapoport SI: Permeability of the blood-brain barrier to macromolecules of different size after osmotic opening. Fed Proc 41:1763, 1982 (abstr).

138

Hyperthermia in the Treatment of Intracranial Tumors

Robert G. Selker

The currently best accepted therapy for glioblastoma provides a median survival period of approximately 55 weeks.[23] Attempts to increase survival time by expanding the limits of current therapy (surgery, radiation, chemotherapy) result in an increase in morbidity and a decrease in overall quality of life. Clearly, one cannot resect the thalamus, the brain stem, the corpus callosum, or the majority of the dominant hemisphere and expect a reasonably functional result. Similarly, radiation dose levels above 6500 rad may result in damage of normal tissue, especially when given as a total head dose. If radiation is confined to the tumor bed plus a 2-cm border (the area of recurrence), viability of surrounding normal tissue still remains an important consideration.[5] Whereas experimentally, cell kill rates may be increased with increasing levels of chemotherapy, systemic toxicity precludes that level of use in the human. Immunotherapy, be it active or passive, specific or nonspecific, cannot control (at least at present) large tumor burdens. Hence, the need for a modality to enhance the effectiveness of currently employed agents, hopefully utilizing inherent biological differences between normal and abnormal tissue to control tumor growth and increase the quality of survival. Such a modality may be hyperthermia.

Before the turn of the century, Coley published a report on the use of a toxin derived from a strain of streptococcus, which, when injected into malignancies of the head and neck, produced fever, chills, and a remarkable reduction in tumor size.[2] Why this occurred remains a subject of much debate. Was the remission, in fact, related to the degree of body temperature elevation? Possibly; patients not experiencing a febrile response seemed destined not to demonstrate a tumor response. Was the beneficial effect of the toxin related to a nonspecific immune response on the part of the host, with invasion of the area by lymphocytes and macrophages? Or, in fact, did this local effect on malignant cells represent suppuration with subsequent cell destruction?

In vitro experiments and some clinical data suggest that the febrile response is important, as evidenced by the relationship of cell kill rates to the degree of temperature elevation and the length of time of application; and that these factors are inversely proportional (i.e., the higher the temperature, the less time required to achieve cell kill) (Fig. 138-1). Furthermore, experimental evidence[19] suggests a synergistic effect when heat is combined with radiation therapy, yielding a therapeutic enhancement ratio (TER), where TER = rad dose/rad dose + heat.

If, then, this combined modality synergism can be demonstrated to occur in tumor tissue, it is proper to inquire as to the effect on surrounding normal tissue. Would, for instance, a differential effect on normal verses abnormal tissue therapeutic gain factor (TGF), where TGF = TER of tumor/TER of normal tissue, subsequently accrue? In point

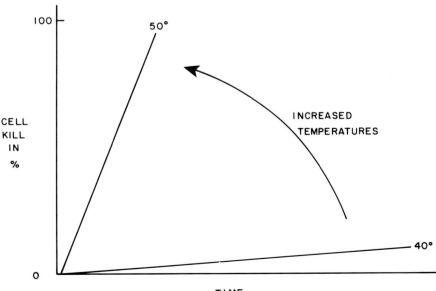

Figure 138-1 Relationship of time and temperature to cell kill rate.

of fact, it would appear that if two modalities (heat and radiation) are delivered simultaneously, a major therapeutic enhancement does occur, but without a normal tissue differential. Hence, the modalities may need to be separated temporally. Which modality (in the case of radiation and heat) is best delivered first remains a matter of conjecture, although most investigators favor a preheating radiation dosage schedule. It must be concluded, then, that an increase in the TER when modalities are employed simultaneously may be achieved at the expense of the TGF (Fig. 138-2). The higher the TGF, the less damage to normal tissue there will be, presumably with less tumor effect as well. The key to success lies in the differential rates of metabolism and DNA repair in normal versus tumor cells.

A similar enhancement effect has been demonstrated in rats when elevated body temperatures are employed with 1, 3-bis(2-chloroethyl)-1-nitrosourea (BCNU), bleomycin, adriamycin, 5-fluorouracil, and methotrexate.[4,5,13] These reports support a therapeutic enhancement ratio of approximately 2, perhaps mandating up to a 50 percent reduction in drug dosage to avoid untoward toxicity. Our own clinical experience, using 75 percent of the usual calculated dose per square meter of body surface and greater than 450°/min of total-body heat, confirms this previously published experimental expectation.[13] (See later explanation of degree/minutes.)

The laboratory evidence is now sufficient to allow the clinical introduction of hyperthermia as an adjuvant to existing treatment modalities. But how should the new tool be applied? How can its possible toxicity be controlled and its potential enhanced? Should it be applied locally, regionally, or as a total body effort? What standard units of dosimetry are applicable? How can these modalities be combined in a hospital setting? Does repeated heating of tumor cells create thermal tolerance and/or resistant mutants in humans? These and other perplexing questions remain only partially answered, creating a technological and biological dilemma.

Methodology

Local Intratumoral Hyperthermia

In many ways the brain tumor lends itself admirably to the application of local intratumoral heating. The glioblastoma is, in most instances, a local infiltrating disease supplied by a well-defined vascular perfusion bed which can be diagnostically imaged by a number of methods. Blood flow within the tumor is, as a rule, slower than in surrounding normal tissue, thereby creating a "heat sink" of poorly dissipated energy. By employing newly advanced microwave, ultrasound, and radio-frequency techniques (some requiring indwelling antennae), temperatures in the range of 45° to 50°C can be produced and monitored by specifically designed thermocouples which do not participate in the created energy field.[12,14,15,20-22] In effect, the physician is committed to heating a geometric volume of tissue which may contain normal and abnormal tissue as well as varying degrees of necrotic central tissue (making uniform intratumoral heating difficult) and yet may not contain an extension of tumor tissue beyond the volume of heating. Some recent work indicates the possibility of a differential effect on normal and abnormal tissue within a heated geometric volume that is subjected to the newer energy sources.[17,21] If this is the case, a major advance in local heating technology will have been made.

Methods of applying local heat energy to the exact con-

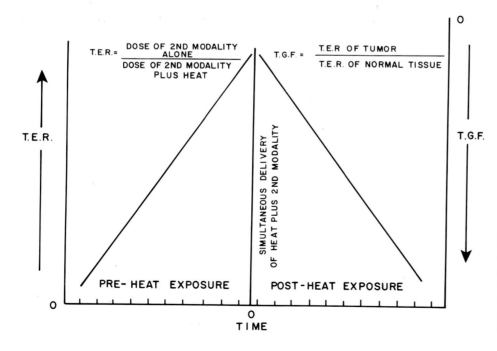

Figure 138-2 Enhancement of a second modality when employed with heat. Presumed effects on therapeutic enhancement ratio (T.E.R.) and therapeutic gain factor (T.G.F.).

fines of the tumor disclosed on computed tomographic (CT) images are currently undergoing study. Since there is often extension of tumor to the opposite hemisphere and a 2-cm border area is also treated, a moderate amount of normal tissue and, more importantly, perhaps, deeper, functionally vital areas will remain within the treatment field. Implantation of antennae, required for some local heat-generation techniques, faces a similar problem in that the surgeon can little afford to thread devices into the brain stem, thalamus, or similar sensitive areas, let alone destroy that volume of tissue.

From a practical point of view, many of the tumors encountered by neurologists and neurosurgeons are metastatic. Once the tumor is palliated by surgery and radiation, the usual cause of death is systemic dissemination and not the intracranial problem. Can a local heating technique be expected to heat all metastatic deposits in bone, brain, lung, marrow, and so forth? With the current state-of-the-art equipment, it seems unlikely. Nevertheless, local intratumoral heating is an attractive technique because it (1) has the ability to achieve intratumoral temperatures much higher than can be tolerated by the human organism as a whole, (2) has the ability to locally enhance the effect of systemic or regionally delivered chemotherapy, (3) requires technology which can be employed without hospitalization or anesthesia, (4) can be repeated on frequent occasions within a short time span, and (5) provides the ability to retreat an area at the time of recurrence without concern for cumulative total body toxicity.

Regional Hyperthermia

Regional hyperthermia for melanoma of the limb, utilizing a closed-circuit system and extracorporeal circulator, has achieved acknowledged success.[7,18] Its application to a similar isolated perfusion area, the brain and/or head and neck, has not been as successful.[16] All perfusion methods involving the intracranial circulation suffer from the inability to restrict the circulatory "leak" of chemotherapeutic agents and from the rapid dissipation of heat from the region as a result of the rapid blood flow perfusing the intra- and extracranial tissue. Total body temperature elevation may occur before any significant intracranial temperature gradient can be achieved. Current work with energy sources in the 13.7 MHz range as used for regional heating elsewhere may show an advantage, but again, blood flow rates and the effect of total brain heating may outweigh the usefulness of the technique.[17]

Thermal Gradient

Popovic and Masironi reported dramatic observations of tumor regression in the experimental animal when tumor tissue was maintained at normothermic or hyperthermic levels while remaining body tissues were cooled to 30°C utilizing systemic hypothermia.[10] Their findings indicate cell kill rates to be dependent upon the length of time the gradient is applied and the span of the gradient between normal and

abnormal tissue temperatures. In attempting to apply this principle to the glioblastoma, the physician is immediately confronted with the same restrictions as outlined for local intracranial-intratumoral heating: the need for an implanted antenna (or similar heating target), the large volume of tissue to be heated, and the inability to be certain of tumor borders. Although it is a method not to be discarded for use in intracranial tumors, a thermal gradient is difficult to effect in a uniform intratumoral manner while sparing areas of functionally significant tissue.

Total Body Hyperthermia

This form of hyperthermia uniformly heats ($\pm 0.05°$ to $0.10°C$ at equilibration) and affects all organ systems of the body. That feature of the procedure is a double-edged sword. On the one hand, the effects of heating and its enhancing capability when combined with other modalities are equally distributed throughout the body (an advantage in metastatic disease). On the other hand, human organ systems cannot withstand total body temperatures much beyond 42°C (a level needed to effect a major cell kill rate when heat is used alone), nor can they withstand heating's potential toxicity when it is employed with simultaneously administered systemic chemotherapy and/or large-volume irradiation. Although much of the literature on total body hyperthermia is concerned with efforts with a single agent (heating), most authors now believe a combined-modality approach to be the most beneficial; that is, radiotherapy, immunotherapy, chemotherapy, and heat in some combination and time relationship. As an adjuvant, the concept of total body heating is based on the assumption that inherent biological differences exist between normal and abnormal cells in pH, oxygen consumption, sugar metabolism, blood flow, and rates of DNA replication and repair. In the glioblastoma, for instance (and in some other solid tumor systems), the inherent phenomenon of anerobic metabolism can be capitalized upon by deliberately creating systemic nonketotic hyperglycemia, resulting in increased levels of intratumoral lactate production and a further decrease in an already lower intratumoral pH, thereby contributing to the differential effect of treatment.[3]

The procedure for total body hyperthermia is technically simple in comparison to the use of electronic instrumentation for local heating. Its potential effects on the organism, however, creates the need for multiparameter physiological monitoring during the procedure. Considering the fine line of normal tissue (brain and liver) temperature tolerance at about 42°C, multisite temperature surveillance must be accurate to within less than 0.1°C, standardized to a recognized international reference probe. Rectal, esophageal, and bladder temperatures have been described[8,9] by various authors; however, our own experience indicates the pulmonary artery temperature, as measured by a Swan-Ganz thermocouple, to be the most predictive of core and brain temperature at equilibration.

The current methods of induction of total body hyperthermia include (1) molten wax immersion,[9] (2) use of an extracorporeal heat exchanger,[8] (3) use of a radiant oven,[11]

(4) use of standard hyperthermia blankets,[6] (5) use of converted space suits or respirator-like devices with hot-air convection heating,[1] and (6) water bath immersion. Some of these methods require general anesthesia; all are inpatient procedures; and all cause changes in basal metabolic rate, cardiovascular physiology, fluid and electrolyte balance, colloid osmotic pressure, peripheral resistance, intracranial pressure, oxygen consumption, liver metabolism, and platelet function. All effects become extremely critical when dealing with intracranial mass effect and increased intracranial pressure.

As with local hyperthermia, dosimetry becomes important in estimation of therapeutic effect. The exact amount of heating required (in time and temperature) to create a response in the glioblastoma is largely unknown. It is assumed to be at least similar to that required in other solid tumor systems and to follow the outlines of previously enumerated time and temperature parameters (Figs. 138-1 and 138-2). Our own experiments indicate glioma cells to be resistant to 2 h of 40.5°C heating when in a sugar-containing tissue culture medium. However, when glioma cells are heated in a non-sugar-containing medium, they cannot be replated and are ultimately determined to be nonviable. At temperatures above 42° to 43°C, cell metabolic rates seem to preclude survival regardless of the sugar content of the medium.

In general, the term *degree/minutes* is used to rate or standardize total body heating dosage. In their simplest form, degree/minutes are calculated by multiplying the number of degrees of body temperature elevation above 40°C by the time that the temperature is maintained at that level. It is, in effect, an expression of the area beneath the described temperature curve. The limit for human tolerance has been quoted as 300°/min, with the highest achieved central temperature being somewhat less than 42°C.[9] Our own experience indicates tolerance to 450°/min when combined with midheating chemotherapy (BCNU) at 50 percent of the usual dose per square meter of body surface. There can be reversible toxicity in the form of platelet loss (<15,000), elevated prothrombin times (>20/10), and major changes in hepatic enzymes. In three patients treated with heat at 450°/min 75 percent of the usual dose per square meter of body surface, proximal myopathy (and/or a Guillain-Barré–like syndrome) has occurred, although some investigators claim to have used a sustained temperature of 41.5°C for as long as 30 hours, apparently without major clinical effect or damage to normal tissue.

Our clinical experience with total body hyperthermia has been exclusively with the use of a water bath immersion technique. It is simple, inexpensive, and easily controlled, does not require anticoagulation (an important feature with intracranial lesions), and reduces insensible fluid loss to a minimum. We have had experience with a number of primary and metastatic lesions to the brain, selecting where possible a target and a control lesion (Fig. 138-3). The target lesion is subjected to preheating sensitizing radiation (500 to 750 R and a presumed TER of 2), thereby making it the object of a three-modality protocol (i.e., midheating chemotherapy, preheating irradiation, and heat), while the control lesion receives only midheating chemotherapy and heat. Our experience thus far in a series of terminal patients, not all of whom could tolerate a planned monthly treatment protocol,

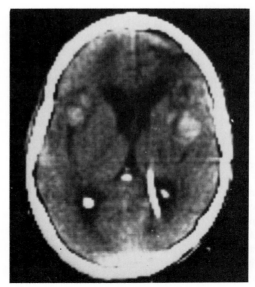

Figure 138-3 CT scan of target (*right hemisphere*) and control (*left hemisphere*) lesions in a patient with metastatic malignant melanoma.

seems to indicate that three modalities are in fact required in order to control tumor growth. If this is true, this requirement could be satisfied with the newly introduced half-body single-fraction low-dose radiation schedule, lending application to patients with widespread dissemination who also harbor an intracranial lesion. Our experience also indicates the need to reduce increased intracranial pressure to normal (or near-normal) levels by some surgical means prior to total body heating. In our hands, this has taken the form of repeat cytoreductive surgery and/or some external ventricular drainage (EVD) device. We suspect the same need is present when local intracranial-intratumoral heating is employed, depending upon the degree of enhanced blood flow and tissue swelling. In patients with an intracranial mass who are undergoing total body heating, vasodilatation and intracranial suffusion have caused recorded pressures as high as 40 torr, necessitating aborting the procedure or controlling the rise by venting CSF through a previously placed reservoir or EVD.

Hyperthermia in Combination with Newer Modalities of Radiation and Drug Delivery

In previous paragraphs the use of heat combined with chemotherapy and external radiation has been described. In the glioblastoma, BCNU remains the drug of choice; the effects of BCNU are fortunately, enhanced by heat. Whether to give the drug before, during, or after the hyperthermia remains a matter of conjecture. Still to be determined is the effect of a single intracarotid injection of the drug during heating verses sustained release throughout the period of heating.

The use of local hyperthermia along with radiation in

nonintracranial lesions is now an acknowledged advantage and is currently employed in many centers, resulting in dramatic reduction of local tumor mass effect. New treatment planners coupled to the computed tomography scanner should promote a greater effect on glioblastoma regardless of the type of heating employed, but their simultaneous use presents a logistical problem in most institutions. The effect of hyperthermia (local or total body) on glioblastoma may be further enhanced with the use of the newly emerging art of interstitial irradiation. Radiation sources implanted stereotactically (by afterloading or permanent implantation) can provide a constant long-term source of therapy to a local area and permit repeated enhancement by multiple heatings, yet confine the main effect to a local intracranial volume. Although complex in its dosimetry requirements, some advantage of using this method should be forthcoming. Again, as with any procedure requiring local implants, tumors in functionally sensitive areas of the brain may be beyond the scope of this procedure.

References

1. Bull JM, Lees D, Schuete W, Whang-Peng J, Smith R, Bynum G, Atkinson R, Gottdiener JS, Gralnick HR, Shawker TH, DeVita VT Jr: Whole body hyperthermia: A phase-I trial of a potential adjuvant to chemotherapy. Ann Intern Med 90:317–323, 1979.
2. Coley WB: The treatment of malignant tumors by repeated inoculations of erysipelas: With a report of 10 original cases. Am J Med Sci 105:487–511, 1893.
3. Duggins EL: Effects of insulin and glucose on the interstitial pH differential between normal and tumor tissues during normo and hyperthermia. In press.
4. Hahn GM, Braun J, Har-Kedar I: Thermochemotherapy: Synergism between hyperthermia (42-43°) and adriamycin (or bleomycin) in mammalian cell inactivation. Proc Natl Acad Sci USA 72:937–940, 1975.
5. Hochberg FH, Pruitt A: Assumptions in the radiotherapy of glioblastoma. Neurology (NY) 30:907–911, 1980.
6. Larkin JM, Edwards WS, Smith DE, Clark PJ. Systemic thermotherapy: Description of a method and physiologic tolerance in clinical subjects. Cancer 40:3155–3159, 1977.
7. Martin H, Oldhoff J, Koops HS: Hyperthermic regional perfusion with melphalan and a combination of melphalan and actinomycin D in the treatment of locally metastasized malignant melanomas of the extremities. J Surg Oncol 20:9–13, 1982.
8. Parks LC, Minaberry D, Smith DP, Neely WA: Treatment of far-advanced bronchogenic carcinoma by extracorporeally induced systemic hyperthermia. J Thorac Cardiovasc Surg 78:883–892, 1979.
9. Pettigrew RT, Galt JM, Ludgate CM, Smith AN: Clinical effects of whole-body hyperthermia in advanced malignancy. Br Med J 4:679–682, 1974.
10. Popovic VP, Masironi R: Disappearance of normothermic tumors in shallow (30°C) hypothermia. Cancer Res 26:863–864, 1966.
11. Robbins HI: Clinical use of a radiant head device (RHD) for whole-body hyperthermia (WBH). Presented at a meeting of the International Clinical Hyperthermia Society, London, June 1982.
12. Salcman M, Samaras GM: Hyperthermia for brain tumors: Biophysical rationale. Neurosurgery 9:327–335, 1981.
13. Selker RG, Bova E, Kristofik M. Jones E, Iannuzzi D, Landay A, Taylor F: Effect of total body temperature on toxicity of 1,3-bis(2-chloroethyl)-1-nitrosourea (BCNU). Neurosurgery 4:157–161, 1979.
14. Selker RG, Wolfson SK Jr: The creation of thermal gradients in primates in the treatment of brain tumors. J Med Primatol 4:351, 1975.
15. Selker RG, Wolfson SK Jr, Medal R, Miller M: Creation of a chemothermal gradient in treatment of brain tumors. Surg Forum 24:461–463, 1973.
16. Shingleton WW, Bryan FA Jr, O'Quinn WL, Krueger LC: Selective heating and cooling of tissue in cancer chemotherapy. Ann Surg 156:408–416, 1962.
17. Silberman AW, Morgan DF, Storm FK, Rand RW, Bubbers JE, Brown WJ, Morton DL: Localized magnetic-loop induction hyperthermia of the rabbit brain. J Surg Oncol 20:174–178, 1982.
18. Stehlin JS Jr, Greeff P, Giovanella BC, Williams LJ Jr: Dramatic response of cancer to localized hyperthermia. NY State J Med 80:70–72, 1980.
19. Stewart FA, Denekamp J: Combined x-ray and heating: Is there a therapeutic gain? in Streffer C, van Beuningen D, Dietzel F, Röttinger E, Robinson JE, Scherer E, Seeber S, Troth KR (eds): *Cancer Therapy by Hyperthermia and Radiation Therapy. Proceedings of Second International Symposium, Essen, June 2–4, 1977.* Baltimore, Urban & Schwarzenberg, 1978, pp 249–250.
20. Sutton CH, Carroll FB: Experimental studies on the use of temperature gradients to increase blood flow in malignant gliomas. Presented at a meeting of the European Association of Neurological Societies, September 1975.
21. Tanaka R: Radiofrequency hyperthermia therapy of experimental brain tumors. Presented at the Brain Tumor Meeting, Nikko, Japan, October 1981.
22. Thackray P, Meiskin ZH, Wolfson SK, Selker RG: Indirect heating source for treatment of malignant brain tumors. Electrocomp Sci Technol 1:91–96, 1974.
23. Walker MD, Green SB, Byar DP, Alexander E Jr, Batzdorf U, Brooks WH, Hunt WE, MacCarty CS, Mahaley MS Jr, Mealey J Jr, Owens G, Ransohoff J, Robertson JT, Shapiro WR, Smith KR Jr, Wilson CB, Strike TA: Randomized comparison of radiotherapy and nitrosoureas for the treatment of malignant glioma after surgery. N Engl J Med 303:1323–1329, 1980.